MacSween's
Pathology of the Liver

Fifth Edition

Commissioning Editor: Michael Houston
Project Development Manager: Sheila Black
Editorial Assistant: Liz Brown
Project Manager: Jess Thompson
Senior Designer: Sarah Russell
Illustration Manager: Bruce Hogarth
Illustrator: Oxford Illustrators
Marketing Managers: Leontine Treur (UK/NL); Katherine Neely (USA)

MacSween's Pathology of the Liver

FIFTH EDITION

Alastair D. Burt BSc MD FRCPath FIBiol
Professor of Pathology and Dean of Clinical Medicine
University of Newcastle upon Tyne;
Honorary Consultant Histopathologist
Royal Victoria Infirmary
Newcastle upon Tyne, UK

Bernard C. Portmann MD FRCPath
Professor of Hepatopathology
King's College London, School of Medicine
at Guy's, King's College and St Thomas' Hospitals;
Consultant Histopathologist
Institute of Liver Studies
King's College Hospital
London, UK

Linda D. Ferrell MD
Professor of Pathology
Vice-Chair of Clinical Affairs
Director of Surgical Pathology
Department of Anatomic Pathology
University of California, San Francisco
San Francisco, CA, USA

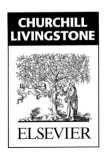

CHURCHILL
LIVINGSTONE

ELSEVIER

CHURCHILL
LIVINGSTONE
ELSEVIER

An imprint of Elsevier Limited

First edition 1979
Second edition 1987
Third edition 1994
Fourth edition 2002
© 2007, Elsevier Limited All rights reserved.

ISBN 13: 978 0 443 10012 3
ISBN 10: 0 443 10012 8

British Library Cataloguing in Publication Data
A catalogue record for this book is available from the British Library

Library of Congress Cataloging in Publication Data
A catalog record for this book is available from the Library of Congress

Notice
Medical knowledge is constantly changing. Standard safety precautions must be followed,
but as new research and clinical experience broaden our knowledge, changes in treatment
and drug therapy may become necessary or appropriate. Readers are advised to check the
most current product information provided by the manufacturer of each drug to be
administered to verify the recommended dose, the method and duration of administration,
and contraindications. It is the responsibility of the practitioner, relying on experience and
knowledge of the patient, to determine dosages and the best treatment for each individual
patient. Neither the Publisher nor the author assume any liability for any injury and/or
damage to persons or property arising from this publication.

The Publisher

Printed in China
Last digit is the print number: 9 8 7 6 5 4 3 2

Contents

List of Contributors

Jorge Albores-Saavedra MD
Professor of Pathology and Director, Division of
Anatomic Pathology
Department of Pathology
LSU Health Sciences Center
Shreveport, LA, USA

Henry C. Bodenheimer MD
Chief, Division of Digestive Diseases
Beth Israel Medical Center—Albert Einstein College
of Medicine
New York, NY, USA

Elizabeth M. Brunt MD
Professor of Pathology
Department of Pathology
Saint Louis University School of Medicine
St Louis University Liver Center
St Louis, MO, USA

Alastair D. Burt BSc MD FRCPath FIBiol
Professor of Pathology and Dean of Clinical
Medicine
University of Newcastle upon Tyne
Honorary Consultant Histopathologist
Royal Victoria Infirmary
Newcastle upon Tyne, UK

Herschel A. Carpenter MD
Professor of Pathology
Department of Pathology
Mayo Clinic College of Medicine
Rochester, MN, USA

James M. Crawford MD PhD
Professor and Chair
Department of Pathology, Immunology & Laboratory
Medicine
University of Florida College of Medicine
Gainesville, FL, USA

Albert J. Czaja MD FACP FACG
Professor of Medicine
Division of Gastroenterology and Hepatology
Mayo Clinic
Rochester, MN, USA

Valeer J. Desmet MD PhD
Emeritus Professor of Histology & Pathology
Department of Pathology
University Hospital St Rafael
Leuven, Belgium

Linda D. Ferrell MD
Professor of Pathology
Vice-Chair of Clinical Affairs
Director of Surgical Pathology
Department of Anatomic Pathology
University of California, San Francisco
San Francisco, CA, USA

Stephen A. Geller MD
Chairman Emeritus, Department of Pathology &
Laboratory Medicine, Cedars-Sinai Medical Center;
Professor of Pathology
Geffen School of Medicine, UCLA
Los Angeles, CA, USA

Zachary D. Goodman MD PhD
Chairman Department of Hepatic and
Gastrointestinal Pathology
Armed Forces Institute of Pathology
Washington, DC, USA

Pauline de la M. Hall MB BSc FRCPA FCPath(SA)
Professor of Pathology
Queensland Health Pathology Service
Department of Anatomical Pathology
Royal Brisbane & Women's Hospital
Herston, Queensland, Australia

Stefan G. Hübscher MBChB FRCPath
Professor of Hepatic Pathology
Department of Pathology
University of Birmingham
Birmingham, UK

Jose Jessurun MD
Professor of Pathology
Department of Pathology
University of Minnesota Medical School
Minneapolis, MN, USA

David E. Kleiner MD PhD
Director, Clinical Operations
Laboratory of Pathology
National Cancer Institute
Bethesda, MD, USA

James H. Lewis MD FACP FACG
Professor of Medicine;
Director, Hepatology
Department of Medicine
Division of Gastroenterology
Georgetown University Medical Center
Washington, DC, USA

Sebastian B. Lucas FRCP FRCPath
Professor of Clinical Histopathology
Department of Histopathology
Guy's & Thomas's NHS Trust
London, UK

Yasuni Nakanuma MD PhD
Professor and Chairman
Department of Human Pathology
Dean
Kanazawa University Graduate School of Medicine
Kanazawa, Japan

W. Stephen Nichols MD
Director, Molecular Pathology
Department of Pathology and Laboratory Medicine
Cedars-Sinai Medical Center
Los Angeles, CA, USA

Alan C. Paterson MB BCh PhD FCPath(SA)
Professor and Head
Division of Anatomical Pathology
School of Pathology
NHLS and University of Witwatersrand
Johannesburg, South Africa

Martha B. Pitman MD
Associate Professor of Pathology, Harvard Medical School;
Assistant Director of Cytopathology
Director of the Fine Needle Aspiration Biopsy Service
Massachusetts General Hospital
Boston, MA, USA

Bernard C. Portmann MD FRCPath
Professor of Hepatopathology
King's College London, School of Medicine
at Guy's, King's College and St Thomas' Hospitals;
Consultant Histopathologist
Institute of Liver Studies
King's College Hospital
London, UK

Eve A. Roberts MD FRCPC
Professor of Paediatrics, Medicine & Pharmacology
Division of Gastroenterology & Nutrition
University of Toronto
Toronto, ON, Canada

Tania Roskams MD PhD
Professor of Pathology
Head, Liver Research Unit
University Hospital, St Rafael
Leuven, Belgium;
Visiting Professor, Faculty of Veterinary Medicine
University of Utrecht
Utrecht, The Netherlands

Luigi Terracciano MD
Professor of Pathology
Department of Pathology
University of Basel
Basel, Switzerland

Neil D. Theise MD
Professor of Pathology
Associate Professor of Medicine (Division of Digestive Diseases)
Beth Israel Medical Center – Albert Einstein College of Medicine
New York, NY, USA

Richard J. Thompson BA BM BCh MRCP MRCPCH
Senior Lecturer in Paediatric Hepatology
Honorary Consultant
Department of Liver Studies and Transplantation
Division of Gene and Cell Based Therapy
King's College London School of Medicine at King's College Hospital
London, UK

Chris Verslype MD PhD
Associate Professor of Medicine
Department of Hepatology
University Hospital Gasthuisberg
Leuven, Belgium

Ian R. Wanless MD CM FRCPC
Professor of Pathology
Dalhousie University
Halifax, Nova Scotia, Canada

Preface

It is now over five years since the last edition of *Pathology of the Liver* was published. It was felt that as the world of hepatology and hepatopathology had continued to advance at an astonishing pace, there was a need to reflect this in a new iteration of the book. The editorial team has changed since the 4th edition. Linda Ferrell has been enlisted as a new editor; she was a major contributor to two previous editions.

Roddy MacSween and Peter Anthony decided to 'close their nibs' on their editorial pens. It was Roddy who had the vision and much of the inspiration for developing an authoritative textbook of liver pathology. We were unanimous that the book should hereafter be known as *MacSween's Pathology of the Liver*. We hope that we can live up to the very high standards set by Roddy and the earlier editorial teams and that 'POL' will continue as a 'household name' among pathologists around the globe.

Very sadly, since the publication of the last edition, two of our previous editors have passed away: Kamal Ishak, who died in 2004 and Peter Scheuer, who died more recently in 2006. Kamal was not only an invaluable editor but had taken on an increasing role as contributor with outstanding chapters on developmental abnormalities, metabolic errors and drug related injury. He had an encyclopaedic knowledge of pathological and clinical aspects of liver disease and an enormous breadth and depth of experience gained from the almost unique resource of the Armed Forces Institute of Pathology collection of liver specimens. He published several landmark papers and was very influential in the development of assessment methods for biopsy changes in chronic hepatitis, the most common international scoring system being (appropriately) named after him. Peter was another of the true great doyens of liver pathology. He was an editor of the first four editions. He too published some of the most quoted and seminal works on liver biopsy interpretation and contributed immensely to the whole modern approach of histopathologists to this diagnostic area. He was also a great mentor to many during their development as liver pathologists. The hepatology and pathology worlds will truly miss the leadership and inspiration of both Kamal and Peter. They were very close friends of ours and we will remember them fondly.

The current editorial team wants to pay tribute to the amazing energy and effort of each of these four gentlemen in the evolution of *Pathology of the Liver*. We have inherited a superbly crafted book which has continued to grow in popularity. The framework developed from earlier editions has meant that for each of the current team, editing has been a labour of love. The goals of this editorial team remain similar to those of the earlier editions. In essence we are seeking to provide, on the one hand an encyclopaedic text of liver pathology ('If it's not in MacSween, it's not in the liver') which is of contemporary relevance to hepatologist and hepatopathologist alike, but on the other hand presenting it in such a way that it is an accessible and frequently used 'bench book' addressing practical issues in everyday hepatopathology.

The layout of the book differs in some respects from that of earlier editions. The first chapter now encompasses structural *and* functional aspects and includes up-to-date coverage of imaging procedures that are being increasingly used in hepatology and of which the twenty-first century hepatopathologist must have a good understanding. The second chapter is a new contribution covering some of the fundamental aspects of injury and repair in the liver. It forms the basis for understanding the principles of specific disease entities covered in later chapters. This is followed by a chapter on diagnostic techniques which we felt logically should come before consideration of disease categories. Chapter 4 is a comprehensive review of developmental abnormalities and owes a great deal to the insightful writing of Kamal Ishak and Harvey Sharp in POL4; Kamal was originally to be the lead contributor in this edition for this chapter. Kamal had also set a magnificent foundation for the current Chapter 5 on genetic and metabolic liver disease. There have been very significant advances in our recent understanding of the genetic basis for many of the rarer (and even not so rare) metabolic disorders and this is reflected in the length of this important chapter; it is also in part because the decision was taken to incorporate diseases related to iron overload into this part of the book, given that the genetic basis of these disorders were now better characterised than hitherto. In relation to fatty liver disease, we have now separated alcoholic liver disease and non-alcoholic fatty liver disease, recognising the importance and prevalence of the latter.

There have been very significant advances in our understanding of, and clinical approach to, infections of the liver with an increasing awareness of viral interactions, most notably co-infections with HIV and hepatitis C. Novel infections continue to afflict humans and the liver is frequently involved; this has most recently been seen in Severe Acute Respiratory Syndrome (SARS) and in this edition we refer to hepatic involvement in the recent Asian epidemic. Special mention should also be made of the updated chapter on injury due to drugs, chemicals and toxins. This was to be led by Kamal Ishak with James Lewis as co-author; we are indebted to him and to David Kleiner for taking on, and so elegantly summarising, one of the fastest moving areas in liver pathology. They particularly wish us to acknowledge their indebtedness to Kamal and Hy Zimmerman for their work on this topic in the 4th edition on which they built and also for their mentorship.

The approach to tumour pathology in the present edition differs from earlier editions in that basic molecular mechanisms and histopathological changes are combined in one chapter; the experimental evidence is more focused on information from human tumours as this has been a major growth area in liver research.

We feel privileged to be working in a field which continues to be both exciting and challenging; we have enjoyed working with our contributors in putting together a text which we hope will be of enduring interest to histopathologists and clinicians alike. It has also been a great pleasure to collaborate with the publishing team in Elsevier.

Alastair D. Burt   Newcastle
Bernard C. Portmann   London
Linda D. Ferrell   San Francisco

2006

Acknowledgements

Acknowledgement of illustrations from previous publications or of modifications to illustrations and diagrams and acknowledgement of original photographic material and microscopic material is appropriately made in each chapter and in figure legends.

We would like to thank our administrative assistants who have helped with the preparation of manuscripts and figures and with some of the chores of proof-reading, notably Emma Reynolds (Newcastle), Elisabeth Portmann (London), Maureen Murphy (San Francisco). As always, preparation of a book of this size and type is a time-consuming business and we would like to thank our respective families for their patience and support during the more fraught times in the development of the 5th edition. We would like to thank our publishers and typesetters for their help and encouragement at all times, and in particular Sheila Black, Michael Houston, Jess Thompson and Richard Lawrence.

Development, structure and function of the liver

1

Tania Roskams   Valeer J. Desmet   Chris Verslype

For a clearer understanding of the mechanisms and expression of pathological processes in the liver, it is important to have an appreciation of the structural and functional properties of the organ. This chapter considers the embryology, macroanatomy, microanatomy and basic functions of the liver; this is followed by a brief section on the clinical investigation of liver disease.

The definition of the structural and functional unit of the liver has been an elusive goal since the first description of liver lobules by Weppler in 1665 (cited by Bloch[1]). Over the years, several concepts of the basic structural organization of the liver have been proposed. The hexagonal lobule (now 'classic lobule') described by Kiernan in 1833[2] has stood the test of time, but its unit organization with a hepatic vein as the centre is not really primary.[3] The portal lobule described by Mall in 1906[4] has been of limited functional significance. More recently attention has been focused on smaller landmarks that could subdivide the classical hexagonal lobule into smaller subdivisions. The liver acinus concept, defined by Rappaport and his colleagues in 1954,[5] regarded the 'terminal portal venule' as the axial vessel of the liver unit. The primary lobule of Matsumoto et al.,[6] described in 1979, regarded the 'vascular septum' as being at the origin of the unit's blood flow. The single-sinusoid hepatic functional unit of Bloch[1] and a refined version by McCuskey in 1988[7] comprises a single sinusoid with its perisinusoidal space and surrounding cylinder of hepatocytes. The metabolic lobulus of Lamers et al.,[8] based on gradients in enzyme-histochemical patterns, and the 'modified' zonal microcirculatory unit (according to Quistorff & Romert[9]) are further proposed concepts. Still the most recent concepts include the choleon (as an exocrine secretory unit) comprising a group of hepatocytes drained by a single bile ductule,[10] the hepatic microcirculatory subunit[3] and a combination of the latter two: the choleohepaton.[3,11]

Most of these concepts represent particular ways of looking at an organ of great structural complexity and with a multitude of functions. However, there is a basic difference between the liver acinus and the other 'lobule-based' concepts, which makes them mutually exclusive. In the second and third editions of this text (in 1979 and 1994) it was stated that the concept of the liver acinus was proving to be of the greatest value to the pathologist in the interpretation of disordered structure and function. It represented the structural and functional liver unit concept that allowed for an explanation of important histopathological features, such as portal-central bridging, hepatic necrosis and fibrosis.[12] However, the concept of the liver acinus was based on injection of coloured gelatin-based infusion fluids, and not on actual vascular reconstruction, in contrast to the proposed primary lobule concept of Matsumoto and his colleagues.[6,13] Because of its meticulously demonstrated angio-architectural base, the primary lobule concept has gradually gained increasing attention, and several other concepts including choleon, hepatic microcirculatory unit, choleohepaton and the single sinusoid hepatic functional unit can be considered as variants of or existing within the primary lobule. For this reason, and in terms of effecting a transition from an acinar to a lobular concept, we will return to a short description of the various proposed hepatic units later in this chapter. However, for a full appreciation of the organization of the liver, an account of the development of this organ before consideration of its apparent definitive structure may be useful.

Development of the liver

General features

In human embryos, the liver first appears at the end of the 3rd week of development. Its parenchyma is of endodermal origin and arises from the liver bud or hepatic diverticulum, which develops as a hollow midline outgrowth from the ventral wall of the future duodenum. Recent evidence suggests that at least in mice, two distinct types of endoderm-progenitor cells, lateral and medial, arising from three spatially separated embryonic domains converge to produce the liver bud.[14] The connective tissue framework of the liver is of mesenchymal origin, and develops from two sources: (i) the septum transversum, a transverse sheet of cells which incompletely separates the pericardial and peritoneal cavities, and (ii) cells derived from the mesenchymal lining of the associated coelomic cavity, which actively invade the septum transversum (Figs 1.1(A) and 1.2(A)).

During the 4th week bud-like clusters of epithelial cells extend forwards and outwards from the hepatic diverticulum into the mesenchymal stroma, in which has appeared a hepatic sinusoidal plexus, fed by a vitelline venous plexus draining blood from the wall of the yolk sac. As the epithelial buds grow into the septum transversum, they break up into thick anastomosing epithelial sheets which meet and enmesh vessels of the hepatic sinusoidal plexus, forming the primitive hepatic sinusoids (Figs 1.1(B) and 1.2(B)). The intimate relation between hepatocytes and sinusoidal capillaries, so characteristic of the adult organ, is therefore, already anticipated in the 4-week-old embryo (Fig. 1.2(C)). The caudal part of the hepatic diverticulum does not contribute to the invading sheets of primitive hepatocytes but forms instead the epithelial primordium of the cystic duct and gallbladder. Once established, the liver grows rapidly and soon extends beyond the confines of the septum transversum in whichever direction it can. It bulges dorsally on each side of the midline, into the peritoneal cavity, as right

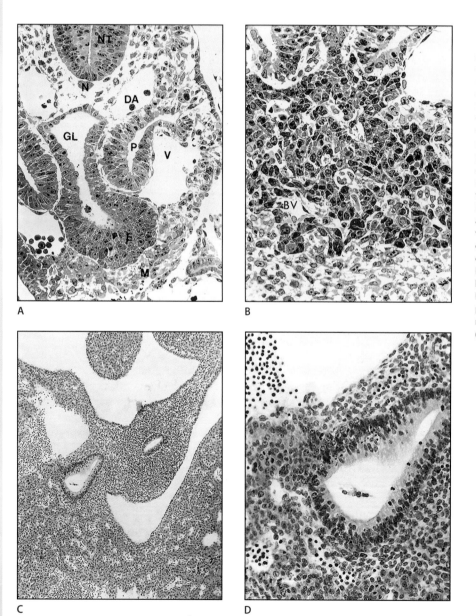

A

B

C

D

Fig. 1.1 • Stages in the early development of the liver in mouse embryos of 14 somites **(A)**, and 26 somites **(B)**; and in a sheep embryo of 10 mm crown rump length **(C)** and **(D)**. **(A)** The hepatic bud appears as a thick-walled hollow diverticulum of the foregut, extending ventrally into the loose mesenchyme of the septum transversum and flanked on each side by a vitelline vein. NT = neural tube; N = notochord; DA = dorsal aorta; GL = gut lumen; P = pericardio-peritoneal canal; V = vitelline vein; E = endodermal component of the developing liver (hepatic bud); M = mesenchyme of the septum transversum. Semi-thin resin section. Toluidine blue. **(B)** The hepatic bud is broken up into thick anastomosing plates between which are blood vessels (BV), the primitive sinusoids. From the deep surface of the thickened mesenchymal epithelium, which lines the coelom, cells are budded off to contribute to the mesenchymal bed of the liver. Semi-thin resin section: Toluidine blue. **(C)** & **(D)** The continuity of the hepatic plates with the hepatic duct in the ventral mesentery (lesser omentum) is shown. **(C)** H&E. **(D)** H&E.

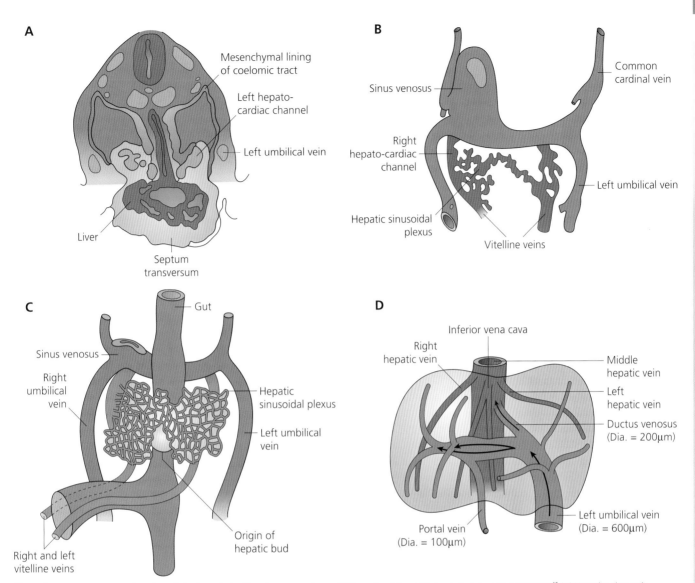

Fig. 1.2• **(A)** Section through region of the hepatic bud in a human embryo of 25 somites (about 26 days). Redrawn from Streeter.[15] **(B)** Vascular channels associated with the developing liver, in a human embryo of 30 somites. Redrawn from Streeter.[15] **(C)** Vascular channels in the human liver at a slightly later stage, showing the further extensive development of the hepatic sinusoidal plexus. Based on Streeter.[16] **(D)** Scheme of the portal hepatic circulation, in a human embryo of 17 mm (about 7 weeks). Redrawn from Lassau & Bastian.[17]

and left lobes, which are initially symmetrical. It also grows ventrally and caudally into the mesenchyme of the anterior abdominal wall, extending down to the umbilical ring. Associated with these changes, the stomach and duodenum, which were initially in broad contact with the septum transversum, draw away from it, thus producing a midsagittal sheet of mesoderm, the ventral mesogastrium or future lesser omentum. As the duodenum withdraws from the septum transversum, the stalk of the original hepatic diverticulum is also drawn out to form, within the lesser omentum, the epithelial elements of the extrahepatic bile ducts (Fig. 1.1(C), (D)). The liver becomes partly freed from its originally broad contact with the septum transversum by extensions of the peritoneal cavity so that, in the adult, direct contact with the diaphragm persists only as the bare area of the liver. This is bounded by the attachments of peritoneal reflexions, which form the coronary and falciform ligaments.

Vascular arrangements

The fetal liver consists of anastomosing sheets of liver cells, each sheet being several cells in thickness and forming a 'muralium multiplex',[15] an arrangement which still pertains, in part at least, in the neonatal liver. By 5 months after birth, the sheets are, in general, two cells thick ('muralium duplex'). The pattern typical of the adult ('muralium simplex') is not established until about 5 years of age. Initially, the hepatic sinusoidal plexus receives blood from symmetrically arranged vitelline veins and is drained into the sinus venosus by similarly symmetrical right and left hepato-cardiac channels[16] (Fig. 1.2(B)). As the developing liver grows, the laterally placed right and left umbilical veins, which run in the body wall and carry oxygenated blood from the placenta to the sinus venosus, also come to supply blood to the hepatic sinusoidal plexus (Fig. 1.2(C)). Once this connection is made (in embryos of 5 mm, 5th week) the circulatory pattern within the liver changes rapidly. The left umbilical vein becomes the principal source of blood entering the liver, partly because it comes to carry all the blood returning from the placenta when the right umbilical vein withers and disappears, and partly because the volume of blood returning from the gut in the vitelline veins is small. The definitive vascular pattern of the fetal liver, already established in embryos of the 7th week (about 17 mm long), is shown in Fig. 1.2(D).[17] The originally paired vitelline veins have given way to a single portal vein which, on entering the liver, divides into right and left branches. Blood in the left umbilical vein has a choice of three routes through the liver: (i) through branches which enter the sinusoidal plexus of the left half of the liver; (ii) through the sinusoidal plexus of the right half of the liver, by retrograde flow through its connection with the left branch of the portal vein; and (iii) through the ductus venosus directly into the inferior vena cava. The ductus venosus is a new venous channel which has developed through the enlargement of pre-existing sinusoidal channels, probably in response to the obliquely directed stream of placental blood. In the fetus, therefore, the umbilical vein is seen as the major contributor to the hepatic circulation, as indeed it must be since the placenta is the sole source of nutrients. Although the flow routes indicated in the embryonic liver in Fig. 1.2(D) are merely inferred from the relative dimensions of the vessels involved, they have been clearly demonstrated by cine-radiography in the late fetal sheep.[18] At birth, a sphincteric mechanism closes the ductus venosus at its proximal end, blood flow ceases in the umbilical vein, and the left side of the liver receives blood which now flows from right to left through the left branch of the portal vein. The closed segment of the umbilical vein between the umbilicus and the liver regresses to form the ligamentum teres; the ductus venosus undergoes fibrosis and becomes the ligamentum venosum.

The embryonic liver appears to develop initially without the presence of a hepatic artery and, in ontogenic development, the artery appears late.[3,11,19] The terminal ramifications of the hepatic artery in the liver during development and postpartum remain controversial, and the topic is further addressed in the section on the hepatic microcirculation.

Hepatocytes and sinusoidal cells

The primitive hepatocytes are derived exclusively from the endodermal outgrowths of the hepatic diverticulum. Synthesis of α-fetoprotein begins at the earliest stage of liver differentiation, some 25–30 days after conception, and continues until birth. Intestinal epithelium and yolk-sac cells also secrete α-fetoprotein. Glycogen granules are present in fetal hepatocytes at 8 weeks; glycogenesis commences at 12–14 weeks, the maximal glycogen reserve is achieved at birth, but the rapid onset of glycogenolysis depletes the storage to approximately 10% within 2–3 days postpartum. Fat accumulation occurs in parallel with glycogenesis.[19]

Haemosiderin deposits appear early in development, become more marked as hepatic haemopoiesis decreases and are then predominantly present in periportal hepatocytes; these are also the storage sites for copper. The sinusoidal endothelial cells, Kupffer cells and hepatic stellate cells appear at 10–12 weeks.[20]

Bile acid synthesis begins at about 5–9 weeks and bile secretion at about 12 weeks.[21] Canalicular transport and hepatic excretory function, however, are still immature at birth and for 4–6 weeks postpartum and, therefore, bile excretion across the placenta is important in the fetus.

The duct system

This is best understood if the liver is regarded as an exocrine gland. The hepatic bud gives rise not only to the epithelial parenchyma—the future hepatocytes—but also to the epithelial lining of the branching duct system, from its main stem, the common bile duct, to its terminal twigs, the smallest ductules, the canals of Hering.

The bile canaliculi are first seen in human embryos of the 6th week, long before bile production begins at 12 weeks. They develop from membrane foldings between junctional complexes, and appear as intercellular spaces within sheets of presumptive hepatocytes, therefore corresponding to the lumens of the secretory elements of any exocrine gland. They have no wall of their own, but simply lie between presumptive hepatocytes. At this early stage the canaliculi resemble those of the adult, except that, in a 'muralium multiplex' each canaliculus is surrounded by several cells, perhaps as many as seven in one sectional profile.

The epithelial lining of the extrahepatic bile ducts develops from the drawn-out stalk of the original hepatic outgrowth. It is continuous at its caudal end with the duodenal epithelium and at the cephalic end with the primitive hepatic sheets. Both hepatic ducts and part of the cystic duct develop from the cephalic end of the diverticulum, while the caudal segment develops into the gallbladder, part of the cystic duct and the common hepatic duct.

The intrahepatic ducts, which link the bile canaliculi and the extrahepatic ducts, develop from the limiting plate of hepatoblasts which surround the branches of the portal vein. This has been known since the 1920s,[22,23] but has been confirmed more recently using immunohistochemical methods and monoclonal antibodies to cytokeratins and cell surface markers.[24-29] Cytokeratins are the intermediate filaments of epithelial cells and 19 different types have been identified.[30] Normal adult hepatocytes express cytokeratins 8 and 18 whereas intrahepatic bile ducts, in addition, express cytokeratins 7 and 19. During the first 7–8 weeks of embryonic development no intrahepatic bile ducts are evident and the epithelial cells express cytokeratins 8, 18 and 19. At about 9–10 weeks (27–30 mm embryos) primitive hepatocytes (hepatoblasts) surrounding large portal vein branches near the liver hilum express these cytokeratins more intensely and form a layer of cells (Fig. 1.3(A)) which ensheaths the mesenchyme of the primitive portal tracts to form the so-called ductal plate.[22,23] This is followed by a second but discontinuous layer of epithelial cells which show a similar phenotypic change and so a segmentally

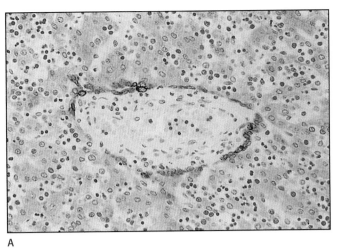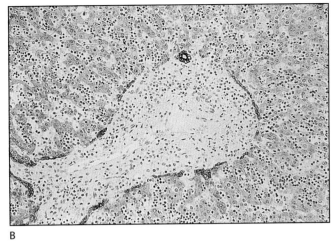

A   B

Fig. 1.3 • Development of the ductal plate and of intrahepatic bile ducts. **(A)** Increased expression of cytokeratins in primitive hepatocytes at the interface with the mesenchyme of the primitive portal tracts; human fetus of 12 weeks' gestation. **(B)** Later stage showing a discontinuous double-layered plate of epithelial cells at the mesenchymal interface; note the formation of tubular structures (upper right) within this plate. Human fetus of 14 weeks gestation. Immunoperoxidase staining; antibody (5D3) to low molecular weight cytokeratins.

double-layered plate is formed. The liver cells which do not form ductal plates lose cytokeratin 19 expression. From 12 weeks onwards a lumen develops in segments of the ductal plates forming double-layered cylindrical or tubular structures (Fig. 1.3(B)). Further remodelling of the plate occurs; invading connective tissue separates it from the liver parenchyma and the tubular structures become incorporated into the mesenchyme surrounding the portal vein branches. Such incorporation of tubules is always preceded by development of a branch of the hepatic artery,[31] suggesting that the hepatic artery branches may be induced by the tubular structures of the ductal plate, whereas the hepatic artery branch in turn plays an inducing role in incorporating the tubule. An anastomosing network of bile ducts is formed, excess ductal epithelium undergoes resorption and bile ducts appear within the definitive portal tracts. Weak immunoreactivity for cytokeratin 7 is present in large bile ducts from about 20 weeks' gestation.

The entire process of duct development progresses centrifugally from the porta hepatis and also from the larger to the smaller portal tracts. However, this process may not be complete at 40 weeks' gestation and full expression of cytokeratin 7 is not found until about 1 month postpartum. Thus, the intrahepatic bile-duct system is still immature at birth.[24] Failure of remodelling and resorption produces the 'ductal plate malformation'[32] and may also be significant in the production of various congenital malformations of the intrahepatic biliary tree. Failure of remodelling has been observed in HNF6 and HNF1β knockout mice, indicating that these transcription factors in tandem play a role in normal remodelling of the ductal plate.[25] Furthermore, injury to or destruction of the ductal plate in utero may be a factor in the development of intrahepatic biliary atresia[29] (see Chapter 4).

It is not known what factors determine whether hepatoblasts differentiate in one direction, to hepatocytes, or in the other, to ductal epithelium. However, differentiation to ductal epithelium is associated, as first noted by Bloom[23] in 1925, with contact of primitive hepatic epithelium with

young connective tissue developing in the portal tracts. There is now experimental evidence to indicate that the association is indeed one of cause and effect: in ectopic grafts of embryonic mouse liver, immature hepatocytes which are in contact with vascular endothelium tend to differentiate into mature hepatocytes, while those in contact with connective tissue cells differentiate into ductal epithelium.[33,34]

Despite their common ancestry, hepatocytes and ductal epithelium have been considered as distinct cell types and the epithelium of the terminal twigs of the biliary tree—the canals of Hering—includes typical hepatocytes and typical ductal cells, but no forms intermediate between the two.[35] However, a change in differentiation from hepatocytes to bile duct cells—ductular metaplasia—occurs in liver injury of various aetiologies and, in particular, contributes to the pattern of so-called ductular reaction seen in cholestatic liver disease. Immunohistochemical investigations have shown that the metaplasia is characterized by a phenotypic change, in which hepatocytes express cytokeratins 7 (CK7) and 19 (CK19) which, in the normal liver, are restricted to bile-duct cells.[35-38] This topic is complicated by the fact that such 'transdifferentiating cells' cannot be distinguished from progenitor cell progeny differentiating towards hepatocytes, resulting in 'transitional cells' expressing both cholangiocellular (CK7, 19) and hepatocellular (CK8, 18) cytokeratins. The topic of bipotential progenitor cells or stem cells is further discussed in the section on hepatic regeneration.

Haemopoiesis

Hepatic haemopoiesis is a feature of the embryonic and fetal liver of mammals including man. It begins at about 6 weeks (10 mm), when foci of haemopoietic cells appear extravascularly among the sheets of hepatocytes. By the 12th week, the liver is the main site of haemopoiesis, having superseded the yolk sac; activity subsides in the 5th month, when the bone marrow becomes haemopoietic, and has normally ceased within a few weeks after birth. It is largely erythropoietic, but the stem cells may also give rise to granulocytes, megakaryocytes and monocytes. When the liver is in the haemopoietic phase it produces a stimulator which can be detected in vitro by its switching of quiescent mouse marrow stem cells into cycle. In mouse liver, declining production of stimulator in late gestation and after birth correlates with a decrease in haemopoietic stem cell numbers in the liver.[39] Recent evidence suggests that *K-Ras* is important in the molecular control of erythropoiesis in the fetus.[40] The source of the stem cells is now well established experimentally in the mouse; they develop de novo in the blood islands of the yolk sac, proliferate and migrate to colonize the fetal liver, and other lymphoid and myeloid organs. Although hepatic haemopoiesis is normally erythropoietic, grafts of fetal mouse hepatic tissue to adult syngeneic hosts show granulopoiesis. The type of haemopoiesis occurring in fetal liver seems to depend therefore, upon factors extrinsic to the liver.[41] Local regulatory effects of macrophages may contribute.[42]

Growth of the liver

In its growth, the liver would seem to favour the traditional view of its structure: it grows by division and growth of constituent 'classic lobules'. Studies in the pig have shown that the average diameter of lobules is 0.33 mm in early fetal life, 0.5 mm at birth, and about 1 mm in the adult. Growth involves increase in number and size of hepatocytes, counter-balanced in part by a reduction in the diameter of sinusoids. New lobules arise by division of existing ones. The process may be understood by reference to Fig. 1.4. The hepatic venule, originally single, has divided, apparently sending out a side branch. This is not, in fact, a new outgrowth, but represents the enlargement of pre-existing sinusoids, as a 'preferred channel' under the moulding influence of increased blood flow.

Factors in early hepatic development

As noted above, the first morphological indication of development of the liver is an endodermal proliferation in the ventral part of the foregut, just cranial to its opening into the yolk sac, at the 18th post-fertilization day in the human embryo (2.5 mm stage). Tissue culture and transplantation experiments have shown that endodermal cells require two inductive interactions to form cells that express hepatocyte morphology ('hepatic specification'). Prehepatic endoderm is induced first by cardiac mesenchyme by fibroblast growth factor signalling, giving rise to proliferation of endodermal cells.[43] These cells then interact with the mesenchyme of the septum transversum and subsequently differentiate into hepatocyte precursors. This was first shown in avian embryos; subsequently similar inductive requirements were observed for mammalian liver development.[44]

Our understanding of the control of this early hepatic development has been enhanced by the use of genetic manipulation in mice and advanced culture techniques (reviewed in reference 44). Thus many of the molecules and receptors involved in regulation of the hepatoblasts and

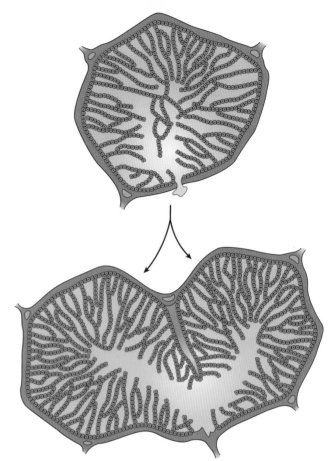

Fig. 1.4 • Diagrammatic illustrations of two stages in the division and growth of a 'classic lobule'.

subsequent hepatocyte and cholangiolar differentiation have now been identified. Furthermore it has become increasingly apparent that cellular interactions with non-parenchymal cells play a key role in early hepatic development.[45,46]

The sheets of hepatoblasts that invade the septum transversum in the developing mouse liver express the transcription factor hepatocyte nuclear factor (HNF) 4α while the surrounding mesenchyme expresses GATA4;[44] the migratory properties of the hepatoblasts appear to require a homeobox gene *Prox1*. GATA6 also appears to be essential in the formation of the early liver bud[47] as does FoxA1 and FoxA2 (previously HNF3β).[48] Some of these factors such as GATA4 appear to be important in early stimulation of hepatocyte specific gene expression including α fetoprotein and albumin; this occurs prior to morphological change toward a hepatocyte phenotype.

Vasculogenic cells (angioblasts) are critical for these earliest stages of organogenesis, prior to blood vessel formation. In the mouse embryo, angioblasts were found as a loose necklace of cells interceding between the thickening hepatically specified endoderm and the mesenchyme of the septum transversum. This mesenchymal–epithelial interaction precedes the emergence of the liver bud and persists throughout further liver development. The essential role of the vascular compartment can be illustrated in the *Flk* knockout mouse which lacks mature endothelial cells and in which there is failure of development of the liver bud.[46]

These interactions are also thought to be important in the development of the human liver.[49]

In the 5 mm embryo, the hepatic diverticulum comprises two parts. The cranial part (pars hepatica) is the one invading the septum transversum. The caudal part (pars cystica) develops into the gallbladder and does not contribute to development of the liver organ. The hepatic primordium consists of a uniform hepatoblast population with a bipotential differentiation capacity into both liver parenchymal cells and biliary epithelial cells. After the liver bud is generated, a different and distinct group of mesenchymal signals and hepatic response pathways (including hepatocyte growth factor/c-met receptor signalling) take over, stimulating further growth and differentiation of hepatoblasts and preventing their apoptosis.

The different vascular compartments in the developing mass of hepatoblasts have different origins. Portal veins derive from the vitelline veins, while the sinusoids derive from the capillary vessels of the septum transversum. Intrahepatic branches of the hepatic artery develop in tandem with the intrahepatic bile ducts in their ductal plate stage, thus progressively extending from the liver hilum along the developing branches of the portal vein. Intraportal capillary vessels derive through vasculogenesis from mesenchymal precursors (angioblasts) from 10 gestational weeks onward. The origin of the centrilobular veins remains unclear. The hepatic sinusoids develop in situ with the invasion of hepatoblasts into the mesenchyme of the septum transversum: the invading cells anastomose around preexisting endothelium-lined vesicles which later coalesce.

The sinusoidal endothelial cells experience a typical differentiation process. By the end of the third month, hepatic stellate cells have developed and contain one or two fat droplets. Kupffer cells originate from primitive macrophages from the yolk sac or develop in situ from hematopoietic stem cells. Their number increases during gestation, reaching adult values in the neonatal period.[50] Within these masses there develop sinusoids, communicating with the vitelline veins.[51] Changes to the surrounding extracellular matrix during fetal development and to the expression of integrin receptor proteins have been well documented and may direct modulation of cellular structure and function.[52] The development of a fenestrated endothelium lacking endothelial cell gaps and devoid of basement membrane is determined by the presence of hepatocytes.[53]

The nature of the signalling pathways involved during hepatogenesis has been elucidated by examining mRNA expression in cultured mouse endoderm; this has demonstrated the importance of the local concentration of FGF1 and FGF2;[54] bone morphogenetic proteins may also be involved.[55] These inductive cues control gene expression in the developing hepatoblasts through transcription factors of which in the mouse Hex appears to be essential.[56] Recent studies utilizing embryonic stem cells and small interfering RNA technology have reinforced the role of FoxA2 in hepatocytic differentiation.[57] The myriad of transcription factors and signalling molecules identified thus far that may be involved are summarised elsewhere;[25,44,58] further insights are likely to be found from analysis of so-called microRNAs[59] and high throughput gene screening in other vertebrates such as zebrafish.[60]

During later fetal liver development there is continued expansion of the parenchymal cell mass. This involves both stimulatory signals and protection from tumour necrosis factor α-mediated apoptosis; these phenomena involve the AP-1 transcription factor cJun, the Wnt signalling pathway, the nuclear factor κB pathway, and the hepatocyte growth factor (HGF)-c-met pathway among others.[44] Development and maintenance of hepatocytic differentiation and function is under the control of HNF4α.[61]

The mechanisms that control differentiation of hepatoblasts towards cholangiocytes (p. 4) is not clearly understood; as discussed in Chapter 4 (p. 166) it appears to involve the Notch-Jagged 1 pathway[62,63] and as noted above may be under the control of HNF6 and HNF1β.

Hepatic regeneration

The liver has a remarkable capacity to regulate its growth and size. This is best demonstrated by the restoration of liver mass that occurs following partial hepatectomy in animals and humans. Liver regeneration is a strictly regulated, nonautonomous process controlled by positive and negative factors which ultimately act to re-establish the appropriate ratio between liver mass and body size.[64] Growth ends when the original liver mass is regained through compensatory hyperplasia of the liver remnant. The signals for the initiation and termination of the process are likely to be related to hepatic function rather than anatomical form, because growth of the liver remnant occurs without morphogenetic restoration of the lobes removed at the operation, but involves enlargement of the remaining part.[65] The growth potential in the liver remnant is retained: after a second or succeeding partial hepatectomies, the liver can be induced to undergo further episodes of regeneration.

Several growth factors are important in liver regeneration.[64,66] These are considered further in Chapter 2. Various serum factors e.g. hepatocyte growth factor (HGF) induce DNA synthesis in hepatocytes as well as in bile-duct epithelial cells. A sharp increase in HGF in the plasma is thought to be the earliest event leading to liver regeneration after partial hepatectomy in the rat. This triggers a cascade of phenomena, leading to early changes in gene expression (so-called immediate early genes c-fos, c-jun, c-myc). Post-translational modification of NFkB-like transcription factor as well as changes in ion flux play a role early in the process. Activated NFkB binds to hepatocyte DNA and initiates transcription of genes, including thymidine kinase and cyclin-dependent kinase which causes transition from a quiescent phase to DNA synthesis. The proteins encoded by these genes act as transactivators of other genes which are then involved in the progression of hepatocytes through the cell cycle.

Regulatory growth factors are expressed by hepatocytes, Kupffer cells, hepatic stellate cells and ductular cells.[67–70] Cytokines, like tumour necrosis factor-alpha (TNFα), interleukin-1 (IL-1) and interleukin-6 (IL-6) produced by

Kupffer cells are also involved. These cytokines and growth factors form complex loops, both stimulatory and inhibitory and autocrine and paracrine: e.g. transforming growth factor beta (TGFβ), produced by hepatic stellate cells, acts as an autocrine stimulator of stellate cells but as a paracrine repressor of hepatocyte proliferation.[71]

Experimental partial hepatectomy in rodents very closely reflects the capacity of the human liver to regenerate after partial hepatectomy.[72] One of the most striking demonstrations of hepatic growth regulation in humans is the observation that transplanted livers which are small for a host will grow until the organ reaches the optimal mass required for this person.[73] This finding has led to the use of split transplants and the increased utilization of living donor transplantation.[74,75] In this latter situation, the liver remnant in the partially hepatectomized donor, as well as the liver transplanted into the new host, grow until they reach the hepatic mass which is appropriate for each of these individuals. The contrary is also true: if an excess of functional liver mass is present, e.g. when a transplant is large for the host, the liver decreases in size (presumably by apoptosis).[76]

Progenitor cells

In the partial hepatectomy model of regeneration, the remaining part of the liver is intact. All differentiated liver-cell compartments are capable of proliferation and can meet replacement demands for cellular loss from these differentiated liver-cell populations. So, in this model there is no need for a progenitor cell compartment. However, where there is extensive hepatocyte injury or when replication of hepatocytes is inhibited, differentiated hepatocytes are unable to assure regeneration. Under these conditions, 'reserve' cells take over. This hypothesis was first postulated by Wilson & Leduc in 1958, based on experiments involving liver regeneration after severe nutritional injury.[77] They concluded that bile ductules (cholangioles) gave rise to hepatocytes in the recovery phase of severe nutritional injury in mice. They proposed that cells of bile ductules formed a reserve compartment that could expand and generate hepatocytes after severe hepatic injury but would not do so after partial hepatectomy.

This theory was subsequently extensively investigated in rodent models of chemical carcinogenesis and chemical injury.[78–87] In these models, a portal population of small primitive epithelial cells with an oval nucleus and scant cytoplasm (so-called oval cells) proliferates in association with or before hepatocyte multiplication. It is generally believed that oval cells are related to terminal biliary ductules, the so-called canals of Hering.[81,88,89,90–94] However, they constitute a heterogeneous population of non-parenchymal epithelial cells and a proportion of these cells expresses phenotypic markers of both immature hepatocytes (like α-fetoprotein) and bile-duct cells.[84,90,91,95–99] At least a subset of oval cells is pluripotent and has the capacity to differentiate towards hepatocytes, bile ductular cells and intestinal epithelium and can give rise to hepatocellular carcinoma and cholangiocellular carcinoma.[83,88,100–104]

A number of recent studies on human liver in different pathological conditions also lend support to the hypothesis that there is a liver progenitor cell in adult human liver.[80,85,105–115] Furthermore, support for the existence of progenitor cells and their location in the canals of Hering has come from a better understanding of normal embryonic development of the liver. As has been described previously the early embryonic liver is composed of progenitor cells (hepatoblasts) that can generate both mature hepatocytes and bile-duct cells.[94,116–119] The hepatoblasts near portal vascular spaces (equivalents of portal tracts in mature liver) form primitive ductular structures, so-called ductal plates. The ductal plates are phenotypically equivalent to oval cells and express markers of both hepatocytes (α-fetoprotein and albumin) and bile-duct cells (cytokeratin 7 and 19, parathyroid hormone-related peptide).[107,120,121] It is likely that a small number of progenitor cells persist in the adult liver and that they are located in the smallest units of the biliary tree, at the transition between portal tracts and the parenchyma. Whether the hepatic progenitor cells are *facultative*[88] (meaning that they are only activated in case of hepatocyte damage or impaired replication), or whether they are part of a *continually renewing stem cell and lineage system*,[122] remains to be elucidated.[94] Recent reports show that in human liver, progenitor cells are not only activated after sub-massive necrosis of parenchyma but also in minimal degrees of chronic hepatitis.[123] Differentiation towards hepatocytes is only seen when a certain threshold of hepatocyte damage is reached. The degree of activation of progenitor cells increases with disease activity (degree of inflammation) and with the stage of the disease (degree of fibrosis). In chronic liver diseases of different aetiology, hepatocyte replication is inhibited due to telomere shortening. Similar to what is seen in animal models, this inhibition of hepatocyte replication is a trigger for progenitor activation in human chronic liver diseases.[80]

Of considerable interest are reports that in rodents[124] and in humans[125,126] hepatocytes and cholangiocytes may be derived from extrahepatic circulating stem cells, probably of bone marrow origin.[127] However, more recent reports indicate that generation of hepatocytes from haematopoietic stem cells does not happen through a process of true differentiation, but rather through a process of cell fusion.[128,129] Overall generation of hepatocytes from bone marrow stem cells is a rare event.[80]

The streaming liver

Studies on cell kinetics in the rat by Zajicek and his colleagues[130–131] suggested that there is a continuous, though extremely slow, production of hepatocytes in the periportal zones and that they move from their site of origin as part of a cell stream, comprising the parenchyma/stromal complex (accompanied by sinusoidal cells, and probably also by its nerve supply). This cell stream advances, at a rate estimated at about 2 μm/day, towards the perivenular zone where its constituents are assumed to undergo apoptosis. Hepatocyte turnover and streaming can be accelerated by liver toxins and slowed down by hypothyroidism.[132]

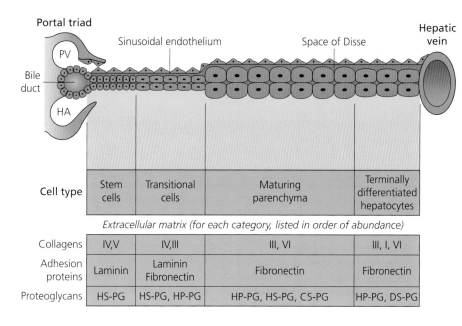

Fig. 1.5 • Model illustrating a stem cell and lineage system in the liver with some details of the extracellular matrix gradient. Within the stem cell compartment in the periportal area cells capable of differentiating into biliary epithelium or hepatocytes are produced. The hepatocytes differentiate as they stream in a periportal to perivenular direction, and this is accompanied by an increase in cell size— < 20 μm in diameter for transitional cells and 30–40 μm for mature cells. The extracellular matrix comprises heparan sulphate (HS), heparin (HP), chondroitin sulphate (CS), dermatan sulphate (DS) and proteoglycans (PG). Modified from Reid et al.[134]

Cell type	Stem cells	Transitional cells	Maturing parenchyma	Terminally differentiated hepatocytes
Extracellular matrix (for each category, listed in order of abundance)				
Collagens	IV,V	IV,III	III, VI	III, I, VI
Adhesion proteins	Laminin	Laminin Fibronectin	Fibronectin	Fibronectin
Proteoglycans	HS-PG	HS-PG, HP-PG	HP-PG, HS-PG, CS-PG	HP-PG, DS-PG

The life expectancy of the hepatocyte in rats was estimated at about 200 days. This concept implies a progenitor zone in the periportal area and, in addition, implies both a chronological and a biological age for the streaming cells, the biological age equating with differentiation and being accompanied by an increased content of DNA. The functional heterogeneity of hepatocytes is discussed below as is the composition of the extracellular matrix, which shows a gradient with different composition in the periportal zone as compared with the mid-zone and perivenular zone. Such matrix gradients may be similar to those identified in the intestine and haemopoietic tissue, and may have an important role in regulating hepatocyte and sinusoidal cell function. Sigal and his colleagues[123,133,134] embraced the concepts of a stem cell compartment, the streaming liver, functional heterogeneity and extracellular matrix gradients to produce a hypothetical model of liver lineage (Fig. 1.5).

However, the concepts of migration of hepatocytes along hepatic plates and of stem cell-fed hepatocyte lineages have been criticized and contradicted by subsequent experiments. Zajicek and his colleagues used tritiated thymidine to tag proliferating hepatocytes. A drawback to the use of tritiated thymidine results from the weak labelling of late replicating hepatocytes due to their re-utilization of labelled thymidine released into the blood when cells of rapidly turning over extrahepatic tissues die, a mechanism which provides labelled DNA substrates for liver cells for several days after a pulse dose of tritiated thymidine.[135] Furthermore, muralia or liver-cell plates cannot serve as radially arranged tracks along which hepatocytes migrate in a linear way, since muralia branch and intersect, mostly in the periportal region, forming a three-dimensional structure that more resembles a sponge than a series of nearly parallel walls.[135] Moreover, studies of hepatic structure in genetically mosaic animals[136] showed that the proliferation of hepatocytes is clonal or quasi-clonal, not only during the growth and regeneration of liver postnatally, but also during hepatic embryogenesis.[137]

Analysis of patches of (immuno) histochemically distinguishable cells in livers of mosaic mice and rats demonstrates that the location of patches is unrelated to hepatic structural landmarks, including portal tracts and liver-cell plates. Individual plates may comprise phenotypically and genetically distinct cells from each of two adjacent patches. This indicates that hepatocyte proliferation occurs in a quasi-clonal pattern in which the newly generated cells are not directionally biased (for instance in a centrilobular direction if liver streaming were to be the case), but instead are sited randomly in relation to their parent cells, including sites within the borders of adjacent patches.[138,139] Several studies in which hepatocyte tagging was performed by the genetic tagging of cells using the *Escherichia coli* β-galactosidase gene coupled to a nuclear localization signal[140,141] produced evidence which contradicted the streaming liver concept. The data were summarized as follows:[142] (i) retroviral marking of hepatocytes in vivo demonstrates that labelled cells do not move, and remain primarily as small clusters of cells for up to 15 months after transduction;[140] (ii) developmental analysis of expression patterns in mosaic livers demonstrates that individual hepatocytes replicate to form a large cluster of hepatocytes during postnatal liver growth;[141] and (iii) the life-span of a differentiated hepatocyte is at least 2 years in rodents.[142]

Is the debate on a stem-cell-fed lineage and streaming liver to be considered closed? The answer is 'yes' for the streaming liver concept in its simplistic form, viewing hepatocytes moving in Indian file-like manner along radially extending liver cell plates towards the hepatic vein. However, accepting the quasi-clonal or 'fractal' pattern of liver cell proliferation, one may consider that instead of single cells streaming, growing clusters of hepatocytes are streaming.[143] This was rejected on the following consideration: in the event that stem cells in Zajicek's postulated periportal proliferative zone of restricted hepatocyte formation[144] were infected by retrovirus as in the experiments of Bralet et al.,[140] tagged progeny cells should have been located all along liver-cell plates at 15 months.[138] However, why in a retroviral infection experiment should 100% of presumed progenitor cells be expected to be tagged, when the present efficiency of gene transduction is such that only a minority of hepatocytes become tagged? Assuming a tagging of only a minority of presumed progenitor cells in periportal locations, one might expect a similar result to that obtained in the studies of Bralet and her colleagues. Indeed, the occasional replication of a tagged progenitor cell would produce from time to time a clone of tagged hepatocytes, whereas the majority of non-tagged progenitor cells would engender a much larger number of non-tagged hepatocyte clones.

A further argument against streaming liver cells was found in studies where hepatocytes were transplanted in transgenic mice suffering from toxic elimination of hepatocytes carrying the transgene, thus resulting in a continuous regenerative stimulus. The transplanted hepatocytes replicated extensively, suggesting that the differentiated hepatocyte itself is capable of many rounds of replication. This, however, does not exclude a role for progenitor cells, and there is even the possibility that occasional 'stem' cells were present in the preparation of hepatocytes which were transplanted.[142] At present it seems unlikely that hepatocytes stream but the debate is not concluded.

Macroanatomy of the liver

This account assumes a knowledge of the macroscopic morphology of the liver, such as could be obtained from a standard undergraduate text, and draws attention only to features of particular interest to the pathologist.

The liver lies almost completely under the protection of the rib-cage, projecting below it and coming into contact with the anterior abdominal wall only below the right costal margin and the xiphisternum. It is moulded to the under surface of the diaphragm, the muscular part of which separates it on each side from the corresponding lung and pleural sac. It is separated by the central tendon of the diaphragm from the pericardium and the heart. The posterior surface of the liver is the least accessible and its relationships are of some clinical importance. It includes the following, from right to left:

1. The 'bare area', which is surrounded by the reflections of peritoneum which form the superior and inferior layers of the coronary ligaments. It lies in direct contact with the diaphragm, except where the inferior vena cava, the right adrenal and the upper part of the right kidney intervene.
2. The caudate lobe, which lies between the inferior vena cava on the right and, on the left, the fissure of the ligamentum venosum and the attachment of the lesser omentum. The caudate lobe projects into the right side of the superior recess of the lesser sac; behind it lies the right crus of the diaphragm, between the inferior vena cava and the aorta.
3. A small area on the left, covered by peritoneum and related to the abdominal oesophagus.

The traditional division into right and left, caudate and quadrate lobes is of purely topographical significance. A more useful and important subdivision is made on the basis of the branching pattern of the hepatic artery, portal vein and hepatic ducts. As these are followed into the liver from the porta hepatis, each branches in corresponding fashion, accompanied by a branching tree of connective tissue, continuous with the external (Glisson) capsule of the liver. On this basis, the liver is divided into right and left 'physiological' lobes of about equal size. The plane of separation between these two 'hemi-livers' corresponds, on the visceral surface of the liver, to a line extending from the left side of the sulcus for the inferior vena cava superiorly, to the middle of the fossa for the gallbladder inferiorly.

On a similar basis each lobe has been further subdivided into portal (or portobiliary-arterial) segments, in studies pioneered by Hjortso[145] and extended by Couinaud[146] and many others. Within each hemi-liver, the primary branches of the portal vein divide to supply two main portal segments, each of which is further divided horizontally into superior and inferior segments. According to this scheme there are, therefore, eight segments, or nine if the caudate lobe is separately designated. In the absence of a fully agreed anatomical nomenclature, the following terms are sufficiently descriptive of the segments: *right lobe*—antero-superior and antero-inferior, postero-superior and medio-inferior; *left lobe*—medio-superior and medio-inferior, latero-superior and latero-inferior. The *caudate lobe* stands at the watershed between right and left vascular and ductal territories; its right portion in particular may be served by right or left vessels and ducts, although its left part is almost invariably supplied by the transverse portion of the left branch of the portal vein.

These nine hepatic segments are separate in the sense that each has its own vascular pedicle (arterial, portal venous and lymphatic) and biliary drainage. There are said to be no intrahepatic anastomoses between the right and left hepatic arteries, a view which is generally supported by injection studies of cadaveric livers. However, Mays & Mays[147] have shown, by selective in vivo hepatic arteriography after ligation of the right or the left hepatic artery in humans, that there exist intrahepatic translobar collateral arteries capable of perfusing the entire occluded arterial system. They found no intermediate filling of sinusoids or of portal venules. However, the virtual vascular independence of each segment has been shown by studies in the living, using computed tomography, magnetic resonance imaging, and ultrasonography together with intravenous contrast injections which allow ready recognition of the liver's major vascular structures.[148,149]

Recognition of this compartmental pattern is of considerable pathological significance: regional degeneration of a lobe or segment may follow disturbance of its blood supply by a particular portal vein branch. While this recognition might be thought to facilitate surgical segmental resection, its usefulness is at present somewhat limited by the absence of defining connective tissue septa between segments and by the topography of the hepatic veins, which run in an intersegmental position and in planes which cross those followed by the portal triad.[150] Moreover, the pattern of segments shows individual variation.

Gupta and his colleagues[151] analysed variations in the segmental pattern of the liver. In nearly one-half of 85 livers examined, the pattern and sizes of segments were similar; in the remainder there were many variants, involving principally increase or decrease in size of one or more segments at the expense of neighbouring segments. There are said to be no anastomoses between the blood vessels or hepatic ducts of adjacent segments.

Anomalous origin of the arterial supply of the liver is very common. In an analysis of more than 2300 cases, Nelson et al.[152] reported a left hepatic artery as arising from the left gastric artery in 14%, a right hepatic from the superior mesenteric artery in 14%, and a common hepatic from the superior mesenteric artery in 3%. Extrahepatic anastomoses have been described between hepatic arteries and a number of other arteries, mostly arising as branches of the common hepatic artery (e.g. right gastric and gastroduodenal arteries). Anastomoses also exist with branches of the superior and inferior phrenic arteries and of the internal thoracic artery and with intercostal arteries. Although normally unimportant, they may constitute the major arterial supply after ligation of the hepatic artery.[153]

Two points should be noted: (i) if, say, the ('physiological') right lobe is supplied by an artery other than the right hepatic, the intrahepatic pattern of branching is usually normal; (ii) a branch of abnormal origin supplying a particular part of the liver is the sole supply of that part: it is aberrant rather than accessory. Similar anomalies not uncommonly affect the duct system. For example, an aberrant segmental duct may leave the liver independently and drain into the extrahepatic duct system, or even directly into the gallbladder.

While the branches of the hepatic artery and portal vein and the tributaries of the hepatic ducts run together and serve segments of liver, the hepatic veins run independently and are intersegmental. Like the portal vein, they lack valves. The three major hepatic veins, the right, intermediate and left (the intermediate and left often forming a common trunk) enter the upper end of the retro-hepatic segment of the inferior vena cava: the terminal portion of each is frequently at least partially exposed above the posterior surface of the liver, where they are vulnerable to trauma. In addition to these major hepatic veins, several (about five per liver) accessory hepatic veins open into the lower part of the hepatic segment of the inferior vena cava.[154] Since the caudate lobe regularly drains directly into the inferior vena cava, it may escape injury from venous outflow block (Chapter 13).

Obstruction of portal venous flow may be compensated for by enlargement of portal-systemic venous anastomoses which occur at several sites: lower oesophagus, anal canal, at the umbilicus, at the bare area of the liver and where parts of the gut, e.g. colon and duodenum, are in direct contact with the posterior abdominal wall. These anastomoses become functionally significant when portal hypertension develops. The effects of increased portal venous pressure are compounded by the absence of valves in the portal system.

Microanatomy of the liver

The hepatic microcirculation
Portal circulation

Within the liver, the portal vein divides into successive generations of distributing or conducting veins, so called because they do not directly feed the sinusoidal circulation. According to their position in the hierarchy of branching, they may be classified as interlobar, segmental and interlobular. The smallest conducting veins are interlobular veins. Further branching of these produces the portal vein branches which distribute their blood into the sinusoids. These succeeding branches are: (i) the pre-terminal portal venules which, microscopically, are found in portal tracts of triangular cross-section; (ii) the terminal portal venules which taper to about 20–30 μm in diameter, and are surrounded by scanty connective tissue in portal tracts of circular rather than triangular cross-section. From the pre-terminal and terminal portal venules there arise very short side branches i.e. the inlet venules, which have an endothelial lining with a basement membrane and scanty adventitial fibrous connective tissue, but no smooth muscle, in their walls. They pass through the periportal limiting plate to open into the sinusoids. These inlets are reported to be guarded by sphincters composed of sinusoidal lining cells— the afferent or inlet sphincters.[155] Some early branching of the smallest conducting veins may produce more than one portal vein within some portal canals and these supply only those sinusoids which abut upon the canal.

Arterial circulation

The hepatic artery branches accompany the portal veins; their number generally equals the number of interlobular ducts in the portal area. The terminal distribution of the arteries is by three routes: into a periportal plexus, into a peribiliary plexus, and into terminal hepatic arterioles.[156]

A periportal plexus is characteristically distributed around portal vein branches within the portal area. It drains into hepatic sinusoids. Occasional arterioportal anastomoses between periportal arterioles and terminal portal venules have been observed but the frequency of these in humans is uncertain.[155,156]

A peribiliary plexus supplies all the intrahepatic bile ducts. Around the larger ducts, the peribiliary plexus is two-layered, with a rich inner, subepithelial, layer of fine capillaries and an outer, periductular, venous network which receives blood from the inner layer. Small bile ducts have only a single layer of fine capillaries. Ultrastructural studies have shown that the capillaries are lined by fenestrated endothelium which contains pinocytic vesicles.[157] The peribiliary plexus drains principally into hepatic sinusoids. This vascular route from a hepatic artery supply through the peribiliary plexus into hepatic sinusoids has been called a 'peribiliary portal system'.[158] The peribiliary plexus develops in parallel with the development of the intrahepatic bile ducts, spreading from the hepatic hilum to the peripheral area of the liver and becoming fully developed with the full maturation of the biliary system.[159] It has been proposed that the peribiliary plexus is involved in reabsorption of bile constituents including bile acids (cholehepatic circulation) and in the uptake of vasoactive substances secreted by cells in the biliary epithelium (see below).[160,161] Rappaport[162] suggested that by providing for countercurrent exchange of ions between blood and bile, the peribiliary plexus was involved in both secretion and resorption of bile constituents; the ultrastructural features are consistent with active transport between the capillaries and biliary epithelial cells, and this activity may be altered to meet increased functional demands in bile duct obstruction.[157]

Terminal hepatic arterioles have an internal elastic lamina and a layer of smooth muscle cells, and open into periportal sinusoids via arteriosinus twigs. Reports of hepatic arterioles which penetrate deeply into the parenchyma before entering sinusoids near to the hepatic veins have been disputed.[163–165] Such vessels may sometimes be seen in liver biopsies. Ekataksin[11] has recently suggested that these vessels, which he refers to as 'the isolated artery (arteriole)', supply isolated vascular beds.

Venous drainage

Having perfused the parenchyma via the sinusoids, the blood enters the terminal hepatic venules (the central veins of the 'classic lobules'). Several collecting venules may drain the blood from individual abutting lobules into the terminal venules. Scanning electron microscopy has clearly demonstrated in the walls of veins the fenestrations through which the sinusoids open.[166] The terminal vein branches unite to form intercalated veins which in turn form larger hepatic vein branches whose macroanatomy has already been described.

Functional histology of the microcirculation

This account is based immediately on the work of McCuskey which has been reviewed by him,[155,165,168,169] but derives ultimately from the pioneering studies of Knisely et al.[170] using quartz rod transillumination of living liver. Arterioportal relationships are summarized in Fig. 1.6, which shows a terminal portal venule from which a series of sinusoids originates, and an accompanying terminal hepatic arteriole (internal diameter approximately 10 μm). There are various kinds of connection between arteriole and sinusoid, all of them being found in the periportal areas, and all of internal diameter no greater than the diameter of an erythrocyte. Approximately two-thirds of the blood supply comes from the portal venules whose inlets are controlled by sphincters—afferent or inlet sphincters—composed of sinusoidal endothelial cells. Flow of arterial blood to the sinusoids is intermittent, and determined by independently contractile smooth muscle sphincters in the walls of hepatic arterioles

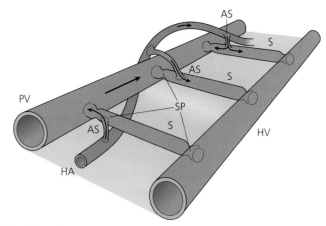

Fig. 1.6 • Scheme to show relationships of hepatic arteriole (HA), portal venule (PV), sinusoids (S) and hepatic venule (HV). Arterio-sinusoidal branches (AS) may open in various ways into the sinusoids and blood flowing to a group of sinusoids could therefore be arterial, venous or mixed. Blood flow through the sinusoids is determined by the activity of 'sphincters' (SP) in the arteriolar wall and of sphincteric mechanisms at the inlet and outlet of the sinusoids. Based on McCuskey.[165]

and their arteriolo-sinusoidal branches. Blood flowing into a group of sinusoids could therefore be arterial, venous or mixed, depending upon sphincteric and contractile activity.

There is heterogeneity in the blood flow through the sinusoids. In the peripheral zones the sinusoids form an interconnecting polygonal network. Downstream, however, they become organized as parallel vessels which open into the terminal hepatic venule; short intersinusoidal sinusoids connect adjacent parallel sinusoids. Blood entering the hepatic venules passes through efferent or outlet sphincters which, like the inlet sphincters, are composed of sinusoidal endothelial cells.

The precise mechanisms which regulate the hepatic microcirculation remain controversial.[155] The potential morphological sites for regulating blood flow through the sinusoids include segments of the portal venules and hepatic arterioles, the sinusoids themselves and the hepatic venules. The portal and hepatic venules and the hepatic arterioles contain some smooth muscle cells in their wall and are therefore contractile. However, the principal site of regulation is thought to reside in the sinusoids themselves. The sinusoidal endothelial cells respond to a variety of vasoactive substances and by contracting or swelling they may vary the diameter of the sinusoid lumen. Thus, blood flow through individual sinusoids is variable. Where the lumen is narrowed, blood flow may be impeded by leucocytes that transiently plug the vessel, a feature which is more common in the narrower more tortuous periportal sinusoids.[171] It seems likely that flow through some sinusoids may be intermittent while others have relatively constant rates of blood flow. Arterial blood flowing into an individual sinusoid through a dilated arteriosinusoid may increase the rate of blood flow.

The Kupffer cells could also affect rate of blood flow through sinusoids.[169] Most recently attention has focused on a possible role for the hepatic stellate cells. Contraction in vitro of hepatic stellate cells in response to agents such as endothelin-1 has been reported.[172] In addition, reduction of the portal blood flow has been shown by in vivo microscopy to reduce sinusoidal blood flow with a considerable reduction in sinusoidal diameter, changes which were reversed on restoring the portal blood flow.[173] It has been suggested that the stellate cells, whose long slender processes surround the sinusoids, may be responsible for producing these changes.

Finally, it is worth pointing out that while the portal vein does supply the larger amount of the blood supply to the liver, the liver is not capable of directly controlling this flow and, thus, the only control of flow within the liver is via the hepatic artery. It has been postulated that the hepatic arterial flow is not regulated by liver metabolic demands but may change inversely in response to altered portal blood flow.[174–176]

Hepatic functional units

Kiernan's concept of the polyhedral or classic lobule has already been mentioned.[2] It is traditionally represented as hexagonal in outline with, at its centre, a central vein, a terminal tributary of the hepatic vein. The boundaries of such a lobule are well-defined in only a few species (e.g. pig, camel, raccoon and polar bear[177]) by interlobular septa of connective tissue. In most other species, including man, connective tissue is sparse, except in the portal canals which lie between the 'corners' of adjacent lobules. It is evident from Fig. 1.7 that the blood from the terminal afferent vessels perfuses through sinusoids which pass into segments only of adjacent hexagonal lobules. It seemed improbable therefore, that such a hexagonal mass of parenchyma could subserve the role of a functional unit and so many other investigators have reported what they regarded as the

hepatic unit. In the second and third editions of this text (in 1987 and 1994) we favoured the concept of Rappaport's hepatic acinus in that it seemed to be of greatest value to the histopathologist in the interpretation of disordered structure and function. However, more recent studies have suggested that the concept of the primary lobule as defined by Matsumoto and his colleagues (and which we described in the third edition) has gained increasing attention. Accordingly, both of these hepatic units are now reviewed, together with other units which have been recently reported, and a critical assessment of the relative merits of these is made.

The hepatic acinus

Rappaport and his colleagues[5] defined a unit or acinus related to the terminal branches of the afferent microcirculation. This concept was extended in subsequent papers and reviews[178–181] in which it was suggested that the hepatic parenchyma is divisible into structural units of first order, second order and third order as illustrated diagrammatically in Fig. 1.8. The division into acini was initially based on the terminal portal circulation as illustrated in Fig. 1.7, but it must be borne in mind that the arterial blood supply and the biliary drainage system follow a similar distribution pattern.

The *simple acinus* was defined as a small parenchymal mass, irregular in size and shape, arranged around a small round portal tract containing a terminal portal vein and its accompanying hepatic arteriole and bile duct: the acinus lies between two (or more) terminal hepatic venules into which it drains: it has no investing capsule: in a two-dimensional view it occupies part only of two adjacent classic lobules (Fig. 1.7) and in a three-dimensional view it

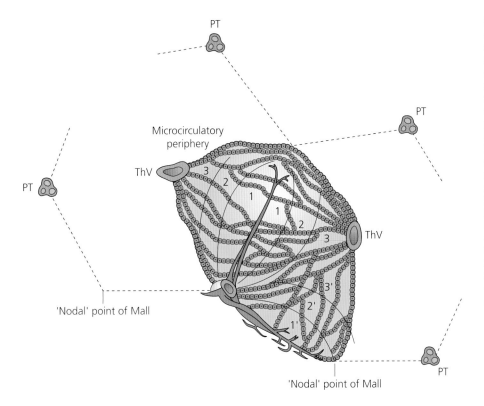

Fig. 1.7 • Diagrammatic representation of the simple acinus and the zonal arrangement of hepatocytes. Two neighbouring classic lobules are outlined by the discontinuous lines, and the acinus occupies adjacent sectors of these. Although only one channel is shown as forming the central core of the acinus, the acinus is arranged round the terminal branches of the portal vein, hepatic artery and bile ductule. Zones 1, 2 and 3 represent areas which receive blood progressively poorer in nutrients and oxygen; zone 3 thus represents the microcirculatory periphery, and the most peripheral portions of zone 3 from adjacent acini form the perivenular area. The nodal points of Mall represent vascular watershed areas where the terminal afferent vessels from neighbouring acini meet. PT = portal tract; ThV = terminal hepatic vein (central vein of 'classic lobule'); 1, 2, 3 = microcirculatory zones; 1', 2', 3' = microcirculatory zones of neighbouring acinus; ----- = outline of 'classic lobule'. Adapted from Rappaport.[179]

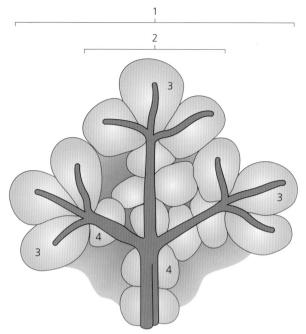

Fig. 1.8 • Diagrammatic representation of the hepatic acinar structure: this shows an acinar agglomerate—1, three complex acini—2, and a number of simple acini—3. The acinar agglomerate is supplied by a portal vein (and hepatic artery) branch which subdivides into three preterminal branches supplying each complex acinus; these branches in turn subdivide into terminal branches supplying the simple acini. The acinuli—4, are arranged as a sleeve around the preterminal and the main supplying vessels. Adapted from Rappaport et al.[182]

appears as a berry-like structure at the end of the terminal vascular/biliary stalk. The simple acini abut against one another and, as shown in Fig. 1.7, the sites where the terminal arterioles and venules from neighbouring acini give out into their final capillaries constitute watershed areas and correspond to the 'nodal' points of Mall.[4] The approximate dimensions of the simple acinus are 1480 μm in length, 1070 μm in width and 800 μm in thickness.[182]

The *complex acinus* comprised at least three simple acini and a sleeve of parenchyma around the pre-terminal portal vein branches and their accompanying arterial and biliary elements. The sleeve of parenchyma around the pre-terminal vessels comprises small clumps—*acinuli*—which are supplied by venular and arteriolar branches from the pre-terminal vessels.

The *acinar agglomerate* comprised three or four complex acini and the acinuli forming the sleeve of parenchyma around the large triangular or oval shaped portal tract supplying the agglomerate. The supplying portal vein is between 300 and 1200 μm in diameter (average 600 μm). The unity of the agglomerate is again determined by the fact that the vascular supply and the biliary drainage are common to the whole agglomerate as well as to its acinar subdivisions.

Within the simple acinus there was further subdivision into zones 1, 2 and 3 (Fig. 1.7) which were related to the zonal heterogeneity of liver tissue. In Fig. 1.7 there is apparent continuity between zone 3 of adjacent simple acini. Although subdivision of the complex acini into circulatory zones is difficult to demonstrate in the normal liver, ischaemic and viral injury extending through adjacent zones

3—pericomplex acinar—provides indirect morphological evidence of continuity between these zones.

The hepatic muralium. Within the acini the hepatocytes appear, in single sections, to form irregularly arranged cords (see Fig. 1.15(A)). The tri-dimensional reconstructions of Elias[183,184] showed that the hepatocytes are in fact arranged in the form of plates or laminae, one cell in thickness, and these studies have been fully confirmed by scanning electron microscopy (SEM).[166,185,186] These hepatic laminae branch and anastomose with one another to form a complicated system of walls, the hepatic muralium, a maze-like arrangement of partitions between which the sinusoids interweave and interconnect in a continuous labyrinth.

Immediately deep to the external capsule of the liver is a single continuous sheet of hepatocytes, forming the external limiting plate. Elias[187] described this as extending inwards at the porta hepatis, to follow the branching of the portal vein and hepatic artery, and forming an internal periportal limiting plate. This bounds the portal tracts and forms an interface between the connective tissue of the tract and the hepatic parenchyma. In similar fashion, the external limiting plate extends into the liver as an investment around the hepatic veins and their tributaries, forming around these an internal perivenular limiting plate. Both the periportal and perivenular limiting plates are discontinuous where perforating vascular and biliary radicles pass through them.

The greatest merit of the acinus concept is that it has drawn attention to the terminal branches of the afferent portal vein, located between the pre-terminal portal tracts of the classical lobule according to Kiernan. The subdivision into three zones (an arbitrary subdivision, which could equally well have included 5 or 10 zones) draws attention to the zonal aspect of heterogeneity of liver tissue, and was welcomed by hepatopathologists as it afforded an explanation for the location and appearance of some histopathological lesions (zonal steatosis, zonal necrosis, bridging necrosis, bridging fibrosis).

Later studies have criticized the concept on the basis of enzyme-histochemical and immunohistochemical investigations,[188,189] which revealed that in microscopic sections of normal liver tissue, zone 1 had a concave rather than convex appearance, and hence rather corresponded with the so-called sickle zone in the primary lobule concept of Matsumoto and colleagues. In contrast with normal liver, the surviving zone 1 parenchyma in liver biopsies with severe portal-central confluent bridging necrosis may appear convex (as in Fig. 1.7). However, and in retrospect, one should keep in mind that in conditions of severe liver necrosis the shape of surviving zone 1 parenchyma may originally have been sickle-shaped, but subsequently become modified to a convex configuration (as in Fig. 1.7) due to intervening hepatocellular regeneration.

The studies of Lamers and his colleagues[188] based on three-dimensional assessment of hepatic enzyme zonation suggested that the perivenular zone was circular and discrete rather than stellate and confluent, whereas the periportal zone was reticular and contiguous between adjacent acini rather than discrete. These results are more consistent with Matsumoto's lobular concept. The 'metabolic lobulus' of Lamers and associates is therefore categorically different from the 'microcirculatory acinus' of Rappaport.

Matsumoto's primary lobule

Matsumoto and colleagues[6,190] performed a detailed study of the angio-architecture of the human liver with graphic reconstructions from thousands of serial sections. They distinguished a conducting and a parenchymal portion of the portal venous tree. The conducting portion should ensure delivery of blood to the parenchyma, with a pressure drop small enough to ensure for the initial parenchymal branch a pressure range sufficient to keep the parenchymal circulation dynamically adapted to any metabolic demand. The conducting portion meets this functional demand by remaining within the macroscopic range throughout its course, thus rendering resistance to flow virtually insignificant.

The parenchymal portion of the portal venous tree follows a strict scheme of ramification in three steps. At the first step, branches arise in orderly rows from every terminal branch of the conducting portion. Each of these first-step branches supplies a fairly definite mass of parenchyma (approximately 1.6 mm wide; 1.2 mm long; and 0.8 mm thick), of themselves representing the central axis of the parenchymal masses. From the conducting portion down to this step, the portal branches of a given order are generally equal in number to the hepatic veins of the corresponding order.

At the second step, every first-step branch gives off at about right angles 11 second-step branches (with an average diameter of 70 μm). This sudden increase in branching frequency (limited to the portal vein, and not observed in corresponding levels of the hepatic vein) engenders a characteristic portohepatic constellation: about six portal vein branches embracing a certain amount of parenchyma with one hepatic vein as the central axis. Evidently, this constellation underscores the time-honoured concept of the classic lobule of Kiernan.[2]

The third-step ramification occurs at about right angles from every second-step branch. At this step all branches virtually lack connective tissue sheets and their wall structure gradually changes over to that of sinusoid. However, they are easily recognizable by their precise interlobular course and their larger lumina. These branches are termed the septal branches.

In this arrangement how do the sinusoidal vascular beds receive their blood supply from the parenchymal portion of the portal vein? The typical lobular patterns (of the classical lobule and of the parenchymal mass embraced by the second-step branches of the parenchymal portion of the portal venous tree) quite naturally lead us to expect that most of the intralobular sinusoids arise from the marginal zone of the lobule and then converge towards the centrilobular area. The important point was to prove this expectation, since such proof had hitherto been lacking. Therefore, Matsumoto and colleagues attempted to clarify the three-dimensional angio-architecture that would mediate the

transit of blood from the parenchymal portal vein to the radial sinusoids. Their observations revealed that the marginal zone that demarcates the lobule comprises two distinct zones in terms of angio-architecture: the septal zone and the portal zone. The septal zone is mainly defined by the above-mentioned septal branches. They not only supply this zone with portal blood, but also support it as a vascular skeleton. The septal branches, located in the plane between two adjacent second-step branches (portal tracts), run a more or less parallel course and are quite regularly spaced about 200 μm apart over the lobular surface. Upwards and downwards, they give off a few branches which all break up into sinusoids, thus forming a septum-like sinusoidal network at the surface of the lobule (Figs 1.9 and 1.10). The septum serves as a starting plane for intralobular radial sinusoids.

The portal zone is part of the marginal zone that is in contact with the portal tract. The vessels that supply this zone are short venules (inlet venules) given off either directly from the portal tract or from the most proximal portion of each septal branch. The characteristic of this vessel is that it soon breaks up into branches of sinusoidal order, which spread in almost transverse direction to the

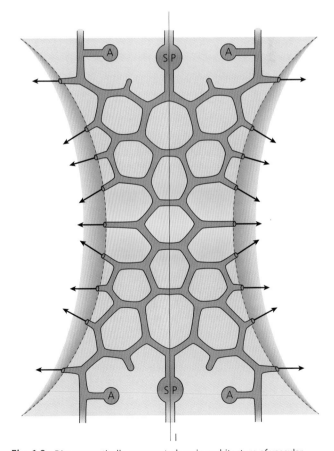

Fig. 1.9 • Diagrammatically represented angio-architecture of vascular septum: a figure generated by sectioning the vascular septum in Fig. 1.10 with a plane perpendicular to both the septal branches and the Y–Z plane. SP: primary septal branch; A: accessory branch; I: line of intersection with the Y–Z plane in Fig. 1.10. Note that each primary septal branch builds (the upper one downward and the lower one upward) 2- to 3-storied (in this figure 2-storied) sinusoidal loops which form the bulk of the septum. Arrows: direction of blood flow. Adapted from Matsumoto & Kawakami.[190]

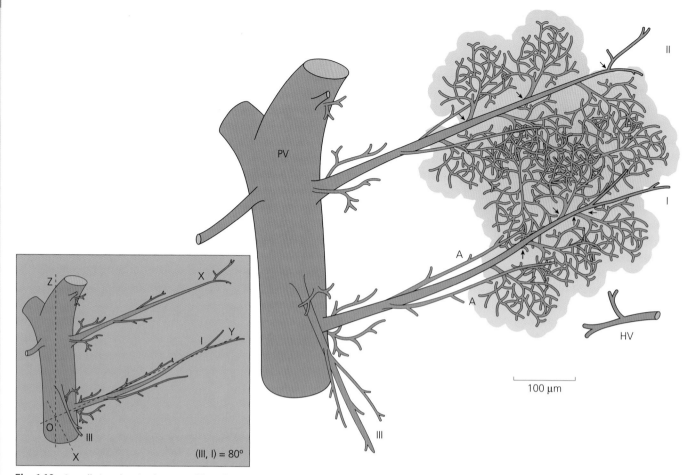

Fig. 1.10 • Overall view showing how septal branches span vascular septum. PV = portal vein; I, II, III = primary septal branches; arrows = secondary septal branches; A = accessory branch; HV = hepatic vein. Inset: diagram indicating the orientation of septal branches relative to their parent portal vein. Adapted from Matsumoto & Kawakami.[190]

original axis of the vessel, thus taking a dish-like form (Fig. 1.11). From this extension blood streams inward into the parenchyma. Although the sinusoids have numerous lateral anastomoses, the preferential paths of blood from the dish-like extension can be followed over some distance until it reaches the surface (surface Fp in Fig. 1.11) where these paths pass into radial sinusoids. Along this course the bundle of preferential sinusoids takes the form of a curved cylinder (Fig. 1.11).

These sinusoidal beds of the septal zone and of the portal zone together constitute a synthetic functional unit: a high potential pool from which portal blood pours uniformly into the radial sinusoids. On lobular cross-sections, this pool space appears as a sickle-shaped area (the sickle zone). The sickle edge represents a cut line of the vertically extending inflow-front, and represents a haemodynamic equipotential surface. The inflow-front appears to be composed of smaller unit areas, each tending to be concave inwards. About six to eight such units cover the entire surface of the lobule. These units of the inflow-front have their counterparts in the draining system: each central vein is found to comprise six to eight draining poles, disposed in such a way that each faces a corresponding unit of the inflow-front across a certain parenchymal distance. The cone-shaped

mass of parenchyma thus sandwiched by this pair is designated *the primary lobule* in the sense that it represents the most elementary parenchymal unit (Fig. 1.12).

All these findings point to a new aspect of the classical lobule: the classical lobule is made up of six to eight primary lobules, and is itself termed *the secondary lobule*. The most important structural feature of the secondary lobule is that the central vein represents its longitudinal axis while the terminal branches of the portal vein form its periphery.[191]

These observations are at variance with the acinus concept in the following ways:[6,190]

1. The lobule has a surface-like inflow-front whereas the acinus is characterized by a linear inflow-source with radial symmetry.
2. The septal branches (conceptual equivalents of the terminal portal venules of the acinus concept) do not run the entire length of the distance between two portal tracts, but taper off into a sinusoidal configuration near the middle of the interportal distance. In other words, the vascular watershed areas are not located at the nodal points of Mall (Fig. 1.7) but at the midpoint of the interportal distance (midseptum M of Zou et al.[191]—Fig. 1.13).

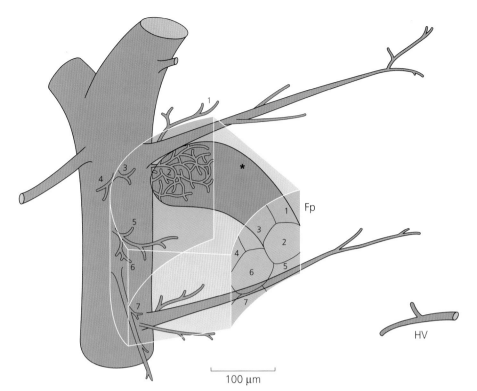

Fig. 1.11 • Vascular beds (*) depending mainly on the inlet venule 2. Fp: inflow-front: equipotential surface that gives rise to typical 'converging sinusoids'. Adapted from Matsumoto & Kawakami.[190]

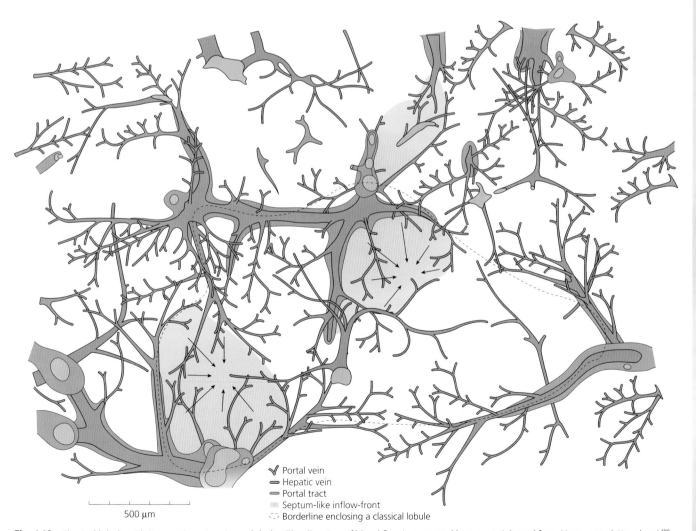

✔ Portal vein
━ Hepatic vein
━ Portal tract
▨ Septum-like inflow-front
◌ Borderline enclosing a classical lobule

Fig. 1.12 • Classical lobule with its constituents, primary lobules. The direction of blood flow is suggested by arrows. Adapted from Matsumoto & Kawakami.[190]

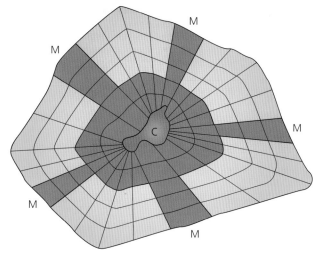

Fig. 1.13 • The vitamin A-low territory (shaded blue) is defined as a compound area comprising centrilobular zones 5 and 4 plus an extension along the midseptal region of intermediate zone 3 and peripheral zones 2 and 1. Roughly the territory appears as a star-shaped area confined to the central vein (C) and extended to the mid-septum (M). If confluent with neighbouring lobules, the territory can create an extensive reticular pattern spanning a number of lobules. Adapted from Zou et al.[191]

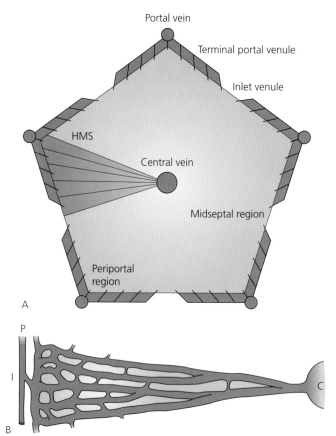

Fig. 1.14 • **(A)** The hepatic lobule is divisible into elementary sectors, the hepatic microcirculatory subunits (HMS), fed by the inlet venules derived from the portal tracts and the terminal portal venules. Note the disparity between the midseptal and periportal regions that comprise the peripheral zones: the latter are proximal to, the former remote from the portal supply. **(B)** A typical HMS is shaped like a cone with a portal (P) inlet venule (I) at the base, where one afferent vessel spreads into many sinusoids. The cross-connecting sinusoids reduce, or 'drop out', while approaching the central vein (C). Adapted from Ekataksin et al.[195]

3. The lines 1, 2 and 3 (Fig. 1.7) represent the borders of the acinar zones in the concept of the liver acinus, in descending order of nutrient level. One can interpret these borderlines of acinar zones as cut lines of haemodynamic equipotential surfaces; hence, any line traversing successively and perpendicularly across these surfaces should represent the potential gradient in that direction. In chronic venous congestion, damage to the hepatocytes starts in the microcirculatory periphery, progressing in all directions up the potential gradient, so that in the case of severe congestion only the zone of highest potential can survive. According to the acinar concept, the surviving parenchyma of acinar zone 1 would appear clover-shaped with the portal tract at its centre. However, Matsumoto et al.[6] claim that this actually never occurs and that, typically in chronic venous congestion, the liver biopsy always shows sickle zones standing in relief.

4. Zonal gradients of metabolic activities and of enzyme histochemical staining patterns also conform with the sickle-zone pattern, and not with the acinus diagram. Matsumoto et al.[6] illustrate this with pictures of peripheral fatty change and the enzyme-histochemical pattern of glucose 6-phosphatase. The sickle-zone pattern has been confirmed by other authors.[188,189,192,193]

Other liver units

The smallest unit ever conceptualized is the *single-sinusoid model* developed by Bloch[1] and refined by McCuskey.[7] However, to make this '*functional microvascular unit*'[7] conceptually valid, the liver should have at the lobular periphery the same number of portal twigs, arterial twigs and biliary tributaries as the number of sinusoids, a context that is unproven and very unlikely.[3]

Hofmann[10] coined the term *choleon* to designate an exocrine secretory unit consisting of the group of hepatocytes drained by a single ductule. Ekataksin & Wake[3] have demonstrated that the most terminal portal vessels, the inlet venules, penetrate the limiting plate and deliver blood by perfusing a preferred column of sinusoids that can be visualized as a conical body; the latter has a broader base at the perimeter and a pointed end tapering toward the centre of the lobule. This pyramidal group of sinusoids is termed the *hepatic microcirculatory subunit* (Fig. 1.14). Ontogenic studies in the rat revealed that the multiple-cell-thick hepatic plates remodel into the one-cell-thick muralium of the adult liver, resulting in elongation of the distance between portal and central vein.[194] Although this provides increased lobular space for more sinusoidal beds to develop, certain sinusoids, and especially the short intersinusoidal sinusoids that communicate between two neighbouring radial sinusoids, are subject to deletion and dropout. The lumina of such dropout sinusoids progressively decrease in calibre and finally disappear. As a result, the hepatic microcirculatory subunits become more clearly defined with little likelihood that blood will cross the streamline when the flow approaches the central vein.[195]

Ekataksin & Wake[3] further showed that the first segment of the biliary passages, that is, the canal of Hering, and the very last segment of the portal venous tree, that is, the inlet venule, are closely co-localized at the lobular periphery. Double injection of coloured media shows that a territory of intralobular bile canaliculi extending through the canal of Hering—a choleon—overlaps spatially with the column of sinusoids of a hepatic microcirculatory subunit extending through the inlet venule. The subpopulation of liver cells associated with such a unit is thus equipped with all of the elementary structures that a liver unit needs to perform its dual exocrine–endocrine functions. This configuration was therefore designated the *choleohepaton* and is believed to represent the elementary morphofunctional unit of the liver.

Comments on liver units

It is well known that in routine histological preparations of normal human liver there are no clear-cut boundaries of structural units, neither lobular nor acinar. In fact, the absence of such boundaries led Elias & Sherrick[14] to state that the liver is an indivisible continuum that has no anatomically definable lobules nor acini, and suggested to Takahashi[197] that the concept of the hepatic lobule as a pre-formed structural unit could not be sustained. Nevertheless, hepatic angio-architecture determines regional directions of blood flow and gradients in oxygen and nutrients in defined territories throughout this parenchymal continuum, resulting in metabolic heterogeneity and varying vulnerability of parenchymal cells. This is clearly demonstrated in a number of studies of enzyme topography and in some pathological lesions. Hence it follows that angio-architectural units are helpful in explaining the normal and deranged functions of the liver organ.

At the present time, the best candidate for the ultimate structural and functional liver unit is the choleohepaton. It represents the smallest mass of liver tissue vascularized by a single, terminal portal venule (inlet venule) and drained by a single hepatic vein (central vein), accounting for the smallest group of cells and sinusoids performing the endocrine (metabolic) functions of the liver. At the same time it also coincides with the smallest group of parenchymal cells producing exocrine secretions that are drained by a single canal of Hering, accounting for the smallest co-operating hepatocellular community responsible for the bile secretory function of the liver. Obviously, the choleohepaton has no clear-cut anatomical borders, and can only be visualized by meticulous investigation.[195] The choleohepaton is part of the primary lobule according to Matsumoto et al.[6,190] A criticism of the primary lobule concept is that structurally it is not a single element, because the primary lobule involves one portal tract and a few portal vein septal branches.[3] Furthermore, the portal vein septal branches (at the origin of the primary lobules) give off inlet venules on both sides of the vascular septum, thus supplying several primary lobules.

For the pathologist, the most important discussion about unit concepts concerns the classical lobule (or the secondary lobule according to Matsumoto and his colleagues) versus the acinus concept. Rappaport et al.[5] formulated the acinus concept after studying the three-dimensional distribution patterns of a gelatin-based fluid coloured with India ink, injected into the portal vein. It was thus realized that the portal tract harbours preterminal (conducting) branches of the portal vein, and that the real terminal branches are located in the borderline between two hexagonal units. In a typical way, a preterminal branch of the portal vein gave off three terminal (parenchymal or distributory) branches. In addition to the observed dye injection patterns, the patterns of hepatic lesions, especially that of central necrosis, led to the definition of the boundaries of zones 1–3.[12] The value of the acinus concept was mainly in hepatopathology, as it explained the topography of important lesions such as portal-central bridging necrosis.

However, careful studies on angio-architecture[6,190,198] and enzyme-histochemical patterns[188,189] re-emphasized the correctness of the lobular relationships in normal liver structure and function. How then does one explain in the lobular concept the so-called portal-central bridging lesions (necrosis, fibrosis), lesions that, par excellence, can be explained on acinar topography? The explanation usually is that the bridging lesions occur in the neighbourhood between pericentral compartments and larger portal tracts, especially near the axis of the branching points of the larger portal veins.[12] As formulated by Matsumoto et al.,[6] points of relatively low potential occur from place to place over the surface of a large portal tract containing a conducting portion of the portal vein.

Nevertheless, many pathologists may have had the impression of looking at portal-central bridging between a portal tract and central vein of the same order. In this respect an interesting remark comes from Lamers et al.:[12] 'that under *physiological* conditions, the boundaries marking regional differences in hepatic microcirculation and metabolism, are most adequately reflected by the boundaries of the (metabolic) lobular concept, whereas under certain *patho(physio)logical* conditions, these boundaries are reduced to those of the acinar concept. A gradual erosion of the periphery of the well oxygenated zone of the liver parenchyma upon introduction of patho(physio)logical conditions can therefore adequately explain observations that, at first glance, appear to support Rappaport's concept of liver architecture. In this respect, it is relevant that the relatively high viscosity of the gelatin-based infusion fluids used by Rappaport to visualize the acini, supports our argument'. Lamers et al.[12] illustrate this statement with the experimental work of Quistorff & Chance,[199] demonstrating a shift from a periportal reticular or continuous appearance of well-oxygenated liver parenchyma into a discrete pattern following ingestion of alcohol, a situation that induces centrilobular hypermetabolism.

A gradual erosion of the periportal zone upon introduction of patho(physio)logical conditions as proposed by Lamers et al.[12] is consistent with several described anatomical details and with the following considerations, although it does not result in a truly acinar pattern:

1. The inlet venules of the portal zone of the sickle area originate directly from the preterminal portal vein in the portal tract, and thus are of an earlier branching order than those arising from the septal branches in the septal zone. In other words, the inlet venules of the septal zone are more peripheral in the microcirculation.

2. The distance between the preterminal conducting portal vein in the portal tract and the sinusoids of the sickle zone is shorter for the sinusoids in the portal zone than for those in the septal zone (Fig. 1.11). Also in this respect, septal sinusoids are more peripheral than portal sinusoids.

3. According to the Zou et al. study[191] in the pig liver the occurrence rate of inlet venules along a side of the lobule between two opposing portal tracts is subject to a regional gradient, with the highest incidence at the proximal periportal and the lowest incidence at the midseptal regions. Hence, a midseptal inlet venule is prone to drain into a larger number of sinusoids than a portal one, and hence is equally prone to a steeper drop in pressure.

4. Furthermore, considering that from a functional point of view, not only is mere angio-architectural anatomy to be considered, but also other factors like intraluminal pressure and flow, so it is acceptable to state that there is a gradual erosion of the periportal zone into an acinar zone 1 pattern (clover-shaped). However, in that case the clover-leaves should not have their axis in the portal-portal line, but in the portal-central line. This also reveals a basic incompatibility between the lobular and acinar concepts.

In relation to bridging hepatic lesions, it is of interest that a recent study on intralobular heterogeneity of liver tissue (in this case, vitamin A storing lipid droplets of hepatic stellate cells in pig liver) revealed a zonal and a regional gradient. The vitamin A-low territory appeared as a star-shaped area confined to the central vein (C) and extended to the mid-septum (M) (the middle of the septum between two adjacent portal tracts) (Fig. 1.13). In several pathological conditions, this C-M-C pattern of fibrosis (that is, central-central fibrosis crossing the midpoint of a portal-portal connecting line) is seen: in pig serum induced rat liver fibrosis, in CCl_4-induced rat liver injury, and in alcoholic liver disease.[191]

It thus appears that there is a basic conflict between the acinar and the lobular concept of liver architecture. All studies since those of Matsumoto et al.[6] in 1979 have supported the lobule concept of liver architecture, resulting in increased acceptance of this concept. The histopathologist should realize, however, that with some exceptions, most studies on fine anatomical details have been performed in species such as rat and pig, and there have been only a few in humans.[6,188] Two recent studies on the rat liver both agreed on rejection of the acinar concept, but amazingly arrived at divergent conclusions about the liver unit: a portal type of lobule (in normal and fibrotic rat liver) according to Bhuncet & Wake[200] and a hepatic (or classic) type of lobule according to Teutsch et al.[201]

Additional problems in the interpretation of liver sections relate to the fact that the liver consists of numerous repeating, but randomly oriented, lobular units.[192] One tends to view such lobules as cylindrical or prismatic; however, in reality the lobules are tortuous, branching structures, which explains why truly sagittal or transverse sections of a lobule are extremely rare.[192]

It is a sobering thought that after more than 300 years since J.J. Wepfer first described liver units in 1665 (cited by Bloch[1]), the quest for the grail of a hepatic structural-functional unit and its application to human liver histopathology is unending. As a transition measure until the time of final consensus and clear comprehension, it is appropriate therefore to retain Table 1.1 as it has appeared in previous editions of this text and outlining a comparison of the acinar and lobular terminologies.

Functional heterogeneity in the liver

Recognition of hepatocyte heterogeneity dates back to as early as the 1850s[202,203] when the heterogeneous contribution of different hepatocytes to bile secretion was described. Anatomical heterogeneity of liver units can be demonstrated in different ways: zonality, regionality, locality and laterality.[194,196] Zonality refers to non-homogeneous distribution patterns of structural features and functional aspects along the portal-central axis, with differences between periportal and centrolobular zones. Concerning regionality, it has been demonstrated that different regions (septal or portal) of the same zone are not functionally identical.[204] Zonation and regionation schematically subdivide lobules into 5 zone/5 region (5 Z/5 R) compartmentalization, which should allow a precise reporting of any morphologically or functionally demonstrable heterogeneity in the liver lobule.[191] Locality in the liver lobe refers to the notion that hepatic lobules are by no means homogeneous. Superficial

Table 1.1	Comparison of lobular and acinar terminologies
Lobular	**Acinar**
Central; centrilobular; centrizonal	Perivenular; acinar zone 3
Mid-zonal	Acinar zone 2
Peripheral; periportal multilobular	Periportal; acinar zone 1
Panlobular	Panacinar
Central/central (necrosis or bridging)	Peri-acinar (complex) (necrosis or bridging)
Central/portal (necrosis or bridging)	Peri-acinar (simple), peripheral acinar, zone 3 (necrosis or bridging)
Portal/portal (necrosis or bridging)	Portal/portal (necrosis or bridging)

lobules (in contact with the capsule of Glisson and its elongation into large portal canals) have a uniform apicobasal arrangement in contrast with the variable orientation of the lobules located elsewhere; furthermore, they are predominantly 'compound' hepatic lobules whereas the deeper ones are preferentially 'simple' hepatic lobules.[194] Finally, laterality refers to a fair possibility of a macroscopic scale of functional heterogeneity in the fetal liver, based on the asymmetrical vascular supply which favours the left lobe of the liver.

The heterogeneity which has been most studied concerns zonality, and to a lesser extent regionality, and these have been summarized in book form.[205] Liver parenchyma shows a remarkable heterogeneity of the hepatocytes along the portocentral axis with respect to ultrastructure and enzyme activities resulting in different cellular functions within different zones of the liver lobules. This resulted in the concept of metabolic zonation, first proposed for carbohydrate metabolism, and implying that opposite metabolic pathways like gluconeogenesis and glycolysis are carried out simultaneously by hepatocytes in the periportal and centrilobular region respectively. It soon became obvious that the concept of metabolic zonation is applicable to all liver functions and indeed reflects an important level of metabolic control. The topic has been reviewed in several publications.[206–208]

Two types of zonal patterns of gene expression in the liver that have been recognized are the gradient versus compartment type of zonation, and the dynamic versus stable type of zonation.[209] In the gradient type of zonation, all hepatocytes are able to express a particular gene, but the level of expression depends on the position of the hepatocyte along the portocentral radius e.g. the key enzymes of carbohydrate metabolism, cytosolic phosphoenol-pyruvate carboxykinase I (PCK) and glucokinase. In the compartment type of zonation, the expression of genes has been thought to be restricted to either the periportal or the pericentral compartment e.g. the key enzymes of ammonia metabolism, carbamoyl phosphate synthetase I (CPS) and glutamine synthetase (GS). The dynamic type of zonation is characterized by adaptive changes in expression in response to changes in the metabolic or hormonal state e.g. PCK, tyrosine aminotransferase, CPS, and ornithine aminotransferase. The stable type of zonation, on the other hand, is characterized by the virtual absence of such adaptive changes e.g. fructose-1,6-biphosphatase and GS. Several studies have been devoted to the determination and the regulation of hepatocyte heterogeneity. As a rule, enzyme proteins and their respective mRNAs are co-localized suggesting that regulation is exerted on the pretranslational level; there are, however, some exceptions like pyruvate kinase L and α-antitrypsin.[206]

In order to unravel the mechanisms underlying heterogeneous gene expression, it is necessary first to establish whether all hepatocytes can express the same spectrum of genes, the evidence for which is succinctly summarized by Christoffels et al.[209] During development of the liver, the emergence of zonal hepatocyte heterogeneity is linked to the establishment of a lobular architectural framework.[210] It

is suggested that factors regulating the onset and the maintenance of hepatocyte heterogeneity originate within the liver and are probably produced by the hepatocytes themselves.[210] The phenotype of upstream, periportal hepatocytes appears to be determined by the concentration of regulatory signals in the afferent blood, whereas the phenotype of the downstream, pericentral hepatocytes is, additionally, determined by changes in blood composition as a result of metabolic and/or biosynthetic activity of the upstream hepatocytes (the 'upstream-downstream' hypothesis).[211]

Christoffels et al.[209] have proposed a model to explain gradients in gene expression in relation to a limited number of signal gradients. The model uses portocentral gradients of signal molecules as input, while the output depends on two gene-specific variables, viz., the affinity of the gene for its regulatory factors and the degree of co-operation that determines the response in the signal-transduction pathways. The diversity in sequence and arrangement of related DNA-response elements of genes appears to account for the gene-specific shape of the portocentral gradients in expression.

In a three-dimensional reconstruction study of parenchymal units in rat liver, Teutsch et al.[201] emphasized the importance of considering three-dimensionality for an adequate functional interpretation of the metabolic heterogeneity of hepatocytes. If the three-dimensionality of the parenchymal units is not taken into consideration, calculations show that it is likely that changes at the origin of sinusoids are under-estimated, whereas those at the termination of sinusoids are over-estimated. This should also apply in the interpretation of sections from pathologically altered liver tissue.[201]

Zonal heterogeneity is a feature that characterizes not only hepatocytes, but other components of liver tissue as well. Sinusoids have a more tortuous course, more frequent intersinusoidal anastomoses, and a narrower lumen in the periportal area, whereas they appear straighter with less intersinusoidal sinusoids and a broader lumen in centrilobular areas.[195] The sinusoidal endothelial cells have higher porosity (by fenestrae) in the centrilobular region, display different wheat-germ agglutinin-binding patterns in periportal versus centrilobular endothelial cells, and show portocentral gradients in mannose receptor-mediated endocytosis, and in production of reactive oxygen metabolites.[212]

The hepatic stellate cells display marked heterogeneity in structure and function based on their zonal (portal-central) and regional (portal versus septal sinusoidal) distribution in the hepatic lobules.[213] They have more cytoplasmic processes with thorn-like microprojections in the centrilobular zone, whereas their desmin immunoreactivity and vitamin A-storage is higher in the periportal zone.

Kupffer cells are located preferentially in periportal regions, and some functional and morphological heterogeneity has been ascribed to their location. Thus, Kupffer cells in periportal zones are larger, contain more heterogeneous lysosomes and are more active in phagocytosis than their centrilobular counterparts.[214] In contrast, in areas around centrilobular veins Kupffer cells are smaller and more active in terms of cytokine production and cytotoxicity.[215]

The extracellular matrix components in the space of Disse may vary along the portal-central axis. Collagens IV and V and laminin may predominate in the area of transition between bile ductules and hepatocytes at the lobular periphery. Fibronectin, and collagens III, IV and VI may be the predominant components throughout the liver cell plate.[207]

The hepatocyte

The hepatocyte is a polyhedral epithelial cell approximately 30 to 40 μm in diameter and, in common with other epithelial cells, it is highly polarized with transport directed from its sinusoidal surface to the canalicular surface (Fig. 1.15). Within its plasma membrane, three specialized regions, or domains, are recognized: *basolateral* (or sinusoidal), which faces the sinusoid and the perisinusoidal space;

canalicular, bounding that part of the intercellular space which constitutes the bile canaliculus, and *lateral*, facing the rest of the intercellular space.[216–219] This polarity is largely maintained by the tight junctions formed between adjacent hepatocytes in the lateral domain and which create a barrier between the two domains and also between the plasma in the intercellular space and the bile in the canaliculus.[220,221] In addition to tight junctions there are also gap junctions and desmosomes in the lateral domain, and it is across this domain that intercellular communication takes place. Stereological studies in the rat have shown that the basolateral, canalicular and lateral domains comprise approximately 70%, 15% and 15% of the total cell surface area.[222] Various techniques (reviewed by Meier[218]) have been used to characterize these domains, mainly in the rat liver, but also more recently in human liver.[223]

The domains of the hepatocyte plasma membrane are not simply topographical entities. They are specialized to subserve different functions and the isolation and study of

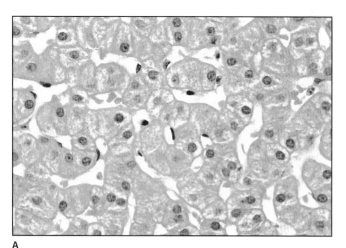

A

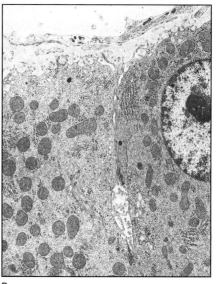

B

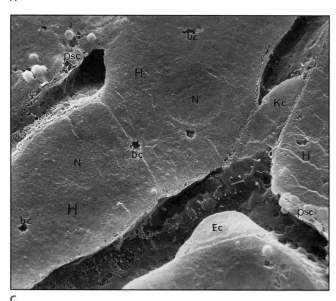

C

Fig. 1.15 • (A) Light microscopy. Liver-cell plates cut longitudinally show: (i) a centrally placed nucleus and occasional binucleate cells, (ii) the sinusoidal surface against which Kupffer-cell nuclei are abutting, (iii) the canalicular pole (arrows), (iv) the intercellular surface. **(B)** Transmission electron micrograph (TEM). Electron micrograph of parts of two hepatocytes, illustrating their three surfaces: sinusoidal (basolateral), canalicular and intercellular. Note the microvilli on the sinusoidal surface projecting into the space of Disse. Baboon liver × 8775. **(C)** Scanning electron micrograph (SEM) showing several cell types. Hepatocytes (H) contain a nucleus (N), and at the junction between cells the bile canaliculus (bc) and the intercellular surface are clearly defined. The sinusoidal surface is seen and in the sinusoidal area a Kupffer cell (Kc), endothelial cell (Ec) and two perisinusoidal cells (psc) are present. This SEM and most of the others shown in this chapter were kindly provided by Professor E Wisse, Brussels. They are all preparations of rat liver.

canalicular and basolateral membrane fractions have shown that there are many differences including differences in protein and lipid composition, fluidity and the presence of various enzymes, receptors and transport systems.[209,213,214,224] The hepatocytes can decrease or increase the concentration of specific proteins in each domain. In addition, recycling of the plasma membrane occurs such that following receptor-mediated endocytosis or 'internalization' the receptor can be recycled back to the cell surface.

Hepatocytes in the limiting plates have a surface which abuts on the adjacent fibrous tissue, and which is irregularly covered with microvilli and may be moulded round connective tissue fibres, producing irregular indentations. The space of Mall, between the hepatocyte in the periportal area and the fibrous tissue, is in continuity with the perisinusoidal space of Disse.

The *basolateral surface* is covered with abundant microvilli (Fig. 1.15(B)) each measuring 0.5 μm long and not evident, even as a brush or striated border, by optical microscopy. Microvilli may protrude through the fenestrae of the endothelial cells and into the sinusoidal lumen. The surface specialization is related here, as elsewhere, to absorptive and/or secretory activity; it obviously increases the surface area, but by a factor (approximately × 6) smaller than one might expect. Between the bases of the microvilli SEM shows small surface indentations or pits.[166] Some of these represent secretory vacuoles discharging into the plasma by a process of exocytosis, and others are clathrin-coated pits involved in selective receptor-mediated endocytosis and further parts of entry for endocytotic pathways called caveolae; the latter are invaginating membrane microdomains enriched in cholesterol and sphingolipids and the cholesterol-binding protein caveolin.[167]

The perisinusoidal space of Disse is a tissue space between the hepatocytes and the endothelial sinusoidal lining cells. Within the space of Disse extracellular matrix proteins are present in low density and they may also have a role in maintaining the polarity of the hepatocyte. However, the hepatocyte has no structured basement membrane.

The basolateral domain of the plasma membrane is the seat of a distinctive set of cell-matrix adhesion molecules. Immunohistochemical investigation revealed that normal human hepatocytes express only two integrin receptors at low level: α1β1 integrin, a receptor for collagens and laminin, and α9β1 integrin.[225]

Canalicular surface: the bile canaliculus has no wall proper to itself. It is an intercellular space (Fig. 1.16(A)), formed by the apposition of the edges of gutter-like hemicanals on the adjacent surfaces of neighbouring hepatocytes (Fig. 1.16(B)). Its diameter varies from 0.5 to 1.0 μm in the perivenular area and from 1 to 2.5 μm in the periportal zone. The surface is unevenly covered by microvilli (Fig. 1.16(A)), which are more abundant along a 'marginal ridge' at each edge of the hemicaniculus. In experimental biliary obstruction the canaliculi become dilated and the microvilli disappear, except along the marginal ridges. Microfilaments are particularly concentrated around the canaliculi forming distinct, organelle-free pericanalicular sheaths and they also extend into the microvilli. The pres-

ence of contractile elements in the pericanalicular zone can be demonstrated by indirect immunofluorescence (Fig. 1.16(C)) using a smooth-muscle antibody-containing serum.[226] The presence of ATPase can be demonstrated histochemically (Fig. 1.16(D)). Accumulations of lipofuscin or haemosiderin (Fig. 1.16(E)) may also outline the canalicular pole of the hepatocyte.

The canalicular surface is isolated from the rest of the intercellular surface by junctional complexes (Fig. 1.16(A)), desmosomes, intermediate junctions, tight junctions and gap junctions. These are discussed further in the section on the bile secretory apparatus below (p. 29). The tight junctions constitute a permeability barrier to macromolecules between the bile canaliculus and the rest of the intercellular space. 'Tightness' is, however, a relative term; there seems to be a positive correlation between degrees of tightness and the number of strands forming the junction. On this basis the canalicular tight junctions are comparable with those elsewhere in the body (e.g. in the rete testis and vasa efferentia), which are regarded as only 'moderately tight'.

The *lateral surface* is the least complex of the three; it extends from the bile canaliculus to the margin of the sinusoidal surface and is specialized for cell attachment and cell–cell communication. It is not entirely flat: microvilli may extend on to it from the sinusoidal surface and protrude into narrow extensions of the space of Disse; there are occasional folds (plicae) and round-mouthed openings, which may represent pinocytic vesicles.[166] There are also seen, by SEM, knob-like protrusions and corresponding indentations which, fitted into one another, would form the 'press-stud' or 'snap fastener' type of intercellular attachment long familiar in transmission electron microscopy (TEM).

There are also specialized areas called gap (or, better, communicating) junctions. These are seen by TEM as patches of close approximation of the two membranes and in freeze-fracture preparations as irregularly shaped aggregates of particles on the P-face. The gap between the two membranes is 2–4 nm wide and is bridged by the intramembrane particles (of protein or lipid), which project like 'bobbins' from the external surface of each of the two membranes. Since each 'bobbin' is perforated by a central pore and apposed 'bobbins' are in contact, communications are established which provide for the transfer of ions or metabolites, or both, between hepatocytes. Such communications have been shown to play a role in the regulation of hepatocyte functions e.g. hepatic carbohydrate metabolism by sympathetic nerve fibres.[227]

Nucleus

This shows the characteristics one would expect in the nucleus of a cell actively engaged in protein synthesis: it is large, occupying 5–10% of the volume of the cell, spherical, with one or more prominent nucleoli, and scattered chromatin. The nuclear membrane is double-layered and contains many pores (Fig. 1.17). There is considerable variation in both number and size of nuclei. About 25% of the cells are binucleate: the two nuclei are similar in size and stain-

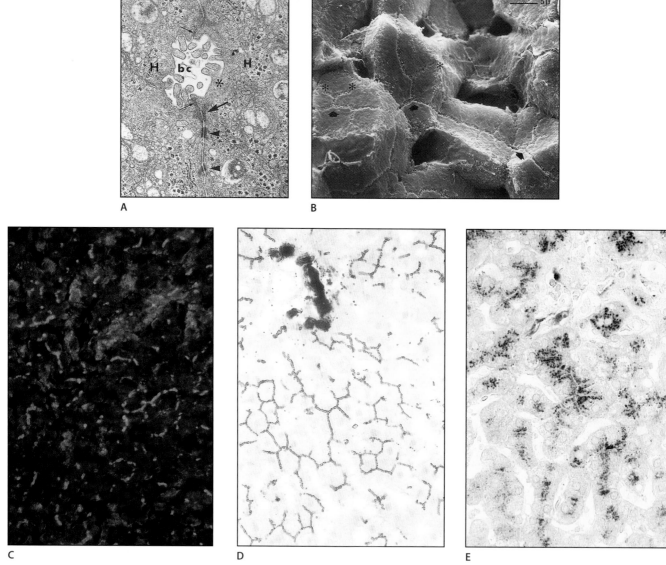

Fig. 1.16 • (A) TEM. Bile canaliculus (bc). Note microvilli projecting into the lumen and the organelle-free pericanalicular cytoplasm (*). Tight junctions (broad arrow), intermediate junctions (thin arrows) and desmosomes (arrowheads) are present between the two adjacent hepatocytes (H). Human liver. Print kindly provided by Professor P Bioulac-Sage. **(B)** SEM. On the surface of a number of neighbouring hepatocytes, an interconnected network of bile hemi-canaliculi show bifurcations (arrows) together with blunt ends (asterisks). **(C)** Bile canaliculi in rabbit liver: immunofluorescence preparation in which the section was reacted with a human serum containing smooth-muscle antibody: the pericanalicular microfilaments have produced strong positive immunofluorescence. **(D)** Pattern of bile canaliculi shown by histochemical demonstration of ATPase in pericanalicular cytoplasm. **(E)** Hepatocytes in iron overload; note how the pericanalicular accumulation of haemosiderin outlines the canalicular network. Perls reaction.

ing properties and they divide simultaneously. At birth, all but a few hepatocytes are mononuclear. Hepatocyte nuclei fall into various sizes, with volumes in the ratio 1 : 2 : 4 : 8. This variation reflects polyploidy, the DNA content increasing correspondingly.[228] At birth, in man, nearly all hepatocytes are diploid (and mononucleate). From the 8th year, when more than 90% of hepatocytes are diploid, the number of tetraploid nuclei (i.e. those with twice the normal DNA content) increases, to reach about 15% in children of 15 years.[229] Tetraploid cells are thought to arise by mitosis of cells with two diploid nuclei. The DNA content of each nucleus doubles, but the chromosomes are then arranged on a single mitotic spindle, so that division produces two daughter cells, each with a single tetraploid nucleus. The

significance of polyploidy in hepatocytes is unknown. Since cell size is proportional to cell ploidy,[230] polyploidy does not provide an increased amount of genetic material per unit volume of cytoplasm.

Mitotic division provides for embryonic and early post-natal growth, but the adult liver has a very low mitotic index with estimates ranging from one mitosis per 10–20 000 cells, to 2.2 mitoses per 1000 cells. The liver has hitherto been classified as a conditional renewal system,[231] and the individual hepatocyte is correspondingly long-lived: cell life may be up to 300 days or even measured in years in laboratory rodents.[232] However, these figures may need downward revision if the liver is shown to be a stem cell and lineage system.

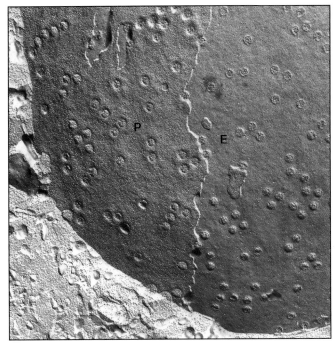

Fig. 1.17 • Freeze-fracture replica illustrating the inner leaflet (P face) and the outer leaflet (E face) of the nuclear membrane of a hepatocyte. Note the numerous nuclear pores. Human liver × 44 800. Supplied by Professor R De Vos.

Endoplasmic reticulum (ER)

This topic has recently been reviewed by Lippincott-Schwarz.[233] Optical microscopy of liver from a well-fed animal shows granular clumps of basophilic material (the 'ergastoplasm') which, like similar material in other cells, was identified on electron microscopy with rough endoplasmic reticulum (RER). This consists of a network of parallel, flattened sacs or cisternae on whose cytoplasmic surfaces are attached polyribosomes (Fig. 1.18(A),(B)). Clusters of RER are scattered randomly throughout the cytoplasm and constitute approximately 60% of the endoplasmic reticulum. The remaining 40% constitutes the smooth endoplasmic reticulum (SER), which also forms anastomosing networks of tubules and vesicles of varying diameter which are continuous with the cisternae of the RER; they lack a ribosomal coating, hence the designation smooth or agranular (Fig. 1.19). The outer nuclear membrane also has attached ribosomes and continuity between the outer nuclear membrane and the outer membrane of the RER has been demonstrated. The SER is often found in the region of the Golgi apparatus and communicates with it; there is frequently a close topographical relationship of the SER with glycogen (Fig. 1.19). Following cell disruption and differential centrifugation the RER is a principal constituent of the so-called microsomal fraction. Studies of isolated rat microsomes suggest that the membrane of the ER comprises about 10% protein and 30% lipid of which 85% is phospholipid. The ER occupies 15% of the total cell volume and its surface area—approximately 60 000 μm^2 per hepatocyte—is more than 35 times the area of the plasma membrane. There is also zonality in the distribution of the ER; the surface area of SER in the centrilobular area is twice that in the periportal zone.

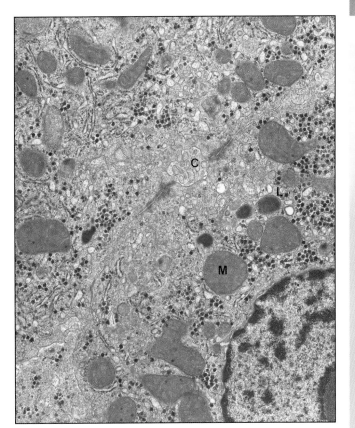

A

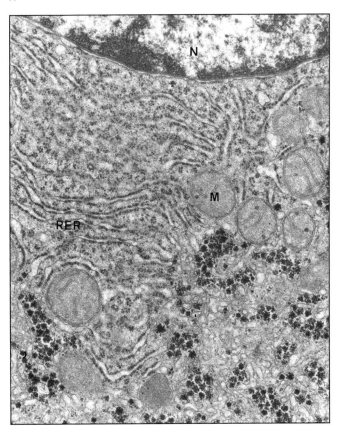

B

Fig. 1.18 • (A) TEM illustrating cytoplasmic organelles, nucleus and bile canaliculus (C) in two adjacent hepatocytes; lysosomes (L); mitochondria (M). Human liver, × 23 000. **(B)** TEM illustrating rough endoplasmic reticulum (RER) and mitochondria (M) with matrix granules; also part of the nucleus (N) with inner and outer membrane. Human liver, × 36 800. Supplied by Professor R De Vos.

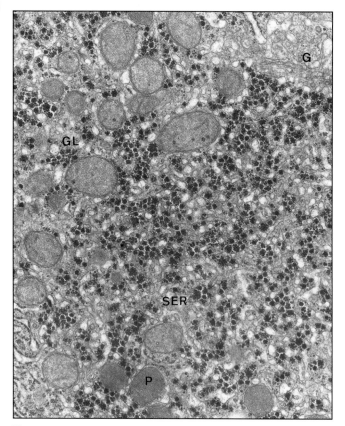

Fig. 1.19 • TEM illustrating networks of smooth endoplasmic reticulum (SER); Golgi apparatus (G) peroxisomes (P). Note also glycogen rosettes (GL). Human liver, × 28 800. Supplied by Professor R De Vos.

A variety of electron microscopic and biochemical techniques has shown the synthesis of protein at the polyribosomes, and its entry into the cisternae of the RER through which it passes via the SER to the Golgi apparatus. It travels from here to be 'packaged for export' in Golgi-derived secretory vesicles.

The cell functions which are associated with the ER include: (i) protein synthesis, both secretory proteins and some of the protein constituents of the cell and organelle membranes; (ii) the metabolism of fatty acids, phospholipids and triglycerides; (iii) the production and metabolism of cholesterol and, possibly, the production of bile acids; (iv) xenobiotic metabolism; (v) ascorbic acid synthesis; and (vi) haem degradation.

Not all protein synthesis in the hepatocyte involves the ER however; some, including structural proteins of the cell itself, are formed by free ribosomes, a process which is particularly active during development and regeneration when the number of these organelles can fluctuate considerably. The cytochrome P-450 system is localized in the ER and this is the system whereby the liver cell functions in the metabolism and detoxification of xenobiotics. This enzyme system can be reversibly induced by certain xenobiotics e.g. phenobarbitol (see Chapter 14) and this is accompanied by the synthesis and hypertrophy of ER; the mechanisms involved in new membrane production are not clear.

Glucose 6-phosphatase is localized on the ER but the role, if any, of the ER in glycogen metabolism is not clear. The SER proliferates during synthesis of glycogen and during

its degradation in fasting animals.[234] However, SER is absent during the period of rapid glycogenolysis, which occurs in mammalian livers just after birth.[235]

Golgi complex

Each hepatocyte contains as many as 50 Golgi zones (which may not be separate but rather form a tri-dimensional continuity) situated most commonly near to the bile canaliculus or beside the nucleus.[236] Each complex appears as a stack of four to six curved, flattened parallel sacs often with dilated bulbous ends containing electron-dense material. The convex or cis surface is directed towards the ER and small vesicles in the cis-Golgi transfer synthesized proteins from the ER. The concave or trans surface is the origin of the secretory vesicles. Vesicles break off from the ends of the sacs, and carry the contained secretory proteins, including lipoproteins, for discharge at the sinusoidal surface. Numerous small primary lysosomes are also present in the vicinity of the Golgi complex. The complex and its associated cytoplasm constitute approximately 2–4% of the cell volume. In addition to its role in the secretion of lipoproteins the Golgi complex is important in the glycosylation of secretory proteins and in the synthesis and recycling of membrane glycoprotein receptors.[236] Its possible role in bile secretion is discussed on p. 31.

Lysosomes

The existence of lysosomes was first predicted by De Duve on the basis of biochemical studies on liver homogenates,[237] and it was he who subsequently identified them with the 'peribiliary dense bodies' found in electron micrographs of liver, and who established them as a new species of cell organelle. Their functions in health and disease have been reviewed,[238,239] and are of particular importance to pathologists because of their involvement in a number of storage diseases (Chapter 5).

Lysosomes present a variety of appearances in electron micrographs of liver, but basically they are vesicles, bounded by a single membrane (Fig. 1.18), containing acid hydrolases: e.g. acid phosphatase, aryl sulphatase, esterase and β-glucuronidase. Their form is so variable that unequivocal identification depends on histochemical demonstration of one of the contained enzymes, most conveniently acid phosphatase.

Lysosomes of this type are essentially storage granules for enzymes, sequestered by membranes from contact with the cytoplasm; the enzymes are elaborated by the usual mechanism of protein synthesis—RER-SER-Golgi complex. Lysosomes number about 30 per hepatocyte[240] and, although they are found particularly in the neighbourhood of the bile canaliculus, there is at present no ultrastructural evidence of their direct involvement in the production or excretion of bile.

Their pleomorphism reflects a variety of functions:

Although the liver cell is long-lived, there is evidence for turnover of its cytoplasm and organelles: e.g. the half-life of hepatocyte mitochondria is estimated at approximately 10 days and of the RER at much less. Cytoplasmic constituents may become incorporated within, and digested by, the primary lysosome, forming with it an *autophagic vacuole*, one variety of secondary lysosome. Autophagic vacuoles therefore show fragments of organelles or of cell inclusions in various stages of digestion. The phenomenon is seen most strikingly in the liver of starving animals when parts of hepatocyte cytoplasm are sacrificed to meet the metabolic needs of the organism. Very rapid glycogenolysis, as in the immediate postnatal period in mammals, is associated with the appearance of 'glycogenosomes'—lysosomes which have incorporated glycogen particles, and, presumably, break them down. Autophagic vacuoles are also conspicuous during periods of rapid growth and differentiation in liver, both in development and in regeneration.

Lysosomes also incorporate lipofuscin pigment, which may accumulate, undigested, over long periods, forming so-called residual bodies and material of exogenous origin, including iron, stored as ferritin, which accumulates in large quantities in iron overload states, and copper which accumulates in copper overload conditions and cholestasis.

Coated vesicles and multivesicular bodies result from receptor-mediated endocytosis.[241] Following aggregation of ligand-receptor complexes in clathrin-coated pits on the basolateral cell surface these coated vesicles are internalized to form endosomes or endocytic vesicles. Ligands which are internalized by hepatocytes in this way include insulin, low-density lipoproteins, transferrin, IgA and asialoglycoproteins. Fusion of endosomes occurs to form multivesicular bodies. Some of these vesicles are responsible for transcytosis or intracellular transport from the basolateral domain to the canalicular domain; others fuse with primary lysosomes and their contents undergo partial degradation before being exocytosed at the canalicular or basolateral domain; still others undergo complete degradation and become increasingly electron dense with the formation of dense bodies.[219,239,241] Microtubules appear to have an important role in sorting the pathways along which endocytic vesicles move within the hepatocyte.[242]

Peroxisomes (microbodies)

These are ovoid single membrane-bound granules 0.2–1.0μm in diameter (Fig. 1.19). They were first described as microbodies by Rouiller & Bernhard in 1956.[243] The properties of peroxisomes in liver have recently been reviewed.[244–246] Each hepatocyte may contain 300–600 peroxisomes and they comprise 1.5–2% of cell volume. There is morphological heterogeneity between species; in the rat, peroxisomes contain a paracrystalline striated core or nucleoid in which urate oxidase is concentrated; human peroxisomes lack a core.[247] Peroxisomes contain oxidases which use molecular oxygen to oxidize a number of substrates with the production of hydrogen peroxide (hence the name of the organelle) which, in turn, is hydrolysed by peroxisomal catalase. Approximately 20% of the oxygen consumption of the liver is used in peroxisomal activity. The energy produced by this oxidation is dissipated as heat. Alcohol

may be metabolized in the liver by peroxisomal catalase. Drugs, such as clofibrate, which lower blood lipids cause a proliferation of peroxisomes, an increase that has been causally linked to the hypolipidaemic action.[248] Alterations in hepatocyte perixosomes have been reported in bacterial infections, viral hepatitis, Wilson disease and alcoholic liver diseases.[249,250] A number of metabolic disorders has been described in which there is either an absence of peroxisomes or a deficiency of peroxisomal enzymes.[246,249] The liver involvement in these is discussed in Chapter 5.

Mitochondria

These are large organelles (1.5 μm in diameter and up to 4 μm long) numbering approximately 1000 per cell, and constitute about 20% of the cytoplasmic volume of hepatocytes.[251] Mitochondria may fuse and are remarkably mobile organelles which move about in the cytoplasm, closely associated with microtubules. They show the features commonly regarded as characteristic of mitochondria in general: an outer membrane, separated by a gap from an inner membrane, from which highly convoluted cristal folds project into the interior of the organelles, to be surrounded by matrix (Fig. 1.18). The cristae considerably increase the area of the inner membrane and, in liver cells, it constitutes about a third of the total membrane of the cell. Stains such as Janus green used to demonstrate mitochondria in living cells by light microscopy do so by virtue of their oxidation by the mitochondria. Fluorescent dyes can also be used to study mitochondria in living cells; these dyes are lipid-soluble cations and accumulate in mitochondria because of the large interior negative membrane potential.[252] The matrix contains electron-dense granules (Fig. 1.18(B)), which may represent concentration of Ca^{2+}, a small circular DNA and ribosomes. Crystalloid structures may also be present but are a non-specific feature and not related to any disease. The DNA codes for some of the mitochondrion's own proteins which are synthesized on the ribosomes within these organelles. The larger proportion of the organelle's protein, however, is encoded by nuclear DNA and then 'imported'. Mitochondria are self-replicating with a half-life of about 10 days.

Mutations in the mitochondrial genome account for various mitochondrial myopathies.[253] More recently it has become apparent that specific biochemical abnormalities of mitochondria may play an important role in the pathogenesis of certain liver diseases and that genetic defects in mitochondrial proteins and enzyme systems may be the underlying cause of other liver and metabolic diseases. Because mitochondria possess a distinct and unique extranuclear genome a new class of maternally, or mitochondrially, inherited diseases has emerged (see p. 246).[254]

In three important papers, Candipan & Sjostrand[255–257] have shown that the methods almost universally used to prepare liver for electron microscopic study may produce appearances in the mitochondria which, though widely accepted as real, are probably artifactual. In particular, their findings suggest that: (i) the inner and outer membranes are closely apposed and that there is no space within the crista;

(ii) the cristal membrane is not simply an infolding of the inner membrane but differs structurally from it; (iii) there is no evidence that the crista undergoes 'conformational changes' in different metabolic states; (iv) the two size classes of mitochondria often referred to as 'condensed' and 'orthodox' are preparative artifacts. These findings, and the knowledge that mitochondria move and change their shape in living cells, make difficult the interpretation of changes in mitochondrial morphology thought to be related to disease processes.

The structural compartmentation of mitochondria provides for topographical localization of various enzyme systems, the details of which form almost a science in themselves. It need only be said here that the outer membrane is relatively unimportant as a locus for enzymes; it keeps the inner membrane together and contains porin, a transport protein which forms channels which are permeable to molecules less than 2 kD.[251] The inner membrane and cristal lamellae support the respiratory chain enzymes concerned with oxidative phosphorylation which generates ATP. The matrix contains most of the components of the citric acid cycle, and the enzymes involved in β-oxidation of fatty acids and in the urea cycle. Mitochondria are randomly distributed within individual hepatocytes but are smaller and less numerous in centrilobular than in periportal cells.[258] These differences may, as already discussed, be of functional significance.

The cytoskeleton

The major components of the cytoskeleton of most eukaryotic cells comprise 6 nm microfilaments, 8–10 nm intermediate filaments and 20 nm microtubules; their structure and function in the hepatocyte has been reviewed by Feldmann.[259] These are structurally, chemically and functionally distinct and are dynamic structures capable of rapid modulation and adaptation in response to functional demands. This is achieved by means of polymerization and depolymerization of their constituent molecules under the influence of various intracellular factors which include free Ca^{2+} ions, high energy compounds and associated proteins. In addition, there are a number of accessory proteins which modulate these components, and which link them to one another, to cell organelles and to the cell membrane; these are part of a microtrabecular lattice or cytomatrix. These structures interact to regulate internal organization, cell shape, movement, secretion and divisions.[216,259–261] They can be visualized on TEM and SEM, but more recently the use of polyclonal and monoclonal antibodies in immunohistochemical methods has allowed their investigation by light microscopy.

Microfilaments are double-stranded molecules of polymerized fibrous (F) actin; the monomeric form of the protein is globular (G) actin and these two forms exist in equilibrium in the cell. The microfilaments are present in bundles and form a three-dimensional intracellular meshwork. There is extensive intracellular binding and cross-linking with other intracellular proteins such as myosin, lamin and spectrin. The filaments are mainly located at the cell periphery; they attach to the plasma membrane and extend into microvilli. They are particularly concentrated in the pericanalicular zone forming a pericanalicular web[216,262] and attach to the junctional complexes which limit the canaliculus. Four main functions are envisaged for the contractile microfilaments of the hepatocyte: (i) translocation of carrier or ferry vesicles implicated in bile secretion; (ii) co-ordinated contraction producing peristaltic movement in the canaliculus;[263] (iii) together with microtubules they exert transmembrane control over the topography of intrinsic proteins in the phospholipid bilayer of the cell membrane, thus influencing the protein mosaic and hence the functional differentiation of a particular membrane domain;[264] (iv) they may modulate the structure and tightness of the so-called tight junction and in this way regulate the permeability of the paracellular pathway.[265,266] The functional roles for microfilaments involve cell membrane motility, endo- and exocytosis, secretion and vesicle transfer.

Microtubules are a family of unbranched rigid tubules of variable length which are structurally similar in all cells. They are polymers composed of two subunits of tubulin, α and β. Polymerization and growth takes place from organizing centres including centrioles. Microtubules are part of the mitotic apparatus and are therefore important in cell division. They are also present in cell cilia. Like the microfilaments, they attach to and cross-link a number of proteins.

The function of microtubules in the liver has been assessed using drugs such as colchicine which causes depolymerization. The precise mechanisms by which they exert their functions have been recently reviewed.[267] They are involved in the blood-bound secretion of several liver-cell products including lipoprotein, albumin, retinol-binding proteins, secretory component, fibrinogen and other glycoproteins.[269] They play a role in the intracellular translocation of vesicles containing IgA and horseradish peroxidase.[268–270] Their role in bile secretion is discussed on p. 32.

Intermediate filaments are a family of self-assembling protein fibres.[270] They can be studied by the quick-freezing and deep etching technique.[271] They are structurally similar in all cells, comprising a central 'backbone' of assembled rods. In addition the individual polypeptidases in intermediate filaments are arranged in an α-helical coiled-coil arrangement which confers tensile strength. Unlike the microtubules and microfilaments, intermediate filaments are heterogeneous in subunit composition and antigenically and are grouped into five immunologically distinct types whose distribution is cell specific:[272] cytokeratin, desmin, vimentin, glial fibrillary acidic protein and neurofilaments.

Cytokeratins are the intermediate filaments of epithelial cells and are present in hepatocytes and, in greater amounts, in bile-duct epithelium. They are thought to act as an intracellular scaffold and are most numerous where there is cellular mechanical stress. In hepatocytes, they are located just inside the plasma membrane and are particularly condensed as a pericanalicular sheath which extends into desmosomes (see p. 32). They are linked to desmosomes on the lateral plasma membrane of hepatocytes. They attach to other components of the cytoskeleton, and to organelles such as the RER and vesicles.

They function as 'the mechanical integrators of cellular space'.[273] Studies using nickel to induce their disorganization indicate that, in the hepatocyte, they maintain structural polarity, provide a scaffolding for the bile canaliculus and provide a framework for the distribution of actin and endocytotic vesicles along the plasma membrane.[270,274]

The cytokeratins were originally divided on the basis of their molecular weight into 19 subtypes.[31] In 1990 a novel type of cytokeratin was added to the catalogue as cytokeratin 20.[275] Most epithelial cells contain at least two, one of which is acidic and the other basic. In hepatocytes, cytokeratins 8 and 18 are present and form an integrated system throughout the cell.[274,252,276,277] Bile-duct epithelium also contain cytokeratins 7 and 19, and in the rat also cytokeratin 20,[278] a phenotypic difference which, as discussed earlier, becomes established during embryogenesis. Intermediate filaments are present in Mallory bodies. In alcoholic liver disease and other types of liver injury, Mallory bodies are thought to form as a result of microtubule depolymerization with a consequent collapse of the intermediate filament network (Fig. 1.20).

The microtrabecular lattice or cytomatrix comprises an extremely fine filamentous network in the cell cytoplasm which, as first suggested by Frey-Wyssling in 1948, confers a 'molecular framework' on it.[279] This microtrabecular lattice divides the cytoplasm into two continuous phases, one protein-rich and the other water-rich.[280] The other cytoskeletal components interact with the microtrabecular lattice which, like them, is readily modulated and altered to ensure normal cell function.

Glycogen

A principal function of liver is the synthesis of glycogen (from glucose, or from lactic and pyruvic acids or glycerol), its storage and its breakdown and release as glucose into the

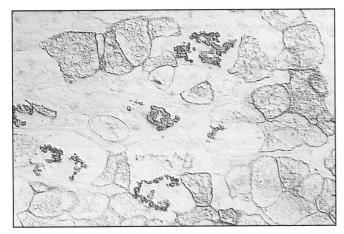

Fig. 1.20 • Liver biopsy from a patient with alcoholic liver disease: immunoperoxidase staining of cytokeratin with antibody CAM 5.2. The cytokeratin microfilaments form a regular network within most of the liver cells but, in some, the network pattern is lost and the microfilaments are aggregated to form coarse, discrete Mallory bodies. Supplied by Professor A D Burt.

circulation. It is depleted in fasting animals, disappearing last from the centrilobular cells; on refeeding, it appears first in periportal cells and in well-fed animals becomes uniformly distributed throughout the lobule. In electron micrographs, glycogen appears as dense granules of two types, β particles, 15–30 nm in diameter and α particles, aggregates of the smaller particles arranged in rosettes (Fig. 1.19). Intranuclear glycogen usually appears as β particles.

The zonal pattern of distribution of glycogen has been demonstrated by using density gradients to separate 'light' and 'heavy' hepatocytes from suspensions of dissociated cells.[281] Glycogen concentrations are similar in the two types, but in the centrilobular ('light') cells, the glycogen granules are dispersed between the SER tubules, whereas in the heavy cells they are packed in large aggregates. It is not clear how far these and other differential characteristics of hepatocytes are a function of their topographical location and how far they depend on intrinsic genetic differences.

The morphological substrate of normal bile secretion ('the bile secretory apparatus')

In earlier studies, the liver cell organelles most obviously involved in bile secretion have been termed 'the bile secretory apparatus'.[282,283] This was originally conceived as comprising mainly the bile canaliculus, the pericanalicular ectoplasm, lysosomes and the Golgi complex. It turned out, however, that the whole liver parenchymal cell is an impressively integrated complex, with several organelles being involved in the process of bile formation and secretion, some of them representing crossroads of internal and external secretory pathways. It is therefore deemed more appropriate to consider the complete hepatocellular machinery involved in bile production as a separate entity, rather than the more restricted concept of 'the bile secretory apparatus'.[284,285] Even the volume of the hepatocyte influences its bile secretory function, in that hypo-osmotic and amino acid-induced cell swelling stimulates taurocholate excretion and bile flow, whereas hyperosmotic cell shrinkage inhibits them.[286]

Bile acids are considered to represent the prime osmotically active solutes responsible for the generation of bile water flow.[287] The mechanism of transport of bile salts by the hepatocyte includes several successive steps: uptake at the sinusoidal membrane domain, vectorial transcellular transport, and concentrative secretion at the canalicular membrane. For recent reviews on the mechanism of bile secretion, see references 287–289.

Basolateral membrane; lobular gradient

The basolateral membrane is the seat of important pumps and transporters involved in bile formation, including Na^+, K^+-ATPase (or sodium) pump, and transport proteins like (i) the sodium taurocholate co-transporting polypeptide (NTCP), (ii) the organic anion transporting polypeptide C (OATPC) also termed organic anion transporting polypeptide 2 (OATP2) or liver specific organic anion transporter 1 (LST-1), the organic anion transporting polypeptide 8 and the organic cation transporter 1 (OCT1). Bile acid uptake at the sinusoidal domain of the plasmalemma is mainly accomplished by periportal hepatocytes[290] so that bile acid transport in the liver follows an intralobular gradient, occurring at a decreasing rate away from the portal tract.[291] However, under conditions of increased bile acid load, additional hepatocytes from midzonal and centrilobular areas become recruited to participate in bile acid transport.[292,293] The transport molecule involved in the uptake of unconjugated bilirubin into the hepatocyte has not yet been definitely identified.[287]

Under normal physiological conditions basolateral efflux of bile salts into the blood is negligible. However, under cholestatic conditions, basolateral bile salt efflux by the multidrug resistance-associated transporter (MRP3) can compensate at least in part, for the disrupted canalicular bile salt secretory pathway.[285]

Vesicle-mediated transport

This topic was thoroughly reviewed by Crawford in 1996.[240] Vesicle-mediated transport plays a role in the transcellular plasma-to-bile trafficking of some biliary solutes and their release into the canaliculus. Most intracellular vesicles are 60–100 nm in diameter, are roughly spherical, are made up of lipids and an ever-changing variety of proteins and contain a mixture of intraluminal contents.

The primary route for bulk fluid movement into and through hepatocytes is fluid-phase endocytosis, a process that starts with pinching off of basolateral membrane patches. Nearly all endocytotic vesicles fuse with intracellular membranous compartments and undergo acidification, before targeting of their contents back to the basolateral surface (about 80%) or to other sites. These vesicles are considerably larger than the clathrin-coated vesicles involved in receptor-mediated endocytosis. Most of the non-regurgitated remaining fluid (about 18%) is directed towards lysosomes. Two per cent of the fluid is secreted into bile. Vesicular trafficking accounts for more than 95% of blood-to-bile transport of large-molecular-weight fluid-phase solutes, and requires intact microtubules.

Substantial quantities of proteins are found in mammalian bile, up to 1 mg/dl. Most biliary proteins are derived from plasma and enter via passive fluid-phase endocytosis. Such proteins include albumin, immunoglobulins, α2-macroglobulin, and α1-acid glycoprotein. Receptor-mediated endocytosis is responsible for the biliary secretion of an IgA-receptor complex, and small amounts of epidermal growth factor, transferrin, haemopexin, and asialoglycoproteins. A much smaller third group of proteins is derived from secretion of lysosomal proteins into bile. The fourth group of biliary proteins is eluted directly from the canalicular membrane, and includes alkaline phosphatase, 5'-nucleotidase and γ-glutamyltranspeptidase. Finally, canalicular membrane proteins (including those partially secreted into bile) reach their apical position via vesicular transport from the basolateral membrane.

A useful experimental serum protein to study fluid-phase transcytosis is horseradish peroxidase, since it can readily be detected in tissue sections. From such experiments it has been postulated that tubular transformation of pericanalicular structures may establish conduits that serve as an alternative to vesicular transport for the delivery of fluid and endocytosed proteins into bile.[294]

Vesicles derived from receptor-mediated endocytosis are initially clathrin-coated and measure 50–100 nm in diameter. After pinching off from the basolateral membrane, they lose their coat and enter the endosomal compartment. This is an anastomosing network of heterogeneous membranous structures which can undergo acidification through the action of membranous proton pumps. The acidification promotes the dissociation of receptors and ligands, permitting the sorting of receptors, ligands and other internalized material for targeting to their respective destinations. These include transport into lysosomes, or back to the cell membrane of origin ('recycling'), and a small proportion toward transcytosis. Transcytotic vesicles seem to enter into a subapical sorting compartment before the insertion of vesicles into the canalicular membrane and release of the vesicle contents. Thus, a small fraction of proteins undergoing receptor-mediated endocytosis is delivered to bile, either directly via transcytosis or after partial degradation in the lysosomal compartment. The ultrastructural correlate for the release of lysosomal contents into bile is not known. Clear-cut fusion of lysosomes with the canalicular membrane has never been documented. The existence of tubular lysosomes and the fusion of tubular structures with the canalicular membrane[295] may constitute an alternative mechanism for microtubule-dependent release of lysosomal contents into bile.

Considerable attention has been given to the question of whether bile salts also traffic via intracellular vesicles into bile. For a time, it was thought that under basal conditions vesicle-mediated transport did not occur, but that such a microtubule-dependent mechanism became additionally operative under conditions of bile salt overload. Numerous investigations have yielded contradictory results; therefore the answer to the question appeared to be a cautious no.[240]

Structural studies have provided evidence that bile salts interact with intracellular organelles such as endoplasmic reticulum and Golgi complex. However, vesicle 'packaging' of bile salts had not been documented, and the question of whether bile salts are carried as cargo through intracellular organelles remained unanswered.[240] It would appear that bile salts are bound to cytosolic proteins and delivered to the canalicular pole of the hepatocyte via diffusion through the cytosol for secretion as monomers across the canalicular membrane. Recent studies indicate that caveolins (located in caveolae and glycolipid-enriched membrane microdomains) may play a role in regulating hepatic bile salt and cholesterol metabolism.[282]

It is probable that bile salt transport at the level of the canalicular membrane is regulated by the retrieval and delivery of transport pumps in a vesicle-mediated fashion, with microtubules playing a role in protein delivery from compartments upstream to the subapical endosomes. It is postulated that exposure of the liver to a physiological bile salt load stimulates the insertion of intracellular vesicles containing bile salt transport proteins into the canalicular membrane, thus enhancing the transport capacity.[240]

Role of the cell organelles in bile secretion

Mitochondria and peroxisomes

Mitochondria are the power plants of the hepatocyte, as in all eukaryotic cells, producing energy in the form of ATP, made available to all energy-consuming functions of the cell, including the bile secretory process.

Peroxisomes are involved in bile acid synthesis. The β-oxidative shortening of the side-chain of cholesterol, in its conversion to C24 bile acids, was shown to be catalysed by the peroxisomal β-oxidation system in rat liver.[245]

Smooth endoplasmic reticulum (SER)

The SER is the site where synthesis of phospholipids takes place, including phospholipids eventually appearing in the bile. It contains 7-α-hydroxylase, which is the rate-limiting enzyme in biotransformation of cholesterol to bile acids, and the enzyme glucuronyltransferase, which conjugates bilirubin to the polar, water-soluble bilirubin diglucuronide.

Studies using the bile acid analogue ^{125}I-cholylglycyltyrosine led to the hypothesis that bile acids coming from the enterohepatic cycle move from the sinusoidal plasma membrane to bile via a pathway that includes the SER and Golgi apparatus.[296-298] Immunoperoxidase studies of taurocholate and ursodeoxycholate have localized these bile acids to vesicles of the SER and Golgi apparatus.[299,300] Furthermore, the SER is the seat of the mixed function oxidase system requiring cytochrome P-450.[301] This is involved in the biotransformation of numerous xenobiotics and carcinogens, forming metabolites which are eliminated in bile. Biotransformation of some xenobiotics that are not cholestatic per se may lead to metabolites with varying degrees of cholestatic potential,[302] depending on individual variations of the enzymatic composition of the SER.[302]

Lysosomes

It has been calculated that acid hydrolases are excreted in bile at a rate corresponding to the daily unloading of about 5% of the hepatic lysosomes.[303] Further studies confirmed that several lysosomal enzymes undergo biliary excretion by a specific mechanism apparently independent of bile acid secretion, consistent with the hypothesis of hepatocellular exocytosis of lysosomal contents.[304-306] Extracellular release through biliary excretion is a major mechanism contributing to the turnover of lysosomal hydrolases.[307]

Although the complete physiological significance of lysosomal discharge into bile remains unclear, this mechanism may provide the hepatocyte with a disposal system for indigestible residues accumulating in lysosomes e.g. copper in Wilson disease and iron in haemochromatosis.[308,309] Previous experiments using tracer substances led to similar conclusions.[310]

Golgi complex

The Golgi complex is involved as an obligatory step in secretion in virtually all secretory cells. A role for the hepatocellular Golgi complex in bile secretion was proposed more than half a century ago but later studies mainly emphasized the involvement of the Golgi system with secretory processes directed towards the sinusoids, such as secretion of albumin, fibrinogen and very low density lipoprotein. However, the close and frequent juxtaposition of Golgi zones and the bile canaliculus is very suggestive of a Golgi role in bile secretion. When hepatocytes are disaggregated by enzyme perfusion, the bile canaliculi disappear and the peripheral location of the Golgi complex is lost; but after 24 hours in vitro in monolayer culture, new bile canaliculi are formed and the Golgi-biliary polarity is restored.[311]

Evidence produced more recently favours the concept that in the hepatocyte the Golgi complex is indeed involved in secretion towards the biliary compartment.[312-317] The Golgi complex was claimed to be involved in intracellular transport of bile acids (at least under high bile acid load) and of lipids.[318] Bile salts have been demonstrated in Golgi vesicles by immunohistochemistry using antibodies against natural bile acids.[319] However, final proof of bile salt transport inside the lumen of Golgi vesicles is lacking.[240]

Cytoskeleton

Contractile actin microfilaments are located mainly in the periphery of the hepatocyte and are concentrated in the pericanalicular zone, forming a pericanalicular web.[238] In this apical portion of the hepatocyte, three actin microfilament regions can be observed: bile canalicular membrane-associated microfilaments, a circumferential pericanalicular actin microfilament band, and actin associated with the core of the canalicular microvilli.[241]

The membrane-associated microfilaments form a network that attaches to the membrane itself. These filaments are associated with myosin II and are likely to be involved in maintaining the elasticity and structural integrity of the membrane, and in the regulation of the vesicle transport processes of the canaliculus.[241]

The circumferential pericanalicular actin microfilament band (contractile pericanalicular actin filament band) comprises filaments that are of mixed polarity, which would enable contractility. The actin-binding proteins, tropomyosin, α-actinin, and myosin II, localize to this pericanalicular actin microfilament band, which is of interest since α-actinin and tropomyosin are control proteins in the regulation of contraction. Also fodrin appears to be located here.[320] Furthermore, this microfilament band is attached to the zonula adhaerens junctions (intermediate junctions), and the proteins actin, vinculin, α-actinin and myosin II are also found in these junctions. There is some evidence that actin filaments from the contractile filament band also insert into the tight junction.[321]

The actin microfilaments in the core of the canalicular microvilli are perpendicularly disposed and arranged in a bundle. Villin, an actin-binding and actin-splicing protein, is found at this site. Transverse cross-linking of the actin core filaments to the microvillar membrane is comparable structurally to similar cross-bridges in intestinal microvilli, which have been shown to be myosin I.

Of the four main functions envisaged for the contractile microfilaments of the hepatocyte those related to bile secretion are: (i) the translocation of carrier or ferry vesicles;[322] (ii) co-ordinated contraction around the canaliculus resulting in a peristalsis-like movement, propelling the secreted bile in the canaliculus; such canalicular contractions have been observed in numerous experiments in vivo and in vitro;[238,323,324] and (iii) possible modulation of the structure and tightness of the so-called tight junctions, thus regulating the permeability of the paracellular pathway.[241,242]

It is not known whether microvilli are static or exhibit motility in response to physiological stimuli. Actin microfilaments undergo continuous assembly and disassembly, which may regulate microvillar length.[324]

Intermediate filaments of the keratin type comprise in the normal hepatocyte the cytokeratins 8 and 18.[276] They form a distinct sheet of matted filaments which envelop the entire hepatocyte and condense around the canaliculus as a 'pericanalicular sheath' which extends into desmosomes (macula adhaerens junctions).[241,325] The cortical intermediate filaments are in continuity with the pericanalicular sheath and the filaments located within the cytoplasm. The function of hepatocellular cytokeratin filaments is to maintain structural polarity, to provide a scaffolding for the bile canaliculus, and to provide a framework for the distribution of actin and endocytotic vesicles along the plasma membrane.[246,274]

Microtubules are involved in the blood-bound secretion of several liver-cell products, including lipoprotein, albumin, retinol-binding protein, secretory component, fibrinogen and other glycoproteins.[235] They play a role in the intracellular translocation of vesicles containing IgA and horseradish peroxidase.[245,246] They are also required for the secretion of bile acids and biliary lipids at the canalicular membrane.[219,318] They appear also to be involved in the canalicular discharge of endogenous and exogenous lysosomal constituents,[326] and in maintaining the structural and functional integrity of the biliary pole of the hepatocyte.[327] High concentrations of bile salts (as in cholestasis) inhibit the function of molecular motors, such as kinesin and dynein, that move vesicles along microtubules.[328]

The microtrabecular lattice[329] plays a role in the spatial positioning and movement of intracellular organelles and vesicles; it appears to represent an extremely dynamic system, in connection with the remaining cytoskeletal components, essential for normal intracellular transport functions. Although not yet studied in hepatocytes, it may be assumed to exert a role similar to that in other cells, and thus to be involved in blood-bound and bile-directed secretions.

Hyaloplasm

The hyaloplasm corresponds to the biochemist's cytosol or supernatant, and represents an apparently structureless gel, corresponding to the cell's cytoplasm in between the organelles. This cellular compartment was, until recently, less attractive to the morphologist because of its apparent lack of structural organization; however, it is the compartment in which the microtrabecular lattice extends. The hyaloplasm is an important molecular traffic zone; cytosolic binding proteins involved in intracellular transport of bile acids are present in this compartment.[219,330]

Junctional complexes

All components of the junctional complexes are to some extent important in relation to bile formation.

The *desmosome (macula adhaerens)* serves as a button-like connector between cytokeratin filament systems of adjacent cells; it thus limits distensibility and prevents excessive deformation and damage from mechanical stress[331] and contributes to the structural stability of the bile canaliculus.[246,274]

The *intermediate junction (zonula adhaerens)* is a continuous belt-like junction immediately below the tight junction. Adhaerens junctions are formed by members of the cadherin family of Ca^{2+}-dependent homotypic adhesion molecules and their cytoplasmic plaque proteins (α-, β- and γ-catenin). Cadherin is bound directly through α-catenin and indirectly through α-actinin, vinculin and radixin to a dense belt of bipolar actin filaments—the pericanalicular actin microfilament band mentioned above. Several lines of evidence suggest that adhaerens junctions and tight junctions are two aspects of a single functional unit.[220] The formation of tight junctions both in developing embryonic tissues and in cultured cell model systems is dependent on the prior formation of cadherin-based contacts. It remains unclear whether cadherin initiates intracellular signals used to instruct the assembly of tight junctions, or whether tight junctions use cadherin as a physical scaffold for assembly, or both.[220]

The *tight junction (zonula occludens)* is the sealing belt which separates the biliary compartment (canaliculus) from the intercellular space. Its structure is more clearly revealed by the freeze-fracture replica technique.[242] The junction is built up by a network of anastomosing junctional lines or fibrils (Fig. 1.21). Each sealing fibril is composed of two firmly attached hemifibrils, located in the plasma membrane of two adjacent hepatocytes. Closer analysis reveals that the hemifibrils in each cell membrane are formed by rows of special tight junctional particles inserted in the phospholipid bilayer of the membrane.[332] This sealing element of the canaliculus allows for the formation of steep ionic and osmotic gradients between the lumen and the interspace. The liver cell tight junction is not as tight as the name implies, and is to some extent a leaky junction, allowing for a paracellular flux of water and solutes, with selectivity for cations, thus establishing a bio-electrical barrier.[242,321,333,334]

The liver-cell tight junction forms a variable network, containing points with lower numbers of junctional fibrils, presumably corresponding to spots of higher conductivity.[242,330] A growing number of tight junction-associated pro-

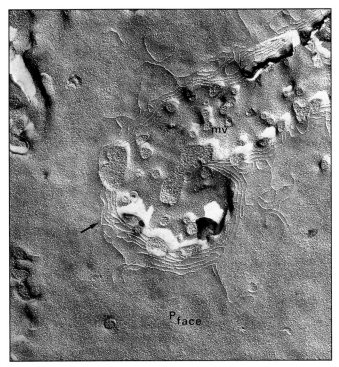

Fig. 1.21 • Freeze-fracture replica of bile canaliculus from normal rat liver. The tight junctions appear as 3–6 more-or-less parallel strands or ridges on the so-called P face (protoplasmic leaflet) of the cleaved intercellular membrane (arrow). Bile canalicular microvilli (mv) can be recognized in the canalicular lumen. 60 000 ×.

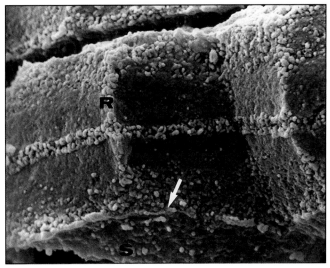

Fig. 1.22 • SEM illustrating bile canaliculus in normal rat liver. The picture shows a broken liver-cell plate; the hemicanaliculus lies in the middle of the intercellular domain; it is provided with numerous microvilli, most numerous near the canalicular margin. The intercellular domain is relatively flat, contrasting with the irregular microvilli of the perisinusoidal recess (R). The sinusoidal lumen (S) is separated from the liver cell's sinusoidal domain by a thin veil of endothelial cytoplasm (arrow). × 10 000.

teins has been identified. The intercellular barrier is formed by rows of the transmembrane protein occludin. Occludin has been shown to localize within the tight junction fibrils. It confers cell–cell adhesion and functions in the permeability barrier.[220] On the cytoplasmic surface, occludin is bound to the cytoplasmic plaque proteins ZO-1 and ZO-2; these proteins are members of the membrane-associated guanylate kinase (MAGUK) protein family and probably have both structural and signalling roles. Additional plaque proteins include cingulin, 7H6 antigen and symplekin, at present without known function. Also localized within the junction are transducing proteins, including both heterotrimeric and rho-related guanosine 5′-triphosphate (GTP)-binding proteins, protein kinase C isoforms and non-receptor tyrosine kinases. The complexity of tight junctions has recently been reviewed.[221]

Although the picture is still incomplete, these findings are of interest in view of the fact that tight junctions are not static structures. Their architecture may be modulated by various factors associated with corresponding variations in permeability. Paracellular permeability is subject to a variety of hormonal, metabolic and drug-related influences,[219,335] and microfilaments and microtubules have been shown to influence tight junctional structure and permeability.[336] Control of perijunctional actin (amongst others in the pericanalicular contractile actin microfilament band) may be the unifying mechanism for regulating paracellular permeability. The tight junctions thus occupy a strategic position: adjacent hepatocytes exert control not only on the transcellular passage of molecules in transepithelial transport, but also regulate the locks of the paracellular pathway, located

at their periphery in the intercellular space. It should be realized, however, that the permeability of the total paracellular pathway depends not only on the tight junctions but also on the configuration and composition of the intercellular space.[337]

The *gap junction (macula communicans)* occurs as larger areas on the intercellular domain of the hepatocellular plasma membrane, but also as small patches between the fibril networks of the tight junctions, i.e. very close to the canaliculus. This suggests that part of the intercellular communication is related to the co-ordination of bile secretory activity between neighbouring hepatocytes.[310]

Canalicular membrane

The bile canalicular membrane represents a specialized domain of the hepatocyte membrane,[310,338] comprising less than 15% of the cell surface and specialized entirely for the purpose of bile formation.[322] The bile canaliculus is formed by a groove (hemicanaliculus) on the lateral plasma membrane (Fig. 1.22). The two hemicanaliculi of adjacent hepatocytes are sealed by tight junctions. Canalicular shape and size may vary to some extent in the normal liver,[339] apparently in relation to secretory activity;[340,341] the normal diameter is about 1 μm.

The canalicular plasma membrane projects into the lumen in the form of numerous finger-like extensions (microvilli) of somewhat variable length and diameter (Fig. 1.22). The spacing of these microvilli is not entirely uniform.[166,342] In the smaller centrilobular canaliculi they appear over the entire canalicular surface; in the broader periportal canaliculi there is a preferential location near the margin.[166] Besides finger-like extensions, diverticulum-like evaginations of the canalicular membrane may be seen, probably representing what have been described as 'intracellular canaliculi'.[166,342]

Techniques for isolation of canalicular subfractions from the liver parenchymal cell membrane have been progressively refined, allowing for ongoing studies on their molecular composition.[343,344] Biochemically, the canalicular domain is a specially differentiated segment of the hepatocyte plasma membrane in terms of phospholipid–cholesterol ratio, content of proteins, presence of specific ecto-enzymes, enrichment of glycosphingolipids[343] and insertion of specific transport molecules.[287–289,345] The histochemically demonstrable bile canalicular ATP-ase (Fig. 1.16(D)) is the Ca^{2+}, Mg^{2+}-ATPase, which is not a transport ATPase but an ecto-enzyme with its active site outside of the cell.[324]

Identity has been confirmed between the ecto-ATPase and the cell adhesion molecule cell—CAM 105,[346] which was demonstrated in the pericanalicular domain of the rat hepatocyte plasma membrane.[347] Besides a role in cell adhesion, the ecto-ATPase is thought to have two functions: (i) hydrolysis of extracellular ATP, which is a ligand for P2-purinergic receptors, to terminate the physiological response, and (ii) protecting cells from deleterious effects of extracellular ATP by acting in concert with 5′-nucleotidase (AMPase), another canalicular ecto-enzyme, to form adenosine, which then interacts with its cell surface receptor or is recaptured by a canalicular nucleoside transporter.[324]

A sodium gradient-energized, concentrative, outside-to-inside orientated nucleoside transport system is present in canalicular membranes. The co-localization of ecto-ATPase, 5′-nucleotidase, and a nucleoside transport system in canalicular membranes suggests a functional link between extracellular nucleotide degradation and nucleoside conservation in hepatocytes.[324]

The canalicular membrane is rich in several other ecto-enzymes, which are all about 100 to 120 kD. Among these are γ-glutamyl-transpeptidase, dipeptidyl peptidase, COOH-terminal peptidases, and leucine aminopeptidase. The ectoenzymes γ-glutamyltranspeptidase and dipeptidyl peptidase degrade extracellular glutathione into cysteine, glutamic acid and glycine, which can be conserved by a sodium gradient-driven amino acid transporter in the bile canalicular membrane. It is likely that the entire repertoire of ecto-enzymes in the canaliculus is linked with unidirectional transporters that conserve amino acids, purines and pyrimidines.[324]

The canalicular membrane is the seat of ATP-dependent export pumps. Under physiological conditions, active solute transport across the canalicular membrane of hepatocytes represents the rate limiting step in overall bile formation. This unidirectional and concentrative transport step is driven by an array of ATP-dependent export pumps that belong to the ABC (ATP-Binding Cassette) family of membrane transporters.[287–289,345,348] These include: (i) the canalicular bile salt transporter (CBST) or bile salt export pump (BSEP), also termed Sister of P Glycoprotein (SPGP), which is the predominant canalicular bile acid export pump, and is deficient in progressive familial intrahepatic cholestasis type 2 (PFIC 2); (ii) a canalicular multispecific organic anion transporter (CMOAT) or MRP2 (isoform 2 of multidrug resistance-associated protein—MRP), involved in transport of non-bile acid organic anions, including conjugated bilirubin[349] as well as sulphated and glucuronidated bile acids. MRP2 is lacking in patients with the Dubin–Johnson syndrome; (iii) multidrug resistance protein MDR3 (human) or mdr2 (rodents), a phospholipid transporter, which functions as a flippase that translocates phosphatidylcholine from the inner to the outer leaflet of the canalicular membrane, where it can be selectively extracted by intracanalicular bile salts and secreted into bile as vesicles[240] and mixed micelles. MDR3 is lacking in patients with progressive familial intrahepatic cholestasis type 3 (PFIC 3), characterized by impaired or absent phosphatidylcholine secretion and elevated serum level of γ-glutamyltranspeptidase; (iv) multidrug resistance protein MDR1 (or P glycoprotein), the first ABC transporter to be localized at the canalicular membrane. Its endogeneous substrate(s) is still unknown.

Phosphotungstic acid staining in electron microscopy shows that the canalicular domain of the membrane is more akin to membranes of the vacuolar apparatus (Golgi complex and lysosomes) than the rest of the cell membrane.[350] The canalicular membrane contains antigens shared by renal proximal tubules and other epithelia involved in absorption or secretion.[351] Bile salt secretion modulates the phospholipid–cholesterol ratio and hence the fluidity and permeability of this membrane.[341] By virtue of their detergent activity, bile salts also elute some glycoprotein ecto-enzymes from the canalicular membrane, explaining the occurrence in bile of such enzymes as 5-nucleotidase, phosphodiesterase, γ-glutamyl transpeptidase and alkaline phosphatase.[240,352–354] Even segments of canalicular membrane may be shed into the lumen during bile secretion.[313] Loss of membrane components from the canalicular domain may be compensated for by insertion of membrane units arriving with transcytotic vesicles.[355,356]

Exactly how the canalicular membrane surface area is maintained in a steady state in the midst of loss of components and insertion of new membrane units remains unknown.[240] The canalicular membrane however turns out to be a crucial structural component involved in bile formation.

The interhepatocellular bile channel or canaliculus (Fig. 1.23)

The bile canalicular network forms a structurally and functionally coherent system; indeed, segments of canaliculi can be isolated as such.[359] Intercellular attachments in the zonulae occludentes, and zonulae and maculae adhaerentes, contribute to the structural cohesion. Its tone is provided by an encircling band of contractile microfilaments inserting on the zonulae adhaerentes. Microfilaments running in the axis of microvilli and connected with the inner leaflet of the microvillous membrane possibly provide microvillar motility. This arrangement appears as a dynamic microequivalent at the subcellular level of the intestinal villous and peristaltic movements, important in the propagation of fluid flow in the system.[360] Co-ordination of bile secretory function between the successive canalicular segments contributed by individual hepatocytes is conceivably important for the

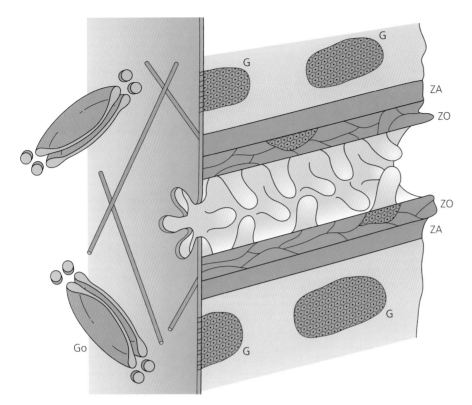

Fig. 1.23 • Schematic representation of the biliary pole of the hepatocyte. The picture shows a hemicaniculus with microvilli, which are more prominent at the margin. The canaliculus is sealed by a tight junction with its characteristic network (zonula occludens—ZO). In some compartments of the tight junctional network, gap junctions are built in. Next to the tight junction lies the intermediate junction (zonula adhaerens—ZA), which is the attachment site for contractile microfilaments. These form a pericanalicular web and also insert on the inner leaflet of the microvillous membrane. Larger gap junctional areas are represented on the intratrabecular cell surface (G). In the vicinity of the bile canaliculus, the liver-cell cytoplasm contains microtubules, pericanalicular vesicles, lysosomes (the latter two not shown in this drawing) and Golgi complexes (Go).

canalicular network to function as a whole. Such integration may be achieved by intercellular communication through maculae communicantes.[361]

The occurrence throughout the liver lobule of a periportal-centrilobular gradient in the concentration of solutes in the sinusoidal plasma[362] and the opposite direction of bile flow to that of plasma flow[361] may further be important in modulating the function of the canalicular network as a whole. Other regulating factors are the type and number of carrier molecules in plasma,[362] the presence of receptors for hormones and metabolites in the sinusoidal plasma membrane domain[363] and the innervation of hepatocytes.[364]

The biliary system

From the complicated polygonal network which has just been described the canaliculi drain into the canals of Hering, partly lined by hepatocytes and partly by cholangiocytes, followed by the bile ductules (cholangioles) which have a basement membrane and are lined by three to six ductal cells or cholangiocytes (Fig. 1.24). The ductules may extend through the limiting plate and join the canals of Hering after a shorter or longer course, bringing the parenchymal-ductular interface for a variable distance into the liver lobule. Some ductules thus are composed of an intralobular and portal segment.[5] In the smaller portal tracts the ductules join the interlobular bile ducts (Fig. 1.25), the smallest branches of which are 15–20 µm in diameter. They are lined by a single layer of flattened cuboidal epithelium, have a basement membrane and are in turn ensheathed in the fibrous tissue of the portal tracts. The interlobular ducts anastomose freely, increase in size and form larger septal or

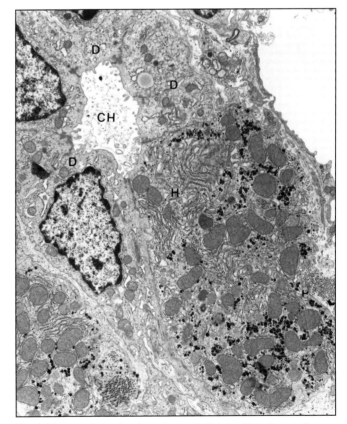

Fig. 1.24 • TEM of a section through a canal of Hering (CH) whose wall shows ductal cells (D) and a hepatocyte (H). Human liver, × 9200. Supplied by Professor R De Vos.

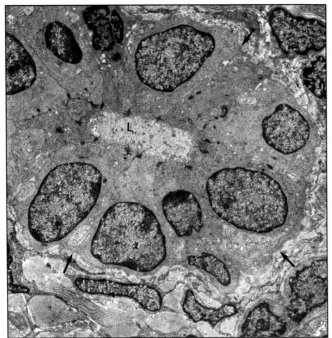

A

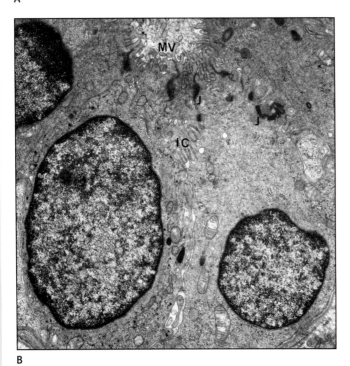

B

Fig. 1.25 • **(A)** TEM of a cross-section of a bile duct. Lumen (L); basement membrane (arrow). Human liver, × 5750. **(B)** TEM of epithelium of a bile duct. Note contorted intercellular space (IC); apical microvilli (MV); junctional complexes (J). Human liver, × 36 800. Supplied by Professor R De Vos.

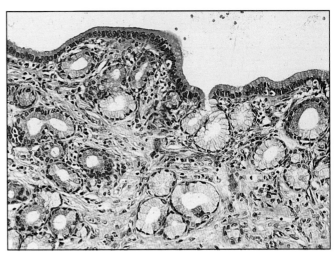

Fig. 1.26 • Large intrahepatic bile duct near the hilum. Note the surrounding mucous and seromucinous peribiliary glands; one mucous gland opens into the duct lumen. H&E.

trabecular ducts which are more than 100 μm in diameter, and which are lined by a simple tall columnar epithelium with basally situated nuclei. The portal tract fibrous tissue shows some condensation round these ducts, but there is no well-marked concentric orientation. The terminology and heterogeneity of the intrahepatic bile ducts as proposed by Desmet, Roskams & De Vos[365] is summarized in Table 1.2. A quantitative computer-aided three-dimensional study of the human biliary system has recently been published.[366]

The larger ducts further anastomose to form the hilar intrahepatic bile ducts, 1–1.5 mm in diameter, which give rise to the main hepatic ducts. Studies by Nakanuma and his colleagues[367–369] have demonstrated the presence of glandular elements around the larger intrahepatic bile ducts (Fig. 1.26). These peribiliary glands are of two types: (i) intramural mucous glands which communicate directly with the bile-duct lumen, and (ii) extramural mixed seromucinous glands which form branching tubulo-alveolar lobules and secretory ducts that drain into the bile-duct lumen. They are found in relation to the common hepatic ducts, the hilar ducts and a proportion of the larger septal ducts. Scanning electron microscopy has shown that hilar ducts may also have irregular side branches and pouches in which bile may be stored and probably modified.[370] As described earlier the intrahepatic bile ducts are supplied by an anastomosing peribiliary vascular plexus derived from the hepatic artery and which drains into periportal sinusoids.

In recent years there has been a considerable increase in our knowledge of the structure and function of bile-duct cells,[29,157,219,371–376] studies which have confirmed the view of Rous & McMaster[377] in 1921 that bile ducts have an important role in modifying canalicular bile, a role to which the intrahepatic peribiliary glands may also contribute. Ultrastructurally, the biliary epithelial cell has a prominent Golgi complex, numerous cytoplasmic vesicles and short luminal microvilli.[378] Studies in the rat suggest that 10–15% of basal bile flow is produced by ductal epithelium[379] and it has been estimated that the corresponding contribution in humans is 40%.[219] Secretion is under hormonal control (secretin and somatostatin); secretin is released from the duodenum following vagal stimulation and the presence of acid in the duodenum, and stimulates the secretion of bicarbonate-rich bile.[371] That the duct epithelium also secretes IgA and IgM (but not IgG) has been shown immunohistochemically on human duct cells.[157,380] Reabsorption involves water, glucose, glutamate and urate.

Table 1.2   Terminology of the biliary tree (adapted from Desmet et al. 1997 and from Roskams et al. 2004)

Generation of branching	Diameter	Terminology	Remarks
Large bile ducts			
First generation	>800 µm	Left and right hepatic duct	Cylindrical epithelium surrounded by dense fibrous tissue and elastic fibres Peribiliary glands
Second generation	400–800 µm	Segmental ducts	Cylindrical epithelium surrounded by dense fibrous tissue and elastic fibres Peribiliary glands
Third generation	300–400 µm	Area ducts	Lower cylindrical epithelium Peribiliary glands
Small intrahepatic bile ducts (not grossly recognizable)	>100 µm 15–100 µm 40–100 µm 15–40 µm	Septal ducts Interlobular ducts Medium-sized Small	Located in periphery of portal tracts Cuboidal epithelium accompanied by artery Lined by 3–4 cuboidal cells
Twelfth generation	<15 µm	Ductules (cholangioles) Canals of Hering	May extend through limiting plate into lobule Lined partly by hepatocytes, partly by biliary epithelial cells

Bile acids are reabsorbed via biliary epithelium and are recirculated by a cholehepatic shunt pathway via the peribiliary plexus and this promotes bile-acid dependent bile flow in the ducts.[10,219,381–383] Immunohistochemical studies localizing ursodeoxycholic acid in bile-duct cells support this concept.[382]

The apical transporter MDR1 and the basolateral transporters MRP1 and MRP3 are expressed in normal bile ducts, suggesting a functional role for these transporters in normal bile formation in both interlobular bile ducts and ductules.[371]

The peribiliary glands share some antigenic determinants with pancreatic exocrine acini. They secrete seromucinous fluid,[366] IgA and secretory piece[380] and contain hormones.[384] The epithelia of large intrahepatic bile ducts and their accompanying peribiliary glands contain pancreatic α-amylase and trypsin.[385]

Bile-duct epithelial cells have phenotypic traits which distinguish them from hepatocytes[378] and display heterogeneity along the different segments of the biliary tree.[372,374,386,387] They express receptors for epidermal growth factor, secretin and somatostatin.[375] Normally they express class I major histocompatibility complex (MHC) antigens but not class II; cytokine-induced expression of class II antigen is seen in graft versus host disease, allograft rejection, primary biliary cirrhosis and primary sclerosing cholangitis and this may be important in the pathogenesis of the bile-duct injury in these diseases (Chapter 11). Bile-duct cells express more cell-matrix adhesion molecules or integrins than hepatocytes, including $\alpha_2 \beta_1$, $\alpha_3 \beta_1$, $\alpha_5 \beta_1$, $\alpha_6 \beta_1$, and $\alpha_6 \beta_4$ concurring with those expressed by most simple epithelial cells.[225] Bile-duct epithelium also expresses glutamyl transpeptidase, carcinoembryonic antigen and epithelial membrane antigen, representing other phenotypic differences when compared with hepatocytes, the precise significance of which is, as yet, uncertain.[157,374,375]

The hepatic sinusoid and the sinusoidal cells

The sinusoids (Fig. 1.27) have an average diameter of about 10 µm, but they may distend to about 30 µm. Periportal sinusoids are more tortuous than the perivenular ones.[390] Four distinct types of sinusoidal cell can be identified (Fig. 1.28), each with its own characteristic morphology, topography and population dynamics:[391] the lining of the sinusoids is formed by endothelial cells; the hepatic stellate cells are found in the space of Disse which lies between the sinusoidal endothelial cells and the hepatocytes; the Kupffer cells and liver-associated lymphocytes lie on the luminal aspect of the endothelium.

Sinusoidal endothelial cells

These form an attenuated cytoplasmic sheet (about 50–80 nm in maximum thickness) perforated by numerous holes (fenestrae) and, unlike endothelial cells elsewhere, they apparently do not form junctions with adjacent endothelial cells (Fig. 1.27(B) and Fig. 1.28(A)). The fenestrae are so abundant that, on SEM, the greater part of the cell has a net-like appearance, forming a tenuous barrier, reinforced here and there where adjacent endothelial cells overlap one another (Fig. 1.27(B)). The fenestrae vary greatly in size, but fall, in general, into two size categories: small (0.1–0.2 µm in diameter), which are grouped in clusters, forming so-called sieve plates, and large (up to 1 µm in diameter) which are more numerous at the distal end of the sinusoid. Thus, endothelial cell porosity is higher in the perivenular zone than in the periportal zone.[392] The smaller fenestrae are intracellular and appear in cultured endothelial cells. The larger are usually intercellular, and some workers consider that they may be artifacts due to fixation.[391] There is evidence that fenestrae are labile structures whose diameter may change in response to endogenous

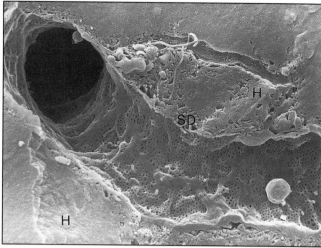

A

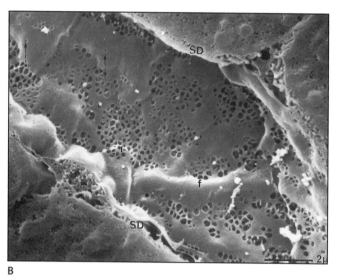

B

Fig. 1.27 • (A) SEM illustrating normal hepatic sinusoid in rat liver. Note the regular distribution of fenestrae in the sieve plates which are separated by intervening cytoplasmic processes. H = hepatocyte; SD = space of Disse. **(B)** SEM. Endothelial fenestrations (f) of about 0.1 µm are grouped together in sieve plates. Processes of endothelial cells show small holes, most probably representing the pinching off of micropinocytotic vesicles (arrows). SD = Space of Disse.

pressure effect of blood cells in the sinusoidal lumen—flexible erythrocytes pressing plasma and small particles into the space of Disse ('forced sieving') and rigid leucocytes squeezing fluid out ('endothelial massage'—see Fig. 1.31).

Sinusoidal endothelial cells show a number of phenotypic differences compared with vascular endothelium. They do not bind the lectin Ulex europaeus and, in most species, do not express factor VIII related antigen (von Willebrand factor),[391] although the cells assume these properties in chronic liver disease.[394,395] Furthermore, they do not normally contain other molecules characteristically found in vascular endothelium, such as GMP-140 and CD34, but do express Fcγ IgG receptors (CD16 and CDw32), CD4, CD14 and amino-peptidase N.[392,396] They also exhibit membrane immunoreactivity for ICAM-1.[396] The natural ligand for this adhesion molecule, LFA-1, is present on Kupffer cells; this receptor may therefore be involved in adhesion of Kupffer cells to the endothelial lining.[396] Up-regulation of intercellular adhesion molecule-1 (ICAM-1) expression in sinusoidal endothelial cells may be important in 'trapping' lymphocyte associated antigen-1 (LFA-1) positive lymphocytes in inflammatory liver diseases.[397] There is also sinusoidal endothelial cell heterogeneity within the acinus: the increased porosity in the perivenular zone has already been mentioned but, in addition, variation in cell size, heterogeneous lectin binding, and expression of various receptors, cytoplasmic density, endocytic capacity and surface glycosylation have also been demonstrated.[396,398–400]

Another unusual feature of sinusoidal endothelial cells is their high endocytotic activity.[393] This process appears to be directed towards uptake and lysosomal degradation of compounds rather than providing an alternative route for their transport from the sinusoidal lumen to the space of Disse. The intracellular handling of denatured proteins such as formaldehyde-treated albumin has been well documented in isolated sinusoidal endothelial cells.[401] Other receptors have now been identified on these cells which may mediate endocytosis of a large number of endogenous compounds, some of which are effete molecules and are cleared from the circulation and others of which are modified and undergo transcytosis to hepatocytes.[378,402] Thus, the sinusoidal endothelial cells have a role in removing soluble immune complexes (like the Kupffer cells) and have also been shown to store and metabolize serum immunoglobulin[398,403,404] and to remove hyaluronic acid/chondroitin sulphate proteoglycans from the circulation.[405] The sinusoidal endothelial cells also have synthetic activity and produce nitrous oxide (NO), endothelins and prostaglandins and possibly cytokines such as interleukin-1 and interleukin-6.[378,406,407]

The space of Disse

The space of Disse (Fig. 1.28(A)) lies primarily between the sinusoidal wall and the outer sinusoidal surface of the hepatocyte, from which abundant microvilli project into the space and may be of importance in keeping the space open. This space is not normally discernible in biopsy material but in autopsy liver the hepatocytes shrink from the sinusoids

mediators (e.g. serotonin)[392] and exogenous agents such as alcohol.[393] The extracellular matrix in the space of Disse also modulates the fenestrae and lack of cell-matrix interaction results in loss of fenestrae in cultured sinusoidal endothelial cells, whereas cells plated on human amnion basement membrane retain their fenestrae.[394] The fenestrae lack diaphragms and since, in most species, a basement membrane is absent on the deep surface of the sinusoidal endothelium, there is continuity between the sinusoidal lumen and the perisinusoidal space of Disse.

This unique structure allows the endothelial cells to filter the sinusoidal blood. Solutes pass freely through the fenestrae from the lumen into the space of Disse and come into contact with the hepatocytes. Large particles such as newly generated chylomicrons, however, are excluded. Wisse and co-workers[393] have postulated that transport of materials through the fenestrae may be facilitated by the

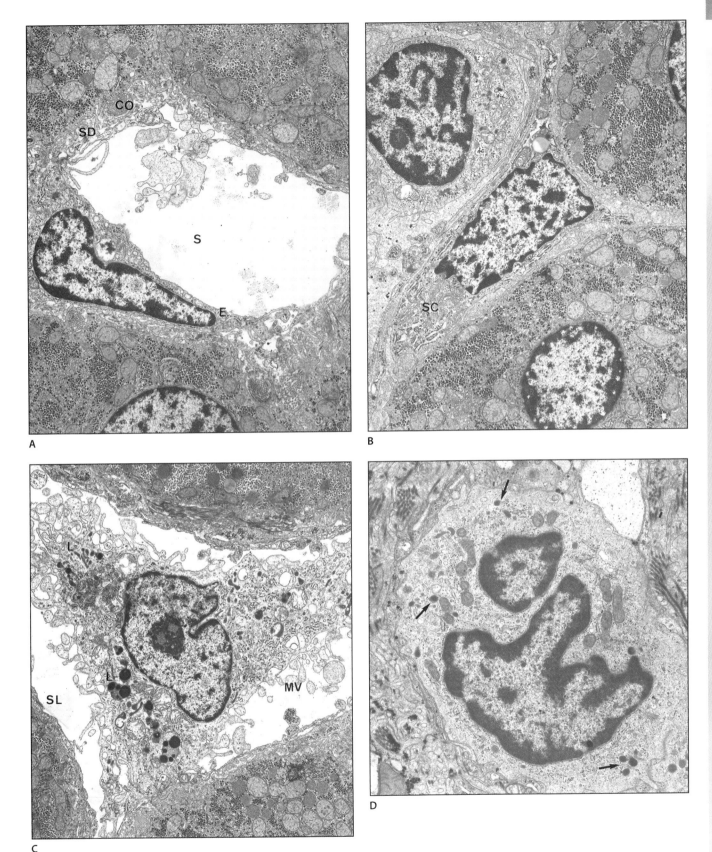

Fig. 1.28 • (A) TEM illustrating a sinusoid (S) with its lining endothelial cells (E); space of Disse (SD); collagen bundles (CO). Human liver, × 11 500. **(B)** TEM showing a stellate cell (SC) in the Disse space. Note cell processes, small fat droplet and rough endoplasmic reticulum (RER). Human liver, × 11 500. **(C)** TEM of a Kupffer cell with numerous cytoplasmic lysosomes (L). Note irregular microvillous projections (MV); sinusoidal lumen (SL). Small rims of endothelial lining cells are observed at both sides of the Kupffer cell. Human liver, × 9200. **(D)** Liver associated lymphocyte within a sinusoid. Note dense granules in the cytoplasm (arrows). Human liver, × 18 400. Supplied by Professor R De Vos.

and the space is then characteristically evident (see Fig. 1.37). Studies with TEM show extensions of the space outwards between adjacent hepatocytes (Fig. 1.15(B)) and this considerably expands the perisinusoidal compartment.[408] It forms, therefore, an extensive and almost unique extravascular space. As noted earlier, the sinusoidal endothelium is not only discontinuous and extensively fenestrated, but in many species (including man) lacks a basement membrane. It is thus freely permeable to blood plasma, which enters the space and comes into direct contact with the hepatocytes and the hepatic stellate cells. This extravascular plasma constitutes the immediate medium of exchange between blood and hepatocytes, whose surface area of contact is increased by the abundant microvilli. The plasma is then presumed to flow towards the hepatic veins; some, however, is taken up by lymphatic spaces in the periportal zone and some may re-enter the sinusoidal blood. The movement of plasma in the space of Disse may in part be due to the 'endothelial massage' effect of leucocytes (see Fig. 1.31). The nature of the anatomical link between the periportal ends of the space of Disse and the lymphatics is discussed later.

The *extracellular matrix*, produced by the hepatic stellate cells, is present within the space of Disse and constitutes the structural 'reticulin' framework of the liver. Hepatocytes may produce some collagen and some proteoglycans; the role of Kupffer cells and sinusoidal endothelial cells is mediated through the production of cytokines which modulate the synthetic activity of the stellate cells, but they may produce small amounts of proteoglycans. The precise structure of the matrix is poorly defined and it is discussed on pp. 98–101. It plays a major role in the normal biology of the liver. It influences hepatocyte, sinusoidal endothelial cell and stellate cell function and interaction between this matrix and these cells is of fundamental importance in maintaining their differentiation, growth and function.[409-411] The importance of altered cell–matrix interactions in chronic liver disease is discussed in Chapter 13.

There is a gradient in the extracellular matrix in the space of Disse (Fig. 1.5) with variation in its amount and composition with increasing distance from the portal tracts.[131,412] Thus, laminin, collagen type IV and heparan sulphate predominate in the periportal zone whereas in the perivenular zones fibronectin, collagen type III and dermatan sulphate are more abundant.[131] In contrast to what happens in other organs the extracellular matrix does not act as a diffusion barrier between the plasma and the hepatocytes. There is no identifiable basement membrane and this facilitates the two-way exchange which has to take place between the hepatocytes and the blood in the sinusoids.

The matrix components interact with the hepatocyte endothelial cell membrane through various surface integrins and other receptors. Hepatocytes have receptors for fibronectin, laminin, type I and type IV collagens,[413-417] and they can also bind proteoglycans.[418] The precise role of the integrins in the cell–matrix interactions is not fully understood. The proteoglycans can also act as adhesion and receptor molecules and act as an important reservoir for cytokines and growth factors.[419-421]

Hepatic stellate cells

Within the space of Disse are stellate cells whose long cytoplasmic processes surround the sinusoids. Originally identified by Boll and von Kupffer in the 1870s they were largely ignored until 1951 when Ito described their morphological features on light microscopy.[422] They were subsequently referred to under a variety of terms—Ito cells, hepatic lipocytes, fat storing cells, stellate cells and parasinusoidal cells.[423-424] The now accepted nomenclature for them is hepatic stellate cells (HSC).[425] Their pathobiology and their role in regulating inflammation in the liver have been extensively reviewed.[426-431] It is of interest that similar stellate cells, and which also share the property of vitamin A storage, have recently been described in rat and human pancreas[432] and there is also evidence that there is a more widespread distribution involving lung, kidney and gut.[433]

Hepatic stellate cells are not readily visualized on light microscopy (Fig. 1.29(A)) but they may be prominent in some pathological conditions.[434-436] They are readily seen in very thin sections or by TEM (Fig. 1.28(B)). The cells resemble pericytes and they establish close contacts with adjacent hepatocytes and (in some species) nerve endings abut on to

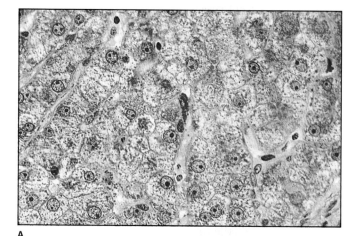

A

B

Fig. 1.29 • Hepatic stellate cells. **(A)** These may occasionally be seen on optical microscopy; the fat globules are phloxinophilic in this section stained by Masson's trichrome and the perisinusoidal location of the cell is readily appreciated. **(B)** Rat liver: immunoperoxidase stain for desmin; the cells show extensive prolongations of their cytoplasm within the space of Disse.

their cytoplasmic processes. They contain many small lipid droplets (Fig. 1.28(B)) which are rich in vitamin A; this can be demonstrated by fluorescence microscopy when excitation light of 328 nm length is used and by gold chloride impregnation. Rough endoplasmic reticulum and Golgi apparatus are well developed in these cells (Fig. 1.28(B)). The type of intermediate filament proteins within the stellate cells shows species variation and changes in their pattern of expression occur when they are activated.[427] Based on their expression of vimentin, desmin (Fig. 1.29(B)) and alpha smooth muscle actin (α-SMA)[437–442] stellate cells have been considered to be of mesenchymal origin. An unusual distribution of the cytoskeletal protein fodrin in stellate cells has been described.[443] In addition, several markers of neural/neuroectodermal differentiation have been found. Stellate cells express the intermediate filament glial fibrillary acidic protein (GFAP)[444–445] and activated rat stellate cells express the intermediate filament nestin.[446] Human stellate cells are immunoreactive with neural cell adhesion molecule (N-CAM) antibody,[447] while rat stellate cells become positive for N-CAM upon activation.[448] Human as well as rat quiescent and activated stellate cells express synaptophysin, a marker of synaptic vesicles containing neurotransmitters.[449] Ultrastructurally, they contain in their processes translucent vesicles, identical to synaptic vesicles seen in neurons. Human and rat hepatic stellate cells express neurotrophins and their receptors.[450] The expression of these neural proteins has led some investigators to suggest that they may at least in part be of neural crest origin;[451] it is of some interest that there may be a contribution from bone marrow derived precursors under some situations.[452]

The hepatic stellate cells have four main functions in the liver:

1. They produce the extracellular matrix proteins both in the normal liver and in the fibrotic liver.[427,428,453–456]
2. They act in a pericyte-like manner around the sinusoids and may have a role in the control of microvascular tone.[454] A contractile role in the normal liver has been suggested[406,457,458] and when activated in response to injury they have been shown to respond to vasoactive agents such as endothelin 1 and nitric oxide.[169,352,427]
3. They are a major site of storage for vitamin A.[198,459] Dietary retinyl esters reach the liver in chylomicron remnants. These pass from the sinusoidal lumen through the endothelial fenestrae and are taken up by hepatocytes. Most of the endocytosed retinol is rapidly transferred to the stellate cells for storage by an as yet poorly defined transport mechanism.[455] The cells contain a high concentration of cellular retinoid-binding protein and cellular retinol-acid binding protein. Their storage of vitamin A, however, shows heterogeneity[191] as indeed does their distribution of intermediate filaments.[444]
4. They play a role in hepatic regeneration both in the normal liver and in response to liver injury.[431] They express hepatocyte growth factor[430,460] and this can be enhanced in human hepatic stellate cells in response to insulin-like growth factor-2.[461]

In response to liver cell necrosis the hepatic stellate cells undergo a process of activation resulting in a number of phenotypic changes. The mechanisms involved in this have been reviewed by Friedman[429] and in Chapter 2.

Kupffer cells

Kupffer cells are hepatic macrophages and are present in the lumen of hepatic sinusoids (Figs 1.28(C) and 1.30). They belong to the mononuclear phagocytic system but manifest phenotypic differences which distinguish them from other macrophages. They are of considerable importance in host defence mechanisms and in addition have an important role in the pathogenesis of various liver diseases.[462] On SEM, Kupffer cells have an irregular stellate shape[463] and within the sinusoidal lumen the cell body rests on the endothelial lining (Fig. 1.30). They are more numerous in the periportal sinusoids[464] and there is some evidence that, like hepatocytes, Kupffer cells also manifest functional heterogeneity in the lobule.[464,465] They never form junctional complexes with endothelial cells, but they may be found in gaps between adjacent endothelial cells and their protoplasmic processes may extend through the larger endothelial fenestrae into the perisinusoidal space. The luminal surface shows many of the structural features associated with macrophages: small microvilli and microplicae and sinuous invaginations of the plasma membrane. These features together give to the surface the appearance of a microlabyrinth (Fig. 1.30).

Kupffer cells have been considered to be fixed tissue macrophages, but they appear capable of actively migrating along the sinusoids, both with and against the blood flow, and can migrate into areas of liver injury and into regional lymph nodes.[466] They contain lysosomes and phagosomes, and the cisternae of their endoplasmic reticulum are rich in peroxidase. Their primary functions include the removal by ingestion and degradation of particulate and soluble

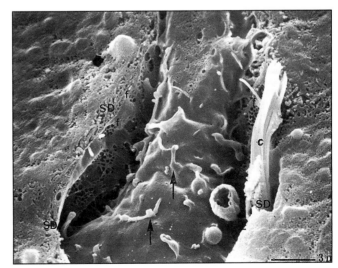

Fig. 1.30 • SEM. Part of Kupffer cell lying in a sinusoid and showing characteristic microvilli projecting at the cell surface (arrows). Small rims of fenestrated endothelium can be observed at both sides of the Kupffer cell—f. A small bundle of collagen fibres—c is situated in the space of Disse (SD) on the right.

material from the portal blood and in this they discriminate between 'self' and 'non-self' particles. They act as scavengers of microorganisms, degenerated normal cells such as effete erythrocytes, circulating tumour cells and various macromolecules. These functions are in part carried out non-specifically, but they are also involved in the initiation of immunological responses and the induction of tolerance to antigens absorbed from the gastrointestinal tract. The efficiency of this clearance function is shown by the fact that removal of particulate material is limited only by the magnitude of hepatic blood flow and that removal of particles may approach single-pass efficiency.

Kupffer cells play a major role in clearance of gut-derived endotoxin from the portal blood[434] and this is achieved without the induction of a local inflammatory response. It has been estimated that the concentrations of endotoxin varies from 100 pg/ml to 1 ng/ml.[467] The precise mechanisms involved are not fully understood, but there appears to be finely balanced autoregulation between the release of proinflammatory and inflammatory mediators such as interleukins 1 and 6, tumour necrosis factor α (TNFα) and interferon gamma, and mediators such as interleukin-10 which suppresses macrophage activation and inhibits their cytokine secretions.[468–470]

Several cytokines released by activated Kupffer cells are also thought to have local effects, modulating microvascular responses[164] and the functions of hepatocytes and the stellate cells[471]. Although Kupffer cells can express class II histocompatibility antigens[472] and can function in vitro as antigen-presenting cells, they appear to be considerably less efficient at this than macrophages at other sites.[473] Their principal roles in the immune response therefore appear to be antigen sequestration by phagocytosis and clearance of immune complexes.[474]

There is firm evidence from bone marrow transplant and liver transplant studies that Kupffer cells are derived, at least in part, from circulating monocytes.[475] However, Kupffer cells are capable of replication and their local proliferation accounts for a substantial part of the expansion of this cell population in response to liver injury.[476,477] Furthermore, Kupffer cells appear in the fetal liver of the mouse before there are circulating monocytes and there is evidence that they are derived from primitive macrophages which first appear in the yolk sac.[478] These data suggest that Kupffer cells may have a dual origin.

Liver-associated lymphocytes

Wisse et al.[479] described so-called pit cells in the sinusoids of rat liver. Similar cells were also identified in the livers of various species including humans.[480,481] These cells were shown to have the morphological features and markers of natural killer (NK) lymphocytes (Fig. 1.28(D)) and to exhibit natural killer activity in vitro.[479–482] Subsequent immunophenotyping studies, however, showed that there was a heterogeneous and large population of lymphocytes in the liver and they are now referred to as liver-associated lymphocytes. The emerging picture suggests that they constitute a lymphoid system which has an innate role specific

for its location and where it comes into early contact with gut-derived antigens. The topic has been reviewed by Doherty & O'Farrelly[483] and the following account draws freely on this review.

It has been estimated that an average normal human liver contains approximately 1×10^{10} lymphoid cells.[484] These lymphocytes are predominantly located around the portal tracts but are also found scattered throughout the parenchyma. They are found in loose contact with Kupffer cells or sinusoidal endothelial cells. In the peripheral blood 85% of the lymphocytes comprise T- and B-cells which possess clonotypic antigen-specific receptors; while significant numbers of T- and B-cells are found in the liver up to 65% of all the lymphocytes present, however, comprise NK cells, T-cells expressing γδ T-cell receptors (TCR) and T-cells expressing NK molecules (NKT cells); these subtypes comprise 13%, 2% and 2%, respectively, of peripheral blood lymphocytes. In addition the CD4/CD8 T-cell ratio of 1 : 3 in the liver contrasts with a 2 : 1 ratio in the peripheral blood.

The hepatic NK cells were indeed those first recognized by Wisse and his colleagues as so-called pit cells. They do not have antigen-specific receptors and are controlled by receptors that mediate activation or inhibition when there is ligation with surface molecules on target cells and by cytokines such as interferon α and some of the interleukins.[485–487] They preferentially kill target cells that lack MHC class 1 molecules. Human NK receptors that mediate activation include the Fcγ receptor for IgG (CD16) and this mediates antibody-dependent cellular cytotoxicity (ADCC). Hepatic NK cells are able to lyse tumour cells and participate in immune responses against certain viruses, intracellular bacteria and parasites.[485,488] The NK cells comprise 50% of the total population of liver-associated lymphocytes and their number is greatly increased when there is hepatic malignancy.[489,490]

The liver contains the largest number of γδ T-cells in the body.[489] γδ T-cells are also found in the skin, gut and respiratory mucosa and in the pregnant uterus, and accumulate at sites of infection.[491] They secrete various cytokines and can lyse antigen-bearing target cells. Their precise function in the liver is not yet clear.

The NKT cells co-express a T-cell receptor and NK activating and inhibitory receptors. They can be further subclassified on the basis of their expressing various types of TCRs and various NK receptors.[483,492] Functional studies have demonstrated that hepatic NKT cells have numerous cytotoxic activities and produce multiple cytokines.[483] Their major role therefore may be to effect local immunological reactions through the production of cytokines.

The relative frequency of the various subpopulations of liver-associated lymphocytes varies between individuals, probably reflecting each individual's immunological status; this in turn is affected by genetic background and both previous and current antigen exposure. It is also possible that the hepatic environment itself may influence the distribution of the various subsets. The presence of these cells in such large numbers indicates that they must subserve important roles in normal hepatic immune responses and immune homeostasis. The liver thus is probably comparable to the gastrointestinal tract which is now regarded as an important lymphoid organ.

Other constituent tissues

The extracellular matrix

The liver normally has only a small amount of connective tissue in relation to its size. Whereas in the human body collagen constitutes about 30% of the total protein, the corresponding figure for the liver is 5–10%. Underlying the visceral peritoneum or serosa there is a layer of dense connective tissue admixed with elastic fibres which varies in thickness from 40 to 70 μm. This constitutes Glisson's capsule, irregular prolongations of which extend into the superficial parenchyma, producing some architectural distortion which must not be misinterpreted when wedge biopsies are examined. Condensation of Glisson's capsule occurs at the porta hepatis, and the fibrous tissue then extends into the liver supporting and accompanying the portal vein, hepatic artery and bile-duct branches and constituting the portal tracts. Some extension of the capsular tissue also accompanies the large hepatic vein branches, but there is no fibrous sheath surrounding the terminal hepatic venules which are in direct contact with perivenular hepatocytes. Within the parenchyma the extracellular matrix is confined to the space of Disse and this so-called reticulin network or framework is usually visualized by silver impregnation staining methods (see Fig. 1.34) and has been discussed earlier.

The extracellular matrix in the liver, in common with that in other organs, serves to provide cohesiveness between cells, induces cell polarization, allows intercellular communication and affects gene expression and cellular differentiation. A brief outline of the extracellular matrix in the normal liver is given in the ensuing paragraphs and is based on detailed reviews which have recently been published.[453,493–495] Hepatic fibrosis and cirrhosis are serious consequences of many types of liver injury and the mechanisms involved in this are discussed in detail in Chapter 2. The components of the extracellular matrix are collagens, glycoproteins and proteoglycans.

Collagens are composed of three identical or similar polypeptide chains folded into a triple helix to give the molecule stability. Numerous types of collagen have been described and of these types I, III, IV, V and VI are found in the liver and most recently collagen XVIII has been reported;[496] types I and III comprise more than 95% of the collagen in normal liver with IV, V and VI contributing approximately 1%, 2 to 5% and 0.1%, respectively.[497]

The matrix glycoproteins are highly cross-linked and insoluble. They are multivalent and have well-defined domains that interact with cell surface receptors and other components of the extracellular matrix. Some are involved in cell adhesion and thus may be present in serum and other body fluids. Laminin is the major glycoprotein in basement membrane and interacts there with type IV collagen; small amounts are normally present in the space of Disse but increased amounts are present in so-called capillarization

of the sinusoids. Fibronectin exists in two isoforms, one of which, plasma fibronectin, is produced by hepatocytes. Fibronectin is also produced by hepatic stellate and sinusoidal endothelial cells. It mediates cell adhesion to collagen. Other glycoproteins present in the liver are vitronectin, which is co-distributed with fibronectin; undulin, which is closely associated with collagen types I and III; nidogen (entactin), which forms a complex with laminin; and elastin, which is found in the walls of blood vessels and in the portal tracts.

The proteoglycans are macromolecules consisting of a central protein core to which glycosaminoglycans and oligosaccharide side-chains are attached. The proteoglycans are classified according to the type of glycosaminoglycan present. They contain specific functional domains which interact with cell surface receptor molecules. In the liver, heparan sulphate is the most abundant and is present in portal tracts, in basement membrane and on the surface of hepatocytes.

The extracellular matrix in the normal liver is considered to be of major importance in regulating and modulating hepatocyte function,[131,498] contributes to the maintenance of hepatocyte polarity[499] and has some regulatory effect on the functional role of non-parenchymal cells. The extracellular matrix is a dynamic structure which also undergoes degradation.[410,500,501] This is a function of various matrix metalloproteinases which include type-specific collagenases which effect degradation in the normal liver.[502]

Lymphatics

The liver is the largest single source of lymph in the body, producing 15–20% of the overall total volume and 25–50% of the thoracic duct flow.[503] Hepatic lymph has an unusually high protein content (about 85–95% of that in plasma) and a high content of cells, of which about 80% are lymphocytes and the remainder macrophages. Indeed it has been calculated that, in the sheep, more lymphocytes migrate through the liver in the lymph than through any other non-lymphoid organ, and that about 2×10^8 macrophages leave the liver in lymph each day.[504]

The terminal twigs of the intrahepatic lymphatic tree are found as a fine, valved plexus of flattened endothelial tubes, associated with terminal branches of the hepatic artery. Traced towards the porta hepatis, the plexus enlarges and remains primarily periarterial, although in the larger portal canals it becomes associated also with portal vein branches and bile-duct tributaries, adding a fourth element to the traditional 'portal triad'. Similar but much smaller and functionally less important lymphatic plexuses are associated with the hepatic vein branches. A third plexus, found in the capsule, forms significant anastomoses with intrahepatic lymphatics. Most of the collecting lymphatics leave the liver at the porta hepatis and drain into hepatic nodes located along the hepatic artery and thence to coeliac nodes. There are other important efferent routes: via the falciform ligament and the superior epigastric vessels to the parasternal nodes; from the bare area to posterior mediastinal nodes; and from the visceral surface to the left gastric nodes.

As efferent collecting lymphatics leave the liver their walls suddenly thicken, through the acquisition of a muscle layer.[505,506] The importance of the anastomoses between intrahepatic and capsular lymphatics is evident when hepatic venous pressure is increased. There follows a great increase in production of hepatic lymph, of protein content identical with that of plasma, indicating unrestricted leakage of protein into Disse space.[507] The capsular efferent lymphatics enlarge in response to the increased lymph flow, and exudation of excess lymph from the capsular plexus forms protein-rich ascitic fluid.[508]

The function of lymphatics is to drain excess fluid and protein from the interstitial spaces of an organ. In the liver the interstitial space of Disse is the most prominent and it is assumed that hepatic lymph is mainly formed there with a small supplement from the peribiliary capillary plexus in the portal tracts. A protein-rich filtrate is produced in the space of Disse because of the free permeability of the sinusoidal endothelium and the consequent absence of a colloid osmotic block.[509,510] A protein-poor filtrate is formed by the less permeable peribiliary capillaries and this may dilute the protein of the sinusoidal filtrate.[503]

The route followed by interstitial fluid formed in Disse's space to its entry into the first-order lymphatic plexus has been controversial.[503,510] It is agreed that lymphatic capillaries are absent within the parenchyma and that there are no direct channels, with a continuous lining, between Disse's space and the primary lymphatics. Wisse and his colleagues[511,512] have suggested that 'endothelial massaging' by blood cells may be of importance in causing fluid movement in the space of Disse (Fig. 1.31). Henriksen et al.[509] suggested that, as in other tissues, the terminal lymphatics in the portal tracts had anchoring filaments between opposing endothelial cells which regulated the direction of flow from the interstitial space into the lymphatics.

An electron microscopic study of rat liver[512] has established the following pathway, by the use of natural markers (precipitated lymph protein and chylomicrons) and artificial tracers injected intravenously (ferritin, pontamine blue and monastral blue). Fluid formed in Disse space escaped at the periphery of the portal tract through gaps between hepatocytes of the limiting plate. These gaps contained hepatocyte microvilli, delicate 'wicks' of collagenous fibres and occasional slender processes of portal tract fibroblasts, extending into the parenchyma from the periportal space

of Mall. Here long flattened processes of fibroblasts formed discontinuous linings of 'spaces' which contained tracer material, occasional lymphocytes and macrophages, and collagen bundles. These 'spaces' were not true lymphatics, since they lacked an endothelial lining, but they appeared to function as prelymphatic channels, leading fluid towards the terminal twigs of the lymphatic tree.

Nerve supply and innervation

Nerve fibres reach the liver in two separate but intercommunicating plexuses around the hepatic artery and portal vein, and are distributed with their branches. They include preganglionic parasympathetic fibres derived from the anterior and posterior vagi, and sympathetic fibres which are mostly postganglionic with cell bodies in the coeliac ganglia, and which receive their preganglionic sympathetic connections from spinal segments T7–T10. The hilar plexuses also include visceral afferent fibres and some phrenic nerve fibres, probably also afferent in character.[512] Current knowledge of the intrahepatic distribution of neural elements and of the various effector humoral mechanisms, including the role of various cytokines, eicosanoids and nitric oxide (NO), has been reviewed.[364,513–518]

It is of historical interest that von Kupffer, in his original study, proposed to examine the nerves within the liver but was unable to demonstrate any. Immunohistochemical studies of human liver, however, using antibodies to common neural proteins such as protein gene product (PGP) 9.5 and N-CAM, have shown that nerve fibres not only are present around vascular structures in portal tracts but extend into the parenchyma (Fig. 1.32), running along the sinusoids. Fluorescence histochemistry[519] and immunohistochemistry using antibodies to dopamine–β-hydroxylase and tyrosine hydroxylase[520] have shown that the majority of intrasinusoidal fibres are sympathetic; many contain neuropeptide tyrosine (NPY), a regulatory peptide commonly found in adrenergic nerves.[520] Unmyelinated nerve fibres can be seen in the space of Disse using TEM.[521] They are frequently surrounded by Schwann-cell processes but a few bare nerve endings or varicosities are found in close apposition to hepatocytes or hepatic stellate cells. Synaptic clefts have been identified at points of contact suggesting that there is direct innervation of these cells, although true synapses are not found.[521]

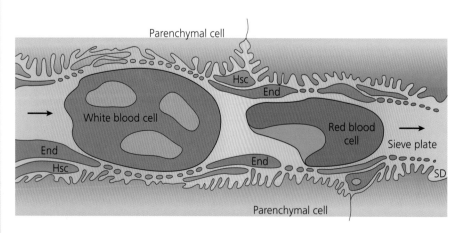

Fig. 1.31 • Diagrammatic reconstruction of a sinusoid. It is proposed that blood cells deform the sinusoidal wall, effectively 'massaging' fluid through the space of Disse (SD). End = endothelial cell; Hsc = hepatic stellate cell. Modified from Wisse & De Leeuw.[388]

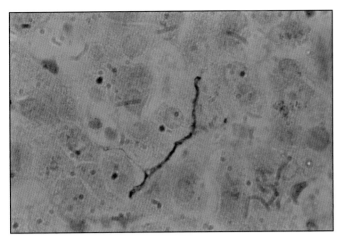

Fig. 1.32 • Neuropeptide tyrosine (NPY) containing nerve fibres in human liver. PAP, nickel DAB counterstain. Supplied by Professor A D Burt.

Release of neurotransmitters from the intrasinusoidal sympathetic fibres may modulate hepatocyte, sinusoidal endothelial cell and hepatic stellate cell function. There is evidence that adrenergic nerves play a role in the control of hepatocyte carbohydrate and lipid metabolism, and in intrahepatic haemodynamics. Stimulation of hepatic sympathetic nerves in vivo produces hyperglycaemia. This effect is caused by enhanced glycogenolysis in hepatocytes and appears to be under α-adrenergic control.[522] The regulation of hepatic carbohydrate metabolism by sympathetic nerve fibres may be mediated by gap junctional communication.[227] Hepatic vascular resistance is increased by hepatic nerve stimulation, but it does not appear to be under sympathetic tone; this response is mediated through adrenergic receptors.[523,524] Bioulac-Sage and co-workers have speculated that adrenergic nerves may induce contraction in hepatic stellate cells, thereby regulating intrasinusoidal blood flow.[521]

An extensive cholinergic (parasympathetic) network is found in rat liver.[525] In human liver, Amenta et al.[526] described parasympathetic cholinergic innervation of portal tract vessels with only limited innervation of the parenchyma. Immunohistochemical studies have also identified intrahepatic fibres containing two neuropeptides—substance P and calcitonin gene-related peptide (CGRP)—which are commonly found in afferent nerves.[527,528] Such afferent fibres may be involved in chemo- and osmoreception as well as in vasomotor regulation.[512] It would seem likely that the liver should have sensory receptors since it is exposed to the nutrient and solute load delivered via the portal circulation from the gut.[524,529-531]

The ability of orthotopic allografts to function satisfactorily suggests that neural mechanisms have only a minor regulatory role, at least under basal conditions; only limited re-innervation occurs in the transplanted human liver.[532,533] However, there is some evidence in experimental animals,[534,535] and possibly in humans,[535] that the liver's normal response to hypovolaemic shock is impaired by denervation and this may result in hepatic ischaemic injury. Loss of intrasinusoidal fibres in the cirrhotic liver may contribute to impaired metabolic function.[536] Whether this loss accounts for some of the abnormalities of portal blood flow is not clear.[536-538]

The liver-specific juxtaposition of diverse cell populations and matrix components in harmony with the angio-architecture results in a delicate bio-ecological system.[539] Investigations in the last decade have provided remarkable new insights into the interactions and feedback loops between the different cell types and the matrix components of the liver, building up a new science of bio-ecology and sociology of liver cells. Striking examples are the multiple metabolic interactions and numerous cytokine networks, and the diversity and complexity of parenchymal and non-parenchymal cell interaction.

Well-coordinated interactions between hepatocytes include: the reciprocal metabolic pathways localized in different lobular territories for carbohydrate[540] and ammonia[541] metabolism; the cell-to-cell communications via gap junctions and the teamwork in the co-ordination of calcium waves;[542,543] and the intercellular signals through surface molecules.[544]

Hepatocyte–Kupffer cell interactions are so manifold that an entire volume was devoted to this subject.[545] Hepatocyte proliferation is controlled by cytokines produced by non-parenchymal cells (Kupffer cells and/or sinusoidal endothelial cells and/or hepatic stellate cells).[546] Kupffer-cell-derived cytokines influence hepatocyte behaviour: interleukin-6 (co-produced by sinusoidal endothelial cells and Kupffer cells) is a typical example for inducing the acute phase reaction.[215,547] Hepatocyte–endothelial interactions involve hepatocellular modulation of the sinusoidal endothelial phenotype[548] and production by endothelial cells of prostaglandins, endothelin and cytokines such as interleukin-1, interleukin-6 and hepatocyte growth factor.[402]

Interplay between hepatocytes and hepatic stellate cells comprises peptides which stimulate hepatic stellate cell proliferation in vitro (hepitoin),[549] and cytokines released from hepatic stellate cell proliferation inhibiting hepatocellular proliferation (TGF-β) as well as cytokines stimulating parenchymal proliferation (e.g. hepatocyte growth factor).[428,550] There may be reciprocal dialogue between hepatocytes and hepatic stellate cells. Insulin-like growth factor-1 (IGF-1) and IGF-1-independent factors from hepatocytes can stimulate hepatocyte growth factor production by hepatic stellate cells, and thus hepatocyte-derived factors may indirectly affect hepatocytes via a paracrine loop.[551] Co-operative interactions between hepatocytes and hepatic stellate cells produce a microenvironment that stimulates the growth and differentiation of small, bipotent, clonogenic hepatocytes,[552] and hepatocytes co-operate with hepatic stellate cells in the deposition of an extracellular matrix in vitro.[553]

Hepatocyte–matrix interactions rely on: (i) adhesion molecules and receptors that mediate cell-matrix binding (the integrin and the non-integrin matrix receptors); (ii) the propensity of the matrix to act as a reservoir and presenter of cell growth factors and cytokines; and (iii) matrix turnover and modification of the matrix (be it by hepatocytes or other cells).[554] Integrins activate intracellular signalling pathways in response to the extracellular matrix. An extracellular matrix protein can be recognized by several integrins, and each integrin can recognize different extracellular matrix proteins. However, particular integrins may play a predominant role in hepatocellular differentiation: in this respect, $\alpha_3 \beta_1$-integrin (with high affinity for laminin) appears to be a critical mediator,[555] and Kupffer cells adhere to endothelial cells through the expression by the latter of the surface receptors CD4 and ICAM-1[396] and initiate activation of hepatic stellate cells by secretion of a hepatic stellate cell stimulating factor.[556]

Sinusoidal endothelial cells secrete a factor that inhibits the growth of hepatic stellate cells.[557] The phenotype of sinusoidal endothelial cells is influenced by hepatocytes as mentioned before[548] but also by components of the extracellular matrix: laminin, for instance, induces the formation of tubes in cultured rat endothelial cells.[547]

Hepatic stellate cells play a primordial role in liver fibrogenesis, and in this cascade-like progressive process are modulated by damaged hepatocytes, Kupffer cells, sinusoidal endothelial cells, platelets and inflammatory cells.[426] A newly described function for hepatic stellate cells is their role in liver morphogenesis through a morphogenic protein termed epimorphin.[558]

The matrix in the space of Disse modulates the phenotype and function of sinusoidal endothelial cells, hepatic stellate cells and hepatocytes.[559] The composition of the matrix at specific points is crucial for finer modulation of intercellular signalling.[560] Nerve fibres contact virtually every parenchymal cell and influence its metabolic activity.[540] Metabolites, hormones and cytokines from the sinusoidal blood influence parenchymal and sinusoidal endothelial cell activity, according to gradients and density of cellular receptors.[207]

Bile-duct epithelial cells may influence differentiated hepatocellular function through direct contact,[561] through the peribiliary portal system[562] and through cholehepatic cycling.[383]

Pathological conditions such as fibrosis and cirrhosis reflect disturbances in the harmonious equilibrium of the innumerable cellular interactions and cytokine networks,[539,563,564] whereas uncontrolled cell growth in neoplasia reflects a breakdown of liver cell sociology.

Each cell type in the liver interacts with all the others and with the extracellular matrix. Therefore, the functional activity of each cell is constantly being modified by the metabolic activities of the others. At the end, liver function is the result of a great number of complex interactions. If any cell fails to perform its role, the functional capacity of the others will be affected. For these reasons, the liver is to be considered as a bio-ecological system, in which the components communicate with each other to maintain homeostasis.[565] However, the liver is only a small bio-ecological system within the universe of an organism composed of several discrete bio-ecological systems. This proposal implies that, for harmonious function of the organism, all bio-ecological systems are interconnected through neurological stimulation and blood-borne products ('milieu interne'). Alterations in any ecological system influence the behaviour of the other ecosystems of the organism. Furthermore, all the interdependent ecosystems are also directly or indirectly connected to the exterior ('milieu externe').[565]

Various compartments can be distinguished in the extracellular space in vertebrates. These compartments are separated by barriers. Special tissues, cells or organs have the function of maintaining homeostasis in extracellular compartments. Examples of such systems, consisting of a specialized paracompartmental tissue and an associated extracellular compartment, are for instance the liver with the bloodstream (extracellular space of the main part of the body), and the choroid plexus with the ventricle system (extracellular space in the brain). The liver is thus the central homeostatic organ for the main extracellular compartment of adult vertebrates. It is involved in maintaining an appropriate environment for the cells of the body, and does so in a number of ways: keeping the concentration of metabolic substrates, intermediates and products in the extracellular fluid within an appropriate range; synthesis and secretion of binding proteins for poorly hydrosoluble compounds; synthesis and secretion of proteins of the blood coagulation system (for rapid sealing of lesions); and synthesis and secretion of proteinase inhibitors (useful in restricting proteolytic breakdown of tissues by proteinases).[566]

The repertoire of functions of liver cells which collectively are termed 'liver function' is of an extraordinary complexity. Nevertheless, additional surprises are still being discovered. Very recently, the homeostatic control of angiogenesis was suggested to be a newly identified function of the liver.[567] Of additional interest is the 'tinkerer' aspect of the story, in that degradation fragments of well-known liver-derived proteins perform the job. Plasminogen, which modulates the breakdown of extracellular matrix through its activation to plasmin, is the precursor of angiostatin, that inhibits angiogenesis. On the other hand, collagen XVIII, which is a basement membrane protein, is the precursor of endostatin. Both endostatin and angiostatin are polypeptides that inhibit endothelial cell proliferation, angiogenesis, and tumour growth in experimental models of cancer. It thus appears that hepatocytes, which are the main source of the proteins plasminogen and collagen XVIII,[496] may influence extrahepatic endothelial growth by the creation of biological response modifiers endowed with functions that appear to be completely different from those of the parent molecule, and with important consequences for tissue repair and cancer.[567]

The liver in biopsy and autopsy specimens

Now that the constituent tissues of the liver have been described in turn (and their interactions discussed in the preceding section), the overall histological patterns and their physiological variations as seen in liver biopsy and autopsy material will be briefly summarized. Details of liver biopsy examination and interpretation are given in Chapter 3.

In the examination of liver tissue attention should be paid to the overall architecture, the portal tracts and their constituent parts, the lobular parenchyma inclusive of hepatocytes, sinusoids and sinusoidal cells, and the hepatic veins. Liver architecture is not homogeneous and the microarchitectural variability at the liver periphery is greater than at deeper sites within the liver.[3] Percutaneous needle biopsy may preferentially sample peripheral tissue. In a recent quantitative reference study of normal human liver,[568] it was found that portal dyads (with only two of three profiles—artery, vein and bile duct) are almost as common as portal triads in normal peripheral liver tissue. However, because of the multiplicity of profiles (more than one arterial branch, venous branch, bile duct) within portal tracts, the average number of profiles per portal tract was 6 ± 5 (range 2–35). One may assume that on average there are two interlobular bile ducts, two hepatic arteries and one portal vein per portal tract, with six full portal triads per linear centimetre of tissue obtained by external Menghini biopsy technique and using a 24 g needle, equivalent to 0.8 ± 0.5 portal triads per mm.[2,568]

The normal portal tract/hepatic vein relationships are as shown in Figure 1.33. Surrounding the hepatic veins the individual hepatocytes tend to have a more regular arrangement resembling cords, and correspondingly the sinusoidal network radiates out for a short distance into the perivenular area with a more regular radial pattern of the reticulin framework. Outside the perivenular zone the liver cell plates are arranged less regularly, and correspondingly the sinu-soidal network and reticulin framework do not demonstrate a distinct radial arrangement. Within the reticulin framework the liver cell plates are two cells thick up to the age of about 5 years (Fig. 1.34(A), (B)); thereafter the normal pattern is for these to be one cell thick (Fig. 1.34(C)). In the adult, the presence of twin-cell liver plates and the formation of rosettes indicates regeneration (Fig. 1.34(D)).

The individual hepatocyte is polygonal in shape and in haematoxylin and eosin preparations the cell margins are clearly outlined. In liver-cell plates cut in a longitudinal plane it is possible to define the sinusoidal margin or pole and also the canalicular pole at the junction between adjacent cells (see Fig. 1.15). The cytoplasm is granular and eosinophilic, but within it basophilic aggregates of RER can be defined in a perinuclear distribution and at the canalicular poles, the intervening cytoplasm tending to be paler in appearance. The nucleus is centrally placed and one or more nucleoli are easily identified. In childhood there is virtually no nuclear pleomorphism. Thereafter, variation in nuclear size develops and, with increasing age, nuclear polyploidy with increased haematoxyphilia is a normal finding, the majority of nuclei being diploid but with a few tetraploid or even larger nuclei being found. This pleomorphism is more marked in the mid-zonal area. The hepatocytes in the portal limiting plates are smaller than other parenchymal cells ($<20 \mu m$ in diameter), show more intense nuclear staining and have a uniform, more basophilic cytoplasm. Binucleate cells may be occasionally found. Mitoses are rarely seen in biopsy material. Nuclear displacement to the sinusoidal pole with hyperchromasia is a cytological indication of regenerative activity (Fig. 1.34(D)).

The liver cell is rich in glycogen, but in routine haematoxylin and eosin preparations its presence is discerned only with difficulty, imparting a fine reticulated and foamy appearance to the cell cytoplasm. Staining by the periodic acid-Schiff (PAS) method readily demonstrates the glycogen (Fig. 1.35(A)) and it is usually uniformly distributed. The amount and distribution, however, shows diurnal and diet-related variations. An irregular distribution pattern may sometimes be found in biopsies and is not of diagnostic significance (Fig. 1.35(B)). Glycogen accumulation in nuclei produces a vacuolated appearance, is common in childhood, may be conspicuous in certain adult conditions (chronic cardiac failure, diabetes and Wilson disease, for example) but is not per se of diagnostic significance.

Lipofuscin forms a further intracytoplasmic inclusion, occurring as fine, light brown, PAS-positive and acid-fast granules at the canalicular pole, predominantly of perivenular hepatocytes. Normally lipofuscin is not abundant until the second decade and thereafter there appears to be a progressive increase in amount both in individual hepatocyte content and also in the extent of hepatocyte involvement. Lipofuscin is a breakdown product of lysosomal material, reflecting cell activity, and is referred to as 'wear and tear' pigment. It is not found in recently regenerated hepatocytes.

It is not unusual in otherwise apparently normal livers to note a very few single hyalinized necrotic liver cells within cell plates, representing apoptosis of hepatocytes;

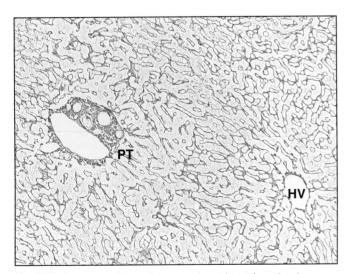

Fig. 1.33 • Low-power view to show normal portal tract/hepatic vein relationships. PT = portal tract; HV = hepatic vein. Gordon & Sweets' reticulin.

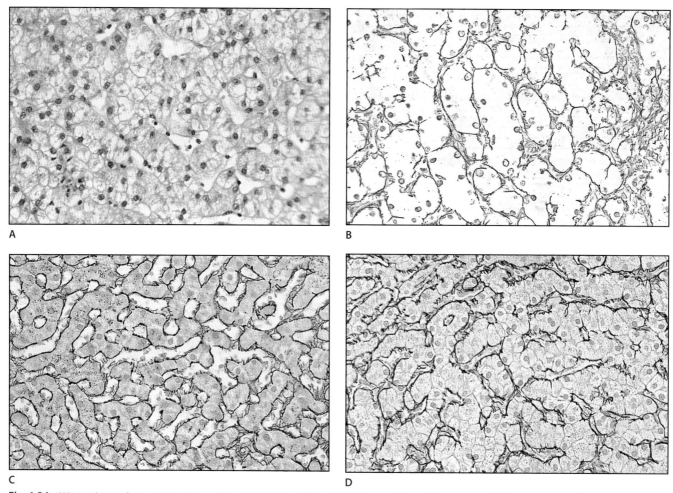

Fig. 1.34 • **(A)** Liver biopsy from a child of 17 months; note the twin-cell liver plates: these are better shown on a reticulin preparation at the same magnification in **(B)**, in which the nuclei are seen in a perisinusoidal position; **(C)** adult liver showing normal single-cell liver plates with centrally placed nuclei; **(D)** adult liver at same magnification as (c) showing a regenerative response with twin-cell liver plates; as in (b) the nuclei tend to be in a perisinusoidal position; there is also rosette formation. Gordon & Sweets' reticulin.

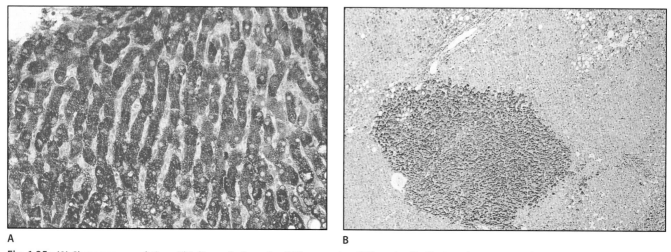

Fig. 1.35 • **(A)** Glycogen accumulation within liver cells shown in a PAS preparation. **(B)** Irregular distribution of PAS-positive glycogen in a wedge biopsy of liver; there are scattered positive cells and also one large positive area.

and also occasional foci where more than one hepatocyte has been lost and is replaced by an aggregate of three or four chronic inflammatory cells. The occasional hepatocyte may also normally contain fat. Stainable iron is absent or demonstrable in only scant amounts.

The sinusoids form an apparently discontinuous system of narrow channels between the liver cell plates, their diameter varying from 4 to 15 μm. Sinusoids in the perivenular area are normally of larger dimension, and with aging and atrophy of liver cell cords there may be apparent dilatation of these sinusoids, a normal variation however. The sinusoids are cylindrical and appear circular in transverse section, running parallel to aligned liver cells. In the normal biopsy specimen the sinusoidal endothelial cells are not conspicuous, and are represented by their flattened elongated nuclei at the sinusoidal margin (Fig. 1.15(A)). Plumper cells containing PAS-positive (diastase resistant), acid-fast granular aggregates of ceroid pigment (similar to lipofuscin) represent Kupffer cells (Fig. 1.36(A)). Their numbers increase with age and, in addition, the presence of aggregates of such cells is a manifestation of liver cell injury (Fig. 1.36(B)). Normal blood cells are present within the sinusoids. Extramedullary haemopoiesis is normal only within the first few weeks of life. Sequestration of lymphocytic or mononuclear cells within sinusoids is abnormal, and may be an early manifestation of some myeloproliferative disorders (Chapter 17).

The perisinusoidal space of Disse is not seen in biopsy material, but in autopsy livers the space becomes dilated, reticulin fibres can be seen traversing it and the sinusoidal lining cells and Kupffer cells now appear to be free and separate from the adjacent hepatocytes (Fig. 1.37). The hepatic stellate cell (Fig. 1.29) cannot be distinguished with certainty on routine stains but can be identified by staining for fat, by demonstration of vitamin A fluorescence, in resin sections and on electron microscopy. In addition immunostaining for synaptophysin marks resting and activated human stellate cells[449] and alpha smooth muscle actin marks activated stellate cells.

The large intrahepatic bile ducts (internal diameter greater than 100 µm)—septal or trabecular ducts—are lined by tall columnar epithelial cells with basally situated nuclei and clear, faintly eosinophilic cytoplasm, which contains granular PAS positive material at their luminal pole (Fig. 1.38). The fibrous tissue of the portal tracts is arranged in a rather irregular circumferential manner round these ducts. Lymphocytes may occasionally be present within the lining epithelium. The small intrahepatic bile ducts—interlobular—are lined by low columnar or cuboidal epithelium, whose cells contain basally situated nuclei in the larger branches; PAS-positive material is also present at the luminal pole. The ducts connect with the bile canaliculi via ductules and canals of Hering. Ductules have a low columnar epithelium; the canals of Hering are in part lined

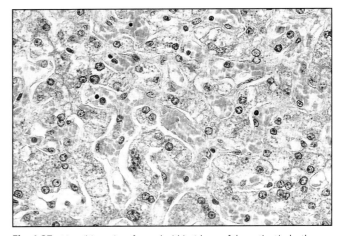

Fig. 1.37 • Liver 'biopsy' performed within 1 hour of the patient's death: note how the sinusoidal endothelium has become separated from the liver-cell plates; the endothelial cells, Kupffer cells and the reticulin framework enclose the intraluminal blood cells and there is 'expansion' of the space of Disse. Masson's trichrome.

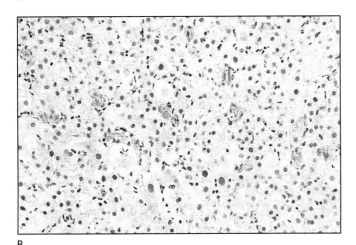

Fig. 1.36 • (A) Kupffer cells in a PAS/diastase preparation: granular aggregates of ceroid pigment are present in a number of cells lying within or at the periphery of sinusoids. (B) Focal aggregates of PAS-positive ceroid-containing Kupffer cells in a liver biopsy from a patient with acute hepatitis.

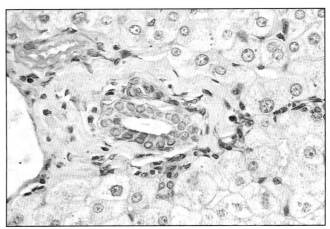

Fig. 1.38 • Septal bile duct lined by cuboidal cells which contain discrete supranuclear PAS-positive granules.

by bile-duct cells and in part by hepatocytes. Biliary cells in canals of Hering, ducts and ductules are readily revealed by immunostaining for bile-duct type cytokeratins 7 and 19.[569]

The microanatomy of the portal vein and hepatic artery has already been described. Progressive hyalinization of the terminal hepatic artery branches is an aging phenomenon occurring even in the absence of systemic hypertension. The type I collagen fibres of portal tracts become denser with age, and in disease processes accompanied by swelling and fibrosis around portal tracts the outlines of the normal tracts can be distinguished because of the increased density of the collagen, its doubly refractile properties and its brownish staining reaction in untoned reticulin preparations contrasting with a yellower staining of young, newly laid-down collagen.

The portal tracts (Fig. 1.39) normally contain a few lymphocytes and macrophages but polymorphs and plasma cells are abnormal findings. Increasing numbers of lymphocytes and macrophages may appear in older persons, the density of their distribution varying between portal tracts. The relationship of such chronic inflammatory cell infiltration of portal tracts to natural wear and tear or undefined hepatotoxins is uncertain. Focal aggregation only within some portal tracts should be regarded as probably not significant, whereas generalized portal tract involvement is abnormal. The differential diagnosis of such infiltrates and non-specific reactive hepatitis is further discussed in Chapter 17.

Normal hepatic function

Introduction

The metabolic activity in the liver is a complex phenomenon, and includes nearly 100 reactions in various fields, taking place virtually at the same time but in separate cellular or subcellular compartments. The different metabolic fields include the synthesis, storage and degradation of proteins, triglycerides, cholesterol, carbohydrates and specific compounds such as haem. In addition, the liver plays a

central role in dealing with endogenous and exogenous toxic compounds. This impressive metabolic activity is regulated by the laws of supply and demand and is controlled by the systemic homeostasis organizers: the endocrine system and the autonomic nervous system. The normal metabolic activity of the liver also depends on a normal blood supply and bile flow, which will be discussed first.

Hepatic circulation

The high level of metabolic activity in the liver is reflected in the magnitude of the blood supply. Total hepatic blood flow in normal adults under resting conditions is between 1500 and 1900 ml/min or approximately 25% of cardiac output.[570] Of this, roughly two-thirds is supplied by the portal vein and the remainder by the hepatic artery. Hepatic blood flow increases after feeding and decreases during exercise and sleep.[571] Arterial and portal venous blood becomes mixed in the sinusoids. The liver normally extracts less than 40% of the oxygen supplied (20 vol.% via the hepatic artery and 15 vol.% via the portal vein) and the extraction rates may be enhanced in situations of increased demand.[572] The principal site of blood flow regulation is thought to reside in the sinusoids itself, where the major blood pressure drop occurs in the liver. The pressure in the hepatic artery is equivalent to the systemic blood pressure while the pressure in the portal system is between 6 and 10 mmHg. In the sinusoids the pressure is estimated to be approximately 3 mmHg higher than the inferior vena cava pressure. It is not clear whether this pressure is influenced mainly by the sinusoidal endothelial cells or the stellate cells or both, or whether there is a level of regulation upstream of the sinusoid or not.[155]

Intrinsic regulation of hepatic blood flow is mediated only through the hepatic artery. The liver is not able to directly regulate portal vein blood flow. The hepatic arterial buffer response is the primary intrinsic regulator of the hepatic artery, which is the inverse response of the hepatic artery to changes in portal vein flow. The mechanism of the hepatic arterial buffer response may be based on adenosine washout.[573,574] Adenosine is produced at a constant rate, independent of oxygen supply or demand, and secreted into a small fluid compartment that surrounds the hepatic arterial resistance vessels. If portal vein flow decreases, less adenosine is washed away into the portal blood and the accumulated adenosine leads to hepatic arterial dilation. These intrinsic regulatory mechanisms maintain total hepatic blood flow at a constant level, thus stabilizing hepatic clearance of hormones, cardiac output and venous return.

Bile flow

The bile secreted at the canalicular membrane (primary, canalicular or hepatocellular bile) is composed of bile salts, phospholipids (lecithin), protein, cholesterol and bilirubin. The canalicular bile flow comprises a bile salt-dependent (250 ml/day) and bile salt-independent fraction (200 ml/day) and is elaborated by a process of osmotic filtration. The

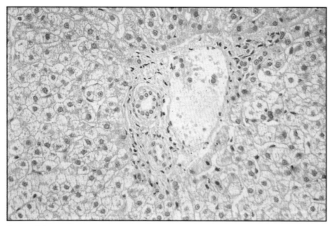

Fig. 1.39 • Normal portal tract containing a portal vein branch, a bile duct and a hepatic arteriole.

formation of bile salt-dependent bile is mainly a function of the periportal zone I, while the bile salt-independent fraction is formed in zone III of the acinus.[575] Different carriers for organic and inorganic anions on the sinusoidal and canalicular membranes are able to transport them against a concentration gradient. Water follows the secretion of anions and cations passively, para- or transcellularly, to keep the bile isotonic. Phospholipids (especially lecithin) are an important constituent of bile and they are translocated across the canalicular membrane. The phospholipids form micellae with bile acids, and hence protect bile-duct epithelial cell membranes from the detergent action of bile acids.

The canaliculus behaves as an active pump with contractile microfilaments (inhibited by phalloidin and cytochalasin B) and microtubules (inhibited by colchicin and vinblastin). The canalicular bile is modified by reabsorption and secretion of organic and inorganic ions in the biliary ductules and ducts. Finally, bile is concentrated up to 20-fold by the gallbladder mucosa before being released in the duodenum, depending upon digestive demands.

Biotransformation and detoxification

Although many bodily tissues have some ability to metabolize drugs, the liver is the main organ involved in drug metabolism, and thus in protecting the body from potentially harmful environmental chemicals. Most orally administered drugs are lipophilic and would therefore remain in the body (especially fat tissue) for a long period of time, if the body did not have the ability to convert drugs into water-soluble metabolites. Biotransformation takes place mainly in the smooth endoplasmic reticulum and in the mitochondria. The process is limited by the hepatic blood flow and by the capacity of the microsomal enzyme systems. Drug metabolism is divided into two categories:[576] phase I (oxidation reactions) and phase II (conjugation with hydrophilic ligands). Phase I drug metabolism is mainly carried out by a distinct repertoire of cytochrome P450 enzymes[577] that insert an oxygen atom into the drug molecule (hydroxylation). In some instances, phase I oxidative metabolism may generate metabolites that are more reactive (and potentially harmful) than the parent compound.[578] These metabolites are rendered unreactive in phase II reactions through the conjugation to polar ligands such as glucuronic acid, sulphate, acetate, amino acids or glutathione. The conjugated metabolite can be eliminated either by the kidneys or via the bile. Moreover, enterohepatic cycling is less likely to occur with the water-soluble metabolite than with the parent lipophilic compound.

Many chemical substances can either enhance (induction) or reduce (inhibition) the activity of drug-metabolizing enzymes. Enzyme induction can be appreciated microscopically by the prominent smooth endoplasmic reticulum and may be accompanied by a rise in serum gamma-glutamyltransferase (GGT).[579,580] The clinical implications of enzyme induction and inhibition will depend on the relative activities of the parent drug and its metabolites and on the presence of other drugs or toxines that need to be metabolized by the induced or inhibited enzymes in parallel.[581]

The phase I oxidative processes described above and the generation of energy in mitochondria through oxidative phosphorylation are vital to the survival of the individual, but also generate side-products: the reactive oxygen species. The liver, more than any other organ, is at risk for damage inflicted by oxidative stress, which is defined as an imbalance between the formation of oxidants and antioxidant defense systems.[582] Because of the variety of oxidants formed and their different subcellular localization and reactivity, a complex network of small antioxidant molecules (glutathion, vitamin C and E) and enzymes (e.g. superoxide dismutase and catalase) is operative in every liver cell.[583,584] Another defence strategy is to keep redox-active metal ions such as copper and iron tightly bound to transport or storage proteins.

Synthesis and degradation of haem: porphyrin and bilirubin metabolism

Haem (ferriprotoporphyrin IX) is the major functional form of iron in eukaryotic cells and an important constituent of haemoglobin, myoglobin, catalase and cytochromes.[585] Biosynthesis of the tetrapyrrole ring of haem (protoporphyrin IX) starts in the mitochondrial matrix by condensing succinyl-CoA (donated from the tricarboxylic acid cycle) with glycine to form aminolevulinic acid (ALA). ALA is exported to the cytoplasm where aminolevulinic acid dehydratase condenses 2 ALAs to porphobilinogen. Four molecules of porphobilinogen are then converted to protoporphyrin IX through decarboxylation and oxidation steps, which begin in the cytosol and return to the mitochondria. Ferrochelatase (FC), located in the inner membrane of the mitochondria, catalyses the last step in haem biosynthesis by inserting iron into protoporphyrin-IX.

Bilirubin is a linear tetrapyrrole that is formed during the process of haem degradation. Haem is metabolized by haem oxygenase to form carbon monoxide, biliverdin, and free iron. Biliverdin is subsequently transformed to bilirubin by biliverdin reductase. About 250–300 mg of bilirubin is produced daily in the spleen by degradation of haemoglobin from red blood cells.[586,587] The bilirubin molecule has two propionic residues and because of the presence of six intramolecular hydrogen bonds its water solubility is very low. Thus, most of bilirubin is transported in blood, forming a complex with albumin; bilirubin is then taken up into hepatocytes for glucuronidation. It is conceivable that there are at least three different pathways utilized for bilirubin uptake in the hepatocytes, through organic anion transporter 2 (or perhaps 8), albumin receptor and a receptor other than albumin.[588]

The major conjugates are bilirubin glucuronides formed by uridine diphosphate (UDP)-glucuronosyltransferase 1 (UGT1). UDP-glucuronosyltransferases (UGTs) catalyse the conjugation of various xenobiotic or metabolic compounds with UDP-glucuronic acid and are classified into two families, UGT1 and UGT2, according to their amino acid sequence.[589] UGT1s mainly catalyse bilirubin and phenol-like compounds, whilst UGT2s catalyse steroids, amines and bile acids. The human genes for the isoenzymes, UGT1A1, A3, A4, A6, A7, A8, A9 and A10, belong to the UGT1 family, and are composed of five exons. The first exon has 10 different tandem arrays whereas the second to fifth exons are conserved. Each first exon has a unique promoter to produce the primary transcripts, and the 10 different mature mRNAs are produced by differential splicing.[590] Bilirubin is conjugated in the form of either mono- or di-glucuronide by UGT1A1 and once conjugated is excreted in the bile through the multidrug-resistance-associated protein 2 (MRP2). In the *UGT1A1* promoter, the number of TA repeats (5, 6, 7, or 8) in the TATA box is inversely correlated with gene transcriptional efficiency. The classical picture of Gilbert syndrome (a harmless bilirubin conjugation deficiency) is usually associated with TA_7 homozygosity (TA_7 allele classified as *UGT1A1*28*).[591]

Within the biliary system, conjugated bilirubin is incorporated into mixed micelles. It is not reabsorbed in/from the small intestine, but hydrolysed by bacterial beta-glucuronidase in the colon, which leads to the formation of urobilinogens. Small amounts of conjugated bilirubin and urobilinogen may then be reabsorbed and re-excreted by the kidneys and the liver.

Metabolism of carbohydrates

Plasma glucose levels are maintained within narrow limits to ensure adequate delivery of glucose to the brain.[592] The main tissues that regulate blood glucose levels are the liver (glucose production and uptake), skeletal muscle (glucose uptake) and kidney (glucose production). The liver can produce glucose from glycogen (glycogenolysis), while both liver and kidney can synthesize glucose via gluconeogenesis. The main gluconeogenic substrates are lactate, pyruvate, glycerol (released from triglyceride) and amino acids (especially alanine). Carbohydrate metabolism is regulated by several hormones and also by the sympathetic and parasympathetic nervous system. The effects of the main hormones affecting the carbohydrate metabolism are summarized in Table 1.3.

After a meal glucose (and fructose) are removed by hepatocytes from the portal venous blood. This has two beneficial effects: it provides a readily accessible energy store and it prevents wide fluctuations in plasma osmolality. The efficiency of first pass uptake of glucose by the liver is disputed; values obtained using different methods range between 25 and 60%.[593] Hepatic uptake is determined by the levels of glucose in sinusoidal blood and by the action of insulin. Hepatic glucose uptake is lower when glucose is infused systemically rather than into the portal vein. In addition, the ratio of insulin to glucagon may be more important and glucocorticoids may play a role. Within the hepatocyte, glucose is converted to glucose 6-phosphate. Priority is given to replenish glycogen stores; thereafter, some glucose is channelled into triglyceride production (discussed below, lipid and lipoprotein metabolism).

During fasting, the liver becomes an essential source of energy for other tissues. Glucose is generated by two routes in the hepatocyte: glycogenolysis and gluconeogenesis. During overnight fasting the former is the more important but its contribution falls rapidly after 24 hours.

Gluconeogenesis in the liver utilizes lactate, pyruvate, amino acids and glycerol. Quantitatively, lactate is the most important precursor. Glycogenolysis and gluconeogenesis are controlled by factors similar to those regulating glucose uptake and glycogen synthesis. Thus autoregulation by the glucose level and insulin, glucagon and other hormones all exert effects through complex interactions. Sympathetic nerves may also play a role.[594] There is evidence for reciprocal heterogeneity within the liver parenchyma in the activity of enzymes involved in glycogen synthesis and gluconeogenesis.[595,596]

The liver is also the predominant site for the metabolism of fructose principally to lactate and glycogen—and of galactose to either glucose or glycogen depending on the nutrient supply.

Lipid and lipoprotein metabolism

Lipids (triglycerides, saturated and unsaturated fatty acids, cholesterol esters) are insoluble in water and depend upon lipoproteins (chylomicrons, very low-density lipoprotein or VLDL, intermediate-density lipoprotein or IDL, low-density lipoprotein or LDL, and high-density lipoprotein or HDL) to allow their transport in the plasma. Lipoproteins consist

Table 1.3	Carbohydrate metabolism: effects of the main hormones (Kruszynska 2005)			
	Liver gluconeogenesis	Glycogenolysis	Hepatic glucose output	Peripheral glucose uptake
Insulin	↓	↓↓	↓↓	↑↑
Glucagon	↑↑°	↑↑	↑↑	—
Growth hormone	↑*	—	↑	↓
Catecholamines	↑*°	↑↑	↑↑	↓
Cortisol	↑*°	—	↑	↓

* Indirect effect due to enhanced lipolysis (increased supply of glycerol and fatty acids)
° Also indirect effect by increased supply of gluconeogenic amino acids

of an outer coat of molecules (apolipoproteins, free cholesterol and phospholipids) and an inner core of hydrophobic molecules (triglycerides, fat-soluble vitamins and cholesterol-esters).[597,598]

Chylomicrons contain the dietary fat that is absorbed in the small intestine. During their passage in the circulation they lose their triglycerides through the actions of lipoprotein lipases. The chylomicron remnant (rich in dietary cholesterol) is taken up by the liver and further metabolized or incorporated in cell membranes. The hepatic cholesterol and triglycerides leave the hepatocytes as VLDL. With a fate similar to that of chylomicrons, the VLDL particles lose their triglycerides and take the shape of cholesterol carrier LDL. LDL receptors on the hepatocytes or peripheral tissues can take up LDL particles. HDL is responsible for the transport of cholesterol from peripheral tissues to the liver (reverse cholesterol transport).[597,575]

Fatty acids

A central metabolic function of the liver is to maintain plasma glucose levels regardless of the nutritional state. In the setting of energy excess, glucose is converted to fatty acids via the conversion of glucose to pyruvate, which enters the Krebs cycle in the mitochondria. Citrate formed in the Krebs cycle is shuttled to the cytosol where it is converted to acetyl-CoA by ATP citrate lyase. Acetyl-CoA carboxylase 1 (ACC1) then converts acetyl-CoA to malonyl-CoA, which is used by fatty acid synthase to form palmitic acid (C16 : 0). Palmitic acid is then either desaturated by stearoyl-CoA desaturase (SCD) to palmitoleic acid, or further elongated by the long-chain fatty acyl elongase to form stearic acid (C18 : 0), which also can be desaturated to form oleic acid (C18 : 1).[598,599] These fatty acids are used to synthesize triglycerides.

Liver cells can also take up exogenous non-esterified fatty acids from the blood. These are principally derived from adipose tissue following triglyceride hydrolysis by a hormone-sensitive lipase. Smaller amounts also come from absorption of dietary non-esterified fatty acids and from circulating triglyceride-rich lipoproteins hydrolysed by the action of lipoprotein lipase. For fatty acids to be metabolized by the hepatocyte, they must first be 'activated' to acyl-CoA esters[600]. These can then be utilized in the formation of triglyceride, phospholipid or cholesterol esters, or alternatively can be oxidized in mitochondria. The latter process is dependent on a specific transporter system involving carnitine palmitoyl transferase I (CPT I) which enables fatty acyl-CoA to gain access to the mitochondrial matrix. This enzyme is inhibited by malonyl CoA, so that in the 'fed' state fatty acid synthesis predominates over oxidation. A small amount of fatty acid oxidation also occurs in peroxisomes.[601]

Triglycerides and phospholipids

Triglycerides represent the primary source of energy storage and transport. They consist of a glycerol molecule, the hydroxy groups of which have been esterified with fatty acids. Triglycerides are formed by esterification of fatty acyl-CoAs with glycerol-3-phosphate. Acyl transferase catalyses the addition of two fatty acyl-CoAs to the 2 free carbons in glycerol-3-phosphate to generate phophatidic acid (PA), which is converted into triglycerides through the action of PA phosphohydrolase and diacylglycerol acyl transferase. The dephosphorylation of PA appears to be the rate-limiting step in triglyceride synthesis with the activity of PA phosphohydrolase tightly regulated by both substrate supply and metabolic hormones.[602] The triglyceride formed by this pathway is either packaged into lipoproteins for export or metabolized within the hepatocyte. This occurs through the action of hepatic lipases located in lysosomes and, to a lesser extent, in the endoplasmic reticulum. Fatty liver or steatosis occurs in circumstances where the synthesis of triglyceride is greater than the capacity of the liver for export or lipolysis.[603]

Phospholipids are more complex compounds than triglycerides and represent pivotal constituents of cell membranes. They also take part in several biochemical reactions. Phospholipid synthesis first requires the activation of specific constituent bases (e.g. inositol, choline and ethanolamine) before their reaction with PA and diacylglycerol to form the various phospholipid classes.

Cholesterol

Cholesterol is a component of all cell membranes, where it exists as free sterol and is a precursor of steroid hormones and bile acids. Cholesterol can be synthesized by most cell types but in the liver synthesis occurs predominantly within hepatocytes. The amount synthesized daily in the liver of normal individuals is approximately twice that obtained from dietary sources (reaching the liver in chylomicron remnants). More than 1 g of cholesterol is lost in the faeces daily in the form of free sterol or as bile acids. In plasma and in some organs such as the liver, cholesterol esters are also found in which a long-chain fatty acid is attached to the 3β-hydroxyl group.

Cholesterol synthesis involves a complex pathway. Mevalonate is initially formed from acetyl coenzyme A (CoA) via 3-hydroxy-3-methylglutaryl-CoA (HMG-CoA) and subsequently phosphorylated and decarboxylated to form isopentenyl pyrophosphate.[604] Condensation of several molecules of this leads to generation of squalene. The subsequent conversion to cholesterol is a multistep process with lanosterol as an intermediate. Cholesterol synthesized in the hepatocyte can be further metabolized by acyl-CoA cholesterol acyl transferase (ACAT) to cholesterol ester which is packaged into lipoproteins and secreted into the bloodstream. Alternatively, it can be excreted via the biliary system either as neutral lipid or following conversion to bile acids.

Bile acids

The primary bile acids, cholic acid and chenodeoxycholic acid, are derived from cholesterol (Fig. 1.40[605]). The biosynthesis takes place primarily in the hepatocytes, through

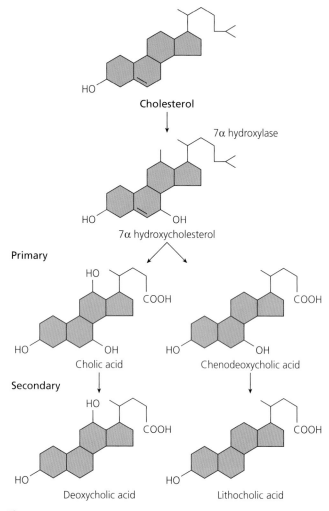

Fig. 1.40 • Pathways of bile acid synthesis.

efflux into the portal circulation, transported by portal vein blood to the liver and extracted from portal blood plasma by hepatocytes.[608] Fasting and postprandial levels of bile acids in the portal venous blood are approximately 0.014 and 0.043 mM, respectively. The liver is efficient in removing bile acids from the circulation, so that peripheral arterial blood serum of healthy individuals has an approximate bile acid concentration of 0.003 mM.[609] Uptake by hepatocytes is an efficient process involving transport systems distinct from those involved in bilirubin uptake, including sodium taurocholate co-transporting protein (NTCP) and organic anion transporting protein (OATP). There are up to 15 enterohepatic circulations per day, so that 20% of the bile acid pool per day enters the colon. Bile acids entering the colon are metabolized by the anaerobic bacterial flora, which carry out two major and a number of minor reactions. The first is deconjugation to release free bile acids, which are only poorly ionized and are lipophilic. The second major reaction is 7-α dehydroxylation to yield deoxycholic and lithocholic acids, respectively, from cholic and chenodeoxycholic acids. Deoxycholic acid is partly absorbed in the colon and enters the enterohepatic circulation, where it is conjugated in the liver and secreted in the bile. Lithocholic acid is only slightly absorbed and mostly excreted in the faeces. The circulating bile acid pool (conjugated when it leaves the gallbladder, and then de-conjugated by action of bacterial enzymes after it enters the colon) is composed of about 30–40% each of cholic acid and chenodeoxycholic acid, about 20–30% of deoxycholic acid, and less than 5% of lithocholic acid.[610] Tertiary bile acids, such as ursodeoxycholic acid, are formed in the liver by epimerization of secondary bile acids and also enter the circulating bile acid pool. However, the latter form of biotransformation is trivial in healthy persons.

Amino acid, protein and ammonia metabolism

Amino acids

In contrast to carbohydrates and fat, there are no specific storage depots of proteins or amino acids. There is an ongoing turnover of body proteins yielding amino acids that are reincorporated into protein, used for the synthesis of other molecules (e.g. neurotramsitters) or oxidized. The liver is of prime importance in amino acid metabolism. Amino acids are removed from the plasma by hepatocytes and are used for protein synthesis or as a source of energy through gluconeogenesis. Under normal circumstances plasma amino acids are derived from intestinal absorption but skeletal muscle becomes the major source when there is dietary protein deprivation.[611]. The 'essential' amino acids (arginine, histidine, isoleucine, leucine, lysine, methionine, phenylalanine, threonine, tryptophan, valine) must be present in the diet as these cannot be synthesized de novo. The liver is the principal site for the synthesis and modification of non-essential amino acids and for the re-amination of most essential amino acids. It may also release amino acids for utilization by peripheral tissues.[612] Furthermore, it

three main pathways involving at least 10 different enzymes and has been reviewed in detail.[605] The rate-limiting step in the conversion of cholesterol to 7α-cholesterol involves 7α-hydroxylase, which is inversely regulated by the bile acids returning to the liver in the enterohepatic circulation. After their synthesis in hepatocytes, bile acids are excreted as C24 carboxylic acids conjugated with glycine or taurine.[606] Other methods of bile acid conjugation (glucuronidation, sulphation) occur to a limited extent in normal individuals but to a greater degree in cholestasis. The bile salts are excreted in the canaliculi against a large concentration gradient, mediated by electrical forces and transporter proteins (mainly the bile salt exporting pump—BSEP). Owing to their osmotic effect they stimulate the bile flow in the biliary system. The conjugated bile salts are excreted from the liver into the gall-bladder, at a concentration of approximately 100 mM[607] and then released into the intestinal tract. Within the small intestine bile acids they are critically important for lipid absorption, through the solubilization of monoglycerides and fatty acids. Bile acids are actively re-absorbed in the terminal ileum, with uptake into ileal columnar epithelium cells, leaving less than 5% of the bile salt pool to enter the colon. After uptake into enterocytes of the ileum, bile salts are shuttled to the basolateral domains of the cells for

plays a major role in the breakdown of amino acids with the production of ammonia and subsequently urea.[613]

While 20 different amino acids are utilized for protein synthesis in man, more than this number are found in proteins since some (e.g. proline) undergo post-translational modifications. The metabolism of the individual amino acids varies considerably. Some (e.g. glycine) can be converted to glucose while others (e.g. leucine) are transaminated or de-aminated to keto-acids. The branched chain essential amino acids leucine, valine and isoleucine are unlike other amino acids in that they are taken up to only a limited extent by the liver, and most are extracted and metabolized by skeletal muscle.[614] The daily turnover of amino acids is high in normal individuals (250–300 g/day in a 70 kg man). Large proportions of those released following protein degradation are re-utilized for synthesis. However, over 30 g per day are irreversibly catabolized and lost to the amino acid/protein pool, and this must be balanced by dietary intake. Nitrogen released from the complete catabolism of amino acids can be removed by a variety of routes but the principal pathway is urea synthesis and excretion. With the exception of the branched chain amino acids, all essential amino acids are degraded in the liver. Non-essential amino acids can be degraded in the liver and skeletal muscle.

Urea, ammonia and nitrogen balance

Catabolism of amino acids yields ammonia. This can be used for the synthesis of other nitrogenous compounds but it is highly toxic and the liver is largely responsible for its removal. Other endogenous sources of ammonia include purines and pyrimidines from nucleic acids and amines such as noradrenaline; up to 25% comes via the portal system from the intestine where it is generated by bacterial ureases. The major pathways of ammonia metabolism are outlined in Fig. 1.41.[614] Over 90% of surplus nitrogen is disposed of by conversion of ammonia to urea which is then excreted by the kidneys. The urea cycle occurs almost exclusively in liver. Two of the key enzymes—carbamyl synthetase I and ornithine transcarbamylase—are found in only trace amounts in other tissues. They are expressed most abundantly by periportal hepatocytes.[615] Urea synthesis is regulated by intrahepatic levels of N-acetylglutamate and is also under hormonal control which involves glucagon and glucocorticoids.[616] The other major pathway for ammonia removal is through the production of glutamine. In contrast to urea cycle enzymes, glutamine synthetase is found only in perivenular liver cells.[617] This is an example of metabolic zonation within the liver parenchyma, which may be modulated by differences in oxygen tension.[595,596]

Protein metabolism and the liver

Hepatic protein synthesis accounts for approximately 15% of total body protein production. A small fraction of this relates to the synthesis of structural proteins and cytoplasmic enzymes but the bulk of it is accounted for by secretory products—the plasma proteins.[618] These are generated on

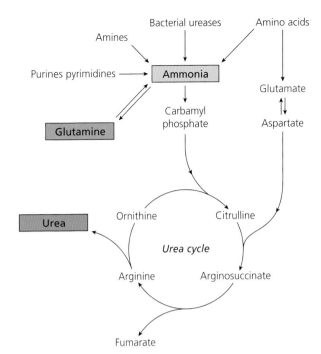

Fig. 1.41 • Major pathways of ammonia metabolism.

the polyribosomes of the rough endoplasmic reticulum of hepatocytes and are released into the circulation at the sinusoidal domain. The multiple steps involved in gene transcription, RNA processing and translation have now been elucidated.[619,620] Some data on transcriptional regulation have come from studies of liver-specific proteins such as albumin. With many genes, there are regulatory sequences upstream from the transcriptional start point which control the rate of transcription. In the case of albumin, this comprises two sequences common to other gene promoters—the TATA- and CAAT-boxes—and two liver-specific control sequences (enhancers).[620] The regulatory function of promoters is mediated by specific proteins—the so-called transcription factors. Newly synthesized protein is transported from the ribosomes into the lumen of the endoplasmic reticulum, a process which involves binding of a signal sequence on the molecule to a signal recognition particle.[621] Once inside the endoplasmic reticulum the signal sequence is cleaved and the protein undergoes further post-translational modifications as it is transported along the secretory pathway via the cis- and trans-Golgi apparatus. These include formation of disulphide bonds and glycosylation. Some blood coagulation proteins synthesized in the liver (factors II, VII, IX, X) contain an N-terminal gamma-carboxyglutamic acid residue which is essential for their normal function. This modification involves a vitamin K-dependent carboxylase. Proteins are finally transported from the trans-Golgi to the cell surface in secretory vesicles by the action of microtubules. The mechanisms responsible for directing secretory proteins to the sinusoidal domain of the cell are thought to involve 'sorting carrier proteins' within the Golgi apparatus.[621,622]

Various factors influence the level of protein synthesis in the liver. Nutritional status is important. In starvation, the rate of synthesis drops owing to decreased availability of amino acids, decreased RNA stability and disaggregation of ribosomes.[623] Several hormones are known to alter hepatic protein synthetic rates. Insulin, for example, increases synthesis whereas glucagon has an inhibitory effect. The synthesis and secretion of some proteins (e.g. C-reactive protein, serum amyloid A, C3) by hepatocytes is increased in the face of tissue injury and inflammation—the so-called acute phase response. Synthesis of serum amyloid A may be increased several hundred-fold. Under such circumstances, however, the rate of synthesis of other proteins such as albumin may decrease. These are referred to as negative acute phase proteins. The acute phase response is mediated principally by cytokines released by lymphocytes and macrophages. Interleukin-1 and tumour necrosis factor-alfa are known to play a role but interleukin-6 is thought to be the most important mediator. These molecules have effects at both transcriptional and post-transcriptional levels.[624] Interleukin-6 induces the interaction of DNA-binding proteins with promoter elements of several acute phase genes. It may also enhance the secretion rate of some proteins including α-macroglobulin.

The major proteins secreted by the hepatocyte are listed in Table 1.4. Albumin is the most abundant with a normal plasma concentration of 40–50 g/l. It has two principal functions: the regulation of plasma oncotic pressure and as a major transport protein.[625] Transferrin is the carrier protein for iron in plasma.[626] Ceruloplasmin is an α-glycoprotein which acts as a specific copper-binding protein. The liver is the sole site of synthesis of all components of the coagulation cascade, apart from factor VIII which is synthesized predominantly by the vascular endothelium. In addition, it produces many of the proteins involved in fibrinolysis, such as plasminogen, although plasminogen activators are mainly synthesized at extrahepatic sites.

The complement system is important in host defence against microorganisms and in inflammation.[627] It can be activated via the classical or alternative pathways and a number of inhibitory control proteins are known to exist. The whole system involves more than 20 proteins, most of which are synthesized by hepatocytes, although other cells, in particular macrophages, also have the capacity to produce complement proteins.[628]

α₁-Antitrypsin is the most abundant of the protease inhibitors (Pi) produced in the liver, with a serum concentration of 2–4 g/l. It is an inhibitor of serine proteases and is mainly involved in inhibiting the activity of neutrophil elastase. There is considerable polymorphism of the α₁-antitrypsin gene; some phenotypes, most notably PiZZ, are associated with reduced serum levels and may be accompanied by panacinar emphysema and cirrhosis. Kupffer cells also produce α₁-antitrypsin and several other plasma proteins such as C3[629] but, in quantitative terms, their contribution is small.

In addition to being a major site of protein production, the liver also plays a role in protein degradation. Endogenous cytoplasmic proteins are degraded by lysosomal proteases, and the amino acids generated are re-utilized for protein synthesis or energy. Circulating glycoproteins are also degraded by hepatocytes, Kupffer cells and sinusoidal endothelial cells following uptake by receptor-mediated endocytosis. A number of elegant studies have characterized the nature and distribution of the asialoglycoprotein receptor present at the sinusoidal domain of hepatocytes and have elucidated the pathways which lead to lysosomal degradation of glycoproteins following their internalization into the cell,[630] the former occurring predominantly in perivenular zones, the latter in periportal zones.

Assessment of hepatic function

A number of blood tests are commonly used to screen for unsuspected liver disease, to confirm its presence, to estimate severity, assess prognosis and evaluate therapy. These do not provide a specific diagnosis but have a high sensitivity and are easy to perform. In most centres a battery of 'liver function tests' (LFTs) is used which normally includes serum bilirubin, aminotransferases, alkaline phosphatase and g-glutamyltransferase (GGT). Strictly speaking, these tests do not assess hepatic function but indicate the pres-

Table 1.4	Plasma proteins synthesized in the liver

Albumin

Transport proteins
Lipoproteins
Transferrin
Transcortin
a₁ Acid glycoprotein
Caeruloplasmin
Thyroid hormone-binding proteins
Retinol-binding proteins
Vitamin D-binding proteins

Coagulation and fibrinolysis proteins
Fibrinogen
Factor II, V, VII–XIII
Prekallikrein
Kininogen
Prothrombin
Protein C
Plasminogen

Complement
C1q,r,s
C2–C9
Factor B
Factor D

Protease inhibitors
α₁-Antitrypsin
α₁-Antichymotrypsin
α₂-Macroglobulin
Antithrombin III
α₂-Antiplasmin
C1 inhibitor

Miscellaneous acute phase proteins
C-reactive protein
Serum amyloid A

ence of hyperbilirubinaemia, hepatocellular necrosis and cholestasis. In addition, serum albumin and prothrombin time (after vitamin K) assess the severity of liver disease.

Any confirmed rise in these blood tests warrants additional investigation for the detection of underlying liver disease. Other biochemical/genetic tests can be used to establish the presence of specific diseases such as haemochromatosis (serum ferritin, serum and hepatic iron, transferrin saturation, HFE genotyping)[631], Wilson disease (ceruloplasmin, serum and hepatic copper, urinary copper, urinary copper excretion, mutation screening of the Wilson gene)[632,633] α_1-antitrypsin deficiency (plasma electrophoresis, genotyping)[634], and hepatocellular carcinoma (a-fetoprotein). Additional methods that can be used to determine the aetiology of liver disease in an individual patient include immunological investigations and imaging techniques. In Table 1.5 possible work-up is illustrated for patients with chronically elevated aminotransferases.

'Conventional' liver function tests

Serum bilirubin
Serum bilirubin estimations are based on the van den Bergh diazo reaction. Conjugated bilirubin may be estimated by a direct reaction at 10 minutes. The total bilirubin is determined by the use of an accelerator. The amount of unconjugated (indirect) bilirubin is calculated by subtracting conjugated from total bilirubin. Other more accurate methods are available (alkaline methanolysis, HPLC). In cholestatic and hepatocellular disease conjugated bilirubin is elevated and associated with a rise in liver enzymes. An isolated rise in serum bilirubin (without enzyme elevation) may be familial (Gilbert, Dubin-Johnson, Rotor) or due to hemolysis.

Serum aminotransferase
The aminotransferases (aspartate aminotransferase or AST, alanine transaminase or ALT) catalyse the reversible transformation of α-ketoacids into amino acids. Their serum levels reflect the amount of hepatocellular injury and death on a day-by-day basis. Aminotransferases (and predominantly AST) are not only found in hepatocytes but also in other tissues (heart and skeletal muscles, kidney, brain, pancreas, lung, and red blood cells). The liver contains 400 U ALT/g protein (mainly cytoplasmic) and 500 U AST/g protein (>80 % contained in mitochondria and endoplasmic reticulum). Damage to one gram of liver tissue (or the membranes of 171 million hepatocytes) results in a significant increase in the serum ALT activity.[635,636] AST responds in the same fashion, especially following liver cell necrosis and destruction of mitochondria and endoplasmic reticulum. Owing to the sudden release of intracellular reservoirs of aminotransferases and their short half-life (1–2 days), the levels of ALT and AST respond quickly to hepatocellular damage or acute bile-duct obstruction. Serum aminotransferase levels can rise to over 10 times the upper limit of normal in hepatic hypoxia or acute bile-duct obstruction. High levels can also be seen in acute hepatitis and toxin-induced necrosis. In chronic hepatitis, the levels are generally less than five times the upper limit of normal. Sensitivity and specificity of ALT for the detection of liver disease is around 83%.[635,636] An isolated rise in ALT is of hepatocellular origin, after exclusion of macroenzyme-I-immune complexes. The diagnostic sensitivity of AST is significantly lower (70%) and less specific. The study of the AST : ALT ratio (or DeRits ratio) can yield some additional information but specific aetiologic diagnosis cannot usually be based on these routine tests or ratios. In alcoholic liver disease the AST : ALT ratio is greater than 2 : 1, owing to an alcohol-related deficiency of pyridoxal 5-phosphate B_6.[637] In contrast, patients with non-alcoholic fatty liver disease (NAFLD) the AST : ALT ratio is said to be less than 1, but this is not invariably the case. An isolated rise in AST is not uncommon in patients with end-stage alcoholic cirrhosis. Serial estimations of transaminases can be used to monitor progress in an individual patient but correlation is poor between absolute values and the extent of necrosis, and values are often normal in patients with compensated cirrhosis.

Alkaline phosphatase and gamma-GT
Alkaline phosphatase is found in the biliary pole of the hepatocytes, the bile-duct epithelia, osteoblasts, kidney, lung, intestine and placenta.[635] The serum activity present in normal individuals is predominantly due to the isoenzymes of the liver, bone and kidney. Thus, an isolated rise in ALP is seen in the third trimester of pregnancy, or during growth (bone ALP) or may be due to intestinal ALP (following ingestion of a fatty meal). Levels of alkaline phophatase rise in cholestasis and to a lesser extent when liver cells are

Table 1.5	Non-invasive evaluation of asymptomatic patients with chronically (>3 months) elevated aminotransferases

1. Clinical history (medication!) and physical examination

2. Excluding liver disease
— Hepatobiliary imaging: liver ultrasound (or if in doubt CT—MRI)
— Liver synthetic and excretory function: prothrombin time, albumin, bilirubin
— Specific tests:
   a. Chronic viral hepatitis B and C: HBsAg, HBcAb, anti-HCV, (HCV-RNA);
   b. Haemochromatosis: serum iron, iron saturation, ferritin, (genetic testing);
   c. Autoimmune disease: antinuclear antibody, antimitochondrial antibody, smooth muscle cell antibody; liver-kidney microsomal antibodies (titres > 1 : 40); immunoglobulins;
   d. α-1-antitrypsin deficiency: protein electrophoresis, (phenotyping);
   e. Wilson disease: caeruloplasmin, urinary copper excretion (<40 yr).

3. Excluding non-hepatic causes of elevated aminotransferases
— Thyroid disorders: TSH
— Coeliac disease: tissue transglutaminase antibodies (endomysium antibodies)
— Muscle pathology: creatine kinase

damaged. In cholestatic liver disease, the elevated bile acids stimulate the synthesis of ALP. Alkaline phosphatase levels are highest in extrahepatic biliary obstruction but may be several times the upper limit of normal in chronic cholestatic conditions such as primary biliary cirrhosis. Increased levels of hepatic alkaline phosphatase are also found with intrahepatic space-occupying lesions and, less frequently, in Hodgkin disease, congestive cardiac failure and some connective tissue disorders. Differentiation between hepatic and non-hepatic causes of ALP elevation can be done by determination of ALP isoenzymes or more easily by testing for GGT, which rises in liver but not in bone disease. GGT is found in hepatocytes, cholangiocytes, kidney, pancreas, epididymis, heart, lung, intestine, bone marrow, salivary glands, thymus, spleen and brain, which is an explanation for the lack of specificity for the diagnosis of hepatobiliary disease. Elevated values of GGT are caused by damage to cellular membranes, cellular regeneration or by enhanced synthesis as a result of induction of the biotransformation enzyme system.[635] Known inducers are bile acids (cholestasis), prolonged regular abuse of alcohol and especially antiepileptic drugs (phenytoin, carbamazepine).[638] A decline in GGT can be observed during oestrogen administration or pregnancy.[639] In contrast to alkaline phosphatase, normal adult levels are found during growth and GGT is used as the principal biochemical marker of cholestasis in children.

Knowledge of enzyme kinetics is important for the correct interpretation of abnormal liver enzymes as predominant hepatocellular or cholestatic patterns. In contrast with serum transaminases, a rise in serum ALP and GGT occurs more slowly in response to cholestasis, and the levels are maintained longer owing to a half-life of more than 4 days.[635,640]

Serum albumin

The measurement of serum levels of this liver-specific protein[641] provides some indication of the synthetic capacity of the liver. The half-life of albumin is about 22 days and thus in acute liver failure a normal serum albumin level may be found. Unfortunately, low levels can be caused by increased loss through the kidneys or gastrointestinal tract, increased catabolism, altered vascular permeability and over-hydration. Alterations in the concentration of serum albumin must therefore be interpreted with caution.

Coagulation tests

As noted above the hepatocyte is the principal site of synthesis of the majority of coagulation proteins. The prothrombin time (after vitamin K administration) represents a good indicator for liver synthetic function, thanks to the short half-life of factor VII (100–300 minutes). Estimation of individual clotting factors is rarely necessary, although the level of factor V (not vitamin K-dependent) is related to outcome in acute liver failure.

Other tests

Plasma bile acid measurements are used in some centres within the battery of first-line liver function tests. Assays have also been developed for the non-invasive assessment

of hepatic fibrosis. There is an unmet need for serum markers that can reliably detect the stage of liver fibrosis. Several serum tests are in development, including the Fibrotest (based on a range of clinical chemistry analyses) and GlycoCirrhoTest (based on profiles of serum protein N-glycans). The combination of both tests achieved a sensitivity for cirrhosis of 75% and a specificity of 100%, obviating the need for biopsy in cirrhotic patients. Further and larger studies are necessary fully to validate these promising results.[642,643]

Dynamic tests of hepatic function

In view of the limitation of conventional tests, additional methods have been developed which provide a more quantitative assessment of hepatic function. These are of potential value in monitoring disease progression in an individual patient and could be used to indicate the need for transplantation. They are, however, more complex than conventional tests. The lack of a major impact above the routine laboratory tests and Child-Pugh grading is reflected in their role in clinical research rather than in daily clinical practice. Most tests involve the administration of a test substance which is known to be taken up, metabolized and/or excreted by the liver with the subsequent collection of serum samples or other body fluids to determine clearance rates. Those used most frequently in clinical studies are the *aminopyrine breath test*, *antipyrine and caffeine clearance tests*, *galactose elimination* and *indocyanine green extraction*.[644,645] A method which may be helpful in assessing function prior to transplantation is formation of monoethylglycinexylidide (MEGX) after the intravenous administration of low concentrations of lignocaine.[646]

Immunological investigations

The detection of auto-antibodies is of value in the differential diagnosis of liver diseases. The earliest methods used for the detection of autoantibodies were based on complement fixation or immunofluorescence. The latter is still widely used in screening but, with the identification of the specific epitopes involved, enzyme immunoassay and immunoblotting are used increasingly for the identification of distinct autoantibody subtypes.

Antinuclear antibodies

These antibodies are present in 80% of patients with type 1 autoimmune hepatitis[647] but are also found in a group of patients with primary biliary cirrhosis who are negative for antimitochondrial antibodies ('autoimmune cholangitis')[648] and in some patients with primary sclerosing cholangitis. Antibodies to nuclear envelope proteins have been described in patients with primary biliary cirrhosis, type I autoimmune hepatitis and hepatitis B with hepatitis D virus (HDV) co-infection; these are directed against lamins and the lamin B receptor.[649]

Smooth muscle antibodies

These are found in 70% of patients with autoimmune hepatitis and in 50% of patients with PBC. The antigen is related to the S-actin of skeletal and smooth muscle. It is also present in the cytoskeleton and cell membrane of the hepatocyte. They are detected using indirect immunofluorescence.

Liver kidney microsomal (LKM) antibodies[647]
Several distinct types of LKM antibody have been described. The target antigen for LKM-1 has been identified as the enzyme cytochrome P-450 2D6; this auto-antibody is characteristic of autoimmune hepatitis types 2a and 2b. LKM-2 reacts against cytochrome P-450 2C9 and occurs exclusively in patients with drug-induced hepatitis caused by tienilic acid. LKM-3 antibodies have been found in the serum of some Italian patients with HDV infection and the microsomal target is uridine diphosphate glucuronyl transferase.[650]

Antimitochondrial antibodies (AMA)
AMA are readily identified in the plasma using indirect immunofluorescence. They are not specific for liver disease and can be found in myocarditis, systemic lupus erythematosus, syphilis, scleroderma and Sjögren syndrome. There are, however, subtypes of AMA which can be considered specific for primary biliary cirrhosis. These antibodies (designated M2) are directed against epitopes on enzymes of the inner mitochondrial membranes, all components of the pyruvate dehydrogenase complex. Further subtypes (M4, M8 and M9), which may react with components of the outer mitochondrial membranes, have been detected by ELISA and complement fixation. It has been suggested that the spectrum of AMA subtypes in an individual patient may relate to the stage of the disease and be of value in prognostication,[651] but this is controversial.[652]

Imaging of the liver

A large number of methods are available which can be used to identify intrahepatic masses, assess liver blood flow and visualize the biliary tract. In many cases a combination of ultrasound, computed tomography (CT) and magnetic resonance imaging (MRI) is required. The choice of method used is determined by the nature of the clinical problem and by the availability of techniques. Radio-isotope scanning, once very popular, retains a limited role for biliary tract imaging or for scanning of metastases using specific ligands. Plain X-ray films are of limited value although they can detect calcified lesions.

Ultrasonography
Real-time ultrasound represents the most widely used imaging method in clinical hepatology. It is the first-line and inexpensive investigation in biliary tract disorders, and the initial examination of choice for the investigation of suspected space-occupying lesions. Traditional grey-scale sonography assesses the degree of echogenicity of a tissue. Cystic lesions are therefore readily demonstrable. The use of Doppler examination in association with conventional ultrasonography (duplex or colour Doppler) provides additional information on blood flow (Fig. 1.42(A)). This approach can be used to identify collateral vessels in portal hypertension, to evaluate the patency of surgical portal-systemic shunts and vascular anastomoses in liver transplants and to examine tumour vascularity. It is also valuable in diagnostic assessment of portal vein or hepatic vein thrombosis.

Computed tomography (CT)
The liver is displayed as a series of adjacent cross-sectional slices. The cross-sectional images obtained by CT scanning are derived from differences in density or attenuation between tissues. This can be enhanced by the prior injection of a contrast agent such as iodine (Fig. 1.42(B)). Conventional CT has been replaced by spiral CT, which offers the advantage that the scan can be completed while there is a peak concentration of contrast medium in the blood vessels of interest.[653] By this methodology, tumour detection is improved.[654]

Magnetic resonance imaging (MRI)
MRI is a recent advance in liver imaging and this technology does not use X-rays to produce images (Fig. 1.43). It represents a powerful imaging technique and relies on the fact that protons behave like small magnets.[655] In an external magnetic field, the protons are forcibly aligned along the direction of the field. After an excitation pulse the magnetization vector is flipped towards the axial plane. During relaxation, the longitudinal magnetization gradually recovers (and is called T1 relaxation), while the transverse magnetization gradually disappears (T2 relaxation). The T1 and T2 relaxation times are tissue-specific and form the basis of image contrast in MRI. In order to obtain an MR signal (also called echo) the transverse magnetization is measured shortly after the radiofrequency pulse. The time interval between the RF pulse and the measurement of the echo is called the echo time (TE). The echo time together with the repetition time (TR), or the time interval between two consecutive pulses, determines which type of MR image is created. To produce a T1-weighted image, short TE and TR values are used. Long TE and TR values result in a T2-weighted image. T1- and T2-weighted images can be distinguished by considering the signal intensity of water: water has a low signal intensity ('black') on T1-weighted images while it has a high signal intensity ('white') on T2-weighted images. No contrast injection is needed for blood vessel or bile duct visualization (Fig. 1.42C) Given the quality of the obtained images MRI-cholangiography has replaced diagnostic ERCP[655]. Using a sequence of moderately and heavily T2-weighted images focal liver lesions can be characterized[656] (Table 1.6). Contrast agents can be used to differentiate among focal liver lesions, such as gadolinium targeting functional hepatocytes or ferumoxides that are taken up by Kupffer cells.

Angiography
With the development of Doppler ultrasonography and MRI scanning, diagnostic angiography (Fig. 1.42(D)) is now less frequently used in hepatology. It remains increasingly used in 'interventional radiology' with the chemo-embolization

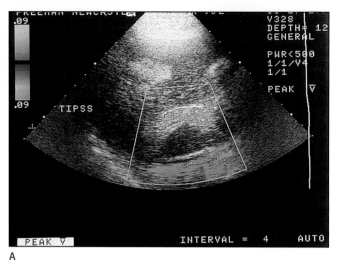

A

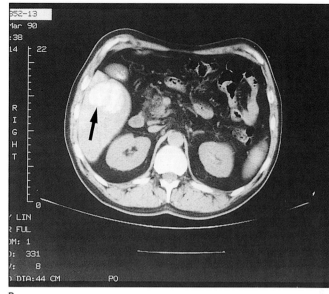

B

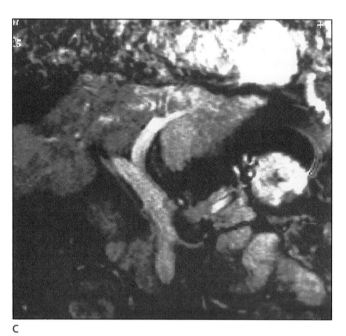

C

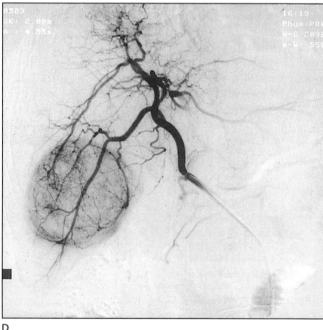

D

Fig. 1.42 • Imaging techniques. **(A)** Colour Doppler ultrasonography. In this case the technique has been used to demonstrate patency of a TIPS stent in a cirrhotic liver (yellow). Flow in the vena cava is seen as a red image. Courtesy of Dr J Rose. **(B)** Lipiodol CT scan of a hepatocellular carcinoma. There is selective uptake by the tumour (arrow). Courtesy of Dr J Rose. **(C)** Magnetic resonance image (MRI) of liver and portal venous system in a patient with cirrhosis undergoing pre-transplant work up. Courtesy of Dr C Baudouin. **(D)** Digital vascular subtraction angiography of tumour depicted in Fig. 2.21b. This shows an abnormal vascular pattern within the lesion characteristic of a hepatocellular carcinoma. The tumour was present in segment VI. Courtesy of Dr J Rose.

of tumours.[657,658] Contrast Lipiodol, mixed with chemotherapeutic agents (doxorubicin, cisplatin) and/or gelfoam, is injected under fluoroscopic control following selective catheterization of the hepatic artery (Fig. 1.44).

Radionuclide investigations

Radio-isotope scanning with ^{99m}Tc-labelled tin colloid and colloids of human albumin, which utilizes the phagocytic ability of Kupffer cells, is now replaced by the above-mentioned new imaging techniques. There remains a limited role for dynamic assessment of biliary excretion by ^{99m}Tc-labelled iminodiacetic acid derivatives (HIDA scanning). The detection of liver metastases from neuroendocrine tumours can be demonstrated by ^{111}In-DTPA octreotide scanning.[628]

Positron emission tomography (PET) is increasingly utilized in clinical practice and research using positron-emitting radionuclides, such as ^{18}F. PET-scanning with ^{18}F-fluoro-2-deoxy-D-glucose measures glucose utilization and can detect metastases from various tumours, although the role is limited for cholangiocarcinoma or hepatocellular carcinoma.[629,630]

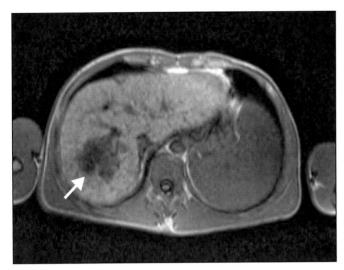

A

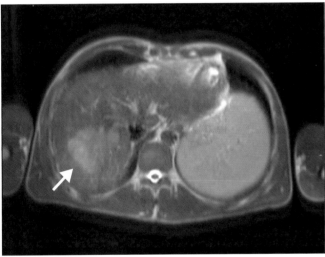

B

Fig. 1.43 • Magnetic resonance imaging (MRI) of the liver in a patient with HBV-related cirrhosis. Lesion with signal characteristics of hepatocellular carcinoma in segment VII-VIII: A. T1-weighted image: hypointense lobulated lesion (arrow); B. T2-weighted image: hyperintense lesion (arrow). Significant signal drop on late echo (not shown) is typical of solid lesion. Marked splenomegaly. Courtesy of Dr D Vanbeckevoort.

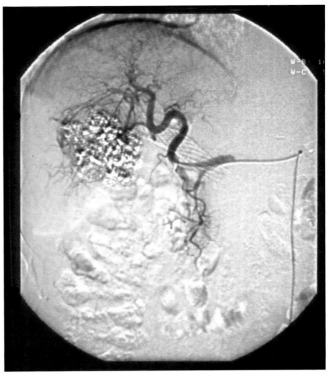

Fig. 1.44 • Chemoembolization of hepatocellular carcinoma: selective catheterization of the feeding vessels of HCC and injection of lipiodol, mixed with chemotherapeutic drug (cisplatin) Courtesy of Dr G Maleux.

Table 1.6	Characterization of focal liver lesions by MRI (snapshot T2-weighted MRI, double echo technique)	
	Signal intensity (relative to normal liver)	
	First echo (Echo time 60 ms—moderately T2-weighted)	**Second echo (echo time 439 ms—heavily T2-weighted)**
Cyst	Hyperintense ++/+++	Hyperintense ++++
Haemangioma	Hyperintense ++	Hyperintense +
Solid lesion	Hyperintense +/++	Isointense

References

1. Bloch EH. The termination of hepatic arterioles and the functional unit of the liver as determined by microscopy of the living organ. Ann N Y Acad Sci, 1970; 170:78–87
2. Kiernan F. The anatomy and physiology of the liver. Philos Trans R Soc Lond, 1833; 123:711–770
3. Ekataksin W, Wake K. New concepts in biliary and vascular anatomy of the liver. In: Boyer JL, Ockner RK, eds. Progress in liver diseases, vol. XV. Philadelphia: WB Saunders, 1997: pp 1–30
4. Mall FP. A study of the structural unit of the liver. Am J Anat, 1906; 5:227–308
5. Rappaport AM, Borowy ZJ, Lougheed WM, Lotto WN. Subdivision of hexagonal liver lobules into a structural and functional unit. Role in hepatic physiology and pathology. Anat Rec, 1954; 119:11–34
6. Matsumoto T, Komori R, Magara T et al. A study on the normal structure of human liver, with special reference to its angioarchitecture. Jikeikai Med J, 1979; 26:1–40
7. McCuskey RS. Hepatic microcirculation. In: Bioulac-Sage P, Balabaud C, eds. Sinusoids in human liver: health and disease. Rijswijk: Kupffer Cell Foundation, 1988: pp 151–164
8. Lamers WH, Hilberts A, Furt E et al. Hepatic enzymic zonation: a reevaluation of the concept of the liver acinus. Hepatology, 1989; 10:72–76
9. Quistorff B, Romert P. High zone-selectivity of cell permeabilization following digitonin-pulse perfusion of rat liver. A re-interpretation of microcirculatory zones. Histochemistry, 1989; 92:487–498
10. Hofmann AF. The choleohepatic circulation of unconjugated bile acids: an update. In: Paumgartner G, Stiehl A, Gerok W, eds. Bile acids and the hepatobiliary system: from basic science to clinical practice. Dordrecht: Kluwer Academic Publishers, 1993: pp 143–160
11. Ekataksin W. Microanatomy of bile secretory epithelium and vasculature: the identification of mammalian livers. In: Manns MP, Boyer JL, Jansen PLM, Reichen J, eds. Cholestatic liver diseases. Dordrecht: Kluwer Academic Publishers, 1998: pp 46–61
12. Lamers WH, Moorman AFM, Charles R. The metabolic lobulus, a key to the architecture of the liver. In: Gumucio JJ, ed. Revisiones sobre biologia cellular. Cell Biology Reviews, vol. 19. Berlin: Springer International, 1989: pp 5–26
13. Matsumoto R, Kawakami M. The unit-concept of hepatic parenchyma—a reexamination based on angioarchitectural studies. Acta Pathol Jpn, 1982; 32:285–314

14. Tremblay KD, Zaret KS. Distinct populations of endoderm cells converge to generate the embryonic liver bud and ventral foregut tissues. Dev Biol, 2005; 280:87–99

15. Elias H, Sherrick JC. Morphology of the liver. Academic Press, New York, 1969

16. Streeter GL. Developmental horizons in human embryos. Age groups XI and XII. Contributions to embryology of the Carnegie Institution of Washington, 1942; 30:213–244

17. Lassau JP, Bastian D. Organogenesis of the venous structure of the human liver. A haemodynamic theory. Anat Clin, 1983; 5:97–102

18. Barclay AE, Franklin FJ, Pritchard MML. The fetal circulation. Oxford: Blackwell Scientific, 1944

19. Ekataksin W. The isolated artery: an intrahepatic arterial pathway that can bypass the lobular parenchyma in mammalian liver. Hepatology 2000; 31:269–279

20. Desmet VJ, Van Eyken P, Roskams T. 'Embryology of the liver and intrahepatic biliary tract'. In Oxford Textbook of Clinical Hepatology, 2nd edition, Section 1: 'Structure of the liver', edited by Bircher J, Benhamou J-P, McIntyre N, Rizzetto M, Rodés J, Oxford University Press, Oxford, 1999, pp 51–61

21. Suchy FJ, Bucuvalas JC, Novak DA. Determinants of bile formation during development: ontogeny of hepatic bile acid metabolism and transport. Semin Liv Dis, 1987; 7:77–84

22. Bloom W. The embryogenesis of human bile capillaries and ducts. Am J Anat, 1925–26; 36:451–466

23. Hammar J. Ueber die erste Entstehung der richt Kappillaren intrahepatischen Gallengänge beim Menschen. Zeitschrift für Mikroskopisch-Anatomische Forschung, 1926; 5:59–89

24. Van Eyken P, Sciot R, Callea V, Van der Steen K, Moerman P, Desmet VJ. The development of the intrahepatic bile ducts in man: a keratin-immunohistochemical study. Hepatology, 1988; 8:1586–1595

25. Lemaigre FP, Zaret KS. Liver development update: new embryo models, cell cineage control and morphongenesis, Curr Opinion Genet Dev, 2004; 285–290

26. Gall JAM, Bhathal PS. Morphological and immunohistochemical assessment of intrahepatic bile duct development in the rat. J Gastroenterol Hepatol, 1989; 4:241–250

27. Shah K, Gerber MA. Development of intrahepatic bile ducts in humans. Immunohistochemical study using monoclonal cytokeratin antibodies. Arch Pathol Lab Med, 1989; 113:1135–1138

28. Desmet VJ. Embryology of the liver and intrahepatic biliary tract, and an overview of malformations of the bile duct. In: MacIntyre N, Benhamou J-P, Bircher J, Rizzetto M, Rodes J, eds. Oxford textbook of clinical hepatology, vol. 1. Oxford, New York, Tokyo: Oxford University Press, 1991; 495–519

29. Desmet VJ. Congenital diseases of intrahepatic bile ducts: variations on the theme 'ductal plate malformation'. Hepatology, 1992; 16:1069–1083

30. Moll R, Franke WW, Schiller DA, Geiger B, Krepler R. The catalog of human cytokeratins: patterns of expression in normal epithelia, tumors and cultured cells. Cell, 1982; 31:11

31. Libbrecht L, Cassiman D, Desmet V, Roskams T. The correlation between portal myofibroblasts and development of intrahepatic bile ducts and arterial branches in human liver. Liver. 2002; 22:252–831

32. Jørgensen MJ. The ductal plate malformation. Acta Path Micr Scand, 1977; 257:1–88

33. Shiojiri N. The origin of intrahepatic bile duct cells in the mouse. J Embryol Exp Morphol, 1984; 79:25–39

34. Lemaigre FP. Development of the biliary tract. Mech Dev, 2003; 120:81–87

35. Roskams TA, Theise ND, Balabaud C et al. Nomenclature of the finer branches of the biliary tree: canals, ductules, and ductular reactions in human livers. Hepatology, 2004; 39:1739–1745

36. Van Eyken P, Sciot R, Van Damme B, De Wolf-Peeters C, Desmet VJ. Keratin immunohistochemistry in normal human liver. Cytokeratin pattern of hepatocytes, bile ducts and acinar gradient. Virchows Arch A, 1987; 412:63–72

37. Van Eyken P, Sciot R, Desmet VJ. A cytokeratin immuno-histochemical study of alcoholic liver disease: evidence that hepatocytes can express 'bile duct-type' cytokeratins. Histopathology, 1988; 13:605–617

38. Van Eyken P, Sciot R, Desmet VJ. A cytokeratin immuno-histochemical study of cholestatic liver disease: evidence that hepatocytes can express 'bile duct-type' cytokeratins. Histopathology, 1989; 15:125–135

39. Dawood KA, Briscoe CV, Thomas DB, Riches AC. Regulation of haematopoietic stem cell proliferation by stimulatory factors produced by murine fetal and adult liver. J Anat, 1990; 168:209–216

40. Khalaf WF, White H, Wenning MJ et al. K-Ras is essential for normal fetal liver erythropoiesis, Blood 2005; 105: 3538–3541

41. Moore MAS, Johnson GR. Hemopoietic stem cells during embryonic development and growth. In: Cairnie AB, Lala PK, Osmond DG, eds. Stem cells of renewing cell populations. New York & London: Academic Press, 1976

42. Li D, Wang GY, Liu ZF et al. Macrophage-associated erythropoiesis and lymphocytopoiesis in mouse fetal liver: ultrastructural and ISH analysis. Cell Biol Int, 2004; 28:457–461

43. Jung J, Zheng M, Goldfarb M, Zaret KS. Initiation of mammalian liver development from endoderm by fibroblast growth factors. Science, 1999; 284:1998–2003

44. Zhao R, Duncan SA. Embryonic development of the liver. Hepatology, 2005; 41:856–967

45. Lammert E, Cleaver O, Melton D. Role of endothelial cells in early pancreas and liver development. Mech Dev, 2003; 120:59–64

46. Matsumoto K, Yoshitomi H, Rossant J, Zaret KS. Liver organogenesis promoted by endothelial cells prior to vascular function. Science, 2001; 294:559–563

47. Zhao R, Watt AJ, Li J et al. GATA6 is essential for embryonic development of the liver but dispensable for early heart formation. Mol Cell Biol, 2005; 25:2622–2631

48. Lee CS, Friedman JR, Fulmer JT, Kaestner KH. The initiation of liver development is dependent on Foxa transcription factors. Nature, 2005; 435:944–947

49. Gouysse G, Couelard A, Frachon S et al. Relationship between vascular development and vascular differentiation during liver organogenesis in humans. J Hepatol, 2002; 367:730–740

50. Enzan H, Hara H, Yamashita Y, Ohkita T, Yamane T. Fine structure of hepatic sinusoids and their development in human embryos and fetuses. Acta Pathol Jpn, 1983; 33:447–466

51. Severn CB. A morphological study of the development of the human liver. II. Establishment of liver parenchyma, extrahepatic ducts and associated venous channels. Am J Anat, 1972; 133:85–108

52. Shiojiri N, Sugiyama Y. Immunolocalisation of extracellular matrix components and integrins during mouse liver development. Hepatology, 2004; 40:346–379

53. Modis L, Martinez-Hernandez A. Hepatocytes modulate the hepatic microvascular phenotype. Lab Invest, 1991; 65:661–669

54. Serls AE, Doherty S, Parvatiyar P, Wells JM, Deutsch GH. Different thresholds of fibroblast growth factors pattern the ventral foregut into liver and lung. Development, 2005; 132:35–47

55. Rossi JM, Dunn RN, Hogan BLM, Zaret KS. Distinct mesodermal signals including BMPs from septum transversum are required for hepatogenesis from the endoderm. Genes Dev, 2001; 15:1998–2009

56. Keng VW, Yagi H, Ikawa M et al. Homeobox gene Hex is essential for onset of mouse embryonic liver development and differentiation of the monocyte lineage Biochem Biophys Res Commun, 2000; 276:1155–1161

57. Zaret KS. Regulatory phases of early liver development: paradigms of organogenesis. Nat Rev Genet, 2002; 3: 499–512

58. Yamamoto Y, Teratani T, Yamamoto H et al. Recapitulation of in vivo gene expression during hepatic differentiation from mature embryonic stem cells. Hepatology, 2005; 42:558–567

59. Fu H, Tie Y, Xu C et al. Identification of human fetal liver miRNAs by a novel method. FEBS Lett, 2005; 579:3849–3854

60. Ober EA, Field HA, Stainer DY. From endoderm formation to liver and pancreas development in zebrafish. Mech Dev, 2003; 120:5–18

61. Parviz F, Matullo, Garrison WD et al. Hepatocyte nuclear factor 4 alpha controls the development of a hepatic epithelium and liver morphogenesis. Nat Genet, 2003; 34:292–296

62. Flynn DM, Nijjar D, Hubscher SG et al. The role of Notch receptor expression in bile duct development and disease. J Pathol, 2004; 204:55–64

63. Kodama Y, Hijikata M, Kageyama R, Shimotohno K, Chiba T. The role of notch signaling in the development of intrahepatic bile ducts. Gastroenterology, 2004; 127:1775–1786

64. Fausto N. Riehle KJ. Mechanisms of liver regeneration and their clinical implications. J Hepatobiliary Pancreat Surg, 2005; 12:181–189

65. Fausto N. Liver regeneration and repair: hepatocytes, progenitor cells, and stem cells. Hepatology, 2004; 39:1477–1487

66. Michalopoulos GK. Liver regeneration: molecular mechanisms of growth control. Faseb J, 1990; 4:176–187

67. Burr AW, Carpenter MR, Hines JE, Gullick WJ, Burt AD. Intrahepatic distribution of transforming growth factor-alpha (TGF alpha) during liver regeneration following carbon tetrachloride-induced necrosis. J Path, 1993; 170:95–100

68. Collier JD, Guo K, Gullick WJ, Bassendine MF, Burt AD. Expression of transforming growth factor-alpha in human hepatocellular carcinoma. Liver, 1993; 13:151–155

69. Hsia CC, Thorgeirsson SS, Tabor E. Expression of hepatitis B surface and core antigens and transforming growth factor-alpha in

'oval cells' of the liver in patients with hepatocellular carcinoma. J Med Virol, 1994; 43:216–221

70. Roskams T, Campos RV, Drucker DJ, Desmet VJ. Reactive human bile ductules express parathyroid hormone-related peptide. Histopathology, 1993; 23:11–19

71. Strain AJ. Transforming growth factor beta: the elusive hepatic chalone? Hepatology, 1992; 16:269–270

72. Nagasue N, Yukaya H, Ogawa Y, Kohno H, Nakamura T. Human liver regeneration after major hepatic resection. A study of normal liver and liver with chronic hepatitis and cirrhosis. Ann Surg, 1987; 206:30–39

73. Van Thiel DH, Gavaler JS, Kam I et al. Rapid growth of an intact human liver transplanted into a recipient larger than the donor. Gastroenterology, 1987; 93:1414–1419

74. Broelsch C, Emond J, Whitington P, Thistlethwaite J, Baker A, Lichtor J. Application of reduced-size liver transplants as split grafts, auxiliary orthotopic grafts, and living-related segmental transplants. Ann Surg, 1990; 212:368–375

75. Strong R, Lynch S, Ong T, Matsunami H, Koido Y, Balderson G. Successful liver transplantation from a living donor to her son. N Engl J Med, 1990; 24:1505–1507

76. Kam I, Lynch S, Svanas G et al. Evidence that host size determines liver size: studies in dogs receiving orthotopic liver transplants. Hepatology, 1987; 7:362–366

77. Wilson JW, Leduc EH. Role of cholangioles in restoration of the liver of the mouse after dietary injury. J Path Bact, 1958; 76:441–449

78. Opie EL. The pathogenesis of tumors of the liver produced by butter yellow. J Exper Med, 1944; 80:231–246

79. Farber E. Similarities in the sequence of early histologic changes induced in the liver of the rat by ethionine, 2-acetylaminofluorene, and 3′-methyl-4-dimethylaminoazobenzene. Cancer Res, 1956; 16:142–148

80. Roskams T, Libbrecht L, Desmet V. Progenitor cells in diseased human liver. Semin Liv Dis, 2003, 23:385–673

81. Grisham JW, Hartroft WS. Morphologic identification by electronmicroscopy of oval cells in experimental hepatic regeneration. Lab Invest, 1961; 10:317–332

82. Lemire JM, Shiojiri N, Fausto N. Oval cell proliferation and the origin of small hepatocytes in liver injury induced by D-galactosamine. Am J Pathol, 1991; 139:535–552

83. Sell S. Is there a liver stem cell? Cancer Res, 1990; 50:3811–3815

84. Dabeva MD, Shafritz DA. Activation, proliferation and differentiation of progenitor cells into hepatocytes in the D-galactosamine model of liver regeneration. Am J Pathol, 1993; 143:1606–1620

85. Sell S. Comparison of liver progenitor cells in human atypical ductular reactions with those seen in experimental models of liver injury. Hepatology, 1998; 27:317–331

86. Sirica AE, Williams TW. Appearance of ductular hepatocytes in rat liver after bile duct ligation and subsequent zone 3 necrosis by carbon tetrachloride. Am J Pathol, 1992; 40:129–136

87. Sirica AE, Gainey TW, Mumaw VR. Ductular hepatocytes: evidence for a bile ductular cell origin in furan-treated rats. Am J Pathol, 1994; 145:375–383

88. Grisham JW. Cell types in long-term propagable cultures of rat liver. Ann N Y Acad Sci, 1980; 349:128–137

89. Paku S, Dezso K, Kopper L, Nagy P. Immunohistochemical analysis of cytokeratin expression in resting and proliferating biliary structures of rat liver. Hepatology, 2005; 42:863–870

90. Germain L, Blouin MJ, Marceau N. Biliary epithelial and hepatocytic cell lineage relationships in embryonic rat liver as determined by the differential expression of cytokeratins, alpha-fetoprotein, albumin, and cell surface-exposed components. Cancer Res, 1988; 48:4909–4918

91. Germain L, Noel M, Gourdeau H, Marceau N. Promotion of growth and differentiation of rat ductular oval cells in primary culture. Cancer Res, 1988; 48:368–378

92. Lenzi R, Liu MH, Tarsetti F et al. Histogenesis of bile duct-like cells proliferating during ethioine hepatocarcinogenesis. Evidence for a biliary epithelial nature of oval cells. Lab Invest, 1992; 66:390–402

93. Petersen B, Zajac VF, Michalopoulos G. Bile ductular damage induced by methylene dianiline inhibits oval cell activation. Am J Pathol, 1997; 151:905–909

94. Fausto N. Liver stem cells. In: Arias IM, Boyer JL, Fausto N, Jacoby WB, Schachter DA, Shafritz DA, eds. The liver: biology and pathobiology, 3rd edn. New York: Raven Press, 1994: pp 1501–1518

95. Germain L, Goyette R, Marceau N. Differential cytokeratin and alpha-fetoprotein expression in morphologically distinct epithelial cells emerging at the early stage of rat hepatocarcinogenesis. Cancer Res, 1985; 45:673–681

96. Hixson DC, Allison JP. Monoclonal antibodies recognizing oval cells induced in the liver of rats by N-2-fluorenylacetamide or ethionine in a choline-deficient diet. Cancer Res, 1985; 45:3750–3760

97. Dunsford HA, Sell S. Production of monoclonal antibodies to preneoplastic liver cell populations induced by chemical carcinogens in rats and to transplantable Morris hepatomas. Cancer Res, 1989; 49:4887–4893

98. Dunsford HA, Karnasuta C, Hunt JM, Sell S. Different lineages of chemically induced hepatocellular carcinoma in rats defined by monoclonal antibodies. Cancer Res, 1989; 49:4894–4900

99. Dabeva MD, Alpini G, Hurston E, Shafritz DA. Models for hepatic progenitor cell activation. Proc Soc Exp Biol Med, 1993; 204:242–252

100. Newsome PN, Hussein MA, Theise ND. Hepatic oval cells: helping redefine a paradigm in stem cell biology. Curr Top Dev Biol, 2004; 61:1–28

101. Evarts RP, Nagy P, Marsden E, Thorgeirsson SS. A precursor-product relationship exists between oval cells and hepatocytes in rat liver. Carcinogenesis, 1987; 8:1737–1740

102. Tatematsu M, Kaku T, Medline A, Farber E. Intestinal metaplasia as a common option of oval cells in relation to cholangiofibrosis in liver of rats exposed to 2-acetylaminofluorene. Lab Invest, 1985; 52:354–362

103. Lee BC, Hendricks JD, Bailey GS. Metaplastic pancreatic cells in liver tumors induced by diethylnitrosamine. Exp Mol Pathol, 1989; 50:104–113

104. Tsao MS, Grisham JW, Nelson KG. Clonal analysis of tumorigenicity and paratumorigenic phenotypes in rat liver epithelial cells chemically transformed in vitro. Cancer Res, 1985; 45:5139–5144

105. De Vos R, Desmet V. Ultrastructural characteristics of novel epithelial cell types identified in human pathological liver specimens with chronic ductular reaction. Am J Pathol, 1992; 140:1441–1450

106. Roskams T, De Vos R, van den Oord JJ, Desmet V. Cells with neuroendocrine features in regenerating human liver. APMIS (Suppl) 1991; 23:32–39

107. Roskams T, Desmet VJ. Parathyroid hormone-related peptide and development of intrahepatic bile ducts in man. Int Hepatol Comm, 1994; 2:121–127

108. Roskams T, De Vos R, Desmet V. 'Undifferentiated progenitor cells' in focal nodular hyperplasia of the liver. Histopathology, 1996; 28:291–299

109. Roskams T, De Vos R, Van Eyken P, Myazaki H, Van Damme B, Desmet V. Hepatic OV-6 expression in human liver disease and rat experiments: evidence for hepatic progenitor cells in man. J Hepatol, 1998; 29:455–463

110. Ruck P, Xiao J-C, Kaiserling E. Small epithelial cells and the histogenesis of hepatoblastoma. Electron microscopic, immunoelectron microscopic and immunohistochemical findings. Am J Pathol, 1996; 148:321–329

111. Hsia CC, Evarts RP, Nakatsukasa H, Marsden ER, Thorgeirsson SS. Occurrence of oval-type cells in hepatitis B virus-associated human hepatocarcinogenesis. Hepatology, 1992; 16:1327–1333

112. Ruck P, Xiao J-C, Pietch T, Schweinitz V, Kaiserling E. Hepatic stem-like cells in hepatoblastoma: expression of cytokeratin 7, albumin and oval cell associated antigens detected by OV-1 and OV-6. Histopathology, 1997; 31:324–329

113. Crosby H, Hubscher S, Joplin R, Kelly D, Strain A. Immunolocalization of OV-6, a putative progenitor cell marker in human fetal and diseased pediatric liver. Hepatology, 1998; 28:980–985

114. Crosby H, Hubscher S, Fabris L et al. Immunolocalization of putative human liver progenitor cells in livers from patients with end-stage primary bilary cirrhosis and sclerosing cholangitis using the monoclonal antibody OV-6. Am J Pathol, 1998; 152:771–779

115. Demetris A, Seaberg E, Wennerberg A, Ionellie J, Michalopoulos G. Ductular reaction after submassive necrosis in humans. Special emphasis on analysis of ductular hepatocytes. Am J Pathol, 1996; 149:439–448

116. Desmet VJ, Van Eyken P, Sciot R. Cytokeratins for probing cell lineage relationships in developing liver. Hepatology, 1990; 12:1249–1251

117. Stosiek P, Kasper M, Karsten U. Expression of cytokeratin 19 during human liver organogenesis. Liver, 1990; 10:59–63

118. Van Eyken P, Desmet VJ. Development of intrahepatic bile ducts, ductular metaplasia of hepatocytes, and cytokeratin patterns in various types of human hepatic neoplasms. In: Sirica AE, ed. The role of cell types in hepatocarcinogenesis. Boca Raton, FL: CRC Press, 1992; pp 227–263

119. Haruna Y, Saito K, Spaulding S, Nalesnik MA, Gerber MA. Identification of bipotential progenitor cells in human liver development. Hepatology, 1996; 23:476–481

120. Roskams T. Progenitor cell involvement in cirrhotic human liver diseases: from controversy to consensus. J Hepatol, 2003 Sep; 39(3):431–434

121. Shiojiri N, Lemire JM, Fausto N. Cell lineages and oval cell progenitors in rat liver development. Cancer Res, 1991; 51:2611–2620

122. Sigal SH, Briss S, Fiorino AS, Reid LM. The liver as a stem cell and lineage system. Am J Physiol, 1992; 263:G139–148

123. Libbrecht L, Desmet V, Van Damme B, Roskams T. Extention of human 'progenitor cells' far into the lobule correlates with parenchymal inflammation in chronic viral hepatitis: can 'progenitor cells' migrate? J Pathol, 2000; 192:373–378

124. Petersen BE, Bowen WC, Patrene KD et al. Bone marrow as a potential source of hepatic oval cells. Science, 1999; 284:1168–1170

125. Theise ND, Nimmakayalu M, Gardner R et al. Liver from bone marrow in humans. Hepatology, 2000; 32:11–16

126. Alison MR, Poulson R, Jeffrey R et al. Hepatocytes from non-hepatic adult stem cells. Nature, 2000; 406:257

127. Grompe M. The role of bone marrow stem cells in liver regeneration. Semin Liver Dis, 2003 Nov; 23(4):363–372

128. Medvinsky A, Smith A. Stem cells: Fusion brings down barriers. Nature, 2003; 422:823–825

129. Vassipoulos G, Wang PR, Russell DW. Transplanted bone marrow regenerates liver by cell fusion. Nature, 2003; 422:901–904

130. Zajicek G, Oren R, Weinreb M Jr. The streaming liver. Liver, 1985; 5:293–300

131. Zajicek G. Hepatocytes and intrahepatic bile duct epithelium originate from a common stem cell. Gastroenterology, 1991; 100:582–583

132. Oren R, Zajicek G, Maaravi Y et al. Methimazole slows down hepatocyte streaming in rats. Dig Dis Sci, 1997; 42:1433–1437

133. Reid LM. Stem cell biology, hormone/matrix synergies and liver differentiation. Curr Opinion Cell Biol, 1990; 2:121–130

134. Reid LM, Fiorino AS, Sigal SH, Brill S, Holst PA. Extracellular matrix gradients in the space of Disse: relevance to liver biology. Hepatology, 1992; 15:1198–1203

135. Grisham JW. Migration of hepatocytes along hepatic plates and stem cell-fed hepatocyte lineages. Am J Pathol, 1994; 144:849–854

136. Iannacone PM. Fractal geometry of mosaic organs: a new interpretation of mosaic pattern. FASEB J, 1990; 1:1508–1512

137. Grisham JW, Hartroft WS. Morphologic identification by electron microscopy of oval cells in experimental degeneration. Lab Invest, 1961; 10:317–332

138. Grisham J. The proliferation of hepatocytes is clonal. Am J Pathol, 1995; 146:773–775

139. Grisham JW. Hepatocyte lineages: of clones, streams, patches, and nodules in the liver. Hepatology, 1997; 25:250–252

140. Bralet MP, Branchereau S, Brechot C, Ferry N. Cell lineage study in the liver using retroviral mediated gene transfer. Evidence against the streaming of hepatocytes in normal liver. Am J Pathol, 1994; 144:896–905

141. Kennedy SC, Rettinger SD, Flye MW, Ponder KP. Experiments in transgenic mice demonstrate that hepatocytes are the source for postnatal liver growth and do not stream. Hepatology, 1995; 22:160–168

142. Ponder KP. Analysis of liver development, regulation, and carcinogenesis by genetic marking studies. FASEB J, 1996; 10:673–682

143. Zajicek G. And the liver streams. Am J Pathol, 1995; 146:772–773

144. Zajicek G. Time dimension in histopathology. Pathol Res Pract, 1992; 188:410–412

145. Hjortso C-H. The topography of the intrahepatic duct systems. Acta Anat, 1951; 11:599–615

146. Couinaud C. Le foie; études anatomiques et chirurgicales. Paris: Masson et Cie, 1957

147. Mays ET II, Mays ET. Are hepatic arteries end arteries? J Anat, 1983; 137:637–644

148. Bismuth H, Aldridge MC, Kunstlinger F. Macroscopic anatomy of the liver. In: McIntyre N, Benhamou JP, Bircher J, Rizzetto M, Rodes J, eds. Oxford textbook of clinical hepatology, vol. 1. Oxford: Oxford University Press, 1991: pp 3–11

149. Menu Y. Modern imaging of the liver and biliary tract. In: McIntyre N, Benhamou JP, Bircher J, Rizzetto M, Rodes J, eds. Oxford textbook of clinical hepatology, vol. 1. Oxford: Oxford University Press, 1991: pp 326–343

150. Ger R. Surgical anatomy of the hepatic venous system. Clin Anat, 1988; 1:15–22

151. Gupta SC, Gupta CD, Arora AK. Subsegmentation of the human liver. J Anat, 1977; 124:413–423

152. Nelson TM, Pollack R, Jonasson O, Abcarian H. Anatomic variants of celiac, superior mesenteric and inferior mesenteric arteries and their clinical relevance. Clin Anat, 1988; 1:75–91

153. Michels NA. Newer anatomy of liver and its variant blood supply and collateral circulation. Am J Surg, 1966; 112:337–347

154. Chang RWH, Quan S-S, Yen WWC. An applied anatomic study of the ostia venae hepaticae and the retrohepatic segment of the inferior vena cava. J Anat, 1989; 164:41–48

155. McCuskey RS. Morphological mechanisms for regulating blood flow through hepatic sinusoids. Liver, 2000; 20:3–7

156. Takasaki S, Hano H. Three dimensional observation of the human hepatic artery (arterial system in the liver). J Hepatol 2001; 34:455–466

157. Kono N, Nakanuma Y. Ultrastructural and immuno-histochemical studies of the intrahepatic peribiliary capillary plexus in normal liver and extrahepatic obstruction in human beings. Hepatology, 1992; 15:411–418

158. Murukami T, Itoshima T, Shimada Y. Peribiliary portal system in the monkey liver as evidenced by the injection replica scanning electron microscopy method. Arch Histol Japan, 1974; 37:245–260

159. Terada T, Nakanuma Y. Development of human peribiliary capillary plexus: a lectin-histochemical and immunohistochemical study. Hepatology, 1993; 18:529–536

160. Tavolini N. The intrahepatic biliary epithelium: an area of growing interest in hepatology. Semin Liv Dis, 1987; 7:280–292

161. Trauner M, Meier PJ, Boyer JL. Molecular regulation of hepatocellular transport systems in cholestasis. J Hepatol, 1999; 31:165–178

162. Rappaport AM. Hepatic blood flow: morphological aspects and physiological regulation. Int Rev Physiol, 1980; 21:1–63

163. Ohtani O, Murakami T, Jones AL. Microcirculation of the liver with special reference to peribiliary portal system. In: Motta PM, Didio LJA, eds. Basic and clinical hepatology. The Hague, Boston, London: Martinus Nijhoff, 1982

164. Yamamoto K, Sherman I, Phillips MJ, Fraser MM. Three dimensional observations of the hepatic arterial termination in rat, hamster and human liver by scanning electron microscopy of microvascular casts. Hepatology, 1985; 5:452–456

165. McCuskey RS. A dynamic and static study of hepatic arterioles and hepatic sphincters. Am J Anat, 1966; 119:455–478

166. Grisham JW, Nopanitaya W, Compagno J. Scanning electron microscopy of the liver: a review of methods and results. In: Popper H, Schaffner F, eds. Progress in liver diseases, vol. V. New York: Grune & Stratton, 1976; pp 1–23

167. Calvo M, Tebar F, Lopes-Iglesias C, Enrich C. Morphologic and functional chracterization of caveolae in rat liver hepatocytes. Hepatology, 2001; 33:1259–1269

168. McCuskey RS, Reilly FD. Hepatic microvasculature: dynamic structure and its regulation. Semin Liv Dis, 1992; 13:1–12

169. McCuskey RS. The hepatic microvascular system. In: Arias IM, Boyer JL, Fausto N, Jakoby WB, Schachter D, Shafritz D, eds. The liver: biology and pathobiology, 3rd edn. New York: Raven Press, 1994: pp 1089–1106

170. Knisely MH, Bloch EH, Warner L. Selective phagocytosis. I. Microscopic observations concerning the regulation of the blood flow through the liver. Kongelige Danske Videnskabernes Selskab Biologiske Skrifter, 1948; 4:1–93

171. Wisse E, McCuskey RS. On the interactions of blood cells with the sinusoidal wall as observed by in vivo microscopy of rat liver. In: Kirn A, Knook DL, Wisse E, eds. Cells of the hepatic sinusoids. Leiden: Kupffer Cell Foundation, 1986; pp 477–482

172. Rockey DC, Raweisiger RA. Endothelin induced contractility of stellate cells from normal and cirrhotic rat liver: implication for regulation of portal pressure and resistance. Hepatology, 1996; 24:233–240

173. McCuskey RS, Ito Y, McCuskey MK, Ekataksin W, Wake K. Morphologic mechanisms for regulating blood flow through hepatic sinusoids: 1998 update and overview. IX Internat Symp Cells of the Hepatic Sinusoid. In: Wisse E, Knook DL, Fraser R, eds. Cells of the hepatic sinusoid, vol. VII. Leiden: Kupffer Cell Foundation, 1999

174. Lautt WW, Greenway CV. Conceptual review of the hepatic vascular bed. Hepatology, 1987; 7:952–963

175. Greenway CV, Lautt WW. Hepatic circulation. In: Schultz SG, Wood JD, Rauner BB, eds. Handbook of physiology—the gastrointestinal system I. American Physiological Society New York: Oxford University Press, 1989; 1:1519–1564

176. Lautt WW, Legare DJ, Ezzat WR. Quantitation of the hepatic arterial buffer response to graded changes in portal blood flow. Gastroenterology, 1990; 98:1024–1098

177. Beresford WA, Henninger JM. A tabular comparative histology of the liver. Arch Histol Jpn, 1986; 49:267–281

178. Rappaport AM. The microcirculatory hepatic unit. Microvasc Res, 1973; 6:218–228

179. Rappaport AM. The microcirculatory acinar concept of normal and pathological hepatic structure. Beitr Pathol, 1976; 157:215–243

180. Rappaport AM. Hepatic blood flow: morphological aspects and physiological regulations. Int Rev Physiol, 1980; 21:1–63

181. Rappaport AM. Physioanatomic considerations. In: Schiff L, Schiff ER, eds. Diseases of the liver, 5th edn. Philadelphia: Lippincott, 1982; pp 1–57

182. Rappaport AM, MacPhee PJ, Fisher MM, Phillips MJ. The scarring of the liver acini (cirrhosis). Virchows Archiv A, 1983; 402:107–137

183. Elias H. A re-examination of the structure of mammalian liver. I. Parenchymal architecture. Am J Anat, 1949; 84:311–334

184. Elias H. A re-examination of the structure of mammalian liver. II. The hepatic lobule and its relation to the vascular and biliary system. Am J Anat, 1949; 85:379–456

185. Grisham JW, Nopanitaya W, Compagno J. Scanning electron microscopy of normal rat liver: the surface structure of its cells and tissue components. Am J Anat, 1976; 144:295–322

186. Motta PM, Muto M, Fujita T. The liver. An atlas of scanning electron microscopy. Tokyo: Igaku-Shoin, 1978

187. Elias H. Anatomy of the liver. In: Rouiller C, ed. The liver: morphology, biochemistry, physiology, vol. 1. New York & London: Academic Press, 1963: p 41

188. Lamers WH, Hilberts A, Furt E et al. Hepatic enzymic zonation: a re-evaluation of the concept of the liver acinus. Hepatology, 1989; 10:72–76

189. Teutsch HF. Regionality of glucose-6-phosphate hydrolysis in the liver lobule of the rat: metabolic heterogeneity of 'portal' and 'septal' sinusoids. Hepatology, 1988; 8:311–317

190. Matsumoto R, Kawakami M. The unit-concept of hepatic parenchyma—a re-examination based on angioarchitectural studies. Acta Pathol Jpn, 1982; 32:285–314

191. Zou Z, Ekataksin W, Wake K. Zonal and regional differences identified from precision mapping of Vitamin A-storing lipid droplets of the hepatic stellate cells in pig liver: a novel concept addressing the intralobular area of heterogeneity. Hepatology, 1998; 27:1098–1108

192. Lamers WH, Geerts WJC, Jonker A, Verbeek J, Wagenaar GTM, Moorman AFM. Quantitative graphical description of porto-central gradients in hepatic gene expression by image analysis. Hepatology, 1997; 26:398–406

193. Quistorff B, Romert P. High zone-selectivity of cell permeabilization following digitonin-pulse perfusion of rat liver. A re-interpretation of microcirculatory zones. Histochemistry, 1989; 92:487–498

194. Ekataksin W, Wake K. Liver units in three dimensions. I. Organization of argyrophylic connective tissue skeleton in porcine liver with particular reference to the 'compound hepatic lobule'. Am J Anat, 1991; 191:113–153

195. Ekataksin W, Zou ZZ, Wake K et al. HMS, hepatic microcirculatory subunits in mammalian species. Intralobular grouping of liver tissue with definition enhanced by drop out sinusoids. In: Wisse E, Knook DL, Wake K, eds. Cells of the hepatic sinusoid. Leiden: Kupffer Cell Foundation, 1995: pp 247–251

196. Ruijter JM, Gieling RG, Markman MM, Hagoort J, Lamers WH. Stereological measurement of porto-central gradients in gene expression in mouse liver. Hepatology, 2004; 39:343–352

197. Takahashi T. Lobular structure of the human liver from the viewpoint of hepatic vascular architecture. Tohoku J Exp Med, 1970; 101:119–140

198. Wünsche A, Preuss F. Pfortaderkörbchen um Leberläppchen beweisen die Läppchengliederung der Leber. Acta Anat, 1986; 125:32–36

199. Quistorff B, Chance B. Redox scanning in the study of metabolic zonation of the liver. In: Thurman RG, Kaufman FC, Jungermann K, eds. Regulation of hepatic metabolism. New York: Plenum Publ. Co, 1986: pp 185–207

200. Bhuncet E, Wake K. The portal lobule in rat liver fibrosis: a re-evaluation of the liver unit. Hepatology, 1998; 27:481–487

201. Teutsch HF, Schuerfeld D, Groezinger E. Three-dimensional reconstruction of parenchymal units in the liver of the rat. Hepatology, 1999; 29:494–505

202. Jones CH. Further enquiries as to the structure, development and function of the liver. Philosophical Transactions of the Royal Society of London Series B: Biological Science, 1853; 143:1–28

203. Beale LS. The minute anatomy of the liver. Med Times Gazette, 1856; 13:82–85

204. Teutsch HF. Regionality of glucose-6-phosphate hydrolysis in the liver lobule of the rat: metabolic heterogeneity of 'portal' and 'septal' sinusoids. Hepatology, 1988; 8:311–317

205. Vidal-Vanaclocha F, ed. Functional heterogeneity of liver tissue: from cell lineage diversity to sublobular compartment-specific pathogenesis. Austin: RG Landes Company, 1997

206. Gebhardt R. Metabolic zonation of the liver: regulation and implications for liver function. Pharmacol Ther, 1992; 53:275–354

207. Gumucio JJ, Bilir BM, Moseley RH, Berkowitz CM. The biology of the liver cell plate. In: Arias IM, Boyer JL, Fausto N, Jakoby WB, Schachter DA, Shafritz DA, eds. The liver: biology and pathobiology, 3rd edn. New York: Raven Press Ltd, 1994: pp 1143–1163

208. Kietzmann T, Jungermann K. Metabolic zonation of liver parenchyma and its short-term and long-term regulation. In: Vidal-Vanaclocha F, ed. Functional heterogeneity of liver tissue. Austin: RG Landes Company, 1997:1–42

209. Christoffels VM, Sassi H, Ruijter JM, Moorman AFM, Grange T, Lamers WH. A mechanistic model for the development and maintenance of portocentral gradients in gene expression in the liver. Hepatology, 1999; 29:1180–1192

210. Notenboom RGE, Lobach H, Moorman AFM, Lamers WH. Gene expression patterns of ammonia-metabolizing enzymes in the developing liver lobule. In: Vidal-Vanaclocha F, ed. Functional heterogeneity of liver tissue. Austin: RG Landes Company, 1997: pp 43–56

211. Wagenaar GTM, Chamuleau RAFM, de Haan JG et al. Experimental evidence that the physiological position of the liver within the circulation is not a major determinant of zonation of gene expression. Hepatology, 1993; 18:1144–1153

212. Vidal-Vanaclocha F. The hepatic sinusoidal endothelium: functional aspects and phenotypic heterogeneity. In: Vidal-Vanaclocha F, ed. Functional heterogeneity of liver tissue. Austin: RG Landes Company, 1997:69–107

213. Wake K. Sinusoidal structure and dynamics. In: Vidal-Vanaclocha F, ed. Functional heterogeneity of liver tissue. Austin: RG Landes Company, 1997: pp 57–67

214. Rømert P, Quistorff B, Behnke O. Histological evaluation of the zonation of colloidal gold uptake by the rat liver. Tissue Cell, 1993; 25:19–32

215. Laskin DL. Role of hepatic macrophages in inflammation and tissue injury. In: Vidal-Vanaclocha F, ed. Functional heterogeneity of liver tissue. Austin: RG Landes Company, 1997: pp 161–176

216. Philips MJ, Satir P. The cytoskeleton of the hepatocyte: organisation, relationships and pathology. In: Arias IM, Jakoby WB, Popper H, Schachter D, Shafritz DA, eds. The liver: biology and pathobiology. New York: Raven Press, 1988: pp 11–27

217. Schachter D. The hepatocyte plasma membrane: organisation and differentiation. In: Arias IM, Jakoby WB, Popper H, Schachter D, Shafritz DA, eds. The liver: biology and pathobiology. New York: Raven Press, 1988: pp 131–140

218. Meier PJ. Transport polarity of hepatocytes. Semin Liver Dis, 1988; 8:293–307

219. Nathanson MH, Boyer JL. Mechanisms and regulation of bile secretion. Hepatology, 1991; 14:551–566

220. Mitic L, Anderson JM. Molecular architecture of tight junctions. Ann Rev Physiol, 1998; 60:121–141

221. Sawada N, Murata M, Kikuchi K et al. Tight junctions and human disease. Med Electron Micros, 2003; 36:157–164

222. Hubbard AL, Wall D, Ma A. Isolation of rat hepatocyte plasma membranes. I. Presence of the three major domains. J Cell Biol, 1983; 96:217–229

223. Wolters H, Spiering M, Gerding A et al. Isolation and characterisation of canalicular and basolateral plasma membrane fractions from human liver. Biochim Biophys Acta, 1991; 1069:61–69

224. Doyle D, Byanover Y, Petill JK. Plasma membrane: biogenesis and turnover. In: Arias IM, Jakoby WB, Popper H, Schachter D, Shafritz DA, eds. The liver: biology and pathobiology. New York: Raven Press, 1988: pp 141–164

225. Scoazec JY. Expression of cell matrix adhesion molecules in the liver and their modulation during fibrosis. J Hepatol, 1995; 22(suppl 2):20–27

226. Armstrong EM, MacSween RNM. Demonstration of bile canaliculi by an immunofluorescent staining technique. Anat Rec, 1973; 177:311–317

227. Seseke FG, Gardemann A, Jungermann K. Signal propagation via gap junctions, a key step in the regulation of liver metabolism by the sympathetic hepatic nerves. FEBS Lett, 1992; 301:265–270

228. Feldmann G. Liver ploidy. J Hepatol, 1992; 16:7–10

229. Adler CP, Ringlage WP, Bohm N. DNA content and cell number in heart and liver of children. Path Res Pract, 1981; 172:25–41

230. Epstein CJ. Cell size, nuclear content and development of polyploidy in mammalian liver. Proc Natl Acad Sci USA, 1967; 57:327–334

231. Wright N, Alison M. The liver. In: Wright N, Alison M, eds. The biology of epithelial cell populations, vol. 2. Oxford: Oxford University Press, 1984: pp 880–956

232. MacDonald RA. 'Lifespan' of liver cells. Arch Int Med, 1981; 107:335–343

233. Lippincott-Schwarz J. The endoplasmic reticulum–Golgi membrane system. In: Arias IM, Boyer JL, Fausto N, Jacoby WB, Schachter DA, Shafritz DA, eds. The Liver, biology and pathobiology, 3rd edn. New York: Raven Press Ltd, 1994: pp 215–228

234. Cardell RR. Action of metabolic hormones on the fine structure of rat liver cells. I. Effects of fasting on the ultrastructure of hepatocytes. Am J Anat, 1971; 131:21–54

235. Philips MJ, Unakar NJ, Doornewaard G, Steiner JW. Glycogen depletion in the new born rat liver. J Ultrastruct Res, 1967; 18:142–165

236. De Pierre JW, Andersson G, Dallner G. Endoplasmic reticulum and Golgi complex. In: Arias IM, Jakoby WB, Popper H, Schachter D, Shafritz DA, eds. The liver: biology and pathobiology. New York: Raven Press, 1988: pp 165–187

237. De Duve. Lysosome concept. In: de Reuck AVJ, Cameron MP, eds. Ciba Foundation Symposium on Lysosomes. Boston: Little Brown, 1963: pp 1–31

238. Bainton DF. The discovery of lysosomes. J Cell Biol, 1981; 91:66s–76s

239. Novikoff AB, Novikoff PM. Lysosomes. In: Arias IM, Jakoby WB, Popper H, Schachter D, Shafritz DA, eds. The liver: biology and pathobiology. New York: Raven Press Ltd, 1988: pp 227–239

240. Crawford J. Role of vesicle-mediated transport pathways in hepatocellular bile secretion. Semin Liver Dis, 1996; 16:169–189

241. Forgac M. Receptor-mediated endocytosis. In: Arias IM, Jakoby WB, Popper H, Schachter D, Shafritz DA, eds. The liver: biology and pathobiology. New York: Raven Press Ltd, 1988: pp 207–225

242. Goltz JS, Wolkoff AW, Novikoff PM, Stockert RJ, Satir P. A role for microtubules in sorting endocytic vesicles in rat hepatocytes. Proc Natl Acad Sci USA, 1992; 89:7026–7030

243. Rouiller C, Bernhard W. 'Microbodies' and the problem of mitochondrial regeneration in liver cells. J Biophys Biochem Cytol, 1956; (suppl) 2:379–358

244. Sotto U, Rapp S, Gorgas K, Just WW. Peroxisomes and lysosomes. In: Le Bouton, ed. Molecular and cell biology of the liver. Boca Raton: CRC Press, 1994: pp 181–262

245. Lazarow PB. Peroxisomes. In: Arias IM, Boyer JL, Fausto N, Jakoby WB, Schachter DA, Shafritz DA, eds. The liver: biology and pathobiology. 3rd edn. New York: Raven Press, 1994: pp 293–307

246. Roels F. Peroxisomes. A personal account. Brussels: VUB Press, 1991

247. Lazarow PB. Peroxisomes. In: Arias IM, Jakoby WB, Popper H, Schachter D, Shafritz DA, eds. The liver: biology and pathobiology. New York: Raven Press Ltd, 1988: pp 241–254

248. Staubli W, Schweizer W, Suter J, Weibel ER. The proliferative response of hepatic peroxisomes of neonatal rats to treatment with SW-13 437 (Nafenopin). J Cell Biol, 1977; 74:665–669

249. Goldfischer SL. Peroxisomal diseases. In: Arias IM, Jakoby WB, Popper H, Schachter D, Shafritz DA, eds. The liver: biology and pathobiology. New York: Raven Press Ltd, 1988: pp 255–267

250. De Creamer D, Pauwels M, Roels F. Peroxisomes in cirrhosis of the human liver: Á cytochemical ultrastructural and quantitative study. Hepatology, 1993; 17:404–410

251. Hinkle PC. Mitochondria. In: Arias IM, Jakoby WB, Popper H, Schachter D, Shafritz DA, eds. The liver: biology and pathobiology. New York: Raven Press Ltd, 1988: pp 269–275

252. Johnson LV, Walsh ML, Chen LB. Localisation of mitochondria in living cells with rhodamine 123. Proc Natl Acad Sci USA, 1980; 77:990–994

253. Lestienne P. Mitochondrial DNA mutations in human disease—a review. Biochemie, 1992; 74:123–130

254. Sokol RJ, Narkewics MR. Mitochondrial hepatopathies. In: Suchy FJ, ed. Liver disease in children. St Louis: Mosby, 1994: pp 888–896

255. Candipan RC, Sjostrand FS. Water movement from intra-cristal spaces in isolated liver mitochondria. J Ultrastruct Res, 1984; 89:249–260

256. Candipan RC, Sjostrand FS. Freeze fracture analysis of isolated liver mitochondria in different metabolic states. J Ultrastruct Res, 1984; 89:274–280

257. Candipan RC, Sjostrand FS. An analysis of the contribution of the preparatory techniques to the appearance of condensed and orthodox conformations of liver mitochondria. J Ultrastruct Res, 1984; 89:281–294

258. Loud AV. A quantitative stereological description of the ultrastructure of normal rat liver parenchymal cells. J Cell Biol, 1968; 37:27–46

259. Feldmann G. The cytoskeleton of the hepatocyte. Structure and functions. J Hepatol, 1989; 8:380–386

260. Lazarides E. Intermediate filaments as mechanical integrators of cellular space. Nature, 1980; 283:249–256

261. Denk H, Franke WW. Cytoskeletal filaments. In: Arias IM, Popper H, Schachter D, Shafritz DA, eds. The liver: pathology and pathobiology. New York: Raven Press Ltd, 1985: pp 57–60

262. Phillips MJ, Oda M. The bile canalicular web. Fed Proc, 1974; 33:626

263. Philips MJ, Oshio C, Miyami M, Katz H, Smith XR. A study of bile canalicular contractions in isolated hepatocytes. Hepatology, 1982; 2:763–768

264. Renaud G, Hamilton RL, Havel RJ. Hepatic metabolism of colloidal gold-low-density lipoprotein complexes in the rat: evidence for bulk excretion of lysosomal contents into bile. Hepatology, 1989; 9:380–392

265. Tsukada N, Ackerley CA, Phillips MJ. The structure and organization of the bile canalicular cytoskeleton with special reference to actin and actin-binding proteins. Hepatology, 1995; 21:1106–1113

266. Desmet VJ, De Vos R. Tight junctions in the liver. In: Popper H, Schaffner F, eds. Progress in liver diseases, vol. 7. New York: Grune and Stratton, 1982: pp 31–50

267. Schroer TA, Sheetz MP. Functions of microtubule-based motors. Ann Rev Physiol, 1991; 53:629–652

268. Kacich RL, Renston RH, Jones AL. Effects of cytochalasin D and colchicine on the uptake, translocation and biliary secretion of horseradish peroxidase and (14G) sodium taurocholate in the rat. Gastroenterology, 1983; 85:385–394

269. Goldman IS, Jones AL, Hradek GT, Huling S. Hepatocyte handling of immunoglobulin A in the rat: the role of microtubules. Gastroenterology, 1983; 85:130–240

270. French SW. Cytoskeleton: intermediate filaments. In: Arias IM, Boyer JL, Fausto N, Jakoby WB, Schachter DA, Shafritz DA, ed. The liver: biology and pathobiology. 3rd edn. New York: Raven Press Ltd, 1994: pp 33–44

271. Furuta K, Ohno S, Gibo Y, Kiyosawa K, Futura S. Three-dimensional ultrastructure of normal rat hepatocytes by quick-freezing and deep-etching method. J Gastroenterol Hepatol, 1992; 7:486–490

272. Wang E, Fischman D, Liem RKH, Sun TT. Intermediate filaments. Ann NY Acad Sci, 1985; 455:32–56

273. Lazarides E. Intermediate filaments as mechanical integrators of cellular space. Nature, 1980; 283:249–256

274. French SW, Cadrin M, Kawahara H, Kachi K. Cytoskeleton. In: Le Bouton AV, ed. Molecular and cell biology of the liver. Boca Raton: CRC Press Inc., 1993: pp 143–180

275. Moll R, Schiller DL, Franke WW. Identification of proteins IT of the intestinal cytoskeleton as a novel type 1 cytokeratin with unusual properties and expression patterns. J Cell Biol, 1990; 3:567–580

276. Van Eyken P, Desmet VJ. Cytokeratins and the liver. Liver, 1993; 13:113–122

277. French SW, Kondo I, Irie T, Ihrig TJ, Benson N, Munn R. Morphologic study of intermediate filaments in rat hepatocytes. Hepatology, 1982; 2:29–38

278. Faa G, van Eyken P, Roskams T et al. Expression of cytokeratin 20 in developing rat liver and in experimental models of ductular and oval cell proliferations. J Hepatol, 1998; pp 29:628–633

279. Frey-Wyssling A. Submicroscopic morphology of protoplasm and its derivatives. New York: Elsevier Publishing Co., 1948

280. Porter KR. Cytomatrix. In: Arias IM, Jakoby WB, Popper H, Schachter D, Shafritz DA, eds. The liver: biology and pathobiology. New York: Raven Press Ltd, 1988: pp 29–45

281. Drochmans P, Wanson JC, Mosselmans R. Isolation and subfractionation on Ficoll gradients of adult rat hepatocytes. J Cell Biol, 1975; 66:1–22

282. Moreno M, Molina H, Amigo L, et al. Hepatic overexpression of caveolins increases bile salt secretion in mice. Hepatology, 2003; 38:1477–1488

283. Schaffner F. Morphologic studies on bile secretion. Am J Dig Dis, 1965; 10:99

284. Desmet VJ. Morphology of bile secretion. In: Gentilini P, Arias IM, Arroyo V, Schrier RW, eds. Liver diseases and renal complications. New York: Raven Press, 1990: pp 93–107

285. Peter J. Meier and B. Stieger, Annu Rev Physiol 2002; 64:635–661

286. Hallbrucker C, Lang F, Gerok W, Häussinger D. Cell swelling increases bile flow and taurocholate excretion into bile in isolated perfused rat liver. Biochem J, 1992; 281:593–595

287. Müller M, Jansen PLM. The secretory function of the liver: new aspects of hepatobiliary transport. J Hepatol, 1998; 28:344–354

288. Arrese M, Ananthananarayanan M, Suchy FJ. Hepatobiliary transport: molecular mechanisms and development of cholestasis. Pediatr Res, 1998; 44:141–147

289. Trauner M, Meier PJ, Boyer JL. Molecular pathogenesis of cholestasis. N Engl J Med, 1998; 339:1217–1227

290. Trauner M, Meier PJ, Boyer JL. Molecular regulation of hepatocellular transport systems in cholestasis. J Hepatol, 1999; 31:165–178

291. Elias HE, Boyer JL. Mechanisms of intrahepatic cholestasis. In: Popper H, Schaffner F, eds. Progress in liver diseases, vol. 6. New York: Grune and Stratton, 1979: pp 457–470

292. Dionne S, Russo P, Tuchweber B, Plaa GL, Yousef IM. Cholic acid and chenodeoxycholic acid transport in the hepatic acinus in rats. Effects of necrosis of zone 3 induced by bromobenzene. Liver, 1990; 10:336–342

293. Buscher HP, Schramm V, MacNelly S, Kurz G, Gerok W. The acinar location of the sodium-independent and the sodium-dependent component of taurocholate uptake. J Hepatol, 1991; 13:169–179

294. Sakisaka S, Harada M, Gondo K, Yoshitake M, Tanikawa K. Tubulovesicular transport of horseradish peroxidase in isolated rat hepatocyte couplets: effects of low temperature, cytochalasin B and bile acids. Hepatology, 1994; 20:1015–1023

295. Sakisaka S, Ng OC, Boyer JL. Tubulovesicular transcytotic pathway in isolated hepatocyte couplets in culture. Effect of colchicine and taurocholate. Gastroenterology, 1988; 95:793–804

296. Goldsmith MA, Huling S, Jones AL. Hepatic handling of bile salts and protein in the rat during intrahepatic cholestasis. Gastroenterology, 1983; 84:978–986

297. Suchy FJ, Balistreri WF, Hung J, Miller P, Garfield SA. Intracellular bile acid transport in rat liver as visualized by electron microscope autoradiography using a bile acid analogue. Am J Physiol, 1983; 245:G681–G689

298. Erlinger S. Regulation of bile secretion. In: Gentilini P, Arias IM, McIntyre N, Rodes J, eds. Cholestasis. Amsterdam: Excerpta Medica, 1994: pp 31–42

299. Lamri Y, Roda A, Dumont M, Feldmann G, Erlinger S. Immunoperoxidase localization of bile salts in rat liver cells. Evidence for a role of the Golgi apparatus in bile salt transport. J Clin Invest, 1988; 82:1173–1182

300. Erlinger S. Intracellular events in bile acid transport by the liver. In: Tavoloni N, Berk PD, eds. Hepatic transport and bile secretion. Physiology and pathophysiology. New York: Raven Press, 1993: pp 467–476

301. Tavoloni N, Boyer JL. Relationship between hepatic metabolism of chlorpromazine and cholestatic effects in the isolated perfused rat liver. J Pharmacol Exp Ther, 1980; 214:269–274

302. Caldwell J. Biological implications of xenobiotic metabolism. In: Arias IM, Jakoby WB, Popper H, Schachter D, Shafritz DA, eds. The liver: biology and pathobiology, 2nd edn. New York: Raven Press, 1988: pp 379–362

303. De Duve C, Wattiaux R. Functions of lysosomes. Annu Rev Physiol, 1966; 28:435–492

304. LaRusso NF, Fowler S. Coordinate secretion of acid hydrolases in rat bile. Hepatocyte excocytosis of lysosomal protein? J Clin Invest, 1979; 64:948–954

305. LaRusso NF, Kost LJ, Carter JA, Barham SS. Triton WR-1339, a lysosomotropic compound, is excreted into bile and alters the biliary excretion of lysosomal enzymes and lipids. Hepatology, 1982; 2:209–215

306. Renaud G, Hamilton RL, Havel RJ. Hepatic metabolism of colloidal gold-low-density lipoprotein complexes in the rat: evidence for bulk excretion of lysosomal contents into bile. Hepatology, 1989; 9:380–392

307. Nakano A, Marks DL, Tietz PS, De Groen PC, LaRusso NF. Quantitative importance of biliary excretion to the turnover of hepatic lysosomal enzymes. Hepatology, 1995; 22:262–289

308. Gross JB, Myers BM, Kost LJ, Kuntz SM, LaRusso NF. Biliary copper excretion by hepatocyte lysosomes in the rat. Major excretory pathway in experimental copper overload. J Clin Invest, 1989; 83:30–39

309. Lévy P, Dumont M, Brissot P, Letreut A, Favier A, Deugnier Y, Erlinger S. Acute infusions of bile salts increase biliary excretion of iron in iron-loaded rats. Gastroenterology, 1991; 101:1673–1679

310. Desmet VJ. Anatomy I: Hepatocyte—Canaliculus. In: Bianchi L, Gerok W, Sickinger K, eds. Liver and bile. Lancaster: MTP Press, 1977:3–31

311. Wanson JC, Drochmans P, Mosselmans R, Ronveaux MF. Adult rat hepatocytes in primary monolayer culture. J Cell Biol, 1977; 74:858–877

312. Desmet VJ. Cholestasis: a problem. In: Csomos G, Thaler H, eds. Clin Hepatol. Berlin: Springer, 1983:299–320

313. Jones AL, Schmucker DL, Renton RH, Murakami T. The architecture of bile secretion. A morphological perspective of physiology. Dig Dis Sci, 1980; 25:609–629

314. Goldsmith MA, Huling S, Jones AL. Hepatic handling of bile salts and protein in the rat during intrahepatic cholestasis. Gastroenterology, 1983; 84:978–986

315. Suchy FJ, Balistreri WF, Hung J, Miller P, Garfield SA. Intracellular bile acid transport in rat liver as visualized by electron microscope autoradiography using a bile acid analogue. Am J Physiol, 1983; 245:G681–G689

316. Jezequel A-M, Bonazzi P, Amabili P, Venturini C, Orlandi F. Changes of the Golgi apparatus induced by diethylmaleate in rat hepatocytes. Hepatology, 1982; 2:856–862

317. Simion FA, Fleischer B, Fleischer S. Two distinct mechanisms for taurocholate uptake in subcellular fractions from rat liver. J Biol Chem, 1984; 259:10874

318. Coleman R, Rahman K. Review. Lipid flow in bile formation. Biochim Biophys Acta, 1992; 1125:113–133

319. Lamri Y, Roda A, Dumont M, Feldmann G, Erlinger S. Immunoperoxidase localization of bile salts in rat liver cells. Evidence for a role of the Golgi apparatus in bile salt transport. J Clin Invest, 1988; 82:1173–1182

320. Sormunen R, Eskelinen S, Lehto V-P. Bile canaliculus formation in cultured HERG2 cells. Lab Invest, 1993; 68:652–662

321. Hardison WGM, Dalle-Molle E, Gosink E, Lowe PJ, Steinbach JH, Yamaguchi Y. Function of rat hepatocyte tight junctions: studies with bile acid infusions. Am J Physiol, 1991; 260:G167–G174

322. Nathanson MH, Boyer JL. Vesicular trafficking in the hepatocyte. In: Arias IM, Boyer JL, Fausto N, Jakoby WB, Schachter DA, Shafritz DA, eds. The Liver: biology and pathobiology. 3rd edn. New York: Raven Press Ltd, 1994: pp 655–664

323. Phillips MJ. Biology and pathobiology of actin in the liver. In: Arias IM, Boyer JL, Fausto N, Jakoby WB, Schachter DA, Shafritz DA, eds. The liver: biology and pathobiology, 3rd edn. New York: Raven Press Ltd, 1994: pp 19–32

324. Gatmaitan ZC, Leveille-Webster CR, Arias IM. The biology of the bile canaliculus. In: Arias IM, Boyer JL, Fausto N, Jakoby WB, Schachter DA, Shafritz DA, eds. The liver: biology and pathobiology, 3rd edn. New York: Raven Press Ltd, 1994: pp 665–675

325. Katsuma Y, Marceau N, Ohta M, French SW. Cytokeratin intermediate filaments of rat hepatocytes: different cytoskeletal domains and their three-dimensional structure. Hepatology, 1988; 8:559–568

326. Sewell RB, Barham SS, Zinsmeister AR, LaRusso NF. Microtubule modulation of biliary excretion of endogenous and exogenous hepatic lysosomal constituents. Am J Physiol, 1984; 246:G8–G15

327. Durand-Schneider AM, Bouanga JC, Feldmann G, Maurice M. Microtubule disruption interferes with the structural and functional integrity of the apical pole in primary cultures of rat hepatocytes. Eur J Cell Biol, 1991; 56:260–268

328. Marks DL, LaRusso NF, McNiven MA. Isolation of the microtubule-vesicle motor kinesin from rat liver: selective inhibition by cholestatic bile acids. Gastroenterology, 1995; 108:824–833

329. Porter KR. Cytomatrix. In: Arias IM, Jakoby WB, Popper H, Schachter D, Shafritz D, eds. The liver: biology and pathobiology, 2nd edn. New York: Raven Press, 1988: pp 29–45

330. Sellinger M, Boyer JL. Physiology of bile secretion and cholestasis. In: Popper H, Schaffner F, eds. Progress in liver diseases, vol. IX. Philadelphia: WB Saunders, 1990:237–260

331. Staehelin LA, Hull BE. Junctions between living cells. Sci Am, 1978; 238:140–152

332. Montesano R, Friend DS, Perrelet A, Orci L. In vivo assembly of tight junctions in fetal rat liver. J Cell Biol, 1975; 67:310–319

333. Hardison WGM, Lowe PJ, Shanahan M. Effect of molecular charge on para- and transcellular access of horseradish peroxidase into rat bile. Hepatology, 1989; 9:866–871

334. Hardison WGM. Hepatocellular tight junctions: role of canalicular permeability in hepatobiliary transport. In: Tavoloni N, Berk PD, eds. Hepatic transport and bile secretion. Physiology and pathophysiology. New York: Raven Press, 1993: pp 571–586

335. Yamaguchi Y, Dalle-Molle E, Hardison WGM. Vasopressin and A23187 stimulate phosphorylation of myosin light chain-1 in isolated rat hepatocytes. Am J Physiol, 1991; 261:G312–G319

336. Rassat J, Robenek H, Themann H. Alterations of tight and gap junctions in mouse hepatocytes following administration of colchicine. Cell Tissue Res, 1982; 223:187–200

337. Kottra G, Frömter E. Functional properties of the paracellular pathway in some leaky epithelia. J Exp Biol, 1983; 106:217–229

338. Meier-Abt PJ. Molecular mechanisms of bile acid transport in hepatocytes. In: Gentilini P, Arias IM, McIntyre N, Rodes J, eds. Cholestasis. Amsterdam: Excerpta Medica, 1994: pp 61–68

339. Cossel L. Die menschliche Leber im Elektronenmikroskop. Jena: Gustav Fischer, 1964

340. Müller O, Mayer D. Die Circadianperiodik der Gallenkanälchen und der Gallesekretion in der Rattenleber. Acta Histochem (suppl.) 1975; XIV:239–246

341. Nemchausky BA, Layden TJ, Boyer JL. Effects of chronic choleretic infusions of bile acids on the membrane of the bile canaliculus: a biochemical and morphologic study. Lab Invest, 1977; 36:259–267

342. Motta P, Fumagalli G. Structure of rat bile canaliculi as revealed by scanning electron microscopy. Anat Rec, 1975; 182:499–513

343. Meier-Abt PJ. Cellular mechanisms of intrahepatic cholestasis. Drugs, 1990; 40:84–97

344. Petzinger E. Canalicular transport: experimental models, morphology requirements and transport processes. In: Siegers CP, Watkins JB, III, eds. Biliary excretion of drugs and other chemicals. Progress in Pharmacology and clinical pharmacology, vol. 8. Stuttgart: Gustaf Fischer, 1991: pp 49–87

345. Jacquemin E, Hadchouel M. Review. Genetic basis of progressive familial intrahepatic cholestasis. J Hepatol, 1999; 31:377–381

346. Lin SH, Gulic O, Flanagan D, Hixson D. Immunochemical characterization of two isoforms of rat liver ecto-ATPase which show structural identity to cell CAM 105. Biochem J, 1991; 278:155–161

347. Mowery J, Hixson DC. Detection of cell-CAM 105 in the pericanalicular domain of the rat hepatocyte plasma membrane. Hepatology, 1991; 13:47–56

348. Meier-Abt PJ. Hepatocellular transport systems involved in bile formation. Hepatol Rapid Lit Rev, 1997; 27(6):XI–XV

349. Kamisako T, Leier I, Cui Y, König J, Buchholz U, Hummel-Eisenbeiss J, Keppler D. Transport of monoglucuronosyl and bisglucuronosyl bilirubin by recombinant human and rat Multidrug Resistance Protein 2. Hepatology, 1999; 30:485–490

350. Daems WT, Wisse E, Brederoo P. Electron microscopy of the vacuolar apparatus. In: Dingle JT, Fell HB, eds. Lysosomes in biology and pathology, vol. I. Amsterdam: North Holland, 1969: pp 64–112

351. Miettinen A, Linder E. Membrane antigens shared by renal proximal tubules and other epithelia associated with absorption and excretion. Clin Exp Immunol, 1976; 23:568–577

352. Godfrey PP, Warner MJ, Coleman R. Enzymes and proteins in bile. Biochem J, 1981; 196:11–16

353. Hatoff DE, Hardison WGM. Bile acid-dependent secretion of alkaline phosphatase in rat bile. Hepatology, 1982; 2:433–439

354. Hirata E, Inoue M, Morino Y. Mechanism of biliary secretion of membranous enzymes: bile acids are important factors for biliary occurrence of gamma-glutamyltransferase and other hydrolases. J Biochem, 1984; 96:289–297

355. Mullock BM, Hinton RH. Transport of proteins from blood to bile. Trends Biochem Sci, 1981; 6:188–190

356. Sztul ES, Howell KE, Palade GE. Intracellular and transcellular transport of secretory component and albumin in rat hepatocytes. J Cell Biol, 1983; 97:1582–1591

357. Phillips MJ, Oda M, Mak E, Edwards V, Yousef I, Fisher MM. The bile canalicular network in vitro. J Ultrastruct Res, 1976; 57:163–167

358. Phillips MJ, Poucell S. Cholestasis: surgical pathology, mechanisms and new concepts. In: Farber E, Phillips MJ, Kaufman N, eds. Pathogenesis of liver diseases. Monograph no. 28 edn, Baltimore: Williams and Wilkins, 1987: pp 65–94

359. Watanabe S, Phillips MJ. Ca^{2+} causes active contraction of bile canaliculi: direct evidence from microinjection studies. Proc Natl Acad Sci USA, 1984; 81:6164–6168

360. Gumucio JJ, Miller DL. Zonal hepatic function: solute–hepatocyte interactions within the liver acinus. In: Popper H, Schaffner F, eds. Progress in liver diseases, vol. VII. New York: Grune & Stratton, 1982:17–30

361. Javitt NB. Hepatic bile formation (first of two parts). N Engl J Med, 1976; 295:1464–1468

362. Gumucio DL, Gumucio JJ, Wilson JAP et al. Albumin influences sulfobromophthalein transport by hepatocytes of each acinar zone. Am J Physiol, 1984; 246:G86–G95

363. Jones EA, Vierling JM, Steer CJ, Reichen J. Cell surface receptors in the liver. In: Popper H, Schaffner F, eds. Progress in liver diseases, Vol. VI. New York: Grune & Stratton, 1979: p 43

364. Metz W, Forssmann WG. Comparative morphology of liver innervation. In: Popper H, Bianchi L, Gudat F, Reutter W, eds. Communications of liver cells. Lancaster: MTP Press, 1980:121–127

365. Desmet VJ, Roskams T, De Vos R. Normal Anatomy in Gallbladder and Bile Ducts. In: LaRusso N, ed. Vol. 6 of the series Gastroenterology and Hepatology: The comprehensive visual reference current medicine. Philadelphia, 1997: pp 1–29

366. Ludwig J, Ritmans EL, LaRusso NF, Sheedy PF, Zumpe G. Anatomy of the human biliary system studied by quantitative computer-aided three-dimensional imaging techniques. Hepatology, 1998; 27:893–899

367. Ishida F, Terada T, Nakanuma Y. Histologic and scanning electron microscopic observations of intrahepatic peribiliary glands in normal human livers. Lab Invest, 1989; 60:260–265

368. Nakanuma Y, Katayanagi K, Terada T, Saito K. Intrahepatic peribiliary glands of humans. I. Anatomy, development and presumed functions. J Gastroenterol Hepatol, 1994; 9:75–79

369. Nakanuma Y, Sasaki M, Terada T, Harada K. Intrahepatic peribiliary glands of humans. II. Pathological spectrum. J Gastroenterol Hepatol, 1994; 9:80–86

370. Yamamoto K, Fisher MM, Phillips MJ. Hilar biliary plexus in human liver. Lab Invest, 1985; 52:103–106

371. Ros JE, Libbrecht L, Geuken M, Jansen PL, Roskams TA. High expression of MDR1, MRP1, and MRP3 in the hepatic progenitor cell compartment and hepatocytes in severe human liver disease. J Pathol, 2003 Aug; 200:553–560

372. Sirica AE. Biology of biliary epithelial cells. In: Boyer JL, Ockner RK, eds. Progress in liver diseases, vol. X. Philadelphia: WB Saunders, 1992: pp 63–87

373. Tarsetti F, Lenzen R, Salvi R, Schuler E, Dembitzer R, Tavoloni N. Biology and pathobiology of intrahepatic biliary epithelium. In: Tavoloni N, Berk PD, eds. Hepatic transport and bile secretion: physiology and pathophysiology. New York: Raven Press Ltd, 1993: pp 619–635

374. Van Eyken P, Desmet VJ. Bile duct cells. In: LeBouton AV, ed. Molecular and cell biology of the liver. Boca Raton: CRC Press, 1993: pp 475–524

375. Alpini G, Phillips JO, La Russo NF. The biology of biliary epithelia. In: Arias IM, Boyer JL, Fausto N, Jakoby WB, Schachter DA, Shafritz DA, eds. The liver: biology and pathobiology, 3rd edn. New York: Raven Press, 1994: pp 623–653

376. Baiocchi L, Le Sage G, Glaser S, Alpini G. Regulation of cholangiocyte bile secretion. J Hepatol, 1999; 31:179–191

377. Rous P, McMaster PD. Physiological causes for the varied character of stasis bile. J Exp Med, 1921; 24:75–95

378. Jezequel AM, Benedetti A, Bassotti C, Rapino K, Orlandi F. Subcellular features of the biliary epithelium in health and disease. In: Alvaro D, Benedetti A, Stazzabosco M, eds. Vanishing bile duct syndrome–pathophysiology and treatment. Dordrecht: Kluwer Academic Publishers, 1997: pp 13–24

379. Alpini G, Lenzi R, Zhai W-R et al. Bile secretory function of intrahepatic biliary epithelium in the rat. Am J Physiol, 1989; 257: G124–G133

380. Sugiura H, Nakanuma Y. Secretory components and immunoglobulins in the intrahepatic biliary tree and peribiliary glands in normal livers and hepatolithiasis. Gastroenterol Jpn, 1989; 24:308–314

381. Yoon YB, Hogey LR, Hofmann AF et al. Effect of side chain shortening on the physiological properties of bile acids: hepatic transport and effect on biliary reaction of 23 ursodeoxycholate in rodents. Gastroenterology, 1986; 90:837–852

382. Lamri Y, Erlinger S, Dumont M, Roda A, Feldmann G. Immunoperoxidase localization of ursodeoxycholic acid in rat biliary epithelial cells. Evidence for a cholehepatic circulation. Liver, 1992; 12:351–354

383. Hofmann AF, Yeh H-Z, Schteingart CD, Bolder U, Ton-Nu H-T, Hagey LR. The cholehepatic circulation of organic anions: a decade of progress. In: Alvaro D, Benedetti A, Strazzabosco M, eds. Vanishing bile duct syndrome–pathophysiology and treatment, pp. 90–103. Dordrecht: Kluwer Academic Publishers, 1997

384. Kurumaya H, Nakanuma Y, Ohta G. Endocrine cells in the intrahepatic biliary tree in normal livers and hepatolithiasis. Arch Pathol Lab Med, 1989; 113:143–147

385. Terada T, Nakanuma Y. Immunohistochemical demonstration of pancreatic α-amylase and trypsin in intrahepatic bile ducts and peribiliary glands. Hepatology, 1991; 14:1129–1135

386. Desmet VJ. Morphology and development of the hepatobiliary system. In: Bock KW, Matern S, Gerok W, Schmid R, eds. Hepatic metabolism and disposition of endo- and xenobiotics. Dordrecht: Kluwer Academic Publishers, 1991:3–17

387. Boyer JL. Vanishing bile duct syndrome—from bench to bedside. In: Alvaro D, Benedetti A, Strazzabosco M, eds. Vanishing bile duct syndrome–pathophysiology and treatment. Dordrecht: Kluwer Academic Publishers, 1997:240–245

388. Wisse E, De Leeuw AM. Structural elements determining transport and exchange processes in the liver. In: Davis SS, Illum L, McVie JG, Tomlinson E, eds. Microspheres and drug therapy. Pharmaceutical, immunological and medical aspects. Amsterdam: Elsevier, 1984: pp 1–23

389. Burt AD, Le Bail B, Balabaud C, Bioulac-Sage P. Morphologic investigation of sinusoidal cells. Semin Liv Dis, 1993; 13:21–38

390. Arias IM. The biology of hepatic endothelial fenestrae. In: Schaffner F, Popper H, eds. Progress in liver diseases, Vol IX. Philadelphia: WB Saunders, 1990: pp 11–26

391. Mak KM, Lieber CS. Alterations in endothelial fenestration in liver sinusoids of baboons fed alcohol. A scanning electron microscopic study. Hepatology, 1984; 4:386–391

392. McGuire RF, Bissell DM, Boyles J, Roll FJ. Role of extracellular matrix in regulating fenestrations of endothelial cells isolated from normal rat liver. Hepatology, 1992; 15:989–997

393. Wisse E, De Zanger RB, Charels K, Van der Smissen M, McCuskey RS. The liver sieve: considerations concerning the structure and function of endothelial fenestrae, the sinusoidal wall and the space of Disse. Hepatology, 1985; 5:683–689

394. Petrovic LM, Burroughs A, Scheuer PJ. Hepatic sinusoidal endothelium: Ulex lectin binding. Histopathology, 1989; 14:233

395. Babbs C, Haboubi NY, Mellor JM et al. Endothelial cell transformation in primary biliary cirrhosis: a morphological and biochemical study. Hepatology, 1990; 11:723–729

396. Scoazec J-Y, Feldmann G. In situ phenotyping study of endothelial cells of the human hepatic sinusoid: results and functional implications. Hepatology, 1991; 14:789–797

397. Volpes R, Van den Oord JJ, Desmet VJ. Immunohisto-chemical study of adhesion molecules in liver inflammation. Hepatology, 1990; 12:65–69

398. Muro H, Shirasawa H, Maeda M, Nakamura S. Fc receptors of liver sinusoidal endothelium in normal rats and humans: a histologic study with soluble immune complexes. Gastroenterology, 1987; 93:1078–1095

399. Vidal-Vanalocha F, Rocha M, Asumendi A, Barbera-Guillem E. Isolation and enrichment of two sublobular compartment-specific endothelial cell subpopulations from liver sinusoids. Hepatology, 1993; 18:328–339

400. Barbera-Guillem E, Rocha M, Alvarez A, Vidal-Vanalocha F. Differences in the lectin-binding patterns of the periportal and perivenous endothelial domains in the liver sinusoids. Hepatology, 1991; 14:131–139

401. Eskild W, Kindberg GM, Smedsrod B, Blomhoff R, Norum KR. Intracellular transport of formaldehyde-treated serum albumin in liver endothelial cells after uptake via scavenger receptor. Biochem J, 1989; 258:511–520

402. Reider H, Meyer zum Buschenfelde KH, Ramadori G. Functional spectrum of sinusoidal endothelial liver cells. Filtration, endocytosis, synthetic capacities and intercellular communication. J Hepatol, 1992; 15:237–250

403. Iwamura S, Enzan H, Saibora T, Onishi S, Yamamoto Y. Appearance of sinusoidal inclusion-containing endothelial cells in liver disease. Hepatology, 1994; 20:604–610

404. Iwamura S, Enzan H, Saibora T, Onishi S, Yamamoto Y. Hepatic sinusoidal endothelial cells can store and metabolize serum immunoglobulins. Hepatology, 1995; 22:456–461

405. McGary CT, Raja RH, Weigel PH. Endocytosis of hyaluronic acid by rat liver endothelial cells. Evidence for receptor recycling. Biochem J, 1989; 257:875–884

406. Rockey D. The cellular pathogenesis of portal hypertension: stellate cell contractility, endothelin and nitric oxide. Hepatology, 1997; 25:2–5

407. Shah V, Garcia-Gardena G, Sessa WC, Groszmann RJ. The hepatic circulation in health and disease: report of a single-topic symposium. Hepatology, 1998; 27:279–288

408. Motta P, Porter K. Structure of rat liver sinusoids and associated tissue spaces as revealed by scanning electron microscopy. Cell Tissue Res, 1974; 148:111–125

409. Kim T-H, Mars WM, Stolz DB, Petersen BE, Michalopoulos GK. Extracellular matrix remodelling at the early stages of liver regeneration in the rat. Hepatology, 1996; 26:896–904

410. Arthur MJP. Matrix degradation in liver: a role in injury and repair. Hepatology, 1997; 26:1069–1071

411. Ashkenaz J, Muschler J, Bissell MJ. The extracellular matrix in epithelial biology: shared molecules and common themes in distant phyla. Dev Biol, 1996; 180:433–444

412. Martinez-Hernandez A, Amenta PS. Morphology, localization and origin of the hepatic extracellular matrix. In: Sern M, Reid L, eds. Extracellular matrix: chemistry, biology, pathology. New York: Marcell Dekker, 1993

413. Hughes RC, Stamatoglou SC. Adhesive interactions and the metabolic activity of hepatocytes. J Cell Sci, 1987; 8(suppl):273–291

414. Johanssen S, Forsberg E, Lundgren B. Comparison of fibronectin receptors from rat hepatocytes and fibroblasts. J Biol Chem, 1987; 262:7819–7824

415. Gullberg D, Terracio L, Borg TK, Rubin K. Identification of integrin-like matrix receptors with affinity for interstitial collagens. J Biol Chem, 1989; 264:12686–12694

416. Clement B, Segui-Real B, Savagner P et al. Hepatocyte attachment to laminin is mediated through multiple receptors. J Cell Biol, 1990; 110:185–192

417. Maher JJ, Bissell DM, Zern M, Reid L, eds. The extracellular matrix and liver disease. In: Cell matrix interactions in liver. New York: Marcell Dekker, 1992

418. Kirch HC, Lammers M, Gresssner AM. Binding of chondroitin sulfate, dermatan sulfate and fat-storing cell-derived proteoglycans to rat hepatocytes. Int J Biochem, 1987; 19:1119–1126

419. Dziadek M, Fujiwara S, Paulsson M et al. Immunological characterization of basement membrane types of heparan sulfate proteoglycan. EMBO J, 1985; 4:1463–1468

420. Andres JL, Stanley K, Cheifetz S, Massague J. Membrane anchored and soluble forms of betaglucan, a polymorphic proteoglycan that binds transforming growth factor-beta. J Cell Biol, 1989; 109:3137–3145

421. Elenius K, Salmvirta, Inki P et al. Binding of human syndecan to extracellular matrix proteins. J Biol Chem, 1990; 265:17837–17843

422. Ito T. Cytological studies on stellate cells of Kupffer and fat-storing cells in the capillary wall of the human liver. Acta Anat Nippon, 1951; 26:2–42

423. Aterman K. The parasinusoidal cells of the liver: a historical account. Histochem J, 1986; 18:279–305

424. Ramadori G. The stellate cell (Ito-cell, fat storing cell, lipocyte, perisinusoidal cell) of the liver. New insights into an intriguing cell. Virchow Archiv (B) Cell Pathol, 1991; 61:147–158

425. Letter. Hepatic stellate cell nomenclature. Hepatology, 1996; 13:193

426. Ratziu V, Friedman SL. Pathobiology of hepatic stellate cells. In: Vidal-Vanaclocha F, ed. Functional heterogeneity of liver tissue. RG Landes Company: Austin, 1997: pp 133–160

427. Burt AD. Pathobiology of hepatic stellate cells. J Gastroenterol, 1999; 34:299–304

428. Marra F. Hepatic stellate cells and the regulation of liver inflammation. J Hepatol, 1999; 31:1120–1130

429. Friedman S. Stellate cells: a moving target in hepatic fibrogenesis. Hepatology 2004; 40:1041–1043

430. Senoo H. Structure and function of hepatic stellate cells. Med Electron Microsc, 2004; 37:3–15

431. Balabaud C, Biolac-Sage P, Demouliere A. The role of hepatic stellate cells in liver regeneration. J Hepatol 2004; 40: 1023–1026

432. Bachem MG, Schneider E, Gross H et al. Identification, culture and characterisation of pancreatic stellate cells in rats and humans. Gastroenterology, 1998; 115:421–432

433. Nagy NE, Holven KB, Roos N et al. Storage of vitamin A in extrahepatic stellate cells in normal rats. J Lipid Res, 1997; 38:645–658

434. Bronfenmajer S, Schaffner F, Popper H. Fat-storing cells (lipocytes) in human liver. Arch Pathol Lab Med, 1966; 82:447–453

435. Wake K. Perisinusoidal stellate cells (fat-storing cells, interstitial cells, lipocytes), their related structure in and around the liver sinusoids and vitamin A-storing cells in extrahepatic organs. Int Rev Cytol, 1980; 66:303–353

436. Cameron RG, Neuman MG, Blendis LM. Multivesicular stellate cells in primary biliary cirrhosis. Hepatology, 1997; 26:550–553

437. Yokoi Y, Namihisa T, Kuroda H et al. Immunocytochemical detection of desmin in fat-storing cells (Ito cells). Hepatology, 1984; 4:709–714

438. Burt AD, Robertson JH, Hair J, MacSween RNM. Desmin-containing stellate cells in rat liver; distribution in normal animals and response to experimental acute liver injury. J Pathol, 1986; 150:29–35

439. Ballardini G, Fallani M, Biagini G, Bianchi FB, Pisi E. Desmin and actin in the identification of Ito cells and in monitoring their evolution to myofibroblasts in experimental liver fibrosis. Virchows Arch (B) Cell Pathol Incl Mol Pathol, 1988; 56:45–49

440. Takase S, Leo MA, Nouchi T, Lieber CS. Desmin distinguishes cultured fat-storing cells from myofibroblasts, smooth muscle cells and fibroblasts in the rat. J Hepatol, 1988; 6:267–276

441. Schmitt Graff A, Kruger S, Bochard F, Gabbiani G, Denk H. Modulation of alpha smooth muscle actin and desmin expression in perisinusoidal cells of normal and diseased human livers. Am J Pathol, 1991; 138:1233–1242

442. Ballardini G, Groff P, Badiali de Giorgi L, Schuppan D, Bianchi FB. Ito cell heterogeneity: desmin-negative Ito cells in normal rat liver. Hepatology, 1994; 19:440–446

443. Aoki T, Hagiawara H, Fujimoto T. Peculiar distribution of fodrin in fat-storing cells. Exp Cell Res, 1997; 234:313–320

444. Neubauer K, Knittel T, Aursch S, Fellmer P, Ramadori G. Glial fibrillary acidic protein—a cell type specific marker for Ito cells in vivo and in vitro. J Hepatol, 1996; 24:719–730

445. Niki T, De Bleser PJ, Xu G, Van Den Berg K, Wisse E, Geerts A. Comparison of glial fibrillary acidic protein and desmin staining

in normal and CC14-induced fibrotic rat livers. Hepatology, 1996; 23:1538–1545

446. Niki T, Pekny M, Hellemans K, Bleser PD, Berg KV, Vaeyens F, Quartier E, Schuit F, Geerts A. Class VI intermediate filament protein nestin is induced during activation of rat hepatic stellate cells. Hepatology, 1999; 29:50–52

447. Nakatani K, Seki S, Kawada N, Kobayashi K, Kaneda K. Expression of neural cell adhesion molecule (N-CAM) in perisinusoidal stellate cells of the human liver. Cell Tissue Res, 1996; 283:159–165

448. Knittel T, Aurisch S, Neubauer K, Eichhorst S, Ramadori G. Cell-type specific expression of neural cell adhesion molecule (N-CAM) in Ito cells of rat liver. Up-regulation during in vitro activation and in hepatic tissue repair. Am J Pathol, 1996; 149:449–462

449. Cassiman D, van Pelt J, De Vos R, Van Lommel F, Desmet V, Yap P, Roskams T. Synaptophysin: a novel marker for human and rat hepatic stellate cells. Am J Pathol, 1999; 155:1831–1839

450. Oakley F, Trim N, Constandinou CM et al. Hepatocytes express nerve growth factor during liver injury: evidence for paracrine regulation of hepatic stellate cell apoptosis. Am J Pathol 2003; 163: 1849–1858

451. Geerts A. On the origin of stellate cells: mesodermal, endodermal or neuro-ectodermal? J Hepatol, 2004; 40:331–334

452. Forbes SJ, Russo FP, Rey V et al. A significant proportion of myofibroblasts are of bone marrow origin in human liver fibrosis. Gastroenterology, 2004; 126:955–963

453. Burt AD. Cellular and molecular aspects of hepatic fibrosis. J Pathol, 1993; 170:105–114

454. Ramadori G. The stellate cell (Ito-cell, fat storing cell, lipocyte, perisinusoidal cell) of the liver. New insights into an intriguing cell. Virchows Archiv (B), 1991; 61:147–158

455. Blomhoff R, Wake K. Perisinusoidal stellate cells of the liver: important roles in retinol metabolism and fibrosis. FASEB J, 1991; 5:271–277

456. Hendriks HFJ, Bosma A, Brouwer A. Fat-storing cells: hyper- and hypovitaminosis A and the relationships with liver fibrosis. Semin Liv Dis, 1993; 13:72–80

457. Rockey DC, Chung JJ. Inducible nitric oxide synthase in rat hepatic lipocytes and the effect of nitric oxide on lipocyte contractility. J Clin Invest, 1995; 95:1199–1206

458. Zhang JX, Pegoli WJ, Cemens MG. Endothelin-1 induces direct constriction of hepatic sinusoids. Am J Physiol, 1994; 266: G624–G632

459. Mathew J, Geerts A, Burt AD. Pathobiology of hepatic stellate cells. Hepatogastroenterology, 1996; 43:72–91

460. Schirmacher P, Geerts A, Pietrangelo A, Dienes HP, Rogler CE. Hepatocyte growth factor/hepatopoietin A is expressed in fat-storing cells from rat liver but not myofibroblast-like cells derived from fat-storing cells. Hepatology, 1992; 15:5–11

461. Skrtic S, Wallenius V, Ekberg S, Brenzel A, Gressner AM, Jansson JO. Insulin-like growth factors stimulate expression of hepatocyte growth factor but not transforming growth factor beta 1 in cultured hepatic stellate cells. Endocrinology, 1997; 138:4683–4689

462. Winwood PJ, Arthur MJP. Kupffer cells: their activation and role in animal models of liver injury and human liver disease. Semin Liv Dis, 1993; 13:50–59

463. Motta PM. A scanning electron microscopic study of the rat liver sinusoid. Cell Tissue Res, 1975; 164:371–385

464. Wake K, Decker K, Kirn A et al. Cell biology and kinetics of Kupffer cells in the liver. Int Rev Cytol, 1990; 118:173–229

465. Te Koppele JM, Thurman RG. Phagocytosis by Kupffer cells predominates in pericentral region of the liver lobule. Am J Physiol, 1990; 259:G814–G821

466. MacPhee PJ, Schmidt EE, Groom AC. Evidence for Kupffer cell migration along liver sinusoids, from high-resolution in vivo microscopy. Am J Physiol, 1992; 263:G17–G23

467. Lumsden A, Henderson J, Kutner M. Endotoxin levels measured by a chromogenic assay in portal, hepatic and peripheral venous blood in patients with cirrhosis. Hepatology, 1988; 8:232–236

468. Mosmann TR. Properties and functions of interleukin-10. Adv Immunol, 1994; 56:1–26

469. Knolle P, Protzer U, Uhrig A, Rose-John S, Meyer zum Büschenfelde K-H, Gerken G. Differential regulation of endotoxin induced IL-6 production in sinusoidal endothelial cells and Kupffer cells. Clin Exp Immunol, 1997; 107:555–563

470. Knolle PA, Uhrig A, Protzer U et al. Interleukin-10 expression is autoregulated at the transcriptional level in human and murine Kupffer cells. Hepatology, 1998; 27:93–99

471. Andus T, Bauer J, Gerok W. Effects of cytokines on the liver. Hepatology, 1991; 13:364–377

472. Barbatis C, Kelly P, Greveson J, Heryet A, McGee JO'D. Immunocytochemical analysis of HLA class II (DR)

antigens in liver disease in man. J Clin Pathol, 1987; 40:879–884

473. Rogoff TM, Lipsky PE. Role of the Kupffer cells in local and systemic immune responses. Gastroenterology, 1981; 80: 854–860

474. Rifai A, Mannik M. Clearance of circulatory IgA immune complexes is mediated by a specific receptor on Kupffer cells in mice. J Exp Med, 1984; 160:125–137

475. Gale RP, Sparkes RS, Golde DW. Bone marrow origin of hepatic macrophages (Kupffer cells) in humans. Science, 1978; 201:937–938

476. Bouwens L, Baekeland M, Wisse E. Cytokinetic analysis of the expanding Kupffer cell population in rat liver. Cell Tissue Kin, 1986; 19:217–226

477. Johnson SJ, Hines JE, Burt AD. Macrophage and peri-sinusoidal cell kinetics in acute liver injury. J Pathol, 1992; 351–358

478. Naito M, Takahashi K, Ohno H, Nishikawa SI. Yolk sac macrophages—a possible Kupffer cell precursor in the fetal mouse liver. In: Wisse E, Knook DL, Decker K, eds. Cells of the Hepatic Sinusoid. Rijswijk: Kupffer Cell Foundation, 1989; 2:419–420

479. Wisse E, van't Noordende JM, van der Meulen J, Daems WTh. The pit cell: description of a new cell type occurring in rat liver and peripheral blood. Cell Tiss Res, 1976; 173:423–435

480. Winnock M, Lafon M-E, Boulard A et al. Characterisation of liver-associated natural killer cells in patients with liver tumours. Hepatology, 1991; 13:676–682

481. Winnock M, Barcina MG, Lukomska B, Bioulac-Sage P, Balabaud C. Liver-associated lymphocytes: role in tumor defense. Semin Liv Dis, 1993; 13:81–92

482. Bouwens L, Remels L, Baekeland M et al. Large granular lymphocytes or 'pit cells' from rat liver: isolation, ultrastructural characterisation and natural killer activity. Eur J Immunol, 1987; 17:37–42

483. Doherty DG, O'Farrelly C. Innate and adaptive lymphoid cells in the human liver. Immunol Rev, 2000; 174:5–20

484. Norris S, Collins C, Doherty DG et al. Resident human hepatic lymphocytes are phenotypically different from circulating lymphocytes. J Hepatol, 1998; 28:84–90

485. Trinchieri G. Biology of natural killer cells. Adv Immunol, 1989; 47:187–376

486. Brown MG, Scalzo AA, Matsumoto K, Yokoyama WM. The natural killer gene complex: a generic basis for understanding natural killer cell function and innate immunity. Immunol Rev, 1997; 155:53–66

487. Lanler II, Corliss B, Phillips JH. Arousal and inhibition of human NK cells. Immunol Rev, 1997; 155:145–154

488. Bancroft GJ. The role of natural killer cells in innate resistance to infection. Curr Opin Immunol, 1993; 5:503–510

489. Shimizu Y, Iwatsuki S, Herberman RB, Whiteside TL. Clonal analysis of tumor-infiltrating lymphocytes from human primary and metastatic liver tumors. Int J Cancer, 1990; 46:878–883

490. Winnock M, Garcia-Barcina M, Huet S et al. Functional characterisation of liver-associated lymphocytes in patients with liver metastasis. Gastroenterology, 1993; 105:1152–1158

491. Modlin RL, Pirmez C, Hoffman FM et al. Lymphocytes bearing antigen-specific γδ T-cell receptors accumulate in human infectious disease lesions. Nature, 1989; 339:544–548

492. Norris S, Doherty DG, Collins C. Natural T cells in the human liver: cytotoxic lymphocytes with dual T cell and natural killer cell phenotype and function are phenotypically heterogeneous and include V24-JQ and T cell receptor bearing cells. Hum Immunol, 1999; 60:20–31

493. Rojkind M. Extracellular Matrix. In: Arias IM, Jakoby WB, Popper H, Schachter D, Shafritz DA eds. The liver: biology and pathobiology. New York: Raven Press Ltd, 1988: pp 707–716

494. Schuppan D. Structure of the extracellular matrix in normal and fibrotic liver: collagens and glycoproteins. Semin Liv Dis, 1990; 10:1–10

495. Friedman SL. Cellular sources of collagen and regulation of collagen production in liver. Semin Liv Dis, 1990; 10:20–29

496. Musso O, Rehn M, Saarela J et al. Collagen XVIII is localized in sinusoids and basement membrane zones and expressed by hepatocytes and activated stellate cells in fibrotic human liver. Hepatology, 1998; 28:98–107

497. Pares A, Caballera J. Metabolism of collagen and other extracellular proteins. In: McIntyre N, Benhamou J-P, Bircher J, Rizzetto M, Rodes J, eds. Oxford textbook of clinical hepatology, vol. 1. Oxford, New York, Tokyo: Oxford University Press, 1991: pp 199–211

498. Bircher N, Robinson G, Farmer S. Effects of extracellular matrix on hepatocyte growth and gene expression: implications for hepatic regulation and the repair of liver injury. Semin Liv Dis, 1990; 10:11–19

499. Murat AI, Sattler CA, Sattler GL, Pitot HC. Reestablishment of cell polarity of rat hepatocytes in primary culture. Hepatology, 1993; 18:198–205

500. Martinez-Hernandez A, Amenta PS. Morphology, localization and origin of the hepatic extracellular matrix. In: Zern M, Reid L, eds. Extracellular matrix: chemistry, biology, pathology. New York: Marcell Dekker, 1993

501. Arthur MJP. Matrix degradation in the liver. Semin Liv Dis, 1990; 10:47–55

502. Kim TH, Mars WM, Stolz DB, Petersen BE, Michalopoulos GK. Extracellular matrix remodelling at the early stages of liver regeneration. Hepatology, 1997; 76:901–999

503. Barrowman JA. Hepatic lymph and lymphatics. In: McIntyre N, Benhamou J-P, Bircher J, Rizzetto M, Rodes J, eds. Oxford textbook of clinical hepatology, vol. 1. Oxford, New York, Tokyo: Oxford University Press, 1991: pp 37–40

504. Smith JB, McIntosh GH, Morris B. The traffic of cells through tissues: a study of peripheral lymph in sheep. J Anat, 1970; 107:87–100

505. Comparini L, Bastianini A. Graphic reconstructions in the morphological study of the hepatic lymph vessels. Angiologica, 1965; 2:81–95

506. Comparini L. Lymph vessels of the liver in man. Angiologica, 1969; 6:262–274

507. Granger DN, Miller T, Allen R, Parker RE, Parker JC, Taylor AE. Permselectivity of cat bloood-lymph barrier to endogenous macromolecules. Gastroenterology, 1979; 77:103–109

508. Witte MH. Ascitic, thy lymph runneth over. Gastroenterology, 1979; 76:1066–1068

509. Henriksen JH, Horn T, Christoffersen P. The blood-lymph barrier in the liver. A review based on morphological and functional concepts of normal and cirrhotic liver. Liver, 1984; 4:221–232

510. Wisse E, de Zanger RB, Jacobs R. Lobular gradients in endothelial fenestrae and sinusoidal diameter favour centro-lobular exchange processes: a scanning EM study. In: Knook DC, Wisse E, eds. Sinusoidal liver cells. Amsterdam: Elsevier, 1982: pp 61–67

511. Wisse E, de Zanger RB, Jacobs R, McCuskey RS. Scanning electron microscope observations on the structure of portal veins, sinusoids and central veins in rat liver. Scanning Electron Microsc, 1983; 3:1441–1452

512. Al-Jomard A, Reid O, Scothorne RJ. An EM study of the route of drainage of interstitial fluid from the space of Disse into portal tract lymphatics. Proceeding of the XIIth International Anatomical Congress, 1985; p. 9 (abstract)

513. Friedman JM. Hepatic nerve function. In: Arias IM, Popper H, Jakoby WB, Schachter D, Shafritz DA, eds. The Liver. Biology and pathobiology. New York: Raven Press, 1988: pp 949–959

514. McCuskey RS Anatomy of efferent hepatic nerves. Anat Rec A Discov Mol Cell Evol Biol 2004; 280:808–820

515. Berthoud HR. Anatomy and function of sensory hepatic nerves. Anat Rec A Discov Mol Cell Evol Biol, 2004; 280:827–835

516. Tiniakos DG, Lee JA, Burt AD. Innervation of the liver: morphology and function. Liver, 1996; 16:151–160

517. Shimazu T. Progress and perspective in neuro-hepatology. In: Shimazu T, ed. Liver innervation. London: John Libbey, 1996

518. Häussinger D, Jungermann K, eds. Liver and nervous system. Dordrecht/Boston/London: Kluwer Academic Publishers, 1998

519. Moghimzadeh E, Nobin A, Rosengren E. Fluorescence microscopical and chemical characterization of the adrenergic innervation in mammalian liver tissue. Cell Tiss Res, 1983; 230:605–613

520. Burt AD, Tiniakos D, MacSween RNM et al. Localization of adrenergic and neuropeptide tyrosine-containing nerves in the mammalian liver. Hepatology, 1989; 9:839–845

521. Bioulac-Sage P, Lafon ME, Saric J, Balabaud C. Nerves and perisinusoidal cells in human liver. J Hepatol, 1990; 10:105–112

522. Hartmann H, Beckh K, Jungermann K. Direct control of glycogen metabolism in the perfused rat liver by the sympathetic innervation. Eur J Biochem, 1982; 123:521–526

523. Lautt WW. Hepatic nerves: a review of their function and effects. Can J Physiol Pharmacol, 1980; 58:105–123

524. Lautt WW. Afferent and efferent neural roles in liver function. Prog Neurobiol, 1983; 21:323–348

525. Skaaring P, Bierring F. On the intrinsic innervation of normal rat liver. Histochemical and scanning electron microscopic studies. Cell Tiss Res, 1976; 171:141–155

526. Amenta F, Cavallotti C, Ferrante F et al. Cholinergic nerves in the human liver. Histochem J, 1981; 13:419–424

527. Goehler LE, Sternini C, Brecha NC. Calcitonin gene-related peptide immunoreactivity in the biliary pathway and liver of the guinea-pig: distribution and colocalization with substance P. Cell Tiss Res, 1988; 277:145–150

528. Feher E, Fodor E, Feher J. Ultrastructural localization of somatostatin- and substance P-immunoreactive nerve fibers in the feline liver. Gastroenterology, 1992; 102:287–294

529. Geary N, Le Sauter J, Noh H. Glucagon acts in the liver to control spontaneous meal size in rats. Am J Physiol, 1993; 264:R116–R122

530. Tanaka K, Inoue S, Saito S, Nagase H, Takamura Y. Hepatic vagal aminoacid sensors modulate amino acid induced insulin and glucagon secretion in the rat. J Autonom Nerv Sys, 1993; 42:225–231

531. Niijima A, Meguid MM. Parenteral nutrients in rat suppresses hepatic vagal afferent signals from portal veins to hypothalamus. Surgery, 1994; 116:294–301

532. Dhillon AP, Sankey EA, Wang JH et al. Immunohistochemical studies on the innervation of human transplanted liver. J Pathol, 1992; 167:211–216

533. Boon AP, Hubscher SG, Lee JL, Hines JE, Burt AD. Hepatic reinnervation following orthotopic liver transplantation in man. J Pathol, 1992; 167:217–222

534. Ozier Y, Braillon A, Gaudia C, Roulat D, Hadengue A, Lebrec D. Hepatic denervation alters haemodynamic response to haemorrhage in conscious rats. Hepatology, 1989; 10:473–476

535. Henderson JM, Mackay GJ, Lumsden AB, Alta HM, Brouillard R, Kutner MH. The effect of liver denervation on hepatic haemodynamics during hypovolaemic shock in swine. Hepatology, 1992; 15:130–133

536. Lee JA, Ahmed Q, Hines JE, Burt AD. Disappearance of hepatic parenchymal nerves in human liver cirrhosis. Gut, 1992; 33:87–91

537. Kanda N, Fukuda Y, Imoto M et al. Localisation of synaptophysin immunoreactivity in the human liver. Scand J Gastroenterol, 1994; 29:275–279

538. Jaskiewicz K, Voigt MD, Robson SC. Distribution of hepatic nerve fibres in liver diseases. Digestion, 1994; 55:247–252

539. Rojkind M. Fibrosis and cirrhosis as alterations in homeostasis of the liver ecosystem. In: Gitnick G, ed. Principles and practice of gastroenterology and hepatology. New York: Elsevier, 1988: pp 1121–1134

540. Jungermann K. Metabolic zonation of liver parenchyma. Semin Liver Dis, 1988; 8:329–341

541. Häussinger D. Nitrogen metabolism in liver: structural and functional organization and physiological relevance. Biochem J, 1990; 267:281–290

542. Burgstahler A, Nathanson MH. Coordination of calcium waves among hepatocytes: teamwork gets the job done. Hepatology, 1998; 27:634–635

543. Tordjmann T, Berthon B, Claret M, Combettes L. Coordinated intercellular calcium waves induced by noradrenaline in rat hepatocytes: dual control by gap junction permeability and agonist. EMBO J, 1997; 16:5398–5407

544. Zaret KS. The touch that hepatocytes seem to like. Hepatology, 1992; 15:1204–1205

545. Billiar TR, Curran RD. Hepatocyte and Kupffer Cell Interactions. London: CRC Press, 1992

546. Maher JJ, Friedman SL. Parenchymal and nonparenchymal cell interactions in the liver. Semin Liver Dis, 1993; 13:13–20

547. Vidal-Vanaclocha F. The hepatic sinusoidal endothelium: functional aspects and phenotypic heterogeneity. In: Vidal-Vanaclocha F, ed. Functional heterogeneity of liver tissue. R.G. Landes Company: Austin, 1997: pp 69–107

548. Modis L, Martinez-Hernandez A. Hepatocytes modulate the hepatic microvascular phenotype. Lab Invest, 1991; 65:661–670

549. Gressner AM, Lofti S, Gressner G, Lahme B. Identification and partial characterization of a hepatocyte-derived factor promoting proliferation of cultured fat-storing cells (parasinusoidal lipocytes). Hepatology, 1992; 16:1250–1266

550. Ramadori G, Neubauer K, Odenthal M et al. The gene of hepatocyte growth factor is expressed in fat-storing cells of rat liver and is downregulated during cell growth and by transforming growth factor-beta. Biochem Biophys Res Commun, 1992; 183:739–742

551. Skrtic S, Wallenius V, Ekberg S, Brenzel A, Gressner AM, Jansson JO. Hepatocyte-stimulated expression of hepatocyte growth factor (HGF) in cultured rat hepatic stellate cells. J Hepatol, 1999; 30:115–124

552. Tateno C, Yoshizato K. Growth and differentiation of adult rat hepatocytes regulated by the interaction between parenchymal and non-parenchymal liver cells. J Gastroenterol Hepatol, 1998; 13(suppl):S83–S92

553. Loréal O, Levavasseur F, Fromaget C, Gros D, Guillouzo A, Clément B. Cooperation of Ito cells and hepatocytes in the

deposition of an extracellular matrix in vitro. Am J Pathol, 1993; 143:538–544

554. Iredale JP, Arthur MJP. Hepatocyte-matrix interactions. Gut, 1994; 35:729–732

555. Lora JM, Rowader KE, Soares L, Giancotti F, Zaret KS. Alpha (3) beta (1)-integrin as a critical mediator of the hepatic differentiation response to the extracellular matrix. Hepatology, 1998; 28:1095–1104

556. Friedman SL. The molecular basis for Kupffer cell/lipocyte interactions. In: Gressner AM, Ramadori G, eds. Molecular and cell biology of liver fibrogenesis. Dordrecht: Kluwer Academic Publishers, 1992: pp 385–392

557. Rosenbaum J, Mavier P, Preaux AM, Lescs MC, Dhumeaux D. Mouse hepatic endothelial cells in culture secrete a growth inhibitor for hepatic lipocytes. In: Wisse E, Knook DL, Decker K, eds. Cells of the hepatic sinusoid, vol. 2. Rijswijk: The Kupffer Cell Foundation, 1989: pp 266–267

558. Hirose M, Watanabe S, Oide H, Kitamura T, Miyazaki A, Sato N. A new function of Ito cells in liver morphogenesis: evidence using a novel morphogenic protein, epimorphin, in vitro. Biochem Biophys Res Commun, 1996; 225:155–160

559. Desmet VJ. Organizational principles. In: Arias I, Boyer J, Fausto N, Jakoby W, Schachter D, Shafritz D, eds. The liver: biology and pathobiology, 3rd edn. New York: Raven Press, 1994: pp 3–14

560. Schuppan D, Milani S. The extracellular matrix in cellular communication. In: Gressner AM, Ramadori G, eds. Molecular and cell biology of liver fibrogenesis. Dordrecht: Kluwer Academic Publishers, 1992: pp 52–71

561. Guguen-Guillouzo C, Clement B, Baffet G et al. Maintenance and reversibility of active albumin secretion by adult rat hepatocytes co-cultured with another liver epithelial cell type. Exp Cell Res, 1983; 143:47–54

562. Ohtani O. The peribiliary portal system in the rabbit liver. Arch Histol Jpn, 1979; 42:153–167

563. Desmet VJ. The hepatocyte: structural specialization and functional integration. In: Molin G, Avagnina P, eds. Systematic and quantitative hepatology. Pathophysiological and methodological aspects. Milan: Masson, 1990: pp 43–50

564. Gressner AM. Liver fibrosis: perspectives in pathobiochemical research and clinical outlook. Eur J Clin Chem Clin Biochem, 1991; 29:293–311

565. Rojkind M, Greenwel P. The liver as a bioecological system. In: Arias JM, Jakoby WB, Popper H, Schachter D, Shafritz DA, eds. The liver: biology and pathobiology. New York: Raven Press, 1988: pp 1269–1285

566. Schreiber G, Aldred AR. Gene activity and regulation. In: Le Bouton AV, ed. Molecular and cell biology of the liver. Boca Raton: CRC Press Inc., 1993: pp 3–29

567. Clément B, Musso O, Liétard J, Theret N. Homeostatic control of angiogenesis: a newly identified function of the liver? Hepatology, 1999; 29:621–623

568. Crawford AR, Lin X-Z, Crawford JM. The normal adult human liver biopsy: a quantitative reference standard. Hepatology, 1998; 28:323–331

569. Roskams T, Desmet VJ. Ductular reaction and its diagnostic significance. Semin Diag Pathol, 1998; 15:159–169

570. Wynne HA, Cope LH, Mutch E, Rawlins MD, Woodhouse KW, James OFW. The effect of age upon liver blood flow in healthy man. Hepatology, 1989; 9:297–301

571. Orrego J, Mena I, Baraona E, Palma R. Modifications in hepatic blood flow and portal pressure produced by different diets. Am J Dig Dis, 1965; 10:239–248

572. Myers JD. The Hepatic blood flow and splanchnic consumption of man—their estimation from urea production or bromsulphthalein excretion during catheterization of the hepatic veins. J Clin Invest, 1947; 26:1130–1137

573. Lautt WW, Legare DJ, D'Almeida MS. Adenosine as putative regulator of hepatic arterial flow (the buffer response). Am J Physiol, 1985; 248:H331–338

574. Ezzat WR, Lautt WW. Hepatic arterial pressure—flow autoregulation is adenosine mediated. Am J Physiol, 1987; 252: H836–H845

575. Sherlock S, Dooley J, eds. Diseases of the liver and biliary system, 11th edn. London: Blackwell Scientific, 2002

576. Correia MA, Castagnoli N. Pharmacokinetics: II. Drug biotransformation. In: Katzung BG, ed. Basic and clinical pharmacology, 3rd edn. Norwalk: Appleton and Lange, 1987: pp 36–43

577. Gonzalez FJ. Molecular genetics of the P-450 superfamily. Pharmacol Ther 1990; 45:1–38

578. Tredger JM, Davis M. Drug metabolism and hepatotoxicity. Gut 1991; 32:S34–S39

579. Rosalki SB, Tarlow D, Rau D. Plasma gamma-glutamyl transpeptidase elevation in patients receiving enzyme-inducing drugs. Lancet. 1971; ii:376–377

580. Okey AB. Enzyme induction in the cytochrome P-450 system. Pharmacol Ther 1990; 45:241–298

581. Zimmerman HJ, Maddrey WC. Acetaminophen (paracetamol) hepatotoxicity with regular intake of alcohol: analysis of instances of therapeutic misadventure. Hepatology 1995; 22:767–773

582. Arthur MJP. Reactive oxygen intermediates and liver injury. J Hepatol 1988; 8:125–131

583. Kaplowitz N, Tsukamoto H. Oxidative stress and liver disease. Prog Liver Dis 1996; 14:131–159

584. Kaplowitz N. Mechanisms of liver cell injury. J Hepatol 2000; 32(suppl I): 39–47

585. Ponka P. Cell biology of heme. Am J Med Sci. 1999; 318:241–256

586. Robinson SH. Formation of bilirubin from erythroid and nonerythroid sources. Semin Hematol, 1972; 9:43–53

587. Fevery J, Vanstapel F, Blackaert N. Bile pigment metabolism. Clin Gastroenterol 1989; 3:283–312

588. Ohta Y, Fukushima S, Yamashita N, Niimi T, Kubota T, Akizawa E, Koiwai O. UDP-glucuronosyltransferase1A1 directly binds to albumin. Hepatol Res. 2005; [Epub ahead of print]

589. Tukey RH, Strassbury CP. Human UDP-glucuronosyltransferase: metabolism, expression and disease. Annu Rev Pharmacol Toxicol 2000; 40:581–619

590. Innocenti F, Ratain MJ 'Irinogenetics' and UGT1A: from genotypes to haplotypes. Clin Pharmacol Ther 2004; 75:495–500

591. Monaghan G, Ryan M, Seddon R, Hume R, Burchell B. Genetic variation in bilirubin UDP-glucuronosyltransferase gene promoter and Gilbert's syndrome. Lancet 1996; 347:578–581

592. Hue L. Gluconeogenesis and its regulation. Diab Metab Rev 1987; 3:111–126

593. Alberti KGM, Taylor R, Johnson DG. Carbohydrate metabolism in liver disease. In: Millward-Sadler GH, Wright R, Arthur MJP, eds. Wright's Liver and biliary disease. London: WB Saunders, 1992: pp 43–60

594. Shimazu T. Reciprocal innervation of the liver: its significance in metabolic control. Adv Metab Dis 1983; 10:379–384

595. Jungermann K, Kietzmann T. Oxygen: modulator of metabolic zonation and disease of the liver. Hepatology 2000; 31:255–260

596. Jungermann K, Kietzmann T. Zonation of parenchymal and non-parenchymal metabolism in liver. Annu Rev Nutr 1996; 16:179–203

597. Harry DS, McIntyre N. Plasma lipoproteins and the liver. In: Millward-Sadler GH, Wright R, Arthur MJP, eds. Wright's Liver and biliary disease. London: WB Saunders, 1992: pp 61–78

598. Kruszynska YT. Nomal metabolism: the physiology of fuel homeostasis. In: Pickup JC, Williams G, eds. Textbook of Diabetes: selected chapters. Oxford: Blackwell Publishing Ltd, 2005: pp. 9.1–9.38

599. Wakil SJ, Stoops JK, Joshi VC. Fatty acid synthesis and its regulation. Annu Rev Biochem 1983; 52:537–579

600. McCarry JD, Foster DW. Regulation of hepatic fatty acid oxidation and ketone body formation. Annu Rev Biochem 1980; 49:395–420

601. Lazarow PB. Rat liver perioxisomes catalyze the β-oxidation of fatty acids. J Biol Chem 1978; 277:1522–1528

602. Day CP, James OFW, Brown ASIJM, Bennett MK, Fleming IN, Yeaman SJ. The activity of the metabolic form of hepatic phosphatidate phosphohydrolase correlates with the severity of alcoholic fatty liver in human beings. Hepatology 1993; 18:832–838

603. Day CP, Yeaman SJ. The biochemistry of alcohol-induced fatty liver. Biochim Biophys Acta 1994; 1215:33–48

604. Preiss B, ed. Regulation of HMG CoA reductase. London: Academic Press, 1985

605. Bjorkhem I, Eggertsen G. Genes involved in initial steps of bile acid synthesis. Curr Opin Lipidol 2001; 12:97–103

606. Kullak-Ublick GA, Stieger B, Meier PJ. Enterohepatic bile salt transporters in normal physiology and liver disease. Gastroenterology 2004; 126:322–342

607. Perwaiz S, Tuchweber B, Mignault D, Gilat T, Yousef IM. Determination of bile acids in biological fluids by liquid chromatography-electrospray tandem mass spectrometry. J Lipid Res 2001; 42:114–119

608. Redinger RN, The coming of age of our understanding of the enterohepatic circulation of bile salts. Am J Surg 2003; 185:168–172

609. Angelin B, Bjorkhem I, Einarsson K, Ewerth S. Hepatic uptake of bile acids in man; fasting and postprandial concentrations of individual bile acids in portal venous and systemic blood serum. J Clin Invest 1982; 70:724–731

610. Bernstein H, Bernstein C, Payne CM, Dvorakova K, Garewal H. Bile acids as carcinogens in human gastrointestinal cancers. Mutat Res 2005; 589:47–65

611. Felig P. Amino acid metabolism in man. Annu Rev Biochem 1975; 44:933–955

612. Christensen HN. Interorgan amino acid nutrition. Physiol Rev 1982; 62:1193–1233

613. Harper AE, Miller RH, Block KP. Branched-chain amino acid metabolism. Annu Rev Nutr 1984; 4:409–454

614. Haussinger D, Lamars WH, Moorman AFM. Metabolism of amino acids and ammonia. Enzyme 1993; 46:72–93

615. Sigsaard I, Almdal T, Hansen BA, Vilstrup H. Dexamethasone increases the capacity of urea synthesis dependently and reduces the body weight of rats. Liver, 1988; 8:193–197

616. Haüssinger D. Hepatocyte heterogeneity in glutamine and ammonia metabolism and the role of an intracellular glutamine cycle during ureogenesis in the perfused rat liver. Eur J Biochem 1983; 133:269–275

617. Haüssinger D. Liver glutamine metabolism. J Parent Ent Nutr 1990; 14:565–625

618. Rothschild MA, Oratz M, Schreiber SS. Serum albumin. Hepatology 1988; 8:385–401

619. Maniatis T, Goodbourn S, Fischer JA. Regulation of inducible and tissue-specific gene expression. Science 1987; 236:1237–1245

620. Moldave K. Eukaryotic protein synthesis. Annu Rev Biochem 1985; 54:1109–1149

621. Kelly RB. Pathways of protein secretion in eukaryotes. Science 1985; 203:25–32

622. Chung KN, Walter P, Aponte GW, Moore H-P. Molecular sorting in the secretory pathway. Science 1989; 243:192–197

623. Tavill AS, McCullough AJ. Protein metabolism and the liver. In: Millward-Sadler GH, Wright R, Arthur MJP, eds. Wright's Liver and biliary disease, 3rd edn. London: WB Saunders, 1992: pp 79–106

624. Andus T, Bauer J, Gerok W. Effects of cytokines on the liver. Hepatology 1991; 13:37–41

625. Peters T. Serum albumin. Adv Clin Chem 1970; 13:37–41

626. Bonkovsky HL. Iron metabolism and the liver. Am J Med Sci 1991; 301:32–45

627. Müller-Eberhard H. Molecular organisation and function of the complement system. Annu Rev Biochem 1988; 57:321–347

628. Hetland G, Johnson E, Falk RJ, Eskeland T. Synthesis of complement components C5, C6, C7, C8 and C9 in vitro by human monocytes and assembly of the terminal complement complex. Scand J Immunol 1986; 24:421–428

629. Burt AD, Geerts A, MacSween RNM, Whaley K, Wisse E. Synthesis of the complement component C3 by isolated rat Kupffer cells. J Hepatol 1986; 3:48

630. Wileman T, Harding C, Stahl P. Review article: receptor-mediated endocytosis. Biochem J 1985; 232:1–14

631. Pietrangelo A. Hereditary hemochromatosis–a new look at an old disease. N Engl J Med. 2004; 350: 2383–2397

632. Walshe JM. Copper: its role in the pathogenesis of liver disease. Semin Liver Dis, 1984; 4:252–263

633. Kenney S, Cox DW. Wilson disease mutation database. http://www.uofa-medical-genetics.org/wilson/index.php, accessed August 2005

634. Eriksson S. Alpha-I-antitrypsin deficiency: lessons learned from the bedside to the gene and back again. Chest, 1989; 95:181–183

635. Kuntz E. Laboratory diagnostics. In: Kuntz E, Kuntz HD, eds. Hepatology, principles and practice. Heidelberg: Springer–Verlag. 2001:78–112

636. Pratt DS, Kaplan MM. Evaluation of abnormal liver-enzyme results in asymptomatic patients. N Engl J Med. 2000; 342:1266–1271

637. Cohen JA, Kaplan MM. The SGOT/SGPT ratio—an indicator of alcoholic liver disease. Dig Dis Sci. 1979; 24:835–838

638. Rosalki SB, Tarlow D, Rau D. Plasma gamma-glutamyl transpeptidase elevation in patients receiving enzyme-inducing drugs. Lancet. 1971; ii:376–377

639. Feldmann HU, Pfeiffer R, Hirche H. Hormonal dependency of gamma-glutamyl transpeptidase. Dtsch Med Wochenschr 1974; 31; 99: 1171–1174

640. Limdi JK, Hyde GM. Evaluation of abnormal liver function tests. Postgrad Med J 2003; 79:307–312

641. Rothschild MA, Oratz M, Schreiber SS. Serum albumin. Hepatology 1988; 8:385–401

642. Rossi E, Adams L, Prins A et al. Validation of the FibroTest biochemical markers score in assessing liver fibrosis in hepatitis C patients. Clin Chem. 2003; 49:450–454

643. Callewaert N, Van Vlierberghe H, Van Hecke A, Noninvasive diagnosis of liver cirrhosis using DNA sequencer-based total serum protein glycomics. Nat Med. 2004; 10:429–434

644. Burt AD. Liver fibrosis: better understanding may help diagnosis and treatment. Br Med J 1992; ii:537–538

645. Schnegg M, Lauterburg BH. Quantitative liver function in the elderly assessed by galactose elimination capacity, aminopyrine demethylation and caffeine clearance. J Hepatol 1986; 3:164–171

646. Ollerich M, Burdelski M, Ringe B et al. Lignocaine metabolic formation as a measure of pre-transplant liver function. Lancet 1989; i:640–642

647. Meyer zum Büschenfelde KH, Lohse AW, Manns M, Poralla T. Autoimmunity and liver disease. Hepatology 1990; 12:354–363

648. Ben-Ari Z, Dhillon AP, Sherlock S. Autoimmune cholangiopathy: part of the spectrum of autoimmune chronic active hepatitis. Hepatology 1993; 18:10–15

649. Worman JH, Courvalin J-C. Autoantibodies against nuclear envelope proteins in liver disease. Hepatology 1991; 14:1269–1279

650. Philipp T, Durazzo M, Trautwein C et al. Recognition of uridine diphosphate glucuronyl transferases by LKM-3 antibodies in chronic hepatitis D. Lancet 1994; 344:578

651. Berg PA, Klein R, Lindenborn-Fotinos J. Antimitochondrial antibodies in primary biliary cirrhosis. J Hepatol 1986; 2:123–131

652. Palmer JM, Yeaman SJ, Bassendine MF, James OFW. M4 and M9 autoantigens in PBC—a negative study. J Hepatol 1991; 18: 251–254

653. El Sherif A, McPherson SJ, Dixon AK. Spiral CT of the abdomen: increased diagnostic potential. Eur J Radiol. 1999; 31:43–52

654. Savci G. The changing role of radiology in imaging liver tumours: an overview. Eur J Radiol 1999; 32:36–51

655. Van Hoe L, Vanbeckevoort D, Van Steenbergen W. Atlas of cross-sectional and projective MR Cholangio-pancreatography. Berlin-Heidelberg: Springer-Verlag, 1999

656. Bosmans H, Gryspeerdt S, van Hoe L, et al. Preliminary experience with a new double echo half-Fourier single-shot turbo spin echo acquisition in the characterization of liver lesions. MAGMA 1997; 5:79–84

657. O'Halpin D, Legge D, MacErlean DP. Therapeutic arterial embolisation: report of five years experience. Clin Radiol 1984; 35:85–93

658. Bruix J, Sala M, Llovet JM. Chemoembolization for hepatocellular carcinoma. Gastroenterology. 2004; 127:S179–188

Basic mechanisms in hepatopathology

2

James M. Crawford

The morphology of liver disease reflects the convergent influences of liver damage and liver recovery. The liver is vulnerable to a wide variety of metabolic, toxic, microbial, circulatory, and neoplastic insults. However, the liver has a remarkable capacity for self repair, including complete restitution of liver mass after loss, either from necroinflammatory events or surgical resection. An understanding of liver pathology requires knowledge of the causes of liver damage and the mechanisms by which the liver responds.

General concepts

Table 2.1 presents the fundamental causes of liver injury. They fall into the general classes of infectious, immune-mediated, drug-induced (including alcohol), metabolic, mechanical, and environmental. This table is not comprehensive, but provides a framework for understanding liver injury. An individual patient is frequently subject to more than one form of liver injury simultaneously. This is due in part to the number of injuries to which the liver is subject, and in part to the remarkable propensity of humans to place their liver at risk for simultaneous injury from multiple sources. Common companion conditions include: viral hepatitis (including simultaneous infection by multiple viruses); drug and environmental toxicity (including alcohol intake); and obesity and/or diabetes with risk for non-alcoholic fatty liver disease.

The enormous functional reserve of the liver masks the clinical impact of early liver damage. With the rare exception of fulminant hepatic failure, liver disease from these various causes is an insidious process in which symptoms of hepatic decompensation may occur weeks, months, or even years after the onset of injury. There is often a long time interval between disease occurrence and detection. Conversely, the liver may be injured and heal without clinical detection. Hence, patients with hepatic abnormalities who are referred to liver disease specialists most frequently have chronic liver disease.

The clinician and liver pathologist alike are therefore obliged to consider a differential diagnosis of multiple potential causes of liver disease, few of which are mutually exclusive. The inciting cause(s) may have begun years previously. When liver tissue is obtained for histological analysis, the liver pathologist's task is further made difficult by the fact that the liver has only a limited repertoire for morphological manifestation of injury, as given in Table 2.2. Specifically, the liver can become inflamed, it can cease to function properly and exhibits morphological manifestations thereof, or portions of the liver can die. Likewise, the hepatic response to injury is quite limited. The liver can regenerate (which it does extremely well), or it can become fibrotic and scarred. The combination of extensive regeneration in the midst of scarring leads to cirrhosis, conceptually the end-stage of chronic liver injury. Interestingly, with cessation of injury and the long passage of time, fibrous tissue can be resorbed and the cirrhosis partially 'reversed'.

For the most part, the events of inflammation, dysfunction, cell death, regeneration, and fibrosis play out on a microscopic scale. The macroscopic anatomy of the liver is usually the lesser consideration in assessment of hepatitic, toxic, cholestatic, or metabolic liver injury. The exception to this statement is when there is mechanical obstruction to larger bile ducts or to major hepatic blood vessels, and when

Table 2.1	Causes of liver injury

Infectious
Viral hepatitis—hepatotropic
Viral hepatitis—opportunistic
Bacterial
Fungal
Parasitic
Helminthic

Immune-mediated
Autoimmune hepatitis
Primary biliary cirrhosis
Primary sclerosing cholangitis
Transplant rejection
Graft-versus-host disease

Drug- and toxin-induced hepatotoxicity
Alcoholic liver disease
Therapeutic agents (including complementary medicines and drugs of abuse)

Metabolic
Inherited metabolic disease
Acquired metabolic derangement
Non-alcoholic fatty liver disease

Mechanical
Obstructive cholestasis
Vascular disorders

Environmental
Environmental toxins
Heat stroke

Table 2.2	Histological manifestations of liver injury

Inflammation
Portal tracts
Interface between portal tracts and parenchyma
Parenchyma (the 'lobule')*

Hepatocellular injury*
Ballooning degeneration
Steatosis
Cholestasis
Inclusions

Necrosis and apoptosis*

Vascular remodelling

Regeneration

Fibrosis*
Cirrhosis

Neoplasia

* The distribution of inflammation, hepatocellular injury, necrosis/apoptosis, and fibrosis within the lobule are critical observations: periportal, mid-zonal, or pericentral

Table 2.3	Well-established risk conditions for liver neoplasia	
Neoplastic condition	**Risk factors**	
Adenoma	Oral contraceptive exposure	
	Glycogen storage disease type 1a (Von Gierke disease)	
Hepatocellular carcinoma	Viral hepatitis	
	Hepatitis B infection	
	Hepatitis C infection	
	Cirrhosis from other causes	
	Alcoholic liver disease	
	Hereditary haemochromatosis	
	Hereditary tyrosinaemia	
	Alpha-1-antitrypsin storage disorder	
	Wilson disease (rare)	
	Primary biliary cirrhosis (rare)	
	Inherited disorders without obligate cirrhosis	
	Glycogen storage disease Type 1a (Von Gierke disease)	
Hepatoblastoma	Familial adenomatous polyposis (FAP)	
Cholangiocarcinoma	Primary sclerosing cholangitis	
	Fluke infection of the biliary tract	
Angiosarcoma	Toxin exposure*	
	Vinyl chloride	
	Arsenic	

* Historically, Thorotrast® exposure was a risk factor for hepatocellular carcinoma, cholangiocarcinoma, and angiosarcoma

macroscopic liver nodules are of concern. In the latter instance, a number of chronic conditions place the liver at risk for neoplastic transformation, as given in Table 2.3.

Interpretation of liver pathology requires rigorous and systematic examination of the microarchitectural compartments of the liver, as given in Table 2.4. Intrinsic changes in native liver elements (hepatocytes, sinusoidal structures, portal tract structures) must be evaluated, and the tissue examined for additional elements that may be present: inflammation, infection, neoplasia. The order in which this is done is a matter of personal preference; that comprehensive examination be performed is imperative (Chapter 3). Such information must be correlated with clinical information on liver status, as optimal interpretation of liver pathology requires all such information.

This chapter will detail the principles of injury and response that are operative in the liver. A constant reference point will be the morphological manifestations of these principles. Mechanisms of carcinogenesis are beyond the scope of this introductory chapter but are considered in Chapter 15.

Inflammation

The predominant form of liver disease throughout the world is hepatitis. Major causes are hepatotropic viral infection,

Table 2.4	Histological examination of liver microarchitecture

Native elements
Hepatic parenchyma
   Hepatocytes
      Hepatocyte cytologic features
      Hepatocyte plate architecture
   Sinusoids
      Endothelial cells
      Kupffer cells
      Stellate cells
      Extracellular matrix
   Zonation
      Periportal zone
         Portal tract interface
      Mid-zonal region
      Perivenous zone ('pericentral zone')
Portal tracts
   Extracellular matrix
   Portal veins
   Hepatic arteries
   Bile ducts
   Lymphatic channels (if visible)

Added elements
Inflammatory cells
Infectious agents
Infiltrating neoplastic cells
Cellular inclusions
   Viral cytopathic change
   Storage disorders

Table 2.5	Inflammatory cells in hepatitis	
Cell type		**Comment**
Antigen-presenting cells		
	Kupffer cells (KC)	When activated, secrete TNF-α, IL-2, IL-12 and leukotriene B3
	Dendritic cells (DC)	Express toll-like receptors (TLR); secrete IL-12, TNF-α, IFN-α, and IL-10
Innate immune system		'Pit cells'; can be Th-1* or Th-2**
Natural killer cells (NK)		
Natural killer T cells (NKT)		
Adaptive immune system		Mature within liver through Th-2** to Th-1* phenotype
B lymphocytes		
T lymphocytes		Secrete immunoglobulin, generate plasma cells
	CD4+ T cells	
	CD4+ CD25+ T cells (T-regs)	Multiple subsets
	CD4+ T helper cells	Regulate activation of CD4+ and CD8+ T cells
	CD8+ T cells	Can be Th-1* or Th-2**
	Cytotoxic T Cells (CTL)	Activity is enhanced by Th-1 cytokines; can be cytolytic or non-cytolytic

* Th-1: proinflammatory, IFN-γ and IL-2 secreting
** Th-2: anti-inflammatory, IL-4 and IL-10 secreting

alcoholic and non-alcoholic steatohepatitis, autoimmune hepatitis, and drug-induced liver injury. All feature inflammation of the liver, either as cause or effect. The inflammatory process will be discussed first, followed by consideration of two of these forms of hepatitis: viral hepatitis and autoimmune hepatitis. A summary of the inflammatory cells that accumulate during hepatic injury (and their abbreviations) is given in Table 2.5.

The innate immune system

Hepatocytes constitute 80% of the cells in the liver. Of the remaining 20%, bile duct epithelial cells comprise 1%, sinusoidal endothelial cells 10%, Kupffer cells (the resident macrophages of the liver) 4%, and lymphocytes 5%. The last include cells of the adaptive immune system (T and B lymphocytes) and innate immune system: natural killer (NK) and natural killer T (NKT) cells.[1] NK cells comprise 31% of hepatic lymphocytes and NKT cells 26%. The liver is thus particularly enriched with cells of the innate immune system, compared to other parenchymal organs. While this has immediate value for dealing with foreign antigens released from the gut into the splanchnic circulation, it also means that the liver is well equipped for an immune response to neoantigens expressed within its substance.

In the normal liver, MHC class I antigens are constitutively expressed on the cells lining the vascular sinusoids (endothelial cells and Kupffer cells), bile duct epithelial cells, and to a lesser extent hepatocytes. MHC class II antigens are normally expressed only by Kupffer cells and by dendritic antigen-presenting cells (APCs) in the portal tracts; bile duct epithelial cells and large vessel endothelial cells express few or no detectable MHC class II antigen. A proinflammatory environment established by such cytokines as tumour necrosis factor-α (TNF-α), interleukin-1β (IL-1β), or IL-6 promotes the expression of HLA class II molecules on cells that do not normally express them, including hepatocytes and bile duct epithelial cells.[2] Aberrant expression of antigens on native liver cells via the MHC class II antigens, especially on hepatocytes and bile duct epithelial cells, makes these native cells targets of the host immune system. Hence, while offending agents such as viruses may be the initial event, it is the activation of cytocidal T lymphocytes that actually causes liver cell death.

NK and NKT cells

Unlike T and B lymphocytes, which require clonotypic antigen receptors to recognize antigens, NK and NKT cells can participate in the immune response without prior antigenic stimulation.[3] NK cells, and potentially NKT cells as well, appear morphologically as 'pit cells'—large granular lymphocytes that reside in the subendothelial interstices of the space of Disse.[4] They both can produce high levels of proinflammatory (Th-1) and anti-inflammatory (Th-2) cytokines.[5] NK cells are major producers of IFN-γ (a proinflammatory cytokine); NKT cells produce IFN-γ or IL-4 (an anti-inflammatory cytokine). The populations of NKT cells can expand locally in regional tissues. Notably, the local hepatic NKT cells include precursor forms which can undergo phenotypic maturation in the liver. Expansion and maturation of NKT precursors is accompanied by conversion from a stage which is Th-2 and IL-4 secreting, to a stage which is Th-1 and hence IFN-γ secreting.[6] IFN-γ enhances the dendritic cell expression of proteins involved in cellular antigen processing and presentation, including proteosome subunits and MHC molecules. In addition, IFN-γ induces additional chemokines that enhance and direct the adaptive immunity of T and B cells.[7] The expanded NKT cell populations are thus a very effective resident proinflammatory effector arm of the host immune system.

After hepatitis B virus (HBV) or hepatitis C virus (HCV) infects the liver, viral replication within hepatocytes occurs and viral particles are continuously released into the circulation.[8] Through the action of antigen-presenting cells (especially dendritic cells), activation of NK and NKT cells occurs, leading to secretion of IFN-γ, inhibiting replication of HBV and HCV through a non-cytolytic mechanism (Fig. 2.1).[9] Expression of IFN-α also occurs (by both NK and NKT cells, and by infected hepatocytes); this interferon initiates intracellular signalling involving the Signal Transducer and Activator of Transcription (STAT) pathway to increase expression of genes that block viral replication. During HBV infection, the innate immune cells contribute significantly to the suppression of viral replication.[10] Unfortunately, the same is not true for HCV infection,[11] as HCV is capable of blocking the antiviral IFN-α effect, through inhibition of STAT signalling within hepatocytes.

Kupffer cells and dendritic cells

The resident macrophages in the liver, Kupffer cells (KC), and circulating blood dendritic cells (DC) take up antigens, process them, and present them to other immune cells.[12] DC express toll-like receptors (TLR) that recognize a particular component of infectious organisms. The activation of TLR signalling pathways results in production of proinflammatory cytokines. It is likely that the TLR pathway plays a role in the liver inflammation, as induced by hepatotropic viruses.[8] DCs then develop a mature phenotype, and stimulate NK cells, NTK cells, T cells, and B cells through secretion of cytokines such as IL-12, TNF-α, IFN-α, and IL-10 (not all of which can be illustrated in Fig. 2.1). The DC subsets that produce IL-12 and TNF-α support generation of cytotoxic T lymphocytes (which are Th-1 with further secretion of IL-2, IFN-γ, and TNF-α). DCs producing IL-10 promote generation of Th-2 T cells, which on further secretion of IL-4, IL-5, IL-10, and IL-13 stimulate B cell antibody production.

Kupffer cells play a role in all forms of hepatitis, as an obligate anatomical companion. Indeed, they comprise 80% of the systemic host mononuclear phagocytic system.[13] They reside normally on the luminal aspect of the sinusoi-

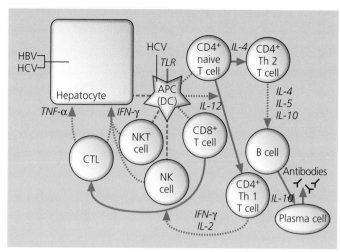

Fig. 2.1 • Schematic of the host immune response to hepatitis viral infection. A hepatocyte infected with either hepatitis B virus (HBV) or hepatitis C virus (HCV) processes and presents antigens, via the major histocompatibility (MHC) proteins expressed on its surface, to antigen-presenting cells (APC), in this case a dendritic cell (DC). The dendritic cell is also capable of taking up HCV directly, and may also respond to chemical products of other infectious agents through its toll-like receptor (TLR). The dendritic cell activates the following lymphocytes: naive CD4+ T cells; CD8+ T cells; natural killer cells (NK); and natural killer T cells (NKT). The naive CD4+ T cell is stimulated by the cytokine interleukin 4 (IL-4) to differentiate into a Th2 CD4+ T cell (denoted by solid line); this T cell secretes cytokines (denoted by dotted line) which stimulate B cells to mature into plasma cells and secrete clonotypic antibodies. Under stimulation by interleukin 12 (IL-12), the activated naive CD4+ T cell differentiates into a Th1 CD4+ T cell; this T cell secretes interferon-γ (IFN-γ) and interleukin 2 (IL-2), which stimulate the activated CD8+ T cells to become cytotoxic lymphocytes (CTL). The activated NK, NKT, and CTL secrete IFN-γ, which has antiviral effects in hepatocytes. These cells can also interact directly with infected hepatocytes to effect cytolysis (not shown). Tumour necrosis factor-α (TNF-α) secreted by CTL also can induce hepatocellular apoptosis through death-signalling pathways. In this fashion, HBV infection can usually be cleared; an inadequate immune response underlies chronic HBV infection. In contrast, HCV infection is usually not cleared successfully, owing both to the genetic instability of HCV and development of quasispecies (which evade the adaptive immune response), and to the inadequacy of the innate immune response to clear virus from infected hepatocytes. Not shown in this schematic is the potential role of CD4+ CD25+ regulatory T cells (T-regs), whose role in the immune response to viral infection is in need of further clarification. Figure courtesy of Aleta R. Crawford. (Adapted from Crawford JM, Immunopathology of the Liver, American Association for the Study of Liver Diseases Post-Graduate Course, 2005, San Francisco, with permission.)

dal endothelium, to engulf particulate material and microorganisms that arrive via the splanchnic circulation from the gut. KCs are potent scavengers for systemic and gut-derived inflammatory mediators and cytokines.[14] Activated KCs release TNF-α, IL-2, IL-12, and leukotriene B3. These mediators are involved in the hepatic recruitment of neutrophils and cytotoxic T lymphocytes (CTL).

Hepatocellular death of any sort is rapidly followed by Kupffer cell phagocytosis of the residual debris. For example, when an isolated hepatocyte undergoes apoptosis, it is routinely engulfed by a nearby Kupffer cell within 2 to 4 hours.[15] With smouldering hepatocellular apoptosis, clumps of macrophages can accumulate in the parenchyma (Fig. 2.2). Such macrophages can persist in the parenchyma for an extended period of time, probably weeks to months, serving as sentinels of prior hepatocellular injury and death.

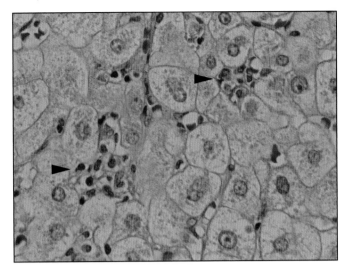

Fig. 2.2 • Lobular inflammation in chronic hepatitis, in which hepatocyte debris has been phagocytosed by resident macrophages, leaving clumps of parenchymal macrophages (arrowheads). H&E stained tissue section, 400× magnification.

Hepatic damage more extensive than just apoptosis of isolated hepatocytes engenders recruitment of circulating macrophages. The most dramatic example is massive hepatic necrosis, in which the vast expanse of the hepatocellular parenchyma undergoes cell death. With survival of the patient over the ensuing hours and days, the hepatic parenchyma becomes a sea of macrophages amidst the cellular debris. Their phagocytic and migratory action facilitates removal of the non-viable material, clearing the way for regeneration and recovery of the liver tissue.

The adaptive immune system

Adaptive immunity plays a critical role in hepatitis. A general principle of inflammation is that leukocytes are recruited to sites of injury in order to perform their normal functions in host defence. This includes activation and proliferation, killing of bacteria and other microbes, and ingestion of offending agents, including the debris of host tissues. The lymphocytes that accumulate in most forms of hepatitis are mobilized to participate in antibody-mediated and cell-mediated immune reactions. Antigen-specific CD4+ and CD8+ T cells are involved in eradication of HBV and HCV infection, during both acute and chronic infection.[16] CD4+ helper T cells recognize short antigenic peptides displayed in the antigen-binding groove of HLA class II molecules; these peptides are derived from intracellular proteolytic cleavage of exogenous antigens such as viruses.[17] CD4+ T cells secrete lymphokines that modulate the activity of antigen specific B cells and CD8+ T cells.[18] A CD4+ T-helper type 1 secretion profile (Th1) consists of antigen-dependent production of IL-2 and IFN-γ. A T-helper type 2 secretion profile (Th2) consists of IL-4 and IL-10 secretion. It is the Th1 cytokine profile which enhances CD8+ T cell cytolytic activity.[19]

Cellular immunity against intracellular viral pathogens involves CD8+ cytotoxic T cells (cytotoxic lymphocytes;

CTL) as the effector arm (see Fig. 2.1). CTL respond to viral peptides presented by infected cells in the antigen-binding groove of HLA class I molecules.[20] CTL-mediated lysis of virus-infected host cells can lead to viral clearances. Cell death is not an obligatory outcome, as CTL can secrete antiviral cytokines to induce non-cytolytic inhibition of viral gene expression and replication.[21,22] Regardless, if the CTL response is incomplete a smouldering infection ensues, with chronic tissue injury.

Regulatory T cells

A population of lymphocytes garnering particular attention are CD4+ T cells constitutively expressing the IL-2-receptor α-chain (CD25): CD4+ CD25+ T-cells or 'T-regs'. T-regs represent about 5 to 10% of peripheral CD4 T cells. They are highly differentiated T cells that have limited proliferative ability and are prone to apoptosis.[23] T-regs regulate the activation of CD4+ and CD8+ T cells by suppressing their proliferation and effector function. This suppressive action is critical in preventing the activation of autoreactive T cells.[24] Suppression occurs both through cell:cell contact and possibly through release of inhibitory cytokines.[25] Once stimulated, T-regs act in an antigen non-specific fashion.[26] Patients with autoimmune hepatitis have a reduced number of circulating T-regs at the time of diagnosis. The numbers are replenished during remission on immunosuppression but never reach normal values.[27] The precise role of T-regs in hepatitis is currently unclear.

Recruitment and influx of inflammatory cells

Over and above the actions of the resident immune system in the liver—innate and adaptive—circulating leukocytes are recruited to the infected liver. Significant numbers of CD4+ T cells, CD8+ T cells, NKT cells and NK cells can accumulate. Their recruitment characteristically is due to aberrant expression of antigens on native liver cells, in this instance hepatocytes. Neutrophilic infiltration of the liver is more characteristic of toxic injury, and is most prominent in alcoholic hepatitis. Neutrophils are also prominently featured in the immediate vicinity of portal tract bile ducts when obstruction to biliary outflow causes leakage of toxic biliary solutes into the portal tract mesenchyme.

The vast circulation of the liver, with both splanchnic influx of venous blood and direct arterial perfusion, gives every opportunity for inflammatory cells to remain in the liver in response to inflammatory stimuli. Unlike most vascular beds elsewhere in the body, however, the most important initial phase of inflammation—vasodilatation—does not appear to be a major regulatory factor in hepatic inflammation. The initial phases of liver inflammation appear to occur virtually independently of blood flow regulation.

Likewise, the second principle of inflammation operative elsewhere in the body, vascular leakage, is almost irrelevant in the liver. The fenestrated sinusoidal endothelium ensures that there is free exchange of plasma fluid with the extravascular space within the hepatic parenchyma. Hence, the liver is not subject to interstitial oedema in the same sense as in other body tissues. Rather, if swelling of the liver occurs during hepatitis, it is due to swelling of hepatocytes themselves. Since hepatocytes comprise over 80% of the liver volume, relatively small changes in hepatocyte volume regulation can have a profound effect on the overall liver size.

The key event in hepatic inflammatory cell recruitment and influx is margination and egress. As is well known, leukocyte extravasation involves the following sequence of events: expression of vascular adhesion molecules by activated endothelial cells; margination and rolling of leukocytes expressing the cognate ligands; adhesion of the leukocytes to the endothelium; transmigration across the endothelium; and migration within the extravascular space towards a chemotactic stimulus. The key intrahepatic endothelium appears to be the activated sinusoidal endothelium.[28] Recruitment of lymphocytes, in particular, may be driven by expression of powerful chemoattractants not only by the sinusoidal endothelium but also by parenchymal hepatocytes.[29] In the case of macrophage recruitment, the chemokine macrophage inflammatory protein-1α (MIP-1α) mediates the recruitment of inflammatory NK cells.[30] Intrahepatic production of MIP-1α is accomplished through IFN-α and IFN-β stimulation of the innate immune system in the liver to generate monocyte chemoattractant protein-1 (MCP-1),[31] which in turn recruits MIP-1α-producing inflammatory macrophages to the liver.[32]

During the acute phase of viral infection, lymphocytes first suffuse the hepatic parenchyma to varying extents; the portal tracts are relatively free of inflammatory cell aggregates (Fig. 2.3A). In the acute phase, the cytolytic action of lymphocytes is exerted on viral peptide-expressing hepatocytes scattered throughout the parenchyma. If viral clearance does not occur, parenchymal cytolysis smoulders on. As the infection settles into a chronic phase, portal tracts characteristically become populated with a mixed inflammatory cell population dominated by lymphocytes, with admixed macrophages and scattered granulocytes (Fig. 2.3B). The portal tract inflammatory infiltrate is capable of generating 'interface hepatitis', whereby destruction of hepatocytes at the interface of the parenchyma with portal tracts occurs (Fig. 2.3C). This is a characteristic feature of progressive chronic hepatitis.

Inflammation of portal tracts

The accumulation of inflammatory cells within portal tracts during chronic hepatitis raises the question of whether leukocytes leave the circulation through the vasculature of the portal tract. In the case of the portal veins, the answer appears to be 'no'. Rather, experimental data indicate that lymphocytes entering the liver via the portal vein undergo adhesion and extravasation at the level of the sinusoids.[33] Their immediate point of arrival is therefore the space of Disse. Definitive evidence is not available on their subsequent journey, but it is reasonable to suggest that the lymphocytes then travel in a retrograde fashion through the

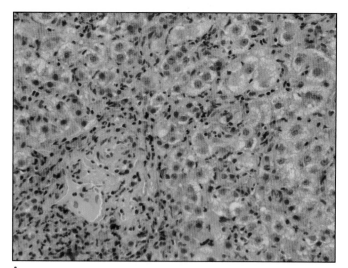

A

B

C

Fig. 2.3 • (A) Acute viral hepatitis (hepatitis A viral infection). The parenchymal sinusoids are suffused with lymphocytes and there is disruption of normal lobular hepatocyte architecture, with ballooning of damaged hepatocytes. The portal tract (lower left) is relatively free of mononuclear inflammation. **(B)** Chronic viral hepatitis (hepatitis C viral infection). A portal tract is expanded by a mononuclear inflammatory infiltrate, consisting almost entirely of lymphocytes. The interface between portal tract and parenchyma is largely intact. **(C)** Chronic viral hepatitis (hepatitis B viral infection). The interface between a portal tract (left) and the parenchyma (right) is extensively disrupted by inflammation, including encirclement of hepatocytes by inflammatory cells. H&E.

space of Disse to the interface of the portal tract; the time frame for such migration is not known.

The principles governing the behaviour of lymphocytes once they arrive at the portal tract are not well understood. On the one hand, it is plausible that fluid and lymphocytes filtered into the space of Disse enter into the hepatic lymphatic system. The elusive space of Mall, a potential space between the portal tract mesenchyme and the limiting plate of hepatocytes at the portal edge, is thought by some to represent the most terminal reaches of the intrahepatic lymphatic system. Alternatively, collagen fibres continuous between the space of Disse and portal tracts may constitute a submicroscopic channel for percolation of lymph from the space of Disse into portal tract lymphatics. Retention of leukocytes within this reticular mesenchyme may then occur.

For those leukocytes that accumulate within portal tracts during chronic hepatitis, a mixture of lymphocytes, plasma cells, macrophages, neutrophils, eosinophils, and even mast cells may occupy an expanded mesenchymal space within the portal tract. The stimuli for their retention are presumably chemotactic factors, although this is a presumption. Evidence is emerging that expression of attractant chemokines, such as CXCL2, on blood vessel endothelial cells within portal tracts, and within the lymphoid aggregates in portal tracts, may promote retention of lymphocytes within portal tracts, and potentially emigration of additional lymphocytes directly into the portal tract.[34] The chronically inflamed liver also expresses mucosal addressin cell adhesion molecules (MAdCAM-1) on the portal vein and sinusoidal endothelium, serving as an additional stimulus for homing of T-lymphocytes directly to the portal tract.[35]

The mechanisms underlying formation of the characteristic portal tract lymphoid aggregates in hepatitis C infection remain unknown. Regardless, it is worth keeping in mind that portal tract inflammation develops and persists over years in these patients, so that there is a prolonged time frame for arrival and organization of leukocytes at their respective destinations.

The accumulation of inflammatory cells in the immediate vicinity of bile ducts and ductules may follow different principles. Throughout the portal tract system, hepatic arteries and bile ducts are paired, travelling in close vicinity and of similar calibre.[36] The blood supply of the biliary tree is arterial, and bile ducts are invested by a hepatic artery-derived capillary bed.[37] Expression of proinflammatory cytokines by damaged bile duct epithelial cells[38] can recruit mononuclear inflammatory cells or neutrophils, depending upon whether the inciting injury is autoimmune or toxic in nature, respectively (Fig. 2.4). In the first instance, aberrant expression of a recently identified CXC3-chemokine, fractaline, by bile duct epithelial cells appears to be capable of recruiting CD4+ and CD8+ T cells, with adhesion to the biliary epithelium and accumulation of intraepithelial lymphocytes.[39] In the second instance, leakage of bile from an obstructed biliary tree appears to be particularly potent in recruiting neutrophils, which accumulate in a periductal location.[40,41] It is plausible to assume that these neutrophils exit from the vascular space in the peribiliary capillary bed

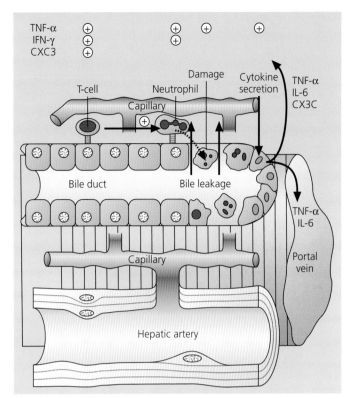

Fig. 2.4 • Schematic of portal tract in longitudinal section, depicting bile duct inflammation. A bile duct, the periductal capillary plexus, the companion hepatic artery, and a portal vein are depicted. First, proinflammatory cytokines tumour necrosis factor-α (TNF-α), interferon-γ (IFN-γ), and the chemokine CXC3 (fractaline) stimulate emigration of CD4+ and CD8+ T cells into the portal tract mesenchyme. Cytotoxic CD4+ T cells may adhere directly to bile duct epithelial cells via cytokine-induced aberrant expression of the major histocompatibility complex class II receptor (MHC-II, not shown). Second, the proinflammatory environment also stimulates emigration of neutrophils into portal tracts; release of noxious chemicals leads to bile duct epithelial cell damage and destruction. TNF-α secreted by portal tract lymphocytes can cause bile duct epithelial cell apoptosis. Third, bile leakage, containing bile salts, is itself proinflammatory, inducing chemotaxis of neutrophils to a periductal location. Lastly, bile duct epithelial cells themselves can secrete TNF-α, interleukin-6 (IL-6), and the chemokine CXC3. These proinflammatory cytokines can enter not only the portal tract space, but also may seep into the portal venous circulation, thus exposing the parenchyma to the deleterious effects of inflammation.

or its immediate postcapillary venules; involvement of the sinusoid and space of Disse seems unlikely. As will be discussed, bile ductules which traverse the portal tract mesenchyme between terminal bile ducts and the canals of Hering can become markedly proliferative under conditions of bile duct obstruction or damage. When such 'bile ductular proliferation' is due to biliary obstruction, neutrophils also accumulate in a periductular location, presumably also in response to the extrusion of bile with its toxic bile salts into the periductal mesenchyme.

Granulomas

Accumulation of activated macrophages into a microscopic focus surrounded by a collar of mononuclear leukocytes or fibrous tissue is termed granulomatous inflammation. The macrophages may exhibit a distinct enlarged cytoplasm with a pale eosinophilic appearance, giving them an 'epithelioid' appearance. Hepatic granulomas may arise in a vast number of clinical settings, including infection (e.g. *Mycobacterium tuberculosis*, with ensuant caseous necrosis of the granuloma centre), foreign body reaction (e.g. talc, with formation of giant cells), drug reaction, and autoimmune disease (especially primary biliary cirrhosis). The mechanisms for formation of granulomas are as diverse as the causes. A key underlying concept is proinflammatory cytokine perpetuation of the immune response, as with chronic local secretion of IL-2 and IFN-γ. This environment keeps the macrophages in an activated state and is capable of transforming them into epithelioid cells and multinucleated giant cells.

Inflammation in specific forms of hepatitis

In addition to the immunologic principles discussed above, specific comments about the main hepatotropic viruses giving rise to chronic hepatitis pertain. General concepts are given in Table 2.6, and are presented schematically in Fig. 2.1.

Hepatitis B viral infection

Patients who control HBV infection after an acute exposure exhibit clearly definable HBV-specific CD4+ and CD8+ T cell responses for a wide range of different HBV epitopes.[42] If present, HBV-specific cytotoxic T cells (CTL) are able to eliminate hepatitis B virus either by inducing apoptosis of infected hepatocytes (the cytolytic mechanism) or by secreting IFN-γ (the non-cytolytic mechanism).[9]

In patients with chronic HBV infection, circulating HBV-specific T cells are hard to find, and when present are specific for few or only single HBV epitopes.[43] A plausible explanation is impaired antigen-presentation by liver dendritic cells (DC). Such defective function can indeed be demonstrated in liver DCs from murine HBV carriers,[44] with production of significantly lower levels of IL-12, TNF-α, IFN-γ, and IL-6 when compared to liver DCs from uninfected mice. This might account for the weak or undetectable HBV-specific immune response in the minority of patients who do develop chronic HBV infection.

Hepatitis C viral infection

Hepatitis C virus (HCV) is not cytopathic for the infected hepatocyte. For example, in HCV-infected patients with or without coinfection with HIV, there is no correlation between HCV viral load and liver disease.[45] Rather, the immune response is the central cause of hepatocyte death.[17] First, in primary HCV infection, hepatocyte damage occurs upon development of the host immune response, and not upon infection and viral replication. Second, viral replication can occur in the absence of evident hepatocyte damage. Third, HCV is non-cytolytic in a number of expression systems, including cell lines and transgenic mice. Fourth, down-regulation of the immune response in patients with chronic HCV infection is usually accompanied by a reduction in serum transaminases and a rise in viral replication. Lastly, hepatocyte damage is associated with an inflammatory infiltrate containing HCV immune-effector cells.

The HCV genome encodes for a polyprotein that contains core, envelope (E1, E2), p7, and non-structural polypeptides (NS2, NS3, NS4A, NS4B, NS5A, NS5B) (Chapter 8). Extensive attention has been given to the core protein, which is the viral nucleocapsid protein. This 191-amino acid protein has RNA-binding activity and regulates a number of important intracellular signalling pathways involving the host interferon response to viral infection, and cellular proliferation and apoptosis. There is controversy as to whether the HCV core protein enhances the sensitivity of hepatocytes to apoptotic events or is antiapoptotic. At the current time, evidence supports a proapoptotic role for this protein. Specifically, the hepatocyte plasma membrane lymphotoxin-B receptor and TNF-receptor 1 can associate with the core protein, which potentiates intracellular proapoptotic signalling. This therefore enhances hepatocellular apoptosis induced by ligands of the TNF family released by intrahepatic lymphocytes, specifically TNF, TNF-related apoptosis-inducing ligand (TRAIL), Fas ligand (FasL), and lymphotoxin αβ complex.[46–48]

The mechanisms by which HCV resists clearance by the host system are not well understood.[11,49] There is a higher propensity for lymphocyte apoptosis during HCV infection,[50] and T cell responses to defined HCV antigens are depressed.[51] There is an enhanced T-regulatory cell response,[52] possibly leading to deletion of T cells which might be otherwise beneficial for clearance of virus.

Table 2.6	The immune response to viral hepatitis
Virus	**Comment**
Hepatitis B virus	
The virus (HBV)	Genetically stable, does not escape adaptive immune system
Dendritic cells (DC)	Process HBV antigens for presentation to lymphocytes
CD4+ and CD8+ T cells	Respond to HBV antigens expressed on infected hepatocytes
Cytotoxic T cells (CTL)	Clear infected hepatocytes through cytolysis or non-cytolytic antiviral action (via secretion of IFN-γ)
Hepatitis C virus	
The virus (HCV)	Genetically unstable, generates numerous quasispecies which escape the adaptive immune system
Hepatocyte changes	Increased sensitivity to apoptosis, decreased responsiveness to antiviral action of IFN-γ
Dendritic cells (DC)	Potentially defective antigen processing and presentation
Innate immune system (NK, NKT)	Contribute to the inflammatory destruction of HCV antigen-expressing hepatocytes
Cytotoxic T cells (CTL)	Chronic infection may arise because CTL response is inadequate to clear infected hepatocytes

HCV has been documented to be taken up by dendritic cells (DC),[53] and defects in DC function in HCV-infected individuals, including impaired DC maturation, have been described.[54] For its part, the HCV NS3 protein is capable of inducing prolonged release of oxygen radicals from mononuclear and polymorphonuclear phagocytes, by activating a key enzyme involved in oxygen radical formation, NADPH oxidase.[55] The NS3-activated phagocytes then induce dysfunction and/or apoptosis in the key major subsets of lymphocytes involved in defence against HCV infection: T cells, NK cells, and NKT cells.

At the risk of oversimplification, the net effect of HCV infection is therefore increased hepatocyte sensitivity to proapoptotic ligands (TNF-α, lymphotoxin-β, TRAIL, FasL) and activation of the innate immune system and recruitment of circulating leukocytes, leading to cytocidal destruction of hepatocytes. Ironically, this occurs in the midst of HCV proteins inducing a relative resistance of hepatocytes to interferon-mediated viral clearance, and down regulation of the cytocidal immune response so that the virus cannot be successfully cleared. Progressive inflammatory liver damage thus occurs.

Autoimmune hepatitis

Several forms of autoimmune hepatitis (AIH) have been identified (Chapter 10). The most common form, Type 1, affects all age groups and features antinuclear antibodies (ANA) and/or antismooth muscle antibodies (SMA). Type 2 AIH exhibits antibodies to liver/kidney microsome 1 (anti-LKM1). Type 3, the least common and thought by some to be a subtype of type 1, is characterized by antibodies to soluble liver antigen (anti-SLA) or a cytoplasmic antigen present in liver and pancreas (anti-LP). Underlying all forms is a loss of immune tolerance against the host liver.[56] The livers of such patients are heavily infiltrated with CD8+ T cells, and the histological features of AIH include infiltration by plasma cells. The histological hallmark of AIH is heavy infiltration of portal tracts with macrophages, plasma cells, and lymphocytes, and periportal interface hepatitis.

The infiltrating lymphocytes are mainly αβ T cells. CD8+ T cells predominate in the area of interface hepatitis, and CD4+ T cells predominate in the more central part of the portal tract.[57] Circulating CD8+ T cells are of the same clonotype as the liver. A key presumption is initiation of autoreactivity by CD4 T cells that recognize self antigen(s),[58] and that antigen-driven expansion of autoreactive CD4+ and CD8+ T cells drives the autoimmune-mediated damage. Noted earlier is a decreased number of circulating T-regs in AIH patients,[27] such that autoreactivity is not adequately down regulated. Not yet known are: how the autoreactive T cells arise; whether molecular mimicry and cross reactivity is involved; and the specific contributions of T cell cytolytic versus antibody-mediated destruction of liver cells.[59]

First, antigens expressed on the surface of hepatocytes are being identified that are targets of the autoreactive antibodies, including: CYP2D6 (to which anti-LKM1 react); and a membrane bound asialoglycoprotein receptor that is unique to hepatocytes and heavily expressed on periportal hepatocytes; a cytosolic UGA-suppressor tRNA protein (recognized by anti-SLA and anti-LP).[56] Second, hepatocytes in AIH patients exhibit aberrant induction of adhesion molecules which recruit inflammatory cells: intercellular adhesion molecule 1/CD54; and lymphocyte function-associated antigen-3 (LFA-3/CD58).[60] Third, polymorphisms are being identified in both the genes for inflammatory cytokines (e.g. TNF-α) and major histocompatibility loci (MHC) which may predispose patients to AIH.[61] What then appears to be operative is initiation of the autoimmune host response through the oligoclonal expansion of a limited number of T cells, potentiated by impaired function of regulatory T cells and inadequate apoptosis and self-deletion of autoreactive T cells. The autoreactive T cells also initiate B cell production of autoantibodies and proinflammatory cytokines. The net outcome is hepatocyte destruction.[59]

Hepatocellular injury

Cellular injury in the liver occurs in the following general settings: oxygen deprivation (either hypoxic or ischaemic); chemical or drug injury; infection; immunological injury; genetic misprogramming; and metabolic imbalance. Examples are given in Table 2.7. Later chapters in this book cover in detail these and related disease conditions. Underlying all of these is a characteristic set of morphological changes in hepatocytes. Short of hepatocellular death, these changes are essentially reversible phenomena, in that with removal of the offending agent or correction of the disease condition hepatocytes presumably can recover both morphologically and functionally. The pathogenesis of these changes is now briefly discussed.

Ballooning degeneration (oncosis)

Hepatocyte volume change (swelling) is part of normal physiology, and plays a critical role in the regulation of hepatocellular metabolism and gene regulation in response to environmental changes such as ambient osmolarity

Table 2.7	Examples of hepatocellular injury	
Form of injury	**Examples of a disease condition**
Oxygen deprivation	
Hypoxia	Shock
Ischaemia	Devascularization during liver transplantation
Ischaemia/reperfusion	Revascularization of organ
Chemical or drug injury	Acetaminophen toxicity
Infection	Cytomegalovirus infection
Immunologic injury	Hepatotropic viral hepatitis: HBV, HCV
Genetic misprogramming	Alpha-1-antitrypsin storage disorder
Metabolic imbalance	Non-alcoholic fatty liver disease

changes, oxidative stress, intracellular substrate accumulation, and hormones such as insulin.[62] However, deranged cellular swelling is a fundamental feature of cellular injury, and is termed 'oncosis'. In the lexicon of liver pathology, 'ballooning degeneration' is the term used. Hepatocyte ballooning is the result of severe cell injury, involving depletion of ATP and a rise in intracellular Ca^{2+}, leading to loss of plasma membrane volume control and disruption of the hepatocyte intermediate filament network.[63] If severe enough, cell death occurs. Oncosis occurs in ischaemic liver cells, cholestasis, and in many other forms of hepatic toxicity.[64]

The morphological manifestation of hepatocellular ballooning degeneration is hepatocellular swelling, vacuolization of the cytoplasm, clumping of intermediate filaments (manifest in haematoxylin and eosin (H & E)-stained tissue sections as clumped strands of eosinophilic cytoplasmic material), swelling of mitochondria, and blebbing of the cell membrane (Fig. 2.5). These features, which affect the entirety of the hepatocyte cytoplasm, are to be distinguished from the well-formed spherical lipid vacuoles of the steatotic hepatocyte (see below).

On a macroscopic scale, with hepatocellular injury and swelling, the liver may be transformed into a swollen and turgid organ. Pallor may be evident both because of the increased intracellular fluid, and because of impending compromise of the hepatic circulation. As sensory innervation of the liver is confined mainly to the liver capsule, it is the swollen liver that, by exerting tension on the liver capsule, engenders localizing right upper quadrant pain.

Steatosis

Accumulation of triglyceride fat droplets within hepatocytes is known as steatosis. Multiple tiny droplets that do not displace the nucleus are known as microvesicular steatosis (Fig. 2.6A), and appear in such conditions as acute fatty liver of pregnancy and valproic acid toxicity. A single large droplet that displaces the nucleus is termed macrovesicular steatosis (Fig. 2.6B), and may be seen in hepatocytes throughout the livers of obese or diabetic individuals, and interestingly in scattered hepatocytes in patients with hepatitis C viral infection. Both microvesicular and macrovesicular steatosis may be present in alcoholic fatty liver, affecting virtually every hepatocyte.

In alcoholic steatohepatitis, hepatocellular steatosis is associated with hepatocyte ballooning degeneration and Mallory body formation (see below), an inflammatory infiltrate of the lobule (neutrophils mixed with lymphocytes, often wrapped around ballooned hepatocytes containing Mallory bodies), and usually brisk sinusoidal fibrosis. Non-alcoholic fatty liver disease (NAFLD) features hepatocellular steatosis; when hepatocyte ballooning degeneration, Mallory body formation, and inflammation are present, the term non-alcoholic steatohepatitis (NASH) is given.[65] In

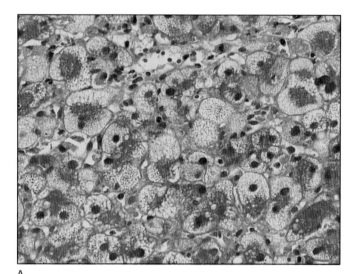

A

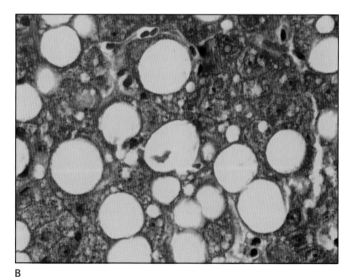

B

Fig. 2.6 • (A) Microvesicular steatosis in the liver of a pregnant woman. Hepatocytes contain innumerable small fat droplets which do not displace the cell nucleus. **(B)** Macrovesicular steatosis in an alcoholic patient. Hepatocytes are distended by single large fat droplets, which displace the cell nucleus to the side. As fat is dissolved during routine tissue processing, a clear space only remains. Masson trichrome.

Fig. 2.5 • Alcoholic hepatitis, in which many hepatocytes are markedly ballooned, with rounded plasma membrane contours, cleared-out cytoplasm, and clumped strands of intermediate filaments (some of which would qualify as Mallory bodies). Interspersed among the ballooned hepatocytes are inflammatory cells and fibrous tissue. H&E.

NASH, the degree of inflammation and fibrosis are usually far less than seen in alcoholic hepatitis.

The accumulation of lipid within hepatocytes is fundamentally a metabolic event. In the normal liver, lipid biosynthesis maintains cellular membranes, supports hepatic bile secretion (which contains bile salts, phospholipids, and cholesterol), and is a key feature of the assembly of very low-density lipoprotein (VLDL) particles, which are exported from the liver into the circulation. The liver does not normally store lipids. During alcohol exposure, hepatocellular metabolism of alcohol to acetaldehyde (via alcohol dehydrogenase), and thence to acetate (via acetaldehyde dehydrogenase) generates reducing equivalents in the form of NADH + H$^+$ (Chapter 6). With excess and/or sustained alcohol exposure, the reducing equivalents cannot be satisfactorily disposed of via mitochondrial oxidative metabolism. The NADH + H$^+$ are therefore diverted into lipid biosynthesis: fatty acids and glycerol. Esterification of fatty acids with glycerol to form triacylglycerols completes the biosynthetic pathway, leading to accumulation of neutral lipid droplets in the cytoplasm of hepatocytes. These droplets can accumulate within hours of a major alcohol exposure. Impaired export of VLDL from the hepatocyte also leads to accumulation of lipoprotein lipid within a distended Golgi apparatus.[66] Regardless of location, these droplets initially are only a micron or two in diameter (microvesicular), with a high surface:volume ratio. These droplets are thus amenable to rapid dissolution through the action of lipases, which occurs at the cytoplasmic interface. Over time (probably days), the droplets coalesce, forming droplets exceeding 20 μm in diameter (macrovesicular), displacing the hepatocyte nucleus. As the surface:volume ratio is exceedingly low, the action of surface lipases is of minimal impact. These macrovesicular lipid droplets can thus remain for months, even in the absence of further alcohol exposure. Eventually, should the alcoholic liver disease progress, the number of steatotic hepatocytes may eventually diminish.

Lipid accumulation in non-alcoholic fatty liver disease (NAFLD) follows a different pathogenetic sequence. Aberrations in insulin-related postprandial lipolysis lead to increased fatty acid delivery to the liver, while excess dietary carbohydrate leads to de novo fatty acid synthesis in the liver. Importantly, mitochondrial β-oxidation of fatty acids is impaired; contributing causes may be increased intrahepatic generation of reactive oxygen species (with lipid peroxidation and oxidative stress), impaired mitochondrial respiratory chain function, and intrahepatic production of proinflammatory cytokines (such as TNF-α).[65,67] The mechanisms underlying these derangements are under intense investigation. The steatosis of NAFLD is predominantly macrovesicular, with one or several lipid droplets occupying the entire cell cytoplasm.

In animal models of hepatic steatosis, accumulation of fat is accompanied by enhanced expression of peroxisome proliferator-activated receptor-γ (PPARγ).[68] This protein is a 'master regulator' of adipogenesis, as it participates in the transcriptional activation of numerous adipogenic and lipogenic genes involved with adipocyte maturation, lipid accumulation, and metabolic coordination of lipid biosynthesis. PPARγ has two major isoforms, γ1 and γ2, generated from the same gene by alternative splicing. PPARγ2 is expressed abundantly in mature adipocytes, and is elevated in fatty livers in animals. When expressed in hepatocytes, PPARγ2 up-regulates expression of adipogenic and lipogenic genes, including: adipose differentiation-related protein (ADRP), adipocyte fatty acid-binding protein 4, sterol regulatory element-binding protein-1, fatty acid synthase, and acetyl-CoA carboxylase.[69] Triacylglyceride biosynthesis and lipid accumulation occur, with uniform coating of the intracellular lipid droplets by ADRP. These findings point towards a potentially key role of PPARγ2 in the development of steatosis in the mammalian liver, whereby events that up-regulate hepatic expression of PPARγ2 would induce hepatic steatosis.

Cholestasis

Bile constitutes the primary pathway for elimination of bilirubin, excess cholesterol (both as free cholesterol and as bile salts), and xenobiotics which are insufficiently water soluble to be excreted into urine. Bile facilitates the digestion and absorption of lipids from the gut. Because bile formation requires well-functioning hepatocytes and an intact biliary tree, this process is readily disrupted.

Physiologically, cholestasis denotes an impairment of bile flow and failure to secrete the inorganic and organic constituents of bile. In particular, cholestasis arises from molecular and ultrastructural changes that impair the entry of small organic molecules, inorganic salts, proteins, and ultimately water into the biliary space. Clinically, the physical findings of jaundice and pruritus are accompanied by elevated serum concentrations of bilirubin, bile salts, and alkaline phosphatase. A general formulation for causes of cholestasis is given in Table 2.8.

Pathologists have marvelled at the profound hepatic alterations in jaundiced patients for almost two centuries,[70] but only in the last 20 years have the molecular secrets of cholestasis been unlocked. A number of key molecular events occur in the hepatocyte in both obstructive and non-obstructive cholestasis.[1,71] These are summarized in Table 2.9. The key conclusion to draw from Table 2.9 is that a strategic subset of the hepatocyte transport system changes during acquired cholestasis. First, expression of the basolateral sodium bile salt transporter, NTCP, is markedly down-regulated. Second, canalicular secretion of bile salts via the bile salt export pump (BSEP) is maintained. However, secretion of other organic anions into bile (especially bilirubin glucuronides via multidrug resistance-associated protein 2; MRP2) is decreased. Meanwhile, canalicular transport systems normally responsible for secretion of other organic anions into bile (MRP1, MRP3) are now expressed on the basolateral plasma membrane. MRP3, in particular, is capable of exporting bile salts into the plasma space. Hence, the hepatocyte adopts a 'cytoprotective' phenotype, whereby bile salt uptake is shut down, and bile salt extrusion is increased through maintenance of canalicular secretion and the addition of basolateral secretion.

Table 2.8	Causes of cholestasis (excludes inherited hyperbilirubinaemic syndromes)*

Cholestasis in the adult or adolescent
  Obstructive cholestasis:
    gallstones
    malignancy: pancreatic cancer, bile duct adenocarcinoma
    stricture of the common bile duct
  Bile duct diseases:
    primary biliary cirrhosis
    primary sclerosing cholangitis
    graft-versus-host disease: acute, chronic
    transplant rejection: acute, chronic
    transplant: infarction of the biliary tree secondary to hepatic artery obstruction
    vanishing bile duct syndromes: ibuprofen, chlorpromazine
  Non-obstructive cholestasis:
    infection: viral hepatitis, endotoxaemia, sepsis
    toxic: drug, total parenteral nutrition
    paraneoplastic syndrome: Hodgkin disease
  Inherited disease: Wilson disease, familial cholestatic syndromes
  Pregnancy: intrahepatic cholestasis of pregnancy
  Infiltrative disorders: amyloidosis, metastatic cancer
  Cirrhosis (any cause)

Cholestasis in the neonate or young child
  Obstructive cholestasis:
    biliary atresia: extrahepatic biliary atresia, 'early severe' biliary atresia
    common bile duct obstruction: biliary sludge, gallstones
    choledochal cyst with biliary sludge
    inspissated bile/mucous plug
  Non-obstructive cholestasis
    bacterial infection: Gram-negative enteric bacteraemia, syphilis, listeria, toxoplasma
    viral infections: cytomegalovirus, herpesvirus (includes simplex, zoster, parvovirus B19, adenovirus), rubella, reovirus, enteroviruses, hepatitis B, hepatitis C
    toxic: total parenteral nutrition, drugs
  Metabolic disease:
    with biliary tract compromise: alpha-1-antitrypsin storage disease, cystic fibrosis
    without biliary tract compromise: galactosaemia, tyrosinaemia, fatty acid oxidation defects, lipid storage disorders, glycogen storage disorders, peroxisomal disorders
    specific defects in biliary function: bile acid biosynthetic defects, PFIC1, PFIC2, PFIC3
  Paucity of bile ducts: Alagille syndrome, non-syndromatic paucity of bile duct syndromes
  Miscellaneous:
    shock/hypoperfusion
    histiocytosis X
  Idiopathic neonatal hepatitis
  Cirrhosis (any cause, as derived from the above specific conditions)

PFIC, progressive familial intrahepatic cholestasis
* Reproduced with permission from Li M, Crawford JM. The pathology of cholestasis. Semin Liver Dis 2004; 24:21–42

Hepatocellular cholestasis, to the pathologist, is the visible manifestation of this broad array of pathophysiological derangements in hepatocellular uptake, transcellular transport, and canalicular secretion of biliary constituents. Notably, hepatocellular changes exhibit considerable overlap between diseases involving bile duct obstruction and those in which the cholestasis is purely hepatocellular in origin. Hence, the features described here for non-obstructive cholestasis are also found in obstructive cholestasis; it is only upon finding additional obstructive changes in portal tracts and bile ducts that the obstruction can be inferred.

The parenchymal morphological changes occurring as a result of non-obstructive or obstructive impairment of hepatocellular bile formation are given in Table 2.10 and illustrated in Fig. 2.7.[72] The dominant themes are accumulation of substances normally secreted in bile and toxic degeneration of hepatocytes, without significant alterations in portal tracts. The most obvious hepatocellular feature is brown pigmentation from retained bilirubin (*bilirubinostasis*). Pigmentation includes accumulation of bilirubin and its glucuronides in hepatocytes, inspissated bile in swollen canaliculi, and bile regurgitation into the sinusoidal space with phagocytosis by Kupffer cells. Such pigmentation occurs predominantly in the perivenular region of the hepatic lobule, as does dilatation of bile canaliculi. During severe cholestasis of long duration, bilirubin deposition and canalicular dilatation may extend into the periportal region.

Necrosis per se is not a prominent feature of cholestatic liver disease, but cell dropout with acidophilic bodies is often present (apoptosis). Hepatocytes undergoing toxic degeneration may appear enlarged with a flocculent cytoplasm, so-called feathery degeneration, also found predominantly in the perivenular zone. When such degeneration leads to confluent necrosis of hepatocytes, *bile infarcts* are produced (also called bile lakes), in which large masses of acellular pigmented material are surrounded by a rim of necrotic hepatocytes or reactive mesenchyme. These are usually encountered only in obstructive cholestasis.

A particular feature of cholestatic periportal hepatocytes is *cholate stasis*. First, periportal hepatocytes may undergo 'ballooning degeneration', evident as cellular swelling with cytoplasmic material clumped around the nucleus, and large lucent peripheral areas of the cell. Second, it is not unusual to find Mallory bodies (intracellular strands of clumped intermediate filaments) in periportal areas, which is in contradistinction to the perivenular Mallory body distribution characteristic of alcoholic liver disease. Lastly, as copper is a heavy metal normally secreted in bile, special stains for copper or copper-associated protein may demonstrate copper accumulation in periportal hepatocytes. All of these changes are attributed to the retention of biliary constituents normally secreted by periportal hepatocytes. In particular, retained bile salts are toxic, both on the basis of their detergent properties and their ability to activate programmed cell death pathways,[73] hence the term 'cholate' stasis. This feature may occur in non-obstructive cholestasis; it is more prominent in obstructive cholestasis.

Table 2.9 Key hepatocyte molecular transport systems, with changes during cholestasis

Transport protein	Transport function	Inherited defect, if known	Phenotype in acquired cholestasis, if known
Basolateral membrane			
NTCP	bile salts	none known	markedly decreased in cholestasis
OATP2	organic anions		modestly decreased in cholestasis
Canalicular membrane			
BSEP	bile salts	PFIC2	modestly decreased during cholestasis
MDR1	multispecific organic solutes		maintained during cholestasis
MDR3	phosphatidylcholines	PFIC3	maintained during cholestasis
ABC1	cholesterol	Tangier disease type 1	
MRP1	organic anions		increased during cholestasis, basolateral expression
MRP2	organic anions, bilirubin glucuronides	Dubin–Johnson syndrome	decreased during cholestasis
MRP3	organic anions, bile salts		increased during cholestasis, basolateral expression
CFTR	chloride	Cystic fibrosis	
FIC1	aminophospholipids	PFIC1	maintained during cholestasis

BSEP, bile salt export pump; MRP, multidrug resistance protein; NTCP, sodium-taurocholate cotransporting polypeptide; PFIC, progressive familial intrahepatic cholestasis
Reproduced with permission from Li M, Crawford JM. The pathology of cholestasis. Semin Liver Dis 2004; 24:21–42

Table 2.10 Histology of cholestasis

Histological feature	Description
Parenchyma	*Morphological features during non-obstructive or obstructive cholestasis*
Bilirubin pigment accumulation	Hepatocyte cytoplasm pigmentation
	Bile canalicular dilatation with inspissated bile
	Regurgitated pigment: Kupffer cell pigmentation
	Acinar distribution: perivenular > periportal
Hepatocellular degeneration	Feathery degeneration with flocculent cytoplasm; perivenular > periportal
	Ballooning degeneration with swollen hepatocytes: periportal > perivenular ('cholate stasis')
	Mallory body formation: periportal
	Bile infarcts: coalescent periportal necrosis with retained pigmented material
Metal accumulation	Accumulation of copper and copper-associated protein: periportal
Liver cell rosettes	Dilated bile canaliculi surrounded by more than two hepatocytes in a pseudotubular arrangement
Giant cell transformation	Coalescence of hepatocytes, with multiple nuclei and free-floating 'canaliculi'
Portal tracts	*Morphological features during obstructive cholestasis*
Portal tract expansion	Oedema, mixed pattern of inflammation with abundant neutrophils
Bile ductular proliferation	Racemose small ductular channels, extending to the periphery of the portal tract, sectioned obliquely in-and-out of the plane of section, with or without inspissated bile
Bile duct dilatation	Prominently dilated marginal bile ductules with inspissated bile ('cholangitis lenta'): occurs in sepsis
	Ectatic interlobular and segmental bile ducts, either with a reactive inflamed epithelium, or an attenuated and potentially ulcerated epithelium with associated neutrophilic abscess
Fibrosis	Broad-based fibrosis expanding portal tracts and creating blunt fibrous septa that subdivide the liver parenchyma in a 'jigsaw' like pattern

Chronic cholestasis of neonates, children, and rarely adults may give rise to so-called cholestatic *liver cell rosettes*, consisting of dilated bile canaliculi surrounded by more than two hepatocytes in a pseudotubular arrangement. These rosettes express some cytokeratins characteristic of biliary epithelium, and by three-dimensional reconstruction they are found to communicate with small bile ducts and ductules.[74] They are thus thought to be an adaptive mechanism to chronic cholestasis.

A further feature of neonatal cholestatic syndromes is the frequent appearance of *giant cells*—foamy-appearing multinucleated hepatocytes with intracellular pigmented inclusions having the appearance of 'floating' bile canaliculi.[75] On occasion, giant cell transformation may be seen in adult cholestatic livers. Although the origin of such cells is unclear, it is thought that the detergent action of retained bile salts leads to dissolution of the lateral plasma membranes and coalescence of adjacent hepato-

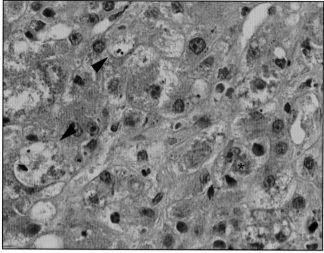

A

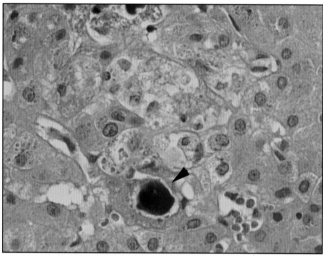

B

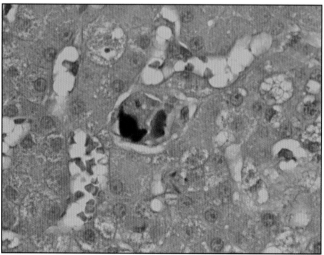

C

Fig. 2.7 • (A) Hepatocellular cholestasis. Numerous hepatocytes are discoloured by brown pigmented material (arrowheads), indicative of retention of biliary constituents within hepatocytes. Note is made that bile salts are colourless; retained bilirubin and bilirubin glucuronides are responsible for the coloration. A Mallory body also is present (*). (B) Hepatocellular and canalicular cholestasis. In addition to the retention of bile by hepatocytes, there is prominent retention of bile in a distended bile canaliculus (arrowhead). (C) A Kupffer cell within a sinusoid has engulfed biliary material that has regurgitated into the circulation, through disruption of the intercellular junctions between hepatocytes. H&E.

cytes. Such giant cell transformation also can occur in biliary atresia.

In non-obstructive cholestasis, there are no distinctive changes in portal tracts other than those associated with the underlying cause (e.g. viral or drug-induced hepatitis). However, with obstructive cholestasis, a distinctive set of portal tract histological features emerge, as detailed in Table 2.10 and illustrated in Fig. 2.8.[40] These features occur upstream to either intrahepatic biliary obstruction (as from primary biliary cirrhosis or primary sclerosing cholangitis) or extrahepatic biliary obstruction (as from gallstone obstruction or pancreatic cancer). Particularly distinctive is proliferation of the small bile ductules (often termed ductular reaction), creating a racemose array of uniformly sized small ductular channels passing in and out of the plane of section, but remaining within the topological space of the portal tract. This response is to be distinguished from the 'ductular reaction' observed during liver regeneration from massive injury, in which irregular partial ductular structures are present at the interface and within the damaged parenchyma. The latter structures represent massive proliferation of the progenitor cell population of the liver.

Mallory bodies

Differentiated hepatocytes exhibit a simple cytokeratin expression pattern: the type I cytokeratin CK8, and the type II cytokeratin CK18.[76] In keeping with the requirement that proper assembly of cytokeratins requires the presence of at least one type I and one type II peptide, CK8 and CK18 assemble in equimolar ratios into intermediate filaments (IF), which form a filamentous network within the cytoplasm of hepatocytes. In a variety of disease conditions, alterations in hepatocellular cytokeratin assembly occur. Ballooning of hepatocytes is accompanied by a reduced density or even loss of the cytoplasmic IF network. Misfolded and aggregated keratins can accumulate, forming Mallory bodies (MBs, Fig. 2.9).[77] MBs exhibit aberrant cross linking, increased phosphorylation, partial proteolytic degradation, and an increase of β-sheet conformation. MBs accumulate in alcoholic and non-alcoholic steatohepatitis, Wilson disease, cholestatic conditions such as primary biliary cirrhosis, and following exposure to certain drugs (such as amiodarone).

A key degradation pathway for misfolded proteins is the ubiquitination–proteasome pathway. By mass spectrometry, MBs consist of keratin, ubiquitinated keratin, the stress-induced and ubiquitin-binding protein p62, heat shock proteins (HSPs) 70 and 25, and other peptides.[78] Hence, antibodies to ubiquitin and p62 highlight MBs in tissue sections.

Interestingly, cytokeratins are able to modulate TNF signalling pathways and the apoptosis pathway. Specifically, cytokeratins can bind to the TNF receptor 2 (TNFR2), thereby influencing TNF-α-induced activation of the death signalling pathway.[79] TNF-α is a potent inducer of neutrophilic inflammation, and ballooned hepatocytes containing MBs are frequently surrounded by neutrophils. Thus, the accumulation of MBs may not simply be a by-

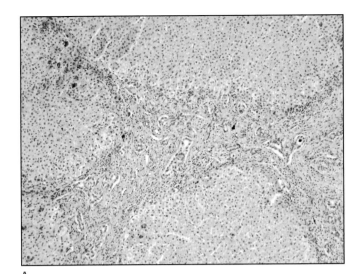

A

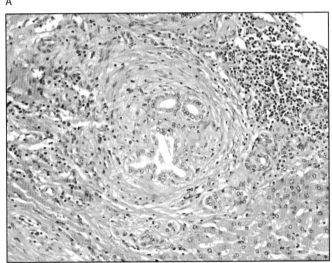

B

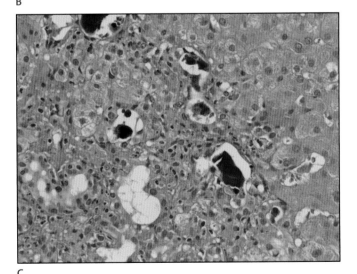

C

Fig. 2.8 • (A) Portal tract in obstructive cholestasis secondary to biliary atresia. There is extensive bile ductular proliferation, evidenced by the racemose ductular structures within the portal tract space. The portal tract is expanded by fibrous tissue, and there is bile retention in the periportal parenchyma. **(B)** Chronic obstructive cholestasis. Bile ducts are surrounded by concentric fibrosis. Peribiliary fibrosis such as this can occur in diseases other than primary sclerosing cholangitis, owing to the brisk fibrogenic response of portal tract myofibroblasts during obstructive cholestasis. **(C)** Cholangitis lenta. A distinctive dilatation of marginal ductules by inspissated bile can occur in the setting of sepsis or endotoxaemia, without there being biliary obstruction. H&E.

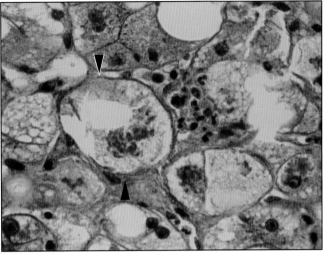

Fig. 2.9 • Mallory body. A ballooned hepatocyte (arrowhead) contains a clumped skein of intermediate filaments, appearing as dense magenta strands of cytoplasmic material. In fact, Mallory bodies are also present in Figs 2.5, 2.7a, and 2.12. Masson trichrome.

product of hepatocellular toxic damage, but may also contribute to the perpetuation or advancement of inflammatory injury.

Apoptosis and necrosis

While the cellular changes described in the previous section may be viewed as reversible, at some point the hepatocyte cannot compensate and recover. The onset of irreversible injury is accompanied by extensive damage to all cellular membranes, swelling of lysosomes, vacuolization of mitochondria, and extensive catabolism of cellular membranes, proteins, ATP, and nucleic acid. Cellular death takes two broad forms: apoptosis and necrosis. Apoptosis is the usual consequence of immunologically-mediated cell death. For the most part, necrosis is a feature of disease processes other than hepatitis, especially injury involving tissue ischaemia. Curiously, despite the past two decades of intense research into the molecular mechanisms of apoptosis and necrosis, there is no specific assay or parameter which allows distinction between the two, other than morphological changes in vivo.[80] In fact, the intracellular signalling pathways overlap to some extent.

Apoptosis

Apoptosis is an active form of cell death in which cells exhibit cytoplasmic shrinkage, cell membrane blebbing, chromatin condensation, and cellular fragmentation into small membrane-bound 'apoptotic bodies'.[81] These characteristic changes are the result of activation of caspases and endonucleases, which induce the cleavage of structural proteins and DNA, respectively.[80] In the liver, apoptotic bodies have long been referred to as acidophilic bodies or Councilman bodies (Fig. 2.10).[82] Identification of apoptotic bodies indicates current and ongoing hepatocellular apoptosis, since apoptotic hepatocytes are engulfed within a

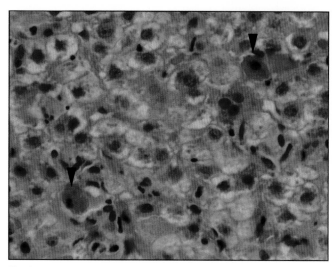

Fig. 2.10 • Hepatocyte apoptosis. Two apoptotic hepatocytes (arrowheads) are present in the parenchyma of an acute hepatitis. H&E.

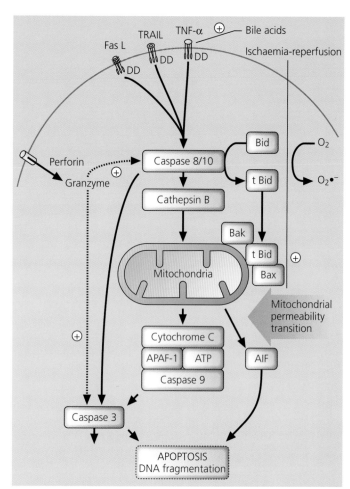

Fig. 2.11 • Schematic overview of receptor-mediated and mitochondria-mediated apoptotic signal transduction pathways. Receptors for Fas-ligand (FasL), tumour necrosis factor-related apoptosis-inducing ligand (TRAIL), and tumour necrosis factor-α (TNF-α) are normally dispersed monomeric subunits in the plasma membrane. Binding of FasL, TRAIL, or TNF-α to their respective receptors induces receptor trimerization and recruitment of accessory intracellular molecules (not shown) to the cytoplasmic 'death domains' (DD) of the receptors. This causes activation of caspases 8 and 10, which then activates a proapoptotic pathway. Both cathepsin and activated Bid (tBid) induce the *mitochondrial permeability transition* (MPT), resulting in release of cytochrome c and apoptosis-inducing factor (AIF) from mitochondria. Assembly of a cytochrome c/Apaf-1/ATP/caspase 9 complex activates caspase 3. Both caspase 3 and AIF converge to cause DNA fragmentation and apoptosis. Caspases 8 and 10 also may activate caspase 3 directly. Additional proapoptotic stimuli include: entry of granzyme into the cell through a perforin pore, following release of perforin/granzyme from T lymphocytes; bile acid induction of trimerization of the cell surface death receptors by ligand-dependent or ligand-independent mechanisms, leading to activation of the proapoptotic pathways; and ischaemia–reperfusion with generation of superoxide radicals ($O_2\cdot^-$), which can activate the MPT directly.

matter of hours by Kupffer cells or other macrophages, as noted earlier. Upon triggering of apoptosis (as by a cytotoxic T cell), a characteristic sequence of down-stream events occurs: translocation of phosphatidylserine to the outer leaflet of the cell plasma membrane; caspase activation; activation of the mitochondrial permeability transition; cytochrome c release from the mitochondrion; and DNA fragmentation. Exposure of phosphatidylserine on the outer leaflet of the cell membrane is an early stimulus for phagocytosis of the apoptotic body. Simply speaking, apoptosis results in elimination of infected host cells from the host organism, and is therefore one mechanism for controlling infection.

Two overlapping signalling pathways lead to apoptosis:[82] the extrinsic 'death receptor' pathway; and the intrinsic 'mitochondrial' pathway (Fig. 2.11).[83,84] The extrinsic pathway is mediated by cell surface receptors such as Fas and the TNF-α receptor-1 (TNF-R1), interacting with cytotoxic T cells expressing Fas-ligand or releasing TNF-α. The downstream signalling involves cross linking of the receptor complexes with adapter proteins and procaspase 8, thereby cleaving procaspase 8 to its active form. Active caspase 8 initiates downstream effector cascades, including caspase 3. The extrinsic pathway may also be initiated by perforin and granzyme B released from activated cytotoxic lymphocytes. Perforin allows granzyme B to enter the cytoplasm of target cells, and directly cleave intracellular proteins such as procaspases. In addition to Fas and the TNF-α receptor-1 mediated pathways, TRAIL-mediated apoptosis can also occur in viral hepatitis and cholestatic liver disease.[85]

The intrinsic pathway for apoptosis arises from mitochondrial dysfunction or possibly endoplasmic reticulum stress.[86] Oxidative damage to the mitochondrial inner membrane leads to the mitochondrial phase transition and release of cytochrome c and apoptosis inducing factor (AIF) from the mitochondrion into the cytosol. Cytochrome c complexes with Apaf-1 to activate procaspase 9, which then activates downstream caspases such as caspase 3, 6, and 7.[82]

Mitochondria also release endo G, which with caspases can cleave chromosomal DNA. Mitochondrial release of cytochrome c is a near-universal event in apoptosis and a key marker of the intrinsic pathway of apoptosis.[87]

Apoptosis is a normal feature of hepatic development and remodelling, both for the parenchyma of the liver and the biliary tree.[82] Notably, hepatocellular apoptosis is also a regular feature of the major inflammatory hepatic diseases: viral hepatitis, autoimmune liver disease, alcoholic liver disease, non-alcoholic liver disease, and drug-induced liver disease,[82,87] attributable to the presence of cytotoxic lymphocytes acting upon hepatocytes. Although apoptosis occurs as part of normal development and tissue remodelling and avoids stimulation of inflammatory pathways, pathological apoptosis may not only result from inflammation but may actually amplify the inflammatory process.[88] In the case of viral hepatitis, a plausible sequence is that viral antigens released from damaged or dead hepatocytes are taken up and processed by dedicated antigen-presenting cells (APC)—dendritic cells or Kupffer cells. These processed antigens are then expressed on the surface of APC in association with class I and class II major histocompatibility antigens (MHC). The T-cell mediated death pathways are then engaged.[89] Apoptosis may also be seen in chronic cholestatic disorders owing to the toxic nature of retained bile salts on the mitochondria and their activation of death-receptor signalling;[90] bile duct epithelial cell apoptosis also occurs in these disorders. While hepatocellular apoptosis can be seen in the alloreactive disorders of graft-versus-host disease and liver allograft rejection, it is bile duct epithelial cell apoptosis which is a key diagnostic feature for these two conditions.[91]

Key regulators of the intracellular apoptotic signalling pathways are antiapoptotic survival proteins and proapoptotic proteins.[92] A key player is nuclear factor-κ B (NFκB), which is activated when the TNF-receptor-1 is ligated by TNF-α.[93] NFκB-induces transcriptional activation of survival factors such as cFLIP, XIAP, c-IAP1, c-IAP2, Bfl-1/A1, Bcl-2, and Bcl-xL. These survival factors down-regulate or inhibit the intracellular apoptotic signalling pathways at a number of points. Paradoxically, activated NFκB can transactivate death receptors such as Fas or tumour necrosis factor-related apoptosis-inducing ligand D5 (TRAIL-D5).[94] TRAIL, which cannot normally induce apoptosis, nevertheless becomes capable of triggering hepatocellular apoptosis during viral infection or under cholestatic conditions when bile acid levels are elevated.[95,96] Under such conditions, there appears to be loss of NFκB-dependent Bcl-xL upregulation.[97] NFκB thus has a dual role as mediator or inhibitor of cell death, whereby the modulation of apoptosis by NFκB appears to be largely determined by the nature of the death stimulus.[97]

Nitric oxide (NO) is capable of protecting the liver against apoptosis,[98] as it is able to inhibit the apoptotic signal transduction cascade at multiple points.[99] As nitric oxide synthase (NOS) is normally expressed by endothelial cells (eNOS, also called NOS3), and may be induced in endothelial cells (iNOS, also NOS2), hepatocytes, and Kupffer cells under a wide variety of conditions, there is ample opportunity for this potent mediator to influence the apoptotic outcomes of hepatic injury.

The mechanisms of hepatocellular death in α$_1$-antitrypsin deficiency are less clear. While retention of the misfolded Z form of α$_1$-antitrypsin, α$_1$-ATZ, in the endoplasmic reticulum is clearly the toxic event, how this retained aggregated mutant leads to hepatocellular injury is unclear. Evidence has been presented that a brisk autophagocytic response is triggered by retention of misfolded α$_1$-antitrypsin, and mitochondria exhibit injury followed by mitochondrial autophagy.[100] The autophagocytic response is associated with activation of caspase signalling cascades and initiation of hepatocellular apoptosis.

Necrosis

Necrosis is different from apoptosis in that it involves cell swelling, vacuolation, karyolysis, and release of cellular contents (Fig. 2.12).[80] In keeping with the earlier discussion on hepatocellular ballooning degeneration (oncosis), the term 'oncotic cell death' is another term for this form of cell death, owing to the loss of osmotic regulation of ion content at the level of the plasma membrane. Necrosis is the predominant mode of death in states of oxidative stress,[99] although apoptosis also may contribute.[101] Accordingly, organ ischaemia due to interruption of blood flow with subsequent reperfusion is a valuable experimental example of injury leading to hepatocyte necrosis. Ischaemia–reperfusion occurs during hepatic resection, liver transplantation, and hypotensive shock followed by recovery.[102] The first key step in the process of injury is depletion of intracellular ATP during the ischaemic period. This then precipitates an increase in intracellular Ca^{2+}, owing to decreased active extrusion of Ca^{2+} from the cell by Ca^{2+}-ATPase, and an opening of voltage-dependent Ca^{2+} channels due to membrane depolarization caused by decreased activity of the Na$^+$-K$^+$ ATPase (the latter of which consumes approximately 25% of cellular ATP under normal conditions).[103] The increase in intracellular Ca^{2+} destroys the cytoskeleton,[104] and plays a critical role in the opening of the mitochondrial permeability transition pore, thereby stimulating the mitochondrial pathway of apoptotic cell death.[105,106]

The second key event in ischaemia–reperfusion injury is the generation of oxygen radicals during reperfusion.[102] As initially hypothesized by McCord in 1985 and Adkins et al. in 1986,[107,108] during the ischaemic interval cytosolic xanthine dehydrogenase is converted to xanthine oxidase. Meanwhile, degradation of adenine nucleotides leads to

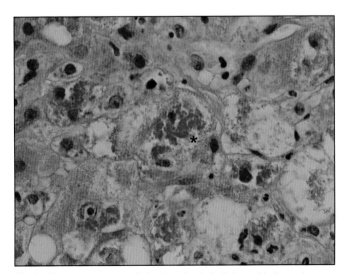

Fig. 2.12 • Oncotic hepatocellular death in alcoholic hepatitis. Severely ballooned hepatocytes have lost their sharply defined cell borders, and have undergone cell death. In the centre of the field a residual Mallory body (*) and brown discoloration of cholestasis is also present. H&E.

accumulation of hypoxanthine in the ischaemic organ. Upon reperfusion and introduction of oxygen substrate, xanthine oxidase generates massive amounts of superoxide anion. The resultant oxidative damage disrupts cytoplasmic and nuclear proteins, organelle membranes and proteins, and DNA. The cytoskeleton also undergoes proteolysis, and mitochondrial oxygen reduction is also impaired. The reactive oxygen species also act as intracellular second messengers, inducing cascade reactions through the transcriptional factors NFκB and AP-1. As the liver has the greatest amount of macrophages of any organ in the body, these macrophages can also secrete oxygen radicals as well as tissue-toxic cytokines such as TNF-α and IL-1; the recruitment of inflammatory cells further exacerbates the tissue injury.

Interestingly, in necrotic death, nitric oxide (NO) potentiates hepatocellular necrosis. This appears to be mediated by an NO-induced decrease in intracellular ATP.[109] As NO is generated by endothelial cells activated during tissue injury and inflammation,[110] the sinusoidal endothelium can be yet another contributor to hepatic injury.

Necrosis frequently exhibits a zonal distribution. The most obvious is necrosis of hepatocytes immediately around the terminal hepatic vein, an injury that is characteristic of ischaemic injury and a number of drug and toxic reactions (Fig. 2.13). Pure midzonal and periportal necrosis are rare; the latter may be seen in eclampsia. Necrosis of entire lobules (submassive necrosis) or of most of the liver (massive necrosis) is usually accompanied by hepatic failure. It should be noted such 'necrosis' is likely to have resulted from apoptosis, as in fulminant viral hepatitis.

Regeneration

Mild injury to hepatocytes, cholangiocytes, or the endothelium and mesenchyme may be met with complete recovery of the organ, and there may be complete recovery of the liver following massive hepatocellular death provided that inflammatory and fibrogenic pathways are not initiated. Regeneration of liver cells is the key step towards recovery from injury. As will be discussed, the rodent liver has a substantive capacity to regenerate from experimental reduction in size. Unfortunately, the human liver recovers its mass slowly, although hepatic function can be maintained despite significantly reduced tissue mass.

Following childhood, the normal liver becomes a stable organ with slow turnover of hepatocytes. However, upon injury or surgical reduction, the liver converts to a proliferative organ that can restore approximately three-quarters of its own mass within 6 months. This is accomplished while maintaining the differentiated functional capacity of its component hepatocytes. Hepatocytes, bile duct epithelial cells, and hepatic progenitor or stem cells maintain the potential to multiply during adult life.[111] Depending on the type of injurious agent, the nature of the liver disease, and the extent of hepatic destruction, liver regeneration may occur by at least two mechanisms (Fig. 2.14).[112-114] First, adult differentiated hepatocytes may undergo division and replication, responding quickly to liver damage associated with mild to moderate hepatocellular loss. Second, more extensive or massive hepatic necrosis stimulates the proliferation of progenitor cells within the periportal region.

Regeneration of mature liver cells

Over-and-above the oft-cited mythological capacity of the liver of Prometheus to regenerate daily,[115-118] the definitive experimental demonstration of liver regeneration was shown in rodents following two-thirds partial hepatectomy.[119] This is not 'regeneration' in the strictest sense, since the lobes of the liver are not regrown. Rather, there is a profound hyperplastic response involving replication of virtually all (95%) of the mature functioning hepatocytes in the residual liver. The regenerative process is compensatory, since it stops once the original mass of the liver has been restored. By far the quickest and most efficient way to restore liver mass is through replication of existing hepatocytes.[120]

These observations have driven the field of liver regeneration ever since, since explanation of both the stimuli for regeneration and for their cessation is considered to have immense value for understanding tissue growth under normal and cancerous conditions (in which failure of 'cessation' is critical). The key questions to be answered are:[116] (i) what are the signals that trigger the early events in the regenerative process? (ii) how are the architecture and function of the liver retained during regeneration? (iii) which signals are responsible for turning off the growth response once the mass of the liver is reconstituted? An extensive literature is reviewed elsewhere,[120-122] and is summarized briefly herein.

In rats, about 12 hours are required for the rate of hepatocyte DNA synthesis to increase, as they move from the G0 phase of the cell cycle (quiescent) to the S phase. Hepatocellular DNA synthesis peaks at around 24 hours. The induction of DNA synthesis occurs later in the non-parenchymal cells: at about 48 hours for Kupffer and biliary

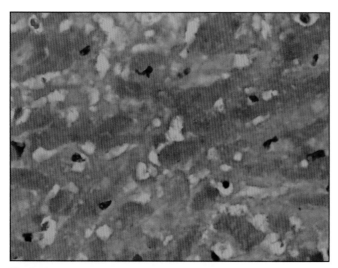

Fig. 2.13 • Ischaemic hepatocyte necrosis. Hepatocyte features are completely lost, leaving only indistinct eosinophilic remnants of the hepatocyte cords, occasional pyknotic hepatocyte nuclei, and partial preservation of some sinusoidal cells such as macrophages. H&E.

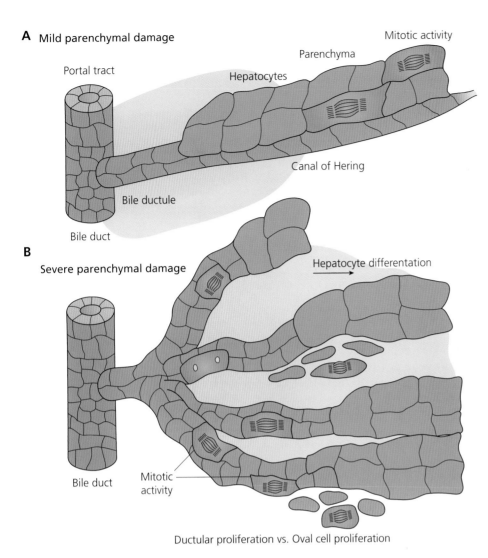

A Mild parenchymal damage

Portal tract

Parenchyma

Mitotic activity

Hepatocytes

Canal of Hering

Bile ductule

Bile duct

B

Severe parenchymal damage

Hepatocyte differentiation

Bile duct

Mitotic activity

Ductular proliferation vs. Oval cell proliferation

Fig. 2.14 • Mechanisms of parenchymal regeneration in the liver. **(A)** With mild-to-moderate parenchymal damage, as in chronic hepatitis, mitotic activity of hepatocytes alone is sufficient to maintain liver mass. The architecture of bile ductules, which bridge between the portal tract bile duct and the canals of Hering, remains normal. **(B)** With severe parenchymal damage, either in the setting of massive hepatic necrosis or during severe bouts of chronic hepatitis, there is proliferation of progenitor cells within the liver. These are thought to be derived from bipotential cells of the bile ductule/canal of Hering compartment, evident histologically as 'ductular reaction' and/or from a stem cell or 'oval cell' compartment. Although the relationship between ductular reaction and oval cell proliferation is not fully established, hepatocyte differentiation of these progenitor cells leads to restitution of liver mass in the unscarred liver, or contributes to the nodular proliferation of the scarred liver characteristic of cirrhosis.

epithelial cells and at about 96 hours for endothelial cells. Complete restoration of liver mass requires about 1.6 cycles of replication in all cells.[116] In mice, the induction of DNA synthesis and cell division occurs slightly later, and varies between strains. It should be noted that the limited number of cell cycles required to restore liver mass does not mean that hepatocytes have limited replication capacity. Serial transplantation experiments demonstrate that hepatocytes can replicate 70 or more times,[123] without depending upon stem cell populations.

The onset of DNA synthesis in hepatocytes begins in the periportal region and expands towards the terminal hepatic vein region. The incidence of mitosis is lower than expected from the levels of DNA synthesis, and is explained by an increase in the ploidy of hepatocytes, thereby limiting further regeneration.[124]

Regenerative signals

Polypeptide growth factors. Early studies by Moolten and Bucher[125] demonstrated that circulating growth factors are present in the serum of hepatectomized rats. These growth factors are capable of inducing hepatocyte replication, and have been demonstrated to be polypeptide growth factors,

including hepatocyte growth factor (HGF), epidermal growth factor (EGF), transforming growth factor alpha (TGFα), heparin-binding growth factors and insulin-like growth factors.

Human hepatocyte growth factor (HGF) is an 85-kD protein, and can act as a mitogen (stimulating proliferation), morphogen (stimulating maturation), or motogen (stimulating cell movement) for many different cell types. HGF is synthesized by non-parenchymal cells, particularly stellate cells, and therefore affects hepatocytes in a paracrine manner.[116] HGF is secreted as a precursor, pro-HGF, and is rapidly activated by proteases—urokinase-type plasminogen activator (uPA) and its downstream effector, plasminogen. HGF is a potent stimulator of DNA and protein synthesis in hepatocytes,[126] and is 10 times more effective than other polypeptide growth factors, such as EGF, in promoting hepatocyte proliferation.[127] On the basis of structural homologies, HGF belongs to the plasminogen-related growth factors (PRGF) family of soluble cytokines. HGF elicits its biological functions upon binding with its membrane receptor, the tyrosine kinase encoded by the c-MET proto-oncogene. The c-Met receptor has a multifunctional docking site on the cytoplasmic domain, enabling the phosphorylation of different intracellular transducers. The balance between proliferation and differentiation elicited by HGF binding to the c-Met receptor depends upon which intracellular signalling pathways are recruited.[128]

Epidermal growth factor (EGF) and transforming growth factor alpha (TGFα) are closely related polypeptides. EGF is synthesized and released by a large number of tissue cells and is mitogenic in many mesenchymal and epithelial structures, including the liver.[129] It is very effective in stimulating liver regeneration and this is considerably enhanced by insulin. Its potency for the liver may be due to the high number of receptors on the hepatocyte plasma membrane. The liver thus has an extraordinary capacity to clear EGF from the blood.[130] EGF stimulates DNA synthesis in hepatocytes in tissue culture, suggesting that it has a direct effect.[131] Although EGF may be a major, primary hepatic growth regulator, blood levels of EGF do not change much immediately after partial hepatectomy[132] and there is no increase in messenger RNA for EGF receptors for the first 24 hours.[133] However, amphiregulin, a ligand for EGF receptor (EGFR) is expressed within 30 min of partial hepatectomy.[134] Amphiregulin is a polypeptide growth factor of the EGF family, and is expressed normally in the human ovary and placenta but not in the healthy and quiescent liver parenchyma.[135] Amphiregulin can be detected in cultured hepatocytes, and is detectable in the cirrhotic liver.[134] In the regenerating liver, tyrosine phosphorylation (and hence activation) of the EGFR is dramatically up-regulated at 60 min despite the absence of an elevation in EGF levels. It appears that amphiregulin is uniquely involved in this activation, as other ligands for EGFR cannot serve as substitutes. Hence, the EGFR may play a key role in initiation of liver regeneration depending upon which agonist ligand is bound, with amphiregulin playing a specific and unique role.[136]

TGFα has approximately 30 to 40% amino acid sequence homology to EGF. It can directly enhance DNA synthesis in hepatocytes in tissue culture. Messenger RNA for TGFα is undetectable in the normal liver but appears within 8 hours of partial hepatectomy and increases rapidly over the next 24 hours in parallel with DNA synthesis.[137] Since release of TGFα may be stimulated by EGF, an early role for EGF in hepatic regeneration cannot be excluded.[138] TGFα also could be derived from extrahepatic sources. Either way, TGFα may act as a potent autocrine regulator in promoting liver regeneration, in the midst of its fibrogenic effects on perisinusoidal stellate cells.

Other polypeptides include heparin-binding growth factors (HBGF) and the insulin-like growth factors (IGF, somatomedins). HBGFs have also been termed fibroblast growth factors (FGF) and are mitogens for a wide variety of cell types. There are two main subtypes, HBGF-1 and HBGF-2, and an increase in both is found in hepatocytes at early, though not the earliest, stages of liver regeneration.[139,140] As with TGFα, they may have an autocrine role in helping to amplify the initial regenerative signals.

Insulin-like growth factors (IGFs) are synthesized in the liver in response to growth hormone and represent the probable mechanisms through which growth hormone influences liver regeneration. A time lag of several hours elapses before enhancement of regeneration occurs in response to growth hormone, and these polypeptides probably have a modulatory rather than an initiating role.[141]

The intracellular signalling pathways induced by these various polypeptide growth factors are complex and highly inter-related; these complex processes are discussed elsewhere.[116,120]

Nutritional and hormonal regulation. Hepatic regeneration depends upon the availability of the basic nutrient building blocks that are usually supplied via the portal venous blood from intestinal digestion and absorption. Nonetheless, the effect of specific dietary deficiencies can be difficult to evaluate because of an ability to mobilize these resources from other cells in the body. Fasting has been shown to delay and diminish regeneration in response to partial hepatectomy, but it does not abolish it.[142] It has also been shown that there is an increase in the amino acid pool following partial hepatectomy[143] and enhanced movement of amino acids occurs across the hepatocellular membrane.[144] Infusions of a branched-chain-enriched mixture of amino acids have been shown to stimulate regeneration[145] although, generally, infusions of amino acids, lipids, or carbohydrate have an inhibitory effect upon the response.[146] However, dietary protein does enhance regeneration as increased mitotic activity can be demonstrated in hepatocytes when experimental animals are transferred from low-protein to normal or high-protein diets.[147] Unfortunately, the very amino acids which may be beneficial to hepatic regeneration in the setting of cirrhosis are likely to tip a human patient into hepatic decompensation due to the amino acid load.

Virtually all hormones have been shown to influence regeneration in the liver. They include insulin and glucagon, thyroid and adrenal cortical hormones, parathyroid hormone, prolactin, vasopressin, prostaglandins, catecholamines, and sex hormones.[148] Of these, the most important seem to be insulin, glucagon, and the catecholamines. In the absence of insulin, regeneration is not diminished but it is delayed in onset and takes much longer.[149–151] Conversely, the presence of insulin has the opposite effect.[152] Glucagon acts synergistically with insulin but neither hormone alone or in concert is able to initiate, or by their absence prevent, regeneration.[148]

Various observations suggest that catecholamines are involved in the early stages of liver regeneration and could play a part in the regulation of liver growth. Blood catecholamine levels are known to increase within 2 hours of partial hepatectomy, and DNA synthesis in the regenerating liver is significantly reduced by chemical or surgical sympathetic denervation.[153] The rich sympathetic nerve supply to portal tracts and sinusoids is also greatly increased in the liver after regeneration.[154] The response appears to be modulated through the α-adrenergic receptors and so β-blockers do not have any influence. The number of $α_1$-adrenergic receptors on hepatocytes decreases by 30 to 40% in the 24 hours after partial hepatectomy while β-receptors increase dramatically.[155,156] Noradrenaline enhances the effects of epidermal growth factor on DNA synthesis in cultured hepatocytes[157] and counteracts the growth inhibitory effects of TGFβ.[158]

Thyroid hormones can also promote regeneration but a combination of triiodothyronine, amino acids, glucagon, and heparin is even more effective.[159]

Cytokines. Cytokines themselves play a critical role in the regulation of liver regeneration. On the positive side, IL-6 is a key effector cytokine, as it acts upon its receptor, IL-6R, to stimulate mitogenic intracellular signalling cascades, and can potentiate signalling induced by growth factors.[160] In mice, normal liver regeneration requires IL-6,[161,162] although whether IL-6 is the major proregeneration cytokine is open to debate.[163,164] Specifically, TNF-α is itself required for a normal proliferative response after partial hepatectomy,[165] as it induces IL-6 expression. However, absence of TNF-α does not impair liver regeneration.[166] Rather, the ability of Kupffer cells to generate IL-6 as the primary source of IL-6 in the liver is a function of stimulation by TNF-α or other agents.[167] As the innate immune system plays a key role in the local generation of TNF-α and IL-6, there is clearly an interplay between the immune response to injury and the initiation of a hepatic regenerative response. Moreover, as liver regeneration in the clinical setting is more often in the setting of inflammation (as opposed to following surgical reduction), it is notable that the NK cells of the innate immune system impede the regenerative response.[168]

Knowledge about cytokines that act as growth inhibitory factors is limited. It has been suggested that they could represent the normal mechanism for regulating liver growth. In this model, inhibitory substances would be produced by the normal liver and their relative absence following hepatic resection or significant hepatocellular damage would release hepatocytes from their effects. Transforming growth factor beta (TGFβ) is the most clearly identified candidate. This is a ubiquitous 25 kD polypeptide whose actions in vivo include stimulation of fibrogenesis by perisinusoidal stellate cells (discussed later). In vitro, TGFβ can inhibit or stimulate cell proliferation, modulate cell differentiation and regulate numerous cellular functions according to the cell type, culture conditions, and presence of other cytokines.[169] However, in an experimental situation TGFβ fails to prevent regeneration after hepatectomy,[170] so its role would seem to be one of modulation rather than primary control.

Maintenance of liver architecture

Insights into how liver architecture is maintained during regeneration are limited. After partial hepatectomy, hepatocytes rapidly proliferate and form cell clusters of 10 to 14 cells.[171] These clusters are devoid of extracellular matrix and vascular channels. Particularly important is the angiogenesis that must occur, whereby ingrowth of epithelial cell buds impales the cell clusters and enables re-establishment of normal sinusoids (Fig. 2.15).[172] This is the result of highly coordinated spatiotemporal expression of angiogenesis growth factor receptors on sinusoidal endothelial cells within the regenerating cell clusters.[173] These include receptors for VEGF, angiopoietin, PDGF, and EGF. As all receptors are tyrosine phosphorylated, they are in a peak state of activation during the angiogenic phase of regeneration.

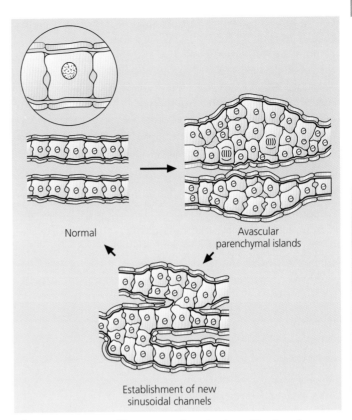

Fig. 2.15 • Schematic of liver regeneration, whereby proliferation of hepatocytes generates avascular parenchymal islands and thickened hepatocyte cords. Angiogenesis with endothelial cell proliferation, infiltration of hepatocyte clusters, and re-establishment of sinusoidal architecture allows return of the parenchyma to a normal vascular architecture. Based on concepts presented in: Ross MA, et al. Hepatology, 2001; 34:1135–1148.

Replicating stellate cells produce extracellular matrix about 4 days after partial hepatectomy, re-establishing the contact between hepatocytes and matrix. The result is re-establishment of sinusoids, although the intervening hepatocyte plates are oversized. Further remodelling is required before the final normal relationships between hepatocytes and the sinusoids are established. This requires elimination of superfluous hepatocytes through apoptosis.[174]

Cessation of the regenerative response

The best known hepatocyte antiproliferative factors are TGFβ and TGFβ-related family members such as activin.[174,175] TGFβ is produced primarily by hepatic stellate cells, and contributes to liver fibrosis (discussed below). Stimulation of the TGFβ signalling pathway can induce G1/S phase arrest and induction of apoptosis.[176] However, hepatocellular responses to TGFβ are complex, in that hepatocytes can exhibit resistance to the antiproliferative effects of TGFβ,[122] most probably through inhibition of the TGFβ-stimulated intracellular SMAD signalling pathways.[177] Activin, in turn, is an apoptogen of the TGFβ family that blocks hepatocyte mitogenesis.[116]

What is most intriguing is how the termination system is engaged. It appears to require, and act in parallel with, restoration of normal sinusoidal architecture and repopulation of the subendothelial space with stellate cells.[174] Stellate cells home to the newly formed space of Disse in response to PDGF, FGF, and EGF. TGFβ augments the chemotactic response of stellate cells to PDGF and FGF. Transient activation of stellate cells to myofibroblasts is required for synthesis of perisinusoidal extracellular matrix and completion of regeneration within the parenchyma.[178] These transiently activated stellate cells are capable of generating TRAIL, thereby generating a TRAIL receptor-dependent apoptosis signal affecting both hepatocytes and stellate cells themselves.[179] There thus appears to be a negative feedback loop which is both autocrine (stellate cell–stellate cell) and paracrine (stellate cell–hepatocyte) to limit the regenerative surge.

Telomere length is important for the replicative potential of hepatocytes, as experimental knockout of telomerase (the enzyme that maintains telomere length) impairs DNA synthesis, shortens the lifespan of hepatocytes, and impairs their ability to regenerate.[180] It is not clear whether relative deficiencies of telomerase both limit the normal regenerative response, and contribute to chronic liver disease through a failure of nascent cells to maintain adequate rates of regeneration.

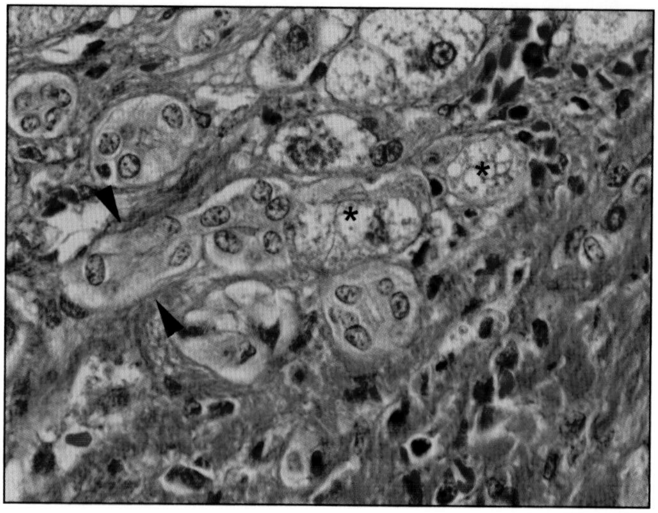

Fig. 2.16 • Ductular hepatocytes. Significant parenchymal destruction, particularly at the interface with the portal tracts, engenders a brisk regenerative response featuring 'ductular reaction'. These ductular structures can differentiate towards a bile ductular phenotype (arrowheads), or acquire the granular and larger cytoplasm of the hepatocellular phenotype (asterisks). In this particular image from autoimmune hepatitis, there is extensive fibrosis as well. Masson trichrome.

The role of progenitor cells

Hepatocytes, bile-duct epithelial cells, and endothelial cells maintain the potential to multiply during adult life.[181] However, certain types of injury render these cells unable to replicate. Toxic injury may diminish or eliminate the capacity of hepatocytes to replicate. Experimental toxins in this category include diplin, retrorsine, galactosamine, and monocrotaline.[182] Above and beyond toxic injury, extensive hepatic necrosis, especially involving the periportal region of the parenchyma, stimulates the proliferation of progenitor cells.[183,184]

Identification of small cells with oval nuclei in rat models of hepatocarcinogenesis and in regenerative responses to liver injury led to the premise that there is a liver progenitor cell compartment.[185] The term 'oval cell' was first coined in 1956 by Farber,[186] to distinguish these cells in different models of rat hepatocarcinogenesis. Similar oval cells have been identified in the human liver,[187] and are capable of differentiating into hepatocytes and bile duct epithelial cells. Similarities to the ductal plate hepatocytes of the fetal liver suggest that adult progenitor cells reside in the periportal region.[181,188] Proliferation of these cells gives rise first to 'ductular hepatocytes', in which ductular structures are present containing cuboidal cells and slightly larger cells with mitochondria-rich cytoplasm (Fig. 2.16). Immunohistochemical stains demonstrate cytokeratin staining characteristic of bile-duct epithelial cells, simultaneously with albumin staining.[181,188] With time, these cells are capable of maturing into definitive hepatocytes on the one hand, and repopulating damaged bile-duct structures on the other.[189] In massive hepatic necrosis, there appears to be an explosive proliferation of ductular structures which are all connected to individual canals of Hering and thence to terminal bile ducts within portal tracts.[190–192] These structures comprise the parenchymal 'ductular reaction' in

massive hepatic necrosis, to be distinguished from the phenomenon observed within portal tracts of the bile duct-obstructed liver (see Fig. 2.8 and Table 2.10).

The hypothesis can thus be advanced that the bipotential progenitor cells reside in, or at least close to, the canals of Hering.[193] The 'ductular' compartment may also serve as a transit point between mature hepatocytes and bile duct epithelial cells, as transdifferentiation of rat hepatocytes into biliary cells has also been demonstrated.[194] Bile ducts themselves may also contain cells phenotypically capable of acting as liver progenitor cells.[195] Clearly, 'plasticity' of the liver may involve the regenerative capacity of progenitor cells within the mature liver parenchyma, an 'oval cell' compartment in, or immediately adjacent to, the canal of Hering, and the biliary tree itself.[196]

There is a growing literature addressing whether hepatic progenitor cells can be derived from non-hepatic precursors, particularly bone marrow stem cells (reviewed in Ref. 120). Initial observations that bone marrow stem cells are capable of populating the liver with hepatocytes, albeit in small numbers,[197,198] have been countered by other observations documenting that: (i) bone marrow stem cell repopulation of the liver parenchyma, if extant, is a rare event;[199,200] and (ii) the possibility of fusion of the bone marrow stem cells with nascent mature cells in the target tissue may explain many of the observations.[201] In one experimental system, the FAH knockout mouse, there may be extensive repopulation of damaged livers by bone marrow-derived stem cells,[202,203] but the kinetics of repopulation are slow and inefficient when compared with hepatocyte transplantation. Alternatively, haematopoietic stem cells have been shown to convert into liver cells within days, without cell fusion, and can contribute to regeneration of the injured liver.[204]

The current research into the biology of hepatic progenitor cells is of extraordinary interest to liver pathobiology. At the very least, ongoing parenchymal destruction in the diseased liver, particularly when it is occurring at the septal interface, appears capable of stimulating proliferation of ductular hepatocytes. The massive expansion of ductular populations in some cases of cirrhosis[188] suggests that activation of at least the bipotential progenitor cell compartment may help maintain hepatic mass. Whether entry of stem cells from the bone marrow into the liver plays a substantive role in liver restitution remains unclear. Comment has also been made that, regardless of whether restitution might involve cell fusion, there may yet be therapeutic benefit in further exploring these biological events.[205]

Fibrosis

While regeneration may be viewed as a beneficial step to recovery, a central and perhaps defining detrimental process in progressive chronic liver disease is fibrosis.[206] Fibrosis may be regarded as the wound-healing response of the liver to repeated injury.[207] Specifically, acute liver injury features regeneration of nascent cell types, associated with an inflammatory response and limited deposition of extracellular matrix. However, if the hepatic injury persists, then eventually the liver regeneration fails and matrix deposition is activated, akin to the formation of scar in the liver.

In the normal liver parenchyma, interstitial collagens (types I and III) are concentrated in portal tracts and around terminal hepatic veins, with occasional bundles in the space of Disse. Delicate strands of type IV collagen (reticulin) course alongside hepatocytes in the space of Disse. In cirrhosis, excess type I and III collagens are laid down not only in portal tracts but also in the lobule, creating delicate or broad septal tracts. Concomitantly, the sinusoids are converted into capillaries with a basement membrane so that blood–hepatocyte solute exchange is impaired despite maintenance of absolute hepatocyte mass.[208] The key events involve stellate cells, deposition of extracellular matrix, and alteration of the parenchymal microvasculature. The mechanisms of hepatic fibrosis will be discussed in this section; discussion of vascular changes follows.

Stellate cells

In the normal liver parenchyma, extracellular matrix may be produced by perisinusoidal stellate cells, hepatocytes, and the sinusoidal endothelial cells.[209–211] Stellate cells, hepatocytes, and sinusoidal endothelial cells are capable of synthesizing types I and IV collagen. Type III collagen and fibronectin can also be elaborated by these cells.[212] Stellate cells have several key functions (Chapter 1): (i) retinoid storage and homeostasis; (ii) remodelling of extracellular matrix by production of both matrix components and matrix metalloproteinases; (iii) production of growth factors and cytokines; and (iv) contraction and dilation of the sinusoidal lumen.[213,214] Stellate cells are present in the subendothelial space of Disse and sometimes in the

perisinusoidal recess between hepatocytes. Stellate cells comprise less than 10% of total resident liver cells under normal conditions, and are regularly spaced along the sinusoids (approximately 40 μm from nucleus to nucleus).[215] Despite their relative scarcity, they have long cytoplasmic processes which can cover the entire perisinusoidal area.[206] It is notable that autonomic nerve endings running in the space of Disse come into contact with stellate cells, and the stellate cells respond to α-adrenergic stimulation.[216]

With repeated injury to the liver parenchyma, stellate cells become activated, lose their retinyl ester stores, and transform into myofibroblast-like cells which are positive immunohistochemically for α-smooth muscle actin (Fig. 2.17).[217] The major parenchymal source of excess collagen under abnormal conditions is stellate cells.[218] The key features of stellate cell activation are: (i) robust mitotic activity in areas developing new parenchymal fibrosis; (ii) a shift from the resting-state lipocyte phenotype to a transitional myofibroblast phenotype; and (iii) increased capacity for synthesis and secretion of extracellular matrix.[218–221] It is predominantly the cytokines secreted by activated Kupffer cells and other inflammatory cells that stimulate the stellate cells to divide and to secrete large amounts of extracellular matrix.[222,223] There is a marked increase in stellate cell expression of messenger RNAs for collagens I, III, IV, and laminin, and no increase of collagen formation by hepatocytes.[224,225] Of interest is recent in vitro data suggesting that activated stellate cells do not necessarily proliferate, but may become polyploid through endoreplication.[226] Although inflammation is a key activator of stellate cells, stellate cells are themselves contributors to the inflammatory response, by acting as antigen-presenting cells.[227] The activated state of stellate cells is maintained by survival factors; apoptosis of the stellate cell population occurs when the state of inflammation and release of proinflammatory cytokines subsides.[228–231] In keeping with the apposition of autonomic nerve endings on stellate cells, the fibrogenic phenotype also is promoted by α-adrenergic stimulation.[216]

The contractile properties of stellate cells have a major impact on liver blood flow and modification of portal resistance during fibrosis and cirrhosis. Endothelin-1 (ET-1) is the key contractile stimulus for activated stellate cells.[206] This system acts in an autocrine loop of stimulation whereby ET-1 synthesis is up-regulated in activated stellate cells, as is expression of its two receptors, ET-A and ET-B.[231] In the normal liver, ET-1 induced vasoconstriction is in balance with nitric oxide (NO) mediated vasodilatation (via antagonism of ET-1). During liver fibrosis, there is an increase in ET-1 expression and a decrease in NO generation by the sinusoidal endothelium, shifting the balance towards stellate cell (myofibroblast) contractility.[232]

The greatest activation of stellate cells is in areas of severe hepatocellular necrosis and inflammation.[233] The activation of stellate cells may exhibit a zonal pattern. Perivenular sinusoidal fibrosis has been well documented in the early stages of liver injury from alcohol[234–238] or toxins,[239] in both animals and humans. This is accompanied by a decrease in sinusoidal density in the perivenular region.[239] Because the size of acini does not change significantly during the

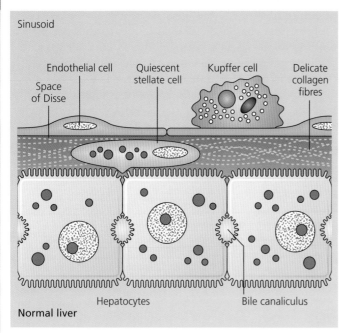 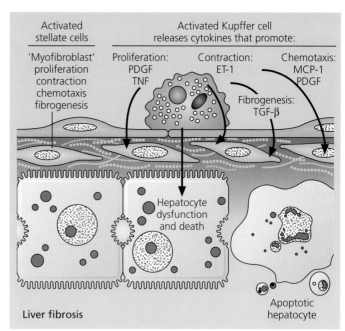

Fig. 2.17 • Stellate cell activation and liver fibrogenesis (right), in comparison to the normal liver sinusoid (left). Inflammatory activation of Kupffer cells leads to secretion of multiple cytokines; cytokines may also be released by endothelial cells, hepatocytes, and other inflammatory cells of the innate immune system within the liver such as T lymphocytes (not shown). These cytokines 'activate' stellate cells, whereby the lipid droplets (present in the quiescent state) are lost, and the stellate cells acquire a myofibroblastic phenotype. Tumour necrosis factor (TNF) is a potent stimulant of the change to a myofibroblastic state. Stellate cell proliferation is stimulated in particular by platelet-derived growth factor (PDGF). Contraction of the activated stellate cells is stimulated by endothelin-1 (ET-1). Deposition of extracellular matrix (fibrogenesis) is stimulated especially by transforming growth factor β (TGF-β). Chemotaxis of activated stellate cells to areas of injury, such as where hepatocytes have undergone apoptosis, is promoted by PDGF and monocyte chemotactic protein-1 (MCP-1). Kupffer cells also are a major source of TNF released into the system circulation. (Schematic based on concepts presented in: Friedman SL. Molecular regulation of hepatic fibrosis: an integrated cellular response to tissue injury. J Biol Chem, 2000; 275:2247–2250; and Crawford JM. Cellular and molecular biology of the liver. Curr Op Gastroenterol, 1997; 13:175–185.)

development of fibrosis/cirrhosis,[219] the reduction in sinusoidal density appears to represent a true loss of microvascular capacity, before complete nodule formation occurs. Moreover, there is an increase in stellate cells in the perivenular region prior to the development of fibrous septa.[219] These findings indicate that simultaneous alterations in stellate cells, extracellular matrix, and the parenchymal microvasculature occur during the evolution of cirrhosis. Put differently, microvascular changes are not merely the consequence of fibrosis and nodule formation, but are part-and-parcel of the evolution of cirrhosis.[239]

Extracellular matrix

There are many different components of the extracellular matrix in the liver, including collagens, glycoproteins, and proteoglycans (Table 2.11); these are all vastly increased in cirrhosis.[240]

Collagens

At least 14 different collagens have been identified, falling broadly into two categories—fibrillar and basement membrane collagens. Types I, III, and V of the fibrillar collagens and types IV and VI of the basement membrane collagens have been identified in the liver. Types I, III and V are confined mainly to the portal tract and terminal hepatic vein wall.[206] Type I collagen corresponds to the doubly refractile mature collagen in portal tracts and around the walls of

Table 2.11	Extracellular matrix components
Component	**Normal distribution**
Collagens	
Type I	Portal tract matrix, hepatic veins, points of inflection in hepatic cords
Type III	Portal tract matrix, space of Disse
Type IV	Portal tract basement membranes, space of Disse
Type V	Portal tract matrix, space of Disse
Type VI	Portal tract matrix, space of Disse
Glycoproteins	
Laminin	Portal tract basement membranes, space of Disse
Fibronectin	Portal tract matrix, space of Disse
Entactin (nidogen)	Portal tract basement membranes
Elastin	Portal tract matrix
Fibrillin	Portal tract matrix
Proteoglycans	
Heparan sulphate	Portal tract basement membranes

(From Virchows Arch A Pathol Anat Histopathol, 423, 1993, 1–11. The hepatic extracellular matrix. I. Components and distribution in normal liver, Martinez-Hernandez A, Amenta PS. With kind permission of Springer Science and Business Media)

hepatic veins, and is evident in tissue sections simply by lowering the substage condenser to increase refraction. Type III collagen also is present in the reticulin framework of the sinusoids, association with type IV collagen, where a two-dimensional lattice is formed.[241] Type IV collagen also forms the basement membranes around bile ducts, arteries, and veins. Type VI collagen, in contrast, is found in the interstitial matrix of the portal tract. It is absent from basement membranes but is frequently present near blood vessels and it may have a role in anchoring vascular tissue to the perivascular matrix.[242]

In fibrotic and cirrhotic livers, total collagen is increased up to eight-fold, mainly because of increased collagen type I deposits.[243] The primary source of collagen is the perisinusoidal stellate cells. Other collagens and non-collagenous extracellular matrix proteins are also deposited in the space of Disse.[244,245] These include collagen types III and IV, laminin, and fibronectin, which are normal components of basement membranes.

Glycoproteins and proteoglycans

The collagens are intimately complexed and interwoven with glycoproteins and the proteoglycans to form the total supporting structure of the liver. The non-collagenous glycoproteins include laminin, fibronectin, entactin–nidogen, and elastin. Laminin is a large glycoprotein (1000 kD) produced by stellate cells and endothelial cells in the normal liver, and in increased quantities by stellate cells and hepatocytes in the diseased liver.[246] Laminin promotes cell adhesion, migration, differentiation, and growth[247–251] and is an important mediator of capillary formation by endothelial cells.[252–254] The fibronectins represent a class of large molecular weight glycoproteins which exist in plasma and cellular forms. In extracellular matrix, fibronectin exists as thin filaments associated with collagen fibres.[255] Entactin, also referred to as nidogen, is a highly sulphated, dumb-bell-shaped glycoprotein restricted to basement membranes, and hence is generally absent from the space of Disse. Elastin fibres are normally scattered throughout portal tracts. Elastin is deposited in fibrous septa of the cirrhotic liver over time; the presence of elastin in fibrous septa thus provides some indication that the fibrous tissue has not been deposited recently. Lastly, von Willebrand factor (vWF), a factor VIII-related antigen, is a large adhesive glycoprotein that mediates the attachment of platelets to the subendothelium in vascular injury.[252,256] vWF is synthesized by the vascular endothelium, being contained in Weibel–Palade bodies prior to release into the bloodstream.[257] Normal hepatic sinusoidal endothelial cells do not contain vWF, but acquire this protein expression during experimental fibrotic injury,[258] suggesting that endothelial cells also alter their phenotype during formation of liver fibrosis.

The proteoglycans include heparan sulphate, chondroitin sulphate, dermatan sulphate, and hyaluronic acid. Proteins in this latter group have a core protein with a variable number of unbranched carbohydrate side chains which are composed of repeating sulphated disaccharide units. For heparan sulphate these are iduronic acid-N-acetylglucosamine, for dermatan sulphate iduronic acid-N-acetylgalactosamine, and for chondroitin sulphate glucuronic acid-N-acetylgalactosamine. Hyaluronic acid is the exception, as it lacks a protein core and is formed as a non-sulphated polysaccharide from glucosamine and glucuronic acid.

The strong anionic charge on the proteoglycans contributes to their binding to the other constituents of the extracellular matrix. Heparan sulphate particularly modulates the proliferative and secretory characteristics of mesenchymal cells[259] and is an essential extracellular component of basement membranes.[260] The proteoglycans can function as adhesion molecules[261] and can act as receptor molecules on cell surfaces.[262] As such, they have been identified as an important reservoir for cytokines and growth factors, by binding up these diffusible substances within the matrix. Remodelling of the extracellular matrix, as during regeneration, can release substantial quantities of cytokines and growth factors.[263] Conversely, deposition of the extracellular matrix during fibrogenesis can increase the reservoir of stored cytokines and growth factors within the liver.

Fibrillin-1 is a more recently described key matrix protein. Fibrillin-1 polymerizes into ordered microfibril aggregates, which form filamentous longer structures that provide much of the biomechanical tensile properties of tissues. Fibrillin microfibrils without associated elastin are found in the extracellular matrix of non-elastic tissues. Fibrillin and elastin form elastic fibres.[264] In the normal human liver, fibrillin-1 and elastin are found in the vessel walls and connective tissue of portal tracts and in the wall of terminal hepatic veins.[265] At the portal:parenchymal interface, only fibrillin-1 is detectable;[266] fibrillin-1 is not found in sinusoids. Under obstructive cholestatic conditions, fibrillin-1 expression increases markedly in the expanded portal tracts. With toxic injury (as from CCl_4), fibrillin-1 is found in perivenular areas.

In the normal liver, the extracellular matrix comprises less than 3% of the relative area on a tissue section.[267] In cirrhosis, all types of collagens, glycoproteins, and proteoglycans can increase to three times or even more the amounts normally found in the liver.[268,269] Aberrant deposition of extracellular matrix within the hepatic parenchyma produces an environment in which: (i) scarring with type I collagen develops; and (ii) extracellular matrix proteins normally present in basement membranes are deposited within the space of Disse, creating a major barrier for solute exchange between hepatocytes and sinusoidal blood.[270] Studies in rats have shown that, on a percentage area basis, total extracellular matrix components can increase to 25 to 40% in cirrhosis.[271] The total matrix in the space of Disse can increase and change its character to the extent that its bulk can be identified by routine light microscopy. In particular, the change of the space of Disse from containing delicate interspersed strands of fibrillar collagen (types III and IV) to a dense matrix of basement membrane-type matrix proteins closes the space of Disse to protein exchange between hepatocytes and plasma. In combination with the loss of fenestrations in the sinusoidal endothelium, this process is called 'capillarization' of the sinusoids

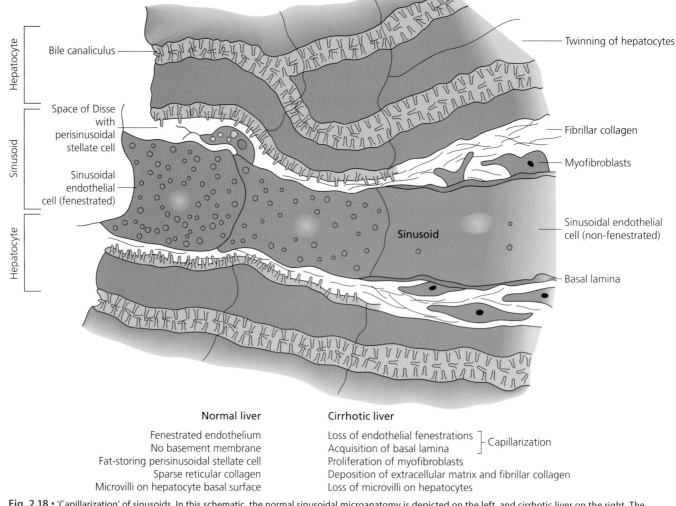

Normal liver
Fenestrated endothelium
No basement membrane
Fat-storing perisinusoidal stellate cell
Sparse reticular collagen
Microvilli on hepatocyte basal surface

Cirrhotic liver
Loss of endothelial fenestrations ⎫
Acquisition of basal lamina ⎬ Capillarization
Proliferation of myofibroblasts
Deposition of extracellular matrix and fibrillar collagen
Loss of microvilli on hepatocytes

Fig. 2.18 • 'Capillarization' of sinusoids. In this schematic, the normal sinusoidal microanatomy is depicted on the left, and cirrhotic liver on the right. The sinusoidal channel is bounded by sinusoidal endothelial cells, which normally are fenestrated but lose their fenestrations in the cirrhotic liver. The space of Disse normally contains scattered fat-storing perisinusoidal stellate cells; these proliferate and become myofibroblasts in the cirrhotic liver. There are normally only delicate reticular collagen fibrils in the space of Disse. Activated myofibroblastic stellate cells are the primary source of fibrillar collagen and other extracellular matrix proteins which are deposited in the space of Disse. Notably, a basal lamina is deposited under the non-fenestrated endothelial cells, completing the process of 'capillarization'. Lastly, hepatocytes lose their abundant basal microvilli (facing the space of Disse); regeneration of hepatocytes leads to thickened hepatocellular plates ('twinning').

(Fig. 2.18).[272] In general, abnormal matrix deposition within the space of Disse occurs in those parts of the parenchyma where cell injury and inflammation are greatest. The extracellular matrix changes have a profound effect on liver cell regeneration and vascular redistribution, as discussed earlier.

Function of the extracellular matrix in the liver

As well as providing the structural framework of the liver, there is evidence that the complex matrix in the space of Disse is essential for maintaining the integrity and function of hepatocytes and sinusoidal cells. In a general sense, the extracellular matrix provides the framework for regulation of cellular polarization, migration, proliferation, differentiation, cell survival, and cell death. This occurs via signalling between the extracellular matrix and cells, via transmembrane receptors such as the integrins or transmembrane proteoglycans. Hepatocyte differentiation in a polarized state requires an extracellular matrix rich in laminin and containing type IV collagen, heparan sulphate, and entactin;[273] contact only with collagen matrix leads to loss of hepatocyte polarity and dedifferentiation as measured by expression of hepatocyte-specific proteins.[249,274,275] Therefore, liver injury that disrupts the sinusoidal subendothelial matrix could result in loss of differentiated hepatocellular function. This has been demonstrated in clinical studies in which the process of capillarization of sinusoids correlated well with impairment of liver function.[268] The sinusoidal subendothelial matrix also helps to preserve the functions and activities of endothelial cells and stellate cells. When stellate cells are maintained on a basement membrane-like gel, they remain spherical with extensive filamentous outbranchings and do not proliferate.[276] When cultured on abnormal substrates, they transform into myofibroblasts and proliferate.[276] Similarly, the fenestrated sinusoidal endothelial cells lose their fenestrations in association with alterations in the extracellular matrix.[251] These events initiate a vicious cycle of reduced porosity of the sinusoidal barrier, impaired movement of solutes and macromolecules into and out of the space of Disse, and hence hepatocellular damage and impaired systemic homeostasis.

Cell–matrix interaction

Receptors for components of the extracellular matrix have been identified on hepatocyte membranes.[277] Amongst these is a family of receptors, the integrins, which possess a recognition site for molecules containing the tripeptide sequence arginine–glycine–aspartic acid (RGD). Laminin, fibronectin, entactin, tenascin, and type I collagen are all known to have RGD sequences. Hepatocytes have integrin receptors for fibronectin and type I collagen,[278,279] and non-integrin receptors for laminin and type IV collagen.[280,281] Hepatocytes also bind proteoglycans and this binding can be saturated, implying a receptor-mediated interaction.[282] As noted, the extracellular matrix serves as a binding reservoir for key fibrogenic cytokines such as TGFβ, TNF-α, PDGF, and IL-6.[283] Release of cytokines by the matrix reservoir facilitates rapid activation of stellate cells, even before cytokine synthesis is up-regulated. The role of integrins in the interaction of stellate cells and sinusoidal endothelial cells with the matrix is poorly understood. Those receptors that have been characterized on these cells seem to be primarily involved in the clearance of ligands.[284]

Regulation of fibrogenesis

The stimuli for synthesis and deposition of collagen may come from several sources:

- chronic inflammation, with production of inflammatory cytokines such as tumour necrosis factor alpha (TNF-α) and beta (TNF-β), interleukin-1 (IL-1), TGFβ, platelet-derived growth factor (PDGF), and insulin-like growth factor (IGF-1);
- cytokine production by injured endogenous cells (Kupffer cells, endothelial cells, hepatocytes, and bile-duct epithelial cells);
- disruption of the extracellular matrix;
- direct stimulation of stellate cells by toxins.

Soluble mediators

The changes in the extracellular matrix may be initiated by proteinases that are produced by stellate cells and Kupffer cells, and a variety of soluble mediators have been identified that are capable of influencing both cell types. These are separated into two broad functional categories of initiation and perpetuation. Proinflammatory cytokines, as released from Kupffer cells, render stellate cells more responsive to soluble factors which may perpetuate liver damage, as in acetaldehyde in alcoholic liver disease,[285,286] and PDGF in many other forms of liver disease.[282] In the latter instance, induction of PDGF receptors on the stellate cells is critical.

The initiating activity of Kupffer-cell medium has been attributed to the release of cytokines and in particular to

TGFβ. The mechanisms controlling the release and activity of cytokines from Kupffer cells are part of a complex cascade of proinflammatory events.[287] The matrix in the space of Disse also provides an extracellular reservoir of TGFβ which can be released and/or activated by matrix proteases. Stellate cells themselves may be capable of producing TGFβ, as the messenger RNA for this cytokine has been identified in these cells.[212] TGFβ can also enhance the proliferation of stellate cells induced by epidermal growth factor (EGF) and PDGF.[288] TGFβ thus would seem to be the most important initiating cytokine so far identified because it can stimulate both stellate cell transdifferentiation into myofibroblasts and collagen synthesis.[289-291] Most of the other soluble cytokines simply modulate proliferation of the stellate cells and have little effect on matrix synthesis. Specifically, cytokines that have been shown to stimulate stellate cells into mitosis and migration include EGF, TGFβ, fibroblast growth factor (FGF), insulin-like growth factor-1 (IGF-1), IL-1, TNF-α, and PDGF.[292]

Retinoids may also play a key role in stellate cell activation. Chronic excess of vitamin A intake is associated with fibrosis and cirrhosis, but cirrhosis from other causes is associated with depletion of hepatic vitamin A.[293] When stellate cells in tissue culture are activated they show a loss of retinoid, but the addition of exogenous retinoid to the tissue culture medium both inhibits cell proliferation and decreases type I collagen synthesis.[294,295] Nuclear receptors for retinoids have now been shown to control expression of many genes within hepatocytes[296] and it stands to reason that gene regulation in stellate cells is likewise regulated. Once stellate cells gain an activated phenotype, it is maintained and amplified through a perpetuation mechanism involving autocrine and paracrine mediators,[206] including a recently described role for osteopontin.[297]

Metalloproteinases

The marked excess of matrix in cirrhosis has meant that matrix formation has received much attention and has been considered to be the key event. Matrix degradation by comparison has been less studied, yet could be a key event in activating stellate cells into both proliferation and matrix synthesis. Likewise, release of soluble cytokines and growth factors from remodelled matrix may have profound effects on proliferation and behaviour of adjacent cells.

In general, matrix may be degraded extracellularly by metalloproteinases and intracellularly by lysosomal cathepsins. The metalloproteinases appear to be important in matrix remodelling in all parts of the body and also play a key role within the liver (Table 2.12). These proteinases are subdivided into collagenases which degrade fibrillar collagens, stromelysins which degrade many protein substrates including type IV collagen, gelatin, laminin, and fibronectin, and the type IV collagenase/gelatinases which have a specificity indicated by the name.

All of the enzymes are closely related[298] and their primary structure contains several well-conserved domains.[299] One of these domains is an 80-amino acid sequence in the propeptide portion of the molecule which is important in

Table 2.12 Matrix metalloproteinases (reproduced from Friedman et al.[240])

Enzyme	Metalloproteinase (MMP) number	Molecular mass (kD)		Substrate specificity
		Proenzyme	Active	
Interstitial collagenase	MMP-1	57, 52	47, 42	Collagen Type III > I > II
Neutrophil collagenase	MMP-8	72, 57	70, 50	Collagen Type I > II > III
72 kD gelatinase/type IV collagenase	MMP-2	72	66	Collagen Type IV, ? V, VII, X, gelatin
92 kD gelatinase/type IV collagenase	MMP-9	92	84	Collagen Type IV, V, gelatin
Stromelysin-1	MMP-3	60, 57	45, 28	Collagen Type III, IV, V, laminin, proteoglycan, fibronectin, gelatins
Stromelysin-2	MMP-10	(53)	47, 28	Collagen Type II, IV, V, fibronectin, gelatins
Stromelysin-3	None	—	—	Not known
PUMP-1	MMP-7	28	21, 19	Collagen Type IV, laminin, fibronectin, gelatin

enzyme activation; another is a catalytic domain containing the highly conserved zinc-binding site. Additionally, individual metalloproteinases have domains that are specific to them. For instance, the 72 kD type IV collagenase/gelatinase has a fibronectin-like gelatin-binding domain.

Interstitial collagenase was first identified in 1962 in tadpole tails undergoing morphogenesis[300] but it has since been identified in a wide variety of cells, including fibroblasts, smooth-muscle cells, mononuclear phagocytes, and capillary endothelial cells. It is synthesized as a preproenzyme which is then activated by proteinases. The activated enzyme cleaves type I collagen at specific Gly–Ile and Gly–Leu bonds. The collagenase can also degrade type II collagen but has no demonstrable activity against type IV basement membrane collagen.

Interstitial collagenase has been identified in the liver but its cellular origin is uncertain. The earliest studies suggested that Kupffer cells were the source,[301] but the techniques used to isolate Kupffer cells resulted in a significant mixture of Kupffer cells with other sinusoidal liver cells. Nonetheless, the identification of this enzyme in peripheral blood monocytes is consistent with Kupffer cells also producing it.[302] The stellate cell in resting conditions does not produce interstitial collagenase, but in tissue culture, fibroblasts prepared from human liver and exposed to IL-1 or TNF-α produce messenger RNA for this enzyme.[303]

A *neutrophil collagenase*, which is very similar to interstitial collagenase, also exists. This also has a substrate specificity for interstitial collagens but has a much greater avidity for degrading type I than type III collagen.[304] The enzyme is released from the cytoplasmic granules of neutrophil polymorphs following activation, and may be relevant to hepatic conditions in which neutrophils are active (e.g. alcoholic hepatitis).

Type IV collagenase/gelatinases—two major proteinases in this category have been described, one is 92 kD and the other 72 kD in size. The larger 92-kD type IV collagenase/gelatinase is synthesized and released predominantly by macrophages and neutrophils.[305,306] As its name implies, it actively degrades gelatin and collagen types IV and V but does not degrade the interstitial fibrillar collagens. The enzyme has been identified in Kupffer cells and is released on their activation.[307] The 72-kD collagenase/gelatinase is synthesized and released by tumour cells, fibroblasts, and osteoblasts, and to a lesser extent by mononuclear phagocytes. The activated enzyme degrades gelatin, collagen types IV and V, and does not cleave the fibrillar collagens. In this respect it is identical to the larger 92-kD proteinase.

The cleavage of type IV collagen is produced by a pepsin-resistant fragment of the molecule which, like interstitial collagenase, cleaves at Gly–Leu and Gly–Ile bonds.[308] The lack of effect of the type IV collagenase on type I and III fibrillar collagens is presumably due to lack of access to these bonds because of the tertiary structure of the fibrillar collagen. In the liver, stellate cells produce and release this enzyme. Stellate cells in tissue culture have been shown to contain messenger RNA for the enzyme, the enzyme has been immunocytochemically demonstrated in these cells, and extracellular release of the enzyme from the cells into the supernatant occurs.[309,310]

Stromelysins—three stromelysins (1, 2, and 3) and a closely related metalloproteinase, PUMP-1, have been identified from a variety of tissues. These enzymes have a broad range of matrix degradation activity but none of them has been clearly identified in the liver.

Metalloproteinase inhibitors

Specific tissue inhibitors of metalloproteinases (TIMPs) have been identified and there are other general proteinase inhibitors such as α$_2$-macroglobulin. TIMP-1 is a small 28-kD glycoprotein secreted by a wide variety of cell types including fibroblasts. It binds irreversibly to active metalloproteinases of all types. Stellate cells have been shown to express the gene for TIMP-1, synthesize the immunoreactive protein, and, in culture, release a protein with TIMP-1 activity into the supernatant.[311,312] Regulation of gene expression is influenced by the same growth factors and cytokines that are involved in the regulation of metalloproteinase gene expression. TIMP-2 is a smaller 21-kD protein with significant homology to TIMP-1 and with many similar properties. Its role in the liver is currently uncertain, as is the role for the other two TIMP inhibitors. α2-Macroglobulin is a high molecular weight plasma glycoprotein (725 kD) that is able to bind both interstitial collagenase and stromelysin.[313] It is synthesized predominantly by hepatocytes but the stellate cell also contains messenger RNA for this proteinase scavenger and can synthesize the molecule.[314]

There is thus a complex interplay of factors involved in the production and maintenance of the liver matrix that is centred around the role of the stellate cell and influenced by the metalloproteinases and their inhibitors. Excess matrix may accumulate in the liver following increased formation of interstitial collagens by stellate cells, from decreased activity of metalloproteinases in their removal, or by increased inhibition of metalloproteinases. The metalloproteinases, specifically type IV collagenase, could potentially disrupt the normal liver matrix and thus create a microenvironment that would enhance stellate cell activation and matrix formation. Conversely, fibrotic liver can degrade type I collagen more readily than normal liver.[315] This collagenase activity seems to be greatest during the development of early and extensive lesions but diminishes with advanced cirrhosis. There is insufficient information on the behaviour of tissue inhibitors of interstitial collagenase in either normal or diseased liver. A full understanding of the interplay of all these factors could lead to treatments that slow or even halt the progression of chronic liver diseases towards cirrhosis.[316]

The portal tract

Virtually all investigations have focused on fibrogenesis from stellate cell-derived myofibroblasts within the parenchyma; examination of portal tract fibrogenesis has received inappropriately little attention. This may be due in part to overconfidence in the fidelity of experimental isolation procedures for hepatic stellate cells; inclusion of fibrogenic cell populations from portal tracts may have led to overlooking them as potential sources of extracellular matrix.[264] However, the potential role of portal tract myofibroblasts and fibroblasts was noted in some key publications over the past 20 years.[317–320]

Portal tracts contain the portal vein, the hepatic artery, and the bile duct. While the portal vein and hepatic artery have walls composed of smooth muscle cells, the bile duct epithelial cells reside on a basement membrane which is surrounded directly by periductular fibroblasts.[264] Biliary fibrosis initiated by bile duct inflammation and obstruction occurs as a result of rapid activation of the peribiliary fibroblasts with acquisition of smooth muscle actin, generating a myofibroblast phenotype.[320] The progressive enlargement of portal tracts in these circumstances involves extensive bile duct proliferation, massive proliferation of peribiliary (myo)fibroblasts and deposition of portal tract collagen, and oedema (Fig. 2.19).[317,321] The fact that it is peribiliary fibroblasts that are primarily responsible for the evolving

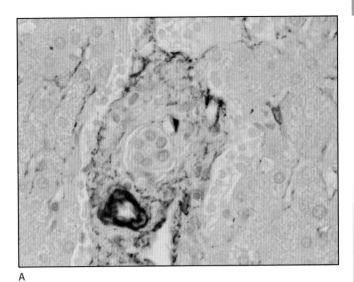

A

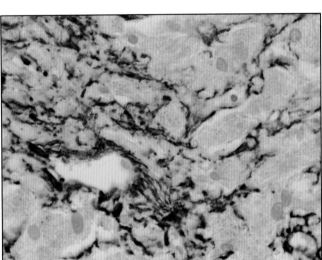

B

Fig. 2.19 • (A) Portal tract and periportal parenchyma, stained immunohistochemically for α-smooth muscle actin. In this mildly activated portal tract, the smooth muscle cells of the hepatic artery are strongly positive, but myofibroblasts within the portal tract and occasional periportal sinusoidal stellate cells also stain positive. **(B)** Portal tract and periportal parenchyma during a brisk fibrotic reaction. The interface between portal tract with its hepatic artery (left) and the parenchyma (right) is indistinct. There are abundant, strongly staining, activated portal tract myofibroblasts and sinusoidal stellate cells. α-Smooth muscle actin immunohistochemistry.

hepatic fibrosis is explanation for the observation that 'biliary fibrosis' does not characteristically subdivide the liver with parenchymal fibrous septa (which would derive from sinusoidal myofibroblasts) until late in the disease. The myofibroblasts of bridging septa in cholestatic fibrotic livers strongly resemble the myofibroblasts of the portal field,[322] suggesting that portal tract myofibroblasts migrate into the developing parenchymal septa.[323] Indeed, fibrillin-1 expression in conjunction with elastin may help distinguish myofibroblasts derived from the portal tract (elastin-positive) versus sinusoidal stellate cells (elastin-negative). Specifically, activated stellate cells acquire smooth muscle actin expression and deposit fibrillin-1-positive but elastin-negative extracellular matrix, whereas portal tract-derived myofibroblasts deposit extracellular matrix containing both fibrillin-1 and elastin.[264] An alternative view, however, is the fact that portal fibroblasts produce significant amounts of TGFβ2 and, unlike activated stellate cells, express all three TGFβ receptors and are growth inhibited by TGFβ1 and TGFβ2.[324] Fibroblast growth factor (FGF)-2, but not PDGF, causes portal fibroblast proliferation. These data suggest a mechanism whereby stellate cells may eventually eclipse portal fibroblasts as the dominant myofibroblast population in biliary fibrosis.

Other populations of fibrogenic cells in portal tracts include myofibroblasts loosely placed around the portal vein and hepatic artery and in the loose connective tissue of the portal field, especially at the interface between the portal tract and parenchyma.[325] These portal myofibroblasts may represent a convergence of phenotype from quiescent portal tract fibroblasts to activated myofibroblasts.[264] However, portal tract-derived myofibroblasts maintain some differences from hepatic stellate cell-derived myofibroblasts, on the basis of protein expression such as cellular retinol-binding protein-1 (CRBP-1).[326] Smooth muscle cells in the wall of the portal tract blood vessels and second layer fibroblasts of the terminal hepatic vein are also capable of synthesizing extracellular matrix proteins, in keeping with the general observation that the main contributors to hepatic matrix production are mesenchymal cells.[327]

Vascular remodelling

Vascular modifications are central to the development of chronic liver damage, leading to the cirrhotic state (see also Chapter 13).[328] Key vascular changes are in endothelial cell porosity, loss of vascular patency owing to thrombosis, and reorganization of the vascular blood flow of the liver at the sinusoidal level and in larger vessels.

Endothelial porosity

In normal liver, sinusoidal endothelial cells lack a basement membrane, and exhibit fenestrations approximately 100 nm in diameter, occupying between 2 and 3% of the area of the endothelial cell ('porosity'). Deposition of extracellular matrix in the space of Disse is accompanied by the loss of fenestrations in the sinusoidal endothelial cells.[329] With progressive fibrosis, the diameter of the endothelial fenestrations slightly decreases, but the area porosity drops to below 0.5%.[330] In combination with the deposition of aberrant extracellular matrix in the space of Disse by stellate cells, the sinusoidal space comes to resemble a capillary rather than a channel for exchange of solutes between hepatocytes and plasma (Fig. 2.20).[329] In particular, hepatocellular secretion of proteins (e.g. albumin, clotting factors, lipoproteins) is greatly impaired.

Vascular thrombosis

The second vascular insult is thrombosis (Fig. 2.21). In angiographic and ultrasonographic studies, portal vein thrombosis has been found in 0.6 to 16.6% of cirrhotic patients,[331] and grossly visible portal vein fibrosis or thrombosis has been found in 39% of cirrhotic livers at autopsy.[332]

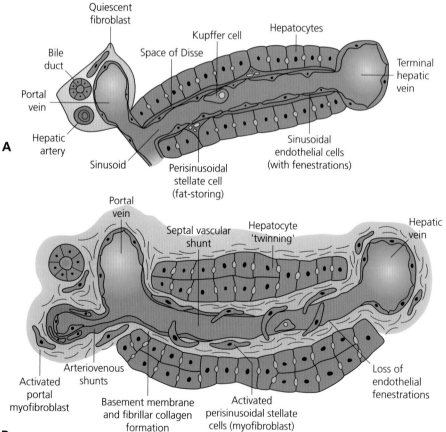

Fig. 2.20 • Key events in the evolution of cirrhosis. **(A)** The normal microanatomy of the liver is depicted, showing especially the channels for flow of portal venous blood through the sinusoids of the parenchyma, and normal sinusoidal architecture. **(B)** With evolution to cirrhosis, the following key events occur. Abnormal arteriovenous shunts and vascular shunts from portal to hepatic veins develop. Portal tract fibroblasts proliferate and become myofibroblasts. Perisinusoidal stellate cells lose their fat stores, proliferate and develop a myofibroblast phenotype. Both populations of cells deposit extracellular matrix, expanding portal tracts and the space of Disse, respectively. Hepatocyte regeneration, leading to 'twinning' of hepatocyte plates, is also shown.

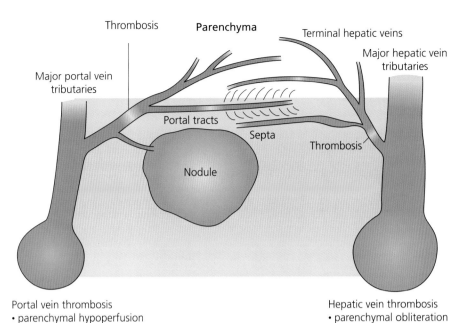

Thrombosis   Parenchyma   Terminal hepatic veins

Major portal vein tributaries

Major hepatic vein tributaries

Portal tracts

Septa

Nodule

Thrombosis

Fig. 2.21 • Vascular thrombosis hypothesis for pathogenesis of cirrhosis.[336,337] Thrombosis of tributary or terminal portal veins alone will lead to atrophy of the downstream parenchyma, and nodular proliferation of residual perfused parenchyma. Thrombosis of terminal hepatic veins or hepatic vein tributaries will lead to formation of venocentric septa and obliteration of the affected parenchyma. Thrombosis of both portal veins and terminal hepatic veins leads to bridging portal-to-central fibrous septa and parenchymal obliteration, alternating with nodular proliferation of residual parenchyma. Propagation of thrombi, with involvement of an increasing percentage of the liver volume, leads to cirrhosis.

Portal vein thrombosis
• parenchymal hypoperfusion
• portal-based fibrous septa
• nodular regeneration of well-perfused areas

Hepatic vein thrombosis
• parenchymal obliteration
• venocentric fibrous septa

Portal vein thrombosis + Hepatic vein thrombosis → Cirrhosis

Veno-occlusive lesions of hepatic veins less than 0.2 mm in diameter have been found in up to 74% of cirrhotic livers examined at autopsy.[333–335] Obliterative lesions in 36% of portal veins and 70% of hepatic veins are found in cirrhotic livers removed at liver transplantation.[336] The distribution of portal vein obliterative lesions was more uniform than those in hepatic veins, each consistent with the concept of propagation of multifocal thrombi downstream from their site of origin. Portal vein lesions were associated with prominent regional variation in the size of cirrhotic nodules. Hepatic vein lesions were associated with regions of confluent fibrosis and parenchymal extinction. The compelling conclusion is that thrombosis of medium and large portal veins and of hepatic veins is a common occurrence in cirrhosis, and that these events are important in causing the propagation of parenchymal extinction to full-blown cirrhosis.

Further support for vascular thrombosis as an origin for cirrhosis has been provided by study of the Budd–Chiari syndrome.[337] In 15 livers resected from patients with the syndrome, six exhibited severe portal vein thrombotic obliteration as well as hepatic vein thrombosis. Each of the livers had venoportal cirrhosis, with fibrous septa bridging hepatic veins to portal tracts. Three livers were free of portal vein thrombosis and exhibited only a venocentric pattern of cirrhosis. The remaining six livers had a mixed venocentric/venoportal pattern of cirrhosis, accompanied by moderate focal portal vein obliteration. Thus, hepatic vein thrombosis alone appears to be insufficient to engender cirrhosis. Superimposed portal vein thrombosis engenders venoportal bridging fibrosis. These authors conclude that vascular thrombosis of medium-to-large sized hepatic veins and portal veins (0.2 to 3.0 mm in diameter) may be a more general causal event in other diseases leading to cirrhosis.

Sinusoidal blood flow

The resultant changes in sinusoidal fluid dynamics during the evolution of cirrhosis are dramatic (Fig. 2.22).[338] First, sclerosis of the portal tracts and their vascular branches increases presinusoidal vascular resistance. Acquisition of myofibres by stellate cells increases sinusoidal vascular resistance, since tonic contraction of these 'myofibroblasts' constricts the sinusoidal vascular channels. Fibrosis in the perivenular region of the lobule may partially obstruct vascular outflow, creating postsinusoidal vascular resistance. Second, with the formation of bona fide bridging fibrous septa between portal tracts and terminal hepatic veins, portovenous and arteriovenous shunting occurs. Specifically, blood entering the liver via portal tracts (portal vein and hepatic artery) is shunted to the terminal hepatic veins through low-resistance high-flow vascular channels, effectively bypassing the parenchymal nodules. These channels may be especially present in the portal–central bridging fibrous septa. As fibrosis progresses to cirrhosis, shunted blood flow through septal 'fast' vascular channels leaves the remainder of the hepatic parenchyma almost bereft of meaningful blood flow.[219]

The fast vascular channels exhibit the endothelial cell defenestration and development of a basal lamina characteristic of capillarization. Progressive fibrosis in the perivenular region of the lobule may partially obstruct vascular outflow, further promoting redistribution of blood to these low resistance pathways. In advanced cirrhosis, most of the hepatic blood supply seems to pass through the liver via fast vascular channels.[219] Supporting these findings in rats, in humans the mean transit time for labelled erythrocytes decreases from 19.9 ± 3.7 s in patients without cirrhosis, to 12.2 ± 4.4 s in patients with cirrhosis.[339] This would explain

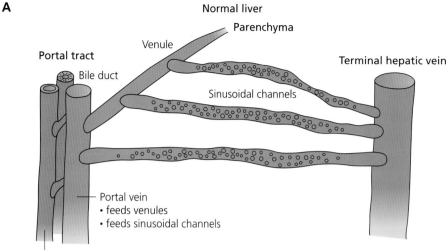

A

Normal liver

Parenchyma

Venule

Portal tract

Bile duct

Terminal hepatic vein

Sinusoidal channels

Portal vein
• feeds venules
• feeds sinusoidal channels

Hepatic artery
• feeds peribiliary capillary plexus
• feeds vasa vasorum (portal vein and terminal hepatic vein)
• feeds capsule

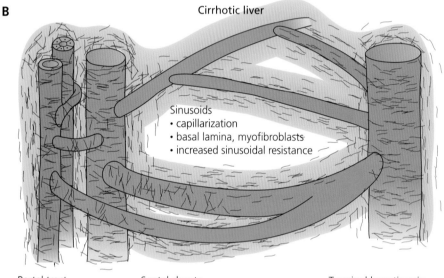

B

Cirrhotic liver

Sinusoids
• capillarization
• basal lamina, myofibroblasts
• increased sinusoidal resistance

Portal tract
• sclerosis
• increased presinusoidal resistance
• arterial-to-venous shunts

Septal shunts
• portal vein-to-terminal hepatic vein
• hepatic artery-to-terminal hepatic vein
• fast transit, bypasses parenchyma

Terminal hepatic vein
• sclerosis
• obstruction to sinusoidal outflow

Fig. 2.22 • Vascular haemodynamics of the cirrhotic liver. **(A)** The normal anatomy is depicted, showing sinusoidal channels emanating from portal vein tributaries (venules) and directly from the portal vein. The hepatic artery primarily feeds the peribiliary capillary plexus, vasavasorum of both portal vein and terminal hepatic vein, and the hepatic capsule. **(B)** In the cirrhotic liver, portal tract extracellular matrix is increased, with sclerosis around portal veins and other structures leading to increased presinusoidal vascular resistance. Abnormal hepatic artery-to-portal vein shunts contribute to increased portal vein pressure. While portal vein-derived venules persist for perfusion of the parenchyma, the sinusoids have lost their fenestrated endothelium and developed a basal lamina with fibrosis in the space of Disse, leading to increased sinusoidal resistance. Concomitantly, abnormal septal vasculature has developed with portal vein-to-terminal hepatic vein and hepatic artery-to-terminal hepatic vein shunting, effectively bypassing the parenchyma. Sclerosis around the terminal hepatic vein increases postsinusoidal resistance, impeding outflow of sinusoidal blood and further promoting shunting of blood around the parenchyma.

the increased blood flow observed in 'fast' sinusoids of the cirrhotic liver, in the midst of relative underperfusion of the liver parenchyma as a whole. Interestingly, sinusoids within the cirrhotic modules may retain much of their normal architecture;[340] they are just not adequately perfused.

Angiogenesis, arterial, and venous changes

Angiogenesis—the formation of new blood vessels—is a key event in chronic liver disease.[341] As a general process, a key stimulus for angiogenesis is hypoxia, which induces hypoxia-inducible transcription factors (HIF) in tissue cells.[342] Generation of nitric oxide (NO) promotes vasodilatation by relaxation of vascular tone;[343] vascular endothelial growth factor (VEFG) increases vascular permeability.

The vascular architecture is thus 'loosened', as a first step in the generation of vascular buds. This is accompanied by enzymatic remodelling of the extracellular matrix through the action of matrix metalloproteinases (discussed above), clearing the path for endothelial cell proliferation. Such proliferation occurs in response to secretion of growth factors by endothelial cells, stellate cells, hepatocytes, Kupffer cells, and infiltrating inflammatory cells. The most studied of these growth factors is VEGF.[344] Endothelial cells proliferate in an ordered manner, with formation of tubular structures with central lumens. The formation of a structured three-dimensional network of vessels is an intricate interplay between signalling pathways that determine branching, stabilization of nascent vessels by recruitment of pericytes, and deposition of basement membranes and extracellular matrix to provide structural stabilization.[345]

Specific mechanisms for angiogenesis in the liver are becoming apparent. Physiological hepatic angiogenesis occurs during liver regeneration, leading to the formation of new functional sinusoids.[341,346] This appears to be a well-orchestrated spatiotemporal expression of angiogenesis-inducing growth factors and growth factor receptors on endothelial cells, ensuring action of vascular growth factors on specific sets of endothelial cells at specific times during revascularization of the regenerating liver.[341,347] In chronic inflammatory liver disease, the fibrosis and inflammation leads to impaired delivery of blood and oxygen to parenchymal tissue, and hence tissue hypoxia. Induction of HIFs initiates angiogenesis and the formation of neovessels.[348] In a non-hypoxic fashion, inflammation also may initiate HIF-1 expression in hepatocytes, Kupffer cells, stellate cells, endothelial cells, and infiltrating leukocytes, leading to secretion of angiogenic factors including VEGF[349] and formation of new vascular structures.[350]

The results can be dramatic. Inflamed portal tracts can develop prominent capillary systems.[348,351] Angiogenesis from the hepatic arterial system may be particularly prominent, particularly if thrombotic occlusion of portal vein tributaries is occurring,[352] which may be both beneficial by enabling tissue repair and regeneration, and detrimental by being a risk factor for the progression of arterial-fed tissue to hepatocellular carcinoma.[353] Neo-vessels may mature into an increased number of vascular structures in chronically inflamed portal tracts,[241,354] including proliferation of the peribiliary vascular plexus.[355] Direct interconnections between arteriolar branches and portal venules in human cirrhosis develop.[356,357] These are noted mainly at the level of relatively small branches of the vascular system, and not at the gross anatomical level.[357]

Of particular impact is the development of vascularized fibrous septa that connect portal tracts to terminal hepatic veins, considered a 'bridge too far' in the development of cirrhosis.[358] Prominent vascular plexuses develop around the regenerative nodules in human cirrhosis, composed of both arterial and portal vein-derived channels.[359,360] A key physiological result of these changes is that hepatic arterial pressures can be transmitted to the portal venous system, contributing to the development of portal hypertension.[361] Afferent blood is shunted through the vascularized septa, leaving the bulk of the hepatocellular parenchyma nearly bereft of blood supply.[219]

Zonation

An under-appreciated physiological change in the damaged liver is alterations in the zonal distribution of hepatocellular metabolism.[362] In the normal liver, heterogeneity in hepatocellular metabolism is observed, with hepatocytes in the periportal region exhibiting different patterns of enzyme complements than those in the perivenular region.[363] During the evolution of cirrhosis, two issues arise. First, does metabolic zonation become altered as a result of hepatocellular injury? Second, do the alterations in vascular architecture translate into altered metabolic zonation? Experimental studies in the rat have shown that the changes in the vascu-

lar architecture of the liver and in the hepatocyte micro-environment induced by liver fibrosis do indeed result in alterations of the metabolic organization of the hepatic parenchyma.[362,364–368] With damage to the pericentral region as with CCl_4, afferent vascular channels penetrate to the centre of parenchymal nodules, and enzymes normally expressed in the perivenular region may be down-regulated.[362] Indeed, the development of penetrating afferent vessels can lead to outright reversal of blood flow, from the centre of parenchymal nodules to the periseptal periphery, which is contrary to what one might expect.[362]

In human studies, reversal of zonation does not appear to occur in biliary patterns of cirrhosis,[367,369,370] and the overall metabolic organization of the acinus is either retained or 'flattened' in cirrhosis from chronic viral hepatitis or alcoholic liver disease, with no zonation at all observed for hepatocellular enzymatic activities.[371] Interestingly, an enzyme with a distribution that is almost exclusively perivenular (and restricted to the layer of two to four hepatocytes around the terminal hepatic vein) is glutamine synthetase. This pattern of enzyme expression is found in fibrotic livers.[372] At this intermediate point during the evolution of cirrhosis, at least, the maintenance of vascular perfusion of the parenchyma appears to be sufficient for the maintenance of metabolic zonation. However, glutamine synthetase is undetectable in cirrhotic nodules and hepatocyte clusters isolated in fibrous septa, regardless of the aetiology of cirrhosis.[371] Given that glutamine synthesis is a critical step in fixing free ammonia for elimination via the urea cycle, the loss of glutamine synthetase expression may contribute to the increased ammonia concentrations found in blood and, hence, indirectly contribute to the pathogenesis of hepatic encephalopathy. Moreover, these findings concur with the lack of terminal hepatic veins in the parenchymal nodules of cirrhosis, and again suggest that the centre of nodules is not an efferent zone (despite the prominence of vascular channels at nodule centres). Conversely, in this study of human livers at least, the periphery of cirrhotic nodules cannot be considered to be homologous to the periportal zone.

Thus, there appear to be profound alterations in the metabolic zonation of parenchymal nodules in the cirrhotic liver. Absolute loss of metabolic function does not appear to occur. Indeed, hepatocytes trapped in nodules or in fibrous septa retain most of their enzymatic activities, and maintain their capacity for protein synthesis (e.g. albumin).[371] These findings support the concept that the impairment of liver function characteristic of advanced liver disease is not caused by a significant and overall decrease in the metabolic activity of residual cells.[372] Rather, it is more likely to be related to the alterations in vascular architecture and impaired exchange of soluble substances between hepatocytes and blood, and only eventually to an absolute loss in hepatocyte mass.

The physiological consequences of these metabolic alterations are not totally clear. However, metabolic zonation of the mammalian hepatic lobule is thought to enable the liver simultaneously to perform anabolic and catabolic activities and to respond quickly to alterations in physiological status.[373-375] Derangement of such zonation may contribute to the pathogenesis of the metabolic disorders associated with advanced liver disease.

Cirrhosis

Cirrhosis is defined anatomically by the presence throughout the liver of fibrous septa that subdivide the parenchyma into nodules,[376] as shown in Fig. 2.23. The required elements of fibrous septa and architectural disturbance each occur in a spectrum from minimal to severe. Several features are critical to the definition. First, the parenchymal architecture of the entire liver is disrupted by interconnecting fibrous scars. Localized hepatic scarring does not constitute fibrosis. Second, the fibrous scars may be present in the form of delicate bands connecting portal tracts and centrilobular terminal hepatic veins in a portal-to-portal, portal-to-central, and/or central-to-central pattern, or may be present as broad fibrous tracts obliterating multiple adjacent lobules. Third, parenchymal nodules are created by fibrotic isolation of islands of hepatic parenchyma. The nodules may vary from micronodules (less than 3 mm in diameter) to macronodules (3 mm to several centimetres in diameter).

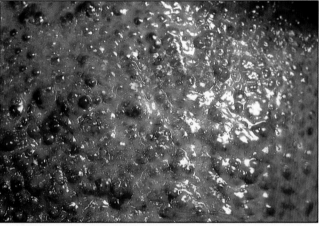

A

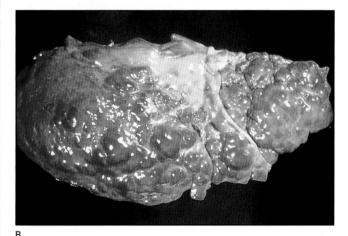

B

Fig. 2.23 • (A) Micronodular cirrhosis: surface of the liver. **(B)** Macronodular cirrhosis.

Some qualifying comments are in order. First, fibrous subdivision of the liver parenchyma into isolated islands is requisite for the diagnosis; regeneration of these islands is not. Hence, fibrosis which evolves rapidly over several months may still produce a cirrhotic organ, even if insufficient time occurs for substantive expansion of the islands into spherical nodules by regeneration. Second, the parenchymal distance from portal tract to terminal hepatic vein is on the order of 0.8 to 1.5 mm, so scarring at the lobular level may produce nodularity on a mm scale. However, the hepatic capacity for regeneration is enormous, and parenchymal regeneration in the face of more slowly developing fibrosis may produce nodules of several cm in diameter. Third, the parenchymal islands do not have to be simple polygons or spheres. Portal tract-based fibrosis may produce a much more coarsely subdivided and irregular cirrhotic liver.

Because of the qualitative nature of the definition for cirrhosis, diagnosis depends on arbitrary limits. Specifically, the point at which a liver with chronic hepatitis and fibrous scarring truly becomes cirrhotic is arbitrary, and cannot easily be established on percutaneous needle biopsy tissue (which represents less than 1 : 10 000th of the liver mass).[377] Moreover, cirrhotic livers exhibit a spectrum of severity, with fibrous septa that are few, numerous, thin, or broad, and with nodules of uniform or variable size and contour. Fortunately, clinical data provide valuable guidance on whether abnormal findings observed in percutaneous liver biopsy tissue are representative of the whole liver. Supporting clinical data include physical examination (e.g. ascites, caput medusa, spider angiomata, gynaecomastia) and impressions gained from imaging studies or intraoperative visualization of the organ. Laboratory data may not reveal abnormalities, in that serum levels for albumin, clotting factors, urea, alkaline phosphatase, aminotransferases, and bilirubin may be normal in a patient who has quiescent cirrhosis with minimal ongoing damage, and who has not yet developed hepatic failure. Conversely, a patient with massive hepatic necrosis and hepatic failure is not cirrhotic, despite profound abnormalities in the above serum parameters. Hence, laboratory data per se do not establish a diagnosis of cirrhosis.

Occasionally, a severe focal injury to the liver results in changes histologically indistinguishable from cirrhosis on percutaneous needle biopsy; this focal change is not considered as true cirrhosis. When this question arises, having definitive information from clinical evaluation and from imaging studies on the general status of the liver, or a biopsy sample from elsewhere in the liver, is critical to determining whether a fibrotic process is focal or diffuse.

Liver cirrhosis is not strictly the end stage of hepatic scarring. Rather, it is a dynamic, biphasic process dominated on the one hand by progressive parenchymal fibrosis, and on the other by severe disruption of vascular architecture and distortion of normal lobular architecture. The three major mechanisms that combine to create cirrhosis are cell death, deposition of aberrant extracellular matrix (fibrosis), and vascular reorganization. The cirrhotic process is usually initiated by hepatocellular death but only after this has occurred consistently and persistently over a long period of time. Cell death can occur in any form of liver injury, and does not define cirrhosis. For example, an acute overdose of paracetamol (acetaminophen) causes severe hepatic necrosis and may kill the patient, but it will not produce chronic liver injury in those who survive. In contrast, small doses of alcohol, which alone are insufficient to cause more than a small degree of hepatic parenchymal injury, are quite capable of producing cirrhosis when imbibed on a daily basis for a number of years. The mechanisms of cell death, fibrosis, and vascular thrombosis have been discussed in earlier sections. A key outcome of all three processes, however, is parenchymal extinction.

Parenchymal extinction

Parenchymal extinction is defined as a focal loss of contiguous hepatocytes (Fig. 2.24).[378] Extinction lesions may involve a small portion of an acinus or larger units of one or more adjacent acini or even a whole lobe. The contiguous cell loss is the result of focal ischaemia resulting from obstruction of veins or sinusoids. The size of extinction lesions depend on the size of the obstructed vessels. Small regions of extinction are most easily recognized by the close approximation of hepatic veins and portal tracts, a lesion called an adhesion (Fig. 2.25). The concept of parenchymal extinction is important because it indicates that: (i) parenchymal extinction is not directly caused by the initial hepatocellular injury but is an epiphenomenon caused by innocent bystander injury of the local vessels; (ii) each parenchymal extinction lesion has its own natural history and may be in an early or late stage of healing; (iii) cirrhosis occurs when numerous independent and discrete parenchymal extinction lesions accumulate throughout the liver; and (iv) the form of cirrhosis is largely determined by the

distribution of the vascular injury. Importantly, parenchymal extinction can continue to occur long after cirrhosis is established, leading to slow conversion of a marginally functional liver into a organ incapable of sustaining life. The pathogenesis of vascular obstruction depends on the size of the vessels. Most small vessel obliteration is secondary to local inflammation.[67,379] Although thrombosis may be important in veins of all sizes, it is the exclusive mechanism for block of medium and large veins. Most parenchymal injury is produced by blocking of veins larger than 100 μm, as obstruction at this site cannot be easily circumvented by collateral flow in sinusoids. Obstruction of several adjacent sinusoids is also difficult to circumvent.

Reversibility of fibrosis/cirrhosis

Although cirrhosis has been traditionally viewed as the end-stage in the evolution of many chronic liver diseases, in recent years, reversal of cirrhosis has been gaining credence.[358] Numerous clinical reports indicate that with cessation of the injurious process, cirrhosis may reverse.[378,380-382] These include patients whose full-blown cirrhosis has subsided to a form of incomplete septal cirrhosis or apparent absence of fibrosis following successful treatment of hereditary haemochromatosis,[383,384] autoimmune hepatitis,[385] and Wilson disease.[386] A reduction in fibrosis has been noted also in primary biliary cirrhosis,[387] schistosomiasis,[388] and extrahepatic biliary obstruction.[389] Of particular interest in recent years has been regression of fibrosis and cirrhosis in patients with hepatitis C.[390] It may take years for significant regression to be achieved, and the time varies depending upon the underlying cause of the liver disease and its severity.[207] Increased collagenolytic activity through the action of matrix metalloproteinases is the major mechanism of fibrosis resolution, accompanied by decreased expression of TIMP-1. Apoptosis of activated stellate cells also favours

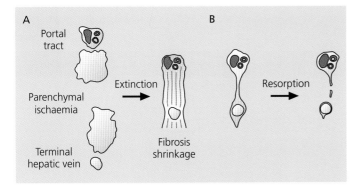

Fig. 2.24 • Diagrammatic depiction of tissue remodelling in chronic hepatitis during the development and regression of cirrhosis. **(A)** With obliteration of small portal and hepatic veins (see Fig. 2.21), the supplied parenchyma becomes ischaemic. The ischaemic parenchyma shrinks and is replaced by fibrosis (process of extinction). The shrinkage is accompanied by close approximation of adjacent vascular structures. **(B)** With time, the fibrous septa are resorbed, becoming progressively thinner and then perforating before disappearing. Small residual tags may extend from portal tracts. Trapped portal structures and hepatic veins are released from the septa and are recognizable as deformed remnants that are irregularly distributed. (Modified from Wanless IR, Crawford JM. Cirrhosis. In: Odze RD, Goldblum JR, Crawford JM, eds. Surgical pathology of the GI tract, liver, biliary tract, and pancreas. Philadelphia: Saunders, 2004; p 866.)

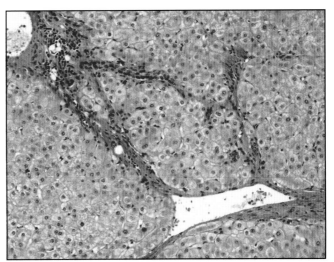

Fig. 2.25 • Chronic hepatitis, with only limited mononuclear inflammation in the portal tract (upper left), but with bridging fibrosis between the portal tract and a terminal hepatic vein (lower right). Such tethering can undergo contraction, bringing the portal tract and terminal hepatic veins into close approximation with one another (adhesion). H&E stained tissue section, 100× magnification.

fibrosis resolution.[391] This is facilitated by stimulation of death receptors in activated stellate cells, and a decrease in the levels of survival factors.

However, even with substantial resorption of fibrous tissue septae, restoration of the hepatic architecture to a normal state does not occur. Rather, depending upon how much extracellular matrix resorbs and where, there may remain incomplete septal cirrhosis, in which there is incomplete resorption of fibrous tissue in both the parenchyma and portal tracts (Fig. 2.26). Alternatively, complete resorption of fibrous tissue from the parenchyma but leaving prominent portal tract fibrosis engenders hepatoportal sclerosis. Resorption of all fibrous tissue but with continuation of irregular vascular supply to the parenchyma engenders nodular regenerative hyperplasia, since hypertrophy occurs in the well-vascularized regions of parenchyma. These latter two conditions are perhaps erroneously viewed as 'vascular' abnormalities.

Non-uniformity of vascular supply to the liver parenchyma is proposed as an underlying cause for de novo development of incomplete septal cirrhosis.[392] The pathogenesis is thought to be the result of recurrent emboli, composed of platelet aggregates and formed within the portal venous system or spleen.[392,393] Collectively, incomplete septal cirrhosis, nodular regenerative hyperplasia, partial nodular transformation, and focal nodular hyperplasia are thought to be interrelated disorders with a common pathogenesis, related to abnormalities in the vascular supply.[394] Obliterative portal venopathy is postulated to produce the hyperplastic lesions by inducing non-uniformity of blood supply to the parenchyma.[393,395,396] The hypothesis is attractive as it unites several entities with similar morphological features but an otherwise poorly understood pathogenesis. It explains the considerable overlap and diagnostic confusion between these entities, provides a mechanism for focality of disease in some instances and diffuse disease in others, and provides a rational explanation for the lack both of any clinically overt disease and of any inflammatory component.

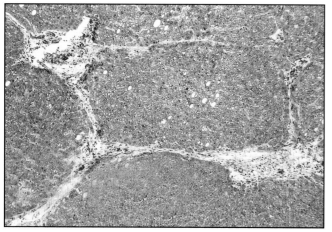

Fig. 2.26 • Incomplete septal cirrhosis. The liver is subdivided by delicate bridging fibrous septa, in the absence of nodule formation. This patient had histologically-demonstrated micronodular cirrhosis at the time of original diagnosis of hereditary haemochromatosis, but following 33 years of phlebotomy treatment had only this residual abnormality. Masson trichrome.

Conclusion

A critical challenge for the interpretation of liver histopathology is to discern the underlying pathophysiology. The current chapter has presented key pathophysiological concepts underlying the many features of hepatic injury. It remains for the pathologist to knit together clinical information and clinical hypotheses, with the pathophysiology deduced on the basis of morphological interpretation of liver findings. At that point, reasonable conclusions can be made about the patient's probable disease course and progression, from which rational clinical management decisions can be made. The great fascination of liver histopathology is that so much can be learned from critical examination of this remarkable tissue.

Acknowledgements

This chapter is drawn in part upon ideas presented in a previous edition (Crawford JM. Cirrhosis. In: MacSween RNM et al. (Eds.), Pathology of the Liver, 4th Edition, Churchill Livingstone, London, 2002; pp. 575–620); a lecture syllabus (Crawford JM, Immunopathology of the Liver, American Association for the Study of Liver Diseases Post-Graduate Course, 2005, San Francisco); and a previous chapter (Wanless IR, Crawford JM, Cirrhosis, In: Odze RD, Goldblum JR, Crawford JM (Eds), Surgical Pathology of the GI Tract, Liver, Biliary Tract, and Pancreas. Saunders, Philadelphia, 2004; pp. 863–884).

References

1. Li Z, Diehl AM. Innate immunity in the liver. Curr Opin Gastroenterol, 2003; 19:565–571
2. Ayres RCS, Neuberger JM, Shaw J, Joplin R, Adams DH. Intercellular adhesion molecule-1 and MHC antigens on human intrahepatic bile duct cells: effect of pro-inflammatory cytokines. Gut, 1993; 34:1245–1249
3. Emoto M, Kaufman SHE. Liver NKT cells: an account of heterogeneity. Trends Immunol, 2003; 24:364–369
4. Nakatani K, Kaneda K, Seki S, Nakajima Y. Pit cells as liver-associated natural killer cells: morphology and function. Med Electron Microsc, 2004; 37:29–36
5. Chen H, Paul W. Cultured NK1.1+ CD4+ T cells produce large amounts of IL-4 and IFN-gamma upon activation by antiCD3 or CD1. J Immunol, 1997; 159:2240–2249
6. Benlagha K, Kyin T, Beavis A, et al. A thymic precursor to the NKT cell lineage. Science, 2002; 296:553–555
7. Bartenschlager R, Frese M, Pietschmann T. Novel insights into hepatitis C virus replication and persistence. Advan Virus Res, 2004; 63:71–180
8. Kanto T, Hayashi N. Measuring immunity in viral hepatitis. J Gastroenterol, 2004; 39:709–716
9. Guidotti LG, Chisari FV. To kill or to cure: options in host defense against viral infection. Curr Opin Immunol, 1996; 8:478–483
10. Kakimi K, Guidotti LG, Koezuka Y, Chisari FV. Natural killer T cell activation inhibits hepatitis B virus replication in vivo. J Exp Med, 2000; 192:921–930
11. Zhu H, Zhao H, Collings CD, et al. Gene expression associated with interferon alfa antiviral activity in an HCV replicon cell line. Hepatology, 2003; 27:1180–1188
12. Bancherau J, Briere F, Caux C, et al. Immunobiology of dendritic cells. Ann Rev Immunol, 2000; 18:767–811
13. Saba TM. Physiology and physiopathology of the reticuloendothelial system. Arch Intern Med, 1970; 126:1031–1052

14. Monshouwer M, Hoebe KHN. Hepatic (dys-)function during inflammation. Toxicology In Vitro, 2003; 17:681–686

15. Gores G, Ren Y, Savill J. Apoptosis: the importance of being eaten. Cell Death Differ, 1998; 5:563–568

16. Day CL, Lauer GM, Robbins GK, et al. Broad specificity of virus-specific CD4+ T-helper-cell responses in resolved hepatitis C virus infection. J Virol, 2002; 76:12584–12595

17. Cerny A, Chisari FV. Pathogenesis of chronic hepatitis C: immunological features of hepatic injury and viral persistence. Hepatology, 1999; 30:595–601

18. Mosmann TR, Sad S. The expanding universe of T-cell subsets: Th1, Th2 and more. Immunol Today, 1996; 17:138–146

19. Bertoletti A, D'Elios MM, Boni C, et al. Different cytokine profiles of intrahepatic T cells in chronic hepatitis B and hepatitis C virus infections. Gastroenterology, 1997; 112:193–199

20. Koszinowski UH, Reddehase MJ, Jonjic S. The role of CD4 and CD8 T cells in viral infections. Curr Opin Immunol, 1991; 3:471–475

21. Guidotti LG, Chisari FV. Noncytolytic control of viral infections by the innate and adaptive immune response. Ann Rev Immunol, 2001; 19:65–91

22. Liu C, Zhu H, Tu Z, Yu YL, Nelson DR. CD8+ T-cell interaction with HCV replicon cells: evidence for both cytokine- and cell-mediated antiviral activity. Hepatology, 2003; 37:1335–1342

23. Akbar AN, Taams LS, Salmon M, et al. The peripheral generation of CD4+ CD25+ regulatory T cells. Immunology, 2003; 109:319–325

24. Shevach EM. CD4+ CD25+ suppressor T cells: more questions than answers. Nat Rev Immunol, 2002; 2:389–400

25. Annacker O, Pimenta-Araujo R, Burelen-Defranoux O, et al. CD25+ CD4+ T cells regulate the expansion of peripheral CD4 T cells through the production of IL10. J Immunol, 2001; 166:3008–3018

26. Thornton AM, Shevach EM. Suppressor effector function of CD4+ CD25+ immunoregulatory T cells is antigen non-specific. J Immunol, 2000; 164:183–190

27. Longhi MS, Ma Y, Bogdanos DP, et al. Impairment of CD4+ CD25+ regulatory T-cells in autoimmune liver disease. J Hepatol, 2004; 41:31–37

28. Butcher EC, Picker LJ. Lymphocyte homing and hemeostasis. Science, 1996; 272:60–66

29. Helbig KJ, Ruszkiewicz A, Semendric L, et al. Expression of the CXCR3 ligand I-TAC by hepatocytes in chronic hepatitis C and its correlation with hepatic inflammation. Hepatology, 2004; 39:1220–1229

30. Salazar-Mather TP, Orange JS, Biron CA. Early murine cytomegalovirus (MCMV) infection induces liver natural killer (NK) cell inflammation and protection through macrophage inflammatory protein 1a (MIP-1a)-dependent pathways. J Exp Med, 1998; 187:1–14

31. Hokeness KL, Kuziel WA, Biron CA, Salazar-Mather TP. Monocyte chemoattractant protein-1 and CCR2 interactions are required for IFN-α/β-induced inflammatory responses and antiviral defense in the liver. J Immunol, 2005; 174:1549–1556

32. Salazar-Mather TP, Lewis CA, Biron CA. Type I interferons regulate inflammatory cell trafficking and macrophage inflammatory protein 1a delivery to the liver. J Clin Invest, 2002; 110:321–330

33. Mehal WZ, Juedes AE, Crispe IN. Selective retention of activated CD8+ T cells by the normal liver. J Immunol, 1999; 163:3202–3210

34. Wald O, Pappo O, Safadi R, et al. Involvement of the CXCL2/CXCR4 pathway in the advanced liver disease that is associated with the hepatitis C virus or hepatitis B virus. Eur J Immunol, 2004; 34:1164–1174

35. Grant AJ, Lalor PJ, Hubscher SG, et al. MAdCAM-1 expressed in chronic inflammatory liver disease supports mucosal lymphocyte adhesion to hepatic endothelium. Hepatology, 2001; 33:1065–1072

36. Crawford JM. Development of the intrahepatic biliary tree. Semin Liver Dis, 2002; 22:213–226

37. Saxena R, Theise ND, Crawford JM. Microanatomy of the human liver: Exploring the hidden interfaces. Hepatology, 1999; 30:1339–1346

38. Crawford JM, Boyer JL. Clinical-Pathologic Conference: Inflammation-induced cholestasis. Hepatology, 1998; 28:253–260

39. Isse K, Harada K, Zen Y, et al. Fractaline and CX3CR1 are involved in the recruitment of intraepithelial lymphocytes of intrahepatic bile ducts. Hepatology, 2005; 41:506–516

40. Li MK, Crawford JM. Pathology of cholestasis. Semin Liver Dis, 2004; 24:21–42

41. Gujral JS, Farhood A, Bajt ML, Jaeschke H. Neutrophils aggravate acute liver injury during obstructive cholestasis in bile duct-ligated mice. Hepatology, 2003; 38:355–363

42. Rehermann B, Folwer P, Signey J, et al. The cytotoxic T lymphocyte response to multiple hepatitis B virus polymerase epitopes during and after acute viral hepatitis. J Exp Med, 1995; 181:1047–1058

43. Chisari FV, Ferrari C. Hepatitis B virus immunopathogenesis. Ann Rev Immunol, 1995; 13:29–60

44. Hasebe A, Akbar SMF, Furukawa S, et al. Impaired functional capacities of liver dendritic cells from murine hepatitis B virus (HBV) carriers: relevance to low HBV-specific immune responses. Clin Exp Immunol, 2004; 139:35–42

45. Marine-Barjoan E, Saint-Paul MC, Pradier C, et al. Impact of antiretroviral treatment on progression of hepatic fibrosis in HIV/hepatitis C virus co-infected patients. AIDS, 2004; 18:2163–2170

46. Zhu NA, Khoshnan A, Schneider R, et al. Hepatitis C virus core protein binds to the cytoplasmic domain of tumor necrosis factor (TNF) receptor 1 and enhances TNF-induced apoptosis. J Virol, 1998; 72:3691–3697

47. Kayagaki N, Yamaguchi N, Nakayama M, et al. Involvement of TNF-related apoptosis-inducing ligand in human CD4+ T cell-mediated cytotoxicity. J Immunol, 1999; 162:2639–2647

48. Chou AH, Tsai HF, Wu YY, et al. Hepatitis C virus core protein modulates TRAIL-mediated apoptosis by enhancing Bid cleavage and activation of mitochondria apoptosis signaling pathway. J Immunol, 2005; 174:2160–2166

49. Eisen-Vandervelde AL, Yao ZQ, Hahan YS. The molecular basis of HCV-mediated immune dysregulation. Clinical Immunol, 2004; 111:16–21

50. Nuti S, Rosa D, Valiante N, et al. Dynamics of intra-hepatic lymphocytes in chronic hepatitis C: enrichment for Va24+ T cells and rapid elimination of effector cells by apoptosis. Eur J Immunol, 1998; 28:3448–3455

51. Chang KM, Thimme R, Melpolder JJ. Differential CD4(+) and CD8(+) T-cell responsiveness in hepatitis C virus infection. Hepatology, 2001; 33:267–276

52. Cabrera R, Tu Z, Xu Y, et al. An immunomodulatory role for CD4(+)CD25(+) regulatory T lymphocytes in hepatitis C virus infection. Hepatology, 2004; 40:1062–1071

53. Barth H, Ulsenheimer A, Paper GR, et al. Uptake and presentation of hepatitis C virus-like particles by human dendritic cells. Blood, 2005; 105:3605–3614

54. Auffemann-Gretzinger S, Keeffe EB, Levy S. Impaired dendritic cell maturation in patients with chronic, but not resolved, hepatitis C virus infection. Blood, 2001; 97:3171–3176

55. Thoren F, Romero A, Lindh M, et al. A hepatitis C virus-encoded, nonstructural protein (NS3) triggers dysfunction and apoptosis in lymphocytes: role of NADPH oxidase-derived oxygen radicals. J Leukocyte Biology, 2004; 76:1180–1186

56. Roskams T. The role of immunohistochemistry in diagnosis. Clin Liver Dis, 2002; 6:571–589

57. Lamps LW, Pinson CW, Raiford DS, et al. The significance of microabscesses in liver transplant biopsies: a clinicopathological study. Hepatology, 1998; 28:1532–1537

58. Diamantis I, Boumpas DT. Autoimmune hepatitis: evolving concepts. Autoimmunity Rev, 2004; 3:207–214

59. Hashimoto E, Lindor KD, Homburger HA, et al. Immunohistochemical characterization of hepatic lymphocytes in primary biliary cirrhosis in comparison with primary sclerosing cholangitis and autoimmune chronic active hepatitis. Mayo Clin Proc, 1993; 68:1049–1055

60. Wen L, Peakman M, Mieli-Vergani G, Vergani D. Elevation of activated gamma delta T cell receptor-bearing T lymphocytes in patients with autoimmune chronic liver disease. Clin Exp Immunol, 1992; 89:78–82

61. Ichiki Y, Aoki CA, Bowlus CL, et al. T cell immunity in autoimmune hepatitis. Autoimmunity Reviews, 2005; 4:315–321

62. Schliess F, Reissman R, Reinehr R, et al. Involvement of integrins and Src in insulin signaling toward autophagic proteolysis in rat liver. J Biol Chem, 2004; 279:21294–21301

63. Farber JL, Kyle ME, Coleman JB. Mechanisms of cell injury by activated oxygen species. Lab Invest, 1990; 62:670–679

64. Ficker P, Trauner M, Fuchsbichler A, et al. Oncosis represents the main type of cell death in mouse models of cholestasis. J Hepatol, 2005; 42:378–385

65. Brunt EM. Nonalcoholic steatohepatitis. Sem Liver Dis, 2004; 24:3–20

66. Mori M. Ultrastructural changes of hepatocyte organelles induced by chemicals and their relation to fat accumulation in the liver. Acta Pathol Jpn, 1983; 911–922

67. Wanless IR, Shiota K. The pathogenesis of nonalcoholic steatohepatitis and other fatty liver diseases: A four-step model including the role of lipid release and hepatic venular obstruction in the progression to cirrhosis. Sem Liver Dis, 2004; 24:99–108

68. Yu S, Matsusue K, Kashireddy P, et al. Adipocyte-specific gene expression and adipogenic steatosis in the mouse liver due to peroxisome proliferator-activated receptor γ1 (PPARγ1) overexpression. J Biol Chem, 2003; 278:498–505

69. Schadinger SE, Bucher NLR, Schreiber BM, Farmer SR. PPARγ2 regulates lipogenesis and lipid accumulation in steatotic hepatocytes. Am J Physiol, 2005; 288:E1195–E1205

70. Anderson J. On hemorrhage from the umbilicus after the separa tion of the fetus. Boston Med Surg J 1850; 41:440–442

71. Trauner M, Boyer JL. Bile salt transporters: molecular characterization, function, and regulation. Physiol Rev, 2003; 83:633–671

72. Green RM, Crawford JM. Hepatocellular cholestasis: Pathobiology and histological outcome. Semin Liver Dis, 1995; 15:372–389

73. Grambihler A, Higuchi H, Bronk SF, Gores GJ. cFLIP-L inhibits p38 MAPK activation: an additional anti-apoptotic mechanism in bile acid-mediated apoptosis. J Biol Chem, 2003; 278:26831–26837

74. Nagore N, Howe S, Boxer L, Scheuer PJ. Liver cell rosettes: structural differences in cholestasis and hepatitis. Liver, 1989; 9:43–51

75. Clayton PT, Casteels M, Mieli-Vergani G, Lawson AM. Familial giant cell hepatitis with low bile acid concentrations and increased urinary excretion of specific bile alcohols: a new inborn error of bile acid synthesis. Pediatr Res, 1995; 37:424–431

76. Zatloukal K, Stumptner C, Fuchsbichler A, et al. The keratin cytoskeleton in liver diseases. J Pathol, 2004; 204:367–376

77. Denk H, Stumptner C, Zatloukal K. Mallory body revisited. J Hepatol, 2000; 32:689–702

78. Zatloukal K, Stumptner C, Fuchsbichler A, et al. p62 is a common component of cytoplasmic inclusions in protein aggregation diseases. Am J Pathol, 2002; 160:255–263

79. Caulin C, Ware CF, Magin TM, Oshima RG. Keratin-dependent, epithelial resistance to tumor necrosis factor-induced apoptosis. J Cell Biol, 2000; 149:17–22

80. Jaeschke H, Gujral JS, Bajt ML. Apoptosis and necrosis in liver disease. Liver Internat, 2004; 24:85–89

81. Kerr JFR. History of the events leading to the formulation of the apoptosis concept. Toxicology, 2002; 181–182:471–474

82. Bai J, Odin JA. Apoptosis and the liver: relation to autoimmunity and related conditions. Autoimmunity Rev, 2003; 2:36–42

83. Yin XM, Ding WX. Death receptor activation-induced hepatocyte apoptosis and liver injury. Curr Mol Med, 2003; 3:491–508

84. Higuchi H, Gores GJ. Mechanisms of liver injury: An overview. Curr Mol Med, 2003; 3:483–490

85. Nakagawa T, Zhu H, Morishma N, et al. Caspase-12 mediates endoplasmic-reticulum-specific apoptosis and cytotoxicity by amyloid-beta. Nature, 2000; 403:98–103

86. Kountouras J, Zavos C, Chatzopoulos D. Apoptosis in hepatitis C. J Viral Hepatitis, 2003; 10:335–342

87. Cambay A, Friedman S, Gores GJ. Apoptosis: the nexus of liver injury and fibrosis. Hepatology, 2004; 39:273–278

88. Lee JY, Chae DW, Kim SM, et al. Expression of FasL and perforin/granzyme B mRNA in chronic hepatitis B infection. J Viral Hepatitis, 2004; 11:130–135

89. Palmeira CM, Rolo AP. Mitochondrially-mediated toxicity of bile acids. Toxicology, 2004; 203:1–15

90. Higuchi H, Gores GJ. Bile acid regulation of hepatic physiology IV. Bile acids and death receptors. Am J Physiol, 2003; 284: G734–G738

91. Demetris AJ, Crawford JM, Nalesnik M, et al. Transplantation pathology of the liver. In: Odze RD, Goldblum JR, Crawford JM, eds. Surgical pathology of the GI tract, liver, biliary tract, and pancreas. Philadelphia: WB Saunders, 2004; pp 909–966

92. Schoemaker MH, Moshage H. Defying death: the hepatocyte's survival kit. Clin Sci, 2004; 107:13–25

93. Locksley RM, Killeen N, Lenardo MJ. The TNF and TNF receptor superfamilies: integrating mammalian biology. Cell, 2001; 104:487–501

94. Ravi R, Bedi GC, Engstrom LW, et al. Regulation of death receptor expression and TRAIL-Apo2L-induced apoptosis by NF-kappaB. Nature Cell Biol, 2001; 3:409–416

95. Janssen HL, Higuchi H, Abdulkarim A, Gores GJ. Hepatitis B virus enhances tumor necrosis factor-related apoptosis-inducing ligand (TRAIL) cytotoxicity by increasing TRAIL-R1/death receptor 4 expression. J Hepatol, 2003; 39:414–420

96. Higuchi H, Yoon JH, Grambihler A, et al. Bile acids stimulate cFLIP phosphorylation enhancing TRAIL-mediated apoptosis. J Biol Chem, 2003; 278:454–461

97. Zender L, Hütker S, Mundt B, et al. NFκB-mediated upregulation of Bcl-xl restrains TRAIL-mediated apoptosis in murine viral hepatitis. Hepatology, 2005; 41:280–288

98. Zeini M, Hortelano S, Través PG, et al. Assessment of a dual regulatory role for NO in liver regeneration after partial hepatectomy: protection against apoptosis and retardation of hepatocyte proliferation. FASEB J, 2005; e-publication March 23, 2005

99. Kim PKM, Zuckerbraun BS, Otterbein LE, et al. 'Til death do us part: nitric oxide and mechanisms of hepatotoxicity. Biol Chem, 2004; 385:11–15

100. Teckman JH, An JK, Blomenkamp K, et al. Mitochondrial autophagy and injury in the liver of a_1-antitrypsin deficiency. Am J Physiol, 2004; 286:G851–G862

101. Jaeschke H, LeMasters JJ. Apoptosis versus oncotic necrosis in hepatic ischemia/reperfusion injury. Gastroenterology, 2003; 125:1246–1257

102. Arii S, Teramoto K, Kawamura T. Current progress in the understanding of and therapeutic strategies for ischemia and reperfusion injury of the liver. J Hepatobiliary Pancreat Surg, 2003; 10:189–194

103. Buck LT, Hochachka PW. Anoxic suppression on Na+-K+-ATPase and constant membrane potential in hepatocytes: support for channel arrest. Am J Physiol, 1993; 265:R1020–R1025

104. Lemasters JJ, Stemkowski CJ, Ji S, Thurman RG. Cell surface changes and enzyme release during hypoxia and reoxygenation in the isolated, perfused rat liver. J Cell Biol, 1983; 97:778–786

105. Gateau-Roesch O, Pavlov E, Lazareva AV, et al. Calcium-binding properties of the mitochondrial channel-forming hydrophobic component. J Bioenerg Biomembr, 2000; 32:105–110

106. Kim JS, He L, Qian T, LeMasters JJ. Role of the mitochrondrial permeability transition in apoptotic and necrotic death after ischemia/reperfusion injury to hepatocytes. Curr Mol Med, 2003; 3:527–535

107. McCord JM. Oxygen-derived free radicals in postischemic tissue injury. N Engl J Med, 1985; 312:159–163

108. Adkins D, Hollwarth ME, Benoit JN, et al. Role of free radicals in ischemia-reperfusion injury to the liver. Acta Physiol Scand Supple, 1986; 548:101–107

109. Lee VG, Johnson ML, Baust J, et al. The roles of iNOS in liver ischemia–reperfusion injury. Shock, 2001; 16:355–360

110. Lin HI, Wang D, Leu FJ, et al. Ischemia and reperfusion of liver induces eNOS and iNOS expression: effects of a NO donor and NOS inhibitor. Chin J Physiol, 2004; 47:121–127

111. Rubin EM, Martin AA, Thung SN, Gerber MA. Morphometric and immunohistochemical characterization of human liver regeneration. Am J Pathol, 1995; 147:397–404

112. Gerber MA, Thung SN. Liver stem cells and development. Lab Invest, 1993; 68:253–254

113. Gerber MA, Thung SN. Sirica AE, eds. The role of cell types in hepatocarcinogenesis. Boca Raton: CRC Press, 1992; Cell lineages in human liver development, regeneration, and transformation; pp 209–226

114. Grisham JW. Migration of hepatocytes along hepatic plates and stem cell-fed hepatocyte lineages. Am J Pathol, 1994; 144:849–854

115. Theise ND, Krause DS. Bone marrow to liver: the blood of Prometheus. Semin Cell Dev Biol, 2002; 13:411–417

116. Taub R. Liver regeneration: from myth to mechanism. Nature Rev, 2004; 5:836–847

117. Michalopoulos GK, DeFrances MC. Liver regeneration. Science, 1997; 276:60–66

118. Reuben A. Prometheus and Pandora—together again. Hepatology, 2004; 39:1460–1463

119. Higgins GM, Anderson RM. Experimental pathology of the liver. I. Restoration of the liver of the white rat following partial surgical removal. Arch Pathol, 1931; 12:186–202

120. Fausto N. Liver regeneration and repair: Hepatocytes, progenitor cells, and stem cells. Hepatology, 2004; 39:1477–1487

121. Black D, Lyman S, Heider TR, Behrns KE. Molecular and cellular features of hepatic regeneration. J Surgical Res, 2004; 117:306–315

122. Koniaris LG, McKillop IH, Schwartz SI, Zimmers TA. Liver regeneration. J Am Coll Surg 2003; 197:634–659

123. Overturf K, al-Dhalimy M, Ou CN, et al. Serial transplantation reveals the stem-cell-like regenerative potential of adult mouse hepatocytes. Am J Pathol, 1997; 151:1273–1280

124. Sigal SH, et al. Partial hepatectomy-induced polyploidy attenuates hepatocyte replication and activates cell aging events. Am J Physiol, 1999; 276:G1260–G1272

125. Moolten FL, Bucher NL. Regeneration of rat liver: transfer of humoral agent by cross circulation. Science, 1967; 158:272–274

126. Ueki T, Kaneda Y, Tsutsui H, et al. Hepatocyte growth factor gene therapy of liver cirrhosis in rats. Nature Med, 1999; 5:226–230

127. Gohda E, Tsubouchi H, Nakayama H, et al. Purification and partial characterisation of hepatocyte growth factor from plasma of a patient with fulminant hepatic failure. J Clin Invest, 1988; 81:414–419

128. Ponzetto C, Bardelli A, Zhen Z, et al. A multifunctional docking site mediates signaling and transformation by the hepatocyte growth factor/scatter factor receptor family. Cell, 1994; 77:261–271

129. Marti U, Burwen SJ, Jones AL. Biological effects of epidermal growth factor, with emphasis on the gastrointestinal tract and liver: an update. Hepatology, 1989; 9:126–138

130. St Hilaire RJ, Hradek GT, Jones AL. Hepatic sequestration and biliary secretion of epidermal growth factors: evidence for a high-capacity uptake system. Proc Natl Acad Sci USA, 1983; 80:3797–3801

131. McGowan JA, Strain AJ, Bucher NLR. DNA synthesis in primary cultures of adult rat hepatocytes in a defined medium: effects of epidermal growth factor, insulin, glucagon and cyclic AMP. J Cell Physiol, 1981; 108:353–363

132. Olsen PS, Boesby S, Kirkegaard P, et al. Influence of epidermal growth factor on liver regeneration after partial hepatectomy in rats. Hepatology, 1988; 8:992–996

133. Johnson AC, Garfield SH, Merlino GT, Patsan I. Expression of epidermal growth factor receptor proto-oncogene mRNA in regenerating rat liver. Biochem Biophys Res Commun, 1988; 150:412–418

134. Beresain C, García-Trevijano ER, Castillo J, et al. Amphiregulin: an early trigger for liver regeneration in mice. Gastroenterology, 2005; 128:424–432

135. Plowman GD, Green JM, McDonald VL, et al. The amphiregulin gene encodes a novel epidermal growth factor-related protein with tumor-inhibitory activity. Mol Cell Biol, 1990; 10:1969–1981

136. Michalopoulos GK, Kahn Z. Liver regeneration, growth factors, and amphiregulin. Gastroenterology, 2005; 128:503–506

137. Mead JE, Fausto N. Transforming growth factor alpha may be a physiological regulator of liver regeneration by means of an autocrine mechanism. Proc Natl Acad Sci USA, 1989; 86:1558–1562

138. Fausto N, Mead JE. Regulation of liver growth: protooncogenes and transforming growth factors. Lab Invest, 1989; 60:4–13

139. Kan M, Huang J, Mansson PE, et al. Heparin-binding growth factor type 1 (acidic fibroblast growth factor): a potential biphasic autocrine and paracrine regulator of hepatocyte regeneration. Proc Natl Acad Sci USA, 1989; 86:7432–7436

140. Presta M, Statuto M, Rusnati M, et al. Characterization of Mr 25,000 basic fibroblast growth factor form in adult, regenerating and fetal rat liver. Biochem Biophys Res Commun, 1989; 164:1182–1189

141. Caro JF, Poulos J, Ittoop O, et al. Insulin-like growth factor 1 binding in hepatocytes from human liver, human hepatoma, and normal regenerating, and fetal rat liver. J Clin Invest, 1988; 81:976–981

142. Stirling GA, Laughlin J, Washington SLA. Effects of starvation on the proliferative response after partial hepatectomy. Exp Mol Pathol, 1973; 19:44–52

143. Ord MG, Stocken LA. Uptake of amino acid and nucleic acid precursors by regenerating rat liver. Biochem J, 1972; 129:175–181

144. LeCam A, Rey JF, Fehlman M, et al. Amino acid transport in isolated hepatocytes after partial hepatectomy in the rat. Am J Physiol, 1979; 236:E594–E602

145. Rigotti P, Peters JC, Tranberg K-G, et al. Effects of amino acid infusions on liver regeneration after hepatectomy in the rat. J Parenter Enteral Nutr, 1986; 10:17–20

146. Talarico KS, Feller DD, Neville ED. Mitotic response to various dietary conditions in the normal and regenerating rat liver. Proc Soc Exp Biol Med, 1971; 136:381–384

147. Schulte-Hermann R. Two-stage control of cell proliferation induced in rat liver by alpha-hexacholorocyclohexane. Cancer Res, 1977; 37:166–171

148. Bucher NLR, Strain AJ. Regulatory mechanisms in hepatic regeneration. In: Millward-Sadler GH, Wright R, Arthur MJP, eds. Wright's liver and biliary disease. London: Saunders, 1992: pp 258–274

149. Barra R, Hall JC. Liver regeneration in normal and alloxan-induced diabetic rats. J Exp Zool, 1977; 201:93–100

150. Johnston D, Johnston M, Alberti KGMM, et al. Hepatic regeneration and metabolism after partial hepatectomy in normal rats: effects of insulin therapy. Eur J Clin Invest, 1986; 16:376–383

151. Johnston D, Johnston M, Alberti KGMM, et al. Hepatic regeneration and metabolism after partial hepatectomy in diabetic rats: effects of insulin therapy. Eur J Clin Invest, 1986; 16:384–390

152. Britton RS, Bacon BR. Intracellular signaling pathways in stellate cell activation. Alcohol Clin Exp Res, 1999; 23:922–925

153. Cruise JL, Knechtle SJ, Bollinger R, et al. Alpha-1-adrenergic effects and liver regeneration. Hepatology, 1987; 7:1189–1194

154. Pietralleli R, Chamuleau RAFM, Speranza V, et al. Immunocytochemical study of the hepatic innervation in the rat after partial hepatectomy. Histochem J, 1987; 19:327–332

155. Okajima F, Ui M. Conversion of the adrenergic regulation of glycogen phosphorylase and synthase from an alpha to a beta type

156. Sandnes D, Sand TE, Sager G, et al. Elevated level of beta-adrenergic receptors in hepatocytes from regenerating rat liver. Exp Cell Res, 1986; 165:117–126

157. Cruise JL, Cotecchia S, Michalopoulos GK. Norepinephrine decreases EGF binding in primary rat hepatocyte cultures. J Cell Physiol, 1986; 127:39–44

158. Houchk KA, Cruise JL, Michalopoulos GK. Norepinephrine modulates the growth-inhibiting effect of transforming growth factor beta in primary rat hepatocyte cultures. J Cell Physiol, 1988; 135:551–555

159. Short J, Brown RF, Husakova A, et al. Induction of the DNA synthesis in the liver of the intact animal. J Biol Chem, 1972; 247:1757–1766

160. Heinrich PC, et al. Principles of interleukin (IL)-6-type cytokine signalling and its regulation. Biochem J, 2003; 374:1–20

161. Cressman DE, et al. Liver failure and defective hepatocyte regeneration in interleukin-6-deficient mice. Science, 1996; 274:1379–1383

162. Sakamoto T, et al. Mitosis and apoptosis in the liver interleukin-6-deficient mice after partial hepatectomy. Hepatology, 1999; 29:403–411

163. Wuestefeld T, et al. Interleukin-6/glycoprotein 130-dependent pathways are protective during liver regeneration. J Biol Chem, 2003; 278:11281–11288

164. Blindenbacher A, et al. Interleukin-6 is important for survival after partial hepatectomy in mice. Hepatology, 2003; 38:674–682

165. Yamada Y, et al. Initiation of liver growth by tumor necrosis factor: defective liver regeneration in mice lacking type 1 tumor necrosis factor receptor. Proc Natl Acad Sci USA, 1997; 94:1441–1446

166. Fujita J, et al. Effect of TNF gene depletion on liver regeneration after partial hepatectomy in mice. Surgery, 2001; 129:48–54

167. Aldeguer X, et al. Interleukin-6 from intrahepatic cells of bone marrow origin is required for normal murine liver regeneration. Hepatology, 2002; 35:40–48

168. Sun R, Gao B. Negative regulation of liver regeneration by innate immunity (natural killer cells/interferon-γ). Gastroenterology, 2004; 127:1525–1539

169. Strain AJ. Transforming growth factor-beta and inhibition of hepatocellular proliferation. Scand J Gastroenterol, 1988; 23 (Suppl. 151):37–45

170. Russell WE, Coffey JR, Ouellette AJ, Moses HL. Type beta transforming growth factor reversibly inhibits the early proliferative response to partial hepatectomy in the rat. Proc Natl Acad Sci USA, 1988; 85:5126–5130

171. Martinez-Hernandez A, Amenta PS. The extracellular matrix in hepatic regeneration. FASEB J, 1995; 9:1401–1410

172. Wack KE, Ross MA, Zegarra V, et al. Sinusoidal ultrastructure evaluated during the revascularization of regenerating rat liver. Hepatology, 2001; 33:363–378

173. Ross MA, Sander CM, Kleeb TB, et al. Spatiotemporal expression of angiogenesis growth factor receptors during the revascularization of regenerating rat liver. Hepatology, 2001; 34:1135–1148

174. Zimmermann A. Regulation of liver regeneration. Nephrol Dial Transplant, 2004; 19 (Suppl 4):iv6–iv10

175. Derynck R, Zhang YE. Smad-dependent and Smad-independent pathways in TGF-β family signaling. Nature, 2003; 425:577–584

176. Romero-Gallo J, Sozmen EG, Chytil A, et al. Inactivation of TGF-β signaling in hepatocytes results in an increased proliferative response after partial hepatectomy. Oncogene, 2005; 24:3028–3041

177. Macias-Silva M, Li W, Leu JI, et al. Up-regulated transcriptional repressors SnoN and Ski bind Smad proteins to antagonize transforming growth factor-β signals during liver regeneration. J Biol Chem, 2002; 277:28483–28490

178. Kalininchencko VV, Bhattacharyya D, Zhou Y, et al. Foxf1 +/- mice exhibit defective stellate cell activation and abnormal liver regeneration following CCl4 injury. Hepatology, 2003; 37:107–117

179. Taimr P, Higuchi H, Kocova E, et al. Activated stellate cells express TRAIL receptor-2/death receptor-5 and undergo TRAIL-mediated apoptosis. Hepatology, 2003; 37:87–95

180. Rudolph KL, et al. Inhibition of experimental liver cirrhosis in mice by telomerase gene delivery. Science, 2000; 287:1253–1258

181. Rubin EM, Martin AA, Thung SN, Gerber MA. Morphometric and immunohistochemical characterization of human liver regeneration. Am J Pathol, 1995; 147:397–404

182. Witek RP, Fisher SH, Petersen BE. Monocrotaline, an alternative to retrorsine-based hepatocyte transplantation in rodents. Cell Transplant, 2004; 14:41–47

during primary culture of rat hepatocytes. Arch Biochem Biophys, 1982; 213:658–668

183. Kofman AV, Morgan G, Kirschenbaum A, et al. Dose- and time-dependent oval cell reaction in acetaminophen-induced murine liver injury. Hepatology, 2005; 41:1252–1261

184. Newsome PN, Hussain MA, Theise ND. Hepatic oval cells: helping redefine a paradigm in stem cell biology. Curr Top Dev Biol, 2004; 61:1–28

185. Sell S. Electron microscopic identification of putative liver stem cells and intermediate hepatocytes following periportal necrosis induced in rats by allyl alcohol. Stem Cells, 1997; 15:378–385

186. Farber E. Similarities in the sequence of early histologic changes induced in the livers of rats by ethionine, 2-acetylamino-azobenzene and 3'-methyl-4-dimethylaminoazobenzene. Cancer Res, 1956; 16:142–148

187. Crosby HA, Hubscher S, Fabris L, et al. Immunolocalization of putative human liver progenitor cells in livers from patients with end-stage primary biliary cirrhosis and sclerosing cholangitis using the monoclonal antibody OV-6. Am J Pathol, 1998; 152:771–779

188. Vandersteenhoven AM, Burchette J, Michalopoulos G. Characterization of ductular hepatocytes in end-stage cirrhosis. Arch Pathol Lab Med, 1990; 114:403–406

189. Eleazar JA, Memeo L, Jhang JS, et al. Progenitor cell expansion: an important source of hepatocyte regeneration in chronic hepatitis. J Hepatol, 2004; 41:983–991

190. Theise ND, Saxena R, Portmann BC, et al. The canals of Hering and hepatic stem cells in humans. Hepatology, 1999; 30:1425–1433

191. Demetris AJ, Seaberg EC, Wennerberg A, et al. Ductular reaction after submassive necrosis in humans. Special emphasis on analysis of ductular hepatocytes. Am J Pathol, 1996; 149:439–448

192. Craig CEH, Quagila A, Selden C, et al. The histopathology of regeneration in massive hepatic necrosis. Semin Liver Dis, 2004; 24:49–64

193. Sell S. Heterogeneity and plasticity of hepatocyte lineage cells. Hepatology, 2001; 33:738–750

194. Michalopoulos GK, Barua L, Bowen WC. Transdifferentiation of rat hepatocytes into biliary cells after bile duct ligation and toxic biliary injury. Hepatology, 2005; 41:535–544

195. Liu C, Schreiter T, Dirsch O, et al. Presence of markers for liver progenitor cells in human-derived intrahepatic biliary epithelial cells. Liver Int, 2004; 24:669–678

196. Laurson J, Selden C, Hodgson HJF. Hepatocyte progenitors in man and in rodents—multiple pathways, multiple candidates. Int J Exp Pathol, 2005; 86:1–18

197. Petersen BE, Bowen WC, Patrene KD, et al. Bone marrow as a potential source of hepatic oval cells. Science, 1999; 284:1168–1170

198. Theise ND, Badve S, Saxena R, et al. Derivation of hepatocytes from bone marrow cells in mice after radiation-induced myeloablation. Hepatology, 2000; 31:235–240

199. Menthena A, Deb N, Oertel M, et al. Bone marrow progenitors are not the normal source of oval cells in the injured liver. Stem Cell, 2004; 22:1049–1061

200. Wang X, Montini E, Muhsen A-D, et al. Kinetics of liver repopulation after bone marrow transplantation. Am J Pathol, 2002; 161:565–574

201. Vassilopoulos G, Wang PR, Russell DW. Transplanted bone marrow regenerates liver by cell fusion. Nature, 2003; 422:897–901

202. Lagasse E, Connors H, Al-Dhalimy M, et al. Purified hematopoietic stem cells can differentiate into hepatocytes in vivo. Nature Med, 2000; 6:1229–1234

203. Austin TW, Lagasse E. Hepatic regeneration from hematopoietic stem cells. Mech Dev, 2003; 120:131–135

204. Jang Y-Y, Collector MI, Baylin SB, et al. Hematopoietic stem cells convert into liver cells within days without fusion. Nature Cell Biol, 2004; 6:532–539

205. Daley GQ. Alchemy in the liver: fact or fusion? Nature Med, 2004; 10:671–672

206. Bedossa P, Paradis V. Liver extracellular matrix in health and disease. J Pathol, 2003; 200:504–515

207. Bataller R, Brenner DA. Liver fibrosis. J Clin Invest, 2005; 115:209–218

208. Ohara N, Schaffner T, Reichen J. Structure-function relationship in secondary biliary cirrhosis in the rat. Stereologic and hemodynamic characterization of a model. J Hepatol, 1993; 17:155–162

209. Eng FJ, Friedman SL. Fibrogenesis I. New insights into hepatic stellate cell activation: the simple becomes complex. Am J Physiol, 2000; 279:G7–G11

210. Arthur MJ. Fibrogenesis II. Metalloproteinases and their inhibitors in liver fibrosis. Am J Physiol, 2000; 279:G245–249

211. Lindquist JN, Marzluff WF, Stefanovic B. Fibrogenesis III. Posttranscriptional regulation of type I collagen. Am J Physiol, 2000; 279:G471–476

212. Geerts A, Geuze JH, Slot JW, et al. Immunogold localisation of procollagen III, fibronectin and heparan sulfate proteoglycan on ultrathin frozen sections of the normal rat liver. Histochemistry, 1986; 84:355–362

213. Sato M, Suzuki S, Senoo H. Hepatic stellate cells: unique characteristics in cell biology and phenotype. Cell Structure Function, 2003; 28:105–112

214. Pinzani M, Failli P, Ruocco C, et al. Fat-storing cells as liver-specific pericytes: spatial dynamics of agonist-stimulated intracellular calcium transient. J Clin Invest, 1992; 90:642–646

215. Pinzani M. Liver fibrosis. Springer Semin Immunopathol, 2000; 21:475–490

216. Dubuisson L, Desmouliere A, Decourt B, et al. Inhibition of rat liver fibrogenesis through noradrenergic antagonism. Hepatology, 2002; 24:325–331

217. Mathew J, Geerts A, Burt AD. Pathobiology of hepatic stellate cells. Hepatogastroenterology, 1996; 43:72–91

218. Friedman SL. Seminars in medicine of the Beth Israel Hospital, Boston: the cellular basis of hepatic fibrosis-mechanisms and treatment strategies. N Engl J Med, 1993; 328:1828–1835

219. Sherman IA, Pappas SC, Fisher MM. Hepatic microvascular changes associated with development of liver fibrosis and cirrhosis. Am J Physiol, 1990; 258:H460–H465

220. Yokoi Y, Namihisa T, Matsuzaki K, Miyazaki A, Yamaguchi Y. Distribution of Ito cells in experimental hepatic fibrosis. Liver, 1988; 8:48–52

221. Ballardini G, Degli Esposti S, Bianchi FB, et al. Correlation between Ito cells and fibrogenesis in an experimental model of hepatic fibrosis. A sequential stereological study. Liver, 1983; 3:58–63

222. Gressner AM, Haarmann R. Regulation of hyaluronate synthesis in rat liver fat storing cell cultures by Kupffer cells. J Hepatol, 1988; 7:310–311

223. Friedman SL, Arthur MJP. Activation of cultured rat hepatic lipocytes by Kupffer cell conditioned medium. Direct enhancement of matrix synthesis and stimulation of cell proliferation via induction of platelet-derived growth factor receptors. J Clin Invest, 1989; 84:1780–1785

224. Nakatsukasa H, Nagy P, Evarts RP, et al. Cellular distribution of transforming growth factor-beta 1 and procollagen types, I, III, IV transcripts in carbon-tetrachloride-induced rat liver fibrosis. J Clin Invest, 1990; 85:1833–1843

225. Milani S, Herbst H, Schuppan D, et al. In situ hybridization for procollagen types I, III and IV RNA in normal and fibrotic rat liver: evidence for predominant expression in non-parenchymal liver cells. Hepatology, 1989; 10:84–92

226. Duda J, Saile B, El Armouche H, et al. Endoreplication and polyploidy in primary culture of rat hepatic stellate cells. Cell Tissue Res, 2003; 313:301–311

227. Viñas O, Bataller R, Ginès P, et al. Human hepatic stellate cells show features of antigen-presenting cells and stimulate lymphocyte proliferation. Hepatology, 2003; 38:919–929

228. Saile B, Matthes N, Knittel T, et al. Transforming growth factor beta and tumor necrosis factor alpha inhibit both apoptosis and proliferation of activated rat hepatic stellate cells. Hepatology, 1999; 30:196–202

229. Saile B, Knittel T, Matthes N, et al. CD95/CD95L-mediated apoptosis of the hepatic stellate cell. A mechanism terminating uncontrolled hepatic stellate cell proliferation during hepatic tissue repair. Am J Pathol, 1997; 151:1265–1272

230. Taimr P, Higuchi H, Kocova E, et al. Activated stellate cells express the TRAIL receptor-2/death receptor-5 and undergo TRAIL-mediated apoptosis. Hepatology, 2003; 37:87–95

231. Housset C, Rockey DC, Bissell DM. Endothelin receptors in rat liver: lipocytes as a contractile target for endothelin 1. Proc Natl Acad Sci USA, 1993; 90:9266–9270

232. Kawada N, Tran-Thi TA, Klein H, Decker K. The contraction of hepatic stellate (Ito) cells stimulated with vasoactive substances: possible involvement of endothelin 1 and nitric oxide in the regulation of sinusoidal tonus. Eur J Biochem, 1993; 213:815–823

233. Enzan H, Himeno H, Iwamura S, et al. Sequential changes in human Ito cells and their relation to postnecrotic liver fibrosis in massive and submassive hepatic necrosis. Virchows Arch, 1995; 426:95–101

234. Worner TM, Lieber CS. Perivenular fibrosis as precursor lesion of cirrhosis. JAMA, 1985; 254:627–630

235. Andrade ZA. Contribution to the study of septal fibrosis of the liver. Int J Exp Pathol, 1991; 72:553–562

236. Nakano M, Lieber CS. Ultrastructure of initial stages of perivenular fibrosis in alcohol-fed baboons. Am J Pathol, 1982; 106:145–155

237. Nakano M, Worner TM, Lieber CS. Perivenular fibrosis in alcoholic liver injury: ultrastructure and histologic progression. Gastroenterology, 1982; 83:777–785

238. Chedid A, Arain S, Snyder A, et al. The immunology of fibrogenesis in alcoholic liver disease. Arch Pathol Lab Med, 2004; 128:1230–1238

239. Vollmar B, Siegmund S, Menger MD. An intravital fluorescence microscopic study of hepatic microvascular and cellular derangements in developing cirrhosis in rats. Hepatology, 1998; 27:1544–1553

240. Friedman SL, Millward-Sadler GH, Arthur MJP. Liver fibrosis and cirrhosis. In: Millward-Sadler GH, Wright R, Arthur MJ, eds. Wright's liver and biliary disease, 3rd edn. London: Saunders, 1992; pp 821–881

241. Timpl R, Wieddemann H, van Delden V, et al. A network model for the organisation of type IV collagen molecules in basement. Eur J Biochem, 1981; 120:203–211

242. Keene DR, Engvall E, Glanville RW. Ultrastructure of type VI collagen in human skin and cartilage suggests an anchoring function for this filamentous network. J Cell Biol, 1988; 107:1995–2006

243. Rojkind M, Ponce-Noyola P. The extracellular matrix of the liver. Coll Relat Res, 1982; 2:151–175

244. Gressner AM, Bachem MG. Cellular sources of noncollagenous matrix proteins: role of fat-storing cells in fibrogenesis. Semin Liver Dis, 1990; 10:30–46

245. Greenwel P, Geerts A, Ogata I, et al. Liver fibrosis. In: Arias I, Boyer J, Fausto N, Jacoby W, Schachter D, et al., eds. The liver: biology and pathobiology. 3rd edn. New York: Raven, 1994; pp 1367–1381

246. Clément B, Rescan P-Y, Baffet G, et al. Hepatocytes may produce laminin in fibrotic liver and in primary culture. Hepatology, 1988; 8:794–803

247. Castronovo V, Taraboletti G, Sobel ME. Laminin receptor complementary DNA-deduced synthetic peptide inhibits cancer cell attachment to endothelium. Cancer Res, 1991; 51:5672–5678

248. Herbst TJ, McCarthy JB, Tsilibary EC, Furcht LT. Differential effects of laminin, intact type IV collagen, and specific domains of type IV collagen on endothelial cell adhesion and migration. J Cell Biol, 1988; 106:1365–1373

249. Kleinman HK, McGarvey ML, Hassell JR, et al. Basement membrane complexes with biological activity. Biochemistry, 1986; 25:312–318

250. Carley WW, Milici AJ, Madri JA. Extracellular matrix specificity for the differentiation of capillary endothelial cells. Exp Cell Res, 1988; 178:426–434

251. McGuire RF, Bissell DM, Boyles J, Roll FJ. Role of extracellular matrix in regulating fenestrations of sinusoidal endothelial cells isolated from normal rat liver. Hepatology, 1992; 15:989–997

252. Kubota Y, Kleinman HK, Martin GR, Lawley TJ. Role of laminin and basement membrane in the morphological differentiation of human endothelial cells into capillary-like structures. J Cell Biol, 1988; 107:1589–1598

253. Grant DS, Tashiro K, Segui-Real B, et al. Two different laminin domains mediate the differentiation of human endothelial cells into capillary-like structures in vitro. Cell, 1989; 58:933–943

254. Grant DS, Lelkes PI, Fukuda K, Kleinman HK. Intracellular mechanisms involved in basement membrane induced blood vessel differentiation in vitro. In Vitro Cell Dev Biol, 1991; 27A:327–336

255. Martinez-Hernandez A, Amenta PS. The hepatic extracellular matrix. I. Components and distribution in normal liver. Virchows Arch A Pathol Anat Histopathol, 1993; 423:1–11

256. Jaffe EA, Hoyer LW, Nachman RL. Synthesis of von Willebrand factor by cultured human endothelial cells. Proc Natl Acad Sci USA, 1974; 71:1906–1909

257. Ewenstein BM, Warhol MJ, Handin RI, Pober JS. Composition of the von Willebrand factor storage organelle (Weibel–Palade body) isolated from cultured human umbilical vein endothelial cells. J Cell Biol, 1987; 104:1423–1433

258. Mori T, Okanoue T, Sawa Y, et al. Defenestration of the sinusoidal endothelial cell in a rat model of cirrhosis. Hepatology, 1993; 17:891–897

259. Fritze LMS, Reille CF, Rosenberg RD. An antiproliferative heparan sulfate species produced by postconfluent smooth muscle cells. J Cell Biol, 1985; 100:1041–1049

260. Dziadek M, Fujiwara S, Paulsson M, et al. Immunological characterization of basement membrane types of heparan sulfate proteoglycan. EMBO J, 1985; 4:1463–1468

261. Elenius K, Salmivirta M, Inki P, et al. Binding of human syndecan to extracellular matrix proteins. J Biol Chem, 1990; 265:17837–17843

262. Andres JL, Stanley K, Cheifetz S, Massague J. Membrane anchored and soluble forms of betaglucan, a polymorphic proteoglycan that binds transforming growth factor-beta. J Cell Biol, 1989; 109:3137–3145

263. Fausto N. Liver regeneration. J Hepatol, 2000; 32:19–31

264. Ramadori G, Saile B. Portal tract fibrogenesis in the liver. Lab Invest, 2004; 84:153–159

265. Lamireau T, Dubuisson L, Lepreux S, et al. Abnormal hepatic expression of fibrillin-1 in children with cholestasis. Am J Surg Pathol, 2002; 26:637–646

266. Dubuisson L, Lepreux S, Bioulac-Sage P, et al. Expression and cellular localization of fibrillin-1 in normal and pathological human liver. J Hepatol, 2001; 34:514–522

267. Lin XZ, Horng MH, Sun YN, et al. Computer morphometry for quantitative measurement of liver fibrosis: comparison with Knodell's score, colorimetry and conventional description reports. J Gastroenterol Hepatol, 1998; 13:75–80

268. Murata K, Ochiai Y, Akaashio K. Polydispersity of acidic glycosaminoglycan components in human liver and the changes at different stages in liver cirrhosis. Gastroenterology, 1985; 89:1249–1257

269. Gressner AM. Hepatic fibrogenesis: the puzzle of interacting cells, fibrogenic cytokines, regulatory loops and extracellular matrix molecules. Z Gastroenterol (Suppl 1), 1992; 30:5–16

270. Martinez-Hernandez A, Martinez J. The role of capillarization in hepatic failure: studies in carbon tetrachloride-induced cirrhosis. Hepatology, 1991; 14:864–874

271. James J, Bosch KS, Zuyderhoudt FM, et al. Histophotometric estimation of volume density of collagen as an indication of fibrosis in rat liver. Histochemistry, 1986; 85:129–133

272. Schaffner F, Popper H. Capillarization of hepatic sinusoids in man. Gastroenterology, 1963; 44:239–242

273. Friedman SL, Rockey DC, McGuire RF, et al. Isolated hepatic lipocytes and Kupffer cells from normal human liver: Morphological and functional characteristics in primary culture. Hepatology, 1992; 15:234–243

274. Bissell DM, Arenson DM, Maher JJ, Roll FJ. Support of cultured hepatocytes by a laminin-rich gel: evidence for a functionally significant subendothelial matrix in normal rat liver. J Clin Invest, 1987; 79:801–812

275. Schuetz EG, Li D, Omiecinski CJ, et al. Regulation of gene expression in adult rat hepatocytes cultured on a basement membrane matrix. J Hepatol, 1988; 134:309–323

276. Friedman SL, Roll FJ, Boyles J, et al. Maintenance of differentiated phenotype of cultured rat hepatic lipocytes by basement membrane matrix. J Biol Chem, 1989; 1264:10756–10762

277. Pinzani M. Liver fibrosis. Semin Immunopathol, 1999; 21:475–490

278. Johanssen S, Forsberg E, Lundgren B. Comparison of fibronectin receptors from rat hepatocytes and fibroblasts. J Biol Chem, 1987; 262:7819–7824

279. Gullberg D, Terracio L, Borg TK, Rubin K. Identification of integrin-like matrix receptors with affinity for interstitial collagens. J Biol Chem, 1989; 264:12686–12694

280. Clement B, Segui-Real B, Savagner P, et al. Hepatocyte attachment to laminin is mediated through multiple receptors. J Cell Biol, 1990; 110:185–192

281. Hughes RC, Stamatoglou SC. Adhesive interactions and the metabolic activity of hepatocytes. J Cell Sci, 1987; 8(suppl):273–291

282. Kirch HC, Lammers M, Gressner AM. Binding of chondroitin sulfate, dermatan sulfate and fat-storing cell-derived proteoglycans to rat hepatocytes. Int J Biochem, 1987; 19:1119–1126

283. Schonherr E, Hausser HJ. Extracellular matrix and cytokines: a functional unit. Dev Immunol, 2000; 7:89–101

284. Laurent TC, Fraser JRE, Pertoft H, Smedsrod B. Binding of hyaluronate and chondroitin sulphate to liver endothelial cells. Biochem J, 1986; 234:653–658

285. Friedman SL. Acetaldehyde and alcoholic fibrogenesis: Fuel to the fire, but not the spark. Hepatology, 1990; 12:609–612

286. Moshage H, Casini A, Lieber CS. Acetaldehyde selectively stimulates collagen production in cultured rat liver fat-storing cells but not in hepatocytes. Hepatology, 1990; 12:511–518

287. Crawford JM. Cellular and molecular biology of the inflamed liver. Curr Op Gastroenterol, 1997; 13:175–185

288. Pinzani M, Weber FL, Gesualdo L, et al. Expression of platelet-derived growth factor (PDGF) in an vivo model of acute liver inflammation. (Abstract) Hepatology, 1990; 12:920

289. Dooley S, Hamzavi J, Breitkopf K, et al. Smad7 prevents activation of hepatic stellate cells and liver fibrosis in rats. Gastroenterology, 2003; 125:178–191

290. Wells RG. The role of matrix stiffness in hepatic stellate cell activation and liver fibrosis. J Clin Gastroenterol, 2005; 39: S158–S161

291. Uemura M, Swenson ES, Gaca MD, et al. Smad2 and Smad3 play different roles in rat hepatic stellate cell function and α-smooth muscle actin organization. Mol Biol Cell, 2005; 16:4214–4224

292. Carloni V, Pinzani M, Giusti S, et al. Tyrosine phosphorylation of focal adhesion inase by PDGF is dependent on ras in human hepatic stellate cells. Hepatology, 2000; 31:131–140

293. Leo MA, Lieber CS. Hepatic vitamin A depletion in alcoholic liver injury. N Engl J Med, 1982; 307:597–601

294. Davis BH, Pratt BM, Madri JA. Retinol and extracellular collagen matrices modulate hepatic Ito cell collagen phenotype and cellular retinol binding protein levels. J Biol Chem, 1987; 262:10280–10286

295. Davis BH, Vucic A. The effect of retinol on Ito cell proliferation in vitro. Hepatology, 1988; 8:788–793

296. Denson LA, Auld KL, Schiek DS, et al. Interleukin-1 beta suppresses retin transactivation of two hepatic transporter genes involved in bile formation. J Biol Chem, 2000; 275:8835–8843

297. Lee SH, Seo GS, Park YN, et al. Effects and regulation of osteopontin in rat hepatic stellate cells. Biochem Pharmacol, 2004; 68:2367–2378

298. Muller D, Quantin B, Gesnel MC, et al. The collagenase gene family in humans consists of at least four members. Biochem J, 1988; 253:187–192

299. Matrisian LM. Metalloproteinases and their inhibitors in matrix remodelling. Trends Genet, 1990; 6:121–125

300. Gross J, Lapiere CM. Collagenolytic activity in amphibian tissues: a tissue culture assay. Proc Natl Acad Sci USA, 1962; 48:1014–1022

301. Bhatnager R, Schade U, Rietschel ET, et al. Involvement of prostaglandin E and adenosine 3'5'-monophosphate in lipopolysaccharide-stimulated collagenase release by rat Kupffer cells. Eur J Biochem, 1982; 124:2405–2409

302. Campbell EJ, Cury JD, Lazarus CJ, Welgus HG. Monocyte procollagenase and tissue inhibitor of metalloproteinases. Identification, characterisation and regulation of secretion. J Biol Chem, 1987; 262:15862–15868

303. Emonard H, Guillouzo A, Lapiere CM, Grimaud JA. Human liver fibroblast capacity for synthesising interstitial collagenase in vitro. Cell Mol Biol, 1990; 36:461–467

304. Hasty KA, Jeffrey JJ, Hibbs MS, Welgus HG. The collagen substrate specificity of human neutrophil collagenase. J Biol Chem, 1987; 262:10048–10052

305. Hibbs MS, Hasty KA, Seyer JM, et al. Biochemical and immunological characterisation of the secreted forms of human neutrophil gelatinase. J Biol Chem, 1985; 260:2493–2500

306. Hibbs MS, Hoidal R, Kang AH. Expression of a metalloproteinase that degrades native type V collagen and denatured collagens by cultured human alveolar macrophages. J Clin Invest, 1987; 80:1644–1650

307. Winwood PJ, Kowalski-Saunders P, Arthur MJP. Kupffer cells release a 95 kD metalloproteinase with degradative activity against gelatin. Gut, 1991; 32:A837–A838

308. Selzter JL, Weingarten H, Akers HT, et al. Cleavage specificity of type IV collagenase (gelatinase) from human skin. Use of synthetic peptides as model substrates. J Biol Chem, 1989; 265:19583–19586

309. Arthur MJP, Friedman SL, Roll FJ, Bissell DM. Lipocytes from normal rat liver release a neutral metalloproteinase that degrades basement membrane (type IV) collagen. J Biol Chem, 1989; 84:1076–1085

310. Arthur MJP, Stanley A, Iredale JP. Release of type IV collagenase by cultured human lipocytes: analysis of gene expression, protein synthesis and protease activity. Gastroenterology, 1991; 100:A716

311. Arthur MJP. Human hepatic lipocytes synthesise and release TIMP-1: An important inhibitor of matrix metalloproteinase activity. Hepatology, 1991; 14:183A

312. Iredale JP, Murphy G, Hembry RM, et al. Human hepatic lipocytes synthesise tissue inhibitor of metalloproteinases-1. Implications for regulation of matrix degradation in liver. J Clin Invest, 1992; 90:282–287

313. Enghild JJ, Salvesen G, Brew K, Nagase H. Interaction of human rheumatoid synovial collagenase (matrix metalloproteinase 1) and stromelysin (matrix metalloproteinase 3) with human alpha-2-macroglobulin and chicken ovostatin. J Biol Chem, 1989; 264:8779–8785

314. Andus T, Ramadori G, Heinrich PC. Cultured Ito cells of rat liver express the alpha 2-macroglobulin gene. Eur J Biochem, 1987; 168:641–646

315. Okazaki I, Maruyama K. Collagenase activity in experimental hepatic fibrosis. Nature, 1974; 252:49–50

316. Peters RL. Viral hepatitis: a pathologic spectrum. Am J Med Sci, 1975; 270:17–32

317. Tuchweber B, Desmoulière A, Bochaton-Piallat ML, Rubbia-Brandt L, Gabbiani G. Proliferation and phenotypic modulation of portal fibroblasts in the early stages of cholestatic fibrosis in the rat. Lab Invest, 1996; 74:265–278

318. Desmouliere A, Darby I, Costa AMA, Raccurt M, Tuchweber B, Sommer P, Gabbiani G. Extracellular matrix deposition, lysyl oxidase expression, and myofibroblastic differentiation during the initial stages of cholestatic fibrosis in the rat. Lab Invest, 1997; 76:765–778

319. Bhunchet E, Wake K. Role of mesenchymal cell populations in porcine serum-induced rat liver fibrosis. Hepatology, 1992; 16:1452–1473

320. Kinnman N, Francoz C, Barbu V, et al. The myofibroblast conversion of peribiliary fibrogenic cells distinct from hepatic stellate cells is stimulated by platelet-derived growth factor during liver fibrogenesis. Lab Invest, 2003; 83:163–173

321. Abdel-Aziz G, Rescan PY, Clement B, et al. Cellular sources of matrix proteins in experimentally induced cholestatic rat liver. J Pathol, 1991; 164:167–174

322. Cassiman D, Libbrecht L, Desmet V, et al. Hepatic stellate cell/myofibroblast subpopulations in fibrotic human and rat livers. J Hepatol, 2002; 36:200–209

323. Lorena D, Darby IA, Reinhardt DP, et al. Fibrillin-1 expression in normal and fibrotic rat liver and in cultured hepatic fibroblastic cells: modulation by mechanical stress and role in cell adhesion. Lab Invest, 2004; 84:203–212

324. Wells RG, Kruglov E, Dranoff JA. Autocrine release of TGF-beta by portal fibroblasts regulates cell growth. FEBS Lett, 2004; 559:107–110

325. Cassiman D, Roskams T. Beauty is in the eye of the beholder: emerging concepts and pitfalls in hepatic stellate cell research. J Hepatol, 2002; 37:527–535

326. Uchio K, Tuchweber B, Manabe N, et al. Cellular retinol-binding protein-1 expression and modulation during in vivo and in vitro myofibroblastic differentiation of rat hepatic stellate cells and portal fibroblasts. Lab Invest, 2002; 82:619–628

327. Schaffner F, Barka T, Popper H. Hepatic mesenchymal cell reaction in liver disease. Exp Mol Pathol, 1963; 31:419–441

328. Rappaport AM, McPhee PJ, Fisher MM, Phillips MJ. The scarring of the liver acini (Cirrhosis). Tridimensional and microcirculatory considerations. Virchows Arch [A], 1983; 402:107–137

329. Bonkovsky HL, Ponka P, Bacon BR, et al. An update on iron metabolism: summary of the Fifth International Conference on Disorders of Iron Metabolism. Hepatology, 1996; 24:718–729

330. Mori T, Okanoue T, Sawa Y, et al. Defenestration of the sinusoidal endothelial cell in a rat model of cirrhosis. Hepatology, 1993; 17:891–897

331. Gaiani S, Bolondi L, Li Bassi S, et al. Prevalence of spontaneous hepatofugal portal flow in liver cirrhosis. Clinical and endoscopic correlation in 228 patients. Gastroenterology, 1991; 100:160–167

332. Hou PC, McFadzean AJS. Thrombosis and intimal thickening in the portal system in cirrhosis of the liver. J Pathol Bact, 1965; 89:473–480

333. Goodman ZD, Ishak KG. Occlusive venous lesions in alcoholic liver disease. A study of 200 cases. Gastroenterology, 1982; 83:786–796

334. Nakanuma Y, Ohta G, Doishita K. Quantitation and serial section observations of focal venocclusive lesions of hepatic veins in liver cirrhosis. Virchows Arch [A], 1985; 405:429–438

335. Burt AD, MacSween RN. Hepatic vein lesions in alcoholic liver disease: retrospective biopsy and necropsy study. J Clin Pathol, 1986; 39:63–67

336. Wanless IR, Wong F, Blendis LM, et al. Hepatic and portal vein thrombosis in cirrhosis: Possible role in development of parenchymal extinction and portal hypertension. Hepatology, 1995; 21:1238–1247

337. Tanaka M, Wanless IR. Pathology of the liver in Budd–Chiari syndrome: portal vein thrombosis and the histogenesis of veno-centric cirrhosis, veno-portal cirrhosis, and large regenerative nodules. Hepatology, 1998; 27:488–496

338. Picchiotti R, Mingazzini PL, Scucchi L, et al. Correlations between sinusoidal pressure and liver morphology in cirrhosis. J Hepatol, 1994; 20:364–369

339. Syrota A, Vinot JM, Paraf A, Roucayrol JC. Scintillation splenoportography: hemodynamic and morphological study of the portal circulation. Gastroenterology, 1976; 71:652–659

340. Schmid C, Meyer H-I, Ringe B, et al. Cystic enlargement of extrahepatic bile ducts. Surgery, 1993; 114:65–70

341. Medina J, Arroyo AG, Sànchez-Madrid F, Moreno-Otero R. Angiogenesis in chronic inflammatory liver disease. Hepatology, 2004; 39:1185–1195

342. Pugh CW, Ratcliffe P. Regulation of angiogenesis by hypoxia: role of the HIF system. Nature Med, 2003; 9:677–684

343. Murohara T, Asahara T, Silver M, et al. Nitric oxide synthase modulates angiogenesis in response to tissue ischemia. J Clin Invest, 1998; 101; 2567–2578

344. Ferrara N, Gerber H, LeCouter J. The biology of VEGF and its receptors. Nature Med, 2003; 9:669–676

345. Jain RK. Molecular regulation of vessel maturation. Nature Med, 2003; 9:685–693

346. Wack KE, Ross MA, Zegarra V, et al. Sinusoidal ultrastructure evaluated during the revascularization of regenerating rat liver. Hepatology, 2001; 33:363–378

347. Ross MA, Sander CM, Kleeb TB, et al. Spatiotemporal expression of angiogenesis growth factor receptors during the revascularization of regenerating rat liver. Hepatology, 2001; 34:1135–1148

348. Garcia-Monzon C, Sànchez-Madrid F, Garcia-Buey L, et al. Vascular adhesion molecule expression in viral chronic hepatitis: evidence of neoangiogenesis in portal tracts. Gastroenterology, 1995; 108:231–241

349. Richard DE, Berra E, Pouyssegur J. Nonhypoxic pathway mediates the induction of hypoxia-inducible factor 1alpha in vascular smooth muscle cells. J Biol Chem, 2000; 275:26765–26771

350. Folkman J. Angiogenesis in cancer, vascular, rheumatoid and other disease. Nature Med, 1995; 1:27–31

351. Mazzanti R, Messerini L, Monsacchi L, et al. CVH induced by hepatitis C but not hepatitis B virus infection correlates with increased liver angiogenesis. Hepatology, 1997; 25:229–234

352. Yokoyama Y, Baveja R, Sonin N, et al. Hepatic neovascularization after partial portal vein ligation: novel mechanism of chronic regulation of blood flow. Am J Physiol, 2001; 280:G21–G31

353. Ohmori S, Shiraki K, Sugimoto K, et al. High expression of CD34-positive sinusoidal endothelial cells is a risk factor for hepatocellular carcinoma in patients with HCV-associated chronic liver diseases. Human Pathol, 2001; 32:1363–1370

354. Medina J, Garcia-Buey L, Moreno-Otero R. Review article: immunopathogenic and therapeutic aspects of autoimmune hepatitis. Aliment Pharmacol Ther, 2003; 17:1–16

355. Masyuk TV, Ritman EL, LaRusso NF. Hepatic artery and portal vein remodeling in rat liver: vascular response to selective cholangiocyte proliferation. Am J Pathol, 2003; 162:1175–1182

356. Popper H, Elias H, Petty D. Vascular pattern of the cirrhotic liver. Am J Clin Path, 1952; 22:717–729

357. Hales MR, Allan JS, Hall EM. Injection-corrosion studies of normal and cirrhotic livers. Am J Pathol, 1959; 35:909–941

358. Desmet VJ, Roskams T. Cirrhosis reversal: a duel between dogma and myth. J Hepatol, 2004; 40:860–867

359. Yamamoto T, Kobayashi T, Phillips MJ. Perinodular arteriolar plexus in liver cirrhosis. Scanning electron microscopy of microvascular casts. Liver, 1984; 4:50–54

360. Hirooka N, Iwasaki I, Horie H, Ide G. Hepatic microcirculation of liver cirrhosis studied by corrosion cast/scanning electron microscope examination. Acta Pathol Jpn, 1986; 36:375–387

361. Koo A, Liang IY, Cheng KK. Effect of the ligation of hepatic artery on the microcirculation in the cirrhotic liver in the rat. Aust J Exp Biol Med Sci, 1976; 54:287–295

362. Sokal EM, Trivedi P, Portmann B, Mowat AP. Adaptive changes of metabolic zonation during the development of cirrhosis in growing rats. Gastroenterology, 1990; 99:785–792

363. Gumucio JJ, Chianale J. Liver cell heterogeneity and liver function. In: Arias IM, Jakoby WB, Popper H, Schachter D, Shafritz DA, eds. The liver: biology and pathobiology, 2nd edn. New York: Raven Press, 1988: pp 931–947

364. Cohen PJ. Change in the distribution of succinic dehydrogenase within the rat hepatic lobule after ligation of the common bile duct. Anat Rec, 1965; 153:429–443

365. Nuber R, Teutsch HF, Sasse D. Metabolic zonation in thioacetamide-induced liver cirrhosis. Histochemistry, 1980; 69:277–288

366. Van Noorden CJ, Frederiks WM, Aronson DC, et al. Changes in the acinar distribution of some enzymes involved in carbohydrate metabolism in rat liver parenchyma after experimentally induced cholestasis. Virchows Arch B Cell Pathol, 1987; 52:501–511

367. Sokal EM, Mostin J, Buts JP. Liver metabolic zonation in rat biliary cirrhosis: Distribution is reverse of that in toxic cirrhosis. Hepatology, 1992; 15:904–908

368. Gebhardt R, Reichen J. Changes in distribution and activity of glutamine synthetase in carbon tetrachloride-induced cirrhosis in the rat: potential role in hyperammonemia. Hepatology, 1994; 20:684–691

369. Sokal EM, Trivedi P, Portmann B, Mowat A. Changes in acinar distribution of microsomal and mitochondrial enzyme activities in cirrhotic livers from infants with biliary atresia (abstract). 23rd meeting of the European Association for the Study of the Liver. J Hepatol, 1988; 7

370. Sokal EM, Collette E, Buts JP. Persistence of a liver metabolic zonation in extra-hepatic biliary atresia cirrhotic livers. Pediatr Res, 1991; 30:286–289

371. Racine-Samson L, Scoazec JY, D'Errico A, et al. The metabolic organization of the adult human liver: A comparative study of normal, fibrotic, and cirrhotic liver tissue. Hepatology, 1996; 24:104–113

372. Wood AJ, Villeneuve JP, Branch RA, Rogers LW, Shand DG. Intact hepatocyte theory of impaired drug metabolism in experimental cirrhosis in the rat. Gastroenterology, 1979; 76:1358–1362

373. Jungermann K, Katz N. Functional specialization of different hepatocyte populations. Physiol Rev, 1989; 69:708–764

374. Gumucio JJ. Hepatocyte heterogeneity: the coming of age from the description of a biological curiosity to a partial understanding of its physiological meaning and regulation. Hepatology, 1989; 9:154–160

375. Gumucio JJ, Bilir BM, Moseley RH, et al. The biology of the liver cell plate. In: Arias IM, Boyer JL, Fausto N, et al., eds. The liver: biology and pathobiology, 3rd edn. New York: Raven Press, 1994: p. 1143

376. Crawford JM. Cirrhosis. In: MacSween RNM, Anthony PP, Scheuer PJ, Burt AD, Portmann BC, eds. Pathology of the liver, 4th edn. Philadelphia, PA: WB Saunders, 2002, pp 575–619

377. Crawford AR, Lin X-Z, Crawford JM. The adult human liver biopsy: a quantitative reference standard. Hepatology, 1998; 28:323–331

378. Wanless IR, Nakashima E, Sherman M. Regression of human cirrhosis: morphologic features and the genesis of incomplete septal cirrhosis. Arch Pathol Lab Med, 2000; 124:1599–1607

379. Wanless IR, Shimamatsu K. Phlebitis in viral and autoimmune chronic hepatitis and primary biliary cirrhosis. Possible role in the histogenesis of cirrhosis. Mod Pathol, 1997; 10:147A

380. Williams R, Smith P, Spicer E, et al. Venesection therapy in idiopathic haemochromatosis. Q J Med, 1969; 38:1–16

381. Bunton GL, Cameron GR. Regeneration of liver after biliary cirrhosis. Ann NY Acad Sci, 1963; 111:412–421

382. Yeong ML, Nicholson GI, Lee SP. Regression of biliary cirrhosis following choledochal cyst drainage. Gastroenterology, 1982; 82:332–335

383. Powell LW, Kerr JF. Reversal of 'cirrhosis' in idiopathic haemochromatosis following long-term intensive venesection therapy. Aust Ann Med, 1970; 19:54–57

384. Blumberg RS, Chopra S, Ibrahim R, et al. Primary hepatocellular carcinoma in idiopathic hemochromatosis after reversal of cirrhosis. Gastroenterology, 1988; 95:1399–1402

385. Dufour JF, DeLellis R, Kaplan MM. Reversibility of hepatic fibrosis in autoimmune hepatitis. Ann Intern Med, 1997; 127:981–985

386. Falkmer S, Samuelson G, Sjolin S. Penicillamine-induced normalization of clinical signs, and liver morphology and histochemistry in a case of Wilson's disease. Pediatrics, 1970; 45:260–268

387. Kaplan MM, DeLellis RA, Wolfe HJ. Sustained biochemical and histologic remission of primary biliary cirrhosis in response to medical treatment. Ann Intern Med, 1997; 126:682–688

388. Dunn MA, Cheever AW, Paglia LM, et al. Reversal of advanced liver fibrosis in rabbits with Schistosomiasis japonica. Am J Trop Med Hyg, 1994; 50:499–505

389. Greenwel P, Geerts A, Ogata I, et al. Liver fibrosis. In: Arias I, Boyer J, Fausto N, et al., eds. The liver: biology and pathobiology, 3rd edn. New York: Raven; 1994, pp 1367–1381

390. Arthur MJ. Reversibility of liver fibrosis and cirrhosis following treatment for hepatitis C. Gastroenterology, 2002; 122:1525–1528

391. Issa R, et al. Spontaneous recovery from micronodular cirrhosis: evidence for incomplete resolution associated with matrix cross-linking. Gastroenterology, 2004; 126:1795–1808

392. Wanless IR, Godwin TA, Allen F, Feder A. Nodular regenerative hyperplasia of the liver in hematologic disorders: A possible response to obliterative portal venopathy. Medicine, 1980; 59:367–379

393. Barnett JL, Appelman HD, Moseley RH. A familial form of incomplete septal cirrhosis. Gastroenterology, 1992; 102:674–678

394. Sciot R, Staessen D, Van Damme B, et al. Incomplete septal cirrhosis: Histopathological aspects. Histopathology, 1988; 13:593–603

395. Wanless IR, Lentz JS, Roberts EA. Partial nodular transformation of liver in an adult with persistent ductus venosus. Arch Pathol Lab Med, 1985; 109:427–432

396. Wanless IR, Mawdsley C, Adams R. On the pathogenesis of focal nodular hyperplasia of the liver. Hepatology, 1985; 5:1194–1200

Cellular and molecular diagnostic techniques

3

Stephen A. Geller   Martha B. Pitman   W. Stephen Nichols

The pioneering work on liver anatomy and pathology was carried out by Vesalius (1514–1564), Fabricius (1537–1619), Harvey (1578–1657), Glisson (1598–1677) and, especially, Malpighi (1628–1694). Malpighi established a firm foundation for our studies of the structure of the liver with the use of a primitive microscope. He recognized the liver lobule, although he was not able to identify individual hepatocytes. Malpighi also identified the liver as the source of bile and suggested, from a series of injection studies, that a sinusoidal network connected portal and hepatic venous systems.[1]

In the 19th century many scientists contributed to our knowledge of the liver. Ehrlich, in 1884, and Lucatello, in 1885, both performed 'puncture' of the liver through laparoscopes for a variety of reasons.[1] Histopathology studies were still in their infancy and tissues were mostly obtained for chemical, rather than morphologic, studies. Ehrlich and others also performed needle puncture of the liver during the latter part of the 19th century and the first third of the 20th century for drainage of hepatic abscesses and hydatid cysts.[2]

In 1938 the Vim–Silverman needle was introduced.[3] Following this, major advances were made in the study of both the pathology and the pathophysiology of the liver. In 1958 the technique of liver biopsy was further refined with the introduction of the Menghini needle,[4] which allowed for the recovery of a core of liver tissue with relatively little artifact. The Menghini needle helped to dramatically expand the use of biopsy, both because it was safer and easier to use than the Vim–Silverman needle and also because it provided tissue of sufficient quality to support sophisticated light microscopic, histochemical, ultrastructural, and immunohistochemical studies. Newer core needle biopsy devices, such as the Tru-Cut biopsy and biopsy guns, have refined the technique.[5] Recent efforts to coat the needles with synthetic materials may contribute to better quality histology with reduced artifact.[6]

The ability to safely and consistently biopsy the liver led to an explosion of our understanding of liver disease, with more information accrued in the years after the Second World War than in all preceding years. In the mid-20th century Popper and co-workers developed the concept of organelle pathology of the liver, based on correlations of clinical observations and light microscopic findings with electron microscopic studies of liver ultrastructure.[7] Seminal studies of the morphological basis of normal liver function followed, as did a greater understanding of the pathophysiology of the hepatocyte, cholangiocyte and other structures of the liver.

In the 1920s Martin and Ellis, at the Memorial Hospital in New York, developed the technique of aspiration cytology.[8] However, this was rarely applied to the study of liver disease, as the core biopsy was preferred in most diagnostic studies. In later years, following the work of Lundquist,[9] who had shown a favourable correlation between cytologic and histologic preparations, there was increasing use of aspiration cytology particularly to study mass lesions. Today, fine needle aspiration biopsy is a well-accepted, safe, easy and accurate diagnostic modality for the evaluation of mass lesions of the liver.

In the last two decades, immunohistochemical approaches have allowed for the identification of specific cellular components, normal and abnormal, including nuclear, cytoplasmic and cell membrane substances. Immunohistochemistry has refined the ability of the pathologist to identify specific pathogens (e.g. hepatitis B core and surface antigens, delta agent, cytomegalovirus, Epstein–Barr virus, adenovirus and many others), normal and abnormal structural components (e.g. various cytokeratins, Mallory bodies and many others), to differentiate primary from metastatic malignant tumours (e.g. antibody directed against polyclonal carcinoembryonic antigen to identify canalicular structures in hepatocellular carcinoma, HMB45 antibody to recognize angiomyolipoma, various vascular markers in epithelioid haemangioendothelioma) and prognostic markers (e.g. hormone receptors and her2/neu in metastatic breast carcinoma, epidermal growth factor receptor in metastatic colon carcinoma).

At the beginning of the 21st century, the techniques of molecular pathology, including polymerase chair reaction (PCR), in situ hybridization, gene array studies, proteomics, and other novel approaches are further revolutionizing our understanding of liver diseases. Time-honoured approaches to the study of the patient with liver disease, including clinical studies, laboratory tests and morphologic observations, are being restudied in the light of newly obtained molecular data.

For most disorders of the liver, percutaneous liver biopsy can yield a satisfactory specimen.[10] Generally, the histopathologist would like to have a specimen at least 2 cm long.[10-14] Ultrasound guidance can be particularly useful in approaching small lesions,[15-18] but can also be of value in obtaining samples in patients with diffuse disease.[19] Laparoscopic biopsy is useful for specific lesions that cannot easily be sampled via the percutaneous route. It is also practical to obtain specimens via the jugular vein passing a venous catheter through the right atrium and inferior vena cava into the hepatic vein.[20,21] Trans-jugular biopsy is particularly useful when the patient has a bleeding diathesis[22,23] or has marked ascites. At first, transjugular biopsies yielded only liver fragments obtained with biopsy forceps, but the technique was refined to allow for the recovery of satisfactory liver cores.[24-26]

Types of biopsy

Liver biopsy samples can be obtained percutaneously as a core with a biopsy needle, as a wedge or a core either during open laparotomy or with the laparoscope, with or without imaging techniques for guidance,[15,16,19,27] or as a core obtained via the jugular vein.[23,27] Alternatively, a fine needle can be used to aspirate clusters of hepatocytes.[5,17,25,26,28-32] Each of these methods has potential limitations and, in order to avoid an unnecessary procedure and/or the preparation of a sample that can not provide the necessary answer, the goal of the biopsy should be determined before deciding upon the method.[33,34] A combination of methods can also be used. The procedure that is followed at our institutions for the diagnosis of mass lesions is to follow a fine needle aspiration biopsy with a percutaneous core needle biopsy. The most common indications for liver biopsy are summarized in Table 3.1.

Newer chemical test panels may eventually allow for evaluation of the degree of fibrosis present in the liver ('stage') without biopsy,[36-45] but refinements and worldwide confirmation of reliability, with clear determination

Table 3.1	Indications for liver biopsy[33-35]

- Abnormal liver function tests
- Fever of unknown origin
- Recognition of systemic disorders
- Evaluation of cholestatic disorders
- Evaluation (diagnosis, grading and staging) of chronic liver disease
  a. Evaluation of the efficacy of therapies for liver disease
- Post-transplant evaluation
- Evaluation of type and extent of liver injury caused by therapeutic drugs
- Diagnosis of space-occupying lesions
- Diagnosis of uninvolved liver in tumour cases to determine feasibility for resection or transplantation
- Patients undergoing bariatric surgery for obesity
- Evaluation of potential living-related donor for transplantation
- Unexplained hepatomegaly and/or mild hepatic dysfunction

of the sensitivity and specificity of biochemical methods, are required before the biopsy is no longer needed for this purpose.[14,46-49] The recognition of the deleterious effects of steatosis in terms of the progression of HCV to cirrhosis has prompted renewed and increased interest in liver biopsy evaluation in HCV patients.[50] Liver biopsy also remains integral in evaluating patients being treated for hepatitis, including hepatitis C (HCV) and hepatitis B (HBV).[51,52]

Clearly, a logical and appropriate goal in hepatology would be to develop non-invasive tests for all liver disorders that would preclude the need for liver biopsy in many cases and thereby reduce the already very low incidence of complications.[10] Although this goal may be reached in the near future in terms of determining the stage in the chronic hepatitides, particularly hepatitis C,[53-55] the liver biopsy will continue to be an indispensable technique in the armamentarium of the hepatologist as liver disease remains a significant world-wide problem.[56]

Liver biopsy is widely used in the evaluation of the patient who has undergone liver transplantation, both in the immediate post-transplant period and later, in identifying acute and chronic rejection, in documenting de novo disease such as post-transplant autoimmune hepatitis in the patient who did not have prior autoimmune hepatitis,[57-59] and in the evaluation of recurrent disease and its differentiation from chronic and acute rejection[60-66] (see Chapter 16).

With increased understanding of the causes and effects of non-alcoholic fatty diseases of the liver (NAFLD), including non-alcoholic steatohepatitis (NASH), liver biopsy has been shown to be invaluable in assessing the degree of steatosis and, more importantly, evidence of liver injury, including hepatocyte necrosis, steatohepatitis and fibrosis.[7-75] It has been well demonstrated that clinical and biochemical data in morbidly obese patients cannot reliably identify those with severe chronic liver disease without liver biopsy.[73]

The effects of potentially hepatotoxic medications similarly can not be completely assessed without liver biopsy.[6-82] As an example, patients with inflammatory bowel disease who were treated with 6-thioguanine developed nodularity and ultrastructural evidence of fibrosis, despite the fact that some of them had no clinical or biochemical evidence of liver disease.[8]

It is becoming increasingly obvious that patients with hepatitis C virus who are co-infected with human immunodeficiency virus (HIV) and who have been treated with highly active antiretroviral therapy (HAART) have a faster progression of their chronic liver disease.[3-90] Furthermore, patients who have demonstrated control of their HIV with HAART are now being accepted for liver transplantation.[91] Severity of disease appears to be related to HCV genotype, with more severe disease in patients with genotype 1.[2,93] Liver biopsies in this group of patients offer new challenges, both because of the nature of the two underlying diseases and also because of the changes potentially induced by ongoing HAART.[94,95]

Liver tissue samples will certainly continue to be invaluable for the further understanding of liver biology and the varied reactions of the liver to injury.[96-101] Increasingly, individuals being considered as potential living donors are biopsied to exclude subclinical abnormalities that could potentially affect graft survival.[102]

The *percutaneous core needle biopsy* technique has proven to be the most useful method for obtaining liver tissue representative of diffuse liver disease as well as for sampling space-occupying lesions when they can be safely approached, and has been the standard for almost 60 years.[103] When combined with a preceding fine needle aspiration biopsy the accuracy in diagnosing focal mass lesions is significantly greater than that obtained with either method alone.[104-108]

The percutaneous core needle biopsy will not provide the sought-after answer in all cases. Although the liver tends to react uniformly to a range of injuries and stimuli, it must be remembered that 'sampling error' can occur in a variety of hepatic disorders.[10,14,109] As an example, the changes of primary sclerosing cholangitis are not uniformly seen throughout the liver and indeed may not be present at all. Two or more biopsies may be required before a portal tract with characteristic bile duct injury and/or periductal concentric fibrosis is identified. Obvious and severe changes of primary sclerosing cholangitis can easily be recognized in imaging studies of the extrahepatic bile ducts, while a series of liver biopsies may fail to demonstrate typical histologic changes. Similarly, characteristic inclusions of cytomegalovirus, in either the post-transplant patient or the AIDS patient, may not be seen in every section of liver prepared. It may be necessary to cut a number of serial sections before the typical structures are identified or to use a more sensitive technique, such as immunocytochemistry or DNA in situ hybridization. Tumour nodules, either deep or superficial, can be missed by the relatively 'blind' percutaneous technique, even when performed with the aid of imaging techniques.

Even in the setting of diffuse disease, the percutaneous needle biopsy sample can sometimes prove insufficient. There are considerable differences in the samples obtained with biopsy needles, since the needles themselves differ in many respects. Biopsy needles vary in terms of the length of the sample obtained, its diameter, and the degree of compression artifact.[5] There are further differences that occur with various pathologic changes of the liver. For example, smaller biopsy needles may not obtain sufficient numbers of portal tracts to evaluate the immune-mediated biliary disorders appropriately or even to grade and stage the chronic hepatitides.[11,14,38] In cirrhosis, a biopsy needle with a small calibre may not obtain any septal structures and may only yield fragments of parenchyma, contributing to difficulty in establishing the correct diagnosis. The Klatskin needle, a variant of the Menghini needle, has been in use for decades and provides an excellent sample in most cases in which percutaneous needle biopsy is indicated. In experienced hands the larger gauge core biopsy needles are not associated with a significant increase in morbidity or mortality.[5,110-112] The most common complications are pain and haemorrhage. The haemorrhage can be intraperitoneal, subcapsular, or intrahepatic and, if intrahepatic, can lead to haemobilia. There is minimal risk of haematogenous dissemination of malignant cells after liver biopsy.[113] Another reported complication in patients with hepatocellular carcinoma is 'seeding' of the biopsy tract, but this is also uncommon.[18,114-117] However, reports have indicated a higher needle tract seeding rate in patients with metastatic colorectal carcinoma (up to 10% in a combination of series evaluating needle track seeding),[118] and investigators have questioned the clinical utility of biopsy documentation of clinically suspicious hepatic metastases as a result of this risk.

Intraoperative biopsies are being obtained more often because of the recent development of laparoscopic (bariatric) surgical techniques for obesity and have been shown to be useful for determining the degree of steatosis and detecting hepatic injury such as steatohepatitis and fibrosis.[67,73,74] In the intraoperative setting the *wedge biopsy* is generally useful for a focal lesion presenting at or immediately below the capsule.[119] In our experience wedge biopsy obtained by the surgeon at the time of an operation performed for another reason, in the absence of a grossly recognizable lesion, and prompted by what the surgeon perceives to be an abnormal appearing liver, is often disappointing. If a primary, generalized liver disorder, such as non-alcoholic steatohepatitis (NASH) or chronic hepatitis C, is suspected, a needle biopsy, rather than a wedge biopsy, should be performed to provide a more representative liver sample.

The interpretation of a wedge biopsy can be erroneous when the capsule is thickened and relatively little diagnostically useful parenchyma is obtained and/or capsule fibrosis extends into the liver mimicking cirrhosis.[120] The same artifact can be found in core needle biopsy samples if the biopsy needle enters the liver at an angle close to that of the capsule (Fig. 3.1). Capsular fibrous tissue can be quite prominent in needle core biopsies. This error can be avoided if the criteria for cirrhosis are adhered to and the presence of elastic-rich vascularized septa and regenerative liver plates is confirmed.

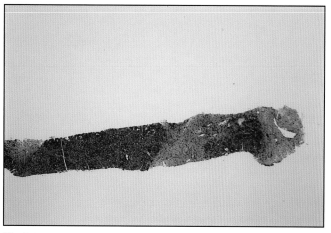

Fig. 3.1 • Capsular fibrous tissue in a core needle liver biopsy sample mimicking the pattern of cirrhosis. H&E.

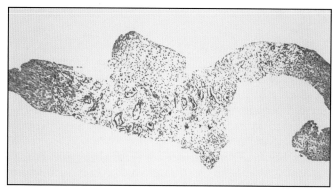

Fig. 3.3 • Bile-duct hamartoma submitted for immediate intraoperative evaluation ('frozen section') showing irregularly branching gland structures with rounded contours in a loosely fibrotic stroma. H&E.

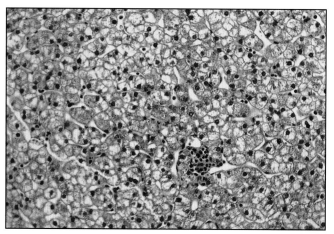

Fig. 3.2 • Clusters of acute inflammatory cells in a liver biopsy obtained immediately before the end of an open abdominal surgical procedure ('surgical hepatitis'). H&E.

Clusters of chronic inflammatory cells in portal areas immediately below the capsule can be misinterpreted as evidence of chronic hepatitis. Finally, clusters of acute inflammatory cells can be seen in the intraoperatively obtained liver biopsy as a non-specific consequence of the laparotomy procedure itself ('surgical hepatitis') (Fig. 3.2).

Bile-duct hamartomas are relatively common and may attract the attention of the surgeon who will biopsy it suspecting a metastasis; this lesion can then be misinterpreted as metastatic carcinoma by the unwary histopathologist. The key to the histological recognition of this lesion is to appreciate the organized, lobular arrangement of the typically rounded (not angulated) glands in a loose fibrotic rather than sclerotic stroma (Fig. 3.3). When bile-duct hamartoma is encountered on fine needle aspiration biopsy, smears contain a disproportionate number of benign-appearing bile-duct epithelial groups relative to the few benign and reactive hepatocytes that usually dominate smears obtained from primary hepatocytic lesions. The unwary pathologist might also misinterpret such a biopsy as metastatic adenocarcinoma.

The principal indication for *laparoscopic biopsy* is to diagnose a focal lesion not easily sampled, because of either location or size, with standard percutaneous liver biopsy or with ultrasound or computed tomography (CT)-guided aspiration. Using the laparoscope, lesions of the left lobe, the dome of both lobes, the undersurface of the liver, and the caudate and quadrate lobes can be biopsied. The samples from relatively difficult-to-reach parts of the liver are often quite small and obtained with a biopsy forceps. Sometimes the sample size, as well as crush artifact (which virtually always occurs to some degree) can make interpretation difficult, and multiple biopsies of a given lesion should be obtained if possible. This is especially true if an unusual diagnosis is suspected in order to provide sufficient material for special studies, such as immunohistochemical markers in the case of lymphoma. The caveats already raised about wedge biopsy clearly hold true for laparoscopic biopsy and are even more pertinent since the usual forceps biopsy obtained with laparoscopic guidance is smaller than the usual wedge taken during laparotomy. Laparoscopic guidance can be combined with a core needle biopsy technique; these samples are usually excellent.

Transjugular biopsy is generally employed for patients with generalized liver disease who have marked ascites, severe thrombocytopenia or another coagulation disorder.[22,23,121] A catheter is passed to the liver via the jugular vein and superior vena cava. A biopsy forceps or core biopsy needle is then inserted into the liver. Less commonly, transjugular biopsy is resorted to for patients with severe cholestasis thought to be due to obstruction about whom there is a concern about the possible development of biliary peritonitis. Transjugular biopsy can also be used for patients in whom there is an infectious peritonitis.

Fine needle aspiration biopsy can be the safest, most efficacious, accurate, and cost-effective means to establish the correct diagnosis in cases of a space-occupying lesion.[15,26,28,29,31,32,122–126] When fine needle aspiration biopsy provides an early diagnosis, the total number of procedures, especially invasive tests, may be reduced, with a decrease in the length of hospital stay.[127] Indeed, the procedure is often performed on an outpatient basis. Pre-biopsy assessment of patients undergoing fine needle aspiration biopsy includes, as for all liver biopsy patients, evaluation of the coagulation system to prevent untoward bleeding. In addition, there is a pre-procedure analysis to determine the optimal imaging modality, the size and location of the lesion(s), and the degree of tumour vascularity. Body habitus and specific patient requirements must be considered. Finally, and importantly, the procedure itself is discussed with the patient, with a clear explanation of the degree of pain to be expected and the likely outcome of the procedure. Reducing patient anxiety, and thereby obtaining full patient co-operation, increases the likelihood of success.[127]

Fine needle aspirations are mostly percutaneous and generally utilize imaging techniques, primarily ultrasound and computed tomography, for localization. Endoscopic ultrasound guided fine needle aspiration biopsies are also employed, particularly for lesions in the left lobe of the liver with the needle easily traversing the stomach wall.[128-131] Among the factors influencing the choice of the guidance system are the size and location of the lesion, as well as the experience and preferences of the operator.[28] Ultrasound provides for rapid localization, flexible patient positioning, and variable imaging of the lesion, and is performed without radiation. Ultrasound is generally used for initial guidance, particularly with multiple and/or large, relatively superficial lesions. Computed tomography, however, has a number of advantages for aspiration biopsy. It allows for optimal resolution of smaller lesions or lesions not visible with ultrasound, for accurate localization of the needle tip immediately prior to sampling, and for improved definition of tissue components and vascularity. There is no transmission of potential imaging impediments such as drains, bone and gas. It also more precisely demonstrates the anatomical relationships of a given lesion.

Multiple biopsies can generally be performed with minimal morbidity. Fine needle aspiration techniques include individual puncture, coaxial biopsy, and tandem needle biopsy.[28] Individual puncture is used with real-time ultrasound only and requires considerable experience and skill. Coaxial biopsy allows for precise needle placement using a stiff cannula for guidance and can be performed

with either ultrasound or computed tomography. Both ultrasound and computed tomography can also be used for the tandem needle biopsy technique; a reference needle serves as a guide for the biopsy needle, making multiple aspirations possible without repeat imaging.[131,132]

In institutions with considerable experience, the sensitivity of fine needle aspiration biopsy is as high as 93% with specificity approaching 100%.[29,106,107,133-136] As with any other form of biopsy, sampling error can occur. This is most often due to inexact needle localization, sometimes reflecting the fact that the sought after lesion is less than 1 cm or, in larger lesions, that there are large areas of necrosis, fibrosis, or a prominent inflammatory rim. For these reasons, the concomitant use of fine needle aspiration biopsy and core biopsy improves accuracy, specificity, and sensitivity.[104-105]

Complications of fine needle aspiration biopsy are uncommon. There may be bleeding, particularly in the case of vascular lesions. This is often dependent on the size of the needle used. The incidence of seeding of the biopsy tract with tumour has been reported to be 0.003% if a small (<23 gauge), non-cutting needle is used.[18,115] With larger needles, especially the Vim–Silverman or other core biopsy needles, seeding may be more common.[137-139] Mortality from fine needle aspiration biopsy is exceedingly uncommon,[140-143] but fatal carcinoid crisis has occurred after biopsy of a metastatic neuroendocrine tumour.[144]

Care and handling of liver biopsy specimens

Tissue biopsy

It can be useful, particularly if a tumour is suspected, to prepare a touch preparation from a tissue biopsy by touching the core or wedge onto a glass slide (Fig. 3.4); the diagnosis can be immediately provided in this way.[145] Despite

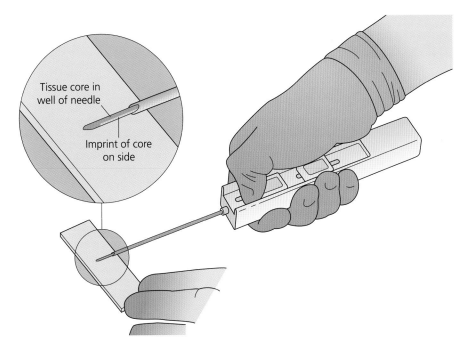

Tissue core in well of needle

Imprint of core on side

Fig. 3.4 • Schematic diagram illustrating technique of core biopsy touch preparation. Redrawn from Hahn et al.[145] with permission from American Journal of Roentology.

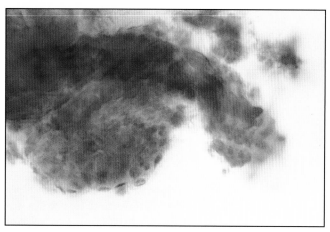

Fig. 3.5 • Hepatocellular carcinoma seen in a touch preparation made from a core needle biopsy. Despite air-drying artifact, the thickened trabeculum and rounded nest with peripherally wrapping endothelium are apparent. H&E.

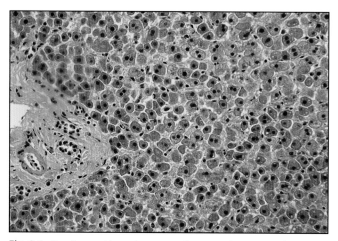

Fig. 3.6 • Needle core biopsy from a post-liver transplant patient showing artifactual discohesion of cells. The specimen was placed in saline solution for approximately 15 minutes before reaching the surgical pathology laboratory. H&E.

the presence of thick, three-dimensional tissue fragments and some air-drying artifact due to the time delay inherent in preparing the slide, architectural clues may be readily apparent and particularly useful (Fig. 3.5).

The way in which the fresh biopsy tissue is handled is important. Biopsy samples should not be placed on dry gauze, which tends to dehydrate cells and make nuclei artifactually prominent. Immersion of biopsies in saline will lead to discohesion of cells (Fig. 3.6). Prompt fixation of liver cores is necessary for high quality histopathology preparations.

In addition to assuring prompt fixation, thought should be given to the goals of the biopsy and the clinician should be consulted. In this way, all studies necessary to arrive at the diagnosis can be performed without the need for a second biopsy solely for the purpose of obtaining appropriately prepared tissue.[34]

In general, the histopathologist decides on the fixative with which he/she is most comfortable. In most laboratories, including our own, the most widely used fixative is 10% neutral buffered formalin. Formalin has many advantages: it is exceedingly stable, it penetrates and adequately

fixes tissues well, and it is inexpensive. Furthermore, formalin allows for the subsequent application of most histochemical, immunohistochemical, and molecular biological procedures. In addition, the characteristics of tissues fixed in formalin are well known and the cytologic alterations subsequent to fixation are familiar. The principal disadvantage of formalin is the relative lack of cytologic detail when compared to some other fixatives. This deficiency is obviated when the core biopsy is accompanied by a touch preparation or fine needle aspiration biopsy. Although RNA can be recovered from formalin-fixed tissue,[146] an alcohol-based fixative is better.[147,148] The usual cytology fixatives contain alcohol and generally do well when RNA recovery is needed.[149]

A core needle biopsy requires at least 2–3 hours of fixation, although microwave processing can be used to reduce this. The wedge biopsy will require fixation for as long as 12 hours unless it is sectioned into 1–2 mm thick portions, in which case satisfactory fixation can be obtained with shorter periods of time. Owing to concern about possible toxic effects of formalin, a variety of other fixatives have been recommended in recent years, but, in settings of adequate ventilation, significant toxicity from formalin has not been documented.

In cases where glycogen storage disease is suspected, the ideal fixative is alcohol. A special fixative for haematopoietic disease that permits optimal cytologic detail in tissue sections, including of lymphomas, should be selected; AZF has replaced B-5 fixative as the most useful fixative for this purpose. In addition, in suspected lymphoma cases, some tissue should also be fixed in neutral buffered formalin, since this provides optimal results for special analyses, such as DNA in situ hybridization and flow cytometry.[150] For some indications, such as the identification of the characteristic lesions of inborn metabolic disorders, tissue should be saved in glutaraldehyde for electron microscopy (EM). It may be particularly important when biopsying children and young adults to fix tissue for possible ultrastructural studies.

There are situations when small portions of tissue should be saved as snap-frozen material and embedded in OCT embedding compound for immunofluorescence analysis. In order to demonstrate the presence of lipids, fresh frozen material may be needed. For example, the microvesicular fat seen in Reye syndrome or acute fatty liver of pregnancy is best seen with a fat stain, such as oil red O or Sudan IV (Fig. 3.7(A)). Alternatively, tissue that has been in formalin, but that has not yet been immersed in lipid solvents, can be post-fixed with osmium tetroxide ('osmic acid') to demonstrate fat droplets (Fig. 3.7(B)).

The hepatologist or surgeon obtaining the biopsy sample should be encouraged to ask questions prior to immersion of the tissue in fixative:[33–35,151]

Do I suspect a lymphoma? If so, I may want to use AZF or some other fixative most useful for the study of haematologic disorders. In these cases it may also be useful to freeze tissues for immunohistochemical study of lymphocyte markers.

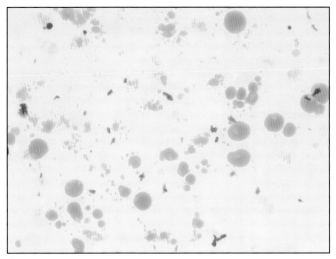

A

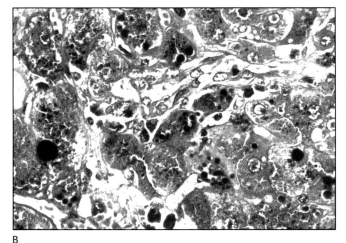

B

Fig. 3.7 • (A) Microvesicular steatosis in a core liver biopsy from a patient with fatty liver of pregnancy, taken three days after caesarean section delivery. Oil red O. **(B)** Microvesicular steatosis in a liver explant from a patient with eclampsia-associated acute hepatic failure, post-fixed with osmic acid and counter-stained with haematoxylin.

Do I suspect Wilson disease? If so, I may want to prepare tissue for electron microscopy. It was once the standard practice to obtain fresh tissue for metal assay purposes from patients suspected of having Wilson disease or genetic haemochromatosis. It has been shown, however, that formalin-fixed, paraffin-embedded tissue is reliable for chemical study in both disorders.[152,153]

Do I suspect a bacterial, fungal or viral disorder? I may want to submit a small portion of tissue for microbiological studies.

Do I want to confirm the presence of hepatitis C/Epstein–Barr virus/other viruses? I may want to save fresh tissue or use formalin-fixed tissue for polymerase chain reaction. *Do I suspect a metabolic disorder? And which metabolic disorder?* I may want to use more than one type of fixative, fresh-freeze some tissue for specialized histochemical studies and also fix tissue in glutaraldehyde for electron microscopy. *Do I suspect a neoplasm?* I may want to prepare a 'touch-preparation' of the specimen for cytologic studies. *What*

kind of neoplasm? Do I need specialized histochemistry? Do I need electron microscopy?

Do I need to talk to the pathologist before I perform the biopsy? The correct answer to this question is often 'yes!'

Fine needle aspiration biopsy

Fine needle aspiration specimens must also be handled properly and promptly. It is desirable to obtain both smears and cell block preparations in all fine needle aspirations. The presence of the cytopathologist at the time of biopsy increases the overall accuracy of the procedure.[135,154–156] This is the optimal time to determine the adequacy of the sample and to decide if special studies, such as flow cytometry and electron microscopy, are needed.

Smears are made from the aspiration part of the biopsy using a small needle tip (22 gauge or higher; 0.7 mm outside diameter). This provides for the immediate evaluation of the specimen to determine adequacy of the sample and may also be diagnostic. A touch preparation from a core biopsy sample serves a similar purpose (Fig. 3.4).

The preparation of a smear requires considerable skill, and is best done by the cytopathologist or cytotechnologist. A wonderfully cellular specimen is useless if it is crushed or, for Papanicolaou staining, air-dried. If a cytopathologist or cytotechnologist cannot be present at the time of aspiration, the radiologist should be taught how to make good-quality smears or cell-rich solutions for the preparation of cytospins, thin-layer preparations and cell blocks.

Smears can be fixed or air-dried. If fixation is the method of choice it must be done immediately after preparing the smear in order to avoid air-drying artifact. In our judgment, fixation is preferred and we use acetic alcohol (5% glacial acetic acid and 95% ethyl alcohol). Air-dried preparations are stained using a Romanowsky method. However, nuclear detail is optimal in rapidly fixed samples.

Papanicolaou is the standard stain for alcohol-fixed material. A number of rapid stains, including modifications of the Papanicolaou method,[157] modifications of haematoxylin-eosin (H&E), and Romanowsky stains such as Diff-Quik® (Baxter Diagnostics, Inc., West Sacramento, CA) or Hema III® (Fisher Scientific, Pittsburgh, PA), are also available for rapid staining of a smear or touch preparation for immediate assessment.

A full range of ancillary studies, including special stains, immunocytochemistry, flow cytometry, image analysis, electron microscopy, and molecular studies can all be performed on aspirated material.

Clotted cell blocks ('buttons') are made from needle rinsings and from any tissue fragments or core biopsies. Sometimes the most useful portion of the aspirate is in the hub of the needle and the needle should always be flushed after each aspirate smear preparation. If a clot forms spontaneously in the needle hub where it joins the syringe, it can be recovered by mechanically scraping it free with either a new needle or an orangewood stick. Clotted cell-rich material is then handled as a routine tissue biopsy with formalin fixation, paraffin embedding and sectioning.[28] Delay in fixation should be avoided to prevent artifactual changes to tissue fragments sitting in saline for too long and also to protect against incomplete recovery of the specimen.

Microbiology sampling

Many microorganisms, including bacteria, fungi, parasites and viruses, can infect the liver (see Chapter 9), and the resultant disease states can be exceedingly complex. Specific aetiologic agents may not always be identified clinically. Whenever liver samples are obtained from a patient in whom the possibility of an infectious agent exists, fresh tissue should be submitted for microbiologic analysis. Tissue can also be submitted for identification using polymerase chain reaction and other molecular approaches.[158]

Molecular pathology sampling

Formalin fixation is satisfactory for DNA studies, including approaches such as determination of loss of heterozygosity (LOH) in tumour tissue. Ethanol (80%) fixation allows for excellent RNA recovery, including after embedding in paraffin, although formalin-fixed tissue is often used for the study of short-fragment (approximately 120 base pairs) mRNA by preparing complementary DNA (cDNA).[159] Fresh, or fresh-frozen, tissue is advisable for protein analyses (proteomics), as well as for some RNA-based determinations.

Common histologic artifacts

Tissue preparation artifacts, particularly in the sectioning of paraffin blocks, are unfortunately common. Staining variability is similarly common. Increasing use of automation for processing prior to sectioning as well as for staining, including common histochemical stains (e.g. trichrome, reticulin, iron, PAS and diastase PAS) and immunohistochemical stains, will allow for more consistency. The tissue sectioning artifacts (e.g. thick sections, folding, chatter) may, however, be more problematic, because of the decreasing numbers of skilled histotechnologists. As one example of the importance of sectioning, quality trichrome stains are not easily obtained if the sections are greater than 5 microns thick.

Squeezing artifacts are seen with some needles (e.g. Vim–Silverman type), as well as with biopsy forceps, sometimes preventing interpretation. Some cellular distortion may be preventable with the use of specially coated biopsy needles.[6] Immersion of tissue for as short a time as 5 minutes in saline solution leads to tissue dissolution (see Fig. 3.6).

General approach to the liver biopsy

A systematic approach to the evaluation of the liver biopsy is vital in order to assure that important diagnostic findings are not overlooked (Table 3.2). Specific histopathological features are generally well recognized, but it is often the topographic and biologic relationships of the morphological changes that contribute to establishing the correct and clinically meaningful diagnosis.

Table 3.2	A method for examination of the liver biopsy

1. Scan entire biopsy at low magnification: assess architecture

2. Portal tracts
   a. portal vein(s)
   b. hepatic artery(ies)
   c. bile duct(s)
   d. mesenchymal structures
   e. lymphatics
   f. nerves (larger portal tracts only)

3. Limiting plate

4. Zone 1 (periportal) hepatocytes

5. Liver plates, sinusoids, sinusoidal cells

6. Zone 3 (pericentral) hepatocytes

7. Terminal hepatic venules (central veins)

8. Focal lesion(s)

9. Histochemical stains
   a. diastase periodic-acid-Schiff (dPAS)
   b. Perls iron or Prussian Blue
   c. trichrome (or Van Gieson)
   d. reticulin
   e. Victoria blue (or orcein or aldehyde fuchsin)

10. Immunohistochemical reactions, as needed

11. Metal assays, as needed (genetic haemochromatosis, Wilson disease)

12. Electron microscopy, as needed

13. Molecular studies, as needed (*in situ* hybridization, polymerase chain reaction)

The biopsy should be examined by first scanning the slide at lowest magnification to determine if there are focal changes. Then, in effect, the flow of blood should be followed for systematic assessment. Start with the portal tracts and their component structures, including portal vein, hepatic artery and bile ducts, as well as the mesenchymal background, remembering that portal tracts can also contain lymphatics and nerves although they are generally only apparent in larger portal areas. Portal tract oedema is one of the earliest signs of large duct obstruction. The number of bile ducts, as well as their pattern, should be studied.[160–162] Ductules may be present in a variety of disorders, for example following large duct obstruction, as a reaction in cholangiopathies, and as a non-specific finding in most cases of cirrhosis.[100] Ductular reaction may itself be chemotactic causing polymorphonuclear leukocytes to accumulate in portal tracts around bile ductules and should not be interpreted as ascending cholangitis. Furthermore, ductular reaction is prominent in many cases of Wilson disease (Fig. 3.8), as was well illustrated in Wilson's original paper.[163] A variety of materials can be seen in the portal tract, including pigment-laden macrophages which may be the only evidence of prior liver cell necrosis. Amyloid, which is usually seen as smudgy eosinophilic deposits in the space

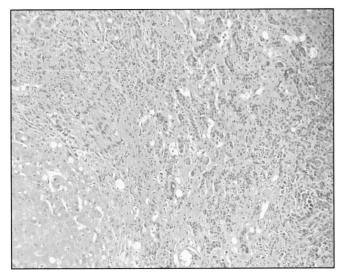

Fig. 3.8 • Portal area showing marked ductular reaction in a case of Wilson disease. H&E.

of Disse, can sometimes be globular in form and localized to the portal tract (Fig. 3.9).[164]

The limiting plate of hepatocytes is reviewed, beginning at an apex of the portal tract and proceeding to the central portion, remembering that the limiting plate includes hepatocytes from all three zones of the liver, with zone 1 extending from the apex of the tract and zone 3 reaching to the central portion of the limiting plate (see Chapter 1). In mild chronic hepatitis C, interface hepatitis may be subtle and focal, and may be better appreciated with a trichrome stain than with haematoxylin-eosin. Study the hepatocytes of the liver plates, the sinusoids and the sinusoidal cells, attempting to identify endothelial cells, Kupffer cells, and stellate cells, all of which may be inconspicuous in the absence of disease. Stellate cells become particularly prominent, with intracytoplasmic fat globules, in patients who have ingested vitamin A to excess.[165] The Disse space is also generally inconspicuous in the healthy liver, but becomes visible with heart failure or outflow obstruction. The zone

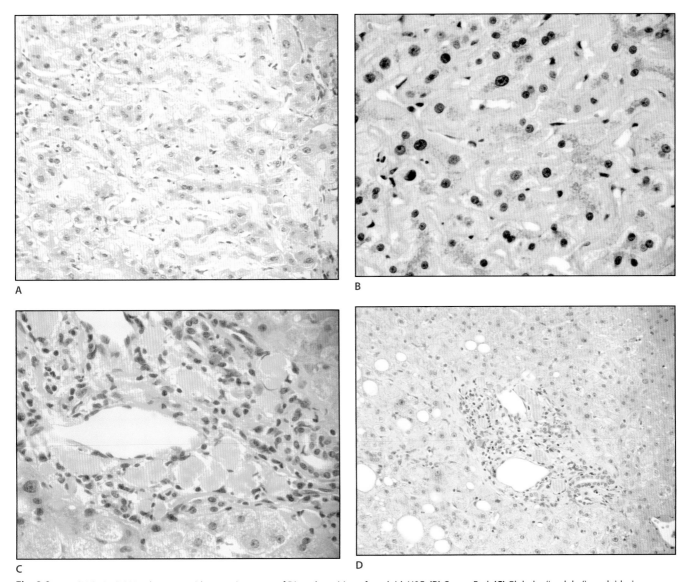

A

B

C

D

Fig. 3.9 • Amyloidosis. **(A)** Usual pattern with extensive space of Disse deposition of amyloid. H&E. **(B)** Congo Red. **(C)** Globular ('nodular') amyloidosis seen as predominantly portal tract deposition. H&E. **(D)** Congo Red.

3 (pericentral) hepatocytes are then examined. Toxic injuries, including those leading to steatosis or cholestasis, often first manifest in this zone. Zone 3 hepatocytic atrophy is characteristic of venous outflow obstruction, as in Budd–Chiari syndrome. Finally, the terminal hepatic venules (central veins), including the junction of sinusoids and venules, are evaluated.

If there are focal changes, examine them with higher magnification only after completing the general study of the liver. In this way, one avoids missing more subtle features by over-concentration on those that are more obvious.

Initial evaluation of the liver biopsy should be carried out without recourse to clinical information. Subsequently, prior to submitting the diagnosis, the morphological observations should be correlated with clinical data. Once the general diagnosis or at least the differential diagnosis has been reached, clinical information is vital. As examples, diagnosis may require knowledge of serologic studies for viral diseases, tests for autoantibodies, and a history of medication usage, as well as findings of imaging studies. When all the available information is put together and special studies (e.g. histochemical, immunohistochemical, ultrastructural, molecular) are performed, the comprehensive interpretation is not only diagnostic, but frequently has prognostic value as well.

General approach to the aspiration biopsy smear

The low magnification objective should be used to scan and evaluate the smear pattern and assess the background for blood, inflammation and necrosis. In many cases the smear pattern is very helpful in the differential diagnosis. For example, many cases of hepatocellular carcinoma show a pattern in which malignant hepatocytes are present in rounded nests and thickened trabecular structures, which can be quite striking at low power (Fig. 3.10). These clusters are often associated with one of two characteristic endothe-

lial patterns. The most specific is the 'peripherally wrapping endothelial pattern', where the sinusoidal endothelial cells wrap around smooth-edged, rounded nests and hepatic trabeculae greater than three cells thick[29,166–168] (Fig. 3.11). This pattern is virtually pathognomonic and particularly useful for the separation of reactive non-neoplastic and benign neoplastic proliferations from well-differentiated hepatocellular carcinoma.[29] Care must be taken to ensure that the endothelial cells fit this pattern and are not sporadic cells embedded with an irregular group of hepatocytes, which is a normal finding. The other pattern, which is not as specific, has been termed 'transgressing',[29] 'arborizing'[169] or central[168] (Fig. 3.12). This pattern can occasionally be seen in cirrhosis and hepatitis.[29]

The background of the smear may also contain valuable information, such as the characteristic 'dirty necrosis' commonly seen with metastatic colonic adenocarcinoma (Fig. 3.13).

After the smear pattern and the background have been evaluated the cytomorphologic features of the cell groups are examined at high power. The section on differential diagnosis, below, will discuss this in greater detail.

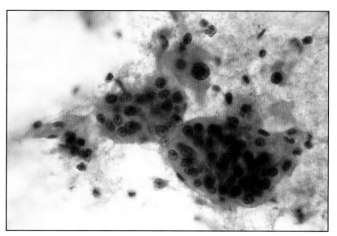

Fig. 3.11 • Aspiration biopsy showing the peripherally wrapping endothelial pattern in well-differentiated hepatocellular carcinoma. Papanicolaou.

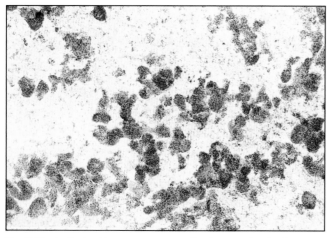

Fig. 3.10 • Aspiration biopsy smear pattern showing smooth-edged, rounded nests and trabecular forms in a case of well-differentiated hepatocellular carcinoma. H&E.

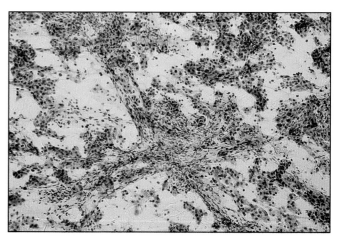

Fig. 3.12 • Aspiration biopsy showing the transgressing endothelial pattern in a case of well-differentiated hepatocellular carcinoma. H&E.

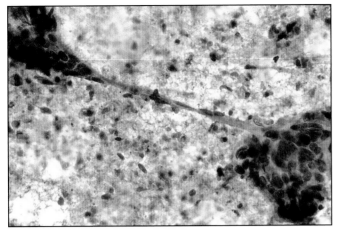

Fig. 3.13 • Aspiration biopsy smear showing 'dirty necrosis' in the background of a metastatic colonic adenocarcinoma. Papanicolaou.

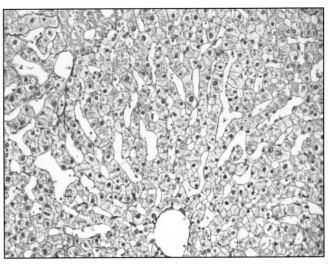

Fig. 3.15 • Reticulin silver impregnation demonstrating the normal pattern of one-cell-thick liver plates. Reticulin.

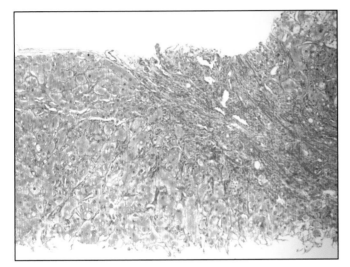

Fig. 3.14 • Trichrome stain demonstrating type I collagen in alcoholic cirrhosis. Note the pericellular ('chicken-wire') pattern of fibrosis. Masson trichrome.

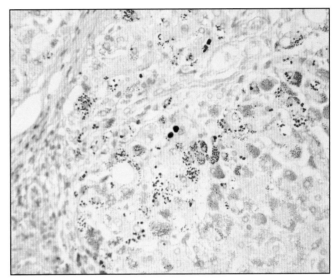

Fig. 3.16 • Diastase-predigested periodic-acid Schiff (dPAS) reaction showing alpha-1-antitrypsin globules in zone 1 hepatocytes. Diastase PAS.

Ancillary techniques

Histochemical stains

Haematoxylin-eosin is the standard stain for the initial study of the liver biopsy. We routinely prepare seven sections, and stain the first and last with H&E. The other sections are stained with: (i) Masson's trichrome to demonstrate type I collagen (Fig. 3.14) (alternative: van Gieson or Sirius red); (ii) reticulin silver impregnation stain to show type III collagen and highlight hepatic plate architecture (Fig. 3.15),[170–173] (iii) periodic acid-Schiff (PAS) after digestion with diastase (dPAS) to show basement membranes, α-1-antitrypsin globules (Fig. 3.16) and phagocytosed ceroid material in Kupffer cells; (iv) Perls stain for haemosiderin (Fig. 3.17) (alternative: Prussian blue) (v) Victoria blue which shows hepatitis B surface antigen (HBsAg) (Fig. 3.18), copper-associated protein (Fig. 3.19), and elastic fibres (Fig. 3.20), as well as phagocytosed material in Kupffer cells and macrophages (alternatives: Shikata orcein, aldehyde-

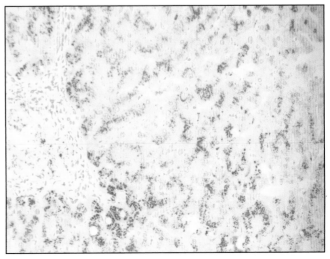

Fig. 3.17 • Genetic haemochromatosis with diffuse hepatocytic haemosiderin deposition. Note the greater intensity of staining in zone 1 hepatocytes at the apex of the portal tract and slightly lesser concentration in zones 2 and 3 at the mid-portion of the limiting plate. Perls iron stain.

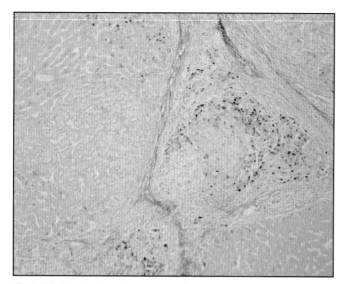

Fig. 3.18 • Hepatitis B surface antigen in hepatocytes in an explant from a patient with chronic hepatitis B cirrhosis. Note the variability of distribution emphasizing the possibility of potential sampling error in a core or aspiration biopsy. Victoria blue.

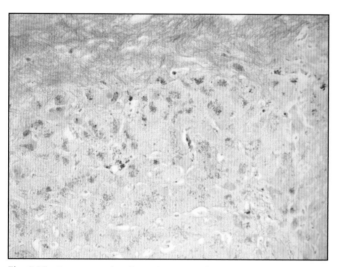

Fig. 3.19 • Copper-associated protein in zone 1 hepatocytes in a patient with chronic cholestasis. Victoria blue.

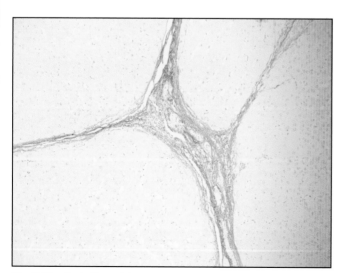

Fig. 3.20 • Elastic fibres of the vascular septa of cirrhosis in an explant from a patient with chronic hepatitis C cirrhosis. Victoria blue.

fuchsin). The same histochemical stains can be used for tissue biopsy and aspiration specimens (Table 3.3).

The trichrome stain also highlights Mallory hyaline and megamitochondria in alcoholic liver disease.[173,174] The trichrome stain is not, however, always sensitive enough for the detection of very early fibrosis for which reticulin silver impregnation is particularly useful (Fig. 3.21). Trichrome can also be misleading if there is parenchymal collapse, simulating septa and leading to a misdiagnosis of cirrhosis. Cirrhotic septa are vascular and contain abundant elastic tissue (Fig. 3.20) that can be demonstrated with stains generally used to detect hepatitis B surface antigen (Victoria blue, orcein, Gomori aldehyde-fuchsin).[35] Reticulin silver is also valuable for the demonstration of abnormal hepatic architecture and can be helpful on either smears[175] or tissue sections, including cell block preparations that may contain only tiny tissue fragments.[126] The two- and three-cell-thick liver cell plates of the regenerative nodules of cirrhosis, as well as the foci of proliferation that characterize nodular (regenerative) hyperplasia (Fig. 3.22), are well demonstrated

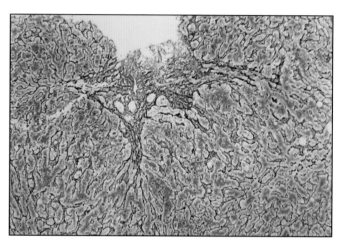

Fig. 3.21 • Needle core biopsy showing increased density of reticulin fibres extending from portal tracts as evidence of early fibrosis (stage 1) in a patient with chronic hepatitis C. Fibrosis was not apparent with either H&E or Masson trichrome stains at this time, but was seen with trichrome in a subsequent biopsy three years later. Reticulin.

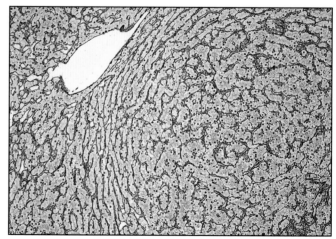

Fig. 3.22 • Needle core biopsy showing early nodular hyperplasia in a patient with primary biliary cirrhosis. The reticulin fibres appear slightly compressed because of the atrophy of liver plates surrounding the nodule. Reticulin.

Stain	Reactive tissue	Source
Trichrome (Van Gieson)	type I collagen	fibrosis
Reticulin	type III collagen	early fibrosis architectural changes: collapse nodule formation
PAS after diastase digestion	non-glycogen carbohydrates	α-1-antitrypsin basement membrane phagocytosed ceroid material
Perls iron or Prussian Blue	haemosiderin	haemosiderosis, genetic haemochromatosis
Victoria blue (orcein, aldehyde fuchsin)	elastic fibres	septa of cirrhosis blood vessels
	copper-associated protein	chronic cholestasis Wilson disease
	hepatitis B surface antigen non-glycogen carbohydrates	hepatitis B surface antigen phagocytosed ceroid material
Emanuele/Goodman	copper	chronic cholestasis Wilson disease
Ziehl–Neelsen	acid-fast bacilli	*M. avium* complex *M. tuberculosis*
Gomori methenamine silver	fungi	fungi

Table 3.3 Histochemical stains and reactions useful in the study of the liver biopsy

with reticulin silver methods. In children, until approximately the age of 5, the hepatic plates are usually two cells thick.

The combination of PAS and dPAS can be helpful in paediatric pathology where it is often necessary to exclude various metabolic diseases. In the glycogenoses, abnormal glycogen can be intensely reactive before diastase digestion and incompletely digested with diastase. PAS is also helpful for the demonstration of bile-duct basement membrane injury, especially in destructive biliary diseases, such as primary biliary cirrhosis. In contrast, there is generally no destruction of the basement membrane in primary sclerosing cholangitis and indeed there may be some increase in thickness. The finding of many PAS-positive Kupffer cells may be the only evidence of a recent, but resolved, hepatitis and can be helpful in correlating a relatively normal-appearing biopsy with recent clinical and biochemical evidence of a hepatitis.

In general, there are few applications for the PAS reaction without diastase digestion in the adult liver. However, PAS without diastase digestion highlights virtually every hepatocyte since they are generally glycogen-rich, and can augment the demonstration of interface hepatitis and parenchymal granulomas.

Perls stain, or Prussian blue, is used for the detection of stainable tissue haemosiderin. In genetic haemochromatosis iron accumulates in hepatocytes, whereas secondary iron deposition mainly occurs in Kupffer cells and macrophages (Chapter 4). The same pattern of iron deposition can also

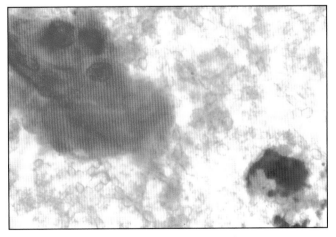

Fig. 3.23 • Aspiration biopsy smear from a patient with genetic haemochromatosis showing pigmented hepatocytes staining blue adjacent to a cluster of unstained well-differentiated hepatocellular carcinoma. Prussian blue. Reproduced from Pitman & Szyfelbein.[28] Reprinted by permission of Edward Hodder.

be seen in alcoholic liver disease and in porphyria cutanea tarda[176,177] and an iron assay with concomitant calculation of hepatic iron index may be needed together with genotyping. The iron stain can also be helpful in fine needle aspiration biopsy samples where malignant hepatocytes are not highlighted by the blue stain because of their inability to store iron. In contrast, the background usually consists of atypical but reactive and heavily pigmented hepatocytes of genetic haemochromatosis that stain intensely blue (Fig. 3.23).

noma (HCC) in liver biopsy samples may not be difficult when the tumour cells are overtly malignant and the tumour architecture recapitulates the normal liver, diagnosis may be less straightforward when HCC is well-differentiated resembling adenoma, poorly differentiated, or even when HCC is moderately differentiated displaying an acinar pattern or an uncommon cytologic feature that is difficult to distinguish from cholangiocarcinoma (CCA) or metastatic adenocarcinoma. In these, and other, instances, immunohistochemistry can be particularly useful to assess histologically problematic liver tumours, including those obtained as core needle biopsies, resection specimens, fine needle aspirate biopsy material, and, of course, tumours in whole livers resected at transplantation or at autopsy.[179]

For example, immunohistochemical studies can be exceedingly helpful in distinguishing between clear cell tumours (Table 3.5). A number of metastatic tumours affecting the liver can have a clear cell appearance (e.g. renal cell carcinoma, adrenocortical carcinoma[4]), as can primary hepatocellular carcinoma. In addition, angiomyolipoma, a usually benign neoplasm, can arise in the liver and may also have clear cell differentiation; this tumour typically is reactive to antibodies directed against markers generally associated with melanoma (e.g. HMB 45, Melan A).

Immunohistochemistry is also indispensable in the study of lymphomas, for both classification and, often, subclassification, and for determining therapy.

Epithelial cell markers

Immunohistochemical reactions for low- and high-molecular weight cytokeratins (CK) are especially helpful in the evaluation of bile ducts and proliferating ductules in a variety of conditions.[185,186] They are also useful markers for differentiating hepatocellular carcinoma from metastatic carcinoma.[187-190] Benign liver, bile-duct epithelium and most carcinomas, including hepatocellular carcinoma, react with antibodies against low-molecular weight keratins (e.g. CAM 5.2). In contrast, almost all cholangiocarcinomas and metastatic carcinomas react with high-molecular weight keratins (e.g. AE 1), but benign liver and most hepatocellular carcinomas do not. Polyclonal CEA (pCEA) is also helpful in this differential diagnosis. In many cases of hepatocellular carcinoma there is a distinct canalicular pattern of reactivity (Fig. 3.26), whereas metastatic adenocarcinomas and cholangiocarcinomas have a more diffuse cytoplasmic staining pattern. The demonstration of a canalicular pattern of reactivity in a tumour with a polyclonal antibody directed against carcinoembryonic antigen is considered pathognomonic for hepatocellular carcinoma. CD10 immunoreactivity may also be helpful in detecting intra-tumoral canalicula.

Antibodies previously used to try to establish the diagnosis of hepatocellular carcinoma, including α-1-antitrypsin, α-1-chymotrypsin and α-fetoprotein,[190] are now considered to be of limited value.[191] Specific cytokeratin antibodies, particularly cytokeratins 7, 19 and 20, can help in distinguishing some non-small-cell carcinomas from each other and from primary hepatic malignan-

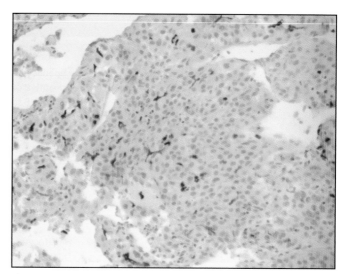

Fig. 3.26 • Sacral biopsy of metastatic hepatocellular carcinoma, two years after liver transplantation showing canalicular pattern demonstrated with polyclonal carcinoembryonic antigen (pCEA) antibody. Immunoperoxidase.

cies.[191-194] Immunostaining for CK 7 and CK 20 is a useful first step in the evaluation of liver tumours of uncertain origin (Tables 3.4, 3.6, 3.7, 3.8, 3.9). Hepatocytes express CK 8 and CK 18, but not CK 7, whereas bile-duct epithelial cells express CK 7, CK 8, CK 18 and CK 19. Neither hepatocytes nor bile ducts express CK 20. Hepatocellular carcinoma is generally cytokeratin 7, 19 and 20 negative, and cholangiocarcinoma cytokeratin 7, 19 and 20 positive. However, as many as 21% of HCC cases react with CK 7 and 5% react with CK 20 (Tables 3.6 and 3.7).[179] In general, breast carcinomas are CK 7 positive and CK 20 negative; ovarian and pancreatic mucinous carcinomas CK 7 and CK 20 positive; and gastrointestinal carcinoma, particularly colorectal carcinoma, CK 7 negative and CK 20 positive.[193] In addition, an increasing range of other antibodies have been applied to the study of liver tumours.[179,195,196]

Hep Par 1 is a mouse monoclonal antibody generated using failed allograft liver tissue as the immunogen.[179,197] Hep Par 1 has proven to be particularly useful in the evaluation of liver tumours, and reacts with most cases of hepatocellular carcinoma. Hep Par 1 does not seem to react with cholangiocarcinoma, but will react with approximately 15% of metastatic adenocarcinomas particularly those with hepatoid differentiation.[179] Hep Par 1 does not distinguish primary ovarian tumours with hepatoid differentiation from metastatic hepatocellular carcinoma.[197]

There is high correlation of Hep Par 1 immunoreactivity with in situ hybridization (ISH) for the detection of albumin in hepatocellular carcinoma.[198] Ninety-three per cent of HCC cases were positive for Hep Par 1 and 93% were positive for albumin ISH, but they were not all the same cases. However, the combined use of Hep Par 1 and albumin ISH detected 100% of cases of hepatocellular carcinoma.

Sinusoidal cell markers

Antibodies to Factor VIII, CD-10, CD-31 and CD-34 can demonstrate vascular endothelial cells, including

Table 3.5 Immunophenotype of clear cell tumours that can involve the liver

	HepPar 1	pcEA (canalicular)	CD34	RCC	Vimentin	HMB45	Melan A	CK 5	CK 8	Chromagranin	Synaptophysin	TTF-1	S-100	EMA
HCC	+	+	+	–	–	–	–	–	–	–	–	–	–	+
Renal CA	–	–	–	+	+	–	–	–	(+)	–	–	–	–	(+)
Adrenal CA	–	–	–	–	+	–	+	–	(+)	+	+	–	–	–
Melanoma	–	–	+	–	+	+	+	–	(+)	–	–	–	+	–
Clear cell sarcoma	–	–	+	–	+	+	+	–	(+)	–	–	–	+	–
Pulmonary	–	–	(+)	–	+	–	–	+	(+)	–	–	(+)	(+)	+
Squamous cell	–	–	–	–	(+)	–	–	+	(+)	–	–	–	(+)	+
Neuroendocrine	–	–	–	–	(+)	–	–	–	+	+	+	–	(+)	(+)
Epithelioid leimyosarcoma	–	–	–	–	+	–	+	–	(+)	–	–	–	–	–
Angiomyo-lipoma	–	–	(+)	–	+	+	+	+	(+)	–	–	–	(+)	–

Table 3.6	Immunhistochemical screening panel for liver malignancy of unknown primary site—adult males (Cedars-Sinai Medical Center)

- Cytokeratin 7 (CK7)—lung, pancreaticobiliary, thyroid, mesothelioma
- Cytokeratin 20 (CK20)—colon, stomach
- Thyroid transcription factor-1 (TTF-1)—lung, thyroid
- Renal cell carcinoma (RCC)—renal cell carcinoma
- Villin—colon, stomach, pancreaticobiliary, hepatocellular carcinoma
- Hep Par 1—hepatocellular carcinoma
- Prostate specific antigen (PSA)—prostate (liver metastases unusual)
- Prostatic alkaline phosphatase (PAP)—prostate (unusual)
- S-100—melanoma, neuroendocrine, lung
- HMB 45—melanoma, angiomyolipoma
- Melan A—melanoma, angiomyolipoma

Table 3.7	Immunohistochemical screening panel for liver malignancy of unknown primary site—adult females (Cedars-Sinai Medical Center)

- Cytokeratin 7 (CK7)—gynaecologic, breast (~15%), lung, pancreaticobiliary, thyroid, mesothelioma
- Cytokeratin 20 (CK20)—colon, stomach
- Estrogen receptor (ER)—breast, gynaecologic
- GCDFP15—breast
- bcl-2—breast, gynaecologic, neuroendocrine, melanoma, thyroid
- Thyroid transcription factor-1 (TTF-1)—lung, thyroid
- Renal cell carcinoma (RCC)—renal cell carcinoma
- Villin—colon, stomach, pancreaticobiliary, hepatocellular carcinoma
- Hep Par 1—hepatocellular carcinoma
- S-100—melanoma, neuroendocrine, lung
- HMB 45—melanoma, angiomyolipoma
- Melan A—melanoma, angiomyolipoma

Table 3.8	Common immunohistochemical patterns in differentiating hepatocellular carcinoma from metastatic adenocarcinoma	
	Hepatocellular carcinoma	Metastatic adenocarcinoma
Hep Par 1	++	−
CEA, monoclonal	−	+/−
CEA, polyclonal	++ (canalicular pattern)	++ (non-canalicular pattern)
CK 7	−	++
CK 20	−	++ (e.g. colon)
CD 10	++ (canalicular pattern)	++ (non-canalicular pattern)
Villin	++ (canalicular pattern)	++ (non-canalicular pattern)
MOC-31	−	++
α-fetoprotein	+/−	−−
CD 34	++ (sinusoidal pattern)	+/−

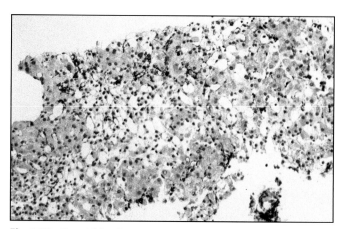

Fig. 3.27 • Sinusoidal stellate cells demonstrated with antibody directed against smooth muscle actin (SMA) in a patient with vitamin A toxicity. Immunoperoxidase. (Slide generously lent by Dr Najeeb S Alshak.)

sinusoidal endothelial cells, as well as the cells of vaso-formative and vascular tumours, such as angiosarcoma and Kaposi sarcoma.[199] CD-10, CD-31 and CD-34 also demonstrate the characteristic sinusoidal pattern of hepatocellular carcinoma, which is not seen in cirrhotic nodules. Adenoma will, however, also show this pattern, and molecular studies may be useful for differentiating adenoma from hepatocellular carcinoma.[200,201] Anti-smooth muscle actin highlights stellate cells (Fig. 3.27). Any of the available histiocytic markers will react with Kupffer cells, but these can usually be easily seen (with less cost) using the periodic-acid Schiff reaction after diastase digestion (dPAS). The presence of many vimentin-positive Kupffer or 'spider cells' on aspirate smears has been suggested to indicate the hepatocytic origin of a tumour, whether in the liver or at a metastatic site.[202]

Immunofluorescence studies

These are only rarely employed. The principal indication is the demonstration of post-transplant humoral allograft rejection using antibodies to C4d but this is, which is exceedingly rare (see Chapter 16). In eclampsia, pre-eclampsia and HELLP syndrome fibrinogen is deposited in sinusoids and immunofluorescence of cryostat-prepared tissue using antibody directed against fibrinogen can be helpful; a reliable antibody for fibrinogen for paraffin embedded tissues is not yet available. Some lymphocyte markers are also best demonstrated with immunofluorescence.

Table 3.9 Immunohistochemical findings in hepatocellular carcinoma, cholangiocarcinoma, and metastatic adenocarcinoma

Antibody	Type		
	Hepatocellular Carcinoma (n = 42)	Cholangiocarcinoma (n = 9)	Metastatic Adenocarcinoma (n = 56)
Hep Par 1	38 (90%)	0 (0%)	8 (14%)
AE1/AE3	19 (45%)	8 (89%)	53 (95%)
CAM 5.2	41 (98%)	8 (89%)	48 (89%)
CK 7	9 (21%)	7 (78%)	20 (36%)
CK 19	4 (10%)	4 (44%)	16 (29%)
CK 20	2 (5%)	1 (11%)	17 (30%)
B72.3	1 (2%)	3 (33%)	7 (13%)
Factor XIIIa	37 (88%)	5 (56%)	22 (43%)
AFP	12 (29%)	0 (0%)	3 (5%)
pCEA	39 (93%)	9 (100%)	54 (96%)
mCEA	0 (0%)	2 (22%)	35 (62%)
Villin	13 (31%)	2 (22%)	22 (39%)
CD10	21 (50%)	1 (11%)	3 (5%)
MOC-31	5 (12%)	6 (67%)	37 (66%)
Inhibin	0 (0%)	0 (0%)	0 (0%)

See reference 179

Other novel techniques

Computer-assisted morphometry, flow cytometry, static cytometry image analysis and neural network analysis can be performed on either fixed or unfixed liver tissue. These methods, however, are not widely available and are more often applied for research purposes,[203–206] although flow cytometry is increasingly available and is used routinely for the study of lymphoid lesions in cytology specimens as well as for the determination of DNA ploidy in certain tumours in many types of specimen preparation.

Molecular pathology of the liver

Remarkably, the liver expresses 25% of the human genome,[207] with alternative splicing yielding as many as forty to fifty thousand different transcripts. New technologies including cDNA-expression microarrays, real-time reverse-transcription mediated polymerase chain reaction (qPCR), FISH, and microsatellite analysis for LOH have invigorated hepatology. These techniques, singly and in combination, are actively addressing both diagnosis and prognosis, and will contribute to the development of targeted, and potentially gene, therapies for hepatitis and HCC. The utility of DNA microarray technology, with emphasis on the liver, has been reviewed.[207] Tissue microarray and a panoply of new tools for protein studies, or proteomics, promise continuing discoveries.[208,209]

Tissue microarray analysis involves placement of dozens to hundreds of 'cores' of tissues (e.g. HCC, pre-neoplastic nodules, etc.) in paraffin for preparation of simultaneous sections of many 'cases'.[208] Candidate proteins are then explored using in situ DNA/RNA probes or antibodies for confirmation of the relative importance of differences identified during expression analysis. A reverse proteomics tool is becoming available, the 'protein microarray', an early example of which is a pattern of antibody spots on a single absorbent surface.[210] As more proteins and antibodies become available, protein microarrays will become available for interrogation of protein extracts of single tissue specimens.

Neoplastic disorders

Studies of loss of heterozygosity (LOH) can be performed with capillary electrophoresis, and other methods, to identify the pattern of LOHs for a given neoplasm via fragment analysis.[211] Comparisons of patterns of LOH are useful for differential diagnosis, for identification of potential second primaries, and for recognition of metastases when staging of HCC is carried out[211,212] (Table 3.10). LOH studies, in particular, are readily applied to paraffin-embedded tissues, including after formalin-fixation, although RNA analysis is more easily performed on fresh or ethanol-fixed tissue. Microdissection of archival materials in paraffin blocks has been extremely productive in both DNA and RNA studies.

Table 3.10	Recurrent losses/gains (LOH) in HCC[212]	
1p, 4q, 6q, 9p, 13q, 16q, 17p		Loss
1q, 6p, 8q, 17q, 20q		Gain
4q, 16q		HBV/HCC*

* Seen in HBV related HCC

Table 3.11	Observations in molecular analysis of HCC
c-met	Increased expression (poor prognosis)[213]
TGF-α	Growth stimulation[214]
TGF-β	Over-expression (inhibitor of immune surveillance?)[215]
c-myc	Poor outcome (younger patients)[216]
p53 (17p)	LOH tumour suppressor[217]
Rb	LOH tumour suppressor[218]
p16[INK4]	Absent protein (poor prognosis)[219]
p27	Increased expression, favourable prognosis[220]
E-cadherin	Reduced expression (LOH)[221]

Table 3.12	Thirteen gene index for prognostication of HCC[222]
TERT	Telomerase reverse transcriptase
IGF2	Insulin-like growth factor 2
Connexin 26/GJB2	Connexin 26
Tie2/TEK	Tie2/TEK tyrosine kinase
TIAM1	T-cell lymphoma invasion and metastasis 1
CXCL12	Chemokine (C-X-C motif) ligand 12
TOP2A	Topoisomerase (DNA) II α
A2M	α-2-macroglobulin
PLG	Plasminogen
p14ARF/CDKN2A	Alternative reading frame p14
PDGFRA	Platelet-derived growth factor receptor α
MKI67	Antigen identified by monoclonal antibody ki-67
THBS1	Thrombospondin 1

Molecular studies of HCC have yielded widely scattered associations, including somewhat 'classical' findings such as abnormalities of gene expression and chromosomal numbers and configurations, microsatellite instability and LOH (Table 3.11).[213–221] What has been needed are molecular 'indexes' for both the more precise diagnosis of lesions that are histologically 'borderline' and the prediction of metastases and intra-hepatic spread[222] (Table 3.12).

A cornerstone in the understanding of hepatocarcinogenesis is the recognition that dysplastic, proliferative nodules in cirrhosis[223] and focal or multi-nodular hyperplasia[224] are generally clonal, even monoclonal, in nature, based on studies using polymorphic markers including the X chromosome and androgen receptor gene. Using microdissection, LOH can be shown to be increased in such nodules, with the demonstration of mild to marked dysplasia.[225]

DNA microarrays are revolutionizing the approach to both understanding and diagnosing HCC. DNA arrays have yielded differential expression analysis for histological subtypes,[226] for HBV and HCV and other aetiologies of HCC,[227] and have provided insights into proangiogenic activity and elements of cross-talk in HCC.[229] Some expression studies have pointed to informative gene expressions, i.e., those that appear in most HCC cases, providing opportunities for improving the diagnosis of borderline lesions, for prognostication and for understanding hepatocarcinogenesis.[222] Although only several thousand genes have been screened to date, when expression microarrays are eventually expanded to tens of thousands of expressions for HCC relevant tissue, a small collection of genes will likely be found informative for diagnosis and prognostication of this cancer,

with acceptable clinical accuracy. In several studies, limited numbers of genes have proven useful in the differential diagnosis of potentially malignant nodules, when expression was quantitated employing the highly sensitive and reproducible technique of real-time RT-PCR (qPCR)[222] and standard cDNA microarray.[207,223,224] The latter is in terms of expression in increasingly poorly differentiated HCC, identifying important genes in this disease. qPCR can be limiting in the number of target genes under analysis; however, the method is relatively straightforward, sensitive and accurate. Gene expressions of interest, as identified from data mining microarray results, may be assayed by qPCR for confirmation of microarray results or for further analysis of diagnostic and prognostic use of a gene or genes of interest. As one example, 219 genes of the metabolic pathways in liver carcinogenesis were assayed for informative value in HCC, with 13 selected for molecular indexing. Subsequently, selected assays correctly ranked 44 of 45 cirrhotic macronodules (including regenerative and dysplastic nodules) as benign or malignant[222] (Table 3.12). Such indexes, when more fully developed, may demonstrate potential for identification of a diversity of hepatic lesions, including borderline and well-differentiated HCCs. Validation of qPCR may be more immediately accessible than cDNA arrays for many clinical laboratories.

Other tools such as transgenic and knockout mice, as well as studies of quick-frozen human liver samples, have yielded useful insights. Potentially relevant observations in HCC are listed (Table 3.13). P21/WAF1 depends on intact p53 expression and, probably, participates widely in hepatic carcinogenesis (p21/WAF1 suppresses cell cycle advance from G_1-S phase).[220] Osteopontin is over-expressed in metastatic HCC, and the demonstration of osteopontin in an apparent primary lesion may be a valuable indicator of possible undetected metastasis and, consequently, prognosis.[228]

Table 3.13	Recent representative molecular markers in HCC*
Assay	**Reference**
LOH	Patterns are diagnostic, prognostic[211]
p21/WAF1	Tumour suppressor—LOH in HCC[220]
Microarray (DNA)	Diagnostic, prognostic RNA signatures[226,227]
Osteopontin	Over-expressed in metastatic HCC[228]
p16	Tumour suppressor—LOH in HCC[229]
H-ras, EGF-R	Oncogenes upregulated in HCC[229]
VEGF	Proangiogenic—prognostic[229]
p53 mutation	DNA damage control[229]
Bcl-2	Paradoxically inhibits HCC development[230]
Rho C (expression)	Prognostic in HCC[231]
Fas (receptor) absence	Suggests immunologic tolerance[232]
IGF axis	Up-regulation in transformation[233]
$(TTAGGG)_n$	Telomeric repeats shortened—risk HCC[234]
IL-1β polymorphisms	Hepatitis C (HCC risk)[235]
HBV-X gene	Integrated (truncated) drives HCC[236]
HBV occult	HCC risk[237]

* Reports of potentially informative DNA/RNA findings and expressions require individual laboratory validation for clinical applications

Matrix metalloproteinase-2 (MMP-2) may prove to be a useful prognostic marker.[229] Other factors positively correlated with invasiveness in HCC include expression and/or up-regulation of H-ras, EGFR, and VEGF, and mutations of p53 and p16, while expression of nm-23-H1 and TIMP-2 (inhibitor of MMP-2) suggest malignancy without 'invasion'.[229] In contrast to lymphoma, where bcl-2 over-expression inhibits apoptosis without affecting cell proliferation, bcl-2 expression opposes hepatic proliferation and hepatocarcinogenesis.[230] Rho C may be prognostic in HCC.[231] Absence of Fas (receptor) expression and generation of soluble Fas may be associated with invasion or metastasis of a suspicious nodule in the liver via HCC escape from immunologic surveillance.[232] The IGF axis, including autocrine production of IGF-II and the over-expression of IGF-I receptor, may be critical in the transformation to HCC.[233]

Other nucleic acid-related findings for HCC have included the reduction of telomeric repeats $(TTAGGG)_n$ in nodular hepatic tissue, indicative of replicative history and increased risk of HCC.[234] Finding simple germ-line polymorphisms in IL-1β, in HCV-related cirrhosis, is evidence for increased risk for development of HCC.[235] An integrated, 3' truncated HBV X gene suggests the likelihood of HCC following HBV infection.[236] Finally, an occult HBV (HBsAg negative) is also a risk factor for HCC.[237] It will continue to be important to examine both HCV- and HBV-related HCC, since the molecular aetiologies of the two appear to be different.[238]

Correlation between DNA microarray results and histological or immunohistological findings is imperative, since for a given gene expression the cell of derivation may be unknown.[239] Molecular analysis interpretation should be validated using both clinical and histological parameters.

The molecular aspects of childhood hepatic neoplasms, including hepatoblastoma and HCC, as well as mesenchymal neoplasms of the liver, have recently been well reviewed.[240]

Non-neoplastic disorders

Since the discovery of hepatitis C virus (HCV) in 1989 by molecular methods,[241] molecular assays for detection and quantization have become integral to the diagnosis and treatment of both HCV and HBV.

Molecular assays address both viral identification and characterization. A useful compendium of molecular assays is available on the world wide web.[242]

Viral load assays, including for HCV, are sensitive and reproducible, and testing kits are widely available.[243] High HCV viral load is more likely to be associated with complications, such as failure to respond to treatment with interferon (IFN).[244,245] Viral loads should be measured early in infection, and may govern the need for therapy, which is expensive and not without serious side-effects.[245] A variety of useful molecular tests for viral load are available, including signal and target amplification.[243] The most sensitive assays for HCV and HBV in the serum are target amplification assays. Such tests are now sensitive to approximately 10–50 copies/ml.

HCV is conveniently typed into six groups, attainable by sequencing or molecular probes available as commercial kits. HCV genotypes 1 and 4 are often associated with complications of chronicity and drug resistance.[246] Type 1 is the most frequent HCV type in the USA. It is on the basis of HCV quasispecies, and rapid adaptation to immune surveillance, that 85% of HCV infections become chronic.[247] Not only are cirrhosis and HCC a complication of HCV infection, but B cell non-Hodgkin lymphoma may also arise secondary to B cell clonal expansions from stimulation by adaptive quasispecies.[248] As a single-stranded RNA virus, HCV may be analysed for active replication (presence of negative strand),[249] which may be important in the future for treatment. It is noteworthy that HIV is known to facilitate HCV replication in macrophages/monocytes.[250]

HBV is now assayable by many of the same technologies as HCV. During treatment, HBV genotype C is aggressive and more refractory to therapy than other types.[251] Type C is associated with chronic disease, including HCC, with greater recurrence of HCC after therapy.[252] Molecular techniques are helping to identify drug resistance mutants, such as emergence of a YMDD polymerase motif during HBV treatment.[253]

DNA microarrays are under development for the molecular identification of cirrhosis. Viral and non-viral expression signatures can be recognized, and development of a chronic hepatitis/cirrhosis DNA 'array' will be useful for diagnosis and may help in the identification of useful therapies.[226,227]

Newer technologies may allow for improved identification of a host of aetiologic factors in chronic liver disease. As an example, HCV and autoimmune hepatitis frequently demonstrate overlapping clinical parameters,[254] and further expression analysis of such diseases may often be warranted.

PCR may be performed for other viruses affecting the liver, commonly Epstein–Barr virus (EBV) and cytomegalovirus (CMV). Importantly, following liver transplantation for any reason, including cirrhosis and HCC, it may be useful to test qualitatively for EBV in the blood, then quantitatively for increasing EBV viral loads if necessary. Post-transplantation lymphoproliferative disorder (PTLD) may follow EBV infection de novo, or reactivation of the virus.[255,256] Reduction of immunosuppression may lead to resolution of the PTLD. Lymphoma occurs in up to 10% of transplant recipients.[257] CMV is a risk factor for chronic allograft rejection,[258] and may be conveniently followed by nucleic acid testing.

Heritable diseases

Inborn errors, or disease gene mutations, may be tested by routine sequencing, restriction fragment length polymorphism, and several other techniques. Most of these tests can be carried out using formalin-fixed tissues. Patients requiring workup for iron overload disorders are now routinely screened for the heritable forms of iron storage disease.[259] There are currently four types of genetic haemochromatosis recognized, with four different genes involved. The most frequent, and classical, form is autosomal recessive and involves the HFE gene (chromosome 6). In most cases genetic haemochromatosis arises from the HFE C282Y substitution. Homozygosity for HFE C282Y is found in roughly 5 of 1000 persons of Northern European descent, although fortunately the gene is relatively low in penetrance. Juvenile haemochromatosis exists (HJV gene), and a transferrin receptor gene mutation is rarely encountered. The classification of haemochromatosis is available online.[260]

Other inborn diseases of the liver include Wilson disease, with mutations of the copper-transporting ATPase gene (Wilson disease protein), the most common mutation within the catalytic site of the protein, the H1069Q substitution.[261]

Occasionally conditions such as Gaucher's disease need confirmation at the time of biopsy. A technique for identifying the common Gaucher mutations in tissue retrieved after paraffin embedding of formalin-fixed tissue has been developed.[262]

Electron microscopy

Electron microscopy (EM) is no longer an integral part of the everyday diagnostic evaluation of liver tissue and is only utilized for certain indications, such as: (i) the study of inherited/metabolic disease (e.g. glycogen storage diseases or the recognition of mitochondrial injury in Wilson disease[263]); (ii) to establish the presence of some viral diseases, even after tissue has been formalin-fixed and embedded in paraffin;[264] (iii) to help define the origin of an otherwise unrecognizable tumour; and (iv) to study the early effects of a variety of medications.[33,78,79,82] EM may sometimes be useful for the study of material obtained as fine needle aspiration biopsy.[33] Electron microscopy, including transmission electron microscopy (TEM), scanning electron microscopy (SEM) and immunoelectron microscopy (IEM), still has considerable utility for studies of the patho-biology of liver cells.[96,97,99,101,265,266]

Horizon techniques

Immunohistochemical studies will continue to be utilized for the evaluation of liver tumours, with newer antibodies directed against a variety of nuclear, cytoplasmic and membrane factors. These include apomucins, beta-catenin, c-myc, epidermal growth factor receptor (EGFR), hepatoma-derived growth factor (HDGF), metastatic tumour antigen-1 (MTA1), somatostatin receptor (SSTR), the anti-apoptosis-related proteins bcl-2 and bcl-xL, telomerase, vascular endothelial growth factor (VEGF) and other angiogenesis factors, to be used for diagnosis, to identify optimal therapy, and for prognostication.

Computer-assisted studies, including morphometric analyses and neural network evaluations,[96] are likely to become more accessible for diagnostic evaluations.

Newer molecular studies, particularly analyses based on protein–protein interactions (proteomics)[267–278] and tissue array analyses,[208] will likely supplement, and perhaps eventually even replace, immunohistochemistry. Proteomics has been coupled with neural network computer analysis to predict liver fibrosis and cirrhosis without liver biopsy.[277] In addition to increasing use of assays of gene expression, there will be important applications for microarray studies to assess variations in RNA concentrations in tissues and cells in various disease processes. Newer microscopy techniques (e.g., confocal microscopy, multiphoton microscopy, spectral analyses) are under evaluation.[265,266] For the present, the standard histological slide remains a key component in the evaluation of patients with liver disease, both primary and secondary, in whom diagnoses, including determination of stage of disease and prognosis, cannot be definitely established with clinical or imaging methods. Furthermore, tissue samples retained in archives may prove invaluable for many patients in helping to understand the aetiology and progress of their disorders as well as identifying novel therapeutic approaches.

Archival tissue for research

Liver samples maintained as paraffin-embedded tissue, particularly if heavy metal fixatives have not been used, are indefinitely useful for the usual histologic and immunohistochemical studies; DNA- and RNA-based studies can also be carried out. Formalin-fixation has generally limited RNA-based detection to short fragments (approximately 120 bp products) although newer techniques may improve RNA fragment-length yield in such tissue.[279] Reliable analysis by microarray can be carried out if, following total

RNA extraction, brief cDNA amplification is employed. Quantitative PCR is easily performed on formalin-fixed paraffin embedded tissue, including for viral and oncogene analysis, again requiring caution in terms of PCR product size. Tissue fixed in alcohol is more suitable for RNA recovery; alcohol fixation preserves full-length mRNA transcripts for RNA expression analysis. Protein studies, utilizing the techniques of proteomics, generally require fresh frozen tissue.

Using laser capture microdissection (LCM), cell populations can be easily obtained from tissue sections, including those that have previously stained, for nucleic acid and protein analyses.[209] Previously, molecular studies have been largely based on samples that included mixed cell populations. With LCM, hepatic-lobule-zone specific cells can be chosen for PCR and other molecular studies.

The US government, among other governments, has mandated that institutional review board (IRB) approval must be obtained for all research based on human material, including histology and cytology samples. Confidentiality and safety issues must be addressed. If possible, patient consent must be obtained. Often, however, an 'expedited' approval process, not necessarily requiring patient consent, can be utilized for the study of archival material, particularly when patient-specific correlations are not made. Pathologists must be 'guardians of the wax', as well as of all other patient samples kept in archives, and therefore need to participate proactively in the establishment of institutional guidelines that determine how such retained materials are preserved for diagnostic and research purposes, and potentially distributed, so that they are not inappropriately exhausted.

Autopsy

Autopsies remain an integral component of quality medical care, as useful and valuable in the study of liver diseases as in any other discipline of medicine. Among the many benefits of autopsy are ongoing education of physicians, including pathologists, assessment of effectiveness and appropriateness of therapies, and detection of unsuspected clinically important conditions (e.g. infectious complications after transplant,[280] previously undiagnosed genetic haemochromatosis, and many others). There is increasing recognition of the important role autopsy can play in assuring quality of care.[281] Institutions with very high autopsy rates tend to have lower rates of significant diagnostic discrepancies ('errors').[281] It has been estimated that there is an approximately 10% decrease in the frequency of major diagnostic errors for every 10% increase in the autopsy rate.[282] There is also considerable benefit to family members and friends who learn of the results of autopsy, often providing relief from unexpressed feelings of guilt and contributing to a shorter and less painful grieving period.

References

1. Chen TS, Chen PS. Understanding the liver. Westport: Greenwood Press, 1984

2. Popper H. Vienna and the Liver. In: Brunner H, Thaler H, eds, Hepatology, A Festschrift for Hans Popper. New York: Raven Press, 1995; pp 1–14
3. Silverman I. A new biopsy needle. Am J Surg, 1938; 40:671–672
4. Menghini G. One-second needle biopsy of the liver. Gastroenterology, 1958; 35:190–199
5. Reddy KR, Jeffers LJ. Liver biopsy and laparoscopy, In: Schiff ER, Sorrell MF, Maddrey WC, eds, Schiff's diseases of the liver, 8th edn, Philadelphia: Lippincott-Raven, 1999; pp 245–266
6. Fukuda H, Inokuti Y. Aspiration biopsy using new ceramic-coated stainless steel puncture needle. J Biomed Mater Res, 2004; 71B:392–397
7. Schaffner F. The history of liver disease at The Mount Sinai Hospital. Mt Sinai J Med, 2000; 67:76–83
8. Martin HE, Ellis EB. Biopsy by needle puncture and aspiration. Ann Surg, 1930; 92:169–181
9. Lundquist A. Fine-needle aspiration biopsy of the liver. Acta med Scand, 1971(Suppl); 520:1–28
10. Kugelmas M. Liver biopsy. Am J Gastroenterol, 2004; 99:1416–1417
11. Bedossa P, Dargere D, Paradis V. Sampling variability of liver fibrosis in chronic hepatitis C. Hepatology, 2003; 38:1449–1457
12. Di Sario A, Feliciangeli G, Bendia E, Benedetti A. Diagnosis of liver fibrosis. Eur Rev Med Pharmacol Sci, 2004; 8:11–18
13. Guido M, Rugge M. Liver fibrosis: natural history may be affected by the biopsy sample. Gut, 2004; 53:1878
14. Scheuer PJ. Liver biopsy size matters in chronic hepatitis: bigger is better. Hepatology, 2003; 38:1356–1358
15. Caturelli E, Solmi L, Anti M et al. Ultrasound guided fine needle biopsy of early hepatocellular carcinoma complicating liver cirrhosis: a multicentre study. Gut, 2004; 53:1356–1362
16. Feld RI. Ultrasound-guided biopsies: tricks, needles tips, and other fine points. Ultrasound Q, 2004; 20:91–99
17. Kaji I, Kasugai H, Takenaka A et al. Outcome of 51 nonmalignant nodules in the liver: usefulness of aspiration cytology for diagnosis of dysplastic nodules. J Exp Clin Cancer Res, 2004; 23:425–431
18. Scholmerich J, Schacherer D. Diagnostic biopsy for hepatocellular carcinoma in cirrhosis: useful, necessary, diagnostic, or academic sport? Gut, 2004; 53:1224–1226
19. Sporea I. Popescu A, Sitrli R, Danila M, Strain M. Ultrasound assisted liver biopsy for the staging of diffuse chronic hepatopathies. Rom J Gastroenterol, 2004; 13:287–290
20. Mc Afee JH, Keeffe EB, Lee RG, Rosch J. Transjugular liver biopsy. Hepatology, 1992; 15:726–732
21. Lebrec D, Goldfarb G, Debott C et al. Transvenous liver biopsy: an experience based on 1000 hepatic tissue samplings with this procedure. Gastroenterology, 1992; 83:338–340
22. Stieltjes N, Ounnoughene N, Sava E et al. Interest of transjugular liver biopsy in adult patients with haemophilia or other congenital bleeding disorders infected with hepatitis C virus. Br J Haematol, 2004; 125:769–776
23. Theodore D, Fried MW, Kleiner DE et al. Liver biopsy in patients with inherited disorders of coagulation and chronic hepatitis C. Haemophilia, 2004; 10:413–421
24. De Hoyos A, Loredo ML, Martinez-Rios MA et al. Transjugular liver biopsy in 52 patients with an automated Trucut-type needle. Dig Dis Sci, 1999; 44:177–180
25. Garcia-Compean D, Cortes C. Transjugular liver biopsy. An update. Ann Hepatol, 2004; 3:100–103
26. Jhala NC, Jhala D, Eltoum I et al. Endoscopic ultrasound-guided fine-needle aspiration biopsy: a powerful tool to obtain samples from small lesions. Cancer, 2004; 102:239–246
27. Applebaum L, Lederman R, Agid R, Libson E. Hepatic lymphoma: an imaging approach with emphasis on image-guided needle biopsy. Isr Med Assoc J, 2005; 7:19–22
28. Pitman MB, Szyfelbein WM. Fine needle aspiration biopsy of the liver. Boston: Butterworth-Heinemann, 1994
29. Pitman MB, Szyfelbein WM. The significance of endothelium in the FNA diagnosis of hepatocellular carcinoma. Diagn Cytopathol, 1995; 12:208–214
30. Kulesza P, Torbenson M, Sheth S, Erozan YS, Ali SZ. Cytopathologic grading of hepatocellular carcinoma on fine-needle aspiration. Cancer, 2004; 102:247–258
31. Lin KJ, Eng HL, Lu Sn, Chiu KW, Kuo FY. Hepatic angiomyolipoma: report of two cases with emphasis on smear cytomorphology and the use of cell block with immunohistochemical stains. Diagn Cytopathol, 2004; 31:263–266
32. Saleh H, Masood S. Value of ancillary studies in fine-needle aspiration biopsy. Diagn Cytopathol, 1995; 13:310–315
33. Desmet VJ. Liver tissue examination. J Hepatol, 2003; 39(Suppl 1): S43–S49

34. Geller SA. Liver biopsy for the nonpathologist. In: Gitnick G, ed. Principles and Practices of Gastroenterology and Hepatology, 2nd edn. Norwalk: Appleton & Lange, 1994; pp 1023–1036

35. Geller SA, Petrovic LM. Biopsy Interpretation of the Liver. Philadelphia: Lippincott Williams & Wilkins, 2004; pp 3–10

36. Adler M, Frotscher B, Thiry P, Gustot T. Non invasive markers of liver fibrosis in hepatitis C. Acta Gastroenterol Belg, 2004; 67:278–281

37. Afdhal NH. Biopsy or biomarkers: is there a gold standard for diagnosis of liver fibrosis? Clin Chem, 2004; 50:1299–1300

38. Afdhal NH, Nunes D. Evaluation of liver fibrosis: a concise review. Am J Gastroenterol, 2004; 99:1160–1174

39. Andriulli A, Persico M, Iacobellis A et al. Treatment of patients with HCV infection with or without liver biopsy. J Viral Hepat, 2004; 11:536–542

40. Callewaert N, Van Vlierberghe H, Van Hecke A et al. Noninvasive diagnosis of liver cirrhosis using DNA sequencer-based total serum protein glycomics. Nature Med, 2004; 10:429–434

41. Campbell MS, Reddy KR. Review article: the evolving role of liver biopsy. Aliment Pharmacol Ther, 2004; 20:249–259

42. Patel K, Gordon SC, Jacobson I et al. Evaluation of a panel of non-invasive serum markers to differentiate mild from moderate-to-advanced liver fibrosis in chronic hepatitis C patients. J Hepatol, 2004; 41:935–942

43. Poynard T, Munteanu M, Imbert-Bismut F et al. Prospective analysis of discordant results between biochemical markers and biopsy in patients with chronic hepatitis C. Clin Chem, 2004; 50:1344–1355

44. Rosenberg WM, Voelker M, Thiel R et al. Serum markers detect the presence of liver fibrosis: a cohort study. Gastroenterology, 2004; 127:1704–1713

45. Tsukamoto T, Yamamoto T, Ikebe T et al. Serum markers of liver fibrosis and histologic severity of fibrosis in resected liver. Hepatogastroenterology, 2004; 51:777–780

46. Bain VG, Bonacini M, Govindarajan S et al. A multicentre study of the usefulness of liver biopsy in hepatitis C. J Viral Hepat, 2004; 11:375–382

47. Rousselet M-C, Michalak S, Dupré F et al. Sources of variability in histologic scoring of chronic viral hepatitis. Hepatology, 2005; 41:257–264

48. Rullier A, Trimoulet P, Neau D et al. Fibrosis is worse in HIV-HCV patients with low-level immunodepression referred for HCV treatment than in HCV-matched patients. Hum Pathol, 2004; 35:1088–1094

49. Ryder SD. Progression of hepatic fibrosis in patients with hepatitis C: a prospective repeat liver biopsy study. Gut, 2004; 53:451–455

50. Westin J, Nordlinder H, Lagging M, Norkrans G, Wejstal R. Steatosis accelerates fibrosis development over time in hepatitis C genotype 3 infected patients. J Hepatol, 2002; 37:837–842

51. Dienstag JL, Goldin RD, Heathcote EJ et al. Histological outcome during long-term lamivudine therapy. Gastroenterology, 2003; 124:105–117

52. Yu AS, Vierling JM, Colquhoun SD et al. Transmission of hepatitis B infection from hepatitis B core antibody-positive liver allografts is prevented by lamivudine therapy. Liver Transpl, 2001; 7:513–517

53. Clouston AD, Jonsson JR, Purdie DM et al. Steatosis and chronic hepatitis C: analysis of fibrosis and stellate cell activation. J Hepatol, 2001; 35:314–320

54. Di Tommaso L, Macchia S, Morandi L et al. Correlation between histologic staging, hepatitis C virus genotypes and clinical features in HCV chronic hepatitis: evidence of a new pattern. Int J Surg Pathol, 2003; 11:197–204

55. Fernandez-Rodriguez CM, Gutierrez ML, Serrano PL et al. Factors influencing the rate of fibrosis progression in chronic hepatitis C. Dig Dis Sci, 2004; 49:1971–1976

56. Vong S, Bell BP. Chronic liver disease mortality in the United States, 1990–1998. Hepatology, 2004; 39:476–483

57. Ogose T, Watanabe T, Suzuya H et al. Autoimmune hepatitis following allogeneic PBSCT from an HLA-matched sibling. Bone Marrow Transplant, 2003; 31:829–832

58. Vergani D, Mieli-Vergani G. Mechanisms of autoimmune hepatitis. Pediatr Transplant, 2004; 8:589–593

59. Kerkar N, Duban C, Rumbo C et al. Rapamycin successfully treats post-transplant autoimmune hepatitis. Am J Transplant, 2005; 5:1085–1089

60. Firpi RJ, Abdelmalek MF, Soldevila-Pico C et al. One-year protocol liver biopsy can stratify fibrosis progression in liver transplant recipients with recurrent hepatitis C infection. Liver Transpl, 2004; 10:1240–1247

61. Neumann UP, Bert T, Bahra M et al. Fibrosis progression after liver transplantation in patients with recurrent hepatitis C. J Hepatol, 2004; 41:830–836

62. Regev A, Molina E, Moura R et al. Reliability of histopathologic assessment for the differentiation of recurrent hepatitis C from acute cell rejection after liver transplantation. Liver Transpl, 2004; 10:1233–1239

63. Rifai K, Sebagh M, Karam V et al. Donor age influences 10-year liver graft histology independently of hepatitis C virus infection. J Hepatol, 2004; 41:446–453

64. Sebach M, Samuel D. Place of the liver biopsy in liver transplantation. J Hepatol, 2004; 41:897–901

65. Shiffman ML, Stravitz RT, Contos MJ et al. Histologic recurrence of chronic hepatitis C virus in patients after living donor and deceased donor liver transplantation. Liver Transpl, 2004; 10:1248–1255

66. Yu YY, Ji J, Zhou GW et al. Liver biopsy in evaluation of complications following liver transplantation. World J Gastroenterol, 2004; 10:1678–1681

67. Abrams GA, Kunde SS, Lazenby AJ, Clements RH. Portal fibrosis and hepatic steatosis in morbidly obese subjects: a spectrum of nonalcoholic fatty liver disease. Hepatology, 2004; 40:475–483

68. Brunt EM, Neuschwander-Tetri BA, Oliver D, Wehrmeier KR, Bacon BR. Nonalcoholic steatohepatitis: histologic features and clinical correlations with 30 blinded biopsy specimens. Hum Pathol, 2004; 35:1070–1082

69. Contos MJ, Choudhury J, Mills AS, Sanyal AJ. The histologic spectrum of nonalcoholic fatty liver diseases. Clin Liver Dis, 2004; 8:481–500

70. Dixon JB, Bhathal PS, Hughes NR, O'Brien PE. Nonalcoholic fatty liver disease: improvement in liver histological analysis with weight loss. Hepatology, 2004; 39:1647–1654

71. Fassio E, Alvarez E, Dominguez N, Landeira G, Longo C. Natural history of nonalcoholic steatohepatitis: a longitudinal study of repeat liver biopsies. Hepatology, 2004; 40:820–826

72. Hubscher SG. Role of liver biopsy in the assessment of non-alcoholic fatty liver disease. Eur J Gastroenterol Hepatol, 2004; 16:1107–1115

73. Papadia FS, Marinari GM, Camerini G et al. Liver damage in severely obese patients: a clinical-biochemical-morphologic study on 1000 liver biopsies. Obes Surg, 2004; 14:952–958

74. Shalhub S, Parsee A, Gallagher SF et al. The importance of routine liver biopsy in diagnosing nonalcoholic steatohepatitis in bariatric patients. Obes Surg, 2004; 14:54–59

75. Sorrentino P, Tarantino G, Conca P et al. Silent non-alcoholic fatty liver disease—a clinical-histologic study. J Hepatol, 2004; 41:751–757

76. Ayoub WS, Geller SA, Tran T et al. Imatinib (Gleevec)-induced hepatotoxicity. J Clin Gastroenterol, 2005; 39:75–77

77. Fernandes NF, Geller SA, Fong TL. Terbinafine hepatotoxicity: case report and review of the literature. Am J Gastroenterol, 1998; 93:459–460

78. Geller SA, Dubinsky MC, Poordad FF et al. Early hepatic nodular hyperplasia and submicroscopic fibrosis associated with 6-thioguanine therapy in inflammatory bowel disease. Am J Surg Pathol, 2004; 28:1204–1211

79. Kamal MA, French SW. Drug-induced increased mitochondrial biogenesis in a liver biopsy. Exp Mol Pathol, 2004; 77:201–204

80. Kremer JM, Lee RG, Tolman KG. Liver histology in rheumatoid arthritis patients receiving long-term methotrexate therapy: a prospective study with baseline and sequential biopsy samples. Arthritis Rheum, 1989; 32:121–127

81. Kremer JM, Kaye GI, Ishak KG et al. Light and electron microscopic analysis of sequential liver biopsy samples from rheumatoid arthritis patients receiving long-term methotrexate therapy. Arthritis Rheum, 1995; 38:1194–2003

82. Ros S, Juanola X, Condom E et al. Light and electron microscopic analysis of liver biopsy samples from rheumatoid arthritis patients receiving long-term methotrexate therapy. Scand J Rheumatol, 2002; 31:330–336

83. Alvarez DF, Latorre JS. Hepatitis C virus and HIV coinfection: clinical management and new strategies. AIDS Read, 2004; 14: S16–S21

84. Anderson KB, Guest JL, Rimland D. Hepatitis C virus coinfection increases mortality in HIV-infected patients in the highly active antiretroviral therapy era: data from the HIV Atlanta VA Cohort Study. Clin Infect Dis 2004; 39:1507–1513

85. Cooper CL. Natural history of HIV and HCV coinfection. J Int Assoc Physicians AIDS Care, 2003; 2:147–151

86. Lewden C, Salmon D, Moriat P et al. Causes of death among human immunodeficiency virus (HIV)-infected adults in the era of potent antiretroviral therapy: emerging role of hepatitis and cancers, persistent role of AIDS. Int J Epidemiol, 2005; 34:121–130

87. Dorruci M, Valdarchi C, Suligoi B et al. The effect of hepatitis C on progression to AIDS before and after highly active retroviral therapy. AIDS, 2004; 18:2313–2318

88. Rockstroh JK, Spengler U. HIV and hepatitis C virus co-infection. Lancet Infect Dis, 2004; 4:437–444

89. Soto B, Sanchez-Quijano A, Rodrigo L et al. HIV infection modifies the natural history of chronic parenterally acquired hepatitis C with an unusually rapid progression to cirrhosis. A multicenter study on 547 patients. J Hepatol, 1997; 26:1–5

90. Verucchi G, Calza L, Manfredi R, Chiodo F. Human immunodeficiency virus and hepatitis C virus coinfection: epidemiology, natural history, therapeutic options and clinical management. Infection, 2004; 32:33–46

91. Neff GW, Bonham A, Tzakis AG et al. Orthotopic liver transplantation in patients with human immunodeficiency virus and end-stage liver disease. Liver Transpl, 2003; 9:239–247

92. Yoo TW, Donfield S, Lail A et al. Effect of hepatitis C virus (HCV) genotype on HCV and HIV-1 diseases. J Infect Dis, 2005; 191:4–10

93. van Asten L, Prins M. Infection with concurrent multiple hepatitis C virus genotypes is associated with faster HIV disease progression. AIDS, 2004; 18:2319–2324

94. Sulkowski MS. Hepatotoxicity associated with antiretroviral therapy containing HIV-1 protease inhibitors. Semin Liver Dis, 2003; 23:183–194

95. Tossing G. Treating hepatitis C in HIV-HCV coinfected patients. Infection, 2002; 30:329–331

96. Chen NL, Bai L, Li L et al. Apoptosis pathway of liver cells in chronic hepatitis. World J Gastroenterol, 2004; 10:3201–3204

97. Cogger VC, Muller M, Fraser R et al. The effects of oxidative stress on the liver sieve. J Hepatol, 2004; 41:370–376

98. Enomoto K, Nishikawa Y, Omori Y et al. Cell biology and pathology of liver sinusoid endothelial cells. Med Electron Microsc, 2004; 208–215

99. Le TH, Caldwell SH, Redick JA et al. The zonal distribution of megamitochondria with crystalline inclusions in nonalcoholic steatohepatitis. Hepatology, 2004; 39:1423–1429

100. Roskams TA, Theise ND, Balabaud C et al. Nomenclature of the finer branches of the biliary tree: canals, ductules, and ductular reactions in human livers. Hepatology, 2004; 39:1739–1745

101. Wilasrusmee C, Sirtheptawee S, Kanchanapanjapon S et al. Ultrastructural changes in cirrhotic and noncirrhotic patients due to hepatectomy. J Hepatobiliary Pancreat Surg, 2004; 11:266–271

102. Tran TT, Changsri C, Shackleton CS et al. Living donor liver transplantation: histologic abnormalities found on liver biopsies of apparently healthy potential donors. J Gastroenterol Hepatol, 2005; in press

103. Hegarty JE, Williams R. Liver biopsy: techniques, clinical applications, and complications. Br Med J, 1984; 288:1254–1256

104. Isler RJ, Ferucci JT, Wittenberg J et al. Tissue core biopsy of abdominal tumors with a 22 gauge cutting needle. AJR Am J Roentgenol, 1981; 136:725–728

105. Bell DA, Carr CR, Szyfelbein WM 1986. Fine needle aspiration cytology of focal liver lesions. Results obtained with examination of both cytologic and histologic preparations. Acta Cytopathol, 1986; 30:397–402

106. Longchampt E, Patriarche C, Fabre M. Accuracy of cytology vs. microbiopsy for the diagnosis of well-differentiated hepatocellular carcinoma and macroregenerative nodule. Definition of standardized criteria from a study of 100 cases. Acta Cytol, 2000; 44:515–523

107. Franca AV, Valerio HM, Trevisan M et al. Fine needle aspiration biopsy for improving the diagnostic accuracy of cut needle biopsy of focal liver lesions. Acta Cytol, 2003; 47:332–336

108. Zainol H, Sumithran E. Combined cytological and histological diagnosis of hepatocellular carcinoma in ultrasonically guided fine needle biopsy specimens. Histopathology, 1993; 22:581–586

109. Maharaj B, Maharaj RJ, Leary WP et al. Sampling variability and its influence on the diagnostic yield of percutaneous needle biopsy of the liver. Lancet, 1986; 1:523–525

110. Perrault J, McGill DB, Ott BJ et al. Liver biopsy: complications in 1000 inpatients and outpatients. Gastroenterology, 1978; 74:103–106

111. Piccinino F, Sagnelli E, Pasquale G et al. Complications following percutaneous liver biopsy: a multicentre retrospective study of 68 276 biopsies. J Hepatol, 1986; 2:165–173

112. Van Thiel DH, Gavaler JS, Wright H et al. Liver biopsy, its safety and complications as seen at a liver transplant center. Transplantation, 1993; 55:1087–1090

113. Yu SCH, Lo DYM, Ip CB et al. Does percutaneous liver biopsy of hepatocellular carcinoma cause hematogenous dissemination? An in vivo study with quantitative assay of circulating tumor DNA using methylation-specific real-time polymerase chain reaction. AJR Am J Roentgenol, 2004; 183:383–385

114. Takamori R, Wong LL, Dang C et al. Needle-tract implantation from hepatocellular cancer: is needle biopsy of the liver always necessary? Liver Transplant, 2000; 6:67–72

115. Smith EH. Complications of percutaneous abdominal fine-needle biopsy. Review. Radiology, 1991; 178:253–258

116. Chapoutot C, Perney P, Fabre D et al. Essaimages tumoraux sur le trajet de ponctions echo-guidées de carcinomas hepatocellulaires. Etude de 150 malades. Gastroenterol Clin Biol, 1999; 23:552–556

117. Kim SH, Lim HK, Lee WJ, Cho JM, Jang HJ. Needle-tract implantation in hepatocellular carcinoma: frequency and CT findings after biopsy with 19.5-gauge automated biopsy gun. Abdom Imaging, 2000; 25:246–250

118. Metcalfe MS, Bridgewater FH, Mullin EJ, Maddern GJ. Useless and dangerous–fine needle aspiration of hepatic colorectal metastases. BMJ, 2004; 328(7438):507–508

119. Clayton RA, Clarker DL, Currie EJ et al. Incidence of benign pathology in patients undergoing hepatic resection for suspected malignancy. Surgeon, 2003; 1:32–38

120. Petrelli M, Scheuer PJ. Variation in subcapsular liver structure and its significance in the interpretation of wedge biopsies. J Clin Pathol, 1967; 20:743–748

121. Corr P, Bennington SJ, Davey N. Transjugular liver biopsy: a review of 200 biopsies. Clin Radiol, 1992; 45:238–239

122. Whitlach S, Nunez C, Pitlik DA. Fine needle aspiration biopsy of the liver; a study of 102 consecutive cases. Acta Cytopathol, 1984; 28:719–725

123. Suen KC. Diagnosis of primary hepatic neoplasm by fine needle aspiration biopsy cytology. Diagn Cytopathol, 1986; 2:99–109

124. Welch TJ, Sheedy PF, Johnson CD et al. CT guided biopsy: prospective analysis of 1000 procedures. Radiology, 1989; 171:493–496

125. Pisharodi ZLR, Lavoie R, Bedrossian CWM. Differential diagnostic dilemmas in malignant fine needle aspirates of liver: a practical approach to final diagnosis. Diagn Cytopathol, 1995; 12:364–371

126. Bergman S, Grame-Cook P, Pitman MB. The usefulness of the reticulin stain in the differential diagnosis of liver nodules on fine needle aspiration biopsy cell block preparations. Mod Pathol, 1997; 10:1–7

127. Bret PM, Fond A, Casola G et al. Abdominal lesions: a prospective study of clinical efficacy of percutaneous fine-needle biopsy. Radiology, 1986; 159:345–346

128. Wiersema MJ, Kochman ML, Cramer HM et al. Endosonography-guided fine-needle aspiration biopsy. Gastrointestinal Endoscopy, 1994; 40:700–707

129. Giovanni M, Seitz JF, Monges G et al. Fine-needle aspiration cytology guided by endoscopic ultrasonography: results in 141 patients. Endoscopy, 1995; 27:171–177

130. Bentz JS, Kochman ML, Faigel DO et al. Endoscopic ultrasound-guided real-time fine-needle aspiration: clinicopathological features of 60 patients. Diagn Cytopathol, 1998; 18:98–109

131. Wittenberg J, Mueller PR, Ferrucci JT et al. Percutaneous core biopsy of abdominal tumors using 22 gauge needles: further observations. AJR A J Roentgenol, 1982; 139:75–80

132. Hollerbach S, Willert J, Topalidis T, Reiser M, Schmiegel W. Endoscopic ultrasound-guided fine-needle aspiration biopsy of liver lesions: histological and cytological assessment. Endoscopy, 2003; 35:743–749

133. Pilotti S, Rilke F, Claron R et al. Conclusive diagnosis of hepatic and pancreatic malignancies by fine needle aspiration. Acta Cytopathol, 1988; 32:27–38

134. Pinto PM, Avila NA, Heller CI, Criscuolo EM. Fine needle aspiration of the liver. Acta Cytopathol, 1988; 32:22–26

135. Fornari F, Buscarini L. Ultrasonically-guided fine-needle biopsy of gastrointestinal organs: indications, results and complications. Dig Dis, 1992; 10:121–133

136. Guo Z, Kurtycz DFI, Salem R, De Las Casas LE, Caya JG, Hoerl HD. Radiologically guided percutaneous fine-needle aspiration biopsy of the liver: retrospective study of 119 cases evaluating diagnostic effectiveness and clinical complications. Diagn Cytopathol, 2002; 26:283–289

137. Vergara V, Garripoli A, Marucci MM et al. Colon cancer seeding after percutaneous fine needle aspiration of liver metastasis. Hepatology, 1993; 18:276–278

138. Yamada N, Shinzawa H, Ukai K et al. Subcutaneous seeding of small hepatocellular carcinoma after fine needle aspiration biopsy. J Gastroenterol Hepatol, 1993; 8:195–198

139. Hamazaki K, Matsubara N, Mori M et al. Needle track implantation of hepatocellular carcinoma after ultrasonically guided needle liver biopsy: a case report. Hepatogastroenterology, 1995; 42:601–606

140. Ferrucci J, Wittenberg J, Mueller PR et al. Diagnosis of abdominal malignancy by radiologic fine-needle aspiration biopsy. AJR A J Roentgenol, 1980; 134:323–330

141. Martino CR, Haaga JR, Bryan PJ et al. CT-guided liver biopsies: eight years' experience. Radiology, 1984; 152:755–757

142. Buscarini L, Fornari F, Bolondi L et al. Ultrasound-guided fine-needle biopsy of focal liver lesions: techniques, diagnostic accuracy and complications. A retrospective study of 2091 biopsies. J Hepatol, 1980; 11:344–348

143. Chawla YK, Ramesh GN, Jaur U et al. Percutaneous liver biopsy: a safe outpatient procedure. J Gastroenterol Hepatol, 1990; 5:94–95

144. Fagelman D, Chess Q. Aspiration fine needle cytology of the liver: a new technique for obtaining diagnostic samples. AJR A J Roentgenol, 1990; 155:1217–1219

145. Hahn PF, Eisenberg PJ, Pitman MB et al. Cytopathologic touch preparations (imprints) from core needle biopsies: accuracy compared with that of fine needle aspirates. AJR Am J Roentgenol, 1995; 165:1277–1279

146. Tyrell L, Elias J, Longley J. Detection of specific mRNAs in routinely processed dermatopathology specimens. Am J Dermatopathol, 1995; 17:476–483

147. Benchekroun M, DeGraw J, Gao J et al. Impact of fixative on recovery of mRNA from paraffin-embedded tissue. Diagn Mol Pathol, 2004; 13:116–112

148. Takamura F, Inaba N, Miyoshi E et al. Optimization of liver biopsy RNA sampling and use of reference RNA for cDNA microarray analysis. Anal Biochem, 2005; 337:224–234

149. Chuaqui R, Cole K, Cuello M et al. Analysis of mRNA quality in freshly prepared and archival Papanicolaou samples. Acta Cytol, 1999; 43:831–836

150. Herbert DJ, Nishiyama RH, Bagwell CD et al. Effects of several commonly used fixatives on DNA and total nuclear protein analysis by flow cytometry. Am J Clin Pathol, 1989; 91:535–541

151. Desmet VJ. What more can we ask from the pathologist? J Hepatol, 1996; 25(Suppl 1):25–29.

152. Ludwig J, Moyer FP, Rakela J. The liver biopsy diagnosis in Wilson diseases; methods in pathology. Am J Clin Pathol, 1994; 102:443–446

153. Olynyk JK, O'Neill R, Britton RS, Bacon BR. Determination of hepatic iron concentration in fresh and paraffin-embedded tissue: diagnostic implications. Gastroenterology, 1994; 106:674–677

154. Pak HY, Yokota S, Teplitz RL et al. Rapid staining techniques employed in fine needle aspirations of the lung. Acta Cytopathol, 1981; 25:178–184

155. Miller DA, Carrasco CH, Katz RL et al. Fine needle aspiration biopsy: the role of immediate cytologic assessment. AJR Am J Roentgenol, 1986; 147:155–158

156. Austin JHM, Cohen MB. Value of having a cytopathologist present during percutaneous fine-needle aspiration of lung: report of 55 cancer patients and metaanalysis of the literature. AJR Am J Roentgenol 1993; 160:175–177

157. Yang GCH. Ultrafast Papanicolaou stain is not limited to rapid assessments: applications to permanent fine-needle aspiration smears. Diagn Cytopathol, 1995; 13:160–162

158. Persing DH, Smith TF, Tenover FC, White TJ (eds). Diagnostic Molecular Microbiology: Principles and Applications. Washington, D.C.: American Society of Microbiology, 1993

159. Byers R, Roebuck J, Sakhinia E, Hoyland J. PolyA PCR amplification of cDNA from RNA extracted from formalin-fixed paraffin-embedded tissue. Diagn Mol Pathol, 2004; 13:144–150

160. Crawford AR, Lin XZ, Crawford JM. The normal adult human liver biopsy: a qualitative reference standard. Hepatology, 1998; 28:323–331

161. Crawford JM. Development of the Intrahepatic biliary tree. Semin Liv Dis, 2002; 22:213–226

162. Awasthi A, Das A, Srinivisan R, Joshi K. Morphological and immunohistochemical analysis of ductal plate malformation: correlation with fetal liver. Histopathology, 2004; 45:260–267

163. Wilson SAK. Progressive lenticular degeneration: a familial disease associated with cirrhosis of the liver. Brain, 1912; 34:295–507

164. Pilgaard J, Fenger C, Schaffalitzky de Muckadell OB. Globular amyloid deposits in the liver. Histopathology, 1993; 23:479–480

165. Fallon MB, Boyer JL. Hepatic toxicity of vitamin A and synthetic retinoids. J Gastroenterol Hepatol, 1990; 5:334–342

166. Tao LC, Ho CS, McLoughlin MJ et al. Cytologic diagnosis of hepatocellular carcinoma by fine needle aspiration biopsy. Cancer, 1984; 53:547–552

167. Cohen MB, Haber MM, Holly EA et al. Cytologic criteria to distinguish hepatocellular carcinoma from nonneoplastic liver. Am J Clin Pathol, 1991; 95:125–130

168. Kung ITM, Chan SK, Fung KH. Fine needle aspiration in hepatocellular carcinoma: combined cytologic and histologic approach. Cancer, 1991; 67:673–680, 1694

169. Noguchi S, Yamamoto R, Tatsuta M et al. Cell features and patterns in fine needle aspirates of hepatocellular carcinomas. Cancer, 1986; 58:321–328

170. Bianchi L. Liver biopsy interpretation in hepatitis. Part I: Presentation of critical morphological features used in diagnosis (glossary). Pathol Res Pract, 1983; 78:2–19

171. Gerber MA, Thung SN: Histology of the liver. Am J Surg Pathol, 1987; 11:709–722

172. Petrovic LM. Benign hepatocellular tumors and tumor-like lesions. In: Ferrell LD, ed, Pathology: state of the art reviews, Philadelphia: Hanley & Belfus, 1994; pp 161–185

173. Scheuer PJ. General considerations. In: Scheuer PJ, Lefkowitch JH, eds: Liver biopsy interpretation. Fifth edn. London: WB Saunders Company Ltd, 1994; pp 1–10

174. Snover DC. Technical aspects of the evaluation of liver biopsies. In: Snover DC, Biopsy diagnosis of liver disease. Baltimore: Williams & Wilkins, 1992; pp 2–23

175. Gagliano EF. Reticulin stain in the fine needle aspiration differential diagnosis of liver nodules. Acta Cytopathol, 1995; 39:596–598

176. Bonkovsky HL, Poh-Fitzpatrick M, Pimstone N et al. Porphyria cutanea tarda, hepatitis C, and HFE gene mutations in North American Hepatology, 1998; 27:1661–1669

177. Elder GH. Porphyria cutanea tarda. Semin Liver Dis,1998; 18:67–75

178. Emanuele P, Goodman ZD. A simple and rapid stain for copper in liver tissue. Ann Diagn Pathol, 1998; 2:125–126

179. Lau SK, Prakash S, Geller SA, Alsabeh R. Comparative immunohistochemical profile of hepatocellular carcinoma, cholangiocarcinoma, and metastatic adenocarcinoma. Hum Pathol, 2002; 33:1175–1181

180. Taylor CR, Shi S-R, Barr NJ, Wu N. Techniques of Immunohistochemistry: principles, pitfalls, and standardization. In: Dabbs D (ed), Diagnostic Immunohistochemistry. New York: Churchill Livingstone, 2002; pp 3–43

181. Raab SS. Cost-effectiveness of Immunohistochemistry. In: Dabbs D (ed), Diagnostic Immunohistochemistry. New York: Churchill Livingstone, 2002; pp 45–55

182. Verslype C, Nevens F, Sinelli N et al. Hepatic immunohistochemical staining with a monoclonal antibody against HCV-E2 to evaluate antiviral therapy and reinfection of liver grafts in hepatitis C viral infection. J Hepatol, 2003; 38:208–214

183. Shiha GE, Zalata KR, Abdalla AF, Mohamed MK. Immunohistochemical identification of HCV target antigen in paraffin-embedded liver tissue: reproducibility and staining patterns. Liver Int, 2005; 25:254–260

184. Ohta M, Marceau N, Perry G et al. Ubiquitin is present on the cytokeratin intermediate filaments and Mallory bodies of hepatocytes. Lab Invest, 1988; 59:848–856

185. Cocjin J, Rosenthal P, Buslon V et al. Bile ductule formation in fetal, neonatal and infant livers compared with extrahepatic biliary atresia. Hepatology, 1996; 24:568–574

186. Shiojiri N. Development and differentiation of bile ducts in the mammalian liver. Micro Res Techn, 1997; 39:328–335

187. Van Eyken P, Sciot R, Paterson A et al. Cytokeratin expression in hepatocellular carcinoma: an immunohistochemical study. Hum Pathol, 1988; 19:562–568

188. Lai Y-S, Thung SN, Gerber MA, Chen M-L, Schaffner F. Expression of cytokeratins in normal and diseased livers and in primary liver carcinomas. Arch Pathol Lab Med, 1989; 113:134–138

189. Johnson DE, Powers CN, Rupp G, Frable WJ. Immunocytochemical staining of fine-needle aspiration biopsies of the liver as a diagnostic tool for hepatocellular carcinoma. Mod Pathol, 1992; 5:117–123

190. Thung SN, Gerber MA, Sarno E, Popper H. Distribution of 5 antigens in hepatocellular carcinoma. Lab Invest, 1979; 41:101–105

191. Bhan AK. Immunohistochemistry of neoplasia: diagnostic strategies on differentiation antigens. In RB Colvin, AK Bhan and RT McCluskey, eds. Diagnostic Immunopathology, 2nd edition, New York: Raven Press, 1995; pp 445–478

192. Berezowski K, Stastny JF, Kornstein MJ. Cytokeratins 7 and 20 and carcinoembryonic antigen in ovarian and colonic carcinoma. Mod Pathol, 1996; 9:426–429

193. Loy TS, Calaluce RD, Keeney GL. Cytokeratin immunostaining in differentiating primary ovarian carcinoma from metastatic colonic adenocarcinoma. Mod Pathol, 1996; 9:1040–1044

194. Maeda T, Kajiyama K, Adachi E et al. The expression of cytokeratins 7, 19, and 20 in primary and metastatic carcinomas of the liver. Mod Pathol, 1996; 9:901–909

195. Fucich LF, Cheles MK, Thung SN et al. Primary vs metastatic hepatic carcinoma. An immunohistochemical study of 34 cases. Arch Pathol Lab Med, 1994; 118:927–930

196. Minervini MI, Demetris AJ, Lee RG et al. Utilization of hepatocyte-specific antibody in the immunocytochemical evaluation of liver tumors. Mod Pathol, 1997; 10:686–692

197. Pitman MB, Triratanachat S, Young RH, Oliva E. Hepatocyte paraffin 1 antibody does not distinguish primary ovarian tumors with hepatoid differentiation from metastatic hepatocellular carcinoma. Int J Gynecol Pathol, 2004; 23:58–64

198. Kakar S, Muir T, Murphy LM, Lloyd RV, Burgart LJ. Immunoreactivity of Hep Par 1 in hepatic and extrahepatic tumors and its correlation with albumin in situ hybridization in hepatocellular carcinoma. Am J Clin Pathol, 2003; 119:361–366

199. Gottschalk-Sabag S, Ron N, Glick T. Use of CD34 and Factor VIII to diagnose hepatocellular carcinoma on fine needle aspirates. Acta Cytopathol, 1998; 42:691–696

200. Chen ZG, Crone KG, Watson MA et al. Identification of a gene expression signature that differentiates hepatocellular adenoma from well differentiated hepatocellular carcinoma. Mod Pathol, 2005; 18(Suppl 1):277A

201. Gabel CC, Ghoshal K, Majunder S et al. Demonstration of metallothionein in hepatocellular carcinomas and hepatocellular adenomas—a molecular and immunohistochemical analysis. Mod Pathol, 2005; 18(Suppl 1):278A

202. Wu HH, Tao L-C, Cramer H. Vimentin-positive spider-shaped Kupffer cells: A new clue to cytologic diagnosis of primary and metastatic hepatocellular carcinoma by fine needle aspiration biopsy. Am J Clin Pathol, 1986; 106:517–521

203. Hata K, Van Thiel DH, Herberman RB, Whiteside TL. Phenotypic and functional characteristics of lymphocytes isolated from liver biopsy specimens from patients with active liver disease. Hepatology, 1992; 15:816–823

204. Orsatti G, Thiese ND, Thung SN, Paronetto F. DNA image cytometric analysis of macroregenerative nodules (adenomatous hyperplasia) of the liver: evidence in support of their preneoplastic nature. Hepatology, 1993; 17:621–627

205. Erler BS, Hsu L, Truong HM, Petrovic L et al. Image analysis and diagnostic classification of hepatocellular carcinoma using neural networks and multivariate discriminant functions. Lab Invest, 1994; 71:446–451

206. Campo-Ruiz V, Lauwers GY, Anderson RR, Delgado-Baeza E, Gonzalez S. In vivo and ex vivo virtual biopsy of the liver with near-infrared, reflectance confocal microscopy. Mod Pathol, 2005; 18:290–300

207. Shackel NA, Gorrell MD, McCaughan GW. Gene array analysis and the liver. Hepatology, 2002; 36:1313–1325

208. Fan Z, van den Rijn M, Montgomery K, Rouse RV. Hep par 1 antibody stain for the differential diagnosis of hepatocellular carcinoma: 676 tumors tested using tissue microarrays and conventional tissue sections. Mod Pathol, 2003; 16:137–144

209. Petricoin EF, Zoon KC, Kahn EC et al. Clinical proteomics: translating benchside promise into bedside reality. Nature Rev (Proteomics Collection), September 2004; 20–30

210. Tannapfel A, Anhalt K, Hausermann P et al. Identification of novel proteins associated with hepatocellular carcinomas using protein microarrays. J Pathol, 2003; 201:238–249

211. Marsh JW, Finkelstein SD, Demetris AJ et al. Genotyping of hepatocellular carcinoma in liver transplant recipients adds predictive power for determining recurrence-free survival. Liver Transpl, 2003; 9:664–671

212. Nishida N, Nishimura T, Ito T et al. Chromosomal instability and human hepatocarcinogenesis. Histol Histopathol, 2003; 18:897–909

213. Ueki T, Fujimoto J, Suzuki T et al. Expression of hepatocyte growth factor and its receptor c-met proto-oncogene in hepatocellular carcinoma. Hepatology, 1997; 25:862–866

214. Kira S, Nakanishi T, Suemori S et al. Expression of transforming growth factor alpha and epidermal growth factor receptor in human hepatocellular carcinoma. Liver, 1997; 17:177–182

215. Ito N, Kawata S, Tamura S et al. Elevated levels of transforming growth factor beta messenger RNA and its polypeptide in human hepatocellular carcinoma. Cancer Res, 1991; 51:4080–4083

216. Peng SY, Lai Pl, Hsu HC. Amplification of the c-myc gene in human hepatocellular carcinoma: biologic significance. J Formos Med Assoc, 1993; 92:866–870

217. Honda K, Sbisa E, Tullo A et al. p53 mutation is a poor prognostic indicator for survival in patients with hepatocellular carcinoma undergoing surgical tumor ablation. Brit J Cancer, 1998; 77:776–782

218. Ashida K, Kishimoto Y, Nakamoto K et al. Loss of heterozygosity of the retinoblastoma gene in liver cirrhosis accompanying hepatocellular carcinoma. J Cancer Res Clin Oncol, 1997; 123:489–495

219. Hui AM, Sakamoto M, Kanai Y et al. Inactivation of p16[INK4] in hepatocellular carcinoma. Hepatology, 1996; 24:575–579

220. Qin LF, Ng IO. Expression of p27(KIP1) and p21 (WAF1/CIP1) in primary hepatocellular carcinoma: clinicopathologic correlation and survival analysis. Hum Pathol, 2001; 32:778–784

221. Kanai Y, Ushimjima S, Hui AM et al. Aberrant DNA methylation precedes loss of heterozygosity on chromosome 16 in chronic hepatitis and liver cirrhosis. Cancer Lett, 2000; 148:73–80

222. Paradis V, Bieche I, Dargere D et al. Molecular profiling of hepatocellular carcinomas (HCC) using a large-scale real-time RT-PCR approach: Determination of a molecular diagnostic index. Am J Pathol, 2003; 163:733–741

223. Aihara T, Noguchi S, Sasaki Y et al. Clonal analysis of precancerous lesion of hepatocellular carcinoma. Gastroenterology, 1996; 111:455–461

224. Gaffey, MJ, Iezzoni JC, Weiss LM. Clonal analysis of focal nodular hyperplasia of the liver. Am J Pathol, 1996; 148:1089–1096

225. Maggioni M, Coggi G, Cassani B et al. Molecular changes in hepatocellular dysplastic nodules on microdissected liver biopsies. Hepatology, 2000; 32:942–946

226. Lee D, Choi SW, Kim M et al. Discovery of differentially expressed genes related to histological subtype of hepatocellular carcinoma. Biotechnol Prog, 2003; 19:1011–1015

227. Kurokawa Y, Matoba R, Takemasa I et al. Molecular features of non-B, non-C hepatocellular carcinoma: a PCR-array gene expression profiling study. J Hepatol, 2003; 39:1004–1012

228. Ye Q, Qin L, Forgues M et al. Predicting hepatitis B virus-positive metastatic hepatocellular carcinomas using gene expression profiling and supervised machine learning. Nature Med, 2003; 9:416–423

229. Zhou XD. Recurrence and metastasis of hepatocellular carcinoma: progress and prospects. Hepatobil Panc Dis Int, 2002; 1:35–41

230. Pierce RH, Vail ME, Ralph L et al. Bcl-2 expression inhibits liver carcinogenesis and delays the development of proliferating foci. Am J Pathol, 2002; 160:1555–1561

231. Wang W, Yang LY, Huang GW et al. Genomic analysis reveals Rho C as a potential marker in hepatocellular carcinoma with poor prognosis. Br J Cancer, 2004; 90:2349–2355

232. Nagao M, Nakajima Y, Hisanaga M et al. The alteration of fas receptor and ligand system in hepatocellular carcinomas: How do hepatoma cells escape from the host immune surveillance in vivo? Hepatology, 1999; 30:413–421

233. Scharf JG, Braulke T. The role of the IGF axis in hepatocarcinogenesis. Hormone Metabol Res, 2003; 35:685–693

234. Isokawa O, Suda T, Aoyagi Y et al. Reduction of telomeric repeats as a possible predictor for development of hepatocellular carcinoma: convenient evaluation by slot-blot analysis. Hepatology, 1999; 30:408–412

235. Wang Y, Kato N, Hoshida Y et al. Interleukin-1β gene polymorphisms associated with hepatocellular carcinoma in hepatitis C virus infection. Hepatology, 2003; 37:65–71

236. Wang Y, Lau SH, Sham JS et al. Characterization of HBV integrants in 14 hepatocellular carcinomas: association of truncated X gene and hepatocellular carcinogenesis. Oncogene, 2004; 23:142–148

237. Pollicino T, Squadrito G, Cerenzia G et al. Hepatitis B virus maintains its pro-oncogenic properties in the case of occult HBV infection. Gastroenterology, 2004; 126:347–350

238. Iizuka N, Oka M, Yamada-Okabe H et al. Comparison of gene expression profiles between hepatitis B virus- and hepatitis C virus-infected hepatocellular carcinoma by oligonucleotide microarray data on the basis of a supervised learning method. Cancer Res, 2002; 62:3939–3944

239. Yerian LM, Anders RA, Tretiakova M et al. Caveolin and thrombospondin expression during hepatocellular carcinogenesis. Am J Surg Pathol, 2004; 28:357–364

240. Finegold MJ. Hepatic tumors in childhood. In Russo P, Ruchelli ED, and Piccoli DA (Eds), Pathology of Pediatric Gastrointestinal and Liver Disease, New York: Springer-Verlag, 2004; pp 300–346

241. Choo Q-L, Kuo G, Weiner AJ et al. Isolation of a cDNA clone derived from a blood-borne non-A, non-B viral hepatitis genome. Science, 1989; 244:359–362

242. http://www.amp.org

243. Lunel F, Cresta P, Vitour D et al. Comparative evaluation of hepatitis C virus RNA quantitation by branched DNA, NASBA, and monitor assays. Hepatology, 1999; 29:528–535

244. Schlaak JF, Trippler M, Ernst I et al. Chronic hepatitis C: the viral load per liver cell before treatment as a new marker to predict long-term response to IFN-a therapy. J Hepatol, 1997; 27:917–921

245. Hofer H, Watkins-Riedel T, Janata O et al. Spontaneous viral clearance in patients with acute hepatitis C can be predicted by repeated measurements of serum viral load. Hepatology, 2003; 37:60–64

246. Khan MH, Farrell GC, Byth K et al. Which patients with hepatitis C develop liver complications? Hepatology, 2000; 31:513–520

247. Eisen-Vandervelde AL, Yao, ZQ, Hahn YS. The molecular basis of HCV-mediated immune dysregulation. Clin Immunol, 2004; 111:16–21

248. Fiorilli M, Meucci C, Farci P et al. HCV-associated lymphomas. Rev Clin Exp Hematol, 2003; 7:406–423

249. Komurian-Pradel F, Perret M, Deiman B et al. Strand specific quantitative real-time PCR to study replication of hepatitis C virus genome. J Virol Meth, 2004; 116:103–106

250. Laskus T, Radkowski M, Jablonska J et al. Human immunodeficiency virus facilitates infection/replication of hepatitis C virus in native human macrophages. Blood, 2004; 103:3854–3859

251. Kao JH, Chen PJ, Lai MY, Chen DS. Hepatitis B virus genotypes and spontaneous hepatitis B e antigen seroconversion in Taiwanese hepatitis B carriers. J Med Virol, 2004; 72:363–369

252. Chen JD, Liu CJ, Lee PH et al. Hepatitis B genotypes correlate with tumor recurrence after curative resection of hepatocellular carcinoma. Clin Gastroenterol Hepatol, 2004; 2:64–71

253. Ohishi W and Chayama K. Rare quasispecies in the YMDD motif of hepatitis B virus detected by polymerase chain reaction with peptide nucleic acid clamping. Intervirol, 2003; 46:355–361

254. Strassburg CP, Vogel A, Manns MP. Autoimmunity and hepatitis C. Autoimmun Rev, 2003; 2:322–331

255. Alshak NS, Jiminez AM, Gedebou M et al. Epstein-Barr virus infection in liver transplant patients: correlation of histopathology and semiquantitative Epstein-Barr virus-DNA recovery using polymerase chain reaction. Hum Pathol, 1993; 24:1306–1312

256. Lones MA, Shintaku IP, Weiss LM et al. Post-transplant lymphoproliferative disorder in liver allograft biopsies: a comparison of three methods for the demonstration of Epstein-Barr virus. Hum Pathol, 1997; 28:533–539

257. Norin S, Kimby E, Ericzon BG et al. Posttransplant lymphoma a single-center experience of 5000 liver transplantations. Med Oncol, 2004; 21:273–284

258. Gao LH and Zheng SS. Cytomegalovirus and chronic allograft rejection in liver transplantation. World J Gastroenterol, 2004; 10:1857–1861

259. Pietrangelo A. Hereditary hemochromatosis—a new look at an old disease. New Engl J Med, 2004; 350:2383–2397

260. Online as Mendelian Inheritance in Man at http://www.ncbi.nlm.nih.gov/omim

261. Tsivkovskii R, Efremov RG, Lutsenko S. The role of the invariant His-1069 in folding and function of the Wilson disease protein, the human copper-transporting ATPase ATP7B. J Biol Chem, 2003; 278:13302–13308

262. Mohan D, Rolston R, Pal R et al. Microdissection genotyping of archival fixative treated tissue for Gaucher disease. Hum Pathol, 2004; 35:482–487

263. Phillips MJ, Purcell S, Patterson J, Valencia P. The Liver. An atlas and text of ultrastructural pathology. New York: Raven Press, 1987

264. Gregor GR, Geller SA, Walker G, Compomanes B. Coxsackie hepatitis in an adult, with ultrastructural demonstration of the virus. M Sinai J Med, 1975; 43:575–580

265. Xiao JC, Jin XL, Ruck P, Adam A, Kaiserling E. Hepatic progenitor cells in human liver cirrhosis: immunohistochemical, electron microscopic and immunofluorescence confocal microscopic findings. World J Gastroenterol, 2004; 10:1208–1211

266. Melling M, Karimian-Teherani D, Mostler S et al. 3-D morphological characterization of the liver parenchyma by atomic force microscopy and by scanning electron microscopy. Microsc Res Teach, 2004; 64:1–9

267. Chignard N, Beretta L. Proteomics for hepatocellular carcinoma marker discovery. Gastroenterology, 2004; 127(5 Suppl 1): S120–S125

268. Marko-Varga G, Berglund M, Malmstrom J, Lindberg H, Fehniger TE. Targeting hepatocytes from liver tissue by laser capture microdissection and proteomics expression profiling. Electrophoresis, 2003; 24:3800–3805

269. Kasinathan C, Vrana K, Beretta L et al. The future of proteomics in the study of alcoholism. Alcohol Clin Exp Res, 2004; 28:228–232

270. Zeindl-Eberhart E, Haraida S, Liebmann S et al. Detection and identification of tumor-associated protein variants in human hepatocellular carcinomas. Hepatology, 2004; 39:540–549

271. Hanash S. Building a foundation for the human proteome: the role of the Human Proteome Organization. J Proteome Res, 2004; 3:197–199

272. Meneses-Lorente G, Gues PC, Lawrence J et al. A proteomic investigation of drug-induced steatosis in rat liver. Chem Res Toxicol, 2004; 17:605–612

273. Yokoyama Y, Kuramitsu Y, Takashima M et al. Proteomic profiling of proteins decreased in hepatocellular carcinoma from patients infected with hepatitis C virus. Proteomics, 2004; 4:2111–2116

274. Cui JF, Liu YK, Pan BS et al. Differential proteomic analysis of human hepatocellular carcinoma cell line metastasis-associated proteins. J Cancer Res Clin Oncol, 2004; 130:615–622

275. Yan W, Lee H, Deutsch EW et al. A dataset of human liver proteins identified by protein profiling via isotope-coded affinity tag (ICAT) and tandem mass spectrometry. Mol Cell Proteomics, 2004; 3:1039–1041

276. Yokoo H, Kondo T, Fujii K et al. Proteomic signature corresponding to alpha fetoprotein expression in liver cancer cells. Hepatology, 2004; 40:609–617

277. Poon TC, Hui AY, Chan HL et al. Prediction of liver fibrosis and cirrhosis in chronic hepatitis B infection by serum proteomic fingerprinting: a pilot study. Clin Chem, 2005; 51:328–335

278. Schwegler EE, Cazares L, Steel LF et al. SELDI-TOF MS profiling of serum for detection of the progression of chronic hepatitis C to hepatocellular carcinoma. Hepatology, 2005; 41:634–642

279. Gloghini A, Canal B, Klein U et al. RT-PCR analysis of RNA extracted from Bouin-fixed and paraffin-embedded lymphoid tissues. J Mol Diag, 2004; 6:290–296

280. Torbenson M, Wang J, Nichols L et al. Causes of death in autopsied liver transplantation patients. Mod Pathol, 1998; 11:37–46

281. Shojania KG, Burton EC, McDonald KM, Goldman L. The Autopsy as an Outcome and Performance Measure. Evidence Report/Technology Assessment no. 58 (Prepared by the University of California at San Francisco-Stanford Evidence-based Practice Center under Contract No. 290-97-0013. AHRQ Publication No. 03-E002.) Rockville, MD: Agency for Healthcare Research and Quality; October 2002

282. Burton EC. The autopsy in performance improvement. Pathol Int, 2004; 54(Suppl. 1): S5–S9

Developmental abnormalities and liver disease in childhood

4

Bernard C. Portmann   Eve A. Roberts

Anatomical anomalies

Agenesis of liver

This condition is incompatible with life. It has been reported in stillborn fetuses, usually in association with other severe anomalies.[1]

Absence (agenesis) of a lobe of the liver

Absence of the left lobe has been described,[2] in one case associated with floating gallbladder.[3] Radin et al. collected 19 cases of absence of the right lobe from the literature.[4] The anomaly was associated with biliary tract disease in 12 patients, portal hypertension in 7 patients, other congenital anomalies in 4 patients, but was an incidental finding in five patients. Inoue et al.[5] reported a case of hypogenesis of the right hepatic lobe associated with portal hypertension and reviewed 31 other cases of agenesis or hypogenesis in the Japanese literature.

Hypoplasia of the right lobe

This rare anomaly has been associated with suprahepatic[6] or retrohepatic[7] gallbladder, the latter complicated by hepatolithiasis and liver abscess.

Anomalies of position

In *situs inversus totalis* or *abdominalis,* the liver is found in the left hypochondrium, with the falciform ligament coursing from the left anterior margin towards the umbilicus. Hepatolithiasis has been reported in a patient with situs inversus.[8] Adenocarcinoma of the distal common bile duct was reported in a 68-year-old woman with total situs inversus.[9] A liver in a left or transverse position is one of the anomalies which may be associated with extrahepatic biliary atresia.[10]

Varying amounts of hepatic tissue may be displaced into congenital diaphragmatic hernias or omphalocoeles. Hepatic tissue was present in 3 of the 19 omphalocoeles studied by Soper and Green.[11] The liver tissue may be the seat of non-parasitic cysts[12] and may be detached from the rest of the liver.[13] Several cases of *hepatic herniation* through defects in the diaphragm have been reported.[14–16] A unique case of a supradiaphragmatic right liver lobe and gallbladder has been reported.[17] Partial eventration of the right hemidiaphragm is a congenital lesion caused by aplasia or hypoplasia of part of the musculature of the diaphragm with resultant bulging of the affected portion from intra-abdominal pressure.[18] The underlying portion of the liver prolapses into the diaphragmatic pouch where it may become strangulated.

Accessory lobes

Riedel lobe is a tongue-like caudal projection from the right lobe of the liver, which may be palpated in the right upper quadrant. In the 31 cases of Reitemeier et al.[19] all the patients except one were women, their ages ranging from 31 to 77 years. Supernumerary lobes are relatively frequent findings, particularly on the inferior surface of the liver. They are connected to the liver by hepatic tissue or by a mesentery containing branches of the portal vein, hepatic vein and hepatic artery, and a bile duct.[20] Intrathoracic accessory lobes, with their vascular supply perforating the diaphragm, have been reported.[21] Accessory lobes may rarely require surgical intervention because of their large size, torsion of a pedicle, or the presence of other associated defects.[22] Pedunculated hepatocellular carcinoma may arise in accessory lobes.

Ectopic hepatic tissue

Ectopic hepatic tissue may be found in the suspensory ligaments of the liver, lung, wall of the gallbladder, splenic capsule, retroperitoneal space, adrenal gland and greater omentum.[23–29] A unique case of ectopic liver in the placenta was reported by Willis.[30] In most instances the hepatic tissue in these ectopic sites is microscopically normal, but when the liver is abnormal (fatty change, chronic hepatitis, cirrhosis) the ectopic liver tissue reflects the same changes.[31,32] Infantile haemangioendothelioma arising in an ectopic intrathoracic liver has been reported.[24] Twenty-three cases of hepatocellular carcinoma, mostly from Japan, have arisen in ectopic livers.[32,33]

Heterotopias of the liver

Most of the so-called adrenal heterotopias are actually examples of *adrenal-hepatic fusion*. Dolan and Janovski made a distinction between 'adhesion' and 'fusion' on the basis of presence or absence of a capsule interposed between the two organs.[34] In both types there was a marked diminution or complete absence of medullary tissue. The fusion is unilateral and is not associated with clinical evidence of adrenal impairment. It was found in 9.9% of unselected autopsy cases in one study.[35] The incidence was much higher in older age groups suggesting that the condition may be an aging phenomenon. There is a single description of hepatolienal fusion.[36]

Pancreatic heterotopias in the liver are rare (Fig. 4.1). In the case reported by Ballinger,[37] an islet cell carcinoma arose in the aberrant pancreatic tissue. Retention cyst has been recorded in an obstructed duct within the heterotopic pancreatic tissue.[38] Foci of exocrine pancreas in the liver of a 41-year-old patient with cirrhosis were attributed to a metaplastic process.[39] Pancreatic acini were found intermingled with peribiliary glandular acini in 4% of autopsy livers, probably representing an intrinsic component of these glands.[40] *Splenic heterotopia* presenting as a mass lesion was reported by Lacerda et al.[41] *Thyroid heterotopia* has been occasionally encountered (Fig. 4.2) and has been reported in a fetus with trisomy 18.[42]

Vascular anomalies

Hepatic artery

Aberrant hepatic arteries occur in a significant proportion of individuals.[43] *Anomalous origin of the hepatic artery* has been described in association with extrahepatic biliary atresia.[44] Congenital duplication of the gallbladder has been reported

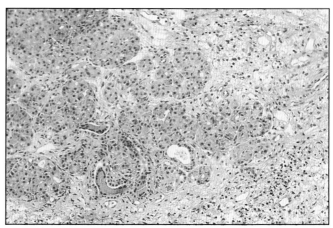

Fig. 4.1 • Pancreatic heterotopia. Pancreatic acini and several small ducts are present but there are no islets of Langerhans. H&E.

Fig. 4.2 • Thyroid heterotopia. Section of nodule in liver **(A)** that is composed microscopically of thyroid acini. H&E **(B)**.

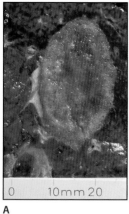

A

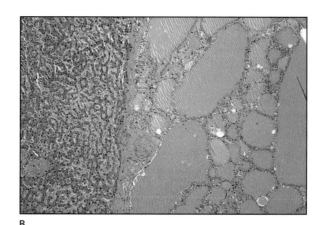

B

in association with an anomalous right hepatic artery.[45] Accessory right hepatic artery (arising from the left and passing behind the portal vein bifurcation) must be recognized and appropriately managed during split liver transplantation, in order to ensure a complete vascular supply to both grafts.[46] Rupture of an aberrant hepatic artery can occur rarely.[47] Congenital hepatoportal arteriovenous fistulas have been reported in infants.[48–50] Surgical correction or embolization using a variety of materials has been followed by reversal of the haemodynamic complications.[50,51]

Portal vein

Anatomical variations of the portal vein are almost as common as those of the hepatic artery, and their recognition is important to radiologists and transplant surgeons.[52] *Preduodenal portal vein* is the result of a variation in the normal developmental pattern of the embryonic precursors of the portal vein, i.e. the right and left vitelline veins and their three anastomotic channels. It may lead to duodenal obstruction[53] and this anomaly was the apparent cause of gastric outlet obstruction in an adult.[54] A vascular complex consisting of absent inferior vena cava, anomalous origin of the hepatic artery and preduodenal portal vein was reported in three children with extrahepatic biliary atresia.[55]

Obstructing valves within the lumen of the splenic vein, the portal vein, or both, may be a rare cause of portal hypertension in children.[56]

A case of *reduplication of the portal vein* was reported by Hsia and Gellis;[56] one branch ran anterior to the pancreas and was obliterated by an old organized thrombus.

Atresia or hypoplasia of the portal vein has been recognized by a number of investigators.[57,58] It may involve the entire length of the vessel or be limited to the point of entrance into the liver, or it may occur just proximal to the division into two branches. Microscopic study of the atretic segments has generally shown no evidence of inflammation.

Congenital absence of the portal vein is rare and is diagnosed mainly in children, although a few cases in adults are reported.[59–62] Cardiac and inferior vena caval anomalies and polysplenia may occur simultaneously. The patient of Marois et al. had an associated hepatoblastoma.[63] Focal nodular hyperplasia,[64] hyperplastic nodules[65] and nodular regenerative hyperplasia[66] have all been reported in association with congenital absence of the portal vein. Another patient presented with hepatopulmonary syndrome.[67] Liver tranplantation is technically possible though more difficult.[68]

Congenital shunts (portocaval, portohepatic and between the left portal vein and internal mammary veins) have been reported.[69–76] Congenital portosystemic venous shunts (PSVS) may lead to hepatic encephalopathy. They can be intra- or extrahepatic. Persistence of the ductus venosus can lead to hypergalactosaemia without an enzyme deficiency in the newborn screen.[74] Patients may present with hepatic impairment associated with a severe steatosis, which is reversed by surgical closure.[75]

Uchino et al.[76] reviewed their experience with 51 cases of portosystemic shunts; 67% were intrahepatic. Twelve patients had hepatic encephalopathy, the frequency of which increased in individuals after 60 years of age. Seventy-five per cent of the newborns had hypergalactosaemia. Children with hepatic encephalopathy had shunt ratios over 60%; no encephalopathy occurred with a shunt ratio less than 30%. Haemangiomas were present in 10% of patients. Ten per cent of patients (all over the age of 20) had a portal vein aneurysm. Twenty per cent of patients had a patent ductus venosus and less than 10% had absence of the portal vein. The extrahepatic PSVS never closed spontaneously. The liver histopathology was usually characterized by steatosis or mild fibrosis. Five patients had hepatic atrophy, and three patients had focal nodular hyperplasia.

A congenital *aneurysmal malformation* of the extrahepatic portal vein was described by Thompson et al.[77] Another *aneurysm* of the left branch of the portal vein was diagnosed in utero by ultrasound examination.[78] An intrahepatic portal vein aneurysm communicating with the hepatic veins was reported by Ito et al.,[79] associated with intrahepatic haemangiomas and an intracranial arteriovenous malformation.

Cavernous transformation of the portal vein ('portal cavernoma') is a condition in which the vein is replaced by a spongy trabeculated venous lake with extension into the gastroduodenal ligament.[80–82] It is a major cause of portal hypertension and may account for as many as 30% of all children with bleeding oesophageal varices.[83] A thrombotic diathesis due to inherited abnormalities of anticoagulant proteins is very rarely a factor in the pathogenesis.[84] Haemorrhage is common but some children present with asymptomatic splenomegaly.[82] An early report of marked growth retardation in children with extrahepatic portal vein obstruction[85] has not been confirmed in subsequent studies.[86] Obstructive jaundice is an uncommon complication.[87–88] It was detected in 8 of 121 children presenting over a 14-year period with cavernous transformation and regressed after surgical decompression.[89] A study in 25 adults with portal cavernoma found that 25% had clinically significant features of biliary obstruction and nearly all patients had cholangiographic evidence of bile duct damage.[90] Pancytopenia of varying degrees occurs in the majority of cases.[91] Colour Doppler ultrasonography, computed tomography, or contrast enhanced magnetic resonance imaging[92,93] obviate the need for splenoportography or angiography. Percutaneous or open liver biopsy specimens are either normal or show minimal fibrosis. Klemperer[80] reported multiple 'adenomas', but the description of the nodules and their designation as 'regenerative formations' suggest that the condition was nodular regenerative hyperplasia.

Two theories have been proposed for the pathogenesis of cavernous transformation, namely a sequel to portal vein thrombosis due to omphalitis, umbilical vein catheterization or intra-abdominal sepsis, or an angiomatous malformation of the portal vein;[94] however, the latter is not supported by hard data and in most instances thrombotic occlusion and recanalization of the vein appears the likely cause. Experimental evidence in support of occlusion of the portal vein and the subsequent opening up of adjacent collateral vessels has been reported by Williams and Johnston.[95]

In a prospective ultrasonographic evaluation of neonates undergoing umbilical catheterization, portal vein thrombosis was detected in 56% of the patients of whom 20% went on to partial or complete resolution.[96] Although not all cases of cavernous transformation have a history of umbilical catheterization, such a procedure, especially when it is prolonged, seems to account for a significant number of cases. Conversely, congenital abnormalities, in particular atrial septal defects, malformations of the biliary tract, and anomalous inferior vena cava, have been observed in 12 of 30 cases studied by Odièvre et al.[97] Several cases of cavernous transformation have also been found associated with congenital hepatic fibrosis.[98] It would appear that in some cases an anatomical anomaly of the portal vein may underpin the thrombotic process. The rapidly changing haemodynamics occurring during birth in regard to the portal circulation may play an additional role.

Hepatic veins

Membranous obstruction of the hepatic portion of the inferior vena cava, which may be associated with occlusion of hepatic veins, was thought to have a congenital aetiology,[99] but this has been disputed.[100,101] Kage et al. have demonstrated histological evidence of thrombus formation and occlusion of hepatic vein orifices in eight cases, suggesting an acquired rather than a congenital lesion.[101] Okuda et al. suggested that membranous obstruction of the vena cava be termed 'obliterative hepatocavopathy' to distinguish it from the classic Budd–Chiari syndrome.[102] The condition is most frequently reported from Japan and South Africa.[101–104] Patients present with the Budd–Chiari syndrome are prone to develop hepatocellular carcinoma.[103,104] Membranous obstruction of the vena cava occurs mainly in adults but a series of nine cases in children was reported from Namibia.[105] Rare instances of congenital Budd–Chiari syndrome, attributed to maternal drug abuse[106] or ingestion of herbal tea[107] or idiopathic,[108,109] have been reported. Veno-occlusive disease in children with cellular and humoral immune deficiency have also been described.[110] In the cases of Mellis and Bale consanguinity and early age of onset suggested an inherited cause for the veno-occlusive disease.[111]

Hereditary haemorrhagic telangiectasia (Osler–Rendu–Weber disease)

Hereditary haemorrhagic telangiectasia (HHT) is an autosomal dominant disorder characterized by an aberrant vascular development.[112,113] The resulting vascular lesions range from smaller mucocutaneous telangiectases to large visceral arteriovenous malformations. The estimated frequency ranges from 1 to 20 per 100 000.[113] Mutations in the genes encoding endoglin (ENG, chromosome 9q34), and activin receptor type-like kinase 1 (ALK-1, chromosome 12q13)[114–116] (both of which mediate signaling by transforming growth factor-β ligands in vascular endothelial cells) are associated with HHT1 and HHT2 subtypes, respectively.[117] The disease is characterized by telangiectases (skin, mucous membranes), arteriovenous fistulas in the liver (30% of cases), lungs and central nervous system, and aneurysms. Hepatic involvement is characterized by pain in the right upper quadrant of the abdomen, and a large, sometimes pulsatile liver. High-output cardiac failure may result from arteriovenous shunting in the liver.[118,119] Portal hypertension and encephalopathy may occur.[120] Intrahepatic lithiasis is a rare complication.[121]

The hepatic lesions can be demonstrated by angiography[122] and colour Doppler ultrasound[123] and are readily visualized during laparoscopy.[124] Arterial embolization has been used successfully in treatment of the disease.[118,119,125] Liver transplantation[126,127] performed in a few patients has been shown to reverse the hyperdynamic circulatory state.

Macroscopically, the liver is nodular, fibrotic or rarely cirrhotic. Spider-like arrangements of minute blood vessels may be noted on the surface. Microscopically, three fibrovascular patterns were reported by Daly & Schiller.[128] One pattern comprises a honeycomb meshwork of dilated sinusoidal channels lined by endothelial cells set either directly upon hepatocyte cords or amid a loose fibrous stroma (Fig. 4.3(A)); the distribution of these foci was haphazard. A second pattern consists of tortuous thick-walled veins flanked by numerous wide-calibre arteries that coursed randomly through the parenchyma amid variable amounts of fibrous tissue. A third pattern is evident in the enlarged portal areas in which numerous dilated vessels (veins, arteries and lymphatics) showed prominently against a background of fibrous tissue (Fig. 4.3(B)). Regenerative nodules (nodular transformation) were described in the cases reported by Zelman[129] and Wanless and Gryfe.[130] One woman treated with ethinyl oestradiol, multiple blood transfusions and iron-dextran developed hepatocellular carcinoma.[131] A high prevalence of focal nodular hyperplasia has been detected by Doppler US in a recent study.[132] Blewitt et al.[133] described marked disruption of the hepatic architecture with hepatocyte necrosis and ischaemic bile duct injury in a patient with HHT and intra-abdominal sepsis. Mouse models have been reported for the two main genomic mutations with histological changes recapitulating those observed in man.[134,135]

Ataxia telangiectasia

This autosomal recessive disorder is characterized by cerebellar ataxia, oculocutaneous telangiectases, IgA and IgE deficiency, recurrent infections, and an increased incidence of cancer. Homozygotes have an incidence of cancer that is 100 times higher than that of unaffected age-matched subjects.[136] There is also an increased incidence (particularly breast cancer) in heterozygotes.[136] Mutations in ATM (ataxia telangiectasia, mutated), a protein kinase shown to be a crucial nexus for the cellular response to DNA double-stranded breaks, have been identified as the underlying cause of the disease.[137] Several cases of hepatocellular carcinoma[138] and two cases of veno-occlusive disease have been reported in patients with this disease.[139] Other hepatic involvement includes hepatitis with periportal fibrosis, telangiectases and cirrhosis.[139]

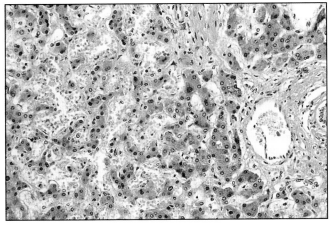

A

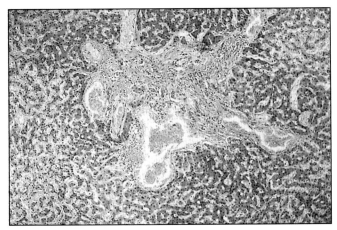

B

Fig. 4.3 • Hereditary haemorrhagic telangiectasia. **(A)** Dilated anastomosing sinusoidal channels, lined by endothelial cells with some subendothelial fibrous tissue. Masson trichrome. **(B)** Same case as (A) showing dilated vessels within a portal tract; foci of dilated sinusoidal vessels are also present (left and upper right). Masson trichrome.

von Hippel–Lindau disease

This autosomal dominant multisystemic cancer syndrome, due to a mutation of the VHL tumor suppressor gene on chromosome 3, rarely involves the liver.[140] Multiple cavernous haemangiomas were reported by Zeitlin,[141] and multiple 'haemangioblastomas' are described.[142,143] Occasionally, pancreatic cysts may lead to jaundice by obstruction of the common bile duct.[144]

Focal nodular hyperplasia

Wanless et al. have shown that focal nodular hyperplasia is a hyperplastic response of the hepatic parenchyma to a pre-existing arterial, spider-like malformation[145] (p. 637). Multiple focal nodular hyperplasia may be associated with haemangioma of the liver, meningioma, astrocytoma, telangiectases of the brain, berry aneurysm, dysplastic systemic arteries and portal vein atresia.[146] Wanless et al. proposed that this was a new syndrome resulting from underlying systemic abnormality of unknown nature.[146] Components of the syndrome (berry aneurysms, cerebral

telangiectases) have subsequently been reported in several patients who only had a solitary focal nodular hyperplasia.[147,148]

Bile-duct anomalies

Congenital abnormalities of the biliary tract are best demonstrated and studied by radiographic methods. In a series of 3845 operative cholangiograms, Puente and Bannura demonstrated anatomical variations (defined as those having no pathological significance) in 24% and congenital abnormalities (defined as pathologically significant deviations from the normal pattern) in 18.4%.[149] The latter included left-sided cystic duct (9.5%), aberrant hepatic ducts (4.6%) and accessory hepatic ducts (1.7%).

Agenesis of the common bile duct

In this very rare anomaly the common hepatic duct empties directly into the gallbladder, while the latter drains by a long cystic duct into the second part of the duodenum.[150]

Agenesis of the common hepatic duct

Three patients with this anomaly were reported by Stellin et al.[151] They presented with obstructive jaundice and at operation were found to have no proximal biliary tree. There were no ductal structures in the hepatic hilum.

Anomalous insertion of the right hepatic duct

Nomura et al. reported a case with this rare anomaly.[152] Cholangiography prior to laparoscopic cholecystectomy demonstrated insertion of the right hepatic duct into the cystic duct.

Anomalous ('accessory') bile ducts

These are found in about 15% of individuals when the bile ducts are dissected.[153] Anomalous hepatic ducts which pass beyond the porta hepatis almost invariably arise from the right lobe and frequently from a dorsal segment. The mode of termination is variable and final entry may be into the gallbladder, cystic duct, right or common hepatic duct, junction of the cystic and common hepatic ducts or even the common bile duct.[154] A rare case of an anomalous right posterior segmental hepatic duct associated with a stricture and hepatolithiases was reported by Cullingford et al.[155] Cholecystohepatic ducts are rare and occur when there is persistence of the fetal connections between the gallbladder and liver parenchyma, with failure of recanalization of the right and left hepatic ducts.[156] Two cases were reported in association with oesophageal atresia.[157] Failure to recognize the presence of cholecystohepatic ducts at cholecystectomy may lead to a persistent biliary fistula, bile peritonitis, stricture or death.[158] Cholangiography is mandatory whenever there is any doubt about the anatomy of the biliary tree in order to avoid the increased morbidity and mortality of reoperation.[159] Anomalous bile ducts may occur in association with biliary cystadenoma of the liver.[160] Two examples of a long accessory hepatic duct have been found among 23 cases of congenital dilatation of the common bile duct.[161] Atresia of the common hepatic duct with an accessory duct has been reported.[162] Accessory hepatic ducts may occasionally contain calculi.[163]

Duplication of the bile ducts

These lesions were reviewed by Swartley & Weeder.[164] One duct may empty into the pylorus or both may drain into the duodenum. In one case a choledochal cyst was associated.[164] Patients are usually free of symptoms until obstruction by stone or infection occurs. A case of congenital duplication involved the cystic duct and the common hepatic duct, which were both lined by gastric mucosa.[165]

Congenital bronchobiliary and tracheobiliary fistulas

Several cases of bronchobiliary and tracheobiliary fistula have been reported.[166] One patient had a bronchobiliary fistula, as well as a tracheo-oesophageal fistula and oesophageal atresia.[167] Another reported case had a bronchobiliary fistula with biliary atresia.[168] The bronchobiliary fistula typically arises from the proximal part of the right main stem bronchus, a short distance below the carina, and generally joins the biliary system at the level of the left hepatic duct. The proximal part of the fistula resembles a bronchus while the distal part is lined by columnar and/or squamous epithelium. Patients present in early infancy with aspiration pneumonia and atelectasis.

Ciliated hepatic foregut cyst

Some 60 cases of this rare cyst have been recently reviewed.[169] The cyst is generally found incidentally at laparotomy or by imaging studies. It occurs more frequently in men and is most commonly in the medial segment of the left hepatic lobe. In one case the cyst appeared closely associated with the left hepatic vein.[170] In most instances the cyst is unilocular (Fig. 4.4). The mean cyst diameter is approximately 3 cm. One large cyst was associated with an elevated serum CA 19–9 level.[171] There have been a few isolated reports of squamous cell carcinoma arising in a ciliated foregut cyst.[172,173]

Histologically, the cyst wall consists of four layers: pseudostratified ciliated columnar epithelium with mucous cells, subepithelial connective tissue, bundles of smooth muscle, and an outermost fibrous capsule (Figs 4.4 and 4.5).[169,174–176] Endocrine cells are present in the cyst epithelium.[175] In all seven cases of Chatelain et al., immunoreactivity of some cells for CD10 suggested the presence of Clara cells.[175] The cysts are believed to arise from the embryonic foregut and to differentiate toward bronchial structures in the liver.

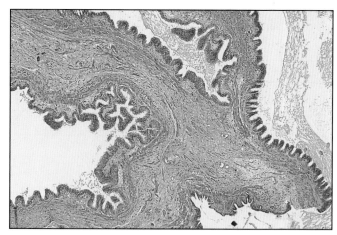

Fig. 4.4 • Ciliated foregut cyst. This multiloculated cyst is very much less common that the unilocular type. H&E.

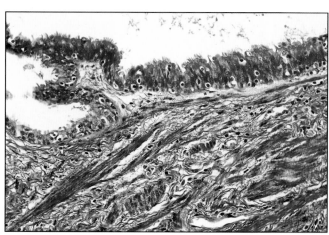

A

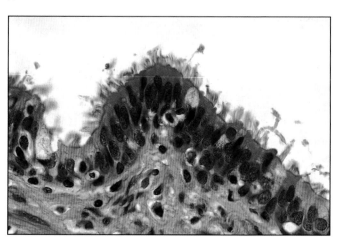

B

Fig. 4.5 • **(A)** Ciliated foregut cyst. The lining of pseudostratified epithelium is supported by fibrous tissue with scattered bundles of smooth muscle. Masson trichrome. **(B)** Cyst lining consists of pseudostratified columnar epithelium. Cilia are clearly seen at high magnification. H&E.

Spontaneous bile-duct perforation

In the first few months of life, spontaneous bile peritonitis may occur from leakage of bile at the junction of the cystic and common bile ducts. In patients without other bile-duct structural lesions, the aetiology is unknown, although congenital weakness of the bile-duct walls, mucous plugs and gallstones have been suggested.[177,178] The clinical presentation consists of jaundice, ascites, failure to thrive, and signs of peritoneal irritation. The diagnosis can be suspected by finding bile on abdominal paracentesis and confirmed by Technetium-99m-labelled hepatobiliary scanning.[179] Treatment is surgical and the prognosis excellent. Pathological descriptions of the liver are usually consistent with obstruction, with ductular reaction and oedematous portal tracts.

Extrahepatic biliary atresia

This is one of the most important causes of severe neonatal liver disease and the major indication for liver transplantation in young children. Initially the extrahepatic biliary tree is affected, evident as an obstuctive picture both clinically and histopathologically. This is the defining lesion of this disorder. Biliary cirrhosis develops early in life. Those children who survive infancy because of having a successful Kasai portoenterostomy continue to have intrahepatic bile duct damage which leads eventually to profound loss of small intrahepatic bile ducts and recurrent cholestasis due to bile duct paucity. Accordingly many experts now prefer calling this hepatobiliary disorder simply *biliary atresia*, without specifying an extrahepatic (or intrahepatic) location. Notably, however, the term 'intrahepatic biliary atresia' to denote intrahepatic bile duct paucity has been obsolete for years. The term 'biliary atresia' is used in this section interchangeably with 'extrahepatic biliary atresia' (EHBA).

Approximately 30% of infants presenting with conjugated hyperbilirubinaemia in the neonatal period have biliary atresia, the overall incidence being approximately 1 in 8000 to 1 in 15 000 live births. There is no clear-cut racial predilection although some ethnicities appear to have a higher incidence: Afro-Americans[180] and Polynesians[181] compared to caucasian infants. Biliary atresia is more common in girls than boys.[44] Seasonal variation in the occurrence of this disease has been suggested in North American studies,[180,182] although it remains somewhat controversial[183] and this pattern has not been confirmed in Europe.[181] Although the pathogenesis remains uncertain, unquestionably there are multiple disease mechanisms since biliary atresia may occur as an isolated lesion or in association with various types of congenital abnormalities or structural chromosomal abnormalties. At the present time biliary atresia is classified in two general patterns: embryonal/fetal or 'early' accounting for 15–35% of cases and perinatal (acquired) or 'late' in 65–85% of cases. This aetiopathogenic heterogeneity of biliary atresia was delineated by a study of 237 children by Silveira et al.[10] Forty-seven of the children (20%) had associated congenital anomalies (28 cardiovascular, 22 digestive and 19 splenic). The splenic malformations included 13 with polysplenia syndrome and two with asplenia. Karyotypic abnormalities were found in two of eight children studied. Silveira et al. divided biliary atresia into four distinct subgroups, three involving a congenital form that could arise through a malformation, a disruption or a chromosomal abnormality, while the fourth is attributable to agents active in the perinatal period (the acquired form).[10] Most infants have this 'late' acquired pattern: their apparently normal biliary system has been subjected to a fibrosing inflammatory process toward the end of gestation or shortly after birth. By contrast, approximately 10–30% of infants with EHBA have extrahepatic congenital abnormalities such as polysplenia, left atrial isomerism, double-sided left lung, pre-duodenal portal vein, intestinal malrotation, and/or congenital heart defects.[44,184,185] These congenital defects are sometimes grouped as a 'laterality complex'. Some infants with biliary atresia have specific chromosomal abnormalties such as trisomy 17–18,[186] or Turner syndrome,[187] or cat-eye syndrome. A lethal autosomal recessive syndrome with intra-uterine growth retardation, intra- and extrahepatic biliary atresia, and oesophageal and duodenal atresia was reported in one family.[188] Familial occurrence has been reported;[189,190] twins concordant for extrahepatic biliary atresia have rarely been reported.

Viral infection in combination with a genetic predisposition may play a role in the development of the perinatal (late) pattern of biliary atresia. Cytomegalovirus (CMV) infection is found in a high proportion of children with extrahepatic biliary atresia. Tarr et al.[191] found evidence for viral infection in 5 of 23 patients with biliary atresia. The diagnosis was based on histopathological evidence of CMV infection, serology (IgM antibodies) or culture. The detection of CMV infection by the polymerase chain reaction (PCR) is higher in neonatal hepatitis than in EHBA.[192] In one family, one twin had biliary atresia and the other had neonatal hepatitis.[193] Reovirus 3 has also been suggested as a cause of EHBA and neonatal hepatitis on the basis of clinical and experimental studies[194-198] but that association was questioned by other investigators.[199,200] More compelling evidence for an aetiological association of biliary atresia and reoviruses was provided by Tyler et al.[201] These investigators detected reovirus RNA from hepatobiliary tissues of 55% of patients with EHBA and 78% of patients with choledochal cysts. A possible relationship between group C rotavirus and biliary atresia was suggested by Riepenhoff-Talty et al.[202] Subsequently however no evidence of group A, B or C rotaviruses was detected by PCR in biliary atresia.[203] Human papilloma virus has been detected in neonatal hepatitis and biliary atresia by nested PCR for DNA,[204] but the role of this virus needs to be clarified.

Recent progress has been made in our understanding of the pathogenesis of biliary atresia, especially the perinatal-acquired form.[205] Genomic studies of liver from infants with biliary atresia showed an upregulation of genes involved in regulating lymphocyte differentiation, mainly of those with Th1-commitment.[206] Upregulation of the expression of interferon-γ and osteopontin was notable. Another study, which included somewhat older patients, also found upregulation of genes involved in morphogenesis, cell signalling and regulation of gene transcription.[207] Further studies suggested that the pattern of regulatory gene expression in perinatal-pattern biliary atresia is not equivalent to that in the embryonic-pattern; these data also failed to show a pattern relating to laterality genes in embryonic-pattern biliary atresia.[208] Nevertheless both forms of biliary atresia appear to induce a strong immunological response. HLA studies relating to this immunological component are confusing. One study showed that infants with perinatal/acquired biliary atresia have a high prevalence of the HLA B12 determinant compared both to normal controls and to infants with EHBA plus congenital anomalies;[209] haplotypes A9-B5 and A28-B35 were also more common in infants with perinatal-pattern EHBA. A more recent study failed to confirm any characteristic HLA pattern in biliary atresia.[210] Studies in liver from infants with biliary atresia showed a Th1-type of cytokine expression pattern with CD4+ and CD8+ lymphocytes, CD68+ macrophages in portal tracts and increased IL-2, IL-12, interferon-γ and tumour necrosis factor-α.[211] Upregulation of osteopontin expression in intrahepatic biliary epithelium correlated with portal fibrosis and bile ductular reaction.[212] Recent work in the rotavirus murine model of biliary atresia indicates that interferon-γ may play an important role in bile duct damage: knockout mice not expressing interferon-γ failed to get severe duct damage after infection with rotavirus despite a brief hepatitis whereas wild type animals did; administration of recombinant interferon-γ abrogated the protective effect of not being able to produce interferon-γ.[213] Thus a complex pattern of immune reactivity appears to be important in the perinatal-acquired type of biliary atresia; in the embryonic form, other genes may play a more direct role.

Other theories regarding the pathogenesis of biliary atresia reflect the dichotomies of clinical findings.[214,215] Landing[216] first proposed that neonatal hepatitis, biliary atresia, infantile choledochal cyst and possibly some instances of 'intrahepatic biliary atresia' (meaning congenital duct paucity syndromes) are all manifestations of a single basic disease process that he named 'infantile obstructive cholangiopathy'. He considered biliary atresia (and choledochal cyst) to be the result of an inflammatory rather than a maldevelopmental process and postulated that the most probable cause was a viral infection. However, the aetiopathogenesis of an important congenital bile duct paucity syndrome, namely Alagille syndrome, has since been elucidated as genetic (p. 166). Nevertheless some cases of biliary atresia have been attributed to congenital rubella, CMV, rotavirus or reovirus 3 infection. Extrahepatic biliary atresia can be simulated in Balb/c-mice which have been infected with rotavirus; most types of biliary atresia can be mimicked in this animal model.[217] Morbidity and mortality are higher in mice lacking interferon-induced protein.[218] Prophylactic interferon alters the clinical course in these mice and their infected progeny. Certain chromosomal abnormalities may give rise to complex syndromes including altered immune reactivity and thus predispose to hepatobiliary disease mediated by viral infection. On the basis of experiments in rats given a drug (1,4-phenylenediisothiocyanate) at different developmental stages, it has been proposed that the various manifestations of infantile obstructive cholangiopathy may depend on the timing of the insult.[219] Thus, rats given the drug during fetal life

developed stenotic or atretic bile ducts due to thickening and fibrosis, whereas those given the drug after birth had dilatation of the ducts with inflammation. It is difficult to generalize from this rat model to human infants. Discordance for biliary atresia in HLA identical twins supports a postnatal event being of primary importance in the pathogenesis of the disorder.[220] Biliary atresia with features of the ductal plate malformation might reflect a different disease mechanism.[221]

Whereas the pathogenesis of the perinatal-pattern biliary atresia probably involves genetic susceptibility and exposure to an instigating factor, such as viral infection, during a limited period of susceptibility, the aetiopathogenesis of the embryonal-pattern EHBA appears to be much more diverse. Extrahepatic congenital abnormalities such as polysplenia, congenital heart defects, and disturbed rotation of the intestines suggest an extensive and early developmental abnormality. Some infants with biliary atresia and these extrahepatic findings show features of the ductal plate lesion on liver biopsy.[215,222] This abnormal configuration of small bile ducts is attributed to disorganization in the fetal development of the biliary tree: failure of remodeling of the ductal plate leads to residual embryonic bile duct structures in this rather striking configuration. Finding the ductal plate lesion in extrahepatic biliary atresia is consistent with a destructive hepatobiliary process beginning early in gestation. Abnormal cilia were reported in a child with the polysplenia syndrome and biliary atresia by Teichberg et al.[223] While the association with abnormal cilia is unclear, ciliary function appears to be important in left/right asymmetry.[224] There is a pathogenic role for multiple defects in the laterality sequence.[225] In the mouse, the c-jun gene is essential for hepatogenesis.[226] Other factors included HLX homeobox gene[227] and HGF gene.[228] The most relevant gene may be the inversion (inv) gene. In the mouse it is one of three genes that control left/right asymmetry.[229,230] Beginning in early embryonic development the liver is a predominant site for this gene expression. A transgenic mouse with recessive deletion of the inversion gene causes situs inversus and jaundice.[231] The early fetal lesion is a complete obstruction with cystic change of the biliary tree.[231] Three children were described with ultrastructural abnormalities of the canalicular microvillus and no expression of villin;[232] phenotypically they had biliary atresia without laterality complex or ductal plate malformation.

The extrahepatic biliary tree in biliary atresia may be totally atretic or the atresia may involve only proximal or distal segments. The intrahepatic bile ducts are gradually destroyed with progression of the disease. Most infants with biliary atresia have conjugated hyperbilirubinaemia from an early age, but clinical jaundice is not always apparent or appreciated; indeed in infants jaundice is initially physiological and merges with the jaundice of advancing liver disease. Infants typically have dark urine and pale stools, but the stools may retain enough colour to be falsely reassuring. The infants look well and generally gain weight adequately. They have hepatomegaly and usually some degree of splenomegaly, unless polysplenia is present. The infant who presents with congenital heart disease and conjugated hyperbilirubinaemia requires intensive evaluation since the leading hepatic diagnoses will be biliary atresia or Alagille syndrome. Untreated biliary atresia rapidly progresses to hepatic fibrosis and cirrhosis with all the complications of portal hypertension, in addition to malnutrition and fat-soluble vitamin deficiency. The median age of death is 12 months if the biliary atresia is not diagnosed and treated.[233]

Clinically, the differential diagnosis is the broad spectrum of disorders constituting the neonatal hepatitis syndrome[234] (p. 159 and Table 4.1). Congenital infection should be excluded, although CMV may be found along with biliary atresia. Systemic bacterial infection should be excluded, including a silent urinary tract infection. Inherited metabolic diseases require specific attention, especially α_1-antitrypsin deficiency, which can be associated with severe cholestasis and acholic stools and very rarely has been associated with biliary atresia; galactosaemia, and cystic fibrosis which can involve a duct lesion indistinguishable clinically from biliary atresia. The last 3 conditions may produce a histological picture closely resembling that of EHBA. Structural abnormalities of the extraheaptic biliary tree cause the clinical presentation like biliary atresia: choledocholithiasis, idiopathic perforation of the biliary tract,[177,178,235,236] true choledochal cyst, and extrahepatic biliary hypoplasia or 'hair-like' bile duct syndrome.

Preoperative diagnosis relies on demonstrating the presence or absence of bile secretion in the intestine. Hepatic sonography may reveal a dilated extrahepatic biliary tree, consistent with distal, 'correctable' atresia, but it is unusual to find dilated intrahepatic bile ducts. Hepatobiliary scanning, using DISIDA or PIPIDA, fails to demonstrate passage of the radiolabelled substance into the intestinal tract over a 24-hour period. Although hepatobiliary scanning has high sensitivity, scanning may appear normal if performed very early in the disease process in late-pattern EHBA.[237,238] Hepatobiliary scanning is informative if it shows that tracer, and thus bile, reaches the intestine; it is objective, recorded, and can be quantified. A negative or non-draining scan does not mean that the disorder is necessarily biliary atresia because non-draining hepatobiliary scans may be found with severe idiopathic neonatal hepatitis, small duct paucity syndromes, such as Alagille syndrome, with severe α1-antitrypsin deficiency or with TPN-associated cholestasis. There is some enthusiasm for direct demonstration of bile or bile products.[239] Endoscopic retrograde cholangio-pancreatography (ERCP) is being utilized for duct visualization.[240,241] Percutaneous liver biopsy is essential and has high diagnostic specificity in the range of 60–95%, depending on the timing of the biopsy, adequacy of the specimen and expertise of the pathologist.[242]

Histological studies of the extrahepatic bile ducts removed at surgery have been carried out by several groups of investigators.[243-246] In a study of 98 cases, Gautier and Eliot[245] classified the biliary remnants into three types: in the first the duct is completely atretic, with little or no inflammatory cells in the surrounding connective tissue (Fig. 4.6(A)); in the second form it is present as a cleft-like lumen lined by occasional cuboidal or low columnar epithelium which is variably necrotic, hyperplastic, or focally absent (Fig. 4.6(B) and 4.6(C)); the altered ducts are sometimes very numerous, usually having lumina of less than 50 µm, periluminal neutrophilic infiltration is characteristic and cellular debris, and less often bile, may be found in the lumen. Epithelial necrosis is evident in ducts with a diameter exceeding 300 µm. The third type consists of altered bile duct incompletely lined by columnar epithelium, in addition to numerous smaller epithelial structures (Fig. 4.6(D)). These histological types were evaluated by Gautier and Eliot[245] at three levels—porta hepatis, junction of the cystic and common hepatic ducts and an intermediate level; completely atretic duct becomes increasingly more frequent from the porta hepatis to the junction of the hepatic duct and cystic ducts. This classification, which may help pathologists to describe the changes observed in the biliary remnants removed at porto-enterostomy, is of limited clinical significance because in individual cases serial sectioning often shows atretic ducts alternating with variably destroyed ducts in a random fashion. In addition the numerous smaller structures intermingled with variably altered ducts are likely to represent anastomosing channels recruited from peribiliary glands, of which effectiveness in by-passing the atretic duct is uncertain; anastomoses between ramified peribiliary glands are well demonstrated in adult livers using injection techniques (see Chapter 11). Correlations between the size and number of residual ducts and establishment of bile flow after surgery have yielded conflicting results. Two groups of investigators believed that bile flow is most likely to occur when the diameter of the residual ducts exceeds 150 µm.[187,243] However, a subsequent study of the extrahepatic biliary remnants of 204 cases of biliary atresia has clearly shown that the patterns of obliteration are not indicative of prognosis.[247]

Portoenterostomy (the Kasai procedure) was introduced in 1959 and remains the only potentially corrective procedure, other than liver transplantation.[248] In this operation, the atretic biliary tree is resected, and bile drainage is re-established via a broad anastomosis of the end of an intestinal Roux-en-Y loop to the bare edge of the transected porta hepatis. The prognosis for a good long-term result from portoenterostomy depends primarily on operation before 60 days of age and the absence of cholangitis,[249-254] but there is potential for reasonable medium-term survival in about one third of infants coming to primary corrective surgery 100 days or older and most centres continue to favour Kasai as the first therapeutic option, rather than subjecting patients to transplant simply on the basis of age.[255] The lack of significant fibrosis at the time of operation may play a role in a good long-term outcome.[256] One group of investigators believes that the histopathology of the initial biopsy can predict the success of portoenterostomy.[257]

Although the Kasai procedure is essentially a palliative operation, many children enjoy prolonged good health afterwards and approximately 20–35% of patients who undergo portoenterostomy will survive more than 10 years without liver transplantation.[225] One-third of the patients drain bile but develop complications of cirrhosis and require liver transplantation before age 10.[258] For the remaining

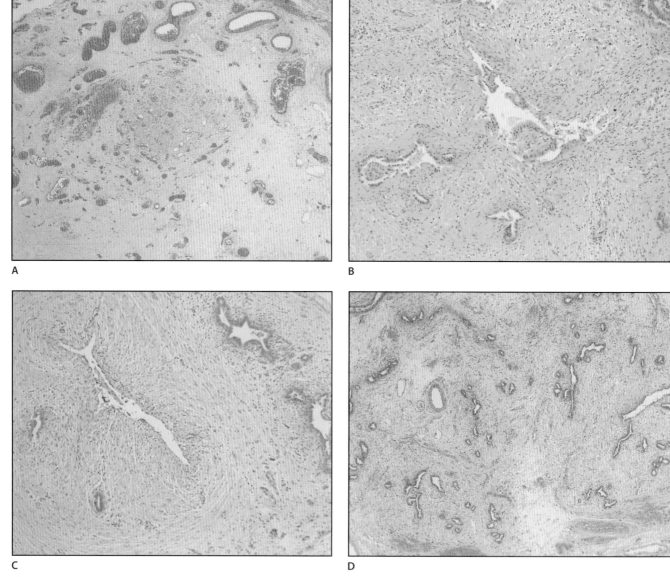

A

B

C

D

Fig. 4.6 • Extrahepatic biliary atresia. Transverse sections of biliary remnants removed at porto-enterostomy. **(A)** Atretic common hepatic duct showing luminal occlusion by vascular fibrous tissue with very few inflammatory cells. **(B)** Distorted bile duct inconsistently lined by desquamated columnar epithelium and surrounding fibroplasia with a light inflammatory cell infiltrate. **(C)** Cleft-like lumen devoid of epithelial lining side by side with duct structures which may represent adjacent segments of the same ducts or hyperplastic peribiliary glands. **(D)** Hilar region close to the surgical resection line showing numerous ducts or glandular structures set in a loose, mildly inflamed fibrous tissue.

one-third of patients, bile flow is inadequate following portoenterostomy and cirrhosis rapidly develops.[214] Survival in biliary atresia with a functioning Kasai portoenterostomy but without orthotopic liver transplantation is 10–20% by the age of 20 years.[259] In a recent survey of 271 patients, 23% were alive with their native liver 20 years after surgery, all but two having signs of cirrhosis; two patients died of liver failure and fourteen underwent or are waiting for a liver transplant.[260] Liver transplantation has become the treatment of choice for infants and children in whom a portoenterostomy has failed.[214] The safety and results of liver transplantation with the use of livers from living related donors and cadaveric donors are excellent. One-year survival is greater than 90%, with better results obtained under elective conditions and in children who are over 10 kg in weight.[259,261,262] Recent data indicate that the overall survival at 10 years for all surgical treatment is 68%.

The macroscopic appearance of the liver in biliary atresia varies according to the stage of the disease. At first it is enlarged and is dark green in colour, becoming finely nodular as cirrhosis develops (Fig. 4.7). In untreated cases the cirrhosis may take between 1 and 6 months from birth to develop. Dilated bile ducts filled with inspissated bile may be seen in sections of large portal areas (Fig. 4.8). The cystically dilated bile ducts may resemble Caroli disease.[263] They only occur after the age of 3 months and are not amenable to surgical drainage procedures. There may be portal lymphadenopathy. The median maximum node dimension in six cases studied by Hubscher and Harrison[264] was 14 mm. These lymph nodes are brown in colour and full of pigment-laden macrophages. Livers removed at transplantation after an apparently successful Kasai procedure (loss of jaundice), but after subsequent development of cirrhosis and portal hypertension, are often coarsely nodular with areas of

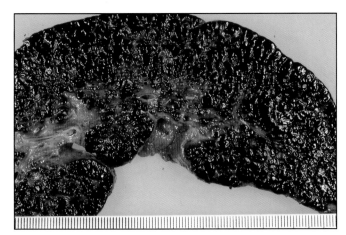

Fig. 4.7 • Liver removed at transplantation 6 months after a failed Kasai procedure. Cirrhosis is characterized by small and dark green parenchymal nodules.

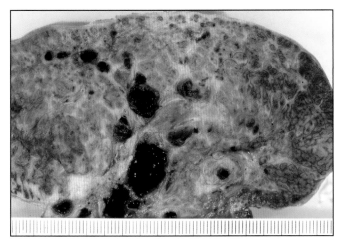

Fig. 4.8 • Bisected liver from patient with extrahepatic biliary atresia. Multiple, dilated bile ducts are filled with black bilirubin casts. Some of the ducts have thick fibrous walls. The hepatic parenchyma is cirrhotic with a periseptal distribution of the cholestasis (right of the field).

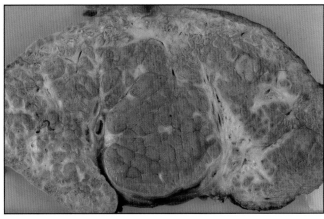

Fig. 4.9 • Liver removed at transplantation 8 years after 'successful' Kasai procedure. Bisected specimen showing macronodular areas of reexpanded parenchyma (centre of the field) with more fibrotic micronodular areas particularly at the periphery. Note the large fibrotic and seemingly stretched portal areas which contain well-identifiable bile duct branches (yellow and light green).

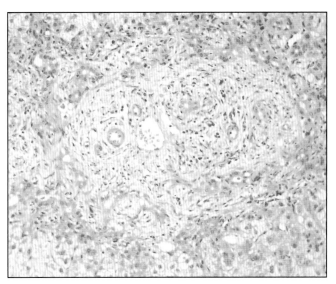

Fig. 4.10 • Extrahepatic biliary atresia, liver biopsy performed at 3 weeks of age. Characteristic portal tract expansion by loose fibrous tissue containing irregularly anastomosing bile ductules at the periphery, some being dilated with inspissated bile in their lumen. H&E.

macronodular hypertrophy and broad intervening or peripherally located scars resembling the gross appearance of 'focal nodular hyperplasia' (Fig. 4.9).

The histological features of biliary atresia include cholestasis, portal tract expansion by oedematous fibroplasia and periportal ductular reaction with the presence of bile plugs in dilated lumens of cholangioles, which are distorted and often form an irregularly anastomosing network at the portal periphery (Figs 4.10 and 4.11). Arterial branches are unusually prominent and portal vein branches appear attenuated. Giant cell transformation of hepatocytes is seen in approximately 15% of cases[265] (Fig. 4.12), and may occasionally be prominent. Loose fibrosis is progressive and periportal/perilobular in location, with linkage of portal areas and eventual development of a secondary biliary cirrhosis (Fig. 4.13). A study of the extracellular and cellular components of the connective tissue matrix in biliary atresia was reported by DeFreitas et al.[266] Activation of a connective tissue cellular clone by the reactive ductules may be responsible for the portal fibroplasia. Ho et al.[267] have reported an arteriopathy (hyperplasia and hypertrophy) of the common hepatic artery and its peripheral branches supplying the entire biliary tree in 11 cases of biliary atresia; the possible pathogenetic significance of their findings remains to be established. Thickening of the medial layer of small hepatic arteries may be present in biliary atresia. Large perihilar bile ducts may show ulceration with loss of epithelial lining, bile impregnation of the wall and bile sludge formation in the lumen. In addition to the severe cholestasis, the cirrhotic stage of biliary atresia is characterized by marked pseudo-xanthomatous transformation, the presence of bile lakes, Mallory bodies and variable accumulation of copper and copper associated protein in liver cells (Figs 4.14–4.15). In one study, copper concentrations were increased in over two-thirds of liver samples obtained during portoenterostomy and decreased in some patients after successful biliary drainage.[268] However, it must be noted that copper deposi-

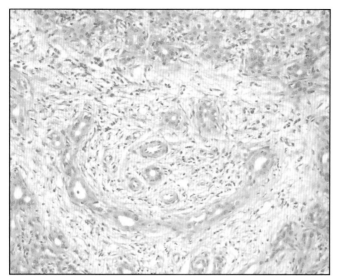

Fig. 4.11 • Extrahepatic biliary atresia. Cholangiolar reaction forming crescent shape profile reminiscent of the embryonal ductal plate. In our experiencee, this pattern may be observed irrespective of the patient having associated extrahepatic malformation. H&E.

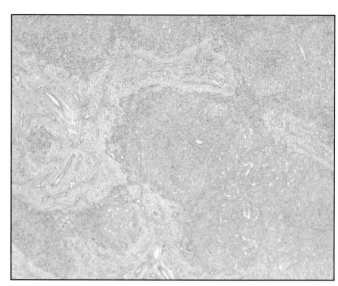

Fig. 4.13 • Extrahepatic biliary atresia, cirrhotic transformation. Porto-portal bridging septa made of oedematous fibrous tissue show a marginal ductular reaction and delineate small and irregularly shaped parenchymal nodules. H&E.

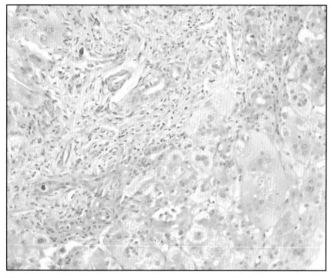

Fig. 4.12 • Extrahepatic biliary atresia. Portal features of distal obstructive cholangiopathy are associated with giant cell transformation in the parenchyma. H&E.

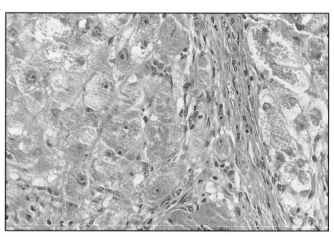

Fig. 4.14 • Extrahepatic biliary atresia. Same case as illustrated in Fig. 4.13. Mallory bodies in ballooned periseptal hepatocytes. H&E.

tion in liver is increased in the first 2 months of life and periportal deposition of copper on liver biopsy specimens does discriminate extra from intrahepatic causes of cholestasis in this age group. Acute and chronic inflammation is noted in portal/periportal areas in biliary atresia in both precirrhotic and cirrhotic stages, and bile-duct degeneration and inflammation may be evident (Fig. 4.16). The mononuclear infiltrate in portal and lobular areas of livers with end-stage biliary atresia is similar to normal adult liver and very different from that associated with autoimmune hepatitis or chronic hepatitis B infection. The growth of large perihilar regenerative nodules, probably as a consequence of functioning intrahepatic ducts in this region, may be important for maintaining biliary drainage after Kasai procedure.[269] Bile lakes occur after the age of 3 months, by which time irreversible hepatic damage has occurred.[270]

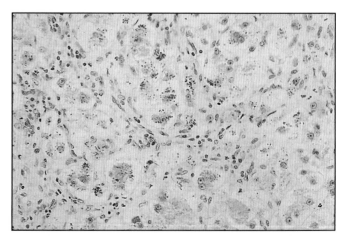

Fig. 4.15 • Extrahepatic biliary atresia. Same case as illustrated in Figs 4.13–4.14. Marked copper accumulation in liver cells (red granules). Rhodanine.

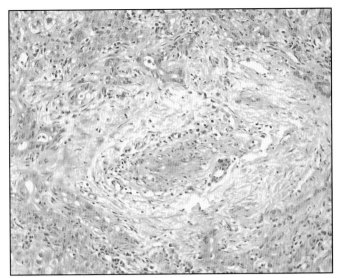

Fig. 4.16 • Extrahepatic biliary atresia. Inflamed and arteriole-rich, lemon-shaped fibrous tissue marks the site of a small, largely destroyed, intrahepatic bile duct. H&E.

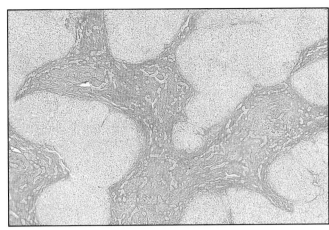

Fig. 4.18 • Extrahepatic biliary atresia. Liver resection one year after porto-enterostomy. Pattern of fibrosis and proliferated small bile ducts is reminiscent of congenital hepatic fibrosis. There were only minimal chronic cholestatic features in this liver. PAS after diastase digestion.

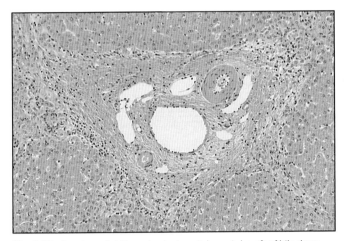

Fig. 4.17 • Extrahepatic biliary atresia. A portal area is bereft of bile ducts. There is periportal cholangiolar reaction with an associated neutrophilic response. H&E.

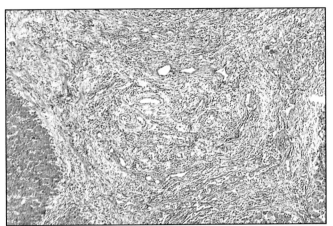

Fig. 4.19 • Extrahepatic biliary atresia. Same liver as illustrated in Fig. 4.18. Note absence of an interlobular bile duct and a pattern of ductular reaction reminiscent of a ductal plate malformation. Masson trichrome.

Interlobular bile ducts become few in number as early as the fourth or fifth month after birth (Fig. 4.17)[271] and advanced duct loss accompanies progressive fibrosis by the age of 8 or 9 months.[216] Activated hepatic stellate cells are responsible for increased collagen production.[272,273] In addition to paucity of ducts, Raweily et al. identified concentric tubular ductal structures in 21.6% of cases of biliary atresia; these bore some resemblance to those seen in ductal plate malformations[222] (Fig. 4.18). Similar observations had been made earlier by Desmet and Callea,[274] who coined the term 'early severe' biliary atresia for that subgroup. It is of interest that children with that subgroup reveal a histopathological picture resembling that of congenital hepatic fibrosis 4 or 5 years after portoenterostomy[274,275] (Figs 4.18–4.19). The interlobular bile ducts continue to disappear and cirrhosis can develop despite satisfactory bile drainage after portoenterostomy.[276] The bile duct loss has been attributed to persistent obstruction of bile flow,[277] recurrent cholangitis or continuation of the initial insult that caused the atresia.

A detailed histopathological study of sequential liver specimens taken at the time of Kasai operation, relaparotomy and/or transplantation has provided evidence that the bile duct loss is due to an unpredictable and uneven obliteration of bile ducts in the porta hepatis during wound healing and scarring after portoenterostomy.

Ultrastructural degenerative changes affecting the intra-hepatic bile ducts and ductules in biliary atresia have been described in detail by Ito et al.[278] The degree of obstruction of the lumen of these ducts appears to be an important determinant of prognosis following corrective surgery.[278]

Malignant epithelial tumours of hepatobiliary origin rarely complicate biliary cirrhosis associated with biliary atresia, but a few have been reported.[279] Also of interest is the development of focal nodular hyperplasia after porto-enterostomy in two children with biliary atresia.[280]

Neonatal hepatitis

Neonatal hepatitis is a term that was coined for presumed viral infections of the liver in early infancy. It has become evident that these disorders are not by any means exclusively viral in aetiology. Neonatal hepatitis represents a clinical pattern of neonatal liver disease, hence the preferred designation 'neonatal hepatitis syndrome'. Other diseases such as galactosaemia, hereditary fructose intolerance, cystic fibrosis[281] and the conditions discussed under biliary atresia and paucity of the intrahepatic bile ducts may also present with pathological changes in the liver resembling an infectious process. Giant-cell transformation, a frequent histological component of neonatal hepatitis, has been seen in all cholestatic conditions in infancy including pure haemolytic anaemias and endotoxic injury.[282] Although clinical jaundice is not present in every case of neonatal hepatitis syndrome, conjugated hyperbilirubinaemia is present. A classification of neonatal hepatitis syndrome is shown in Table 4.1. In the past twenty years the proportion of cases with no known aetiology has fallen substantially from 50–60%[283] to approximately 30%. Many of the disorders dissected out of the idiopathic category are inherited metabolic diseases, discussed in detail in Chapter 5.

Nomenclature for neonatal liver disease is problematic. The simplest term 'neonatal jaundice' may be confused with physiological jaundice in the newborn. The term 'neonatal cholestasis' is not precise since in the first 3–4 months of life every infant has some degree of cholestasis physiologically. This physiological cholestasis occurs because uptake of bile acids and other organic anions by hepatocytes is immature and thus inefficient, leading to high concentrations of bile acids in blood. In addition, hepatocellular pathways for bile acid conjugation and biliary secretion are also immature, in part because bile canalicular transporters are also regulated developmentally. The circulating bile acid pool is contracted, and ileal uptake of bile acids is underdeveloped. The term 'neonatal hepatitis' is imprecise because hepatic inflammation is not a feature of every condition. The term 'neonatal hepatitis syndrome' emphasizes the uniformity of the clinical presentation and similarity of pathological findings as well as the broad spectrum of causative disease processes.

The spectrum of diseases causing neonatal hepatitis syndrome embraces numerous infections, usually congenital. Implicated infectious agents include CMV, rubella virus, hepatitis B virus, herpes simplex virus, herpes zoster virus, Coxsackie and Echo viruses, toxoplasma and *Treponema pallidum*. An unusually high incidence of CMV infection (49%) was reported in a series of 45 cases from Taiwan.[284] Herpes simplex virus, enteroviruses, adenovirus and hepatitis B virus may cause neonatal liver failure. In addition to genetic metabolic disorders, endocrine disorders may cause neonatal hepatitis syndrome. An association with hypopituitarism was reported in two infants by Herman et al.,[285] and later Sheehan et al.[286] Immunological disorders may cause neonatal hepatitis syndrome: neonatal lupus erythematosus is most common. Rarely a Coombs positive haemolytic anaemia defines a severe form of giant cell hepatitis which rapidly progresses to cirrhosis or death.[287] Early and sustained immunosuppressive therapy may control the disease in some patients.[288] The liver lesion has been shown to recur in the allograft of the few cases transplanted.[289,290] Infants

with birth asphyxia may develop severe neonatal hepatitis syndrome.[291,292] Conjugated hyperbilirubinaemia typically occurs at 1 week of age, lasts 3–4 months, and the hepatomegaly and liver tests return to normal by 1 year of age. Various hepatobiliary structural abnormalities, of which the most important is biliary atresia, are associated with the neonatal hepatitis syndrome. Furthermore certain chromosomal defects predispose to the neonatal heptitis syndrome.

A proportion of cases of neonatal hepatitis syndrome (around 30%) are considered idiopathic. The prognosis for idiopathic neonatal hepatitis is generally good; mortality runs at 13–25%.[284,293] In the study of Dick and Mowat,[283] two of 29 patients with idiopathic neonatal hepatitis died, and only a further two had signs of persisting liver disease. Overall, predictors of poor prognosis include persisting severe jaundice, acholic stools, prominent hepatomegaly, severe inflammation on liver biopsy, and familial occurrence. Numerous inherited disorders causing the neonatal hepatitis syndrome have recently been described in terms of gene defect, such as the bile canalicular transporter disorders and bile acid synthesis disorders, and these had previously been classified as idiopathic neonatal hepatitis. Undoubtedly other such disorders remain to be delineated. A hereditary form with *giant-cell transformation and lymphoedema* resulting from abnormal deep lymphatics has been reported but the gene abnormality has not yet been determined.[294] A further identified aetiology is *adenosine deaminase deficiency*, with recovery after enzyme replacement.[295] Citrullinaemia type 2 due to deficiency of citrin can cause neonatal hepatitis syndrome.[296–298] 'Le foie vide' describes a severe neonatal liver disorder characterized by failure of hepatocellular regeneration.[299]

Liver biopsy specimens are characterized by varying degrees of cholestasis (with or without pseudoglandular structures), giant cell transformation, ballooning, apoptotic bodies, extramedullary haemopoiesis, lobular and portal inflammation, and progressive fibrosis in some cases. Unusually severe inflammation and hepatocellular damage may be found in α_1-antitrypsin deficiency, hereditary tyrosinemia type 1, Niemann–Pick disease type C, syncytial giant cell hepatitis, citrullinaemia type 2, primary disorders of bile acid synthesis (mainly Δ^4-3-oxosteroid 5β-reductase deficiency), bile salt export pump (BSEP) deficiency (progressive familial intrahepatic cholestasis type 2) and idiopathic neonatal hepatitis. Associated macrovesicular steatosis favours a metabolic disorder, e.g. tyrosinaemia. Confluent hepatocyte necrosis or loss with bridging collapse is seen in the rare patients presenting with acute-pattern neonatal liver failure or having a subacute clinical course associated with perinatal haemochromatosis, non-Wilsonian copper load, or other metabolic disorders such as tyrosinaemia (Chapter 5), occasionally viral hepatitis, in particular infants born to mothers carrying the precore mutant of hepatits B, and seronegative (idiopathic) neonatal hepatitis.

The pathological aspects of giant-cell transformation, a frequent and often dominant finding in neonatal hepatitis, have been reviewed extensively in the past.[300,301] The change

Table 4.1 Classification of neonatal hepatitis syndrome with major histological and diagnostic investigations

Categories	Specfic diseases/causes	Comments	Liver histology	Diagnostic investigations
Infection	Toxoplasmosis (congenital)		NSH (calcifications)	Maternal infection/IgM specific Abs; PCR on amniotic fluid
	Rubella (congenital)		NSH	IgM specific Abs
	Cytomegalovirus (congenital)	Acute-pattern neonatal liver failure	NSH ± 'owl-eye' nuclear inclusions	Urine for viral culture, IgM Abs, PCR
	Herpes simplex (congenital)		Necrotizing hepatitis/viral inclusions (IHC)	Liver biopsy; Viral culture (Scrapings from skin vesicles)
	Syphilis (congenital)		Diffusely fibrosing hepatitis	Standard test, VDRL, florescent treponema Abs
	Human herpesvirus-6	Acute-pattern neonatal liver failure	Necrotizing hepatitis/viral inclusions (rare)	Serology, PCR
	Herpes zoster		NSH	Serology, PCR
	Hepatitis B (mainly vertical)	Acute-pattern neonatal liver failure	Severe hepatitis	Mother's serum eAg positive (or negative due to precore mutant)
	Hepatitis C (mainly vertical)	Rarely cause of NHS		Screening of infants born to HCV +ve mothers by RT PCR
	Human immunodeficiency virus (vertical)	Rarely cause of NHS	NSH (opportunistic infections, in particular CMV)	Anti-HIV, CD4 count
	Parvovirus 19 infection	Chronic-pattern neonatal liver failure	NSH, marked haemopoiesis, siderosis, perisinusoidal fibrosis, few GC	Severe anaemia
	Syncytial giant cell hepatitis (?paramyxovirus)		NSH, prominent syncytial GC (EM paramyxovirus-like inclusions)	IgM Abs, PCR; Liver ultrastructure (no supportive serology)
	Enteric viral sepsis (echoviruses, Coxsackie viruses, adenoviruses)	Acute-pattern neonatal liver failure	NSH ± GC/cholestasis	Appropriate serology, viral culture or direct fluorescent assay
	Bacterial infection (extrahepatic or sepsis)	Acute-pattern neonatal liver failure	Non-specific hepatitis/cholestasis (ductular bile casts)	Blood, urine or CNS culture
	Listeriosis		NSH, focal necrosis ± granulomas	*Listeria m.* isolation from blood, CSF or liver; High index of suspicion
	Tuberculosis		Caseating granulomas (±acid-fast bacilli)	Mantoux test
Structural	Extrahepatic biliary atresia		Biliary features: loose portal fibroplasia, ductular reaction and cholestasis including ductular bile plugs/GC (15%); DPM-like (20%)	Acholic stools/Liver histology; No excretion on hepatobiliary scan; ERCP; Laparotomy
	Choledochal cyst	*Differentiate from biliary atresia*	Biliary features	Ultrasound, cholangiography
	Caroli disease/syndrome	*Differentiate from biliary atresia*	Biliary features/DPM	Ultrasound, cholangiography
	Choledocholithiasis	*Differentiate from biliary atresia*	Biliary features	Ultrasound, cholangiography
	Neonatal sclerosing cholangitis		Biliary features/periductal fibrosis inconstant	Cholangiography
	Extrahepatic biliary hypoplasia ('hair-like bile duct syndrome')	*Differentiate from biliary atresia*	Biliary features	Cholangiography

Table 4.1 Classification of neonatal hepatitis syndrome with major histological and diagnostic investigations—cont'd

Categories	Specific diseases/causes	Comments	Liver histology	Diagnostic investigations
	Spontaneous perforation of common bile duct	*Differentiate from biliary atresia*	Biliary features	Imaging Bile stained ascites (paracentesis)
	Non-syndromic duct paucity (idiopathic)		Paucity of intrahepatic bile ducts Cholestasis	Liver biopsy
	Alagille syndrome	*Differentiate from biliary atresia*	Paucity of intrahepatic bile ducts Cholestasis/identifiable bile ducts ± mild ductular reaction occasionally seen in early biopsy	Extrahepatic syndromic features High serum cholesterol Liver biopsy *JAG1* mutations (20p)
Metabolic genetic (Ch. 5)	α_1-antitrypsin deficiency	*Differentiate from biliary atresia*	Variable. Biliary features mimicking EHBA, duct paucity or NSH (DPAS not diagnostic before 8–12 weeks of age); GC rare; periportal steatosis	Serum alpha$_1$-antitrypsin concentration Alpha1-antitrypsin phenotype (Pi type)
	Cystic fibrosis	*Differentiate from biliary atresia*	Steatosis/cholestasis/biliary features (focal fibrosis)/cholangiolar eosinophilic casts	Sweat chloride/extrahepatic complications Gene mutation (7q31.2—CFTR protein)
	Galactosaemia	Acute- or chronic-pattern neonatal liver failure	Steatosis/biliary features/fibrosis Severe parenchymal damage and loss Later cirrhosis (now rare)	Galactose-1-6-phosphate uridyl transferase assay Erythrocyte galactose-1-phosphate level
	Tyrosinaemia, type 1	Acute- or chronic-pattern neonatal liver failure	Severe parenchymal injury and loss, steatosis, GC, regenerative nodules ± cell dysplasia; fibrosis, cirrhosis	Elevated serum tyrosine, phenylalanine, methionine/ elevated succinylacetone in urine/FAA activity in fibroblasts or lymphocytes Gene mutation (15q23–25)
	Hereditary fructosaemia	Chronic-pattern neonatal liver failure	Steatosis, biliary rosettes, GC, fibrosis, later cirrhosis	Liver biopsy (enzyme analysis) Gene mutation (9q22)
	Glycogen storage disease, type IV	Early perinatal variant, very rare	Eosinophilic ('ground glass') cytoplasmic inclusions, PAS positive, diastase resistant (amylopectin-like)	Liver biopsy Brancher enzyme in liver, white blood cells or cultured fibroblasts
	Niemann–Pick, Type A		Hepatocyte and macrophage storage (lipidic, microvesicular/foamy)	Sphingomyelinase assay (peripheral blood cells or liver)
	Niemann–Pick, Type C	Chronic-pattern neonatal liver failure	Hepatocytic/macrophage storage as type A, but few cells; biliary features	Storage cells in bone marrow aspirate Cultured fibroblasts/cholesterol esterification studies
	Wolman disease		Cholesterol ester stored mainly in macrophages (cholesterol crystals)/neutral lipids in hepatocytes	Liver biopsy Lysosomal acid lipase activity
	Gaucher disease		Macrophage storage (foamy/striated cytoplasm)/ variable perisinusoidal fibrosis	Liver biopsy Acid β-glucosidase activity (white blood cells or cultured fibroblasts)
	FIC-1 deficiency (PFIC type 1)		Bland cholestasis, mild disease EM: granular bile ('Byler bile')	Low GGT cholestatic syndrome Liver biopsy (EM) Genomic mutation (18q21–22)
	Bile salt export pump (BSEP) deficiency (PFIC type 2)		Severe parenchymal injury, ballooned (cholate-static) hepatocytes/GC/ +absent canalicular BSEP (IHC staining)	Low GGT cholestatic syndrome Liver biopsy Genomic mutation (2q24)

		Histology	Diagnosis
Multidrug resistant 3 (MDR3) deficiency (PFIC type 3)		Biliary features; progressive fibrosis; absent canalicular MDR3 (IHC staining)	High GGT cholestatic syndrome; Histology + IHC; Genomic mutation (7q21)
North American Indian familial cholestasis		Bland cholestasis; Later progressive fibrosis	Gene mutation (16q22/cirhin)
Aagenaes syndrome	Very rare		Cholestatic syndrome; Lymphoedema (lower limb)
Primary disorders of bile acid synthesis: — 3β-hydroxy-Δ^5-C_{27}-steroid dehydrogenase/isomerase deficiency — Δ^4-3-oxosteroid 5β-reductase deficiency		Resemble PFIC type 2, but canalicular BSEP present (IHC)	Cholestasis; Low GGT cholestatic syndrome; Urine and plasma bile acids
Peroxisomal disorders (e.g., Zellweger syndrome)		Variable; Cholestasis/fibrosis/haemosiderosis; Absence of peroxisomes on EM	Dysmorphic features; Very long chain fatty acid study/red cell plasmalogens
X-linked adrenoleukodystrophy	Chronic-pattern neonatal liver failure	Absent or reduced peroxisomes on EM	Dysmorphic features (less striking than Zellweger)
Perinatal haemochromatosis	Chronic-pattern neonatal liver failure	Severe parenchymal injury and loss; ± GC—haemosiderin pigment in hepatocytes	High serum ferritin, TIBC; Iron accumulation in heart and/or pancreas on computerized tomography or magnetic resonance imaging; Liver biopsy/Lip biopsy for extrahepatic iron storage (accessory salivary glands)
Mitochondrial DNA depletion syndrome	Chronic-pattern neonatal liver failure	Microvesicular steatosis, oxyphilic cells, siderosis, cirrhosis; Mitochondrial anomalies (EM)	Lactic acidosis ± hypoglycemia; Abnormally low ratio of mtDNA/nDNA in tissue
Citrullinaemia, type II Adenosine deaminase deficiency	Mainly Asian descent Very rare	Cholestasis/steatosis/siderosis	Gene mutation (SLC25A13)
Panhypopituitarism (septo-optic dysplasia)		NS hepatitis/no distinctive features	Low cortisol, TSH and T4
Hypothyroidism		NSH/cholestasis	High TSH titre, low T4, free T4, T3
Genetic (gross chromosomal abnormalities)			
Trisomy 18	Associated with biliary atresia	Biliary features	Karyotype
Cat-eye syndrome	Associated with biliary atresia	Biliary features	Karyotype
Trisomy 21	Chronic-pattern neonatal liver failure (rare); associated biliary atresia (occasional)	Fibrosing hepatitis with leukaemoid cell infiltration	Karyotype
Kabuki syndrome[a,b]	Rarely associated with biliary atresia	Biliary features	Congenital anomalies/mental retardation

Table 4.1 Classification of neonatal hepatitis syndrome with major histological and diagnostic investigations—cont'd

Categories	Specific diseases/causes	Comments	Liver histology	Diagnostic investigations
Neoplasia (Ch15)	Neonatal leukaemia	Acute-pattern neonatal liver failure	Leukaemic infiltration	Peripheral blood, bone marrow aspirate
	Neuroblastoma	Acute-pattern neonatal liver failure	Small cell tumour ± rosettes; IHS, EM	Imaging; Urinary vanilylmandelic and homovanillic acid
	Langerhans cell histiocytosis		Biliary features similar to sclerosing cholangitis/Langerhans cells (CD1a) inconstant	Involvement of other systems (skin, bone, lung)
	Haemophagocytic lymphohistiocytosis	Chronic-pattern neonatal liver failure	Haemophagocytic activity	High level of macrophage derived cytokines in serum; Elevated ferritin; elevated triglycerides
Toxic	Total parenteral nutrition-associated cholestasis	Differentiate from biliary atresia	Biliary features, cholestasis	
	Drug-induced (via breast-milk or other)			
Vascular	Budd–Chiari syndrome	Rare	Features of venous outflow block	
	Severe congestive heart failure		Perivenular cell dropout/congestion	
	Perinatal/neonatal asphyxia	Differentiate from biliary atresia	Ischaemic necrosis	
Immune	Inspissated bile syndrome associated with ABO incompatibility	Differentiate from biliary atresia	Biliary features	Coombs test
	Neonatal lupus erythematosus		NSH; Anti-Ro—anti-La in liver tissue (IHC)	Maternal history/congenital heart block/skin rash (discoid lupus); Anti-Ro and anti-La antibodies
	Neonatal hepatitis with autoimmune haemolytic anaemia	Acute or chronic pattern liver disease	Prominent syncytial GC, necrosis, inflammation, fibrosis	Coombs positive haemolytic anaemia
Idiopathic	Idiopathic neonatal hepatitis (sero-negative)	Differentiate from biliary atresia	GC, parenchymal loss with stromal collapse of variable severity	Liver biopsy
	'Le foie vide' (infantile hepatic non-regenerative disorder)	Chronic-pattern neonatal liver failure	Total parenchymal cell dropout, scant ductular reaction	Liver biopsy

Notes: Acute-pattern neonatal liver failure denotes metabolic instability, coagulopathy, and extremely elevated serum aminotransferases in a neonate; chronic-pattern neonatal liver failure denotes metabolic instability, coagulopathy, hypoalbuminaemia, near-normal serum aminotransferases in a neonate; conditions which require specific consideration vis-à-vis biliary atresia are denoted 'Differentiate from biliary atresia'

Abbreviations: NSH, non-specific hepatitis; GC, multinucleated giant cells; IHC, immunohistochemistry; Abs, antibodies; EM, electron microscopy; DPM, ductal plate malformation; PFIC, progressive familial intrahepatic cholestasis; FAA, fumaryl acetoacetase; GGT, gamma-glutamyl-transpeptidase; TIBC, total iron binding capacity; mtDNA, mitochondrial DNA; nDNA nuclear DNA; T3, triiodothyronine; T4, thyroxine; TSH, thyroid-stimulating hormone

a Selicorni, A, Colombo C, Bonato S, Milani D, Giunta AM, Bedeschi MF. Biliary atresia and Kabuki syndrome: another case with long-term follow-up. (Letter) Am. J. Med. Genet, 2001; 100:251

b van Haelst MM, Brooks AS, Hoogeboom J, Wessels MW, Tibboel D, de Jongste JC et al. Unexpected life-threatening complications in Kabuki syndrome. Am. J. Med. Genet, 2000; 94:170–173

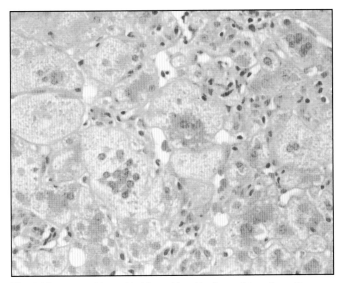

Fig. 4.20 • Neonatal hepatitis, idiopathic, with giant cell transformation. H&E.

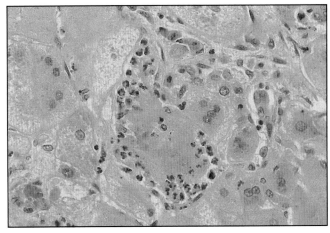

Fig. 4.22 • Same case as illustrated in Figs. 4.20 and 4.21. Neutrophilic satellitosis of degenerated giant cell. H&E.

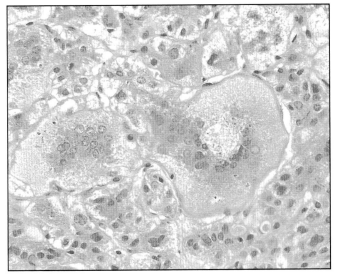

Fig. 4.21 • Same case as illustrated in Fig. 4.20. Detail of multinucleated giant hepatocyte. Periphery of cell (left) suggests fusion with several smaller cells. H&E.

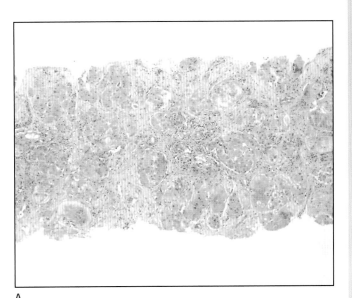

A

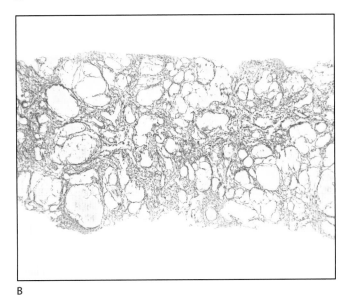

B

Fig. 4.23 • Severe neonatal hepatitis of undetermined cause. Extensive bridging parenchymal loss with concomitant reticulin collapse divides the parenchyma into minutes nodules with prominent giant cell transformation. (A) H&E; (B) Gordon-Sweet reticulin.

is seen throughout the parenchyma but it is often more marked in the perivenular areas. The giant cells contain four or more nuclei, sometimes as many as 40 per cell, have ill-defined outlines and may be detached from other cells in the hepatic plate (Figs 4.20 and 4.21). The cytoplasm of some giant cells may contain remnants of cell membranes. It is partially rarefied and often contains bile and/or haemosiderin. The cells may have more glycogen than normal hepatocytes and a greater activity of a variety of enzymes, such as glucose 6-phosphatase, acid phosphatase and succinic dehydrogenase. Death of the giant cells is associated with a neutrophilic inflammatory response (Fig. 4.22). In severe forms, extensive bridging cell loss may divide the parenchyma into micronodules which are highlighted by a reticulin stain (Fig. 4.23(A) and (B)). The number of giant cells decreases as patients grow older, and are rare after the age of 1. Formation of giant cells is considered to be a characteristic change resulting from mitotic inhibition of the young, growing liver tissue by a number of agents such as viruses, drugs, or hereditary abnormalities,[302] or from dissolution of cell membranes, as suggested by Craig and Landing,[303] who first described this entity. Negative nuclear staining for cell proliferation markers and the demonstration of canalicular remnants using carcino-embryonic antigen (CEA) immunostaining support a fusion of rosette-forming hepatocytes as the likely mechanism of giant-cell formation.[304]

Paucity of the intrahepatic bile ducts

Paucity of the intrahepatic bile ducts has been reported in many conditions, either congenital or acquired, affecting all age groups, but especially infants and children. The relevant finding is a reduction in the number of interlobular bile ducts, that is, in the small bile ducts with portal tracts. The normal ratio of small bile ducts per portal tract in full-term infants, children and adults is 0.9–1.8 ducts per tract. In duct paucity syndromes this ratio is <0.5 bile ducts per portal tract, given an adequate number of portal tracts (at least 10) examined on biopsy. Premature infants have a reduced number of small bile ducts per portal tract and if they have duct paucity with cholestasis, it may be physiological. In addition, it must be noted that early biopsy specimens in a few cases of clinically undisputed paucity of the intrahepatic bile ducts have shown not only identifiable ducts, but significant ductular reaction. Liver disorders with paucity of the intrahepatic bile ducts are generally divided into two groups: 'syndromic', which refers to Alagille syndrome (AGS, arteriohepatic dysplasia), and 'non-syndromic', which refers to all the rest of these diseases. The non-syndromic duct paucity conditions include numerous diseases where portal small duct paucity is associated with another identifiable disease. These include infection (congenital rubella or cytomegalovirus infection), immune abnormality (graft-versus-host disease, liver allograft chronic rejection), and hepatotoxicity (due to carbamazepine or amoxicillin-clavulinic acid),[305] the latter two groups being generally referred to as ductopenia, formerly vanishing bile duct syndromes (see Chapter 11). Various inherited metabolic diseases such as Zellweger syndrome, α_1-antitrypsin deficiency, and inborn errors of bile acid metabolism (discussed in Chapter 5) may display paucity of the intrahepatic ducts. Chromosomal defects, such as 45XO Turner syndrome[306], trisomy 17–18, trisomy 21[307], and prune belly syndrome[308] may have duct paucity. More importantly, the term *non-syndromic duct paucity* may be used to refer to isolated, idiopathic paucity of interlobular bile ducts in infancy and childhood; this condition may be the same as idiopathic adult ductopenia. Finally, paucity of the intrahepatic ducts or ductopenia is frequently found as a late feature of certain chronic diseases such as extrahepatic biliary atresia, sclerosing cholangitis, Langerhans cell histiocytosis, and primary biliary cirrhosis (Chapter 11).

Patients in the *syndromic group* have Alagille syndrome, also known as arteriohepatic dysplasia.[309] Comprehensive descriptions have been reported by Alagille and colleagues[310,311] and others.[312–315] It is due to mutations in *JAG 1* (which encodes ligand for this NOTCH1 receptor) on chromosome 20p[316,317] and may be associated with a macroscopic deletion of the short arm of chromosome 20 in some patients or microdeletions of 20p in others. The pattern of genetic transmission is autosomal dominant due to haploinsufficiency or dominant negative effect:[317] gene penetrance is high but expression is extremely variable.[318] The reported incidence of arteriohepatic dysplasia is 1:70 000 live births, but this may be an underestimate. Approximately 50–70% of patients have new mutations, rather than genetic transmission within the family. Crosnier et al.[319] found mutations of the *JAGGED 1* gene in 69 of 109 patients (63%) with Alagille syndrome, and transmission analysis showed a high frequency of sporadic cases (70%). Numerous mutations have now been defined.[320]

The common clinical findings in Alagille syndrome include cholestatic liver disease due to paucity of the intrahepatic bile ducts (94%); congenital heart disease, usually peripheral pulmonary stenosis although complex congenital heart disease may occur (92%); a typical facies (91%); posterior embryotoxon in the eye (80–93%); and butterfly-shaped vertebral arch deficits (40–67%)[315] The facies of arteriohepatic dysplasia consists of an inverted triangle shape, slight hypertelorism, deep-set eyes, broad and rather prominent forehead, and beak-like nose. Although the specificity of the facies was questioned,[321] now the facies is accepted as a typical finding, better appreciated in the actual clinical setting than in photographs. The facies is sometimes not evident in the first months of life, and in adults the facies is somewhat different from that described in children (longer face, rather coarse features, prominent forehead, comparatively small nose). Most patients have a systolic murmur related to stenosis of the pulmonary arterial system. More severe conditions include: tetralogy of Fallot, pulmonary valve stenosis, aortic stenosis, ventricular septal defect, atrial septal defect, anomalous pulmonary venous return, and complex problems involving a single right ventricle with pulmonary valve atresia.[322,323] Up to 15% of patients may have life-threatening cardiac complications.[311] In addition to posterior embryotoxon or Axenfeld anomaly, abnormal retinal pigmentation may be found.[324] Strabismus, ectopic pupil, and hypotrophic optic discs have also been reported. Optic disc drusen, which are calcified deposits in the extracellular space of the optic nerve head, occur commonly in Alagille syndrome. These can be found by ocular ultrasound examination and it may facilitate the diagnosis.[325] Other skeletal abnormalities include short distal phalanges and clinodactyly.[326–328]

Other systems apart from those in the cardinal criteria for the syndrome may be affected. Renal abnormalities, such as tubulo-interstitial nephropathy, membranous nephropathy, single kidney and renovascular hypertension, may be prominent. The most frequent finding is mesangiolipidosis.[220,329] Nephrolithiasis may occur, and various types of renal cystic disease have been reported.[330] Skin changes relate mainly to formation of xanthomas which regress after successful liver transplantation.[331] Systemic vascular disease appears to be more prevalent than originally appreciated. Several cases of moya-moya disease in association with Alagille syndrome have been reported.[332,333] The propensity to intracranial bleeding found in the first few years of life in Alagille syndrome may be due to abnormal intracranial vessels.[334-336] Abnormalities in the large intra-abdominal vessels have been found, and these abnormalities may complicate liver transplantation.[337]

Abnormalities of the biliary tract include hypoplasia of the extrahepatic bile ducts,[338-342] hypoplasia of the gall-bladder[327] and cholelithiasis.[338] Endoscopic retrograde cholangiopancreatography has demonstrated narrowing of the intrahepatic ducts, reduced arborization and focal areas of dilatation, as well as narrowing of the extrahepatic ducts.[338-340] Portal venous disease may also be present, specifically hypoplasia of the portal vein.[343]

Many patients develop growth retardation prior to adolescence,[337] especially if they have persisting clinical jaundice. Short stature is found in some affected children whose nutrition is normal. Although some display some degree of mental retardation, in general children with Alagille syndrome show a broad range of cognitive and intellectual ability. Nearly all patients have pruritus, although it may be mild. They have elevated serum bile acids, the levels of cholic acid being greater than those of chenodeoxycholic acid. Variable hyperlipidaemia (sometimes severe, with xanthomas) is frequent. Treatments for the pruritus include cholestyramine, rifampicin or surgical diversion of bile flow.[344]

In general the prognosis is good for children whose jaundice resolves; however, approximately 25% of patients succumb in childhood to severe cardiac disease or progressive liver disease. The outcome in 92 patients in the series of Emerick et al.[315] was as follows: the 20-year predicted life expectancy was 75% for all patients, 80% for those not requiring liver transplantation, and 60% for those who required transplantation. Liver transplantation has been reserved for patients with chronic liver failure, intolerable pruritus unresponsive to medical treatment, and severe growth failure. Transplantation for hepatic decompensation was necessary in 19 of 92 cases (21%) with 79% survival 1 year post-transplantation; the mortality was 17%. The mortality is higher among patients who have more severe cardiac disease or intracranial bleeding, or who had previously undergone porto-enterostomy.[345] Catch-up growth after transplantation has been reported[346] but is variable.[347] Long-term complications of Alagille syndrome not requiring liver transplant have been reported including renal failure and intracranial bleeding or stroke.[314,315,342] Hepatocellular carcinoma has been reported in children and adults with Alagille syndrome.[348-351] Hepatic malignancy may occur in childhood and rarely in infancy.

Pathological aspects of arteriohepatic dysplasia are described in various reports and reviews.[310-312,340,352-360] The major finding is absence of bile ducts from portal areas (Figs 4.24 and 4.25). According to Alagille,[358] the ratio of interlobular bile ducts to the number of portal areas is between 0.0 and 0.4 compared to 0.9 and 1.8 in normal children. A reduced number of portal areas has been noted.[354] The loss

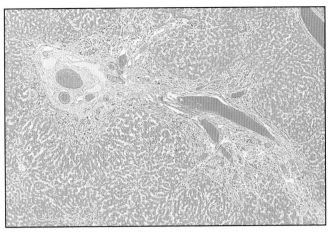

Fig. 4.24 • Arteriohepatic dysplasia. Two fused portal areas lack bile ducts. H&E.

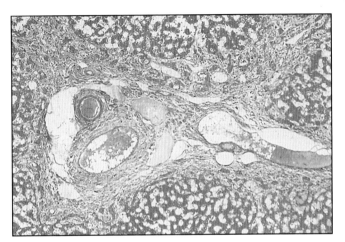

Fig. 4.25 • Same case as illustrated in Fig. 4.24. Portal area contains vessels but no ducts. There is patchy periportal fibrosis but no cholangiolar proliferation. Masson trichrome.

of bile ducts is progressive from early infancy to childhood.[315,340,359,360,362] Cholangiodestructive lesions have been observed in infants between 3 and 6 months of age.[340,360] The degree of cholestasis is variable in intensity and is especially prominent in the first 12 months of life. Giant cell transformation may be seen in early infancy.[340,359,360] There is usually patchy pseudoxanthomatous change[359] and accumulation of stainable copper in periportal hepatocytes.[340,352,359,360] The latter has also been demonstrated by quantitative methods in both syndromatic and non-syndromatic types of paucity of the intrahepatic bile ducts.[352] Periportal fibrosis is mild, and, when present, remains unchanged in long-term follow-up studies.[310] This may be partly explained by the absence of ductular reaction, which is known to play a major role in periportal fibrogenesis. Nonetheless, although progression to cirrhosis is rare, occasional patients do develop extensive fibrosis or cirrhosis (Fig. 4.26). Portal inflammation and periportal ductular reaction, when present, are seen mainly in early infancy and can suggest the presence of distal duct obstruction.[340,360]

Ultrastructural studies of the intrahepatic bile ducts in Alagille syndrome have been reported.[353,359-361] Bile canalicular changes are controversial. In one study of 12 biopsies

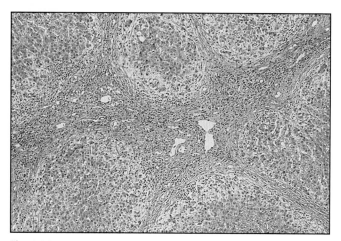

Fig. 4.26 • Arteriohepatic dysplasia. Micronodular cirrhosis. Note ductopenia, moderate septal inflammation and cholate stasis. H&E.

from 10 patients, distinctive ultrastructural changes were noted.[353] Bile pigment retention was found in the cytoplasm of liver cells, especially in lysosomes and in vesicles of the cis-Golgi, but only rarely in bile canaliculi or the immediate pericanalicular region. It was suggested that the basic defect in arteriohepatic dysplasia involves the bile secretory apparatus.[353] The aetiopathogenesis of the cholangiodestructive lesions described histopathologically and ultrastructurally remains to be elucidated, but the possibility of 'disuse atrophy' has been raised by two groups of investigators.[353,360] Recent studies suggest defective branching of intrahepatic bile ducts in the postnatal period.[363]

Alagille syndrome is the first childhood disorder identified with a mutation in a ligand for a Notch protein. *JAG 1* is the human homologue of the rat gene *Jagged 1*. It encodes a ligand of Notch 1, one of a family of transmembrane proteins with epidermal growth factor (EGF)-like motifs. These highly conserved proteins have a role in determining cell fate during differentiation, especially in tissues where epithelial-mesenchymal interactions are important. Cell–cell Jagged/Notch interactions are known to be critical for determination of cell fates in early development. Notch 4 expression during embryogenesis is seen in endothelial cells of vessels forming the dorsal aorta, intersegmental vessels, cephalic vessels and the heart. The expression of Notch 1 and its ligand includes many of the organs potentially abnormal in Alagille syndrome. *JAG 1* is expressed in adult heart and kidney; it is not expressed in adult liver, but in fetal liver[364] it is expressed in portal venous tissue and ductal plate and later in postnatal bile duct epithelial cells. Jagged 1 on ductal plate and Notch 3 on portal tract mesenchyme and hepatic arterial endothelium interact for ductal plate remodeling and development of intrahepatic bile ducts.[365,366] Mice with defects in murine *Jagged 1* and *Notch 2* expression have abnormalities similar to human Alagille syndrome; zebrafish with knockdowns of *jagged* ± *notch* genes have biliary, pancreatic, cardiac, renal, and craniofacial developmental abnormalities; these studies suggest that Notch may promote biliary epithelial cell evolution from a bipotential precursor cells.[367] In humans, mutations in *JAG1* result in truncated, and inactive proteins; since residual gene expression cannot compensate, there is hap-

loinsufficiency.[320] Dose of Notch ligands is critical and this may contribute to the clinical diversity of Alagille syndrome. No clear relationship between genotype and phenotype has been found, but the Delta/Serrate/Lag-2 (DSL) domain in the JAG1 protein may influence the severity of liver disease.[368–370]

In contrast to patients with Alagille syndrome, those with non-syndromic bile duct paucity do not have a constellation of extrahepatic disorders. Children with non-syndromic bile duct paucity are supposed to have a less favorable outlook than children with Alagille syndrome. They present with persistent cholestasis and severe pruritus. Growth retardation is common. No associated aetiological agent, defined genetic factors or congenital anomalies have been found in this group, except for one study of 10 patients with a high rate of consanguinity.[371] A chronic cholestatic disease with duct paucity, called idiopathic adult ductopenia, has been described in adults.[372–374] Most of these patients are young adults, although patients over 60 have been reported.[375] Non-syndromatic paucity of bile ducts in infancy and idiopathic adulthood ductopenia may be related diseases. The outlook for younger patients with idiopathic adult ductopenia is poor; approximately 50% succumb to progressive liver disease or require transplantation.

A histopathological study of 17 children with non-syndromic paucity of bile ducts was reported by Kahn et al.[376] Before 90 days of age there was paucity of ducts and periportal fibrosis as well as non-specific parenchymal changes (cholestasis, giant cell transformation, perisinusoidal fibrosis and haematopoiesis). After 90 days the duct paucity and fibrosis persisted but cholestasis was mild or no longer apparent. Kahn et al.[376] suggested that the paucity in non-syndromic cases may result from a primary ductal insult with destruction and disappearance of the ducts. The differential diagnosis of paucity of the intrahepatic bile ducts in children and adults has been reviewed by West & Chatila.[377]

Congenital dilatations of the bile ducts

Congenital dilatations of the bile ducts are classified into five types, both extrahepatic and intrahepatic:[378]

- Type I—a dilatation of the common bile duct which may present three anatomical variations:
  a. large saccular,
  b. small localized, and
  c. diffuse fusiform.
- Type II—diverticulum of the common bile duct or the gallbladder.
- Type III—choledochocele.
- Type IV—multiple intrahepatic and extrahepatic dilatations (Caroli disease).
- Type V—fusiform intrahepatic and extrahepatic dilatations.

Types I and IV account for the majority of reported cases although types IV and V may prevail in the Far East, where the disease occurs more frequently. Type IV cysts are more frequent in adults than in children.[379] Although this classification remains in common use, its value has been questionned by Visser et al.,[380] who consider the distinction between type I and IV arbitrary; they suggest that the term 'choledochal cyst' should be reserved for congenital dilatation of the extrahepatic and intrahepatic bile ducts, other forms being referred to by their name, for example choledochocoele and bile duct diverticulum. Caroli disease, assimilated to type IV in Hadad's classification, is not clearly related to 'choledochal cyst', given its common association with both congenital hepatic fibrosis and fibrocystic lesions in the kidney and its distinct morphological features (see below).

Choledochal cyst

The classic clinical triad of pain, a mass in the right upper quadrant and jaundice, occurs in less than a third of patients with a choledochal cyst.[381,382] In children, jaundice is the most common presentation, while in adults the signs and symptoms are those of ascending cholangitis.[383] In the early years of life cholestasis is usually associated with cystic dilatation of the common bile duct and accounts fo 2% of infants presenting with cholestasis. Up to 60% of choledochal cysts are diagnosed before age 10, but diagnosis can be made at any age and some cases may present for the first time at as late as the eighth decade of life.[384] Several cases have been diagnosed antenatally.[385,386] Eighty per cent of the patients are female. Differences in presentation between children and adults with choledochal cysts have been emphasized in two large series.[387,388] The preoperative diagnosis can be made in the majority of patients by cholangiographic studies, ultrasound and isotope scanning.[389] Dynamic magnetic resonance cholangiopancreatography (MRCP), including secretion stimulation, contributes to the understanding of the pathophysiology.[390]

Complications include perforation, liver abscesses, stone formation, secondary biliary cirrhosis, pancreatitis, amyloidosis and carcinoma of the biliary tree.[381,391–395] Regression of biliary cirrhosis following drainage of a choledochal cyst has been reported.[396] One case presented with anaemia secondary to bleeding from erosions of the duodenal mucosa between the ampullary sphincter and the sphincters of the common bile duct and pancreatic duct.[397]

Biliary tract anomalies reported in association with a choledochal cyst include double common bile duct, double gallbladder, absent gallbladder, annular pancreas, biliary atresia or stenosis,[398] anomalies of the pancreatico-biliary junction and stenoses of the intrahepatic bile ducts.[399–401] In a series of 104 choledochal cysts from Japan, 25% were found to have co-existing biliary anomalies.[402] Differences between (i) choledochal cysts and (ii) choledochal cysts with biliary atresia have been noted by ultrasonography. In the former the cysts are larger, intrahepatic ducts are dilated and the gallbladder is not atretic as compared to those with choledochal cysts and biliary atresia.[403] In general, the apparent choledochal cyst associated with biliary atresia is actually proximal duct dilatation associated with focal atresia of the distal common bile duct, so-called correctable atresia.

Maljunction of the pancreatico-biliary ductal system (common channel) remains the most plausible aetiopathogenetic mechanism for choledochal cysts, and this is supported by experimental studies.[404] Reovirus 3 RNA sequences have been recovered from resected choledochal cysts,[201] but the implication of reovirus infection in the aetiology of choledochal cyst is unclear. A single report of choledochal cysts in association with familial adenomatous polyposis raises the possibility of a genetic basis for the cysts.[405]

Treatment is by complete cyst resection, cholecystectomy and Roux-en-Y hepaticojejunostomy as a preventive measure for the subsequent development of carcinoma.[406,407] Dilemmas may arise when the cysts involve the intrahepatic or intrapancreatic segments, requiring more extensive surgery, given the small risk of malignancy developing in cystic remnant at the anastomotic site or in the dilated intrahepatic bile duct of type IV or V cysts.[382,408] In a report of 48 Japanese patients treated by total or subtotal excision, no malignant change occurred after a mean follow up of 9.1 years.[409] Choledochal cysts vary greatly in size with some of the larger ones containing 5–10 litres of bile (Figs 4.27 and 4.28). Histopathologically, the wall is usually thickened by inflammation and fibrosis, and is bile stained. Smooth muscle fibres may be identified in the lower portion of the cyst but not in the narrow (intrapancreatic) portion.[410] There is generally no epithelial lining but islets of cylindrical or columnar epithelium may be preserved (Fig. 4.29). Intestinal metaplasia with mucous gland proliferation, as well as the presence of goblet and Paneth cells and neuroendocrine differentiation, have been reported.[411,412] According to Komi et al.[412] the intestinal metaplasia increases with age, so that cysts from almost all patients over 15 years of age contain it. Kusunoki et al. noted the absence of ganglion cells in the narrow portion of a choledochal cyst, and suggested that the cyst could be the result of postganglionic neural dysfunction.[413]

The majority of tumours arising in congenital cystic dilatations of the bile ducts are adenocarcinomas, but some anaplastic and a several squamous carcinomas have been reported[414–416] one report mentioned sarcomatous changes.[417]

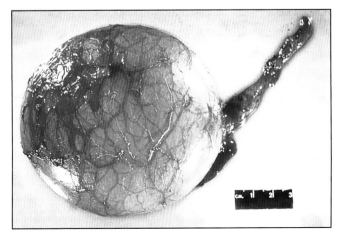

Fig. 4.27 • Choledochal cyst measuring about 10 cm in diameter. Note numerous vessels over the surface.

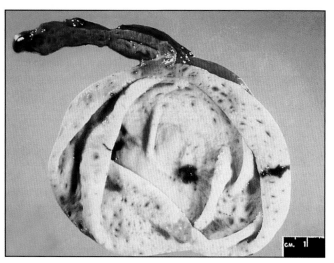

Fig. 4.28 • Same cyst as illustrated in Fig. 4.27. Opened, collapsed cyst has a smooth inner lining. It did not contain bile.

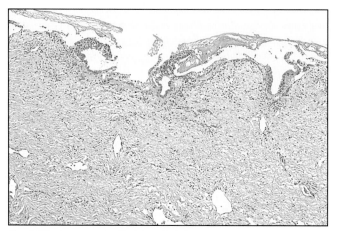

Fig. 4.29 • Segment of wall of choledochal cyst shows inflammation and focal epithelial ulceration. H&E.

The overall incidence of carcinoma arising in all cystic dilatations of the bile ducts is about 3%.[414] The risk is age-related, increasing from 0.7% in the first decade to 6.8% in the second decade to 14.3% in later decades.[416] The complication is thus usually seen in adults; only 3 patients reviewed by Iwai et al. were under 18 years of age.[418] Reveille et al.[419] found that stasis of bile in the choledochal cyst contributes to bacterial overgrowth and the generation of unconjugated secondary bile acids, a possible cause of biliary metaplasia and carcinoma. Interestingly, bile from congenital choledochal cyst patients is shown to promote the proliferation of human cholangiocarcinoma QBC939 cells.[420] Some bile acid fractions and reflux of pancreatic enzymes may play a primary role as pancreaticobiliary maljunction is associated with an increased risk of biliary tree malignancy irrespective of the presence of cysts.[421]

Hereditary fibro-polycystic disease of the liver (ductal plate malformation)

The term *fibropolycystic diseases* of the liver—not to be confused with cystic fibrosis—is used to describe a heterogeneous group of genetic disorders in which segmental dilatations of the intrahepatic bile ducts and associated fibrosis can be interpreted as sequelae of persistence and/or aberrant remodelling of the embryonal ductal plate (p. 4). They represent a merging spectrum of microscopic and/or macroscopic cystic lesions often associated with fibrocystic anomalies in the kidneys. The severity of the renal lesions may overshadow the liver disease, as in the early presentation of *autosomal recessive polycystic kidney disease*. Conversely, portal hypertension with a preserved liver function may later in life dominate the picture as exemplified by *congenital hepatic fibrosis*. Cholangitis may develop, especially when the cysts communicate with the biliary system. These abnormalities are classified as ductal plate malformation,[422,423] a term which refers to the histological changes of circumferentially disposed and variably ectatic bile ducts, often directly abutting the hepatocytic plates, which resemble an exuberant embryonal ductal plate. The main disorders, in particular autosomal recessive polycystic kidney disease, the closely associated congenital hepatic fibrosis and Caroli disease, and autosomal dominant polycystic kidney disease, are discussed in detail, whereas the rarer associated syndromes, which have been comprehensively reviewed by Knisely,[424] are briefly mentioned.

Autosomal recessive polycystic kidney disease (ARPKD)

Infantile presentation

This disease is inherited in an autosomal recessive manner. The prevalence is estimated to be between 1 : 10 000 and 1 : 60 000.[425] The gene for this disorder, PKHD1 (polycystic kidney and hepatic disease 1), has been mapped to chromosome 6p 21.2–p12,[426,427] both severe and mild form of the disease being mapped to the same locus.[428,429] The gene encodes a 4074-amino-acid protein, called fibrocystin[430] or polyductin;[431] this large transmembrane polypeptide may be a receptor that acts in collecting-duct and biliary differentiation. An animal model has been described.[432] There is an equal sex incidence. Depending on the age of presentation and the degree of renal involvement, ARPKD has been divided into four types by Blyth and Ockenden[433]—perinatal, neonatal, infantile and juvenile. These authors proposed that four different mutant alleles are responsible, and that there may be a fifth group in which the onset of symptoms is later than juvenile. ARPKD has been reviewed by a number of authors.[215,434,435]

The *perinatal* type is the most severe form. Fifty per cent of patients are diagnosed perinatally and die shortly after birth.[436] In the series of Blyth and Ockenden,[433] no infant survived beyond 6 weeks of age. The majority of patients were admitted with signs of respiratory distress and had marked abdominal distension due to huge symmetrical renal masses. Liver function test abnormalities were uncommon. Surviving patients with the *neonatal* type of the disease develop gradually increasing renal insufficiency and systemic hypertension. Pyelonephritis is common. Portal fibrosis and cystic dilatation of bile ducts are severe, and cholangitis is a frequent complication. In the *infantile* group the clinical picture is either of chronic renal failure or of increasing portal hypertension. Portal fibrosis is moderate. The *juvenile* group of Blyth and Ockenden[433] typically includes children (1 to 5 years old) who present with portal hypertension. Liver histopathological changes are marked. It is likely that this group represents cases of congenital hepatic fibrosis, as suggested by Landing et al.[437]

Gang and Herrin[438] have found that ARPKD has a spectrum of phenotype expression with prognostic implications, but suggest that not all cases fit into the sharply defined subgroups of Blyth and Ockenden. In their study of 11 patients, four had 90% or more renal cystic change; these patients did not survive beyond 20 days of birth. In contrast, five of the seven less severely diseased patients with a 20–75% range of cystic changes in the kidneys were all alive at 6 to 21 years of age.

The liver in ARPKD does not appear abnormal macroscopically, although it may be enlarged and firm. Histologically, the changes range from a persistent, circular ductal plate (Fig. 4.30) to a striking increase in the number of biliary channels which arise in portal areas and extend irregularly and deeply into the parenchyma (Fig. 4.31(A)). They appear to branch or 'anastomose' and often show polypoid projections (Fig. 4.31(B)). Normal interlobular ducts with corresponding arteries are not seen. According to Witzleben,[434] the biliary channels are in continuity with the rest of the biliary system, similar to the cystic space of Caroli disease ('communicating' cystic disease), in contrast to the non-communicating ADPKD. The supporting connective tissue is very scanty and, in the intralobular extensions, the basement membrane of the epithelium appears to be in direct contact with the liver cell plates. The epithelial lining consists of a single layer of low columnar to cuboidal cells. Cyst formation is uncommon. The dilated channels may contain a small quantity of a pink or orange-coloured material or, rarely, pus. Reconstruction studies by Adams et al.[439] have shown irregularly dilated ducts running longitudinally at the periphery of the portal tract and anastomosing so extensively that they formed a single annular channel; no main interlobular duct could be identified in that portal tract or in several others from the same liver. A

stereological study of 10 cases by Jörgensen[440] showed ductal structures that could be divided into two groups: one consisted of irregular tubular structures shaped like circular cylinders, and the other of elliptical cylinders (the 'ductal plates'). These were dilated but cysts were rare. In patients who survive for months or years there is marked fibrosis in the liver as well as kidney lesions which appear to have been progressive lesions.

Juvenile and adult presentation—congenital hepatic fibrosis (CHF)

Congenital hepatic fibrosis is considered a variant of ARPKD affecting predominantly children and adolescents, some cases being identical to the 'juvenile' form. The inheritance pattern is not a simple autosomal recessive one. It may be associated with dilatation of the intra- or extrahepatic bile ducts,[441,442] so-called Caroli syndrome (see below), the intrahepatic cysts being detectable by sonography or magnetic resonance cholangiography.[443] Infants present with abdominal distension from enlarged organs, respiratory distress and systemic hypertension. Older patients come to medical attention because of hepatosplenomegaly or

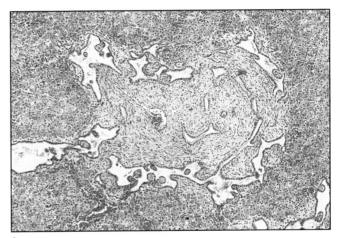

A

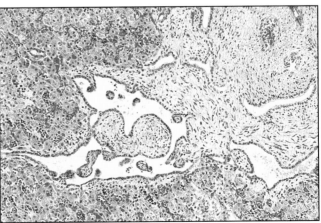

B

Fig. 4.31 • Autosomal recessive polycystic kidney disease. **(A)** The bile ducts form an interrupted ring at the periphery of what should eventually become a portal area. There is no interlobular bile duct. Note branch of portal vein, as well as smaller vessels. H&E. **(B)** Same case, higher magnification of part of the ductal plate showing irregularity in outline of the ducts with polypoid projections into a dilated lumen. The lining epithelium is low cuboidal. H&E.

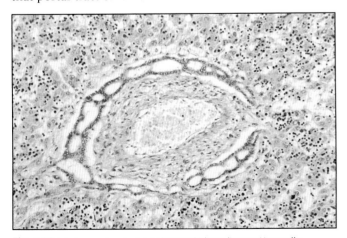

Fig. 4.30 • Autosomal recessive polycystic kidney disease: Unusually prominent ductal plate in the liver of a stillborn foetus with huge polycystic kidneys.

bleeding from oesophageal varices,[444] but asymptomatic cases have been reported.[445] Cholangitis as a manifestation of CHF has been emphasized by Fauvert and Benhamou,[445] who recognized four clinical forms —portal hypertensive, cholangitic, mixed portal hypertensive-cholangitic and latent forms. The pure cholangitic form is rare. In the mixed form patients suffer from recurrent bouts of cholangitis, with or without jaundice, in addition to the manifestations of portal hypertension. In one series of 42 children from 20 sibships, 12 patients presented in the perinatal period, 9 in the neonatal period, 13 in the infantile period, and 8 in the juvenile period; the presentation and course of the disease was disparate in over 50% of patients.[446] The organ predominantly affected, may vary within the same family. Routine liver function tests are usually normal, although alkaline phosphatase levels may be increased.

When present, the usual renal disease is medullary tubular ectasia, a fusiform or cystic dilation of tubules (particularly the collecting ducts). Occasionally, patients have cystic kidneys typical of adult-type polycystic disease, an autosomal dominant disease, and others may have nephronophthisis.[447–450]

The prognosis in patients surviving beyond the neonatal period is generally good and depends on the extent of hepatic and renal disease. Death related to renal failure or uncontrollable variceal bleed is now exceptional.[451] The combination of a patent portal vein and well-preserved liver function makes patients with CHF ideal candidates for portosystemic shunt surgery. Follow-up examination of 16 patients who underwent portosystemic shunt surgery by Alvarez et al.[452] revealed no impairment of liver function or hepatic encephalopathy. Development of cholangiocarcinoma in an adult may have been a chance occurrence in cases not associated with Caroli disease.[453,454]

Pathological descriptions of CHF have been published by many authors.[434,445,455] Grossly, the liver is enlarged, has a firm to hard consistency, and shows a fine reticular pattern of fibrosis; no cysts are visible to the naked eye. Although the entire liver is usually involved, occasional lobar cases of CHF are described.[452]

Microscopically, there is diffuse periportal fibrosis, the bands of fibrous tissue varying in thickness. Irregularly shaped islands of hepatic tissue, some incorporating several lobules, may be seen (Fig. 4.32). When the bands of fibrous tissue are thick, hepatic venules may be encroached upon and become incorporated within the fibrous tissue; thus, portal hypertension in this condition may not always be presinusoidal. The fibrous bands may encircle single or groups of lobules; occasionally, a small islet of hepatic tissue becomes separated from an acinus and becomes encircled by fibrous tissue. Numerous uniform and generally small bile ducts are scattered in the fibrous tissue (Fig. 4.33). An interrupted circular arrangement of the ducts (ductal plate malformation) is often recognizable (Fig. 4.34). The ducts are lined by cuboidal to low columnar epithelium and may contain bile or traces of mucin. They may be slightly dilated and irregular in outline. Cholestasis is not a feature of the uncomplicated case of CHF. Reduction in the number of portal vein branches is often apparent, the likely cause of

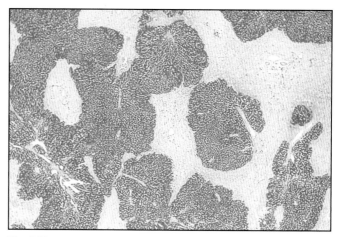

Fig. 4.32 • Congenital hepatic fibrosis. Jigsaw pattern of hepatic parenchyma and fibrous tissue. PAS.

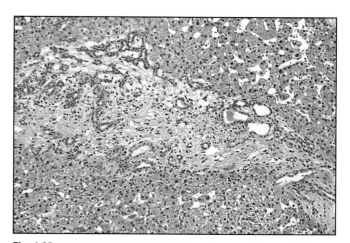

Fig. 4.33 • Congenital hepatic fibrosis. Fibrous tissue contains small bile ducts, a few of which are dilated and contain bile. Note absence of inflammation. The adjacent hepatic parenchyma shows no evidence of cholestasis and the patient is jaundice-free. H&E.

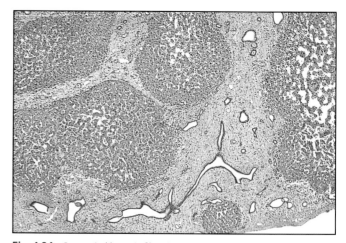

Fig. 4.34 • Congenital hepatic fibrosis. Same case as illustrated in Fig. 4.33. Appearance of ducts suggests part of a ductal plate malformation. H&E.

the portal hypertension. There is generally little inflammation in CHF except in cases associated with cholangitis, when numerous neutrophils infiltrate the ducts and surrounding connective tissue (Fig. 4.35); rupture of the ducts can result in micro-abscess formation. Histopathologically,

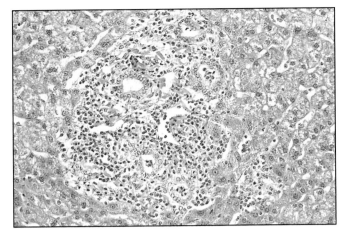

Fig. 4.35 • Congenital hepatic fibrosis, 'cholangitic type'. The ducts are involved by an acute cholangitis. H&E.

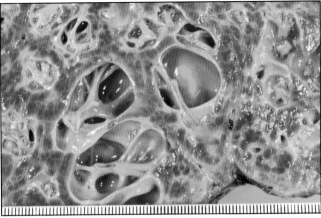

Fig. 4.36 • Caroli disease. Section of liver shows cystically dilated bile ducts. The cystic cavities are traversed by fibrous cords, known to contain the portal vessels. The lining of the ducts is bile stained.

the latter cases may be difficult to differentiate from extra-hepatic biliary obstruction with ascending infection, particularly since there may be an associated tissue cholestasis. The correct diagnosis must be based on the history, clinical findings and the results of radiographic studies. Cholestasis is particularly prominent in those cases associated with microscopic dilatation of the larger intrahepatic bile ducts, too subtle to be seen on imaging ('microscopical Caroli'). Recurrent cholangitis may lead to progressive fibrosis with functional impairment similar to cirrhosis.

- A number of malformation syndromes, characterized by hepatic morphological changes which resemble those of CHF (ductal plate malformation), can be differentiated by the associated findings. They include:
- *Medullary cystic kidney disease 1* (MCKD1), which has an autosomal dominant inheritance, has been mapped to chromosome 1q21;[456]
- *Medullary cystic kidney disease 2*—via uromodulin (UMOD 2), also autosomal dominant, mapped to chromosome 16p12;[457]
- *Nephronophthisis—congenital hepatic fibrosis,*[449] a recessive disorder, whose gene *NPHP1* has been mapped to chromosome 16p12;[458]
- *Meckel syndrome* with encephalocoele, polydactyly and cystic kidneys;[459]
- *Asplenia with cystic liver, kidney and pancreas,* which represents Ivemark syndrome with variants;[460]
- *Ellis–van Creveld syndrome or chondroectodermal dysplasia*[461] with polydactyly, short limbs, short ribs, postaxial polydactyly, and dysplastic nails and feet, which has been mapped to chromosome 4p16;
- *Asphyxiating thoracic dystrophy (Jeune syndrome)* with skeletal dysplasia, pulmonary hypoplasia and retinal lesions;[462]
- *Congenital disorder of glycosylation, type Ib (phosphomannose isomerase deficiency),*[463] sometimes with protein-losing enteropathy (see Chapter 5);
- *Joubert syndrome* with cerebellar vermis hypoplasia/aplasia, colobomata, and psychomotor retardation;[464]
- *Vaginal atresia syndrome;*[437]
- *Tuberous sclerosis.*[437]

Caroli disease

This disease generally involves the entire liver, but it may be segmental or lobar.[465–467] The inheritance is autosomal recessive. By 1982 some 99 cases had been reported; they were evaluated together with 10 personally studied cases by Mercadier et al.[468] Since then many other case reports, as well as small series, have been reported.[469,470] Clinically, patients suffer from bouts of recurrent fever and pain.[467] Jaundice occurs only when sludge or stones block the common bile duct. Liver function tests are generally normal except during episodes of biliary obstruction. The diagnosis is established by a variety of imaging modalities including ERCP, ultrasonography, computed tomography, and MRCP.[471–474]

The complications of Caroli disease resemble those of choledochal cyst and include recurrent cholangitis, abscess formation, septicaemia, intrahepatic lithiasis and amyloidosis. Spontaneous rupture of a bile duct was reported by Chalasani et al.[475] Adenocarcinomas, including some arising in cases with a lobar distribution, have also been reported;[454,476] their incidence is 7%.[477] Hepatocellular carcinoma occurs rarely.[478] Medical treatment consists of symptomatic, or prophylactic, treatment of cholangitis and promotion of bile flow with ursodiol. Surgical treatment includes internal or external drainage procedures.[468] Transhepatic decompression has been advocated.[479] Segmental or lobar forms of Caroli disease can be treated by partial hepatectomy.[468,480] Extracorporeal shock wave lithotripsy has been utilized for disintegration of intrahepatic bile-duct stones.[481] Macroscopically, the intrahepatic cystic dilatations are round or lanceolate, 1.0 to 4.5 cm in diameter, and may be separated by stretches of essentially normal duct (Fig. 4.36).[465] Transluminal fibro-vascular bridges are reminiscent of the periportal location of the cysts (ductal plate) and explain in part the central dot sign observed on computed tomography.[473] Inspissated bile or soft and friable bilirubin calculi may be found in the lumen. Microscopically, the dilated ducts usually show severe chronic inflammation, with or without superimposed acute inflammation, and varying degrees of fibrosis (Fig. 4.37).

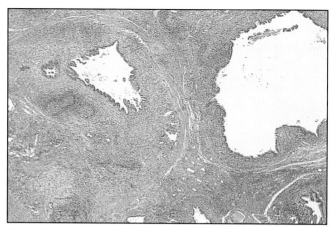

Fig. 4.37 • Caroli disease. Dilated bile ducts have thickened walls due to marked chronic inflammation. Note lymphoid follicles in the wall of one duct (left). H&E.

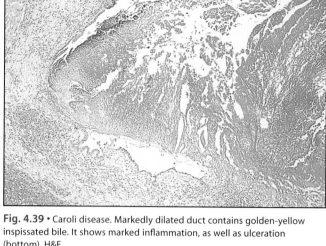

Fig. 4.39 • Caroli disease. Markedly dilated duct contains golden-yellow inspissated bile. It shows marked inflammation, as well as ulceration (bottom). H&E.

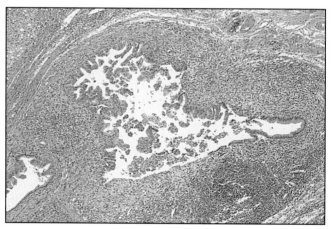

Fig. 4.38 • Caroli disease. The thickened bile duct wall reveals marked chronic inflammation. The lining epithelium is hyperplastic, except for a small segment of the duct (right). There is an area of ulceration (bottom). H&E.

The epithelium may appear normal (cuboidal to tall columnar), partly or completely ulcerated, or focally hyperplastic; all of these changes can be found in different ducts in the same liver (Fig. 4.38). Mucous glands (sometimes in abundance) may be present in the fibrotic and inflamed wall. Areas of severe epithelial dysplasia are seen rarely.[482] The lumen contains admixtures of inspissated mucin and bile, calcareous material, or frank pus during bouts of acute cholangitis (Fig. 4.39). Caroli disease is frequently associated with congenital hepatic fibrosis (in which case it is termed Caroli syndrome), rarely with infantile polycystic disease[483] and even adult polycystic disease.[484]

According to Desmet[422] the pathogenesis of Caroli disease seems to involve total or partial arrest of remodelling of the ductal plate of the larger intrahepatic bile ducts. In Caroli syndrome the hereditary factor causing the arrest of remodelling seems to exert its influence not only during the early period of bile duct embryogenesis, but also later on during development of the more peripheral biliary ramifications (the interlobular bile ducts).

There is a single case described of *Marfan syndrome with diffuse ectasia of the biliary tree.*[485] The authors suggested that the defect of connective tissue in that disease could have led to weakness of the wall of the bile ducts with resultant ectasia.

Autosomal dominant polycystic kidney disease (ADPKD)

Mutations mainly in two different genes *PKD1* and *PKD2* can lead to ADPKD, one of the most common genetic disorders worldwide. The *PKD1* gene lies on the short arm of chromosome 16 (16p 13.3), immediately adjacent to the TSC2, a gene responsible for approximately 50% of tuberous sclerosis.[486,487] The incidence of this mutant gene, comprising 90% of cases, is 1 in 1000. The *PKD1* gene encodes a protein called polycystin.[488] It is present in plasma membranes of renal tubular cells, bile ductules and pancreatic ducts.[489] A subsequent study documents its presence also in hepatocytes and cells of large bile ducts and, in the kidney, an intense reaction at the contact points (only between neighbouring cells) indicating its main function is cell to cell interaction with loss of function contributing to cyst formation.[490] The *PKD2* gene is located on chromosome 4 (4q 21–23) and encodes a 100 kd protein, polycystin 2 with sequence homology to α subunits of voltage-activated calcium channels.[491] Recent studies, one localizing polycystin-1 and polycystin-2 to primary cilia in cultured renal epithelial cells,[492] the other showing that the protein function as a ciliary flow-sensitive mechanosensors,[493] implicate defects in ciliary structure and function as posible mechanism of cyst formation.[494] There is at least one unmapped focus, which accounts for 5% of the disease population.[495] Although PKD2 is clinically milder than PKD1 it does have a deleterious impact on overall life expectancy and cannot be regarded as a benign disorder.[496] The mean age to death or end-stage renal disease is 53 years in PKD1, 69 years in PKD2 and 78 years in controls. PKD2 patients are less likely to have systemic hypertension, urinary tract infections and haematuria.[496] Cerebral aneurysms are found in 10–15% of patients with PKD1. Associated conditions in patients with

PKD2 include colonic diverticula, aortic aneurysm and mitral valve prolapse.

ADPKD is a multisystem disease with cysts and connective-tissue abnormalities involving multiple organs.[497] The renal disease can be present at birth but hepatic manifestations are rare before 16 years of age.[498] The average age at first admission for liver-related problems was 52.8 years with an average duration of symptoms of 3 years.[499] The symptoms included a gradually enlarging abdominal mass, upper abdominal pain or discomfort, and rare episodes of severe pain with or without nausea, vomiting, and occasionally fever. The most frequent physical finding is hepatomegaly, which can be massive.[500] Liver tests are often normal. Jaundice is unusual,[501,502] and portal hypertension is rare.[503] At times this can be related to hepatic outflow obstruction.[504,505] There is an increased risk of gallstones in patients with hepatic cysts.[506] Rarely is treatment needed by excision[507] or a combination of excision and fenestration.[508] Liver or combined liver and renal transplantation has been performed successfully in patients with ADPKD.[509]

The incidence of liver involvement and its complications have been reviewed in a large series including 132 patients on, and 120 patients not on, haemodialysis.[510] Liver cysts were found by non-invasive radiological procedures in 85 of 124 patients on dialysis; sex distribution was equal. In contrast, the non-dialysed population demonstrated a 75% incidence of liver cysts in females and 44% incidence in males, the peak incidence occurring 10 years sooner in females. The cysts were larger and greater in number in that population, and there was a correlation with the number of pregnancies. Nineteen autopsies were reported in which five deaths were liver-related. Risk factors for the development of hepatic cysts in ADPKD were also examined in 39 patients and 189 unaffected family members by Gabow.[511] The hepatic expression of the disease was found to be modulated by age, female gender, pregnancy, and severity of the renal lesion and function. In a recent study Sherstha et al. found that oestrogen treatment of postmenopausal women with ADPKD is associated with selective liver enlargement and abdominal symptoms.[512]

The leading complication in ADPKD is infection of the liver cysts, with cholangiocarcinoma the second most common complication. A study examining hepatic cyst infection suggested that the incidence increases from 1 to 3% during end-stage renal failure.[513] Enterobacteriaceae were cultured from the infected cysts in 9 of 12 patients. In the case of Ikei et al., *Pseudomonas aeroginosa* was cultured from the infected cysts.[514]

Hepatic cysts are rarely detected before puberty and increase with age (ultimately to 75%) in individuals over 70.[515] However, cysts have been found in early childhood and even in the first year of life.[516,517] Prior to availability of a genetic probe, the criteria for identification of this disorder in children included a positive paternal history, cysts in any portion of the renal tubule or Bowman space, macroscopic cysts in the liver and cerebral aneurysms. Associated conditions in ADPKD include colonic diverticula (70%), cardiac valve complications (25%), ovarian cysts (40%), inguinal hernia (15%), and intracranial aneurysms (10%),

suggesting a diffusely abnormal matrix. ADPKD is the cause of end-stage renal disease in 8–10% of adults; the number of cysts is age related.[518,519]

Grossly, the liver in ADPKD is enlarged and diffusely cystic, the cysts varying from <1 mm to 12 cm or more in diameter (Fig. 4.40). One liver reported by Kwok and Lewin weighed 7.7 kg.[500] Occasionally one lobe, usually the left, is affected. Diffuse dilatation of the intra- and extrahepatic bile ducts has been reported in some cases.[520] The cysts contain a clear, colourless or yellow fluid. Analysis of cyst fluid in one case disclosed similarities to the 'bile salt-independent' fraction of human bile, suggesting that such cysts are lined by a functioning secretory bile duct epithelium.[521]

Microscopically, the cysts are lined by columnar or cuboidal epithelium, but the larger cysts have a flat epithelium (Fig. 4.41). Collapsed cysts resemble corpora atretica of the ovary (Fig. 4.42). The supporting connective tissue is scanty except in relation to von Meyenburg complexes (Fig. 4.41), a frequently associated lesion, where it may be dense and hyalinized. A small number of inflammatory cells, usually lymphocytes, may infiltrate the supporting stroma. Infected

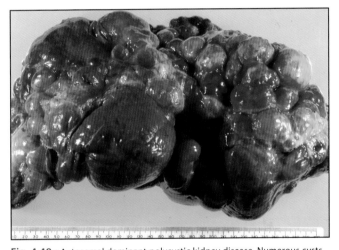

Fig. 4.40 • Autosomal dominant polycystic kidney disease. Numerous cysts of varied size are studded throughout the liver. They contained clear fluid.

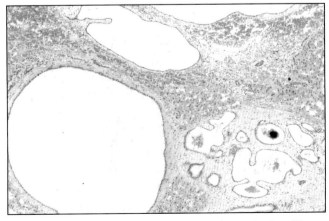

Fig. 4.41 • Autosomal dominant polycystic kidney disease. Section of liver shows multiple cysts of varied size that are lined by a flattened epithelium adjacent to a von Meyenburg complex. H&E.

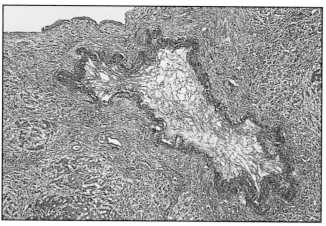

Fig. 4.42 • Autosomal dominant polycystic kidney disease. Collapsed cyst has a corrugated wall and the lumen is filled in with a loose connective tissue. Masson trichrome.

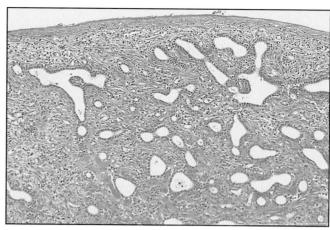

Fig. 4.44 • von Meyenburg complex. Small bile ducts are embedded in a fibrous stroma. Note irregular shape of two of the ducts, each of which contains a polypoid projection. H&E.

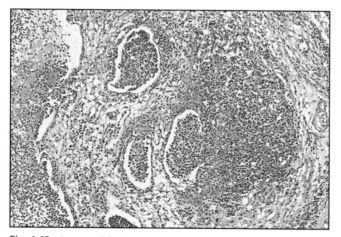

Fig. 4.43 • Autosomal dominant polycystic kidney disease. Infected cysts are filled with pus. The cyst to the right has ruptured with formation of a small cholangitic abscess. H&E.

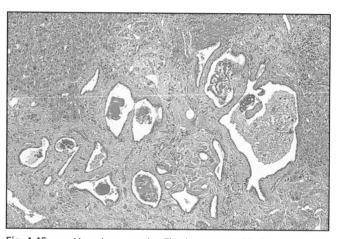

Fig. 4.45 • von Meyenburg complex. The ducts are variably dilated and contain altered bile. H&E.

cysts contain pus and may rupture (Fig. 4.43). Calcification of the wall of hepatic (and renal) cysts in ADPKD has been reported.[522]

Von Meyenburg complexes are considered part of the spectrum of adult polycystic disease, and Melnick was of the opinion that polycystic disease of the liver develops progressively over the years by gradual cystic dilatation of these complexes.[523] That view is supported by a histomorphometric and clinicopathological study of 28 cases of ADPKD reported by Ramos et al.[524] Kida et al. have suggested that cystic dilatation of peribiliary glands also may lead to formation of the cysts in ADPKD.[525] Von Meyenburg complexes are small (less than 0.5 cm in diameter), greyish white or green, and are usually scattered in both lobes.[526] They are occasionally associated with cavernous haemangiomas, and have an abnormal vascular pattern in angiographic studies. Microscopically, the lesions are discrete, round to irregular in shape and typically periportal in location. The constituent ducts are embedded in a collagenous stroma and are often round (but may be irregular in shape) and have a slightly dilated lumen (Fig. 4.44). They are lined by low columnar or cuboidal epithelium and contain pink

amorphous material that may be bile-stained, or actual bile (Fig. 4.45). Cholangiocarcinomas have been reported in association with von Meyenburg complexes,[527,528] as well as with multiple hepatic cysts considered part of the spectrum of ADPKD.[529,530] Congenital hepatic fibrosis has been found in some cases.[531] Mitral valve prolapse was found in 12% of affected children.[532]

Isolated polycystic liver disease (PCLD), not linked to *PKD1* or *PKD2*, has been reported.[533-535] Recently, germline mutations in *PRKCSH*, a known gene encoding for a previously described human protein 'noncatalytic beta-subunit of glucosidase II' have been associated with ADPKD.[536] This protein, now renamed hepatocystin, seems to segregate in families with PCLD.

Solitary (non-parasitic) bile-duct cyst

Solitary bile-duct cyst is defined as a unilocular cyst lined by a single layer of columnar or low cuboidal epithelium resting on a basement membrane and a layer of fibrous tissue. The cysts occur at all ages though the majority present in the fourth to the sixth decades. They are rare in the paediatric age group; in the Boston Children's Hospital 31 solitary nonparasitic cysts (26 unilocular and 5 multilocular) were diagnosed in 63 years.[537] The female to male ratio is 4 : 1.[538] Cysts smaller than 8–10 cm rarely cause symptoms. When present, symptoms include fullness or an upper abdominal mass, nausea and occasional vomiting. Rapid enlargement has been reported in infancy.[539] Jaundice occurs infrequently.[540] An acute abdominal crisis may result from torsion, strangulation, haemorrhage into the cyst or rupture.[541] Diagnosis is usually established by ultrasonography, computed tomography or other imaging modalities. Solitary bile-duct cysts involve the right lobe twice as often as the left. Rarely, they can arise in the falciform ligament.[542] They are usually round and rarely are pedunculated; the lining is typically smooth (Fig. 4.46). The larger ones may contain one to several litres of fluid which is usually clear, but may be mucoid, purulent (if the cyst is infected), haemorrhagic or rarely bile-stained.

Microscopically, the cyst lining usually consists of a single layer of columnar, cuboidal or flat epithelium (Fig. 4.47). The epithelium rests on a basement membrane that in turn is supported by a layer of fibrous tissue. Adenocarcinomas may arise in the cyst.[543] Other malignancies reported to arise in solitary cysts include squamous cell carcinoma.[544] carcinosarcoma[545] and carcinoid tumour.[546]

The pathogenesis of solitary bile-duct cyst is unknown. A congenital origin is supported by the occurrence of the cysts in fetuses and newborns,[539] by a case presenting as a congenital diaphragmatic hernia,[547] and the association of another case with the Peutz–Jeghers syndrome.[548]

In the past, the treatment of choice of solitary cysts was excision,[549] but this has been supplanted by aspiration and sclerotherapy,[550,551] or laparoscopic fenestration.[552,553]

Reye syndrome

The syndrome of fatty liver and encephalopathy, first described in 1963 by Reye et al.,[554] based on post-mortem findings in 17 children from Australia, was soon recognized to have a worldwide distribution.[555] The original observation of an association between aspirin and Reye syndrome,[556] subsequent advice from the Surgeon General of the USA[557] that the use of salicylates be avoided in children suffering from influenza or varicella and confirmation by a pilot prospective study suggested similar results[558,559] and have been followed by a steady decline in the incidence of 'classic' or 'idiopathic' Reye syndrome worldwide.[560,561] At the present time, all patients presenting with a 'Reye-like syndrome' are presumed to have an inherited metabolic disorder unless there is clear evidence of the classical combination of a flu-like illness and salicylate therapy (see p. 247). In addition, metabolic disorders have been subsequently diagnosed in many patients who had survived an acute disease attributed to Reye syndrome.[562]

With few exceptions,[563,564] idiopathic Reye syndrome occurs almost exclusively in children, has no sex predilection, and is usually preceded by a resolving viral illness, particularly influenza B or varicella. Initial symptoms include vomiting (usually repetitive), lethargy and changes in mental status. Hepatic dysfunction can be overlooked since the liver is minimally enlarged, and there is no jaundice or splenomegaly. Subsequent symptoms and signs are predominantly neurological and terminate in coma. Seizures sometimes occur, particularly in younger children with hypoglycaemia. Most patients have received multiple medications, including aspirin, for the symptoms of the viral illness. Initial laboratory screening tests disclose elevated serum aminotransferase levels, hyperammonaemia and coagulopathy. Although the liver disease is benign and transient, the encephalopathy (secondary to a hypoxic/metabolic insult resulting in cerebral oedema) can be life-threatening and results in permanent neurological disability.[555]

Grossly, liver biopsy or autopsy specimens from patients with Reye syndrome are yellow. The major histopathological finding is diffuse microvesicular steatosis.[565] In the typical case the hepatocytes are swollen and packed with multiple small vacuoles (Fig. 4.48); neutral lipid can be demonstrated in frozen sections stained with oil red-O or Sudan black B (Fig. 4.49(A)). The lipid droplets are consistently smaller in the perivenular zone than in other areas.[565] Vacuolization

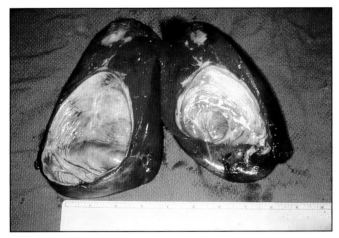

Fig. 4.46 • Solitary bile-duct cyst. The sectioned cyst has a smooth lining.

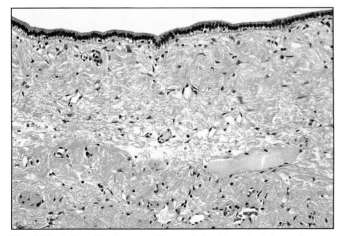

Fig. 4.47 • Solitary bile-duct cyst. The cyst is lined by a single layer of columnar cells. H&E.

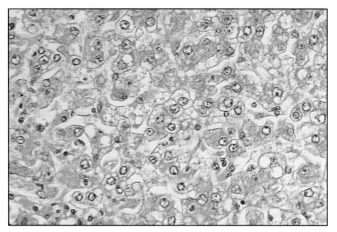

Fig. 4.48 • Reye syndrome. Liver cells show microvesicular steatosis. H&E.

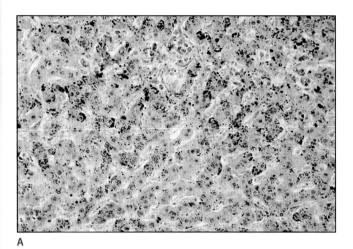

A

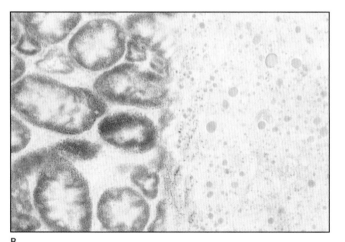

B

Fig. 4.49 • Reye syndrome. **(A)** Microvesicular steatosis is shown in this frozen section stained with Sudan black B. **(B)** Succinyl dehydrogase is absent in the liver (right of the field), contrasting with the finely granular staining in the tubules of a control rat kindney (left of the field), in which the liver biopsy specimen has been embedded.

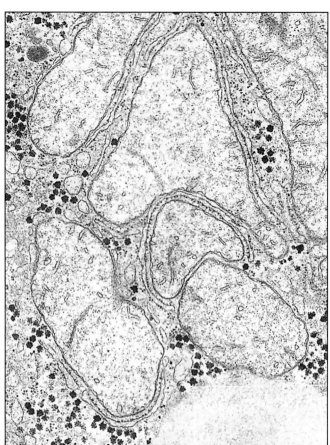

Fig. 4.50 • Reye syndrome. Electron micrograph showing swollen mitochondria with loss of matrix density and both fragmentation and reduction in the number of cristae. Note absence of dense granules in the mitochondria. × 20 000. Courtesy of Dr Cynthia C Daugherty, Children's Hospital Medical Center, Cincinnati, Ohio, USA.

may not be evident in biopsy material obtained less than 24 hours after the onset of encephalopathy, even though appropriately stained frozen sections will reveal an abundance of fat. Nuclei of the liver cells are enlarged and centrally located. Mitotic activity of variable degree may be seen. Hepatocellular necrosis is generally absent or is mild and spotty. Periportal necrosis is occasionally found,[566] preceded by ballooning degeneration of periportal hepatocytes. Variation in the severity of glycogen depletion of liver cells in early biopsies correlates with other histological measures of severity, and with the occurrence of hypoglycaemia, severity of encephalopathy at the time of admission, and the mortality rate. Portal inflammation is either minimal or absent. Cholestasis is rarely observed; in some instances it may be related to an associated pancreatitis.[567] Reduction of succinic dehydrogenase and cytochrome oxidase activities (and other mitochondrial enzymes) has been demonstrated by enzymatic stains and is most helpful in confirming the diagnosis[568] (Fig.4.49(B)).

At the ultrastructural level, the most dramatic changes are seen in hepatocellular mitochondria,[568,569] which are enlarged and misshapen. The degree of enlargement correlates to some extent with the stage of encephalopathy.[569] The severity of the disease may also be correlated with lucency of the mitochondrial matrix and loss of matrical dense bodies (Fig. 4.50). Other mitochondrial changes in initial hepatic biopsy specimens from patients who die or have severe neurological sequelae include a decrease in size and number of cristae (Fig. 4.50). There may be an increase in the amount of smooth endoplasmic reticulum with varying degrees of dilatation, and 50% of hepatic biopsy specimens reveal flocculent peroxisomes.[570]

Microvesicular steatosis has been reported in several inherited metabolic disorders (Chapter 5) and in drug- and toxin-induced liver injury, such as with tetracycline, nucleoside analogues, aflatoxin, pyrrolizidine alkaloids, margosa oil, hypoglycin A, pentenoic acid and valproic acid (Chapter 14). Aspirin toxicity may mimic Reye syndrome.[571] At the light microscopic level, the liver findings in children with fatal salicylate intoxication resemble those of Reye syndrome,[572] but the ultrastructural changes appear to be different.[569]

Animal models of Reye syndrome with encephalomyocarditis virus[573] or influenza B[574] infection, treatment with 4-pentenoic acid,[575] and the spontaneous 'Reye-like syndrome' in BALB/c ByJ mice have been developed.[576]

Kawasaki disease

First described as acute febrile mucocutaneous lymph node syndrome in 1967,[577] the clinical features, diagnostic criteria and management of Kawasaki disease have been recently reviewed.[578] The principal diagnostic criteria of this acute, self-limited vasculitis of childhood are fever; bilateral non-exudative conjunctivitis; erythema of lips and oropharyngeal cavitiy; changes in the extremities, an erythematous rash; and cervical lymphadenopathy.[579] Gastrointestinal signs and symptoms include abdominal tenderness, vomiting, diarrhoea, bloody stools and mild jaundice. Hepatobiliary complications comprise hepatosplenomegaly, mild ascites and hydrops of the gallbladder. Painless jaundice is rarely the first symptom.[580] The laboratory data include abnormal electrocardiograms, neutrophil leucocytosis with a shift to the left, thrombocytosis and an increased erythrocyte sedimentation rate. Mortality is twice the normal rate in boys during the first 2 months of the illness.[581] Coronary aneurysms and myocarditis occur in 10–20% of patients, with a higher incidence in boys.[582] Early therapy with high-dose intravenous γ-globulin and perhaps aspirin has proved beneficial, the former seemingly reducing the frequency of coronary artery abnormalities.[583,584] Atypical cases not fulfilling these diagnostic criteria have a much higher mortality rate, perhaps because of the lack of therapy.[585]

The hepatobiliary complications of Kawasaki disease have been underestimated in the past. The most common problem results from a hydrops of the gallbladder, which is detectable by sonography with an incidence ranging from 2.5 to 13.7%.[586] Prolonged pain has been attributed to poor emptying of the gallbladder.[587] The patients have right upper quadrant pain sometimes associated with vomiting. A majority have hepatomegaly and, at times, a palpable gallbladder. Resolution usually occurs in 4 weeks. Perforation is a rare complication. Cholangitis with bile duct injury and ductular reaction has been observed on liver biopsy in 3 cases.[588] Pathological findings at laparotomy include inflammation of the gallbladder, with or without evidence of vasculitis, and occasionally cystic duct obstruction due to inflammatory oedema or lymph node compression.

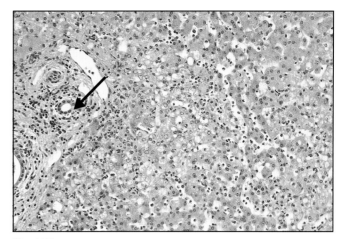

Fig. 4.51 • Kawasaki disease. Portal inflammation (left) with an acute cholangitis (arrow). Note presence of neutrophils in sinusoids and periportal steatosis. H&E.

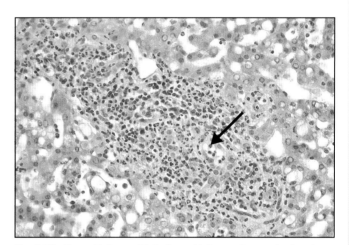

Fig. 4.52 • Kawasaki disease. Marked portal inflammation, predominantly neutrophilic, and acute cholangitis (arrow). H&E.

In addition to vasculitis, inflammation has been noted in autopsy cases in the oral cavity (including ductal structures), small bowel, and the pancreas (including the ducts);[589] acute cholangitis or bile-duct damage has also been observed.[589–591] Slight bile ductular reaction has been noted but, to date, ductopenia has not been a feature. Cholangitis may be associated with sinusoidal neutrophilic infiltrates (Figs 4.51 and 4.52), and proliferation and swelling of Kupffer cells are commonly seen.

Similarities between this condition and leptospirosis have been pointed; although the Weil–Felix reaction may be positive, tests for leptospirosis are negative.[592] The close resemblance of fatal cases to infantile periarteritis nodosa has also been emphasized in several studies.[589,593] Affected vessels include the larger coronary arteries, splenic, renal, pulmonary, pancreatic, spermatic, periadrenal, hepatic and mesenteric vessels. Microscopically, the vessels show periarterial inflammation, necrosis and destruction of the media, and intimal inflammation. Lesions of varying stages can be observed in different vessels in the same patient and in different areas of the same type of vessel (e.g. coronary arteries), suggesting that the inflammatory process continues over a period of time during the course of the disease.

Aneurysmal dilatation of coronary and other vessels (brachial, iliac, renal and pulmonary) may occur.[589,594] A case of a 4-year-old boy with a hepatic artery aneurysm that caused obstructive jaundice was reported by Marks et al.[595]

Other than leptospirosis, *Propionobacterium acnes*,[596] toxin-secreting *Staphylococcus aureus*,[597] HIV,[598] Epstein–Barr virus (EBV),[599] parvovirus B19,[600] *Yersinia* infection,[601] and an unusual response in a susceptible individual to an infectious agent such as the measles virus[602] have all been proposed as causes of Kawasaki disease but are not supported by hard data.

Langerhans cell histiocytosis

This rare disorder, previously termed histiocytosis X or Langerhans cell granulomatosis, is characterized by infiltration of various tissues and organs by Langerhans cell histiocytes. Langerhans cell histiocytosis (LCH) primarily affects bone, but lung, skin and lymph node involvement is not uncommon. Hepatic involvement is also well recognized, especially in children, with sclerosing cholangitis occurring in 10–15% of those with multisystemic involvement,[603,604] whereas LCH confined to the liver appears very unusual.[605,606] Kaplan et al. reported 9 cases of hepatobiliary LCH and found another 85 acceptable cases in the literature.[607] Ages ranged from 7 days to 62 years of age, with a median of 18 months, and a 2 to 1 female preponderence. Hepatosplenomegaly, jaundice, liver dysfunction and ascites were the most common clinical presentations.

Gross findings vary with the stage of disease and type of hepatic involvement. Large aggregates of Langerhans cells, eosinophils and other inflammatory cells may form tumour-like masses. Infiltration of large ducts may lead to grossly visible cystic dilatation and rupture. Other cases show irregularly distributed biliary fibrosis, while a biliary cirrhosis is already present in a few cases.[607]

The diagnostic feature of all cases was the presence of Langerhans cells.[608] They typically have an abundant pink cytoplasm, lobulated, coffee-bean shaped or contorted nuclei with a fine chromatin pattern and no discernible nucleoli (Figs 4.53 and 4.54). In the vast majority of cases the Langerhans cells are accompanied by varying numbers of eosinophils (Fig. 4.55), lymphocytes, neutrophils, plasma cells, non-Langerhans histiocytes, and occasional multinucleated giant cells. Immunostains were useful in confirming the nature of the Langerhans cells using antibodies to S-100 protein, CD1a (Fig. 4.56)[609,610] and CD31.[611] CD1a is important as activated Kupffer cells may acquire S100 positivity.[612] CD101 is a new phenotypic marker that might be useful in combination with other markers of Langerhans histiocytes, but it can only be used in frozen sections.[613] Typical Birbeck granules may be found ultrastructurally in Langerhans cell histiocytes.

Many with disseminated disease have aggregates of Langerhans cells that ranged from granulomatous foci to large nodules in the liver (Figs 4.57 and 4.58) with eosinophils present in abundance in these lesions.[607,614] The majority of cases show some degree of active bile-duct infiltration, injury and destruction by Langerhans cells (Figs 4.59 and 4.60); this is the most characteristic feature of hepatic involvement. Small and medium-size bile ducts are often infiltrated by the Langerhans cells with displacement of the epithelial cells. Some ducts may be entirely replaced by masses of Langerhans cells within the pre-existing basement membrane. Injury to large bile ducts by the Langerhans

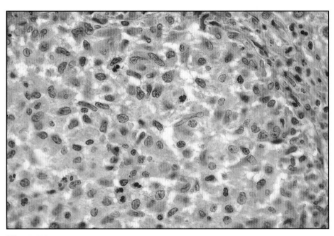

Fig. 4.54 • Langerhans cell histiocytosis. Higher magnification of Langerhans cell. H&E.

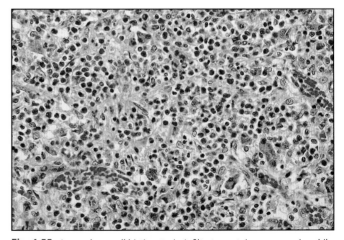

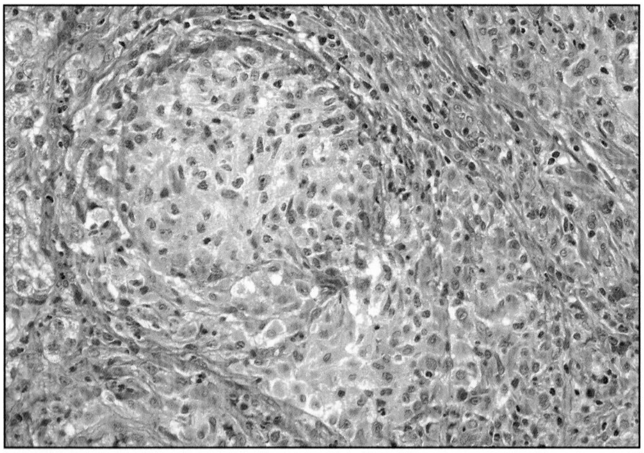

Fig. 4.55 • Langerhans cell histiocytosis. Infiltrate contains many eosinophils. H&E.

Fig. 4.53 • Langerhans cell histiocytosis. Granulomatoid aggregate of Langerhans cell. H&E.

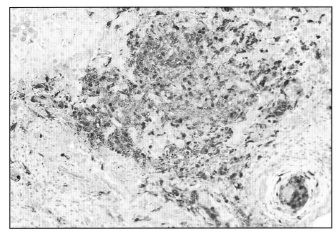

Fig. 4.56 • Langerhans cell histiocytosis. Langerhans cells are strongly immunoreactive to anti-CD1a.

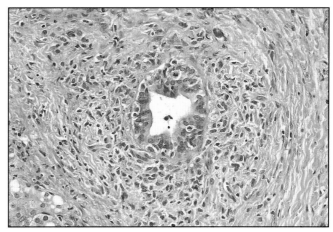

Fig. 4.59 • Langerhans cell histiocytosis. Bile duct showing degenerative changes is surrounded by Langerhans cells. H&E.

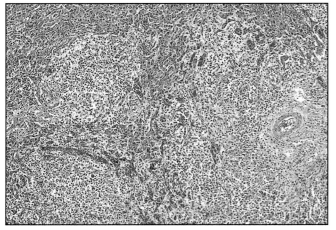

Fig. 4.57 • Langerhans cell histiocytosis. The section is from a case that had a grossly visible tumour. H&E.

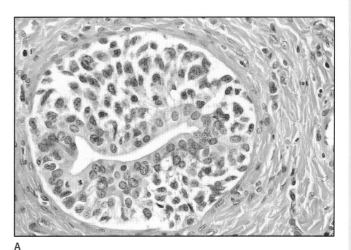

A

B

Fig. 4.60 • Langerhans cell histiocytosis. **(A)** High magnification of degenerating bile duct surrounded by a cuff of Langerhans cells. H&E. **(B)** Bile duct is heavily infiltrated by Langerhans cells that are strongly immunoreactive to anti-CD1a.

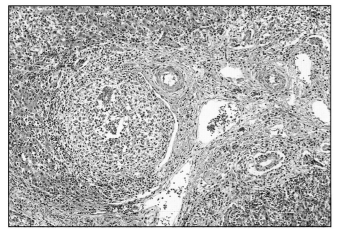

Fig. 4.58 • Langerhans cell histiocytosis. Same case depicted in Fig. 3.56 showing heavy infiltration of portal area and bile duct necrosis (left). H&E.

cells may produce cystic dilatation and rupture with a xanthogranulomatous inflammatory response.

Concentric periductal fibrosis is a prominent feature in the majority of cases. When the ductal infiltration by Langerhans cells is pronounced, there is often marked surrounding fibrosis with demonstrable Langerhans cells in the fibrous tissue. Ducts at a distance from the Langerhans cell lesions may also show epithelial injury and periductal fibrosis, indicating a secondary sclerosing cholangitis.

Changes secondary to the bile-duct lesions include periportal ductular reaction, ductopenia (Fig. 4.61), chronic cholestatic features with periportal cholate stasis ('pseudo-

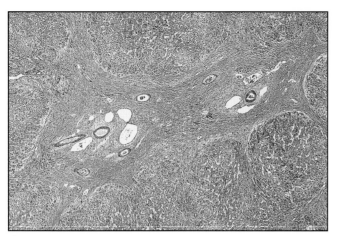

Fig. 4.61 • Langerhans cell histiocytosis. Two fused portal areas are bereft of bile ducts. Masson trichrome.

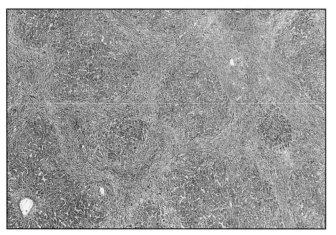

Fig. 4.62 • Langerhans cell histiocytosis. End-stage micronodular cirrhosis. Masson trichrome.

of human cytomegalovirus,[621] Epstein–Barr virus[622] and human herpes virus 6[623] have been detected by immunohistochemistry, in situ hybridization and PCR in LCH tissue, but whether these represent causal agents or opportunistic infections secondary to immune dysregulation remains uncertain.

Although patients with LCH have a good overall prognosis,[624] approximately 20% of patients with multisystem involvement will show a progressive disease course despite treatment.[625,626] In particular, patients with hepatic involvement have a worse prognosis with survival at 3 years of 96.7% for those without, but only 51.8% for those with liver involvement.[627] In patients with liver cirrhosis and failure secondary to LCH sclerosing cholangitis, orthotopic liver transplantation has been proven a successful therapeutic option[615,628] with 67% of patients living long-term after surgery (median follow-up 5.8 years, range 2.1 to 7.5 years).[629] A significant number of LCH patients have developed post-transplant lymphoproliferative disorders, which seems related to a higher incidence of refractory rejection.[629] Disease recurrence in the liver allograft occurs in some 30% of patients and seems easily managed.[629,630]

Juvenile xanthogranuloma, a histiocytic disorder, primarily but not exclusively seen throughout the first two decades of life and principally as a solitary cutaneous lesion, can manifest with multiple small systemic lesions—xanthoma disseminatum—in which case the liver can occasionally be involved.[631] The infiltrating cells are factor XIIIa, fascin and CD68 positive, but S100 and CD1a negative.[631] Touton cells are rarely seen in extracutaneous sites. There appears to be an overlap with LCH since skin lesions with characteristics of juvenile xanthogranuloma may be found in children with LCH.[604]

Sinus histiocytosis with massive lymphadenopathy (Rosai–Dorfman disease)

This disorder was first reported by Rosai & Dorfman[632] and has been reviewed by Foucar et al.[633] It usually affects patients between the ages of 10 and 20 years. In addition to massive enlargement of cervical and other lymph nodes, there is fever, leucocytosis, an elevated sedimentation rate and hyperglobulinaemia. The course is protracted, lasting from 3 to 9 months, but the prognosis is usually excellent. The disease can involve extranodal sites, including soft tissues, the oral cavity, lower respiratory tract, genitourinary system, and the liver. Involvement of the last 3 organs is associated with a poor prognosis.[633] Lauwers et al. studied 11 patients in whom the disease involved the intestinal tract (5 cases), liver (5 cases) and pancreas (one case).[634] Most patients also had evidence of disease in other extranodal sites, as well as in one or more lymph node groups.

In the review of Foucar et al., hepatomegaly was noted in 27 of 157 cases.[633] Four patients had histopathological evidence of hepatic involvement. In most instances gross evidence of disease is lacking, except for one case in which a

xanthomatous change') and deposition of copper and copper-binding protein. Some degree of periportal or bridging fibrosis is common and progress to a biliary cirrhosis (Fig. 4.62). It must be noted that needle biopsy specimens may show changes secondary to a distal cholangiopathy only, without demonstration of Langerhans cells, despite direct LCH infiltration of the major bile ducts.[615]

The differential diagnosis of LCH in childhood includes *primary sclerosing cholangitis*, with or without chronic inflammatory bowel disease (See Chapter 11). In view of the morphological overlap with LCH it is recommended that immunostains for S-100 and CD1a be performed in all cases clinically and/or morphologically diagnosed as primary sclerosing cholangitis in children.

The aetiology and pathogenesis of LCH remain undetermined. Evidence suggests an immune dysregulation with uncontrolled clonal proliferation of dendritic cells exhibiting Langerhans cell characteristics. A low susceptibility to apoptosis[616] and high level of diverse cytokines production by Langerhans cells,[617] with sustained stimulation of T cells, lead to the unique pathological picture, which combines features of a neoplasm and chronic inflammation.[618] The demonstrated clonality of LCH does not prove the neoplastic nature of the lesion.[619,620] Viral proteins and DNA seqences

1.5 cm, well-circumscribed white nodule was found in the right lobe of the liver.[633] The hallmark of the disease is the proliferation of histiocytes which have an abundant cytoplasm and normal-appearing nuclei (Figs 4.63 (A), (B)). The cells are seen in portal areas and in hepatic sinusoids. They display avid leucophagocytosis, but can also phagocytose red cells. According to Eisen et al.,[635] the cells express: S-100

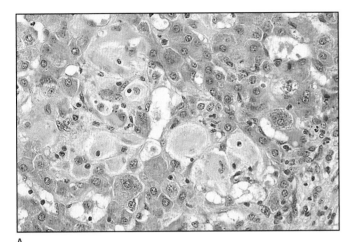

A

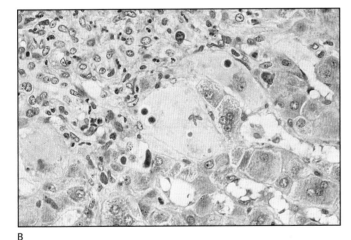

B

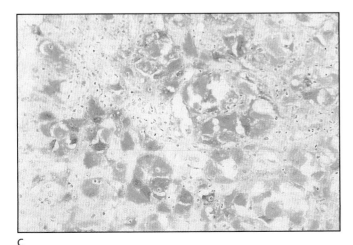

C

Fig. 4.63 • Rosai–Dorfman disease. **(A)** Sinusoids are filled with large histiocytes showing leucophagocytosis. H&E. **(B)** Same case as illustrated in (A). Histiocytes display both erythro- and leucophagocytosis. H&E. **(C)** Same case as illustrated in (A),(B). Histiocytes are immunoreactive for S-100 protein.

protein (Fig. 4.63(C)); pan-macrophage antigens such as EBM11, HAM56 and Leu-M3; antigens functionally associated with phagocytosis (Fc receptor for IgG and complement receptor); antigens functionally associated with lysosomal activity (lysozyme, α_1-antitrypsin and α_1-antichymotrypsin); antigens associated with early inflammation (Mac-387, 27E10); antigens commonly found on monocytes, but not tissue macrophages (OKM5, Leu-M1); and activation antigens (Ki-1 and receptors for transferrin and interleukin-2). The cells thus appear to be true, functionally activated macrophages derived recently from circulating monocytes.[635]

The haemophagocytic syndromes

Haemophagocytic lymphohistiocytosis (familial haemophagocytic reticulosis)

Familial haemophagocytic lymphohistiocytosis (FLH), a fatal inherited form of haemophagocytic lymphohistiocytosis (HLH) syndrome, is a defect in cell-mediated cytotoxicity characterized by the overwhelming activation of T lymphocytes and macrophages. FLH is a heterogeneous autosomal recessive disorder; one causative gene (PFR1, localized to chromosome 10q21–22) encoding for perforin, a cytotoxic effector protein, is identified in a subset of patients.[636,637] FLH can usually be distinguished from other infantile causes of histiocytosis by the absence of skin lesions and the high incidence of central nervous system involvement. The disease is characterized by fever, anorexia, irritability and pallor in infancy and early childhood. Jaundice and hepatosplenomegaly may develop later.[638] FLH may present as acute liver failure in early childhood, and due to very high serum ferritin levels in this condition, distinction from so-called perinatal haemochromatosis can be difficult.[639,640] Tissue specimens are critical in distinguishing these two diseases as liver transplantation is contraindicated in FHL, whereas it might be life-saving in perinatal haemochromatosis.[640] Markedly abnormal coagulation studies reflect low fibrinogen levels and thrombocytopenia, but other coagulation factors are normal. Neurological symptoms may develop from histiocytic involvement of the brain. Although clinical manifestations may remit temporarily, the disease is eventually fatal. The diagnosis is based on identifying erythrophagocytosis by histiocytes in bone marrow biopsy material, or occasionally on liver biopsy. Perforin expression by peripheral lymphocytes, assessment of 2B4 lymphocyte receptor and natural killer (NK) cell activity have been proposed as rapid tests to assist differentiating FLH from HLH subtypes, therefore highlighting patients with a poor prognosis who may benefit from bone marrow transplantation.[636]

In an autopsy series haemophagocytosis was most commonly observed in the spleen, lymph nodes and bone marrow.[641] Hepatic involvement is characterized by hypertrophy of Kupffer cells and portal macrophages which manifest striking erythrophagocytosis[642] (Fig. 4.64), but this may be inconspicuous or even absent.[643] Portal areas show lymphohistiocytic infiltrates with a predominance of T-

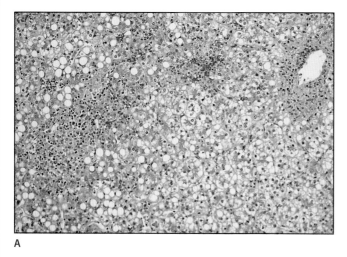

A

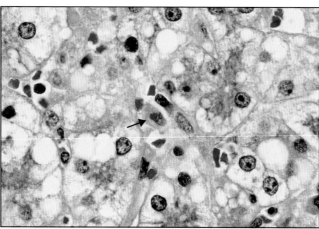

B

Fig. 4.64 • Haemophagocytic lymphohistiocytosis. **(A)** Portal area (left) infiltrated by lymphocytes. H&E. There is mild periportal steatosis. **(B)** Higher magnification showing erythrophagocytosis by a Kupffer cell (arrow). H&E.

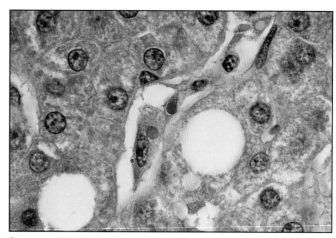

A

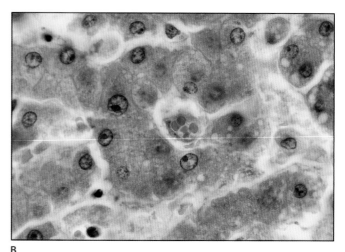

B

Fig. 4.65 • Reactive haemophagocytosis in a patient with AIDS. **(A)** Kupffer cell has phagocytosed two erythrocytes. H&E. **(B)** Kupffer cell contains three erythrocytes. Biebrich scarlet.

lymphocytes, in a pattern reminiscent of chronic hepatitis (Fig. 4.64). In some cases there is striking enlargement of endothelial cell nuclei and perivenous erythropedesis resembling graft rejection.[643] Other changes include mild hepatocellular damage in the vicinity of the lymphohistiocytic infiltrates, variable cholestasis and epithelioid granulomas.[643]

Infection-associated (reactive) haemophagocytic syndrome

In this condition there is proliferation of morphologically non-malignant histiocytes showing phagocytosis of haemopoietic cells, with associated fever and pancytopenia. There is a wide range of clinical severity from the incidental observation during infection or at autopsy that macrophages throughout the body are large and activated to the full-blown haemophagocytic syndrome (HLH) that includes fever, hepatosplenomegaly, coagulopathy, and various cytopaenias.[604] Epstein–Barr virus infection (virus-associated haemophagocytic syndrome) remains the most frequent association, but since the first report in 1979, many other viruses[644] and other infectious agents have been incrimi-

ated.[645] Patients with rheumatic disorders, especially juvenile chronic arthritis, appear particularly at risk.[646,647] Haemophagocytic features are often seen in livers of patients with AIDS (Fig. 4.65). The syndrome may also develop in diseases other than infections, such as lymphoma and disseminated carcinoma.[648] Common to the macrophage activation syndrome with reactive (secondary), HLH is a massive cytokine and chemokine release, mostly TNF-alpha, interferon (IFN)-gamma, soluble interleukin-2 (IL-2) receptor, IL-6, and other cytokines whose levels in the blood may have a prognostic value.[649] This cytokine profile distinguishes HLH from the primary familial conditions in which an underlying genetic defect is identified. In contrast, natural killer cell function is preserved in the reactive form but defective in the inherited syndromes.[604]

Histologically, there is infiltration of the portal tracts with normal-appearing histiocytes, lymphocytes and plasma cells, together with marked hypertrophy of Kupffer cells displaying prominent haemophagocytosis. The Kupffer cells are only weakly stained with PAS, a feature helpful in distinguishing this change from a response to necroinflammatory conditions, in which the Kupffer cells are often strongly PAS positive.[650] Additionally, Kupffer cells frequently show siderosis, possibly related to the erythrophagocytosis itself or to blood transfusions.[650] There is a lack of correlation between the degree of peripheral cytopenia and the degree of hepatic haemophagocytosis.[650] The hepatic manifestations in 30 patients with haemophagocytic syndrome were reviewed.[651] Recently, immunohistochemical findings on liver tissues have provided direct evidence for the involvement of activated CD8(+) lymphocytes through the production of IFN-gamma, and of macrophages through the haemophagocytosis and production of both interleukin 6 and TNF-alpha, irrespective of the associated condition.[652]

Down syndrome

Severe liver disease can occur in Down syndrome or trisomy 21 mosaicism.[653,654] Stillbirth, hydrops fetalis, or liver failure at or within a few weeks of birth are recognized presentations.[655-659] Morphologically, there is diffuse fibrosis surrounding reactive bile ductules and residual hepatocytes.[653] Extensive hepatic necrosis has also been observed.[656] In most livers a large number of megakaryocytes or megakaryoblasts, staining positively for factor VIII-related antigen and binding to Ulex europaeus 1, as well as other haematopoietic elements, are present in the sinusoids.[653,655] Parenchymal iron deposition of variable degree was noted in most of the cases studied by Ruchelli et al.[653] Arai et al. have suggested that megakaryocyte-derived $TGF\beta_1$ is one of the candidates in the activation of stellate cells leading to the hepatic fibrosis.[659] High levels of N-terminal peptide of procollagen III, type IV collagen, and hyaluronic acid were found in the serum of a lethal case at 5 days of life.[660]

The liver disease generally accompanies a haematological disorder unique to Down syndrome called transient abnormal myelopoiesis or transient leukaemia.[661,662] The condition consists of a clonal proliferation of blast cells exhibiting megakaryocytic features and historically associated with a high rate of spontaneous remission. Its true incidence remains to be determined. A number of cases may occur as an incidental finding of abnormal cell counts and blast cells in the peripheral blood in an otherwise well child, but in approximately 20% of cases the disease is manifest as hydrops fetalis and liver or multi-organ failure resulting in death. Of those children who enter a spontaneous remission, 13-33% have been found to develop acute megakaryoblastic leukemia, usually within the first 3 years of life, which if left untreated is fatal.[662] One study suggests that early treatment with cytosine-arabinoside of neonates presenting with severe liver disease is beneficial.[661]

Neonatal lupus erythematosus

Hepatic involvement may occur as part of the spectrum of neonatal lupus erythematosus (NLE), which is due to passage of maternal anti-Ro and anti-La antibodies across the placenta. Fetal tissues expressing Ro and La antigenic determinants may be damaged. The heart, skin and liver are most likely to be involved, rarely with thrombocytopaenia and leukopaenia.[663] Congenital heart block is the most important cardiac manifestation, and some infants develop a rash which resembles discoid lupus erythematosus in the newborn period or some weeks later. In approximately 10% hepatic disease occurs, usually typical neonatal hepatitis syndrome.[664-666] Occasionally it is severe enough to suggest extrahepatic biliary tract obstruction, with acholic stools and non-draining hepatobiliary scan.[667,668] One infant had severe liver disease with features of perinatal haemochromatosis,[669] and increased iron accumulation in the liver may be a finding on liver biopsy. Transient elevation of serum aminotransferases only or unexplained isolated conjugated hyperbilirubinaemia in the perinatal period and later presentation at 2 to 3 months of age with transient elevations of serum aminotransferases are recognized.[670] In most infants the liver disease resolves completely between 6 to 12 months of age, as the maternal antibodies are degraded. Mild fibrosis was found in one child with NLE on repeat liver biopsy.

The diagnosis of NLE is difficult in absence of congenital heart block or typical skin rash. Some infants have only transient jaundice and myocarditis with abnormal electrocardiogram. The diagnosis should be suspected if the mother is known to have systemic lupus erythematosus or Sjögren syndrome. Frequently, however, the mother is asymptomatic with respect to rheumatological disease. Routine methods may fail to detect anti-Ro and anti-La in the infant; these studies should be performed at as young an age as possible. Very high titres of ANA in the infant may be due to NLE. Deposits of associated antibodies (Anti-Ro and/or anti-La) may be found in affected liver tissue by immunofluorescence.[671] Most infants with unexplained neonatal hepatitis syndrome do not have NLE.[672] One infant was reported with neonatal hepatitis syndrome and transplacental transfer of anti-mitochondrial antibodies.[673]

References

1. Grosfeld JL, Clatworthy HW. Hepatic agenesis. In: Bergsma D, editor. Birth defects. Atlas and compendium. New York: Alan R Liss; 1973. p. 517
2. Belton RL, Van Zandt TF. Congenital absence of the left lobe of the liver: A radiologic diagnosis. Radiology, 1983; 147:184
3. Maeda N, Horie Y, Shiota G, et al. Hypoplasia of the left hepatic lobe associated with floating gallbladder. A case report. Hepatogastroenterology, 1998; 45:1100-1103
4. Radin DR, Colletti PM, Ralls PW, Boswell WD, Jr., Halls JM. Agenesis of the right lobe of the liver. Radiology, 1987; 164:639-642
5. Inoue T, Matsuzaki Y, Okauchi Y, et al. Hypogenesis of right hepatic lobe accompanied by portal hypertension: Case report and review of 31 Japanese cases. J Gastroenterol, 1997; 32:836-842
6. Faintuch J, Machado MCC, Raia AA. Suprahepatic gallbladder with hypoplasia of the right lobe of the liver. Arch Surg, 1980; 115:658-659
7. Hsu KL, Cheng YF, Ko SF. Hypoplastic right hepatic lobe with retrohepatic gallbladder complicated by hepatolithiasis and liver abscess: A case report. Hepatogastroenterology, 1997; 44:803-807
8. Sato M, Watanabe Y, Iseki S, et al. Hepatolithiasis with situs inversus: First case report. Surgery, 1996; 119:534-537
9. Organ BC, Skandalakis LJ, Gray SW, Skandalakis JE. Cancer of the bile duct with situs inversus. Arch Surg, 1991; 126:1150-1153
10. Silveira TR, Salzano FM, Howard ER, Mowat AP. Congenital structural abnormalities in biliary atresia: evidence for

etiopathogenic heterogeneity and therapeutic implications. Acta Paediatr Scand, 1991; 80:1192–1199

11. Soper RT, Green EW. Omphalocele. Surg Gynecol Obstet, 1961; 113:501–508

12. Desser PL, Smith S. Nonparasitic liver cysts in children. J Pediatr, 1956; 49:297–305

13. Fock G. Ectopic liver in omphalocele. Acta Paediatr, 1963; 52:288–292

14. Rendina EA, Venuta F, Pescarmona EO, Martelli M, Ricci C. Intrathoracic lobe of the liver: Case report and review of the literature. Eur J Cardiothorac Surg, 1989; 3:75–78

15. Feist JH, Lasser EC. Identification of uncommon liver lobulations. JAMA, 1959; 169:1859–1862

16. Korobkin MT, Miller SW, deLorimier AA, Gordon LS, Palubinskas AJ. Hepatic herniation through the Morgagni foramen. Am J Dis Child, 1973; 126:217–219

17. Organ CH, Hayes DF. Supradiaphragmatic right liver lobe and gallbladder. Arch Surg, 1980; 115:989–990

18. Vogel A, Small A. Partial eventration of the right diaphragm (congenital diaphragmatic herniation of the liver). Ann Intern Med, 1955; 43:63–82

19. Reitemeier RJ, Butt HR, Baggenstoss AH. Riedel's lobe of the liver. Gastroenterology, 1958; 34:1090–1095

20. Cullen TSL. Accessory lobes of the liver. Arch Surg, 1925; 11:718–764

21. Naganuma H, Ishida H, Niizawa M, Morikawa P, Masamune O, Kato T. Intrathoracic accessory lobes of the liver. J Clin Ultrasound, 1993; 21:143–146

22. Peter H, Strohm WD. Torquierter akzessorischer Leberlappen als Ursache eines akuten Abdomens. Leber Magen Darm, 1980; 4:203–206

23. Mendoza A, Voland J, Wolf P, Benirschke K. Supradiaphragmatic liver in the lung. Arch Pathol Lab Med, 1986; 110:1085–1086

24. Shah KD, Beck AR, Jhaveri MK et al. Infantile hemangioendothelioma of heterotopic intrathoracic liver associated with diaphragmatic hernia. Hum Pathol, 1987; 18:754–756

25. Buck FS, Koss MN. Heterotopic liver in an adrenal gland. Pediatr Pathol, 1988; 8:535–540

26. Tejada E, Danielson C. Ectopic or heterotopic liver (choristoma) associated with the gallbladder. Arch Pathol Lab Med, 1989; 113:950–952

27. Shapiro JL, Metlay LA. Heterotopic supradiaphragmatic liver formation in association with congenital cardiac anomalies. Arch Pathol Lab Med, 1991; 115:238–240

28. Boyle L, Gallivan MVE, Chan B, Lack EE. Heterotopia of gastric mucosa and liver involving the gallbladder. Arch Pathol Lab Med, 1992; 116:138–142

29. Ikoma A, Tanaka K, Hamada N et al. Left-sided gallbladder with accessory liver accompanied by intrahepatic cholangiocarcinoma. J Jpn Surg Soc, 1992; 93:434–436

30. Willis RA. Some unusual developmental heterotopias. Br Med J, 1968; 2:267–272

31. Lieberman MK. Cirrhosis in ectopic liver tissue. Arch Pathol, 1966; 82:443–446

32. Arakawa M, Kimura Y, Sakata K, Kubo Y, Fukushima T, Okuda K. Propensity of ectopic liver to hepatocarcinogenesis: Case reports and a review of the literature. Hepatology, 1999; 29:57–61

33. Le Bail B, Carles J, Saric J, Balabaud C, Bioulac-Sage P. Ectopic liver and hepatocarcinogenesis. Hepatology, 1999; 30:585–586

34. Dolan MF, Janovski NA. Adreno-hepatic union (adrenal dystopia). Arch Pathol, 1960; 86:22–24

35. Honma K. Adreno-hepatic fusion: an autopsy study. Zentralb Pathol, 1991; 137:117–122

36. Cotelingam JD, Saito R. Hepatolienal fusion: Case report of an unusual lesion. Hum Pathol, 1978; 9:234–236

37. Ballinger J. Hypoglycemia from metastasizing insular carcinoma of aberrant pancreatic tissue in liver. Arch Pathol, 1941; 32:277–285

38. Schaefer B, Meyer G, Arnholdt H, Hohlbach G. Heterotope Pankreaspseudocyste in der Leber. Chirurg, 1989; 60:556–558

39. Wolf H, Burshette J, Garcia J, Michalopoulos G. Exocrine pancreatic tissue in human liver: a metaplastic process? Am J Surg Pathol, 1990; 14:590–595

40. Terada T, Nakanuma Y, Kakita A. Pathologic observations of intrahepatic peribiliary glands in 1000 consecutive autopsy livers. Heterotopic pancreas in the liver. Gastroenterology, 1990; 98:1333–1337

41. Lacerda MA, Ludwig J, Ward EM. Intrahepatic spleen presenting as a mass lesion. Am J Gastroenterol, 1993; 88:2116–2117

42. Sekine S, Nagata M, Hamada H, Watanabe T. Heterotopic thyroid tissue at the porta hepatis in a fetus with trisomy 18. Virchows Arch, 2000; 436:498–501

43. Michels N. The hepatic, cystic and retroduodenal arteries and their relation to the biliary ducts. Ann Surg, 1951; 133:503–524

44. Carmi R, Magee CA, Neill CA, Karrer FM. Extrahepatic biliary atresia and associated anomalies: etiologic heterogeneity suggested by distinctive patterns of associations. Am J Med Genet, 1993; 45:683–693

45. Udelsman R, Sugarbaker PH. Congenital duplication of the gallbladder associated with an anomalous right hepatic artery. Am J Surg, 1985; 149:812–815

46. Rela M, McCall JL, Karani J, Heaton ND. Accessory right hepatic artery arising from the left. Implications for split liver transplantation. Transplantation, 1998; 66:792–794

47. Perea A, Tinsley EA, Mason LB. Abdominal apoplexy due to spontaneous rupture of an aberrant accessory hepatic artery. South Med J, 1982; 75:234–235

48. Helikson MA, Shapiro DL, Seashore JH. Hepatoportal arteriovenous fistula and portal hypertension in an infant. Pediatrics, 1977; 60:921–924

49. Vauthey J-N, Tomczak RJ, Helmberger T et al. The arterioportal fistula syndrome: clinicopathologic features, diagnosis and therapy. Gastroenterology, 1997; 113:1390–1401

50. Lamireau T, Chateil JF, Portier F, Manuel M, Grenier N. Successful embolization of congenital intrahepatic arterioportal fistula in two infants. J Pediatr Gastroenterol Nutr, 1999; 29:211–214

51. Bilbao JM, Longo JM, Aquerreta J, Rodriguez-Cabello J, Fernandez A. Platinum wire embolization of an intrahepatic arterioportal fistula. Am J Gastroenterol, 1990; 85:859–860

52. Covey AM, Brody LA, Getrajdman GI, Sofocleous CT, Brown KT. Incidence, patterns, and clinical relevance of variant portal vein anatomy. AJR Am J Roentgenol, 2004; 183:1055–1064

53. Boles ET, Jr., Smith B. Preduodenal portal vein. Pediatrics, 1978; 28:805–809

54. John AK, Gur U, Aluwihare A, Cade D. Pre duodenal portal vein as a cause of duodenal obstruction in an adult. ANZ J Surg, 2004; 74:1032–1033

55. Lilly JR, Starzl TE. Liver transplantation in children with biliary atresia and vascular anomalies. J Pediatr Surg, 1974; 9:707–714

56. Hsia DYY, Gellis SS. Portal hypertension in infants and children. Am J Dis Child, 1955; 90:290–298

57. Bell JW. Portal-vein hypoplasia with inferior mesenteric hypertension. N Engl J Med, 1970; 283:1149–1150

58. Raffensperger JG, Shkolnik AA, Boggs JD, Swenson O. Portal hypertension in children. Arch Surg, 1972; 105:249–254

59. Matsuoka Y, Ohtomo K, Okubo T et al. Congenital absence of the portal vein. Gastrointest Radiol, 1992; 17:31–33

60. Morgan G, Superina R. Congenital absence of the portal vein: two cases and a proposed classification system for portasystemic vascular anomalies. J Pediatr Surg, 1994; 29:1239–1241

61. De Gaetano AM, Gui B, Macis G, Manfredi R, Di Stasi C. Congenital absence of the portal vein associated with focal nodular hyperplasia in the liver in an adult woman: imaging and review of the literature. Abdom Imaging, 2004; 29:455–459

62. Appel H, Loddenkemper C, Schirmacher P et al. Congenital absence of the portal vein with splenomegaly and hypersplenism in a young woman. Digestion, 2003; 67:105–110

63. Marois D, van Heerden JA, Carpenter HA, Sheedy PF. Congenital absence of the portal vein. Mayo Clin Proc, 1979; 54:55–59

64. Guariso G, Fiorio S, Altavilla G et al. Congenital absence of the portal vein associated with focal nodular hyperplasia of the liver and cystic dysplasia of the kidney. Eur J Pediatr, 1998; 157:287–290

65. Tanaka Y, Takayanagi M, Shiratori Y et al. Congenital absence of portal vein with multiple hyperplastic nodular lesions in the liver. J Gastroenterol, 2003; 38:288–294

66. Tsuji K, Naoki K, Tachiyama Y et al. A case of congenital absence of the portal vein. Hepatol Res, 2005; 31:43–47

67. Cheung KM, Lee CY, Wong CT, Chan AK. Congenital absence of portal vein presenting as hepatopulmonary syndrome. J Paediatr Child Health, 2005; 41:72–75

68. Andreani P, Srinivasan P, Ball CS, Heaton ND, Rela M. Congenital absence of the portal vein in liver transplantation for biliary atresia. Int J Surg Investig, 2000; 2:81–84

69. Ozbek SS, Killi MR, Pourbagher MA, Katranci N, Solak A. Portal venous system aneurysms: Report of five cases. J Ultrasound Med, 1999; 18:417–422

70. Shawker TH, Chang R, Garra B, Edelstein RA et al. An unusual anomalous intrahepatic connection between the left portal vein and internal mammary veins. J Clin Ultrasound, 1988; 16:425–435

71. Lewis AM, Aquino NM. Congenital portohepatic vein fistula that resolved spontaneously in a neonate. AJR Am J Roentgenol, 1992; 159:837–838

72. Fiane AE, Gjestvang FT, Smevik B. Hepatoportal arteriovenous fistula and bleeding oesophageal varices in a child. Eur J Surg, 1993; 159:185–186

73. Raskin NK, Price JB, Fishman RA. Portal-systemic encephalopathy due to congenital intrahepatic shunts. N Engl J Med, 1964; 270:225–229

74. Gitzelmann R, Arbenz OU, Willi UV. Hypergalactosemia and portosystemic encephalopathy due to persistence of the ductus venosus Aranti. Eur J Pediatr, 1992; 151:564–568

75. Uchino T, Endo F, Ikeda S, Sheraki Y, Sera Y, Matsuda I. Three brothers with progressive hepatic dysfunction and severe hepatic steatosis due to a patent ductus venosus. Gastroenterology, 1996; 110:1964–1968

76. Uchino T, Matsuda I, Endo F. The long-term prognosis of congenital portosystemic venous shunt. J Pediatr, 1999; 135:254–256

77. Thompson PB, Oldham KT, Bedi DG, Guice KS, Davis M. Aneurysmal malformation of the extrahepatic portal vein. Am J Gastroenterol, 1986; 81:695–697

78. Gallagher DM, Leiman S, Hux CH. In utero diagnosis of a portal vein aneurysm. J Clin Ultrasound, 1993; 21:147–151

79. Ito Y, Tarao K, Tamai S et al. Portal vein aneurysm in the liver associated with multiple vascular malformations. J Gastroenterol, 1994; 29:776–781

80. Klemperer P. Cavernous transformation of the portal vein. Arch Pathol, 1928; 6:353–377

81. Myers NA, Robinson MJ. Extrahepatic portal hypertension in children. J Pediatr Surg, 1973; 8:467–473

82. Berdon WE, Baker DH, Casarella W. Liver disease in children: portal hypertension, hepatic masses. Semin Roentgenol, 1975; 10:207–214

83. Maksoud JG, Goncalves ME, Porta G, Miura I, Velhote MC. The endoscopic and surgical management of portal hypertension in children: analysis of 123 cases. J Pediatr Surg, 1991; 26:177–181

84. Pinto RB, Silveira TR, Bandinelli E, Roehsig L. Portal vein thrombosis in children and adolescents: the low prevalence of hereditary thrombophilic disorders. J Pediatr Surg, 2004; 39:1356–1361

85. Sarin SK, Bansal A, Sasan S, Nigem A. Portal-vein obstruction in children leads to growth retardation. Hepatology, 1992; 15:229–233

86. Bellomo-Brandao MA, Morcillo AM, Hessel G, Cardoso SR, Servidoni Mde F, da-Costa-Pinto EA. Growth assessment in children with extra-hepatic portal vein obstruction and portal hypertension. Arq Gastroenterol, 2003; 40:247–250

87. Chandra R, Kapoor D, Tharakan A, Chaudhary A, Sarin SK. Portal biolopathy. J Gastroenterol Hepatol, 2001; 16:1086–1092

88. Perlemuter G, Béjanin H, Fritsch J et al. Biliary obstruction caused by portal cavernoma: Study of 8 cases. J Hepatol, 1996; 25:58–63

89. Gauthier-Villars M, Franchi S, Gauthier F, Fabre M, Pariente D, Bernard O. Cholestasis in children with portal vein obstruction. J Pediatr, 2005; 146:568–573

90. Condat B, Vilgrain V, Asselah T et al. Portal cavernoma-associated chaloangiopathy: a clinical and MR cholangiography couped with MR portography imaging study. Hepatology, 2003; 37:1302–1308

91. Voorhees AB, Jr, Harris RD, Britton RC, Price JB, Santulli TV. Portal hypertension in children: 98 cases. Surgery, 1965; 58:540–549

92. Ros PR, Viamonte M, Soila K et al. Demonstration of cavernomatous transformation of the portal vein by magnetic resonance imaging. Gastrointest Radiol, 1986; 11:90–92

93. Bradbury MS, Kavanagh PV, Chen MY, Weber TM, Bechtold RE. Noninvasive assessment of portomesenteric venous thrombosis: current concepts and imaging strategies. J Comput Assist Tomogr, 2002; 26:392–404

94. Marks C. Developmental basis of the portal venous system. Am J Surg, 1969; 117:671–681

95. Williams AO, Johnston GV. Cavernous transformation of the portal vein in rhesus monkeys. J Pathol Bacteriol, 1965; 90:613–618

96. Kim JH, Lee YS, Kim SH, Lee SK, Lim MK, Kim HS. Does umbilical vein catheterization lead to portal venous thrombosis? Prospective US evaluation in 100 neonates. Radiology, 2001; 219:645–650

97. Odievre M, Pige G, Alagille D. Congenital abnormalities associated with extrahepatic portal hypertension. Arch Dis Child, 1977; 52:383–385

98. Bayraktar Y, Balkanci F, Kayhan B et al. Congenital hepatic fibrosis associated with cavernous transformation of the portal vein. Hepatogastroenterology, 1997; 44:1588–1594

99. Yamamoto S, Yokoyama Y, Takeshige K, Iwatsuki S. Budd-Chiari syndrome with obstruction of the inferior vena cava. Gastroenterology, 1968; 54:1070–1084

100. Terabayashi H, Okuda K, Nomura F et al. Transformation of inferior vena caval thrombosis to membranous obstruction in a patient with the lupus anticoagulant. Gastroenterology, 1986; 91:219–224

101. Kage M, Arakawa M, Kojiro M, Okuda K. Histopathology of membranous obstruction of the inferior vena cava in the Budd-Chiari syndrome. Gastroenterology, 1992; 102:2081–2090

102. Okuda K, Kage M, Shrestha SM. Proposal of a new nomenclature for Budd-Chiari syndrome: hepatic vein thrombosis versus thrombosis of the inferior vena cava at its hepatic portion. Hepatology, 1998; 28:1191–1198

103. Okuda K. Membranous obstruction of the inferior vena cava: etiology and relation to hepatocellular carcinoma. Gastroenterology, 1982; 82:376–379

104. Simson IW. Membranous obstruction of the inferior vena cava and hepatocellular carcinoma in South Africa. Gastroenterology, 1982; 82:171–178

105. Hoffman HD, Stockland B, von der Heyden U. Membranous obstruction of the inferior vena cava with Budd-Chiari syndrome in children: A report of nine cases. J Pediatr Gastroenterol Nutr, 1987; 6:878–884

106. Jaffe R, Yunis EJ. Congenital Budd-Chiari syndrome. Pediatr Pathol, 1983; 1:187–192

107. Roulet M, Laurini R, Rivier L, Calame A. Hepatic veno-occlusive disease in newborn infant of a woman drinking herbal tea. J Pediatr, 1988; 112:433–436

108. Gentil-Kocher S, Bernard O, Brunelle F et al. Budd-Chiari syndrome in children: report of 22 cases. J Pediatr, 1988; 113:30–38

109. Sergi C, Beedgen B, Linderkamp O, Hofmann WJ. Fatal course of veno-occlusive disease of the liver (endophlebitis hepatica obliterans) in a preterm infant. Pathol Res Pract, 1999; 195:847–851

110. Etzioni A, Benderly A, Rosenthal E et al. Defective humoral and cellular immune functions associated with veno-occlusive disease of the liver. J Pediatr, 1987; 110:549–554

111. Mellis C, Bale PM. Familial hepatic veno-occlusive disease with probable immune deficiency. J Pediatr, 1976; 88:236–242

112. Haitjema T, Westermann CJ, Overtoom TT et al. Hereditary hemorrhagic telangiectasia (Osler-Weber-Rendu disease). New insights in pathogenesis, complications, and treatment. Arch Intern Med, 1996; 156:714–719

113. Sharma VK, Howden CW. Gastrointestinal and hepatic manifestations of hereditary hemorrhagic telangiectasia. Dig Dis, 1998; 16:169–174

114. McAllister KA, Grogg KM, Johnson DW et al. Endoglin, a TGF-b binding protein of endothelial cells, in the gene for hereditary hemorrhagic telangiectasia type 1. Nat Genet, 1994; 8:345–351

115. Vincent P, Plauchu H, Hazan J et al. A third locus for hereditary haemorrhagic telangiectasia maps to chromosome 12q. Hum Mol Genet, 1995; 4:945–949

116. Harrison RE, Flanagan JA, Sankelo M et al. Molecular and functional analysis identifies ALK-1 as the predominant cause of pulmonary hypertension related to hereditary haemorrhagic telangiectasia. J Med Genet, 2003; 40:865–871

117. Letteboer TG, Zewald RA, Kamping EJ et al. Hereditary hemorrhagic telangiectasia: ENG and ALK-1 mutations in Dutch patients. Hum Genet, 2005; 116:8–16

118. Caselitz M, Wagner S, Chavan A et al. Clinical outcome of transfemoral embolisation in patients with arteriovenous malformations of the liver in hereditary haemorrhagic telangiectasia (Weber-Rendu-Osler disease). Gut, 1998; 42:123–126

119. Trotter JF, Suhocki P, V, Lina JR et al. Hereditary hemorrhagic telangiectasia causing high output failure: Treatment with transcatheter embolization. Am J Gastroenterol, 1998; 93:1569–1571

120. Fagel WJ, Perlberger R, Kauffmann RH. Portosystemic encephalopathy in hereditary hemorrhagic telangiectasia. Am J Med, 1988; 85:858–860

121. Mendoza A, Oliff S, Elias E. Hereditary haemorrhagic telangiectasia and secondary biliary cirrhosis. Eur J Gastroenterol Hepatol, 1995; 7:999–1002

122. Hashimoto M, Tate E, Nishii T, Watarai J, Shioya T, White RI. Angiography of hepatic vascular malformations associated with hereditary hemorrhagic telangiectasia. Cardiovasc Intervent Radiol, 2003; 26:177–180

123. Ralls PW, Johnson MB, Radin R et al. Hereditary hemorrhagic telangiectasia: Findings in the liver with color Doppler sonography. Am J Roentgenol, 1992; 159:59–61

124. Solis-Herruzo JA, Garcia-Cabezudo J, Santalla-Pecina F et al. Laparoscopic findings in hereditary haemorrhagic telangiectasia (Osler-Weber-Rendu disease). Endoscopy, 1984; 16:137–139

125. Chavan A, Caselitz M, Gratz KF et al. Hepatic artery embolization for treatment of patients with hereditary hemorrhagic

telangiectasia and symptomatic hepatic vascular malformations. Eur Radiol, 2004; 14:2079–2085

126. Boillot O, Bianco F, Viale J-P et al. Liver transplantation resolves the hyperdynamic circulation in hereditary hemorrhagic telangiectasia with hepatic involvement. Gastroenterology, 1999; 116:187–192

127. Azoulay D, Precetti S, Emile JF et al. Liver transplantation for intrahepatic Rendu–Osler–Weber's disease: the Paul Brousse hospital experience. Gastroenterol Clin Biol, 2002;26: 828–883

128. Daly JJ, Schiller AL. The liver in hemorrhagic telangiectasia (Osler–Weber–Rendu disease). Am J Med, 1976; 60:723–726

129. Zelman S. Liver fibrosis in hereditary hemorrhagic telangiectasia. Fibrosis of diffuse insular character. Arch Pathol, 1962; 74:66–72

130. Wanless IR, Gryfe A. Nodular transformation of the liver in hereditary hemorrhagic telangiectasia. Arch Pathol Lab Med, 1986; 110:331–335

131. Sussman EB, Sternberg SS. Hereditary hemorrhagic telangiectasia, a case with hepatocellular carcinoma and acquired hepatocerebral degeneration. Arch Pathol, 1975; 99:95–100

132. Buscarini E, Danesino C, Plauchu H et al. High prevalence of hepatic focal nodular hyperplasia in subjects with hereditary hemorrhagic telangiectasia. Ultrasound Med Biol, 2004; 30:1089–1097

133. Blewitt RW, Brown CM, Wyatt JI. The pathology of acute hepatic disintegration in hereditary haemorrhagic telangiectasia. Histopathology, 2003; 42:265–269

134. Torsney E, Charlton R, Diamond AG, Burn J, Soames JV, Arthur HM. Mouse model for hereditary hemorrhagic telangiectasia has a generalized vascular abnormality. Circulation, 2003; 107:1653–1657

135. Srinivasan S, Hanes MA, Dickens T et al. A mouse model for hereditary hemorrhagic telangiectasia (HHT) type 2. Hum Mol Genet, 2003; 12:473–482

136. Swift M, Morrell D, Massey RB, Chase CL. Incidence of cancer in 161 families affected by ataxia-telangiectasia. N Engl J Med, 1991; 325:1831–1836

137. McKinnon PJ. ATM and ataxia telangiectasia. EMBO Rep, 2004; 5:772–776

138. Weinstein S, Scottolini AG, Loo SYT, Caldwell PC, Bhagavan NV. Ataxia telangiectasia with hepatocellular carcinoma in a 15-year-old girl and studies of her kindred. Arch Pathol Lab Med, 1985; 109:1000–1004

139. Srisirirojanakorn N, Finegold MJ, Gopalakrishna GS, Klish WJ. Hepatic veno-occlusive disease in ataxia telangiectasia. J Pediatr, 1999; 134:786–788

140. Joerger M, Koeberle D, Neumann HP, Gillessen S. Von Hippel–Lindau disease—a rare disease important to recognize. Onkologie, 2005; 28:159–163

141. Zeitlin H. Hemangioblastomas of the meninges and their relationship to Lindau's disease. J Neuropathol Exp Neurol, 1942; 1:14–23

142. Rojiani AM, Owen DA, Berry K et al. Hepatic hemangioblastoma: an unusual presentation in a patient with von Hippel–Lindau disease. Am J Surg Pathol, 1991; 15:81–86

143. McGrath FP, Gibney RG, Morris DC et al. Case report: Multiple hepatic and pulmonary hemangioblastomas—a new manifestation of von Hippel–Lindau disease. Clin Radiol, 1992; 42:37–39

144. Deboever G, Dewulf P, Maerteus J. Common bile duct obstruction due to pancreatic involvement in the von Hippel–Lindau syndrome. Am J Gastroenterol, 1992; 87:1866–1868

145. Wanless IR, Mawdsley C, Adams R. On the pathogenesis of focal nodular hyperplasia of the liver. Hepatology, 1985; 5:1194–1200

146. Wanless IR, Albrecht S, Bilbao J et al. Multiple focal nodular hyperplasia of the liver associated with vascular malformations of various organs and neoplasia of the brain: A new syndrome. Mod Pathol, 1989; 3:456–462

147. Goldin RD, Rose DSC. Focal nodular hyperplasia of the liver associated with intracranial vascular malformations. Gut, 1990; 31:554–555

148. Forns X, Castella A, Bruix J, Solé M, Rodés J. Hiperplasia nodular focal associada a malformaciones vasculares cerebrales. Gastroenterol Hepatol, 1992; 15:405–407

149. Puente SG, Bannura GC. Radiological anatomy of the biliary tract: Variations and congenital abnormalities. World J Surg, 1983; 7:271–276

150. Markle GB. Agenesis of the common bile duct. Arch Surg, 1981; 116:350–352

151. Stellin GP, Karner FM, Toyama WM, Lilly JR. Biliary agenesis. Hepatology, 1986; 6:1218

152. Nomura T, Shirai Y, Sasagawa M, Wakai T, Hatakeyama K. Anomalous insertion of the right hepatic duct into the cyst duct: Report of a case before laparoscopic cholecystectomy. Surg Laparosc Endosc, 1999; 9:211–212

153. Dowdy GS, Waldron GW, Brown WG. Surgical anatomy of the pancreaticobiliary system: Observations. Arch Surg, 1962; 84:229–246

154. Hand BH. Anatomy and function of the extrahepatic biliary system. Clin Gastroenterol, 1973; 2:3–29

155. Cullingford G, Davidson B, Dooley J, Habit N. Hepatolithiasis with anomalous biliary anatomy and a vascular compression. HPB Surg, 1991; 3:129–137

156. Jackson JB, Kelly TB. Cholecystohepatic ducts: Case report. Ann Surg, 1964; 159:581–584.

157. Redkar R, Davenport M, Myers N, Howard ER. Association of oesophageal atresia and cholecystohepatic duct. Pediatr Surg Int, 1999; 15:21–23

158. Stokes TL, Old L. Cholecystohepatic duct. Ann Surg, 1978; 135:703–705

159. Benson MD. Aberrant hepatic ducts. Australas Radiol, 1988; 32:348–355

160. Ishak KG, Willis GW, Cummins SD, Bullock AA. Biliary cystadenoma and cystadenocarcinoma. Report of 14 cases and review of the literature. Cancer, 1977; 39:322–338

161. Ng JWT, Wong MK, Kong CK. Long accessory hepatic duct with congenital dilation of the common bile duct. Am J Gastroenterol, 1993; 88:619–621

162. Nygren EJ, Barnes WA. Atresia of the common hepatic duct with shunt via an accessory duct: Report of a case. Arch Surg, 1954; 68:337–343

163. Walters W. Surgical lesions of the biliary tract. Arch Surg, 1960; 81:1–13

164. Swartley WB, Weeder SD. Choledochus cyst with a double common bile duct. Ann Surg, 1935; 101:912–920

165. Lee CMJ. Duplication of the cystic and common hepatic ducts, lined with gastric mucosa: A rare congenital anomaly. N Engl J Med, 1957; 256:927–931

166. Hourigan JS, Carr MG, Burton EM, Ledbetter JC. Congenital bronchobiliary fistula: MRI appearance. Pediatr Radiol, 2004; 34:348–350

167. Kalayoglu M, Olcay I. Congenital bronchobiliary fistula associated with esophageal atresia and tracheoesophageal fistula. J Pediatr Surg, 1976; 11:463–464

168. Chan YT, Ng WD, Mak WP et al. Congenital bronchobiliary fistula associated with biliary atresia. Br J Surg, 1984; 71:240–241

169. Jakowski JD, Lucas JG, Seth S, Frankel WL. Ciliated hepatic foregut cyst: a rare but increasingly reported liver cyst. Ann Diagn Pathol, 2004; 8:342–346

170. Momin TA, Milner R, Sarmiento JM. Ciliated hepatic foregut cyst of the left hepatic vein. J Gastrointest Surg, 2004; 8:601–603

171. Wu MLC, Abecassis MM, Rao MS. Ciliated hepatic foregut cyst mimicking neoplasm. Am J Gastroenterol, 1998; 93:2212–2214

172. Vick DJ, Goodman ZD, Ishak KG. Squamous cell carcinoma arising in a ciliated hepatic foregut cyst. Arch Pathol Lab Med, 1999; 23:1115–1117

173. Furlanetto A, Dei Tos AP. Squamous cell carcinoma arising in a ciliated hepatic foregut cyst. Virchows Arch, 2002; 441:296–298

174. Vick DJ, Goodman ZD, Devers MT et al. Ciliated hepatic foregut cyst: A study of six cases and review of the literature. Am J Surg Pathol, 1999; 23:671–677

175. Chatelain D, Chailley-Heu B, Terris B et al. The ciliated hepatic foregut cyst, an unusual bronchiolar foregut malformation: A histological, histochemical, and immunohistochemical study of 7 cases. Hum Pathol, 2000; 31:241–246

176. Terada T, Nakanuma Y, Kono N, Ueda K, Kadoya M, Matsui O. Ciliated hepatic foregut cyst. A mucus histological, immunohistochemical, and ultrastructural study in three cases in comparison with normal bronchi and intrahepatic bile ducts. Am J Surg Pathol, 1990; 14:356–363

177. Haller JO, Condon VR, Berdon WE et al. Spontaneous perforation of the common bile duct in children. Radiology, 1989; 172:621–624

178. Davenport M, Heaton N, Howard ER. Spontaneous perforation of the bile duct in infants. Br J Surg, 1991; 78:1068–1070

179. So SKS, Lindahl J, Sharp HL et al. A case report of bile ascites during infancy diagnosed by Tc-99m-disofenin sequential scintiphotography. Pediatrics, 1983; 71:402–405

180. Yoon PW, Bresee JS, Olney RS, James LM, Khoury MJ. Epidemiology of biliary atresia: a population-based study. Pediatrics, 1997; 99:376–382

181. Chardot C, Carton M, Spire-Bendelac N, Le Pommelet C, Golmard J-L, Auvert B. Epidemiology of biliary atresia in France: A national study 1986–96. J Hepatol, 1999; 31:1006–1013

182. Strickland AD, Shannon K. Studies in the etiology of extrahepatic biliary atresia: Time-space clustering. J Pediatr, 1982; 100:749–753

183. Ayas MF, Hillemeier AC, Olson AD. Lack of evidence for seasonal variation in extrahepatic biliary atresia during infancy. J Clin Gastroenterol, 1996; 22:292–294

184. Chandra RS. Biliary atresia and other structural anomalies in the congenital polysplenic syndrome. J Pediatr, 1974; 85:649–655

185. Davenport M, Mowat AP, Howard ER. Biliary atresia splenic malformation syndrome: An etiology and prognostic subgroup. Surgery, 1993; 113:662–668

186. Alpert LI, Strauss L, Hirschorn K. Neonatal hepatitis and biliary atresia associated with trisomy 17–18. N Engl J Med, 1969; 280:16–20

187. Kasai M, Watanabe I, Ohi R. Follow-up studies of long-term survivors after hepatic portoenterostomy for 'non-correctable' biliary atresia. J Pediatr Surg, 1975; 10:173–182

188. Annéren G, Mearling S, Lilja H, Wallander J, von Döbelm U. Lethal autosomal recessive syndrome with intrauterine growth retardation, intra- and extra-hepatic biliary atresia and esophageal and duodenal atresia. Am J Med Genet, 1998; 78:306–309

189. Lachaux A, Descos B, Plauchu H et al. Familial extrahepatic biliary atresia. J Pediatr Gastroenterol Nutrit, 1988; 7:280–283

190. Smith BM, Laberge J-M, Schreiber R, Weber AM, Blanchard H. Familial biliary atresia in three siblings including twins. J Pediatr Surg, 1991; 26:1331–1333

191. Tarr PI, Haas JE, Christie DL. Biliary atresia, cytomegalovirus, and age at referral. Pediatrics, 1996; 97:828–831

192. Chang MH, Huang HH, Huang ES, Kao CL, Hsu HY, Lee CY. Polymerase chain reaction to detect human cytomegalovirus in livers of infants with neonatal hepatitis. Gastroenterology, 1992; 103:1022–1025

193. Hart MH, Kaufman SS, Vanderhoof JA et al. Neonatal hepatitis and extrahepatic biliary atresia associated with cytomegalovirus infection in twins. Am J Dis Child, 1991; 145:302–305

194. Bangaru S, Morecki R, Glaser LM, Horwitz MS. Comparative studies in the human newborn and reovirus-induced cholangitis in weanling mice. Lab Invest, 1980; 43:456

195. Morecki R, Glaser JH, Cho S, Balistreri WF, Horwitz MS. Biliary atresia and reovirus type 3 infection. N Eng J Med, 1982; 307:481–484

196. Rosenberg DP, Morecki R, Lollini LO, Glaser J, Cornelius CE. Extrahepatic biliary atresia in a Rhesus monkey (Macaca mulatta). Hepatology, 1983; 3:577–580

197. Glaser JH, Balistreri WF, Morecki R. Role of reovirus type 3 in persistent infantile cholestasis. J Pediatr, 1984; 105:912–915

198. Morecki R, Glaser JH, Johnson AB, Kress Y. Detection of reovirus type 3 in the porta hepatis of an infant with extrahepatic biliary atresia: ultrastructural and immunocytochemical study. Hepatology, 1984; 4:1137–1142

199. Brown WR, Sokol RJ, Levin MJ et al. Lack of correlation between infection with reovirus 3 and extrahepatic biliary atresia or neonatal hepatitis. J Pediatr, 1988; 113:670–676

200. Steele MI, Marshall CM, Lloyd RE, Randolph VE. Reovirus 3 not detected by reverse transcriptase-mediated polymerase chain reaction analysis of preserved tissue from infants with cholestatic liver disease. Hepatology, 1995; 21:697–702

201. Tyler KL, Sokol RJ, Oberhaus SM et al. Detection of reovirus RNA in hepatobiliary tissues from patients with extrahepatic biliary atresia and choledochal cysts. Hepatology, 1998; 27:1475–1482

202. Riepenhoff-Talty M, Gouvea V, Evans MJ et al. Detection of group C rotavirus in infants with extrahepatic biliary atresia. J Infect Dis, 1996; 174:8–15

203. Saito T, Shinozaki K, Matsunaga T et al. Lack of evidence for reovirus infection in tissues from patients with biliary atresia and congenital dilatation of the bile duct. J Hepatol, 2004; 40:203–211

204. Drut R, Drut RM, Gomez MA, Rua EC, Lojo MM. Presence of human papilloma virus in EBA. J Pediatr Gastroenterol Nutr, 1998; 27:530–535

205. Mack CL, Sokol RJ. Unraveling the pathogenesis and etiology of biliary atresia. Pediatr Res, 2005; 57:87R–94R

206. Bezerra JA, Tiao G, Ryckman FC et al. Genetic induction of proinflammatory immunity in children with biliary atresia. Lancet, 2002; 360:1653–1659

207. Chen L, Goryachev A, Sun J et al. Altered expression of genes involved in hepatic morphogenesis and fibrogenesis are identified by cDNA microarray analysis in biliary atresia. Hepatology, 2003; 38:567–576

208. Zhang DY, Sabla G, Shivakumar P et al. Coordinate expression of regulatory genes differentiates embryonic and perinatal forms of biliary atresia. Hepatology, 2004; 39:954–962

209. Silveira TR, Salzano FM, Donaldson PT, Mieli-Vergani G, Howard ER, Mowat AP. Association between HLA and extrahepatic biliary atresia. J Pedaitr Gastroenterol Nutr, 1993; 16:114–117

210. Donaldson PT, Clare M, Constantini PK et al. HLA and cytokine gene polymorphisms in biliary atresia. Liver, 2002; 22:213–219

211. Mack CL, Tucker RM, Sokol RJ et al. Biliary atresia is associated with CD4+ Th1 cell-mediated portal tract inflammation. Pediatr Res, 2004; 56:79–87

212. Whitington PF, Malladi P, Melin-Aldana H, Azzam R, Mack CL, Sahai A. Expression of osteopontin correlats with portal biliary proliferation and fibrosis in biliary atresia. Pediatr Res, 2005; 57:837–844

213. Shivakumar P, Campbell KM, Sabla GE et al. Obstruction of extrahepatic bile ducts by lymphocytes is regulated by IFN-gamma in experimental biliary atresia. J Clin Invest, 2004; 114:322–329

214. Balistreri WF, Grand R, Hoofnagle JH et al. Biliary atresia: Current concepts and research directions. Summary of a symposium. Hepatology, 1996; 23:1682–1692

215. Desmet VJ. Congenital diseases of intrahepatic bile ducts: variations on the theme 'ductal plate malformation'. Hepatology, 1992; 16:1069–1083

216. Landing BH. Considerations of the pathogenesis of neonatal hepatitis, biliary atresia and choledochal cyst—the concept of infantile obstructive cholangiopathy. Prog Pediatr Surg, 1974; 6:113–139

217. Petersen C, Grasshoff S, Luciano L. Diverse morphology of biliary atresia in an animal model. J Hepatol, 1998; 28:603–607

218. Petersen C, Kuske M, Bruns E, Biermanns D, Wussow PV, Mildenberger H. Progress in developing animal models for biliary atresia. Eur J Pediatr Surg, 1998; 8:137–141

219. Ogawa T, Suruga K, Kojima Y et al. Experimental study of the pathogenesis of infantile obstructive cholangiography and its clinical evaluation. J Pediatr Surg, 1983; 18:131–135

220. Hyams JS, Berman MM, Davis BH. Tubulointerstitial nephropathy associated with arteriohepatic dysplasia. Gastroenterology, 1983; 85:430–434

221. Desmet VJ. Cholangiopathies: Past, present and future. Semin Liver Dis, 1987; 7:67–76

222. Raweily EA, Gibson AAM, Burt AD. Abnormalities of intrahepatic bile ducts in extrahepatic biliary atresia. Histopathology, 1990; 17:521–527

223. Teichberg S, Markowitz J, Silverberg M et al. Abnormal cilia in a child with the polysplenic syndrome and extrahepatic biliary atresia. J Pediatr, 1982; 100:399–401

224. Chen J, Knowles IFU, Herbert JL, Hackett BP. Mutations of the mouse hepatocyte nuclear factor 1 fork head homologue 4 gene results in absence of cilia and random left/right asymmetry. J Clin Invest, 1998; 102:1077–1082

225. Bates MD, Bucuvales JC, Alonso W, Ryckman FC. Biliary atresia: Pathogenesis and treatment. Semin Liver Dis, 1998; 18:281–293

226. Hillberg F, Aguzzi A, Howets IN, Wagner EF. cJun is essential for normal mouse development and hepatogenesis. Nature, 1993; 365:179–181

227. Hentsch B, Lyons I, Li R et al. HLX homeo box gene is essential for an inductive tissue interaction that drives expansion of embryonic liver and gut. Genes Dev, 1996; 10:70–79

228. Schmidt C, Bladt F, Goedecke S et al. Scatter factor/hepatocyte growth factor is essential for liver development. Nature, 1995; 373:699–702

229. Mochizuki T, Yukio S, Tsuchiya K et al. Cloning of inv, a gene that controls left/right asymmetry and kidney development. Nature, 1998; 395:177–181

230. Morgan D, Turnpenny L, Goodslub J et al. Inversion, a novel gene in the vertebrate left—right axis pathway is partially deleted in the inv mouse. Nat Genet, 1998; 20:149–156

231. Mazotti MV, Willis LK, Huckeroth RO et al. Anomalous development of the hepatobiliary system in the Inv mouse. Hepatology, 1999; 30:372–378

232. Phillips MJ, Azuma T, Meredith S-LM et al. Abnormalities in villin gene expression and canalicular microvillus structure in progressive cholestatic liver disease of childhood. Lancet, 2003; 362:1112–1119

233. Adelman S. Prognosis of uncorrected biliary atresia: an update. J Pediatr Surg, 1978; 13:389–391

234. Roberts EA. Neonatal hepatitis syndrome. Semin Neonatol, 2003; 8:357–374

235. Howard ER, Johnston DI, Mowat AP. Spontaneous perforation of the common bile duct in infants. Arch Dis Child, 1976; 51:883–886

236. Lloyd DA, Mickel RE. Spontaneous perforation of the extra-hepatic bile ducts in neonates and infants. Br J Surg, 1980; 67:621–623

237. Gilmour SM, Hershkop M, Reifen R, Gilday D, Roberts EA. Outcome of hepatobiliary scanning in neonatal hepatitis syndrome. J Nucl Med, 1997; 38:1279–12782

238. Clarke B, O'Donovan AN, Coates G. Delayed excretion of radionuclide in scanning with diisopropyl iminodiacetic acid does not exclude the possibility of primary biliary atresia: case report. Can Assoc Radiol J, 1997; 48:42–43

239. Fawega AG, Akinjunka O, Sodeende O. Duodenal intubation and aspiration test: Utility in the differential diagnosis of infantile cholestasis. J Pediatr Gastroenterol Nutr, 1991; 13:290–292

240. Wilkinson ML, Mieli-Vergani G, Ball C, Portmann B, Mowat AP. Endoscopic retrograde cholangiopancreatography in infantile cholestasis. Arch Dis Child, 1991; 66:121–123

241. Derkx HH, Huibregste K, Taminiau JA. The role of endoscopic retrograde cholangiopancreatography in cholestatic infants. Endoscopy, 1994; 26:724–728

242. Manolaki AG, Larcher VF, Mowat AP, Barrett JJ, Portmann B, Howard ER. The prelaparotomy diagnosis of extrahepatic biliary atresia. Arch Dis Child, 1983; 58:591–594

243. Chandra RS, Altman RP. Ductal remnants in extrahepatic biliary atresia: A histopathological study with clinical correlation. J Pediatr, 1978; 93:196–200

244. Witzleben CL, Buck BE, Schnaufer L, Brzosko WJ. Studies on the pathogenesis of biliary atresia. Lab Invest, 1978; 38

245. Gautier M, Eliot N. Extrahepatic biliary atresia. Morphological study of 98 biliary remnants. Arch Pathol Lab Med, 1981; 105:397–402

246. Ohi R, Shikes RH, Stellin GP, Lilly JR. In biliary atresia duct histology correlates with bile flow. J Pediatr Surg, 1984; 19:467–470

247. Tan CE, Davenport M, Driver M, Howard ER. Does the morphology of the extrahepatic biliary remnants in biliary atresia influence survival? A review of 205 cases. J Pediatr Surg, 1994; 29:1459–1464

248. Kasai M, Suzuki S. A new operation for 'non-correctable' biliary atresia, hepatic protoenterostomy (In Japanese). Shijutsu, 1959; 13:733–739

249. Kasai M. Advances in treatment of biliary atresia. J Pediatr Surg, 1983; 13:265–276

250. Mieli-Vergani G, Howard ER, Portmann B, Mowat AP. Late referral for biliary atresia—missed opportunities for effective surgery. Lancet, 1989; i:421–423

251. Ohi R, Nio M, Chiba T, Endo N, Goto M, Ibrahim M. Long-term follow-up after surgery for patients with biliary atresia. J Pediatr Surg, 1990; 25:442–445

252. Karrer FM, Price MR, Bensard DD et al. Long-term results with the Kasai operation for biliary atresia. Arch Surg, 1996; 131:493–496

253. Valayer J. Conventional treatment of biliary atresia: Long-term results. J Pediatr Surg, 1996; 31:1546–1551

254. Chardot C, Carton M, Spire-Bendelac N, Le Pommelet C, Golmard JL, Auvert B. Prognosis of biliary atresia in the era of liver transplantation: French national study from 1986 to 1996. Hepatology, 1999; 30:606–611

255. Davenport M, Puricelli V, Farrant P et al. The outcome of the older (> or =100 days) infant with biliary atresia. J Pediatr Surg, 2004; 39:575–581

256. Schweizer P, Lunzmann K. Extrahepatic bile duct atresia: How efficient is hepato-porto-enterostomy? Eur J Pediatr Surg, 1998; 8:150–154

257. Azarow KS, Phillips MJ, Sandler AD, Hagerstrand I, Superina RA. Biliary atresia: Should all patients undergo portoenterostomy? J Pediatr Surg, 1997; 32:168–170

258. Matsuo S, Suita S, Kubota M, Shono K. Long-term results and clinical problems after portoenterostomy in patients with biliary atresia. Eur J Pediatr Surg, 1998; 8:142–145

259. Ryckman FC, Alonso MH, Bucavalas JC, Balistreri WF. Biliary atresia—surgical management and treatment options as they relate to outcome. Liver Transpl Surg, 1998; 4 (suppl 1):S24–S33

260. Lykavieris P, Chardot C, Sokhn M, Gauthier F, Valayer J, Bernard O. Outcome in adulthood of biliary atresia: a study of 63 patients who survived for over 20 years with their native liver. Hepatology, 2005; 41:366–371

261. Otte JB, de Ville de Goyet J, Reding R et al. Sequential treatment of biliary atresia with Kasai portoenterostomy and liver transplantation: a review. Hepatology, 1994; 20:41S–48S

262. Avitzur Y, DeLuca E, Cantos M et al. Health status ten years after pediatric liver transplantation—looking beyond the graft. Transplantation, 2004; 78:566–573

263. Fain JS, Lewin KJ. Intrahepatic biliary cysts in congenital biliary atresia. Arch Pathol Lab Med, 1989; 113:1383–1386

264. Hübscher SG, Harrison RF. Portal lymphadenopathy associated with lipofuscin in chronic cholestatic liver disease. J Clin Pathol, 1989; 42:1160–1165

265. Landing BH, Wells TR, Reed GB, Natayan MS. Diseases of the bile ducts in children. Baltimore MD: Williams and Wilkins; 1973

266. de Freitas LA, Chevallier M, Louis D, Grimaud JA. Human extrahepatic biliary atresia: portal connective tissue activation related to ductular proliferation. Liver, 1986; 6:253–261

267. Ho CW, Shioda K, Shirasaki K, Takahashi S, Tokimatsu S, Maeda K. The pathogenesis of biliary atresia: a morphological study of the hepatobiliary system and the hepatic artery. J Pediatr Gastroenterol Nutr, 1993; 16:53–60

268. Ohi R, Lilly JR. Copper kinetics in infantile hepatobiliary disease. J Pediatr Surg, 1980; 15:509–512

269. Hussein A, Wyatt J, Guthrie A, Stringer MD. Kasai portoenterostomy—new insights from heaptic morphology. J Pediatr Surg, 2005; 40:322–326

270. Fonkelsrud EW, E A. Bile lakes in congenital biliary atresia. Surgery, 1975; 77:384–390

271. Kasai M. Intra- and extrahepatic bile ducts in biliary atresia. Washington DC: US Government Printing Press; 1979

272. Ramm GA, Nair VG, Bridle KR, Shepherd RW, Crawford DH. Contribution of hepatic parenchymal and nonparenchymal cells to hepatic fibrogenesis in biliary atresia. Am J Pathol, 1998; 153:527–535

273. Lamireau T, Le Bail B, Broussarie L et al. Expression of collagens type I and IV, osteonectin and transforming growth factor beta-1 (TGF 1) in biliary atresia and paucity of intrahepatic bile ducts during infancy. J Hepatol, 1999; 31:248–255

274. Desmet VJ, Callea F. Cholestatic syndromes of infancy and childhood. In: Zakim D, Boyer TD, eds. Hepatology: A textbook of liver disease, vol.2, 2nd edn. Philadelphia: W B Saunders; 1990 pp 1355–1395

275. Callea F, Facchetti F, Lucini L et al. Liver morphology in anicteric patients at long-term follow-up after Kasai operation: A study of 16 cases. Tokyo: Professional Postgraduate Services; 1987

276. Alagille D. Extrahepatic biliary atresia. Hepatology, 1984; 4:7S–10S

277. Nietgen GW, Vacanti JP, Perez-Atayde AR. Intrahepatic bile duct loss in biliary atresia despite portoenterostomy: a consequence of ongoing obstruction? Gastroenterology, 1992; 102:2126–2133

278. Ito T, Horisawa M, Ando H. Intrahepatic bile ducts in biliary atresia—a possible factor determining prognosis. J Pediatr Surg, 1983; 18:124–130

279. Kulkarni PB, Beatty E, Jr. Cholangiocarcinoma associated with biliary cirrhosis due to congenital biliary atresia. Am J Dis Child, 1977; 131:442–444

280. Ohtomo K, Itai Y, Hasizume K, Kosaka N, Iio M. CT and MR appearance of focal nodular hyperplasia of the liver in children with biliary atresia. Clin Radiol, 1991; 43:88–90

281. Rosenstein BJ, Oppenheimer EH. Prolonged obstructive jaundice and giant cell hepatitis in an infant with cystic fibrosis. J Pediatr, 1977; 91:1022–1023

282. Campbell LV, Jr., Gilbert EF. Experimental giant cell transformation in the liver induced by E. coli endotoxin. Am J Pathol, 1967; 51:855–864

283. Dick MC, Mowat AP. Hepatitis syndrome in infancy—an epidemiological survey with 10 year follow-up. Arch Dis Child, 1985; 60:512–516

284. Chang MH, Hsu HC, Lee CY, Wang TR, Kao CL. Neonatal hepatitis: a follow-up study. J Pediatr Gastroenterol Nutr, 1987; 6:203–207

285. Herman SP, Baggenstoss AH, Cloutier MD. Liver dysfunction and histologic abnormalities in neonatal hypopituitarism. J Pediatr, 1975; 87:892–895

286. Sheehan AG, Martin SR, Stephure D, Scott RB. Neonatal cholestasis, hypoglycemia and congenital hypopituitarism. J Pediatr Gastroenterol Nutr, 1992; 14:426–430

287. Bernard O, Hadchouel M, Scotto J, Odievre M, Alagille D. Severe giant cell hepatitis with autoimmune hemolytic anemia in early childhood. J Pediatr, 1981; 99:704–711

288. Brichard B, Sokal E, Gosseye S, Buts JP, Gadisseux JF, Cornu G. Coombs-positive giant cell hepatitis of infancy: effect of steroids and azathioprine therapy. Eur J Pediatr, 1991; 150:314–317

289. Pappo O, Yunis E, Jordan JA et al. Recurrent and de novo giant cell hepatitis after orthotopic liver transplantation. Am J Surg Pathol, 1994; 18:804–813

290. Vilca Menedez H, Rela M, Baker A et al. Liver transplant for giant cell hepatitis with autoimmune haemolytic anaemia. Arch Dis Child, 1997; 7:249–251

291. Vajro P, Amelio A, Stagni A et al. Cholestasis in newborn infants with perinatal asphyxia. Acta Paediatr, 1997; 86:895–898

292. Jacquemin E, Lykavieris P, Chaoui N, Hadchouel M, Bernard O. Transient neonatal cholestasis: origin and outcome. J Pediatr, 1998; 133:563–567

293. Suita S, Arima T, Ishii K, Yakabe S, Matsuo S. Fate of infants with neonatal hepatitis: pediatric surgeons' dilemma. J Pediatr Surg, 1992; 27:696–699

294. Aagenaes O. Hereditary cholestasis with lymphoedema (Aagenaes syndrome, cholestasis- lymphoedema syndrome). New cases and follow-up from infancy to adult age. Scand J Gastroenterol, 1998; 33:335–345

295. Bollinger ME, Arredondo-Vega F, Santisteban I, Schwarz K, Hershfield MS, Lederman HM. Brief report: Hepatic dysfunction as

a complication of adenosine deaminase deficiency. N Eng J Med, 1996; 334:1367–1371

296. Tazawa Y, Kobayashi K, Ohura T et al. Infantile cholestatic jaundice associated with adult-onset type II citrullinemia. J Pediatr, 2001; 138:735–740

297. Ben-Shalom E, Kobayashi K, Shaag A et al. Infantile citrullinemia caused by citrin deficiency with increased dibasic amino acids. Mol Genet Metab, 2002; 77:202–208

298. Saheki T, Kobayashi K. Mitochondrial aspartate glutamate carrier (citrin) deficiency as the cause of adult-onset type II citrullinemia (CTLN2) and idiopathic neonatal hepatitis (NICCD). J Hum Genet, 2002; 47:333–341

299. Gilmour SM, Hughes-Benzie R, Silver MM, Roberts EA. Le foie vide: a unique case of neonatal liver failure. J Pediatr Gastroenterol Nutr, 1996; 23:618–623

300. Montgomery CK, Ruebner BH. Neonatal hepatocellular giant cell transformation: A review. Perspect Pediatr Pathol, 1976; 3:85–101

301. Ruebner B, Thaler MM. Giant cell transformation in infantile liver disease. In: Javitt NB, editor. Neonatal hepatitis and biliary atresia. Washington DC: US Government Printing Press; 1979. p. 299–311

302. Oledzka-Slotwinska H, Desmet V. Morphologic study on neonatal liver 'giant' cell transformation. Exp Mol Biol, 1969; 10:162–175

303. Craig JM, Landing BH. Form of hepatitis in neonatal period simulating biliary atresia. Arch Pathol, 1952; 54:321–333

304. Koukoulis G, Mieli-Vergani G, Portmann B. Infantile liver giant cells: immunohistological study of their proliferative state and possible mechanisms of formation. Pediatr Dev Pathol, 1999; 2:353–359

305. Richardet JP, Mallat A, Zafrani ES, Blazquez M, Bognel JC, Campillo B. Prolonged cholestasis with ductopenia after administration of amoxicillin/clavulanic acid. Dig Dis Sci, 1999; 44:1997–2000

306. Gardner LJ. Intrahepatic bile stasis in 45/X Turner's syndrome. N Eng J Med, 1974; 290:406

307. Puri P, Guiney EJ. Intrahepatic biliary atresia in Down's syndrome. J Pediatr Surg, 1975; 10:423–424

308. Aanpreung P, Beckwith B, Galansky SH, Koyle MA, Sokol RJ. Association of paucity of interlobular bile ducts with prune belly syndrome. J Pediatr Gastroenterol Nutr, 1993; 16:81–86

309. Watson GH, Miller V. Arteriohepatic dysplasia. Familial pulmonary arterial stenosis with neonatal liver disease. Arch Dis Child, 1973; 48:459–466

310. Alagille D, Odievre M, Gautier M, Dommergues JP. Hepatic ductular hypoplasia associated with characteristic facies, vertebral malformations, retarded physical, mental, and sexual development, and cardiac murmur. J Pediatr, 1975; 86:63–71

311. Alagille D, Estrada A, Hadchouel M et al. Syndromatic paucity of interlobular bile ducts Alagille syndrome or arteriohepatic dysplasia: Review of 80 cases. J Pediatr, 1987; 110:195–200

312. Henriksen NT, Langmark F, Sorland SJ, Fausa O, Landaas S, Aagenaes O. Hereditary cholestasis combined with peripheral pulmonary stenosis and other anomalies. Acta Paediatr Scand, 1977; 66:7–15

313. Riely CA, Collier E, Jensen P, Klatskin G. Arteriohepatic dysplasia: A benign syndrome of intrahepatic cholestasis with multiple organ involvement. Ann Intern Med, 1979; 91:520–527

314. Deprettere A, Portmann B, Mowat AP. Syndromic paucity of the intrahepatic bile ducts: diagnostic difficulty; severe morbidity throughout early childhood. J Pediatr Gastroenterol Nutr, 1987; 6:865–871

315. Emerick KM, Rand EB, Goldmuntz E, Krantz ID, Spinner NB, Piccoli DA. Features of Alagille syndrome in 92 patients: frequency and relation to prognosis. Hepatology, 1999; 29:822–829

316. Oda T, Elkahloun AG, Pike BL et al. Mutations in the human Jagged 1 gene are responsible for the Alagille syndrome. Nat Genet, 1997; 16:235–242

317. Boyer J, Crosnier C, Driancourt C et al. Expression of mutant JAGGED1 alleles in patients with Alagille syndrome. Hum Genet, 2005; 116:445–453

318. LaBrecque DR, Mitros FA, Nathan RJ et al. Four generations of arteriohepatic dysplasia. Hepatology, 1982; 2:467–474

319. Crosnier C, Driancourt C, Raynaud N et al. Mutations in JAGGED1 gene are predominantly sporadic in Alagille syndrome. Gastroenterology, 1999; 116:1141–1148

320. Spinner NB, Colliton RP, Crosnier C, Krantz ID, Hadchouel M, Meunier-Rotival M. Jagged1 mutations in alagille syndrome. Hum Mutat, 2001; 17:18–33

321. Sokol RJ, Heubi JE, Ballistreri WF. Intrahepatic 'cholestasis facies': Is it specific for Alagille syndrome? J Pediatr, 1983; 103:205–208

322. Silberbach M, Lashley D, Reller MD, Kinn WFJ, Terry A, Sunderland CO. Arteriohepatic dysplasia and cardiovascular malformations. Am Heart J, 1991; 127:695–699

323. McElhinney DB, Krantz ID, Bason L et al. Analysis of cardiovascular phenotype and genotype-phenotype correlation in individuals with a JAG1 mutation and/or Alagille syndrome. Circulation, 2002; 106:2567–2574

324. Hingorani M, Nischal KK, Davies A et al. Ocular abnormalities in Alagille syndrome. Ophthalmology, 1999; 106:330–337

325. Nischal KK, Hingorani M, Bentley CR et al. Ocular ultrasound in Alagille Syndrome. A new sign. Ophthalmology, 1997; 104:79–85

326. Rosenfield NS, Kelley MJ, Jensen PS et al. Arteriohepatic dysplasia: Radiologic features of a new syndrome. Am J Roentgenol, 1980; 135:1217–1223

327. Levin SE, Zarvos P, Milner S, Schmaman A. Arteriohepatic dysplasia: Association of liver disease with pulmonary arterial stenosis as well as facial and skeletal abnormalities. Pediatrics, 1980; 66:876–883

328. Sanderson E, Newman V, Haigh SF, Baker A, Sidhu PS. Vertebral anomalies in children with Alagille syndrome: an analysis of 50 consecutive patients. Pediatr Radiol, 2002; 32:114–119

329. Russo PA, Ellis E, Hashida Y. Renal histopathology in Algille's syndrome. Pediatr Pathol, 1987; 7:557–568

330. Martin SR, Garel L, Alvarez F. Alagille's syndrome associated with cystic renal disease. Arch Dis Child, 1996; 74:232–235

331. Garcia MA, Ramonet M, Ciocca M et al. Alagille syndrome: cutaneous manifestations in 38 children. Pediatr Dermatol, 2005; 22:11–14

332. Woolfenden AR, Albers GW, Steinberg GK, Hahn JS, Johnston DC, Farrell K. Moyamoya syndrome in children with Alagille syndrome: additional evidence of a vasculopathy. Pediatrics, 1999; 103:505–508

333. Connor SE, Hewes D, Ball C, Jarosz JM. Alagille syndrome associated with angiographic moyamoya. Childs Nerv Syst, 2002; 18:186–190

334. Berard E, Triolo V. Intracranial hemorrhages in Alagille syndrome. J Pediatr, 2000; 136:708–710

335. Lykavieris P, Crosnier C, Trichet C, Meunier-Rotival M, Hadchouel M. Bleeding tendency in children with Alagille syndrome. Pediatrics, 2003; 111:167–170

336. Emerick KM, Krantz ID, Kamath BM et al. Intracranial vascular abnormalities in patients with Alagille syndrome. J Pediatr Gastroenterol Nutr, 2005; 41:99–107

337. Kamath BM, Spinner NB, Emerick KM et al. Vascular anomalies in Alagille syndrome: a significant cause of morbidity and mortality. Circulation, 2004; 109:1354–1358

338. Gorelick FS, Dobbins JW, Burrell M, Riely CA. Biliary tract abnormalities in patients with arteriohepatic dysplasia. Dig Dis Sci, 1982; 27:815–820

339. Markowitz J, Daum F, Kahn FI et al. Arteriohepatic dysplasia. I. Pitfalls in diagnosis and management. Hepatology, 1983; 3:74–76

340. Kahn EI, Daum F, Markowitz J et al. Arteriohepatic dysplasia. II. Hepatobiliary morphology. Hepatology, 1983; 3:77–84

341. Morelli A, Pelli AA, Vedovelli A et al. Endoscopic retrograde cholangiopancreatography study in Alagille's syndrome: First report. Am J Gastroenterol, 1983; 78:241–244

342. Schwarzenberg SJ, Grothe RM, Sharp HL, Snover DC, Freese D. Long-term complications of arteriohepatic dysplasia. Am J Med, 1992; 93:171–176

343. Cruz M, Corretger LM, Arquer A. Hypoplasie veineuse portale intrhepatique dans le syndrome d'Alagille. Arch Fr Pediatr, 1985; 42:107–109

344. Emerick KM, Whitington PF. Partial external biliary diversion for intractable pruritus and xanthomas in Alagille syndrome. Hepatology, 2002; 35:1501–1506

345. Tzakis AG, Reyes J, Tepetes K et al. Liver transplantation for Alagille's syndrome. Arch Surg, 1993; 128:337–339

346. Cardona J, Houssin D, Gauthier F et al. Liver transplantation in children with Alagille syndrome—a study of twelve cases. Transplantation, 1995; 60:339–342

347. Quiros-Tejeira RE, Ament ME, Heyman MB et al. Does liver transplantation affect growth pattern in Alagille syndrome? Liver Transpl, 2000; 6:582–587

348. Adams PC. Hepatocellular carcinoma associated with arteriohepatic dysplasia. Dis Dig Sci, 1986; 31:438–442

349. Rabinowitz M, Imperial JC, Schade R et al. Hepatocellular carcinoma in Alagille's syndrome. J Pediatr Gastroenterol Nutr, 1989; 8:26–30

350. Bach N, Kahn H, Thung S et al. Hepatocellular carcinoma in a long-term survivor of intrahepatic biliary hypoplasia. Am J Gastroenterol, 1991; 86:1527–1530

351. Kim B, Park SH, Yang HR, Seo JK, Kim WS, Chi JG. Hepatocellular carcinoma occurring in Alagille syndrome. Pathol Res Pract, 2005; 201:55–60

352. Perrault J. Copper overload in paucity of interlobular bile ducts syndrome. Gastroenterology, 1980; 75:875–878

353. Valencia-Mayoral P, Weber J, Cutz E, Edwards VD, Phillips MJ. Possible defect in the bile secretory apparatus in arteriohepatic dysplasia (Alagille's syndrome): a review with observations on the ultrastructure of liver. Hepatology, 1984; 4:691–698

354. Hadchouel M, Hugon RN, Gautier M. Reduced ratio of portal tracts to paucity of intrahepatic bile ducts. Arch Pathol Lab Med, 1978; 102:402–403

356. Witzleben CL. Bile duct paucity ('intrahepatic atresia'). Perspect Pediatr Pathol, 1982; 7:185–201

357. Hashida Y, Yunis EJ. Syndromatic paucity of inter-lobular bile ducts: Hepatic histopathology of the early and endstage liver. Pediatr Pathol, 1988; 8:1–15

358. Alagille D, editor. Intrahepatic biliary atresia (hepatic ductular hypoplasia). Baltimore: Williams & Wilkins; 1976

359. Berman MD, Ishak KG, Schaefer EJ, Barnes S, Jones EA. Syndromatic hepatic ductular hypoplasia (arteriohepatic dysplasia): A clinical and hepatic histologic study of three patients. Dig Dis Sci, 1981; 26:485–497

360. Dahms B, Petrelli M, Wyllie R et al. Arteriohepatic dysplasia in infancy and childhood: A longitudinal study of six patients. Hepatology, 1982; 2:350–358

361. Witzleben CL, Finegold M, Piccoli DA, Treem WR. Bile canalicular morphometry in arteriohepatic dysplasia. Hepatology, 1987; 7:1262–1266

362. Kahn E. Paucity of interlobular bile ducts. Arteriohepatic dysplasia and nonsyndromic duct paucity. Perspect Pediatr Pathol, 1991; 14:168–215

363. Libbrecht L, Spinner NB, Moore EC, Cassiman D, Van Damme-Lombaerts R, Roskams T. Peripheral bile duct paucity and cholestasis in the liver of a patient with Alagille syndrome: further evidence supporting a lack of postnatal bile duct branching and elongation. Am J Surg Pathol, 2005; 29:820–826

364. Pollet N, Boccaccio C, Dhorne-Pollet S et al. Construction of an integrated physical and gene map of human chromosome 20p12 providing candidate genes for Alagille syndrome. Genomics, 1997; 42:489–492

365. Flynn DM, Nijjar S, Hubscher SG et al. The role of Notch receptor expression in bile duct development and disease. J Pathol, 2004; 204:55–64

366. Kodama Y, Hijikata M, Kageyama R, Shimotohno K, Chiba T. The role of notch signaling in the development of intrahepatic bile ducts. Gastroenterology, 2004; 127:1775–1786

367. Lorent K, Yeo SY, Oda T et al. Inhibition of Jagged-mediated Notch signaling disrupts zebrafish biliary development and generates multi-organ defects compatible with an Alagille syndrome phenocopy. Development, 2004; 131:5753–5766

368. Crosnier C, Driancourt C, Raynaud N, Hadchouel M, Meunier-Rotival M. Fifteen novel mutations in the JAGGED1 gene of patients with Alagille syndrome. Hum Mutat, 2001; 17:72–73

369. Yuan ZR, Okaniwa M, Nagata I et al. The DSL domain in mutant JAG1 ligand is essential for the severity of the liver defect in Alagille syndrome. Clin Genet, 2001; 59:330–337

370. Colliton RP, Bason L, Lu FM, Piccoli DA, Krantz ID, Spinner NB. Mutation analysis of Jagged1 (JAG1) in Alagille syndrome patients. Hum Mutat, 2001; 17:151–152

371. Kocak N, Gurukun F, Yuce A, Cagler M, Kale G, Gogus S. Non-syndrome paucity of the interlobular bile ducts: Clinical and laboratory findings in 10 cases. J Pediatr Gastroenterol, Nutr 1997; 24:44–48

372. Ludwig J, Wiesner RH, LaRusso NF. Idiopathic adulthood ductopenia: a cause of chronic cholestatic liver disease and biliary cirrhosis. J Hepatol, 1988; 7:193–199

373. Zafrani ES, Metreau JM, Douvin C et al. Idiopathic biliary ductopenia in adults: a report of five cases. Gastroenterology, 1990; 99:1823–1828

374. Bruguera M, Llach J, Rodes J. Nonsyndromic paucity of intrahepatic bile ducts in infancy and idiopathic ductopenia in adulthood: the same syndrome? Hepatology, 1992; 15:830–834

375. Muller C, Ulrich W, Penner E. Manifestation late in life of idiopathic adulthood ductopenia. Liver, 1995; 15:213–218

376. Kahn E, Daum F, Markowitz J et al. Nonsyndromatic paucity of interlobular bile ducts: light and electron microscopic evaluation of sequential liver biopsies in early childhood. Hepatology, 1986; 6:890–901

377. West AB, Chatila R. Differential diagnosis of bile duct injury and ductopenia. Semin Diagn Pathol, 1998; 15:270–284

378. Hadad AR, Westbrook KC, Campbell GS, Caldwell FT, Morris WD. Congenital dilatation of the bile ducts. Am J Surg, 1976; 132:799–804

379. Soreide K, Korner H, Havnen J, Soreide JA. Bile duct cysts in adults. Br J Surg, 2004; 91:1538–1548

380. Visser BC, Suh I, Way LW, Kang SM. Congenital choledochal cysts in adults. Arch Surg, 2004; 139:855–860

381. Sherman P, Kolster E, Davies C, Stringer D, Weber J. Choledochal cysts: heterogeneity of clinical presentation. J Pediatr Gastroenterol Nutr, 1986; 5:867–872

382. Metcalfe MS, Wemyss-Holden SA, Maddern GJ. Management dilemmas with choledochal cysts. Arch Surg, 2003; 138:333–339

383. Shukri N, Hasegawa T, Wasa M, Higaki J, Nakamura T, Okada A. Characteristics of infantile cases of congenital dilatation of the bile duct. J Pediatr Surg, 1998; 33:1794–1797

384. Sela-Herman S, Scharschmidt BF. Choledochal cyst: A disease for all ages. Lancet, 1996; 347:779

385. Bancroft JD, Bucuvalas JC, Ryckman FC, Dudgeon DL, Saunders RC, Schwarz KB. Antenatal diagnosis of choledochal cyst. J Pediatr Gastroenterol Nutr, 1994; 18:142–145

386. Hamada V, Tanano A, Sato K et al. Rapid enlargement of a choledochal cyst: Antenatal diagnosis and delayed primary excision. Pediatr Surg Int, 1998; 5–6:419–421

387. Lipsett PA, Pitt HA, Colombani PM, Boitnott JK, Cameron JL. Choledochal cyst disease. A changing pattern of presentation. Ann Surg, 1994; 220:644–652

388. Chaudhary A, Dhar P, Sachdev A et al. Choledochal cysts—differences in children and adults. Br J Surg, 1996; 83:186–188

389. Takaya J, Muneyuki M, Tokuhara D, Takada K, Hamada Y, Kobayashi Y. Congenital dilatation of the bile duct: changes in diagnostic tools over the past 19 years. Pediatr Int, 2003; 45:383–387

390. Matos C, Nicaise N, Deviere J et al. Choledochal cysts: comparison of findings at MR cholangiopancreatography and endoscopic retrograde cholangiopancreatography in eight patients. Radiology, 1998; 209:443–448

391. Robertson JFR, Raine PAM. Choledochal cyst: A 33-year review. Br J Surg, 1988; 75:799–801

392. Swisher SG, Cates JA, Hunt KK et al. Pancreatitis associated with adult choledochal cysts. Pancreas, 1994; 9:633–637

393. Karnak I, Tanyei FC, Buyukpamukcu N, Hicsonmez A. Spontaneous rupture of choledochal cyst: An unusual cause of acute abdomen in children. J Pediatr Surg, 1997; 32:736–738

394. Tomomasa T, Tabata K, Myashite M, Itoh K, Kuroume T. Acute pancreatitis in Japanese and Western children; etiologic comparisons. J Pediatr Gastroenterol Nutr, 1994; 19:109–110

395. Bismuth H, Krissat J. Choledochal cystic malignancies. Ann Oncol, 1999; 10 (Suppl 4):94–98

396. Yeong ML, Nicholson GI, Lee SP. Regression of biliary cirrhosis following choledochal cyst drainage. Gastroenterology, 1982; 82:332–335

397. Krepel HP, Siersema PD, Tilanus HW et al. Choledochocele presenting with anaemia. Eur J Gastroenterol Hepatol, 1997; 9:641–643

398. Barlow B, Tabor E, Blanc WA et al. Choledochal cyst: A review of 19 cases. J Pediatr, 1976; 89:934–940

399. Okada A, Nakamura T, Okumura K, Okumara K, Kamata S, Oguchi Y. Surgical treatment of congenital dilatation of bile duct (choledochal cyst) with technical considerations. Surgery, 1987; 101:239–243

400. Young WT, Thomas GV, Blethyn AJ, Lawrie BW. Choledochal cyst and congenital anomalies of the pancreatico-biliary junction: The clinical findings, radiology and outcome in nine cases. Br J Radiol, 1992; 65:33–38

401. Ando H, Takahiro I, Kaneko K et al. Congenital stenosis of the intrahepatic bile duct associated with choledochal cysts. J Am Coll Surg, 1995; 181:426–430

402. Todani T, Watanabe Y, Toki A, Ogura K, Wang ZQ. Co-existing biliary anomalies and anatomical variants in choledochal cyst. Br J Surg, 1998; 85:760–763

403. Kim WS, Kim ID, Yeon KM et al. Choledochal cyst with or without biliary atresia in neonates and young infants: US differentiation. Radiology, 1998; 209:465–469

404. Yamashiro Y, Mijano T, Suruga K et al. Experimental study of the pathogenesis of choledochal cyst and pancreatitis, with special reference to the role of bile acids and pancreatic enzymes in the anomalous choledocho-pancreatico ductal junction. J Pediatr Gastroenterol Nutr, 1984; 3:721–727

405. Behrns KE, Shaheen NJ, Grimm IS. Type 1 choledochal cyst in association with familial adenomatous polyposis. Am J Gastroenterol, 1998; 93:1377–1379

406. Miyano T, Yamataka A, Koto Y et al. Hepaticoenterostomy after excision of choledochal cyst in children: A 30-year experience with 180 cases. J Pediatr Surg, 1996; 31:1417–1421

407. de Vries JS, de Vries S, Aronson DC et al. Choledochal cysts: age of presentation, symptoms, and late complications related to Todani's classification. J Pediatr Surg, 2002; 37:1568–1573

408. Goto N, Yasuda I, Uematsu T et al. Intrahepatic cholangiocarcinoma arising 10 years after the excision of

congenital extrahepatic biliary dilation. J Gastroenterol, 2001; 36:856–862

409. Ishibashi T, Kasahara Y, Yasuda Y et al. Malignant change in the biliary tract after excision of choledochal cyst. Br J Surg, 1997; 84:1687–1691

410. Ando H, Ito T, Sugito T. Histological study of the choledochal cyst wall. Jpn J Gastroenterol, 1987; 84:1797–1801

411. Kozuka S, Kurashima M, Tsubone M, Hachisuka K, Yasui A. Significance of intestinal metaplasia for evolution of cancer in the biliary tract. Cancer, 1984; 54:2277–2285

412. Komi N, Tamura T, Tsuge S, Miyoshi Y, Udaka H, Takehara H. Relation of patient age to premalignant changes in choledochal cyst epithelium: Histochemical and immunohistochemical studies. J Pediatr Surg, 1986; 21:430–433

413. Kusunoki M, Yamamura T, Takahashi T, Kautoh M, Ishikawa M, Utsunomiya J. Choledochal cyst: Its possible autonomic involvement in the bile duct. Arch Surg, 1987; 122:997–1000

414. Kagawa Y, Kashihara S, Kuramoto S, Maetani S. Carcinoma arising in a congenitally dilated biliary tract. Report of a case and review of the literature. Gastroenterology, 1978; 74:1286–1294

415. Gallagher PJ, Mills RR, Mitchinson MJ. Congenital dilatation of the intrahepatic bile ducts with cholangiocarcinoma. J Clin Pathol, 1972; 25:804–808

416. Voyles CR, Smadja C, Shands C, Blumgart LH. Carcinoma in choledochal cysts: Age-related incidence. Arch Surg, 1983; 118:986–988

417. Nonomura A, Mizukami Y, Matsubara F, Ueda H. A case of choledochal cyst associated with adenocarcinoma exhibiting sarcomatous features. J Gastroenterol, 1994; 29:669–675

418. Iwai N, Deguchi E, Yanagihara J et al. Cancer arising in a choledochal cyst in a 12-year-old girl. J Pediatr Surg, 1990; 25:1261–1263

419. Reveille RM, Van Stiegmann G, Everson GT. Increased secondary bile acids in a choledochal cyst. Possible role in biliary metaplasia and carcinoma. Gastroenterology, 1990; 99:525–527

420. Wu GS, Zou SQ, Luo XW, Wu JH, Liu ZR. Proliferative activity of bile from congenital choledochal cyst patients. World J Gastroenterol, 2003; 9:184–187

421. Matsumoto Y, Fujii H, Itakura J, Matsuda M, Nobukawa B, Suda K. Recent advances in pancreaticobiliary maljunction. J Hepatobiliary Pancreat Surg, 2002; 9:45–54

422. Desmet VJ. What is congenital hepatic fibrosis? Hepatology, 1992; 20:465–477

423. Desmet VJ. Ludwig symposium on biliary disorders—part I. Pathogenesis of ductal plate abnormalities. Mayo Clin Proc, 1998; 73:80–89

424. Knisely AS. Biliary tract malformations. Am J Med, 2003; 122:343–350

425. McDonald RA, Avner EA. Inherited polycystic kidney disease in childhood. Semin Nephrol, 1991; 11:632–642

426. Zerres K, Mucher G, Bachner L et al. Mapping the gene for autosomal recessive polycystic kidney disease (ARPKD) to chromosome 6p21cm. Nat Genet, 1994; 7:429–432

427. Mucher G, Wirth B, Zerres K. Refining the map and defining flanking markers of the gene for autosomal recessive polycystic kidney on chromosome 6p 21.2–p12. Am J Hum Genet, 1994; 55:1281–1284

428. Guay-Woodford LK, Meucha G, Hopkins SD. The severe perinatal form of autosomal recessive polycystic kidney disease. Am J Hum Genet, 1995; 56:1101–1107

429. Park JH, Dixit MP, Onuchic LF et al. A 1-Mb BAC/PAC-based physical map of the autosomal recessive polycystic kidney disease gene (PKHD1) region on chromosome 6. Genomics, 1999; 57:249–255

430. Ward CJ, Hogan MC, Rossetti S et al. The gene mutated in autosomal recessive polycystic kidney disease encodes a large, receptor-like protein. Nat Genet, 2002; 30:259–69

431. Onuchic LF, Furu L, Nagasawa Y et al. PKHD1, the polycystic kidney and hepatic disease 1 gene, encodes a novel large protein containing multiple immunoglobulin-like plexin-transcription-factor domains and parallel beta-helix 1 repeats. Am J Hum Genet, 2002; 70:1305–1317

432. Moyer JH, Lee-Tischler MJ, Kwon HY et al. Candidate gene associated with a mutation causing recessive polycystic kidney disease in mice. Science, 1994; 264:1329–1333

433. Blyth H, Ockenden BG. Polycystic disease of kidneys and liver presenting in childhood. J Med Genet, 1971; 81:257–284

434. Witzleben CL. Cystic diseases of the liver. In: Zakim D BT, editor. Hepatology. A textbook of liver disease. Philadelphia: WB Saunders; 1990. p. 1395–1411

435. Lonergan GJ, Rice RR, Suarez ES. Autosomal recessive polycystic kidney disease: Radiologic-pathologic correlation. Radiographics, 2000; 20:837–855

436. Lens XM, Onuchie LF, Wu G et al. An integrated genetic and physical map of the autosomal recessive polycystic kidney disease region. Genomics, 1997; 41:463–466

437. Landing BH, Walls TR, Claireaux AE. Morphometric analysis of liver lesions in cystic diseases of childhood. Hum Pathol, 1980; 11:549–560

438. Gang DL, Herrin JT. Infantile polycystic disease of the liver and kidneys. Clin Nephrol, 1986; 25:28–36

439. Adams CM, Danks DM, Campbell PE. Comments upon the classification of infantile polycystic diseases of the liver and kidney, based upon three dimensional reconstruction of the liver. J Med Genet, 1974; 11:234–243

440. Jörgensen MJ. The ductal plate malformation. APMIS (Suppl), 1977; 257:1–88

441. Nakanuma Y, Terada T, Ohta G. Caroli's disease in congenital hepatic fibrosis and infantile polycystic disease. Liver, 1982; 2:346–354

442. Summerfield JA, Nagafuchi Y, Sherlock S et al. Hepatobiliary fibropolycystic diseases. A clinical and histological review of 51 patients. J Hepatol, 1986; 2:141–156

443. Jung G, Benz-Bohm G, Kugel H, Keller KM, Querfeld U. MR cholangiography in children with autosomal recessive polycystic kidney disease. Pediatr Radiol, 1999; 29:463–466

444. Averback P. Congenital hepatic fibrosis: asymptomatic adults without renal anomaly. Arch Pathol Lab Med, 1977; 101:260–261

445. Fauvert R, Benhamou JP. Congenital hepatic fibrosis. In: Schaffner F, Sherlock S, Leevy CM, editors. The liver and its diseases. New York: Intercontinental Medical Book; 1974. p. 283–288

446. Deget F, Rudnik-Schoneborn S, Zerres K. Course of autosomal recessive polycystic kidney disease (ARPKD) in siblings: a clinical comparison of 20 sibships. Clin Genet, 1995; 47:248–253

447. Kerr DNS, Harrison CV, Sherlock S, Walker RM. Congenital hepatic fibrosis. Q J Med, 1960; 30:91–117

448. Sommerschild HC, Langmark F, Maurseth K. Congenital hepatic fibrosis: report of two new cases and review of the literature. Surgery, 1973; 73:53–58

449. Boichis H, Passwell J, David R, Miller H. Congenital hepatic fibrosis and nephronophthisis. Q J Med, 1973; 42:221–233

450. Cobben JM, Breuning MH, Schoots C, ten Kate LP, Zerres K. Congenital hepatic fibrosis in autosomal-dominant polycystic kidney disease. Kidney Int, 1990; 38:880–885

451. Roy S, Dillon MJ, Trompeter RS, Barratt TM. Autosomal recessive polycystic kidney disease: long-term outcome of neonatal survivors. Pediatr Nephrol, 1997; 11:302–306

452. Alvarez F, Bernard O, Brunelle F et al. Congenital hepatic fibrosis in children. J Pediatr, 1981; 99:370–375

453. Scott J, Shousha S, Thomas HC, Sherlock S. Bile duct carcinoma: a late complication of congenital hepatic fibrosis. Case report and review of literature. Am J Gastroenterol, 1980; 73:113–119

454. Chen KTK. Adenocarcinoma of the liver: association with congenital hepatic fibrosis and Caroli's disease. Arch Pathol Lab Med, 1981; 105:294–295

455. De Vos BF, Cuvelier C. Congenital hepatic fibrosis. J Hepatol, 1988; 6:222–228

456. Christodoulou K, Tsingis M, Stavrou C et al. Chromosome 1 localization of a gene for autosomal dominant medullary cystic kidney disease. Hum Mol Genet, 1998; 7:905–911

457. Hart TC, Gorry MC, Hart PS et al. Mutations of the UMOD gene are responsible for medullary cystic kidney disease 2 and familial juvenile hyperuricaemic nephropathy. J Med Genet, 2002; 39:882–892

458. Donaldson JC, Dise RS, Ritchie MD, Hanks SK. Nephrocystin-conserved domains involved in targeting to epithelial cell-cell junctions, interaction with filamins, and establishing cell polarity. J Biol Chem, 2002; 277:29028–29035

459. Blankenberg TA, Ruebner BH, Ellis WG, Bernstein J, Dimmick JE. Pathology of renal and hepatic anomalies in Meckel syndrome. Am J Med Genet, 1987; Suppl 3:395–410

460. Torra R, Alos L, Ramos J, Estivill X. Renal-hepatic-pancreatic dysplasia: an autosomal recessive malformation. J Med Genet, 1996; 33:409–412

461. Böhm N, Fukuda M, Staudt R, Helwig H. Chondroectodermal dysplasia (Ellis–van Creveld syndrome) with dysplasia of the renal medulla and bile ducts. Histopathology, 1978; 2:267–281

462. Labrune P, Fabre M, Trioche P et al. Jeune syndrome and liver disease: report of three cases treated with ursodeoxycholic acid. Am J Med Genet, 1999; 87:324–328

463. Freeze HH. New diagnosis and treatment of congenital hepatic fibrosis. J Pediatr Gastroenterol Nutr, 1999; 29:104–106

464. Lewis SM, Roberts EA, Marcon MA et al. Joubert syndrome with congenital hepatic fibrosis: an entity in the spectrum of oculo-encephalo-hepato-renal disorders. Am J Med Genet, 1994; 52:419–426

465. Caroli J. Diseases of the intrahepatic biliary tree. Clin Gastroenterol, 1973; 2:147–161

466. Ramond MJ, Huguet C, Danan G, Rueff B, Benhamou J-P. Partial hepatectomy in the treatment of Caroli's disease. Report of a case and review of the literature. Dig Dis Sci, 1984; 29:367–370

467. Sandle GI, Lodge JPA. A 32-year-old man with recurrent cholangitis. Lancet, 1997; 350:408

468. Mercadier M, Chigot JP, Clot JP, Langlois P, Lansieux P. Caroli's disease. World J Surg, 1984; 8:22–29

469. Nagusue N. Successful treatment of Caroli's disease by hepatic resection. Ann Surg, 1984; 200:718–723

470. Tandon RK, Grewal H, Amand AC, Vashisht S. Caroli's syndrome: A heterogeneous entity. Am J Gastroenterol, 1990; 85:170–173

471. Marchal GJ, Desmet VJ, Proesmans WC et al. Caroli's disease: high-frequency US and pathologic findings. Radiology, 1986; 158:507–511

472. Hopper KD. The role of computed tomography in the evaluation of Caroli's disease. Clin Imaging, 1989; 13:68–73

473. Choi BI, Mo-Yeon K, Kim SH, Han MC. Caroli disease: Central dot sign in CT. Radiology, 1990; 174:161–163

474. Asselah T, Ernst O, Sergent G et al. Caroli's disease: A magnetic resonance cholangiopancreatography diagnosis. Am J Gastroenterol, 1998; 93:109–110

475. Chalasani N, Nguyen C, Gitlin N. Spontaneous rupture of a bile duct and its endoscopic management in a patient with Caroli's syndrome. Am J Gastroenterol, 1997; 92:1062–106

476. Chevillotte G, Sastre B, Sahel J, Payan H, Michotey G, Sarles H. Maladie de Caroli localisée et associée à un adénocarcinome papillaire mucosécrétant: interêt de la résection hépatique. Presse Med, 1984; 13:1137–1139

477. Taylor ACF, Plamer K. Caroli's disease. Eur J Gastroenterol Hepatol, 1998; 10:105–108

478. Kchir N, Haouet S, Boubaker S et al. Caroli's disease associated with hepatocarcinoma. A case report and review of the literature. Arch Anat Cytol Pathol, 1990; 38:95–99

479. Witlin LT, Gadacz TR, Zuidema GD, Kridelbaugh WW. Transhepatic decompression of the biliary tree in Caroli's disease. Surgery, 1982; 91:205–209

480. Giovanardi RO. Monolobar Caroli's disease in an adult. Case report. Hepatogastroenterology, 2003; 50:2185–2187

481. Lointier PH, Kauffmann P, Francannet P, Dezet D, Chipponi J. Management of intrahepatic calculi in Caroli's disease by extracorporeal shock wave lithotripsy. Br J Surg, 1980; 77:987–988

482. Fozard JBJ, Wyatt JI, Hall RI. Epithelial dysplasia in Caroli's disease. Gut, 1989; 30:1150–1153

483. Hussman KL, Friedwald JP, Gollub MJ, Melamed J. Caroli's disease associated with infantile polycystic kidney disease: Prenatal sonographic appearance. J Ultrasound, 1991; 10:235–237

484. Jordon D, Harpaz N, Thung SN. Caroli's disease and adult polycystic kidney disease: A rarely recognized association. Liver, 1989; 9:30–35

485. Merza AP, Raiser MW. Biliary tract manifestations of the Marfan syndrome. Am J Gastroenterol, 1987; 82:779–782

486. Consortium EPKD. The polycystic kidney disease 1 gene encodes a 14 kb transcript and lies within a duplicated region on chromosome 16. Cell, 1994; 77:881–894

487. Ong AC, Harris PC. Molecular pathogenesis of ADPKD: The polycystin complex gets complex. Kidney Int, 2005; 67:1234–1247

488. Hughes J, Ward CJ, Peral B et al. The polycystic kidney disease 1 (PKD1) gene encodes a novel protein with multiple cell recognition domains. Nat Genet, 1995; 10:151–160

489. Geng L, Segal Y, Peissel B et al. Identification and localization of polycystin, the PKD1 gene product. J Clin Invest, 1996; 98:2674–2682

490. Peters DJM, van DeWall A, Spruit L et al. Cellular localization and tissue distribution of polycystin-1. J Pathol, 1999; 188:439–446

491. Mochizuki T, Wu G, Hayashi T et al. PKD2, a gene for polycystic kidney disease that encodes an integral membrane protein. Science, 1996; 272:1339–1342

492. Yoder BK, Hou X, Guay-Woodford LM. The polycystic kidney disease proteins, polycystin-1, polycystin-2, polaris, and cystin, are co-localized in renal cilia. J Am Soc Nephrol, 2002; 13:2508–2516

493. Nauli SM, Alenghat FJ, Luo Y et al. Polycystins 1 and 2 mediate mechanosensation in the primary cilium of kidney cells. Nat Genet, 2003; 33:129–137

494. Bacalloa RL, Carone FA. Recent advances in the understanding of polycystic kidney disease. Curr Opin Nephrol Hypertens, 1997; 6:377–383

495. Daoust MC, Reynold DM, Bichet DO, Somlo S. Evidence for a third genetic locus for autosomal dominant kidney disease. Genomics, 1995; 25:733–736

496. Hateboer N, v Dijk MA, Bogdanova N et al. Comparison of phenotypes of polycystic kidney disease types 1 and 2. Lancet, 1999; 353:103–107

497. Gabow PA. Autosomal dominant polycystic kidney disease. N Eng J Med, 1993; 329:332–342

498. Fick GM, Johnson AM, Strain JD et al. Characteristics of very early onset autosomal dominant polycystic kidney disease. J Am Soc Nephrol, 1993; 3:1863–1876

499. Henson SW, Jr., Gray HK, Dockerty MB. Benign tumours of the liver III. Solitary cysts. Surg Gynecol Obstet, 1956; 103:607–612

500. Kwok MK, Lewin KJ. Massive hepatomegaly in adult polycystic liver disease. Am J Surg Pathol, 1988; 12:321–324

501. Dumot JA, Fields MS, Meyer RA, Shay SS, Conwell DL, Brzezinski A. Alcohol sclerosis for polycystic liver disease and obstructive jaundice: use of a nasobiliary catheter. Am J Gastroenterol, 1994; 89:1555–1557

502. Garber S, Mathieson J, Cooperberg PL. Percutaneous sclerosis of hepatic cysts to treat obstructive jaundice in a patient with polycystic liver disease. AJR Am J Roentgenol, 1993; 161:77–78

503. van Erpecum KJ, Janssens AR, Terpstra JL, Tjon A, T. TR. Highly symptomatic adult polycystic disease of the liver. A report of fifteen cases. J Hepatol, 1987; 5:109–117

504. Torres VE, Rastogi S, King BF, Stanson AW, Gross JB, Jr., Nogorney DM. Hepatic venous outflow obstruction in autosomal dominant polycystic kidney disease. J Am Soc Nephrol, 1994; 5:1186–1192

505. Uddin W, Ramage JK, Portmann B et al. Hepatic venous outflow obstruction in patients with polycystic liver disease: pathogenesis and treatment. Gut, 1995; 36:142–145

506. Harris RA, Gray DW, Britton BJ, Toogood GJ, Morris PJ. Hepatic cystic disease in an adult polycystic kidney disease transplant population. Aust N Z J Surg, 1996; 66:166–168

507. Vons C, Chauveau D, Martinod E et al. Résection hépatique chez les malades atteints de polykystose hépatique [Liver resection in patients with polycystic liver disease]. Gastroenterol Clin Biol, 1998; 22:50–54

508. Que F, Nagorney DM, Gross JB, Jr., Torres VE. Liver resection and cyst fenestration in the treatment of severe polycystic liver disease. Gastroenterology, 1995; 108:487–494

509. Everson GT, Taylor MR. Management of polycystic liver disease. Curr Gastroenterol Rep, 2005; 7:19–25

510. Starzl TE, Reyes J, Tzakis A, Mieles L, Todo S, Gordon R. Liver transplantation for polycystic liver disease. Arch Surg, 1990; 125:575–577

511. Gabow PA. Autosomal dominant polycystic kidney disease: more than a renal disease. Am J Kidney Dis, 1990; 16:403–413

512. Sherstha R, McKinley C, Russ P et al. Postmenopausal estrogen therapy selectively stimulates hepatic enlargement in women with autosomal dominant polycystic kidney disease. Hepatology, 1997; 26:1282–1286

513. Telenti A, Torres VE, Gross JB, Jr., Van Scoy RE, Brown ML, Hattery RR. Hepatic cyst infection in autosomal dominant polycystic kidney disease. Mayo Clin Proc, 1990; 65:933–942

514. Ikei S, Yamaguchi Y, Mori K. Infection of hepatic cysts with Pseudomonas aeroginosa in polycystic liver disease. Dig Surg, 1990; 7:117–121

515. Kaehny WD, Everson GT. Extrarenal manifestations of autosomal dominant polycystic kidney disease. Semin Nephrol, 1991; 11:661–670

516. Milutinovic J, Schabel SI, Ainsworth SK. Autosomal dominant polycystic kidney disease with liver and pancreatic involvement in early childhood. Am J Kidney Dis, 1989; 13:340–344

517. Cole BR, Conley SB, Stapleton FB. Polycystic kidney disease in the first year of life. J Pediatr, 1987; 111:693–699

518. Perron RD. Extrarenal manifestations of autosomal dominant polycystic kidney disease. Kidney Int, 1997; 51:2022–2036

519. Thomsen H, J T. Frequency of hepatic cysts in adult polycystic kidney disease. Acta Med Scand, 1998; 224:381–384

520. Terada T, Nakanuma Y. Congenital biliary dilatation in autosomal dominant adult polycystic disease of the liver and kidneys. Arch Pathol Lab Med, 1988; 112:1113–1116

521. Patterson M, Gonzalez-Vitale JC, Fagan CJ. Polycystic liver disease: a study of cyst fluid constituents. Hepatology, 1982; 2:475–478

522. Coffin B, Hadengue A, Gegos F, Benhamou J-P. Calcified hepatic and renal cysts in adult dominant polycystic kidney disease. Dig Dis Sci, 1990; 35:1172–1175

523. Melnick PJ. Polycystic liver. Arch Pathol, 1955; 59:162–172

524. Ramos A, Torres VE, Holley KE et al. The liver in autosomal dominant polycystic kidney disease. Arch Pathol Lab Med, 1990; 114:180–184

525. Kida T, Nakanuma Y, Terada T. Cystic dilatation of peribiliary glands in livers with adult polycystic disease and livers with solitary nonparasitic cysts: an autopsy study. Hepatology, 1992; 16:334–340

526. Redston MS, Wanless IR. The hepatic von Meyenburg complex: prevalence and association with hepatic and renal cysts among 2843 autopsies [corrected]. Mod Pathol, 1996; 9:233–237

527. Honda N, Cobb C, Lechago J. Bile duct carcinoma associated with multiple von Meyenburg complexes in the liver. Hum Pathol, 1986; 17:1287–1290

528. Bruns CD, Kuhms JG, Wieman J. Cholangiocarcinoma in association with multiple biliary microhamartomas. Arch Pathol Lab Med, 1990; 114:1287–1289

529. Rossi RL, Silverman ML, Braasch JW, Munson JL, ReMine SG. Carcinomas arising in cystic conditions of the bile ducts. Ann Surg, 1987; 205:377–384

530. Theise N, Miller F, Worman HJ et al. Biliary cystadenocarcinoma arising in a liver with fibropolycystic disease. Arch Pathol Lab Med, 1993; 117:163–165

531. Coffen T, Breuning M, Shoots C, Tinkate L, Zerbes K. Congenital hepatic fibrosis in ADPKD. Kidney Int, 1990; 38:880–885

532. Ivy D, Shaffer E, Johnson A, Kimberling W, Dobin A, Gabow P. Cardiovascular abnormalities in children with austosomal dominant polycystic kidney disease. J Am Soc Nephrol, 1995; 5:2032–2036

533. Iglesias DM, Palmitano JA, Arrizurieta E et al. Isolated polycystic liver disease not linked to polycystic kidney disease 1 and 2. Dig Dis Sci, 1999; 44:385–388

534. Pirson Y, Lannoy N, Peters D et al. Isolated polycystic liver disease as a distinct genetic disease, unlinked to polycystic kidney disease 1 and polycystic kidney disease 2. Hepatology, 1996; 23:249–252

535. Qian Q, Li A, King BF et al. Clinical profile of autosomal dominant polycystic liver disease. Hepatology, 2003; 37:164–171

536. Li A, Davila S, Furu L et al. Mutations in PRKCSH cause isolated autosomal dominant polycystic liver disease. Am J Hum Genet, 2003; 72:691–703

537. Donovan MJ, Kozakewich H, Perez-Atayde A. Solitary non parasitic cysts of the liver. The Boston Children's Hospital experience. Pediatr Pathol Lab Med, 1995; 15:419–428

538. Geist DC. Solitary nonparasitic cyst of the liver; review of the literature and report of two patients. Arch Surg, 1955; 71:867–880

539. Byrne WJ, Fonkalsrud EW. Congenital solitary nonparasitic cyst of the liver: a rare cause of rapidly enlarging abdominal mass in infancy. J Pediatr Surg, 1982; 17:316–317

540. Cappell MS. Obstructive jaundice from benign, nonparasitic hepatic cysts: identification of risk factors and percutaneous aspiration for diagnosis and treatment. Am J Gastroenterol, 1988; 83:93–96

541. Akriviadis EA, Steindel H, Ralls P, Redeker AG. Spontaneous rupture of nonparasitic cyst of the liver. Gastroenterology, 1989; 97:213–215

542. Brock JS, Pachter HL, Schreiber J, Hofstetter SR. Surgical diseases of the falciform ligament. Am J Gastroenterol 1992; 67:757–758

543. Kashima S, Asanuma Y, NwA M, Koyama K. A case of true hepatic cyst with malignant change. Acta Hepatol Jpn, 1988; 29:1265–1268

544. Pliskin A, Cualing H, Stenger RJ. Primary squamous cell carcinoma originating in congenital cysts of the liver. Arch Pathol Lab Med, 1992; 166:105–107

545. Terada T, Notsumata K, Nakanuma Y. Biliary carcinosarcoma arising in nonparasitic simple cyst of the liver. Virchows Arch, 1994; 424:331–335

546. Ueyama T, Ding J, Hashimoto H, Tsuneyoshi M, Enjoji M. Carcinoid tumor arising in the wall of a congenital bile duct cyst. Arch Pathol Lab Med, 1992; 116:291–293

547. Chu DY, Olson AL, Mishalany HG. Congenital liver cyst presenting as congenital diaphragmatic hernia. J Pediatr Surg, 1986; 21:897–899

548. Thrasher S, Adelman S, Chang C-H. Hepatic cyst associated with Peutz-Jeghers syndrome. Arch Pathol Lab Med, 1990; 114:1278–1280

549. Deziel DJ, Rossi RL, Munson JL et al. Management of bile duct cysts in adults. Arch Surg, 1986; 121:410–415

550. Furuta T, Yoshida Y, Saku M et al. Treatment of symptomatic non-parasitic liver cysts—surgical treatment versus alcohol injection therapy. HPB Surg, 1990; 2:269–277

551. Pozniczek M, Wysocki A, Bobrzynski A, Krzywon J, Kostarczyk W, Budzynski P. Sclerosant therapy as first-line treatment for solitary liver cysts. Dig Surg 2004; 21:452–454

552. Fabiani P, Mazza D, Toouli J et al. Laparoscopic fenestration of symptomatic non-parasitic cysts of the liver. Br J Surg, 1997; 84:321–322

553. Fiamingo P, Tedeschi U, Veroux M et al. Laparoscopic treatment of simple hepatic cysts and polycystic liver disease. Surg Endosc, 2003; 17:623–626

554. Reye RDK, Morgan G, Baral J. Encephalopathy and fatty degeneration of the viscera, a disease entity in childhood. Lancet, 1963; ii:749–752

555. Crocker JF. Reye's syndrome. Semin Liver Dis, 1982; 2:340–352

556. Starko KM, Ray CG, Dominguez LB, Stromberg WL, Woodall DF. Reye's syndrome and salicylate use. Pediatric, 1980; 66:859–864

557. SurgeonGeneral. Surgeon General's advisory on the use of salicylates and Reye's syndrome. MMWR, 1982; 31:289–290

558. Hurwitz ES, Barrett MJ, Bregman D et al. Public Health Service study on Reye's syndrome and medications. Report of the pilot phase. N Engl J Med, 1985; 313:849–857

559. Hurwitz ES, Barrett MJ, Bregman D et al. Public Health Service study of Reye's syndrome and medications. Report of the main study. JAMA, 1987; 257:1905–1911

560. Belay ED, Bresee JS, Holman RC, Khan AS, Shahriari A, Schonberger LB. Reye's syndrome in the United States from 1981 through 1997. N Engl J Med, 1999; 340:1377–1382

561. Hall SM, Lynn R. Reye's syndrome. N Engl J Med, 1999; 341:845–846

562. Orlowski JP. Whatever happened to Reye's syndrome? Did it ever really exist? Crit Care Med, 1999; 27:1582–1587

563. Varma RR, Riedel DR, Komorowski RA, Harrington GJ, Nowak TV. Reye's syndrome in nonpediatric age groups. JAMA, 1979; 242:1373–1375

564. Stillman A, Gitter H, Shillington D et al. Reye's syndrome in the adult: case report and review of the literature. Am J Gastroenterol, 1983; 78:365–368

565. Bove KE, McAdams AJ, Partin JC, Partin JS, Hug G, Schubert WK. The hepatic lesion in Reye's syndrome. Gastroenterology, 1975; 69:685–697

566. Bentz MS, Cohen C. Periportal hepatic necrosis in Reye's syndrome. One case in a review of eight patients. Am J Gastroenterol, 1980; 73:49–53

567. Ellis GH, Mirkin LD, Mills MC. Pancreatitis and Reye's syndrome. Am J Dis Child, 1979; 133:1014–1016

568. Phillips MJ, Poucell S, Patterson J, Valencia P. The Liver. An Atlas and Text of Ultrastructural Pathology. New York: Raven Press; 1987

569. Partin JC, Schubert WK, Partin JS. Mitochondrial ultrastructure in Reye's syndrome (encephalopathy and fatty degeneration of the viscera). N Engl J Med, 1971; 285:1339–1343

570. Bradel EJ, Reiner CB. The fine structure of hepatocytes in Reye's syndrome. In: D PJ, editor. Reye's syndrome. New York: Grune & Stratton; 1975. p. 147–158

571. Baboolal R, Monaghan H, Ward OC. Reye's syndrome in a boy treated with salicylates for Reiter's disease. Ir Med J, 1986; 79:289–291

572. Starko KM, Mullick FG. Hepatic and cerebral pathology findings in children with fatal salicylate intoxication: further evidence for a causal relation between salicylate and Reye's syndrome. Lancet, 1983; 1:326–329

573. Hug G, Bosken J, Bove K, Linnemann CC, Jr., McAdams L. Reye's syndrome simulacra in liver of mice after treatment with chemical agents and encephalomyocarditis virus. Lab Invest, 1981; 45:89–109

574. Davis LE, Cole LL, Lockwood SJ, Kornfeld M. Experimental influenza B virus toxicity in mice. Lab Invest, 1983; 48:140–147

575. Sakaida N, Senzaki H, Shikata N, Morii S. Microvesicular fatty liver in rats with resembling Reye's syndrome induced by 4-pentenoic acid. Acta Pathol Jpn, 1990; 40:635–642

576. Brownstein DG, Johnson EA, Smith AL. Spontaneous Reye's-like syndrome in BALB/cByJ mice. Lab Invest, 1984; 51:386–395

577. Kawasaki T. Acute febrile mucocutaneous syndrome with lymphoid involvement with specific desquamation of the fingers and toes in children. Arerugi, 1967; 16:178–222

578. Royle J, Burgner D, Curtis N. The diagnosis and management of Kawasaki disease. J Paediatr Child Health, 2005; 41:87–93

579. Melish ME, Hicks RV. Kawasaki syndrome: clinical features. Pathophysiology, etiology and therapy. J Rheumatol, 1990; 24(Suppl):2–10

580. Granel B, Serratrice J, Ene N et al. Painful jaundice revealing Kawasaki disease in a young man. J Gastroenterol Hepatol, 2004; 19:713–715

581. Nakamura Y, Yanagawa H, Kawasaki T. Mortality among children with Kawasaki disease in Japan. N Engl J Med, 1992; 326:1246–1249

582. Nakamura Y, Fujita Y, Nagai M et al. Cardiac sequelae of Kawasaki disease in Japan: statistical analysis. Pediatrics, 1991; 87:1144–1147

583. Newburger JW, Takahashi M, Burns JC et al. The treatment of Kawasaki syndrome with intravenous gamma globulin. N Engl J Med, 1986; 315:341–347

584. Onouchi Z, Hamaoka K, Sakata K et al. Long-term changes in coronary artery aneurysms in patients with Kawasaki disease: comparison of therapeutic regimens. Circ J, 2005; 69:265–272

585. Levy M, Koren G. Atypical Kawasaki disease; analysis of clinical presentation and diagnostic clues. Pediatr Infect Dis J, 1990; 9:122–126

586. Suddleson EA, Reid B, Woolley MM, Takahashi M. Hydrops of the gallbladder associated with Kawasaki syndrome. J Pediatr Surg, 1987; 22:956–959

587. Bishop WP, Kao SC. Prolonged postprandial abdominal pain following Kawasaki syndrome with acute gallbladder hydrops: association with impaired gallbladder emptying. J Pediatr Gastroenterol Nutr, 1991; 13:307–311

588. Bader-Meunier B, Hadchouel M, Fabre M, Arnoud MD, Dommergues JP. Intrahepatic bile duct damage in children with Kawasaki disease. J Pediatr, 1992; 120:750–752

589. Amano S, Hazama F, Kubagawa H, Tasaka K, Haebara H, Hamashima Y. General pathology of Kawasaki disease. On the morphological alterations corresponding to the clinical manifestations. Acta Pathol Jpn, 1980; 30:681–694

590. Edwards KM, Glick AD, Greene HL. Intrahepatic cholangitis associated with mucocutaneous lymph node syndrome. J Pediatr Gastroenterol Nutr, 1985; 4:140–142

591. Gear JH, Meyers KE, Steele M. Kawasaki disease manifesting with acute cholangitis. A case report. S Afr Med J, 1992; 81:31–33

592. Bergeson PS, Serlin SP, Corman LI. Mucocutaneous lymph-node syndrome with positive Weil-Felix reaction but negative Leptospira studies. Lancet, 1978; 1:720–721

593. Ahlström H, Lundstrom NR, Mortensson W, Ostberg G, Lantorp K. Infantile periarteritis nodosa or mucocutaneous lymph node syndrome. A report on four cases and diagnostic considerations. Acta Paediatr Scand, 1977; 66:193–198

594. Kato H, Koike S, Yamamoto M, Ito Y, Yano E. Coronary aneurysms in infants and young children with acute febrile mucocutaneous lymph node syndrome. J Pediatr, 1975; 86:892–898

595. Marks WH, Coran AG, Wesley JR et al. Hepatic artery aneurysm associated with the mucocutaneous lymph node syndrome. Surgery, 1985; 98:598–601

596. Kato H, Fujimoto T, Inoue O et al. Variant strain of Propionobacterum acnes: A clue to the aetiology of Kawasaki disease. Lancet, 1983; ii:1383–1388

597. Leung DY, Meissner HC, Fulton DR, Murray DL, Kotzin BL, Schlievert PM. Toxic shock syndrome toxin-secreting Staphylococcus aureus in Kawasaki syndrome. Lancet, 1993; 342:1385–1388

598. Viraben A, Dupre A. Kawasaki disease associated with HIV infection. Lancet, 1987; 1:1430–1431

599. Kikuta H, Taguchi Y, Tomizawa K et al. Epstein–Barr virus genome-positive T-lymphocytes in a boy with chronic active EBV infection associated with Kawasaki-like disease. Nature, 1988; 333:455–457

600. Nigro G, Zerbini M, Krzysztofiak A et al. Active or recent parvovirus B19 infection in children with Kawasaki disease. Lancet, 1994; 343:1260–1261

601. Chou CT, Chang JS, Ooi SE et al. Serum anti-Yersinia antibody in chinese patients with Kawasaki disease. Arch Med Res, 2005; 36:14–18

602. Whitby D, Hoad JG, Tizard EJ et alolation of measles virus from child with Kawasaki disease. Lancet, 1991; 338:1215

603. Pagnoux C, Hayem G, Roux F, Palazzo E, Meyer O. Sclerosing cholangitis as a complication of Langerhans'cell histiocytosis. Rev Med Interne, 2003; 24:324–332

604. Jaffe R. Liver involvement in the histiocytic disorders of childhood. Pediatr Dev Pathol, 2004; 7:214–225

605. Finn LS, Jaffe R. Langerhans' cell granuloma confined to the bile duct. Pediatr Pathol Lab Med, 1997; 17:461–468

606. Buza N, Lagarde DC, Dash S, Haque S. Langerhans cell histiocytosis: report of a single organ involvement in a child. J Cell Mol Med, 2004; 8:397–401

607. Kaplan KJ, Goodman ZD, Ishak KG. Liver involvement in Langerhans' cell histiocytosis. A study of nine cases. Mod Pathol, 1999; 12:370–378

608. Favara BE, Jaffe R, Egeler RM. Macrophage activation and hemophagocytic syndrome in Langerhans cell histiocytosis: report of 30 cases. Pediatr Dev Pathol, 2002; 5:130–140

609. Emile JF, Wechsler J, Brousse N et al. Langerhans' cell histiocytosis: Definitive diagnosis with the use of monoclonal antibody O10 on routinely paraffin-embedded samples. Am J Surg Pathol, 1995; 19:636–641

610. Krenacs L, Tiszaluicz L, Krenacs T, Boumsell L. Immunohistochemical detection of CD1a antigen in formalin-fixed and paraffin-embedded tissue sections with monoclonal antibody 010. J Pathol, 1993; 171:99–104

611. Slone SP, Fleming DR, Buchino JJ. Sinus histiocytosis with massive lymphadenopathy and Langerhans cell histiocytosis express the cellular adhesion molecule CD31. Arch Pathol Lab Med, 2003; 127:341–344

612. Niki T, Oka T, Shiga J, Takahashi K, Geerts A, Machinami R. Increased S-100 protein-immunoreactivity of Kupffer cells is associated with lymphohematological malignancy. Pathol Int, 1995; 45:742–747

613. Bouloc A, Boulland M-L, Geissmann F et al. CD101 expression by Langerhans' cell histiocytosis cells. Histopathology, 2000; 36:229–232

614. Cavazza A, Pasquinelli G, Carlinfante G et al. Nodular Langerhans' cell histiocytosis of the liver in an adult with colonic adenocarcinoma. Histopathology, 1999; 34:273–275

615. Braier J, Ciocca M, Latella A, de Davila MG, Drajer M, Imventarza O. Cholestasis, sclerosing cholangitis, and liver transplantation in Langerhans cell Histiocytosis. Med Pediatr Oncol, 2002; 38:178–182

616. Marchal J, Kambouchner M, Tazi A, Valeyre D, Soler P. Expression of apoptosis-regulatory proteins in lesions of pulmonary Langerhans cell histiocytosis. Histopathology, 2004; 45:20–28

617. Annels NE, Da Costa CE, Prins FA, Willemze A, Hogendoorn PC, Egeler RM. Aberrant chemokine receptor expression and chemokine production by Langerhans cells underlies the pathogenesis of Langerhans cell histiocytosis. J Exp Med, 2003; 197:1385–1390

618. Laman JD, Leenen PJ, Annels NE, Hogendoorn PC, Egeler RM. Langerhans-cell histiocytosis 'insight into DC biology'. Trends Immunol, 2003; 24:190–196

619. Willman CL, Busque L, Griffith BB et al. Langerhans'-cell histiocytosis (histiocytosis X)—a clonal proliferative disease. N Eng J Med, 1994; 331:154–160

620. Yu RC, Chu C, Buluwela L, Chu AC. Clonal proliferation of Langerhans cells in Langerhans cell histiocytosis. Lancet, 1994; 343:767–768

621. Kawakubo Y, Kishimoto H, Sato Y et al. Human cytomegalovirus infection in foci of Langerhans cell histiocytosis. Virchows Arch, 1999; 434:109–115

622. Shimakage M, Sasagawa T, Kimura M et al. Expression of Epstein–Barr virus in Langerhans' cell histiocytosis. Hum Pathol, 2004; 35:862–868

623. Glotzbecker MP, Carpentieri DF, Dormans JP. Langerhans cell histiocytosis: a primary viral infection of bone? Human herpes virus 6 latent protein detected in lymphocytes from tissue of children. J Pediatr Orthop, 2004; 24:123–129

624. Lieberman PH, Jones CR, Steinman RM et al. Langerhans cell (eosinophilic) granulomatosis: A clinicopathologic study encompassing 50 years. Am J Surg Pathol, 1996; 20:519–522

625. Howarth DM, Gilchrist GS, Mullan BP et al. Langerhans cell histiocytosis. Diagnosis, natural history, management and outcome. Cancer, 1999; 85:2278–2290

626. Jubran RF, Marachelian A, Dorey F, Malogolowkin M. Predictors of outcome in children with Langerhans cell histiocytosis. Pediatr Blood Cancer, 2005; 45:37–42

627. Anonymous. A multicentre retrospective survey of Langerhans' cell histiocytosis: 348 cases observed between 1983 and 1993. The French Langerhans' Cell Histiocytosis Study Group. Arch Dis Child, 1996; 75:17–24

628. Zandi P, Panis Y, Debray D, Bernard O, Houssin D. Pediatric liver transplantation for Langerhans' cell histiocytosis. Hepatology, 1995; 21:129–133

629. Newell KA, Alonso EM, Kelly SM, Rubin CM, Thistlethwaite JR, Jr., Whitington PF. Association between liver transplantation for Langerhans cell histiocytosis, rejection, and development of posttransplant lymphoproliferative disease in children. J Pediatr, 1997; 131:98–104

630. Hadzic N, Pritchard J, Webb D et al. Recurrence of Langerhans cell histiocytosis in the graft after pediatric liver transplantation. Transplantation, 2000; 70:815–819

631. Dehner LP. Juvenile xanthogranulomas in the first two decades of life: a clinicopathologic study of 174 cases with cutaneous and extracutaneous manifestations. Am J Surg Pathol, 2003; 27:579–593

632. Rosai J, Dorfman RF. Sinus histiocytosis with massive lymphadenopathy: A newly recognized benign clinicopathological entity. Arch Pathol, 1969; 87:63–70

633. Foucar E, Rosai J, Dorfman R. Sinus histiocytosis with massive lymphadenopathy (Rosai–Dorfman disease): review of the entity. Semin Diagn Pathol, 1990; 7:19–73

634. Lauwers GY, Perez-Atayde A, Dorfman RF, Rosai J. The digestive system manifestations of Rosai-Dorfman disease (sinus

histiocytosis with massive lymphadenopathy): Review of 11 cases. Hum Pathol, 2000; 31:380–385

635. Eisen R, Buckley PJ, Rosai J. Immunophenotypic characterization of sinus histiocytosis with massive lymphadenopathy (Rosai-Dorfman disease). Semin Diagn Pathol, 1990; 7:74–82

636. Arico M, Allen M, Brusa S et al. Haemophagocytic lymphohistiocytosis: proposal of a diagnostic algorithm based on perforin expression. Br J Haematol, 2002; 119:180–188

637. Feldmann J, Le Deist F, Ouachee-Chardin M et al. Functional consequences of perforin gene mutations in 22 patients with familial haemophagocytic lymphohistiocytosis. Br J Haematol, 2002; 117:965–972

638. Favara BE. Hemophagocytic lymphohistiocytosis: a hemophagocytic syndrome. Semin Diagn Pathol, 1992; 9:63–74

639. Parizhskaya M, Reyes J, Jaffe R. Hemophagocytic syndrome presenting as acute hepatic failure in two infants: clinical overlap with neonatal hemochromatosis. Pediatr Dev Pathol, 1999; 2:360–366

640. Natsheh SE, Roberts EA, Ngan B, Chait P, Ng VL. Liver failure with marked hyperferritinemia: 'ironing out' the diagnosis. Can J Gastroenterol, 2001; 15:537–540

641. Ost A, Nilsson-Ardnor S, Henter J-I. Autopsy findings in 27 children with haemophagocytic lymphohistiocytosis. Histopathology, 1998; 32:310–316

642. Hsu TS, Kemp DM. Clinical features of familial histiocytosis. Am J Pediatr Hematol Oncol, 1981; 3:61–65

643. Favara BE. Histopathology of the liver in histiocytosis syndromes. Pediatr Pathol Lab Med, 1996; 16:413–433

644. Imashuku S, Ueda I, Teramura T et al. Occurrence of haemophagocytic lymphohistiocytosis at less than 1 year of age: analysis of 96 patients. Eur J Pediatr, 2005; 164:315–319

645. Woda BA, Sullivan JL. Reactive histiocytic disorders. Am J Clin Pathol, 1993; 99:459–463

646. Sawhney S, Woo P, Murray KJ. Macrophage activation syndrome: a potentially fatal complication of rheumatic disorders. Arch Dis Child, 2001; 85:421–426

647. Stephan JL, Kone-Paut I, Galambrun C, Mouy R, Bader-Meunier B, Prieur AM. Reactive haemophagocytic syndrome in children with inflammatory disorders. A retrospective study of 24 patients. Rheumatology (Oxford) 2001; 40:1285–1292

648. Chan JKC, Ng CS, Law CK, Ng WF, Wong KF. Reactive hemophagocytic syndrome. A study of 7 fatal cases. Pathology, 1987; 19:43–50

649. Fujiwara F, Hibi S, Imashuku S. Hypercytokinemia in hemophagocytic syndrome. Am J Pediatr Hematol Oncol, 1993; 15:92–98

650. Tsui WMS, Wong KF, Tse CCH. Liver changes in reactive haemophagocytic syndrome. Liver, 1992; 12:363–367

651. de Kerguenec C, Hillaire S, Molinie V et al. Hepatic manifestations of hemophagocytic syndrome: A study of 30 cases. Am J Gastroenterol, 2001; 96:854–857

652. Billiau AD, Roskams T, Van Damme-Lombaerts R, Matthys P, Wouters C. Macrophage activation syndrome: characteristic findings on liver biopsy illustrating the key role of activated, IFN-gamma-producing lymphocytes and IL-6- and TNF-alpha-producing macrophages. Blood, 2005; 105:1648–1651

653. Ruchelli ED, Uri A, Dimmick JE et al. Severe perinatal liver disease and Down syndrome: an apparent relationship. Hum Pathol, 1991; 22:1274–1280

654. Schwab M, Niemeyer C, Schwarzer U. Down syndrome, transient myeloproliferative disorder, and infantile liver fibrosis. Med Pediatr Oncol, 1998; 31:159–165

655. Becroft DMO, Zwi J. Perinatal visceral fibrosis accompanying the megakaryoblastic leukemoid reaction of Down syndrome. Pediatr Pathol, 1990; 10:397–406

656. Tsuda T, Komiyama A, Aonuma K, Akabane T, Nakayama M. Transient abnormal myelopoiesis and diffuse hepatic necrosis in Down's syndrome with bleeding diathesis. Acta Paediatr Scand, 1990; 79:241–244

657. Gilson JP, Bendon RW. Megakaryocytosis of the liver in a trisomy 21 stillbirth. Arch Pathol Lab Med, 1993; 117:738–739

658. Zipursky A, Rose T, Skidmore M, Thorner P, Doyle J. Hydrops fetalis and neonatal leukemia in Down syndrome. Pediatr Hematol Oncol, 1996; 13:81–87

659. Arai H, Ishida A, Nakajima W, Nishinomiya F, Yamazoe A, Takada G. Immunohistochemical study on transforming growth factor-beta 1 expression in liver fibrosis of Down's syndrome. Hum Pathol, 1999; 30:474–476

660. Shiozawa Y, Fujita H, Fujimura J et al. A fetal case of transient abnormal myelopoiesis with severe liver failure in Down syndrome: prognostic value of serum markers. Pediatr Hematol Oncol, 2004; 21:273–278

661. Dormann S, Kruger M, Hentschel R et al. Life-threatening complications of transient abnormal myelopoiesis in neonates with Down syndrome. Eur J Pediatr 2004; 163:374–377

662. Massey GV. Transient leukemia in newborns with Down syndrome. Pediatr Blood Cancer, 2005; 44:29–32

663. Silverman ED, Laxer RM. Neonatal lupus erythematosus. Rheum Dis Clin N A, 1997; 23:599–618

664. Lin SC, Shyur SD, Huang LH, Wu JY, Chuo HT, Lee HC. Neonatal lupus erythematosus with cholestatic hepatitis. J Microbiol Immunol Infect, 2004; 37:131–134

665. Laxer RM, Roberts EA, Gross KR et al. Liver disease in neonatal lupus erythematosus. J Pediatr, 1990; 116:238–242

666. Evans N, Gaskin K. Liver disease in association with neonatal lupus erythematosus. J Paediatr Child Health, 1993; 29:478–480

667. Rosh JR, Silverman ED, Groisman G, Dolgin S, LeLeiho NS. Intrahepatic cholestasis in neonatal lupus erythematosus. J Pediatr Gastroenterol Nutr, 1993; 17:310–312

668. Kanitkar M, Rohini KP, Puri B, Nair MN. Neonatal lupus mimicking extrahepatic biliary atresia. Indian Pediatr, 2004; 41:1252–1254

669. Schoenlebe J, Buyon JP, Zitelli BJ, Friedman D, Greco MA, Knisely AS. Neonatal hemochromatosis associated with maternal antibodies against Ro/SS-A and La/SS-B ribonucleoproteins. Am J Dis Child, 1993; 147:1072–1075

670. Lee LA, Sokol RJ, Buyon JP. Hepatobiliary disease in neonatal lupus: prevalence and clinical characteristics in cases enrolled in a national registry. Pediatrics, 2002; 109:E11

671. Selander B, Cedergren S, Domanski H. A case of severe neonatal lupus erythematosus without cardiac or cutaneous involvement. Acta Paediatr, 1998; 87:105–107

672. Burch JM, Sokol RJ, Narkewicz MR et al. Autoantibodies in mothers of children with neonatal liver disease. J Pediatr Gastroenterol Nutr, 2003; 37:262–267

673. Hannam S, Bogdanos D-P, Davies ET et al. Neonatal liver disease associated with placental transfer of anti-mitochondrial antibodies. Autoimmunity, 2002; 35:545–550

Genetic and metabolic liver disease

5

Bernard C. Portmann   Richard J. Thompson   Eve A. Roberts   Alan C. Paterson

The list of identified inherited metabolic disorders continues to expand, many having immediate or long-term relevance to the liver. For example, liver histology is usually normal in primary hyperoxaluria while the kidneys and other organs may be irreparably damaged; however, despite medical management, dialysis, and repetitive kidney transplants, cure is only obtained with a liver transplant.[1] In other inherited disorders, the liver disease may remain asymptomatic until precipitous acute liver failure develops; the classical example is Wilson disease.[2] In many instances, the clinical diagnosis of an inherited disorder may not be evident, and thus diagnosis becomes the responsibility of the histopathologist, who may save not only the life of the patient but that of other family members. Steady advances in molecular genetics constantly improve our understanding of the biological basis of many metabolic diseases. Prenatal detection is available for more families. In the long-term, these techniques may lead to gene therapy, which is already under evaluation to treat some of these disorders.

The effect of the inherited metabolic disorders on the liver may be considered *primary*, i.e. due to the accumulation of a metabolite resulting from an enzyme defect (e.g. sphingomyelin in Niemann–Pick disease), or *secondary*, when the major changes in the liver are the result of a primarily extrahepatic defect (e.g. steatosis of the liver secondary to pancreatic insufficiency in Shwachman syndrome).

Unfortunately, many metabolic disorders of diverse aetiologies manifest similar morphological findings. Numerous conditions are characterized by neonatal cholestasis and giant cell transformation of liver cells, e.g. α_1-antitrypsin deficiency, Niemann–Pick disease type C, progressive familial intrahepatic cholestasis type 2 (BSEP deficiency), to name but a few. Steatosis is one of the most frequent abnormalities, either alone (e.g. in the urea cycle disorders, homocystinuria, lipoprotein disorders, the mitochondrial cytopathies and Shwachman syndrome) or in combination with other changes such as cholestasis, pseudogland formation and fibrosis (e.g. in galactosaemia, tyrosinaemia and hereditary fructose intolerance). Furthermore, neutral lipid may be stored in combination with other metabolites such as cholesterol (e.g. in Wolman disease, cholesterol ester storage disease) or glycogen (e.g. in type I and III glycogenosis). Most of the disorders of lipid metabolism are expressed morphologically by 'foam' cells (e.g. in Niemann–Pick disease and the gangliosidoses),[3] but the ultimate diagnosis is dependent on the clinical and laboratory data and identification of the specific enzyme defect. While histological changes may not lead to a specific diagnosis, their characteristics may add to the phenotypic expression of individual disorders and help selecting further investigations, in particualar enzymatic assays and genomic studies. In that respect, the following discussion includes the major clinical, laboratory and genomic features, in the context of which histological changes should be evaluated.

The histopathologists have at their disposal many special stains and techniques, both at the light microscopic and ultrastructural level. The best all-round fixative for light microscopy remains 10% buffered formalin, but some metabolic diseases (e.g. the mucopolysaccharidoses, cystinosis and the glycogenoses) may require special fixatives to prevent leaching of metabolites that are water soluble. Special stains for lipid, cholesterol and sphingomyelin must be performed on frozen sections cut from formalin-fixed or fresh material since routine processing will extract the lipid material from the cells. Familiarity is required with the many special stains that can be used on formalin-fixed and routinely processed material for the demonstration of uroporphyrin, haemosiderin, copper, copper binding protein, bile, lipofuscin, lipomelanin (the pigment in the Dubin–Johnson syndrome), carbohydrates, mucopolysaccharides and other substances that need to be identified. Immunohistochemical stains are useful in a number of diseases, for example in the identification of catalase in patients with peroxisomal diseases, or identifying the presence of α_1-antitrypsin, α_1-antichymotrypsin or fibrinogen in eosinophilic globules in various storage diseases. The repertoire of specific antibodies working on paraffin sections is continuously broadening (e.g. antibodies reacting with bile salt export protein, BSEP, or with cMOAT).

Special microscopy should be utilized whenever necessary. The porphyrins can be demonstrated by their autofluorescence in frozen sections made from unfixed hepatic biopsy or autopsy material. Polarizing microscopy is especially useful for the identification of various crystals such as cholesterol, cystine, calcium oxalate, uroporphyrin and protoporphyrin. Transmission electron microscopy (TEM) is very important in the diagnosis of many inherited metabolic diseases.[4–7] According to Phillips et al.[5] the findings are diagnostic in α_1-antitrypsin deficiency, Farber disease, glycogenoses types II and IV, hereditary fructose intolerance, Gaucher disease, metachromatic leucodystrophy, the gangliosidoses, the Dubin–Johnson syndrome, erythropoietic protoporphyria, Wilson disease, Zellweger syndrome and infantile Refsum disease. In other disorders, electron microscopy, although not diagnostic, can help to categorize the disease (e.g. as a glycogenosis, phospholipidosis, or oligosaccharidosis) or to suggest the correct diagnosis (e.g. Byler disease, arteriohepatic dysplasia, cholesterol ester storage disease). The role of scanning electron microscopy (SEM) is much more limited.[3]

In summary, histopathological studies contribute significantly to the diagnosis of metabolic disorders. Selection of appropriate pathological studies must be made before liver biopsy, to ensure appropriate fixation and handling of samples. In general a portion of the biopsy core at least 5 mm in length should be snap frozen using OCT compound which does not interfere with most enzyme assays and allows subsequent frozen sectioning for microscopy. Ideally a few bits (1 mm^3) should be immersed in a fixative appropriate for electron microscopy. Tissue freezing and EM fixative, in addition to usual fixation and paraffin processing should be applied to all biopsy specimens taken from children or older patients in whom a metabolic disorder is suspected. Prebiopsy consultation with a histopathologist, and at times with laboratory staff of a centre dealing with highly specialized techniques, may preclude the loss of diagnostic information.

Disorders of porphyrin metabolism

The porphyrias are disorders of the biosynthesis of porphyrins and haem that lead to the excessive accumulation and excretion of porphyrins and porphyrin precursors. Only two of the porphyrias which importantly affect the liver are discussed in this chapter.

Porphyria cutanea tarda

The classification, clinical aspects and therapy of porphyria cutanea tarda (PCT) and other porphyrias are covered in several comprehensive reviews.[8–12] Most patients with PCT have the *sporadic type (type I)*. Decreased activity of uroporphyrinogen decarboxylase is restricted to the liver and the family history is negative. *Familial (type II)* PCT, comprising about 20% of cases of PCT, is inherited as an autosomal dominant trait. The gene is located on chromosome 1p34. The enzyme defect (50% reduction of activity) is present in all tissues. Clinical penetrance is low, with less than 10% of affected persons developing symptoms.

Sporadic (type I) PCT occurs typically in male patients between 40 and 50 years of age. Familial (type II) PCT has an earlier onset, with some cases presenting in childhood. Precipitating factors in the sporadic form include toxins (e.g. hexachlorobenzene), oestrogens, alcohol, mutations in the *HFE* gene and viral infection.[13,14] The interaction of the *HFE* mutation and susceptibility to sporadic PCT has been discussed in several studies.[15–17] Mild to moderate iron overload is found in 60–70% of patients with PCT; 10% have increases in the range of hereditary haemochromatosis.[18] In almost all studies, a high prevalence of HFE gene mutations has been detected with differences between patients of northern European ancestry and those of Mediterranean origin.[19] In a study performed in the USA, 19% of the PTC patients tested were homozygous for the C282Y mutation and 7% were compound heterozygous (respectively 0.5 and 1.0% in the general population).[15]

Viral infections have been considered PCT triggering factors. Initial reports of a high incidence of hepatitis B serological markers in PCT[20–22] and anecdotal cases of HIV infection[23] have been later overwhelmed by the evidence of a strong association between hepatitis C and PCT.[20,24–26] In the series reviewed by Elder,[10] the prevalence of antibodies to hepatitis C virus in PCT has ranged from 9 to 79%. This is broadly related to the level of endemicity of hepatitis C virus infection in the general population in various countries. More recently, a meta-analysis led Gisbert et al.[25] to conclude that the mean prevalence of HCV using polymerase chain reaction in PCT patients is approximately 50%, much higher than that reported in the general population; the prevalence similarly varied depending on the country and the type of PCT (57% in the sporadic and 25% in the familial form). It must be noted that HCV in itself is unlikely to derange the haem synthesis pathway since only a small proportion of HCV-infected patients show an increase in urinary porphyrins and the prevalence of PCT among HCV-infected patients has been reported between 1 and 5%.[24,27]

Histopathological findings in the liver in PCT include the accumulation of uroporphyrin in the cytoplasm of liver cells. Needle-shaped cytoplasmic inclusions have been identified in hepatocytes by light, fluorescent and electron microscopy in biopsy specimens; the crystals are also birefringent under polarizing light.[28,29] According to Cortes et al.[28] the inclusions are best seen by light microscopy in unstained paraffin sections. The crystals can be specifically stained in paraffin sections by the ferric ferricyanide reduction test (Fig. 5.1).[30] They are often found close to ferritin-like deposits.[29] Morphometric studies have shown significantly higher amounts of uroporphyrin crystals in familial than sporadic PCT.[29] The crystals have been induced experimentally in mice by iron overload.[31] Ultrastructurally, they reveal alternating areas of differing electron density. The crystals appear to be a mixture of porphyrinogens and porphyrins surrounding uroporphyrin crystals.[31] Other changes in liver biopsy specimens from patients with PCT have been described in several series.[28,32,33] They include steatosis, variable haemosiderosis in periportal hepatocytes and fibrosis. Cortes et al.[28] found periductal lymphoid aggregates in 43% of their cases. The incidence of cirrhosis in two series was 33% and 34%.[28,33] It should be emphasized that tests for chronic viral hepatitis, particularly chronic hepatitis C, were not performed in the above-mentioned series.

Hepatocellular carcinoma has been reported in association with PCT[28,29,34–36] and also in patients with acute intermittent porphyria, variegate porphyria and hereditary coproporphyria.[37–43] Factors related to an increased risk of hepatocellular carcinoma in PCT are a long symptomatic period before start of therapy, and the presence of chronic hepatitis (particularly hepatitis C), iron overload and advanced fibrosis or cirrhosis. In one series there was a direct relationship between increasing age and extent of

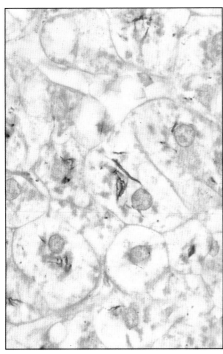

Fig. 5.1 • Porphyria cutanea tarda. Needle-shaped crystals of varied length are present in the cytoplasm of liver cells. Ferric ferricyanide.

liver damage, with fibrosis present at a mean of 48 years, cirrhosis at 57 years and hepatocellular carcinoma at 66 years.[28]

Erythropoietic protoporphyria

Erythropoietic protoporphyria (EPP) was first reported in 1926[44] with further definition of the dermatological manifestations in 1961[45] and the first liver disease reported 35 years ago.[46] Presentation begins with photosensitivity, usually before 6 years of age; patients have an extreme burning sensation with erythema and swelling. Onset of liver disease is usually later; most cases are diagnosed after 30 years of age, although presentation of liver disease can begin in the teenage years. Males are affected twice as often as females. Patients often present with right upper quadrant pain radiating to the back. Cirrhosis develops in only 1–10% of patients.[47–49] There is no evidence of biliary obstruction.[50] Death occurs within 3 to 5 months (range 1 month to 2 years) following the development of jaundice. A few patients have exhibited haemolysis and neurological dysfunction.

Ferrochelatase, the defective enzyme, catalyses the insertion of iron into protoporphyrin as the final step in haem synthesis.[51] Functional enzyme levels are usually less than 50%, allowing diagnosis by measurement of elevated plasma, erythrocyte, and/or faecal protoporphyrin. The bone marrow contributes 80% of the protoporphyrins and the liver up to 20%.[52] Protoporphyrin is poorly water soluble and is only secreted by hepatocytes into bile. When this hepatobiliary transport is overwhelmed, insoluble aggregates of protoporphyrin form crystals in hepatocytes, canaliculi and proximal bile ducts, resulting in 'black liver disease'.[53] Autosomal dominant inheritance is found in most families, but autosomal recessive inheritance has been documented.[54] The incidence of the disease is 1 in 75 000 to 1 in 200 000 world-wide.

Up to 90 different mutations have been identified in the ferrochelatase gene, localized on chromosome 18, including point mutations, nucleotide deletions and a partial chromosome deletion.[12,55–58] The ferrochelatase gene is composed of 11 exons and 10 introns with a size of approximately 4.5 kb, and the enzyme is localized to the matrix side of the inner mitochondrial membrane. Patients with EPP who develop liver disease usually have a mutation in one ferrochelatase allele that alters enzyme function, together with a polymorphism in the nonmutant allele that causes low gene expression. This results in significant increase in the hepatobiliary excretion of protoporphyrin, which can damage the liver through both cholestatic injury and oxidative stress.[59]

Haematin has been the most successful medical therapy.[60,61] Liver transplantation is appropriate for patients with liver failure or end-stage cirrhosis.[62,63] However, recurrence of protoporphyric liver disease has been reported.[63–65] Bone marrow transplantation is needed after liver transplantation to prevent disease recurrence in younger patients.[66] A mouse model is available for future evaluation of therapy.[67–69] The hepatobiliary alterations in this murine model have been reversed by bone marrow transplantation.[70] It has thus been suggested that bone marrow transplantation may be an option for EPP patients at risk of developing hepatic complications.[70]

Macroscopically, the liver affected by EPP is generally black. The first description of the characteristic, if not pathognomonic changes was published by Cripps & Scheuer.[46] Sections from percutaneous hepatic biopsy specimens from five patients showed focal accumulations of a dense, dark brown pigment in canaliculi, interlobular bile ducts, connective tissue and Kupffer cells (Fig. 5.2). The pigment had an intense red autofluorescence in frozen sections examined by fluorescence microscopy with an iodine tungsten quartz light source. Two of the patients had portal and periportal fibrosis and, in one case, the portal areas were infiltrated by mononuclear cells. Cholelithiasis occurs in some patients with EPP, and the calculi contain protoporphyrin.[71] Crystals isolated from the liver in one case of EPP had the same fluorescence spectrum as protoporphyrin.[71]

The deposits in canaliculi, bile ducts and Kupffer cells display bright red birefringence with a centrally located dark maltese cross (Fig. 5.3).[72] Some of the larger deposits and most of the smaller ones in the cytoplasm of hepatocytes and Kupffer cells appear as clusters of brilliantly illuminated granules on polarizing microscopy.

Transmission electron microscopic studies have demonstrated that the deposits of protoporphyrin in EPP consist of numerous, slender, electron-dense crystals arranged singly in sheaves or in a 'star-burst' pattern (Fig. 5.4).[5,72–78] The crystals are straight or slightly curved and are 43–646 nm in length and 6.1–22.0 nm in width. The crystalline accumulations in the cytoplasm of liver cells are not surrounded by a membrane, but in Kupffer cells they are intralysosomal. Non-membrane-bound crystals have also been

demonstrated in the cytoplasm of bile-duct cells.[76] The protoporphyrin casts in canaliculi are readily visualized by scanning electron microscopy (Fig. 5.5).

As already noted, the liver disease in EPP may progress to cirrhosis, although the overall incidence of significant hepatic disease is probably small.[53,79–82] Hepatic failure may be precipitated by viral infection (e.g. Epstein–Barr virus) or by alcohol.[19,83] A direct toxic effect of protoporphyrin in the pathogenesis of liver disease is suggested by the changes

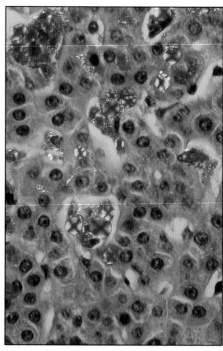

Fig. 5.3 • Protoporphyrin deposits have a red to yellow birefringence with a maltese cross configuration. H&E.

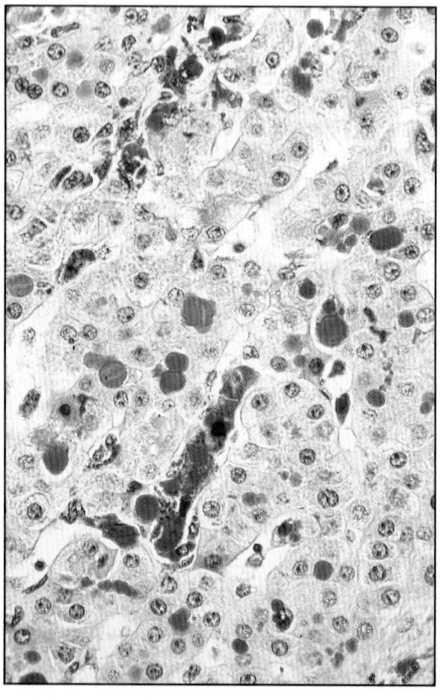

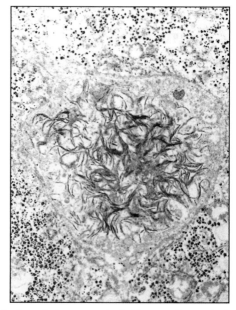

Fig. 5.4 • Erythropoietic protoporphyria. Electron micrograph showing a mass of radiating, hair-like pigment crystals in a dilated canaliculus. ×1800. Courtesy of the late Dr G Klatskin.

Fig. 5.2 • Erythropoietic protoporphyria. Brown deposits are present in canaliculi, hepatocytes and Kupffer cells. H&E.

observed in protoporphyrin-perfused rat livers.[84] The occurrence of cirrhosis in two sisters with EPP also raises the possibility of a genetic predisposition for hepatic disease.[85] A unique association of two rare diseases, Langerhans cell histiocytosis and EPP, has been reported.[86]

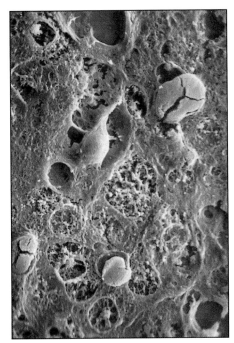

Fig. 5.5 • Erythropoietic protoporphyria. Rounded protoporphyrin casts in canaliculi show fracture lines. Casts are solid and have a granular structure at higher magnifications. Hypertrophied Kupffer cell (upper left) probably contains phagocytosed protoporphyrin. SEM × 1250.

Disorders of carbohydrate metabolism and related conditions

Glycogen storage diseases

Type I glycogen storage diseases

The various glycogen storage diseases that have been characterised are outlined in Table 5.1. Glycogen storage disease (GSD) type I is caused by deficiency of glucose-6-phosphatase, the enzyme catalysing the conversion of glucose-6-phosphate (G6P) to glucose, resulting in decreased hepatic production of glucose and accumulation of glycogen in liver, kidney and intestine. Von Gierke described type 1a glycogen storage disease (GSD) in 1929.[87] The incidence of the disease is 1 : 100 000. Inheritance is autosomal recessive. The gene is located on chromosome 17q21 for type Ia[88] and on chromosome 11q23 for type 1b.[89] Over 70 gene mutations have been identified and a number of ethnic-specific mutations have been described.[90] The diagnosis can be made prenatally.[91] The only available animal model is the glucose-6-phosphatase (G6P) knockout mouse.[92]

Hypoglycaemia in the presence of a markedly enlarged liver is the usual presentation in type I glycogen storage disease in the first year of life. Additional features associated with type 1b GSD include neutropaenia, recurrent infections and inflammatory bowel disease which may resemble Crohn disease, often accompanied by oral, perioral and perianal ulcers, infections, abscesses and fistulae.[93–97]

Usually, patients survive into adulthood if death does not occur in the first year of life. All type 1a adults have

Table 5.1	Glycogen storage disease: enzyme defects, gene locations, diagnostic tests and major histological features			
Type	**Enzyme**	**Gene**	**Enzymatic test**	**Liver abnormalities**
0	Glycogen synthase	12p12.2	Liver	Steatosis
Ia	Glucose-6-phosphatase	17q21	Liver	Steatosis and GHD Adenoma, later HCC
Ib (non-a)	Glucose-6-phasphate translocase	11q23	Freshly removed liver	Steatosis and GHD Adenoma, later HCC
II	Lysosomal-γ1-4 and-γ1-6- glucosidase	17q25	Leukocytes, liver, muscle, amniocytes	Cytoplasmic vacuoles Lysosomal monoparticulate glycogen in EM
IIIa / b	Amylo-1-6 glycosidase (debrancher)	1p21	a. Liver, muscle, heart b. Liver	GHD and steatosis, fibrosis, rarely cirrhosis
IV	Amylo-1-4 glycan6- glycosyltransferase	3p12	Leukocytes, liver, amniocytes	Ground-glass, diastase resistant inclusions Non-membrane bound fibrillar material on EM
VI	Liver phophorylase E	14q21-22	Liver	GHD, steatosis, fibrosis, rarely cirrhosis
IX	Liver phosphorylase kinase	Xp22.1-22.2 16q12–13 16p11.2-12.1	Liver, muscle, erythrocytes, leukocytes	Non-uniform GHD, steatosis
XI	GLUT2 transporter	3q26.1-q26.3	Liver	GHD

Abbreviations: GHD glycogenic hepatocyte distension; EM electron microscopy

hepatomegaly.[98] Other findings include: short stature in 90%; hepatocellular adenomas in 75%, the majority being multiple; iron deficiency in 81%; proteinuria from focal glomerulosclerosis in 67%; renal calcification in 65%; and fractures in 27% of patients. Hypertriglyceridaemia occurs in 100% of patients, hypercholesterolaemia in 76% and hyperuricaemia in 89% of patients. Rarer complications include pancreatitis (thought to be secondary to high lipid levels) and myocardial infarction (from coronary artery disease). Pericardial effusion with valvular disease has been reported.[98] It is evident that a number of complications develop from childhood to adulthood, often despite medical therapy. In children, epistaxis and bleeding during invasive procedures is associated with long bleeding times. Studies indicate a decrease in platelet adhesion, aggregation and ATP release associated with hypoglycaemia, with improvement following normalization of blood glucose levels.[99,100] Von Willebrand factor may be deficient. Correction has been documented with intravenous 1-deamino-8-D-arginine vasopressin (DDAVP).[101]

Two serious complications of this disorder may develop by the time adulthood is reached. One is the development of focal segmental glomerulosclerosis without immune deposits (and presumably not related to renal tubular problems), and uric acid nephropathy occurring prior to this complication.[102] The amount of interstitial fibrosis correlates with the degree of renal insufficiency. Hyperfiltration occurs throughout childhood.[103] The second major complication is the development of hepatocellular adenomas.[104–106] In all series, the male to female ratio is at least 2 : 1. Adenomas are seen as early as 3 years of age and as late as 40 years of age, the vast majority developing in the second decade. Most adenomas take between 2 and 7 years to develop into carcinomas, with a patient mean age of 23 years.[104] Compared to patients without adenomas, the serum concentrations of C-reactive protein, fibrinogen, prealbumen, fibronectin, and retinal binding protein are higher. More importantly, α-fetoprotein levels are often not elevated; thus, the diagnosis depends on the presence of poorly defined nodules on liver imaging. Hepatocellular carcinoma has been seen after 4 years of dietary management despite evidence of adenoma regression.[107,108] There is an isolated publication of type 1a GSD with multiple adenomas associated with Niemann–Pick disease.[109]

In 1952, Cori & Cori reported that G6P activity was virtually absent in the livers of affected individuals.[110] The enzyme is necessary for gluconeogenesis and glycogenolysis, in order to provide 80% of the normal hepatic glucose production. This enzyme also resides in the kidney, pancreas and intestinal epithelium but not in white blood cells.[111] The enzyme is absent in type Ia GSD. A transmembrane transport protein (glucose-6-phosphatase translocase) is defective in type Ib GSD[112] which is currently referred to as type I non-a. Previous denomination of type Ib, Ic, Id followed the belief that different proteins carried out these transport reactions, but recent evidence suggests that GSD type Ib, Ic and Id do not differ from GSD type Ib clinically, enzymatically or genetically.[113] To perform its function of transporting G6P, the enzyme must be active.

This transporter is present in many organs and is active in neutrophils and monocytes. It is a G6P receptor/sensor that regulates calcium sequestration, glycolysis, and the hexose monophosphate activity in white blood cells.[87,114] A deficiency of a 21 kD stabilizing protein (which stabilizes the catalytic enzyme activity) also presents as type 1 GSD in the first year of life.[115,116]

The goal of therapy in infancy and childhood is to keep the glucose level at 70 g/dl. This can be achieved by nocturnal gastric infusions of glucose-containing solution or by the administration of uncooked cornstarch around the clock or by a combination of both.[117,118] Considerable family commitment is required. Death and severe neurological disease have resulted from feeding pump failure.[119] Liver transplantation has been successful in curing GSD type 1a but does not alter the course of the renal disease.[120–122] Combined liver–kidney transplantation has been successful.[123,124] Management of hepatocellular adenomas includes resection or hepatic transplantation.[105,125,126]

With reference to long-term follow-up, 17 patients were followed from infancy in one study, with close to normal growth achieved; however, puberty was delayed in five of the patients. Five patients also received allopurinol for hyperuricaemia, while two were treated for hypertriglyceridaemia. Thirty-five per cent of the patients were anaemic. Hepatocellular adenomas developed in 29%. All but one patient had glomerular hyperfiltration, with protein loss in two.[118] Infections and inflammatory bowel disease in type 1b can be improved by granulocyte colony stimulating factor,[127] which seems to ameliorate neutrophil membrane function,[128] but does not reduce the number of apoptotic neutrophils in the circulation.[129] Despite the persistence of neutropenia after liver transplantation[130] dramatic catch-up growth and reduced infections has been observed.[131] In one patient surgery was followed by an increase in neutrophil counts with a normalization of neutrophil function tests.[132]

Type II glycogen storage disease (acid maltase deficiency, Pompe disease)

Type II glycogen storage disease (GSD), first described by Pompe,[133] is due to a deficiency of the lysosomal enzyme acid alpha-glucosidase (GAA, acid maltase). It includes a generalized infantile type[134] and a milder forms that present during childhood (juvenile) or adulthood.[135,136] The fatal infantile disease presents as a 'floppy baby' with massive cardiomegaly, macroglossia, and progressive muscle weakness leading to death at a median age of 6 to 8 months.[137] Hepatomegaly is mild, without dysfunction and hypoglycaemia is absent.

The milder forms with a late onset present with exercise intolerance, myalgia, varying weakness with or without rhabdomyolysis and myoglobinuria; contractures develop eventually.[135] The juvenile form also involves respiratory muscles and death may result from respiratory failure.[135,136,138] The adult form presents from the second to the sixth decade without cardiac involvement. Creatinine phosphokinase is usually elevated. There is no abnormality in glucose metabolism. Vacuolated lymphocytes are found in the peripheral blood and bone marrow. All organs show vacuolated cells due to enlarged lysosomes containing glycogen. They are particularly prominent in routine histology of autopsy material as a result of the disappearance of extra-lysosomal glycogen. Skeletal, cardiac and smooth muscle fibres contain glycogen-filled vacuoles. In the kidneys, glycogen accumulation is primarily in the loops of Henle and collecting tubules, a location that distinguishes this variety from GSD type I.[139,140]

The prevalence of type II GSD is 1 in 100 000 live births (infantile form), 1/720 000 (juvenile form) and 1/53 000 (adult form).[141] The defect in acid maltase can be demonstrated in all cells including fibroblasts, lymphocytes, amniotic cells, and chorionic villi. The milder forms have more enzyme activity. The gene is localized to chromosome 17q25.[142] There are over 40 mutations,[143] which largely dictate the clinical phenotypes.[144] There are a number of animal models, some of which, e.g. the Japanese quail[145] and a knockout mouse model,[146] are used for studying the possible reversal of tissue pathology and symptomatology under different therapeutic regimens.[147] Clinical trials using recombinant human-glucosidase (rhAGLU) from rabbit milk have produced encouraging results in both infantile and late onset GSD II.[137,148]

Type III glycogen storage disease (Forbe disease, limit dextrinosis)

This autosomal recessive disease is caused by a deficiency in amylo-1,6-glucosidase, 4-alpha-glucanotransferase (AGL or glycogen debranching enzyme), whose gene is located on chromosome 1p21.[149,150] Multiple mutations have been identified which mirror the biochemical and clinical heterogeneity of the disease.[151,152] Presentation may be similar to type I GSD; growth failure is less severe with better resolution at puberty. Hepatocellular adenomas may occur in up to 25% of patients.[153] Type IIIb is characterized by liver involvement alone, whereas type IIIa involves muscle as well as liver, type IIIb being specifically associated with mutations in exon 3.[154] Adults may develop cirrhosis, adenomas and, rarely, hepatocellular carcinoma.[155] Portal hypertension can be present despite normal liver enzymes.[156] Muscle involvement, including cardiac, can become an increasing problem in adulthood.[157] Treatment consists of a high protein diet and uncooked cornstarch.[158,159] Prenatal diagnosis is available.[160]

Type IV glycogen storage disease (branching enzyme deficiency; amylopectinosis; Anderson disease)

Type IV GSD is a rare autosomal recessive disorder caused by a deficiency of glycogen branching enzyme (GBE) leading to the accumulation of amylopectin-like polysaccharides in affected tissues. The deficient enzyme can be measured in the liver, white blood cells, or cultured fibroblasts and prenatal diagnosis is available. The gene localizes to chromo-

some 3p12; multiple defects have been described[161,162] which may correlate with clinical heterogeneity.[163]

The prenatal course may be complicated by polyhydramnios, decreased fetal movement, and dilated cardiomyopathy.[164] A rare congenital variant with early perinatal death is well recognosed.[165–167] Infantile presentation includes hepato-splenomegaly and failure to thrive. Some patients may have arthrogryphosis of the lower limbs.[162] Hypoglycaemia is rare except as a feature of liver failure. Occasionally, patients may not have progression of the liver disease.[168] Later presentation includes congestive cardiac failure, skeletal muscle weakness and nerve involvement.[169,170] In adults progressive involvement of the upper and lower motor neurons, sensory loss, early neurogenic bladder and, in some patients, late dementia may be presenting features.[163] Adult cases are often referred to as adult proteoglucosan body disease.[171,172]

Liver transplantation is an effective treatment for those patients who develop liver failure.[173–175] Out of fourteen reported patients, death from cardiac failure has occurred in a single case,[176] nine of the survivors seem not to have developed any neurological, muscular or cardiac complications up to 13.5 years after transplantation.[90] A reduction in myocardial amylopectin storage has been reported by one group,[175] but not found by others.[174]

Type VI and IX glycogen storage disease and related subtypes (phosphorylase system deficiency)

Defects in the phosphorylase system are due to either deficiencies of phosphorylase enzymes or in the phosphorylase activating system—phosphorylase kinase. These systems are enzymatically distinct in the liver and skeletal muscle. Muscle phosphorylase deficiency (GSD V) does not involve the liver and is not discussed further. Of the liver phosphorylase system defects, phosporylase kinase defects (GSD IX)[177] are much more common than liver phosphorylase deficiency (GSD VI).[178]

The liver phosphorylase gene (PYGL) is localized on chromosome 14q21-22. Glycogen storage disease type VI is a relatively benign disease. The first year may be complicated by hypoglycaemia, hyperlipidaemia and hyperketosis which are generally mild. Growth failure is not uncommon during childhood. The prognosis for most patients is good, with reduction of hepatomegaly after puberty and abnormalities improving with age; adults are usually asymptomatic. Deficient activities of liver phosphorylase in type VI GSD (Hers disease) leads to glycogen accumulation because of a decreased ability to degrade glycogen by cleavage of the α1,4 glycosidic bonds to form glucose 1-phosphate. There is an isoform of phosphorylase in muscle (deficient in McArdle, type VI GSD, gene on chromosome 11) and in brain (gene on chromosome 20).

The genetics of the phosphorylase kinase is more complex, as the enzyme consists of four tissue specific subunits encoded on different genes (including chromosome X) and differentially expressed in different tissues. The phosphorylase kinase liver alpha subunit gene is on chromosome

Xp22.1-22.2, the beta subunit gene is on 16q12-13 and the gamma-subunit is on 16p11.2-12.1. Gene defects include splice and mis-sense mutations.[178]

Phosphorylase kinase activates phosphorylase and is itself activated by a cAMP dependent protein which can be stimulated by glucagon or adrenaline.[179] The alpha and beta subunits modulate the gamma subunit which contains the catalytic portion of the enzymes. The delta subunit is an isoform of calmodulin; an indication that calcium activation can occur.[180]

Phosphorylase kinase deficiency (GSD IX) is clinically and genetically more heterogeneous than phosphorylase deficiency (GSD VI). Seventy-five percent of all cases have X-linked phosphorylase kinase deficiency (GSD IXa), which manifests between the age of 1 and 5 years with hepatomegaly (92%), growth retardation (68%), hypercholesterolaemia (76%), hypertriglycaeridemia (70%) and mild elevation in transaminases (56%); hypoglycaemia and metabolic acidosis are rare.[181] Hepatomegaly and growth retardation usually resolve at puberty. Autosomal recessive forms of phosphorylase kinase deficiency (GSD IXb, c) present with more severe liver disease, which may progress to cirrhosis.[182-184] Renal tubular acidosis or neurological complications, including peripheral sensory neuropathy, are seen.[185]

Enzyme activity is measured most accurately in liver tissue. Blood cells may or may not demonstrate these deficiencies. Therapy is usually not necessary in type VI and IX GSD; uncooked cornstarch may be helpful. The animal model for the disease is the gsd/gsd rat.[186]

Fanconi–Bickel syndrome (glycogen storage disease type XI)

This rare form of glycogen storage disease is characterized by hepatorenal glycogen accumulation, fasting hypoglycaemia, hypergalactosaemia and renal tubular acidosis. It is due to defective function of GLUT2[187] which is the most important glucose transporter in hepatocytes, pancreatic β-cells, enterocytes and renal tubular cells.[188] The GLUT2 gene has been localized to chromosome 3q26.1-q26.3, and 34 different mutations have been reported.[189] Deficiency results in impaired import and export of glucose and galactose in affected tissues. Renal glycogen accumulation leads to impaired tubular function, Fanconi nephropathy and rickets. Patients may be picked up by the galactosaemia screen test since galactose, as well as glucose, are transported by GLUT2.[190] Untreated, the disease can be compatible with survival into adulthood, but patients continue to be symptomatic even after hepatomegaly recedes.[187]

Synthase deficiency (glycogen storage disease type 0)

Synthase deficiency is a rare inborn error of metabolism leading to fasting hypoglycaemia in infancy or early childhood and accompanied by high blood ketones and low alanine and lactate concentrations.[191] The liver GS gene (GYS2) has been localized to chromosome 12p12.2.[192] Modes of presentation of GS deficiency include non-specific symptoms after overnight fasting, an incidental finding or positive family history. The diagnosis is based on the characteristic biochemical profile and the demonstration of absent synthase activity and slightly reduced glycogen content in liver tissue which is frequently steatotic.[193]

Gross, light microscopic and ultrastructual features of the glycogenoses

Grossly, the liver in the glycogenoses is enlarged, smooth and paler than normal. Type IV livers have a tan and waxy appearance with myriad tiny nodules that occasionally aggregate into larger nodules.[194] A reticular pattern of fibrosis or, rarely, a micronodular or mixed type of cirrhosis may be seen in some types, for example types III and IV. Tumour nodules of varied size (representing either adenomas or carcinoma) may be visible macroscopically in glycogenosis type I.

The diagnosis of a specific type of glycogen storage disease requires biochemical determination of the enzyme defect. Although subtle differences have been described by McAdams et al.[139] the pathological features are distinctive in only a few of the glycogenoses, e.g. the light microscopic appearance of the liver in glycogenosis type IV, and the ultrastructural features of types II and IV.

In the majority of the glycogenoses, hepatocytes are two to several times the normal size and are rarefied, with wisps of pinkish material in an otherwise empty cytoplasm (Fig. 5.6). Cell membranes appear thickened due to peripheral displacement of organelles by the stored glycogen. The overall appearance of hepatocytes has been likened to that of plant cells. The presence of sharply defined vacuoles in the cytoplasm, particularly in glycogenosis type I and III, indicates the simultaneous accumulation of neutral lipid. Nuclei of liver cells are centrally placed, and those in the periportal zone may be glycogenated. The excess cytoplasmic glycogen is stained with periodic acid-Schiff (PAS), ideally in alcohol fixed specimens, and readily digested by diastase (Fig. 5.7), but pathologists should be aware that it is highly soluble and often removed in formalin-fixed and routinely processed tissue. The absence of G6P activity in glycogenosis type Ia, in contrast to its presence in type Ib,

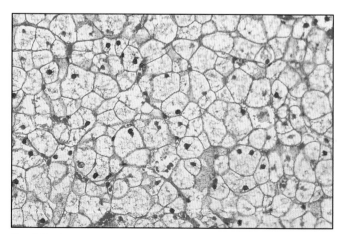

Fig. 5.6 • Glycogenosis type III. Liver cells are swollen and have pyknotic centrally or eccentrically-located nuclei. The cytoplasm is rarefied. H&E.

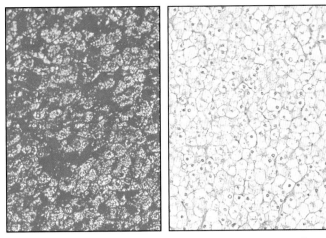

Fig. 5.7 • Glycogenosis type III. A large quantity of glycogen in liver cells (left) has been digested by diastase (right). PAS before and after diastase.

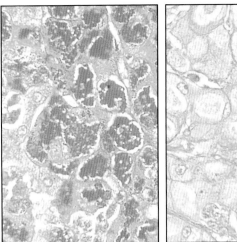

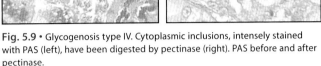

Fig. 5.9 • Glycogenosis type IV. Cytoplasmic inclusions, intensely stained with PAS (left), have been digested by pectinase (right). PAS before and after pectinase.

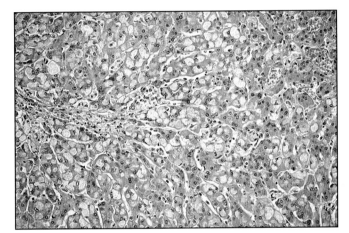

Fig. 5.8 • Glycogenosis type IV. Lightly eosinophilic (ground glassy) inclusions are present in many liver cells. H&E.

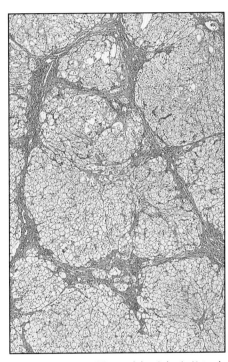

Fig. 5.10 • Glycogenosis type III. Micronodular cirrhosis. Note absence of inflammation and interface hepatitis. H&E.

has been demonstrated by histochemical staining.[195] Perivenular Mallory bodies and periportal fibrosis have been reported in glycogenosis type Ia.[196] Another unusual finding is the occurrence of localized peliosis hepatis in an adult patient with glycogenosis type I.[197]

The histopathology of the liver in glycogenosis type IV is markedly different from that of the other glycogenoses.[198–200] The changes closely resemble those of Lafora disease[201] but in Lafora disease progression to cirrhosis does not occur. Typically, hepatocytes in glycogenosis type IV are enlarged and contain colourless or lightly eosinophilic ground-glass inclusions that are round, oval or bean-shaped (Fig. 5.8). An artifactual space may surround the inclusions. They are most heavily concentrated in the periportal zone, but can be found in other zones.

Both the inclusions and the rest of the hepatocytic cytoplasm in type IV glycogenosis are stained deeply with periodic acid-Schiff (PAS) (Fig. 5.9); diastase treatment removes the normal glycogen but not the abnormal amylopectin-like material in the inclusions. The latter can, however, be digested by pectinase (Fig. 5.9) and α- or β-amylase.[198,201] The inclusions can be non-specifically stained with colloidal iron (green), Best's carmine (red) and Lugol's iodine

(mahogany brown).[201] Globular, PAS-positive inclusions with a Maltese cross birefringence have been reported in the liver, skeletal muscle and central nervous system in several congenital cases.[167]

Fibrosis, which can progress to cirrhosis, is a frequent finding in glycogenosis type IV, but can also occur in glycogenosis types III[155] and IXb, c[182,183] (Fig. 5.10). As already noted, patients with glycogenosis type I may develop hepatocellular adenoma or carcinoma. The hepatocellular adenomas are often multiple and arise in a non-cirrhotic parenchyma. Unusual histological features in the adenomas have been described in two cases.[202] They included marked steatosis, Mallory bodies, lamellar fibrosis and, in one case, amyloidosis.

The ultrastructural features of the glycogenoses are quite comparable, with the exception of types II and IV. In the cytoplasm of liver cells there are large pools of glycogen rosettes that displace organelles, such as mitochondria and the endoplasmic reticulum, to the periphery of the cell. The glycogen may be associated with vesicles of smooth endoplasmic reticulum or it may assume a starry-sky pattern, as observed in glycogenosis types III, VI and IX.[5] Morphometric analysis in glycogenosis type I has shown an increased volume of glycogen per unit volume of the hepatocytic cytoplasm.[203] Additionally, there is marked reduction (by 50%) of the rough endoplasmic reticulum per unit volume of liver tissue. Double-contoured vesicles in the endoplasmic reticulum are characteristic of glycogenosis type I.[203] Lipid droplets of varied size are seen in most of the glycogenoses, but appear to be more prominent in types I, II and VI.[5] Nuclear glycogenation is minimal or absent in glycogenosis type Ib in comparison to type Ia.[204] Increased collagen deposition in the space of Disse is observed in the glycogenoses types I, III, IV, VI and XI.[5]

Glycogenosis type II differs from the other types in the accumulation of monoparticulate glycogen in lysosomes that vary from 1 to 8 μm in diameter (Fig. 5.11).[205] Increased accumulation of glycogen rosettes may also be noted in the cytoplasm.[5] The ultrastructural features of glycogenosis type IV are pathognomonic.[5] The inclusions noted by light microscopy consist ultrastructurally of undulating, randomly-oriented, delicate fibrils that measure up to 5 nm in diameter; these accumulations are not membrane bound (Fig. 5.12).

Myoclonus epilepsy (Lafora disease)

Lafora disease is an autosomal recessive and fatal form of epilepsy with onset in late childhood or adolescence. One of the characteristic features of the disease is the presence of periodic acid-Schiff positive inclusion bodies which in the liver are morphologically and immunohistochemically similar to those of glycogenosis type IV. Two genes causing Lafora disease, *EPM2A* on chromosome 6q24 and *NHLRC1*

(*EPM2B*) on chromosome 6p22.3 have been identified.[206,207] The *EPM2A* gene product, laforin, is a protein tyrosine phosphatase with a carbohydrate-binding domain in the N-terminus. *NHLRC1* encodes a protein named malin, containing a zinc finger of the RING type in the N-terminal half and 6 NHL-repeat domains in the C-terminal direction. To date 43 different variations in *EPM2A* and 23 in *NHLRC1* are known.[208] Laforin through its phosphorylase activity and malin, possibly through binding to and inactivation of glycogen synthase seem to have an inhibitory activity to polyglucosan accumulation, their deficiency leading to an accumulation of insufficiently branched and hence insoluble glycogen molecules in the form of polyglucosan or Lafora bodies.[209]

The disease begins in adolescence with epileptic seizures (grand mal attacks being the most common) followed by myoclonus (beginning in the face and extremities, but progressively involving other muscles), and dementia. Atypical cases without myoclonus or epilepsy have been reported. Axillary skin biopsy is the simplest and least invasive diagnostic procedure, with characteristic inclusion bodies reliably found in duct cells of eccrine sweat glands. Most patients die between the ages of 16 and 24. A late onset and slowly progressive form, possibly related to a distinctive mutation has been reported.[210]

The histological hallmark of the disease is the presence of distinctive intraneuronal inclusions (Lafora bodies) which are most frequently found in the substantia nigra, globus pallidus, dentate nucleus, parts of the reticular system and cerebral cortex. In the central nervous system Lafora bodies vary in size from dot-like to as large as 35 μm. They stain positively with PAS, Best's carmine, Lugol's iodine (dark brown), colloidal iron and methenamine silver nitrate.[211–215] Three types have been described.[216] With the PAS stain, type I bodies (the most common) are granular and red, type II bodies have a densely stained peripheral zone, and type III bodies (the least common) are homogeneously bright red.[216] The bodies are digested by α-amylase,

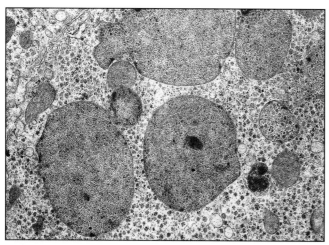

Fig. 5.11 • Glycogenosis type II. Electron micrograph reveals accumulation of monoparticulate glycogen in enlarged lysosomes. Note glycogen rosettes between the lysosomes. ×15 000.

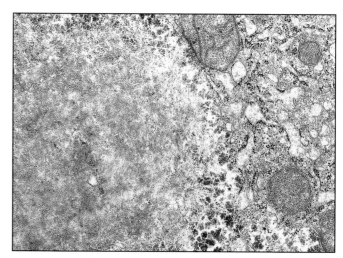

Fig. 5.12 • Glycogenosis type IV. Electron micrograph shows segment of inclusion (left) consisting of non-membrane-bound fibrillar material; some glycogen rosettes are present between the inclusion and the hepatocyte cytoplasm (right). ×21 130.

amyloglucosidase and pectinase. On the basis of histochemical and chemical studies, Yokoi et al.[215] have concluded that Lafora bodies are composed predominantly of an unusual branched polyglucosan. Ultrastructurally, they are not membrane-bound and are composed of varying proportions of fibrillar and granular material. The core is usually granular while the fibrils, which measure from 6 to 13 nm, radiate outwards and branch repeatedly.[199,211,213,216,217]

Extraneural deposits of abnormal material are frequently found when searched for. The histochemical and ultrastructural characteristics of these deposits in skeletal and smooth muscle, myocardium, liver and other organs resemble those of Lafora bodies in the brain, with minor differences. Hepatic involvement has been reported by a number of investigators.[218-223] In haematoxylin and eosin (H&E) preparations, liver cells contain round, oval or kidney-shaped inclusions that are sharply circumscribed, homogeneous or finely granular and lightly eosinophilic; they may be surrounded by a 'halo' that is probably artifactual[221] (Fig. 5.13). The nuclei of hepatocytes are frequently displaced to the periphery.

Affected cells in Lafora disease are predominantly periportal in location. They resemble those seen in type IV glycogenosis and show identical staining reactions, with the exception of the colloidal iron stain; the cytoplasm in Lafora disease is homogeneous (Fig. 5.14) while the stored material in type IV glycogenosis is coarse and clumped. Hepatocytes not harbouring Lafora bodies contain a large quantity of glycogen. According to Yokota et al.[223] antibodies prepared against Lafora bodies are immunoreactive to deposits of glycogenosis type IV. The inclusions also bear a resemblance to ground-glass hepatocytes of hepatitis B antigen carriers (but do not stain with the orcein, Victoria blue or aldehyde fuchsin stains), as well as to liver cells injured by cyanamide, a drug used in alcohol aversion therapy. Lafora body-like inclusions were also reported in patients who did not have myoclonus or epilepsy.[224] They have also been observed following chemotherapy, in particular in the liver of leukaemic children treated with 6-thioguanine.[225] Cirrhosis has not been reported in myoclonus epilepsy, but there may be slight periportal fibrosis.[221]

Galactosaemia

This autosomal recessive disorder caused by deficiency of galactose-1-phosphate uridyl transferase was first described by Von Ruess in 1908.[226] The deficient enzyme was identified by Isselbacher et al. in 1956.[227] The incidence is 1 : 45 000 births. Several allelic variants have been reported in the gene, located on chromosome 9q13, resulting in varying degree of residual enzyme activity.[228] Mis-sense mutations are associated with low to undetectable enzymatic producing the most profound symptoms. The 'Duarte' variant produces some active enzyme and patients with this allele have a better prognosis.[229] Compound heterozygotes (for example, a classic allele with a Duarte allele) can be affected, although again, less severely.[230] Much more rarely a defect in the epimerase enzyme produce the same neonatal symptoms.[231-233]

Common symptoms in early infancy are failure to thrive, vomiting and diarrhoea following galactose ingestion.[234] Newborns are predisposed to overwhelming sepsis, most commonly from *Escherichia coli*.[235] Haemolytic anaemia may occur early.[234] Increased intracranial pressure and cerebral oedema may be presenting features.[236] Other signs include lethargy, jaundice and cataracts, with severe cases manifesting oedema, ascites, and bleeding.[237,238] Long-term complications such as mental disability, speech defects, ataxia[239-241] and ovarian failure[242] may occur despite dietary restriction.

The diagnosis is classically suggested by the detection of urinary, non-glucose, reducing substances, which is neither sensitive nor specific, or by assaying galactose-1-phosphate uridyl transferase, or erythrocyte galactose 1-phosphate levels in Guthrie spots.[243,244] Testing for the main genomic mutation or measurement of parental-erythrocyte galactose-1-phosphate uridyl transferase may be confirmatory. Prenatal diagnosis is done by assaying chorionic villus biopsies or amniotic cells for the enzyme deficiency.[245]

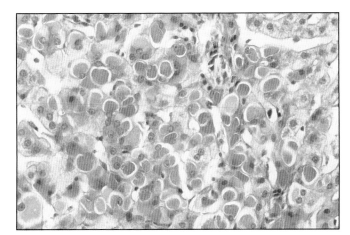

Fig. 5.13 • Lafora disease. More or less rounded pink inclusions in the cytoplasm of periportal hepatocytes; note artefactual 'halo' around the inclusions. H&E.

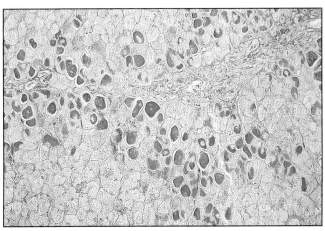

Fig. 5.14 • Lafora bodies are positively stained with colloidal iron. Note varied shapes and location in periportal hepatocytes. Rinehart–Abul Haj stain.

Complete dietary restriction of galactose is the only available therapy. The liver disease undergoes remarkable recovery[246] but neurodevelopmental complications are not necessarily avoided by dietary therapy. Dietary therapy is difficult, since fruits and vegetables contain significant amounts of soluble galactose.[247] In addition, there is an endogenous synthesis of galactose.[248] Long-term follow-up should be considered in peripheral epimerase deficiency. Dietary restriction is recommended during an affected pregnancy; but whether this will prevent or reduce neurological damage is unknown.

Of the pathological changes, those in the liver are the most distinctive, although they are not pathognomonic.[249,250] The earliest, which may appear within 10 or 11 days of birth, is marked steatosis and periportal ductular reaction; the cholangioles usually contain bile plugs and may be surrounded and infiltrated by neutrophils. Fibrosis can already be present at this early stage (Fig. 5.15(A), (B)). The next change, which begins as early as 2 weeks and is fully developed by 4–6 weeks, is a striking pseudoglandular (pseudoacinar) transformation of the hepatic plates. The hepatocytes surround dilated canaliculi that are either empty or contain bile or some pink or orange-coloured material. During this and the preceding phase, extramedullary haemopoiesis and haemosiderosis, which are common findings in the infant liver, may at times be prominent (Fig. 5.15(C)). Fibrosis, which is significant by the age of 6 weeks and culminating in cirrhosis at 3–6 months, spreads from portal areas. As this progresses, the portal areas become linked together and fibrous septa reach in to connect them to terminal hepatic venules. Hyperplasia of segments of lobular parenchyma carved out by the fibrous septa, leads to a micronodular cirrhosis. While it is doubtful that established cirrhosis is ever reversible, Appelbaum & Thaler[246] have documented the regression of extensive liver damage in an infant 5 months after the institution of a galactose-free diet. One patient who survived to the age of 52 years with established cirrhosis has been reported.[251] Occasional findings in the liver in galactosaemia include giant-cell transformation[247] and hepatocellular adenomas.[252] In today's terminology, the 'adenomas' described by Edmonds et al.[252] would be called macrogenerative nodules (or dysplastic nodules) since they occurred in a cirrhotic liver and measured 2.9, 1.5 and 1.0 cm in diameter.

The pathogenesis of both liver and neurological disease in this disorder remains controversial; a good review of the issues has been published by Segal.[243]

Hereditary fructose intolerance

Hereditary fructose intolerance is caused by deficiency of aldolase B resulting in an inability to convert fructose-1-phosphate into dihydroxyacetone and glyceraldehyde. This may result in acute liver failure or in cirrhosis. The disorder was first described by Hers & Joassin in 1961.[253] The presentation is quite variable, with liver disease appearing in infants upon introduction of fructose in the diet at the time of weaning. The predominant symptoms are poor feeding,

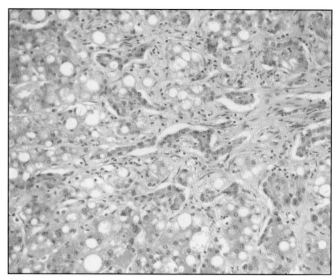

A

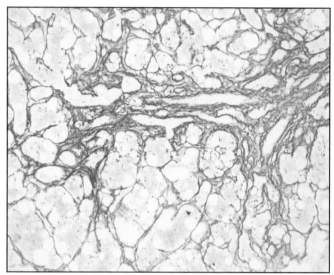

B

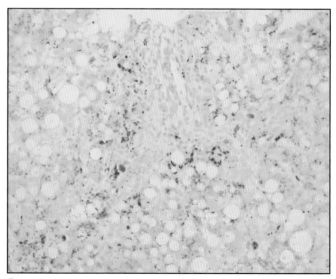

C

Fig. 5.15 • Galactosaemia. Steatosis, cholestasis and fibrous expansion of the portal tract are associated with mild ductular reaction and conspicuous periportal haemosiderosis in this liver biopsy specimen taken from a 3 week old baby. **(A)** H&E. **(B):** reticulin. **(C)** Perls method for iron.

vomiting and failure to thrive.[254,255] Other findings may include hepatomegaly, pallor, haemorrhage, trembling and jerkiness, shock, jaundice, oedema, tachypnoea, ascites, splenomegaly, fever and rickets. Patients who survive beyond infancy develop an aversion to sweet foods, and characteristically have caries-free teeth. Some present later with cirrhosis.

Laboratory tests may reveal fructosaemia and fructosuria after recent fructose administration, together with hypophosphataemia, metabolic acidosis and abnormal liver function tests. Uric acid levels may be elevated. A generalized amino aciduria with excretion of organic acids, as well as elevated serum levels of tyrosine and methionine, can simulate the findings in tyrosinaemia. None of these findings is diagnostic.[254]

Diagnosis is made unequivocally by mutational analysis of the *aldolase B* gene. The *aldolase B* gene is located on chromosome 9q22.[256] More than 30 mutations have been identified.[257,258] The A150P (65%), A175D (11%) and N335K (8%) were the most common mutated alleles in a recent series from Europe, where the disease occur in an estimated 1 in 26 000 births.[259] Analysis of liver or intestinal tissue for aldolase B enzyme activity can also confirm the diagnosis.[260]

Dietary treatment with restriction of fructose, sorbitol and sucrose may lead to full restoration of normal health, growth and development, provided liver and renal diseases are not advanced at the time of starting treatment.[255] Life-threatening acute liver failure may develop on the reintroduction of fructose, sucrose or sorbitol.

Pathological findings in hereditary fructose intolerance include neonatal hepatitis with giant-cell transformation,[261] steatosis,[255,262,263] fibrosis and cirrhosis.[255,262,264–266] Quantification of the amount of glycogen showed a high level in one case, but microscopic findings were not documented.[267] The resemblance of the lesions to those of galactosaemia has been noted.[262,268] As pointed out by Hardwick & Dimmick,[269] most descriptions of the histopathology of the liver in hereditary fructose intolerance refer to changes consistent with the early phases of cirrhosis rather than with an established cirrhosis. Hepatocellular carcinoma has been reported in a 49-year-old man suspected of having hereditary fructose intolerance.[270]

Ultrastructural changes in hepatic biopsy material were described by Phillips et al.[271] Concentric and irregularly disposed membranous arrays are present in the glycogen areas of most hepatocytes and are associated with marked rarefaction of the hyaloplasm (Fig. 5.16). Many of the membranous formations resemble cytolysosomes. It has been suggested that these changes are related to the intracellular accumulation of substrates. Similar ultrastructural changes have been reproduced in rats whose livers were infused with fructose via the portal vein.[271] Survival of injured cells is thought to be dependent on the sequestration of damaged areas (cytolysosome formation), as might occur with minimal or mild exposure to fructose. Larger quantities of fructose, particularly if repeated, may lead to more severe liver injury with necrosis and ultimately, to cirrhosis.

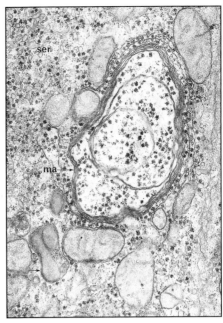

Fig. 5.16 • Hereditary fructose intolerance. Electron micrograph of liver from a patient prior to instituting a fructose-free diet. Note the prominence of the smooth endoplasmic reticulum (ser) and the formation of membranous arrays (ma). Glycogen particles are aligned between the layers of the smooth membranes, and the enclosed cytoplasm is rarefied and watery. A cytolysosome (arrow) is also illustrated. ×28 200. Courtesy of Dr M J Phillips.

Disorders of glycoprotein and glycolipid metabolism

The diseases in this section involve systemic disorders resulting from deficient activity of enzymes mediating the catabolism of glycosaminoglycans (mucopolysaccharidoses), or the synthesis or degradation of glycoproteins and glycolipids (mannosidosis, fucosidosis, aspartylglycosaminuria, mucolipidoses, and the carbohydrate deficient glycoprotein syndrome).

Mucopolysaccharidoses

In the mucopolysaccharidoses (MPS), excessive amounts of mucopolysaccharides accumulate in somatic and visceral tissues, and their partial degradation products are excreted in the urine; in addition, there may be accumulation of gangliosides. These disorders are all extremely rare. The mucopolysaccharidoses are distinguished by clinical manifestations and by two-dimensional electrophoresis and specific enzyme assay. Enzyme analysis is performed in white blood cells and fibroblasts. The selective measurement of glycosaminoglycan-derived oligosaccharides in urine provides a sensitive method for the early identification of individuals with MPS and allows the determination of oligosaccharide profiles which not only characterize subtype but also can be used for the biochemical monitoring of therapies.[272] Except for type II, which is X-linked, all MPS are inherited as autosomal recessive traits. The six mucopolysaccharidoses (Hurler syndrome, Hunter syndrome,

Sanfilippo syndrome, Morquio syndrome, Maroteaux-Lamy syndrome and type VII β-glucuronidase deficiency), which are associated with variable degree of enlargement of the liver and spleen, are discussed in this chapter.

Mucopolysaccharidoses type I (MPS I); Hurler (H); Scheie (S); Hurler–Scheie (H/S)

MPS type I (MPS I), due to deficiency of the degradative lysosomal enzyme α-L-iduronidase, results in a wide range of clinical symptoms from mild somatic complications and a normal lifespan to severe central nervous system involvement and a significantly shortened lifespan. The leucocytes of obligate heterozygotes have about half the mean specific enzyme activity of normal controls.[273] The gene is located on chromosome 4q16;[274] multiple mutations have been characterized, with disease severity linked to the specific mutation.[275,276] Scheie and Hurler–Scheie are subtypes associated with less severe clinical disease.[277] Patients with the most severe phenotype (Hurler subtype) manifest developmental delay by 12–14 months of age. Features include corneal clouding, dysostosis multiplex, organomegaly, macroglossia, a prominent forehead and stiff joints. Death occurs by 10 years of age, usually from obstructive airway disease, respiratory infections or cardiac complications. Prenatal diagnosis by amniocentesis is now routine, and in utero therapy has been attempted. Bone marrow transplantation is very effective if performed before significant loss of cognitive function, usually at under 2 years of age.[278-283] Cord blood[284] or haemopoietic stem cells transplant[285] can achieve a favourable outcome in Hurler syndrome, with improved cognitive function, but with a limited effect on corneas and skeleton.[286] Enzyme replacement with intravenous laronidase therapy is well tolerated and effective for patients who do not have neuronal pathology.[287,288]

Mucopolysaccharidoses type II (MPS II); Hunter syndrome

MPS type II (MPS II) is caused by a deficiency of α-L-iduronidate sulphatase and is the only X-linked MPS. The gene has been localized to Xq27.3-28. Affected children have coarse facies, deafness, cognitive deterioration, growth failure, joint contractures, severe hepatosplenomegaly and chronic diarrhoea; death usually occurs before age 15 years. A milder form of this disease exists with complications that include hearing impairment, and papilloedema resulting from local infiltration in the eye. Death is usually from airway obstruction or cardiac failure. Bone marrow transplantation does not prevent the severe cognitive deterioration and is not currently recommended.[283,289]

Mucopolysaccharidoses type III (MPS III); Sanfilippo disease

This comprises four phenotypically identical subtypes with different enzyme defects. All forms are characterized by coarse features, hepatomegaly, variable splenomegaly and mental retardation, but there is no corneal clouding. Type A results from deficiency of heparan-N-sulphatase; type B from deficiency of N-acetyl α-D-glucosidase; type C from deficiency of acetyl CoA: α-glucosaminide acetyltransferase; type D from deficiency of N-acetylglucosamine 6-sulphatase.[290] The gene for type A has been cloned and several mutations associated with Sanfilippo disease have been described.[291] A locus for type C has been mapped to the pericentromeric region of chromosome 8.[292] The gene for type D has been cloned and localized to chromosome 16q24. Prenatal diagnosis is available.[293,294] There is no known therapy.

Mucopolysaccharidoses type IV (MPS IV); Morquio syndrome

MPS type IV (MPS IV) is due to deficiency in N-acetyl-glucosamine 6-sulphate sulphatase (type A) or β-galactosidase (type B), both type being phenotypically similar with severe skeletal deformities and growth retardation, cervical myelopathy, mild corneal clouding, hepatomegaly, but no mental retardation. A late onset characterizes type B.[295]

Mucopolysaccharidoses type VI (MPS VI); Maroteaux-Lamy syndrome

Deficiency of N-acetylgalactosamine 4-sulphatase (arylsulphatase B) is the cause of MPS type VI (MPS VI) which has three clinical subtypes (infantile, intermediate and adult) which vary in severity. The infantile form is characterized by growth retardation, dysostosis multiplex, coarse facial features, restricted movement, hepatosplenomegaly and corneal clouding. Death in the second and third decades is the result of cardiac failure. Intellect is not compromised in any form of the disease. The gene has been localized to chromosome 5q13-14; several mutations in the *arylsulphatase* gene have been found but clear mutational-phenotype correlations are not yet possible.[290,296] Sensitive immune assays to detect 4-sulfatase activity may allow an early detection of MPS VI on blood-spots.[297] Bone marrow transplantation has been helpful in this disorder.[298] Recent studies have concentrated on recombinant enzyme therapy[299] which is well-tolerated, reduce lysosomal storage as evidenced by reduction in urinary glycosaminoglycan, with clinical responses in all patients, the largest gains occurring in patients with advanced disease receiving high-dose recombinant enzyme.[300]

Mucopolysaccharidosis type VII (MPS VII); Sly syndrome

MPS type VII (MPS VII) is due to a deficiency of β-glucuronidase. This rare disorder is characterized by dysostosis multiplex, hepatosplenomegaly, mental retardation, and frequent pulmonary infections. It is one of the storage disorders that can present with hydrops fetalis. One patient had isolated neonatal ascites as first manifestation.[301] The gene has been localized to chromosome 7q21.1-22; it appears that more than one mutation can result in MSP VII[290] Prenatal diagnosis is possible using amniotic fluid.[302] In one case, bone marrow transplantation resulted in improved motor function and fewer infections.[303]

Pathological changes in the mucopolysacharidoses

Macroscopically, the liver in the MPS is enlarged, firm or hard and has a pale, slightly yellowish or greyish colour.[304] There may be extensive fibrosis or cirrhosis. Microscopically, both hepatocytes and Kupffer cells are swollen and have an empty or faintly vacuolated cytoplasm (Fig. 5.17) Since much of the stored acid mucopolysaccharide is leached out by aqueous fixatives, other methods of fixation, such as Lindsay's dioxane picrate solution,[305] are preferable. Alternatively, addition of a 10% solution of acetyl trimethylammonium bromide to the formalin fixative is said to preserve acid mucopolysaccharide in the cells.[306] The stored acid mucopolysaccharide is best demonstrated by a colloidal iron stain, and most of it can be digested with hyaluronidase (Fig. 5.18). It is weakly positive with the PAS stain but cannot be digested by diastase. Acid mucopolysaccharide is metachromatic when stained with toluidine blue. Little or no neutral lipid can be demonstrated in frozen sections of the liver stained with the sudanophilic dyes.

When fibrosis is present in the MPS it is diffuse, with heavy deposition of collagen bundles in the space of Disse and gradual microdissection of the parenchyma into nodules (Fig. 5.19). Periportal bridging fibrosis has been emphasized by Parfrey & Hutchins.[307] The type of cirrhosis associated with the MPS may be macronodular or micronodular.[308] When it supervenes, it generally does so in older children and adults.[308–310]

Ultrastructural studies of the liver in MPS I, MPS II and MPS III have demonstrated the presence of vacuoles of varied size in both hepatocytes and Kupffer cells; these are bounded by a single membrane and contain some electron-dense, poorly structured material.[5,304,311,312] It is now generally accepted that the clear vacuoles represent lysosomes filled with acid mucopolysaccharide. It has been suggested that cytoplasmic vacuoles may form by mitochondrial 'budding' in the hepatocytes of patients with MPS I and MPS III.[313] A peculiar crystalloid structure has been described in mitochondria of hepatocytes in MPS III.[314] In MPS IV, Kupffer cells but not hepatocytes contain clear vacuoles.[315] The ultrastructural changes in MPS V are similar to those of MPS I and MPS II.[316] In MPS VI there is moderate storage of electron-lucent material in lysosomes of hepatocytes, but Kupffer cells and hepatic fibroblasts contain as much acid mucopolysaccharide as in MPS I.[315]

Non-cirrhotic portal hypertension and nodular regenerative hyperplasia of the liver have been reported in dogs with MPS-1.[317] The nodular regenerative hyperplasia is associated with a venopathy of small portal veins but the pathogenesis of these lesions is undetermined.

Aspartylglucosaminuria

The deficient enzyme, aspartylglucosaminidase, is normally present in the liver and brain as well as other tissues. Several different mutations in the gene, located on chromosome 4q32-33.2, can result in clinical disease.[318–321] Peripheral blood and bone marrow examinations show vacuolated

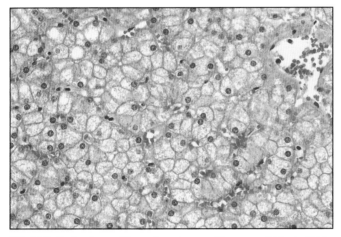

Fig. 5.17 • Hurler disease. Liver cells are large and have a rarefied cytoplasm. H&E.

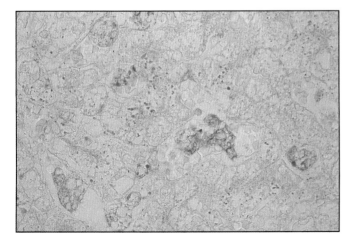

Fig. 5.18 • Hurler disease. Greenish-blue, punctate mucopolysaccharide is present in the cytoplasm of hepatocytes and Kupffer cells. Rinehart–Abul Haj stain.

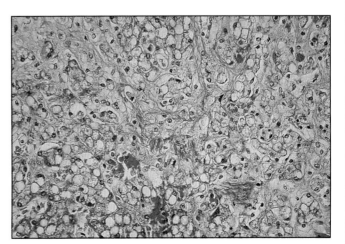

Fig. 5.19 • Hurler disease. Perisinusoidal fibrosis in the hepatic parenchyma. Note also the swollen vacuolated appearance of the hepatocytes. Masson trichrome.

lymphocytes that do not stain with Best's carmine or PAS. The urine contains large quantities of 2-acetamide-1 (B-L-aspartamide 1)-1,2-dideoxy B-D-glucose.[322]

The diagnosis should be considered in children who present with a mucopolysaccharide-like disorder but with negative urinary screens.[323] Clinical signs include coarse facial features, (which increase with age), a protuberant abdomen with an umbilical defect, hepatosplenomegaly (which regresses with age), and the heart murmur of mitral insufficiency. Other features may include acne, macroglossia causing tooth malocclusion, hoarseness and short stature. Oral complications include dental cavities, gingivitis, candidiasis, extensive gingival overgrowth, benign odontogenic tumours or tumour-like lesions and reduced maxillary sinuses.[324]

Appearing normal at birth, patients have accelerated growth through early puberty but end up short in stature. Mental development may be normal except for delayed speech until 5 years of age. Deterioration is noted between 6 and 15 years of age with development of clumsiness and hyperkinesia. Rapid mental and somatic deterioration occurs in adulthood; adults usually have an IQ under 40 along with uncontrollable behaviour and seizures.[325] Patients seldom reach the age of 45 years. The neurological abnormalities are related to significant changes in the grey matter; the white matter is characterized by delayed myelination.[326]

The incidence of this disorder is highest in Finland[327] where the frequency of carriers is $1/36$[328] and DNA testing is available.[319] Prenatal diagnosis is achieved by enzyme assay in amniotic cells.

Bone marrow transplantation may be beneficial; no loss of capabilities and an improvement in biochemical markers and MRI white-matter signals were observed in 2 siblings followed up for five years after bone marrow transplantation.[329]

Histopathologically, liver cells contain large and small vacuoles that stain variably with PAS;[323] Kupffer-cell vacuoles do not react with PAS. There is no increase in fibrous tissue. Ultrastructurally, enlarged lysosomes are present in hepatocytes and Kupffer cells.[330,331] The fine matrix background is similar to that of the mucopolysaccharidoses. Membranous structures are found in these large lysosomes as well as electron-lucent lipid droplets. Round, electron-dense structures and, less frequently, single membranous structures of varied sizes are also present.

α-Mannosidosis

This rare autosomal recessive disease is due to deficiency in acidic α-mannosidase A and B in various tissues and in leucocytes, which leads to the tissue accumulation and abnormally high urinary excretion of mannose-rich oligosaccharides. Diagnosis is established by analysing urinary oligosaccharides by thin layer chromatography to demonstrate increased mannose enrichment, or by assaying α-mannosidase activity level in leukocytes. Prenatal diagnosis is made by measurement of α-mannosidase in chorionic villi or trophoblast biopsy.[332] The gene for acidic α-man-

nosidase has been localized to chromosome 19p13.2-q12[327] and several mutations have been identified.[333]

Patients present with psychomotor retardation. They have a distinctive coarse facies, corneal and lenticular opacities, hearing loss, hepatosplenomegaly (usually early in the course of the disease) and symptoms and signs of recurrent infection.[334] Dysostosis multiplex is demonstrated by skeletal radiology in the majority of patients. Vacuolated lymphocytes are seen in the peripheral blood. About half the patients have decreased levels of serum IgG. The susceptibility to infection may be a direct consequence of impaired leukocyte membrane recognition processes, which result from defective catabolism of substrates with α-D-mannose residues.[334] The disorder may contribute to the onset of systemic lupus erythematosus in predisposed patients.[335]

Two types are recognized. Type I is the more severe infantile type with death between 3 and 10 years of age, while type II is a milder disease with a juvenile or adult onset. There is no known treatment but, despite recurrent infections, some patients may survive into adulthood.[336] Allogeneic hematopoietic stem cell or T-cell-depleted peripheral blood stem cell transplantation may halt the progressive cognitive loss and reverse the pattern of urinary oligosaccharides.[337,338]

Hepatocytes in mannosidosis contain PAS-negative vacuoles in the cytoplasm. Ultrastructurally, the vacuoles are bounded by a single membrane and contain amorphous and occasionally membranous and/or filamentous material.[332,339] Vacuoles may also be present in sinusoidal lining cells.[339] Light microscopic changes, which are non-specific, include vacuolization of liver cells, steatosis and perisinusoidal fibrosis.[339]

Fucosidosis

Fucosidosis is caused by a profound deficiency of tissue α₁-fucosidases resulting in storage of fucose-containing glycolipids, glycoproteins and polysaccharides or oligosaccharides. There seems to be no biochemical difference in α₁-fucosidase between the phenotypically different, type I and II disease.[340] The gene has been localized to chromosome 1q34. The disease results from several different mutations in one subunit of the α-fucosidase gene.[341]

Type I is rapidly progressive and fatal between 4 and 6 years of age. Type II pursues a much slower course with survival into adolescence and beyond. Common to both variants are psychomotor retardation, neurological deficits and skeletal abnormalities, Hurler-syndrome-like features, hepatosplenomegaly, thickness of the skin, tendency to hernias and cardiomegaly. Almost all patients experience repeated bouts of respiratory infection.[342,343] The patients with the slower evolution are characterized by angiokeratoma corporis diffusum.[344] Diagnosis is made by thin-layer chromatography of urine. Prenatal diagnosis has been made both by DNA analysis and by enzyme analysis, but requires an experienced laboratory.[341] Bone marrow transplantation in one patient has been followed by progressive rise of enzymatic levels and some improvement in psychomotor development.[345]

The gross and light microscopic changes are similar to those of Hurler disease.[327,341] Both hepatocytes and Kupffer cells are vacuolated. Ultrastructurally, hepatocytes show membrane-bound vacuoles representing lysosomes that contain granular or reticulogranular material suggesting polysaccharide, as well as lamellar bodies which indicate the accumulation of complex lipids.[304,346] Kupffer cells contain similar material but the vacuoles are smaller and are poor in lipid content. Bile-duct cells are markedly vacuolated by light microscopy and contain numerous clear vacuoles by electron microscopy.[346]

Mucolipidoses

This is a group of diseases with features overlapping those of the mucopolysaccharidoses and sphingolipidoses. They are lysosomal storage diseases with evidence of multiple primary defects of mucopolysaccharide, lipid and glycoprotein metabolism in various combinations.[327,347-349]

Mucolipidosis I (sialidosis)

This rare syndrome is due to a deficiency in lysosomal sialidase (neuraminidase) resulting in defective intralysosomal catabolism of sialylated glycoconjugates and sialic acid transport out of the lysosomes. Mutations in the sialidase gene *NEU1*, located on chromosome 6p21.3, result in the progressive lysosomal storage of sialylated glycopeptides and oligosaccharides.[350] Two major forms are recognized. Sialidosis type I (Salla disease) is a milder, late-onset, non-dysmorphic form of the disorder; patients develop visual defects, myoclonus syndrome, cherry-red macular spots, ataxia, hyperreflexia, and seizures. Type II, the severe infantile form, is characterized by gargoyle-like facial dysmorphism and dysostosis is apparent by 4 or 5 years of age. Peripheral neuropathy develops, with muscular weakness and difficulties in co-ordination. Findings include corneal opacities, and impaired hearing, and hepatosplenomegaly. Vacuolated lymphocytes are found in all cases. An increased amount of bound sialic acid is excreted in the urine, a finding that can be used as a simple screening test.[348,351] Definitive diagnosis is established by demonstration of a deficiency of sialidase in peripheral leucocytes or cultured fibroblasts of both type I and type II patients. Some patients with similar features appear deficient in both sialidase and β-galactosidase, a disease termed galactosialidosis (gene map locus 20q13).[352] Sialidase can also be measured in cells from amniotic fluid, but special fresh preparations are necessary.[353] A mouse model of sialidosis is currently used to evaluate enzyme replacement therapy.[354]

Light microscopy of the liver reveals marked enlargement of portal macrophages and Kupffer cells, both of which have a foamy cytoplasm.[5,349,355] Ultrastructurally, hepatocytes contain membrane-bound vacuoles that are electron-lucent. The vacuoles frequently contain numerous osmiophilic droplets as well as a reticulogranular or flocculent material. Riches & Smuckler[355] also described multilamellar bodies and fragments of membrane-like material in the vacuoles. Similar vacuoles are found in Kupffer cells, and to a lesser extent in endothelial cells, stellate cells and biliary epithelial cells.[5]

Mucolipidosis II (I-cell disease) and mucolipidosis III (pseudo-Hurler polydystrophy)

Mucolipidosis II and III (MLII and MLIII) are biochemically related diseases with different clinical manifestations. These disorders of lysosomal enzyme targeting are due to a defective N-acetylglucosamine 1-phosphotransferase (termed phosphotransferase) activity in Golgi compartments of the cells and leads to the impaired formation of mannose 6-phosphate recognition markers in soluble lysosomal enzymes followed by their defective transport to lysosomes and increased excretion into the serum.[356-358] The diseases are autosomal recessive and linked to chromosome 4q21-23.[359]

MLII presents in the first year of life, with severe psychomotor retardation, early growth retardation, facial dysmorphism with characteristic gingival hyperplasia, equivocal or absent corneal clouding, hepatomegaly, skeletal dysplasia and severe dysostosis multiplex[360-362] which may resemble Pacman dysplasia.[363] MLIII has similar symptoms, but they are milder and present later in life. Patients may survive into adulthood with the milder form of the disease.

Fibroblasts cultured from patients with MLII contain numerous dense inclusions (hence the term 'I-cell') which are best seen on phase contrast microscopy.[315] Vacuolated lymphocytes of B-cell lineage in lymph nodes, spleen and kidney have been found to contain large amounts of hexosamine.[364] Cytoplasmic vacuoles were also noted in Kupffer cells, fibroblasts in the myocardium, renal podocytes and in acinar cells of the pancreas. The vacuolated cells stain positively with Hale's colloidal iron method.

Diagnosis is made by measurement of the activity of the phosphotransferase in fibroblasts, or by demonstration of elevated levels of serum lysosomal enzymes (as a result of hypersecretion rather than targeting into the lysosomes). Prenatal diagnosis is possible by measurement of lysosomal enzymes or phosphotransferase activity on cultured amnion cells. There is no definitive treatment, although bone marrow transplantation in one MLII patient has been followed by neurodevelopmental gains and prevention of cardiopulmonary complications.[365]

Light microscopy may show no changes in hepatocytes but there is enlargement of Kupffer cells and portal macrophages that have a foamy cytoplasm, and granulomas composed of finely vacuolated epithelioid cells may be seen in portal areas.[366] The vacuoles are limited by single membranes and contain either fibrillo-granular material, membranous lamellae or lipid globules.[366] Hepatocytes are generally only slightly affected but may contain different types of dense polymorphic inclusions.[315,361,367] Vacuoles in hepatocytes correspond to triglyceride droplets and membranous inclusions, as well as enlarged lysosomes containing granular material by electron microscopy. Kupffer cells contain electron-dense membranous lamellae.

Vacuolated cells (leucocytes and, in MLIII, bone marrow cells), similar to those of mucolipidosis I, are present.

Cultured fibroblasts show inclusions resembling those of the I-cells of MLII. Ultrastructural findings in the liver include slightly enlarged secondary lysosomes without storage of any abnormal material, while Kupffer cells are relatively rich in unstructured osmiophilic material.[315]

Mucolipidosis IV (sialolipidosis)

This rare disease is postulated to be due to a defect in intracellular packaging or transport of lysosomal enzymes.[368] Chromosome assignment is to 19p13.3-13.2.[369,370]

The disease, which is most common among Ashkenazi Jews, is characterized by an early onset of corneal opacification and psychomotor retardation; a small head circumference is frequent. Gargoyle-like facies, skeletal deformities and organomegaly are absent.[371,372] Diagnosis is made by demonstration of characteristic inclusions in epithelial cells and conjunctival biopsies. Biochemically, the disease is characterized by the accumulation of gangliosides, phospholipids and acidic mucopolysaccharides in skin fibroblasts.[373] The heterogeneity of the store material accounts for cell vacuoles being variably stain with periodic acid Schiff, Soudan black and/or Luxol fast blue.[368] Prenatal diagnosis of mucolipidosis IV is performed using transmission electron microscopy to demonstrate lamellar bodies in endothelial cells of chorionic villi.[374,375]

Ultrastructural studies of conjunctival biopsies from four patients have shown two types of abnormal inclusion bodies, both in stromal fibroblasts and in epithelial cells: (i) single membrane-limited cytoplasmic vacuoles containing both fibrillo-granular material and membranous lamellae; and (ii) lamellar and concentric bodies similar to those found in Tay–Sachs disease.[372] In liver biopsy material, Berman et al.[376] have shown that hepatocytes contain inclusions composed predominantly of concentric lamellae, whereas vacuoles in Kupffer cells have clear contents. The prenatal diagnosis of mucolipidosis IV was reported by Kohn et al.[374] A partial ganglioside sialidase deficiency has been found in cultured fibroblasts, but it is doubtful that that is the primary enzyme defect.[377]

Congenital disorders of glycosylation

The congenital disorders of glycosylation (CDG) were previously referred to as the carbohydrate-deficient glycoprotein syndrome (CDGS). They result from a heterogeneous group of metabolic defects in the synthesis of N-linked glycosylation residues; six types have been described to date.[378] In the common form of this disease (CDG Type Ia), patients present with neurodevelopmental delay, hypotonia, diarrhoea leading to poor weight gain, and dysmorphism (esotropia, inverted nipples, and a peculiar distribution of fat). Cerebellar hypoplasia is seen on computed axial tomography. Patients have deficiencies in many serum proteins and elevated hepatocellular enzymes. The illness may progress to death in infancy, usually from infections, stroke and/or inanition.[379]

If patients survive early childhood without diagnosis, many of the characteristic dysmorphisms become less apparent and it becomes more difficult to recognize older patients with this disease. Older patients are characterized by non-progressive neuro-developmental delay, with or without seizures, a stooped posture and a high risk of thrombosis. Ataxia is present in most patients. Some patients have progressive retinitis pigmentosa.[380] Puberty is delayed in females, but not in males.[381] Impaired linear growth is common.[382]

The characteristic serological findings are the result of deficiencies in a wide spectrum of serum proteins, all of which are normally glycosylated. Glycosylation residues on secretory proteins perform several essential functions: they assist in achieving proper three-dimensional conformation, facilitate secretion of mature protein, protect the polypeptide from degradation, and serve as recognition sites for some receptors.[383,384] In all forms of CDG, the failure of normal glycosylation leads to deficiencies in the glycoproteins essential for coagulation and inhibition of coagulation (including factor XI, antithrombin III, proteins C and S, and heparin cofactor II).[385–387] These defects contribute to the significant potential for strokes and transient stroke-like episodes. Defective synthesis of hormonal binding proteins or receptors cause the abnormal endocrine findings.[379,388,389]

There is no specific screening test for CDG. The disease should be suspected in a patient with the characteristic clinical findings and/or an unexplained deficiency of more than one glycosylated serum protein, particularly albumin, transferrin, antithrombin III and α_1-antitrypsin. Studies for several different diseases which depend on the absence of a glycosylated protein may be abnormal, suggesting several different unrelated diseases.

Diagnosis is made by isoelectric focusing of serum transferrin, with quantitation of the glycosylation variants. The absence of sialic acid residues in transferrin from patients with CDG results in a more cathodal migration of serum transferrin. The test is simple, easily available, and relatively inexpensive. Patterns of transferrin isoelectric focusing are used to determine the type of CDG, in combination with the clinical presentation.[390,391] False positives in the transferrin assay are not common: hypoglycosylation of serum proteins can occur in chronic alcoholism, in classic galactosaemia or in hereditary fructose intolerance. In these cases, treatment of the primary disease and clearance of the abnormal metabolic byproducts results in resolution of the glycosylation abnormalities.[392–395] All patients with positive transferrin assays should have galactose-1-phosphate uridyl transferase testing, and also diagnostic testing for hereditary fructose intolerance.

In a patient with abnormal glycosylation of transferrin, the exact enzyme defect must be determined, if possible. The syndrome is typed by a combination of the clinical presentation and the pattern of glycosylation present in isoelectric focused transferrin. Type Ia, the most common form, presents as described previously. Most, but not all patients with the type Ia phenotype have a deficiency in the enzyme phosphomannomutase.[380,396,397] Type Ib has the same pattern of isoelectric focusing as Ia, but patients present with cyclic vomiting, failure to thrive, protein-losing enteropathy and congenital hepatic fibrosis, without the neuro-developmental delays and dysmorphic features of type Ia. This defect is the result of a deficiency in phosphomannose isomerase.[398–400] Patients with abnormal isoelectric focusing patterns of transferrin in whom both the defined types of CDG and known secondary disturbances of glycosylation have been ruled out are classified as CDG Ix.[401,402]

The remaining four types are each known only from case reports. Type II CDG presents with coarse facies, widely spaced nipples, and severe neuro-developmental delay. The deficient enzyme is N-acetylglucosaminyl transferase II. Serum liver enzyme values are normal.[403–406] Types III, IV and V, and several case reports of non-classical CDG have been described. Most have abnormalities of serum glycosylation, but few have significant liver disease.[380,407]

The incidence of the disease has been difficult to determine; estimates have ranged from 1 : 50 000 to 80 000 live births,[408,409] although they may be low.[410] Cases of CDG have been described world-wide. Gene localization for the CDG varies according to types. Phosphomannomutase (type Ia, PMM2 gene) has been localized to chromosome 16p13,[410,411] phosphomannose isomerase (type Ib) to 15q22-qter and N-acetyl glucosaminyltransferase II (type II) to chromosome 14q21.[380,405] Further gene loci are expected as identification of mutant genes continues.

There is no reliable method for prenatal diagnosis in CDG; a combination of enzymology and genetic linkage analysis may allow prenatal diagnosis.[412–414] Therapy in CDG is symptomatic. Oral mannose supplementation has been successful in treating several cases of CDG Ib.[400,415]

Histopathological features in the liver in CDG appear to be non-specific. Conradi et al.[416] studied liver biopsies from seven children and found slight to moderate fibrosis and steatosis. In the case report by Jaeken et al.[399] a biopsy at the age of 5.5 months showed microvesicular steatosis and periportal fibrosis. A second biopsy at the age of 1 year revealed more pronounced fibrosis and ductular reaction, a picture resembling congenital hepatic fibrosis. Postmortem findings in two twins with the deficiency included diffuse steatosis (particularly in periportal areas) and fibrosis in one, and cirrhosis in the other.[417] Ultrastructural findings in the cases of Conradi et al.[416] included lysosomal vacuoles with concentric electron-dense membranes, and variable electron-lucent and electron-dense material in liver cells.

Endoplasmic reticulum storage diseases

The term endoplasmic reticulum storage disease was first used by Callea et al.[418] for a group of inborn errors of metabolism to convey the message that the site of protein retention is one common denominator. The disorders affect secretory proteins, some of them, in particular α-antitrypsin, α-antichymotrypsin and C1 inhibitor,[419] belonging to the serine proteinase inhibitors (serpins), a superfamily of proteins whose encoding gene cluster on chromosome 14q 31.2.[420,421] The storage results from a molecular abnormality leading to misfolding that prevents the transfer of the protein from the rough to the smooth endoplasmic reticulum, with consequent accumulation in hepatocyte endoplasmic reticulum and low levels of the corresponding protein in the plasma.

α₁-Antitrypsin deficiency

The association of panlobular emphysema with α₁-antitrypsin (α₁-AT) deficiency was recognized by Laurell and Eriksson in 1963.[422] Subsequently, Sharp et al.[423] reported cirrhosis in 10 children from six different kindreds with α₁-AT deficiency. Liver disease was subsequently shown to be most commonly associated with the α₁-AT variant Z or protease inhibitor (Pi) Z, and cholestasis during infancy was soon recognized as the most common presentation.[424–426]

The diagnosis of α₁-AT deficiency should be sought in all patients with undefined liver disease by measuring the serum level of α₁-AT. In homozygotes low levels of serum α₁-AT (normal (>1.0 g/L) suggests the diagnosis, but serum levels of α₁-AT, which is an acute-phase reactant, may increase secondary to hepatic inflammation and may lead to normal values in heterozygotes. The diagnosis is confirmed by protease inhibitor (Pi) typing of the patient, and of the parents if they are available. Pi typing is based on amino acid variations which produce differently charged proteins that can be detected by isoelectric focusing in polyacrylamide gels. ELISA procedure may be used, and recently allele specific PCR technique has been proposed to detect the Z and S variants.[427] At least 90 allelic variants of α₁-AT have been described by isoelectric focusing or DNA sequencing.[428] The most common deficiency alleles are PiZ and PiS. Hepatic pathology is predominantly seen in individuals carrying the Z allele, of whom only a relatively small proportion ever develops liver disease.

The PiZ allele is found in approximately 1–2% of Caucasians of northern European ancestry, being highest in Scandinavian populations; it is virtually absent in black and Oriental populations, but a review of epidemiologic surveys shows that it can affect individuals in all racial subgroups worldwide.[429] In the West, α₁-AT deficiency is estimated to affect about one in 2000–5000 individuals.[430] The α₁-AT gene is located on chromosome 14q31-32.3.[431] The phenotypic expression of α₁-AT involves the protein production of both alleles, i.e., it is co-dominant. Most allelic variants are the result of an amino acid substitution in the polypeptide chain. In the Z allele the substitution of Lys342 for Glu342 directly affects secretion of α₁-AT which then accumulates in the endoplasmic reticulum.[432] The secretory defect, the mechanism of aggregation of α₁-AT, and the pathogenetic hypotheses underlying the hepatic injury in the homozygote and heterozygote were reviewed by Eriksson[428] and Perlmutter.[433] The marked variation in phenotypical expression of the liver disease is believed to be determined by genetic modifiers and/or environmental factors that influence the intracellular disposal of the mutant glyco-protein or the signal transduction pathways that are activated.[434]

α_1-AT is a plasma glycoprotein of approximately 52 kD which is synthesized mainly by hepatocytes,[435] although several other tissues produce small amounts. α_1-AT is a competitive inhibitor of leucocyte elastase with reaction kinetics favouring elastase complexing with α_1-AT rather than with its substrate elastin.[435–437] The major factors controlling serum levels of α_1-AT are inflammatory stimuli, although oestrogenic and androgenic hormones and some liver diseases alter serum levels.[423,436,437]

Clinically, neonates who develop liver disease present with conjugated hyperbilirubinaemia. Severe cholestasis may be associated with acholic stools and has to be differentiated from extrahepatic biliary atresia. Cholestasis usually resolves by 6 months of age without therapy[438] but a certain proportion of infants develop chronic liver disease. Up to 10% may have paucity of the intrahepatic bile ducts with prolongation of cholestasis and the development of pruritus.

In prospective studies on the incidence of liver disease in PiZ individuals, Sveger[439] followed 127 homozygous PiZ children and 54 PiSZ children into adolescence by physical examinations and routine liver function tests. Initially, symptomatic liver disease was found in 11% of infants. Follow-up revealed the development of chronic liver disease leading to death in only 2.5% of PiZ individuals by age 12.[426,439] Despite the absence of clinical liver disease, 75% of all PiZ infants had an elevated serum alanine transferase (ALT). By the age of 12 years, only 33% of the infants who presented with liver disease had ALT elevation, while 14% of patients, who had had no clinical liver disease in infancy, had an elevated ALT. Thus, evidence of hepatocyte injury decreased as the children approached the teenage years. PiSZ children with serum α_1-AT levels that were 40% of normal did not have abnormal ALT levels.[440]

In a survey of α_1-AT liver disease in children from the UK outcome fell into four categories. Approximately 25% of the infants gradually improve and appear normal at ages ranging from 3–10 years, 25% have persistently abnormal serum aminostransferase, 25% die of cirrhosis or require transplantation at ages ranging from 6 months to 17 years, in the remaining 25% jaundice resolved but raised aminotransferase with enlarged liver and spleen persist.[441] A retrospective study of 85 children with neonatal hepatitis and α_1-AT showed that ALT greater than 260 U/L, a prothrombin time greater than 16 seconds, and a α_1-AT concentration less than 0.25 g/L were associated with a poor outcome.[424] On follow-up, serum bilirubin elevations and abnormal coagulation tests associated with factor V levels below normal predicted death within 1 year, and were used as criteria for liver transplant evaluation.[424,442]

α_1-AT-deficient individuals who escape severe liver disease in childhood generally are free of clinical liver disease until late in life.[443] From the ages of 20–40, the incidence of liver disease in the α_1-AT-deficient population is approximately 2%. From 41–50 years of age, the incidence increases to approximately 5%, with a 2 : 1 male predominance. Between 51 and 60 years of age, there is a 15% incidence in males and 0% in females. In an autopsy series of 246 Swedish PiZ patients, the incidence of cirrhosis was 12%, but this increased to 19% in individuals over 50 years of age.[443] Male gender and obesity, but not alcohol or viral hepatitis, predispose to advanced liver disease in adults with α_1-AT.[444] Registry data show that emphysema and cirrhosis were the most common underlying causes of death (72% and 10%, respectively), with malignancy and diverticulitis accounting for 3% of deaths each.[445] Death usually occurs within 2 years of the clinical diagnosis of cirrhosis. Rare cases of liver disease have been reported in adults with PiMMalton and PiMDuarte.[446,447]

Prospective, non-disease-oriented population surveys do not demonstrate a risk in heterozygotes (PiMZ) for either liver or lung disease.[448] Liver disease population studies in England, Sweden and Norway have shown an increased frequency of the PiMZ phenotype in patients with cryptogenic cirrhosis.[449–451]

Glomerulonephritis occurs in about 17% of patients with liver disease but may be subtle in its presentation. The clinical hallmarks of proteinuria and haematuria may not be present, particularly if the serum albumin is below 20 g/L. Immunofluorescence studies of α_1-AT deficiency-associated membranoproliferative glomerulonephritis have revealed the presence of immunoglobulins, complement and α_1-AT in the subendothelial region of the glomerular basement membrane.[452] α_1-AT appears not associated with the risk of primary IgA nephropathy, but might have an impact on disease outcome as well as on the risk of secondary IgA nephropathy.[453]

Swedish investigators have documented an increased incidence of malignancy with or without cirrhosis in adult homozygous PiZ patients. They have determined that the odds ratio in α_1-AT deficiency for cirrhosis was 7.8 and for hepatocellular carcinoma was 20, compared to age-matched control subjects.[454] The topic of malignant liver disease in α_1-AT deficiency has been reviewed.[455] Recent studies suggest that hepatocytes with marked accumulation of α_1-ATZ-containing globules engender a cancer-prone state, by surviving with intrinsic damage and by chronically stimulating in 'trans' adjacent relatively undamaged hepatocytes that have a selective proliferative advantage.[434]

In a study from the USA, heterozygosity for α_1-AT Pi types was not associated with an increased risk for hepatocellular carcinoma or bile-duct carcinoma.[456] However, a study from Germany established an association between PiZ heterozygosity and hepatocellular carcinoma.[457] In this series of 317 consecutive cancers the PiZ detected immunohistochemically was 5.99% (3.43% the biopsy and 1.84% in the autopsy series acting as control). The α_1-AT zygosity status was verified by analysis of single strand conformational polymorphism and by sequencing DNA extracted from paraffin embedded tissue. Cholangiocarcinomas and/or combined hepatocholangiocarcinomas were seen significantly more frequently in PiZ-associated carcinoma (57.9%) than in non-PiZ-associated carcinoma (27.2%). Cirrhosis was found in only 3 of the 19 PiZ-associated carcinomas.

Morphologically, the finding of PAS-positive, diastase-resistant globules in periportal hepatocytes is the hallmark of Z-type α_1-AT (Figs 5.20 and 5.21) They represent the retention of the abnormal enzyme within the rough endoplasmic reticulum or its transition zone as demonstrated by immunohistochemical methods (Fig. 5.22). Immuno-electronmicroscopic studies have confirmed the localization of amorphous α_1-AT material to the endoplasmic reticulum[458] (Fig. 5.23). Globules have subsequently been found in the livers of individuals homozygous and heterozygous for α_1-AT deficiency, but without liver disease (as discussed later), and in chronic liver disease unrelated to α_1-AT deficiency in all age groups.[459,460] Similar globules have also been seen in patients with other α_1-AT alleles which lead to unsecretable protein, such as PiMMalton and PiMDuarte.[446,461] In illness associated with inflammation, large areas of hepatic parenchyma may be immunopositive for α_1-AT in PiMZ persons.[462] The positivity appears in the form of crescents or rectilinear arrays in the cytoplasm of liver cells; these patients also have the usual globular inclusions. It should be noted that α_1-AT globules, in the absence of the Z allele, may be found in elderly patients who are severely ill and have high plasma concentrations of the enzyme.[463] In some instances, a person with a PiM pheno-type and an acute inflammatory lesion has had typical globules.[464] This is thought to be due to overproduction of α_1-AT exceeding the capacity of the endoplasmic reticulum to process the protein for secretion. In one case, hepatocyte globules were acquired in a 60-year-old man with the Pi Elemberg M phenotype and primary biliary cirrhosis.[465] This phenotype is not associated with very low serum α_1-AT levels. Globules of α_1-AT are not uncommonly found in cells of hepatocellular carcinoma, but the majority of these patients have a normal phenotype for α_1-AT.

The eosinophilic globules of α_1-AT may not be readily apparent with H&E staining. They are difficult to detect in infants less than 12 weeks of age.[446] Immunoperoxidase staining for α_1-AT can be helpful in ambiguous cases; it has been found to be positive as early as 19 weeks of

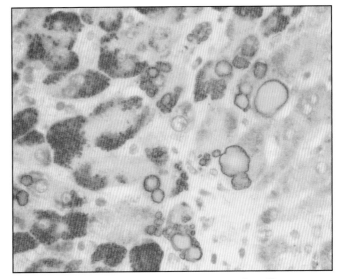

Fig. 5.22 • The presence of α_1-AT in the globules is confirmed by immunohistochemistry. Note that the periphery of the larger globules is more intensely stained than the centre. PAP technique.

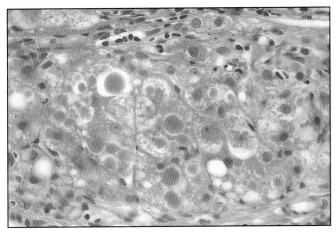

Fig. 5.20 • Homozygous α_1-antitrypsin (PiZZ) deficiency. Eosinophilic globules of varied size are present in the cytoplasm of periportal liver cells. H&E.

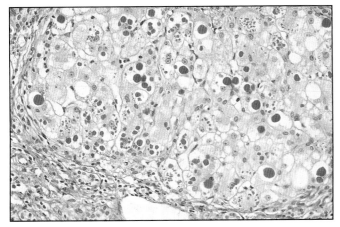

Fig. 5.21 • α_1-antitrypsin (α_1-AT) deficiency. The globules are intensely PAS-positive. PAS after diastase digestion.

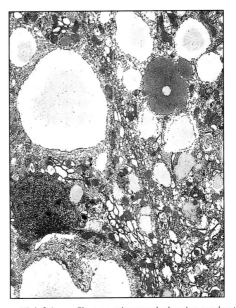

Fig. 5.23 • α_1-AT deficiency. Electron micrograph showing moderately electron-dense amorphous material in the cisterns of the dilated endoplasmic reticulum of a hepatocyte. The larger deposits have a serrated edge. Note the 'halo' surrounding the deposits. ×6500.

sequencing,[457] allowing differentiation between heterozygous and homozygous PiZ status. Antenatal diagnosis by chorionic villus sampling is available using synthetic probes specific for the Z and M gene or by restriction fragment length polymorphism.[473]

Medical therapy is mainly supportive. Breast feeding should be encouraged although no prospective studies validate its value in the prevention of chronic liver disease.[424,474,475] Liver transplantation corrects the genetic defect and cures the patient.[442,469] α_1-AT deficiency is the second most frequent indication for this procedure in children and the most common inherited disease for which liver transplantation is performed.[469,476]

Transgenic mice, constructed using either the M or the Z human genomic clones, express these proteins in liver, as well as in several other organs. Mice constructed using the M allele secrete the human α_1-AT protein from the liver normally, while the Z protein accumulates in the liver of mice transgenic for this allele. There have been histological abnormalities noted in animals transgenic for the Z α_1-AT gene, but they are not the pathological features of human α_1-AT liver disease.[477,478] Transgenic mouse models are used to study gene delivery and potential therapy.[479,480]

α_1-Antichymotrypsin deficiency

In a study of adults, Eriksson et al.[481] established that low α_1-antichymotrypsin (α_1-ACT) levels (with normal levels of α_1-AT) could be associated with cryptogenic chronic hepatitis. Among relatives with the α_1-ACT deficiency, there is an increased incidence of cryptogenic liver and lung disease.[481] In a study from the USA a surprisingly strong association was found between α_1-ACT deficiency and cirrhosis, particularly HCV-related cirrhosis.[482] Thus, 34% of patients with HCV-related cirrhosis were α_1-ACT deficient as compared with 11% of patients with cirrhosis of other aetiologies. Of interest is a report of two siblings, ages 42 and 47, who were heterozygous for both PiSZ α_1-AT and α_1-ACT deficiencies, suggesting that combined deficiency of these two major serine protease inhibitors may enhance the risk of developing liver disease.[483]

The deficiency is familial, with a gene frequency of up to 0.003. Deficient individuals described thus far are heterozygotes; homozygosity may be incompatible with life.[454] Diagnosis is by quantification of serum α-ACT, with demonstration of a level of approximately 64% of normal.[454] The inheritance is autosomal co-dominant. The α_1-ACT gene maps to chromosome 14q31–32.3, the protease inhibitor gene, which is the same site as the α_1-antitrypsin locus.[484,485] The gene has been cloned and at least one deficiency allele sequenced.[486] Treatment at present is supportive.

Liver biopsy in reported cases has shown cirrhosis and granular inclusions that are slightly positive in the DPAS-stained section.[482,486] Immunohistochemical staining discloses granular inclusions in liver cells, particularly those adjacent to portal areas and fibrous bands.[482,487] A fluffy material has been noted in dilated cisterns of the endoplasmic reticulum ultrastructurally.[487]

Afibrinogenaemia and hypofibrinogenaemia

Afibrinogenaemia and hypofibrinogenemia (Type I fibrinogen deficiencies) are rare congenital disorders characterized by unmeasurable or low plasma fibrinogen levels. Their genetic bases are represented by mutations of one or another of the three fibrinogen genes localized to chromosome 4. In afibrinogenaemia, a rare autosomal recessive disorder, complete absence of detectable fibrinogen often presents with umbilical bleeding. Other complications include intracranial haemorrhage following mild trauma, severe epistaxis, gingival and gastrointestinal bleeding, ecchymoses and spontaneous splenic rupture. Affected females may experience menorrhagia, recurrent abortions and postpartum haemorrhage.[488,489] Treatment consists of administration of fibrinogen or cryoprecipitate either prophylactically or on demand.

In hypofibrinogenaemia fibrinogen levels are low, yet variable, which account for the difference in symptomatology. The majority of patients are asymptomatic. Elevated serum aminotransferase levels may be the only manifestation of liver disease in these patients. Some patients progress to cirrhosis, although in afibrinogenaemia the bleeding diathesis is the more common cause of death[490] Prothrombin, partial thromboplastin and thrombin times are markedly prolonged. Plasma will not clot in these patients. Fibrinogen is the primary factor affecting the erythrocyte sedimentation rate, which is therefore very low. Plasma fibrinogen, levels are low or absent. Differentiation from secondary hypofibrinogenaemia (e.g. secondary to drugs) or dysfibrinogenaemia is important. Diagnosis can be made by liver biopsy with immunohistochemistry for fibrinogen, however the procedure may be followed by life-threatening haemorrhage. Mild thrombocytopenia is present in about 25% of patients.[491]

The disease is very rare, approximately 1–2 per million population. Consanguinity is common. The inheritance of afibrinogenaemia is likely to be autosomal recessive, but hypofibrinogenaemia may be either autosomal recessive or dominant.[491] The fibrinogen gene cluster is located on chromosome 4q28–31.[492] It consists of three related fibrinogen genes: alpha (FGA); beta (FGB), or gamma (FGG). Mutations in the α-fibrinogen gene (FGA) account for the majority of cases of congenital afibrinogenaemia, though mutations in all 3 fibrinogen genes, FGG, FGA, and FGB, can cause congenital afibrinogenemia.[493–495]

DNA sequencing of fibrinogen from patients with hypofibrinogenaemia and fibrinogen storage have showed single heterozygous mutations of the gamma-chain[496,497] and beta-chain genes.[496] Round and elongated inclusions may be present in the liver in patients with familial hypofibrinogenaemia (Figs 5.31–5.33).[498–500] The small inclusions in 'fibrinogen storage disease' are irregular in outline, while the large inclusions are spherical and often vacuolated. They are strongly positive with the phosphotungstic acid-haematoxylin stain but are only weakly PAS-positive, and some have a darker core. Immunoreactivity to fibrinogen antibody can be demonstrated (Fig. 5.33). Ultrastructurally, the cisterns of the rough endoplasmic reticulum are filled

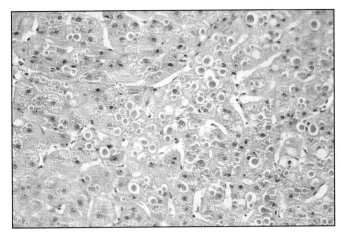

Fig. 5.31 • Fibrinogen storage disease: hepatocytes contain eosinophilic globules of varied size. H&E.

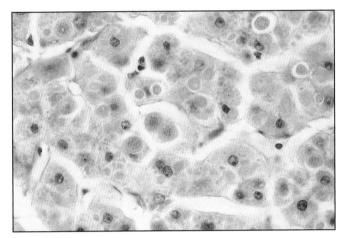

Fig. 5.32 • Same case as illustrated in Fig. 5.31. Some globules are vacuolated and others have a dark core. PAS after diastase digestion.

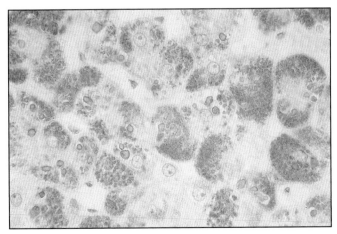

Fig. 5.33 • Same case as illustrated in Figs 5.31 and 5.32. Globules are immunoreactive to fibrinogen antibodies. PAP technique.

with densely packed, curved tubular structures arranged in a fingerprint-like pattern[498,499,501] (Fig. 5.34). Fibrinogen inclusions may resemble the ground-glass inclusions seen in carriers of hepatitis B surface antigen, or the Lafora-like bodies, but they are orcein negative, only weakly PAS positive and their fibrinogen content is demonstrable by

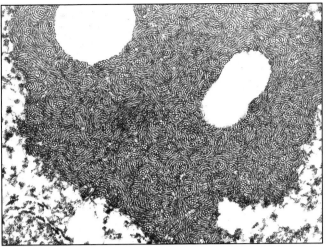

Fig. 5.34 • Electron micrograph of the same case as illustrated in Figs 5.31–5.33. The fibrinogen inclusion in the liver cell has a fingerprint-like pattern. ×31 700.

immunohistochemistry.[418] They may be found incidentally in patients without evidence of hypofibrinogenaemia and in whom mutational analysis have not been found or investigated.[502–505] Conversely, an afibrinogenic patient with proven mutation has shown no evidence of storage in liver.[506] Proliferation of catalase-positive peroxisomes, interpreted as an adaptation response, was reported in liver cells in a case of fibrinogen storage disease[507] In some patients, cirrhosis may occur.

Antithrombin III deficiency

This uncommon disorder has an autosomal dominant inheritance with complete penetrance. The gene for antithrombin III is located at chromosome 1q 23–25.[508] There is a propensity for venous thrombo-embolism ranging from superficial thrombophlebitis to pulmonary embolism.[509,510] The deficiency may be complicated by the Budd–Chiari syndrome.[511,512] The deficiency does not lead to excess mortality, according to Rosendaal et al.[513] who do not recommend prophylactic anticoagulation. An 8-month-old infant with antithrombin III deficiency developed multiple large venous and arterial thromboses and *E. coli* sepsis.[514] He had a micronodular cirrhosis, and liver cells contained multiple, eosinophilic, PAS-positive globules resembling those of α_1-AT deficiency. However, the globules failed to react with anti-α_1-AT or with antithrombin III antisera.

Disorders of amino acid metabolism

Tyrosinaemia

Tyrosinaemia is caused by a deficiency of fumarylacetoacetate hydrolase (FAH), the last enzyme in the tyrosine degradation pathway (Fig. 5.35).[515] This leads to accumulation of highly reactive intermediate metabolites like maleyl- and fumaryl-acetoacetate, that are toxic and mutagenic within the liver. The secondary metabolite succinylacetone is

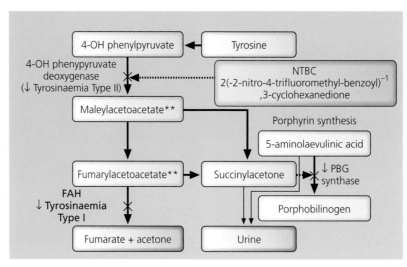

Fig. 5.35 • Tyrosine metabolic pathway. In tyrosinaemia type 1, deficient fumarylacetoacetate hydrolase (FAH) leads to accumulation of highly reactive intermediate metabolites (**) and the production of succinylacetone, which is both excreted in urine (diagnostic test) and has an inibitory effect on porphobilinogen (PBG) synthase (acute porphyria crisis and urinary excretion of 5-aminolaevulinic acid). NTBC therapy blocks the degradation pathway, preventing reactive metabolite formation.

excreted in the urine; a high urinary level is a diagnostic feature.[516] Succinylacetone has also an inhibitory effect on porphobilinogen synthase, accounting for episodes similar to acute hepatic porphyria, with neurological crises and excretion of 5-aminolaevulinic acid in the urine (Fig. 5.35).

Clinical presentation is heterogeneous even within the same family. Progressive liver damage is often not reflected in routine liver tests.[517] The earlier the presentation, the worse the prognosis.[518] Patients present with vomiting, diarrhoea, failure to thrive, abdominal distension, anaemia, bleeding and rickets. Common findings include ascites, hepatosplenomegaly, peripheral oedema, hypoglycaemia, urinary findings compatible with the renal tubular changes of Fanconi syndrome, hypoproteinaemia and severe coagulopathy. Liver crisis, often precipitated by an infection, typically presents in the first 2 years of life and is characterized by increased severity of hepatic dysfunction. Coagulation tests (prothrombin and partial thromboplastin times) worsen and are not responsive to vitamin K; jaundice heralds the terminal event.[517,519]

Neurological crisis may also be precipitated by infection. Children become irritable, less active, and develop severe pain, often localized to the legs. Paraesthesias, hypertension, tachycardia, and paralysis may develop. The paralysis may progress to complete flaccid quadriplegia, including paralysis of the diaphragm and may require mechanical ventilation. Cerebrospinal fluid analysis is unremarkable. This complication may account for 10% of deaths but the incidence varies greatly.[516,520,521] Nerve toxicity due to delta-aminolaevulinic acid retention is thought responsible (see Fig. 5.35).

More than 80% of patients have renal tubular defects. Histologically, 25% have some degree of glomerulosclerosis and 50% have mild to moderate interstitial nephritis and fibrosis. Nephrocalcinosis can be detected by ultrasound in a third of the patients. Fifty per cent of the patients may have an abnormal glomerular filtration rate.[522] Hypertrophic cardiomyopathy has been documented.[523,524]

Hepatocellular carcinoma (HCC) occurs in 10–37% of cases.[194,525] It is associated with cirrhosis, and may occur as early as the first year of life or in adulthood. α-Fetoprotein screening may be helpful, but the complication has been seen with normal α-fetoprotein levels.[526]

Hereditary tyrosinaemia occurs world-wide, although it is particularly common in individuals of French-Canadian descent and is most common in the Canadian province of Quebec. A variety of mutations in the FAH gene have been described. One hundred per cent of patients in the province of Quebec and 28% elsewhere carry a splice mutation in intron 12 of the FAH gene.[527,528] The gene is found on chromosome 15q 23–25.[529] Prenatal diagnosis is available.[530,531] Interestingly, many patients with tyrosinaemia have a mosaic pattern of fumarylacetoacetase (FAH) expression in liver tissue. This phenomenon has been explained by a spontaneous reversion of the mutation in one allele to a normal genotype.[532] There seems to be no evidence that it could be of maternal origin due to transplacental cell trafficking and subsequent fusion.[533] In one study, the extent of mutation reversion of the FAH gene in the liver correlated inversely with the clinical severity of the disease, suggesting that the corrected hepatocytes play a substantial protective role in liver function.[534]

NTBC (2-(2-nitro-4-trifluoromethyl-benzoyl)-1, 3-cyclohexanedione) inhibits 4-hydroxyphenylpyruvate, the enzyme deficient in tyrosinaemia type II, and prevents the accumulation of toxic metabolities (see Fig. 5.36). Since the first clinical trial of NTBC therapy in 1991, over 220 tyrosinaemia patients have been treated by the drug.[535] Only 10% of patients appear not to respond. Of the patients started on NTBC early in life, 2 cases (1%) have developed HCC during the first year of treatment, but no further cases

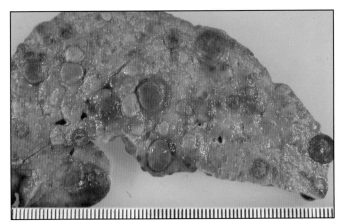

Fig. 5.36 • Tyrosinaemia. Section of explanted liver showing cirrhotic nodules of varied size and colour.

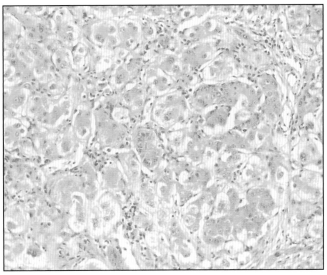

Fig. 5.38 • Tyrosinaemia. Same case as illustrated in Fig. 5.36. Higher magnification to show disruption of the liver cell plates with rosette formation, varied cell ballooning or eosinophilic shrinkage and a light inflammatory cell infiltration throughout. H&E.

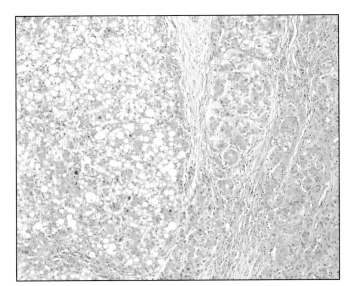

Fig. 5.37 • Tyrosinaemia. Same case as illustrated in Fig. 5.36. A segment of a macroregenerative nodule shows marked steatosis. H&E.

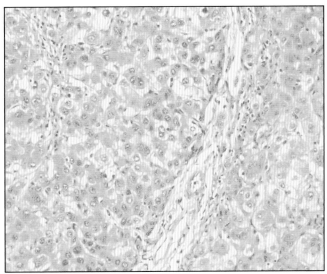

Fig. 5.39 • Tyrosinaemia. Same case as illustrated in Fig. 5.36. Another macroregenerative nodule shows dysplastic changes with increased cell basophilia and nucleo-cytoplasmic ratio. H&E.

have occurred among patients followed for up to 9 years. However, with late onset of treatment, the risk of malignancy remains despite NTBC therapy.[536] Corneal lesions reported in 13% of patients can be controlled by using a low-tyrosine, low-phenylalanine diet.

Dietary therapy must be maintained despite NTBC therapy. The unique renal tubular dysfunction resulting in hypophosphataemic rickets is usually responsive to dietary therapy.[537] However, the marked coagulopathy,[538] neurological complications simulating porphyria,[521] and development of hepatocellular carcinoma[525] are not responsive to dietary therapy alone. Liver transplantation remains the treatment of choice for medical treatment failures. Renal disease does not progress after liver transplantation.[539] Mouse models of the disease are used to study mechanism of injury and potential therapy.[540–542]

Pathological aspects of tyrosinaemia have been described in several reports.[543–549] The liver at autopsy or removed at transplantation is slightly to moderately enlarged, yellow, firm and nodular (Fig. 5.36). The microscopic features include fatty change, cholestasis, pseudoacinar transforma-

tion of hepatic plates, pericellular and periportal fibrosis, variable haemosiderosis, extramedullary haemopoiesis, and varying-sized foci of nodular regeneration, some qualifying as macroregenerative nodules (Figs 5.37 and 5.38). The regenerating nodules, which appear as high attenuation foci on CT scans, are difficult to differentiate from multifocal hepatocellular carcinoma.[550] The nodules often show more fat accumulation than the adjacent liver (Fig. 5.37) and some may exhibit dysplastic changes (Fig. 5.39). Periportal ductular reaction, although present, is usually not striking. Cirrhosis may be micronodular, macronodular or mixed.[547,551] The prominence and variegated colours of the macronodules (yellow, tan, green) have been commented on by Jaffe[194] (Fig. 5.36). Transition from a micronodular to a macronodular cirrhosis has been documented.[544] Liver-cell dysplasia (liver-cell change), both the large and small cell varieties, are commonly observed and the distinction between dysplastic nodules and hepatocellular carcinoma may be difficult if not impossible.[194]

Cytogenetic studies on skin fibroblasts from a patient with tyrosinaemia and hepatocellular carcinoma have demonstrated chromosome breakages in 71% of cells.[552] DNA ploidy abnormalities detected in three cases[549] may be a useful marker for early malignant transformation. Ultrastructural studies have confirmed the presence of fat in hepatocytes and the cholestasis, as well as a number of non-specific changes.[5,547] In the case studied by Jevtic et al.,[553] hepatocytes surrounded a central canaliculus forming tubules; the cells were joined by many desmosomes. The basal portions of the cells were not covered by microvilli or a space of Disse, and basement membrane-like material was present. Mitochondria of liver cells can be markedly increased in number in tyrosinaemia and may show mild to moderate pleomorphism with randomly oriented cristae. Peroxisomes are frequently enlarged and may contain nucleoids or small lipid droplets.[5]

In the pancreas, about 50% of patients have hyperplasia of the islets of Langerhans.[554] Renal changes include interstitial oedema, tubular dilatation with vacuolar and granular degeneration, loss of glomeruli, and hypertrophy and hyperplasia of the juxtaglomerular complex.[553]

Congenital hyperammonaemia syndromes and urea cycle disorders

Defects in any of the enzymes of the urea cycle may lead to hyperammonaemia and encephalopathy at any age, although presentation is commonly in the neonatal period.[555,556] Such patients are normal at birth but by 24 hours of age develop irritability, poor feeding, vomiting, lethargy and respiratory distress. This is quickly followed by hypotonia, seizures, coma and respiratory arrest. If treatment is not instituted early, long-term neurological function may be irreversibly compromised.[557] Patients may be misdiagnosed as having respiratory distress syndrome, sepsis, or intraventricular haemorrhage in the newborn period, or Reye-like syndrome when presentation is delayed. Thus, in evaluating a patient the possibility of a hyperammonaemia syndrome should be considered in families that have lost children to one of these more common disorders. These disorders are autosomal recessive apart from ornithine transcarbamylase (OTC), which is X-linked.

The urea cycle disorders have been comprehensively reviewed.[555,558,559] The only urea cycle defect in which there is significant liver disease is argininosuccinic aciduria (ASA).[560] The urea cycle enzyme which is deficient in this disorder, argininosuccinic lyase, is located on chromosome 7.[561] Several mutations within this gene may result in argininosuccinate lyase deficiency.[562] The enzyme protein may be absent in the liver;[563] it can also be measured in red blood cells, fibroblasts, and amnion cells with substrate accumulation occurring in the fluid of cultured cells. Liver disease is manifested clinically by hepatomegaly, and serum ALT elevation, and severe fibrosis on liver biopsy.[560] Marked macrovesicular steatosis has been noted.[564] Ultrastructural changes include dilatation of the rough or smooth endo-plasmic reticulum[560,564,565] and the presence of megamito-chondria in zones affected by steatosis.[564]

Despite the structural changes, survival figures in these patients and in those with argininosuccinate synthetase deficiency (citrullinaemia) are much better than in those with ornithine transcarbamylase (OTC) and carbamyl phosphate synthetase (CPS) deficiencies.

Pathological studies of the liver in males with OTC deficiency have generally been normal. Occasional case reports suggest some mitochondrial and peroxisomal changes.[566] Acquired abnormalities, more likely to be seen with the passage of time, are documented in females who have varying degrees of deficiency. At the light microscopic level, the mild changes include fat accumulation, inflammation, interface hepatitis and mild periportal fibrosis.[566,567] Organelles in the hepatocytes usually are normal.

In the neonatal period intensive care management of hyperammonaemia is often necessary. Long-term treatment consists of a combination of dietary restriction of protein, bypassing the defect by administering arginine and, on occasion, the use of ammonia scavengers.[558,568] Liver transplantation is the definitive treatment for patients with severe variants, progressive liver disease, and for some patients whose disease manifestations have proved very difficult to control with conventional therapy.[569,570]

Cystinosis

Cystinosis is a rare autosomal recessive disease (1 in 100 000–200 000 live births).[571] It is characterized by the accumulation of L-cystine crystals in lysosomes due to a defective carrier-mediated transport system for cystine. The cystine accumulates in the eye, reticuloendothelial system, kidney and other internal organs. The gene responsible for this disease, located on chromosome 17p13, is called *CTNS*; it encodes a lysosomal membrane protein named cystinosin, whose cysteine transport activity is H$^+$-driven.[572] Several mutations of this gene are associated with cystinosis.[573,574]

The most severe clinical form is nephrogenic (infantile) cystinosis. Patients are normal at birth, but symptoms of renal tubular dysfunction (Fanconi syndrome) develop by 6 to 12 months and progress to renal failure by 10 years of age. This tubular defect accounts for the presenting symptoms of polyuria, polydypsia and failure to thrive. Affected children are often hospitalized because of dehydration, acidosis resulting from potassium and bicarbonate urinary loss, vomiting and electrolyte imbalance. Renal phosphate loss causes the subsequent development of vitamin D-resistant rickets. Mental development is normal.[571] Patients develop photophobia from accumulation of cystine crystals in the cornea and conjunctiva. The crystals can be detected by slit lamp examination and are diagnostic of the disease.[575] Hot weather accentuates symptoms because of a decreased ability to sweat. Crystal accumulation in the thyroid may lead to hypothyroidism.[576]

Dialysis or renal transplantation is usually undertaken between 6 and 12 years of age. Although the disease does not recur in the donor kidney storage continues in other organs resulting in blindness, corneal erosions, diabetes and neurological deterioration between 13 and 30 years of age.[577] Medical therapy consists of fluid and electrolyte replacement for the renal tubular defects and carnitine to replace urinary losses. Cysteamine has been given both systemically and topically (in the eyes). While there is significant toxicity involved in using this drug, large-scale trials have shown that it delays loss of renal function, particularly in patients treated very early in their disease course.[578]

Massive hepatomegaly has been reported in this disorder with the incidence of detectable hepatomegaly as high as 42% in patients over 10 years of age. Most patients do not have significant liver dysfunction.

There are adolescents and adults with more benign forms of cystinosis; a late form, not associated with symptoms before the 5th year of life, is compatible with survival well into the second decade. Clinical manifestations include retinal depigmentation, rickets, mild renal failure, and the accumulation of cystine crystals in the conjunctiva and bone marrow. In benign cystinosis patients are asymptomatic and have a normal life expectancy, presumably because substantially less cystine accumulates within cells than in the nephropathic or intermediate forms.[579] This form of the disease is diagnosed only by slit lamp examination of the eyes.

Diagnosis in all forms is made by identification of crystals in polymorphonuclear leucocytes or by slit lamp examination to identify corneal crystals. The latter procedure may give false negative results in infants. Prenatal diagnosis is available by measurement of cystine in amniotic cells or chorionic villi.[580,581] The diagnosis of cystinosis is established by visualization of the rectangular and hexagonal crystals in bone marrow aspirates, in conjunctival, rectal or renal biopsy tissue, or by ophthalmological examination. Phase contrast and polarizing microscopy are especially useful in searching for the crystals in biopsy material. Because of the solubility of the crystals in water, all tissues should be fixed in alcohol, and aqueous stains should be avoided.[582] The crystals are therefore best seen in unstained frozen sections or in sections made from alcohol-fixed tissue, and examined by phase or polarizing microscopy. Electron microscopy is a useful method of diagnosis if light microscopic examination of biopsy tissue fails to reveal the crystals.[583] The diagnosis has been made before birth by light and electron microscopic examination of fetal tissues.[584,585] Other methods of diagnosis include the determination of the amount of cystine in white blood cells or in cultured skin fibroblasts. A non-invasive method of diagnosis based on infra-red spectroscopy of hair, was reported by Lubec et al.[586] Fluorescence in situ hybridization (FISH) may provide a rapid detection of the 57-kb deletion in CTNS.[587]

The cystine crystals accumulate within lysosomes.[588,589] The most severely affected organ is the kidney.[582,590] Most of the cells containing the crystals are of reticuloendothelial origin. Crystals in many organs, such as the cornea, conjunctiva, bone marrow, spleen and liver, excite little or no reaction. In the liver, markedly hypertrophied Kupffer cells packed with cystine are located mainly in perivenular zones

(Fig. 5.40). They have a brilliant silvery birefringence when viewed under polarized light (Fig. 5.41). The spaces made by the crystals in Kupffer cells can be seen by electron microscopy[591,592] (Fig. 5.42) and the crystals have a characteristic appearance by scanning electron microscopy (Fig. 5.43).

Hepatic fibrosis in cystinosis was reported in one case.[593] The patient, who died at the age of 24 years after multiple renal transplants, presented with portal hypertension. In addition to massive crystal accumulation, the liver showed

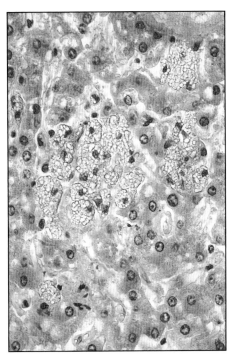

Fig. 5.40 • Cystinosis. Cystine crystals are packed in the cytoplasm of hypertrophied Kupffer cells. H&E.

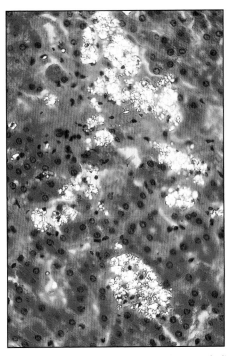

Fig. 5.41 • Same case as illustrated in Fig. 5.40. Cystine crystals display brilliant silvery birefringence. H&E.

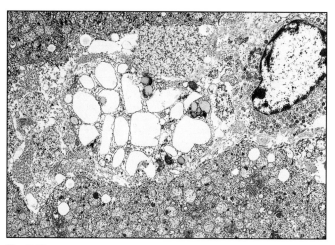

Fig. 5.42 • Electron micrograph shows spaces created by cystine crystals that were dissolved during processing. Several have rectangular shapes. ×32 000.

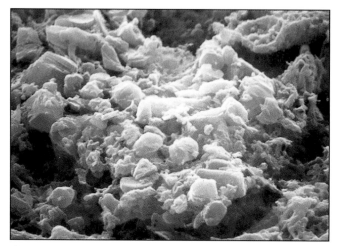

Fig. 5.43 • Three-dimensional appearance of cystine crystals, some having a hexagonal shape. Scanning electron micrograph, ×5000.

extensive fibrosis without cirrhosis, and numerous hepatic stellate cells were seen in association with the fibrous tissue. The authors suggested that the stellate cells were activated by injured cystine-laden Kupffer cells, but cannot dismiss a possible role of the multiple renal transplants in the fibrosis. A patient with cystinosis treated with oral cysteamine developed veno-occlusive disease that eventually required transplantation.[594] The hepatectomy specimen disclosed many cystine crystals in the fibrous scars around terminal hepatic venules.[194] Ten years later, after a kidney transplant that failed because of disease recurrence, the patient presented with hepatic dysfunction, once again with veno-occlusive disease and crystal reaccumulation.[194] Additional cases of non-cirrhotic portal hypertension have been ascribed to cystine accumulation in Kupffer cells.[595,596]

Cystathionine β-synthase deficiency (homocystinuria)

Patients with this condition present with ectopia lentis, osteoporosis, genu valgum, pes cavus, kyphoscoliosis,

and progressive mental retardation.[597] In addition, arterial thrombosis is common; however, most patients with homocystinuria and strokes have a concurrent factor V Leiden mutation.[598] Hepatomegaly with normal liver enzymes is common. Screening is by detection of high levels of methionine and homocystine in urine. Diagnosis includes evaluation for other causes of homocystinuria, including vitamin B_{12} or an abnormality in its processing. Cystathionine β-synthase (CBS) can be measured in cultured fibroblasts.[599]

The disease has an estimated worldwide frequency of 1 in 344 000 but the frequency is higher in Ireland (1 in 65 000).[600] The cystathionase gene is found on chromosome 21q-22.3;[601] it has been cloned.[602] Several different defects have been found to be associated with homocystinuria.[603,604] Prenatal diagnosis can be performed. Treatment is with supplementation with folic acid and betaine.[605,606]

Light microscopic studies of the liver in homocystinuria have shown steatosis, more prominent in the perivenular regions.[607-609] Mild to moderate portal fibrosis and thickened arterioles with intimal hyperplasia or fibrosis have been observed in some patients.[608] Ultrastructural studies have demonstrated mitochondria with unusual shapes, increased smooth endoplasmic reticulum and numerous pericanalicular lysosomes.[610,611] Hyperhomocysteinemia in liver of CBS-deficient mice has been shown to promote oxidative stress, leading to fibrosis and steatosis.[612]

Disorders of lipoprotein and lipid metabolism

Abetalipoproteinaemia

The disease was first described by Bassen & Kornzweig[613] Patients with abetalipoproteinaemia have malabsorption of fat, acanthocytosis, retinitis pigmentosa and ataxic neuropathic disease. Symptoms usually begin in infancy with steatorrhoea and failure to thrive. Acanthocytes are evident by 12 months of age. Neurological abnormalities causing an unsteady gait develop between 2 and 17 years of age. Degenerative changes affect the posterior and lateral columns of the spinal cord, spinocerebellar pathways and peripheral nerves[613,614] The diagnosis is suspected by the clinical features, a serum cholesterol level of less than 1.3 mmol/L (50 mg/dL) and an extremely low serum triglyceride value. The diagnosis is confirmed by determination of the β-lipoprotein value using lipoprotein electrophoresis, ultracentrifugation, or immunochemical methods. Small bowel biopsies reveal fat droplets in the epithelium (Fig. 5.44).

The inheritance is autosomal recessive. The defective gene codes for the microsomal triglyceride transfer protein (MTP). This protein is essential for the transport of triglyceride, cholesteryl ester, and phospholipid from phospholipid surfaces. It is synthesized as a heterodimer; in abetalipoproteinaemia the large subunit of the protein is absent.[615] Subsequently, mutations in the large subunit gene were demonstrated in two patients with abetalipoproteinaemia.[616]

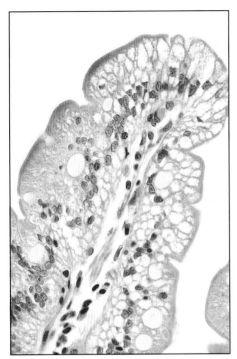

Fig. 5.44 • Abetalipoproteinaemia. Intestinal microvillus reveals marked vacuolization of epithelial cells. H&E.

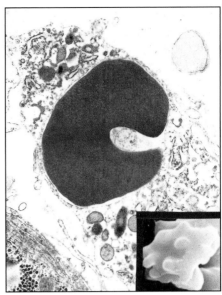

Fig. 5.45 • Abetalipoproteinaemia. Transmission electron micrograph shows Kupffer cell with phagocytosed acanthocyte. ×40 000. Scanning electron micrograph (inset) shows a sinusoidal acanthocyte. ×5000.

Treatment consists of a low fat diet and replacement of vitamins A and E.[617] Late manifestations include essential fatty acid deficiency and peripheral vascular disease. Supplementation with medium chain triglycerides for calories was a common recommendation in the past; this therapy has been implicated as the cause of cirrhosis in some patients and is no longer recommended.[618] Liver transplantation cures the liver disease and corrects the serum lipid profile, but it does not cure the steatorrhoea as the mutation in the MTP gene is also present in the intestine.[619]

Liver transplantation in a 20-year-old woman with untreated abetalipoproteinaemia who had developed cirrhosis[620] was followed by a dramatic rise in cholesterol and triglycerides, and a rise in apo B from barely measurable (<1) to 76. Studies of apo B and apo B mRNA in cultured liver and intestinal cells suggested that the defect in abetalipoproteinemia does not involve the apolipoprotein B gene or the synthesis/glycosylation of the apolipoprotein, but rather some aspect of lipoprotein assembly or secretion.

Histological studies of the liver in several cases of abetalipoproteinaemia have shown variable steatosis.[621,622] The patient studied by Partin et al.[622] underwent biopsies prior to and after 2, 14 and 20 months of therapy with medium chain triglycerides. Before treatment, hepatocytes contained large fat droplets which had ruptured to form perivenular 'fatty lakes'. Ultrastructurally, the Golgi apparatus was nearly completely deficient in trans-Golgi vacuole formation. Endogenous triglyceride particles could not be found and the circum-Golgi smooth endoplasmic reticulum was absent. During the 14 months of dietary treatment, the fat droplets in hepatocytes became smaller and less numerous, but there was progression of initially mild hepatic fibrosis to a micronodular cirrhosis. Mallory bodies were identified in hepatocytes of the cirrhotic liver by electron microscopy. Clinically, the patient had substantial hepatomegaly and a persistent increase of serum aminotransferase activity. Whether the hepatic lesions were part of the natural course of the disease or related to therapy remains undetermined. The ultrastructural findings of one reported case included fatty change, a normal Golgi apparatus and endoplasmic reticulum, acanthocytes in sinusoids, and phagocytosis of deformed erythrocytes by Kupffer cells[621] (Fig. 5.45). An ultrastructural study of another case by Collins et al.[623] demonstrated striking changes in hepatocellular peroxisomes. They included pleomorphism and a broadened range of size, often larger than normal with marginal bars in some. Whether the changes were those of a peroxisomal disorder or a reflection of the disturbed lipid metabolism remains undetermined.

Familial hypobetalipoproteinaemia (FHBL)

This disorder is characterized by reduced levels of β and apo β-containing lipoprotein.[624,625] A mutation of the apolipoprotein apo B gene leading to synthesis of a truncated form of apo B (apo B-38.95) was reported by Taruji et al.[626] Many other truncations of apo B have been identified and are reviewed by Kane & Havel.[624] Sporadic cases of FHBL with an apparently recessive transmission may be caused by de novo mutations of apo B gene.[627]

Patients with *heterozygous-betalipoproteinaemia* are usually asymptomatic, and have low plasma levels of total cholesterol (45–150 mg/dL) and low to normal levels of triglycerides (11–140 mg/dL).[625] Mild to moderate increases in the levels of the serum aminotransferases have been reported.[626] Ultrasound examination discloses a hyperechoic liver. Liver biopsies have revealed mild to moderate steatosis without necroinflammatory changes or fibrosis.[626,628–632] The long-term prognosis is excellent; patients may actually be protected from developing coronary atherosclerotic disease.[625]

In *homozygous hypobetalipoproteinaemia*, apo B and low-density lipoprotein (LDL)-cholesterol levels are very low or undetectable.[624,625] When β-lipoproteins are absent the clinical phenotype is indistinguishable from that of abetalipoproteinaemia, with fat malabsorption, acanthocytosis, retinitis pigmentosa and neuromuscular degeneration. Liver biopsies also reveal marked steatosis.[633,634] Perisinusoidal fibrosis in one case was attributed to hypervitaminosis A.[634] A mouse model may provide new insights into apoB metabolism.[635] Treatment is similar to that of abetalipoproteinaemia, namely restriction of dietary fat and intensive supplementation of vitamin E.

Familial high density lipoprotein deficiency (Tangier disease)

This rare autosomal recessive disease is caused by a mutation in the ATP-binding cassette-1 gene[636–638] on chromosome 9q31.[639] The ATP-binding cassette-1 protein is also called the cholesterol efflux regulatory protein.[637,640] In the absence of this regulatory protein, apolipoprotein-mediated cholesterol removal from cells is blocked, leading to the characteristic accumulation of cholesterol esters in reticuloendothelial cells[641] and low or absent plasma high density lipoprotein, low plasma cholesterol levels.[642]

Patients present with a striking tonsillar enlargement with orange discolouration, lymphadenopathy, hepatosplenomegaly and peripheral neuropathy. Thrombocytopenia, corneal opacities and xanthomas are less frequent. Some patients have hyperbilirubinaemia.[643,644]

The pathological aspects of the disease have been comprehensively discussed in two publications.[642,644] Deposition of cholesterol esters is widespread, with involvement of tonsillar and adenoidal tissue, liver, spleen, lymph nodes, bone marrow, thymus, intestinal mucosa, skin and cornea. The foam cells contain birefringent, needle-shaped cholesterol crystals, are sudanophilic and PAS-negative, and stain positively with the Schultz modification of the Lieberman–Burchard reaction. Involvement of the liver by clusters of cholesterol containing cells has been noted in patients studied by a number of investigators.[642,645,646] The differential diagnosis from other cholesterol storage diseases is discussed by Bale et al.[642]

Familial hypercholesterolaemia

Patients with this disease have an elevated concentration of cholesterol, which is deposited in tendons and skin, cornea and arteries. The severity of disease is related to the gene dosage, i.e. this is an autosomal dominant trait with homozygotes affected more severely than heterozygotes.[647] Heterozygotes have a two-fold elevation of plasma cholesterol from birth, with onset of tendon xanthomas and coronary atherosclerosis after the age of 20 years. Homozygotes have severe hypercholesterolaemia with complications developing in the first decade of life; xanthomas may be present at birth. Coronary heart disease begins in child-hood and frequently leads to death before the age of 20 years.

Patients have elevated concentrations of low density lipoprotein, the major cholesterol transport lipoprotein in plasma. The incidence of heterozygotes is about 1 in 500 and of homozygotes about 1 per 1 000 000. The defect is an abnormal low density lipoprotein receptor gene.[648] Several different mutations have been described.[649] The gene is on chromosome 19p.[650,651] Therapy is directed at lowering plasma cholesterol to control complications.[652] Homozygotes have been managed by combined liver–heart transplantation.[653]

Reported pathological findings in homozygous familial hypercholesterolaemia have been reviewed by Buja et al.[654] In addition to atherosclerosis of the aorta and coronary vessels there is neutral lipid accumulation in extravascular sites that include the skin, tendons, spleen, thymus and other organs. In the liver, there is accumulation of lipid in hepatocytes and Kupffer cells. Ultrastructurally, accumulation of both neutral lipid and cholesterol has been observed in hepatocytes.[5]

Wolman and cholesterol ester storage diseases

Wolman disease and cholesterol ester storage disease (CESD) are two disorders caused respectively by an absent or a reduced (3–8%) activity of the enzyme lysosomal acid lipase.[655,656] The enzyme is essential for the intralysosomal metabolism of cholesterol esters and triglycerides, namely their uptake by receptor mediated endocytosis into lipoprotein particles.[655] The enzyme is trafficked to the lysosome via the mannose-6-phosphate receptor systems.[656,657] The gene encoding the lipase is on chromosome 10q23.2–q23.3 and contains 10 exons spread over 36 kb.[658]

Wolman disease was first described in 1956.[659] Patients may present with hydrops fetalis or congenital ascites.[660] However, the usual presentation is failure to thrive with vomiting, frequently with severe diarrhoea accompanied by steatorrhoea. Physical findings include severe malnutrition, hepatosplenomegaly, ascites, pallor and mild lymphadenopathy.[661] Neurological development is abnormal. Radiological studies reveal large adrenals with calcification. Examination of the peripheral blood smear reveals vacuolated lymphocytes, while bone marrow examination discloses foam cells which stain positively for cholesterol and neutral fat or triglyceride. Serum lipid levels are usually low or normal, but in rare instances they are elevated. Adrenal responses become depressed with time. Death usually occurs in the first year of life despite aggressive nutritional support.[661]

The milder form of the disease, cholesterol ester storage disease (CESD), presents at any age with hepatomegaly, and variable splenomegaly secondary to portal hypertension and/or lipid retention.[655,662–664] In children, diarrhoea may occur due to small intestinal lipid retention; resulting malnutrition may lead to short stature.[665] Recurrent abdominal pain may be a feature. There have been reports of premature atherosclerosis,[666–668] pulmonary vascular obstruction,[669] and mesenteric lipodystrophy.[670] An asymptomatic 51-year-old man with CESD and accelerated atherosclerosis developed cholangiocarcinoma and died of liver failure as a result of extensive tumour infiltration.[671] Cholangiocarcinoma had similarly developed in a 51-year-old lady with CESD referred to our centre (unpublished observation). Jaundice suggests the development of cirrhosis which may be followed by liver failure. Laboratory abnormalities in CESD include elevated levels of the aminotransferases, cholesterol and its esters, LDL, triglycerides and bile acids. Sea-blue histiocytes have been noted in the liver, small bowel and bone marrow.[672] Prenatal diagnosis is available.[660,673]

Wolman disease can result from a number of mutations in the lysosomal acid lipase gene, all resulting in the absence of enzyme activity.[674] CESD seems distinct from Wolman in that at least one mutant allele has the potential to produce enough residual enzymatic function to ameliorate the phenotype.[675] The most common mutation in CESD is an aberrant splicing of exon 8.[676] This nucleotide substitution results in the production of a shortened lysosomal acid lipase mRNA lacking 72 nucleotides, and in the synthesis of an enzyme missing 24 amino acids. Compound heterozygosity for a mutation causing Wolman disease is common among CESD patients.[677]

Nutritional therapy in Wolman disease is difficult. Wolman[678] suggested avoidance of lipid esters despite the presence of an essential fatty acid deficiency. Also, the role of antioxidant therapy remains unclear, although vitamin E has been routinely used. Bone marrow transplantation corrects the enzyme defect.[679] Bone marrow transplantation performed early in the course of the disease preserved the life of one patient with Wolman disease; growth and mental development have improved over the years.[680] In another patient successful long-term engraftment was followed by continued normalization of acid lipase enzyme activity in peripheral leukocytes, weight gain, and normal cholesterol, tryglyceride and liver enzymes levels at 4 year of age.[681] Previous attempts had been unsuccessful, presumably because of advanced liver disease at the time of bone marrow transplantation.

In CESD, a favourable clinical response has been seen with a stage I American Heart Association diet and large doses of cholestyramine at the University of Minnesota. Medical therapy with an HMG CoA reductase inhibitor has been utilized in the past 10 to 15 years with reasonable success, though its effect on lipid levels and liver tests has been variable.[667,682–685] Success with liver transplantation has been reported.[686,687] End-stage renal disease has developed in one liver transplant patient.[688]

Rat[689–691] and mouse[692] models are available to study experimental therapies of acid lipase deficiency. In vitro correction of fibroblasts in the two human diseases was successful.[692–695]

The adrenal glands in Wolman disease are grossly enlarged, hard and bright yellow. They cut with a gritty sensation and have a yellow cortex and an inner calcified zone. The surface of the small intestine, particularly the duodenum and ileum, has a yellow velvety appearance. The liver in CESD is enlarged, yellow–orange and greasy (Fig. 5.46).

In Wolman disease all affected organs, particularly the liver, spleen, adrenals, haemopoietic system and the intestines, are infiltrated by numerous foamy macrophages that contain cholesterol and/or cholesterol esters.[659,696–699] Stains for lipid (oil red O, Sudan black) are positive, as is the Schultz modification of the Lieberman–Burchard reaction for cholesterol; these stains must be performed on frozen sections, either of fresh or of formalin-fixed tissue. Frozen sections examined by polarizing microscopy reveal numerous anisotropic acicular crystals in the foamy histiocytes. In the liver, cholesterol and cholesterol ester are mainly stored in Kupffer cells and portal macrophages, while hepatocytes contain increased neutral lipid. Reticuloendothelial cells may also contain free fatty acids.[700] There may be marked pericellular fibrosis and varying degrees of periportal cholangiolar proliferation and fibrosis.[700] Ultrastructurally, the enlarged Kupffer cells contain peripheral vacuoles, sometimes within lysosomes, and large central crystal clefts of cholesterol ester.[701] Lake & Patrick[700] observed that the crystals are membrane-bound. Hepatocytes contain many lipid droplets but only occasional crystal clefts.[700] It has been suggested that the cholesterol esters are discharged from the hepatic parenchymal cells in an insoluble form and then are taken up by the Kupffer cells where crystallization occurs.[701]

The light microscopic and ultrastructural changes in the liver of patients with CESD are similar to those of Wolman disease.[664,670,682] A highly characteristic feature of CESD is the presence of markedly hypertrophied Kupffer cells and portal macrophages with a foamy, tan-coloured cytoplasm that stains strongly with PAS (Figs 5.47(A) and 5.47(B)).[682] The birefringent cholesterol crystals are demonstrated as shown in Fig. 5.47(C). Periportal fibrosis of varied degree is present in most of the cases, but cirrhosis is rare.[666,670,682] Ultrastructurally, triglyceride droplets are noted in abundance in hepatic and reticuloendothelial cells; most are surrounded by a single membrane. Many of the lysosomal lipid droplets have a 'moth-eaten' appearance due to the

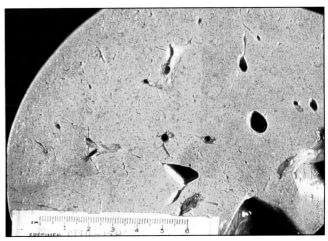

Fig. 5.46 • Cholesterol ester storage disease. This section of liver has a yellow colour and is faintly nodular.

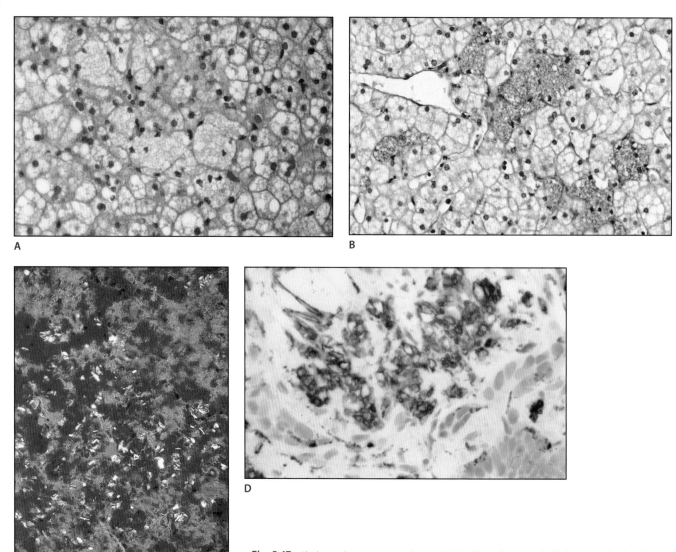

Fig. 5.47 • Cholesterol ester storage disease. **(A)** Kupffer cells are markedly hypertrophied and have a foamy, light tan-coloured cytoplasm; their nuclei are pyknotic. Hepatocytes show microvesicular steatosis. H&E. **(B)** Foamy Kupffer cells in the perivenular zone are PAS-positive. PAS after diastase digestion. **(C)** Cholesterol crystals display brilliant silvery birefringence. There is a large amount of fat (red) in liver cells. Oil red O stain of frozen section. **(D)** CD68 immunostain of macrophages hightlights negatively stained lipids and needle-shaped cholesterol crystals. PAP method.

inclusion of cholesterol within them (Fig. 5.48).[682] Cholesterol crystals are also seen lying free in the cytoplasm, as demonstrated in a case of Wolman disease (Fig. 5.49). A recent study of both liver and intestinal biopsy specimens in Wolman and CESD diseases is reemphasizing the diagnostic role of morphological findings.[702]

The gangliosidoses

GM₁ gangliosidosis

Three subtypes of this disorder are recognized.

Type I, the infantile form

This manifests during the first 6 months of life. Patients present with progressive psychomotor retardation, seizures, hepatosplenomegaly, oedema of the extremities, and failure to thrive. The appetite is poor and sucking is weak, in part because of the infant's hypotonia. By the first year of life

patients are blind, deaf and in decerebrate rigidity. Death, usually from bronchopneumonia, occurs within 2 years of age.

Facial abnormalities include frontal bossing, a depressed nasal bridge, large low-set ears, an increased distance between the nose and upper lip, and downy hirsutism of the forehead and neck. The gums are hypertrophied and there is mild to moderate macroglossia. The corneas are clear. Cherry-red spots are present in the macula in half the patients;[703,704] dermal melanosis may be prominent.[705]

Ganglioside accumulates in neurons, liver, spleen and in histiocytes in other tissues, as well as in the epithelial cells of the kidney.[706] This is a result of a deficiency in all three isoenzymes of lysosomal β-galactosidase-1 (A, B and C), located on chromosome 3p21.[707] The mutations in the infantile form of GM₁-gangliosidosis interfere with phosphorylation of precursor β-galactosidase which as a result is secreted instead of being further processed in the lysosomes.[708]

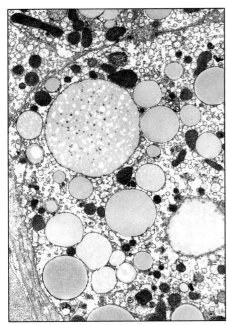

Fig. 5.48 • Cholesterol ester storage disease. Electron micrograph of liver cell containing triglyceride droplets of varied size. 'Moth-eaten' appearance of several droplets is due to the presence of cholesterol crystals within them. ×10 000.

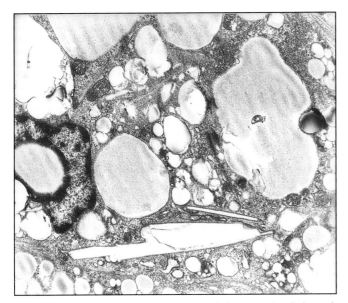

Fig. 5.49 • Wolman disease. Electron micrograph demonstrating cholesterol crystals in the cytoplasm of a liver cell (×11 000). Electron micrograph donated by Dr J E Dimmick, Vancouver, Canada.

Foam cells are seen in bone marrow preparations. Lymphocytes are vacuolated. Mild radiological abnormalities consist of inferior beaking of the lumbar vertebrae and proximal pointing of the metacarpal bones. Neurons are ballooned and contain cytoplasmic membranous inclusions similar to those of Tay–Sachs disease. Lipid laden histiocytes are found throughout the reticuloendothelial system. Renal glomerular epithelial cells, hepatocytes and Kupffer cells are finely vacuolated. Ultrastructurally, the vacuoles in affected cells in GM$_1$-gangliosidosis are empty or contain fibrillar or granular material.[706] Kupffer cells may also contain membrane-bound fibrillary structures[709] (Fig. 5.50).

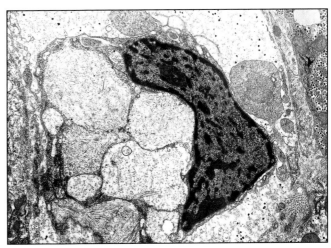

Fig. 5.50 • GM$_1$ gangliosidosis, type I. The cytoplasm of a Kupffer cell is replaced by single membrane-bound vacuoles. Some of the vacuoles contain amorphous material, while others are filled with irregularly arranged fibrillar material. ×300. Courtesy of Dr M Petrelli.

Most affected systemic cells, including hepatocytes and phagocytic cells, bind WGA lectin, and to a lesser extent other lectins such as ConA, S-WGA, DSA and BS-1.[706] Enzyme analysis indicates almost complete absence of β-galactosidase A, B and C in skin fibroblasts and leucocytes.

Type II, the juvenile form

This presents at about 1 year of age. Clinical findings are primarily neurological and include seizures, spasticity, ataxia and mental retardation. Radiological changes are minimal. Facial abnormalities, visceromegaly and macular cherry-red spots are absent. Death occurs between 3 and 8 years of age.[710] This disease is also caused by a mutation in the β-galactosidase-1 gene, but only isoenzymes B and C are deficient.[704] Successful bone marrow engraftment in a pre-symptomatic patient with type II GM$_1$ normalized white cell β-galactosidase levels, but did not influence long-term clinical outcome.[711] In common with type I, there is neuronal storage and foamy histiocytes are present in various organs (Fig. 5.51). Hepatocytes are only slightly vacuolated and Kupffer cells stain intensely with the PAS reagent (Fig. 5.52). Ultrastructurally, the Kupffer cells contain a distinctive granulofibrillar material[709] (Fig. 5.53), or membrane-bound inclusions may be seen in both Kupffer cells and hepatocytes.[712] Two canine models of GM$_1$ gangliosidosis have been described.[713]

Type III, the adult form

This is much less severe than the other two forms and is associated with little or no visceromegaly. While mutations in the β-galactosidase-1 gene are described, the cause of the phenotypic differences from types I and II is as yet undetermined.[714,715]

GM$_2$ gangliosidosis

These are a group of disorders having primarily neurological manifestations. They result from defects in the

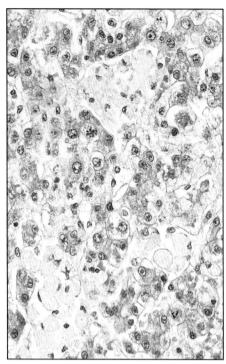

Fig. 5.51 • GM₁ gangliosidosis, type II. Clusters of pale-staining foamy Kupffer cells that have eccentric nuclei. H&E.

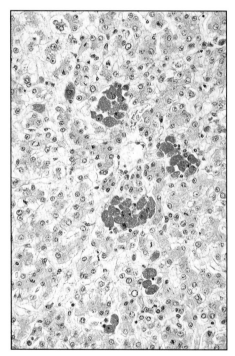

Fig. 5.52 • Same case as illustrated in Fig. 5.50. Ganglioside-laden Kupffer cells are intensely PAS-positive. PAS after diastase digestion.

lysosomal enzyme hexosaminidase leading to the accumulation of glycolipids, particularly GM_2 gangliosidase. Hexosaminidase consists of two major isozymes, hexosaminidase A, composed of an alpha and beta subunit, and hexosaminidase B, composed of two beta subunits. The alpha subunit has been localized to chromosome 15 and the beta subunit to chromosome 5. A lysosomal enzyme, GM_2 activator protein, also localized to chromosome 5,

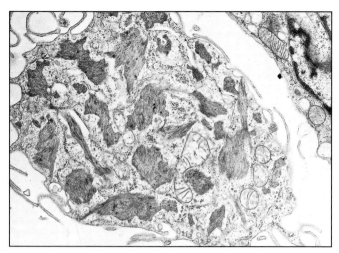

Fig. 5.53 • GM₁ gangliosidosis, type II. A Kupffer cell contains several angulated and focally membrane-bound inclusions. The inclusions are composed of granulofibrillar material and a few osmiophilic granules. ×13 500. Courtesy of Dr M Petrelli.

complexes with the lipid substrate for presentation to hexosaminidase for cleavage hydrolysis. Inheritance of all the variants is autosomal recessive. Prenatal diagnosis is available for all types.

Hexosaminidase alpha subunit defect or deficiency (Tay–Sachs disease; infantile Tay–Sachs disease)

These patients present at 3–6 months of age with motor weakness, apathy and feeding problems. The most common initial sign is the startle response to sound that is characterized by upper and lower extremity extension, often associated with a myoclonic jerk. Progressive weakness and hypotonia develop, with definite neurologic regression by 10–12 months of age. The mental and motor deterioration continue with death from bronchopneumonia, usually by 4 years of age. The typical, but not specific, cherry-red spot is observed in the macula during the early stages of the disease. Degeneration of the optic nerve is common and results in blindness. Megalocephaly may develop during the second year of life.

Tay–Sachs disease has a carrier frequency of 1 : 30 for Ashkenazi Jews and 1 : 300 for non-Jewish persons.[716] The diagnosis is based on the absence or near absence of hexosaminidase A in serum or fibroblast cell cultures. The deficiency allows massive accumulation of GM_2 ganglioside and asialo-GM_2 in enlarged cerebral neurons, retinal ganglion cells and autonomic ganglia.[716] Electron microscopy shows concentrically laminated inclusions or membranous cytoplasmic bodies in affected neurons, and somewhat more pleomorphic inclusions in the glia. Although hepatocytes appear normal by light microscopy, they may contain similar bodies by electron microscopic examination.[712]

Over 70 mutations in the hexosaminidase A gene, which is located on chromosome 15, have been described.[717] Prenatal diagnosis is performed in most centres.

Juvenile GM₂ gangliosidosis

This disorder presents with motor ataxia between 2 and 6 years of age followed by progressive dementia. Optic atrophy and retinitis pigmentosa occur late in the course of the disease without cherry-red spots. Decerebrate rigidity is present by 10–12 years of age and death from infection occurs between 10 to 15 years of age. Patients have a form of hexosaminidase A which cannot be activated.[718]

Hexosaminidase B subunit deficiency or defect (Sandhoff disease; infantile Sandhoff disease)

Previously, infants with Sandhoff disease were misdiagnosed as having Tay–Sachs disease because the clinical features and course are similar. In the first few months of life subtle signs of delayed motor development are noted. Cardiovascular symptoms may be observed early in the course of the disease along with minimal hepatosplenomegaly. During the second half of the first year little if any progress is made in motor or mental development. Cherry-red spots and early optic atrophy are evident by ophthalmoscopic examination. By 12 months of age the patients no longer use pincer grasp and develop bilateral pyramidal tract abnormalities, including increased deep tendon reflexes, spasticity and positive Hoffman and Babinski signs. In addition, there is regression in sitting, smiling and laughing appropriately. The psychomotor deterioration is progressive, with death resulting from aspiration pneumonia, usually between 22 and 36 months of age.[719] A juvenile form of this disease exists, but it lacks hepatic involvement.[720]

There are mild skeletal abnormalities in Sandhoff disease, and ECG changes range from mild left ventricular hypertrophy to severe abnormalities compatible with endocardial fibroelastosis. Vacuolated lymphocytes may be present in the peripheral blood. Markedly increased levels of globoside in the urinary sediment and plasma differentiate Sandhoff from Tay–Sachs disease.

This disease results from the deficient activity of both hexosaminidase A and B.[721] Decreased activities of both enzymes are found in biopsy specimens, peripheral leucocytes, platelets, cerebrospinal fluid, cultured skin fibroblasts and plasma. There is neural and visceral deposition of GM_2 ganglioside, its asialo derivative, and tetrahexosyl ceramide in affected infants.[719] The gene is found on chromosome 5q11.[722] It may be the case that only the hexosaminidase B gene is defective in the disease; the requirement for shared subunits between A and B may result in the complete absence of hexosaminidase activity.[723] Heterozygosity in the parents is more reliably established by examination of tissue specimens than of serum.[724]

Sandhoff disease shows no ethnic predilection.[725] The diagnosis can be made in utero by demonstration of deficient hexosaminidase levels in amniotic fluid.[726] Patients with Sandhoff disease were previously missed at autopsy because routine formalin fixation obscured the visceral lipid accumulation. However, 1 mm sections of Epon-embedded material reveal the lipid deposition when studied by light microscopy. Lysosomal lipid accumulation in the liver progresses with age; the lysosomes are twice the normal size at 3 months of age, and by 1 year many are distended by membranous lipid deposits to a diameter equal to that of the liver cell nucleus.[724,727] (Fig. 5.54). The extent, size and variation of the membranous deposits within lyso-

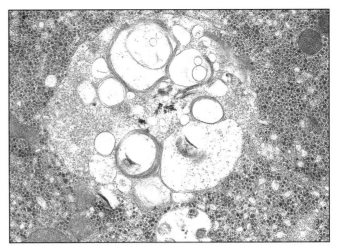

Fig. 5.54 • Sandhoff disease. Electron micrograph showing a large cytoplasmic lysosome containing single and laminated membranous structures within a finely particulate matrix. Note the size of the lysosome in comparison to the other cytoplasmic organelles. ×13 500.

somes are characteristic but not pathognomonic of Sandhoff disease. Kupffer cells are also involved and stain positively with the PAS reagent. Periportal fibrosis has been reported.[728]

Alpha-galactosidase A deficiency (Fabry disease)

Fabry disease is an X-linked disorder of glycosphingolipid metabolism. Hemizygous males are variably affected, while heterozygous females are often asymptomatic, but may develop significant clinical features with advancing age.[729,730] The disease is caused by a defect in the lysosomal hydrolase, α-galactosidase A[731] which results in accumulation of globotriaosylceramide in tissue lysosomes throughout the body. The gene localizes to chromosome Xq22.[732] The α-galactosidase gene has been cloned and several mutations are associated with Fabry disease.[733]

Clinical disease usually begins during childhood or adolescence with pain and paraesthesias in the extremities secondary to vascular substrate accumulation that affects peripheral nerves. Nausea, vomiting and diarrhoea are common.[734] Hypohidrosis results from vascular lesions in the autonomic nervous system. Skin signs include angiokeratomas.[735,736] Renal lipid deposition leads to proteinuria and gradual deterioration of renal function. Hypertension, left ventricular hypertrophy, myocardial ischaemia or infarction, and cerebral vascular disease may develop. Some patients have lymphoedema and mild anaemia. Death is usually from renal or cardiovascular complications. Atypical variants affecting predominantly the heart[737] or the kidneys[738,739] are well recognized. The diagnosis may be suspected by the combined findings of corneal dystrophy, lipid-laden and PAS-positive macrophages in the bone marrow, and birefringent Maltese crosses in the urinary sediment. Measurement of alpha-GLA enzyme activity in blood leukocytes is confirmatory. Examination of urinary sediment can be used as non-invasive method for early diagnosis and monitoring the effect of therapy.[740,741]

Phenytoin or carbamazepine are administered for the symptomatic relief of the neurologic problems. Renal transplantation may be required for kidney failure.[724] Two recombinant enzymes agalsidase-beta and agalsidase-alpha have been used clinically with significant long-term benefit, particularly when started before permanent tissue damage has occurred.[734,737,741,742]

The substance that accumulates in the tissues is globotriaosylceramide (GL-3). Pathological findings in Fabry disease have been reviewed in detail.[743] In the liver there is accumulation of GL-3 and cholesterol in Kupffer cells, portal macrophages and the endothelial cells of blood vessels. The cells are swollen and light tan in H&E preparations (Fig. 5.55). They contain birefringent crystals in frozen sections, and the Schultz modification of the Lieberman–Burchard reaction is moderately positive. The stored material is intensely PAS-positive and resists diastase digestion (Fig. 5.56). Ultrastructurally, the stored material in Fabry disease consists of concentrically laminated lysosomal inclusions with a periodicity of 5–6 nm (Figs 5.57 and 5.58). Lipid accumulations consisting of amorphous material as well as stacks of lamellar leaflets may be seen in hepatocytes, Kupffer cells and portal tract macrophages.[744] Two peroxidase-labelled lectins are found to be strongly reactive with the storage material of Fabry disease.[745] This observation has diagnostic implications since lectin binding is more specific than any other histochemical method. Lectin histochemistry with enzyme digestion enabled Kanda et al.[746] to detect α-galactosyl, β-galactosyl and glucosyl sugar residues in the lysosomal deposits at the ultrastructural level in Fabry disease. This technique has potential for the investigation of other glycolipid and glycoprotein storage diseases. The stored material is demonstrable by light and electron microscopy using a mouse monoclonal anti-GL-3 antibody.[747]

Sulphatide lipidosis (metachromatic leucodystrophy)

Metachromatic leukodystrophy (MLD) is a lysosomal lipid storage disorder caused by mutations in the gene for

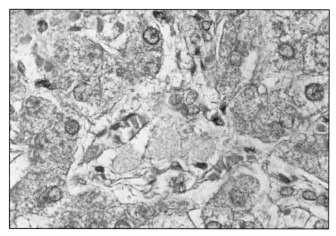

Fig. 5.55 • Fabry disease. Several portal macrophages are hypertrophied and have a tan-coloured cytoplasm. H&E.

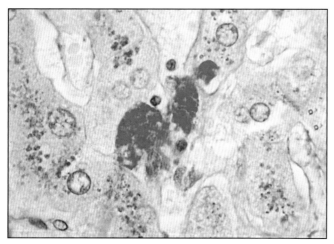

Fig. 5.56 • Fabry disease. Kupffer cells contain a granular material that stains intensely with PAS after diastase digestion.

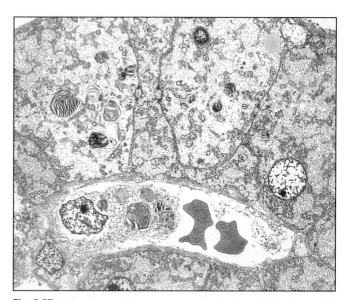

Fig. 5.57 • Fabry disease. Electron micrograph showing multiple dense and often laminated inclusions in hepatocytes and in a Kupffer cell. ×8800.

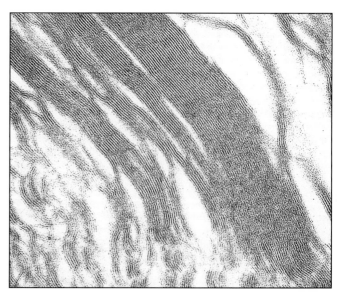

Fig. 5.58 • Fabry disease. Concentric lamination of inclusion material, with periodicity of 5–6 nm. ×170 000.

arylsulphatase A (ASA), an enzyme involved in the degradation of the sphingolipid 3-O-sulphogalactosylceramide (sulphatide). Sphingolipid storage results in progressive demyelination and severe neurologic symptoms. The ASA gene localized to chromosome 22q13;[748] multiple mutations which cause MLD have been described.[749]

Clinically, MLD is a group of disorders, differentiated by the time of onset of the symptoms.[750] Symptoms are worse the younger the presentation. Late infantile MLD presents between 1 and 2 years of age with developmental delay. Signs of neurological deterioration include progressive mental retardation, optic atrophy, loss of speech, hypertonic quadriplegia, ataxia and absent tendon reflexes. Pain in the extremities and unexplained fever are common. In the terminal stages of the disease, the patient loses sensory contact with the surroundings. Death results from infection or hyperpyrexia.

Early and late juvenile MLD present between 4 and 6 and 6 and 12 years, respectively. The neurological progression described above proceeds at a slower pace.[751] The adult form of MLD presents after 16 years of age and the mean duration of the disease is 15 years.[752] Most patients present with psychological problems, dementia or paralysis. Progressive neurological abnormalities develop during the course of the disease and include incoordination, ataxia, spastic paresis, visual disorders, tremors and athetotic movements. Death occurs from cachexia or pneumonia.[752]

Diagnosis is made by detection of sulphatide in peripheral nerves and urinary sediment. Deficiency of ASA can be demonstrated in leucocytes, cultured skin fibroblasts and amniotic cells. The latter was used as the basis for prenatal diagnosis, but the presence of a pseudodeficiency allele of ASA made diagnosis difficult by this method.[753,754] Bone marrow transplantation has produced minor, if any clinical improvement, in selected patients.[755,756]

Histologically, sulphatide accumulation has been demonstrated in the central nervous system, liver, gallbladder, pancreas and other organs.[757–759] The gallbladder is small and fibrotic and may show multiple polyps or papillomas, and contain calculi.[758,760–765] Microscopic examination reveals large foamy macrophages in the tunica propria (Fig. 5.59) that stain positively with cresyl violet, toluidine blue, the PAS reagent and the Hirsch–Pfeiffer stain[766] (Fig. 5.60).

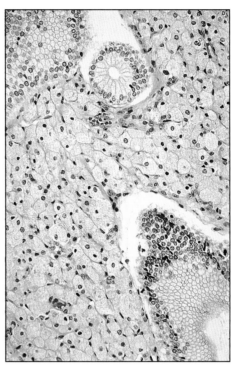

Fig. 5.59 • Metachromatic leucodystrophy. Foamy macrophages in the tunica propria of the gallbladder. H&E.

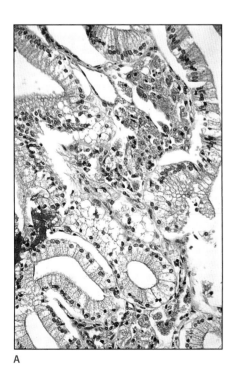

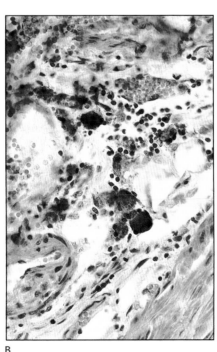

Fig. 5.60 • Metachromatic leucodystrophy. (A) Macrophages in gallbladder are PAS-positive after diastase digestion. (B) Macrophages are positive (brown) with the Hirsch–Pfeiffer stain.

A

B

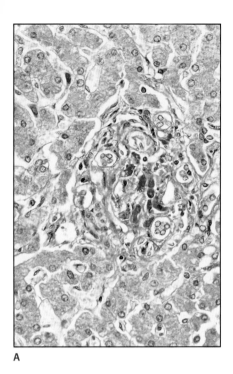
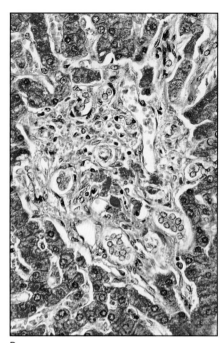

Fig. 5.61 • Metachromatic leucodystrophy. **(A)** A cluster of macrophages is present in a portal area. PAS after diastase digestion. **(B)** The macrophages have a bright-red colour with Masson trichrome stain.

A

B

In frozen sections they contain sudanophilic material that is anisotropic and can also be stained with the Schultz modification of the Lieberman–Burchard reaction due to simultaneous accumulation of cholesterol.[762] Metachromatic granules can be demonstrated in epithelial cells of the gall-bladder and to a lesser extent in those of the intrahepatic bile ducts.[758] In the liver, metachromatic granules may be seen in some portal macrophages, and less often in Kupffer cells and hepatocytes[759] (Fig. 5.61). Ultrastructurally, prismatic lysosomes are found in epithelial cells of the gallbladder. They are composed of periodic leaflets which appear tubular in cross section.[5]

Cerebrotendinous xanthomatosis

Cerebrotendinous xanthomatosis (CTX) is a rare autosomal recessive metabolic disease due to deficiency of mitochondrial C27-steroid 26-hydroxylase on the inner mitochondrial membrane which can be demonstrated in liver and cultured fibroblasts,[767–769] leading to tissue accumulation of cholestanol, a minor component in the human body. The defective gene, *sterol 27-hydroxylase*, localized to chromosome 2q33, has been cloned, and mutations associated with the disease have been described.[770,771]

The symptoms of this disease often begin with chronic diarrhoea in infancy. Neonatal hepatitis has been recorded in a few patients.[772–774] Juvenile cataracts develop during childhood,[775] as do tuberous xanthomas (particularly over the Achilles tendons). The neurological manifestations vary from mental retardation developing during adolescence to normal intelligence throughout adult life.[776,777] Spasticity and ataxia are usually detected in the second and third decades. Progression results in dementia, spinal cord paresis and peripheral neuropathy. Less frequent findings include gallstones and osteoporosis. Death in the fourth to sixth decades is usually related to neurological deterioration;

however, some patients develop early heart disease and/or atheroma.[778]

The 5-α-dihydro derivative of cholesterol, cholestanol (but not cholesterol), is elevated in serum. There is excessive deposit of cholestanol and cholesterol in tissues. Bile acid concentrations are low in bile, with high bile alcohol levels in bile and urine.[718] Heterozygotes can be detected by measurement of urinary bile alcohol levels following administration of a bile-salt-binding agent, cholestyramine.[719]

A combination of chenodeoxycholic acid and pravastatin (an inhibitor of 3-hydroxy-3-methylglutaryl coenzyme A, HMG-CoA reductase)[779] has reduced serum cholestanol and prevented an increase of total cholesterol. The therapy has stopped disease progression, but has not reversed clinical manifestations. Low density lipoprotein (LDL)-apharesis has been added to the regimen in a few patients.[780]

Liver specimens from two patients revealed intracellular inclusions that appeared either as amorphous pigment or had a crystalloid form.[781] The pigment is usually found in association with the smooth endoplasmic reticulum but occasionally lies free in the cytosol. An ultrastructural study of four cases revealed perisinusoidal fibrosis, bile canalicular changes (dilatation, distortion and loss of microvilli and an increase in microfilaments), fatty change, proliferation of smooth endoplasmic reticulum, accumulation of lipofuscin, focal cytoplasmic degeneration, proliferation of microbodies and prominent mitochondrial changes.[782] One patient had crystalloid cores in microbodies that disappeared after therapy.[782] The accumulated material may indicate the presence of non-metabolizable bile alcohols resulting from a defect of bile-acid synthesis.[781]

Ceramidase deficiency (Farber disease)

The disease is due to a deficit in acid ceramidase (AC), the lysosomal enzyme that degrades ceramide into sphingosine and fatty acid. The mode of inheritance is autosomal recessive. The acid ceramidase gene has been mapped to the chromosomal region 8p21.3–p22, and mutations responsible for Farber disease described.[783,784]

In the most common and classic form of the disease, *type I*, patients present between 2 weeks and 4 months of age. A triad of symptoms including joint disease, erythematous subcutaneous nodules (particularly at the wrists) and a hoarse cry, have been described. Aphonia may result from swelling and granuloma formation in the epiglottis and larynx. Other symptoms include poor feeding and difficult respiration, which results in poor weight gain, fever, and pneumonia.[785] Patients with severe involvement have generalized lymphadenopathy, an enlarged tongue, cardiac valve granulomas and hepatomegaly. Nerve involvement is common particularly in the lower motor neurons.

Milder forms of the disease, *types II and III*, have been described with no significant liver, lung, or brain involvement. *Type IV* ceramidase deficiency resembles a histiocytic disorder with neonatal hepatosplenomegaly progressing to death by 6 months of age.[786] *Type V* presents with psychomotor deterioration before 3 years of age with sparing of the viscera; findings include subcutaneous nodules, joint disease and macular cherry-red spots.[787] No therapy is available.

The diagnosis depends on demonstration of deficiency of acid ceramidase (less than 8% of normal) in cultured skin fibroblasts, white blood cells, or amniocytes.[788] Excess gangliosides are found in the granulomatous lesions and neurons of the cerebral cortex while lymph nodes, liver, kidney and lung (as well as the subcutaneous nodules) contain very high levels of free ceramide.[785]

Histological studies have shown granulomatous infiltrates in the subcutaneous nodules, periarticular and synovial tissue, lymph nodes, and to a lesser extent in the lungs, liver, spleen and other viscera.[785,789] They consist of lymphocytes, histiocytes and foam cells which contain PAS-positive material. Necrosis and dense fibrosis may develop in older lesions.[789] In one case, a liver biopsy revealed numerous atypical histiocytes with cytoplasmic vacuolization which filled the sinusoids and distorted the liver architecture. Post-mortem examination revealed massive histiocytic infiltration of the liver, spleen, lymph nodes, thymus and lungs.[790]

The granulomatous lesions of Farber disease have been reproduced experimentally by injection of ceramide from a patient and by commercial ceramide.[788] In patients, neurons of the central and autonomic nervous systems are distended with PAS-positive cytoplasmic material,[791] considered to be a mucopolysaccharide–polypeptide complex to which lipid was later added.[789] Ultrastructurally, the histiocytes contain rectilinear and curvilinear structures in the cytoplasm, inclusions that are sometimes referred to as Farber bodies.[792–794] Cross sections strongly suggest a tubular disposition of the stored material, the diameter being 20–23 nm. The Farber bodies have also been reproduced experimentally in mice by injection of ceramides and related sphingolipids.[795] Hepatocytic dense bodies and clear vacuoles have been described in a case studied by electron microscopy.[794] The former were generally round, osmiophilic deposits that surrounded electron-lucent material in a dense granular matrix. The clear vacuoles, which were also noted in cells lining intrahepatic bile ducts, resembled those seen in the mucopolysaccharidoses. Banana-like bodies have been seen in Schwann cells ultrastructurally.[796] They resemble miniature bananas and seem to arise from needle-like, membrane-bound inclusions. On average, they are about 1.6 µm long and have a diameter of 0.23 µm.

Glycosyl ceramide lipidosis (Gaucher disease)

Gaucher disease, the most common lysosomal disorder, is caused by deficiency in acid β-glucosidase (glucocerebrosidase) resulting in lysosomal accumulation of glucosylceramide (glucocerebroside), mainly in macrophages.[797,798]

There are three major phenotypes of Gaucher disease (Table 5.2).[799]

Type I (chronic non-neuronopathic) can be detected at any age including the ninth decade. The usual presentation is

Table 5.2	Gaucher disease—major clinical phenotypes		
Clinical features	**Type I**	**Type II**	**Type III**
Onset	Childhood/adulthood	Infancy	Childhood/adolescence
Hepatosplenomegaly	Mild to severe	Moderate	Mild to severe
Skeletal disease	Mild to severe	Minimal	Mild to severe
Neurodegeneration	Absent	++++	+ to ++++
Survival	<5 to >80 years	~2 years	<5 to ~50 years
Ethnic predilection	Ashkenazi Jews	Pan-ethnic	Swedish
Frequency estimates	~1/40 000 to 1/300 000 1/400–1/800 in Ashkenazi Jews	<1/100 000	<1/100 000
Relative frequency	94%	<1%	5%

hepatosplenomegaly in late childhood or adolescence. Over 50% of patients have mild haemorrhagic phenomenon associated with thrombocytopenia.[800] Variable skin pigmentation is recorded.[801] Adolescent patients may have aseptic necrosis of the metaphyseal areas, and 10% of patients have skeletal symptoms that include bone pain, spontaneous fractures, degenerative hip disease, or pseudo-osteomyelitis. Sixty per cent of patients have abnormal skeletal radiographs including the classic 'Erlenmeyer flask' deformity.[802] Bone symptoms and radiograph anomalies seem more likely to occur in splenectomized patients.[803] The lungs are rarely affected by infiltration by storage cells.[804] Hepatomegaly is common, often without significant clinical consequences. However, massive hepatic fibrosis with portal hypertension does occur[805]and has required liver transplantation in a 15 year old girl, despite 6 years of enzyme replacement therapy.[806] One patient presented with neonatal cholestasis.[807] Partial or complete splenectomy is often performed for pancytopenia.[808,809] Splenic infarctions may cause severe left upper quadrant pain.[810] Renal failure is rare. According to data from the International Gaucher Registry, Gaucher patients have an increased risk of developing multiple myeloma, but no other tumours.[811]

Type II (infantile disease) presents during the first 3 months of life with hepatosplenomegaly, cough, and neurological signs. Patients may present with hydrops fetalis, ichthyosis, or collodion skin.[812–816] Late manifestations include laryngeal stridor and pulmonary infiltrates. Physical findings include hepatosplenomegaly, lymphadenopathy, opisthotonic posturing, spasticity, and cranial nerve involvement. Death usually occurs by 3 years of age.

Type III (juvenile disease) presents with hepatosplenomegaly followed by gradual mental deterioration any time after the first year of life. Initial evidence of neurological involvement may not present until adulthood with supranuclear oculomotor deficits.[817] Death occurs in the second to fourth decades. Three subtypes are now described: (i) *Type IIIa* is primarily a neurological disorder in adolescence with mild visceral involvement. Death is from slowly progressive neurologic degeneration. Myoclonic seizures are common. (ii) *Type IIIb* has the severe visceral involvement with massive hepatomegaly, oesophageal varices, and severe skeletal involvement. Horizontal supranuclear gaze paresis is the major neurological finding.[818] Death is from hepatic or pulmonary complications. Hepatocytes rarely accumulate glucocerebroside because of bile excretion.[819] Disease is accelerated by splenectomy. (iii) *Type IIIc* is an unusual variant with calcification of the left-sided heart valves and corneal opacifications.[820] Other visceral involvement is mild. In type III typical complications of portal hypertension occur if cirrhosis develops.[821] Hepatic calcification is rare.[822] Pulmonary arteriovenous shunts causing hypoxia and cyanosis occur mainly in patients with liver disease.[804] There is also infiltration of the lungs with storage cells. The pulmonary shunts as well as the cirrhosis respond to liver transplantation. Based on the clinical presentation along with the detected genotypic heterogeneity Goker-Alpan et al.[823] have suggested that neuronopathic Gaucher disease is more likely to be a continuum of phenotypes from type II

with severe perinatal presentation to mild type III with oculomotor problems.

The gene for acid β-glucosidase is on chromosome 1q21.[824,825] Nearly 200 mutations in this gene have been described.[826] Although there is a trend for the *N370S* allele to be associated with milder and non-neuronopathic disease and the *L444P* allele to be strongly associated with neuronopathic forms, genotype-phenotype correlations are poor,[827] implicating that if a mutation in the glucocerebrosidase gene is required, other factors play an important role in the manifestation of the disease. Glucocerebrosidase is synthesized on endoplasmic reticulum (ER)-bound polyribosomes and translocated into the ER. Following N-linked glycosylations, it is transported to the Golgi apparatus, from where it is trafficked to the lysosomes. The degree of ER retention and proteasomal degradation and impaired trafficking of the mutants are likely factors that determine disease severity.[828,829]

A rare variant of Gaucher disease is due to deficiency in small acidic protein activator, saposin C, which is required for optimal hydrolysis of sphingolipids. Mutation in the saposin gene localized to chromosome 10, leads to a variant with a normal acid β-glucosidase enzyme activity which will not be influenced by enzyme therapy.[830,831]

Diagnosis of Gaucher disease is made by assay of acid β-glucosidase enzyme in white blood cells or cultured fibroblasts. Prenatal diagnosis is by assay of enzyme activity in amniocytes or chorionic villi; polymerase chain reaction can be performed when the genetic mutation is known in both parents.[799]

Therapy for type I disease is intravenous recombinant enzyme replacement (ERT) designed to be taken up by the mannose receptor on macrophages.[832,833] This results in rapid reversal of liver, splenic and bone marrow pathology with clinical improvement, but skeletal disease responds more slowly or may be resistant[834,835] the poorest responses were in splenectomized patients, or patients with advanced liver, splenic and bone marrow disease. As an alternative to ERT, substrate reduction using oral miglustat, an inhibitor of glucosylceramide synthase, a key enzyme in glycosphingolipid synthesis, has been shown to produce slower and less robust responses than those obtained with enzyme replacement.[836] Neurological disease does not respond as the enzyme does not cross the blood-brain barrier, although stabilization or some improvement may be achieved with intravenous treatment in very high dose in type III disease.[837]

Bone marrow transplantation has been successful but with significant morbidity. Liver transplantation is rarely indicated and must be accompanied by other therapy in order to obtain a cure.[838] Chimerism following hepatic transplantation will not reliably produce a cure.[839] Gene therapy is being pursued vigorously. A knockout mouse model is available to assist in these studies.[840]

Histiocytes containing glycocerebroside (Gaucher cells) are dispersed throughout the reticuloendothelial system. A full surface marker study of the splenic storage cells in a case of Gaucher disease has largely substantiated the monocyte/histiocyte nature of Gaucher cells.[841] Scanning electron

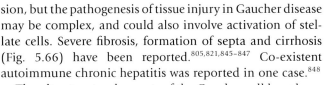

microscopy reveals microvilli, ruffles, ridges and blebs of varying number and shape on their surface.[842] In the liver, Kupffer cells and portal macrophages are primarily affected. The distribution may be focal or zonal, with the perivenular zone being mainly affected. The cells, which can measure up to 100 μm, in maximum dimension are lightly stained with eosin, have a faintly striated or crinkled cytoplasm and pyknotic, eccentric or centrally located nuclei (Fig. 5.62). The striations are best demonstrated with the Masson trichrome or a PAS stain (Fig. 5.63). Intense acid phosphatase (Fig. 5.64) and lysozyme activity are found by histochemical or immunohistochemical methods respectively. Gaucher cells are also strongly immunoreactive to anti-KP-1 (Fig. 5.65). They usually contain a small amount of iron that is derived both from ingested erythrocytes and from the labile plasma pool.[843] Other staining reactions of Gaucher cells have been reviewed.[843,844]

Gaucher cells in the liver may enlarge to such an extent that they completely block sinusoidal spaces. They also compress hepatocytes with progressive atrophy and disruption of the hepatic plates. There is a variable increase in the number of reticulin and collagen fibres in the space of Disse. Perisinusoidal fibrosis and mechanical blockage of sinusoidal spaces are presumed to be the cause of portal hyperten-

sion, but the pathogenesis of tissue injury in Gaucher disease may be complex, and could also involve activation of stellate cells. Severe fibrosis, formation of septa and cirrhosis (Fig. 5.66) have been reported.[805,821,845–847] Co-existent autoimmune chronic hepatitis was reported in one case.[848]

The ultrastructural aspects of the Gaucher cell have been described in detail.[5,843,844,849] The cytoplasm is filled with

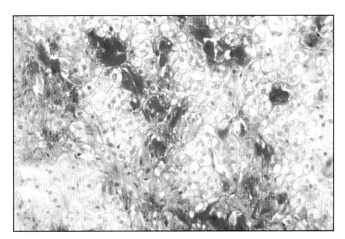

Fig. 5.64 • Gaucher cells exhibit marked acid phosphatase activity (red). Phenylphosphate Mx acid phosphatase reaction.

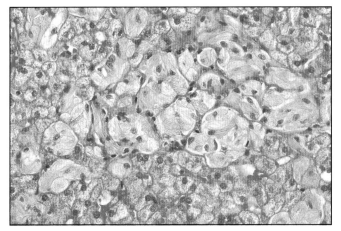

Fig. 5.62 • Pale-staining Gaucher cells have a faintly striated cytoplasm. H&E.

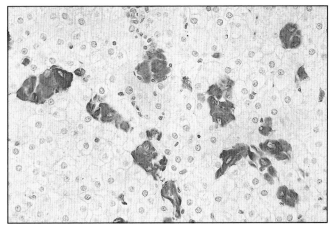

Fig. 5.65 • Gaucher cells are strongly immunoreactive to KP-1 antibody.

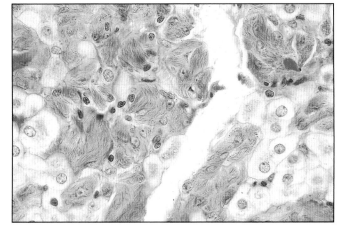

Fig. 5.63 • Gaucher disease. Striations are well visualized in a PAS after diastase digestion.

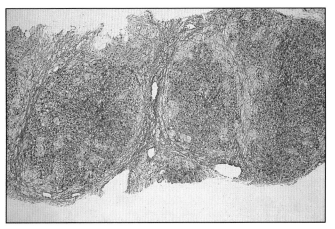

Fig. 5.66 • Gaucher disease. Section of needle biopsy specimen reveals established cirrhosis. Masson trichrome.

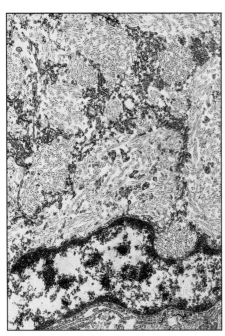

Fig. 5.67 • Electron micrograph showing cytoplasm of a Gaucher cell that is packed with tubules cut tangentially or in cross section. ×8475.

spindle or rod-shaped inclusion bodies bounded by a limiting membrane; they measure 0.6 μm in diameter (Fig. 5.67). In cross section the inclusions contain numerous small tubules, 13–75 nm in diameter. Acid phosphatase activity has been localized to the inclusions by electron microscopic histochemistry.[849] Freeze-fracture and X-ray diffraction analysis of the purified deposits have shown them to consist of twisted membranous bilayers 6 μm in thickness.[850] The iron in the Gaucher cell is dispersed as individual micelles of ferritin.[851]

Sphingomyelin-cholesterol lipidosis (Niemann–Pick disease)

Niemann–Pick disease[852,853] refers to a group of storage disorders with characteristic foamy storage cells currently grouped into type A, B and C. Type A and B are the 2 phenotypic variants caused by mutation in the sphingomyelin phosphodiesterase-1 gene *(SMPD1)* localized to chromosome 11p15.4. The gene encodes acid sphingomyelinase (ASM) whose deficiency leads to sphingomyelin accumulation in both types which are markedly different clinically. Mutations in both type A and B have been documented and may bear some correlation with phenotype.[854] *Type A Niemann–Pick disease* (NPA) begins in utero and is detected after birth by massive hepatosplenomegaly; severe disease presents as hydrops fetalis.[855,856] Placental ultrasonic abnormalities caused by storage cells can be detected in the first two trimesters.[857] Paucity of the intrahepatic bile ducts has been reported, and giant cell transformation with pruritus has been observed in infants.[858] Abnormal neurological development may not be detected until 3 months of age; developmental regression occurs by 1 year of age. Moderate lymphadenopathy may be present. Malnutrition, weakness

and hypotonia lead to death between 2 and 5 years of age. Macular cherry-red spots are found in 50% of patients.[859]

Although fatal liver failure has been documented in two children with *Type B Niemann–Pick disease* (NPB),[860] and cirrhosis with complications of portal hypertension has been reported in a number of adults,[861–863] the natural history of type B patients is characterized by hepatosplenomegaly with stable liver dysfunction and progressive hypersplenism, worsening atherogenic lipid profile and gradual deterioration in pulmonary function due to foam cell infiltration.[864] The latter has more clinical relevance than in type A and can result in death. Rupture of the spleen is another cause of death. Abnormal linear growth and delayed skeletal maturation are common in children and adolescents.[865] Macular cherry-red spots are detected in less than 10% of patients. Cerebellar ataxia may be present.

The finding of large foamy macrophages in bone marrow, liver or spleen may be the initial clue to the diagnosis. The diagnosis of NPA and NPB is confirmed by sphingomyelinase assay in leukocytes, lymphocytes or skin fibroblasts. Antenatal diagnosis is possible by assaying ASM activity in chorionic villi or cultured amniocytes.[866]

Type C Niemann–Pick disease (NPC) is clinically, biochemically and genetically distinct from type A and B. It is caused by a defect in intracellular cholesterol and glycosphingolipid trafficking which leads to the accumulation of unesterified cholesterol and other lipids in endo/lysosomal compartments.[867] Approximately 95% of patients have mutations in *NPC 1* gene (mapped to chromosome 18q11–12) which encode a large endosomal membrane glycoprotein. The remainder have mutations in the *NPC 2/ HE1* gene (mapped at 14q24.3) which encodes a small soluble lysosomal protein with cholesterol-binding properties.[866,868] The identical biochemical patterns observed in NPC1 and NPC2 mutants suggest that the two proteins function in a coordinate fashion. Numerous mutations have been identified,[869] with the recent finding that the Q775P mutation may correlate with a severe infantile neurological form and the C177Y mutation with a late infantile clinical phenotype.[870]

NPC presents anytime between the perinatal period and adulthood. There may be foetal ascites.[871] Two-thirds of patients present with neonatal hepatitis syndrome. Most patients clear their cholestasis but have residual mild hepatosplenomegaly. However, liver failure with cholestasis develops in 10% of cases.[872] Two reported patients had biliary atresia and meconium ileus.[873] Severe forms of the disease result in death by 3 to 5 years of age. Other patients present later with mild splenomegaly which regresses with aging.[872,874] All patients develop neurological complications. The most consistent finding is vertical supranuclear gaze palsy. Other manifestations include cerebellar involvement, cataplexy with or without narcolepsy, and learning difficulties. Late changes include mental regression, seizures and neurological pyramidal signs.[874] One patient with sea-blue histiocytes developed hepatocellular carcinoma with recurrence in the transplanted liver along with further neurological deterioration.[875]

As for NPA and NPB, the finding of large foamy macrophages in bone marrow, liver or spleen may be the initial clue to the diagnosis. The foam cells can resemble sea-blue histiocytes in 50% of cases. The diagnosis of NPC is further suspected by normal sphyngomyelinase levels. The accumulation of unesterified cholesterol in lysosomes is confirmatory. Specialized laboratories prefer to work with cultured fibroblasts for diagnosis. Filipin staining demonstrates the intense staining of unesterified cholesterol. By this technique, lysosomal cholesterol may not be deemed abnormal in 15% of cases. Challenging fibroblasts with purified human LDL 3 days after culture in lipoprotein deficient media provides more consistent results.[876] Cholesterol ester measurements can be performed. LDL cholesterol accumulates in lysosomes; transport to other sites is retarded. There is no repression of cholesterol and LDL receptor synthesis. For the prenatal diagnosis, demonstration of an abnormal intracellular cholesterol trafficking is a complex procedure, and mutational analysis (*NPC1* or *NPC2/HE1* gene), whenever feasible, represents a major advance.[877]

Therapeutic trials with low cholesterol diets, cholestyramine, niacin, and lovastatin have been unsuccessful in altering the course of NPC.[878] At the present time no specific therapy has emerged for the treatment of NPA, NPB or NPC.

Spontaneous mouse models of NPC[879,880] have been used to study cholesterol accumulation and cell death;[881] other studies of NPC gene function are performed on fibroblast cell lines.[868] A sphyngomyelinase knock-out mice for NPA/NPB is a model used to evaluate hepatic gene transfer by means of recombinant encoding sphingomyelinase.[882] A study of pulmonary macrophages from the same model suggests that macrophage lipid accumulation leads to abnormalities in mannose 6-phosphate receptor trafficking and/or degradation, resulting in reduced enzyme uptake.[883]

Both the liver and the spleen are enlarged in Niemann–Pick disease. The characteristic finding is the presence of large macrophages with a foamy or microvesicular cytoplasm. These are least conspicuous and easily overlooked in type C, particularly in the liver with associated hepatitis, but generally obvious in a bone marrow smear (Fig. 5.68). In the liver, Kupffer cells are markedly hypertrophied and have a vacuolated cytoplasm (Fig. 5.69(A)). They are often lighttan in colour due to their content of lipofuscin (ceroid). A single small eccentric or centrally placed nucleus is generally found in each cell. Hepatocytes also contain sphingomyelin, and their cytoplasm shows progressive loss of eosinophilia with increasing vacuolization, until they become indistinguishable from affected Kupffer cells. The foam cells are autofluorescent but have a nodular pattern, in contrast to the uniform fluorescence of Gaucher cells.[884] The cells are positively stained with oil red O, Luxol fast

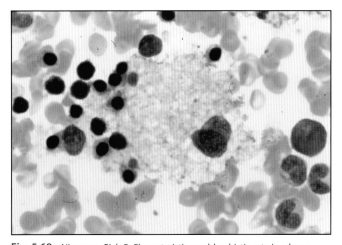

Fig. 5.68 • Niemann–Pick C. Characteristic sea-blue histiocyte in a bone marrow smear.

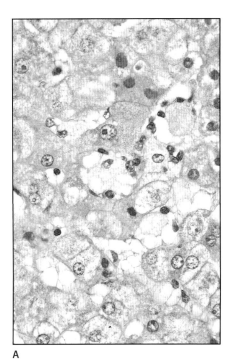

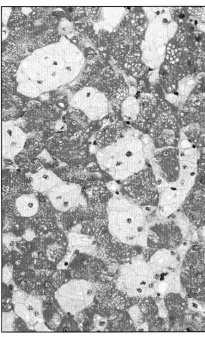

Fig. 5.69 • Niemann–Pick disease. **(A)** Kupffer cells storing sphingomyelin are foamy. H&E. **(B)** Pale-staining clusters of foam cells containing sphingomyelin stand out in sharp contrast to glycogen-containing (purple) liver cells. PAS.

A

B

blue and Baker's acid haematin stain in frozen sections; the latter stain becomes negative after pyridine extraction. The cytoplasm is variably PAS-positive or negative, depending on the quantity of lipofuscin (Fig. 5.69(B)). The presence of the cholesterol-containing sea-blue histiocytes in Niemann–Pick type C has already been touched upon. Intrahepatic cholestasis is found in some infants, and a number of cases with giant-cell transformation have been reported in both NPC and NPB disease.[858,885–888] As is the case in Gaucher disease and other metabolic disorders, there may be varying degrees of atrophy of hepatic plates and parenchymal fibrosis (Fig. 5.70). A true cirrhosis has been reported in both children and adults.[863] Fibrosis in type B Niemann–Pick disease may depend on the phenotype.[862]

Ultrastructurally, the foam cells contain dense mixed lipid inclusions or lipid cytosomes; these are polymorphic and range from less than 1 μm to 5 μm in diameter.[884] The inclusions consist of concentrically laminated myelin-like figures with a periodicity of roughly 5 nm (Fig. 5.71).[5,889] Typical lipofuscin bodies, lipid droplets and cholesterol clefts may also be observed.[5]

Peroxisomal disorders

Peroxisomes may form by synthesis of their membranes followed by importation of enzymes synthesized elsewhere in the cell, or by budding from pre-existing peroxisomes. They perform numerous functions including catabolism of glyoxylate, α-oxidation of phytanic acid, biosynthesis of bile acids, biosynthesis of ether phospholipids (plasmalogens), biosynthesis of docosahexaenoic acid, and β-oxidation of fatty acids; they are essential for β-oxidation of very long chain (C:24 or 26) fatty acids. The peroxisomal disorders are usually subdivided into two subgroups including: (i) *the peroxisomal biogenesis disorders*, in which an absence or decreased number of peroxisomes results in multiple functional defects (Zellweger syndrome, neonatal adrenoleucodystrophy, infantile Refsum disease, referred to as the Zellweger spectrum, and rhizomelic chondrodysplasia punctata, which is clearly distinct from the others); and (ii) *the single peroxisomal (enzyme-) protein deficiencies* with decreased or absent activity of one peroxisomal enzyme (X-linked adrenoleucodystrophy, di- and trihydroxycholestanoic acidaemia, mevalonate kinase deficiency, adult Refsum disease, hyperoxaluria type I, and others).[890] At least 21 genetic disorders have now been found that are linked to peroxisomal dysfunction.[891] Only the peroxisomal disorders that result in liver disease, namely Zellweger syndrome, di- and trihydroxycholestanoic acidaemia and mevalonate kinase deficiency, are discussed.

Peroxisomal biogenesis disorders

Diseases of the Zellweger spectrum represent a continuum of clinical disorders with Zellweger syndrome having the most severe phenotype, and neonatal adrenoleukodystrophy and infantile Refsum disease having progressively milder phenotypes. The Zellweger syndrome spectrum is caused by defects in any of at least 12 peroxin (PEX) genes required for normal organelle assembly. Most common are mutations in *PEX1*, which encodes a 143-kDa AAA ATPase protein needed for peroxisome biogenesis, followed by *PEX26, PEX6, PEX12, PEX10,* and *PEX2*.[892] The *PEX1* mutations identified to date comprise insertions, deletions, nonsense, missense, and splice site mutations. Mutations that produce premature truncation codons (PTCs) are distributed throughout the *PEX1* gene, whereas the majority of missense mutations segregate with the two essential AAA domains of the PEX1 protein. Severity at the two ends of the Zellweger spectrum (ZS) correlates broadly with mutation type and impact (i.e., the severe ZS correlates with PTCs on both alleles, and the milder phenotypes correlate

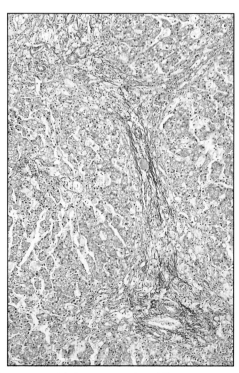

Fig. 5.70 • Niemann–Pick disease. Parenchymal fibrosis is associated with the foam cells. Masson trichrome.

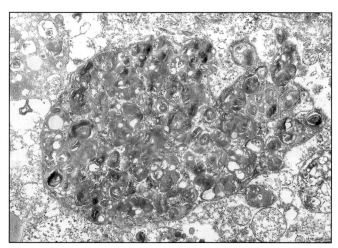

Fig. 5.71 • Niemann–Pick disease. Electron micrograph showing electron-opaque laminated inclusions densely packed in the cytoplasm of a Kupffer cell. ×7900.

with missense mutations), but exceptions to these general correlations exist.[893] Chromosomes 12, 8, 7 and 6 contain loci associated with Zellweger disease spectrum.[894–900]

Zellweger syndrome

Patients present at birth with a characteristic facial dysmorphia, severe hypotonia, hepatomegaly, renal cysts, optic atrophy, seizures and severe neurological impairment.[901] Diagnosis is made through a combination of studies. These include serum plasma quantitation of very long chain fatty acids, pipecolic acid and phytanic acid, and measurement of red cell plasmalogens.[902–904] Liver biopsy with electron microscopy establishes the absence of peroxisomes.[905,906] Peroxisomal enzymes and structure can be studied in cultured fibroblasts.[907]

The incidence of Zellweger syndrome is estimated at 1 in 25 000 to 1 in 100 000 births.[908] Inheritance is autosomal recessive. Prenatal diagnosis in affected families is possible using techniques to assess adequate peroxisomal function. Referral to a qualified centre is essential. Therapy is supportive.

Less severe variants of classic Zellweger syndrome include *neonatal adrenoleucodystrophy and infantile Refsum disease.*[901] The dysmorphic features are less striking than those of classic Zellweger syndrome, and the peroxisomes in the liver are not as markedly diminished.[909] Inasmuch as these diseases are milder, with some hope for neurological development, controlled clinical trials of therapies to bypass the deficient peroxisomal enzymes have been initiated.[910]

Whereas much progress has been made in biochemistry and genetics of peroxisomal disorders, the pathophysiology and therapy has been slow.[890] The increasing availability of mouse models for these disorders is in this respect a major step forward.[911,912]

Autopsy findings in Zellweger syndrome include cerebral anomalies (abnormal convolutional pattern, heterotopic cortex, olivary dysplasia), renal glomerular microcysts, cardiovascular defects (patent ductus and patent foramen ovale), thymic anomalies and pancreatic islet cell hyperplasia.[913]

The hepatic histopathological findings in Zellweger syndrome have not been consistent, and some cases have shown no or only minimal, non-specific alterations. Portal inflammation, periportal fibrosis, focal necrosis with progression to parenchymal fibrosis, cholestasis and haemosiderosis have been recorded.[913–918] In a survey of the literature, Gilchrist et al.[915] found reduction of 'cholangioles' in 23% of cases. Cases with severe fibrosis and disruption of the parenchyma[917–921] and even cirrhosis[906,922,923] have been described.

The absence of peroxisomes in liver cells, first described by Goldfischer et al.,[924] has been a consistent finding in subsequent ultrastructural studies.[5,905,917,918] In some cases, however, small bodies resembling incompletely developed peroxisomes could be found.[5] A variant of the disease with detectable hepatic peroxisomes has also been reported.[925] Another ultrastructural feature is the occurrence within macrophages of large angulate lysosomes filled with fine

double lamellae.[917] Mitochondria show disarrangement and twisting of their cristae and have a dense matrix.[5,917,926] The absence of catalase, a peroxisomal enzyme, was demonstrated at the ultrastructural level in a liver biopsy specimen from a patient with Zellweger syndrome. It is also possible to demonstrate several other peroxisomal enzymes by immunogold labelling.[927]

In adrenoleucodystrophy, there is variable fibrosis and irregular nodularity of the hepatic parenchyma.[928,929] Cirrhosis was reported in one case.[930] PAS-positive macrophages and Kupffer cells were identified in another.[931] Ultrastructurally, hepatic peroxisomes are either absent or markedly reduced in number and size[909,930] and may contain electron-dense cores.[932] Lamellar cytoplasmic inclusions are found in Kupffer cells and hepatocytes.[931,932] Mitochondria with crystalline inclusions and/or abnormal cristae have also been noted.[932]

An accentuated lobular architecture, with fibrous bands linking portal areas together, has been observed in Refsum disease.[933] A micronodular cirrhosis was found in a patient who died at the age of 12 years.[933] A deficiency of hepatic peroxisomes has been detected ultrastructurally and cytochemically.[934–936] Phillips et al.[5] believe that while some hepatocytes totally lack peroxisomes, others contain very small underdeveloped ones that sometimes have a very dense matrix. They have also noted the presence of numerous angulate lysosomes in Kupffer cells in this disorder.

Disorders with a single peroxisomal functional deficiency

Di- and trihydroxycholestanoic acidaemia

Patients with this rare disease present with severe cholestasis and obstructive jaundice. Trihydroxy-coprostanic acid coenzyme A (THCA-CoA) a bile acid ester, is converted to δ4-THCA initiated by a specific THCA-CoA oxidase. Similarly, dihydroxycoprostanic acid is also processed in the peroxisomes. In di- and trihydroxycholestanoic acidaemia (alligator bile syndrome), serum levels of these precursors are high, as either transport of the CoA ester into the peroxisome or subsequent processing are deficient.[937–939] An isolated case of THCA-CoA has been subsequently reallocated to a peroxisomal biogenesis disorder on the basis of mutations in the *PEX12* gene, although all peroxisomal functions in cultured skin fibroblasts were normal leading the author to question the existence of THCA-CoA as an entity.[940]

Mevalonate kinase deficiency

The gene encoding mevalonate kinase (MVK) was mapped by fluorescence in situ hybridization to chromosome 14q24.[941] Gene mutations lead to two groups of disorders, *mevalonate aciduria* the first recognized defect in the biosynthesis of cholesterol and isoprenoids, a consequence of severe deficiency in MVK,[942] and *hyper IgD syndrome (HIDS)/periodic fever* seemingly associated with mild deficiency.[943]

The clinical spectrum of mevalonate aciduria shows varying degrees of severity despite absent MVK activity in all. Severely affected patients have profound developmental delay, dysmorphic facies, cataracts, hepatosplenomegaly, lymphadenopathy, and anaemia, as well as diarrhoea and malabsorption, and died in infancy. Less severely affected patients have psychomotor retardation, hypotonia, myopathy, and ataxia. All patients will have recurrent crises in which there was fever, lymphadenopathy, increase in size of liver and spleen, arthralgia, oedema, and a morbilliform rash.[942,944] Anaemia, petechiae, hepatosplenomegaly, leukocytosis, and recurrent febrile episodes, and facial rashes, in cases without significant neurologic abnormalities raise the differential diagnosis of congenital infections, myelodysplastic syndromes, or chronic leukemia.[945] Mevalonic acid concentrations are grossly elevated in body fluids in all patients, because of disordered biosynthesis of cholesterol. Mevalonic acid can be detected clinically by urinary organic acid analysis. Prenatal diagnosis is possible by measurement of mevalonic acid in amniotic fluid.[942]

Hyper IgD syndrome (HIDS)/periodic fever is characterized by recurrent attack of spiking fever with early onset before one year of age, associated with abdominal pains (72%), vomiting (56%), diarrhoea (82%), poly-arthralgia (80%) non-destructive arthritis (68%). Eighty-two percent of patients report skin lesions, with vasculitis histologically. Swollen, tender lymph nodes, are noted most often in the cervical region. Serum IgD levels (more than 100 U/mL) remain elevated during the attack, most often associated with raised IgA levels.[943] The diagnosis is confirmed by MVK gene screening, in particular the V377I mutation which has been identified exclusively in HIDS patients.[946,947] Hepatomegaly is common, cholestatic liver disease is recorded,[945] but detailed histological changes in these disorders are not available.

Mitochondrial cytopathies and related conditions

Primary mitochondrial disorders

Mitochondrial disorders comprise an extremely broad array of diseases affecting multiple organ systems.[948–951] Mitochondriopathies include many disorders which affect the neuromuscular system with no known hepatic involvement.[952] A disorder in mitochondrial function or structure may result in a combination of many diverse symptoms, including hepatic failure, or cholestasis with preserved liver function, cardiomyopathy, pigmentary retinopathy, myoclonic seizures, hypotonia, proximal tubular disorder, endocrinopathies or pancytopenia. Disease severity is highly variable, as are the time of presentation and rate of disease progression. Inherited hepatic mitochondriopathies tend to present clinically in infancy or childhood; late hepatic involvement is less common.

Classification of the mitochondriopathies is also challenging, especially as the number of known mitochondrial cytopathies continues to expand. Diseases can be classified by the genetic defect (autosomal or mitochondrial) or by the affected enzyme system (oxidative phosphorylation or fatty acid oxidation). A comprehensive classification of mitochondrial disease has recently been proposed.[953] In this section, we will focus on mitochondrial disorders in which liver disease is an important clinical feature. Acquired hepatic mitochondrial disorders, for example, associated with toxicity of nucleoside analogue retroviral drugs or with alcoholic liver disease, are discussed in other chapters.

Mitochondria produce ATP within cells and, coincidentally, activated oxygen species; in hepatocytes mitochondria play an important role in β-oxidation. Mitochondria are unique among cell organelles in having their own complement of DNA, which encodes some of the proteins in the respiratory chain responsible for oxidative phosphorylation, as well as specific RNAs critical to protein synthesis in mitochondria. Inheritance of mitochrondrial DNA (mtDNA) is along maternal lines. Mitochondria are derived almost exclusively from the ovum, since sperm contain very few mitochondria. Mitochondria have their own DNA polymerase, polymerase γ, for production of mtDNA. Proofreading and DNA repair capacities are extremely limited in mitochondria. Tissue expression of mtDNA abnormalities is complex, depending on the population of mitochondria in each cell. Gene localization and determination of specific genetic defects are available for some of the mitochondriopathies. Lack of simple one-to-one correspondence of a certain mtDNA mutation to a clinical disease pattern has made genotype-phenotype correlations difficult.

Defects originating from mutations in nuclear DNA are inherited as autosomal traits whereas defects in mitochondrial DNA are inherited maternally. Mitochondrial disorders are rare, but their exact incidence is undetermined, mainly because until recently accurate diagnosis was difficult. Genetic mitochondrial disorders can be classified on the basis of whether the mutations affect a single protein in the mitochondrion or production of mtDNA. Mutations affecting single proteins in the repiratory chain have been described in detail. The usual clinical features are either severe neonatal hepatitis syndrome or else neonatal liver failure.[954–961] Children with mitochondrial respiratory chain defects may be at increased risk to develop hepatocellular carcinoma.[962] A cytochrome c oxidase deficiency found in Quebec kindreds may be associated with fatty liver.[963] Abnormalities in proteins vital to the assembly of respiratory chain proteins can also cause liver disease.[964] GRACILE syndrome is a severe multisystem autosomal recessive disorder with features including cholestasis and hepatic iron overload and lactic acidsosis; the mutation is in the gene for the protein *BCS1L* which is required for assembly of complex III.[965] Liver failure due to *BCS1L* mutations has also been described.[966] Another important group of mitochondrial disorders display mtDNA depletion. Dysfunction of the respiratory chain may occur as a consequence. Two specific gene defects are known to be associated with mtDNA depletion; of these mutations in *deoxyguanosine kinase (dGK or DGOUK)* is the abnormality more frequently associated with liver disease.[967–971] Recent studies have shown that Alpers syndrome, which typically follows a relatively more chronic course, is associated with mutations in DNA polymerase γ.[972–975] Mutations in polymerase γ can lead to a diverse spectrum of clinical disease, and this may account for some of the heterogeneity of Alpers syndrome.[976]

Clinically, the mitochondrial cytopathies with liver disease present in one of two ways.[960] The first group is characterized by severe liver disease during the first week of life. The infant may die suddenly or may appear to be septic. Patients have transient hypoglycaemia, severe neurological involvement (hypotonia, myoclonic seizures, and developmental delay), and hepatic failure with a rapidly fatal clinical course.[960,977,978] In the second group, the onset of symptoms is delayed from 2 to 18 months of age. Liver disease is less severe initially (although hepatic failure occurs progressively), neurological involvement is more variable and some patients survive. This second group includes *Alpers progressive infantile poliodystrophy.*[979] Patients with Alpers disease have diffuse cerebral degeneration and progressive neuromuscular deterioration which leads to death, often in the first 2 years of life.[980] The initial presentation is usually neurological, with myoclonic seizures and developmental delay; hepatic failure occurs late, and frequently heralds death. Mitochondrial cytopathies, particularly Alpers syndrome, are a risk factor for valproate-induced fulminant liver failure, which may obscure the underlying diagnosis.[981–985]

Fatty acid oxidation disorders represent a broad spectrum of defects in β-oxidation.[986] Hepatocellular fatty acid metabolism involves complex processes in both the cytoplasm and mitochondria. Long-chain acyl-coenzyme A (CoA) esters are transported into mitochondria via a carnitive-dependent mechanism; these esters are then metabolized by β-oxidation within the mitochondria. Some of these processes take place at the inner mitochondria membrane and others within the mitochondrial matrix. Defects in fatty acid oxidation compromise energy production and interfere with formation of ketone bodies; production of dicarboxylic acids becomes a dominant alternate pathway. Hepatic clinical presentation often mimics Reye syndrome.[987] Disorders which are especially likely to cause liver disease include: defects in carnitine handling, especially carnitine uptake (OCTN2) and carnitine palmitoyl transferase (CPT1, CPT2) defects; medium-chain acyl-CoA dehydrogenase (MCAD) deficiency; LCHAD deficiency in that fatty liver of pregnancy occurs in a heterozygote mother carrying a homozygote-affected fetus and because affected indiviuals may develop neonatal liver failure or have a delayed hepatic presentation with cholestatic liver disease or cirrhosis.[988] Diagnosis and treatment of these disorders is difficult.[986,987] Carnitine supplementation may be effective in some of these disorders and indeed life-saving in carnitine uptake deficiency (OCTN2 defects), and avoiding fasting is critically important for all.

Screening for a mitochondrial disorder includes a careful history and physical examination to uncover any subtle supporting signs and symptoms. Lactic acidosis is an important finding. Hypoglycaemia may be the only sign of a mitochondrial disorder.[989] Laboratory findings which support a diagnosis of mitochondrial respiratory chain

defect include elevated plasma lactate, arterial plasma lactate/pyruvate ratio, and arterial α-hydroxybutyrate/acetoacetate. These abnormalities may be exaggerated after a meal or oral glucose load. Urine organic acids, serum carnitine levels or renal tubular function may also be abnormal in disorders of fatty acid oxidation. Confirming the diagnosis of a mitochondriopathy can be difficult. Histopathological study of liver and muscle, with electron microscopy, may reveal characteristic abnormalities. Some respiratory chain subunits can be detected by immunohistochemistry. Molecular biological techniques permit quantification of mtDNA as well as detection of some deletions and/or mutations in either nuclear or mitochondrial DNA. Some centres have developed polarographic or enzymatic methods of measuring respiratory chain activity. These and newer diagnostic modalities have been reviewed.[990–992] If fresh tissue is required for these studies, patients may need to go to centres specializing in mitochondrial disorders. Assays of fatty acid oxidation can be performed in skin fibroblasts, either enzymatically or functionally.[948] Liver biopsy tissue may be informative regarding repiratory chain defects even in the absence of obvious liver disease.[993]

Accumulating evidence indicates that many infants with mitochondrial disorders exhibit abnormalities before birth.[994] Prenatal diagnosis is dependent on identification and cloning of mutant genes or direct measurement of mitochondrial metabolism in cultured chorionic villus cells or amniocytes.[995] If the gene involved in the mitochondriopathy of a previously affected sibling has been identified, the family can benefit from prenatal diagnosis.

Therapy varies with the disease. Intensive supportive care is required for the neonate with hepatic failure, especially to permit accurate diagnosis and meticulous global evaluation of extrehepatic involvement. Patients with the more delayed form of liver disease are supported clinically; neurological features may require anti-epileptic medication. In some cases, use of a 'mitochondrial cocktail' has improved a patient's clinical condition.[996] Treatment for fatty acid oxidation disorders is customized to the actual defect.[987,997] Liver transplantation is controversial. Several authors have reported successful resolution of liver disease with transplantation. However, in patients with Alpers disease or other mitochondriopathies with neurological involvement, transplantation does not slow the progression of the neurological disease. Careful patient selection is crucial; liver tranplantion is not indicated for those patients with clinically-evident extrahepatic disease.[998,999]

In nine cases of *fatty acid oxidation disorders, medium chain (MCAD) and long chain (LCHAD) acyl-CoA dehydrogenase*, the histopathological findings were mainly those of microvesicular steatosis.[1000] In the case reported by Amirkhan[1001] there was severe ballooning degeneration of liver cells, mild cholestasis and marked bridging fibrosis. Ultrastructurally, large, oval, membrane-bound vesicles containing a loose, flocculent material and irregular internal membrane profiles were noted. Histopathological changes in defects of *mitochondrial oxidative phosphorylation* have been described by numerous investigators.[954,957,977,1002,959,961,1001,1003–1005] All have been characterized by microvesicular steatosis (Fig. 5.72), variable cholestasis and ductular proliferation, variable and sometimes progressive fibrosis, and in some cases by cirrhosis (Figs 5.73 and 5.74). The most detailed descriptions, including ultrastructural studies, were reported in a series of 10 cases by Bioulac-Sage et al.[1002] and in another series of five cases by Morris et al.[1003] Additional histopathological features have included haemosiderosis,[1002] and an oncocytic appearance of liver cells (due to an increased number of mitochondria) (Fig. 5.74).[1004] Changes at the ultrastructural level include pleomorphic mitochondria with few or no cristae and a granular fluffy matrix (Fig. 5.75).[957,1002] Morphological findings in Alpers syndrome are very similar to those of other mitochondrial cytopathies (Figs 5.76 and 5.77). Correlation of hepatic changes with those in other organ systems may be useful.[1006]

Pearson syndrome

This syndrome consists of refractory sideroblastic anaemia with vacuolization of marrow precursors, and exocrine pancreatic dysfunction.[1007] Patients have large deletions or rearrangements of the mitochondrial genome.[1008] A recently reported patient had predominantly hepatic manifestations, such as microvesicular steatosis, massive haemosiderosis and a rapidly developing cirrhosis.[1009] That patient had a 7436 bp deletion of the mitochondrial genome in all tissues investigated, compatible with Pearson syndrome. He died within 3 months of birth from liver failure. This patient's haemosiderosis may have been due to heterozygosity

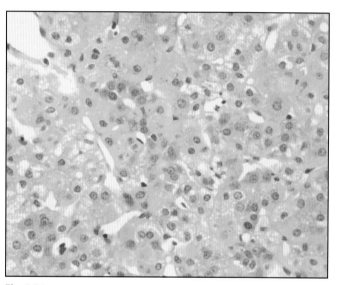

Fig. 5.74 • Same case as Illustrated In Fig. 5.73. Oxyphilic and microvesiculated hepatocytes are intermingled with groups of smaller hepatocytes with basophilic cytoplasm.

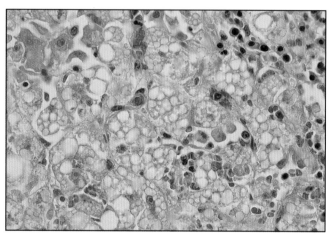

Fig. 5.72 • Mitochondrial cytopathy. Neonatal liver failure in patient with disorder of oxidative phosphorylation complex I. Liver biopsy shows marked microvesicular steatosis. H&E.

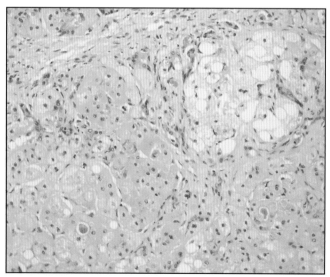

Fig. 5.73 • Mitochondrial cytopathy. The parenchyma, which is dissected by thin fibrous septa with subtle ductular reaction shows variable steatosis and oxyphilic transformation. H&E.

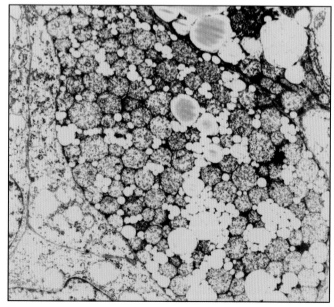

Fig. 5.75 • Mitochondrial cytopathy. Electron micrograph showing densely packed mitochondria separated by small lipid droplets. Note the mitochondrial granular appearance and loss of cristae. ×5800. Courtesy of Professor P Bioulac-Sage.

(C282Y and H63D) in mutations of the hereditary haemochromatosis gene, but other infants with Pearson syndrome also have had hepatic haemosiderosis.[1010]

Navajo neurohepatopathy

This autosomal recessive disorder is a sensorimotor neuropathy in full-blooded Navajo Indian children (of the southwestern USA) that was first described by Appenzeller et al.[1011] in 1976, and further characterized by Singleton et al. in 1990,[1012] and by Holve et al. in 1999;[1013] the latter authors suggested changing the name from neuropathy to neurohepatopathy since liver involvement is an important component of the disease. They described three clinical phenotypes, based on age at presentation and course:[1013] an *infantile type,* presenting before 6 months of age with jaundice and failure to thrive; a *childhood type* presenting between 1 and 5 years of age with liver dysfunction that progressed to liver failure and death within 6 months; and a *classic type* with variable onset of liver disease but progressive neurological deterioration.

Liver histopathological findings are characterized by multinucleated giant cells, mixed macro- and microvesicular steatosis, pseudoacini, cholestasis, inflammation, bridging fibrosis, and cirrhosis in some cases. Ultrastructural findings in four patients have included abnormalities of mitochondria (ringed cristae, swelling and loss of cristae, pleomorphic contour), effacement of canalicular microvilli, and accumulation of intracellular bile pigments and fat-containing vesicles.[1013]

The nature of the defect in Navajo neurohepatopathy remains unknown. The infantile form has some similarities to progressive familial intrahepatic cholestasis, whereas the childhood form suggests a mitochondrial disorder,[1013] hence its inclusion in this section.

Disorders of copper metabolism

Wilson disease

Wilson disease (previously referred to as hepatolenticular degeneration) is an autosomal recessive disease, with an incidence of 1 in 30 000 individuals. The implicated gene, localized to chromosome 13q-14.3, encodes a P-type ATPase which transports copper. Over 280 mutations in this gene have been identified. The symptoms and signs of Wilson disease are the result of copper overload in various tissues and organs. The disease is rarely symptomatic before 3 years of age and usually is manifested by signs of liver disease during adolescence.[1014] The diagnosis is occasionally made in patients who are over 50 years of age. The diagnosis should be considered in any child or adult with hepatocellular disease of undetermined cause, namely with elevated

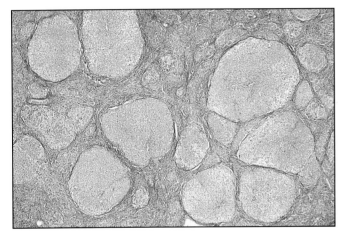

Fig. 5.76 • Alpers syndrome. Low power view showing a micronodular cirrhosis.

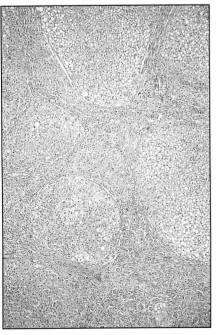

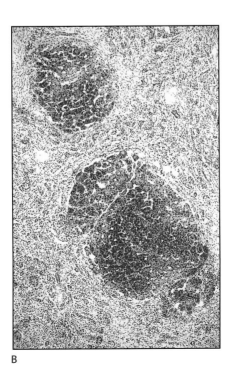

Fig. 5.77 • Alpers syndrome. Same case as illustrated in Fig. 5.76. **(A)** Micronodules show marked steatosis. H&E. **(B)** Marked steatosis (orange), predominantly microvesicular, of liver cells in the micronodules. Frozen section, oil red-O stain.

A   B

serum aminotransferases.[1015] Wilson disease may present as a non-infectious recurrent hepatitis or may mimic autoimmune hepatitis, the findings including a rash, arthropathy, elevated γ-globulin levels and positive anti-nuclear or anti-smooth muscle antibodies.[1014,1015] A Coombs-negative intravascular hemolyis is commonly seen when the presentation is that of acute liver failure (which occurs more often in females); other findings include an extremely low alkaline phosphatase level, comparatively low serum aminotransferases, and a low uric acid level prior to renal failure. The ratio of serum alkaline phosphatase (in IU/L) to serum bilirubin (in mg/dL) is typically <2 in Wilsonian liver failure.[1016] More recently, in children with Wilsonian fulminant hepatic failure this ratio, in units IU/μmol, was <2 and distinguished Wilson disease patients from those with fulminant hepatic failure due to other causes.[1017] Fulminant liver failure in Wilson disease may sometimes be precipitated by viral hepatitis.[1018] Neuropsychiatric signs are the predominant presentation in adults, but they may be present in up to 50% of teenagers. Tremors, dysarthria, drooling and gait disturbances are commonly observed. Psychiatric manifestations include personality changes and irritability, frank psychosis and depression; some patients may present with only psychiatric symptoms.[1019]

Low-grade haemolysis or bouts of jaundice due to intermittent haemolysis occur in some patients. Bilirubinate gallstones may develop. Eye findings include the Kayser–Fleischer ring, due to copper accumulation in Descemet's membrane, and sunflower cataracts, due to copper accumulation in the lens. Relatively common complications include gynaecomastia in males and amenorrhoea in females. Although pregnancy is still possible, repeated spontaneous abortion may occur in untreated women with Wilson disease. Cardiac complications include electrocardiographic abnormalities in 33% of patients.[1020] Ventricular fibrillation is rare, with or without cardiomyopathy. Orthostatic hypotension occurs in 19% of patients, with a third having an abnormal vascular response.[1020] Urolithiasis is a rare initial presentation.[1021] Renal tubular disease is common and may be either proximal or distal dysfunction. Less well-known complications include hyperpigmentation in Asians, hypoparathyroidism, and pancreatic insufficiency from pancreatitis.[1022,1023] Although considered generally rare in Wilson disease, hepatocellular carcinoma has been reported in more than 15 cases.[1024-1027] Hepatocellular carcinoma is a common complication in the Long–Evans Cinnamon rat, the animal model of the disease, but this rat also has hepatic iron overload and abnormalties in p53 function. A recent report suggests that liver and gastrointrointestinal malignancies may be more common than previously appreciated.[1028]

Correlation of phenotype with specific mutations (genotype) is difficult in Wilson disease because the vast majority of affected individuals are compound heterozygotes, possessing one copy each of two different mutations. In general those mutations which abrogate production of an intact functional Wilson ATPase protein cause more severe disease with an earlier, and typically hepatic, presentation.[1029-1031] Differences in clinical manifestations of various mutations between siblings and even identical twins suggests that other genes or environmental factors are important.[1015,1032-1034] The only modifying gene thus far identified is apolipoprotein E.[1035]

The diagnosis is not necessarily easy even when the disease is under consideration. In a patient in the age range 5–45 years, who has hepatic disease or typical neurological symptoms, finding serum caeruloplasmin below 5 mg/dL is highly consistent with Wilson disease; finding a Kayser–Fleischer ring as well confirms the diagnosis. A serum caeruloplasmin below 20 mg/dL is seen in up to 95% of patients but is not diagnostic of the disease. (The copper oxidase method is more reliable than the immunoassay which also measures apocaeruloplasmin as well as holocaeruloplasmin.) Kayser–Fleischer rings are diagnostic, except in patients who have chronic cholestasis of other aetiology. Absence of Kayser–Fleischer rings occurs in 50% of adult patients with liver disease and thus does not rule out Wilson disease. Rarely, Kayser–Fleischer rings may not be present even when there is neurological involvement.[1036]

In Wilson disease, the 24 hour urine copper excretion is usually greater than 100 μg and almost always exceeds 40 μg. When penicillamine 500 mg is administered by mouth every 12 hours during a 24-hour urine collection, copper excretion greater than 25 μmol (1587 μg) per 24 hours is taken as diagnostic.[1037] This test has been validated only in children. With compatible pathological changes, a liver copper concentration over 250 μg/g dry weight is diagnostic; however, lower values may be found if the sample is too small or there is variable distribution of parenchymal copper. Liver copper less than 55 μg/g dry weight is within normal range.[1038] Screening other members in the propositus family should include serum aminotansferases (AST and ALT), serum copper and caeruloplasmin determinations, slit-lamp examination for Kayser–Fleischer rings, and a basal 24-hour urinary copper determination. Liver biopsy is appropriate for subjects with abnormal findings.

Mutational analysis can be difficult for several reasons: patients are usually compound heterozygotes; some mutations may be in the promoter region; mutations must be shown to lead to a non-functional Wilson ATPase, a criterion not met currently by all proposed mutations. The role of mutational analysis is critically important in identifying affected first-degree relatives if the genotype of the propositus is established. It can also be useful in ethnicities known to have a limited spectrum of *ATP7B* mutations, for example, in Iceland, Sardinia, the Canary Islands, and possibly in northern Europe. However, high-throughput detection methods for analysing DNA are improving rapidly. These include denaturing high-performance liquid chromatography (DHPLC),[1039] automated single strand conformation polymorphism (SSCP) analysis,[1040] and direct sequencing.[1041]

Dietary copper is taken up by the intestinal cell, transported to copper-containing cellular proteins, including metallothionein, or exported from the cell across the basolateral membrane by a process involving the Menkes ATPase (ATP7A). The protein normally resides in the trans-Golgi network and in cell culture moves to the cell surface under conditions of high cellular copper concentrations.[1042,1043] The *ATP7A* gene is expressed in most tissues except the liver. An X-linked copper deficiency disorder, *Menkes disease*, results from mutations in this gene.[1044,1045] The gene abnormal in Wilson disease (*ATP7B*) shows 56% homology to *ATP7A* and has 21. exons.[1046–1048] Its product, the Wilson ATPase, has six copper binding sites with a CXXC amino acid motif. Like the Menkes ATPase, this copper-transporting ATPase is also located in the trans-Golgi network. Since crystallographic data are not yet available, the structure of the Wilson ATPase has recently been determined by homology mapping using Serca1, the sarcoplasmic Ca^{2+} P-type ATPase, as a model.[1049] More than 280 mutations in *ATP7B* have been reported. These are listed comprehensively, with all relevant references, in the HUGO Wilson Disease Database maintained at the University of Alberta (http://www.medicalgenetics.med.ualberta.ca/wilson/index.php). The overall pattern of *ATP7B* mutations (mainly missense) in Wilson disease differs from the *ATP7A* mutational spectrum found in Menkes disease.

Copper disposition in hepatocytes is complicated. Available copper in the plasma compartment is bound to albumin or histidine and undergoes reduction to the cuprous form before being transported into hepatocytes by the transmembrane transport hCtr1, encoded by the gene *SLC31A1*, which appears to span the hepatocellular plasma membrane as a trimer to form a channel. Near the amino terminus, hCtr1 has copper-binding domain which contains a methionine cluster (MXXM).[1050–1052] A second copper transporter, hCtr2, is involved in low-affinity copper uptake by hepatocytes. The action of hCtr1 does not regulate hepatocellular copper homeostasis; however, when copper concentrations are elevated, hCtr1 is degraded. Inside the hepatocyte, little if any copper exists as free copper, apparently because it is a pro-oxidant. Cellular copper toxicity can be prevented by binding to polypeptides particularly metallothionein.[1053,1054] Small proteins called metallochaperones mediate delivery of copper to specific sites within the cell.[1055,1056] CCS1 directs copper to SOD1 in the cytoplasm. Cox17 supplies copper to cytochrome c oxidase in mitochondria. Sco1 and Sco2 mediate the transfer of copper to subunit II of cytochrome c oxidase, and other metallochaperones might be involved. ATOX1 transports copper to the Wilson ATPase, which is located in the trans-Golgi network region.[1057,1058] ATOX1 has a single MXCXXC copper-binding unit; it interacts directly with the Wilson ATPase to transfer copper.[1059,1060] The Wilson ATPase has dual functions: incorporating copper into ceruloplasmin and in facilitating excretion of copper into the bile. Studies using various cell lines have shown that the intracellular location of the Wilson ATPase changes with increased intracellular copper concentration. When intracellular copper concentration is elevated, the Wilson ATPase redistributes to the vicinity of the bile canalicular membrane.[1061–1065] Details of the cellular mechanism of biliary excretion of copper remain unknown. Lysosomal function relating biliary excretion in the Long–Evans Cinnamon (Wilsonian) rat is normal.[1066] Murr1 (renamed as COMMD1) is a ubiquitously expressed protein encoded by *MURR1*, the gene which is abnormal in

Bedlington terrier hereditary copper toxicosis. Murr1 is multifunctional but likely plays a role in the biliary excretion of copper, although the exact mechanism remains unclear. Studies have shown that Murr1 can interact with the Wilson ATPase.[1067]

Based on clinical experience, the therapeutic strategy of choice remains chelating agents, particularly penicillamine.[1068] In the Long–Evans cinnamon rat the drug dissolves copper-rich granules in hepatic lysosomes and prevents the development of fulminant hepatitis.[1069] Alternatives to penicillamine include trientine[1070,1071] and zinc.[1072] Trientine is a chelator which has an entirely different structure from that of penicillamine whereas the mechanism of action of zinc involves competition for copper uptake. It entails induction of enterocyte metallothioneins which have greater affinity for copper than for zinc: consequently copper taken up by enterocytes is bound and excreted with normal enterocyte turnover. In addition to blocking uptake, this leads to total body depletion of copper by interfering with reabsorption of copper recycled though bile and other fluids draining into the intestinal tract. Zinc treatment may also cause hepatic copper to be stabilized by induction of hepatocellular metallothioneins. The effect of zinc is independent of which salt is administered. Compliance remains a major issue since dosage is thrice daily away from food, but effectiveness can be monitored by a decrease in non-caeruloplasmin-bound copper, regression of Kayser–Fleischer rings, improving liver tests, and 24-hour urinary excretion of copper. On chelator treatment this is expected to run in the 3 to 8 µmol per day range, but on zinc it should diminish toward normal (<1.2 µmol per day as target), as a reflection of decreased total body copper load. Antioxidants (mainly vitamin E) may be used as adjunctive therapy. Dietary therapy includes avoidance of liver, shellfish, mushrooms, chocolate and nuts, but dietary treatment alone will not control the disease.

Liver transplantation is reserved for disease unresponsive to medical therapy or for fulminant liver failure. One year survival is excellent at approximately 90%.[1073,1074] Living donor transplantation from an individual obliged to be a heterozygote with one *ATP7B* mutation (for example, a first-degree relative) is physiologically acceptable.[1075,1076] Liver transplantation for neurological complications is highly controversial and generally not recommended.[1077–1079] Experimental therapies include ammonium tetrathiolmolybdate (mainly used in patients with central nervous system involvement),[1080] and a combination therapy with zinc and trientine adminsitered indiviually in a temperally-dispersed pattern every 5–6 hours through the day (for clinically severe disease, usually decompensated cirrhosis).[1081] Introduction of *ATB7B* into the Long–Evans Cinnamon rat (the animal model of the disease) by recombinant adenovirus mediated gene delivery restores normal hepatic copper secretion into the serum and bile.[1082–1084]

The pathological effects of Wilson disease are considered to be directly related to the accumulation of copper in the brain, cornea, liver and kidneys, but pathogenetic mechanisms are unknown. Oxidative stress appears to play an important role since copper is a redox-active pro-oxidant. In severe liver disease requiring liver transplantation, functional abnormalities in hepatic mitochondria have been detected.[1085] The findings may also provide additional rationale for the use of antioxidants in Wilson disease.

Patients presenting with acute hepatitis are rarely biopsied. According to Scheinberg and Sternlieb,[1015] the livers of these patients show ballooning of hepatocytes, apoptotic bodies, cholestasis and a sparse lymphocytic infiltrate. Typically the biopsy in the precirrhotic stage is characterized by variable portal inflammation, moderate anisonucleosis, focal necrosis, scattered sinusoidal apoptotic bodies and moderate to marked steatosis[1086] (Figs 5.78 and 5.79). Glycogenated nuclei are a fairly constant finding in periportal hepatocytes (Fig. 5.78). Lipofuscin accumulates in periportal areas and some of the granules are large, irregular in shape and vacuolated.[1086] Kupffer cells may be slightly enlarged and laden with haemosiderin, presumably as a result of the acute haemolytic crises that may complicate the disease. There is a progressive increase in periportal cholangiolar proliferation and fibrosis. Variable numbers of inflammatory cells, chiefly lymphocytes and plasma cells, are seen in the connective tissue of portal areas. Changes indistinguishable from those of chronic hepatitis due to other aeti-

ologies, in particular autoimmune hepatitis, may be seen (Figs 5.80 and 5.81).[1087–1089] In our experience, helpful differential clues in the diagnosis of Wilson disease (in addition to portal inflammation and interface hepatitis) include steatosis, periportal glycogenated nuclei, moderate to marked copper storage (Fig. 5.82), and the presence of Mallory bodies in periportal liver cells.

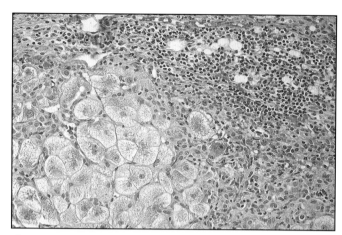

Fig. 5.80 • Wilson disease, chronic hepatitis. Marked portal inflammation and interface hepatitis. H&E.

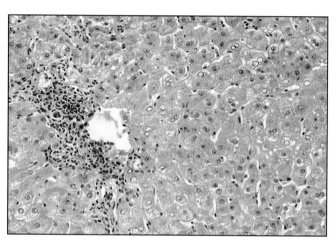

Fig. 5.78 • Wilson disease. Biopsy from a 6-year-old child. Pre-cirrhotic stage exhibiting mild portal inflammation and periportal glycogenated nuclei. H&E.

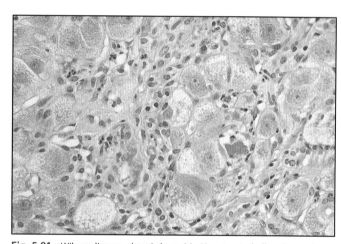

Fig. 5.81 • Wilson disease, chronic hepatitis. Hepatocyte ballooning and apoptotic bodies in an area of interface hepatitis. H&E.

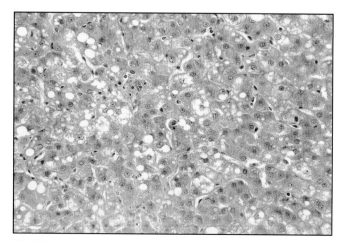

Fig. 5.79 • Wilson disease. Same case as illustrated in Fig. 5.78 showing patchy steatosis and occasional apoptotic bodies. H&E.

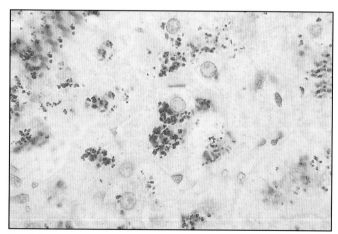

Fig. 5.82 • Wilson disease, chronic hepatitis. Marked copper accumulation (red granules) in periportal liver cells. Rhodanine.

Cytochemically demonstrable copper is usually confined to periportal hepatocytes in the precirrhotic stage of Wilson disease. With the use of special stains (Timm's stain) and electron probe microanalysis, Goldfischer and Sternlieb[1090] showed that in young, asymptomatic patients copper is diffusely distributed in the cytoplasm of hepatocytes. In slightly older patients who exhibit early symptoms or signs of the disease, the metal is both diffusely distributed and intralysosomal, while in patients with advanced disease all the copper is confined to lysosomes (Fig. 5.82). The various staining methods for the demonstration of copper in tissue sections have been reviewed by Lindquist[1091] and Irons et al.[1092] In our experience and that of others[1092] the p-dimethylaminobenzylidene rhodanine method gives the most reproducible results (Fig. 5.82); both it and the rubeanic acid method are specific for copper. There is a linear relationship between microscopical evaluation of the stain and actual tissue copper levels.[1092] Copper-binding protein can be stained by orcein in Wilson disease and other conditions (e.g. chronic cholestatic disorders),[1092–1095] as well as by aldehyde fuchsin and Victoria blue. The granules also stain with a variety of stains for lipofuscin that is aggregated in the same lysosomes.[1086] It must be pointed out that negative staining for both copper and copper-associated protein does not exclude the diagnosis of Wilson disease. At an early stage essentially cytosolic copper is highly soluble, particularly in poorly buffered formalin, and lysosomal copper-binding protein may also be absent at this stage.

Both caeruloplasmin and metallothionein have been demonstrated immunohistochemically in the liver in Wilson disease. Graul et al.[1096] found no difference in the pattern of staining of caeruloplasmin in the livers of patients with Wilson disease and normal adults or neonates. The distribution of metallothionein in Wilson disease was studied by Nartey et al.[1097] In sections with minimal tissue damage, there was intense cytoplasmic staining for metallothionein in liver cells, whereas in sections with extensive necrosis and fibrosis there was both nuclear and cytoplasmic staining.

The Wilson ATPase has been examined in the human liver by immunoblotting, immunohistochemistry, and double-label confocal scanning laser microscopy.[1063,1065] It is present predominantly in trans-Golgi vesicles in the pericanalicular area, but relatively small amounts of the protein appear to localize to the canalicular membrane, consistent with a dual function of the protein in holocaeruloplasmin synthesis and biliary copper excretion. Defective trafficking within hepatocytes is a functional characteristic of some mutations.

The cirrhosis of Wilson disease is usually macronodular, but can be mixed or even micronodular in type.[1086] Microscopically, it is characterized by varying-sized nodules separated by fibrous septa that may be wide or very thin, with minimal cholangiolar proliferation and variable inflammation (Fig. 5.83). All changes in the precirrhotic stage are also seen in the cirrhotic liver. In addition, Mallory bodies can be identified frequently at the periphery of the cirrhotic nodules (Fig. 5.84). Variable numbers of apoptotic

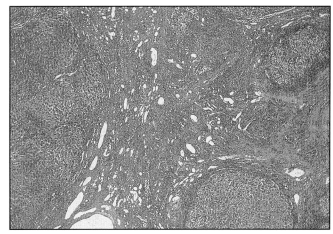

Fig. 5.83 • Wilson disease. Cirrhotic nodules are separated by wide bands of fibrous tissue with many vessels and chronic inflammation. H&E.

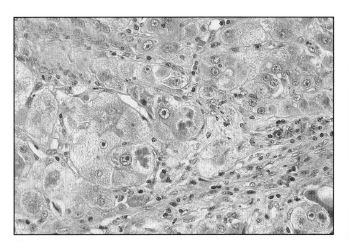

Fig. 5.84 • Wilson disease. Periseptal liver cells contain Mallory bodies. H&E.

bodies may be present. Clusters of large hepatocytes with a granular eosinophilic cytoplasm (oncocytic or oxyphil cells), due to an increased number of mitochondria, are often seen. The distribution of copper is quite variable, with some of the cirrhotic nodules containing a lot and others containing little or none.[1086] Copper is rarely demonstrable in Kupffer cells or portal macrophages in the cirrhotic stage, but is frequently encountered in cases of submassive or massive necrosis in patients who present with fulminant liver failure (Figs 5.85 and 5.86). Davies et al.[1098] also noted the presence of copper in hepatic parenchymal and mononuclear phagocytic cells in 11 cases of Wilson disease which although presenting as fulminant hepatic failure were cirrhotic. Another case was described recently.[1099]

Ultrastructural findings in the precirrhotic stage of Wilson disease have been described in detail by a number of investigators.[1015,1100,1101] Of these, the mitochondrial changes are the most distinctive and pathogenetically significant; they include heterogeneity of size and shape, increased matrix density, separation of inner from outer membranes, enlarged intercristal spaces and various types of inclusions (Fig. 5.87). In a recent study, Sternlieb[1102] described three distinct patterns of structural abnormalities of the mitochondria in hepatocytes of 40 of 42 asymptomatic and 8 of 32 symptomatic patients with Wilson disease prior to therapy. There

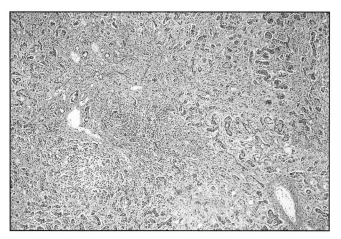

Fig. 5.85 • Wilson disease. Massive necrosis (cell dropout) and prominent ductular reaction. H&E.

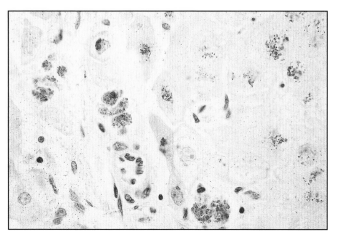

Fig. 5.86 • Wilson disease. Same case as illustrated in Fig. 5.85 showing accumulation of copper in Kupffer cells as well as in hepatocytes. Rhodanine.

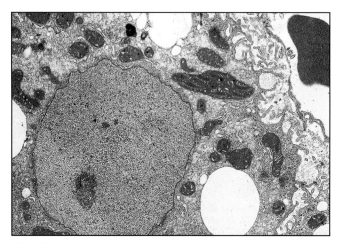

Fig. 5.87 • Wilson disease. Mitochondria show a denser than normal matrix, enlarged and occasionally vacuolated granules, vacuoles with granular contents, crystalline inclusions and separation of the outer from the inner membranes. Electron micrograph ×16 275.

mitochondria, include an increase in the number of peroxisomes (which may appear heterogeneous and denser and larger than normal), lipofuscin granules and multivesicular bodies. Mallory bodies appear as masses of randomly oriented and densely packed fibrils (each about 15 μm in diameter), which are partially rimmed by bundles of finer filaments but are not limited by membranes.[1103,1104] Lipolysosomes, which constitute 1–2% of the lipid droplets in hepatocytes in Wilson disease, may represent a nonspecific alternate route for the mobilization of excess lipid from hepatocytes.[1105] An ultrastructural study of liver tissue from a family of nine siblings has demonstrated that this method is not useful in distinguishing the presymptomatic affected person from the homozygous one.[1106] It should be noted at this juncture that ultrastructural mitochondrial changes in Wilson disease cannot be considered pathognomonic.[1107]

The long-term effects of D-penicillamine therapy on the structure and function of the liver in patients with Wilson disease were reported by Sternlieb and Feldmann.[1108] Liver biopsy specimens from seven patients, obtained before and after 3–5 years of therapy, were studied by electron microscopy and stereology. The characteristic mitochondrial abnormalities encountered in the hepatocytes of untreated patients were less pronounced or disappeared after treatment in five of the seven patients. Simultaneously, relative mitochondrial volume, surface density of the external mitochondrial membranes, and the number of these profiles per unit area increased, whereas abnormal elevations of serum aminotransferases returned to normal.

Indian childhood cirrhosis (ICC)

This hepatic copper toxicosis has been most prevalent in the Indian subcontinent.[1109] However, ICC, or a liver disorder strongly resembling it, has been reported from numerous countries, including a few cases from the USA.[1110–1112] ICC should not be confused with North American Indian cirrhosis (or cholestasis) which is due to mutations in the cirhin gene.[1113–1115]

In India, ICC was formerly a significant cause of morbidity and mortality amongst children below the age of 5 years.[1116] The incidence in India has declined sharply after recognition of the role of copper overload in its pathogenesis.[1117,1118] Epidemiological and clinical aspects of ICC are covered in a number of publications.[1116,1119] The age range is from 6 months to 5 years with a peak around 2 years. In 30–50% of cases of ICC there is a history of sibling disease and death, but Mendelian inheritance is not apparent. Evidence against a genetic background for the disease is its apparent absence in Indian expatriates in the UK, Africa and North America.[1120] Three clinical stages of ICC have been recognized:[1119] (i) an *early stage* with an insidious onset characterized by disturbances of appetite and bowel movement, slight enlargement of the liver and occasional jaundice; (ii) an *intermediate stage* characterized by irritability, minimal jaundice, marked hepatomegaly, splenomegaly and occasionally, subcutaneous oedema, ascites and susceptibility to infection; (iii) a *late stage* with increasing

was no correlation between the type of abnormality and the patient's age, hepatic copper concentration, degree of hepatic steatosis or the serum aminotransferase levels. There was, however, a high degree of fraternal concordance, indicating that the structural changes are genetically determined. Alterations in Wilson disease, other than those affecting

jaundice, hepatosplenomegaly, and progression to hepatic failure and death.

One of the earliest and most comprehensive microscopic descriptions of the liver in ICC was reported by Smetana et al.[1121] in 1961. Other contributions were made by a number of investigators.[1116,1119] The earliest changes are ballooning degeneration and focal necrosis, followed by formation of Mallory bodies,[1104] sometimes with neutrophilic satellitosis. Steatosis is conspicuously absent (Fig. 5.88(A), (B)). The mesenchymal reaction is characterized by inflammatory cell infiltration (lymphocytes, histiocytes, neutrophils and a few plasma cells), variable periportal ductular proliferation, progressive fibrosis and eventually, development of a micronodular cirrhosis (Fig. 5.89). Smetana et al.[1121] emphasized the absence of regenerative activity.

ICC is associated with marked hepatic copper overload (Fig. 5.90). The copper storage has been demonstrated histochemically (by staining tissue sections with orcein for copper-binding protein and the rhodanine method for copper), and by quantitative techniques such as atomic absorption spectrophotometry.[1117,1118,1122,1123] It is now generally accepted that the copper storage is directly responsible for the histopathological lesions in ICC. The copper accumulates first in periportal hepatocytes and then extends towards the terminal hepatic venules. Orcein stain may also have diagnostic utility.[1124]

Tanner et al.[1125] proposed that increased dietary copper (from copper-contaminated milk stored in brass and copper containers) could be of aetiological significance in ICC. Subsequently, O'Neill and Tanner[1126] demonstrated experimentally that copper (but not zinc) is avidly taken up from brass and bound to casein from which it is completely removable by picolinate chelation. They concluded that milk is an effective carrier of copper from a brass utensil to the infant enterocyte. Lending support to a direct cytopathic effect of copper are several studies of clinical recovery, improved long-term survival and even reversal of the hepatic histological lesions by penicillamine therapy in infants with ICC.[1127–1129] Cases of an ICC-like disease caused by chronic ingestion of water with high levels of copper ('hepatic copper toxicosis') are discussed in the chapter on drug-induced injury (Chapter 14). The decline in the incidence of ICC since feeding practices have been changed to avoid the use of copper vessels for infants and young

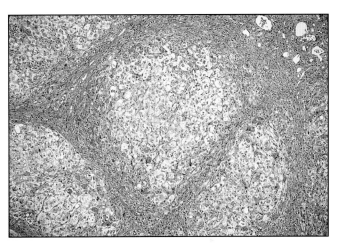

Fig. 5.89 • Indian childhood cirrhosis, same case as illustrated in Fig. 5.88. Micronodular cirrhosis. H&E.

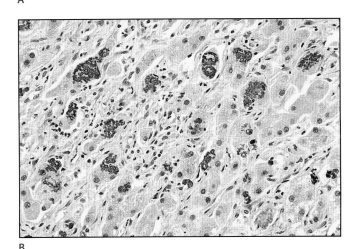

A

B

Fig. 5.88 • Indian childhood cirrhosis. (A) Hepatocyte ballooning without significant steatosis is associated with Mallory bodies which are highlighted by immunostaining for ubiquitin (B).

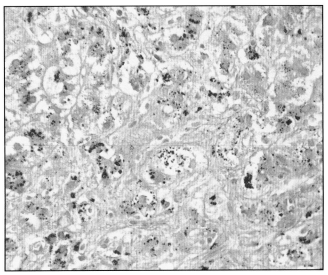

Fig. 5.90 • Indian childhood cirrhosis. Same case as illustrated in Fig. 5.88. Marked accumulation of copper-binding protein. Orcein.

children and the continued remission of affected children after discontinuing penicillamine once sufficient hepatic copper has been removed suggest that environmental factors are important in the development of ICC. Devleopmental and genetic factors cannot be entirely excluded.[1130] Recent studies indicate that *Murr1*, the gene abnormal in Bedlington terrier hereditary copper toxicosis, does not play a role in either Indian childhood cirrhosis or in Tyrolean infantile cirrhosis.[1131,1132]

Endemic Tyrolean infantile cirrhosis

This disease, clinically and pathologically indistinguishable from Indian childhood cirrhosis, was reported from a circumscribed rural area of Western Austria between 1900 and 1974.[1133] One hundred and thirty-eight infants and young children died from the disease. The frequency of the disease peaked between 1930 and 1960; it has disappeared from that area since 1974. The inheritance was autosomal recessive. Cow's milk, contaminated with copper from untinned copper or brass vessels, may have contributed to the development of copper toxicosis. Replacement of untinned copper cooking utensils by modern industrial vessels eradicated the disease. Tyrolean infantile cirrhosis is believed to be an ecogenetic disorder requiring the involvement of both genetic and environmental factors for its manifestation.[1133,1134] It is not an allelic variant of Wilson disease.[1135] Histopathlgical changes includes micronodular cirrhosis with copper overload in the most severely affected children.[1136]

Disorders of iron metabolism

Iron is a transition metal that is essential for the survival of most organisms, particularly those existing in an environment that is rich in oxygen. The principal role for iron in mammalian homeostasis is via the oxygen transport system of the haemoglobin molecule. However, iron is also a crucial component in the development of the central nervous system as well as many essential biochemical reactions including DNA synthesis, oxidative phosphorylation, and host defence. There is a requirement for exquisite conservation and regulation of body iron, given both the body's absolute need for iron and the fact that the human does not have a physiological iron excretion mechanism. Thus a variety of abnormal states may arise, namely iron deficiency in the form of anaemia, and excess or maldistribution of iron stores with consequent organ loading and maldistribution, as typified by hereditary haemochromatosis. Together these reflect two of the more common disease states of humans. Disorders associated with iron overload in the liver are summarized in Table 5.3.

There have been recent major advances in the understanding of the handling of iron and iron overload disorders since the identification of the gene responsible for classic HFE-hereditary haemochromatosis,[1137] largely afforded by in vivo transgenic and knockout techniques as well as positional cloning in humans. Furthermore, it is increasingly apparent that the liver plays a crucial role in the control of iron homeostasis.

Metabolism of iron

Total body iron content ranges from 3 to 5 g, mostly in haemoglobin or as storage iron in the liver and spleen, with smaller amounts in myoglobin and various enzymes. Under physiological conditions, there must be carefully regulated absorption of iron with minimal loss of less than 0.1% daily through menstrual bleeding and cellular desquamation. The daily requirement for iron in the adult is 20 to 25 mg, mainly for erythopoiesis,[1138] but only 1 to 2 mg of dietary iron are required daily in a healthy individual as the reticuloendothelial system recovers the remainder via the efficient phagocytosis of effete red cells.[1139]

Iron absorption and transport

The two major sources of dietary iron are ionic iron and haem. In the West, over half of dietary iron comes from haem whereas, worldwide, most is ingested in its ionic form.[1140,1141] Dietary iron is digested in the acidic environment of the stomach and taken up by the apical brush border of the small intestine, principally the duodenum. Various active uptake pathways have been identified.[1142]

In the case of ionic iron, the ingested ferric form must be reduced to its ferrous state through the action of a brush border ferrireductase, DcytB.[1143] It is then actively transported through the apical membrane of the duodenal enterocyte by the divalent metal transporter DMT1, formerly Nramp2 or DCT1, that is also capable of transporting other divalent metals.[1144] Dietary haem, after its dissociation from globin, is transported across the brush border and released within the enterocyte by haem oxygenase or transported to plasma as an intact porphyrin.[1141] Although the mechanism for haem import is not confirmed, a human intestine brush border haem receptor/transporter on the apical membrane has been postulated, with haem being acquired and transported via an active metabolic/transport process.[1145] A putative haem exporter, FLVCR, a member of the major facilitator superfamily of transporter proteins, has been recently isolated.[1146] A third conduit, the so-called integrin and mobilferrin pathway (IMP) for uptake of ferric iron is also identified.[1140,1147] The absorbed iron, from either ionic or haem pathways, may also be retained within the enterocyte as ferritin and eventually lost through desquamation. Otherwise, the metal is transported actively through the basolateral membrane.

The only transporter protein currently identified is ferroportin, also known as Ireg1 or MTP1.[1148–1150] Ferroportin is similar to DMT1 in that it is a transmembranous segment protein that preferentially transports ferrous iron but there is no sequence homology between the two proteins.[1151] The export is facilitated by an accessory protein, hephaestin, a ferroxidase and caeruloplasmin homologue, thus returning the iron to the ferric state and promoting its binding to transferrin.[1152] Indeed, caeruloplasmin per se is also required for the export of iron from nonintestinal cells.[1153] The crucial

Table 5.3	Hepatic iron overload states

Disorder	Inheritance (OMIM[1195])
Primary/hereditary—haemochromatosis	
Haemochromatosis (haemochromatosis type 1)	
HFE-associated	6p21.3 (HFE)
• C282Y homozygote	
• C282Y/H63D heterozygote	
• H63D homozygote	
Juvenile haemochromatosis (haemochromatosis type 2)	1q21 (hemojuvelin)
	19q13 (hepcidin)
TFR2-associated haemochromatosis (haemochromatosis type 3)	7q22
Ferroportin (haemochromatosis type 4)	2q32
Neonatal haemochromatosis	Unknown but variable inheritance from recessive to non-Mendelian. Alloimmunity queried.
Other non-HFE-related haemochromatosis (haemochromatosis type 5)	Hyperferritinaemia. See text. (Unknown, polygenic)
African/American iron overload	Possible environmental and genetic influences. 2q32 (ferroportin) mutation. See text.
Primary/inherited—disorders of iron balance/distribution	
Atransferrinaemia	3q21
Acaeruloplasminaemia	3q23-24
Secondary/acquired iron overload	
Iron-loading anaemias	
• Thalassaemia major	11p.15.5
• Sideroblastic anaemia (including X-linked)	Various (Xp11.21)
Porphyria cutanea tarda	1p34
Parenteral iron overload	
Anaemia of inflammation	
Iron overload in other chronic liver diseases	
Hepatitis B and C viruses	
Alcoholic siderosis	
Insulin resistance (NAFL/NASH)	
End-stage cirrhosis	
Portocaval shunt	

relationship between ferroportin and the regulatory peptide hormone hepcidin is discussed later.

Transferrin (Tf) is the major iron-binding glycoprotein in plasma. The Tf molecule allows for high affinity binding of two atoms of ferric iron with transferrin iron-binding sites and is normally about 30% saturated in the physiological state. Given the potentially toxic nature of iron, Tf allows the iron to remain soluble and non-reactive in the aqueous environment, and facilitates the cellular importation of iron into cells.[1154] The latter occurs via the Tf cycle whereby the two diferric Tf molecules bind with a high affinity transferrin receptor (TfR1) that is ubiquitously expressed on most cell surfaces.[1155] All nucleated cells have TfR1 on their cell surfaces, most importantly the developing red cells in bone marrow, syncytotrophoblast and both Kupffer cells and hepatocytes, which receive first pass blood from the portal circulation.[1156] The Tf-TfR1complex is internalized and, after endocytosis, the endosome is acidified by proton pumps and the iron is released from Tf into the cytoplasm via a process that also requires DMT1. The unbound Tf, apotransferrin, and TfR1 recycle to the cell membrane to again participate in the transport pathway.[1154]

A second transferrin receptor (TfR2), which is localized to chromosome 7q22 and is cell-cycle dependent, has also been identified.[1157–1159] The TfR2 protein is a membrane glycoprotein with at least 2 alternatively spliced transcripts, α and β, the former representing the membrane-bound form, while TfR2-β comprises only the extracellular domain of the protein. TfR2 shows moderate homology to TfR1, reaching 45% in the extracellular region but there are many functional differences between the two. Although both TfR1 and 2 are competent transporters of transferrin-bound iron into the cell, TfR2 mRNA is quite distinct from TfR1 in that it is expressed at much higher levels in liver when compared with other tissues, whereas the TfR1 gene demonstrates little hepatic expression. TfR1 and TfR2 differ also in their response to changes in cellular iron status with TfR1 containing multiple iron-responsive elements (IREs) in its 3′-untranslated region (see later) but with TfR2 showing low affinity for transferrin. TfR2 does not contain IREs and its message and protein levels vary little with changes in iron status. TfR2 is unable to bind HFE, although this is a constitutive feature of TfR1, but it co-localizes with HFE in duodenal crypt cells.[1160] Furthermore, while functional loss of TfR1 in knockout mice produces an lethal embryonic phenotype,[1161] targeted mutagenesis of TfR2 in the mouse causes a phenotype analogous to hereditary haemochromatosis.[1162] While the current function of TfR2 in the iron regulatory pathway is uncertain, it is suggested that TfR2 may act as a sensor of iron-saturated Tf in the liver in vivo although this is currently not borne out in vitro.[1163,1164]

Cycling and storage of iron

Tissue macrophages are primarily responsible for scavenging and phagocytosing effete erythrocytes.[1165] After the red cell is degraded, iron is released from haem via haem oxygenase and may be stored as ferritin or efficiently mobilized and exported as required to the bone marrow for purposes of erythropoiesis.[1151] While the export process is incompletely understood, it would appear that it again occurs via the action of ferroportin and haephestin.[1152,1166] This is, in turn, controlled by the peptide hormone hepcidin, as reviewed later. Under normal physiological conditions, hepatocytes and macrophages store iron to an amount of 0.5 to 1 g. The hepatocyte is the major storage facility for iron and, after endocytosis and acidification of the Tf-TfR1 complex, it may be incorporated into enzymes or stored either as ferritin or, far less efficiently, haemosiderin.

Ferritin is the most important mechanism by which cells store iron. This large and complex protein comprises 24 similar subunits that sequester up to 4500 iron atoms in a central core, thus isolating the metal from the cellular environment. Ferritin is highly conserved across all organisms, thus indicating a critical function in iron homeostasis. Human ferritin comprises H (active) and L (inactive) subunits whose relative proportions vary according to cell-specific iron and oxygen homeostasis, tissue type, development and, in animal models, iron overload. The H subunit carries a ferroxidase site that allows rapid oxidation of $Fe2+$ with the formation of diferroxo-mineral precursors at the expense of generating hydrogen.[1151,1156,1167] When compared to the efficiency of the ferritin system in iron cycling and storage, degradation of the protein leads to the accumulation of haemosiderin that is, by contrast, a potentially pathological non-homogeneous conglomerate of iron, protein and membrane breakdown products that is mobilized poorly if at all.[1151]

Regulation of iron homeostasis

As noted, iron is a critical nutrient and there is no physiological pathway for iron excretion in man. Hence there must be meticulous coordination of the uptake, storage and utilization of the metal. To accomplish this, cells contain proteins that have the ability to register the presence or absence of iron, identified in mammalian cells as two homologous iron regulatory proteins, IRP1 and IRP2. These discern cytosolic iron levels and alter the expression of proteins involved in iron metabolism, including ferritin, TfR1 (but not TfR2), DMT1 and ferroportin. IRP1 and IRP2 share extensive sequence homology.[1168] However, there are significant differences between the two, as reviewed by Rouault.[1169] Sensing of iron levels is coupled to availability of oxygen and other oxidants. The proteins involved in iron metabolism have motifs called iron responsive elements (IREs), which are stem loop structures in their 3' or 5' untranslated regions.[1142,1168] When, for example, the IRP binds to the 5' untranslated region of the ferritin mRNA transcript, ferritin synthesis is halted whereas binding at the 3' untranslated region allows translation to proceed.[1170]

Storage iron in hepatocytes and tissue macrophages must be mobilized in response to need and the concept of store and erythroid 'regulators' was originally conceived by Finch.[1171] The store regulator would control duodenal iron uptake by means of a tightly regulated feedback mechanism to prevent iron overload. The erythroid regulator would enhance intestinal absorption in response to erythroid demand when there is an increased requirement for iron but the capacity of storage cells is insufficient. In addition, iron could be regulated at the level of the duodenum by the amount of iron recently consumed, thus invoking a dietary regulator, probably resulting from the build-up of intracellular iron. Even in systemic iron deficiency, a bolus of iron may cause a so-called mucosal block.[1172] Furthermore, iron homeostasis is also modified in conditions of hypoxia, via a humoral hypoxia regulator, and cellular iron may be retained and its absorption interrupted by infection, the inflammatory regulator, presumably to withhold iron from the pathogen.[1168]

Such 'regulators' were largely theoretical until the discovery of the 25 amino acid peptide, hepcidin (hepatic bactericidal protein) or LEAP-1 (liver expressed antimicrobial peptide 1).[1173,1174] Originally identified as a type II acute phase protein produced by the liver, it is a 25-amino acid peptide containing four disulphide bonds that forms a hairpin stabilized by these bonds.[1175] Hepcidin is induced by infection and inflammation, and plays a central role in the anaemia and hypoferraemia of chronic disease, alternatively called anaemia of inflammation. IL-6 and, possibly, IL-1 are identified as the key mediators of hepcidin activation.[1176,1177] The evolutionarily conserved hepcidin gene (HAMP) maps to the long arm of chromosome 19 (19q13) and its mRNA expression is almost entirely restricted to the liver.

Pigeon and co-workers then identified murine hepcidin gene mRNA by subtractive hybridization of iron-overloaded versus normal livers, identifying the mRNA as being predominantly expressed by hepatocytes,[1178] while Nicolas et al. fortuitously removed the murine hepcidin gene while generating upstream stimulatory factor 2 (USF2 null) knockout mice.[1179] This resulted in spontaneous iron loading analogous to the pattern seen in hereditary haemochromatosis, with elevated Tf saturation and reticuloendothelial sparing. Transgenic mice constitutively overexpressing hepcidin conversely died perinatally of severe iron deficiency anaemia with concomitant reticuloendothelial iron overload[1180] while transgenic overexpression of hepcidin prevented hepatic iron deposition in the mouse model of haemochromatosis.[1181]

In addition to its role as an inflammatory regulator, hepcidin functions at the point of convergence of the erythroid and store regulators as a key regulator of iron absorption and iron homeostasis, controlled by both hypoxia and iron.[1182–1184] Hepcidin is an inhibitor of iron absorption in the duodenum and of iron release from placenta, hepatic stores and macrophages.[1179,1185] The hormone is identified to inhibit the efflux of cellular iron by binding with and inducing the internalization and degradation of ferroportin.[1186] As noted, while cytokines are responsible for the production of hepcidin in inflammatory states, they can be blocked by inactivation of Kupffer cells. However, their synthesis in iron overload states does not appear to require functional Kupffer cells, at least in vitro.[1187]

The molecular control of iron metabolism was further advanced by the identification of an association between hepcidin and TfR2,[1164] as well as mutations of the gene coding for hemojuvelin (*HJV*) on chromosome 1q,[1188] and it is currently held that both TfR2 and HJV have a putative erythroid regulatory role in hepcidin expression. It is likely that the identification of yet other regulators will be required in order to fully explain the regulatory process, but it is believed that most forms of hereditary haemochromatosis are due to hepcidin deficiency with the remainder due to disruption of ferroportin, the main target for the hepcidin protein. Taken together with its putative relationships to TfR2 and HJV, a significant role for hepcidin in iron overload states is thus stressed although it is currently incompletely understood.[1183,1185,1189]

In summary, iron homeostasis requires specific transportation across membranes and meticulous intracellular storage. Diminution of iron stores due to dietary deficiency, iron loss, or infection gives rise to eventual iron restriction and progression to anaemia. However the converse may arise whereby the large ionic iron molecule, in excess and in solution with oxygen, may generate free radical formation via Fenton and Haber-Weiss chemistry, with hydrogen peroxide (H_2O_2), being changed into its radical (HO). This leads to consequent damage to DNA, proteins and membranes.[1190,1191] The classic example of iron overload in human pathology is HFE-hereditary haemochromatosis but numerous other entities are now identified to cause pathological iron overload.[1192] Some are well described and have a verified hereditary basis, while in others the genetic and hereditary basis is still speculative. A further percentage reflect iron overload on an inflammatory or infectious basis or as a reactive response to systemic or, as yet, unknown disease processes.

There is controversy regarding nomenclature of these iron overload states.[1193] Haemochromatosis, as identified in the liver, has previously related to iron loading in primary liver cells, hepatocytes and biliary epithelium, whereas haemosiderosis, iron staining in tissues, was employed by some as the terminology of choice when the overload was predominantly within Kupffer cells. Many overload states may show elements of both, however. As such, it may be appropriate to consider all as hepatic iron overload disorders, reserving the term 'haemochromatosis' to those conditions in which there is an established or implied primary or genetic aetiology.

Thus hereditary haemochromatosis may be defined as an inherited disorder resulting from an inborn error of iron metabolism that leads to progressive loading of parenchymal cells including liver, pancreas, heart and endocrine organs.[1194] These iron overload states, as currently identified, are summarized in Table 1. The caveat, however, is that current classifications, including the Online Mendelian Inheritance in Man database,[1195] are founded on the basis of single-gene defects and have significant shortcomings in that numbers of atypical cases are increasingly identified that relate to multiple gene mutations.[1196]

Hereditary iron overload disorders

Historical perspective

Trousseau first described a diabetic patient with an 'almost bronzed' appearance in 1865,[1197] while Emile Troisier shortly afterwards detailed the first autopsied case of a diabetic patient with cirrhosis and a red-brown liver containing clumps of pigment.[1198] von Recklinghausen later termed the condition 'haemochromatosis'.[1199] Two main theories grew out of subsequent reports, namely that the primary disease was diabetes that then gave rise to cirrhosis and pigmentation or, alternatively, that the pigment was primarily derived from the blood.[1200] After years of dispute as to its pathogenesis, Sheldon consolidated the existing knowledge of haemochromatosis with its classic triad of diabetes, cirrhosis and melanin-based pigmentation.[1201] He described the entity as 'an inborn error of metabolism, which has an overwhelming incidence in males and which at times has a familial incidence'.

The autosomal recessive inheritance pattern of classic hereditary haemochromatosis was thereafter established, but it was only in 1976 that Simon and co-workers confirmed an association between the disorder and the HLA antigens A3 and B14.[1202,1203] The subsequent discovery that β_2-microglobulin knockout mice developed iron overload analogous to human haemochromatosis raised the postulate that the defective gene would be within an MHC molecule.[1204,1205] Positional cloning experiments using linkage disequilibrium and haplotype analysis allowed the identification of the affected gene, an atypical class 1 HLA molecule originally designated HLA-H and subsequently redefined as *HFE*.[1137] Subsequent knockout of the mouse *HFE* gene confirmed iron overload, thus confirming *HFE* to be the defective gene in classic hereditary haemochromatosis.[1206,1207]

In the wake of these crucial experiments, it rapidly became clear that the HFE mutation did not explain all cases of iron overload[1192] and major advances in the understanding of iron overload disorders, including the discovery and elucidation of TfR2, hepcidin and hemojuvelin, have allowed greater insight into the pathogenesis of these disorders as well as identifying many of the additional genes involved in inherited iron storage disorders (Table 5.3).

HFE-associated haemochromatosis (Haemochromatosis type 1)

An autosomal recessive disease, classical HFE-associated hereditary haemochromatosis is the most common monoallelic inherited disorder in Western society. The dominant missense mutation identified in 80% of cases, C282Y, is characterized by a single nucleotide change, G to A, resulting in a Cys → Tyr at position 282 of the unprocessed protein, occurring in a highly conserved region involved in the disulphide bridge in the MHC class 1 protein. A less common missense mutation is a C to G change resulting in a Hys → Asp substitution at amino acid 63, showing limited clinical effects although compound heterozygosity for C282Y and H63D may cause disease expression.[1137] Of several other uncommon mutations, S65C, in which cysteine replaces serine at position 65, has been associated with compound heterozygosity for either C282Y or H63D. It has been related to the development of a mild form of haemochromatosis with mild to moderate hepatic iron overload but without clinical manifestations. Its significance is still controversial.[1208,1209]

The C282Y mutation is most prevalent amongst populations of northern European origin with over 90% of patients with clinically penetrant haemochromatosis in the United Kingdom being homozygous for C282Y. Worldwide allele frequencies are calculated at 1.9% for C282Y and 8.1% for H63D with highest frequencies being 10% for C282Y in Irish chromosomes and 30.4% for H63D in Basque chromosomes.[1210] The origin of the genetic mutation was thought to represent a unique event in chromosome HLA-A3 and -B7 originating from the Celts in central Europe between 65 and 70 generations ago and spreading north and west by population migration.[1211] However an alternative Viking origin has been postulated and it is recently proposed that the initial C282Y mutation occurred in mainland Europe before 4000 BC, earlier than both the Celtic and Viking periods.[1212]

The pathogenetic mechanism that leads to the gradual accumulation of body iron stores is identified as a persistent small increase in ingested dietary iron that overrides the dietary regulator over the lifetime of the patient. The normal HFE protein, as demonstrated immunohistochemically, is present in most human tissues, including all liver cells, and, while localizing throughout the gastrointestinal tract,[1213] shows high affinity with the crypt cells of the duodenum. There it physically associates with both TfR1 and β2-microglobulin and the possibility was suggested that normal HFE protein may play a role in down-regulating TfR-mediated iron uptake.[1214]

However, the precise mechanism leading to excessive dietary iron absorption in hereditary haemochromatosis is still unknown and two hypotheses are currently advanced to explain the mechanism.[1215,1216] The first involves programming of the duodenal crypt cell. The demonstration of both the mutant HFE protein and TfR1 in these cells raises the postulate that mutant HFE protein decreases the regulatory iron pool in the undifferentiated crypt.[1214] These cells are not exposed to dietary iron and normally require uptake of iron from the bloodstream, via normal HFE and TfR1, to sustain growth and function, hence the hypothesis that HFE is involved in the sensing of circulating iron levels. In hereditary haemochromatosis, the mutation results in an iron-deficient crypt enterocyte, which results in the daughter villus enterocytes having a relatively iron deficient state. They are thus programmed to increase expression of the iron transporter genes including *DMT1* and *ferroportin*. This would result in increased dietary iron uptake and transfer into the bloodstream regardless of body iron requirements. The crypt programming hypothesis would be supported by the observation that iron uptake from plasma Tf by the duodenum is impaired in Hfe knockout mice.[1217]

The second hypothesis involves the action of hepcidin, which acts as a negative regulator of dietary iron absorption. Hepcidin expression is either inappropriately low or has decreased efficacy in both Hfe knockout mice and patients with hereditary haemochromatosis.[1218-1220] Furthermore, hepcidin knockout mice develop a very similar phenotype to the Hfe knockout model, with hepatic iron loading, an elevated Tf saturation, and reticuloendothelial iron sparing.[1179] It is thus apparent that abnormally low levels of hepcidin play an important role in the pathogenesis of HFE-related hereditary haemochromatosis although the cause of this under-expression is still unknown. In classic hereditary haemochromatosis, the mutant HFE may alter iron sensing upstream from hepcidin,[1168] possibly by loss of complexing with TfR1 on the cell surface, or other currently unknown factors, that could then lead to down-regulation of hepcidin by the hepatocyte regardless of circulating iron levels. This, in turn, may cause the aberrant release of iron from duodenal enterocytes and macrophages via iron exporting proteins such as ferroportin, resulting in excessive iron ingress into the circulation. The hepcidin model is further supported by the similar but more rapid loading of body iron in younger patients with juvenile haemochromatosis in which the *HAMP* gene, responsible for hepcidin synthesis, is mutated (see later).

The ultimate mechanisms whereby HFE and hepcidin interact are thus still uncertain and require further study. While the concept of crypt sensing as an important mechanism in the regulation of iron absorption has been challenged by the discovery of hepcidin,[1221] both of these paradigms may not be mutually exclusive and further studies are necessary to refine or refute these hypotheses.[1215,1216]

Four clinical stages of the disorder exist: genetic predisposition without any abnormality, asymptomatic iron overload of 2 to 5 g, iron overload with early symptoms, and iron overload with organ damage. The clinical presentation in patients who are homozygous for C282Y is highly variable with general signs of weakness in 60% of patients, arthralgia/arthritis (30–40%), hepatomegaly/cirrhosis (13–60%), diabetes mellitus (10–30%), sexual dysfunction (10–40%), and cardiac symptoms with arrhythmia (20–29%) and cardiac failure (15–35%).[1194] Skin pigmentation is estimated to occur in 47% of proband cases.[1193] However modern studies tend to downplay the importance of extrahepatic disease, including diabetes mellitus, arthritis and heart disease. The initial presentation is often vague and non-specific in many patients and a high index of suspicion is required to diagnose the condition.

Furthermore, while patients with defined HFE-haemochromatosis will test positively for the C282Y mutation, a significant proportion do not develop significant hepatic iron overload. Gene penetrance is not obligatory and recent large population-based studies confirm that penetrance is low in HFE-hereditary haemochromatosis, implying that C282Y homozygosity is necessary but not sufficient on its own to cause clinically manifesting disease.[1222,1223] Ethnicity, environmental factors including blood loss, which is an important modifier in females, dietary intake, alcohol and other as yet unknown genetic modulators may play a part in this differential expression.[1194,1215] It is likely that these disease frequencies will change further with increased awareness of the disease and the development of screening techniques.

In proband cases in whom the diagnosis is suspected, serum testing for iron overload forms the cornerstone of initial identification, namely transferrin saturation (TS), unbound iron binding capacity (UIBC) and serum ferritin. Consensus is that TS of >45%, UIBC <28 µmol/L and ferritin >300 µg/L (>200 in women) identifies hereditary haemochromatosis, although these values may not be appropriate for all populations. Ferritin in isolation is highly sensitive and its normality rules out iron overload, but it is an acute phase protein that is also elevated in inflammatory states.[1194]

Prior to the discovery of *HFE* gene mutations, liver biopsy confirmed diagnosis, identifying the typical histological features and allowing for grading and determination of the hepatic iron index (ratio of hepatic iron concentration divided by age), as discussed later. However, subsequent to the development of genotyping, the necessity for liver biopsy is now dependent on clinical status. If inflammation and other confounding factors are excluded, then serum ferritin correlates well with the level of iron excess. Magnetic-susceptibility measurement or magnetic resonance imaging (MRI) may act as a second accurate estimation of iron overload.[1224-1226] If iron load is moderate and other diagnostic parameters are normal, including serum aminotransferases, fasting blood glucose, hormonal evaluation, cardiogram, and joint and bone x-rays, then therapy by venesection may commence. In cases of heavy iron overload, when one or more of these parameters are abnormal, then liver biopsy is mandatory. In particular, this is to evaluate the presence of cirrhosis, other hepatic pathology, or iron-free foci and, at this stage, the biopsy is performed as a prognostic marker.[1194] The current gold standard in the case of hereditary haemochromatosis is thus genetic testing. The relevance of the H63D mutation as well as C282Y/H63D compound heterozygosity is still uncertain as a small percentage may develop clinically significant haemochromatosis.[1154]

The macroscopic and microscopic features of penetrant HFE-haemochromatosis are highly characteristic in the liver. The classic description is one of a brown to rusty colour, staining intense blue with the Perls stain (Fig. 5.91), with or without the naked eye appearance of cirrhosis. Histologically, the progression of the disease is again char-

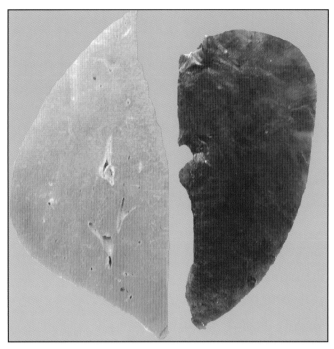

Fig. 5.91 • Post-mortem liver from a patient with hereditary haemochromatosis confirmed by HLA-A3/B7 testing. The liver has an orange-brown colour that, when dipped in Perls solution, demonstrates the characteristic Prussian-blue reaction.

acteristic. Iron deposition begins in the periportal hepatocytes (zone 1) (Fig. 5.92) and extends progressively to involve all zones of the liver (Fig. 5.93). The iron has a characteristic pericanalicular pattern when observed under high power (Fig. 5.94). With progression of the disease, there is deposition of iron in the biliary epithelium (Fig. 5.95) and, in a percentage of cases, transfer into Kupffer cells and portal macrophages with sideronecrosis (Fig. 5.96). Progressive portal fibrosis may evolve to cirrhosis that has a stellate to biliary appearance (Fig. 5.97). Of importance is the identification of iron free foci in histologically advanced liver disease, which may foretell the development of hepatocellular carcinoma, as discussed later.[1227]

Venesection forms the foundation of successful therapy for hereditary haemochromatosis. Ideally, this entails weekly phlebotomy (400–500 mL) until ferritin is <20–50 µg/L and transferrin saturation is <30%, after which maintenance venesections are carried out for the lifetime of the patient according to the above guidelines. If biopsy has been performed, the hepatic iron index can be calculated as well as a 'body iron ratio', which estimates total iron removed based on phlebotomies and related to age. Abstinence from iron-rich foods, supplements and vitamins is recommended. Chelation therapy is not warranted unless there are contraindications to venesection.[1194]

Fully penetrant hereditary haemochromatosis carries with it significant potential for morbidity and mortality, including cirrhosis and hepatocellular carcinoma, diabetes mellitus, cardiac failure, and impotence. The prevalence of alcohol abuse and chronic hepatitis C virus infections appears increased in patients with haemochromatosis, as discussed later, but sepsis secondary to bacterial infection

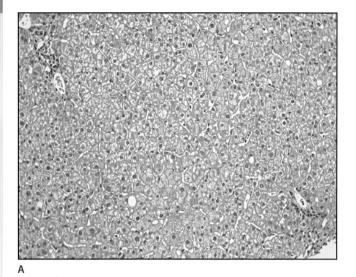

A

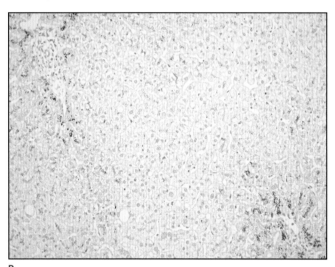

B

Fig. 5.92 • Male of 38 years with deranged liver function tests. He was subsequently identified as homozygous for the C282Y mutation on the basis of the biopsy finding. **(A)** Liver biopsy is histologically unremarkable on routine staining. H&E. **(B)** However there is grade 1 iron deposition in periportal hepatocytes. Perls stain.

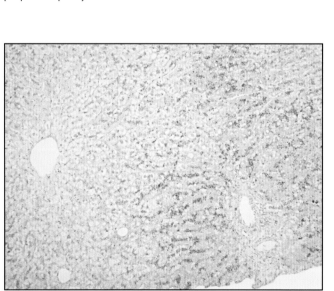

Fig. 5.93 • Male of 45 years homozygous for C282Y with abnormal liver function tests. There is grade 3 iron overload although a hepatic iron gradient is still identified. Perls stain.

Fig. 5.94 • The pericanalicular pattern of iron distribution that is characteristic of hereditary haemochromatosis. Perls stain.

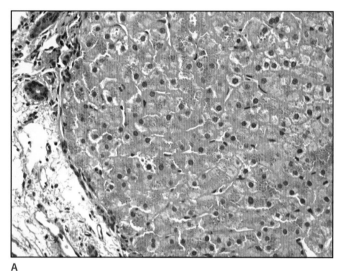

A

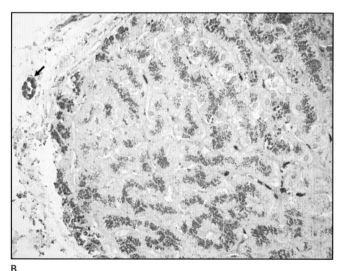

B

Fig. 5.95 • C282Y homozygote with grade 4 haemochromatosis. **(A)** Iron accumulation can be appreciated on H&E staining. **(B)** There is loss of the gradient pattern and marked iron overload in the original bile duct (arrow).

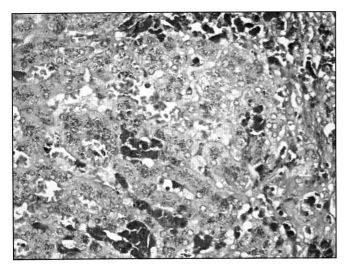

Fig. 5.96 • Male of 45 years confirmed to be homozygous for the C282Y mutation and with a history of alcohol abuse. A cirrhosis with grade 4 iron overload was confirmed histologically. Sideronecrosis is identified by large globules of haemosiderin associated with aggregates of heavily iron-laden Kupffer cells, both periportal and within the lobular parenchyma. PAS stain.

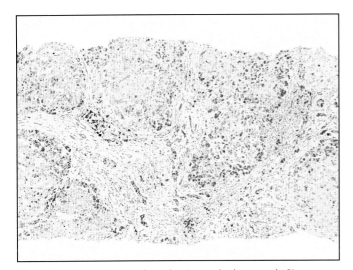

Fig. 5.97 • Patient with oesophageal varices and splenomegaly. Biopsy demonstrates established cirrhosis with periportal sideronecrosis and haemosiderin deposition in bile ducts and portal macrophages. Perls stain.

does not appear to be a significant problem, with the exception of cases of Yersinia infections. Hepatocellular carcinoma is identified as a significant cause of mortality in HFE-hereditary haemochromatosis,[1228] although its prevalence is not as high as was previously thought. The risk of developing other extrahepatic cancers is still debated. This anticipates the potential role of iron as a putative carcinogen as discussed later.[1229]

However, quantification of these factors is confounded by the prevalence of the C282Y mutation when measured against the penetrance of the gene. Few of the genetic factors influencing the expression of clinical haemochromatosis phenotype in C282Y homozygotes are currently established but polymorphisms of the major genes such as *TfR2*, *hepcidin* and *HJV* may play a role.[1196,1230] Furthermore, many common entities classically identified in patients with hereditary haemochromatosis, including diabetes and

arthritis, are also frequent in the general population. Earlier series demonstrated significant morbidity and mortality in both untreated and treated patients. Bomford and Williams identified poor survival amongst untreated patients of 18 and 6% at 5 and 10 years, respectively.[1231] Similarly, for treated cases, Niederau et al. identified a cumulated survival of 93% at 5 years and 77% at 10 years, significantly reduced when compared with the expected survival rates for a normal population.[1232] However, more modern series identify that, although most C282Y homozygotes have increased levels of transferrin saturation and serum ferritin, symptoms associated with iron overload are no greater in C282Y homozygotes when compared with sex- and age-matched controls and life expectancy is not significantly curtailed.[1194,1233]

Juvenile haemochromatosis (Haemochromatosis type 2)

Sheldon almost certainly described patients having the characteristics of juvenile haemochromatosis.[1201] However, the entity was only formally recognized after the case study and literature review of Lamon and co-workers.[1234] They described a female patient of 36 years with heart failure, diabetes mellitus, hepatomegaly and secondary amenorrhoea and reviewed another 52 cases published over the previous 85 years. Essential differences between these cases and classic hereditary haemochromatosis are notable, when compared with the large series of Finch and Finch,[1235] namely that it is a rare form of iron overload with rapid and severe progression of disease leading to significant complications before the age of 30 years. Lamon also noted the inherited nature of this rare disease and favoured an autosomal recessive inheritance.[1234] Subsequent genotyping identified the disorder to be distinct from HFE-linked iron overload. A high frequency of consanguinity is observed in patients with juvenile haemochromatosis, with the disease occurring in siblings but not parents.[1236]

A human-genome search demonstrated linkage between the disease and numerous markers on the long arm of chromosome 1q.[1237] Subsequent analysis of Greek, Canadian and French families carrying the disorder identified multiple deleterious mutations at LOC148738, whose protein product is identified as hemojuvelin (*HJV*), previously *HFE2*.[1188] A G320V substitution was identified in the *HJV* gene product in approximately two thirds of the cohort. Numerous other mutations have subsequently been identified.[1238,1239] More recent analysis of patients from the central and northern parts of Europe, specifically Germany, Slovakia, Croatia, and Ireland has also identified the G320V mutation in the majority.[1240,1241]

In addition, the investigation of juvenile haemochromatosis identified a second cohort that is even more rare, demonstrating a mutation, C70R, on *19q13*, the gene encoding hepcidin.[1240-1243] Thus classical juvenile haemochromatosis comprises a more common mutation, *HJV*, formerly *HFE2*, that causes *juvenile haemochromatosis type 2A* and a less frequent mutation, *HAMP*, formerly *HFE2B*, causing *juvenile haemochromatosis type 2B*.[1154] While hepcidin is now well recognized to play a crucial role in all aspects of iron metabolism, as already discussed, the function of hemojuvelin is uncertain. It is possible that hemojuvelin could regulate the synthesis of hepcidin. This has to be confirmed although low levels of hepcidin production are identified in patients with *HJV* mutations.[1185,1196,1244] The severe and rapid clinical course identified in juvenile haemochromatosis, when compared to haemochromatosis types 1 and 3, further emphasizes the importance of hepcidin and, almost certainly, hemojuvelin in the regulation of iron metabolism.[1239]

The concept and spectrum of juvenile haemochromatosis has been further extended by the recent identification of two young patients presenting with typical features of the disease, namely severe endocrinopathy and cardiomyopathy, but testing positively for combined mutations for C282Y/H63D and TfR2.[1196] In addition, there is evidence that selected *HJV* and *HAMP* mutations, when carried simultaneously with mutant *HFE* genes, may influence iron status in older patients being evaluated for a molecular diagnosis of haemochromatosis because of increased transferrin saturation and/or serum ferritin.[1230,1245,1246] This further challenges the current classification system for hereditary haemochromatosis in that juvenile haemochromatosis does not represent a distinct monogenic disorder but may be linked to the adult-onset form of hereditary haemochromatosis.[1196]

Juvenile haemochromatosis otherwise differs considerably from HFE-hereditary haemochromatosis with respect to age, an almost equal ratio between sexes, greater frequency of cardiac and endocrine disturbances and lower frequency of diabetes and hepatic involvement.[1234,1237] The patient usually presents in the second decade, typically with hypogonadism that manifests as primary infertility in the female. A dilated cardiomyopathy that often becomes refractory to treatment is a common complication and the untreated patient usually dies of cardiac disease by the 30th year. The hepatic complications of iron overload in juvenile haemochromatosis are not as common as in the case of hereditary haemochromatosis despite the fact that iron indices are usually far higher in these younger patients. The hepatic pathology may be profound, however, with histologically diagnosed cirrhosis developing even at a young age in up to 40% of patients.[1247] However, the clinical diagnosis of juvenile haemochromatosis is often coincidental, relating to investigation of endocrine or cardiac abnormalities including cardiac shock.[1248] Glucose intolerance is manifest in almost two-thirds of patients and there may be presentation due to arthropathy or skin changes.[1247] As noted, iron indices are often considerably higher than in the case of hereditary haemochromatosis.

The histological features of juvenile haemochromatosis are similar to those of hereditary haemochromatosis in that there is progressive zonal iron loading with typical sparing of the reticuloendothelial system.

As with hereditary haemochromatosis, aggressive venesection remains the cornerstone of therapy. Depending on the extent of progression of the disease, there may be a place for chelating therapy,[1247] with successful cardiac transplants performed in some patients.[1249]

TfR2-associated haemochromatosis (Haemochromatosis type 3)

TfR1 is ubiquitously expressed on most cell surfaces and the Tf/TfR1 pathway is critical to the normal development of erythroid precursors.[1168] However, a second receptor, TfR2 that maps to chromosome 7q22, is restricted to the liver, lacks IREs and is constitutively unable to bind HFE.[1159,1163] Rare cases of autosomal recessive iron overload in patients who are HFE-negative have been identified as being due to mutations of the TfR2 receptor.[1250]

TfR1 is consistently absent in patients with classical HFE-hereditary haemochromatosis.[1251–1253] Hepatic iron-loading continues unabated in these patients, however. In murine models of dietary iron overload and iron deficiency, as well as Hfe/mice, TfR2 expression in liver persists regardless of the model and it appears that TfR2 allows continued uptake of Tf-bound iron by hepatocytes even after TfR1 has been down-regulated by iron overload, and that this uptake contributes to the susceptibility of liver to iron loading in hereditary haemochromatosis.[1254] In addition, *TfR2*-mutant mice demonstrate low levels of expression of hepcidin mRNA, but higher levels of duodenal DMT1,[1164] which is analogous to the situation in humans with *TfR2* mutations where urinary hepcidin is measured as low or absent.[1255] However, the TfR1-deficient mouse dies in the embryonic stage of severe iron deficiency anaemia, which implies that TfR2 cannot compensate for the lack of TfR1.[1161] TfR2 may act to sense transferrin saturation, thus acting as a modulator of hepcidin in situations of iron overload, with the protein acting upstream of hepcidin in the regulatory pathway.[1163] The role of HFE and its interaction with TfR2 is still controversial, but it is postulated that these two molecules may be independent but complementary upstream modulators of hepcidin activity.[1216]

While the *TfR2* mutation is rare, at least nine individual *TfR2* mutations have been identified.[1163] With the exception of one patient of Portuguese descent with a c2069 A→C, Q690P mutation in the *TfR2* gene mutation and two affected homozygous female siblings,[1256] most represent largely inbred families of Italian extraction with various mutations of the *TfR2* gene with consanguinity being a common feature.[1257–1259] However, the AVAQ 594–597 deletion originally described by Girelli and co-workers in their Italian cohort[1258] has also been identified in three members of a Japanese family.[1260] Subsequent investigation of a further nine unrelated Japanese patients with haemochromatosis of unknown origin described two more novel *TfR2* mutations, L490R and V561X. The patient with the V561X mutation, aged 58 years, was a member of a consanguineous family.[1261] Both of these patients had cirrhosis and diabetes, one with associated skin pigmentation. Haemochromatosis is rare in the Far East, particularly amongst the Japanese, with only one patient with HFE-hereditary haemochromatosis currently described. It would thus appear that TfR2-hereditary haemochromatosis is the most common form of hereditary iron overload amongst Japanese patients although iron loading secondary to acaeruloplasminaemia is also identified in this population.[1163]

The clinical appearance of these patients mimics that of HFE-hereditary haemochromatosis, namely patients with high transferrin saturation and serum ferritins and low penetrance in premenopausal women. Age range is somewhat younger, but with slow progression of iron overload thus differing it from juvenile haemochromatosis.[1258] Occasional patients also tested heterozygous for the H63D mutation with some also exhibiting a thalassaemic trait. That the latter may contribute to the phenotypic sensitivity is not ruled out.[1256,1259]

Furthermore, analysis of a family of southern Italian lineage with features of juvenile haemochromatosis has recently demonstrated combined mutations for C282Y/H63D (compound heterozygosity) and TfR2 (Q317X) homozygosity while failing to show mutations for either HJV or hepcidin. Two siblings, male and female, diagnosed with severe endocrinopathy and cardiomyopathy at ages of 24 and 25 years respectively. Both showed cirrhosis with massive loading of iron in hepatocytes while a younger brother, aged 21 years, demonstrated a milder phenotype resembling the iron distribution of classic adult-onset hereditary haemochromatosis but carrying only the Q317X serum TfR2 homozygote mutation.[1196]

While relatively few cases have been documented, the liver pathology is again described as strongly resembling HFE-hereditary haemochromatosis with early iron deposition in periportal hepatocytes. Most demonstrate a milder degree of iron overload than those with HFE-hereditary haemochromatosis although there is progression to cirrhosis in some published cases.

Treatment, as for classic hereditary haemochromatosis, is by venesection although there is often a persistence of transferrin saturation after phlebotomy.[1255] The diagnosis is made by clinical presentation, serum iron indices and elimination of the HFE genotype. Although TfR2 hereditary haemochromatosis is even rarer than juvenile haemochromatosis, both stand to be of considerable importance in the understanding of the molecular pathogenesis of iron regulation.

Ferroportin-associated iron overload (haemochromatosis Type 4)

After the identification of the HFE gene it rapidly became apparent that significant numbers of iron overload disorders could not be explained by HFE mutations, particularly in Europe where C282Y homozygosity was responsible for 90% of cases in the United Kingdom and Brittany but only 64% and 30% in the southern European countries of Italy and Greece respectively.[1262] Occasional cases could be explained by mutations of TfR2 or HJV/HAMP but a more common disease related to abnormalities of the iron exporter ferroportin.[1148–1150]

Previous studies had identified an autosomal dominant iron overload condition in a large family from Italy.[1263] In the wake of the discovery of ferroportin, genome-wide screening procedures confirmed that these same patients were affected by a candidate gene on 2q32, SLC40A1, previously named SLC11A3. All were heterozygous for a c. 230

C→A substitution resulting in the replacement of alanine 77 with aspartate.[1264] At the same time a different heterozygosity was identified in a Dutch pedigree, c. 430 A→C (N144H),[1265] This was subsequently known as ferroportin disease.[1262]

Ferroportin encodes a transmembrane transporter with IRE function that acts as an iron exporter. The pathogenesis is thus quite different from that of hereditary haemochromatosis although the protein is situated at the membranes of the same cell types as HFE, including placental syncytiotrophoblasts, duodenal enterocytes, reticuloendothelial cells and liver, particularly Kupffer cells. Ferroportin is directly involved in the release of iron from macrophages and mutations of SLC40A1 represent the mechanism leading to the ferroportin disease. Various mutations of the gene have been identified with similar outcomes, leading to the conclusion that the basic mechanism is a net loss of protein function.[1238,1262]

In an elegant in vitro study,[1266] ferroportin was identified as multimeric and mutant ferroportin can multimerize with the normal thus affecting its function. All mutations are of missense type and, depending on the mutation, the mutant ferroportin can affect the cellular location of the wild type protein and/or its responsiveness to hepcidin. Two pathogenetic groups are recognized. In one, there is loss of iron export function due to mislocalization of the mutant protein with the protein localizing in an intracellular distribution as opposed to the normal membranous display. In this situation, there is no binding to hepcidin or hepcidin-induced degradation. The resultant reduction in iron efflux causes a bottleneck in macrophages, which generate the largest iron flows, resulting in iron accumulation in Kupffer cells and macrophages with high ferritin levels and low to normal transferrin saturation.

The second group retains full iron export capability with the mutation localized to the membrane but resistant to hepcidin. The authors surmise that the mutation affects domains required for internalization and degradation; the lack of ferroportin regulation by hepcidin thus mimics hepcidin deficiency and causes a phenotype similar to classic haemochromatosis, with inappropriately high duodenal absorption, increased transferrin saturation, and iron deposition in hepatocytes.[1266] These in vitro findings explain the variable clinical and histological findings of the disease.

Numerous mutations of the ferroportin gene have been identified,[1238,1267] with divergent findings with respect to the pattern of ferritin/transferrin dissociation in probands of French-Canadian, Melanesian, Thai and European heritage,[1268–1272] which explains the in vitro findings discussed above.[1266] Clinical presentation thus appears heterogeneous. Ferroportin disease, as originally described, may manifest with the same features of haemochromatosis including glucose intolerance, arthropathy and skin pigmentation. The associated liver disease is usually not as severe. Dependent on the mutation, serum ferritin rises early in the disease in spite of low to normal transferrin saturation, the opposite picture to classic haemochromatosis. Hypochromic anaemia is common and may require iron supplementation, which may further exacerbate the iron overload. There may be poor tolerance to phlebotomy. If the mutation retains full iron export capability, however, the clinical picture is analogous to hereditary haemochromatosis with high duodenal absorption and increased transferrin saturation and the disease may present at a younger age.

Equally, two patterns of histology are identified (Fig. 5.98). In the ferroportin disease, as originally described, the early stage of the disease demonstrates Kupffer cell iron overload, increasing over time with often large and coalescent deposits in Kupffer cells and macrophages and some deposition in hepatocytes. In the second pattern, there is evidence of primary hepatocyte loading. In a family of European heritage described by Sham and co-workers, with a unique mutation, 977 GYC(Cys326Ser), there was hepatocyte rather than Kupffer cell accretion,[1267] and in patients first described as having an autosomal dominant form of haemochromatosis, from the Solomon islands, the histology resembles the gradient pattern of hepatocyte described for classic hereditary haemochromatosis.[1268,1269]

Although venesection is again the cornerstone of therapy, it may not be tolerated equally in all patients and low transferrin saturation with anaemia may be rapidly established despite serum ferritin still being elevated. If phlebotomy is discontinued, there is a rapid rise in the ferritin level and both oral chelation and erythropoietin may be of some benefit.[1262] The disease must be suspected in any individual with unexplained hyperferritinaemia, and investigated with serum iron studies and genetic testing, if available, of the immediate family.

A possible role for a common ferroportin polymorphism (Q248H) identified in African and African-American iron overload, and that may act as a modifying factor in this disease, is discussed later.

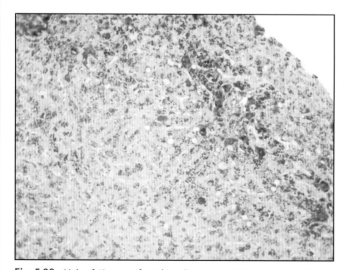

Fig. 5.98 • Male of 43 years of southern European origin presenting with arthritis and mildly deranged liver function tests. Serum ferritin was 4150 ng/mL with transferrin saturation of 63.7%. No demonstrable cause for the iron overload was identified and C282Y and H63D mutations were not detected. In view of the marked iron deposition in hepatocytes and Kupffer cells, a diagnosis of ferroportin disease was considered although definitive genetic testing was not available. Perls stain.

Neonatal haemochromatosis

A disorder characterized by stillbirth or hepatic failure during the first days to, rarely, weeks of life, neonatal haemochromatosis demonstrates accumulation of heavy iron overload in the liver and other organs including pancreas and heart in a distribution similar to that identified in HFE-hereditary haemochromatosis but not demonstrating HLA serotypes.[1273] The syndrome is extremely rare with little more than 100 cases being described,[1274] and is the most poorly understood of the putative genetic iron overload disorders.

Various theories exist to explain the aetiology of neonatal haemochromatosis including fetal liver injury causing abnormalities of iron handling or, alternatively, abnormalities of iron handling by the maternofetal unit, with the possibility existing that they are not mutually exclusive.[1275] An alloimmune mechanism for the disease is recently postulated.[1276] The inheritance is not confirmed in all cases and transmission has been variably reported as autosomal recessive, codominant and dominant with variable penetrance with reports of recurrence in siblings and half-siblings.[1274] However, in these sibships, the recurrence is at a rate higher than may be predicted for simple Mendelian autosomal-recessive inheritance,[1275] and the disease has also occasionally been reported in consanguineous families.[1277,1278] Patients and parents may carry an *HFE* gene, but homozygosity to C282Y or compound heterozygosity for C282Y/H63D is not yet reported.[1247]

The neonatal phenotype may also present in patients with other metabolic, genetic and infectious disorders including tyrosinaemia, Down Syndrome, tricho-hepato-enteric and GRACILE syndromes, cytomegalovirus and non-A, non-B hepatitis.[1275] Kelly and co-workers have identified three modes of disease transmission: (i) infection acquired in pregnancy or infectious diseases namely Coxsackie viral infection, E coli bacteraemia, Candidiasis, Staphylococcus aureus, and Herpes simplex virus; (ii) maternal transmission with the appearance of maternal antinuclear factor and ribonuclear antibodies, mitochondria harbouring pathogenic mutations in the organellar genome, or gonadal mosaicism for a new dominant gene mutation in the mother; and (iii) transmission suggesting autosomal recessive inheritance.[1278]

The neonate suffering from neonatal haemochromatosis is often stillborn or premature, exhibiting intrauterine growth retardation and, often, associated placental oedema and either oligohydramnios or polyhydramnios. The overriding presentation in patients is one of chronic-pattern neonatal liver failure in the antenatal or early neonatal period, usually within a period of hours to days post-delivery. Jaundice with coagulopathy, hypoglycaemia and hypoalbuminaemia are common with transferrin saturation, low iron-binding capacity and high serum ferritin. The latter may reflect non-specific liver disease or inflammation. Thus diagnosis is made after exclusion of other causes of liver failure and may be confirmed by salivary gland biopsy, which demonstrates excess iron,[1279] and magnetic resonance imaging, which typically shows iron deposition in liver, pancreas and heart but with sparing of the spleen.[1280,1281]

Autopsy findings include a shrunken liver usually with cirrhosis. At histology, there is framework collapse with giant cell transformation, stem cell proliferation and bile plugging with diffuse haemosiderin deposition in hepatocytes and, sometimes, bile duct cells (Fig. 5.99). Regenerative nodules may show severe atypism.[1275] There is often sparing of the reticuloendothelial system. Extensive haemosiderin deposition is also inevitably identified in many other organs including myocardium, pancreas, thymus, thyroid and salivary glands.[1278]

The prognosis of neonatal haemochromatosis is generally poor. Antioxidant therapy and chelation may be of limited value,[1278,1282] and orthototopic liver transplantation has been identified as a viable therapeutic option. In this case, there may be re-accumulation of hepatic iron, probably from mobilization of general iron stores, and post-transplantation chelation may thus be of value.[1283] Spontaneous remissions have been reported in two patients.[1284,1285]

Of note is a recent study by Hibbard and Whitington who administered high dose intravenous immunoglobulin derived from pooled serum of multiple donors to 15 women whose most recent pregnancy ended in neonatal haemochromatosis.[1276] Twelve babies had evidence of liver involvement with neonatal haemochromatosis but all survived with medical or no treatment and were healthy at follow-up at 6 months. The authors postulate that treatment with high-dose IVIG during gestation appears to have modified recurrent neonatal haemochromatosis, thus further supporting an alloimmune mechanism for the disease.

African (-American) iron overload

Strachan originally identified iron overload in black African patients in 1929, based on a necropsy study of 876 individuals. These patients were from several parts of southern and central Africa, dying in Johannesburg, South Africa from 1925 to 1928. He noted its commonality, postulated a dietary origin and identified changes ranging from mild pigmentation to established cirrhosis and 'bronzed diabetes'.[1286] Although declining in urbanized communities in south Africa,[1287] African iron overload (AIO), formerly called 'Bantu siderosis', is still an important pathology in rural society where up to 15% of adult males may be affected.[1288–1290] Traditional teaching is that the condition is the consequence of consumption of food or and, more significantly, large quantities of traditional beer prepared in iron pots or drums.[1291,1292] During cooking or brewing in these iron pots, the pH falls to acidic levels thus leeching an ionized and bio-available iron into the food or beverage.[1293]

AIO was originally considered to reflect a disease exclusively related to surplus dietary iron. There is no evidence that it relates to HFE mutations.[1294] However, more recent and discordant data imply that not all drinkers, and some nondrinkers, acquire the disease. This has led to the postulate that AIO may have both dietary and genetic components.[1289,1295,1296] There has been recent interest in iron overload amongst African-American patients who present with mild anaemia and possible tendency to iron loading that is thought to be underdiagnosed in that population.[1297] Its relationship to AIO is unclear although a mutation of the ferroportin gene (Q248H) has recently been identified in a minority of Africans and African-Americans with iron overload.[1298,1299] However, its significance in the pathogenesis of these disorders is currently unknown and, in a study of black African patients with dietary iron overload, the mutation was not detected more often in the index patients than in unaffected family members.[1300]

In southern Africa, more than two-thirds of the rural adult population consumes traditional beverages. These are mostly male patients and the result is often an iron overload state with hepatic iron concentrations that may be as high as are identified in hereditary haemochromatosis. The

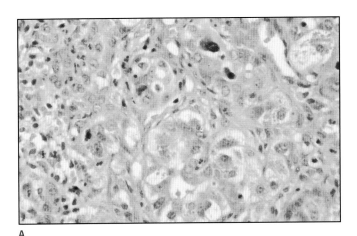

A

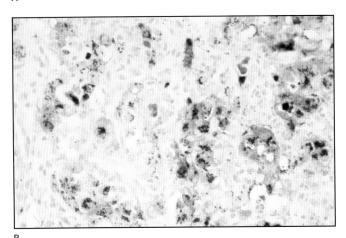

B

Fig. 5.99 • Neonatal haemochromatosis. Liver removed from a baby boy aged 4 weeks at the time of transplantation. (A) Parenchymal damage with extensive bridging cell loss, ballooning and pigmentation associated with severe canalicular cholestasis. H&E. (B) Same case to show that the pigment consists largely of haemosiderin. Perls stain.

patient with advanced AIO may develop a constellation of features including cirrhosis[1291,1301,1302] and diabetes mellitus,[1303] together with ascorbic acid deficiency[1304] and osteoporosis.[1305]

The liver pathology in AIO has traditionally been described as a primary reticuloendothelial disease with secondary involvement of the hepatocytes.[1306] However, a review of patients in later years has identified a range of morphological changes ranging from primary deposition in hepatocytes, having the typical pericanalicular deposition of hereditary haemochromatosis (Figs 5.100 and 5.101), through a mixed pattern to the predominant reticulo-endothelial pattern described by earlier workers (Fig. 5.102).[1307] This bears a resemblance to the patterns of alternate Kupffer cell and hepatocyte dominance identified in ferroportin-linked haemochromatosis.[1266] Despite the alcoholic connotation of AIO, there is very rarely evidence of acute or chronic alcoholic liver disease. Steatosis, alcoholic hepatitis and perivenular fibrosis are not identified and the pattern of fibrosis is characteristically one of progressive portal-portal linking with normal hepatic veins identified until late in the disease after cirrhosis has intervened.

Survival in patients with established AIO is poor. In a series of 22 patients, 14 of whom originally presented to hospital because of liver disease, serum ferritin was elevated in all and the transferrin saturation was greater than 60% in 93% of cohort. Three quarters of the patients had hepatic iron concentration greater than 350 µg/g dry weight, an extreme elevation associated with a high risk of fibrosis and cirrhosis. Six patients (26%) had died after a median follow-up of 19 months.[1308] A lethal outcome is the development of hepatocellular carcinoma.[1309]

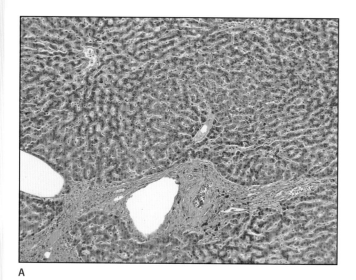

A

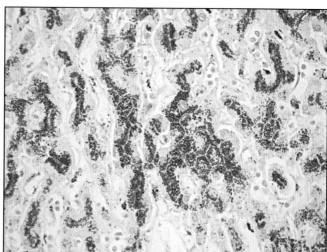

Fig. 5.101 • Same patient as is illustrated in Fig. 5.100. A high power photomicrograph demonstrates the pericanalicular iron distribution for comparison with Fig. 5.94. Perls stain.

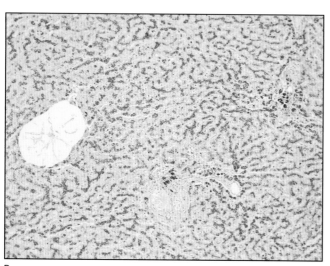

B

Fig. 5.100 • Black male patient 72 years of age from a region of South Africa noted for African iron overload. Post mortem liver tissue was submitted from a rural hospital. **(A)** Identifiable hepatocyte iron overload with mild portal fibrosis. H&E. **(B)** Grade 4 hepatocyte iron overload with focal deposition in portal macrophages. The pattern bears striking resemblance to HFE-hereditary haemochromatosis. Perls stain.

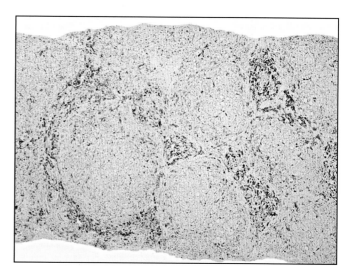

Fig. 5.102 • The pattern of mesenchymal iron overload and portal fibrosis is that typically illustrated in earlier publications dealing with African iron overload. Perls stain.

Hereditary hyperferritinaemia

Elevation of serum ferritin results from a variety of causes that can be either acquired or hereditary. The former is caused by a plethora of conditions including inflammation and malignancy, alcohol, insulin resistance and other primary liver diseases, while the latter encompasses the various types of hereditary haemochromatosis. After eliminating the former, most variants of haemochromatosis are confirmed by symptomatology, a biochemical profile including ferritin and transferrin saturation, visceral iron overload and genotyping. A high serum ferritin in the face of high transferrin saturation would suggest hereditary haemochromatosis that may be HFE-related, juvenile or the *TfR2* variant. Conversely, a high serum ferritin without an in increase transferrin saturation may imply the Ferroportin disease or African iron overload. However, in the absence of an identifiable cause, the presence of a high to very high serum ferritin with normal to only moderately raised transferrin saturation may suggest a hereditary hyperferritinaemia.[1196,1310]

The hereditary hyperferritinaemias, excluding ferroportin disease, are mostly related to mutations in the L-ferritin gene, which causes the hereditary hyperferritinaemia cataract syndrome (HHCS), or the caeruloplasmin gene as discussed later. HHCS is characterized by an elevation of serum ferritin with early onset cataract formation. The hyperferritinaemia is due to the aberrant regulation of L-ferritin translation caused by mutations throughout the 5′-untranslated region of the IRE of L-ferritins.[1311,1312] This rare condition is not associated with visceral iron overload.

However, another mutation of H-ferritin, with hyperferritinaemia and concomitant iron overload, is described in four of seven members of a Japanese family.[1313] It is a dominantly inherited iron overload with a heterozygous single point mutation (A49U) in the IRE motif of H-ferritin mRNA. The proband, a female of 56 years, was coincidentally identified during workup for gastric cancer and had a serum ferritin of 1654 µg/L and a moderately raised transferrin saturation of 58%. Liver biopsy demonstrated a pattern of iron overload similar to hereditary haemochromatosis in addition to heavy loading of iron in splenic macrophages. No further cases have been identified since the original series, and the results are not reproduced in the heterozygous H-ferritin knockout mouse that demonstrates iron overload in the spleen but not the liver.[1314] This entity has been identified as haemochromatosis type 5[1315] but not in the OMIM database,[1316] where the cohort is identified at OMIM No. 134770.

Summary

Current understanding of the group of conditions that may be considered within the spectrum of hereditary haemochromatosis is that HFE-hereditary haemochromatosis is the most common and dominant mutation worldwide, but largely within populations of northern European heritage. Lesser but significant numbers of cases due to the various ferroportin mutations are identified in southern Europe and in other populations including French-Canadian, Melanesian and Thai. Africans and African-Americans show a specific ferroportin mutation although an identifiable hereditary basis still has to be confirmed for AIO. Juvenile and *TfR2* variants are extremely rare, the former confined to Europe and the latter identified in both Japan and Europe. Neonatal haemochromatosis is, again, rare and genetically undefined at present time while hereditary hyperferritinaemia is currently confined to a single Japanese family.

Hepcidin is considered pivotal to the understanding of most of these variants of iron overload although, and as noted, it is likely that the identification of yet other regulators will be required in order to fully explain the regulatory process. To this end, mutation of DMT1 is recently reported in humans, again associated with hypochromic anaemia and hepatic iron overload.[1317] Furthermore, animal models hold significant promise in further elucidating the molecular pathogenesis of iron overload, including the recent development of a mouse model of juvenile haemochromatosis.[1318] Numerous extensive reviews offer further insight into the subject.[1154,1156,1168,1193,1215,1216,1319,1320]

Primary/inherited disorders of iron balance and distribution

Atransferrinaemia/hypotransferrinaemia

Hypotransferrinaemia may be acquired in cases of infection, primary liver disease and malignant tumours.[1156] An extremely rare hereditary disorder, atransferrinaemia was first described in a young girl with severe hypochromic anaemia and marked, generalized iron overload[1321] and has since been described in less than 10 families worldwide with molecular characterization in two individuals.[940,1322,1323] An autosomal recessive inheritance is postulated,[1324] with possible consanguinity identified in one patient.[1323] It is also considered that the mutation may be slightly 'leaky' with a small amount of gene product being produced in mouse models and some patients.[1322]

Transferrin delivers iron to the erythroid precursors and the defect leads to decreased haemoglobin synthesis resulting in a severe microcytic, hypochromic anaemia. However, this in turn leads to increased intestinal absorption that, although inefficiently handled in the plasma, is efficiently imported by parenchymal cells leading to often severe parenchymal iron overload at sites including liver, myocardium, pancreas and thyroid.

Clinical presentation and features of the deficiency include pallor and fatigue with high serum ferritin, serum iron and decreased TIBC with absent to low transferrin saturation.[1154] Treatment may be relatively effective, at least in some patients, via combined infusion of fresh frozen plasma, and subsequent phlebotomy or chelation therapy.[1154,1322] A spontaneous form of hypotransferrinaemia has been identified in mice, resulting in circulating levels of transferrin at about 1% of normal and animals that survive for short periods of time unless treated with transfusions and transferrin replacement. Development is then normal apart from iron overload in multiple organs and subtle architectural changes in the central nervous system.[1325]

Acaeruloplasminaemia

Caeruloplasmin is a serum glycoprotein and a copper-containing ferroxidase mapping to chromosome 3q21-24.7.[1326] It is synthesized by hepatocytes and catalyses the oxidation of ferrous to ferric iron, this being necessary for the release of iron to plasma transferrin. Recognition of this role came with the identification of patients with aceruloplasminemia,[1327,1328] an extremely rare autosomal recessive disease described mainly in Japanese patients. Loss of function mutations in the ceruloplasmin gene result in iron overload in the liver and pancreas and progressive neurodegeneration.

Patients develop diabetes mellitus, retinal degeneration, ataxia, and dementia late in life.[1329] A mild-to-moderate degree of anaemia with low serum iron and elevated serum ferritin is a constant feature and the pattern of hepatic iron overload is reminiscent of hereditary haemochromatosis.[1330,1331] As noted by Bosio and colleagues, although rare in Caucasians, acaeruloplasminaemia is sometimes identified and should be included in the differential diagnosis of anaemia with high serum ferritin.[1330]

Acquired/secondary iron overload

Hypochromic anemia is common and generally caused by iron deficiency with numerous well-defined causes. However, less common genetic causes are identified and, within the spectrum of these hereditary anaemias, variable iron overload in the liver may be identified as the result of mechanisms that are variably understood. These include the iron loading anaemias, Thalassaemia major and sideroblastic anaemia.

Thalassaemia

The thalassaemias represent the major cause of iron overload in Mediterranean countries and constitute the most common single gene inherited disorder in the world. The disease comprises a defect of synthesis of either the alpha or beta globin chains of haemoglobin, transmitted by Mendelian recessive inheritance.[1332] Beta-thalassaemia is the more severe and clinically important type, in particular the homozygote and compound heterozygote (thalassaemia major and intermedia).

Beta-thalassaemia requires constant transfusions from shortly after birth and iron starts to accumulate at a relatively young age. The extent of body iron overload is the most important determinant of clinical outcome in thalassaemia major with the metal starting to accumulate after a year of regular transfusions.[1333] The number of transfusions is often inadequate to account for the iron overload and the disease is characterized by mild, ineffective erythropoiesis that can also induce excess iron absorption via provocation of the dietary pool.[1334] Thus chelation forms a major part of its management. However, the burden of disease is often in less developed countries where these conventional therapies are often unavailable and, even in developed first world countries such as the UK, up to 50% of patients with beta-

thalassaemia major die before the age of 35 years, mainly because conventional iron-chelation therapy is too taxing for full adherence (Fig. 5.103).[1335]

That thalassaemic patients may be burdened by a second form of iron overload is thus significant. Longo and co-workers concluded that a single mutation in the *HFE* gene does not influence the severity of iron loading in thalassaemia patients following a regular transfusion and chelation program, although their solitary patient with H63D homozygosity was severely iron-loaded.[1336] Conversely, Riva et al. described clinical, biochemical and histopathological findings of a patient with type 3 haemochromatosis associated with the beta-thalassaemia trait and concluded that, as observed in HFE haemochromatosis, the beta-thalassaemia trait seems to aggravate the clinical picture of patients lacking TFR2, favouring higher rates of iron accumulation probably by activation of the erythroid iron regulator.[1337] In their study of 101 individuals heterozygous for beta-thalassaemia, Martins et al. suggested that the

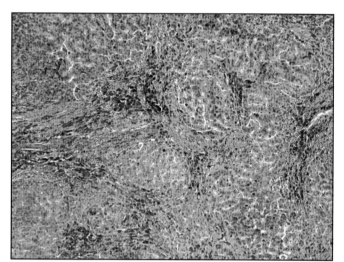

A

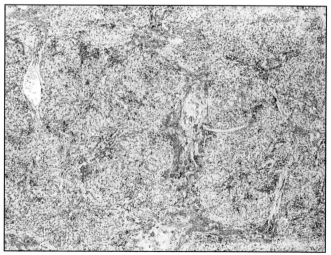

B

Fig. 5.103 • (A) Beta thalassaemia. Male patient died aged 17 years despite chelation and venesection once the diagnosis was confirmed. The post mortem liver specimen demonstrates advanced portal fibrosis and identifiable pigmentation. H&E. **(B)** There is massive iron overload of both hepatocytes and Kupffer cells. Perls stain.

beta-thalassemia trait tends to be aggravated with the coinheritance of H63D mutation, even when present in heterozygosity.[1334] Thus the relationship between the disease and other forms of haemochromatosis is still somewhat contentious, although a current review supports the concept of increased iron burden and more severe clinical phenotype in C282Y homozygotes with beta-thalassaemia.[1319]

Sideroblastic anaemias

The sideroblastic anaemias comprise a heterogeneous group of haemopoietic disorders, both hereditary and acquired, characterized by anaemia with ringed sideroblasts in the bone marrow. The sideroblast is an erythroid precursor that shows excessive deposition of mitochondrial iron, mostly in the form of the recently identified mitochondrial ferritin (m-Ferr), encoded by a gene on chromosome 5q23,[1338] and whose discovery may influence the understanding of entities such as X-linked sideroblastic anaemia and Friedreich ataxia.[1339,1340] Features of the X-linked disorder and its numerous allelic variants include: (i) anaemia detected first in childhood in some cases; (ii) death from haemochromatosis at a relatively young age, with the number of transfusions inadequate to account for the iron overload; (iii) hyperferricaemia; and (iv) abundance of siderocytes in peripheral blood after splenectomy.[1341]

The reason for the excessive iron overload in patients with sideroblastic anaemia is currently uncertain. Peto and co-workers identified a middle-aged female with a very mild form of familial sideroblastic anaemia dying from cardiac iron overload. They assumed excessive absorption of dietary iron to be the mechanism.[1342] Subsequently, study of the family of a patient with idiopathic refractory sideroblastic anaemia and haemochromatosis revealed that 2 of 5 first-degree relatives had significant elevations of serum ferritin and shared a human leucocytic antigen haplotype, supporting the concept that patients with idiopathic refractory sideroblastic anaemia and significant iron overload have at least one allele for haemochromatosis.[1343] Conversely, Beris and colleagues investigated forty Caucasian patients with acquired sideroblastic anaemia and concluded that ineffective erythropoiesis without associated mutation in the *HFE* gene can lead to iron overload in these patients.[1344]

Porphyria cutanea tarda

The porphyrias, as discussed earlier in this chapter, are a group of metabolic disorders that demonstrate defects in the haem synthetic pathway, classified as hepatic or erythroid. PCT is the most common porphyria associated with iron overload. Hepatic steatosis on liver biopsy is a near-universal finding with varying degrees of iron overload identified in approximately 80% of patients. Cirrhosis develops in 30 to 40% of cases and the incidence of hepatocellular carcinoma is also increased, as well as a high prevalence of hepatitis virus antibodies, the latter having significant geographic variability.[1345]

As mentioned earlier there is an apparent association between PCT and hereditary haemochromatosis with carriage of the C282Y and H63D mutations in ranges ranging from 17 to 47% in various parts of the world, which may serve to explain the poor response of some patients with PCT to appropriate phlebotomy.[17] It is postulated that inheritance of one or more HFE mutations is an important susceptibility for sporadic PCT.[1346] There is also debate regarding a relationship between PCT, HFE and chronic hepatitis C viral infection (Fig. 5.104), with the recommendation that all patients with PCT should be tested for chronic HCV infection and HFE mutations.[27]

Parenteral iron overload

The absolute need for long-term transfusion for diseases such as thalassaemia or the various causes of bone marrow failure is long established. As there is no physiological mechanism for the excretion of iron, the result is an

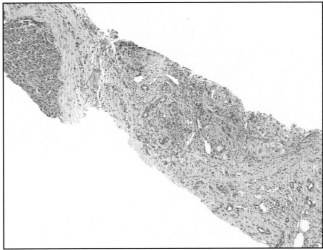

A

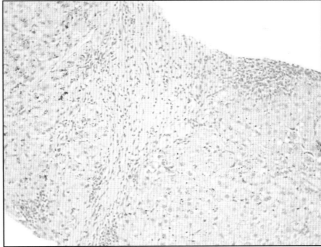

B

Fig. 5.104 • Female of 72 years with porphyria cutanea tarda and chronic hepatitis C virus infection. The patient was clinically cirrhotic. HFE status was unknown. (A) A broad, inflamed fibrous septum traverses the biopsy and focus of hepatocellular carcinoma is identified in a portal vessel. H&E. (B) There is mild haemosiderin deposition in the surrounding parenchyma, which could be explained by either the PCT or the chronic viral infection. Perls stain.

accumulation of iron, each unit of transfused blood containing 200 to 250 mg of iron.[1139] The iron excess is derived from senescent red blood cells and will thus be sequestered in Kupffer cells and macrophages. This is associated with minimal architectural disturbance in the liver (Fig. 5.105).

In excess, transfusional iron will also deposit in other organs including spleen, endocrine organs and heart. Cardiomyopathy is more likely in transfusional iron overload than hereditary haemochromatosis, possibly due to the rapidity of loading. Routine serum ferritin measurements are indicated and liver biopsy or magnetic imaging studies[1225] may be necessary for more accurate quantitation of the body iron burden. As phlebotomy is usually not a treatment option, chelation therapy may have to be instituted in such patients.[1139]

Anaemia of inflammation

Alternatively known as anaemia of chronic disease, this condition commonly accompanies many chronic infectious and inflammatory states as well as certain malignant diseases. Iron is a prerequisite for all systems and a decrease in serum iron in infectious states, for example, may actively contribute to the host defence system by withholding iron from invading pathogens. Hepcidin was originally identified as a microcidal agent although the extent of its efficacy in vivo is uncertain.[1347] Evidence from animal models now confirms the dominant role played in these conditions by the mediation of hepcidin by interleukin-6 and possibly interleukin-1.[1176,1177]

It is held that such states, typified by chronic hypoferraemia, are reflected in the liver by the sequestration of iron in Kupffer cells (Fig. 5.106). This is borne out in animal models but recent murine models of hepcidin-producing tumours demonstrate predominant hepatocyte overload when compared to reticuloendothelial sites.[1348] Hepatocytes may thus play a previously unappreciated role in the sequestration of iron in anaemia of inflammation. However,

detailed human studies of hepatic iron stores in chronic inflammation in are currently unavailable and it remains to be seen whether the mouse model is predictive of the cellular and organ distribution of iron in human anaemia of inflammation.

Iron overload in other chronic liver diseases

Common chronic liver diseases including viral hepatitis, alcoholic liver disease and the non-alcoholic fatty liver are often associated with hepatic iron overload. This is usually of low grade, but is sometimes sufficiently severe as to mistakenly identify hereditary haemochromatosis although this is less of a problem after the introduction of genotyping.[1349] Important questions still have to be answered, however. These include the relationship between iron and the primary disease as well as well as its possible association with the various types of hereditary haemochromatosis. Is iron a bystander or does it contribute to the pathogenesis and outcome of these diseases? In the light of modern advances in the molecular pathogenesis of iron overload, there is a need for re-evaluation.

Hepatitis B and C viruses

Research conducted before genotyping was available documented the deposition of iron in the livers of patients with chronic hepatitis B virus (HBV) infection and supported the observation that the amount of iron accumulated in these patients related to severity of the inflammation rather than the duration of infection or degree of fibrosis, as summarized by Bonkovsky and colleagues.[1350] An association between HBV and HFE mutations is more contentious in recent studies, however, either supporting or refuting a relationship.[1351,1352] This may, in part, reflect the ethnic and geographic differences that exist with respect to both diseases. In southern Africa, for example, chronic HBV infection and African iron overload are both associated with

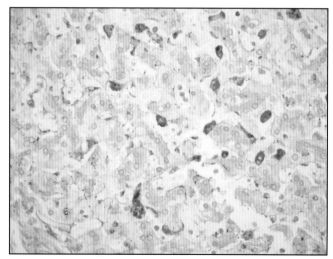

Fig. 5.105 • Parenteral iron overload. Male patient with sideroblastic anaemia requiring regular blood transfusions. There is haemosiderin deposition in Kupffer cells. Occasional granules are identified in hepatocytes. Perls stain.

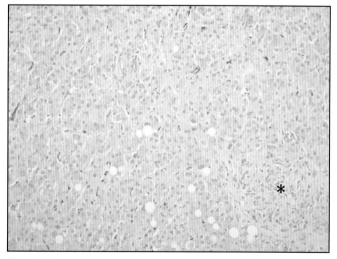

Fig. 5.106 • Patient of 36 years with anaemia of inflammation. A granulomatous hepatitis was identified and tuberculosis was thereafter confirmed. Excess iron is noted in Kupffer cells as well as the epithelioid cells of the granuloma (asterisk). Perls stain.

fibrosis, cirrhosis and hepatocellular carcinoma (Fig. 5.107).[1309] Such studies are infrequent when compared to those pertaining to the more ubiquitous hepatitis C virus (HCV) infection based, at least, on numbers of current publications.

Chronic virus C infection often results in elevation of serum ferritin levels and build-up of iron in the liver (Fig. 5.108).[1353] The accumulation of iron is typically mild but tends to increase with progression of the disease and iron indices may ultimately approximate that equivalent to hereditary haemochromatosis.[1349,1354] Levels of inflammation and stage of disease may also correlate with the build-up of iron,[1355,1356] and numerous studies have demonstrated that therapeutic phlebotomy may decrease alanine aminotransferase, as summarized by Eisenbach et al.[1357] Furthermore, recent studies from Japan indicate that histological staging may improve with the institution of long-term phlebotomy.[1358,1359] That therapy and sustained viral response may relate to iron overload and iron depletion remains disputed.[1357]

The presence of iron is critical for both host and pathogen and the possibility that iron overload gives a selective advantage to replication of the virus has been supported by in vitro experiments.[1360] Of interest, too, is the association between chronic HVC infection and the expression of hepcidin. Aoki and co-workers studied hepcidin RNA extracted from the livers of patients chronically infected with HCV and identified its expression to be independent of markers of inflammation, genotype and viral load, but strongly associated with hepatic iron concentrations and ferritin levels. They note that HCV is a cell-mediated immune response characterized by a TH1 immune response, as opposed to the IL-6 and IL-1 driven acute phase response that stimulates hepcidin. These workers did not identify the HFE status of their patients.[1361]

A relationship between HCV infection and hereditary haemochromatosis would appear apparent, as is the case with PCT. Given the relatively high global prevalence of HFE mutations, there is clear evidence for a higher frequency of stainable iron amongst C282Y carriers and, possibly, H63D heterozygotes with chronic HCV infection. However, the relationship between disease severity and HFE mutations is less clear-cut with numerous groups producing discrepant results. In a recent, large study of 316 patients with chronic HCV infection, 57 having an HFE mutation, it was concluded that HFE mutations are independently associated with hepatic iron concentration and advanced fibrosis in patients with compensated liver disease from chronic hepatitis C, especially after controlling for duration of disease.[1362] The authors suggest that HFE mutations accelerate hepatic fibrosis in hepatitis C but may not be responsible for progression to end-stage liver disease. Conversely, Eisenbach and colleagues, summarizing numerous other recent studies, conclude that the virus alters iron homeostasis in the liver and accelerates and aggravates liver injury,

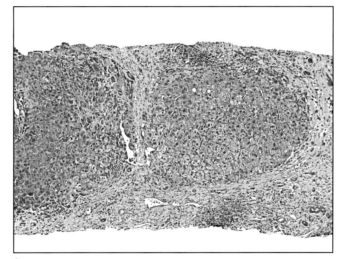

A

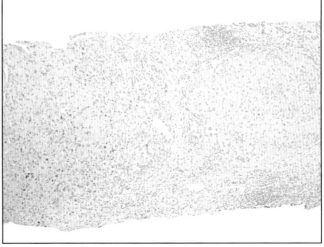

B

Fig. 5.108 • Hepatitis C virus and iron. Caucasian female of 68 years with chronic hepatitis C virus infection. HFE status is unknown. **(A)** Established cirrhosis with lymphocytic inflammatory aggregates. Masson trichrome. **(B)** Moderate haemosiderin deposition without the pericanalicular accentuation that is typical of hereditary haemochromatosis. The haemosiderin is more prominent in one of two cirrhotic nodules. Perls stain.

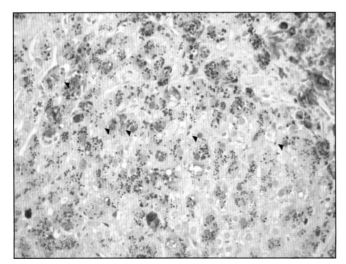

Fig. 5.107 • Hepatitis B virus and iron. Black South African male of 46 years with chronic hepatitis B virus infection and a history of traditional beer usage. There is nuclear hepatitis B core antigen (arrowed), implying on-going viral replication, and marked iron overload. Marked portal fibrosis with imminent cirrhosis was noted on the biopsy. Immunostaining for HBcAg with Perls counterstaining.

and, furthermore, that patients carrying heterozygous C282Y or C282Y/H63D mutations are at substantial risk for acceleration of disease.[1357] Furthermore, there is putative interaction between chronic HCV infection, PCT and the HFE mutation as summarized by Bonkovsky and co-workers.[27]

Certainly a percentage, but not, all cases of chronic HCV infection and iron overload can be explained by HFE mutations. Other co-factors, including patient demographics, genotype, duration of disease and alcohol consumption, have to be factored into the pathogenesis,[1354] and further analysis and larger series are required to confirm or refute these relationships.[1357,1363]

Alcoholic siderosis

Varying degrees of iron overload are common in the livers of patients with alcoholic liver disease. Most tend to be relatively mild and confined to periportal hepatocytes and Kupffer cells (Fig. 5.109). Levels of iron sometimes parallel those seen in hereditary haemochromatosis, particularly where there is established cirrhosis. This led previously to debate as to whether hereditary haemochromatosis was a variant of alcoholic liver disease.[1364–1367] The hepatic iron index (HHI) was originally conceived and developed for precisely this discrimination.[1368] Nevertheless, a percentage of such patients are not carriers of the HFE mutation and, as in the cases of PCT and chronic HCV infection, both cause and implications of this observation are controversial. Two questions are only partially answered at present. The first is the role of iron as an independent factor in alcoholic liver disease, regardless of the patient's HFE mutational status. The second is the relationship itself between the HFE mutation and alcohol (Fig. 5.110).

Oxidative stress is considered crucial to the pathogenesis of alcoholic liver disease.[1369] In addition, iron induces oxidative stress by catalysing the conversion of superoxide and hydrogen peroxide to more potent oxidants such as hydroxyl radicals. These may cause tissue injury by initiating lipid peroxidation and causing oxidation of proteins and nucleic acids. Increasing evidence indicates that iron plays a significant role in the pathogenesis of alcoholic liver disease by exacerbating existing oxidative stress. Further data demonstrate a correlation between body iron burden and extent of fibrosis, as reviewed by Tavill and Qadri.[1370] These authors summarize evidence for a final common pathway of liver fibrogenesis as first put forward by Pietrangelo. In this scenario, iron may be either the primary hepatotoxin or a secondary catalyst in conjunction with alcohol, or hepatotropic viruses.

Powell and co-workers originally identified a significant correlation between alcohol and hereditary haemochromatosis, prior to the discovery of HFE. Over 40% of patients

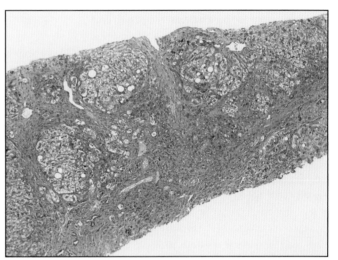

A

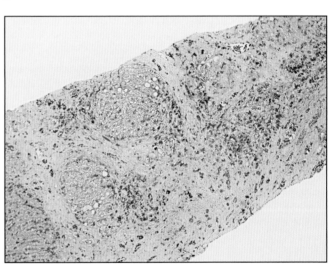

B

Fig. 5.110 • HFE-hereditary haemochromatosis and alcohol. Liver biopsy from a male of 42 years and of Irish pedigree. He is a C282Y homozygote, admitting to >80 g of alcohol daily at time of biopsy. Initial serum ferritin was 3140 ng/mL with transferrin saturation of 100%. He thereafter abstained from alcohol and now has normal ferritin and saturation and is asymptomatic 5 years later. **(A)** Biopsy after commencement of venesection demonstrates an established micronodular cirrhosis with mild steatosis. Masson trichrome. **(B)** There is marked haemosiderin deposition that is most prominent in zone 1 and fibrous septa. Perls staining.

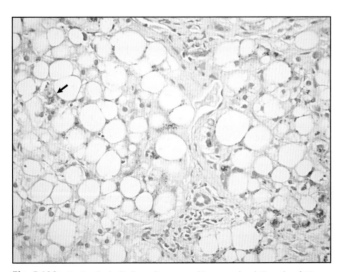

Fig. 5.109 • Acute alcoholic liver disease and iron overload. Female of 42 years presenting with peripheral neuropathy and with acknowledged alcoholic liver disease. The liver biopsy is not cirrhotic but demonstrates grade 3 macrovesicular steatosis with a Mallory body (arrowed). Immunostaining for ubiquitin with Perls counterstaining.

in their earlier series who presented with overt symptomatic hereditary haemochromatosis were noted to consume more than 100 g of alcohol daily, this being significantly higher than controls.[1371] After genotyping was introduced, a study of the effect of alcohol in C282Y homozygotes from the same population group confirmed that alcohol consumption exacerbates liver disease. Cirrhosis was confirmed in 7% of patients consuming less than 60 g of alcohol per day when compared with 66% in those imbibing more than 60 g of alcohol.[1372] Fletcher and Powell suggest an additive effect of iron and alcohol, both of which being able to cause oxidative stress, stellate cell activation, and hepatic fibrogenesis. They considered an increase in dietary iron or increased iron absorption to be unlikely.[1373]

It is not fully apparent how alcohol intake influences iron stores. It is also unclear as to how diet and dietary supplements may influence the progression of the disease. In a study of iron overload amongst elderly subjects, three dietary factors were associated with elevated iron stores, namely the use of iron supplements with or without supplemental vitamin C, frequent consumption of red meat, and frequent intake of fruit or fruit juices presumably rich in organic acids such as vitamin C.[1374] Furthermore the role of newly identified iron regulatory molecules have yet to be investigated in alcoholic liver disease.[1375]

Non-alcoholic fatty liver disease

Non-alcoholic fatty liver disease (NAFLD) is amongst the most common liver diseases identified in many societies and is a hepatic manifestation of the insulin resistance or metabolic syndrome.[1376] Biochemically, elevations in serum ferritin, iron, and transferrin saturation are common, together with mild increases in hepatic iron on histology (Fig. 5.111).

Controversy surrounds both the role of iron in the pathogenesis of the disease and the relationship between NASH and HFE mutations. In countries where there is a significant population of northern European or Celtic origin, there appears to be a positive relationship between the two conditions, with increased stainable hepatic iron and fibrosis, when compared with community controls.[1377,1378] Moreover, it is postulated that the mild iron overload associated with heterozygosity for the C282Y mutation may confer susceptibility to NAFLD, causing relative insulin deficiency.[1379]

Conversely, other studies from North America failed to demonstrate an increase in hepatic iron in patients demonstrating increased liver fibrosis, although HFE status was not assessed in these series.[1380,1381] This was further supported by two groups who genotyped their cohorts but failed to identify a relationship. Chitturi and co-workers noted that previous studies positively associating the two disorders were from centres with a special interest in iron storage disorders and, furthermore, that the ethnic origins of these patients were not identified.[1382] They thus factored ethnicity into their study of an Australian population and asserted that hepatic iron is not linked to hepatic fibrosis and that HFE mutations do not confer an additional risk of fibrosis in NAFLD. Bugianesi et al. identified insulin resistance as an independent risk factor for fibrosis and increased ferritin levels as markers of severe histological damage, while discounting iron burden and HFE.[1383] Similarly, in countries such as India where there is a significant variant NAFLD phenotype, 'the lean Asian male',[1384] there is no evidence that iron overload and HFE status are important pathogenetic mechanisms in the development of NAFLD.[1385]

In studies where an association between the *HFE* gene and NAFLD is considered likely, the explanation for the relationship between iron and fibrosis is again one of oxidative stress.[1386] However it is apparent that further multicentre studies that take factors such as ethnicity into account, as well as further molecular insights into the mechanisms at play in these patients, are necessary to confirm the molecular pathogenesis and importance of iron overload in NAFLD.

End-stage cirrhosis

Iron overload is not uncommon in patients with end-stage liver disease, with hepatic iron index elevated beyond 1.9 in 8.5% of patients with end-stage liver disease in one series (Fig. 5.112).[1349] While most of those patients did not have hereditary haemochromatosis, an increased prevalence of heterozygosity for H63D or C282Y is to be expected in view of the prevalence of HFE mutations in many populations. In addition, there is co-morbidity due to insults such as alcohol, NASH and HCV, all putatively iron-related disorders.[1387] Thus the extent to which excess hepatic iron contributes to hepatic failure and need for liver transplantation in patients with end-stage liver disease is currently unknown.[1355]

Portocaval shunting

Iron deposition is observed in many patients undergoing portosystemic shunt procedures,[1388] with greater annual accumulation of iron in patients who have undergone

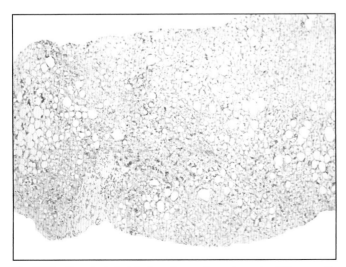

Fig. 5.111 • Non-alcoholic fatty liver disease. Caucasian male of 42 years with severe NAFLD. The patient had a BMI of 36 kg/m² and type 2 diabetes mellitus. C282Y and H63D mutations were not detected. Grading of iron is extremely difficult in the presence of such severe steatosis. Perls stain.

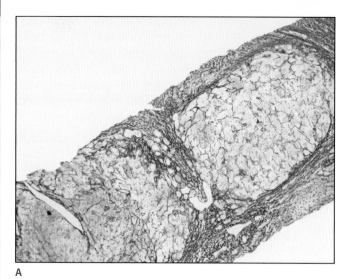

A

B

Fig. 5.112 • End-stage cryptogenic cirrhosis. **(A)** Broad fibrous bands traverse the biopsy, with central regenerating nodules. Reticulin stain. **(B)** There is mild to moderate haemosiderin deposition in hepatocytes and Kupffer cells throughout a lobule. A pericanalicular distribution is not identified. Perls stain.

portosystemic shunt than controls, although the hepatic iron concentrations in both groups may remain within normal limits.[1389–1391] The reason for this phenomenon is unknown but increased absorption of iron from the duodenum is postulated as well as other mechanisms including relative hepatic hypoxia, and pancreatic insufficiency with decreased bicarbonate secretion, as summarized by Bonkovsky et al.[1355]

Miscellaneous

Iron overload and hepatocellular carcinoma

Clinical observation, in vitro studies and biochemical data have long associated iron overload states and hepatocellular carcinoma (HCC). Furthermore, there is evidence, albeit controversial, that iron alone may confer an increased risk of extrahepatic malignancies.[1194] The relationship between iron and HCC has been most extensively studied in patients with hereditary haemochromatosis where HCC is identified

as a common and sinister complication, with a risk of premature death in these patients being primarily due to intervention by the tumour.[1392]

Earlier studies recognized a risk ranging from 93 to in excess of 200 for the development of HCC, with the tumour complicating an estimated 10% of patients,[1393–1395] carrying the highest risk for the development of HCC of any of the known hepatocarcinogenic factors, including HBV and aflatoxin.[1392,1394] However, as observed by Kowdley, these earlier studies were retrospective and open to bias, being mostly carried out in referral and transplant centres.[1229] Thus the prevalence may somewhat lower, although still significant, accounting for up to 45% of deaths in some series.[1232,1396] Fracanzani and colleagues calculate a relative risk of 1.8 (95% confidence interval, 1.1–2.9) for hereditary haemochromatosis with HCC, when compared with other chronic liver diseases.[1397]

The risk of development of HCC in hereditary haemochromatosis is most strongly associated with both long-standing disease and existing cirrhosis although the tumour is also recognized against a background of normal or only fibrotic liver.[1398–1402] Furthermore, the risk may persist in patients with haemochromatosis who are therapeutically iron-depleted.[1396,1403,1404] This, according to Deugnier, may not eliminate iron as a direct carcinogen as patients who are insufficiently treated and may have low serum ferritin but persistently elevated transferrin saturation, which is known to be carcinogenic via the production of reactive oxygen species and free radicals.[1405] Similarly, other potential iron overload states, including HCV and PCT, that may also be associated with *HFE* gene mutations, also show increased risk for the development of HCC.[1397,1406]

African dietary iron overload (AIO) was originally believed not to be complicated by HCC.[1407] However, as more recently reviewed by Gordeuk and co-workers, a statistical reappraisal of Strachan's original thesis that first described the condition has demonstrated an increase in incidence of HCC in the iron overloaded livers of southern and central African black patients.[1286] These authors calculated a risk for HCC of 23.5 (95% confidence limits 2.1, 225) with the highest grades of hepatic iron after allowing for the confounding effect of cirrhosis. More recently Moyo et al. documented a relative risk of 3.1 (95% confidence limits 1.05, 9.4) in Zimbabwean Blacks with dietary iron overload after adjusting for the confounding effect of cirrhosis.[1408] However, neither study addressed the major risk factors for the tumour in Black Africans, namely, hepatitis B virus infection and dietary exposure to aflatoxin B_1. Thus, in a later case/control study, Mandishona et al. reported a relative risk for HCC of 10.6 (95% confidence limits 1.5, 76.8) and a population attributable risk of 29 in rural South African Blacks after adjusting for the possible confounding effects of other risk factors, namely chronic HBV and HCV infections, aflatoxin B_1, and alcohol, but not of cirrhosis (Fig. 5.113).[1309]

Many hepatocellular carcinomas related to iron overload states are identified against the background of a cirrhotic liver, which, in itself, is considered a carcinogenic precursor, or against other confounding factors including

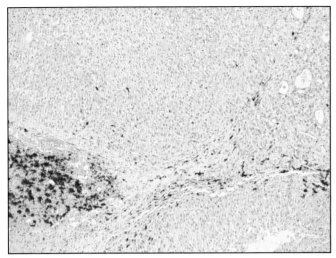

A

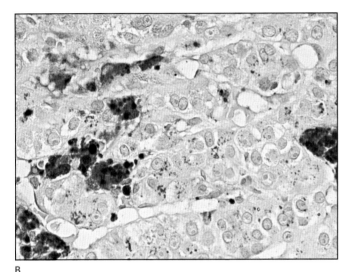

B

Fig. 5.113 • Hepatocellular carcinoma in a patient with African iron overload. **(A)** The tumour is well differentiated and typically iron-free, with iron-laden macrophages in fibrous septa. Perls stain. **(B)** Haemosiderin granules are also identified in the neoplastic cells. This is unusual in human hepatocellular carcinoma and may relate to the well differentiated nature of the tumour. Perls stain.

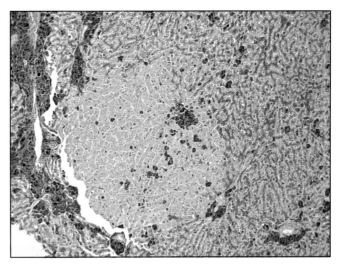

Fig. 5.114 • Iron free focus in a patient with severe African iron overload. Large aggregates of iron-laden Kupffer cell are identified within the focus. This was considered analogous to the situation in hereditary haemochromatosis and hepatocellular carcinoma was confirmed on re-biopsy. Perls stain.

hepatotropic viruses, alcohol and mycotoxins. Biochemically, iron is associated with the production of reactive oxygen species and free radicals, via the Fenton reaction that may promote tissue damage, including lipid peroxidation with consequent DNA and protein injury,[1190,1191] which may in turn be carcinogenic.[1409]

Although the spontaneous development of both altered hepatic foci and HCC is observed in various species, the results of in vivo data in many murine models are mixed. Smith and Yeoh reported oval cell proliferation in rats that were chronically fed an iron-overloaded diet,[1410] while Pigeon and co-workers identified hepatocyte nuclear changes, mitosis and iron free hepatocytes in similarly iron supplemented BALB/CJ mice.[1411] Furthermore, 7% of β_2 knockout mice that were maintained for up to two years developed hepatocellular carcinomas.[1412] Of note in human hepatocellular carcinoma is the recognition by Deugnier and colleagues of iron-free-foci (IFF) in the livers of patients with hereditary haemochromatosis (Fig. 5.114).[1227,1404,1413] These foci showed immunohistochemical evidence of proliferative activity with half of their cases demonstrating liver cell dysplasia. In addition, IFF were identified in 83% of patients with hereditary haemochromatosis and hepatocellular carcinoma.[1404] This phenomenon has also been identified in the rat model (Figs 5.115 and 5.116).[1414,1415] Conversely, other workers did not identify a role for iron in the development of murine HCC[1416] although these authors used the Salt–Farber model of chemical carcinogenesis with subsequent dietary iron supplementation. Thus, while various authorities do not discount iron as a putative carcinogen,[1229,1405,1417,1418] whether iron per se is a direct carcinogen, co-carcinogen or a bystander is currently unresolved.

Liver transplantation in iron overload states

The subject is discussed in Chapter 16. Although based on limited number of cases, the overall outcome of haemochromatotic patients is poorer than that of patients transplantated due to other causes, recurrence of HCC or arrhythmias and cardiac failure being mostly responsible for this shortcoming.[1419] Reaccumulation of iron in the transplanted liver is somewhat controversial but would appear to be insignificant in the majority of patients with pre-transplantation iron overload due to hereditary haemochromatosis or other causes.[1419,1420] The converse situation of an iron loaded donor liver is considered in Chapter 16 (and see Fig. 5.117).

The role of the liver biopsy in iron overload

Iron overload syndromes are not synonymous with hereditary haemochromatosis. However, the role of the liver biopsy has changed in recent years, mostly with the evolution of genotyping for HFE-related hereditary haemochromatosis. Currently a biopsy is no longer obligatory for

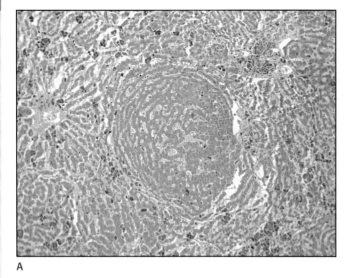

A

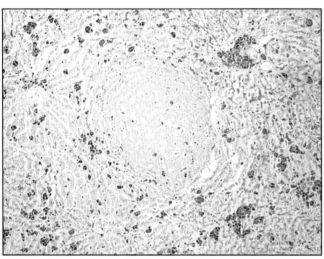

B

Fig. 5.115 • Animal model of dietary iron overload. **(A)** Altered hepatic focus in a 28 week Wistar rat. H&E. **(B)** The focus is largely iron-free apart from occasional Kupffer cells. For comparison with Fig. 5.114. Perls stain.

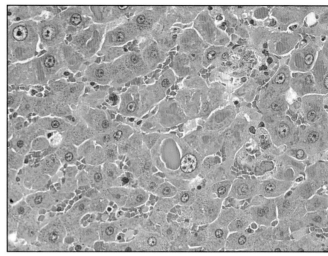

A

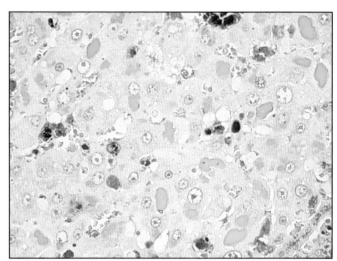

B

Fig. 5.116 • Iron free focus in a 32 week rat model of iron overload. **(A)** Individual hepatocytes demonstrate large nuclei with prominent and often multiple nucleoli. Intracytoplasmic globes are present. H&E. **(B)** The globules stain for haemosiderin and are morphologically similar to those described in human hereditary haemochromatosis by Deugnier et al.[1227] Perls stain.

diagnosis but remains an invaluable tool with respect to prognosis.[1194] The otherwise uncomplicated C282Y homozygote patient without hepatomegaly and having serum ferritin levels lower than 1000 ng/mL together with normal serum aspartate aminotransferase levels, is not considered to be at risk for bridging fibrosis, cirrhosis or iron-free foci, and thus does not require liver biopsy. Conversely, liver biopsy is often a critical adjunct in those patients who do not fulfil these three criteria because 50% thereof have been shown to have bridging fibrosis or cirrhosis and may be at risk for the development of HCC.[1421,1422]

Elsewhere, the liver biopsy is deemed by many investigators to be the gold standard in patients with evidence of iron overload but a genotype that is not informative, or without other apparent aetiology. The biopsy then allows detailed morphological assessment that, apart from confirming the degree of iron overload, also identifies, localizes and grades inflammation, as well as noting presence or absence of steatosis, Mallory bodies and other morphological features of steatohepatitis. Finally, it allows for staging of hepatic

fibrosis. As discussed previously, assessment of hepatic iron content may also serve as a prognostic adjunct in patients with chronic HCV infection and may have therapeutic implications.

Staining for hepatic iron should be a routine procedure in all liver biopsies (Chapter 3), in view of the numerous conditions where iron may be identified. Perls stain is most commonly used although it suffers the disadvantage of only identifying ferric iron whereas the Tirmann Schmeltzer stain recognizes both ferric and ferrous forms of the metal.[1418] An immunohistochemical system is also described, the Perls DAB technique, that identifies both haemosiderin and ferritin and that may have greater research application than is currently identified.[1318]

Two practical issues then arise, namely the distribution of iron within the various cells of the liver, and the grading of iron overload. The distribution of iron, hepatocyte vs. reticuloendothelial, may serve as a clue towards diagnosis. Typically a predominant hepatocyte loading with pericanal-

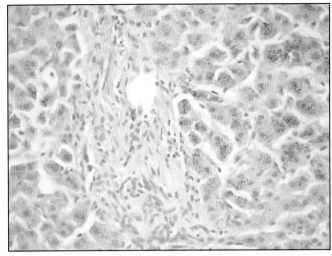

A

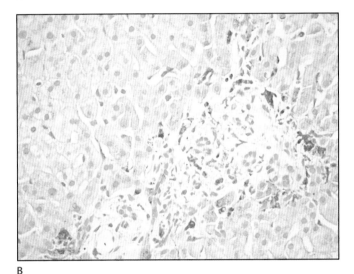

B

Fig. 5.117 • Liver transplantation with an iron overloaded donor liver. The HFE status of the donor was not known. **(A)** Donor liver demonstrating a grade 2 iron overload in periportal hepatocytes at time of transplant. Perls stain. **(B)** Liver biopsy at 100 days showing mobilization of iron to periportal Kupffer cells and portal tract macrophages. Perls stain.

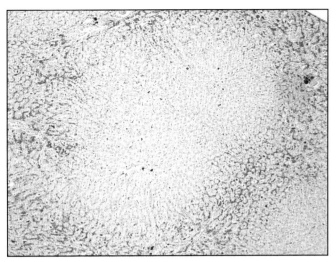

Fig. 5.118 • Scheuer grade 2 iron overload in a rat dietary iron overload model. The typical gradient is identified with maximum iron in periportal (zone 1) hepatocytes. Perls stain.

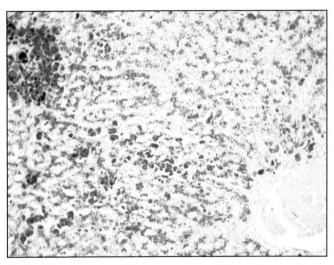

Fig. 5.119 • Scheuer grade 4 iron overload in a rat dietary iron overload model. There is uniform distribution of hepatocyte iron across all zones of the liver. The marked Kupffer cell and macrophage iron deposition is not catered for in the Scheuer system, however. Perls stain.

icular localization and acinar gradient would favour most types of hereditary haemochromatosis, the exception being ferroportin disease that, together with many forms of secondary iron overload, may have a predominantly, though not exclusively, reticuloendothelial distribution.[1266]

Grading systems serve as an indirect measure of hepatic iron stores. The first attempt at grading was published by Scheuer and co-workers in 1962.[1423] Since that time, many authorities have put forward various systems, as summarized by Turlin and Deugnier.[1418] Few, however, could be totally validated by alternative techniques including image analysis and/or biochemistry.[1413,1424] Two distinct approaches have been identified. The first is essentially an acinar overview usually with a simple 1 to 4 scoring system with grade 1 representing minimal deposition and grade 4 characterized by deposition of iron throughout all zones of the liver and consequent loss of the acinar gradient (Figs 5.118 and 5.119).[1425] The most obvious disadvantage of such systems is that they do not differentiate hepatic from reticuloen-

dothelial iron. The second approach is thus more detailed and comprehensive, assigning a numerical score to all of the tissues represented in the biopsy, including hepatocytes, bile ducts, Kupffer cells and vessels.[1426] It is consequently more accurate and reproducible but more time-consuming. Thus, in general, the Scheuer grading system is more accessible for routine histopathology while that of Deugnier and co-workers has obvious advantages in experimental situations.

The liver biopsy specimen also allows for the calculation of liver iron concentration (LIC) by atomic absorption spectrometry, expressed in µg/g (or µmol) of dry weight liver tissue, where levels <400 µg/g weight (<30 µmol/g) are considered to be within normal limits.[1368] The hepatic iron index (HII), namely liver iron concentration in micromoles per gram dry weight divided by age in years, may then also be calculated.[1427] In the past, this served to further assist in distinguishing patients with HFE-homozygous hereditary haemochromatosis, in whom the HII is usually greater than

1.9 when compared with values lower than 1.5 in heterozygotes or those with secondary iron overload disorders.[1427] However, subsequent experience with HII is that there are numerous exceptions to this rule and calculation of the HII would not appear as reliable as earlier thought.[1349,1354,1418] A further drawback to LIC is that it implies destruction of the sample if the same block is used for histology.[1418] It has thus been discontinued in many centres, especially those with access to genotyping.[1413] Furthermore, iron stains are a more sensitive indicator of very mild hepatic tissue iron abnormalities than chemical studies although this may sometimes be an inconsequential observation.[1349]

Before leaving this section, it must be stressed that the liver in infant is physiologically iron loaded and periportal haemosiderin deposition is a common histological finding during the first 10 days of life. This may be prominent and prolonged in relation to non-specific injuries, and has been emphasized in numerous studies dealing in particular with metabolic disorders such as tyrosinaemia,[544] Zellweger syndrome,[914,1428] mitochondriopathies[1002] and galactosaemia (see Fig. 5.15(C)) to name but a few. The transient increase in iron may raise the differential diagnosis of neonatal haemochromatosis when patients with these varied conditions present as severe neonatal syndrome.[1428]

Inborn errors of bile acid synthesis

Patients with bile acid synthetic defects present with neonatal cholestasis. There are no distinguishing features other than age-related normal levels of gamma glutamyl transpeptidase (γGT). Patients presenting with cholestasis of infancy and normal γGT should be screened for elevated cholenoic bile acids in the urine by a colour reaction with the Lifshütz reagent. (This reagent is prepared by mixing 10 mL glacial acetic acid and 1mL concentrated H_2SO_4; when 200 μL of reagent are added to 25 mL of dried urine extract a purple colour is produced when cholenoic acids are present.)

Diagnosis is by assaying urine or bile by mass spectrometry of bile acids. Analysis can also be performed by fast atom bombardment or gas liquid chromatography. Three enzyme deficiencies have been described: (i) delta 4-3-oxosteroid, 5β-reductase in liver; (ii) 3 β-hydroxy delta 5-C_{27} steroid dehydrogenase/isomerase in liver or fibroblasts; and (iii) oxysterol 7α hydroxylase in liver and fibroblasts.

Delta 4-3-oxosteroid, 5β-reductase deficiency

The responsible enzyme is found only in the liver[1002,1429,1430] and not in fibroblasts. It is the enzymatic step in the primary pathway from cholesterol to cholic and chenodeoxycholic acid, involved in the saturation of the steroid ring. A deficiency would result in the decreased formation of these primary bile acids with an elevation of cholenoic bile acids. This enzyme was not detectable in the original patients presenting with neonatal hepatitis who were evaluated in follow-up after bile acid therapy.[1431-1433] Enzyme analysis of the liver in a subsequent patient did not verify that this is a specific genetic defect, i.e. no mutation was present.[1434]

A tentative diagnosis is presently based on greater than 70% of the urinary bile acids being 3-oxo delta 4 and significant detection of allo-(5aH)-bile acids.[1433,1435] Elevation of primary bile acids should raise doubts concerning a diagnosis of a bile acid synthetic defect and other aetiologies should be sought. Why these patients might respond to ursodeoxycholic acid is unclear other than by a decrease in the levels of the offending bile acids. Certainly, lack of response can occur, yet improvement subsequently can be observed with chenodeoxycholic acid and cholic acid therapy.[1436]

Light microscopic and ultrastructural findings in 5β-reductase deficiency (and other bile acid synthetic defects) are discussed in detail by Bove et al.[1437] Light microscopic changes in most reported cases resemble non-specific neonatal hepatitis, with prominent cholestasis, giant cell transformation and erythropoiesis. Interlobular bile ducts are consistently normal. Ultrastructurally, injury patterns common to other forms of cholestasis are seen, as well as features that may be specific for the defect. Thus, there is a non-uniform mosaic of normal and abnormal canaliculi, often in adjacent clusters of hepatocytes, but there is no canalicular dilatation. However, some canaliculi show diverticula, and junctional complexes are extraordinarily convoluted, often enclosing pockets of dense granular material presumed to be bile residue.

3β-hydroxy delta 5-C_{27} steroid dehydrogenase (3βHSD) deficiency

This seems to be a more definitive inborn error of primary bile acid metabolism, which is involved in the conversion of 7α-hydroxy-cholesterol to the primary bile acid pathways.[1438] The first patient reported was a 3-month-old infant with cholestasis. Early biopsies of the liver in the patient and siblings demonstrated giant-cell hepatitis. Primary bile acids were not detected. The natural substrate, unesterified 7α-hydroxy-cholesterol, was elevated in the serum. Fibroblasts from this patient demonstrated complete absence of the enzyme. The parents' fibroblasts demonstrated reduced 3βHSD activity.[1439] The patient responded to chenodeoxycholic acid, including relief from pruritus.[1440] The presentation during childhood may be quite variable.[1441] Five patients had hepatomegaly, of whom four had jaundice and two had fatty stools. Microcysts were found in the kidney in two patients. All patients responded to ursodeoxycholic acid.[1441] In both of these disorders, the abnormal bile acids that are formed inhibit the canalicular ATP dependent bile acid transporter.[1442]

Hepatic histopathological changes in 3βHSD deficiency depend on the age of the patient and rate of progression of the liver disease. Two of the three patients reported by Clayton et al.[1438] who were biopsied at 6 weeks and 18 months of age had giant cell hepatitis, and giant cell hepatitis with bridging fibrosis, respectively. Similarly, Jacquemin et al.[1441] found giant cell hepatitis in young patients (4 and 6 months of age) and portal and perilobular fibrosis in older patients (36–46 months). Three patients studied by Bove et al.[1437] had portal and intralobular fibrosis with 'pseudoductular metaplasia' and cholangiolar proliferation; there was no paucity of interlobular bile ducts.

One infant was described who not only presented with cholestasis but had liver disease that had already advanced to cirrhosis.[1443] There was no response to either ursodeoxycholic acid or cholic acid by clinical indicators or alterations in the measured bile acids. The patient demonstrated a homozygous mutated oxysterol 7α-hydroxylase gene. Since this is one of the alternate pathways more important in early bile acid synthesis, the deficiency results in the accumulation of 3β-hydrocholenoic and 3β-hydroxy-5-cholestenoic acids. Because of the early lack of development of *oxysterol 7α-hydroxylase,* serum levels of 27-hydroxy cholesterol were greater than 4500 times normal. Both parents had an exon 5 premature terminated codon (R388X) as a heterozygous defect. Histopathologically, the liver showed giant-cell transformation, bile-duct proliferation, and canalicular and bile-duct plugging; no specific ultrastructural changes were noted.[1443] This first reported patient underwent a liver transplant from a cadaver donor and had problems with acute rejection. Death occurred on postoperative day 19 from Epstein–Barr virus-related disseminated lymphoproliferative disease.

It seems reasonable to expect other rare defects in bile acid metabolism as it is a complex pathway; alternate pathways may be more prominent in the fetus, and newborn infant. For instance, a 25-hydroxylation pathway exists to a small extent normally that may contribute to cholic acid production.[1444] A family with two children presenting with giant cell hepatitis indicated in the evaluated child that conversion of 5β cholestane 3α, 7α, 12α, 24S 25 pentol to cholic acid and acetone was defective.[1445] Improvement in liver tests occurred when cholic acid was added to the treatment regimen. Although clinically well, including improvement in pruritus, normal liver function tests, and physical examination, the patients developed cirrhosis.

In general, therapy is with ursodeoxycholic acid initially, but this may not be curative. It would be preferable to treat patients with primary bile acids—chenodeoxycholic acid—when levels are not elevated, or with cholic and chenodeoxycholic acids. However, these bile acids are not available commercially. Liver transplantation has been performed for alternate pathway enzyme deficiency. A recent comprehensive review of diseases of bile acid synthesis is recommended for further reading.[1446]

Progressive familial intrahepatic cholestasis (PFIC) and benign recurrent intrahepatic cholestasis (BRIC)

Progressive familial intrahepatic cholestasis was originally described in 1965 in a Pennsylvanian Amish kindred named Byler, but it is now recognized world wide,[1446–1448] and although widely referred to as being split into types I, II and III, these terms are confusing an should be avoided. It has been reclassified according to the molecular basis, with designation based on the protein that is deficient. Genetic testing is not always immediately available: a clinically helpful subdivision is, however, possible into diseases

manifesting normal (or low) levels of serum γGT and those with elevated levels. Two low γGT forms of PFIC are now termed FIC1 deficiency[1449] and BSEP deficiency.[1450] The best characterized form with a high γGT is termed MDR3 deficiency.[1451] All three are caused by recessive mutations in different genes.

Benign recurrent intrahepatic cholestasis was also described in 1965.[1452] Although the name and original description suggest a distinct condition, it is now understood that this condition is really a milder form of PFIC. In fact there are less severe, and later presenting forms, of all three of the major genetic diseases referred to above. Furthermore they should not be seen as distinct entities as there is a whole spectrum of severity between the two originally described conditions. The neonatal presentations of all conditions are the best studied. Later onset disease may not be recognized as such, unless features indicating similarity to neonatal disease is noted. This applies particularly to the histological features.

FIC1 deficiency (familial intrahepatic cholestasis protein 1) deficiency

This is caused by mutations in the gene *ATP8B1*.[1449] Most recognized patients present in the first 6 months of life with a bland cholestasis (Fig. 5.120), without significant giant cell transformation or cellular infiltrate.[1453] The identification of canaliculi filled with pale-appearing bile is not infrequent. Diarrhoea and growth failure are major complications. Sensineural deafness requiring hearing aids develops in some 30% of patients. There is a slow progression to cirrhosis. Over 30 years ago, Linarelli et al.[1454] suggested that the ultrastructure of canalicular bile was coarsely granular in PFIC and called it 'Byler's bile' (Fig. 5.121). Subsequently, this type of bile was found to be characteristic of FIC1 deficiency, from which members of the Amish Byler family suffer.[1449,1453] The function of the FIC1 protein is still not clear, as is the mechanism by which a lack may lead to cholestasis, and extra hepatic manifestations.

The diagnostic criteria for BRIC, summarized by Luketic and Shiffman,[1455] include: (i) at least two episodes of

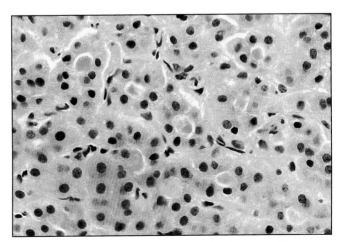

Fig. 5.120 • FIC1 deficiency. Prominent canalicular cholestasis with pseudoglandular formation. H&E.

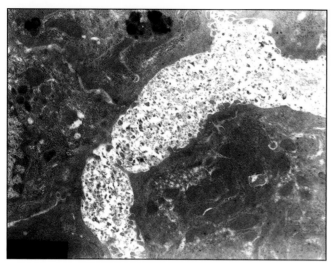

Fig. 5.121 • FIC1 deficiency. Dilated canaluculus with loss of microvilli Is filled with characteristically loose coarsely granular bile. Courtesy of Dr Alex Knisely.

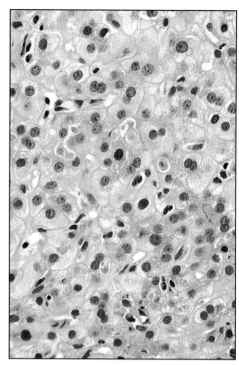

Fig. 5.122 • Benign recurrent intrahepatic cholestasis. Bland canalicular cholestasis. H&E.

jaundice separated by a symptom-free interval lasting several months to years; (ii) laboratory values consistent with intrahepatic cholestasis; (iii) severe pruritus secondary to cholestasis; (iv) normal intra- and extrahepatic bile ducts confirmed by cholangiography; and (v) absence of factors known to be associated with cholestasis, e.g. drugs, pregnancy. Early onset was associated with a more severe course, in terms of frequency and duration of attacks, in one series; some patients developed kidney stones, pancreatitis and diabetes.[1456] The same authors proposed dropping the adjective 'benign' because of the profound effect that the disease has on the long-term quality of life of the patients. There is no specific treatment; various modalities are discussed in detail by Luketic and Shiffman.[1455] Liver transplantation in one case produced good short-term results.[1456] The vast majority of the patients in these series undoubtedly had a form of FIC1 deficiency (Fig. 5.122). The suggestion that BRIC is in fact not benign is borne out by the finding that some cases do progress, albeit slowly.[1457,1458] In fact there is a whole spectrum of severity, with some degree of phenotype/genotype correlation.[1459]

Histopathological observations of biopsy specimens from 22 patients at the milder end of the spectrum were detailed by Brenard et al.[1460] During attacks of jaundice there was cholestasis (hepatocellular and canalicular) in all patients, and infiltration of portal areas with mononuclear cells in seven patients. Other findings included focal mononuclear cell infiltration with or without focal necrosis, infiltration of portal areas with many eosinophils, ductular proliferation (one patient) and periportal fibrosis (one patient).

A form of cholestatic syndrome was reported as being specific to inhabitants of Greenland.[1461] Jaundice, bleeding, pruritus, malnutrition, steatorrhoea, osteodystrophy and dwarfism were typical clinical features. Eight of the children died between the ages of 6 weeks and 3 years from bleeding or infections. Hyperbilirubinaemia, profound hypoprothrombinaemia, thrombocytosis and elevated alkaline phosphatase values were evident. 'Greenland familial cholestasis' has now been shown to be FIC1 deficiency with all affected individuals carrying two copies of the same missense mutation.[1462] The liver biopsies from the 16 children were studied by Ornvold et al.[1463] The changes were characterized as early, intermediate and late. Early changes (up to 5 months of age) were restricted to the perivenular zone and consisted of cholestasis with rosette formation. Intermediate stage changes (5–14 months) included perivenular and then periportal fibrosis in addition to persistent cholestasis. Changes in the late stage (17–60 months) included progressive cholestasis and portal-portal and portal-central fibrosis in seven patients, and cirrhosis in two of the patients. Inflammation and paucity of bile ducts were not seen.

BSEP deficiency

This is caused by mutations in *ABCB11*, which encodes the human bile salt export pump.[1450,1464,1465] The severe form presents in infancy, with a marked hepatitis usually with obvious giant cell transformation (Figs 5.123 and 5.124), and eventually cirrhosis. There is usually marked intracellular retention of biliary pigment, and considerable hepatocyte disarray, Byler bile is not seen; instead, the bile is amorphous or finely filamentous, Mallory bodies may be present.[1453,1466,1467] Milder forms of BSEP deficiency do not seem to constitute as large a proportion of later onset disease as is FIC1 deficiency, however there is also clearly a spectrum of disease,[1468] which may be considerably underestimated. Two cases of hepatocellular carcinoma developed in the cirrhotic liver of patients with PFIC;[1469,1470] these were reported prior to the characterization of the various subtypes. However, BSEP deficiency seems to be the main risk

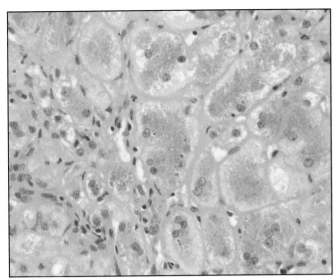

Fig. 5.123 • BSEP deficiency. Multinucleated giant hepatocytes are variably pale or heavily loaded with bile pigment. H&E.

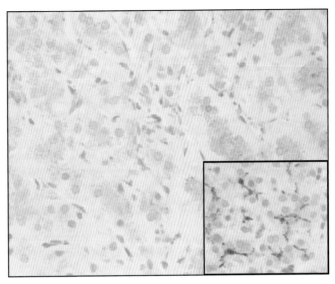

Fig. 5.125 • BSEP deficiency. Same case as Figs 5.123 and 5.124. Immunohistochemistry for BSEP shows wholly absent marking at canalicular margins while the control (inset) stains adequately. PAP method.

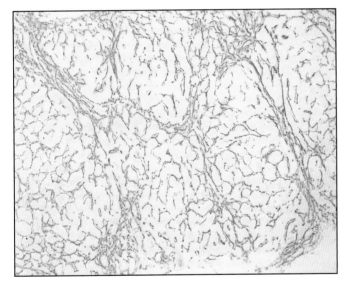

Fig. 5.124 • BSEP deficiency. Same case as illustrated in Fig. 5.123 showing early porto-portal and porto-central bridging fibrosis. Reticulin.

factor.[1471] The histological features of BSEP deficiency are not specific. In an attempt to improve this, immunohistochemistry using a number of anti-BSEP antibodies has been developed (Fig. 5.125). The specificity has not yet been proven, but it is a useful guide.

MDR3 deficiency

This has previously been termed 'Type III PFIC'. The disease has been shown to be caused by a deficiency in the multidrug-resistance 3 (MDR3) protein due to mutations in the encoding gene *ABCB4*.[1472] This protein is essential for the entry of the main phospholipid, phosphatidylcholine, into bile. In the absence of phospholipids, bile acids cannot form mixed micelles, and the bile is extremely hydrophobic.[1473] Much, or all, of the phenotype is probably induced by this bile. In the severe cases the features seen include portal inflammation, proliferation of the bile ducts and subsequent fibrosis[1472] (Fig. 5.126(A)). The result of partial loss of function of MDR3 may turn out to be of more widespread clinical importance than that of the early onset disease. Furthermore a reduction in biliary phospholipid does not only result in parenchymal damage, but also reduces the amount of cholesterol that may be maintained in solution.[1474,1475] As with BSEP, anti MDR3 antibodies have been raised. Although this may be a useful method of establishing a complete loss of protein (Fig. 5.126(B)), it is less clear cut in milder cases. Partial loss of MDR3 function may lead to more slowly progressive disease (Figs 5.127–5.129), but may still require liver transplantation.

The primary medical therapies utilized in PFIC include ursodeoxycholic acid, phenobarbital and rifampicin; response to medical therapy occurs but is unusual. Some investigators have found ursodeoxycholic acid to be more beneficial in PFIC.[1476,1477] Ursoedoxycholic acid feeding may be of particular benefit in MDR3 deficiency, where bile salt hydrophobocity is thought to be particularly important in the disease pathogenesis. Certainly the mouse model supports this concept.[1478]

Partial bile diversion by a cholecystojejunal cutaneous conduit and/or ileal diversion produces complete resolution of the liver disease, but the results are variable from one institution to another. The surgery must be performed before significant fibrosis has developed.[1479–1481]

Cholestasis during pregnancy has also been reported in individuals heterozygous for mutations in *ABCB4* (MDR3 deficiency).[1472,1482] Histopathological findings include bile ductular proliferation with inflammation, resembling the changes in the mouse model. One diagnostic test is the detection of low bile phospholipids (less than 1 mM) in the face of normal bile salt concentrations.

In one series hepatic transplantation was performed in 14 children with 'Byler disease'.[1483] One patient died postoperatively from arterial thrombosis. In the remaining 13 patients graft function, growth, and quality of life were

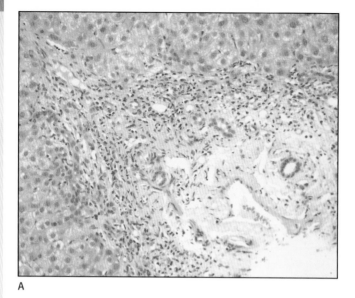

A

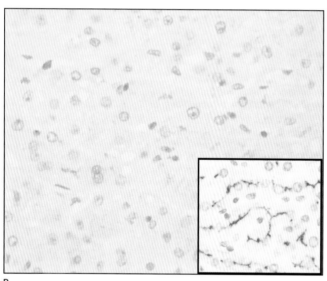

B

Fig. 5.126 • MDR3 deficiency, liver biopsy form a 4 year old boy. **(A)** The portal tract is expanded due to inflammation, ductular reaction and increased similar to the changes seen with a chronic cholangiopathy. **(B)** Immunohistochemistry for MDR3 shows complete absence of staining at canalicular margins. The normal control illustrates adequate labelling (Inset). PAP method.

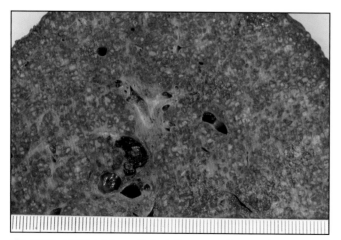

Fig. 5.127 • MDR3 deficiency. Cirrhotic liver removed at transplantation show a green discoloration and inspissated bile within dilated intrahepatic bile ducts.

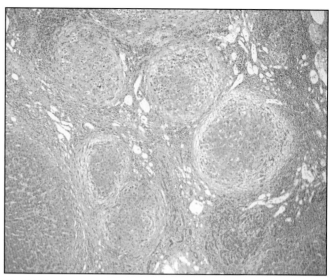

Fig. 5.128 • MDR3 deficiency. Same case as illustrated In Fig. 5.127. A micronodular pattern with perinodular halo is in keeping with an advanced biliary cirrhosis.

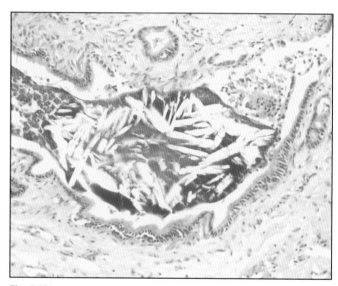

Fig. 5.129 • MDR3 deficiency. Same case as illustrated In Fig. 5.127. Intraductal bile sludge showing a mixed bilirubin and cholesterol composition in keeping with phospholipid deficiency.

good after an average follow up of 17 months, without evidence of disease recurrence. A wealth of, as yet, unpublished data transplant in PFIC exists. It appears to show excellent results in both BSEP deficiency and MDR3 deficiency. The results in FIC1 deficiency are less clear, in-keeping with the widespread expression of the gene. One frequently encountered post transplant feature in FIC1 deficiency is steatosis.[1484]

Other diseases causing progressive intrahepatic cholestasis

North American Indian childhood cirrhosis

Weber et al.[1485] studied 14 North American Indian children, all from the Cree and Ojibwa-Cree tribes, with a severe familial cholestasis. Jaundice occurred neonatally in nine children but disappeared before the end of the first year. Light microscopy revealed that there was giant cell transformation and bilirubinostasis. Progressive liver damage was documented by persistently high levels of alkaline phosphatase, moderate elevation of aminotransferases, severe pruritus and morphologically, by fibrosis and cirrhosis. Early portal hypertension and variceal bleeding necessitated portal-systemic shunts in seven children. Ultrastructural and immunohistochemical studies suggested that this group of children might represent a human model of microfilament dysfunction-induced cholestasis. The disease locus was mapped to chromosome 16q22.[1114] A single mutation was identified in all affected individuals in a gene labelled CIRH1A.[1115] The function of the encoded protein (cirhin) is unknown.

Familial benign chronic intrahepatic cholestasis

Three of four adult siblings in a family studied for three generations had clinical and/or laboratory evidence of slowly progressive intrahepatic cholestasis.[1486] Slight hyperpigmentation, facial hypertrichosis and hypothyroidism were seen in affected individuals, who also had prolonged increases in serum aminotransferases, GGT and alkaline phosphatase activities. A biopsy of one patient who was jaundiced showed cholestasis and other changes indistinguishable from those of extrahepatic obstruction. Asymptomatic intervals were characterized by abnormal BSP retention, reduced N-demethylation capacity, elevated fasting total bile acid levels, and normal light microscopic findings. A high serum α-lipoprotein level was found in affected individuals. The inheritance is believed to be autosomal recessive. A defect in prekeratin–keratin metabolism is postulated to account for the lesions in liver and other tissues.

Progressive cholestasis in the McCune–Albright syndrome

This syndrome is characterized by café-au-lait spots, polyostotic fibrous dysplasia and sexual precocity. Two patients with the syndrome, who presented with neonatal cholestasis, were reported by Silva et al.[1487] Despite the severity of presentation, both patients cleared their jaundice in 6 months but continued to have mild abnormalities of liver function tests. The two patients showed an activating mutation of codon 201 in the gene encoding the α-subunit of the G-protein that stimulates adenylcyclase in liver tissue, suggesting that this metabolic defect could be responsible for their cholestatic syndrome.

Hereditary defects of bilirubin metabolism

Patients present with asymptomatic jaundice and elevations of unconjugated or conjugated serum bilirubins. For excel-lent coverage of bilirubin metabolic pathways see reviews by Sauter et al.[1488] and Nowicki & Poley.[1489]

Crigler–Najjar disease type I

Crigler–Najjar disease is characterized by severe non-haemolytic jaundice beginning in the newborn peroid.[1490] Patients with Crigler–Najjar type I can develop kernicterus at any age. The diagnosis should be entertained in the first 3 days of life. Levels of unconjugated bilirubin are usually over 20 mg/dL and may be as high as 50 mg/dL before therapy. Routine liver function tests are in the normal range. Crigler–Najjar disease is rare, with an incidence of about one per million. Inheritance is autosomal recessive. Patients lack the enzyme uridine diphosphate-glucuronosyltransferase completely, and consequently are unable to conjugate bilirubin.[1491] The gene for the deficient enzyme has been cloned and sequenced;[1492] it is localized to chromosome 2. Mutations have been found in exons 1–5.

Therapy is difficult and limited. Patients do not respond to phenobarbital. Phototherapy has been utilized long term with plasmapheresis for acute bilirubin elevations and, if initiated promptly, can reverse early bilirubin encephalopathy.[1493,1494] Therapeutic effectiveness decreases during adolescence.[1495,1496] Liver transplantation results in a cure.[1495–1497] Experimental hepatocyte transplantation has decreased the hours needed for phototherapy.[1498] Gene therapy is under investigation. The Gunn rat has been a valuable animal model.[1499] The histopathology of the liver in Criglar–Najjar type I is characterized by intrahepatic cholestasis,[5,1500–1502] but the liver may be normal.[5]

Gilbert syndrome and Crigler–Najjar disease type II

These two diseases are likely the same disease with differences only in the severity of manifestations. They are characterized by unconjugated hyperbilirubinaemia, but with a milder phenotype than Crigler–Najjar type I. Both are the result of mutations in the same gene; differences may be related to the severity of the resulting deficiency of the enzyme.

Gilbert syndrome is a mild form of unconjugated hyperbilirubinaemia. Patients often present at puberty, when jaundice is first noticed. Bilirubin levels increase following starvation or other stress.[1503] In newborns it can exacerbate neonatal jaundice in the first two days, and can contribute to higher bilirubin levels in patients with concomitant glucose-6-phosphate dehydrogenase deficiency.[1504] Mild haemolysis and hepatocyte bilirubin uptake defects have been found.[1505,1506] Liver enzymes are in the normal range.

Arias et al.[1507] described Crigler–Najjar disease type II in 1969. Patients present with neonatal jaundice but the jaundice is less severe than in patients with Crigler–Najjar type I. Bilirubin levels fluctuate between 7 and 20 mg/dL. These patients generally do not suffer the severe intellectual compromise of type I patients, although, during illness, bilirubin levels may rise to 40 mg/dL and cause kernicterus.

In both Gilbert syndrome and Crigler–Najjar disease type II, analysis of bile before administration of phenobarbital demonstrates the presence of significant quantities of bilirubin monoglucuronide, which are not seen in type I disease. Patients with Crigler–Najjar type II and significant bilirubin elevations can be distinguished from type I patients by the response to phenobarbital; in the former the drug lowers the bilirubin by 30%.

Gilbert syndrome is the most common genetic bilirubin defect in Caucasians.[1508,1509] The incidence is 3–16% of the population; inheritance is autosomal recessive. Hepatic bilirubin uridine diphosphate-glucuronosyltransferase-1 activity may be 25% of normal. Mutations have been found in both the promoter and coding regions of the uridine diphosphate-glucuronosyltransferase-1 gene in patients with Gilbert syndrome, resulting in reduced enzyme expression.[1510–1512]

Inheritance of Crigler–Najjar type II appears to be autosomal dominant, although occasional patients with autosomal recessive inheritance have been reported.[1513–1516] Type II patients also have significantly reduced levels of bilirubin uridine diphosphate-glucuronosyltransferase-I.

No therapy is necessary for Gilbert syndrome. A primate animal model has been reported.[1517] Increased lipofuscin pigment accumulation in liver cells has been described in Gilbert syndrome.[1518] The pigment granules do not exhibit the coarse granularity of those of the Dubin–Johnson syndrome. Ultrastructurally, hepatocytes reveal hypertrophy of the smooth endoplasmic reticulum.[1519]

Dubin–Johnson syndrome

Dubin–Johnson syndrome was first described in 1954 by Dubin & Johnson[1520] and Sprinz & Nelson.[1521] Dubin[1522] subsequently reviewed in detail 50 cases reported up to 1958. Patients present with conjugated hyperbilirubinaemia, but have normal liver enzymes and no other evidence of hepatic dysfunction. Some patients have hepatomegaly and abdominal pain. Age of onset may be up to 56 years.

Elevations of predominantly conjugated bilirubin range from 2 to 5 mg/dL. Sulphobromophthalein is retained in these patients, with levels increased at 60–90 minutes over those at 45 minutes after intravenous administration.[1523] In urine, the total coproporphyrin level is normal but isomer I is greater than 80%, which is characteristic of the syndrome.

Dubin–Johnson syndrome is rare in infancy[1524,1525] except in an inbred population of Iranian Jews, where the incidence is as high as 1 in 1300.[1523] Inheritance is autosomal recessive, with reduced penetrance in females.[1526] The underlying defect is complete absence of the canalicular multispecific organic anion transporter (CMOAT). The gene is localized to chromosome 10q24.[1527] It was cloned in humans in 1996.[1528] Multiple gene mutations have been documented and can be detected in fibroblasts.[1529] The most common mutation is R1066X which leads to a premature termination of the canalicular transporter.[1530] Human multidrug-resistance protein 2 (MRP2) is encoded by the same gene (ABBC2) with 32 exons.[1531] Animal models include the Corriedale sheep[1532] and TR (−) rat.[1533] Pigment accumulation resembling that of the Dubin–Johnson syndrome has been described in the Howler monkey.[1534]

An increased amount of a coarsely granular brown pigment in liver cells is diffuse, though more heavily concentrated in the perivenular zone, is characteristic of the Dubin–Johnson syndrome.[1520,1522] (Fig. 5.130(A)). The accumulation of the pigment in hepatocytes gives the liver a grey to black colour grossly. The pigment shares some of its physicochemical properties with lipofuscin and melanin in that it is oil red-O positive (in frozen sections), stains black with the Fontana stain (Fig. 5.130(B)), is variably PAS-positive, and is autofluorescent when examined by violet microscopy.[1535] Ultrastructurally, the Dubin–Johnson pigment is lysosomal and thought to differ from lipofuscin in being pleomorphic and having a more variegated appearance and less lipid.[5,1536] Phillips et al.[5] believe that the lysosomes are distinctive in having very dense areas as well as moderately electron-dense, finely stippled areas. An electron spin resonance spectroscopy study suggested that the pigment is not melanin but rather is a stable free radical with unusual properties.[1537]

Rotor syndrome

This form of conjugated hyperbilirubinaemia was reported in 1948.[1538] Although clinically similar to the Dubin–Johnson syndrome there is no abnormal liver pigmentation.[1539] Total coproporphyrin excretion in the urine is increased and isomer I is elevated, but is less than 80% of the total. Inheritance is autosomal recessive, but the genetic defect is unknown. Cholescintigraphy reveals no minimal visualization.[1540] There is no pigment storage or other morphologic change in Rotor syndrome. A number of ultrastructural changes were described by Phillips et al.[5] that included distinctive 'two-tone' lysosomes.

Miscellaneous disorders

Cystic fibrosis

Cystic fibrosis, the most common recessive disorder with an estimated incidence of approximately 1 : 2500 live births, has a worldwide distribution. The disease was first recognized as a pancreatic disease distinct from coeliac disease in 1938.[1541] Formerly known as CF of the pancreas (mucoviscidosis), the disease was soon labelled simply cystic fibrosis (CF) with the recognition that not only the exocrine pancreas, but also bronchial glands (obstructive bronchopulmonary disease), the intestinal glands (meconium ileus), the sweat glands (high sweat electrolytes) and the biliary tree (focal biliary cirrhosis) may be main manifestations of the disease.

The gene was localized at chromosome 7q31.2 in 1989.[1542–1544] It codes for a large protein named CF transmembrane regulator (CFTR) whose key role is in maintaining the fluid balance across epithelial cells. CFTR belongs to the ABC-cassette family of ATP-dependent channels and

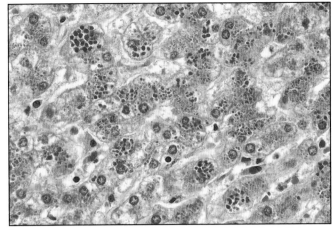

A

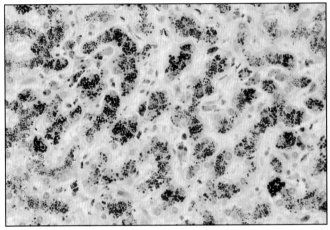

B

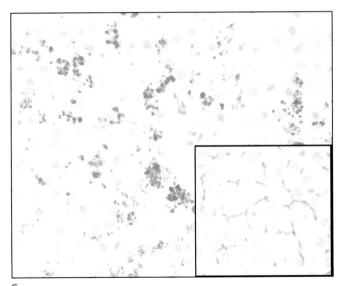

C

Fig. 5.130 • Dubin–Johnson syndrome. Liver cells contain an abundance of a brown, coarsely-granular pigment. **(A)** H&E. **(B)** Fontana stain. **(C)** Immunostain for canalicular multiple organic anion transporter (cMOAT) showing no specific staining, only the coarsely granular pigment which is still to be seen; the normal control (inset) shows the expected pattern of canalicular staining. PAP method.

transporters and functions mainly as a cAMP-dependent chloride channel in the apical membrane of secretory epithelial cells of many tissues, where it promotes transmembrane efflux of chloride ions.[1545-1548] The receptor protein is abundantly present in the branching ducts of the pancreas, intestinal epithelium and testes, and to a lesser degree in respiratory tissue.[1549] It is expressed at the apical membranes of the epithelium of branching hepatic bile ducts and the gallbladder, but not on cells of the common hepatic bile duct or hepatocytes.[1550,1551] The CF secretory defect consists of inability to maintain the luminal hydration of ducts, leading to physicochemical abnormalities of secretions and duct obstruction.[1552] More than 1000 different disease causing mutations have been identified that are distinguished in severe and mild on the basis of the residual activity of the codified protein.[1553,1554] The most common mutation is deltaF508, a three bp deletion in CFTR, resulting in loss of phenylalanine from the protein with subsequent retention in the endoplasmic reticulum.[1555]

Since liver disease in CF is often subclinical, its prevalence is uncertain and to some extent depends on definition, type of screening and age. Based on prospective studies, significant clinical liver disease is seen in 4–6% of the patients,[1556-1558] but biochemical evidence of liver involvement without clinical symptoms occurs in 20–50%.[1559] Autopsy series in the 1950s found an incidence of multifocal biliary cirrhosis of 22–25%.[1560,1561] The liver disease usually become apparent in the first decade with sharp decline after the age of 10 years.[1556,1559] The mode of presentation of the liver disease is variable. There may be transient neonatal cholestasis. In one series the majority of cholestatic infants had meconium ileus, 28% had mucus plugs, and 11% had focal biliary cirrhosis.[1562] Paucity of the intrahepatic bile ducts has been reported in one patient who presented with cholestasis of infancy.[1563] Obstruction by pancreatic fibrosis has been reported but is much more common beyond infancy.[1564] In late childhood, intermittent elevation of transaminases and alkaline phosphatase, asymptomatic hepatomegaly, hepatosplenomegaly, hypersplenism or variceal haemorrhage might be the first indications of liver involvement. The unique liver lesion, termed focal biliary fibrosis (or 'cirrhosis') is found in over 70% of adults who die after 24 years of age.[1565] A prospective study of 183 CF patients followed for a mean of 10 years revealed an incidence of liver disease of 17%.[1566] Clinically relevant disease suggests an incidence of 1.4–2.7%, with a peak in adolescence.[1565] Rare and unusual manifestations of liver disease in CF include common bile-duct involvement proximal to the pancreas,[1567] obstruction by pancreatic fibrosis, and nodular regenerative hyperplasia of the liver in CF-associated colitis with fibrosing colonopathy.[1568] At times, endoscopic retrograde cholangiopancreatography (ERCP) and liver biopsy findings may mimic those of primary sclerosing cholangitis.[1569] Irrespective of relatively rare chronic progressive liver disease, steatosis (macrovesicular) is the most common pathological finding in the liver and is present in over 50% of autopsy cases.[1570] Steatosis is likely related to malnutrition[1571] and essential fatty acid deficiency.[1572] Death from liver disease occurs in some 3.4% of patients,[1573] whereas lung disease accounts for 78% of CF related deaths.

Factors that contribute to the variability in incidence and severity of the liver disease are unknown. Some studies have found significant association with meconium ileus,[1558,1574] male sex, meconium ileus and severe genotype,[1556] or meconium ileus and pancreatic insufficiency,[1559] but such risk factors were not identified in a Swedish cohort.[1557] There is no close correlation between particular CFTR mutations and liver disease.[1555,1575] Kinnman et al.[1551] examined the expression of CFTR and its relationship to histopathological changes in CF. They found impairment of deltaF508 CFTR processing in intrahepatic biliary epithelium. However, intercellular adhesion molecule type 1 (ICAM)-1 expression on bile-duct epithelial cells and inflammatory infiltrates were rare findings, indicating that immunological mechanisms are unlikely to be involved in initiation of CF-associated liver disease. There is generally discordance for liver disease within sibships,[1576,1577] but this is not uniform.[1555] These observations have intensified the search for modifier genes which may in part explain the lack of genotypic/phenotypic correlations.[1578,1579] The mannose binding lectin gene,[1580] a relation with HLA-DQ6 in males,[1581] and the PiZ allele of alpha1-antitrypsin[1582] have already been proposed as potential candidates. The development of the sweat chloride test[1583] followed the observations of salt depletion through sweat during summer heat waves.[1584] Values greater than 60 meq/L are diagnostic of CF. There are unusual CF patients with sweat chloride values between 40 and 60 meq/L or even in the normal range.[1585,1586] In such patients, abnormal bio-electric potential or immunoreactive trypsinogen screen can confirm the diagnosis.[1587,1588] Recently, extensive CFTR gene sequencing has been proposed to detect rare mutations and to established a definite diagnosis in symptomatic patients with previously negative results.[1589] An elevated serum collagen type VI has been suggested as a screening test for detection of liver disease.[1590] Newborn screening using elevated serum trypsin (trypsinogen) by radioimmunoassay at 3–5 days of age or mutational analysis on Guthrie spots is followed by substantial and prolonged health gain when compared with children clinically diagnosed at a later stage.[1591]

Most investigations have shown improved liver enzymes, lipid profiles, and vitamin A levels with ursodeoxycholic acid therapy.[1572,1592–1595] One report documents normalization of liver function tests and improvement in the portal tract inflammation on pathological examination.[1596] The same authors also noted improvement in ultrastructural abnormalities of bile ducts.

In CF, ursodeoxycholic acid is not effective for gallstone disease,[1597] whose incidence may be 12% in older patients.[1598] Although the stones are often radiolucent, they contain calcium bilirubinate instead of increased cholesterol.[1599] A transjugular intrahepatic portosystemic shunt (TIPS) procedure is rarely utilized in CF liver disease because sclerotherapy or banding therapy has been reasonably successful for treating bleeding varices.[1600,1601] Because of rebleeds, some surgeons still advocate portosystemic shunts for patients with a good synthetic function.[1601] Liver trans-

plantations has been successful,[1602,1603] with long-term survival comparable to that of liver transplantation for other causes.[1604] Postoperative death has been due mainly to lung complications. A few combined liver–heart–lung, liver–pancreas and liver–intestine transplantations have been reported.[1604–1606]

Pathological studies of the liver have been described in a number of reports.[1541,1570,1607–1610] The changes include steatosis, periportal fibrosis with cholangiolar reaction and dilatation (with or without inspissation of secretions) (Fig. 5.131), focal biliary fibrosis ('cirrhosis') and multinodular biliary fibrosis ('cirrhosis'). Steatosis is probably the most frequent lesion. It was present in 121 of 198 cases (61%) reported by Craig et al.[1570] The fat was located most frequently in periportal hepatocytes, but was unevenly distributed throughout when severe. No positive correlations could be made between the presence of fat in the liver and the general nutritional status of the patient. An incidental finding in infant livers is the deposition of haemosiderin in periportal hepatocytes.[1609] This finding is presumably related to the increased iron transport from the gut in pancreatic insufficiency.[1611]

The characteristic if not pathognomonic lesion is focal biliary fibrosis, found in 22 to 33% of patients in 3 early series.[1561,1570,1607] An increasing frequency with duration of survival was noted.[1609] Thus, it was found at post-mortem examination in 10.6% of infants younger than 3 months, in 15.6% of infants from 3 to 12 months, and in 26.9% of children older than 1 year.

Macroscopically, the liver with focal biliary fibrosis shows multiple, depressed, greyish-white scars that are triangular or stellate in shape.[1561,1570] As already noted, there is variable ductular reaction and periportal fibrosis. The ductules are generally dilated and show varying degrees of atrophy of the lining cells (Fig. 5.132). The lumen contains the pathognomonic pink to light orange rounded masses (concretions) or amorphous material (Fig. 5.133), first described by Farber in 1944.[1612] The inspissated secretions in the cholangioles stain intensely with PAS and resist diastase digestion; they do not stain positively with mucicarmine or Alcian blue, but there may be some mucin in the interlobular bile ducts. Some greatly dilated ductules eventually rupture with

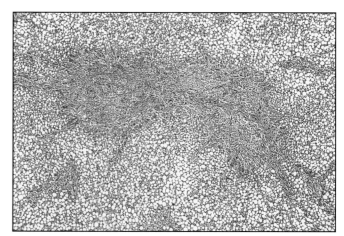

Fig. 5.131 • Cystic fibrosis. Periportal bridging fibrosis and ductular reaction. Note marked steatosis. Masson trichrome.

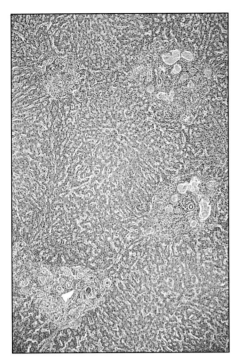

Fig. 5.132 • Cystic fibrosis. Expanded and moderately inflamed portal areas contain markedly dilated bile ductules. Ductular lumens are filled with pink inspissated secretion. H&E.

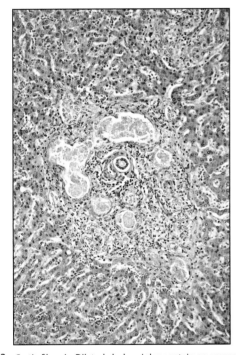

Fig. 5.133 • Cystic fibrosis. Dilated cholangioles contain an amorphous, pink secretion. Note absence of lining cells. H&E.

extrusion of their contents and induction of an acute inflammatory response.[1561] The cholangitis is thus 'chemical' but it may be complicated by bacterial infection.[1613] Chronic inflammatory cells may also be present in the fibrous tissue. It is important to emphasize that periportal fibrosis may occur in the absence of cholangiolar proliferation and inspissation of secretion,[1570,1608] this non-specific change being only found in infants less than 3 months of age.

With the passage of time the focal biliary lesions may coalesce, with extension of fibrosis, atrophy of the intervening parenchyma and entrapment and encirclement of groups of hepatic lobules.[1561] This type of lesion, referred to as 'multilobular biliary cirrhosis with concretions' or 'multilobular cirrhosis', occurs in 6% of patients who are over 1 year of age.[1608] Large irregular nodules are produced and the deep clefts between the nodules may resemble hepar lobatum.[1561]

In addition to the presence of excessive mucus in extrahepatic bile ducts in occasional patients, there may be excessive mucus accumulation in intrahepatic bile ducts, particularly those adjacent to the porta hepatis.[1608] This change occurs in 23.4% of infants under 3 months of age and in 12.5% of patients from 3 to 12 months of age. In two-thirds of the patients less than 3 months of age with mucus in their ducts histological cholestasis is seen, and a history of jaundice is noted. The gallbladder in up to 30% of patients is hypoplastic, and contains mucoid material and a small amount of viscid bile. Mucous cysts are seen in the wall and stones may be present in the lumen.[1614]

Liver biopsy material from 11 patients with cystic fibrosis was examined ultrastructurally by Arends et al.[1615] A finding unique to this disease was the presence of filamentous material, with an average diameter of 15 nm, in the lumen of bile ductules and ducts. Bile granules were scattered between the filaments. A reaction product of carbohydrates was found in the filaments by histochemical techniques. It was suggested that the typical mucus deposits in bile ducts are built up from these filaments. Similar ultrastructural findings were noted by others.[5,1616] Bradford et al.[1616] studied the ultrastructure of liver cells in detail and described the presence of membrane-bound deposits of electron-lucent material containing electron-dense cores resembling mucus. Bile duct cells with irregular shapes, protruding into the lumen, and the presence of necrotic cells have been observed.[1617] An increase in the number of hepatic stellate cells (HSC) around portal areas, with deposition of collagen around bile ducts and ductules, has been noted.[1617,1618] A definitive role for hepatic stellate cells has been shown and transforming growth factor (TGF-β1) produced by bile duct epithelial cells demonstrated as inducer of HSC collagen gene expression.[1619]

Shwachman syndrome

Shwachman–Diamond syndrome (SDS) is an autosomal recessive disorder[1620] characterized by pancreatic exocrine insufficiency, bone marrow dysfunction and skeletal abnormalities. The Shwachman locus has been mapped to chromosome 7q11.[1621] Disease-associated mutations have been identified in this as-yet uncharacterized gene.[1622]

SDS was differentiated from cystic fibrosis by Shwachman et al. in 1964.[1623] The syndrome may begin in utero; the average birth weight is 25% of normal. By 6 months of age patients are below the fifth percentile. The apparent causes of the poor growth, pancreatic insufficiency and fat malabsorption, may improve with age.[1624–1626] Haematological abnormalities occur in 100% of patients with neutropenia in up to 95%, thrombocytopenia in up to 70% and anaemia in over 50%.[1625,1627–1629] The neutropenia can be intermittent, and abnormal chemotaxis may be present temporarily. Bone marrow biopsy may reveal hypoplasia with fat replacement and myeloid maturation arrest.[1630] Electron microscopic examination of cartilage reveals material retained in the rough endoplasmic reticulum.[1631] At least half the patients have metaphyseal dysostosis.[1631] Hepatomegaly is present in 15% of patients, and the aspartate aminotransferase (AST) and ALT are elevated in up to 60% of patients; there is a tendency for liver improvement with age.[1632–1634]

Some patients have responded to treatment with granulocyte colony-stimulating factor.[1635] There is an increased risk of haematological malignancies similar to those that occur with Fanconi anemia.[1636] Nineteen patients with myelodysplastic syndrome and leukaemia have been reported.[1637] Bone marrow transplantation has been attempted; only two of eight patients are disease free, including one who has required liver transplantation for veno-occlusive disease.[1638,1639]

The pancreas in Shwachman syndrome shows replacement of exocrine tissue by fat with preservation of the endocrine islets.[1560,1623] According to Burke et al.[1640] the degeneration of pancreatic exocrine tissue is progressive. Cardiomegaly and testicular fibrosis were reported in one case.[1641] The liver shows variable steatosis.[1560,1623] Some of the patients in the series of Bodian et al.[1560] also had portal fibrosis or 'cirrhosis', but detailed histological descriptions of the hepatic changes were not reported.

Familial and genetic non-alcoholic steatohepatitis and cirrhosis

Non-alcoholic steatohepatitis (NASH) with or without cirrhosis, or with cryptogenic cirrhosis, was reported by Struben et al.[1642] in 18 members of eight kindreds. Fifteen (83%) of the 18 subjects were obese and 11 (31%) had type 2 diabetes mellitus. The occurrence of these disorders within kindreds suggested a common pathogenesis and possible genetic risk. Other cases of familial cirrhosis[1643] or cryptogenic cirrhosis with a family history of unexplained liver disease (19% of the patients in the series of Caldwell et al.[1644]) have been reported. Steatohepatitis[1645] and cirrhosis[1646] have been reported in patients with *partial lipodystrophy*. NASH is also reported in children with *Bardet–Biedl syndrome* and both children and adults with *Alström syndrome*,[1647–1649] in which cirrhosis may occur. Steatohepatitis (sclerosing hyaline necrosis) was also described in a patient with *Bloom syndrome*.[1650] This autosomal recessive disorder is characterized by a normally proportioned but strikingly small body size, characteristic facies, photosensitive skin lesions, immunodeficiency and marked predisposition to a variety of cancers. Of relevance to this section are reports of marked hepatic steatosis (but no steatohepatitis or cirrhosis) in patients with the *Dorfman–Chanarin syndrome*, an autosomal recessive disorder characterized by marked hepatic steatosis, ichthyosis and variable involvement of muscle and the central nervous system.[1651,1652]

Hepatotoxicity and other known genetic/metabolic diseases that can cause fatty liver, such as Wilson disease and cystic fibrosis, must be excluded since treatment is radically different.[1653]

Congenital total lipodystrophy

This disease is characterized by near absence of adipose tissue, severe insulin-resistant diabetes, hyperlipidaemia, hepatomegaly, muscular hypertrophy, hypertrichosis and acanthosis nigricans.[1654] Inheritance is believed to be autosomal recessive. A disease locus has been identified on chromosome 11q13 (Magre J 2001), with some families having linkage to 9q34.[1655] An association with peripheral pulmonary artery stenosis was reported in three children by Uzon et al.[1656]

The liver is enlarged and grossly yellow or light yellow–brown in colour. Light microscopic changes have been described in a number of case reports.[1657–1664] They include steatosis and periportal fibrosis, with portal to portal bridging. Ductular proliferation was noted in several cases.[1661] Cirrhosis was present in some patients.[1657–1659,1662] Hepatocytes in one case were described as 'plant-like' with prominent cell walls, a pale vacuolated cytoplasm and pale, centrally placed nuclei; the presence of fat and glycogen was demonstrated in the cytoplasm of liver cells by special stains.

Ultrastructural abnormalities have been described in several reports.[5,1659,1660,1662] In addition to numerous lipid droplets, there are many lysosomes containing variable quantities of lipofuscin and lipolysosomes.[5] Peroxisomes are said to be increased[1659,1661] or reduced in number[5] and they contain dense matrix granules. Mitochondria are misshapen and, contain distinctive, elongated, crystal-like matrical inclusions that adopt various geometric configurations.[5] They possibly represent cholesterol or other lipid material. Partial lysis of swollen and irregular mitochondria was described in one case.[1657]

Chronic granulomatous disease

Chronic granulomatous disease (CGD) is characterized by recurrent purulent infections caused by bacteria (usually catalase-positive) or fungi. The onset is generally before 1 year of age, although milder forms may present in adulthood. Marked lymphadenopathy, hepatomegaly and splenomegaly are common findings.[1665] In this disorder antimicrobial activity of phagocytes is impaired due to the lack of reactive oxygen species, or oxidative burst, normally produced by NADPH oxidase. The most common X-linked form of CGD represents 70% of all cases.[1666] There are autosomal recessive forms which are considerably rarer. The disease is caused by mutations in the cytochrome b beta subunit (*CYBB*) gene, which maps to chromosome Xp21,[1667] which was cloned in 1986,[1668] encodes the gp91-phox (for phagocyte oxidase) protein, a necessary component in the NADPH oxidase pathway.[1669,1670] Mutations in the *CYBB* gene responsible for chronic granulomatous disease have been described and permit prenatal diagnosis.[1671] Assessment of defective granulocyte function by flow cytometry can be used in neonates.[1672] Patients are screened for the disease by the nitroblue tetrazolium dye reduction assay.[1673]

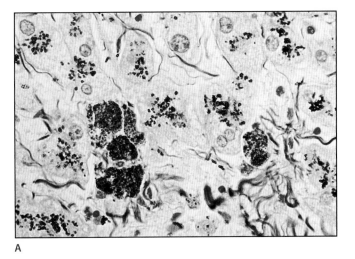

A

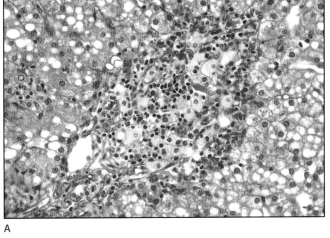

A

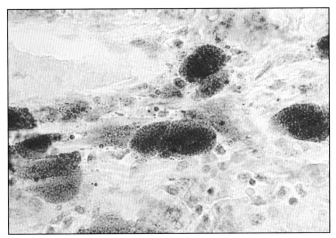

B

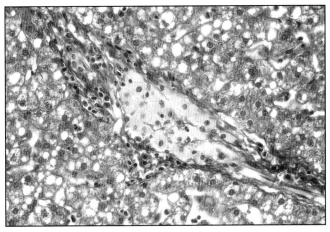

B

Fig. 5.134 • Chronic granulomatous disease. **(A)** Markedly hypertrophied Kupffer cells contain lipofuscin (black). Fontana stain. **(B)** Portal area macrophages contain orange-coloured lipofuscin. Oil red-O stain of frozen section.

Fig. 5.135 • Chronic granulomatous disease. **(A)** Macrovesicular steatosis. Portal area is inflamed and contains several large macrophage cells. H&E. **(B)** Same case as illustrated in Fig. 5.93(A) demonstrating a cluster of macrophage cells in a portal area at higher magnification. Masson trichrome.

While some patients respond to interferon-γ therapy, this has not been a useful long-term treatment.[1674] Radical surgery is recommended for liver abscess.[1675] Bone marrow transplantation was helpful in one case.[1676] Granulocytes transfusions from healthy donors given granulocyte colony-stimulating factor subcutaneously and dexamethasone orally 12 h before collection have helped eradication of invasive aspergillosis.[1677] Recently, stem cell transplantation with a reduced intensity conditioning protocol has been followed by full donor chimerism and normalization of superoxide production.[1678] Gene therapy, including ex-vivo protocols, are promising[1679] and the object of intense investigation in murine models.[1680,1681]

The characteristic pathological features are the granulomatous response to infection and the widespread accumulation of lipofuscin pigment in reticuloendothelial cells[1682–1685] (Fig. 5.134). Small granulomas consist of rings of mononuclear cells which surround an area of homogeneous eosinophilic material, and are associated with many plasma cells and a few giant cells.[1686] Confluent granulomas may show larger areas of necrosis and suppuration. Palisading granulomas with central necrosis and associated giant cells were

noted in four of seven cases reported by Nakhleh et al.[1687] Special stains for microorganisms are usually negative, unless the granulomas are caused by fungi.[1688] The pigmented histiocytes have a light-tan colour and are PAS-positive, argentaphilic, sudanophilic (in frozen sections), and autofluorescent (Fig. 5.134). The accumulation of the pigment is thought to be a secondary phenomenon.[1689] In the liver, most of the lipofuscin is found in clusters of markedly hypertrophied portal macrophages or Kupffer cells. Portal areas are infiltrated by plasma cells and lymphocytes, and there may be minimal to moderate fibrosis. A hepar lobatum-like cirrhotic process was described in one patient.[1690] Varying numbers of granulomas and/or microabscesses may be scattered within the parenchyma and there may be slight to moderate portal inflammation and fatty change (Fig. 5.135).

Liver disease in X-linked hyper-IgM syndrome

The largest study with the rare, X-linked hyper-IgM syndrome (XHIM) was reported by the Registry of Primary

Immunodeficiencies of the European Society for Immune Deficiency.[1691] The study comprised the clinical, immunological features and outcome of 56 patients with this syndrome. The defect is caused by mutations in the gene encoding for CD40 ligand, located on chromosome Xq 26.3–27. It is a cellular immunodeficiency characterized by disruption of multiple cellular interactions (T-cells and B-cells; T-cells and macrophages). Patients are unable to mount IgG, IgA and IgE responses to T-cell dependent antigens and lack germinal centres, but their ability to produce IgM is preserved. Infections are the most prominent clinical manifestations of XHIM. Upper and lower respiratory tract infections (the latter frequently caused by *Pneumocystis carinii*), chronic diarrhoea and liver involvement (both caused by *Crystosporidium* infections) are common.[1691] Many patients have chronic neutropenia associated with oral and rectal ulcers. An example of cryptosporidiosis in a 15-year-old male with XHIM (diagnosed at the age of 18 months) is illustrated in Fig. 5.136; ERCP revealed sclerosing cholangitis. In the series of Levy et al.[1691] 19.6% of patients had sclerosing cholangitis and 55% of those patients had concomitant cryptosporidiosis. In another series of 20 children (all boys) from 16 families, 45% had sclerosing cholangi-

tis.[1692] Liver tests are persistently abnormal, with a median AST of 117 IU/l and a γGT of 182 IU/l in one series.[1692]

Patients with XHIM have developed carcinomas of the liver (hepatocellular carcinoma or bile-duct carcinoma), pancreas or gallbladder, and of neuroectodermal endocrine cells.[1691,1693,1694] The tumours were fatal in eight of nine cases in one series[1693] and in most instances were preceded by a chronic cholangiopathy and/or cirrhosis.

Survival in XHIM is poor—20% at 26 years in the series of Levy et al.[1691] The treatment of choice is intravenous immune globulin.[1691] Liver transplantation has been associated with a high rate of recurrence of cryptosporidiosis although long-term survivors have been reported.[1691,1695] Bone marrow transplantation is curative but its success is hampered by conditioning-related liver complications (such as veno-occlusive disease and graft-versus-host disease).[1692] Allogeneic haemopoietic stem cells from HLA matched related or unrelated donors is feasible and curative if performed before significant infections and organ damage occur.[1696] Successful sequential liver and bone marrow transplantation have been reported.[1692,1695]

Aarskog syndrome

The salient features of this syndrome include short stature and facial, digital and genital malformations.[1697] The inheritance is X-linked.[1698] The gene has been mapped to chromosome Xq13.[1698–1700] One reported patient had a slightly elevated total serum bilirubin, and needle biopsy of the liver revealed haemosiderosis and a micronodular cirrhosis.[1701]

Leprechaunism (Donohue syndrome)

This is a rare disorder characterized by a grotesque elfin facies with a flat nasal bridge and flaring nostrils, thick lips and large low-set ears. Patients have hirsutism, enlargement of the breasts and external genitalia, motor and mental retardation, failure to thrive and progressive marasmus. Death occurs before 2 years of age.[1702,1703] The disease is autosomal recessive. Patients have mutations in the high-affinity insulin-receptor. At least two mutations in this gene leading to leprechaunism have been described.[1703]

A consistent pathological feature of the syndrome in females is follicular maturation of the ovaries with cyst formation. Some patients have hyperplasia of the islets of Langerhans and severe malformations of the brain and heart. Other associated findings have been reviewed.[1704] The liver has been reported to be histologically normal in some patients,[1705,1706] or to show non-specific changes such as an increased glycogen content,[1705,1707] mild fatty change,[1707] or haemosiderosis.[1708] Haemosiderosis, both hepatocellular and reticuloendothelial, was also present in the cases reported by Donohue & Uchida,[1702] and Ordway & Stout[1709] in combination with other changes. Both these reports described multiple small nodules in the liver that were composed of large, pale, foamy hepatocytes containing much glycogen and a little fat, with occasional fusion of cells and formation of syncytial masses. Ordway & Stout[1709]

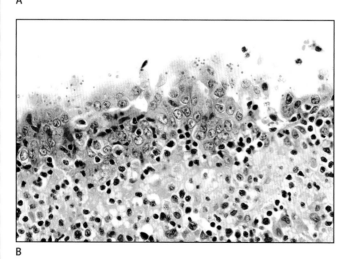

A

B

Fig. 5.136 • (A) X-linked hyper-IgM syndrome. Prominent perivenular cholestasis in patient who had sclerosing cholangitis. H&E. **(B)** Same case showing spherical cryptosporidia attached to the epithelium of a large bile duct. H&E.

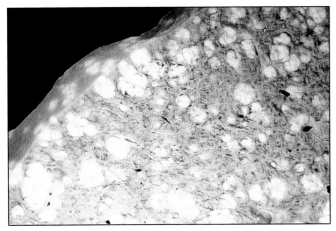

Fig. 5.137 • Leprechaunism. This section of liver is green and studded with pale, white nodules of varied size.

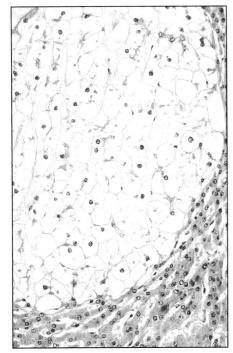

Fig. 5.138 • Leprechaunism. Segment of regenerative nodule is composed of large, empty hepatocytes. A PAS-stained section (not shown) confirmed the presence of glycogen in these cells. H&E.

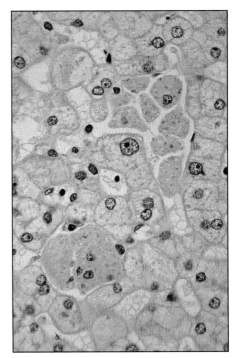

Fig. 5.139 • Hermansky–Pudlak syndrome. Kupffer cells are markedly hypertrophied and contain a light tan pigment. H&E.

interpreted these foci as regenerative nodules. An example is illustrated in Figs 5.137 and 5.138. Intrahepatic cholestasis has been reported in several cases[1704] and bile-duct proliferation in one case.[1709]

Albinism

Of the several forms of oculocutaneous albinism which are known, only two involve the liver: Chediak–Higashi syndrome and Hermansky–Pudlak syndrome.

Chediak–Higashi syndrome

Patients with this syndrome are distinctive, with a light cream to slate grey skin and hair that has a metallic, frosted-grey sheen. Other findings include photophobia, squint,

nystagmus and decreased pigment in the retina. Patients suffer from recurrent infections, most often by Gram-positive organisms. A progressive neuropathy, usually noted at about 5 years of age, involves cranial and peripheral nerves. Rarely, adults with a less severe form of the disease have findings consistent with either spinocerebellar degeneration or Parkinsonian disease. Hepatosplenomegaly is common, particularly in the accelerated phase of the disease,[1710] which is heralded by fever, lymphadenopathy, hepatosplenomegaly, pancytopenia, hyperlipidaemia and coagulopathy. Tissue infiltrates consist of benign-appearing histiocytes showing haemophagocytosis, plus lymphocytes and plasma cells which, in the liver, are found in portal areas and sinusoids.[1711]

Diagnosis is based on the presence of characteristic giant, eosinophilic, peroxidase-positive inclusions in leucocytes which do not degranulate. The disease is autosomal recessive and is caused by a defect in the lysosomal trafficking gene *LYST*, which is essential for the function of natural killer cells.[1712] Treatment has included chemotherapeutic agents, particularly during the accelerated phase, but the only cure has been bone marrow transplantation.[1711]

Hermansky–Pudlak syndrome

This disorder is characterized by oculocutaneous albinism, a mild bleeding diathesis due to a storage pool platelet defect, and widespread deposition of ceroid pigment in cells of the reticuloendothelial system.[1713,1714] Complications include pulmonary fibrosis, renal failure, cardiomyopathy and a granulomatous colitis.[1713] The disease is autosomal recessive. It maps to chromosome 10q.[1715] The gene has been identified, but its function is as yet undetermined.[1716,1717]

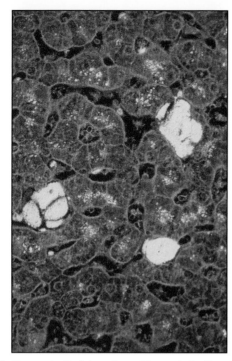

Fig. 5.140 • Hermansky–Pudlak syndrome. Pigment in Kupffer cells displays bright yellow autofluorescence. Unstained section, examined under ultraviolet light.

Involvement of the liver in this syndrome is limited to the presence of a light-tan, granular pigment in hypertrophied Kupffer cells and portal macrophages (Fig. 5.139). The pigment has all the characteristics of ceroid or lipofuscin, being PAS-positive and diastase-resistant, sudanophilic and argentaphilic, and it reveals bright-yellow autofluorescence when viewed by ultraviolet microscopy (Fig. 5.140). Ultrastructurally, the pigment is granular, intermingled with lipid and bounded by a single membrane. Occasionally; it shows a finger-print pattern of concentric light and dark bands which have a periodicity of approximately 20 nm.[1718]

References

1. Watts RW, Morgan SH, Danpure CJ et al. Combined hepatic and renal transplantation in primary hyperoxaluria type I: clinical report of nine cases. Am J Med, 1991; 90:179–188
2. Stein C, Gieselmann V, Kreysing J et al. Cloning and expression of human arylsulfatase A. J Biol Chem, 1989; 264:1252–1259
3. Ishak KG. Hepatic morphology in the inherited metabolic diseases. Semin Liver Dis, 1986; 6:246–258
4. Gilbert-Barness E, Barness L. Metabolic diseases. Foundations of clinical management, genetics, and pathology. 2000, Natick, MA: Eaton Publishing
5. Phillips MJ, Poucell S, Patterson J, Valencia P. The liver. An atlas and text of ultrastructural pathology. 1987, New York: Raven Press
6. Spycher MA. Electron microscopy: A method for the diagnosis of inherited metabolic storage disease. Pathol Res Pract, 1980; 167:118–135
7. Tanikawa K. Ultrastructural aspects of the liver and its disorders. 2nd edn ed. 1979, Tokyo: Igaku-Shoin
8. Badminton MN, Elder GH. Molecular mechanisms of dominant expression in porphyria. J Inherit Metab Dis, 2005; 28:277–286
9. Bloomer J, Bruzzone C, Zhu L, Scarlett Y, Magness S, Brenner D. Molecular defects in ferrochelatase in patients with protoporphyria requiring liver transplantation. J Clin Invest, 1998; 102:107–114
10. Elder GH. Porphyria cutanea tarda. Semin Liver Dis, 1998; 18:67–75
11. Nordmann Y, Puy H, Deybach JC. The porphyrias. J Hepatol, 1999; 30:12–16
12. Scarlett YV, Brenner DA, Bloomer JR. Hepatic porphyrias. Clin Liver Dis, 1998; 2:77–102
13. Egger NG, Goeger DE, Payne DA, Miskovsky EP, Weinman SA, Anderson KE. Porphyria cutanea tarda: multiplicity of risk factors including HFE mutations, hepatitis C, and inherited uroporphyrinogen decarboxylase deficiency. Dig Dis Sci, 2002; 47:419–426
14. Roberts AG, Whatley SD, Morgan RR, Worwood M, Elder GH. Increased frequency of the haemochromatosis Cys282Tyr mutation in sporadic porphyria cutanea tarda. Lancet, 1997; 349:321–323
15. Bulaj ZJ, Phillips JD, Ajioka RS et al. Hemochromatosis genes and other factors contributing to the pathogenesis of porphyria cutanea tarda. Blood, 2000; 95:1565–1571
16. Hift RJ, Corrigall AV, Hancock V, Kannemeyer J, Kirsch RE, Meissner PN. Porphyria cutanea tarda: the etiological importance of mutations in the HFE gene and viral infection is population-dependent. Cell Mol Biol (Noisy-le-grand), 2002; 48:853–859
17. Mehrany K, Drage LA, Brandhagen DJ, Pittelkow MR. Association of porphyria cutanea tarda with hereditary hemochromatosis. J Am Acad Dermatol, 2004; 51:205–211
18. Bonkovsky HL, Lambrecht RW. Iron-induced liver injury. Clin Liver Dis, 2000; 4:409–429
19. Bonkovsky HL, Schned AR. Fatal liver failure in protoporphyria. Synergism between ethanol excess and the genetic defect. Gastroenterology, 1986; 90:191–201
20. Fargion S, Piperno A, Capellini MD et al. Hepatitis C virus and porphyria cutanea tarda: evidence of a strong association. Hepatology, 1992; 16:1322–1326
21. Rocchi E, Gibertini P, Cassanelly M, Pietrangelo A, Jensen J, Ventura E. Hepatitis B virus infection in porphyria cutanea tarda. Liver, 1986; 6:153–157
22. Valls V, de Salamanca RE, Lapena L et al. Hepatitis B serum markers in porphyria cutanea tarda. J Dermatol, 1986; 15:24–29
23. Boisseau AM, Couzigou P, Forestier JF et al. Porphyria cutanea tarda associated with human immunodeficiency virus infection. Dermatologica, 1991; 182:155–159
24. El-Serag HB, Hampel H, Yeh C, Rabeneck L. Extrahepatic manifestations of hepatitis C among United States male veterans. Hepatology, 2002; 36:1439–1445
25. Gisbert JP, Garcia-Buey L, Pajares JM, Moreno-Otero R. Prevalence of hepatitis C virus infection in porphyria cutanea tarda: systematic review and meta-analysis. J Hepatol, 2003; 39:620–627
26. Herrero C, Vicente A, Bruguera M et al. Is hepatitis C virus infection a trigger of porphyria cutanea tarda? Lancet, 1993; 341:288–289
27. Bonkovsky HL, Poh-Fitzpatrick M, Pimstone N et al. Porphyria cutanea tarda, hepatitis C, and HFE gene mutations in North America. Hepatology, 1998; 27:1661–1669
28. Cortes JM, Oliva H, Paradinas FJ, Hernandez-Guio C. The pathology of the liver in porphyria cutanea tarda. Histopathology, 1980; 4:471–485
29. Siersema PD, Rademakers LHPM, Cleton MI et al. The difference in liver pathology between sporadic and familial forms of porphyria cutanea tarda: the role of iron. J Hepatol, 1995; 23:259–267
30. Fakan F, Chlumska A. Demonstration of needle-shaped hepatic inclusions in porphyria cutanea tarda using the ferric ferricyanide reduction test. Virchows Arch [A], 1987; 411:365–368
31. Siersema PD, Van Helvoirt RP, Ketelaars DAM et al. Iron and uroporphyrin in hepatocytes of inbred mice in experimental porphyria: a biochemical and morphological study. Hepatology, 1991; 14:1179–1188
32. Campo E, Bruguera M, Rodes J. Are there diagnostic histologic features of porphyria cutanea tarda in liver biopsy specimens? Liver, 1990; 10:185–190
33. Lefkowitch JH, Grossman ME. Hepatic pathology in porphyria cutanea tarda. Liver, 1983; 3:19–29
34. Salata H, Cortes JM, de Salamanca RE et al. Porphyria cutanea tarda and hepatocellular carcinoma. Frequency of occurrence and related factors. J Hepatol, 1985; 1:477–487
35. Siersema PD, Kate FJW, Mulder PGH, Wilson JHP. Hepatocellular carcinoma in porphyria cutanea tarda: frequency and factors related to its occurrence. Liver, 1992; 12:56–61
36. Solis JA, Betancor P, Campos R et al. Association of porphyria cutanea tarda and primary liver cancer. Report of ten cases. J Dermatol, 1982; 9:131–137
37. Andant C, Puy H, Bogard C et al. Hepatocellular carcinoma in patients with acute hepatic porphyria: frequency of occurrence and related factors. J Hepatol, 2000; 32:933–939

38. Andant C, Puy H, Deybach JC, Soule JC, Nordmann Y. Occurrence of hepatocellular carcinoma in a case of hereditary coproporphyria. Am J Gastroenterol, 1997; 92:1389–1390

39. Hardell L, Bengtsson NO, Jonsson U, Eriksson S, Larsson LG. Aetiological aspects on primary liver cancer with special regard to alcohol, organic solvents and acute intermittent porphyria—an epidemiological investigation. Br J Cancer, 1984; 50:389–397

40. Kauppinen R, Mustajoki P. Acute hepatic porphyria and hepatocellular carcinoma. Br J Cancer, 1988; 57:117–120

41. Lithner F, Wetterberg L. Hepatocellular carcinoma with acute intermittent porphyria. Acta Med Scand, 1984; 215:271–274

42. Thunissen PLM, Meyer J, de Koning RW. Acute intermittent porphyria and primary liver-cell carcinoma. Nether J Med, 1991; 38:171–174

43. Tidman MJ, Higgins EM, Elder GH, Macdonald DM. Variegate porphyria associated with hepatocellular carcinoma. Br J Dermatol, 1989; 121:503–505

44. Gray AMH. Haematoporphyria congenita with hydrovacciniforme and hirsuties. Q J Med, 1926; 19:381

45. Mangus IA, Jarrett A, Prankerd TAJ. Erythrocyte protoporphyrin P: A new porphyria syndrome with solar urticaria due to protoporphyrinaemia. Lancet, 1961; ii:448

46. Cripps DJ, Scheuer PJ. Hepatobiliary changes in erythropoietic protoporphyria. Arch Pathol, 1965; 80:500–508

47. Baart de la Faille H, Bijlmer-Iest JC, van Hattum J, Koningsberger J, Rademakers LH, van Weelden H. Erythropoietic protoporphyria: clinical aspects with emphasis on the skin. Curr Probl Dermatol, 1991; 20:123–134

48. Gross U, Frank M, Doss MO. Hepatic complications of erythropoietic protoporphyria. Photodermatol Photoimmunol Photomed, 1998; 14:52–57

49. Nordmann Y. Erythropoietic protoporphyria and hepatic complications. J Hepatol, 1992; 16:4–6

50. Rank JM, Straka JG, Bloomer JR. Liver in disorders of porphyrin metabolism. J Gastroenterol Hepatol, 1990; 5:573–585

51. Bonkowsky HL, Bloomer JR, Ebert PS, Mahoney MJ. Heme synthetase deficiency in human protoporphyria. Demonstration of the defect in liver and cultured skin fibroblasts. J Clin Invest, 1975; 56:1139–1148

52. Poh-Fitzpatrick MB. Protoporphyrin metabolic balance in human protoporphyria. Gastroenterology, 1985; 88:1239–1242

53. Bloomer JR. The hepatic porphyrias. Pathogenesis, 1976; 71:689–701

54. Sarkany RP, Alexander GJ, Cox TM. Recessive inheritance of erythropoietic protoporphyria with liver failure. Lancet, 1994; 344:958–959

55. Di Pierro E, Cappellini MD, Mazzucchelli R et al. A point mutation affecting an SP1 binding site in the promoter of the ferrochelatase gene impairs gene transcription and causes erythropoietic protoporphyria. Exp Hematol, 2005; 33:584–591

56. Goerz G, Bolsen K, Bunselmeyer S, Schurer NY. Recessive inheritance of erythropoietic protoporphyria with liver failure. Lancet, 1994; 344:337

57. Imoto S, Tanizawa Y, Sato Y, Kaku K, Oka Y. A novel mutation in the ferrochelatase gene associated with erythropoietic protoporphyria. Br J Haematol, 1996; 94:191–197

58. Taketani S, Inazawa J, Nakahashi Y, Abe T, Tokunaga R. Structure of the human ferrochelatase gene. Exon/intron gene organization and location of the gene to chromosome 18. Eur J Biochem, 1992; 205:217–222

59. Bloomer J, Wang Y, Singhal A, Risheg H. Molecular studies of liver disease in erythropoietic protoporphyria. J Clin Gastroenterol, 2005; 39:S167–S175

60. Bloomer JR, Pierach CA. Effect of hematin administration on patients with protoporphyria and liver disease. Hepatology, 1982; 2:817–821

61. Potter C, Tolaymat N, Bobo R, Sharp H, Rank J, Bloomer J. Hematin therapy in children with protoporphyric liver disease. J Pediatr Gastroenterol Nutr, 1996; 23:402–407

62. Bloomer JR, Rank JM, Payne WD et al. Follow-up after liver transplantation for protoporphyric liver disease. Liver Transpl Surg, 1996; 2:269–275

63. Meerman L, Haagsma EB, Gouw AS, Slooff MJ, Jansen PL. Long-term follow-up after liver transplantation for erythropoietic protoporphyria. Eur J Gastroenterol Hepatol, 1999; 11:431–438

64. De Torres I, Demetris AJ, Randhawa PS. Recurrent hepatic allograft injury in erythropoietic protoporphria. Transplantation, 1996; 61:1412–1413

65. Dellon ES, Szczepiorkowski ZM, Dzik WH et al. Treatment of recurrent allograft dysfunction with intravenous hematin after liver transplantation for erythropoietic protoporphyria. Transplantation, 2002; 73:911–915

66. Kauffman L, Evans DI, Stevens RF, Weinkove C. Bone-marrow transplantation for congenital erythropoietic porphyria. Lancet, 1991; 337:1510–1511

67. Boulechfar S, Lamoril J, Montagutelli X et al. Ferrochelatase structural mutant (Fechm1Pas) in the house mouse. Genomics, 1993; 16:645–648

68. Libbrecht L, Meerman L, Kuipers F, Roskams T, Desmet V, Jansen P. Liver pathology and hepatocarcinogenesis in a long-term mouse model of erythropoietic protoporphyria. J Pathol, 2003; 199:191–200

69. Tutois S, Montagutelli X, Da Silva V et al. Erythropoietic protoporphyria in the house mouse. A recessive inherited ferrochelatase deficiency with anemia, photosensitivity, and liver disease. J Clin Invest, 1991; 88:1730–1736

70. Fontanellas A, Mazurier F, Landry M et al. Reversion of hepatobiliary alterations by bone marrow transplantation in a murine model of erythropoietic protoporphyria. Hepatology, 2000; 32:73–81

71. Bloomer JR, Enriquez R. Evidence that hepatic crystalline deposits in a patient with protoporphyria are composed of protoporphyrin. Gastroenterology, 1982; 82:569–572

72. Klatskin G, Bloomer JR. Birefringence of hepatic pigment deposits in erythrohepatic protoporphyria. Gastroenterology, 1974; 67:294–302

73. Bloomer JR, Phillips MJ, Davidson DL, Klatskin G. Hepatic disease in erythropoietic protoporphyria. Am J Med, 1975; 58:869–882

74. Bruguera M, Esquerada JE, Mascaro JM, Pinol J. Erythropoietic protoporphyria. A light, electron, and polarization microscopical study of the liver in three patients. Arch Pathol Lab Med, 1976; 100:587–589

75. Matilla A, Molland EA. A light and electron microscopic study of the liver in case of erythropoietic protoporphyria and in griseofulvin-induced porphyria in mice. J Clin Pathol, 1974; 27:698–709

76. Nakanuma Y, Wada M, Kono N, Miyamura H, Ohta G. An autopsy case of erythropoietic protoporphyria with cholestatic jaundice and hepatic failure, and a review of the literature. Virchows Arch Pathol Anat, 1998; 393:123–132

77. Rademakers LHPM, Cleton MI, Kooijman C, Kooijman C, de la Faille HB, Van Hattum J. Early involvement of hepatic parenchymal cells in erythrohepatic protoporphyria—An ultrastructural study of patients with and without overt liver disease and the effect of chenodeoxycholic acid treatment. Hepatology, 1990; 11:449–457

78. Wolff K, Wolff-Schreiner E, Gschnait F. Liver inclusions in erythropoietic protoporphyria. Eur J Clin Invest, 1975; 5:21–26

79. Cripps DJ, Gilbert LA, Goldfarb SS. Erythropoietic protoprophyria. Juvenile protoporphyrin hepatopathy, 1977; 91:744–748

80. DeLeo VA, Mathews-Roth M, Harber LC. Erythropoietic protoporphyria. 10 years experience. Am J Med, 1976; 60:8–22

81. Singer JA, Plant AG, Kaplan MM. Hepatic failure and death from erythropoietic protoporphyria. Gastroenterology, 1978; 74:588–591

82. Wagner S, Doss MO, Wittkind C, Backer U, Meassen D, Schmidt FW. Erythrohepatische Protoporphyria mit rasch progredienter Leberzirrhose. Dtsch Med Wschr, 1989; 114:1837–1841

83. Poh-Fitzpatrick MB, Whitlock RT, Lefkowitch JH. Changes in protoporphyrin distribution dynamics during liver failure and recovery in a patient with protoporphyria and Epstein–Barr viral hepatitis. Am J Med, 1986; 80:943–950

84. Lee RG, Avner DL, Berenson MM. Structure-function relationship of protoporphyrin-induced liver injury. Arch Pathol Lab Med, 1984; 108:744–746

85. Thompson RPH, Molland EA, Nicholson DA, Nicholson DA, Gray CH. Erythropoietic protoporphyria and cirrhosis in sisters. Gut, 1973; 14:934–1038

86. Graham-Brown RAC, Scheuer PJ, Sarkany I. Histiocytosis X and erythropoietic protoporphyria. J Roy Soc Med, 1984; 77:238–240

87. von Gierke E. Hepato-nephro-megale glycogenica (Glykogenspeicher-Krankheit der Leber und Nieren). Beitr Pathol Anat, 1929; 82:497

88. Leik J, Pan CJ, Shelly LL, Chou JY. Mutations in the gene for glucose-6-phosphatase. The enzyme deficient in glycogen storage disease 1a. J Clin Invest, 1994; 93:1994–1999

89. Annabi B, Hiraiwa H, Mansfield BC et al. The gene for glycogen-storage disease type 1b maps to chromosome 11q23. Am J Hum Genet, 1998; 62:400–405

90. Chen Y-T. Glycogen storage disease. In: Metabolic and Molecular Bases of Inherited Diseases. C.R. Scriver, A.L. Beaudet, W.S. Sly, J. Valle, Editors. 2001, McGraw-Hill New York. p. 1521–1552

91. Parvari R, Hershkovitz E, Carmi R, Moses S. Prenatal diagnosis of glycogen storage disease type 1a by single stranded conformation polymorphism (SSCP). Prenat Diagn, 1996; 16:862–865

92. Lei KJ, Chen H, Pan CJ et al. Glucose-6-phosphatase dependent substrate transport in the glycogen storage disease type-1a mouse. Nat Genet, 1996; 13:203–209

93. Couper R, Kapelushnik J, Griffiths AM. Neutrophil dysfunction in glycogen storage disease Ib: association with Crohn's-like colitis. Gastroenterology, 1991; 100:549–554

94. Gitzelman R, Bosshard NU. Defective neutrophil and monocyte functions in glycogen storage disease type 1b: a literature review. Eur J Pediatr, 1993; 152 (suppl 1):S33–S38

95. Melis D, Parenti G, Della Casa R et al. Crohn's-like ileo-colitis in patients affected by glycogen storage disease Ib: two years' follow-up of patients with a wide spectrum of gastrointestinal signs. Acta Paediatr, 2003; 92:1415–1421

96. Sanderson IR, Bisset WM, Milla PJ, Leonard JV. Chronic inflammatory bowel disease in glycogen storage disease type 1B. J Inherit Metab Dis, 1992; 14:771–776

97. Wendel U, Schroten H, Burdach S, Wahn V. Glycogen storage disease type Ib: infectious complications and measures for prevention. Eur J Pediatr, 1993; 152(suppl 1):S49–S51

98. Talente GM, Coleman RA, Alter C et al. Glycogen storage disease in adults. Ann Intern Med, 1994; 120:218–226

99. Gilchrist GS, Fine RN, Donnell GN. The hemostatic defect in glycogen storage disease, type 1. Acta Paediatr Scand, 1968; 57:205–208

100. Hutton RA, Macnab AJ, Rivers RP. Defect of platelet function associated with chronic hypoglycaemia. Arch Dis Child, 1976; 51:49–55

101. Marti GE, Rick ME, Sidbury J, Gralnick HR. DDAVP infusion in five patients with type Ia glycogen storage disease and associated correction of prolonged bleeding times. Blood, 1986; 68:180–184

102. Chen YT, Coleman RA, Scheinman JI, Kolbeck PC, Sidbury JB. Renal disease in type I glycogen storage disease. N Engl J Med, 1988; 318:171–175

103. Baker L, Dahlem S, Goldfarb S et al. Hyperfiltration and renal disease in glycogen storage disease, type I. Kidney Int, 1989; 35:1345–1350

104. Bianchi L. Glycogen storage disease I and hepatocellular tumours. Eur J Pediatr, 1993; 152 (suppl 1):S63–S70

105. Franco LM, Krishnamurthy V, Bali D et al. Hepatocellular carcinoma in glycogen storage disease type Ia: a case series. J Inherit Metab Dis, 2005; 28:153–162

106. Labrune P, Trioche P, Duvaltier I, Chevalier P, Odièvre M. Hepatocellular adenomas in glycogen storage disease type I and III: a series of 43 patients and review of the literature. J Pediatr Gastroenterol Nutr, 1997; 24:276–279

107. Michels VV, Beaudet AL, Potts VE, Montandon CM. Glycogen storage disease: long-term follow-up of nocturnal intragastric feeding. Clin Genet, 1982; 21:136–140

108. Parker P, Burr I, Slonim A, Ghishan FK, Greene H. Regression of hepatic adenomas in type Ia glycogen storage disease with dietary therapy. Gastroenterology, 1981; 81:534–536

109. Narita T, Nakazawa H, Hizawa Y, Kudo H. Glycogen storage disease associated with Niemann–Pick disease: Histochemical, enzymatic, and lipid analysis. Mod Pathol, 1994; 7:416–421

110. Cori GI, Cori CF. Glucose-6-phosphatase of the liver glycogen storage disease. J Biol Chem, 1952; 199:661

111. Pan CJ, Lei KJ, Annabi B, Chou JY. Transmembrane topology of glucose-6-phosphatase. J Biol Chem, 1998; 273:6144–6148

112. Hiraiwa H, Pan CJ, Lin B, Moses SW, Chou JY. Inactivation of the glucose 6-phosphate transporter causes glycogen storage disease type 1b. J Biol Chem, 1999; 274:5532–5536

113. Moses SW. Historical highlights and unsolved problems in glycogen storage disease type 1. Eur J Pediatr, 2002; 161 (Suppl 1): S2–S9

114. Korchak HM, Garty BZ, Stanley CA, Baker L, Douglas SD, Kilpatrick L. Impairment of calcium mobilization in phagocytic cells in glycogen storage disease type 1b. Eur J Pediatr, 1993; 152 (Suppl 1):S39–S43

115. Burchell A, Waddell I. Diagnosis of a novel glycogen storage disease: type 1aSP. J Inherit Metab Dis, 1990; 13:247–249

116. Lei KJ, Shelly LL, Lin B et al. Mutations in the glucose-6-phosphatase gene are associated with glycogen storage disease types 1a and 1a but not 1b and 1c. J Clin Invest, 1995; 95:234–240

117. Rake JP, Visser G, Labrune P, Leonard JV, Ullrich K, Smit GP. Glycogen storage disease type I: diagnosis, management, clinical course and outcome. Results of the European Study on Glycogen Storage Disease Type I (ESGSD I). Eur J Pediatr, 2002; 161 (Suppl 1):S20–S34

118. Wolfsdorf JI, Crigler JF Jr. Effect of continuous glucose therapy begun in infancy on the long-term clinical course of patients with type I glycogen storage disease. J Pediatr Gastroenterol Nutr, 1999; 29:136–143

119. Dunger DB, Sutton D. Hypoglycemia complicating treatment regimen for glycogen storage disease. Arch Dis Child, 1995; 72:274

120. Faivre L, Houssin D, Valayer J, Brouard J, Hadchouel M, Bernard O. Long-term outcome of liver transplantation in patients with glycogen storage disease type Ia. J Inherit Metab Dis, 1999; 22:723–732

121. Malatack JJ, Finegold DN, Iwatsuki S et al. Liver transplantation for type I glycogen storage disease. Lancet, 1983; i:1073–1075

122. Sokal EM, Lopez-Silvarrey A, Buts JP, Otte JB. Orthotopic liver transplantation for type I glycogenosis unresponsive to medical therapy. J Pediatr Gastroenterol Nutr, 1993; 16:465–467

123. Lee PJ, Muiesan P, Heaton N. Successful pregnancy after combined renal-hepatic transplantation in glycogen storage disease type Ia. J Inherit Metab Dis, 2004; 27:537–538

124. Panaro F, Andorno E, Basile G et al. Simultaneous liver-kidney transplantation for glycogen storage disease type IA (von Gierke's disease). Transplant Proc, 2004; 36:1483–1484

125. Leese T, Farges O, Bismuth H. Liver cell adenomas. A 12 year surgical experience from a specialist hepatobiliary unit. Ann Surg, 1988; 208:558–564

126. Rosh JR, Collins J, Groisman GM et al. Management of hepatic adenoma in glycogen storage disease 1a. J Pediatr Gastroenterol Nutr, 1995; 20:225–228

127. Visser G, Rake JP, Labrune P et al. Granulocyte colony-stimulating factor in glycogen storage disease type 1b. Results of the European Study on Glycogen Storage Disease Type 1. Eur J Pediatr, 2002; 161 (Suppl 1):S83–S87

128. Lesma E, Riva E, Giovannini M, Di Giulio AM, Gorio A. Amelioration of neutrophil membrane function underlies granulocyte-colony stimulating factor action in glycogen storage disease 1b. Int J Immunopathol Pharmacol, 2005; 18:297–307

129. Kuijpers TW, Maianski NA, Tool AT et al. Apoptotic neutrophils in the circulation of patients with glycogen storage disease type 1b (GSD1b). Blood, 2003; 101:5021–5024

130. Lachaux A, Boillot O, Stamm D et al. Treatment with lenograstim (glycosylated recombinant human granulocyte colony-stimulating factor) and orthotopic liver transplantation for glycogen storage disease type Ib. J Pediatr, 1993; 123:1005–1008

131. Bhattacharya N, Heaton N, Rela M, Walter JH, Lee PJ. The benefits of liver transplantation in glycogenosis type Ib. J Inherit Metab Dis, 2004; 27:539–540

132. Adachi M, Shinkai M, Ohhama Y et al. Improved neutrophil function in a glycogen storage disease type 1b patient after liver transplantation. Eur J Pediatr, 2004; 163:202–206

133. Pompe JC. Over idopatische hypertrophie van het hart. Ned tijdschr Gen eeskd, 1932; 76:304–314

134. Hers HG. alpha-glucosidase deficiency in generalized glycogen-storage disease (Pompe's Disease). Biochem J, 1963; 86:11–16

135. DiMauro S, Bruno C. Glycogen storage diseases of muscle. Curr Opin Neurol, 1998; 11:477–484

136. Hirschhorn R. Glycogen storage disease type II: Acid alpha-glucosidase (acid maltase) deficiency. In: The metabolic and molecular basis of inherited disease. C.R. Scriver et al., Editors. 1997, McGraw-Hill: New York. p. 2443–2464

137. Van den Hout JM, Kamphoven JH, Winkel LP et al. Long-term intravenous treatment of Pompe disease with recombinant human alpha-glucosidase from milk. Pediatrics, 2004; 113:e448–e457

138. de Jager AE, van der Vliet TM, van der Ree TC, Oosterink BJ, Loonen MC. Muscle computed tomography in adult-onset acid maltase deficiency. Muscle Nerve, 1998; 21:398–400

139. McAdams AJ, Hug G, Bove KE. Glycogen storage disease, types I to X: criteria for morphologic diagnosis. Hum Pathol, 1974; 5:463–487

140. Potter EL, Craig JM. Pathology of the fetus and the infant. 3rd edn ed. 1975, Chicago: Year Book Medical

141. Ausems MG, ten Berg K, Kroos MA et al. Glycogen storage disease type II: birth prevalence agrees with predicted genotype frequency. Community Genet, 1999; 2:91–96

142. Kuo WL, Hirschhorn R, Huie ML, Hirschhorn K. Localization and ordering of acid alpha-glucosidase (GAA) and thymidine kinase (TK1) by fluorescence in situ hybridization. Hum Genet, 1996; 97:404–406

143. Huie ML, Shanske AL, Kasper JS, Marion RW, Hirschhorn R. A large Alu-mediated deletion, identified by PCR, as the molecular basis for glycogen storage disease type II (GSDII). Hum Genet, 1999; 104:94–98

144. Hermans MM, van Leenen D, Kroos MA et al. Twenty-two novel mutations in the lysosomal alpha-glucosidase gene (GAA) underscore the genotype-phenotype correlation in glycogen storage disease type II. Hum Mutat, 2004; 23:47–56

145. Kikuchi T, Yang HW, Pennybacker M et al. Clinical and metabolic correction of Pompe disease by enzyme therapy in acid maltase-deficient quail. J Clin Invest, 1998; 101:827–833

146. Bijvoet AG, van de Kamp EH, Kroos MA et al. Generalized glycogen storage and cardiomegaly in a knockout mouse model of Pompe disease. Hum Mol Genet, 1998; 7:53–62

147. Bijvoet AG, van Hirtum H, Vermey M et al. Pathological features of glycogen storage disease type II highlighted in the knockout mouse model. J Pathol, 1999; 189:416–424

148. Winkel LP, Van den Hout JM, Kamphoven JH et al. Enzyme replacement therapy in late-onset Pompe's disease: a three-year follow-up. Ann Neurol, 2004; 55:495–502

149. Chen YT, Burchell A. Glycogen storage disease. In: The metabolic and molecular basis of inherited disease. C.R. Scriver et al., Editors. 1997, McGraw-Hill: New York. p. 935–966

150. Yang-Feng TL, Zheng K, Yu J, Yang BZ, Chen FT, Kao FT. Assignment of the human glycogen debrancher gene to chromosome 1p21. Genomics, 1992; 13:931–934

151. Lam CW, Lee AT, Lam YY et al. DNA-based subtyping of glycogen storage disease type III: mutation and haplotype analysis of the AGL gene in Chinese. Mol Genet Metab, 2004; 83:271–275

152. Lucchiari S, Donati MA, Melis D et al. Mutational analysis of the AGL gene: five novel mutations in GSD III patients. Hum Mutat, 2003; 22:337

153. Smit GP, Fernandes J, Leonard JV et al. The long-term outcome of patients with glycogen storage diseases. J Inherit Metab Dis, 1990; 13:411–418

154. Shen JJ, Chen YT. Molecular characterization of glycogen storage disease type III. Curr Mol Med, 2002; 2:167–175

155. Haagsma EB, Smit GP, Niezen-Koning KE, Gouw AS, Meerman L, Slooff MJ. Type IIIb glycogen storage disease associated with end-stage cirrhosis and hepatocellular carcinoma. Hepatology, 1997; 25:537–540

156. Hashimoto M, Watanabe G, Yokoyama T et al. Case report: rupture of a gastric varix in liver cirrhosis associated with glycogen storage disease type III. J Gastroenterol Hepatol, 1998; 13:232–235

157. Coleman RA, Winter HS, Wolf B, Gilchrist JM, Chen YT. Glycogen storage disease type III (glycogen debranching enzyme deficiency): correlation of biochemical defects with myopathy and cardiomyopathy. Ann Intern Med, 1992; 116:896–900

158. Gremse DA, Bucuvalas JC, Balistreri WF. Efficacy of cornstarch therapy in type III glycogen-storage disease. Am J Clin Nutr, 1990; 52:671–674

159. Ullrich K, Schmidt H, van Teeffelen-Heithoff A. Glycogen storage disease type I and III and pyruvate carboxylase deficiency: results of long-term treatment with uncooked cornstarch. Acta Paediatr Scand, 1988; 77:531–536

160. Yang BZ, Ding JH, Brown BI, Chen YT. Definitive prenatal diagnosis for type III glycogen storage disease. Am J Hum Genet, 1990; 47:735–739

161. Bao Y, Kishnani P, Wu JY, Chen YT. Hepatic and neuromuscular forms of glycogen storage disease type IV caused by mutations in the same glycogen-branching enzyme gene. J Clin Invest, 1996; 97:941–948

162. Moses SW, Parvari R. The variable presentations of glycogen storage disease type IV: a review of clinical, enzymatic and molecular studies. Curr Mol Med, 2002; 2:177–188

163. Bruno C, van Diggelen OP, Cassandrini D et al. Clinical and genetic heterogeneity of branching enzyme deficiency (glycogenosis type IV). Neurology, 2004; 63:1053–1058

164. Alegria A, Martins E, Dias M, Cunha A, Cardoso ML, Maire I. Glycogen storage disease type IV presenting as hydrops fetalis. J Inherit Metab Dis, 1999; 22:330–332

165. Giuffre B, Parinii R, Rizzuti T et al. Severe neonatal onset of glycogenosis type IV: clinical and laboratory findings leading to diagnosis in two siblings. J Inherit Metab Dis, 2004; 27:609–619

166. Janecke AR, Dertinger S, Ketelsen UP et al. Neonatal type IV glycogen storage disease associated with "null" mutations in glycogen branching enzyme 1. J Pediatr, 2004; 145:705–709

167. van Noort G, Straks W, van Diggelan OP, Henne Kam RCM. A congenital variant of glycogenosis type IV. Pediatr Pathol, 1993; 13:685–698

168. McConkie-Rosell A, Wilson C, Piccoli DA et al. Clinical and laboratory findings in four patients with the non-progressive hepatic form of type IV glycogen storage disease. J Inherit Metab Dis, 1996; 19:51–58

169. Greene GM, Weldon DC, Ferrans VJ et al. Juvenile polysaccharidosis with cardioskeletal myopathy. Arch Pathol Lab Med, 1987; 111:977–982

170. Servidei S, Riepe RE, Langston C et al. Severe cardiopathy in branching enzyme deficiency. J Pediatr, 1987; 111:51–56

171. Sindern E, Ziemssen F, Ziemssen T et al. Adult polyglucosan body disease: a postmortem correlation study. Neurology, 2003; 61:263–265

172. Ubogu EE, Hong ST, Akman HO et al. Adult polyglucosan body disease: a case report of a manifesting heterozygote. Muscle Nerve, 2005; 32:675–681

173. Matern D, Starzl TE, Arnaout W et al. Liver transplantation for glycogen storage disease types I, III, and IV. Eur J Pediatr, 1999; 158 (Suppl 2):S43–S48

174. Rosenthal P, Podesta L, Grier R et al. Failure of liver transplantation to diminish cardiac deposits of amylopectin and leukocyte inclusions in type IV glycogen storage disease. Liver Transpl Surg, 1995; 1:373–376

175. Selby R, Starzl TE, Yunis E, Brown BI, Kendall RS, Tzakis A. Liver transplantation for type IV glycogen storage disease. N Engl J Med, 1991; 324:39–42

176. Sokal EM, Van Hoof F, Alberti D, de Ville de Goyet J, de Barsy T, Otte JB. Progressive cardiac failure following orthotopic liver transplantation for type IV glycogenosis. Eur J Pediatr, 1992; 151:200–203

177. Schippers HM, Smit GP, Rake JP, Visser G. Characteristic growth pattern in male X-linked phosphorylase-b kinase deficiency (GSD IX). J Inherit Metab Dis, 2003; 26:43–47

178. Burwinkel B, Bakker HD, Herschkovitz E, Moses SW, Shin YS, Kilimann MW. Mutations in the liver glycogen phosphorylase gene (PYGL) underlying glycogenosis type VI. Am J Hum Genet, 1998; 62:785–791

179. van den Berg IE, van Beurden EA, Malingre HE et al. X-linked liver phosphorylase kinase deficiency is associated with mutations in the human liver phosphorylase kinase alpha subunit. Am J Hum Genet, 1995; 56:381–387

180. Kilimann MW. Molecular genetics of phosphorylase kinase: cDNA cloning, chromosomal mapping and isoform structure. J Inherit Metab Dis, 1990; 13:435–441

181. Willems PJ, Gerver WJ, Berger R, Fernandes J. The natural history of liver glycogenosis due to phosphorylase kinase deficiency: a longitudinal study of 41 patients. Eur J Pediatr, 1990; 149:268–271

182. Burwinkel B, Shiomi S, Al Zaben A, Kilimann MW. Liver glycogenosis due to phosphorylase kinase deficiency: PHKG2 gene structure and mutations associated with cirrhosis. Hum Mol Genet, 1998; 7:149–154

183. Kagalwalla AF, Kagalwalla YA, al Ajaji S, Gorka W, Ali MA. Phosphorylase b kinase deficiency glycogenosis with cirrhosis of the liver. J Pediatr, 1995; 127:602–605

184. van Beurden EA, de Graaf M, Wendel U, Gitzelmann R, Berger R, van den Berg IE. Autosomal recessive liver phosphorylase kinase deficiency caused by a novel splice-site mutation in the gene encoding the liver gamma subunit (PHKG2). Biochem Biophys Res Commun, 1997; 236:544–548

185. Burwinkel B, Amat L, Gray RG et al. Variability of biochemical and clinical phenotype in X-linked liver glycogenosis with mutations in the phosphorylase kinase PHKA2 gene. Hum Genet, 1998; 102:423–429

186. Clark D, Haynes D. The glycogen storage disease (gsd/gsd) rat. Curr Top Cell Regul, 1988; 29:217–263

187. Santer R, Schneppenheim R, Suter D, Schaub J, Steinmann B. Fanconi–Bickel syndrome—the original patient and his natural history, historical steps leading to the primary defect, and a review of the literature. Eur J Pediatr, 1998; 157:783–797

188. Brown GK. Glucose transporters: structure, function and consequences of deficiency. J Inherit Metab Dis, 2000; 23:237–246

189. Santer R, Steinmann B, Schaub J. Fanconi–Bickel syndrome—a congenital defect of facilitative glucose transport. Curr Mol Med, 2002; 2:213–227

190. Muller D, Santer R, Krawinkel M, Christiansen B, Schaub J. Fanconi–Bickel syndrome presenting in neonatal screening for galactosaemia. J Inherit Metab Dis, 1997; 20:607–608

191. Gitzelmann R, Spycher MA, Feil G et al. Liver glycogen synthase deficiency: a rarely diagnosed entity. Eur J Pediatr, 1996; 155:561–567

192. Orho M, Bosshard NU, Buist NR et al. Mutations in the liver glycogen synthase gene in children with hypoglycemia due to glycogen storage disease type 0. J Clin Invest, 1998; 102:507–515

193. Laberge AM, Mitchell GA, van de Werve G, Lambert M. Long-term follow-up of a new case of liver glycogen synthase deficiency. Am J Med Genet A, 2003; 120:19–22

194. Jaffe R. Liver transplant pathology in pediatric metabolic disorders. Pediatr Develop Pathol, 1998; 1:102–117

195. Kuzuya T, Matsuda A, Yoshida S et al. An adult case of type Ib glycogen-storage disease. Enzymatic and histochemical studies. N Engl J Med, 1983; 308:566–569

196. Itoh S, Ishida Y, Matsuo S. Mallory bodies in a patient with type Ia glycogen storage disease. Gastroenterology, 1987; 92:520–523

197. Eising EG, Auffermann W, Peters PE, Schmidt H, Ullrich K. Fokale peliosis der Leber im Erwachsenenalter in Kombination mit Glycogenose Typ I (V. Gierke) Radiologe, 1990; 30:428–432

198. Bannayan GA, Dean WJ, Howell RR. Type IV glycogen-storage disease. Light-microscopic, 1976; 66:702–709

199. Ishihara T, Yokota T, Yamashita Y et al. Comparative study of the intracytoplasmic inclusions in Lafora disease and type IV glycogenesis by electron microscopy. Acta Pathol Jpn, 1987; 37:1591–1601

200. Reed GB, Dixon JEP, Neustein HB, Donnell GN, Landing BH. Type IV glycogenosis. Lab Invest, 1968; 19:546–557

201. Ishak KG, Sharp HL. Metabolic errors and liver disease. In: Pathology of the liver. R.N.M. MacSween, P.J. Anthony, and P.J. Scheuer, Editors. 1987, Churchill Livingstone: Edinburgh. p. 99–180

202. Poe R, Snover DC. Adenomas in glycogen storage disease Type 1. Two cases with unusual histologic features. Am J Surg Pathol, 1998; 12:477–483

203. Riede UN, Spycher MA, Gitzelmann R. Glycogenosis type I (glucose G-phosphatase deficiency. I. Ultrastructural morphometric analysis of juvenile liver cells. Pathol Res Pract, 1980; 167:136–150

204. Buchino, II, Brown BI, Volk DM. Glycogen storage disease type IB. Arch Pathol Lab Med, 1983; 107:283–285

205. Bandhuin P, Hers HG, Loeb H. An electron microscopic and biochemical study of type II glycogenosis. Lab Invest, 1964; 13:1139–1152

206. Chan EM, Young EJ, Ianzano L et al. Mutations in NHLRC1 cause progressive myoclonus epilepsy. Nat Genet, 2003; 35:125–127

207. Ianzano L, Zhao XC, Minassian BA, Scherer SW. Identification of a novel protein interacting with laforin, the EPM2a progressive myoclonus epilepsy gene product. Genomics, 2003; 81:579–587

208. Ianzano L, Zhang J, Chan EM et al. Lafora progressive Myoclonus Epilepsy mutation database-EPM2A and NHLRC1 (EMP2B) genes. Hum Mutat, 2005; 26:397

209. Lohi H, Ianzano L, Zhao XC et al. Novel glycogen synthase kinase 3 and ubiquitination pathways in progressive myoclonus epilepsy. Hum Mol Genet, 2005; 14:2727–2736

210. Baykan B, Striano P, Gianotti S et al. Late-onset and slow-progressing Lafora disease in four siblings with EPM2B mutation. Epilepsia, 2005; 46:1695–1697

211. Gambetti P, DiMauro S, Hirt L, Blume RP. Myoclonic epilepsy with Lafora bodies. Some ultrastructural, 1971; 25:483–493

212. Janeway R, Ravens JR, Pearce LA, Odar DL, Suzuki K. Progressive myoclonus epilepsy with Lafora inclusion bodies. Arch Neurol, 1967; 16:565–582

213. Ota T, Hisatomi Y, Kashiwamura K et al. Histochemistry and substructure of atypical myoclonus body (type II). Acta Neuropathol, 1974; 28:45–54

214. Schwarz GA, Yanoff M. Lafora's disease. Distinct clinicopathologic forms of Univerricht's syndrome. Arch Neurol, 1965; 12:172–188

215. Yokoi S, Austin J, Witmer F et al. Studies on myoclonus epilepsy (Lafora body form). Arch Neurol, 1968; 19:15–33

216. Van Hoof F, Hageman-Bal M. Progressive familial myoclonic epilepsy with Lafora bodies. Electronmicroscopic and histochemical study of a cerebral biopsy. Acta Neuropathol, 1967; 7:315–326

217. Jenis EH, Schochet SS, Earle KM. Myoclonus epilepsy with Lafora bodies. Case report with electron microscopic observations. Milit Med, 1970; 135:116–119

218. Collins GH, Cowden RR, and Nevis AH. Myoclonus epilepsy with Lafora bodies. Arch Pathol, 1968; 86:239–254

219. Edgar GWF. Progressive myoclonus epilepsy as an inborn error of metabolism comparable to storage disease. Epilepsia, 1963; 4:120–137

220. Harriman DGF, Miller JHD. Progressive familial myoclonic epilepsy in three families. Its clinical features and pathological basis. Brain, 1955; 78:325–349

221. Nishimura RN, Ishak KG, Reddick R, Porter R, James S, Barranger JA. Lafora disease: Diagnosis by liver biopsy. Ann Neurol, 1979; 8:409–415

222. Seitelberger F. Myoclonus body disease. In: Pathology of the nervous system. J. Minckler, Editor. 1968, McGraw-Hill: New York. p. 1121–1134

223. Yokota T, Ishihara T, Kawano H et al. Immunological homogeneity of Lafora body, corpora amylacea, basophilic degeneration in heart, and intracytoplasmic inclusions of liver and heart in type IV glycogenosis. Acta Pathol Jpn, 1987; 37:941–946

224. Ng IOL, Sturgess RP, Williams R, Portmann B. Ground-glass hepatocytes with Lafora body like inclusions—histochemical, immunohistochemical and electron microscopic characterization. Histopathology, 1990; 17:109–115

225. De Bruyne R, Portmann B, Samyn M et al. Chronic liver disease related to 6-thioguanine in children with acute lymphoblastic leukaemia. J Hepatol, 2006; 44:407–410

226. Von Ruess A. Zuckerausscheidung im Säuglingsalter. Wien Med Wochenschr, 1908; 18:799–804

227. Isselbacher KJ, Anderson EP, Koski K et al. Congenital galactosemia, a single enzyme block in galactose metabolism. Science, 1956; 123:635–636

228. Reichardt JK. Genetic basis of galactosemia. Hum Mutat, 1992; 1:190–196

229. Elsas LJ, Dembure PP, Langley S, Paul KEM, Hjelm LN, Fridovich-Keil J. A common mutation associated with the Duarte galactosemia allele. Am J Hum Genet, 1994; 54:1030–1036

230. Elsevier JP, Wells L, Quimby BB et al. Heterodimer formation and activity in the human enzyme galactose-1-phosphate uridylyltransferase. Proc Natl Acad Sci USA, 1996; 93:7166–7171

231. Alano A, Almashanu S, Chinsky JM et al. Molecular characterization of a unique patient with epimerase-deficient galactosemia. J Inherit Metab Dis, 1998; 21:341–350

232. Henderson MJ, Holton JB, MacFaul R. Further observations in a case of uridine diphosphate galactose-4-epimerase deficiency with a severe clinical presentation. J Inherit Metab Dis, 1983; 6:17–20

233. Walter JH, Roberts RE, Besley GT et al. Generalised uridine diphosphate galactose-4-epimerase deficiency. Arch Dis Child, 1999; 80:374–376

234. Nadler HL, Inouye T, Hsia DYY. Clinical galactosemia. In: Galactosemia. D.Y.Y. Hsia, Editor. 1969, Charles C Thomas: Springfield IL. p. 127–132

235. Levy HL, Sepe SJ, Shih VE, Vawter GF, Klein JO. Sepsis due to Escherichia coli in neonates with galactosemia. N Engl J Med, 1977; 297:823–825

236. Belman AL, Moshe SL, Zimmerman RD. Computed tomographic demonstration of cerebral edema in a child with galactosemia. Pediatrics, 1986; 78:606–609

237. Donnell GN, Bergen WR. Galactosemia. In: Birth defects. Atlas and compendium. D. Bergsma, Editor. 1973, Williams & Wilkins: Baltimore. p. 422

238. Komrower GM, Lee DH. Long-term follow-up of galactosaemia. Arch Dis Child, 1970; 45:367–373

239. Ridel KR, Leslie ND, Gilbert DL. An updated review of the long-term neurological effects of galactosemia. Pediatr Neurol, 2005; 33:153–161

240. Schweitzer S, Shin Y, Jacobs C, Brodehl J. Long-term outcome in 134 patients with galactosemia. Eur J Pediatr, 1993; 152:36–43

241. Waggoner DD, Buist NRM, Donnell GN. Long-term prognosis in galactosemia from infancy to childhood. J Inher Metab Dis, 1990; 13:802–808

242. Xu YK, Ng WG, Kaufman FR, Lobo RA, Donnell GN. Galactose metabolism in human ovarian tissue. Pediatr Res, 1989; 25:151–155

243. Segal S. Galactosaemia today: the enigma and the challenge. J Inherit Metab Dis, 1998; 21:455–471

244. Service UPH. Newborn screening. Am Fam Physician, 1994; 50:354–355

245. Rolland MO, Manden G, Farriaiax JP, Porche C. Galactose-1-phosphate uridyl transferase activity in chorionic villi. A first trimester prenatal diagnosis of galactosemia. J Inherit Metabol Dis, 1986; 9:284

246. Applebaum MD, Thaler MM. Reversibility of extensive liver damage in galactosemia. Gastroenterology, 1975; 69:496–502

247. Gross KC, Acosta PB. Fruits and vegetables are a source of galactose: Implications in planning the diets of patients with galactosemia. J Inherit Metab Dis, 1991; 14:253–255

248. Berry GT, Nissim I, Lin Z, Mazure AT, Gibson JB, Segal S. Endogenous synthesis of galactose in normal men and patients with hereditary galactosemia. Lancet, 1995; 346:1073–1074

249. Buyssens N. Cholestasis and regeneration of the liver in congenital galactosemia. Tijdschr Gastroenterol, 1964; 76:125–132

250. Smetana HF, Olen E. Hereditary galactose disease. Am J Clin Pathol, 1962; 38:3–25

251. Gitzelman R. Galactosaemia and other inherited disorders of galactose metabolism. In: Liver in metabolic diseases. L. Bianchi et al., Editors. 1983, MTP Press: Lancaster. p. 235–238

252. Edmonds AM, Hennigar CR, Crooks R. Galactosemia. Pediatrics, 1952; 10:40–47

253. Hers HG, Joassin G. Anomalie de l-aldolase h,patique dans l-intol,rance au fructose. Enzymol Biol Clin, 1961; 1:4–14

254. Baerlocher K, Gitzelmann R, Steinmann B, Gitzelmann-Cumarasamy N. Hereditary fructose intolerance in early childhood: a major diagnostic challenge. Survey of 20 symptomatic cases. Helv Paediatr Acta, 1978; 33:465–487

255. Odièvre M, Gentil C, Gautier M, Alagille D. Hereditary fructose intolerance in childhood. Diagnosis, 1978; 132:605–608

256. Tolan DR, Penhoet EE. Characterization of the human aldolase B gene. Mol Biol Med, 1986; 3:245–264

257. Ali M, Rellos P, Cox TM. Hereditary fructose intolerance. J Med Genet, 1998; 35:353–365

258. Esposito G, Santamaria R, Vitagliano L et al. Six novel alleles identified in Italian hereditary fructose intolerance patients enlarge the mutation spectrum of the aldolase B gene. Hum Mutat, 2004; 24:534

259. Santer R, Rischewski J, von Weihe M et al. The spectrum of aldolase B (ALDOB) mutations and the prevalence of hereditary fructose intolerance in Central Europe. Hum Mutat, 2005; 25:594

260. Gitzelmann R, Steinmann B, Tuchschmid P. Patients with hereditary fructose intolerance have normal erythrocyte aldolase activity. Clin Chim Acta, 1989; 181:163–166

261. Black JA, Simpson K. Fructose intolerance. Br Med J, 1967; 2:138–141

262. Levin B, Snodgrass GJ, Oberholzer VG, Brugess EA, Dobbs RH. Fructosemia. Am J Med, 1968; 45:826–838

263. Phillips MJ, Little JA, Ptak TW. Subcellular pathology of hereditary fructose intolerance. Am J Med, 1968; 44:910–921

264. Jeune M, Planson E, Cotte J, Bonnefoy S, Nivelon JL, Skosowskv J. L'intolérance héréditaire au fructose. A propos d-un cas. Pediatrie, 1961; 16:605–613

265. Lelong M, Alagille D, Gentil J et al. L'intolérance héréditaire au fructose. Arch Franc Pediatr, 1962; 19:841–866

266. Perheentupa J, Pitkanen E, Nikkila EA, Somersalo O, Hakosalo J. Hereditary fructose intolerance: a clinical study of four cases. Ann Pediatr Fenn, 1962; 8:221–235

267. Cain ARR, Ryman BE. High liver glycogen in hereditary fructose intolerance. Gut, 1971; 12:929–932

268. Royer P, Lestradet H, Habib R, Lardinosis R, Debuquois B. L'intolérance héréditaire au fructose. Bull Mem Soc Med Hop Paris, 1964; 115:805–823

269. Hardwick DF, Dimmick JE. Metabolic cirrhosis of infancy and early childhood. Persp Pediatr Pathol, 1976; 3:103–144

270. See G, Marchal G, Odievre M. Hépatocarcinome chez un adulte suspect d'une intolérance héréditaire au fructose. Ann Pediatr (Paris), 1984; 31:49–51

271. Phillips MJ, Hetenyi G, Adachi F. Ultrastructural hepatocellular alterations induced by in vivo fructose infusion. Lab Invest, 1970; 22:370–379

272. Fuller M, Rozaklis T, Ramsay SL et al. Disease-specific markers for the mucopolysaccharidoses. Pediatr Res, 2004; 56:733–738

273. Dulaney JT, Milunsky A, Moser HW. Detection of the carrier state of Hurler's syndrome by assay of alpha-L-iduronidase in leukocytes. Clin Chim Acta, 1976; 69:305–310

274. Scott HS, Ashton LJ, Eyre HJ et al. Chromosomal localization of the human alpha-L-iduronidase gene (IDUA) to 4p16.3. Am J Hum Genet, 1990; 47:802–807

275. Bunge S, Kleijer WJ, Steglich C et al. Mucopolysaccharidosis type I: identification of 8 novel mutations and determination of the frequency of the two common alpha-L-iduronidase mutations (W402X and Q70X) among European patients. Hum Mol Genet, 1994; 3:861–866

276. Terlato NJ, Cox GF. Can mucopolysaccharidosis type I disease severity be predicted based on a patient's genotype? A comprehensive review of the literature. Genet Med, 2003; 5:286–294

277. McKusick VA, Howell RR, Hussels IE, Neufeld EF, Stevenson RE. Allelism, non-allelism, and genetic compounds among the mucopolysaccharidoses. Lancet, 1972; i:993–996

278. Conway J, Dyack S, Crooks BN, Fernandez CV. Mixed donor chimerism and low level iduronidase expression may be adequate for neurodevelopmental protection in Hurler Syndrome. J Pediatr, 2005; 147:106–108

279. Guffon N, Souillet G, Maire I, Straczek J, Guibaud P. Follow-up of nine patients with Hurler syndrome after bone marrow transplantation. J Pediatr, 1998; 133:119–125

280. Hendriksz CJ, Moss GM, Wraith JE. Pregnancy in a patient with mucopolysaccharidosis type IH homozygous for the W402X mutation. J Inherit Metab Dis, 2004; 27:685–686

281. Hobbs JR, Hugh-Jones K, Barratt A et al. Reversal of clinical features of Hurler's disease and biochemical improvement after treatment by bone marrow transplantation. Lancet, 1981; ii:709

282. Peters C, Balthazor M, Shapiro EG et al. Outcome of unrelated donor bone marrow transplantation in 40 children with Hurler syndrome. Blood, 1996; 87:4894–4902

283. Vellodi A, Young E, Cooper A, Lidchi V, Winchester B, Wraith JE. Long-term follow-up following bone marrow transplantation for Hunter disease. J Inherit Metab Dis, 1999; 22:638–648

284. Staba SL, Escolar ML, Poe M et al. Cord-blood transplants from unrelated donors in patients with Hurler's syndrome. N Engl J Med, 2004; 350:1960–1969

285. Souillet G, Guffon N, Maire I et al. Outcome of 27 patients with Hurler's syndrome transplanted from either related or unrelated haematopoietic stem cell sources. Bone Marrow Transplant, 2003; 31:1105–1117

286. Grigull L, Beilken A, Schrappe M et al. Transplantation of allogeneic CD34-selected stem cells after fludarabine-based conditioning regimen for children with mucopolysaccharidosis 1H (M. Hurler). Bone Marrow Transplant, 2005; 35:265–269

287. Miebach E. Enzyme replacement therapy in mucopolysaccharidosis type I. Acta Paediatr Suppl, 2005; 94:58–60; discussion 57

288. Wraith JE, Clarke LA, Beck M et al. Enzyme replacement therapy for mucopolysaccharidosis I: a randomized, double-blinded, placebo-controlled, multinational study of recombinant human alpha-L-iduronidase (laronidase). J Pediatr, 2004; 144:581–588

289. McKinnis EJ, Sulzbacher S, Rutledge JC, Sanders J, Scott CR. Bone marrow transplantation in Hunter syndrome. J Pediatr, 1996; 129:145–148

290. Neufeld E, Muenzer J. The mucopolysaccharidoses. In: The metabolic and molecular basis of inherited disease. C.R. Scriver et al., Editors. 1995, McGraw-Hill: New York. p. 2465–2494

291. Scott HS, Blanch L, Guo XH et al. Cloning of the sulphamidase gene and identification of mutations in Sanfilippo A syndrome. Nature Genet, 1995; 11:465–467

292. Ausseil J, Loredo-Osti JC, Verner A et al. Localisation of a gene for mucopolysaccharidosis IIIC to the pericentromeric region of chromosome 8. J Med Genet, 2004; 41:941–945

293. Hopwood JJ. Prenatal diagnosis of Sanfilippo syndrome. Prenat Diagn, 2005; 25:148–150

294. Kleijer WJ, Karpova EA, Geilen GC et al. Prenatal diagnosis of Sanfilippo A syndrome: experience in 35 pregnancies at risk and the use of a new fluorogenic substrate for the heparin sulphamidase assay. Prenatal Diag, 1996; 16:829–835

295. Beck M, Glossl J, Grubisic A, Spranger J. Heterogeneity of Morquio disease. Clin Genet, 1986; 29:325–331

296. Litjens T, Hopwood JJ. Mucopolysaccharidosis type VI: Structural and clinical implications of mutations in N-acetylgalactosamine-4-sulfatase. Hum Mutat, 2001; 18:282–295

297. Hein LK, Meikle PJ, Dean CJ et al. Development of an assay for the detection of mucopolysaccharidosis type VI patients using dried blood-spots. Clin Chim Acta, 2005; 353:67–74

298. Herskhovitz E, Young E, Rainer J et al. Bone marrow transplantation for Maroteaux-Lamy syndrome (MPS VI): long-term follow-up. J Inherit Metab Dis, 1999; 22:50–62

299. Harmatz P, Kramer WG, Hopwood JJ, Simon J, Butensky E, Swiedler SJ. Pharmacokinetic profile of recombinant human N-acetylgalactosamine 4-sulphatase enzyme replacement therapy in patients with mucopolysaccharidosis VI (Maroteaux-Lamy syndrome): a phase I/II study. Acta Paediatr Suppl, 2005; 94:61–68; discussion 57

300. Harmatz P, Whitley CB, Waber L et al. Enzyme replacement therapy in mucopolysaccharidosis VI (Maroteaux-Lamy syndrome). J Pediatr, 2004; 144:574–580

301. Saxonhouse MA, Behnke M, Williams JL, Richards D, Weiss MD. Mucopolysaccharidosis Type VII presenting with isolated neonatal ascites. J Perinatol, 2003; 23:73–75

302. Natowicz MR, Isman F, Prence EM, Cedrone P, Allen JJ. Rapid prenatal testing for human beta-glucuronidase deficiency (MPS VII). Genet Test, 2003; 7:241–243

303. Yamada Y, Kato K, Sukegawa K et al. Treatment of MPS VII (Sly disease) by allogeneic BMT in a female with homozygous A619V mutation. Bone Marrow Transplant, 1998; 21:629–634

304. Van Hoof F. Mucopolysaccharidoses. In: Lysosomes and storage disease. H.A. Hers and F. Van Hoof, Editors. 1973, Academic Press: New York. p. 217–259

305. Lindsay S, Reilly WA, Gotham TJ, Skahen R. Gargoylism. II. Study of pathologic lesions and clinical review of twelve cases. Am J Dis Child, 1948; 76:239–306

306. Wolfe HJ, Blennerhauser JB, Young GF, Cohen RB. Hurler's syndrome. A histochemical study. New techniques for localization of very water soluble acid mucopolysaccharides. Am J Pathol, 1964; 45:1007–1027

307. Parfrey NA, Hutchins GM. Hepatic fibrosis in the mucopolysaccharidoses. Am J Med, 1986; 81:825–829

308. Schwarz H, Cagne R. A case of gargoylism. Can Med Assoc J, 1952; 66:375–377.

309. Henderson JL, MacGregor AP, Thanhauser SJ, Holden R. The pathology and biochemistry of gargoylism. A report of three cases with a review of the literature. Arch Dis Child, 1952; 27:230–253

310. Strauss R, Merlin R, Reiser R. Gargoylism. Review of the literature and report of the sixth autopsied case with chemical studies. Am J Clin Pathol, 1947; 17:671–691

311. Callahan WP, Lorincz AE. Hepatic ultrastructure in the Hurler syndrome. Am J Pathol, 1966; 48:277–298

312. Loeb H, Jonniaux G, Resibois A et al. Biochemical and ultrastructural studies in Hurler's syndrome. J Pediatr, 1968; 72:860–874

313. Haust MD. Mitochondrial budding and morphogenesis of cytoplasmic vacuoles in hepatocytes of children with Hurler's syndrome and Sanfilippo disease. Exper Mol Biol, 1968; 9:242–257

314. Haust MD. Crystalloid structure of hepatic mitochondria in children with heparitin sulfate mucopolysaccharidosis (Sanfilippo type). Exp Mol Biol, 1968; 8:123–134

315. Van Hoof F. Mucopolysaccharidoses and mucolipidoses. J Clin Pathol, 1974; 27(Suppl 8):64–93

316. Dekaban AS, Constantopoulos G, Herman MM, Stensing JK. Mucopolysaccharidosis type V (Scheie syndrome). Arch Pathol Lab Med, 1976; 100:237–245

317. McEntee MF, Wright KN, Wanless I, De Novo R, Schneider JF, Shull R. Noncirrhotic portal hypertension and nodular regenerative hyperplasia of the liver in dogs with mucopolysaccharidosis type 1. Hepatology, 1998; 28:385–390

318. Guan C, Cui T, Rao V et al. Activation of glycosylasparaginase. Formation of active N-terminal threonine by intramolecular autoproteolysis. J Biol Chem, 1996; 271:1732–1737

319. Ikonen E, Julkunen I, Tollersrud OK, Kalkkinen N, Peltonen L. Lysosomal aspartylglucosaminidase is processed to the active subunit complex in the endoplasmic reticulum. Embo J, 1993; 12:295–302

320. Morris C, Heisterkamp N, Groffen J, Williams JC, Mononen I. Chromosomal localization of the human glycoasparaginase gene to 4q32–q33. Hum Genet, 1992; 88:295–297

321. Saarela J, von Schantz C, Peltonen L, Jalanko A. A novel aspartylglucosaminuria mutation affects translocation of aspartylglucosaminidase. Hum Mutat, 2004; 24:350–351

322. Jenner FA, Pollitt RJ. Large quantities of 2-acetamido-1-(B-L-aspartamido)-1,2-dideoxyglucose in the urine of mentally retarded siblings. Biochem J, 1967; 103:48–49

323. Isenberg JN, Sharp HL. Aspartylglucosaminuria: psychomotor retardation masquerading as a mucopolysaccharidosis. J Pediatr, 1975; 86:713–717

324. Arvio P, Arvio M, Wolf J, Lukinmaa PL, Saxen L, Pirinen S. Impaired oral health in patients with aspartylglucosaminuria. Oral Surg Oral Med Oral Pathol Oral Radiol Endod, 1998; 86:562–568

325. Arvio P, Arvio M. Progressive nature of aspartylglucosaminuria. Acta Paediatr, 2002; 91:255–257

326. Autti T, Raininko R, Haltia M et al. Aspartylglucosaminuria: radiologic course of the disease with histopathologic correlation. J Child Neurol, 1997; 12:369–375

327. Thomas GH, Beaudet AL. Disorders of glycoprotein degradation and structure: α-mannosidosis, β-mannosidoses, fucosidosis, sialidosis, aspartylglucosaminuria and CDGS. In: The metabolic and molecular basis of inherited disease. C.R. Scriver, A.L. Beaudet, W.S. Sly et al., Editors. 1995, McGraw-Hill: New York. p. 2529–2561

328. Syvanen AC, Ikonen E, Manninen T et al. Convenient and quantitative determination of the frequency of a mutant allele using solid-phase minisequencing: application to aspartylglucosaminuria in Finland. Genomics, 1992; 12:590–595

329. Malm G, Mansson JE, Winiarski J, Mosskin M, Ringden O. Five-year follow-up of two siblings with aspartylglucosaminuria undergoing allogeneic stem-cell transplantation from unrelated donors. Transplantation, 2004; 78:415–419

330. Isenberg JN, Sharp HL. Aspartylglucosaminuria. Biochemical and ultrastructural characteristics unique to this visceral storage disease. Hum Pathol, 1976; 7:469–481

331. Palo J, Rickkinen P, Arstila A, Autio S. Biochemical and fine structural studies on brain and liver biopsies in aspartylglucosaminuria. Neurology, 1971; 21:1198–1204

332. Petushkova NA. First-trimester diagnosis of an unusual case of alpha-mannosidosis. Prenat Diagn, 1991; 11:279–283

333. Beccari T, Bibi L, Ricci R et al. Two novel mutations in the gene for human alpha-mannosidase that cause alpha-mannosidosis. J Inherit Metab Dis, 2003; 26:819–820

334. Desnick RJ, Sharp HL, Grabowski GA et al. Mannosidosis: clinical, morphologic, immunologic, and biochemical studies. Pediatr Res, 1976; 10:985–996

335. Urushihara M, Kagami S, Yasutomo K et al. Sisters with alpha-mannosidosis and systemic lupus erythematosus. Eur J Pediatr, 2004; 163:192–195

336. Montgomery TR, Thomas GH, Valle DL. Mannosidosis in an adult. Johns Hopkins Med J, 1982; 151:113–121

337. Albert MH, Schuster F, Peters C et al. T-cell-depleted peripheral blood stem cell transplantation for alpha-mannosidosis. Bone Marrow Transplant, 2003; 32:443–446

338. Grewal SS, Shapiro EG, Krivit W et al. Effective treatment of alpha-mannosidosis by allogeneic hematopoietic stem cell transplantation. J Pediatr, 2004; 144:569–573

339. Gordon BA, Carson R, Haust MD. Unusual clinical and ultrastructural features in a boy with biochemically typical mannosidosis. Acta Paediatr Scand, 1980; 69:787–792

340. Peratis NG, Turner BM, Labadie G, Hirschhorn K. Alpha-L-fucosidase in cultured skin fibroblasts from normal subjects and fucosidosis patients. Pediatr Res, 1977; 11:862–866.

341. Beaudet AL, Thomas GH. Disorders of glycoprotein degradation and structure: α-mannosidosis, β-mannosidosis, fucosidosis, sialidosis, aspartylglucosaminuria, and carbohydrate-deficient glycoprotein syndrome. In: The metabolic and molecular basis of inherited disease. C.R. Scriver, A.L. Beaudet, W.S. Sly, J. Valle et al., Editors. 1989, McGraw-Hill: New York. p. 603–621

342. Kornfeld M, Snyder RD, Wenger DA. Fucosidosis with angiokeratoma. Electron microscopic changes in the skin. Arch Pathol Lab Med, 1977; 101:478–485

343. Koussef BG, Beratis NG, Strauss L et al. Fucosidosis type II. Pediatrics, 1976; 57:205–213

344. Kanitakis J, Allombert C, Doebelin B et al. Fucosidosis with angiokeratoma. Immunohistochemical & electronmicroscopic study of a new case and literature review. J Cutan Pathol, 2005; 32:506–511

345. Miano M, Lanino E, Gatti R et al. Four year follow-up of a case of fucosidosis treated with unrelated donor bone marrow transplantation. Bone Marrow Transplant, 2001; 27:747–751

346. Freitag F, Kuchemann K, Flumcke S. Hepatic ultrastructure in fucosidosis. Virchows Arch, 1971; 7:99–113

347. Kornfeld S, Sly WS. I-cell disease and pseudo-Hurler polydystrophy: Disorders of lysosomal enzyme phosphorylation and localization. In: The metabolic and molecular basis of inherited disease. C.R. Scriver, A.L. Beaudet, W.S. Sly, J. Valle et al., Editors. 1995, McGraw-Hill: New York. p. 2495–2508

348. Lowden JA, O'Brien JS. Sialidosis: a review of human neuraminidase deficiency. Am J Hum Genet, 1979; 31:1–18

349. Spranger J, Mucolipidosis I. In: Disorders of connective tissue. D. Bergsma, Editor. 1975, Stratton Intercontinental: New York. p. 279–282

350. Seyrantepe V, Poupetova H, Froissart R, Zabot MT, Maire I, Pshezhetsky AV. Molecular pathology of NEU1 gene in sialidosis. Hum Mutat, 2003; 22:343–352

351. Gravel RA, Lowden JA, Callahan JW, Wolfe LS, Ng Yin Kin NMK. Infantile sialidosis: a phenocopy of type 1 GM1 gangliosidosis distinguished by genetic complementation and urinary oligosaccharides. Am J Hum Genet, 1979; 31:669–679

352. Rothschild CB, Akots G, Hayworth R et al. A genetic map of chromosome 20q12–q13.1: multiple highly polymorphic microsatellite and RFLP markers linked to the maturity-onset diabetes of the young (MODY) locus. Am J Hum Genet, 1993; 52:110–123

353. Sasagasako N, Miyahara S, Saito N, Shinnoh N, Kobayashi T, Goto I. Prenatal diagnosis of congenital sialidosis. Clin Genet, 1993; 44:8–11

354. Wang D, Bonten EJ, Yogalingam G, Mann L, d'Azzo A. Short-term, high dose enzyme replacement therapy in sialidosis mice. Mol Genet Metab, 2005; 85:181–189

355. Riches WG, Smuckler EA. A severe infantile mucolipidosis: clinical, biochemical and pathologic features. Arch Pathol Lab Med, 1983; 107:147–152

356. Nolan CM, Sly WS. I-cell disease and pseudo-Hurler polydystrophy: disorders of lysosomal enzyme phosphorylation and localizatio. In: The metabolic and molecular basis of inherited disease. C.R. Scriver, A.L. Beaudet, W.S. Sly, J. Valle et al., Editors. 1989, McGraw-Hill: New York. p. 1589–1601

357. Tiede S, Muschol N, Reutter G, Cantz M, Ullrich K, Braulke T. Missense mutations in N-acetylglucosamine-1-phosphotransferase alpha/beta subunit gene in a patient with mucolipidosis III and a mild clinical phenotype. Am J Med Genet A, 2005; 137:235–240

358. Tiede S, Storch S, Lubke T et al. Mucolipidosis II is caused by mutations in GNPTA encoding the alpha/beta GlcNAc-1-phosphotransferase. Nat Med, 2005; 11:1109–1112

359. Mueller OT, Wasmuth JJ, Murray JC, Lozzio CB, Lovrien EW, Shows TB. Chromosomal assignment of N-acetylglucosaminylphospho-transferase, the lysosomal hydrolase targeting enzyme deficient in mucolipidosis II and III. (abstract) Cytogenet Cell Genet, 1987; 46:664

360. Amato RSS. Mucolipidosis II. In: Birth defects encyclopedia. M.L. Buyse, Editor. 1989, Center for Birth Defects Information Services: Dover MA. p. 1157–1158

361. Leroy JG, Martin JJ. Mucolipidosis II. In: Disorders of connective tissue. D. Bergsma, Editor. 1975, Stratton International: New York. p. 283–293

362. Patriquin HB, Kaplan P, Kind HP, Giedion A. Neonatal mucolipidosis II (I-cell disease): clinical and radiologic features in three cases. Am J Roentgenol, 1977; 129:37–43

363. Saul RA, Proud V, Taylor HA, Leroy JG, Spranger J. Prenatal mucolipidosis type II (I-cell disease) can present as Pacman dysplasia. Am J Med Genet A, 2005; 135:328–332

364. Kitagawa H, Toki J, Morimoto T et al. An autopsy case of I-cell disease. Ultrastructural and biochemical analyses. Am J Clin Pathol, 1991; 96:262–266

365. Grewal S, Shapiro E, Braunlin E et al. Continued neurocognitive development and prevention of cardiopulmonary complications after successful BMT for I-cell disease: a long-term follow-up report. Bone Marrow Transplant, 2003; 32:957–960

366. Kenyon KR, Sensenbrenner JA, Wyllie RG. Hepatic ultrastructure and histochemistry in mucolipidosis II (I-cell disease). Pediatr Res, 1973; 7:560–568

367. Tondeur M, Vamos-Hurwitz E, Mockel-Pohl S et al. Clinical, biochemical and ultrastructural studies in a case of chondrodystrophy presenting the I-cell phenotype in tissue culture. J Pediatr, 1971; 79:366–378

368. Folkerth RD, Alroy J, Lomakina I, Skutelsky E, Raghavan SS, Kolodny EH. Mucolipidosis IV: morphology and histochemistry of an autopsy case. J Neuropathol Exp Neurol, 1995; 54:154–164

369. Goldin E, Stahl S, Cooney AM et al. Transfer of a mitochondrial DNA fragment to MCOLN1 causes an inherited case of mucolipidosis IV. Hum Mutat, 2004; 24:460–465

370. Slaugenhaupt SA, Acierno JS, Helbling LA et al. Mapping of the mucolipidosis type IV gene to chromosome 19p and definition of founder haplotypes. Am J Hum Genet, 1999; 65:773–778

371. Amir N, Zlotogora J, Bach G. Mucolipidosis type IV: Clinical spectrum and natural history. Pediatrics, 1987; 79:953–959

372. Merin S, Livni N, Berman ER et al. Mucolipidosis IV: ocular, systemic, and ultrastructural findings. Invest Ophthalmol, 1975; 14:437–448

373. Caimi L, Tettamanti G, Berra B et al. Mucolipidosis IV, a sialolipidosis due to ganglioside sialidase deficiency. J Inherit Metab Dis, 1982; 5:218–224

374. Kohn G, Livni N, Onoy A et al. Prenatal diagnosis of mucolipidosis IV by electron microscopy. J Pediatr, 1977; 90:62–66

375. Ornoy A, Arnon J, Grebner EE, Jackson LG, Bach G. Early prenatal diagnosis of mucolipidosis IV. Am J Med Genet, 1987; 27:983–985

376. Berman ER, Livni N, Shapira E, Merin S, Levy IS. Congenital corneal clouding with abnormal systemic storage bodies. A new variant of mucolipidosis. J Pediatr, 1974; 84:519–526

377. Crandall B, Philipart M. Mucolipidosis IV. In: Birth defects encyclopedia. M.L. Buyse, Editor. 1989, Center for Birth Defects Information Services Dover MA. p. 1159–1160

378. Orlean P. Congenital disorders of glycosylation caused by defects in mannose addition during N-linked oligosaccharide assembly. J Clin Invest, 2000; 105:131–132

379. Petersen MB, Brostrom K, Stibler H, Skovby F. Early manifestations of the carbohydrate-deficient glycoprotein syndrome. J Pediatr, 1993; 122:66–70

380. Krasnewich D, Gahl WA. Carbohydrate-deficient glycoprotein syndrome. Adv Pediatr, 1997; 44:109–140

381. Stibler H, Blennow G, Kristiansson B, Lindehammer H, Hagberg B. Carbohydrate-deficient glycoprotein syndrome: clinical expression in adults with a new metabolic disease. J Neurol Neurosurg Psychiatry, 1994; 57:552–556

382. Kristiansson B, Borulf S, Conradi N, Erlanson-Albertsson C, Ryd W, Stibler H. Intestinal, pancreatic and hepatic involvement in carbohydrate-deficient glycoprotein syndrome type I. J Pediatr Gastroenterol Nutr, 1998; 27:23–29

383. Kottgen E, Buchsel R, Bauer C. Glycoproteins in liver disease. In: Liver in metabolic disease. L. Bianchi, W. Gerok, L. Landmann, K. Sickinger, G.A. Stalder, Editors. 1983, MTP Press: Lancaster. p. 145–153

384. Lippincott-Schwartz J. The endoplasmic reticulum-Golgi membrane system. In: The liver: biology and pathobiology. I.M. Arias, J.L. Boyer, N. Fausto, W.B. Jakoby, D. Schachter, D.A. Shafritz, Editors. 1994, Raven Press: New York. p. 215–224

385. Iijima K, Murakami F, Nakamura K et al. Hemostatic studies in patients with carbohydrate-deficient glycoprotein syndrome. Thromb Res, 1994; 76:193–198.

386. Okamoto N, Wada Y, Kobayashi M et al. Decreased blood coagulation activities in carbohydrate-deficient glycoprotein syndrome. J Inherit Metab Dis, 1993; 16:435–440

387. Van Geet C, Jaeken JA. unique pattern of coagulation abnormalities in carbohydrate-deficient glycoprotein syndrome. Pediatr Res, 1993; 33:540–541

388. de Zegher F, Jaeken J. Endocrinology of the carbohydrate-deficient glycoprotein syndrome type 1 from birth through adolescence. Pediatr Res, 1995; 37:395–401

389. Macchia PE, Harrison HH, Scherberg NH, Sunthornthepfvarakul T, Jaeken J, Refetoff S. Thyroid function tests and characterization of thyroxine-binding globulin in the carbohydrate-deficient glycoprotein syndrome type I. J Clin Endocrinol Metab, 1995; 80:3744–3749

390. Jaeken J, van Eijk HG, van der Heul C, Corbeel L, Eeckels R, Eggermont E. Sialic acid-deficient serum and cerebrospinal fluid transferrin in a newly recognized genetic syndrome. Clin Chim Acta, 1984; 144:245–247

391. Stibler H, Borg S, Joustra M. A modified method for the assay of carbohydrate-deficient transferrin (CDT) in serum. Alcohol Alcohol, 1989; 24:388

392. Adamowicz M, Pronicka E. Carbohydrate deficient glycoprotein syndrome-like transferrin isoelectric focusing pattern in untreated fructosaemia. Eur J Pediatr, 1996; 155:347–348 (letter)

393. Jaeken J, Carchon H. The carbohydrate-deficient glycoprotein syndromes: an overview. J Inherit Metab Dis, 1993; 16:813–820

394. Jaeken J, Pirard M, Adamowicz M, Pronicka E, van Schaftingen E. Inhibition of phosphomannose isomerase by fructose 1-phosphate: an explanation for defective N-glycosylation in hereditary fructose intolerance. Pediatr Res, 1996; 40:764–766

395. Stibler H, Borg S, Joustra M. Micro anion exchange chromatography of carbohydrate-deficient transferrin in serum in relation to alcohol consumption. Alcoholism: Clin Exp Res, 1986; 10:535–544

396. Acarregui MJ, George TN, Rhead WJ. Carbohydrate-deficient glycoprotein syndrome type 1 with profound thrombocytopenia and normal phosphomannomutase and phosphomannose isomerase activities. J Pediatr, 1998; 133:697–700

397. Van Schaftingen E, Jaeken J. Phosphomannomutase deficiency is a cause of carbohydrate-deficient glycoprotein syndrome type I. FEBS Lett, 1995; 377:318–320

398. de Koning TJ, Dorland L, van Diggelen OP et al. A novel disorder of N-glycosylation due to phosphomannose isomerase deficiency. Biochem Biophys Res Commun, 1998; 245:38–42

399. Jaeken J, Matthijs G, Saudubray JM et al. Phosphomannose isomerase deficiency: a carbohydrate-deficient glycoprotein syndrome with hepatic-intestinal presentation. Am J Hum Genet, 1998; 62:1535–1539

400. Niehues R, Hasilik M, Alton G et al. Carbohydrate-deficient glycoprotein syndrome type Ib. Phosphomannose isomerase deficiency and mannose therapy. J Clin Invest, 1998; 101:1414–1420

401. de Lonlay P, Seta N, Barrot S et al. A broad spectrum of clinical presentations in congenital disorders of glycosylation I: a series of 26 cases. J Med Genet, 2001; 38:14–19

402. Prietsch V, Peters V, Hackler R et al. A new case of CDG-x with stereotyped dystonic hand movements and optic atrophy. J Inherit Metab Dis, 2002; 25:126–130

403. Charuk JH, Tan J, Bernardini M et al. Carbohydrate-deficient glycoprotein syndrome type II. An autosomal recessive N-acetylglucosaminyltransferase II deficiency different from typical hereditary erythroblastic multinuclearity, 1995; 230:797–805

404. Jaeken J, De Cock P, Stibler H et al. Carbohydrate-deficient glycoprotein syndrome type II. J Inherit Metab Dis, 1993; 16:1041

405. Jaeken J, Schachter H, Carchon H, De Cock P, Coddeville B, Spik G. Carbohydrate deficient glycoprotein syndrome type II: a deficiency in Golgi localised N-acetyl-glucosaminyltransferase II. Arch Dis Child, 1994; 71:123–127

406. Ramaekers VT, Stibler H, Kint J, Jaeken J. A new variant of the carbohydrate deficient glycoprotein syndrome. J Inherit Metab Dis, 1991; 14:385–388

407. Korner C, Knauer R, Holzbach U, Hanefeld F, Lehle L, von Figura K. Carbohydrate-deficient glycoprotein syndrome type V: deficiency of dolichyl-P-Glc:Man9GlcNAc2-PP-dolichyl glucosyltransferase. Proc Natl Acad Sci USA, 1998; 95:13200–13205

408. Bjursell C, Stibler H, Wahlstrom J et al. Fine mapping of the gene for carbohydrate-deficient glycoprotein syndrome, type I (CDG1): linkage disequilibrium and founder effect in Scandinavian families. Genomics, 1997; 39:247–253

409. Kristiansson B, Stibler H, Hagberg B, Wahlstrom J. CDGS-1-a recently discovered hereditary metabolic disease. Multiple organ manifestations, 1998; 95:5742–5748

410. Martinsson T, Bjursell C, Stibler H et al. Linkage of a locus for carbohydrate-deficient glycoprotein syndrome type I (CDG1) to chromosome 16p, and linkage disequilibrium to microsatellite marker D16S406. Hum Mol Genet, 1994; 3:2037–2042.

411. Matthijs G, Schollen E, Pardon E et al. Mutations in PMMM2, a phosphomannomutase gene on chromosome 16p13, in carbohydrate-deficient glycoprotein type I syndrome (Jaeken syndrome) published erratum appears in Nat Genet 1997 Jul;16:316. Nat Genet, 1997; 16:88–92

412. Clayton P, Winchester B, Di Tomaso E, Young E, Keir G, Rodeck C. Carbohydrate-deficient glycoprotein syndrome: normal glycosylation in the fetus. Lancet, 1993; 341:956 (letter)

413. Matthijs G, Schollen E, Cassiman JJ, Cormier-Daire V, Jaeken J, van Schaftingen E. Prenatal diagnosis in CDGS families: beware of heterogeneity. Eur J Hum Genet, 1998; 6:99–104

414. Stibler H, Cederberg B. Diagnosis of the carbohydrate-deficient glycoprotein syndrome by analysis of transferrin in filter paper blood spots. Acta Paediatr, 1993; 82:55–59

415. de Lonlay P, Cuer M, Vuillaumier-Barrot S et al. Hyperinsulinemic hypoglycemia as a presenting sign in phosphomannose isomerase deficiency: a new manifestation of carbohydrate-deficient glycoprotein syndrome treatable with mannose. J Pediatr, 1999; 135:379–383

416. Conradi N, De Vos R, Jaeken J, Lunden P, Kristiansson B, Van Hoof F. Liver pathology in the carbohydrate-deficient glycoprotein syndrome. Acta Paediatr Scand, 1991; (suppl) 375:50–54

417. Stromme P, Maehlin J, Strom EH, Torvik A. Postmortem findings in two patients with the carbohydrate-deficient glycoprotein syndrome. Acta Paediatr Scand, 1991; (Suppl) 375:55–62

418. Callea F, De Vos R, Tagni R, Tardanico R, Vanstapel MJ, Desmet VJ. Fibrinogen inclusions in liver cells a new type of ground-glass hepatocyte; Immune, light and electron microscopic characterization. Histopathology, 1986; 10:65–73

419. Cicardi M, Zingale L, Zanichelli A, Pappalardo E, Cicardi B. C1 inhibitor: molecular and clinical aspects. Springer Semin Immunopathol, 2005; 27:286–298

420. Marsden MD, Fournier RE. Chromosomal elements regulate gene activity and chromatin structure of the human serpin gene cluster at 14q32.1. Mol Cell Biol, 2003; 23:3516–3526

421. Whisstock JC, Bottomley SP, Bird PI, Pike RN, Coughlin P. Serpins 2005—fun between the beta-sheets. Meeting report based upon presentations made at the 4th International Symposium on Serpin Structure, Function and Biology (Cairns, Australia). Febs J, 2005; 272:4868–4873

422. Laurell CB, Ericksson S. The electrophoretic a1-1-globulin pattern of serum alpha-1-antitrypsin deficiency. Scand J Clin Lab Invest, 1963; 15:132–140

423. Sharp HL, Bridges RA, Krivit W, Freier EF. Cirrhosis associated with alpha-1-antitrypsin deficiency: a previously unrecognized inherited disorder. J Lab Clin Med, 1969; 73:934–939

424. Ibarguen E, Gross CR, Savik SK, Sharp HL. Liver disease in alpha-1-antitrypsin deficiency: prognostic indicators. J Pediatr, 1990; 117:864–870

425. Moroz SP, Cutz E, Cox DW, Sass-Kortsak A. Liver disease associated with alpha 1-antitrypsin deficiency in childhood. J Pediatr, 1976; 88:19–25

426. Sveger T. Liver disease in alpha 1-antitrypsin deficiency detected by screening of 200,000 infants. N Engl J Med, 1976; 294:1316–1321

427. Ghebranious N, Mallum J. A Single multiplexed allele-specific polymerase chain reaction for simultaneous detection of alpha1-antitrypsin S and Z mutations. Genet Test, 2005; 9:185–189

428. Eriksson S. Alpha 1-antitrypsin deficiency. J Hepatol, 1999; 30 (Suppl 1):34–39

429. de Serres FJ. Worldwide racial and ethnic distribution of alpha1-antitrypsin deficiency: summary of an analysis of published genetic epidemiologic surveys. Chest, 2002; 122:1818–1829

430. Stoller JK, Aboussouan LS. Alpha1-antitrypsin deficiency. Lancet, 2005; 365:2225–2236

431. Schroeder WT, Miller MF, Woo SL, Saunders GF. Chromosomal localization of the human alpha 1-antitrypsin gene (PI) to 14q31–32. Am J Hum Genet, 1985; 37:868–872

432. Jeppsson JO. Amino acid substitution Glu leads to Lys alpha 1-antitrypsin PiZ. FEBS Lett, 1976; 65:195–197

433. Perlmutter DH. Alpha-1-antitrypsin deficiency: diagnosis and treatment. Clin Liver Dis, 2004; 8:839–59, viii–ix

434. Rudnick DA, Perlmutter DH. Alpha-1-antitrypsin deficiency: a new paradigm for hepatocellular carcinoma in genetic liver disease. Hepatology, 2005; 42:514–521

435. Carrell RW, Jeppsson JO, Laurell CB et al. Structure and variation of human alpha 1-antitrypsin. Nature, 1982; 298:329–334

436. Gadek JE, Crystal RG. Alpha-1-antitrypsin deficiency. In: Metabolic basis of inherited disease. J.B. Stanbury, J.B. Wyngaarden, D.S. Fredrickson, J.L. Goldstein, M.S. Brown, Editors. 1983, McGraw-Hill: New York. p. 1450–1467

437. Johnson DA, Travis J. Human alpha-1-proteinase inhibitor mechanism of action: evidence for activation by limited proteolysis. Biochem Biophys Res Commun, 1976; 72:33–39

438. Schwarzenberg SJ, Sharp HL. Alpha-1-antitrypsin deficiency. In: Diseases of the liver. L. Schiff and E.R. Schiff, Editors. 1993, Lippincott: New York. p. 692–706

439. Sveger T. Prospective study of children with a-1-antitrypsin deficiency: eight-year-old follow-up. J Pediatr, 1989; 104:91–94

440. Sveger T. The natural history of liver disease in alpha 1-antitrypsin deficient children. Acta Paediatr Scand, 1988; 77:847–851

441. Psacharopoulos HT, Mowat AP, Cook PJ, Carlile PA, Portmann B, Rodeck CH. Outcome of liver disease associated with alpha 1 antitrypsin deficiency (PiZ). Implications for genetic counselling and antenatal diagnosis. Arch Dis Child, 1983; 58:882–887

442. Esquivel CO, Vicente E, Van Thiel D et al. Orthotopic liver transplantation for alpha-1-antitrypsin deficiency: an experience in 29 children and ten adults. Transplant Proc, 1987; 19:3798–3802

443. Larsson C. Natural history and life expectancy in severe alpha 1-antitrypsin deficiency, Pi Z. Acta Med Scand, 1978; 204:345–351

444. Bowlus CL, Willner I, Zern MA et al. Factors associated with advanced liver disease in adults with alpha1-antitrypsin deficiency. Clin Gastroenterol Hepatol, 2005; 3:390–396

445. Stoller JK, Tomashefski J, Jr., Crystal RG et al. Mortality in individuals with severe deficiency of alpha1-antitrypsin: findings from the National Heart, Lung, and Blood Institute Registry. Chest, 2005; 127:1196–1204

446. Crowley JJ, Sharp HL, Freier E, Ishak KG, Schow P. Fatal liver disease associated with alpha 1-antitrypsin deficiency PiM1/PiMduarte. Gastroenterology, 1987; 93:242–244

447. Reid CL, Wiener GJ, Cox DW, Richter JE, Geisinger KR. Diffuse hepatocellular dysplasia and carcinoma associated with the Mmalton variant of alpha 1-antitrypsin. Gastroenterology, 1987; 93:181–187

448. Morse JO. Alpha 1-antitrypsin deficiency. N Engl J Med, 1978; 299:1099–1105

449. Bell H, Schrumpf E, Fagerhol MK. Heterozygous MZ alpha-1-antitrypsin deficiency in adults with chronic liver disease. Scand J Gastroenterol, 1990; 25:788–792

450. Carlson J, Eriksson S. Chronic -cryptogenic- liver disease and malignant hepatoma in intermediate alpha 1-antitrypsin deficiency identified by a Pi Z-specific monoclonal antibody. Scand J Gastroenterol, 1985; 20:835–842

451. Hodges JR, Millward-Sadler GH, Barbatis C, Wright R. Heterozygous MZ alpha 1-antitrypsin deficiency in adults with chronic active hepatitis and cryptogenic cirrhosis. N Engl J Med, 1981; 304:557–560

452. Davis ID, Burke B, Freese D, Sharp HL, Kim Y. The pathologic spectrum of the nephropathy associated with alpha 1-antitrypsin deficiency. Hum Pathol, 1992; 23:57–62

453. Szonyi L, Dobos M, Vasarhelyi B et al. Prevalence of alpha1-antitrypsin phenotypes in patients with IgA nephropathy. Clin Nephrol, 2004; 62:418–422

454. Eriksson S, Carlson J, Velez R. Risk of cirrhosis and primary liver cancer in alpha 1-antitrypsin deficiency. N Engl J Med, 1986; 314:736–739

455. Poley JR. Malignant liver disease in alpha1-antitrypsin deficiency. Acta Paediatr, 1994; 393(Suppl):27–32

456. Berkowitz M, Gavalier JS, Kelly RH, Prieto M, Van Thiel DH. Lack of increased heterozygous alpha-1-antitrypsin deficiency phenotypes among patients with hepatocellular and bile duct carcinoma. Hepatology, 1992; 15:407–410

457. Zhou H, Ortiz-Pallardo ME, Ko Y, Fischer HP. Is heterozygous alpha-1-antitrypsin deficiency type PIZ a risk factor for primary liver carcinoma? Cancer, 2000; 88:2668–2676

458. Feldmann G, Bignon J, Chahinian P, Degott C, Benhamou JP. Hepatocyte ultrastructural changes in alpha 1-antitrypsin deficiency. Gastroenterology, 1974; 67:1214–1220

459. Iezzoni JC, Gaffey MJ, Stacy EK, Normansell DE. Hepatocytic globules in end-stage hepatic disease. Relationship to alpha 1-antitrypsin phenotype. Am J Clin Pathol, 1997; 107:692–697

460. Ishak KG, Sharp HL. Metabolic errors and liver disease. In: Pathology of the liver. R.N.M. MacSween, P.J. Anthony, P.J. Scheuer, A.D. Burt, B.C. Portmann, Editors. 1994, Churchill Livingstone: Edinburgh. p. 123–218

461. Fabbretti G, Sergi C, Consales G et al. Genetic variants of alpha-1-antitrypsin (AAT). Liver, 1992; 12:296–301

462. Callea F, Fevery J, Massi G, Lievens C, de Groote J, Desmet VJ. Alpha-1-antitrypsin (AAT) and its stimulation in the liver of PiMZ phenotype individuals. A -recruitment-secretory block- (-R-SB-) phenomenon. Liver, 1984; 4:325–337

463. Carlson J, Eriksson S, Hagerstrand I. Intra- and extracellular alpha 1-antitrypsin in liver disease with special reference to Pi phenotype. J Clin Pathol, 1981; 34:1020–1025

464. Bradfield JWB, Blankinsopp WK. Alpha-1-antitrypsin globules in the liver and PiM phenotype of alpha-1-antitrypsin. Am J Clin Pathol, 1977; 30:579–584

465. Berninger RW, DeLellis RA, Kaplan MM. Liver disease and the Pi Elemberg M phenotype of alpha-1-antirypsin. Am J Clin Pathol, 1985; 83:559–563

466. Malone M, Mieli-Vergani G, Mowat AP, Portmann B. The fetal liver in (Pizz) a1-antitrypsin deficiency: A report of five cases. Pediatr Pathol, 1989; 9:623–631

467. Janciauskiene S, Eriksson S, Callea F et al. Differential detection of PAS-positive inclusions formed by the Z, Siiyama, and Mmalton variants of alpha1-antitrypsin. Hepatology, 2004; 40:1203–1210

468. Takahashi H, Crystal RG. Alpha-1-antitrypsin Nullisola di procida: alpha-1-antitrypsin deficiency allele caused by deletion of all alpha-1-antitrypsin coding exons. Am J Hum Genet, 1990; 47:403–413

469. Francavilla R, Castellaneta SP, Hadzic N et al. Prognosis of alpha-1-antitrypsin deficiency-related liver disease in the era of paediaric liver transplantation. J Hepatol, 2000; 32:986–992

470. Rubel LR, Ishak KG, Benjamin SB, Knuff TE. a1-antitrypsin deficiency and hepatocellular carcinoma: association with cirrhosis, copper storage and Mallory bodies. Arch Pathol Lab Med, 1982; 106:678–681

471. Triger DK, Milward-Sadler GH, Czaykowski AA, Trowell J, Wright R. Alpha-1-antitrypsin deficiency and liver disease in adults. Q J Med, 1976; 45:351–372

472. Ortiz-Pallardo ME, Ko Y, Sachinidis A, Vetter H, Fischer HP, Zhou H. Detection of alpha-1-antitrypsin PiZ individuals by SSCP and DNA sequencing in formalin-fixed and paraffin-embedded tissue: a comparison with immunohistochemical analysis. J Hepatol, 2000; 32:406–411

473. Povey S. Genetics of alpha 1-antitrypsin deficiency in relation to neonatal liver disease. Mol Biol Med, 1990; 7:161–172

474. Sveger T. Breast-feeding, alpha-1-antitrypsin deficiency. A retrospective analysis of the influence of early breast-vs bottle-feeding. JAMA, 1985; 253:2679–2682

475. Udall JN, Jr, Dixon M, Newman AP, Wright JA, James B, Bloch KJ. Liver disease in alpha 1-antitrypsin deficiency. A retrospective analysis of the influence of early breast- vs bottle-feeding. JAMA, 1985; 253:2679–2682

476. Schwarzenberg SJ, Sharp HL. Pathogenesis of alpha 1-antitrypsin deficiency-associated liver disease, 1990. J Pediatr Gastroenterol Nutr, 1990; 10:5–12

477. Dycaico MJ, Grant SGN, Felts K et al. Neonatal hepatitis induced by a1-antitrypsin: a transgenic mouse model. Science, 1988; 242:1409–1411

478. Geller SA, Nichols WS, Dycaico MJ, Felts KA, Sorge JA. Histopathology of a1-antitrypsin liver disease in a transgenic mouse model. Hepatology, 1990; 12:40–47

479. Conlon TJ, Cossette T, Erger K et al. Efficient hepatic delivery and expression from a recombinant adeno-associated virus 8 pseudotyped alpha1-antitrypsin vector. Mol Ther, 2005; 12:867–875

480. Duan YY, Wu J, Zhu JL et al. Gene therapy for human alpha1-antitrypsin deficiency in an animal model using SV40-derived vectors. Gastroenterology, 2004; 127:1222–1232

481. Eriksson S, Lindmark B, Lilja H. Familial alpha 1-antichymotrypsin deficiency. Acta Med Scand, 1986; 220:447–453

482. Thomas RM, Schiano TD, Kueppers F, Black M. Alpha-antichymotripsin globules within hepatocytes in patients with chronic hepatitis C and cirrhosis. Hum Pathol, 2000; 31:575–577

483. Yoon D, Kueppers F, Genta RM, Klintmalm GB, Khaoustov VI, Yoffe B. Role of alpha-1-antichymotrypsin deficiency in promoting cirrhosis in two siblings with heterozygous alpha-1-antitrypsin deficiency phenotype SZ. Gut, 2002; 50:730–732

484. Kelsey GD, Abeliovich D, McMahon CJ et al. Cloning of the human alpha-1 antichymotrypsin gene and genetic analysis of the gene in relation to alpha-1 antitrypsin deficiency. J Med Genet, 1988; 25:361–368

485. Rabin M, Watson M, Kidd V, Woo SLC, Breg WR, Ruddle FH. Regional location of alpha-1-antichymotrypsin and alpha-1-antitrypsin genes on human chromosome 14. Somat. Cell Mol Genet, 1986; 12:209–214

486. Lindmark B, Millward-Sadler H, Callea F, Eriksson S. Hepatocyte inclusions of a1-antichymotrypsin in a patient with partial deficiency of a1-antichymotrypsin and chronic liver disease. Histopathology, 1990; 16:221–225

487. Yoon DK, Kueppers F, Genta RM et al. Alpha-1-antichymotrypsin deficiency in two siblings with end-stage liver disease and phenotype SZ alpha-1-antitrypsin deficiency. Hepatology, 2000; 32:488A

488. Fried KKS. Congenital afibrinogenemia in 10 offsprings of uncle-niece marriages. Clin Genet, 1980; 17:223–227

489. Grech H, Majamdar G, Lawril AS, Savidge GF. Pregnancy in congenital afibrinogenemia: Report of a successful case and review of the literature. Br J Haematol, 1991; 78:571–572

490. Callea F, Lucini L, Bonetti M, Togni R, Kojima T, Favret M. Chronic cryptogenic liver disease and hepatocyte endoplasmic reticulum

491. storage of fibrinogen in hereditary hypofibrinogenemia. Hepatology, 1988; 8:1419

491. Al-Mondhiry H, Ehmann WC. Congenital afibrinogenemia. Am J Hematol, 1994; 46:343–347

492. Kant JA, Fornace AJ, Jr, Saxe D, Simon MI, McBride OW, Crabtree GR. Evolution and organization of the fibrinogen locus on chromosome 4: gene duplication accompanied by transposition and inversion. Proc Natl Acad Sci USA, 1985; 82:2344–2348

493. Duga S, Asselta R, Santagostino E et al. Missense mutations in the human beta fibrinogen gene cause congenital afibrinogenemia by impairing fibrinogen secretion In Process Citation. Blood, 2000; 95:1336–1341

494. Neerman-Arbez M, de Moerloose P, Bridel C et al. Mutations in the fibrinogen aalpha gene account for the majority of cases of congenital afibrinogenemia. Blood, 2000; 96:149–152

495. Neerman-Arbez M, de Moerloose P, Honsberger A et al. Molecular analysis of the fibrinogen gene cluster in 16 patients with congenital afibrinogenemia: novel truncating mutations in the FGA and FGG genes. Hum Genet, 2001; 108:237–240

496. Brennan SO, Maghzal G, Shneider BL, Gordon R, Magid MS, George PM. Novel fibrinogen gamma375 Arg-> Trp mutation (fibrinogen aguadilla) causes hepatic endoplasmic reticulum storage and hypofibrinogenemia. Hepatology, 2002; 36:652–658

497. Brennan SO, Wyatt J, Medicina D, Callea F, George PM. Fibrinogen Brescia: Hepatic endoplasmic reticulum storage and hypofibrinogenemia due to a y284Gly'Arg mutation. Am J Pathol, 2000; 157:189–196

498. Callea F, De Vos R, Pinackay J et al. Hereditary hypofibrinogenaemia with hepatic storage of fibrinogen. Ital J Gastroenterol, 1987; 19:304–305 (abstract)

499. Pfeifer U, Ormanns W, Klinge O. Hepatocellular fibrinogen storage in familial hypofibrinogenemia. Virchows Arch (Cell Pathol), 1981; 36:247–255

500. Wehinger H, Klinge O, Alexandrakis E, Schurman J, Witt J, Seydewitz HH. Hereditary hypofibrinogenemia with fibrinogen storage in the liver. Eur J Pediatr, 1983; 141:109–112

501. Ishak KG, Sharp HL, Schwarzenberg SJ. Metabolic errors and liver disease. In: Pathology of the Liver. R.N.M. MacSween, A.D. Burt, B.C. Portmann, K.G. Ishak, P.J. Scheuer, P.P. Anthony, Editors. 2002, Harcourt Health Sciences: London. p. 155–255

502. Abukawa D, Tazawa Y, Noro T et al. Cytoplasmic inclusion bodies and minimal hepatitis: fibrinogen storage without hypofibrinogenemia. Pediatr Dev Pathol, 2001; 4:304–309

503. Marucci G, Morandi L, Macchia S et al. Fibrinogen storage disease without hypofibrinogenaemia associated with acute infection. Histopathology, 2003; 42:22–25

504. Mitsui H, Miyauchi E, Miyahara J, Wada K, Yamakawa M, Kawata S. A case of primary biliary cirrhosis accompanied with fibrinogen storage disease. Pathol Res Pract, 2005; 201:341–345

505. Ng IOL, Ng M, Lai ECS et al. Endoplasmic storage disease of liver: Characterization of intracytoplasmic hyaline inclusions. Histopathology, 1989; 15:473–481

506. Duga S, Braidotti P, Asselta R et al. Liver histology of an afibrinogenemic patient with the Bbeta-L353R mutation showing no evidence of hepatic endoplasmic reticulum storage disease (ERSD); comparative study in COS-1 cells of the intracellular processing of the Bbeta-L353R fibrinogen vs. the ERSD-associated gamma-G284R mutant. J Thromb Haemost, 2005; 3:724–732

507. De Craemer D, Pipeleers-Marichal M, Vandenplas Y, Van den Branden C. Peroxisome proliferation associated with fibrinogen storage in the liver. Histopathology, 1996; 29:171–173

508. Lane DA, Olds RJ, Thein SL. Antithrombin III: summary of first database update. Nucleic Acids Res, 1994; 22:3556–3559

509. Demers C, Ginsberg JS, Hirsh J, Henderson P, Blajchman MA. Thrombosis in antithrombin-III-deficient persons. Report of a large kindred and literature review. Ann Intern Med, 1992; 116:754–761

510. Sharon BI. Antithrombin III deficiency. In: Birth defects encyclopedia. M.L. Buyse, Editor. 1990, Center for Birth Defects Information Services Inc: Dover MA. p. 152–154

511. Das M, Carroll SF. Antithrombin III deficiency: an etiology of Budd–Chiari syndrome. Surgery, 1985; 97:242–245

512. McClure S, Dincsoy HP, Glueck H. Budd–Chiari syndrome and antithrombin III deficiency. Am J Clin Pathol, 1982; 78:236–241

513. Rosendaal FR, Heijboer H, Briet E et al. Mortality in hereditary antithrombin-II deficiency—1830 to 1989. Lancet, 1991; 337:260–262

514. Mendelsohn G, Gomperts ED, Gurwitz D. Severe antithrombin III deficiency in an infant associated with multiple arterial and venous thrombosis. Thromb Haemost, 1976; 36:495–502

515. Lindblad B, Lindstedt S, Steen G. On the enzymic defects in hereditary tyrosinemia. Proc Natl Acad Sci USA, 1977; 74:4641–4645

516. Mitchell GA, Lambert M, Tanguay RM. Hypertyrosinemia. In: The metabolic and molecular basis of inherited disease. C.R. Scriver, A.L. Beaudet, W.S. Sly, J. Valle, Editors. 1995, McGraw-Hill: New York. p. 1077–1106

517. Freese DK, Tuchman M, Schwarzenberg SJ et al. Early liver transplantation is indicated for tyrosinemia type I. J Pediatr Gastroenterol Nutr, 1991; 13:10–15

518. van Spronsen FJ, Thomasse Y, Smit GP et al. Hereditary tyrosinemia type I: a new clinical classification with difference in prognosis on dietary treatment. Hepatology, 1994; 20:1187–1191

519. Paradis K. Tyrosinemia: the Quebec experience. Clin Invest Med, 1996; 19:311–316

520. Kvittingen EA. Tyrosinaemia type I—an update. J Inherit Metab Dis, 1991; 14:554–562

521. Mitchell G, Larochelle J, Lambert M et al. Neurologic crises in hereditary tyrosinemia. N Engl J Med, 1990; 322:432–437

522. Paradis K, Mitchell G, Russo P. Tyrosinemia. In: Liver disease in children. F.J. Suchy, Editor. 1994, Mosby: St. Louis. p. 203

523. Edwards MA, Green A, Colli A, Rylance G. Tyrosinaemia type I and hypertrophic obstructive cardiomyopathy. Lancet, 1987; i:1437–1438

524. Lindblad M, Fallstrom SP, Hoyer S, Nordborg C, Solynar L, Velander H. Cardiomyopathy in fumarylacetoacetase deficiency (hereditary tyrosinaemia: a new feature of the disease). J Inhert Metab Dis, 1987; 10:319.

525. Weinberg AG, Mize CE, Worthen HG. The occurrence of hepatoma in the chronic form of hereditary tyrosinemia. J Pediatr, 1976; 88:434–438

526. Paradis K, Weber A, Seidman EG et al. Liver transplantation for hereditary tyrosinemia. The Quebec experience. Am J Hum Genetics, 1990; 47:338

527. Grompe M, St-Louis M, Demers SI, al-Dhalimy M, Leclerc B, Tanguay RM. A single mutation of the fumarylacetoacetate hydrolase gene in French Canadians with hereditary tyrosinemia type I. N Engl J Med, 1994; 331:353–357

528. St-Louis M, Tanguay RM. Mutations in the fumarylacetoacetate hydrolase gene causing hereditary tyrosinemia type I: overview. Hum Mutat, 1997; 9:291–299

529. Phaneuf D, Labelle Y, Berube D et al. Cloning and expression of the cDNA encoding human fumarylacetoacetate hydrolase, the enzyme deficient in hereditary tyrosinemia: assignment of the gene to chromosome 15. Am J Hum Genet, 1991; 48:525–535

530. Demers SI, Phaneuf D, Tanguay RM. Hereditary tyrosinemia type I: strong association with haplotype 6 in French Canadians permits simple carrier detection and prenatal diagnosis. Am J Hum Genet, 1994; 55:327–333

531. Ploos van Amstel JK, Jansen RP, Verjaal M, van den Berg IE, Berger R. Prenatal diagnosis of type I hereditary tyrosinaemia. Lancet, 1994; 344:336

532. Kvittingen EA, Rootwelt H, Berger R, Brandtzaeg P. Self-induced correction of the genetic defect in tyrosinemia type I. J Clin Invest, 1994; 94:1657–1661

533. Bergeron A, Lettre F, Russo P, Morissette J, Tanguay RM. No evidence of maternal cell colonization in reverted liver nodules of tyrosinemia type I patients. Gastroenterology, 2004; 127:1381–1385

534. Demers SI, Russo P, Lettre F, Tanguay RM. Frequent mutation reversion inversely correlates with clinical severity in a genetic liver disease, hereditary tyrosinemia. Hum Pathol, 2003; 34:1313–1320

535. Holme E, Lindstedt S. Tyrosinaemia type I and NTBC (2-(2-nitro-4-trifluoromethylbenzoyl)-1,3-cyclohexanedione). J Inherit Metab Dis, 1998; 21:507–517

536. Holme E, Lindstedt S. Nontransplant treatment of tyrosinemia. Clin Liver Dis, 2000; 4:805–814

537. Suzuki Y, Konda M, Imai I, Imamura H, Shimao S, Okaka T. Effect of dietary treatment on the renal tubular function in a patient with hereditary tyrosinemia. Int J Pediatr Nephrol, 1987; 8:171–176

538. Evans DI, Sardharwalla IB. Coagulation defect of congenital tyrosinaemia. Arch Dis Child, 1984; 59:1088–1090

539. Laine J, Salo MK, Krogerus L, Karkkainen J, Wahlroos O, Holmberg C. The nephropathy of type I tyrosinemia after liver transplantation. Pediatr Res, 1995; 37:640–645

540. Grompe M, Lindstedt S, al-Dhalimy M et al. Pharmacological correction of neonatal lethal hepatic dysfunction in a murine model of hereditary tyrosinaemia type I. Nat Genet, 1995; 10:453–460

541. Kubo S, Sun M, Miyahara M et al. Hepatocyte injury in tyrosinemia type 1 is induced by fumarylacetoacetate and is inhibited by caspase inhibitors. Proc Natl Acad Sci U S A, 1998; 95:9552–9557

542. Vogel A, van Den Berg IE, Al-Dhalimy M et al. Chronic liver disease in murine hereditary tyrosinemia type 1 induces resistance to cell death. Hepatology, 2004; 39:433–443

543. Carson NAJ, Biggart JD, Bittles AH, Donovan D. Hereditary tyrosinaemia. Clinical, 1976; 51:106–113

544. Dehner LP, Snover DC, Sharp HL, Ascher N, Nakhleh R, Day DL. Hereditary tyrosinemia type I (chronic form): pathologic findings in the liver. Hum Pathol, 1989; 20:149–159

545. Manowski Z, Silver MM, Roberts EA, Superina RA, Phillips MJ. Liver cell dysplasia and early liver transplantation in hereditary tyrosinemia. Mod Pathol, 1990; 3:694–701

546. Mieles LA, Esquivel CO, Van Thiel DH et al. Liver transplantation for tyrosinemia. A review of 10 cases from the University of Pittsburgh. Dig Dis Sci, 1990; 35:153–157

547. Partington MW, Haust MD. A patient with tyrosinaemia and hypermethioninemia. Can Med Assoc J, 1967; 97:1059–1067

548. Perry TL. Tyrosinemia associated with hypermethioninemia and islet cell hyperplasia. Can Med Assoc J, 1967; 97:1067–1072

549. Zerbini C, Weinberg DS, Hollister KA, Perez-Atayde AR. DNA ploidy abnormalities on the liver of children with hereditary tyrosinemia type I. Correlation with histopathologic features. Am J Pathol, 1992; 140:1111–1119

550. Day DL, Letourneau JG, Allan BT et al. Hepatic regenerating nodules in hereditary tyrosinemia. Am J Roentgenol, 1987; 149:391–393

551. Scriver CR, Silverberg M, Clow CL. Hereditary tyrosinemia and tyrosyluria: clinical report of four patients. Can Med Assoc J, 1967; 97:1047–1050

552. Gilbert-Barness E, Barness LA, Meisner LF. Chromosomal instability in hereditary tyrosinemia type I. Pediatr Pathol, 1990; 10:243–252

553. Jevtic MM, Thorp FK, Hruban Z. Hereditary tyrosinemia with hyperplasia and hypertrophy of juxtaglomerular apparatus. Am J Clin Pathol, 1974; 61:423–437

554. Prive L. Pathological findings in patients with tyrosinemia. Can Med Assoc J, 1967; 97:1054–1056

555. Burton BK. Urea cycle disorders. Clin Liver Dis, 2000; 4:815–830, vi

556. Smith W, Kishnani PS, Lee B et al. Urea cycle disorders: clinical presentation outside the newborn period. Crit Care Clin, 2005; 21(4 Suppl):S9–S17.

557. Rowe PC, Newman SL, Brusilow SW. Natural history of symptomatic partial ornithine transcarbamylase deficiency. N Engl J Med, 1986; 314:541–547

558. Brusilow SW, Maestri NE. Urea cycle disorders: diagnosis, pathophysiology, and therapy. Adv Pediatr, 1996; 43:127–170

559. Nassogne MC, Heron B, Touati G, Rabier D, Saudubray JM. Urea cycle defects: management and outcome. J Inherit Metab Dis, 2005; 28:407–414

560. Zimmermann A, Bachmann C, Baumgartner R. Severe liver fibrosis in argininosuccinic aciduria. Arch Pathol Lab Med, 1986; 110:136–140

561. Naylor SL, Klebe RJ, Shows TB. Argininosuccinic aciduria: assignment of the argininosuccinate lyase gene to the pter to q22 region of human chromosome 7 by bioautography. Proc Natl Acad Sci USA, 1978; 75:6159–6162

562. McInnes RR, Shih V, Chilton S. Interallelic complementation in an inborn error of metabolism: genetic heterogeneity in argininosuccinate lyase deficiency. Proc Natl Acad Sci USA, 1984; 81:4480–4484

563. Kobayashi K, Itakura Y, Saheki T et al. Absence of argininosuccinate lyase protein in the liver of two patients with argininosuccinic aciduria. Clin Chim Acta, 1986; 159:59–67

564. Jorda A, Portoles M, Rubio V. Liver fibrosis in arginase deficiency. Arch Pathol Lab Med, 1987; 111:691–692

565. Travers H, Reed JS, Kennedy JA. Ultrastructural study of the liver in argininosuccinase deficiency. Pediatr Pathol, 1986; 5:307–318

566. Tallen H, Schaffner F, Taffet S, Schneidman K, Gaul G. Ornithine carbamyl-1 transferase deficiency in an adult male patient: significance of hepatic ultrastructure in clinical diagnosis. Pediatr Res, 1983; 71:224–232

567. Aida S, Ogata T, Kamoto et al. Primary ornithine transcarbamylase deficiency. A case report and electron microscopic study. Acta Pathol Jpn, 1985; 39:451–456

568. Rutledge SL, Havens PL, Haymond MW, McLean RH, Kan JS, Brusilow SW. Neonatal hemodialysis: effective therapy for the encephalopathy of inborn errors of metabolism. J Pediatr, 1990; 116:125–128

569. Leonard JV, McKiernan PJ. The role of liver transplantation in urea cycle disorders. Mol Genet Metab, 2004; 81(Suppl 1):S74–S78

570. Morioka D, Kasahara M, Takada Y et al. Current role of liver transplantation for the treatment of urea cycle disorders: a review of the worldwide English literature and 13 cases at Kyoto University. Liver Transpl, 2005; 11:1332–1342

571. Gahl WA, Schneider JA, Aula PP. Lysosomal transport disorders: Cystinosis and sialic acid storage disorders. In: The metabolic and

molecular basis of inherited disease. C.R. Scriver, A.L. Beaudet, W.S. Sly, J. Valle, Editors. 1995, McGraw-Hill: New York. p. 3763–3797

572. Kalatzis V, Antignac C. New aspects of the pathogenesis of cystinosis. Pediatr Nephrol, 2003; 18:207–215

573. Shotelersuk V, Larson D, Anikster et al. CTNS mutations in an American-based population of cystinosis patients. Am J Hum Genet, 1988; 63:1352–1362

574. Town M, Jean G, Cherqui S et al. A novel gene encoding an integral membrane protein is mutated in nephropathic cystinosis. Nature Genet, 1998; 18:319–324

575. Wong VG. The eye in cystinosis. In: Cystinosis. J.D. Schulman, Editor. 1973, Government Printing Office: Washington, DC. p. 23–35

576. Chan AM, Lynch MJ, Bailey JD et al. Hypothyroidism in cystinosis. A clinical, endocrinologic and histologic study involving sixteen patients with cystinosis. Am J Med, 1970; 48:678–692

577. Malekzadeh MH, Nurstein HB, Schneider JA et al. Cadaver renal transplantation in children with cystinosis. Am J Med, 1977; 63:525–533

578. Markello TC, Bernardini IM, Gahl WA. Improved renal function in children with cystinosis treated with cysteamine. N Engl J Med, 1993; 238:1157

579. Brubaker RF, Wong WG, Schulman JD, Seegmiller JE, Kawabare T. Benign cystinosis: The clinical, biochemical and morphological findings in a family with two affected siblings. Am J Med, 1970; 49:546–550

580. Schneider JA, Verroust FM, Kroll WA et al. Prenatal diagnosis of cystinosis. N Engl J Med, 1974; 290:878–882

581. Smith ML, Pellett OL, Cass MM et al. Prenatal diagnosis of cystinosis utilizing chorionic villus sampling. Prenatal Diag, 1987; 7:23–26

582. Seegmiller JE. Cystinosis. In: Lysosomes and storage diseases. H.G. Hers and F. Van Hoof, Editors. 1973, Academic Press: New York. p. 485–513

583. Witzleben CL, Monteleone JA, Rejent AJ. Electron microscopy in the diagnosis of cystinosis. Arch Pathol, 1972; 94:362–365

584. Boman H, Schneider JA. Prenatal diagnosis of nephropathic cystinosis. Acta Paediatr Scand, 1981; 70:389–393

585. Haynes ME, Carter RF, Pollard AC, Carey WF. Light and electron microscopy of infants and foetal tissus in cystinosis. Micron, 1980; 11:443–444

586. Lubec G, Nauer G, Pollack A. Non-invasive diagnosis of cystinosis by infra-red spectroscopy of hair. Lancet, 1983; i:623

587. Bendavid C, Kleta R, Long R et al. FISH diagnosis of the common 57-kb deletion in CTNS causing cystinosis. Hum Genet, 2004; 115:510–514

588. Harms E. Cystinosis and liposomal free amino acids. In: Liver in metabolic diseases. L. Bianchi et al., Editors. 1983, MTP Press: Lancaster. p. 129–136

589. Schulman JD, Wong V, Olson WH, Seegmiller JE. Lysosomal site of crystalline deposits in cystinosis as shown by ferritin uptake. Arch Pathol, 1970; 90:259–284

590. Spears GS. Pathology of the kidney in cystinosis. Pathol Annu, 1974; 9:81–92

591. Roels H. Pathology of aminoacidurias. In: Monographs in human genetics. L. Beckman and M. Hauge, Editors. 1972, Karger: Basel. p. 79–80

592. Scotto JM, Stralin HG. Ultrastructure of the liver in a case of childhood cystinosis. Virchous Arch A Pathol Anat Histol, 1977; 377:43–48

593. Klenn PJ, Rubin R. Hepatic fibrosis associated with hereditary cystinosis: novel form of noncirrhotic portal hypertension. Mod Pathol, 1994; 7:879–882

594. Avner ED, Ellis D, Jaffe R. Veno-occlusive disease of the liver associated with cysteamine treatment of nephropathic cystinosis. J Pediatr, 1983; 102:793–796

595. DiDomenico P, Berry G, Bass D, Fridge J, Sarwal M. Noncirrhotic portal hypertension in association with juvenile nephropathic cystinosis: case presentation and review of the literature. J Inherit Metab Dis, 2004; 27:693–699

596. Rossi S, Herrine SK, Navarro VJ. Cystinosis as a cause of noncirrhotic portal hypertension. Dig Dis Sci, 2005; 50:1372–1375

597. Mudd SH, Skovby F, Levy HL et al. The natural history of homocystinuria due to cystathionine beta-synthase deficiency. Am J Hum Genet, 1985; 37:1–31

598. Mandel H, Brenner B, Berant M et al. Coexistence of hereditary homocystinuria and factor V Leiden-effect on thrombosis. N Engl J Med, 1996; 343:763–768

599. Uhlendorf BW, Mudd SH. Cystathionine synthase in tissue culture derived from human skin: enzyme defect in homocystinuria. Science, 1968; 160:1007–1009

600. Yap S, Naughten E. Homocystinuria due to cystathionine beta-synthase deficiency in Ireland: 25 years' experience of a newborn screened and treated population with reference to clinical outcome and biochemical control. J Inherit Metab Dis, 1998; 21:738–747

601. Munke M, Kraus JP, Ohura T, Francke U. The gene for cystathionine beta-synthase (CBS) maps to the subtelomeric region on human chromosome 21q and to proximal mouse chromosome 17. Am J Hum Genet, 1988; 42:550–559

602. Chasse JF, Paul V, Escanez R, Kamoun P, London J. Human cystathionine beta-synthase: gene organization and expression of different 5-prime alternative splicing. Mamm Genome, 1997; 8:917–921

603. Fowler B, Kraus J, Packman S, Rosenberg LE. Homocystinuria. Evidence for three distinct classes of cystathionine beta-synthase mutants in cultured fibroblasts. J Clin Invest, 1978; 61:645–653

604. Kraus JP, Janosik M, Kozich V et al. Cystathionine beta-synthase mutations in homocystinuria. Hum Mutat, 1999; 13:362–375

605. Carey MC, Fennelly JJ, FitzGerald O. Homocystinuria. II. Subnormal serum folate levels, increased folate clearance and effects of folic acid therapy. Am J Med, 1968; 45:26–31

606. Wilcken DE, Dudman NP, Tyrrell PA. Homocystinuria due to cystathionine beta-synthase deficiency—the effects of betaine treatment in pyridoxine-responsive patients. Metabolism, 1985; 34:1115–1121

607. Carson NAJ, Dent CE, Field CMB, Gaull GE. Homocystinuria; clinical and pathological review of ten cases. J Pediatr, 1965; 66:565–583

608. Gibson JB, Carson NAJ, Neill DW. Pathological findings in homocystinuria. J Clin Pathol, 1964; 17:427–437

609. Schimke RN, McKusick VA, Huang T et al. Homocystinuria. Studies of 20 families with 38 affected members. JAMA, 1963; 193:711–719

610. Gaull GE, Schaffner F. Electron microscopic changes in hepatocytes of patients with homocystinuria. Pediatr Res, 1971; 5:23–32

611. Gaull GE, Sturman JA, Schaffner F. Homocystinuria due to cystathionine synthase deficiency: enzymatic and ultrastructural studies. J Pediatr, 1974; 84:381–390

612. Robert K, Nehme J, Bourdon E et al. Cystathionine beta synthase deficiency promotes oxidative stress, fibrosis, and steatosis in mice liver. Gastroenterology, 2005; 128:1405–1415

613. Bassen FA, Kornzweig AL. Malformation of the erythrocytes in a case of atypical retinitis pigmentosa. Blood, 1950; 5:381–387

614. Sobrevilla LA, Goodman ML, Kane CA. Demyelinating central nervous system disease, macular atrophy and acanthocytosis (Bassen–Kornzweig syndrome). Am J Med, 1964; 37:821–832

615. Wetterau JR, Aggerbeck LP, Bouma ME et al. Absence of microsomal triglyceride transfer protein in individuals with abetalipoproteinemia. Science, 1992; 258:999–1001

616. Sharp D, Blinderman L, Combs KA et al. Cloning and gene defects in microsomal triglyceride transfer protein associated with abetalipoproteinaemia. Nature, 1993; 365:65–69

617. Bieri JG, Hoeg JM, Schafer J, Zech LA, Brewer HB. Vitamin A and vitamin E replacement in abetalipoproteinemia. Ann Intern Med, 1984; 100:238–239

618. Illingworth DR, Connor WE, Miller RG. Abetalipoproteinemia: report of two cases and review of therapy. Arch Neurol, 1980; 37:659–662

619. Braegger CP, Belli DC, Mentha G, Steinmann B. Persistence of the intestinal defect in abetalipoproteinaemia after liver transplantation. Eur J Pediatr, 1998; 157:576–578

620. Black DD, Hay RV, Rohwer-Nutter PL et al. Intestinal and hepatic apolipoprotein 13 gene expression in abetalipoproteinemia. Gastroenterology, 1991; 101:520–528

621. Avigan MI, Ishak KG, Gregg RE et al. Morphologic features of the liver in abetalipoproteinemia. Hepatology, 1984; 4:1223–1226

622. Partin JS, Partin JC, Schubert WK, McAdams J. Liver ultrastructure in abetalipoproteinemia: Evolution of micronodular cirrhosis. Gastroenterology, 1974; 67:107–118

623. Collins JC, Scheinberg H, Giblin DR, Sternlieb I. Hepatic peroxisomal abnormalities in abetalipoproteinemia. Gastroenterology, 1989; 97:766–770

624. Kane JP, Havel RJ. Disorders of the biogenesis and secretion of lipoproteins containing the B apolipoproteins. In: The metabolic and molecular basis of inherited disease. C.R. Scriver et al., Editors. 1995, McGraw-Hill: New York. p. 1853–1885

625. Linton MF, Farese RV, Jr., Young SG. Familial hypobetalipoproteinemia. J Lipid Res, 1993; 34:521–541

626. Tarugi P, Lonardo A, Ballarini G et al. Fatty liver in heterozygous hypobetalipoproteinemia caused by a novel truncated form of apolipoprotein B. Gastroenterology, 1996; 111:1125–1133

627. Lancellotti S, Di Leo E, Penacchioni JY et al. Hypobetalipoproteinemia with an apparently recessive inheritance

due to a 'de novo' mutation of apolipoprotein B. Biochim Biophys Acta, 2004; 1688:61–67

628. Ahmed A, Keeffe EB. A symptomatic elevation of aminotransferase levels and fatty liver secondary to heterozygous hypobetalipoproteinemia. Am J Gastroenterol, 1998; 93:2598–2599

629. Castellano G, Garfia C, Gomez-Coronado D et al. Diffuse fatty liver in familial heterozygous hypobetalipoproteinemia. J Clin Gastroenterol, 1997; 25:379–382

630. Hagve TA, Myrseth LE, Schrumpf E et al. Liver steatosis in hypobetalipoproteinemia. A case report. J Hepatol, 1991; 13:104–111

631. Ogata H, Akagi K, Baba M et al. Fatty liver in a case with heterozygous familial hypobetalipoproteinemia. Am J Gastroenterol, 1997; 92:339–342

632. Wishingrad M, Paaso B, Garcia G. Fatty liver due to heterozygous hypobetalipoproteinemia. Am J Gastroenterol, 1994; 89:1106–1107

633. Cottrill C, Glueck J, Partin J, Leuba V, Puppione D, Brown WV. Familial homozygous hypobetalipoproteinemia. Metabolism, 1974; 23:779–791

634. Scoazec JY, Bouma ME, Roche JF et al. Liver fibrosis in a patient with familial homozygous hypobetalipoproteinaemia: possible role of vitamin supplementation. Gut, 1992; 33:414–417

635. Kim E, Cham CM, Veniant MM, Ambroziak P, Young SG. Dual mechanisms for the low plasma levels of truncated apolipoprotein B proteins in familial hypobetalipoproteinemia. Analysis of a new mouse model with a nonsense mutation in the Apob gene. J Clin Invest, 1998; 101:1468–1477

636. Bodzioch M, Orso E, Klucken J et al. The gene encoding ATP-binding cassette transporter 1 is mutated in Tangier disease. Nature Genet, 1999; 22:347–351

637. Brooks-Wilson A, Marcil M, Clee SM et al. Mutations in ABC1 in Tangier disease and familial high-density lipoprotein deficiency. Nature Genet, 1999; 22:336–345

638. Rust S, Rosier M, Funke H et al. Tangier disease is caused by mutations in the gene encoding ATP-binding cassette transporter 1. Nature Genet, 1999; 22:352–355

639. Rust S, Walter M, Funke H et al. Assignment of Tangier disease to chromosome 9q31 by a graphical linkage exclusion strategy. Nature Genet, 1998; 20:96–98

640. Knight BL. ATP-binding cassette transporter A1: regulation of cholesterol efflux. Biochem Soc Trans, 2004; 32(Pt 1):124–127

641. Lawn RM, Wade DP, Garvin MR et al. The Tangier disease gene product ABC1 controls the cellular apolipoprotein-mediated lipid removal pathway. J Clin Invest, 1999; 104:R25–R31

642. Bale PM, Clifton-Bligh P, Benjamin BNP et al. Pathology of Tangier disease. J Clin Pathol, 1971; 24:609–616

643. Brook JG, Lees RS, Yules JH et al. Tangier disease (alpha-lipoprotein deficiency). Jama, 1977; 238:332–334

644. Ferrans VJ, Fredrickson DS. The pathology of Tangier disease. Am J Pathol, 1975; 78:101–136

645. Dechelotte P, Kantelip B, de Laguillamie BV. Tangier disease. A histological and ultrastructural study. Pathol Res Pract, 1985; 180:424–430

646. Labbe A, Dechelotte P, Meyer M et al. La maladie de Tangier. Une th,saurismose rare. Presse Med, 1985; 14:1189–1192

647. Goldstein JL, Brown MS. Familial hypercholesterolemia: identification of a defect in the regulation of 3-hydroxy-3-methylglutaryl coenzyme A reductase activity associated with overproduction of cholesterol. Proc Natl Acad Sci USA, 1973; 70:2804–2808

648. Brown MS, Goldstein JL. Familial hypercholesterolemia: defective binding of lipoproteins to cultured fibroblasts associated with impaired regulation of 3-hydroxy-3-methylglutaryl coenzyme A reductase activity. Proc Natl Acad Sci USA, 1974; 71:788–792

649. Hobbs HH, Russell DW, Brown MS, Goldstein JL. The LDL receptor locus in familial hypercholesterolemia: mutational analysis of a membrane protein. Annu Rev Genet, 1990; 24:133–170

650. Beekman M, Heijmans BT, Martin NG et al. Evidence for a QTL on chromosome 19 influencing LDL cholesterol levels in the general population. Eur J Hum Genet, 2003; 11:845–850

651. Lindgren V, Luskey KL, Russell DW, Francke U. Human genes involved in cholesterol metabolism: chromosomal mapping of the loci for the low density lipoprotein receptor and 3-hydroxy-3-methylglutaryl-coenzyme A reductase with cDNA probes. Proc Natl Acad Sci USA, 1985; 82:8567–8571

652. Tonstad S, Knudtzon J, Sivertsen M, Refsum H, Ose L. Efficacy and safety of cholestyramine therapy in peripubertal and prepubertal children with familial hypercholesterolemia. J Pediatr, 1996; 129:42–49

653. Starzl TE, Bilheimer DW, Bahnson HT et al. Heart-liver transplantation in a patient with familial hypercholesterolaemia. Lancet, 1984; i:1382–1383

654. Buja M, Kovanen PT, Bilheimer DW. Cellular pathology of homozygous familial hypercholesterolemia. Am J Pathol, 1979; 97:327–345

655. Assman G, Seedorf U. Acid lipase deficiency Wolman disease and cholesterol ester storage disease. In: The metabolic and molecular basis of inherited disease. C.R. Scriver, B.L. Beaudet, W.S. Sly, D. Valle, Editors. 1995, McGraw-Hill: New York. p. 2563–2587

656. Pagani F, Pariyarath R, Garcia R et al. New lysosomal acid lipase gene mutants explain the phenotype of Wolman disease and cholesteryl ester storage disease. J Lipid Res, 1998; 39:1382–1388

657. Neufeld EF, Sando GN, Garvin AJ, Rome LH. The transport of lysosomal enzymes. J Supramol Struct, 1977; 6:95–101

658. Anderson RA, Rao N, Byrum RS et al. In situ localization of the genetic locus encoding the lysosomal acid lipase/cholesteryl esterase (LIPA) deficient in Wolman disease to chromosome 10q23.2–q23.3. Genomics, 1993; 15:245–247

659. Abramov A, Schorr S, Wolman M. Generalized xanthomatosis with calcified adrenals. Am J Dis Child, 1956; 91:282–286

660. Machim GA. Hydrops revisited: Literature review of 1,414 cases published in the 1980's. Am J Med Genet, 1989; 34:366–390

661. Meyers WF, Hoeg JM, DeMosky SJ, Herbst JJ, Brewer HB. The use of parenteral hyperalimentation and elemental formula feeding in the treatment of Wolman disease. Nutr Res, 1988; 5:423–429

662. Hoeg JM, Demosky SJ, Jr, Pescovitz OH, Brewer HB, Jr. Cholesteryl ester storage disease and Wolman disease: phenotypic variants of lysosomal acid cholesteryl ester hydrolase deficiency. Am J Hum Genet, 1984; 36:1190–1203

663. Philippart M, Durand P, Borrone C. Neutral lipid storage with acid lipase deficiency: a new variant of Wolman's disease with features of the Senior syndrome. Pediatr Res, 1982; 16:954–959

664. Schiff L, Schubert WK, McAdams AJ, Spiegel EL, O'Donnell JF. Hepatic cholesterol ester storage disease, a familial disorder. I. Clinical aspects. Am J Med, 1968; 44:538–546

665. Partin JC, Schubert WK. Small intestinal mucosa in cholesterol ester storage disease. A light and electron microscope study. Gastroenterology, 1969; 57:542–558

666. Beaudet al., Ferry GD, Nichols BL, Jr, Rosenberg HS. Cholesterol ester storage disease: clinical, biochemical, and pathological studies. J Pediatr, 1977; 90:910–914

667. Gasche C, Aslanidis C, Kain R et al. A novel variant of lysosomal acid lipase in cholesteryl ester storage disease associated with mild phenotype and improvement on lovastatin. J Hepatol, 1997; 27:744–750

668. Sloan HR, Fredrickson DS. Enzyme deficiency in cholesteryl ester storage disease. J Clin Invest, 1972; 51:1923–1926

669. Michels VV, Driscoll DJ, Ferry GD, Duff DF, Beaudet AL. Pulmonary vascular obstruction associated with cholesteryl ester storage disease. J Pediatr, 1979; 94:621–623

670. Dincsoy HP, Rolfes DB, McGraw CA, Schubert WK. Cholesterol ester storage disease and mesenteric lipodystrophy. Am J Clin Pathol, 1984; 81:263–269

671. Elleder M, Chlumska A, Hyanek J et al. Subclinical course of cholesterol ester storage disease in an adult with hypercholesterolemia, accelerated atherosclerosis, and liver cancer. J Hepatol, 2000; 32:528–534

672. Besley GT, Broadhead DM, Lawlor E et al. Cholesterol ester storage disease in an adult presenting with sea-blue histiocytosis. Clin Genet, 1984; 26:195–203

673. Coates PM, Cortner JA, Mennuti MT, Wheeler JE. Prenatal diagnosis of Wolman disease. Am J Med Genet, 1978; 2:397–407

674. Anderson RA, Byrum RS, Coates PM, Sando GN. Mutations at the lysosomal acid cholesteryl ester hydrolase gene locus in Wolman disease. Proc Natl Acad Sci USA, 1994; 91:2718–2722

675. Anderson RA, Bryson GM, Parks JS. Lysosomal acid lipase mutations that determine phenotype in Wolman and cholesterol ester storage disease. Mol Genet Metab, 1999; 68:333–345

676. Klima H, Ullrich K, Aslanidis C, Fehringer P, Lackner KJ, Schmitz G. A splice junction mutation causes deletion of a 72-base exon from the mRNA for lysosomal acid lipase in a patient with cholesteryl ester storage disease. J Clin Invest, 1993; 92:2713–2718

677. Lohse P, Maas S, Lohse P et al. Compound heterozygosity for a Wolman mutation is frequent among patients with cholesteryl ester storage disease. J Lipid Res, 2000; 41:23–31

678. Wolman M. Wolman disease and its treatment. Clin Pediatr (Phila), 1995; 34:207–212

679. Hobbe JR. Wolman's disease corrected by displacement bone marrow transplantation with immunoprophylaxis. Plasma Ther Transfusion Technology, 1985; 6:221–246

680. Krivit W, Freese D, Chan KW, Kulkarni R. Wolman's disease: a review of treatment with bone marrow transplantation and

considerations for the future. Bone Marrow Transplant, 1992; 10(Suppl 1):97–101

681. Krivit W, Peters C, Dusenbery K et al. Wolman disease successfully treated by bone marrow transplantation. Bone Marrow Transplant, 2000; 26:567–570

682. Di Bisceglie AM, Ishak KG, Rabin L, Hoeg JM. Cholesteryl ester storage disease: hepatopathology and effects of therapy with lovastatin. Hepatology, 1990; 11:764–772

683. Glueck CJ, Lichtenstein P, Tracy T, Speirs J. Safety and efficacy of treatment of pediatric cholesteryl ester storage disease with lovastatin. Pediatr Res, 1992; 32:559–565

684. Iverson SA, Cairns SR, Ward CP, Fensom AH. Asymptomatic cholesteryl ester storage disease in an adult controlled with simvastatin. Ann Clin Biochem, 1997; 34:433–436

685. Tarantino MD, McNamara DJ, Granstrom P et al. Lovastatin therapy for cholesterol ester storage disease in two sisters. J Pediatr, 1991; 118:131–135

686. Arterburn JN, Lee WM, Wood RP, Shaw BW, Markin RS. Orthotopic liver transplantation for cholesteryl ester storage disease. J Clin Gastroenterol, 1991; 13:482–485

687. Ferry GD, Whisennand HH, Finegold MJ, Alpert E, Glombicki A. Liver transplantation for cholesteryl ester storage disease. J Pediatr Gastroenterol Nutr, 1991; 12:376–378

688. Kale AS, Ferry GD, Hawkins EP. End-stage renal disease in a patient with cholesterol ester storage disease following successful liver transplantation and cyclosporine immunosuppression. J Pediatr Gastroenterol Nutr, 1995; 20:95–97

689. Honda Y, Kuriyama M, Higuchi I, Fujiyama J, Yoshida H, Osame M. Muscular involvement in lysosomal acid lipase deficiency in rats. J Neurol Sci, 1992; 108:189–195

690. Kuriwaki K, Yoshida H. Morphological characteristics of lipid accumulation in liver-constituting cells of acid lipase deficiency rats (Wolman's disease model rats). Pathol Int, 1999; 49:291–297

691. Nakagawa H, Matsubara S, Kuriyama M et al. Cloning of rat lysosomal acid lipase cDNA and identification of the mutation in the rat model of Wolman's disease. J Lipid Res, 1995; 36:2212–2218

692. Du H, Heur M, Witte DP, Ameis D, Grabowski GA. Lysosomal acid lipase deficiency: correction of lipid storage by adenovirus-mediated gene transfer in mice. Hum Gene Ther, 2002; 13:1361–1372

693. Brown MS, Sobhani MK, Brunschede GY, Goldstein JL. Restoration of a regulatory response to low density lipoprotein in acid lipase-deficient human fibroblasts. J Biol Chem, 1976; 251:3277–3286

694. Kyreakecks EC, Paul B, Balient JA. Lipid accumulation and acid lipase deficiency in fibroblasts from a family with Wolman's disease and their apparent correction in vitro. J Clin Med, 1992; 80:810–816

695. Poznansky MJ, Hutchison SK, Davis PJ. Enzyme replacement therapy in fibroblasts from a patient with cholesteryl ester storage disease. Faseb J, 1989; 3:152–156

696. Crocker AC, Vawter GW, Neuhauser EBD, Bonkowsky A. Wolman's disease: three new patients with a previously described lipidosis. Pediatrics, 1965; 35:627–640

697. Marshall WC, Ockenden BG, Fosbrooke AS, Cumings JN. Wolman's disease. A rare lipidosis with adrenal calcification. Arch Dis Child, 1969; 46:331–341

698. Miller R, Bialer MG, Rogers F, Johnson HT, Allen RV, Hennigar GR. Wolman's disease: report of a case with multiple studies. Arch Pathol Lab Med, 1982; 106:41–45

699. Wolman M, Sterk VV, Gatt S, Frenkel M. Primary familial xanthomatosis with involvement and calcification of the adrenals. Pediatrics, 1961; 28:742–745

700. Lake BD, Patrick AD. Wolman's disease: deficiency of E600 resistant acid esterase with storage of lipids in lysosomes. J Pediatr, 1970; 76:262–266

701. Lough J, Fawcett J, Wiegensberg B. Wolman's disease. An electron microscopic, histochemical, and biochemical study. Arch Pathol, 1970; 89:103–110

702. Boldrini R, Devito R, Biselli R, Filocamo M, Bosman C. Wolman disease and cholesteryl ester storage disease diagnosed by histological and ultrastructural examination of intestinal and liver biopsy. Pathol Res Pract, 2004; 200:231–240

703. Landing BH, Silverman FN, Craig JM, Jacoby MD, Lahey ME, Chadwick DL. Familial neurovisceral lipidosis. An analysis of eight cases of a syndrome previously reported as 'Hurler-variant', 'pseudo-Hurler,' and 'Tay-Sachs disease with visceral involvement'. Am J Dis Child, 1964; 108:503–522

704. O'Brien JS. Generalized gangliosidosis. J Pediatr, 1969; 75:167–186

705. Hanson M, Lupski JR, Hicks J, Metry D. Association of dermal melanocytosis with lysosomal storage disease: clinical features and hypotheses regarding pathogenesis. Arch Dermatol, 2003; 139:916–920

706. Folkerth RD, Alroy J, Bhan I, Kaye EM. Infantile GM1 gangliosidosis: Complete morphology and histochemistry of two autopsy cases, with particular reference to delayed central nervous system myelination. Pediatr Develop Pathol, 2000; 3:73–86

707. Takano T, Yamanouchi Y. Assignment of human beta-galactosidase-A gene to 3p21.33 by fluorescence in situ hybridization. Hum Genet, 1993; 92:403–404

708. Hoogeveen AT, Reuser AJJ, Kroos M, Galjaard H. GM1-gangliosidosis: defective recognition site on beta-galactosidase precursor. J Biol Chem, 1986; 261:5702–5704

709. Petrelli M, Blair JD. The liver in GM gangliosidosis types 1 and 2. Arch Pathol, 1975; 99:111–116

710. O'Brien JS. Ganglioside-storage diseases. N Engl J Med, 1971; 284:893–896

711. Shield JP, Stone J, Steward CG. Bone marrow transplantation correcting beta-galactosidase activity does not influence neurological outcome in juvenile GM1-gangliosidosis. J Inherit Metab Dis, 2005; 28:797–798

712. Volk BW, Wallace BJ. The liver in lipidosis. An electron microscopic and histochemical study. Am J Pathol, 1966; 49:203–225

713. Alroy J, Orgad U, DeGasperi R et al. Canine G1M1-gangliosidosis: a clinical, morphologic, histochemical and biochemical comparison of two different models. Am J Pathol, 1992; 140:675–689

714. Taylor HA, Stevenson RE, Parks SE. Beta-galactosidase deficiency: studies of two patients with prolonged survival. Am J Med Genet, 1980; 5:235–245

715. Wenger DA, Goodman SI, Myers GB. Beta-galactosidase deficiency in young adults. Lancet, 1974; ii:1319–1320 (letter)

716. Kaback MM, Rimoin DL, O'Brien JS. Tay-Sachs disease: screening and prevention. 1977, New York: Alan R Liss

717. Myerowitz R. Tay–Sachs disease-causing mutations and neutral polymorphisms in the Hex A gene. Hum Mutat, 1997; 9:195–208

718. Inui K, Grebner EE, Jackson LG, Wenger DA. Juvenile GM2 gangliosidosis (A(M)B variant): inability to activate hexosaminidase A by activator protein. Am J Hum Genet, 1983; 35:551–564

719. Sandhoff K, Andreae U, Jatzkewitz H. Deficient hexosaminidase activity in an exceptional case of Tay–Sachs disease with additional storage of kidney globoside in visceral organs. Life Sci, 1968; 7:283–288

720. Wood S, MacDougall BG. Juvenile Sandhoff disease: some properties of the residual hexosaminidase in cultured fibroblasts. Am J Hum Genet, 1976; 28:489–495

721. Neufeld EF. Natural history and inherited disorders of a lysosomal enzyme, beta-hexosaminidase. J Biol Chem, 1989; 264:10927–10930

722. Mattei JF, Balestrazzi P, Baeteman MA, Mattei MG. De novo balanced translocation (5;13)(q11;p11) in a child with Franceschetti syndrome and significant decrease of hexosaminidase B (abstract). Cytogenet Cell Genet, 1984; 37:532

723. O'Dowd BF, Klavins MH, Willard HF, Gravel R, Lowden JA, Mahuran DJ. Molecular heterogeneity in the infantile and juvenile forms of Sandhoff disease (0-variant G(M2) gangliosidosis). J Biol Chem, 1986; 261:12680–12685

724. Desnick RJ, Simmons RL, Allen KY et al. Correction of enzymatic deficiencies by renal transplantation: Fabry's disease. Surgery, 1972; 72:203–211

725. Cantor RM, Kaback MM. Sandhoff disease (SHD) heterozygote frequencies (HF) in North American (NA) Jewish (J) and non-Jewish (NJ) populations: implications for carrier (C) screening. Am J Hum Genet, 1985; 37:A48. (Abstract)

726. Desnick RJ, Krivit W, Sharp HL. In utero diagnosis of Sandhoff's disease. Biochem Biophys Res Commun, 1973; 51:20–24

727. Krivit W, Desnick RJ, Lee J et al. Generalized accumulation of neutral glycosphingolipid with GM1 ganglioside accumulation in the brain, Sandhoff's disease (variant of Tay-Sach's disease). Am J Med, 1972; 52:763–770

728. Hadfield MG, Mammes P, David PB. The pathology of Sandhoff's disease. J Pathol, 1977; 123:137–144

729. Lukacs Z, Keil A, Kohlschutter A, Beck M, Mengel E. The ratio of alpha-galactosidase to beta-glucuronidase activities in dried blood for the identification of female Fabry disease patients. J Inherit Metab Dis, 2005; 28:803–805

730. Masson C, Cisse I, Simon V, Insalaco P, Audran M. Fabry disease: a review. Joint Bone Spine, 2004; 71:381–383

731. Brady RO, Gal AE, Bradley RM, Martensson E, Warshaw AL, Laster L. Enzymatic defect in Fabry's disease, Ceramide trihexosidase deficiency. N Engl J Med, 1967; 276:1163–1167

732. Shows TB, Brown JA, Haley LL et al. Assignment of alpha-galactosidase (alpha GAL) to the q22 leads to qter region of the X chromosome in man. Cytogenet Cell Genet, 1978; 22:541–544

733. Schafer E, Baron K, Widmer U et al. Thirty-four novel mutations of the GLA gene in 121 patients with Fabry disease. Hum Mutat, 2005; 25:412

734. Banikazemi M, Ullman T, Desnick RJ. Gastrointestinal manifestations of Fabry disease: clinical response to enzyme replacement therapy. Mol Genet Metab, 2005; 85:255–259

735. Desnick RJ, Bishop DF. Fabry disease; alpha-galactosidase deficiency; Shindler Disease; alpha-N acetylgalactosaminidase deficiency. In: The metabolic and molecular basis of inherited disease. C.R. Scriver, A.L. Beaudet, W.S. Sly, J. Valle, Editors. 1989, McGraw-Hill: New York. p. 1751–1796

736. Rodriquez FH, Hoffman EO, Ordinario AT et al. Fabry's disease in a heterozygous woman. Arch Pathol Lab Med, 1985; 109:89–91

737. Shah JS, Elliott PM. Fabry disease and the heart: an overview of the natural history and the effect of enzyme replacement therapy. Acta Paediatr Suppl, 2005; 94(447):11–14; discussion 9–10

738. Ichinose M, Nakayama M, Ohashi T, Utsunomiya Y, Kobayashi M, Eto Y. Significance of screening for Fabry disease among male dialysis patients. Clin Exp Nephrol, 2005; 9:228–232

739. Nakao S, Kodama C, Takenaka T et al. Fabry disease: detection of undiagnosed hemodialysis patients and identification of a 'renal variant' phenotype. Kidney Int, 2003; 64:801–807

740. Kitagawa T, Ishige N, Suzuki K et al. Non-invasive screening method for Fabry disease by measuring globotriaosylceramide in whole urine samples using tandem mass spectrometry. Mol Genet Metab, 2005; 85:196–202

741. Utsumi K, Mitsuhashi F, Asahi K et al. Enzyme replacement therapy for Fabry disease: morphologic and histochemical changes in the urinary sediments. Clin Chim Acta, 2005; 360:103–107

742. Clarke JT, Iwanochko RM. Enzyme replacement therapy of Fabry disease. Mol Neurobiol, 2005; 32:43–50

743. Brady RO, King FM. Fabry's disease. In: Peripheral neuropathy. P.J. Dyck, P.K. Thomas, and E.H. Lambert, Editors. 1975, Saunders: New York. p. 914–927

744. Meuwissen SGM, Dingemans KP, Stryland A, Taer JM, Ooms BCM. Ultrastructural and biochemical liver analyses in Fabry's disease. Hepatology, 1982; 2:263–268

745. Faraggiana T, Churg J, Grishman E et al. Light-and electron-microscopic histochemistry of Fabry's disease. Am J Pathol, 1981; 103:247–262

746. Kanda A, Nakao S, Tsuyama S, Murata F, Kanazaki T. Fabry's disease: ultrastructural lectin histochemical analyses of lysosomal deposits. Virchows Arch, 2000; 436:36–42

747. Kanekura T, Fukushige T, Kanda A et al. Immunoelectron-microscopic detection of globotriaosylceramide accumulated in the skin of patients with Fabry disease. Br J Dermatol, 2005; 153:544–548

748. Geurts van Kessel AHM, Westerveld A, de Groot PG, Meera Khan P, Hagemeijer A. Regional localization of the genes coding for human ACO2, ARSA, and NAGA on chromosome 22. Cytogenet. Cell Genet, 1980; 28:169–172

749. Gieselmann V, Zlotogora J, Harris A, Wenger DA, Morris CP. Molecular genetics of metachromatic leukodystrophy. Hum Mutat, 1994; 4:233–242

750. Kihara H. Genetic heterogeneity in metachromatic leukodystrophy. Am J Hum Genet, 1982; 34:171–181

751. von Figura K, Steckel F, Conary J, Hasilik A, Shaw E. Heterogeneity in late-onset metachromatic leukodystrophy: effect of inhibitors of cysteine proteinases. Am J Hum Genet, 1986; 39:371–382

752. Betts TA, Smith WT, Kelly RE. Adult metachromatic leukodystrophy (sulphatide lipidosis) simulating acute schizophrenia: report of a case. Neurology, 1968; 18:1140–1142

753. Baldinger S, Pierpont ME, Wenger DA. Pseudodeficiency of arylsulfatase A: a counseling dilemma. Clin Genet, 1987; 31:70–76

754. Greene H, Hug G, Schubert WK. Arylsulfatase A in the urine and metachromatic leukodystrophy. J Pediatr, 1967; 71:709–711

755. Kapaun P, Dittmann RW, Granitzny B et al. Slow progression of juvenile metachromatic leukodystrophy 6 years after bone marrow transplantation. J Child Neurol, 1999; 14:222–228

756. Malm G, Ringden O, Winiarski J et al. Clinical outcome in four children with metachromatic leukodystrophy treated by bone marrow transplant. Bone Marrow Transplant, 1996; 17:1003–1008

757. Austin J. Metachromatic leukodystrophy (sulfatide lipidosis). In: Lysosomes and storage diseases. H.G. Hers and F. Van Hoof, Editors. 1973, Academic Press: New York. p. 411–437

758. Hagberg B, Sourander P, Svennerholm L. Sulfatide lipidosis in childhood. Am J Dis Child, 1962; 104:644–656

759. Wolfe HJ, Pietra GG. The visceral lesions of metachromatic leukodystrophy. Am J Pathol, 1964; 44:921–930

760. Burgess JH, Kalfayan B, Shingaard RK, Gilbert E. Papillomatosis of the gallbladder associated with metachromatic leukodystrophy. Arch Pathol Lab Med, 1985; 109:79–81

761. Dalinka MK, Rosen RA, Kurth RJ, Hemming VG. Metachromatic leukodystrophy, a cause of cholelithiasis in childhood. Am J Dig Dis, 1969; 14:603–606

762. Dische MR. Metachromatic leukodystrophic polyposis of the gallbladder. J Pathol Bacteriol, 1969; 97:388–390

763. Kohn R. Papillomatosis of the gallbladder in metachromatic leukodystrophy. Am J Clin Pathol, 1969; 52:737–740

764. Tesluk H, Munn RJ, Schwartz MZ, Ruebner BH. Papillomatous transformation of the gallbladder in metachromatic leukodystrophy. Pediatr Pathol, 1989; 9:741–746

765. Warfel KA, Hull MT. Villous papilloma of the gallbladder in association with leukodystrophy. Hum Pathol, 1984; 15:1192–1194

766. Prophet EB, Mills B, Arrington JB, Sobin LS. Laboratory methods in histotechnology. 1992, American Registry of Pathology: Washington, D.C. p. 97

767. Bjorkhem I, Fausa O, Hopen G, Oftebro H, Pedersen JI, Skrede S. Role of the 26-hydroxylase in the biosynthesis of bile acids in the normal state and in cerebrotendinous xanthomatosis: an in vivo study. J Clin Invest, 1983; 71:142–148

768. Oftebro H, Bjorkhem I, Skrede S, Schreiner A, Pedersen JI. Cerebrotendinous xanthomatosis: a defect in mitochondrial 26-hydroxylation required for normal biosynthesis of cholic acid. J Clin Invest, 1980; 65:1418–1430

769. Skrede S, Bjorkhem I, Kvittingen EA et al. Demonstration of 26-hydroxylation of C27-steroids in human skin fibroblasts, and a deficiency of this activity in cerebrotendinous xanthomatosis. J Clin Invest, 1986; 78:729–735

770. Cali JJ, Hsieh CL, Francke U et al. Mutations in the bile acid biosynthetic enzyme sterol 27-hydroxylase underlie cerebrotendinous xanthomatosis. J Biol Chem, 1991; 266:7779–7783

771. Lee MH, Hazard S, Carpten JD et al. Fine-mapping, mutation analyses, and structural mapping of cerebrotendinous xanthomatosis in U.S. pedigrees. J Lipid Res, 2001; 42:159–169

772. Clayton PT, Verrips A, Sistermans E, Mann A, Mieli-Vergani G, Wevers R. Mutations in the sterol 27-hydroxylase gene (CYP27A) cause hepatitis of infancy as well as cerebrotendinous xanthomatosis. J Inherit Metab Dis, 2002; 25:501–513

773. Moghadasian MH. Cerebrotendinous xanthomatosis: clinical course, genotypes and metabolic backgrounds. Clin Invest Med, 2004; 27:42–50

774. von Bahr S, Bjorkhem I, Van't Hooft F et al. Mutation in the sterol 27-hydroxylase gene associated with fatal cholestasis in infancy. J Pediatr Gastroenterol Nutr, 2005; 40:481–486

775. Cruysberg JRM, Wevers RA, Tolboom JJM. Juvenile cataract associated with chronic diarrhea in pediatric cerebrotendinous xanthomatosis. Am J Ophthal, 1991; 112:606–607 (letter)

776. Berginer VM, Salen G, Shefer S. Long-term treatment of cerebrotendinous xanthomatosis with chenodeoxycholic acid. N Engl J Med, 1984; 311:1649–1652

777. Mosbach EH. Cerebrotendinous xanthomatosis. In: Liver in metabolic diseases. L. Bianchi, W. Gerok, L. Landmann, K. Sickinger, G.A. Stalder, Editors. 1983, MTP Press: Boston. p. 65–71

778. Valdivielso P, Calandra S, Duran JC, Garuti R, Herrera E, Gonzalez P. Coronary heart disease in a patient with cerebrotendinous xanthomatosis. J Intern Med, 2004; 255:680–683

779. Kuriyama M, Tokimura Y, Fujiyama J, Utatsu Y, Osame M. Treatment of cerebrotendinous xanthomatosis: effects of chenodeoxycholic acid, pravastatin, and combined use. J Neurol Sci, 1994; 125:22–28

780. Ito S, Kuwabara S, Sakakibara R et al. Combined treatment with LDL-apheresis, chenodeoxycholic acid and HMG-CoA reductase inhibitor for cerebrotendinous xanthomatosis. J Neurol Sci, 2003; 216:179–182

781. Salen G, Zaki G, Sobesin S, Boehme D, Shefer S, Mosbach EH. Intrahepatic pigment and crystal forms in patients with cerebrotendinous xanthomatosis (C7X). Gastroenterology, 1978; 74:82–89

782. Boehme DH, Sobel HJ, Marquet E, Salen G. Liver in cerebro-tendinous xanthomatosis (CTX): a histochemical and EM study of four cases. Pathol Res Pract, 1980; 170:192–201

783. Koch J, Gartner S, Li CM et al. Molecular cloning and characterization of a full-length complementary DNA encoding human acid ceramidase: identification of the first molecular lesion causing Farber disease. J Biol Chem, 1996; 271:33110–33115

784. Li CM, Park JH, He X et al. The human acid ceramidase gene (ASAH): structure, chromosomal location, mutation analysis, and expression. Genomics, 1999; 62:223–231

785. Moser HW, Moser AB, Chen WW, Schram AW. Ceramidase deficiency: Farber lipogranulomatosis. In: The metabolic basis of inherited disease. C.R. Scriver et al., Editors. 1989, McGraw-Hill: New York. p. 1645–1654

786. Nowaczyk MJM, Feigenbaum A, Silver MM, Callahan J, Levin A, Jay V. Bone marrow involvement and obstructive jaundice in Farber lipogranulomatosis: clinical and autopsy report of a new case. J Inherit Metab Dis, 1996; 19:655–660

787. Zarbin MA, Green WR, Moser HW, Morton SJ. Farber's disease: light and electron microscopic study of the eye. Arch Ophthal, 1985; 103:73–80

788. Rutsaert J, Tondeur M, Vamos-Hurwitz E, Dustin P. The cellular lesions of Farber's disease and their experimental reproduction in tissue culture. Lab Invest, 1977; 36:474–480

789. Abul-Haj SK, Martz DG, Douglas WF, Geppert LJ. Farber's disease. Report of a case with observations and notes on the nature of the stored material. J Pediatr, 1962; 61:221–232

790. Antonarakis S, Valle D, Moser HW, Moser A, Qualinan SJ, Zinkham WH. Phenotypic variability in siblings with Farber's disease. J Pediatr, 1984; 104:406–409

791. Crocker AC, Cohen J, Farber S. The 'lipogranulomatosis' syndrome: review with report of patient showing milder involvement. In: Inborn diseases of sphingolipid metabolism. S.M. Aronson and B.W. Volk, Editors. 1967, Pergamon: Oxford. p. 485–503

792. Burck U, Moser HW, Goebel HH, Gruttner R, Held KR. A case of lipogranulomatosis Farber: some clinical and ultrastructural aspects. Eur J Pediatr, 1985; 143:203–208

793. Tanaka T, Takahashi K, Hakozaki H, Kimoto H, Suzuki Y. Farber's disease (disseminated lipogranulomatosis): a pathological histochemical and ultrastructural study. Acta Pathol Jpn, 1979; 29:135–155

794. Van Hoof F, Hers HG. Other lysosomal storage disorders. In: Lysosomes and storage diseases. H.G. Hers and F. Van Hoof, Editors. 1973, Academic Press: New York. p. 553–573

795. Koga M, Ishihara T, Uchino F. Farber bodies found in murine phagocytes after injection of ceramides and related sphingolipids. Virchows Arch B Cell Pathol, 1992; 82:297–302

796. Rauch HJ, Aubock L. 'Banana bodies' in disseminated lipogranulomatosis (Farber's disease). Am J Dermatopathol, 1983; 5:263–266

797. Brady RO, Kanfer JN, Bradley RM, Shapiro D. Demonstration of a deficiency of glucocerebroside-cleaving enzyme in Gaucher's disease. J Clin Invest, 1966; 45:1112–1115

798. Cox TM, Schofield JP. Gaucher's disease: clinical features and natural history. Baillieres Clin Haematol, 1997; 10:657–689

799. Beutler E. Gaucher's disease. N Engl J Med, 1991; 325:1354–1360

800. Zimran A, Kay A, Gelbart T et al. Gaucher disease. Clinical, 1992; 71:337–353

801. Goldblatt J, Beighton P. Cutaneous manifestations of Gaucher disease. Br J Dermatol, 1984; 111:331–334

802. Lanir A, Hadar H, Cohen I et al. Gaucher disease: assessment with MR imaging. Radiology, 1986; 161:239–244

803. Charrow J, Andersson HC, Kaplan P et al. The Gaucher registry: demographics and disease characteristics of 1698 patients with Gaucher disease. Arch Intern Med, 2000; 160:2835–2843

804. Schneider EL, Epstein CJ, Kaback MJ, Brandes D. Severe pulmonary involvement in adult Gaucher's disease. Report of three cases and review of the literature. Am J Med, 1977; 63:475–480

805. Lachmann RH, Wight DGD, Lomas DJ et al. Massive hepatic fibrosis in Gaucher's disease: Clinicopathological and radiological features. Q J Med, 2000; 93:237–244

806. Perel Y, Bioulac-Sage P, Chateil JF et al. Gaucher's disease and fatal hepatic fibrosis despite prolonged enzyme replacement therapy. Pediatrics, 2002; 109:1170–1173

807. Barbier J, Devisme L, Dobbelaere D, Noizet O, Nelken B, Gottrand F. Neonatal cholestasis and infantile Gaucher disease: a case report. Acta Paediatr, 2002; 91:1399–1401

808. Cohen IJ, Katz K, Freud E, Zer M, Zaizov R. Long-term follow-up of partial splenectomy in Gaucher's disease. Am J Surg, 1992; 164:345–347

809. Rubin M, Yampolski I, Lambrozo R, Zaizov R, Dintsman M. Partial splenectomy in Gaucher's disease. J Pediatr Surg, 1986; 21:125–128

810. Hill SC, Damaska BM, Ling A et al. Gaucher disease: abdominal MR imaging findings in 46 patients. Radiology, 1992; 184:561–566

811. Rosenbloom BE, Weinreb NJ, Zimran A, Kacena KA, Charrow J, Ward E. Gaucher disease and cancer incidence: a study from the Gaucher Registry. Blood, 2005; 105:4569–4572

812. Ginsburg SJ, Groll M. Hydrops fetalis due to infantile Gaucher's disease. J Pediatr, 1973; 82:1046–1048

813. Lui K, Commens C, Choong R, Jaworski R. Collodion babies with Gaucher's disease. Arch Dis Child, 1988; 63:854–856

814. Sidransky E, Ginns EI. Clinical heterogeneity among patients with Gaucher's disease clinical conference. Jama, 1993; 269:1154–1157

815. Sidransky E, Sherer DM, Ginns EI. Gaucher disease in the neonate: a distinct Gaucher phenotype is analogous to a mouse model created by targeted disruption of the glucocerebrosidase gene. Pediatr Res, 1992; 32:494–498

816. Sun CC, Panny S, Combs J, Gutberlett R. Hydrops fetalis associated with Gaucher disease. Pathol Res Pract, 1984; 179:101–104

817. Stowens DW, Chu FC, Cogan DG, Barranger JA. Oculomotor deficits in Gaucher disease. In: Gaucher disease: A century of delineation and research. R.J. Desnick, S. Gait, and G.A. Grabowski, Editors. 1982, Alan R Liss: New York. p. 131–142

818. Brady RO, Barton NW, Grabowski GA. The role of neurogenetics in Gaucher disease. Arch Neurol, 1993; 50:1212–1224

819. Tokoro T, Gal AE, Gallo LL, Brady RO. Studies of the pathogenesis of Gaucher's disease: tissue distribution and biliary excretion of 14C L-glucosylceramide in rats. J Lipid Res, 1987; 28:968–972

820. Abrahamov A, Elstein D, Gross-Tsur V et al. Gaucher's disease variant characterised by progressive calcification of heart valves and unique genotype. Lancet, 1995; 346:1000–1003

821. James SP, Stromeyer FW, Chang C, Barranger JA. Liver abnormalities in patients with Gaucher's disease. Gastroenterology, 1981; 80:126–133

822. Stone R, Benson J, Tronic B, Brennan T. Hepatic calcifications in a patient with Gaucher's disease. Am J Gastroenterol, 1982; 77:95–98

823. Goker-Alpan O, Schiffmann R, Park JK, Stubblefield BK, Tayebi N, Sidransky E. Phenotypic continuum in neuronopathic Gaucher disease: an intermediate phenotype between type 2 and type 3. J Pediatr, 2003; 143:273–276

824. Barneveld RA, Keijzer W, Tegelaers FP et al. Assignment of the gene coding for human beta-glucocerebrosidase to the region q21–q31 of chromosome 1 using monoclonal antibodies. Hum Genet, 1983; 64:227–231

825. Horowitz M, Wilder S, Horowitz Z, Reiner O, Gelbart T, Beutler E. The human glucocerebrosidase gene and pseudogene: structure and evolution. Genomics, 1989; 4:87–96

826. Jmoudiak M, Futerman AH. Gaucher disease: pathological mechanisms and modern management. Br J Haematol, 2005; 129:178–188

827. Grabowski GA, Horowitz M. Gaucher's disease: molecular, genetic and enzymological aspects. Baillieres Clin Haematol, 1997; 10:635–656

828. Ron I, Horowitz M. ER retention and degradation as the molecular basis underlying Gaucher disease heterogeneity. Hum Mol Genet, 2005; 14:2387–2398

829. Schmitz M, Alfalah M, Aerts JM, Naim HY, Zimmer KP. Impaired trafficking of mutants of lysosomal glucocerebrosidase in Gaucher's disease. Int J Biochem Cell Biol, 2005; 37:2310–2320

830. Christomanou H, Chabas A, Pampols T, Guardiola A. Activator protein deficient Gaucher's disease. A second patient with the newly identified lipid storage disorder. Klin Wochenschr, 1989; 67:999–1003

831. Pampols T, Pineda M, Giros ML et al. Neuronopathic juvenile glucosylceramidosis due to sap-C deficiency: clinical course, neuropathology and brain lipid composition in this Gaucher disease variant. Acta Neuropathol (Berl), 1999; 97:91–97

832. Barton NW, Brady RO, Dambrosia JM et al. Replacement therapy for inherited enzyme deficiency-macrophage-targeted glucocerebrosidase for Gaucher's disease. N Engl J Med, 1991; 324:1464–1470

833. Grabowski GA, Barton NW, Pastores G et al. Enzyme therapy in type 1 Gaucher disease: comparative efficacy of mannose-terminated glucocerebrosidase from natural and recombinant sources. Ann Intern Med, 1995; 122:33–39

834. Germain DP. Gaucher's disease: a paradigm for interventional genetics. Clin Genet, 2004; 65:77–86

835. Grabowski GA, Leslie N, Wenstrup R. Enzyme therapy for Gaucher disease: the first 5 years. Blood Rev, 1998; 12:115–133

836. Weinreb NJ, Barranger JA, Charrow J, Grabowski GA, Mankin HJ, Mistry P. Guidance on the use of miglustat for treating patients with type 1 Gaucher disease. Am J Hematol, 2005; 80:223–229

837. Vellodi A, Bembi B, de Villemeur TB et al. Management of neuronopathic Gaucher disease: a European consensus. J Inherit Metab Dis, 2001; 24:319–327

838. Carlson DE, Busuttil RW, Giudici TA, Barranger JA. Orthotopic liver transplantation in the treatment of complications of type 1 Gaucher disease. Transplantation, 1990; 49:1192–1194

839. Starzl TE, Demetris AJ, Trucco M et al. Chimerism after liver transplantation for type IV glycogen storage disease and type 1 Gaucher's disease. N Engl J Med, 1993; 328:745–749

840. Liu C, Bahnson AB, Dunigan JT, Watkins SC, Barranger JA. Long-term expression and secretion of human glucocerebrosidase by primary murine and human myoblasts and differentiated myotubes. J Mol Med, 1998; 76:773–781

841. Burns GF, Cawley JC, Flemans RJ et al. Surface marker and other characteristics of Gaucher's cells. J Clin Pathol, 1977; 30:981–983

842. Djaldetti M, Fishman P, Bessler H. The surface ultrastructure of Gaucher cells. Am J Clin Pathol, 1979; 71:146–150

843. Peters SP, Lee RE, Glen RH. Gaucher's disease. A review. Medicine, 1977; 56:425–442

844. Brady RO, King FM. Gaucher's disease. In: Lysosomes and storage diseases. H.G. Hers and F. Van Hoof, Editors. 1973, Academic Press: New York. p. 381–394

845. Benita Leon V, Garcia Cabezudo J, Gomex Tabera C et al. Enfermedad de Gaucher con cirrosis y gammapetia monoclonal benigna. Gastroenterol Hepatol, 1985; 8:354–357

846. Cadaval RL, Gonzalez-Campora R, Davidson HG, Vicente AM. Cirrosis hepatica en la enfermedad de Gaucher. Gastroenterol Hepatol, 1983; 6:299–301

847. Pastores GM, Barnett NL, Kolodny EH. An open-label, noncomparative study of miglustat in type I Gaucher disease: Efficacy and tolerability over 24 months of treatment. Clin Ther, 2005; 27:1215–1227

848. Patel SC, Davis GL, Barranger JA. Gaucher's disease in a patient with chronic active hepatitis. Am J Med, 1986; 80:523–525

849. Hibbs RG, Ferrans VJ, Cipriano PR, Tardiff KJ. A histochemical and electron microscopic study of Gaucher cells. Arch Pathol, 1970; 89:137–153

850. Lee RL. The bilayer nature of deposits occurring in Gaucher's disease. Arch Biochem Biophys, 1973; 159:259–266

851. Lorber M, Niemes JL. Identification of ferritin within Gaucher cells. An electron microscopic and immunofluorescent study. Acta Haematol, 1967; 37:18

852. Niemann A. Ein unbekanntes Krankenheitsbild. Jaherb Kinderheilkd, 1914; 79:1–10

853. Pick L. Uber die lipoidzellige Splenohepatomegalie Typus Niemann–Pick als Stoffwechselerkrankung. Med Klin, 1927; 23:1483–1488

854. Simonaro CM, Desnick RJ, McGovern MM, Wasserstein MP, Schuchman EH. The demographics and distribution of type B Niemann–Pick disease: novel mutations lead to new genotype/phenotype correlations. Am J Hum Genet, 2002; 71:1413–1419

855. Crocker AC, Farber S. Niemann–Pick disease: a review of eighteen patients. Medicine (Baltimore), 1958; 37:1–95

856. Meizner I, Levy A, Carmi R, Robinson C. Niemann–Pick disease associated with nonimmune hydrops fetalis. Am J Obstet Gyn, 1990; 163:128–129

857. Schoenfeld A, Abramovici A, Klibanski C et al. Placental ultrasonographic biochemical and histochemical studies in human fetuses affected with Niemann–Pick disease type A. Placenta, 1985; 6:33–43

858. Ashkenzi A, Yarom R, Gutman A et al. Niemann–Pick disease and giant cell transformation of the liver. Acta Paediatr Scand, 1971; 60:285–289

859. Schuchman ED, Desnick RJ. Niemann–Pick disease types A and B: acid sphingomyelinase deficiencies. In: The metabolic and molecular bases of inherited disease. C.R. Scriver, A.L. Beaudet, W.S. Sly et al., Editors. 1994, McGraw-Hill: New York. p. 2625–2639

860. LaBrune P, Bedossa P, Huguet P, Roset F, Vanier MT, Odièvre M. Fatal liver failure in two children with Niemann–Pick disease type B. J Pediatr Gastroenterol Nutr, 1991; 13:104–109

861. Smanik EJ, Tavill AS, Jacobs GH et al. Orthotopic liver transplantation in two adults with Niemann–Pick and Gaucher's disease. Implications for the treatment of inherited metabolic disease. Hepatology, 1993; 17:42–49

862. Takahashi T, Akiyama K, Tomihara M. Heterogeneity of liver disorder in type B-Niemann–Pick disease. Hum Pathol, 1997; 28:385–388

863. Tassoni JP, Fawaz KA, Johnston DE. Cirrhosis and portal hypertension in a patient with adult Niemann–Pick disease. Gastroenterology, 1991; 100:567–569

864. Wasserstein MP, Desnick RJ, Schuchman EH et al. The natural history of type B Niemann–Pick disease: results from a 10-year longitudinal study. Pediatrics, 2004; 114:e672–e677

865. Wasserstein MP, Larkin AE, Glass RB, Schuchman EH, Desnick RJ, McGovern MM. Growth restriction in children with type B Niemann–Pick disease. J Pediatr, 2003; 142:424–428

866. Vanier MT, Millat G. Niemann–Pick disease type C. Clin Genet, 2003; 64:269–281

867. Mukherjee S, Maxfield FR. Lipid and cholesterol trafficking in NPC. Biochim Biophys Acta, 2004; 1685:28–37

868. Willenborg M, Schmidt CK, Braun P et al. Mannose 6-phosphate receptors, Niemann–Pick C2 protein, and lysosomal cholesterol accumulation. J Lipid Res, 2005; 46:2559–2569

869. Park WD, O'Brien JF, Lundquist PA et al. Identification of 58 novel mutations in Niemann–Pick disease type C: correlation with biochemical phenotype and importance of PTC1-like domains in NPC1. Hum Mutat, 2003; 22:313–325

870. Fernandez-Valero EM, Ballart A, Iturriaga C et al. Identification of 25 new mutations in 40 unrelated Spanish Niemann–Pick type C patients: genotype-phenotype correlations. Clin Genet, 2005; 68:245–254

871. Maconochie IK, Chong S, Mieli-Vergani G, Lake BD, Mowat AP. Fetal ascites as an unusual presentation of Niemann–Pick disease type C. Arch Dis Child, 1989; 64:1391–1393

872. Kelly DA, Portmann B, Mowat AD, Sherlock S, Lake BD. Niemann–Pick Disease Type C. Diagnosis and outcome in children with particular reference to liver disease. J Pediatr, 1993; 123:242–247

873. Adam G, Breton RJ, Arawal M, Lake BD. Biliary atresia and meconium ileus associated with Niemann–Pick disease. J Pediatr Gastroenterol Nutr, 1988; 7:128–131

874. Vanier MT. Phenotypic and genetic heterogeneity in N-P disease type C: current knowledge and practical implications. Wien Klin Wochenschr, 1997; 109;3:68–73

875. Gartner JC, Jr., Bergman I, Malatuck JJ et al. Progression of neurovisceral storage disease with supranuclear ophthalmoplegia following orthotopic liver transplantation. Pediatrics, 1986; 77:104–106

876. Vanier MT, Pentchev P, Rodriguez-LaFrasse C, Rousson R. Niemann–Pick disease Type C an update. J Inherit Metab Dis, 1991; 14:580–595

877. Vanier MT. Prenatal diagnosis of Niemann–Pick diseases types A, B and C. Prenat Diagn, 2002; 22:630–632

878. Schiffmann R. Niemann–Pick disease Type C from bench to bedside. Jama, 1996; 276:561–564

879. Kruth HS, Weintraub H, Stivers T, Brady RO. A genetic storage disorder in BALB/c mice with a metabolic block in esterification of exogenous cholesterol. J Biol Chem, 1984; 259:5784–5791

880. Loftus SK, Morris JA, Castea ED et al. Murine model of Niemann–Pick C disease; mutation in a cholesterol homeostasis gene. Science, 1997; 277:232–235

881. Beltroy EP, Richardson JA, Horton JD, Turley SD, Dietschy JM. Cholesterol accumulation and liver cell death in mice with Niemann–Pick type C disease. Hepatology, 2005; 42:886–893

882. Barbon CM, Ziegler RJ, Li C et al. AAV8-mediated hepatic expression of acid sphingomyelinase corrects the metabolic defect in the visceral organs of a mouse model of Niemann–Pick disease. Mol Ther, 2005; 12:431–440

883. Dhami R, Schuchman EH. Mannose 6-phosphate receptor-mediated uptake is defective in acid sphingomyelinase-deficient macrophages: implications for Niemann–Pick disease enzyme replacement therapy. J Biol Chem, 2004; 279:1526–1532

884. Brady RO, King FM. Niemann–Pick disease. In: Lysosomes and storage diseases. H.G. Hers and F. Van Hoof, Editors. 1973, Academic Press: New York. p. 439–452

885. Elleder M, Smid F, Hymova H. Liver findings in Niemann–Pick disease type C. Histochem J, 1984; 16:1147–1170

886. Jaeken J, Proesmans W, Eggermont E et al. Niemann–Pick type C disease and early cholestasis in three brothers. Acta Paediatr Belg, 1980; 33:43–46

887. Rutledge JC. Case 5 Progressive neonatal liver disease due to Type C Niemann–Pick disease. Pediatr Pathol, 1989; 9:779–784

888. Semeraro LA, Riely CA, Kolodny EH, Dickerson GR, Gryboski JD. Niemann–Pick variant lipidosis presenting as -neonatal hepatitis. Gastroenterol Nutr, 1986; 5:492–500

889. Lynn R, Terry RD. Lipid histochemistry and electron microscopy in adult Niemann–Pick disease. Am J Med, 1964; 37:987–994

890. Wanders RJ, Waterham HR. Peroxisomal disorders I: biochemistry and genetics of peroxisome biogenesis disorders. Clin Genet, 2005; 67:107–133

891. Poggi-Travert F, Fournier B, Poll-The BT, Saudubray JM. Clinical approach to inherited peroxisomal disorders. J Inherit Metab Dis, 1995; 18 Suppl 1:1–18

892. Steinberg S, Chen L, Wei L et al. The PEX Gene Screen: molecular diagnosis of peroxisome biogenesis disorders in the Zellweger syndrome spectrum. Mol Genet Metab, 2004; 83:252–263

893. Crane DI, Maxwell MA, Paton BC. PEX1 mutations in the Zellweger spectrum of the peroxisome biogenesis disorders. Hum Mutat, 2005; 26:167–175

894. Chang CC, Gould SJ. Phenotype-genotype relationships in complementation group 3 of the peroxisome-biogenesis disorders. Am J Hum Genet, 1988; 63:1294–1306

895. Dodt G, Braverman N, Wong C et al. Mutations in the PTS1 receptor gene, PXR1, define complementation group 2 of the peroxisome biogenesis disorders. Nature Genet, 1995; 9:115–125

896. Fukuda S, Shimozawa N, Suzuki Y et al. Human peroxisome assembly factor-2 (PAF-2): a gene responsible for group C peroxisome biogenesis disorder in humans. Am J Hum Genet, 1996; 59:1210–1220

897. Moser AB, Rasmussen M, Naidu S et al. Phenotype of patients with peroxisomal disorders subdivided into sixteen complementation groups. J Pediatr, 1995; 127:13–22

898. Naritomi K, Hyakuna N, Suzuki Y, Orii T, Hirayama K. Zellweger syndrome and a microdeletion of the proximal long arm of chromosome 7. Hum Genet, 1988; 80:201–202

899. Reuber BE, Germain-Lee E, Collins CS et al. Mutations in PEX1 are the most common cause of peroxisome biogenesis disorders. Nature Genet, 1997; 17:445–448

900. Shimozawa N, Tsukamoto T, Suzuki Y et al. A human gene responsible for Zellweger syndrome that affects peroxisome assembly. Science, 1992; 255:1132–1134

901. Lazarow PB, Moser HW. Disorders of peroxisome biogenesis. In: The metabolic and molecular basis of inherited disease. C.R. Scriver, A.L. Beaudet, W.S. Sly, J. Valle, Editors. 1995, McGraw-Hill: New York. p. 2287–2324

902. Gootjes J, Mooijer PA, Dekker C et al. Biochemical markers predicting survival in peroxisome biogenesis disorders. Neurology, 2002; 59:1746–1749

903. Moser AE, Singh I, Brown FR et al. The cerebrohepatorenal (Zellweger) syndrome: increased levels and impaired degradation of very-long-chain fatty acids and their use in prenatal diagnosis. N Engl J Med, 1984; 310:1141–1146

904. Peduto A, Baumgartner MR, Verhoeven NM et al. Hyperpipecolic acidaemia: a diagnostic tool for peroxisomal disorders. Mol Genet Metab, 2004; 82:224–230

905. Depreter M, Espeel M, Roels F. Human peroxisomal disorders. Microsc Res Tech, 2003; 61:203–223

906. Versmold HT, Bremer HJ, Herzog V et al. A metabolic disorder similar to Zellweger syndrome with hepatic acatalasia and absence of peroxisomes, altered content and redox state of cytochromes, and infantile cirrhosis with hemosiderosis. Eur J Pediatr, 1977; 124:261–275

907. Santos MJ, Ojeda JM, Garrido J, Leighton F. Peroxisomal organization in normal and cerebrohepatorenal (Zellweger) syndrome fibroblasts. Proc Natl Acad Sci USA, 1985; 82:6556–6560

908. Martinez RD, Martin-Jimenez R, Matalon R. Zellweger syndrome. Pediatrics, 1991; 6:91–93

909. Vamecq J, Drayl JP, Van Hoof F et al. Multiple peroxisomal enzymatic deficiency disorders: A comparative biochemical, and morphological study of Zellweger cerebro-hepato-renal syndrome and neonatal adrenoleukodystrophy. Am J Pathol, 1986; 125:525–535

910. Wanders RJA, Barth PG, Schutgens RBH, Heymans HSA. Peroxisomal disorders: Post- and prenatal diagnosis based on a new classification with flow charts. Int Pediatr, 1996; 11:203–214

911. Dirkx R, Vanhorebeek I, Martens K et al. Absence of peroxisomes in mouse hepatocytes causes mitochondrial and ER abnormalities. Hepatology, 2005; 41:868–878

912. Faust PL, Banka D, Siriratsivawong R, Ng VG, Wikander TM. Peroxisome biogenesis disorders: the role of peroxisomes and metabolic dysfunction in developing brain. J Inherit Metab Dis, 2005; 28:369–383

913. Patton RG, Christie DL, Smith DW, Beckwith JB. Cerebro-hepatorenal syndrome of Zellweger. Am J Dis Child, 1972; 124:840–844

914. Danks DM, Tippett P, Adams C, Campbell P. Cerebro-hepato-renal syndrome of Zellweger: a report of eight cases with comments upon the incidence, the liver lesion, and a fault of pipecolic acid metabolism. J Pediatr, 1975; 86:382–387

915. Gilchrist RW, Gilbert EG, Goldfarb S et al. Studies of malformation syndromes of man. IIB. Cerebro-hepato-renal syndrome of Zellweger: comparative pathology. Eur J Pediatr, 1976; 122:99–118

916. Jan JE, Hardwick DF, Lowry RB, McCormick AQ. Cerebro-hepatorenal syndrome of Zellweger. Am J Dis Child, 1970; 119:274–277

917. Mooi WJ, Dingemans KP, Weerman MAVB, Jobsis AC, Heymans HSA, Barth PG. Ultrastructure of the liver in the cerebrohepatorenal syndrome of Zellweger. Ultrastruct Pathol, 1983; 5:135–144

918. Pfeifer U, Sandhage K. Licht- und Elekron microscopische Leberfunde beim Cerebro-Hepato-Renalen Syndrom nach Zellweger (Peroxisomen-Defizienz). Virch Arch A Pathol Anat Histol, 1979; 384:269–284

919. Goldfischer SL. Peroxisomal diseases. In: The liver. Biology and pathobiology. I.M. Arias, W.B. Jakoby, H. Popper, D. Schachter, Editors. 1988, Raven Press: New York. p. 255–265

920. Powers JM, Moser HW, Moser AB et al. Fetal cerebrohepatorenal (Zellweger) syndrome. Dysmorphic, 1985; 16:610–620

921. Smith DW, Opitz JM, Inhorn SL. A syndrome of multiple developmental defects including polycystic kidneys and intrahepatic dysgenesis in two siblings. J Pediatr, 1965; 67:617–624

922. Nakamura K, Takenouchi T, Aizawa M et al. Cerebro-hepato-renal syndrome of Zellweger. Clinical and autopsy findings and a review of previous cases in Japan. Acta Pathol Jpn, 1986; 36:1727–1735

923. Passarge E, McAdams AJ. Cerebro-hepato-renal syndrome: a newly recognized hereditary disorder of multiple congenital defects, including sudanophilic leukodystrophy, cirrhosis of the liver, and polycystic kidneys. J Pediatr, 1967; 71:691–702

924. Goldfischer S, Moore CL, Johnson AB et al. Peroxisomal and mitochondrial defects in the cerebro-hepato-renal syndrome. Science, 1973; 182:6264

925. Suzuki Y, Shimozawa N, Orii T et al. Zellweger-like syndrome— Deficiencies in several peroxisomal oxidative activities. J Pediatr, 1986; 108:25–32

926. Mathis RK, Watkins JB, Szczepanik-Van Leeuwen P, Lott IT. Liver in the cerebro-hepato-renal syndrome: defective bile acid synthesis and abnormal mitochondria. Gastroenterology, 1980; 79:1311–1317

927. Litwin JQ, Volki A, Muller-Hocker J, Hashimoto T, Fahimi HD. Immunohistochemical localization of peroxisomal enzymes in human liver biopsies. Am J Pathol, 1987; 128:141–150

928. Jaffe R, Crumrine P, Hashida Y, Moser HW. Neonatal adrenoleukodystrophy. Clinical, pathologic, and biochemical delineation of a syndrome affecting both males and females. Am J Pathol, 1982; 108:100–111

929. Moser HW, Moser AB, Chen WW, Watkins PA. Adrenoleukodystrophy and Zellweger syndrome in fatty acid oxidation: clinical, biochemical and molecular aspects. In: Progress in clinical and biological research. K. Tanaka, Editor. 1990, Alan R Liss: New York. p. 511–535

930. Dimmick JE. Liver pathology in neonatal adrenoleukodystrophy. Lab Invest, 1984; 50:3P (abstract)

931. Haas JE, Johnson ES, Farrell DL. Neonatal-onset adrenoleukodystrophy in a girl. Ann Neurol, 1982; 12:449–457

932. Hughes JL, Poulos A, Robertson E et al. Pathology of hepatic peroxisomes and mitochondria in patients with peroxisomal disorders. Virchows Arch A Pathol Anat, 1990; 416:255–264

933. Torvik A, Torp S, Kase BF, Skjeldal O, Stokke O. Infantile Refsum's disease. A generalized peroxisomal disorder. Case with postmortem examination. J Neurol Sci, 1988; 85:39–53

934. Budden SS, Kennaway NG, Buist NRM, Poulos A, Weleber RG. Dysmorphic syndrome with phytanic acid oxidase deficiency, abnormal very long chain fatty acids, and pipecolic acidemia: studies in four children. J Pediatr, 1986; 108:33–39

935. Roels F, Cornelis A, Poll-The BT et al. Hepatic peroxisomes are deficient in infantile Refsum disease. A cytochemical study of four cases. Am J Med Genet, 1986; 25:257–271

936. Scotto JM, Hadchouel M, Odievre M et al. Infantile phytanic acid storage disease, a possible variant of Refsum's disease: three cases, including ultrastructural studies of the liver. J Inherit Metab Dis, 1982; 5:83–90

937. Eyssen H, Parmentier G, Campernolle F, Boon J, Eggermont E. Trihydroxycoprostanic acid in the duodenal fluid of two children with intrahepatic bile duct anomalies. Biochim Biophys Acta, 1972; 273:212–221

938. Hanson RF, Isenberg JN, Williams GC. The metabolism of 3 alpha, 7 alpha 12 alpha-trihydroxy-5 beta-cholestan-26-oic acid in two siblings with cholestasis due to intrahepatic bile duct anomalies: an apparent inborn error of cholic acid synthesis. J Clin Invest, 1975; 56:577–587

939. Isenberg JN, Hanson RF, Williams G et al. A clinical experience with familial paucity of intrahepatic bile ducts associated with defective metabolism of trihydroxycoprostanic acid to cholic acid. In: Liver diseases in children. D. Alagille, Editor. 1976, Institut National de la Santé et de la Recherche Médicale: Paris. p. 43–56

940. Gootjes J, Skovby F, Christensen E, Wanders RJ, Ferdinandusse S. Reinvestigation of trihydroxycholestanoic acidemia reveals a peroxisome biogenesis disorder. Neurology, 2004; 62:2077–2081

941. Gibson KM, Hoffmann GF, Tanaka RD, Bishop RW, Chambliss KL. Mevalonate kinase map position 12q24. Chromosome Res, 1997; 5:150

942. Hoffmann GF, Charpentier C, Mayatepek E et al. Clinical and biochemical phenotype in 11 patients with mevalonic aciduria. Pediatrics, 1993; 91:915–921

943. Drenth JP, Haagsma CJ, van der Meer JW. Hyperimmunoglobulinemia D and periodic fever syndrome. The clinical spectrum in a series of 50 patients. International Hyper-IgD Study Group. Medicine (Baltimore), 1994; 73:133–144

944. Prietsch V, Mayatepek E, Krastel H et al. Mevalonate kinase deficiency: enlarging the clinical and biochemical spectrum. Pediatrics, 2003; 111:258–261

945. Hinson DD, Rogers ZR, Hoffmann GF et al. Hematological abnormalities and cholestatic liver disease in two patients with mevalonate kinase deficiency. Am J Med Genet, 1998; 78:408–412

946. D'Osualdo A, Picco P, Caroli F et al. MVK mutations and associated clinical features in Italian patients affected with

autoinflammatory disorders and recurrent fever. Eur J Hum Genet, 2005; 13:314–320

947. Houten SM, van Woerden CS, Wijburg FA, Wanders RJ, Waterham HR. Carrier frequency of the V377I (1129G > A) MVK mutation, associated with Hyper-IgD and periodic fever syndrome, in the Netherlands. Eur J Hum Genet, 2003; 11:196–200

948. Sokol RJ, Treem WR. Mitochondria and childhood liver diseases. J Pediatr Gastroenterol Nutr, 1999; 28:4–16

949. Morris AA. Mitochondrial respiratory chain disorders and the liver. Liver, 1999; 19:357–368

950. Zeviani M, Spinazzola A, Carelli V. Nuclear genes in mitochondrial disorders. Curr Opin Genet Dev, 2003; 13:262–270

951. Taylor RW, Turnbull DM. Mitochondrial DNA mutations in human disease. Nat Rev Genet, 2005; 6:389–402

952. Munnich A, Rotig A, Chretien D et al. Clinical presentation of mitochondrial disorders in childhood. J Inherit Metab Dis, 1996; 19:521–527

953. Naviaux RK. Developing a systematic approach to the diagnosis and classification of mitochondrial disease. Mitochondrion, 2004; 4:351–361

954. Boustany RN, Aprille JR, Halperin J, Levy H, DeLong GR. Mitochondrial cytochrome deficiency presenting as a myopathy with hypotonia, external ophthalmoplegia, and lactic acidosis in an infant and as fatal hepatopathy in a second cousin. Ann Neurol, 1983; 14:462–470

955. Sperl W, Ruitenbeek W, Trijbels JM, Sengers RC, Stadhouders AM, Guggenbichler JP. Mitochondrial myopathy with lactic acidaemia, Fanconi–De Toni–Debre syndrome and a disturbed succinate: cytochrome c oxidoreductase activity. Eur J Pediatr, 1988; 147:418–421

956. Parrot-Roulaud F, Carre M, Lamirau T et al. Fatal neonatal hepatocellular deficiency with lactic acidosis: a defect of the respiratory chain. J Inherit Metab Dis, 1991; 14:289–292

957. Fayon M, Lamireau T, Bioulac-Sage P et al. Fatal neonatal liver failure and mitochondrial cytopathy: an observation with antenatal ascites. Gastroenterology, 1992; 103:1332–1335

958. Edery P, Gerard B, Chretien D et al. Liver cytochrome c oxidase deficiency in a case of neonatal-onset hepatic failure. Eur J Pediatr, 1994; 153:190–194

959. Goncalves I, Hermans D, Chretien D et al. Mitochondrial respiratory chain defect: a new etiology for neonatal cholestasis and early liver insufficiency. J Hepatol, 1995; 23:290–294

960. Cormier-Daire V, Chretien D, Rustin P et al. Neonatal and delayed-onset liver involvement in disorders of oxidative phosphorylation. J Pediatr, 1997; 130:817–822

961. Mazzella M, Cerone R, Bonacci W et al. Severe complex I deficiency in a case of neonatal-onset lactic acidosis and fatal liver failure. Acta Paediatr, 1997; 86:326–329

962. Scheers I, Bachy V, Stephenne X, Sokal EM. Risk of hepatocellular carcinoma in liver mitochondrial respiratory chain disorders. J Pediatr, 2005; 146:414–417

963. Merante F, Petrova-Benedict R, MacKay N et al. A biochemically distinct form of cytochrome oxidase (COX) deficiency in the Saguenay-Lac-Saint-Jean region of Quebec. Am J Hum Genet, 1993; 53:481–487

964. Valnot I, Osmond S, Gigarel N et al. Mutations of the SCO1 gene in mitochondrial cytochrome c oxidase deficiency with neonatal-onset hepatic failure and encephalopathy. Am J Hum Genet, 2000; 67:1104–1109

965. Fellman V. The GRACILE syndrome, a neonatal lethal metabolic disorder with iron overload. Blood Cells Mol Dis, 2002; 29:444–450

966. de Lonlay P, Valnot I, Barrientos A et al. A mutant mitochondrial respiratory chain assembly protein causes complex III deficiency in patients with tubulopathy, encephalopathy and liver failure. Nat Genet, 2001; 29:57–60

967. Bakker HD, Scholte HR, Dingemans KP, Spelbrink JN, Wijburg FA, Van den Bogert C. Depletion of mitochondrial deoxyribonucleic acid in a family with fatal neonatal liver disease. J Pediatr, 1996; 128:683–687

968. Salviati L, Sacconi S, Mancuso M et al. Mitochondrial DNA depletion and dGK gene mutations. Ann Neurol, 2002; 52:311–317

969. Labarthe F, Dobbelaere D, Devisme L et al. Clinical, biochemical and morphological features of hepatocerebral syndrome with mitochondrial DNA depletion due to deoxyguanosine kinase deficiency. J Hepatol, 2005; 43:333–341

970. Mancuso M, Ferraris S, Pancrudo J et al. New DGK gene mutations in the hepatocerebral form of mitochondrial DNA depletion syndrome. Arch Neurol, 2005; 62:745–747

971. Slama A, Giurgea I, Debrey D et al. Deoxyguanosine kinase mutations and combined deficiencies of the mitochondrial respiratory chain in patients with hepatic involvement. Mol Genet Metab, 2005; 86:462–465

972. Naviaux RK, Nyhan WL, Barshop BA et al. Mitochondrial DNA polymerase gamma deficiency and mtDNA depletion in a child with Alpers' syndrome. Ann Neurol, 1999; 45:54–58

973. Tesarova M, Mayr JA, Wenchich L et al. Mitochondrial DNA depletion in Alpers syndrome. Neuropediatrics, 2004; 35:217–223

974. Davidzon G, Mancuso M, Ferraris S et al. POLG mutations and Alpers syndrome. Ann Neurol, 2005; 57:921–923

975. Ferrari G, Lamantea E, Donati A et al. Infantile hepatocerebral syndromes associated with mutations in the mitochondrial DNA polymerase-gammaA. Brain, 2005; 128:723–731

976. Longley MJ, Graziewicz MA, Bienstock RJ, Copeland WC. Consequences of mutations in human DNA polymerase gamma. Gene, 2005; 354:125–131

977. Cormier V, Rustin P, Bonnefont JP et al. Hepatic failure in disorders of oxidative phosphorylation with neonatal onset. J Pediatr, 1991; 119:951–954

978. Mazziotta MR, Ricci E, Bertini E et al. Fatal infantile liver failure associated with mitochondrial DNA depletion. J Pediatr, 1992; 121:896–901

979. Narkewicz MR, Sokol RJ, Beckwith B, Sondheimer J, Silverman A. Liver involvement in Alpers disease. J Pediatr, 1991; 119:260–267

980. Wilson DC, McGibben D, Hicks EM, Allen IV. Progressive neuronal degeneration of childhood (Alpers syndrome) with hepatic cirrhosis. Eur J Pediatr, 1993; 152:260–262

981. Bicknese AR, May W, Hickey WF, Dodson WE. Early childhood hepatocerebral degeneration misdiagnosed as valproate hepatotoxicity. Ann Neurol, 1992; 32:767–775

982. Schwabe MJ, Dobyns WB, Burke B, Armstrong DL. Valproate-induced liver failure in one of two siblings with Alpers disease. Pediatr Neurol, 1997; 16:337–343

983. Krahenbuhl S, Brandner S, Kleinle S, Liechti S, Straumann D. Mitochondrial diseases represent a risk factor for valproate-induced fulminant liver failure. Liver, 2000; 20:346–348

984. Delarue A, Paut O, Guys JM et al. Inappropriate liver transplantation in a child with Alpers-Huttenlocher syndrome misdiagnosed as valproate-induced acute liver failure. Pediatr Transplant, 2000; 4:67–71

985. Kayihan N, Nennesomo I, Ericzon BG, Nemeth A. Fatal deterioration of neurological disease after orthotopic liver transplantation for valproic acid-induced liver damage. Pediatr Transplant, 2000; 4:211–214

986. Sim KG, Hammond J, Wilcken B. Strategies for the diagnosis of mitochondrial fatty acid beta-oxidation disorders. Clin Chim Acta, 2002; 323:37–58

987. Saudubray JM, Martin D, de Lonlay P et al. Recognition and management of fatty acid oxidation defects: a series of 107 patients. J Inherit Metab Dis, 1999; 22:488–502

988. den Boer ME, Wanders RJ, Morris AA, Heymans HS, Wijburg FA. Long-chain 3-hydroxyacyl-CoA dehydrogenase deficiency: clinical presentation and follow-up of 50 patients. Pediatrics, 2002; 109:99–104

989. Mochel F, Slama A, Touati G et al. Respiratory chain defects may present only with hypoglycemia. J Clin Endocrinol Metab, 2005; 90:3780–3785

990. Munnich A, Rotig A, Chretien D, Saudubray JM, Cormier V, Rustin P. Clinical presentations and laboratory investigations in respiratory chain deficiency. Eur J Pediatr, 1996; 155:262–274

991. Thorburn DR, Chow CW, Kirby DM. Respiratory chain enzyme analysis in muscle and liver. Mitochondrion, 2004; 4:363–375

992. Rotig A, Lebon S, Zinovieva E et al. Molecular diagnostics of mitochondrial disorders. Biochim Biophys Acta, 2004; 1659:129–135

993. Panetta J, Gibson K, Kirby DM, Thorburn DR, Boneh A. The importance of liver biopsy in the investigation of possible mitochondrial respiratory chain disease. Neuropediatrics, 2005; 36:256–259

994. von Kleist-Retzow JC, Cormier-Daire V, Viot G et al. Antenatal manifestations of mitochondrial respiratory chain deficiency. J Pediatr, 2003; 143:208–212

995. Blake JC, Taanman JW, Morris AM et al. Mitochondrial DNA depletion syndrome is expressed in amniotic fluid cell cultures. Am J Pathol, 1999; 155:67–70

996. Przyrembel H. Therapy of mitochondrial disorders. J Inherit Metab Dis, 1987; 10 (Suppl 1):129–146

997. Ogier de Baulny H, Superti-Furga A. Disorders of mitochondrial datty acid oxidation and ketone body metabolism. In: Physician's Guide to the treatment and Follow-Up of Metabolic Diseases. N. Blau, G.F. Hoffman, J.V. Leonard, J.T.R. Clarke, Editors. 2006, Springer Verlag: Heidelberg. p. 147–160

998. Sokal EM, Sokol R, Cormier V et al. Liver transplantation in mitochondrial respiratory chain disorders. Eur J Pediatr, 1999; 158 Suppl 2:S81–S84

999. Rake JP, van Spronsen FJ, Visser G et al. End-stage liver disease as the only consequence of a mitochondrial respiratory chain deficiency: no contra-indication for liver transplantation. Eur J Pediatr, 2000; 159:523–526

1000. Boles RG, Martin SK, Blitzer MG, Rinaldo P. Biochemical diagnosis of fatty acid oxidation disorders by metabolite analysis of postmortem liver. Hum Pathol, 1994; 25:735–741

1001. Amirkhan RH, Timmons CF, Brown KO, Weinberger MJ, Bennett MJ. Clinical, biochemical, and morphologic investigations of a case of long-chain 3-hydroxyacyl-CoA dehydrogenase deficiency. Arch Pathol Lab Med, 1997; 121:730–734

1002. Bioulac-Sage P, Parrot-Roulaud F, Mazat JP et al. Fatal neonatal liver failure and mitochondrial cytopathy (oxidative phosphorylation deficiency): a light and electron microscopic study of the liver. Hepatology, 1993; 18:839–846

1003. Morris AA, Taanman JW, Blake J et al. Liver failure associated with mitochondrial DNA depletion. J Hepatol, 1998; 28:556–563

1004. Ducluzeau PH, Lachaux A, Bouvier R, Streichenberger N, Stepien G, Mousson B. Depletion of mitochondrial DNA associated with infantile cholestasis and progressive liver fibrosis. J Hepatol, 1999; 30:149–155

1005. Muller-Hocker J, Muntau A, Schafer S et al. Depletion of mitochondrial DNA in the liver of an infant with neonatal giant cell hepatitis. Hum Pathol, 2002; 33:247–253

1006. Chow CW, Thorburn DR. Morphological correlates of mitochondrial dysfunction in children. Hum Reprod, 2000; 15 (Suppl 2):68–78

1007. Pearson HA, Lobel JS, Kocoshis SA et al. A new syndrome of refractory sideroblastic anemia with vacuolization of marrow precursors and exocrine pancreatic dysfunction. J Pediatr, 1979; 95:976–984

1008. Kleinle S, Wiesmann U, Superti-Furga A et al. Detection and characterization of mitochondrial DNA rearrangements in Pearson and Kearns-Sayre syndromes by long PCR. Hum Genet, 1997; 100:643–650

1009. Krahenbuhl S, Kleinle S, Henz S et al. Microvesicular steatosis, hemosiderosis and rapid development of liver cirrhosis in a patient with Pearson's syndrome. J Hepatol, 1999; 31:550–555

1010. Gurakan B, Ozbek N, Varan B, Demirhan B. Fatal acidosis in a neonate with Pearson syndrome. Turk J Pediatr, 1999; 41:361–364

1011. Appenzeller O, Kornfeld M, Snyder R. Acromutilating, paralyzing neuropathy with corneal ulceration in Navajo children. Arch Neurol, 1976; 33:733–738

1012. Singleton R, Helgerson SD, Snyder RD et al. Neuropathy in Navajo children: clinical and epidemiologic features. Neurology, 1990; 40:363–367

1013. Holve SA, Hu D, Shub M, Tyson RW, Sokol RJ. Liver disease in Navajo neuropathy. J Pediatr, 1999; 135:482–493

1014. Roberts EA, Cox DW. Wilson disease. Baillieres Clin Gastroenterol, 1998; 12:237–256

1015. Scheinberg IH, Sternlieb I. Wilson's disease. 1984, Philadelphia: WB Saunders

1016. Sallie R, Katsiyiannakis L, Baldwin D et al. Failure of simple biochemical indexes to reliably differentiate fulminant Wilson's disease from other causes of fulminant liver failure. Hepatology, 1992; 16:1206–1211

1017. Tissieres P, Chevret L, Debray D et al. Fulminant Wilson's disease in children: appraisal of a critical diagnosis. Pediatr Crit Care Med, 2003; 4:338–343

1018. Sallie R, Chiyende J, Tan KC et al. Fulminant hepatic failure resulting from coexistent Wilson's disease and hepatitis E. Gut, 1994; 35:849–853

1019. Rathbun JK. Neuropsychological aspects of Wilson's disease. Int J Neurosci, 1996; 85:221–229

1020. Kuan P. Cardiac Wilson's disease. Chest, 1987; 91:579–583

1021. Nakada SY, Brown MR, Rabinowitz R. Wilson's disease presenting as symptomatic urolithiasis: a case report and review of the literature. J Urol, 1994; 152:978–979

1022. Carpenter TO, Carnes DL, Jr., Anast CS. Hypoparathyroidism in Wilson's disease. N Engl J Med, 1983; 309:873–877

1023. Weizman Z, Picard E, Barki Y, Moses S. Wilson's disease associated with pancreatitis. J Pediatr Gastroenterol Nutr, 1988; 7:931–933

1024. Cheng WS, Govindarajan S, Redeker AG. Hepatocellular carcinoma in a case of Wilson's disease. Liver, 1992; 12:42–45

1025. Guan R, Oon CJ, Wong PK, Foong WC, Wee A. Primary hepatocellular carcinoma associated with Wilson's disease in a young woman. Postgrad Med J, 1985; 61:357–359

1026. Polio J, Enriquez RE, Chow A, Wood WM, Atterbury CE. Hepatocellular carcinoma in Wilson's disease. Case report and review of the literature. J Clin Gastroenterol, 1989; 11:220–224

1027. Sternlieb I. Wilson's disease. Clin Liver Dis, 2000; 4:229–239, viii–ix

1028. Walshe JM, Waldenstrom E, Sams V, Nordlinder H, Westermark K. Abdominal malignancies in patients with Wilson's disease. QJM, 2003; 96:657–662

1029. Wilson DC, Phillips MJ, Cox DW, Roberts EA. Severe hepatic Wilson's disease in preschool-aged children. J Pediatr, 2000; 137:719–722

1030. Thomas GR, Forbes JR, Roberts EA, Walshe JM, Cox DW. The Wilson disease gene: spectrum of mutations and their consequences. Nat Genet, 1995; 9:210–217

1031. Panagiotakaki E, Tzetis M, Manolaki N et al. Genotype-phenotype correlations for a wide spectrum of mutations in the Wilson disease gene (ATP7B). Am J Med Genet A, 2004; 131A:168–173

1032. Bonne-Tamir B, Frydman M, Agger MS et al. Wilson's disease in Israel: a genetic and epidemiological study. Ann Hum Genet, 1990; 54:155–168

1033. Maier-Dobersberger T, Ferenci P, Polli C et al. Detection of the His1069Gln mutation in Wilson disease by rapid polymerase chain reaction [see comments]. Ann Intern Med, 1997; 127:21–26

1034. Shah AB, Chernov I, Zhang HT et al. Identification and analysis of mutations in the Wilson disease gene (ATP7B): population frequencies, genotype-phenotype correlation, and functional analyses. Am J Hum Genet, 1997; 61:317–328

1035. Schiefermeier M, Kollegger H, Madl C et al. The impact of apolipoprotein E genotypes on age at onset of symptoms and phenotypic expression in Wilson's disease. Brain, 2000; 123 Pt 3:585–590

1036. Ross ME, Jacobson IM, Dienstag JL et al. Late-onset Wilson's disease with neurological involvement in the absence of Kayser-Fleischer rings. Ann Neurol, 1985; 17:411–413

1037. Martins da Costa C, Baldwin D, Portmann B, Lolin Y, Mowat AP, Mieli-Vergani G. Value of urinary copper excretion after penicillamine challenge in the diagnosis of Wilson's disease. Hepatology, 1992; 15:609–615

1038. Nuttall KL, Palaty J, Lockitch G. Reference limits for copper and iron in liver biopsies. Ann Clin Lab Sci, 2003; 33:443–450

1039. Weirich G, Cabras AD, Serra S et al. Rapid identification of Wilson's disease carriers by denaturing high-performance liquid chromatography. Prev Med, 2002; 35:278–284

1040. Butler P, McIntyre N, Mistry PK. Molecular diagnosis of Wilson disease. Mol Genet Metab, 2001; 72:223–230

1041. Waldenstrom E, Lagerkvist A, Dahlman T, Westermark K, Landegren U. Efficient detection of mutations in Wilson disease by manifold sequencing. Genomics, 1996; 37:303–309

1042. Yamaguchi Y, Heiny ME, Suzuki M, Gitlin JD. Biochemical characterization and intracellular localization of Menkes disease protein. Proc Natl Acad Sci USA, 1996; 93:14030–14035

1043. Petris M, Mercer JFB, Culvenor JG, Lockhart P, Gleeson PA, Camakaris J. Ligand-regulated transport of the Menkes copper P-type ATPase from the Golgi apparatus to the plasma membrane; a novel mechanism of regulated trafficking. EMBO J, 1996; 15:6084–6095

1044. Vulpe C, Levinson B, Whitney S, Packman S, Gitschier J. Isolation of a candidate gene for Menkes disease and evidence that it incodes a copper-transporting ATPase. Nature Genet, 1993; 3:7–13

1045. Danks DM. Disorders of copper transport. In: The Metabolic Basis of Inherited Disease. C.R. Scriver, A.L. Beaudet, W.S. Sly, D. Valle, Editors. 1995, McGraw-Hill: New York. p. 4125–4158

1046. Bull PC, Thomas GR, Rommens JM, Forbes JR, Cox DW. The Wilson disease gene is a putative copper transporting P-type ATPase similar to the Menkes gene. Nat Genet, 1993; 5:327–337

1047. Tanzi RE, Petrukhin K, Chernov I et al. The Wilson disease gene is a copper transporting ATPase with homology to the Menkes disease gene. Nat Genet, 1993; 5:344–350

1048. Petrukhin K, Fischer SG, Pirastu M et al. Mapping, cloning and genetic characterization of the region containing the Wilson disease gene. Nat Genet, 1993; 5:338–343

1049. Fatemi N, Sarkar B. Structural and functional insights of Wilson disease copper-transporting ATPase. J Bioenerg Biomembr, 2002; 34:339–349

1050. Klomp AE, Juijn JA, van der Gun LT, van den Berg IE, Berger R, Klomp LW. The N-terminus of the human copper transporter 1 (hCTR1) is localized extracellularly, and interacts with itself. Biochem J, 2003; 370(Pt 3):881–889

1051. Guo Y, Smith K, Lee J, Petris MJ. Identification of methionine-rich clusters that regulate copper-stimulated endocytosis of the human Ctr1 copper transporter. J Biol Chem, 2004; 279:17428–17433

1052. Petris MJ. The SLC31 (Ctr) copper transporter family. Pflugers Arch, 2004; 447:752–755

1053. Harris ED. Cellular copper transport and metabolism. Annu Rev Nutr, 2000; 20:291–310

1054. Kelly EJ, Palmiter RD. A murine model of Menkes disease reveals a physiological function of metallothionein. Nat Genet, 1996; 13:219–222

1055. Huffman DL, O'Halloran TV. Function, structure, and mechanism of intracellular copper trafficking proteins. Annu Rev Biochem, 2001; 70:677–701

1056. Field LS, Luk E, Culotta VC. Copper chaperones: personal escorts for metal ions. J Bioenerg Biomembr, 2002; 34:373–379

1057. Larin D, Mekios C, Das K, Ross B, Yang AS, Gilliam TC. Characterization of the interaction between the Wilson and Menkes disease proteins and the cytoplasmic copper chaperone, HAH1p. J Biol Chem, 1999; 274:28497–28504

1058. Hamza I, Schaefer M, Klomp LW, Gitlin JD. Interaction of the copper chaperone HAH1 with the Wilson disease protein is essential for copper homeostasis. Proc Natl Acad Sci U S A, 1999; 96:13363–13368

1059. Wernimont AK, Huffman DL, Lamb AL, O'Halloran TV, Rosenzweig AC. Structural basis for copper transfer by the metallochaperone for the Menkes/Wilson disease proteins. Nat Struc Biol, 2000; 7:766–771

1060. Walker JM, Huster D, Ralle M, Morgan CT, Blackburn NJ, Lutsenko S. The N-terminal metal-binding site 2 of the Wilson's Disease Protein plays a key role in the transfer of copper from Atox1. J Biol Chem, 2004; 279:15376–15384

1061. Nagano K, Nakamura K, Urakami KI et al. Intracellular distribution of the Wilson's disease gene product (ATPase7B) after in vitro and in vivo exogenous expression in hepatocytes from the LEC rat, an animal model of Wilson's disease. Hepatology, 1998; 27:799–807

1062. Schaefer M, Hopkins RG, Failla ML, Gitlin JD. Hepatocyte-specific localization and copper-dependent trafficking of the Wilson's disease protein in the liver. Am J Physiol, 1999; 276:G639–G646

1063. Schaefer M, Roelofsen H, Wolters H et al. Localization of the Wilson's disease protein in human liver. Gastroenterology, 1999; 117:1380–1385

1064. Harada M, Kumemura H, Sakisaka S et al. Wilson disease protein ATP7B is localized in the late endosomes in a polarized human hepatocyte cell line. Int J Mol Med, 2003; 11:293–298

1065. Huster D, Hoppert M, Lutsenko S et al. Defective cellular localization of mutant ATP7B in Wilson's disease patients and hepatoma cell lines. Gastroenterology, 2003; 124:335–345

1066. Schilsky ML, Stockert RJ, Sternlieb I. Pleiotropic effect of LEC mutation: a rodent model of Wilson's disease. Am J Physiol, 1994; 266:G907–G913

1067. Tao TY, Liu F, Klomp L, Gitlin JD. The copper toxicosis gene product Murr1 directly interacts with the Wilson disease protein. J Biol Chem, 2003; 278:41593–41596

1068. Walshe JM. Wilson's disease. New oral therapy. Lancet, 1956; i:25–26

1069. Klein D, Lichtmannegger J, Heinzmann U, Summer KH. Dissolution of copper-rich granules in hepatic lysosomes by D-penicillamine prevents the development of fulminant hepatitis in Long-Evans cinnamon rats. J Hepatol, 2000; 32:193–201

1070. Walshe JM. Treatment of Wilson's disease with trientine (triethylene tetramine) dihydrochloride. Lancet, 1982; 1:643–647

1071. Dahlman T, Hartvig P, Lofholm M, Nordlinder H, Loof L, Westermark K. Long-term treatment of Wilson's disease with triethylene tetramine dihydrochloride (trientine). Q J Med, 1995; 88:609–616

1072. Brewer GJ. Zinc acetate for the treatment of Wilson's disease. Expert Opin Pharmacother, 2001; 2:1473–1477

1073. Emre S, Atillasoy EO, Ozdemir S et al. Orthotopic liver transplantation for Wilson's disease: a single-center experience. Transplantation, 2001; 72:1232–1236

1074. Sutcliffe RP, Maguire DD, Muiesan P et al. Liver transplantation for Wilson's disease: long-term results and quality-of-life assessment. Transplantation, 2003; 75:1003–1006

1075. Asonuma K, Inomata Y, Kasahara M et al. Living related liver transplantation from heterozygote genetic carriers to children with Wilson's disease. Pediatr Transplant, 1999; 3:201–205

1076. Wang XH, Cheng F, Zhang F et al. Copper metabolism after living related liver transplantation for Wilson's disease. World J Gastroenterol, 2003; 9:2836–2838

1077. Bax RT, Hassler A, Luck W et al. Cerebral manifestation of Wilson's disease successfully treated with liver transplantation. Neurology, 1998; 51:863–865

1078. Schumacher G, Platz KP, Mueller AR et al. Liver transplantation: treatment of choice for hepatic and neurological manifestation of Wilson's disease. Clin Transplant, 1997; 11:217–224

1079. Kassam N, Witt N, Kneteman N et al. Liver transplantation for neuropsychiatric Wilson disease. Can J Gastroenterol, 1998; 12:65–68

1080. Brewer GJ, Hedera P, Kluin KJ et al. Treatment of Wilson disease with ammonium tetrathiomolybdate: III. Initial therapy in a total of 55 neurologically affected patients and follow-up with zinc therapy. Arch Neurol, 2003; 60:379–385

1081. Askari FK, Greenson J, Dick RD, Johnson VD, Brewer GJ. Treatment of Wilson's disease with zinc. XVIII. Initial treatment of the hepatic decompensation presentation with trientine and zinc. J Lab Clin Med, 2003; 142:385–390

1082. Terada K, Nakako T, Yang XL et al. Restoration of holoceruloplasmin synthesis in LEC rat after infusion of recombinant adenovirus bearing WND cDNA. J Biol Chem, 1998; 273:1815–1820

1083. Ha-Hao D, Merle U, Hofmann C et al. Chances and shortcomings of adenovirus-mediated ATP7B gene transfer in Wilson disease: proof of principle demonstrated in a pilot study with LEC rats. Z Gastroenterol, 2002; 40:209–216

1084. Meng Y, Miyoshi I, Hirabayashi M et al. Restoration of copper metabolism and rescue of hepatic abnormalities in LEC rats, an animal model of Wilson disease, by expression of human ATP7B gene. Biochim Biophys Acta, 2004; 1690:208–219

1085. Gu M, Cooper JM, Butler P et al. Oxidative-phosphorylation defects in liver of patients with Wilson's disease. Lancet, 2000; 356:469–474

1086. Stromeyer FW, Ishak KG. Histology of the liver in Wilson's disease: a study of 34 cases. Am J Clin Pathol, 1980; 73:12–24

1087. Sternlieb I, Scheinberg IH. Chronic hepatitis as a first manifestation of Wilson's disease. Ann Intern Med, 1972; 76:59–64

1088. Scott J, Gollan JL, Samourian S, Sherlock S. Wilson's disease, presenting as chronic active hepatitis. Gastroenterology, 1978; 74:645–651

1089. Milkiewicz P, Saksena S, Hubscher SG, Elias E. Wilson's disease with superimposed autoimmune features: report of two cases and review. J Gastroenterol Hepatol, 2000; 15:570–574

1090. Goldfischer S, Sternlieb I. Changes in the distribution of hepatic copper in relation to the progression of Wilson's disease (hepatolenticular degeneration). Am J Pathol, 1968; 53:883–901

1091. Lindquist RR. Studies on the pathogenesis of hepatolenticular degeneration. II. Cytochemical methods for the localization of copper. Arch Pathol, 1969; 87:370–379

1092. Irons RD, Schenk EA, Lee JCK. Cytochemical methods for copper. Arch Pathol Lab Med, 1977; 101:298–301

1093. Salospuro M, Sipponen P. Demonstration of an intracellular copper-binding protein by orcein staining. Gut, 1976; 13:787–790

1094. Jain S, Scheuer PJ, Archer B, Newman SP, Sherlock S. Histological demonstration of copper and copper-associated protein in chronic liver diseases. J Clin Pathol, 1978; 31:784–790

1095. Sumithran E, Looi LM. Copper-binding protein in liver cells. Hum Pathol, 1985; 16:677–682

1096. Graul RS, Epstein O, Sherlock S, Scheuer PJ. Immunocytochemical identification of caeruloplasmin in hepatocytes of patients with Wilson's disease. Liver, 1982; 2:207–211

1097. Nartey N, Cherian MG, Banerjee D. Immunohistochemical localization of metallothionein in human thyroid tumors. Am J Pathol, 1987; 129:177–182

1098. Davies SE, Williams R, Portmann B. Hepatic morphology and histochemistry of Wilson's disease presenting as fulminant hepatic failure: a study of 11 cases. Histopathology, 1989; 15:385–394

1099. Ferlan-Marolt V, Stepec S. Fulminant Wilsonian hepatitis unmasked by disease progression: report of a case and review of the literature. Dig Dis Sci, 1999; 44:1054–1058

1100. Phillips MJ, Poucell S, Patterson J, Valencia P. The Liver. An Atlas and Text of Ultrastructural Pathology. 1987, New York: Raven Press

1101. Sternlieb I. Mitochondrial and fatty changes in hepatocytes of patients with Wilson's disease. Gastroenterology, 1968; 55:354–367

1102. Sternlieb I. Fraternal concordance of types of abnormal hepatocellular mitochondria in Wilson's disease. Hepatology, 1992; 16:728–732

1103. Sternlieb I. Evolution of the hepatic lesion in Wilson's disease (hepatolenticular degeneration). Prog Liver Dis, 1972; 4:511–525

1104. Muller T, Langner C, Fuchsbichler A et al. Immunohistochemical analysis of Mallory bodies in Wilsonian and non-Wilsonian hepatic copper toxicosis. Hepatology, 2004; 39:963–969

1105. Hayashi H, Sternlieb I. Lipolysosomes in human hepatocytes. Ultrastructural and cytochemical studies of patients with Wilson's disease. Lab Invest, 1975; 33:1–7

1106. Lough J, Wiglesworth FW. Wilson disease. Comparative ultrastructure in a sibship of nine. Arch Pathol Lab Med, 1976; 100:659–653

1107. Geubel AP, Gregoire V, Rahier J, Lissens W, Dive C. Hypoceruloplasminemia and ultrastructural changes resembling Wilson's disease in nonalcoholic liver steatosis. A clinical and pathological study of five cases. Liver, 1988; 8:299–306

1108. Sternlieb I, Feldmann G. Effects of anticopper therapy on hepatocellular mitochondria in patients with Wilson's disease: an ultrastructural and stereological study. Gastroenterology, 1976; 71:457–461

1109. Pankit AN, Bhave SA. Copper metabolic defects and liver disease: Environmental aspects. J Gastroenterol Hepatol, 2002; 17 Suppl 3: S403–S407

1110. Bhagwat AG, Walia BN, Koshy A, Banerji CK. Will the real Indian childhood cirrhosis please stand up? Cleve Clin Q, 1983; 50:323–337

1111. Lefkowitch JH, Honig CL, King ME, Hagstrom JW. Hepatic copper overload and features of Indian childhood cirrhosis in an American sibship. N Engl J Med, 1982; 307:271–277

1112. Adamson M, Reiner B, Olson JL et al. Indian childhood cirrhosis in an American child. Gastroenterology, 1992; 102:1771–1777

1113. Drouin E, Russo P, Tuchweber B, Mitchell G, Rasquin-Weber A. North American Indian cirrhosis in children: a review of 30 cases. J Pediatr Gastroenterol Nutr, 2000; 31:395–404

1114. Betard C, Rasquin-Weber A, Brewer C et al. Localization of a recessive gene for North American Indian childhood cirrhosis to chromosome region 16q22-and identification of a shared haplotype. Am J Hum Genet, 2000; 67:222–228

1115. Chagnon P, Michaud J, Mitchell G et al. A missense mutation (R565W) in cirhin (FLJ14728) in North American Indian childhood cirrhosis. Am J Hum Genet, 2002; 71:1443–1449

1116. Nayak NC, Ramalingaswami V. Indian childhood cirrhosis. Clin Gastroenterol, 1975; 4:333–349

1117. Portmann B, Tanner MS, Mowat AP, Williams R. Orcein-positive liver deposits in Indian childhood cirrhosis. Lancet, 1978; 1:1338–1340

1118. Tanner MS, Portmann B, Mowat AP et al. Increased hepatic copper concentration in Indian childhood cirrhosis. Lancet, 1979; 1:1203–1205

1119. Joshi VV. Indian childhood cirrhosis. Perspect Pediatr Pathol, 1987; 11:175–192

1120. Tanner MS, Portmann B. Indian childhood cirrhosis. Arch Dis Child, 1981; 56:4–6

1121. Smetana BF, Hadley GG, Sirsat SM. Infantile cirrhosis. An analytic reivew of the literature and a report of 50 cases. Pediatics, 1961; 28:107–127

1122. Popper H, Goldfischer S, Sternlieb I, Nayak NC, Madhavan TV. Cytoplasmic copper and its toxic effects. Studies in Indian childhood cirrhosis. Lancet, 1979; 1:1205–1208

1123. Mehrotra R, Pandey RK, Nath P. Hepatic copper in Indian childhood cirrhosis. Histopathology, 1981; 5:659–665

1124. Sethi S, Khodaskar MB. Diagnostic potential of histochemical demonstration for copper-orcein stain. J Indian Med Assoc, 2000; 98:434–435, 438

1125. Tanner MS, Kantarjian AH, Bhave SA, Pandit AN. Early introduction of copper-contaminated animal milk feeds as a possible cause of Indian childhood cirrhosis. Lancet, 1983; 2:992–995

1126. O'Neill NC, Tanner MS. Uptake of copper from brass vessels by bovine milk and its relevance to Indian childhood cirrhosis. J Pediatr Gastroenterol Nutr, 1989; 9:167–172

1127. Tanner MS, Bhave SA, Pradhan AM, Pandit AN. Clinical trials of penicillamine in Indian childhood cirrhosis. Arch Dis Child, 1987; 62:1118–1124

1128. Bhusnurmath SR, Walia BN, Singh S, Parkash D, Radotra BD, Nath R. Sequential histopathologic alterations in Indian childhood cirrhosis treated with d-penicillamine. Hum Pathol, 1991; 22:653–658

1129. Bavdekar AR, Bhave SA, Pradhan AM, Pandit AN, Tanner MS. Long term survival in Indian childhood cirrhosis treated with D-penicillamine. Arch Dis Child, 1996; 74:32–35

1130. Tanner MS. Role of copper in Indian childhood cirrhosis. Am J Clin Nutr, 1998; 67:1074S–1081S

1131. Muller T, van de Sluis B, Zhernakova A et al. The canine copper toxicosis gene MURR1 does not cause non-Wilsonian hepatic copper toxicosis. J Hepatol, 2003; 38:164–168

1132. de Bie P, van de Sluis B, Klomp L, Wijmenga C. The Many Faces of the Copper Metabolism Protein MURR1/COMMD1. J Hered, 2005; 96:803–811

1133. Muller T, Feichtinger H, Berger H, Muller W. Endemic Tyrolean infantile cirrhosis: an ecogenetic disorder. Lancet, 1996; 347:877–880

1134. Dieter HH, Schimmelpfennig W, Meyer E, Tabert M. Early childhood cirrhoses (ECC) in Germany between 1982 and 1994 with special consideration of copper etiology. Eur J Med Res, 1999; 4:233–242

1135. Wijmenga C, Muller T, Murli IS et al. Endemic Tyrolean infantile cirrhosis is not an allelic variant of Wilson's disease. Eur J Hum Genet, 1998; 6:624–628

1136. Muller-Hocker J. Pathomorphology of the liver in exogenic infantile copper intoxication in Germany. Eur J Med Res, 1999; 4:229–232

1137. Feder JN, Gnirke A, Thomas W, Tsuchihashi Z, Ruddy DA, Basava A. A novel MHC class 1-like gene is mutated in patients with hereditary haemochromatosis. Nat Genet, 1996; 13:399–408

1138. Cook JD, Barry WE, Hershko C, Fillet G, Finch CA. Iron kinetics with emphasis on iron overload. Am J Pathol, 1973; 72:337–343

1139. Andrews NC. Disorders of iron metabolism. N Engl J Med, 1999; 341:1986–1995

1140. Conrad ME, Umbreit JN. Pathways of iron absorption. Blood Cells Mol Dis, 2002; 29:336–355

1141. Fleming RE. Advances in understanding the molecular basis for the regulation of dietary iron absorption. Curr Opin Gastroenterol, 2005; 21:201–206

1142. Roy CN, Enns CA. Iron homeostasis: new tales from the crypt. Blood, 2000; 96:4020–4027

1143. McKie AT, Latunde-Dada GO, Miret S, McGregor JA, Anderson GJ, Vulpe CD. Molecular evidence for the role of a ferric reductase in iron transport. Biochem Soc Trans, 2002; 30:722–724

1144. Grushin H, Mackenzie B, Berger UV, Gunshin Y. Cloning and characterisation of a mammalian proton-coupled metal-iron transporter. Nature, 1997; 388:482–488

1145. Uc A, Stokes JB, Britigan BE. Haem transport exhibits polarity in Caco-2 cells: evidence for an active and membrane protein-mediated process. Am J Physiol Gastrointest Liver Physiol, 2004; 287:G1150–G1157

1146. Quigley JG, Yang Z, Worthington MT et al. Identification of a human haem exporter that is essential for erythropoiesis. Cell, 2004; 118:757–766

1147. Umbreit JN, Conrad ME, Moore EG, Latour LF. Iron absorption and cellular transport: the mobilferrin/paraferritin paradigm. Semin Hematol, 1998; 35:13–26

1148. Aboud S, Haile DJ. A novel mammalian iron-regulated protein involved in intracellular iron metabolism. J Biol Chem, 2000; 275:19906–19912

1149. Donovan A, Brownlie A, Zhou Y et al. Positional cloning of zebrafish ferroportin1 identifies a conserved vertebrate iron exporter. Nature, 2000; 403:776–781

1150. McKie AT, Marciani P, Rolfs A et al. A novel duodenal iron-regulated transporter, IREG1, implicated in the basolateral transfer of iron to the circulation. Mol Cell, 2000; 5:299–309

1151. Andrews NC. Molecular control of iron metabolism. Best Prac Res Clin Haematol, 2005; 18:159–169

1152. Vulpe CD, Kuo YM, Murphy TL et al. Hephaestin, a caeruloplasmin homologue implicated in intestinal iron transport, is defective in the sla mouse. Nat Genet, 1999; 21:195–199

1153. Harris ZL, Durley AP, Man TK, Gitlin JD. Targeted gene disruption reveals an essential role for ceruloplasmin in cellular iron efflux. Proc Natl Acad Sci U S A, 1999; 96:10812–10817

1154. Heeney MM, Andrews NC. Iron homeostasis and inherited iron overload disorders: an overview. Hematol Oncol Clin North Am, 2004; 18:1–20

1155. Cheng Y, Zak O, Alsen P, Harrison LC, Walz T. Structure of the transferrin receptor-transferrin complex. Cell, 2004; 116:565–576

1156. Hagar W, Theil E, Vichinsky EP. Diseases of iron metabolism. Pediatr Clin North Am, 2002; 49:893–909

1157. Glockner G, Scherer S, Schattevoy R, Brennan K, Wehr K, Barrow D. Large-scale sequencing of two regions in human chromosome 7q22: analysis of 650 kb of genomic sequence around the EPO and CUTL1 loci reveals 17 genes. Genome Res, 1998; 8:1060–1073

1158. Kawabata H, Germain RS, Vuong PT, Nakamaki T, Said JW, Koeffler HP. Transferrin receptor 2-alpha supports cell growth in both iron-chelated cultured cells and in vivo. J Biol Chem, 2000; 275:16618–16625

1159. Kawabata H, Yang R, Hirama T et al. Molecular cloning of transferrin receptor 2. A new member of the transferrin receptor-like family. J Biol Chem, 1999; 274:20826–20832

1160. Griffiths WJ, Cox TM. Co-localization of the mammalian hemochromatosis gene product (HFE) and a newly identified transferrin receptor (TfR2) in intestinal tissue and cells. J Histochem Cytochem, 2003; 51:613–624

1161. Levy JE, Jin O, Fujiwara Y, Kuo F, Andrews NC. Transferrin receptor is necessary for development of erythrocytes and the nervous system. Nat. Genet, 1999; 21:396–399

1162. Fleming RE, Ahmann JR, Migas MC et al. Targeted mutagenesis of the murine transferrin receptor-2 gene produces hemochromatosis. Proc Natl Acad Sci U S A, 2002; 99:10653–10658

1163. Camaschella C. Why do humans need two types of transferrin receptor? Lessons from a rare genetic disorder. Haematologica, 2005; 90:296

1164. Kawabata H, Fleming RE, Gui D et al. Expression of hepcidin is down-regulated in TfR2 mutant mice manifesting a phenotype of hereditary hemochromatosis. Blood, 2005; 105:376–381

1165. Bratosin D, Mazurier J, Tissier JP et al. Cellular and molecular mechanisms of senescent erythrocyte phagocytosis by macrophages A review. Biochimie, 1998; 80:173–195

1166. Knutson MD, Vafa MR, Haile DJ, Wessling-Resnick M. Iron loading and erythrophagocytosis increase ferroportin 1 (FPN1) expression in J774 macrophages. Blood, 2003; 102:4191–4197

1167. Thiel E. Ferritin: at the crossroads of iron and oxygen metabolism. J Nutr, 2003; 133:1549S–1553S

1168. Hentze MW, Muckenthaler MU, Andrews NC. Balancing acts: molecular control of mammalian iron metabolism. Cell, 2004; 117:285–297

1169. Rouault TA. Post-transcriptional regulation of mammalian iron metabolism by iron regulatory proteins. Blood Cells Mol Dis, 2002; 29:309–314

1170. Beutler E. 'Pumping' iron: the proteins. Science, 2004; 306:2051–2053

1171. Finch C. Regulators of iron balance in humans. Blood, 1994; 84:1697–1702

1172. Andrews NC. Iron metabolism: iron deficiency and iron overload. Annu Rev Genomics Hum Genet, 2000; 1:75–98

1173. Krause A, Neitz S, Magert HJ et al. LEAP-1, a novel highly disulphide-bonded human peptide, exhibits antimicrobial activity. FEBS lett, 2000; 480:147–150

1174. Park CH, Valore EV, Waring AJ, Ganz T. Hepcidin, a urinary antimicrobial protein synthesized by the liver. J Biol Chem, 2001; 276:7806–7810

1175. Hunter HN, Fulton GB, Ganz T, Vogel HJ. The solution structure of hepcidin, a peptide hormone with antimicrobial activity that is involved in iron uptake and hereditary haemochromatosis. J Biol Chem, 2002; 277:37597–37603

1176. Lee P, Peng H, Gelbart T, Wang L, Beutler E. Regulation of hepcidin transcription by interleukin-1 and interleukin-6. Proc Natl Acad Sci U S A, 2005; 102:1906–1910

1177. Nemeth E, Valore EV, Territo M, Schiller G, Lichtenstein A, Ganz T. Hepcidin, a putative mediator of anemia of inflammation is a type II acute-phase protein. Blood, 2002; 101:2461–2463

1178. Pigeon C, Ilyin G, Courselaud B et al. A new mouse liver specific gene, encoding a protein homologous to human antimicrobial peptide hepcidin, is overexpressed during iron overload. J Biol Chem, 2001; 276:7811–7819

1179. Nicolas G, Bennoun M, Devaux I et al. Lack of hepcidin gene expression and severe tissue iron overload in Upstream Stimulator knockout mice. Proc Natl Acad Sci U S A, 2001; 98:8780–8785

1180. Nicolas G, Bennoun M, Porteu A et al. Severe iron deficiency anemia in transgenic mice expressing liver hepcidin. Proc Natl Acad Sci U S A, 2002; 99:4596–4601

1181. Nicolas G, Viatte L, Lou DQ et al. Constitutive hepcidin expression prevents iron overload in a mouse model of hemochromatosis. Nat Genet, 2003; 34:97–101

1182. Ganz T. Hepcidin, a new key regulator of iron metabolism and mediator of anaemia of inflammation. Blood, 2003; 102:783–788

1183. Ganz T. Hepcidin—a regulator of intestinal iron and iron recycling by macrophages. Best Prac Res Clin Haematol, 2005; 18:171–182

1184. Robson KJ. Hepcidin and its role in iron absorption. Gut, 2004; 53:617–619

1185. Papanikolaou G, Tzilianos M, Christakis JI et al. Hepcidin in iron overload disorders. Blood, 2005; 105:4103–4105

1186. Nemeth E, Tuttle MS, Powelson J et al. Hepcidin regulated cellular iron efflux by binding to ferroportin and inducing its internalization. Science, 2004; 306:2090–2093

1187. Montosi G, Corradini E, Garuti C et al. Kupffer cells and macrophages are not required for hepatic hepcidin activation during iron overload. Hepatology, 2005; 41:545–552

1188. Papanikolaou G, Samuels ME, Ludwig MLE et al. Mutations in HFE2 cause iron overload in chromosome 1q-linked juvenile hemochromatosis. Nat Genet, 2004; 36:77–82

1189. Ganz T. Hepcidin in iron metabolism. Curr Opin Hematol, 2004; 11:251–254

1190. McCord JM. Iron, free radicals, and oxidative injury. Semin Haematol, 1998; 35:5–12

1191. Papanikolaou G, Pantopolous K. Iron metabolism and toxicity. Toxicol Appl Pharm, 2005; 202:199–211

1192. Pietrangelo A. Hemochromatosis 1998. Is one gene enough? J Hepatol, 1998; 29:502–509

1193. Adams PC. Hemochromatosis. Clin Liv Dis, 2004; 8:735–753

1194. Adams P, Brissot P, Powell LW. EASL international consensus conference on haemochromatosis. J Hepatol, 2000; 33:487–496

1195. Hemochromatosis. In: Online Mendelian Inheritance in Man (OMIM). Baltimore: McKusick Nathans Institute for Genetic Medicine 2000; Available from: http://www.ncbi.nlm.nih.gov/omim/

1196. Pietrangelo A, Caleffi A, Henrion J et al. Juvenile hemochromatosis associated with pathogenic mutations of adult hemochromatosis genes. Gastroenterology, 2005; 128:470–479

1197. Trousseau A. Glycosurie: diabète sucré. In: Clinique médicale de l'Hôtel Dieu de Paris. 1865, J.-B. Bailliere: Paris. p. 663–698

1198. Troisier M. Diabète sucré. Bull Soc Anat Paris, 1871; 44:231–235

1199. von Recklinghausen FD. Uber Haemochromatose. Tageblatt Versammlung Dtsche Naturforscher Arzte Heidelberg, 1889; 62:324–325

1200. Reuben A. Landmarks in Hepatology: praise ye the god of iron. Hepatology, 2004; 40:1231–1234

1201. Sheldon JH. Haemochromatosis. The Bradshaw lecture. Lancet, 1934; 2:1031–1036

1202. Simon M, Alexandre JL, Bourel M, Le Marec B, Scordia C. Heredity of idiopathic hemochromatosis: a study of 106 families. Clin Genet, 1977; 11:327–341

1203. Simon M, Bourel M, Fauchet R, Genetet B. Association of HLA A3 and HLAB14 antigens with idiopathic hemochromatosis. Gut, 1976; 17:332–334

1204. de Sousa M, Reimao R, Lacerda R et al. Iron overload in beta 2-microglobulin-deficient mice. Immunol Lett, 1994; 39:105–111

1205. Santos M, Schilham MW, Rademakers LH, Marx JJ, de Sousa M, Clevers H. Defective iron homeostasis in beta2-microglobulin knockout mice recapitulates hereditary hemochromatosis in man. J Exp Med, 1996; 184:1975–1985

1206. Levy JE, Montross LK, Cohen DE, Fleming MD, Andrews NC. The C282 mutation causing hereditary hemochromatosis does not produce a null allele. Blood, 1999; 94:9–11

1207. Xhou XY, Tomatsu S, Fleming RE, Parkilla S, Waheed A, Jiang J. HFE knockout produces mouse model of hereditary hemochromatosis. Proc Natl Acad Sci U S A, 1998; 95:2492–2497

1208. Holmstrom P, Marmur J, Eggertsen G, Gafvels M, Stal P. Mild iron overload in patients carrying the HFE S65C gene mutation: a retrospective study in patients with suspected iron overload and healthy controls. Gut, 2002; 51:723–730

1209. Mura COR, Ferec C. HFE mutation analysis in hemochromatosis probands: evidence of S65C implication in mild form of hemochromatosis. Blood, 1999; 711:2502–2505

1210. Merryweather-Clarke AT, Pointon JJ, Shearman JD, Robson KJ. Global prevalence of putative haemochromatosis mutations. J Med Genet, 1997; 34:275–278

1211. Lucotte G. Celtic origin of the C282Y mutation of hemochromatosis. Blood, 1998; 24:433–438

1212. Distante S, Robson KJH, Graham-Campbell J, Arnaiz-Villena A, Brissot P, Worwood M. The origin and spread of the HFE-C282Y haemochromatosis mutation. Hum Genet, 2004; 115:269–279

1213. Parkkila S, Waheed A, Britton RS et al. Immunohistochemistry of HLA-H, the protein defective in patients with hereditary haemochromatosis, reveals unique pattern of expression in gastrointestinal tract. Proc Natl Acad Sci U S A, 1997; 94:2534–2539

1214. Waheed A, Parkkila S, Saarnio J et al. Association of HFE protein with transferrin receptor in crypt enterocytes of human duodenum. Proc Natl Acad Sci U S A, 1999; 96:1579–1584

1215. Fleming RE, Britton RS, Waheed A, Sly WS, Bacon BR. Pathogenesis of hereditary hemochromatosis. Clin Liv Dis, 2004; 8:755–773

1216. Pietrangelo A. Hereditary hemochromatosis—a new look at an old disease. N Engl J Med, 2004; 350:2383–2397

1217. Trinder D, Olynyk JK, Sly WS, Morgan EH. Iron uptake from plasma transferrin by the duodenum is impaired in the Hfe knockout mouse. Proc Natl Acad Sci U S A, 2002; 99:5622–5626

1218. Ahmad KA, Ahmann JR, Migas MC et al. Decreased liver hepcidin expression in the hfe knockout mouse. Blood Cells Mol Dis, 2002; 29:361–366

1219. Bridle KR, Frazer DM, Wilkins SJ et al. Disrupted hepcidin regulation in HFE associated haemochromatosis and the liver as a regulator of body iron homoeostasis. Lancet, 2003; 361:669–673

1220. Muckenthaler M, Roy CN, Custodio AO et al. Regulatory defects in liver and intestine implicate abnormal hepcidin and Cybrd1 expression in mouse hemochromatosis. Nat Genet, 2003; 34:102–107

1221. Frazer DM, Anderson GJ. The orchestration of body iron intake: how and when do enterocytes receive their cues? Blood Cells Mol Dis, 2003; 30:288–297

1222. Adams PC, Reboussin DM, Barton JC et al. Hemochromatosis and iron-overload screening in a racially diverse population. N Engl J Med, 2005; 352:1769–1778

1223. Beutler E, Felitti VJ, Koziol JA, Ho NJ, Gelbart T. Penetrance of the 845G to A (C282Y) HFE hereditary haemochromatosis mutation in the USA. Lancet, 2002; 359:211–218

1224. Brittenham GM, Farrell DE, Harris JW et al. Magnetic-susceptibility measurement of human iron stores. N Engl J Med, 1982; 307:1671–1675

1225. Pietrangelo A. Non invasive assessment of hepatic iron overload: are we finally there? Journal of Hepatology, 2005; 42:153–154

1226. St Pierre TG, Clark PR, Chua-anusorn W et al. Noninvasive measurement and imaging of liver iron concentrations using proton magnetic resonance. Blood, 2005; 105:855–861

1227. Deugnier YM, Charalambous P, Le Quilleuc D et al. Preneoplastic significance of hepatic iron-free foci in genetic hemochromatosis: a study of 185 patients. Hepatology, 1993; 18:1363–1369

1228. Fargion S, Fracanzani AL, Piperno A et al. Prognostic factors for hepatocellular carcinoma in genetic haemochromatosis. Hepatology, 1994; 20:1426–1431

1229. Kowdley KV. Iron, hemochromatosis, and hepatocellular carcinoma. Gastroenterology, 2004; 127:S79–S86

1230. Biasiotto G, Roetto A, Daraio F et al. Identification of new mutations of hepcidin and hemojuvelin in patients with HFE C282Y allele. Blood Cells Mol Dis, 2004; 33:338–343

1231. Bomford A, Williams R. Long term results of venesection therapy in idiopathic haemochromatosis. Q J Med, 1976; 45:611–623

1232. Niederau, Fischer R, Pürschel A, Stremmel W, Haussinger D, Strohmeyer G. Long-term survival in patients with hereditary hemochromatosis. Gastroenterology, 1996; 110:1107–1119

1233. Waalen J, Nordestgaard BG, Beutler E. The penetrance of hereditary hemochromatosis. Best Pract Res Clin Haem, 2005; 18:203–220

1234. Lamon JM, Marynick SP, Rosenblatt R, Donnelli S. Idiopathic hemochromatosis in a young female: a case study and review of the syndrome in young people. Gastroenterology, 1979; 76:178–183

1235. Finch SC, Finch CA. Idiopathic hemochromatosis, an iron storage disease. Medicine, 1955; 34:381–430

1236. Camaschella C, Roetto A, Cicilano M et al. Juvenile and adult haemochromatosis are distinct genetic disorders. Eur J Hum Genet, 1997; 5:371–375

1237. Roetto A, Totaro A, Gazzola M et al. Juvenile hemochromatosis locus maps to chromosome 1q. Am J Hum Genet, 1999; 64:1388–1393

1238. Beutler J, Beutler E. Hematologically important mutations: iron storage diseases. Blood Cells Mol Dis, 2004; 33:40–44

1239. Lanzara C, Roetto A, Daraio F et al. Spectrum of hemojuvelin gene mutations in 1q-linked juvenile haemochromatosis. Blood, 2004; 103:4317–4321

1240. Daraio F, Ryan E, Gleeson A, Roetto A, Crowe J, Camaschella C. Juvenile haemochromatosis due to G320V/Q116X compound heterozygosity of hemojuvelin in an Irish patient. Blood, Cells Mol Dis, 2005; 35:174–176

1241. Gehrke SG, Pietrangelo A, Kascak M et al. HJV gene mutations in European patients with juvenile hemochromatosis. Clin Genet, 2005; 67:425–438

1242. Roetto A, Daraio F, Poporato P et al. Screening hepcidin for mutations in juvenile hemochromatosis: identification of a new mutation (C70R). Blood, 2004; 103:2407–2409

1243. Roetto A, Papanikolaou G, Politou M, Alberti F, Girelli D, Christakis J. Mutant antimicrobial polypeptide hepcidin is associated with severe juvenile hemochromatosis. Nat Genet, 2003; 33:21–22

1244. Matthes T, Aguilar-Martinez P, Pizzi-Bosman L et al. Severe hemochromatosis in a Portuguese family associated with a new mutation in the 5'-UTR of the HAMP gene. Blood, 2004; 104:2181–2183

1245. Jacolot S, Le Gac G, Scotet V, Quere I, Mura C, Ferec C. HAMP as a modifier gene that increases the phenotypic expression of the HFE pC282Y homozygous genotype. Blood, 2004; 103:2835–2840

1246. Le Gac G, Scotet V, Ka C et al. The recently identified type 2A juvenile haemochromatosis gene (HJV), a second candidate modifier of the C282Y homozygous phenotype. Hum Mol Gen, 2004; 13:1913–1918

1247. Cox TM, Halsall DJ. Hemochromatosis—neonatal and young subjects. Blood Cells Mol Dis, 2002; 29:411–417

1248. Filali M, Le Jeunne C, Durand E et al. Juvenile hemochromatosis JHV-related revealed by cardiac shock. Blood Cells Mol Dis, 2004; 33:120–124

1249. Kelly AL, Rhodes DA, Roland JM, Schofield P, Cox TM. Hereditary juvenile hemochromatosis: a genetically heterogeneous life-threatening iron storage disease. Q J Med, 1998; 91:607–618

1250. Camaschella C, Roetto A, Cali A et al. The gene TFR2 is mutated in a new type of haemochromatosis mapping to 7q22. Nat Genet, 2000; 25:14–15

1251. De Vos R, Sciot R, van Eyken P, Desmet VJ. Immunoelectron microscopic localization of hepatic transferrin receptors in human liver with and without iron overload. Virchows Arch B Cell Pathol Incl Mol Pathol, 1988; 55:11–17

1252. Lombard M, Bomford A, Hynes M et al. Regulation of the hepatic transferrin receptor in hereditary hemochromatosis. Hepatology, 1989; 9:1–5

1253. Sciot R, Paterson AC, Van den Oord JJ, Desmet VJ. Lack of transferrin receptor in hemochromatosis. Hepatology, 1987; 7:831–837

1254. Fleming RE, Migas MC, Holden CC et al. Transferrin receptor 2: Continued expression in mouse liver in the face of iron overload and in hereditary hemochromatosis. Proc Natl Acad Sci U S A, 2000; 97:2214–2219

1255. Nemeth E, Roetto A, Garozzo G, Ganz T, Camaschella C. Hepcidin is decreased in TFR2 hemochromatosis. Blood, 2005; 105:1803–1806

1256. Mattman A, Huntsman D, Lockitch G et al. Transferrin receptor 2 (TfR2) and HFE mutational analysis in non-C282Y iron overload: identification of a novel TfR2 mutation. Blood, 2002; 100:1075–1077

1257. Camaschella C, Fargion S, Sampietro M et al. Inherited HFE-unrelated hemochromatosis in Italian families. Hepatology, 1999; 29:1563–1564

1258. Girelli D, Bozzini C, Roetto A et al. Clinical and pathologic findings in hemochromatosis type 3 due to a novel mutation in transferrin receptor 2 gene. Gastroenterology, 2002; 122:1295–1302

1259. Roetto A, Totaro A, Piperno A et al. New mutations inactivating transferrin receptor 2 in hemochromatosis type 3. Blood, 2001; 97:2555–2560

1260. Hattori A, Wakusawa S, Hayashi H et al. AVAQ 594–597 deletion of the TfR2 gene in a Japanese family with hemochromatosis. Hepatol Res, 2003; 26:154–156

1261. Koyama C, Wakusawa S, Hayashi H et al. Two novel mutations, L490R and V561X, of the transferrin receptor 2 gene in Japanese patients with haemochromatosis. Haematologica, 2005; 90:302–307

1262. Pietrangelo A. The ferroportin disease. Blood Cells Mol Dis, 2004; 32:131–138

1263. Pietrangelo A, Montosi G, Totaro A et al. Hereditary hemochromatosis in adults with pathogenic mutations in the hemochromatosis gene. N Engl J Med, 1999; 341:725–732

1264. Montosi G, Donovan A, Totaro A et al. Autosomal-dominant hemochromatosis is associated with a mutation in the ferroportin (SLC11A3) gene. J Clin Invest, 2001; 108:619–623

1265. Njajou N, Vaessen M, Joosse B et al. Mutation in SLC11A3 is associated with autosomal dominant haemochromatosis. Nat Genet, 2001; 28:213–214

1266. De Domenico I, Ward DM, Nemeth E et al. The molecular basis of ferroportin-linked hemochromatosis. Proc Natl Acad Sci U S A, 2005; 102:8955–8960

1267. Sham RL, Pradyumna D, Phataka PD, Lee P, Andrews C, Beutler E. Autosomal dominant hereditary hemochromatosis associated with a novel ferroportin mutation and unique clinical features. Blood Cells Mol Dis, 2005; 34:157–161

1268. Arden KE, Wallace DF, Dixon JL et al. A novel mutation in ferroportin1 is associated with hemochromatosis in a Solomon Islands patient. Gut, 2003; 52:1215–1217

1269. Eason RJ, Adams PC, Aston CE, Searle J. Familial iron overload with possible autosomal dominance. Aust NZ Med J, 1990; 20:226–230

1270. Rivard SR, Lanzara C, Grimard D et al. Autosomal dominant reticuloendothelial iron overload due to a new missense mutation in the FERROPORTIN 1 gene (SLC11A3) in a large French-Canadian family. Haematologica, 2003; 88:824–826

1271. Viprakasit V, Merryweather-Clarke A, Chinthammitr Y et al. Molecular diagnosis of the first ferroportin mutation (C326Y) in the far east causing a dominant form of inherited iron overload. Blood, 2004; 104:3204

1272. Wallace DF, Clark RM, Harley HAJ, Subramaniam VN. Autosomal dominant iron overload due to a novel mutation of ferroportin1 associated with parenchymal iron loading and cirrhosis. J Hepatol, 2004; 40:710–713

1273. Hardy L, Hansen JL, Kushner JP, Knisely AS. Neonatal hemochromatosis: genetic analysis of transferrin-receptor, H-apoferritin, and L-apoferritin loci and of the human leukocyte antigen class 1 region. Am J Pathol, 1990; 137:149–153

1274. Murray KF, Kowdley KV. Neonatal hemochromatosis. Pediatrics, 2001; 108:960–964

1275. Knisely AS, Mieli-Vergani G, Whitington PF. Neonatal hemochromatosis. Gastroenterol Clin North Am, 2003; 32:877–889

1276. Whitington PF, Hibbard JU. High dose immunoglobulin during pregnancy for recurrent neonatal haemochromatosis. Lancet, 2004; 364:1690–1698

1277. Flynn DM, Mohan N, McKiernan P et al. Progress in treatment and outcome for children with neonatal haemochromatosis. Arch Dis Child Fetal Neonatal Ed, 2003; 88:124–127

1278. Kelly AL, Lunt PW, Rodrigues F et al. Classification and genetic features of neonatal haemochromatosis: a study of 27 affected pedigrees and molecular analysis of genes implicated in iron metabolism. J Med Genet, 2001; 38:599–610

1279. Knisely AS, O'Shea PA, Stocks JF, Dimmick JE. Oropharyngeal and upper respiratory gland mucosal-gland siderosis in neonatal hemochromatosis: an approach to biopsy diagnosis. J Pediatr, 1988; 113:871–874

1280. Andrews NC, Anupindi S, Badizadegan K. Case records of the Massachusetts General Hospital. Case 21–2005. A four-week-old male infant with jaundice and thrombocytopenia. N Engl J Med, 2005; 353:189–198

1281. Oddone M, Bellini C, Bonacci W, Bartocci M, Toma P, Serra G. Diagnosis of neonatal hemochromatosis with MR imaging and duplex Doppler sonography. Eur Radiol, 1999; 9:1882–1885

1282. Sigurdsson L, Reyes J, Kocoshis SA, Hansen TW, Rosh J, Knisely AS. Neonatal hemochromatosis: outcomes of pharmacologic and surgical therapies. J Pediatr Gastroenterol Nutr, 1998; 26:85–89

1283. Egawa H, Bergquist W, Garcia-Kennedy R, Cox K, Knisely AS, Esquivel CO. Rapid development of hepatocellular siderosis after transplantation for neonatal hemochromatosis. Transplantation, 1996; 62:1511–1513

1284. Bellini C, Mazzella M, Scopesi F, Serra G. Spontaneous recovery in neonatal hemochromatosis. J Hepatol, 2004; 41:882–883

1285. Inui A, Fujisawa T, Kubo T, Sogo T, Komatsu H, Kagata Y. A Case of Neonatal Hemochromatosis-Like Liver Failure with Spontaneous Remission. J Pediatr Gastroenterol Nutr, 2005; 40:374–377

1286. Gordeuk VR, McLaren CE, MacPhail AP, Deichsel G, Bothwell TH. Associations of iron overload in Africa with hepatocellular carcinoma and tuberculosis: Strachan's 1929 thesis revisited. Blood, 1996; 87:3470–3476

1287. MacPhail AP, Simon MO, Torrance JD, Charlton RW, Bothwell TH, Isaacson C. Changing patterns of dietary iron overload in black South Africans. Am J Clin Nutr, 1979; 32:1272–1278

1288. Friedman BM, Baynes RD, Bothwell TH et al. Dietary iron overload in southern African rural blacks. S Afr Med J, 1990; 78:301–305

1289. Gordeuk VR. African iron overload. Semin Hematol, 2002; 39:263–269

1290. Gordeuk VR, Boyd RD, Brittenham GM. Dietary iron overload persists in rural sub-Saharan Africa. Lancet, 1986; 1:1310–1313

1291. Bothwell TH, Bradlow BA. Siderosis in the Bantu. A combined histopathological and chemical study. Arch Path, 1960; 70:279–292

1292. Walker ARP, Arvidsson UB. Iron overload in the South African Bantu. Tr Roy Soc Trop Med Hyg, 1953; 47:536–548

1293. Bothwell TH, Seftel H, Jacobs P, Torrance JD, Baumslag N. Iron overload in Bantu subjects. Studies on the availability of iron in bantu beer. Am J Clin Nutrit, 1964; 14:47–51

1294. McNamara L, MacPhail AP, Gordeuk VR, Hasstedt SJ, Rouault T. Is there a link between African iron overload and the described mutations of the hereditary haemochromatosis gene? Br J Haematol, 1998; 102:1176–1178

1295. Moyo VM, Gangaidzo IT, Gomo ZA et al. Traditional beer consumption and the iron status of spouse pairs from a rural community in Zimbabwe. Blood, 1997; 89:2159–2166

1296. Moyo VM, Mandishona E, Hasstedt SJ et al. Evidence of genetic transmission in African iron overload. Blood, 1998; 91:1076–1082

1297. Wurapa RK, Gordeuk VR, Brittenham GM, Khiyami A, Schechter GP, Edwards CQ. Primary iron overload in African Americans. Am J Med, 1996; 101:9–18

1298. Beutler E, Barton JC, Felitti VJ et al. Ferroportin 1 (SCL40A1) variant associated with iron overload in African-Americans. Blood Cells Mol Dis, 2003; 31:305–309

1299. Gordeuk VR, Caleffi A, Corradini E et al. Iron overload in Africans and African-Americans and a common mutation in the SCL40A1 (ferroportin 1) gene. Blood Cells Mol Dis, 2003; 31:299–304

1300. McNamara L, Gordeuk VR, MacPhail AP. Ferroportin (Q248H) mutations in African families with dietary iron overload. J Gastroenterol Nutr, 2005; 20:1855–1858

1301. Bothwell TH, Isaacson C. Siderosis in the Bantu. A comparison of incidence in males and females. Br Med J, 1962; 1(5277):522–524

1302. Isaacson C, Seftel HC, Keeley KJ, Bothwell TH. Siderosis in the Bantu: The relationship between iron overload and cirrhosis. J Lab Clin Med, 1962; 58:845–853

1303. Seftel HC, Keeley KJ, Isaacson C, Bothwell TH. Siderosis in the Bantu: The clinical incidence of hemochromatosis in diabetic subjects. J Lab Clin Med, 1961; 58:837–844

1304. Seftel HC, Malkin C, Schmaman A et al. Osteoporosis, scurvy and siderosis in Johannesburg Bantu. Br Med J, 1966; 1:642–646

1305. Wapnick AA, Lynch SR, Seftel HC, Charlton RW, Bothwell TH, Jowsey J. The effect of siderosis and ascorbic acid depletion on bone metabolism with special reference to osteoporosis in the Bantu. Br J Nutr, 1971; 25:367–376

1306. Bothwell TH, Abrahams C, Bradlow BA, Charlton RW. Idiopathic and Bantu hemochromatosis. Arch Pathol, 1965; 79:163–168

1307. Paterson AC, MacPhail AP, Gordeuk VR. African iron overload revisited: histology in relation to measurements of iron status (abstract). Hepatology, 1999; 30(Suppl):382A

1308. MacPhail AP, Mandishona EM, Bloom PD, Paterson AC, Rouault TA, Gordeuk VR. Measurements of iron status and survival in African iron overload. S Afr Med J, 1999; 89:966–972

1309. Mandishona E, MacPhail PA, Gordeuk VR et al. Dietary iron overload as a risk factor for hepatocellular carcinoma in Black Africans. Hepatology, 1998; 27:1563–1566

1310. Aguilar-Martinez P, Schved JF, Brissot P. The evaluation of hyperferritinemia: an updated strategy based on advances in detecting genetic abnormalities. Am J Gastroenterol, 2005; 100:1185–1194

1311. Allerson CR, Cazzola M, Rouault TA. Clinical severity and thermodynamic effects of iron-responsive element mutations in Hereditary Hyperferritinemia-Cataract Syndrome. J Biol Chem, 1999; 274:26439–26447

1312. Beaumont C, Leneuve P, Devaux I et al. Mutation in the iron responsive element of the L ferritin mRNA in a family with dominant hyperferritinaemia and cataract. Nat Genet, 1995; 11:444–446

1313. Kato J, Fujikawa K, Kanda M et al. A mutation in the iron-responsive element of H ferritin mRNA, causing autosomal dominant iron overload. Am J Hum Genet, 2001; 69:191–197

1314. Ferreira C, Santambrogio P, Martin ME et al. H ferritin knockout mice: a model of hyperferritinemia in the absence of iron overload. Blood, 2001; 98:525–532

1315. Siah CW, Trinder D, Olynyk JK. Iron overload. Clin Chim Acta, 2005; 358:24–36

1316. Online Mendelian Inheritance in Man O, Ferritin Heavy Chain 1, in Ferritin Heavy Chain. 2000, McKusick-Nathans Institute for Genetic Medicine

1317. Mims MP, Guan Y, Pospisilova D et al. Identification of a human mutation of DMT1 in a patient with microcytic anemia and iron overload. Blood, 2005; 105:1337–1342

1318. Huang FW, Pinkus JL, Pinkus GS et al. A mouse model of juvenile hemochromatosis. J Clin Invest, 2005; 115:2187–2191

1319. Camaschella C. Understanding iron homeostasis through genetic analysis of hemochromatosis and related disorders. Blood 2005; 106:3710–3717

1320. Pietrangelo A. Non-HFE hemochromatosis. Hepatology, 2004; 39:21–29

1321. Heilmeyer L, Keller W, Vivell O, Betke K, Wöhler F, Keiderling W. Die kongenitale Atransferrinämie. Schweiz Med Wochenschr, 1961; 91:1203

1322. Beutler E, Gelbart T, Lee P, Fernandez MA, Fairbanks VF. Molecular characterization of a case of atransferrinemia. Blood, 2000; 96:4071–4074

1323. Knisely AS, Gelbart T, Beutler E. Molecular characterization of a third case of human atransferrinaemia (letter). Blood, 2004; 104:2607

1324. Hayashi A, Wada Y, Suzuki T, Shimizu A. Studies on familial hypotransferrinemia: a unique clinical course and molecular pathology. Am J Hum Genet, 1993; 53:201–213

1325. Trenor CC, Campagna DR, Sellers VM, Andrews NC, Fleming MD. The molecular defect in hypotransferrinemic mice. Blood, 2000; 96:1113–1118

1326. Royle NJ, Irwin DM, Koschinsky ML, MacGillivray RT, Hamerton JL. Human genes encoding prothrombin and ceruloplasmin map to 11p11–q12 and 3q21–24, respectively. Somat Cell Mol Genet, 1998; 13:285–292

1327. Harris ZL, Takahashi Y, Miyajima H, Serizawa M, MacGillivray RTA, Gitlin JD. Aceruloplasminemia: molecular characterization of this disorder of iron metabolism. Proc Natl Acad Sci U S A, 1995; 92

1328. Yoshida K, Furihata K, Takeda S et al. A mutation in the ceruloplasmin gene is associated with systemic hemosiderosis in humans. Nat Genet, 1995; 9:267–272

1329. Hellman NE, Schaefer M, Gehrke S et al. Hepatic iron overload in aceruloplasminemia. Gut, 2000; 47:858–860

1330. Bosio S, De Gobbi M, Roetto A et al. Anemia and iron overload due to compound heterozygosity for novel ceruloplasmin mutations. Blood, 2002; 100:2246–2248

1331. Hellman NE, Kono S, Miyajima H et al. Biochemical analysis of a missense mutation in aceruloplasminemia. J Biol Chem, 2002; 277:1375–1380

1332. Lo L, Singer ST. Thalassemia: current approach to an old disease. Pediatr Clin N Am, 2002; 49:1165–1191

1333. Brittenham GM, Griffith PM, Nienhuis AW et al. Efficacy of deferroxamine in preventing complications of iron overload in patients with thalassaemia major. N Engl J Med, 1994; 331:567–573

1334. Martins R, Picanco I, Fonseca A et al. The role of HFE mutations on iron metabolism in beta thalassemia carriers. J Hum Genet, 2004; 49:651–655

1335. Modell B, Khan M, Darlison M. Survival in beta-thalassaemia major in the UK: data from the UK Thalassaemia Register. Lancet, 2000; 355:2051–2052

1336. Longo F, Zecchina G, Sbaiz L, Fischer R, Piga A, Camaschella C. The influence of hemochromatosis mutations on iron overload of thalassemia major. Haematologica, 1999; 84:799–803

1337. Riva A, Mariani R, Bovo G et al. Type 3 hemochromatosis and beta-thalassemia trait. J Haematol, 2004; 72:370–374

1338. Levi S, Corsi B, Bosisio M et al. A human mitochondrial ferritin encoded by an intronless gene. J Biol Chem, 2001; 276:24437–24440

1339. Napier I, Ponka P, Richardson DR. Iron trafficking in the mitochondrion: novel pathways revealed by disease. Blood, 2005; 105:1867–1874

1340. Roy CN, Andrews NC. Recent advances in disorders of iron metabolism: mutations, mechanisms and modifiers. Hum Mol Genet, 2001; 10:2181–2186

1341. Online Mendelian Inheritance in Man, OMIM, X linked sideroblastic anemia. 2000, McKusick Nathans Institute for Genetic Medicine

1342. Peto TE, Pippard MJ, Weatherall DJ. Iron overload in mild sideroblastic anaemias. Lancet, 1983; 1:375–378

1343. Barron R, Grace ND, Sherwood G, Powell LW. Iron overload complicating sideroblastic anemia is the gene for hemochromatosis responsible? Gastroenterology, 1989; 96:1204–1206

1344. Beris P, Samii K, Darbellay R et al. Iron overload in patients with sideroblastic anaemia is not related to the presence of the haemochromatosis Cys282Tyr and His63Asp mutations. Br J Haematol, 1999; 104:97–99

1345. Chemmanur AT, Bonkovsky HL. Hepatic porphyrias: diagnosis and management. Clin Liv Dis, 2004; 8:807–838

1346. Sampietro M, Fiorelli G, Fargion S. Iron overload in porphyria cutanea tarda. Haematologica, 1999; 84:248–253

1347. Walker AP, Partridge J, Srai SK, Dooley JS. Hepcidin: what every gastroenterologist should know. Gut, 2004; 53:624–627

1348. Rivera S, Liu L, Nemeth E et al. Hepcidin excess induces the sequestration of iron and exacerbates tumor-associated anemia. Blood, 2005; 105:1797–1802

1349. Ludwig J, Hashimoto E, Porayko MK, Moyer TP, Baldus WP. Hemosiderosis in cirrhosis: a study of 447 native livers. Gastroenterology, 1997; 112:882–888

1350. Bonkovsky HL, Banner BF, Rothman AL. Iron and chronic viral hepatitis. Hepatology, 1997; 25:759–768

1351. Mah YH, Kao JH, Liu CJ et al. Prevalence and clinical implications of HFE gene mutations (C282Y and H63D) in patients with chronic hepatitis B and C in Taiwan. Liv Int, 2005; 25:214–219

1352. Uraz S, Aygun C, Sonsuz A, Ozbay G. Serum iron levels and hepatic iron overload in nonalcoholic steatohepatitis and chronic viral hepatitis. Dig Dis Sci, 2005; 50:964–969

1353. Di Bisceglie AM, Axiotis CA, Hoofnagle JH, Bacon BR. Measurements of iron status in patients with chronic hepatitis. Gastroenterology, 1992; 102:2108–2113

1354. Cotler SJ, Bronner MP, Press RD, Carlson TH, Perkins JD, Edmond MJ. End-stage liver disease without hemochromatosis associated with elevated hepatic iron index. J Hepatol, 1998; 29:257–262

1355. Bonkovsky HL, Lambrecht RW, Shan Y. Iron as a co-morbid factor in nonhaemochromatotic liver disease. Alcohol, 2003; 30:137–144

1356. Hezode C, Cazeneuve C, Coue O, Roudot-Thoraval F, Lonjon I, Bastie A. Liver iron accumulation in patients with chronic active hepatitis C: prevalence and role of hemochromatosis gene mutations and relationships with hepatic histological lesions. J Hepatol, 1999; 31:979–984

1357. Eisenbach C, Gehrke SG, Stremmel W. Iron, the HFE gene, and hepatitis C. Clin Liv Dis, 2004; 8:775–785

1358. Kato J, Kobune M, Nakamura T, Kuroiwa G, Takada K, Takimoto R. Normalization of elevated hepatic 8-hydroxy-2′-deoxyguanosine levels in chronic hepatitis C patients by phlebotomy and low iron diet. Cancer Res, 2001; 61:8697–8702

1359. Yano M, Hayashi H, Wakusawa S, Sanae F, Takikawa T, Shiono Y. Long term effects of phlebotomy on biochemical and histological parameters of chronic hepatitis C. Am J Gastroenterol, 2002; 97:13 133–137

1360. Kakizaki S, Takagi H, Horiguchi N, Toyoda M, Takayama H, Nagamine T. Iron enhances hepatitis C virus replication in cultured hepatocytes. Liver, 2000; 20:125–128

1361. Aoki CA, Rossaro L, Ramsamooj R, Brandhagen D, Burritt MF, Bowlus CL. Liver hepcidin mRNA correlates with iron stores, but not inflammation, in patients with chronic hepatitis C. J Clin Gastroenterol, 2005; 39:71–74

1362. Tung BY, Emond MJ, Bronner MP, Raaka SD, Cotler SJ, Kowdley KV. Hepatitis C, iron status, and disease severity: relationship with HFE mutations. Gastroenterology, 2003; 124:318–326

1363. Bataller R, North KE, Brenner DA. Genetic polymorphisms and the progression of liver fibrosis: a critical appraisal. Hepatology, 2003; 37:493–503

1364. Conrad ME, Berman A, Brosby WH. Iron kinetics in Laennec's cirrhosis. Gastroenterology, 1962; 43:386–390

1365. Gilbert A, Grenet A. Cirrhose alcoolique hypertrophique pigmentaire. Compte Rendus Soc de Biol, 1896; 10:1078–1081

1366. MacDonald RA. Prog Hematol. Primary hemochromatosis: inherited or acquired?, 1966; 5:324–353

1367. Sabesin SM, Thomas LB. Parenchymal siderosis in patients with preexisting portal cirrhosis. A pathological entity simulating idiopathic and transfusional hemochromatosis. Gastroenterology, 1964; 46:477–485

1368. Bassett ML, Halliday JW, Powell LW. Value of hepatic iron measurements in early hemochromatosis and determination of the critical iron level associated with fibrosis. Hepatology, 1986; 6:24–29

1369. Arteel GE. Oxidants and antioxidants in alcohol-induced liver disease. Gastroenterology, 2003; 124:778–790

1370. Tavill AS, Qadri AM. Alcohol and iron. Semin Liv Dis, 2004; 24:317–325

1371. Powell LW. Iron storage in relatives of patients with haemochromatosis and in relatives of patients with alcoholic cirrhosis and haemosiderosis. A comparative study of 27 families. Q J Med, 1965; 34:427–442

1372. Fletcher LM, Dixon JL, Purdie DM, Powell LW, Crawford DHG. Excess alcohol greatly increases the prevalence of cirrhosis in hereditary hemochromatosis: quantifying the risk. Gastroenterology, 2002; 122:281–289

1373. Fletcher LM, Powell LW. Hemochromatosis and alcoholic liver disease. Alcohol, 2003; 30:131–136

1374. Swanson CA. Iron intake and regulation: implications for iron deficiency and iron overload. Alcohol, 2003; 30:99–102

1375. Rouault TA. Hepatic iron overload in alcoholic liver disease: why does it occur and what is its role in pathogenesis? Alcohol, 2003; 30:103–110

1376. Ludwig J, Yiggiano TR, McGill DB, Ott BJ. Nonalcoholic steatohepatitis. Mayo Clinic experiences with a hitherto unnamed disease. Mayo Clin Proc, 1980; 55:434–438

1377. Bonkovsky HL, Jawaid Q, Tortorelli K et al. Non-alcoholic steatohepatitis and iron: increased prevalence of mutations of the HFE gene in non-alcoholic steatohepatitis. J Hepatol, 1999; 31:421–429

1378. George DK, Goldwurm S, MacDonald GA et al. Increased hepatic iron concentration in nonalcoholic steatohepatitis is associated with increased fibrosis. Gastroenterology, 1998; 114:311–318

1379. Valenti L, Dongiovanni P, Fracanzani AL et al. Increased susceptibility to nonalcoholic fatty liver disease in heterozygotes for the mutation responsible for hereditary haemochromatosis. Dig Liv Dis, 2003; 35:172–178

1380. Angulo P, Keach JC, Batts KP, Lindor KD. Independent predictors of liver fibrosis in patients with nonalcoholic steatohepatitis. Hepatology, 1999; 30:1356–1362

1381. Younossi ZM, Gramlich T, Bacon BR et al. Hepatic iron and nonalcoholic fatty liver disease. Hepatology, 1999; 30:847–850

1382. Chitturi S, Weltman M, Farrell GC et al. HFE mutations, hepatic iron, and fibrosis: ethnic-specific association of NASH with C282Y but not with fibrotic severity. Hepatology, 2002; 36:142–149

1383. Bugianesi E, Manzini P, D'Antico S et al. Relative contribution of iron burden, HFE mutations, and insulin resistance to fibrosis in nonalcoholic fatty liver. Hepatology, 2004; 39:179–187

1384. Marchesini G, Forlani G. NASH: from liver diseases to metabolic disorders and back to clinical hepatology. Hepatology, 2002; 35:497–499

1385. Duseja A, Das R, Nanda M, Das A, Garewal G, Chalwa Y. Nonalcoholic steatohepatitis is neither associated with iron overload nor with HFE gene mutations. World J Gastroenterol, 2005; 11:393–395

1386. Weltman MD, Farrell GC, Hall P, Ingelman-Sundberg M, Liddle C. Hepatic cytochrome P450 2E1 is increased in patients with nonalcoholic steatohepatitis. Hepatology, 1998; 27:128–133

1387. Brandhagen DJ, Alvarez W, Therneau TM et al. Iron overload in cirrhosis; HFE genotypes and outcome after liver transplantation. Hepatology, 2000; 31:456–460

1388. Brodanova M, Hoenig V. Iron metabolism in patients with porta-caval shunts. Scand J Gastroenterol, 1966; 1:167–172

1389. Adams PC, Bradley C, Frei JV. Hepatic iron and zinc concentrations after portacaval shunting for nonalcoholic cirrhosis. Hepatology, 1994; 19:101–105

1390. Coder SJ, Bronner MEPRD et al. End-stage liver disease without hemochromatosis associated with elevated hepatic iron index. J Hepatol, 1998; 29:257–262

1391. Conn HO. Portacaval anastomosis and hepatic hemosiderin deposition: a prospective, controlled investigation. Gastroenterology, 1972; 62:61–72

1392. Niederau C, Fischer R, Sonnenberg A, Stremmel W, Trampisch, HJ, Strohmeyer, G. Survival and causes of death in cirrhotic and noncirrhotic patients with primary hemochromatosis. N Engl J Med, 1985; 313:1256–1262

1393. Adams PC. Hepatocellular carcinoma in hereditary hemochromatosis. Can J Gastorenterol, 1993; 7:37–41

1394. Bradbear RA, Bain C, Siskind V et al. Cohort study of internal malignancy in genetic hemochromatosis and other chronic nonalcoholic liver diseases. J Natl Cancer Inst, 1985; 75:81–84

1395. Hsing AW, McLaughlin JK, Olsen JH, Mellemkjar L, Wacholder S, Fraumeni JF. Cancer risk following primary hemochromatosis: a population-based cohort study in Denmark. Int J Cancer, 1995; 60:160–162

1396. Fargion S, Mandelli C, Piperno A et al. Survival and prognostic factors in 212 Italian patients with genetic hemochromatosis. Hepatology, 1992; 15:655–659

1397. Fracanzani AL, Conte D, Fraquelli M et al. Increased cancer risk in a cohort of 230 patients with hereditary hemochromatosis in comparison to matched control patients with non-iron-related chronic liver disease. Hepatology, 2001; 33:647–651

1398. Britto MR, Thomas LA, Balaratnam N, Griffiths AP, Duane PD. Hepatocellular carcinoma arising in non-cirrhotic liver in genetic haemochromatosis. Scand J Gastroenterol, 2000; 35:889–893

1399. Deugnier Y, Charalambous P, Le Quilleuc D et al. Primary liver cancer in genetic hemochromatosis: a clinical, pathological and pathogenetic study of 54 cases. Gastroenterology, 1993; 104:228–234

1400. Fellows IW, Stewart M, Jeffcoate WJ, Smith PG, Toghill PJ. Hepatocellular carcinoma in primary haemochromatosis in the absence of cirrhosis. Gut, 1988; 29:1603–1606

1401. Goh J, Callagy G, McEntee G, O'Keane JC, Bomford A, Crowe J. Hepatocellular carcinoma arising in the absence of cirrhosis in genetic haemochromatosis: three case reports and review of literature. Eur J Gastroenterol Hepatol, 1999; 11:915–919

1402. Morcos M, Dubois S, Bralet MP, Belghiti J, Degott C, Terris B. Primary carcinoma in genetic hemochromatosis reveals a broad genetic spectrum. Am J Clin Pathol, 2001; 116:738–843

1403. Blumberg RS, Chopra S, Ibrahim R et al. Primary hepatocellular carcinoma in idiopathic hemochromatosis after reversal of cirrhosis. Gastroenterology, 1988; 95:1399–1402

1404. Deugnier YM, Guyader D, Crantock L et al. Primary liver cancer in genetic hemochromatosis: a clinical, pathological and pathogenetic study of 54 cases. Gastroenterology, 1993; 104:228–234

1405. Deugnier Y. Iron and liver cancer. Alcohol, 2003; 30:145–150

1406. Linet MS, Gridley G, Nyren O et al. Primary liver cancer, other malignancies, and mortality risks following porphyria: a cohort study in Denmark and Sweden. Am J Epidemiol, 1999; 149:1010–1015

1407. Higginson J. Primary carcinoma of the liver in Africa. Br J Cancer, 1956; 10:609–622

1408. Moyo VM, Makunike R, Gangaidzo IT et al. African iron overload and hepatocellular carcinoma. Eur J Hematol, 1998; 60:28–34

1409. Toyokuni S. Iron induced carcinogenesis: the role of redox regulation. Free Radical Biology & Medicine, 1996; 20:553–566

1410. Smith PG, Yeoh GCT. Chronic iron overload in rats induces oval cells in the liver. Am J Pathol, 1996; 149:389–398

1411. Pigeon C, Turlin B, Iancu TC et al. Carbonyl-iron supplementation induces hepatocyte nuclear changes in BALB/CJ male mice. J Hepatol, 1999; 30:926–934

1412. Rothenberg BE, Voland JR. β2 Knockout mice develop parenchymal iron overload: a putative role for class I genes of the major histocompatibility complex in iron metabolism. Proc Natl Acad Sci U S A, 1996; 93:1529–1534

1413. Deugnier Y, Loréal O, Turlin B et al. Liver pathology in genetic hemochromatosis: a review of 135 homozygous patients and their bioclinical correlations. Gastroenterology, 1992; 102:2050–2059

1414. Asare G, Paterson AC, Kew MC, Khan S, Mossanda KS. Development of iron free foci and hepatocellular carcinoma in the absence of cirrhosis in rats fed a diet high in iron. Submitted

1415. Williams G, Yamamoto R. Absence of stainable iron from preneoplastic and neoplastic lesions in rat liver with 8-hydroxyquinolone-induced siderosis. J Natl Cancer Inst, 1972; 49:685–692

1416. Stål P, Hultcrantz R, Moller L, Eriksson LC. The effects of dietary iron on initiation and promotion in chemical hepatocarcinogenesis. Hepatology, 1995; 21:521–528

1417. Harrison SA, Bacon BR. Relation of hemochromatosis with hepatocellular carcinoma: epidemiology, natural history, pathophysiology, screening, treatment, and prevention. Med Clin N Am, 2005; 89:391–409

1418. Turlin B, Deugnier Y. Evaluation and interpretation of iron in the liver. Sem Diagn Pathol, 1998; 15:237–245

1419. Crawford DHG, Fletcher LM, Hübscher SG et al. Patient and graft survival after liver transplantation for hereditary haemochromatosis: implications for pathogenesis. Hepatology, 2004; 39:1655–1662

1420. Parolin MB, Batts KP, Weisner RH et al. Liver allograft iron accumulation in patients with and without pretransplantation hepatic hemosiderosis. Liver Transpl, 2002; 8:331–339

1421. Guyader D, Jacquelinet C, Moirand R et al. Noninvasive prediction of fibrosis in C282Y homozygous hemochromatosis. Gastroenterology, 1998; 115:929–936

1422. Turlin B, Deugnier Y. Iron overload disorders. Clin Liv Dis, 2002; 6:481–496

1423. Scheuer PJ, Williams R, Muir A. Hepatic pathology in relatives of patients with hemochromatosis. J Pathol Bacteriol, 1962; 84:53–64

1424. Brissot P, Bourel M, Herry D et al. Assessment of liver iron content in 271 patients: reevaluation of direct and indirect methods. Gastroenterology, 1981; 80:557–565

1425. Scheuer PJ, Lefkowitch JH. Liver biopsy interpretation. 6th ed. 2000, London: WB Saunders pp. 274–275

1426. Deugnier YM, Turlin B, Powell LW et al. Differentiation between heterozygotes and homozygotes hemochromatosis by means of a histological hepatic iron index: a study of 192 cases. Hepatology, 1993; 17:30–34

1427. Adams PC, Bradley C, Henderson AR. Evaluation of the hepatic iron index as criterion for genetic hemochromatosis a diagnostic criterion for genetic hemochromatosis. J Lab Clin Med, 1997; 130:509–514

1428. Sharma R, Hudak ML, Perszyk AA, Premachandra BR, Li H, Monteiro C. Perinatal lethal form of Gaucher's disease presenting with hemosiderosis. Am J Perinatol, 2000; 17:201–206

1429. Onishi Y, Noshiro M, Shimosato T, Okuda K. Molecular cloning and sequence analysis of cDNA encoding delta 4-3-ketosteroid 5 beta-reductase of rat liver. FEBS Lett, 1991; 283:215–218

1430. Onishi Y, Noshiro M, Shimosato T et al. delta 4-3-Oxosteroid 5 beta-reductase. Structure and function. Biol Chem Hoppe Seyler, 1991; 372:1039–1049

1431. Daugherty CC, Setchell KD, Heubi JE, Balistreri WF. Resolution of liver biopsy alterations in three siblings with bile acid treatment of an inborn error of bile acid metabolism (delta 4-3-oxosteroid 5 beta-reductase deficiency). Hepatology, 1993; 18:1096–1101

1432. Kondo KH, Kai MH, Setoguchi Y et al. Cloning and expression of cDNA of human delta 4-3-oxosteroid 5 beta-reductase and substrate specificity of the expressed enzyme. Eur J Biochem, 1994; 219:357–363

1433. Setchell KD, Suchy FJ, Welsh MB, Zimmer-Nechemias L, Heubi J, Balistreri WF. Delta 4-3-oxosteroid 5 beta-reductase deficiency described in identical twins with neonatal hepatitis. A new inborn error in bile acid synthesis. J Clin Invest, 1988; 82:2148–2157

1434. Sumazaki R, Nakamura N, Shoda J, Kurosawa T, Tohma M. Gene analysis in delta 4-3-oxosteroid 5 beta-reductase deficiency. Lancet, 1997; 349:329 (letter)

1435. Russell DW, Setchell KD. Bile acid biosynthesis. Biochemistry, 1992; 31:4737–4749

1436. Clayton PT, Mills KA, Johnson AW, Barabino A, Marazzi MG. Delta 4-3-oxosteroid 5 beta-reductase deficiency: failure of ursodeoxycholic acid treatment and response to chenodeoxycholic acid plus cholic acid. Gut, 1996; 38:623–628

1437. Bove KE, Daugherty CC, Tyson W et al. Bile acid synthetic defects and liver disease. Pediatr Develop Pathol, 2000; 3:1–16

1438. Clayton PT, Leonard JV, Lawson AM et al. Familial giant cell hepatitis associated with synthesis of 3b, 7 a-dihydroxy-and 3b, 7 a, 12 a-trihydroxy-5-cholenoic acids. J Clin Invest, 1987; 79:1031–1038

1439. Buchmann MS, Kvittingen EA, Nazer H et al. Lack of 3 beta-hydroxy-delta 5-C27-steroid dehydrogenase/isomerase in fibroblasts from a child with urinary excretion of 3 beta-hydroxy-delta 5-bile acids. A new inborn error of metabolism. J Clin Invest, 1990; 86:2034–2037

1440. Ichimiya H, Nazer H, Gunasekaran T, Clayton P, Sjovall J. Treatment of chronic liver disease caused by 3 beta-hydroxy-D5-

C27-steroid dehydrogenase deficiency with chenodeoxycholic acid. Arch Dis Child, 1990; 65:1121–1124

1441. Jacquemin E, Setchell KD, NC OC et al. A new cause of progressive intrahepatic cholestasis: 3 beta-hydroxy-C27- steroid dehydrogenase/isomerase deficiency. J Pediatr, 1994; 125:379–384

1442. Stieger B, Zhang J, O'Neill B, Sjovall J, Meier PJ. Differential interaction of bile acids from patients with inborn errors of bile acid synthesis with hepatocellular bile acid transporters. Eur J Biochem, 1997; 244:39–44

1443. Setchell KD, Schwarz M, NC OC et al. Identification of a new inborn error in bile acid synthesis: mutation of the oxysterol 7a-hydroxylase gene causes severe neonatal liver disease. J Clin Invest, 1998; 102:1690–1703

1444. Shefer S, Cheng FW, Dayal B et al. A 25-hydroxylation pathway of cholic acid biosynthesis in man and rat. J Clin Invest, 1976; 57:897–903

1445. Clayton PT, Casteels M, Mieli-Vergani G, Lawson AM. Familial giant cell hepatitis with low bile acid concentrations and increased urinary excretion of specific bile alcohols: a new inborn error of bile acid synthesis? Pediatr Res, 1995; 37:424–31

1446. Whitington PF, Freese DK, Alonso EM, Schwarzenberg SJ, Sharp HL. Clinical and biochemical findings in progressive familial intrahepatic cholestasis. J Pediatr Gastroenterol Nutr, 1994; 18:134–141

1447. Maggiore G, Bernard O, Riely CA, Hadchouel M, Lemonnier A, Alagille D. Normal serum gamma-glutamyl-transpeptidase activity identifies groups of infants with idiopathic cholestasis with poor prognosis. J Pediatr, 1987; 111:251–252

1448. Riely CA. Familial intrahepatic cholestatic syndromes. Semin Liver Dis, 1987; 7:119–133

1449. Bull LN, van Eijk MJ, Pawlikowska L et al. A gene encoding a P-type ATPase mutated in two forms of hereditary cholestasis. Nat Genet, 1998; 18:219–224

1450. Strautnieks SS, Bull LN, Knisely AS et al. A gene encoding a liver-specific ABC transporter is mutated in progressive familial intrahepatic cholestasis. Nat Genet, 1998; 20:233–238

1451. de Vree JM, Jacquemin E, Sturm E et al. Mutations in the MDR3 gene cause progressive familial intrahepatic cholestasis. Proc Natl Acad Sci USA, 1998; 95:282–287

1452. Summerskill WH. The Syndrome of Benign Recurrent Cholestasis. Am J Med, 1965; 38:298–305

1453. Bull LN, Carlton VE, Stricker NL et al. Genetic and morphological findings in progressive familial intrahepatic cholestasis (Byler disease [PFIC-1] and Byler syndrome): evidence for heterogeneity. Hepatology, 1997; 26:155–164

1454. Linarelli LG, Williams CN, Phillips MJ. Byler's disease: fatal intrahepatic cholestasis. J Pediatr, 1972; 81:484–492

1455. Luketic VA, Shiffman ML. Benign recurrent intrahepatic cholestasis. Clin Liver Dis, 1999; 3:509–528

1456. Tygstrup N, Steig BA, Juijn JA, Bull LN, Houwen RH. Recurrent familial intrahepatic cholestasis in the Faroe Islands. Phenotypic heterogeneity but genetic homogeneity. Hepatology, 1999; 29:506–508

1457. van Mil SW, Klomp LW, Bull LN, Houwen RH. FIC1 disease: a spectrum of intrahepatic cholestatic disorders. Semin Liver Dis, 2001; 21:535–544

1458. van Ooteghem NA, Klomp LW, van Berge-Henegouwen GP, Houwen RH. Benign recurrent intrahepatic cholestasis progressing to progressive familial intrahepatic cholestasis: low GGT cholestasis is a clinical continuum. J Hepatol, 2002; 36:439–443

1459. Klomp LW, Vargas JC, van Mil SW et al. Characterization of mutations in ATP8B1 associated with hereditary cholestasis. Hepatology, 2004; 40:27–38

1460. Brenard R, Geubel AP, Benhamou JP. Benign recurrent intrahepatic cholestasis. A report of 26 cases. J Clin Gastroenterol, 1989; 11:546–551

1461. Nielsen IM, Ornvold K, Jacobsen B, Ranek L. Fatal familial cholestatic syndrome in Greenland Eskimo children. Acta Pediatr Scand, 1986; 75:1010–1016

1462. Klomp LW, Bull LN, Knisely AS et al. A missense mutation in FIC1 is associated with greenland familial cholestasis. Hepatology, 2000; 32:1337–1341

1463. Ornvold K, Nielsen IM, Poulsen H. Fatal familial cholestatic syndrome in Greenland Eskimo children. A histomorphological analysis of 16 cases. Virchows Archiv A Pathol Anat, 1989; 415:275–281

1464. Byrne JA, Strautnieks SS, Mieli-Vergani G, Higgins CF, Linton KJ, Thompson RJ. The human bile salt export pump: characterization of substrate specificity and identification of inhibitors. Gastroenterology, 2002; 123:1649–1658

1465. Noe J, Stieger B, Meier PJ. Functional expression of the canalicular bile salt export pump of human liver. Gastroenterology, 2002; 123:1659–1666

1466. Knisely AS. Progressive familial intrahepatic cholestasis: a personal perspective. Paediatr Dev Pathol, 2000; 3:113–125

1467. Naveh Y, Bassan L, Rosenthal et al. Progressive familial intrahepatic cholestasis among the Arab population in Israel. J Pediatr Gastroenterol Nutr, 1997; 24:548–554

1468. van Mil SW, van der Woerd WL, van der Brugge G et al. Benign recurrent intrahepatic cholestasis type 2 is caused by mutations in ABCB11. Gastroenterology, 2004; 127:379–384

1469. Dahms BB. Hepatoma in familial cholestatic cirrhosis of childhood. Arch Pathol Lab Med, 1979; 103:30–33

1470. Ugarte N, Gonzalez-Crussi F. Hepatoma in siblings with progressive familial cholestatic cirrhosis of childhood. Am J Clin Pathol, 1981; 76:172–177

1471. Strautnieks S, Knisely AS, Scheimann A et al. Bile salt export pump (BSEP) deficiency is a significant risk factor for both paediatric and adult hepatobiliary malignancy. Hepatology, 2005; 42(Suppl 1):380A

1472. de Vree JM, Jacquemin E, Sturm E et al. Mutations in the MDR3 gene cause progressive familial intrahepatic cholestasis. Proc Natl Acad Sci USA, 1998; 95:282–287

1473. Elferink RP, Tytgat GN, Groen AK. Hepatic canalicular membrane 1:The role of mdr2 P-glycoprotein in hepatobiliary lipid transport. Faseb J, 1997; 11:19–28

1474. Jacquemin E, De Vree JM, Cresteil D et al. The wide spectrum of multidrug resistance 3 deficiency: from neonatal cholestasis to cirrhosis of adulthood. Gastroenterology, 2001; 120:1448–1458

1475. Lucena JF, Herrero JI, Quiroga J et al. A multidrug resistance 3 gene mutation causing cholelithiasis, cholestasis of pregnancy, and adulthood biliary cirrhosis. Gastroenterology, 2003; 124:1037–1042

1476. Deleuze JF, Jacquemin E, Dubuisson C et al. Defect of multidrug-resistance 3 gene expression in a subtype of progressive familial intrahepatic cholestasis. Hepatology, 1996; 23:904–908

1477. Jacquemin E, Dumont M, Bernard O, Erlinger S, Hadchouel M. Evidence for defective primary bile acid secretion in children with progressive familial intrahepatic cholestasis (Byler disease). Eur J Pediatr, 1994; 153:424–428

1478. Van Nieuwkerk CM, Elferink RP, Groen AK et al. Effects of Ursodeoxycholate and cholate feeding on liver disease in FVB mice with a disrupted mdr2 P-glycoprotein gene. Gastroenterology, 1996; 111:165–171

1479. Hollands CM, Rivera-Pedrogo FJ, Gonzalez-Vallina R, Loret-de-Mola O, Nahmad M, Burnweit CA. Ileal exclusion for Byler-s disease: an alternative surgical approach with promising early results for pruritus. J Pediatr Surg, 1998; 33:220–224

1480. Meller M, Rodeck B, Kardorff R et al. Progressive familial intrahepatic cholestasis: partial biliary diversion normalizes serum lipids and improves growth in noncirrhotic patients. Am J Gastroenterol, 2000; 95:3522–3528

1481. Whitington PF, Whitington GL. Partial external diversion of bile for the treatment of intractable pruritus associated with intrahepatic cholestasis. Gastroenterology, 1988; 95:130–136

1482. Jacquemin E, Crestell D, Manouvrier OB, Hadchouel M. Heterozygous non-sense mutation of the MDR 3 gene in familial intrahepatic cholestasis of pregnancy. Lancet, 1999; 353:210–211

1483. Sanbrane O, Gauthier F, Devictor D et al. Orthotopic liver transplantation for Byler disease. Transplantation, 1990; 50:804–806

1484. Lykavieris P, van Mil S, Cresteil D et al. Progressive familial intrahepatic cholestasis type 1 and extrahepatic features: no catch-up of stature growth, exacerbation of diarrhea, and appearance of liver steatosis after liver transplantation. J Hepatol, 2003; 39:447–452

1485. Weber AM, Tuchweber B, Yousef I et al. Severe familial cholestasis in North American Indian children: a clinical model of microfilament dysfunction? Gastroenterology, 1981; 81:653–662

1486. Eriksson S, Larsson C. Familial benign chronic intrahepatic cholestasis. Hepatology, 1983; 8:391–398

1487. Silva ES, Lumbroso S, Medina M, Gillerot Y, Sultan C, Sokal EM. Demonstration of McCune-Albright mutations in the liver of children with high gGT progressive cholestasis. J Hepatol, 2000; 32:154–158

1488. Sauter BV, Chowdhury NR, Chowdhury JR. Bilirubin metabolism and jaundice. In: Clinical practice of gastroenterology. L.J. Brand, Editor. 1999, Churchill Livingston: Philadelphia. p. 795–803

1489. Nowicki MJ, Poley JR. The hereditary hyperbilirubinaemias. Baillieres Clin Gastroenterol, 1998; 12:355–367

1490. Crigler JF, Najjar VA. Congenital familial nonhemolytic jaundice with kernicterus. Pediatrics, 1952; 10:169–179

1491. Szabo L, Kovacs Z, Ebrey P. Congenital non-haemolytic jaundice. Lancet, 1962; 1:322

1492. Jackson MR, McCarthy LR, Harding D, Wilson S, Coughtrie MW, Burchell B. Cloning of a human liver microsomal UDP-glucuronosyltransferase cDNA. Biochem J, 1987; 242:581–588

1493. Jansen PL, Mulder GJ, Burchell B, Bock KW. New developments in glucuronidation research: report of a workshop on - glucuronidation, its role in health and disease. Hepatology, 1992; 15:532–544

1494. Karon M, Imach D, Schwartz A. Effective phototherapy in congenital nonobstructive, nonhemolytic jaundice. N Engl J Med, 1970; 282:377–380

1495. Shevell MI, Bernard B, Adelson JW, Doody DP, Laberge JM, Guttman FM. Crigler-Najjar syndrome type 1: treatment by home phototherapy followed by orthotopic hepatic transplantation. J Pediatr, 1987; 110:429–431

1496. Sokal EM, Silva ES, Hermans D et al. Orthotopic liver transplantation for Crigler-Najjar Type I disease in six children. Transplantation, 1995; 60:1095–1098

1497. van der Veere CN, Sinaasappel M, McDonagh AF et al. Current therapy for Crigler-Najjar syndrome type 1: report of a world registry. Hepatology, 1996; 24:311–315

1498. Fox IJ, Chowdhury JR, Kaufman SS et al. Treatment of the Crigler-Najjar syndrome type I with hepatocyte transplantation. N Engl J Med, 1998; 338:1422–1426

1499. Ilan Y, Attavar P, Takahashi M et al. Induction of central tolerance by intrathymic inoculation of adenoviral antigens into the host thymus permits long-term gene therapy in Gunn rats. J Clin Invest, 1996; 98:2640–2647

1500. Huang PWH, Rozdilsky B, Gerrard JW, Goluboff N, Holman GH. Crigler-Najjar syndrome in four of five siblings with postmortem findings in one. Arch Pathol, 1970; 90:536–542

1501. Kaufman SS, Wood RP, Shaw BW et al. Orthotopic liver transplantation for Type I Crigler-Najjar syndrome. Hepatology, 1986; 6:1259–1262

1502. Wolkoff AW, Chowdhury JR, Gartner LA et al. Crigler-Najjar syndrome (type I) in an adult male. Gastroenterology, 1979; 76:840–848

1503. Felsher BF, Rickard D, Redeker AG. The reciprocal relation between caloric intake and the degree of hyperbilirubinemia in Gilbert's syndrome. N Engl J Med, 1970; 283:170–172

1504. Bancroft JD, Kreamer B, Gourley GR. Gilbert syndrome accelerates development of neonatal jaundice. J Pediatr, 1998; 132:656–660

1505. Berk PD, Bloomer JR, Howe RB, Berlin NI. Constitutional hepatic dysfunction (Gilbert's syndrome). A new definition based on kinetic studies with unconjugated radiobilirubin. Am J Med, 1970; 49:296–305

1506. Billing BH, Williams R, Richards TG. Defects in hepatic transport of bilirubin in congenital hyperbilirubinaemia: an analysis of plasma bilirubin disappearance curves. Clin Sci, 1964; 27:245–257

1507. Arias IM, Gartner LM, Cohen M, Ezzer JB, Levi AJ. Chronic nonhemolytic unconjugated hyperbilirubinemia with glucuronyl transferase deficiency. Clinical, 1969; 47:395–409

1508. Powell LW, Hemingway E, Billing BH, Sherlock S. Idiopathic unconjugated hyperbilirubinemia (Gilbert's syndrome). A study of 42 families. N Engl J Med, 1967; 277:1108–1112

1509. Sleisenger MH. Nonhemolytic unconjugated hyperbilirubinemia with hepatic glucuronyl transferase deficiency: a genetic study in four generations. Trans Assoc Am Physicians, 1967; 80:259–266

1510. Bosma PJ, Chowdhury JR, Bakker C et al. The genetic basis of the reduced expression of bilirubin UDP-glucuronosyltransferase 1 in Gilbert's syndrome. N Engl J Med, 1995; 333:1171–1175

1511. Koiwai O, Nishizawa M, Hasada K et al. Gilbert's syndrome is caused by a heterozygous missense mutation in the gene for bilirubin UDP-glucuronosyltransferase. Hum Mol Genet, 1995; 4:1183–1186

1512. Maruo Y, Wada S, Yamamoto K, Sato H, Yamano T, Shimada M. A case of anorexia nervosa with hyperbilirubinaemia in a patient homozygous for a mutation in the bilirubin UDP-glucuronosyltransferase gene. Eur J Pediatr, 1999; 158:547–549

1513. Guldutuna S, Langenbeck U, Bock KW, Sieg A, Leuschner U. Crigler-Najjar syndrome type II. New observation of possible autosomal recessive inheritance. Dig Dis Sci, 1995; 40:28–32

1514. Hunter JO, Thompson RP, Dunn PM, Williams R. Inheritance of type 2 Crigler-Najjar hyperbilirubinaemia. Gut, 1973; 14:46–49

1515. Labrune P, Myara A, Hennion C, Gout JP, Trivin F, Odièvre M. Crigler-Najjar type II disease inheritance: a family study. J Inherit Metab Dis, 1989; 12:302–306

1516. Seppen J, Bosma PJ, Goldhoorn BG et al. Discrimination between Crigler-Najjar type I and II by expression of mutant bilirubin uridine diphosphate-glucuronosyltransferase. J Clin Invest, 1994; 94:2385–2391

1517. Portman OW, Chowdhury JR, Chowdhury NR, Alexander M, Cornelius CE, Arias IM. A nonhuman primate model of Gilbert-s syndrome. Hepatology, 1984; 4:175–179

1518. Barth RF, Grimely PM, Berk PD, Bloomer JR, Howe PB. Excess lipofuscin accumulation in constitutional hepatic dysfunction (Gilbert's syndrome). Arch Pathol, 1971; 91:41–47

1519. Dawson J, Carr-Locke DL, Talbot IC, Rosenthal FD. Gilbert's syndrome: Evidence of morphological heterogeneity. Gut, 1979; 20:848–853

1520. Dubin IN, Johnson FB. Chronic idiopathic jaundice with an unidentified pigment in liver cells; new clinicopathologic entity with report of 12 cases. Medicine, 1954; 33:155–158

1521. Sprinz H, Nelson RS. Persistent nonhemolytic hyperbilirubinemia associated with lipochrome-like pigment in liver cells: report of four cases. Ann Intern Med, 1954; 41:952–962

1522. Dubin IN. Chronic idiopathic jaundice. A review of 50 cases. Am J Med, 1958; 24:268–291

1523. Shani M, Seligsohn U, Gilon E, Sheba C, Adam A. Dubin-Johnson syndrome in Israel. I. Clinical, laboratory, and genetic aspects of 101 cases. Q J Med, 1970; 39:549–567

1524. Kimura A, Ushijima K, Kage M et al. Neonatal Dubin-Johnson syndrome with severe cholestasis: Effective phenobarbital therapy. Acta Paediatr Scand, 1991; 80:381–385

1525. Nakata F, Oyanagi K, Fujiwara M et al. Dubin-Johnson syndrome in a neonate. Eur J Pediatr, 1979; 132:299–301

1526. Wolkoff AW, Cohen LE, Arias IM. Inheritance of the Dubin-Johnson syndrome. N Engl J Med, 1973; 288:113–117

1527. van Kuijck MA, Kool M, Merkx GF et al. Assignment of the canalicular multispecific organic anion transporter gene (CMOAT) to human chromosome 10q24 and mouse chromosome 19I32 by fluorescent in situ hybridization. Cytogenet Cell Genet, 1997; 77:285–287

1528. Wada M, Toh S, Taniguchi K et al. Mutations in the canalicular multispecific organic anion transporter (cMOAT) gene, a novel ABC transporter, in patients with hyperbilirubinemia II/Dubin-Johnson syndrome. Hum Mol Genet, 1998; 7:203–207

1529. Paulusma CC, Kool M, Bosma PJ et al. A mutation in the human canalicular multispecific organic anion transporter gene causes the Dubin-Johnson syndrome. Hepatology, 1997; 25:1539–1542

1530. Kagawa T, Sato M, Hosoi K et al. Absence of R1066X mutation in six Japanese patients with Dubin-Johnson syndrome. Biochem Mol Biol Int, 1999; 47:639–644

1531. Tsujii H, Konig J, Rost D, Stockel B, Leuschner U, Keppler D. Exon-intron organization of the human multidrug-resistance protein 2 (MRP2) gene mutated in Dubin Johnson syndrome. Gastroenterology, 1999; 117:653–660

1532. Cornelius CE, Arias IM, Osburn BI. Hepatic pigmentation with photosensitivity: A syndrome in Corriedale sheep resembling Dubin-Johnson syndrome in man. J Am Vet Med Assoc, 1965; 146:709–713

1533. Paulusma CC, Bosma PJ, Zaman GJ et al. Congenital jaundice in rats with a mutation in a multidrug resistance-associated protein gene. Science, 1996; 271:1126–1128

1534. Maruppo CA, Malinow MR, Depaoli JR, Katz S. Pigmentary liver disease in Howler monkeys. Am J Pathol, 1966; 49:445–456

1535. Barone P, Inferrera C, Carrozza G. Pigments in the Dubin-Johnson syndrome. In: Pigments in pathology. M. Wolman, Editor. 1969, Academic Press: New York. p. 307–325

1536. Toker C, Trevino N. Hepatic ultrastructure in chronic idiopathic jaundice. Arch Pathol, 1965; 80:454–460

1537. Swartz HM, Sarna T, Varma RR. On the nature and excretion of the hepatic pigment in the Dubin-Johnson syndrome. Gastroenterology, 1979; 76:958–964

1538. Rotor AB, Manahan L, Florentin A. Familial nonhemolytic jaundice with direct van den Bergh reaction. Acta Med Phil, 1948; 5:37

1539. Pereira Lima JE, Utz E, Roisenberg I. Hereditary nonhemolytic conjugated hyperbilirubinemia without abnormal liver cell pigmentation. A family study. Am J Med, 1966; 40:628–633

1540. Fretzayas AM, Garoufi A, Moutsouris CX, Karpathios TE. Cholescintigraphy in the diagnosis of Rotor syndrome. J Nucl Med, 1994; 35:1048–1050

1541. Anderson DH. Cystic fibrosis of the pancreas and its relationship to celiac disease: A clinical and pathologic study. Am J Dis Child, 1938; 56:344–399

1542. Kerem BS, Rommens JM, Buchanan JA et al. Identification of the cystic fibrosis gene: genetic analysis. Science, 1989; 245:1073–1080

1543. Riordan JR, Rommens JM, Kerem BS et al. Identification of the cystic fibrosis gene: Cloning and characterization of complementary DNA. Science, 1989; 245:1066–1073

1544. Rommens JM, Iannuzzi MC, Kerem BS et al. Identification of the cystic fibrosis gene. Chromosome walking and jumping. Science, 1989; 245:1059–1065

1545. Ratjen F, Doring G. Cystic fibrosis. Lancet, 2003; 361:681–689

1546. Reisin IL, Prat AG, Abraham EH et al. The cystic fibrosis transmembrane conductance regulator is a dual ATP and chloride channel. J Biol Chem, 1994; 269:20584–20591

1547. Schwilbert EM, Egan ME, Hwang TH et al. CFTR regulates outwardly rectifying chloride channels through an autocrine mechanism involving ATP. Cell, 1995; 81:1063–1073

1548. Thelin WR, Kesimer M, Tarran R et al. The Cystic Fibrosis Transmembrane Conductance Regulator Is Regulated by a Direct Interaction with the Protein Phosphatase 2A. J Biol Chem, 2005; 280:41512–41520

1549. Engelhart JF, Yankaskas JR, Ernst SA et al. Submucosal glands are the predominate site of CFTR expression in the human bronchus. Nat Genet, 1992; 2:240–247

1550. Cohn JA, Strong TV, Picciotto MR, Nairn AC, Collins FS, Fitz JC. Localization of the cystic fibrosis transmembrane conductance regulator in human bile duct epithelial cells. Gastroenterology, 1993; 105:1857–1864

1551. Kinnman N, Lindbald A, Housset C et al. Expression of cystic fibrosis transmembrane conductance regulator in liver tissue from patients with cystic fibrosis. Hepatology, 2000; 32:334–340

1552. Knowles MR, Durie PR. What is cystic fibrosis? N Engl J Med, 2002; 347:439–42

1553. Kerem B, Kerem E. The molecular basis for disease variability in cystic fibrosis. Eur J Hum Genet, 1996; 4:65–73

1554. Tsui LC. The spectrum of cystic fibrosis mutations. Trends Genet, 1992; 8:392–398

1555. Duthie A, Doherty DC, Williams C et al. Genotype analysis for DF 508, G551D and R553V mutations in children and young adults with CF with and without liver disease. Hepatology, 1992; 15:660–664

1556. Colombo C, Battezzati PM, Crosignani A et al. Liver disease in cystic fibrosis: A prospective study on incidence, risk factors, and outcome. Hepatology, 2002; 36:1374–1382

1557. Lindblad A, Strandvik B, Hjelte L. Incidence of liver disease in patients with cystic fibrosis and meconium ileus. J Pediatr, 1995; 126:155–156

1558. Psacharopoulos HT, Howard ER, Portmann B, Mowat AP, Williams R. Hepatic complications of cystic fibrosis. Lancet, 1981; ii:78–80

1559. Lamireau T, Monnereau S, Martin S, Marcotte JE, Winnock M, Alvarez F. Epidemiology of liver disease in cystic fibrosis: a longitudinal study. J Hepatol, 2004; 41:920–925

1560. Bodian M, Sheldon W, Lightwood R. Congenital hypoplasia of the exocrine pancreas. Acta Paediatr, 1964; 53:582–593

1561. di Sant-Agnese PA, Blanc WA. Distinctive type of biliary cirrhosis of the liver associated with cystic fibrosis of the pancreas. Pediatrics, 1956; 18:387–409

1562. Roy CC, Weber AM, Morin CL, LePage G, Youssef I, LaSalle R. Hepatobiliary disease in cystic fibrosis: a survey of current issues and concepts. J Pediatr Gastroenterol Nutr, 1982; 1:469–475

1563. Furuja KW, Roberts EA, Camy GJ, Phillip MJ. Neonatal hepatitis with paucity of interlobular bile ducts in CF. J Pediatr Gastroenterol Nutr, 1991; 2:127–130

1564. Vitullo BB, Rocher L, Seemage TA, Beardmore H, DeBelle RC. Intrapancreatic compression of the common bile duct in cystic fibrosis. J Pediatrics, 1978; 93:1060–1061

1565. Durie PR. Cystic fibrosis: gastrointestinal and hepatic complications and their management. Semin Pediatr Gastroenterol Nutr, 1993; 4:2

1566. Colombo C, Apostolo MG, Ferrari M et al. Analysis of risk factors for the development of liver disease associated with cystic fibrosis. J Pediatrics, 1994; 124:393–399

1567. Waters DL, Dorney SFA, Gruca MA et al. Hepatobiliary disease in CF patients with pancreatic sufficiency. Hepatology, 1995; 21:963–969

1568. Schwarzenberg SJ, Wielinksi CL, Shamieh I et al. Cystic fibrosis-associated colitis and fibrosing colonopathy. J Pediatrics, 1995; 127:565–570

1569. Benett I, Sahl B, Haboubi NY, Braganza JM. Sclerosing cholangitis with hepatic microvesicular steatosis in cystic fibrosis and chronic pancreatitis. J Clin Pathol, 1989; 42:466–469

1570. Craig JM, Haddad H, Schwachman H. The pathological changes in the liver in CF of the pancreas. Am J Dis Child, 1957; 93:357–369

1571. Wilroy RS, Crawford SE, Johnson WW. Cystic fibrosis with extensive fat replacement of the liver. J Pediatr, 1966; 68:67–73

1572. Strandvik B, Hulterantz R. Liver function and morphology during long term fatty acid supplementation in cystic fibrosis. Liver, 1994; 14:32–36

1573. Fitz-Simmons SC. The changing epidemiology of cystic fibrosis. J Pediatr, 1993; 122:1–9

1574. Lykavieris P, Bernard O, Hadchouel M. Neonatal cholestasis as the presenting feature of cystic fibrosis. Arch Dis Child, 1996; 75:67–70

1575. The Cystic Fibrosis Genotype-Phenotype Consortium. Correlation between gentoype and phenotype in patients with cystic fibrosis. N Engl J Med, 1993; 329:1308–1313

1576. Castaldo G, Fuccio A, Salvatore D et al. Liver expression in cystic fibrosis could be modulated by genetic factors different from the cystic fibrosis transmembrane regulator genotype. Am J Med Genet, 2001; 98:294–297

1577. Scott-Jupp R, Lama M, Tanner MS. Prevalence of liver disease in cystic fibrosis. Arch Dis Child, 1991; 66:698–701

1578. Salvatore F, Scudiero O, Castaldo G. Genotype-phenotype correlation in cystic fibrosis: the role of modifier genes. Am J Med Genet, 2002; 111:88–95

1579. Sontag MK, Accurso FJ. Gene modifiers in pediatrics: application to cystic fibrosis. Adv Pediatr, 2004; 51:5–36

1580. Gabolde M, Hubert D, Guilloud-Bataille M, Lenaerts C, Feingold J, Besmond C. The mannose binding lectin gene influences the severity of chronic liver disease in cystic fibrosis. J Med Genet, 2001; 38:310–311

1581. Duthie A, Doherty DG, Donaldson PT et al. The major histocompatibility complex influences the development of chronic liver disease in male children and young adults with CF. J Hepatol, 1995; 23:532–537

1582. Tanner MS. Current clinical management of hepatic problems in cystic fibrosis. J R Soc Med, 1986; 79 Suppl 12:38–43

1583. Gibson LE, Cooke RE. A test for concentration of electrolytes composition in the sweat in cystic fibrosis of the pancreas utilizing pilocarpine by iontophoresis disease. Pediatrics, 1959; 23:545–549

1584. di Sant-Agnese PA, Darling RC, Perera GA, Shea E. Abnormal electrolyte composition in the sweat in cystic fibrosis of the pancreas. Clinical significance and relationship of the disease. Pediatrics, 1993; 12:549–563

1585. Augarten A, Kerem BS, Yahavy Y et al. Mild cystic fibrosis and normal or borderline sweat test in patients with the 3849 plus 10kbc to T mutation. Lancet, 1993; 342:25–26

1586. Stern RC, Boat TF, Abramowsky CR, Mathews LW, Wood RF, Doershuk CR. Intermediate-range sweat chloride content ratios and pseudomonas bronchitis. A CF variant with preservation of exocrine pancreatic function. JAMA, 1978; 239:2676

1587. Gowen CW, Lawson EE, Gingras-Leatherman J, Gatzy JT, Boucher RC, Knowles MR. Increased nasal potential difference and amiloride sensitivity in neonates with cystic fibrosis. J Pediatrics, 1986; 108:512–521

1588. Sander RA, Chesrown SE, Loughlin G. Clinical application of transepithelial potential difference measurements in cystic fibrosis. J Pediatr, 1987; 111:353–358

1589. McGinniss MJ, Chen C, Redman JB et al. Extensive Sequencing of the CFTR gene: lessons learned from the first 157 patient samples. Hum Genet, 2005:1–8

1590. Gerling B, Becker M, Stalab D, Schuppan D. Prediction of liver fibrosis according to serum collagen VI level in children with cystic fibrosis. N Engl J Med, 1997; 336:1611–1612 (letter)

1591. Dankert-Roelse JE, Merelle ME. Review of outcomes of neonatal screening for cystic fibrosis versus non-screening in Europe. J Pediatr, 2005; 147:S15–S20

1592. Colombo C, Battezzati PM, Podda C et al. Ursodeoxycholic acid for liver disease associated with cystic fibrosis. A double blind multicenter trial. Hepatology, 1996; 23:1484–1490

1593. Colombo C, Battezzati PM, Strazzabosco M, Podda M. Liver and biliary problems in cystic fibrosis. Semin Liver Dis, 1998; 18:227–236

1594. LePage G, Paradis K, Lacaille F et al. Ursodeoxycholic acid improves the hepatic metabolism of essential fatty acids and retinol in children with cystic fibrosis. J Pediatr, 1997; 130:52–58

1595. Narkewicz MR, Smith D, Gregory C, Lear J, Osberg I, Sokol RJ. Effects of ursodeoxycholic acid therapy on hepatic function in children with intrahepatic cholestasis. J Pediatr Gastroenterol Nutr, 1998; 26:49–50

1596. Lindblad A, Glaumann H, Strandvik B. A two year prospective study of the effect of ursodeoxycholic acid on urinary bile acid excretion and liver morphology in cystic fibrosis associated liver disease. Hepatology, 1998; 27:166–174

1597. Colombo C, Bertolini E, Assaisso ML, Berttinadi N, Giunta A, Podda M. Failure of ursodeoxycholic acid to dissolve radiolucent gall stones in patients with cystic fibrosis. Acta Paediatr, 1993; 82:562–565

1598. L'Heureux PR, Isenberg JN, Sharp HL, Warwick WJ. Gallbladder disease in cystic fibrosis. Am J Roentgenol, 1977; 128:953–956

1599. Angelico M, Gandin C, Canuzzi P et al. Gallstones in cystic fibrosis. A critical reappraisal. Hepatology, 1991; 14:68–75

1600. Berger KJ, Schreiber RA, Tcherenkov J, Kopelman H, Brassard R, Stern L. Decompression of portal hypertension in a child with cystic fibrosis after transjugular intrahepatic porto-systemic shunt placement. J Pediatr Gastroenterol Nutr, 1994; 19:322–325

1601. Debray D, Lykavieris P, Gauthier F et al. Outcome of cystic fibrosis—associated liver cirrhosis: management of portal hypertension. Hepatology, 1999; 31:77–83

1602. Molmenti EP, Squires RH, Nagata D et al. Liver transplantation for cholestasis associated with cystic fibrosis in the pediatric population. Pediatr Transplant, 2003; 7:93–97

1603. Sharp HL. Cystic fibrosis liver disease and transplantation. J Pediatr, 1995; 127:944–946

1604. Fridell JA, Mazariegos GV, Orenstein D, Sindhi R, Reyes J. Liver and intestinal transplantation in a child with cystic fibrosis: a case report. Pediatr Transplant, 2003; 7:240–242

1605. Couetil JPA, Soubrane O, Houssin DP et al. Combined heart-lung-liver double lung-liver and isolated liver transplantation for cystic fibrosis in children. Transplant Int, 1997; 10:33–39

1606. Fridell JA, Vianna R, Kwo PY et al. Simultaneous liver and pancreas transplantation in patients with cystic fibrosis. Transplant Proc, 2005; 37:3567–3569

1607. Bodian MM. Fibrocystic disease of the pancreas: a congenital disorder of mucus production-mucosis. 1952, London: William Heinemann Medical Books

1608. Oppenheimer EH, Esterly JR. Hepatic changes in young infants with cystic fibrosis: possible relation to focal biliary cirrhosis. J Pediatr, 1975; 86:683–689

1609. Oppenheimer EH, Esterly JR. Pathology of cystic fibrosis: review of the literature and comparison with 146 autopsied cases. Persp Pediatr Pathol, 1975; 2:244–278

1610. Porta EA, Stein AA, Patterson D. Ultrastructural changes of the pancreas and liver in cystic fibrosis. Am J Clin Pathol, 1964; 41:451–465

1611. Isenberg JN. Cystic fibrosis. Its influence on the liver, 1982; 2:301–313

1612. Farber S. Pancreatic function and disease in early life. V Pathologic changes associated with pancreatic insufficiency in early life. Arch Pathol, 1944; 37:238–250

1613. Dominick HC Cystic fibrosis. In: Liver in metabolic diseases. L. Bianchi, W. Gerok, L. Landmann, K. Sickinger, G.A. Stalder, Editors. 1983, MTP Press: Lancaster. p. 283–290

1614. Esterly JR, Oppenheimer EH. Observations in cystic fibrosis of the pancreas. I. The gallbladder. Bull Johns Hopkins Hosp, 1962; 110:247–255

1615. Arends P, von Bassewitz DB, Dominick HC. Ultrastructure of liver biopsies in cystic fibrosis. Cystic Fibrosis Q Annot Ref, 1974; 13:13 (abstract)

1616. Bradford W, Allen D, Sheburne J, Spock A. Hepatic parenchymal cells in cystic fibrosis: ultrastructural evidence for abnormal intracellular transport. Pediatr Pathol, 1983; 1:269–279

1617. Lindblad A, Hulternaz R, Strandvik B. Bile-duct destruction and collagen deposition: a prominent ultrastructural feature of the liver in cystic fibrosis. Hepatology, 1992; 16:372–381

1618. Hultcrantz R, Mengarelli S, Strandvik B. Morphological findings in the liver of children with cystic fibrosis: a light and electron microscopical study. Hepatology, 1986; 6:881–889

1619. Lewindon PJ, Pereira TN, Hoskins AC et al. The role of hepatic stellate cells and transforming growth factor-beta(1) in cystic fibrosis liver disease. Am J Pathol, 2002; 160:1705–1715

1620. Ginzberg H, Shin J, Ellis L et al. Segregation analysis in Shwachman-Diamond syndrome: evidence for recessive inheritance. Am J Hum Genet, 2000; 66:1413–1416

1621. Popovic M, Goobie S, Morrison J et al. Fine mapping of the locus for Shwachman-Diamond syndrome at 7q11, identification of shared disease haplotypes, and exclusion of TPST1 as a candidate gene. Eur J Hum Genet, 2002; 10:250–258

1622. Boocock GR, Morrison JA, Popovic M et al. Mutations in SBDS are associated with Shwachman-Diamond syndrome. Nat Genet, 2003; 33:97–101

1623. Shwachman H, Diamond LK, Oski FA, Khaw KT. The syndrome of pancreatic insufficiency and bone marrow dysfunction. J Pediatr, 1964; 65:645–663

1624. Cipolli M, C DO, Delmarco A, Marchesini C, Miano A, Mastella G. Shwachman's syndrome: pathomorphosis and long-term outcome. J Pediatr Gastroenterol Nutr, 1999; 29:265–272

1625. Mack DR, Forstner GG, Wilschanski M, Freedman MH, Durie PR. Shwachman syndrome: exocrine pancreatic dysfunction and variable phenotypic expression. Gastroenterology, 1996; 111:1593–1602

1626. Moore DJ, Forstner GG, Largman C, Cleghorn GJ, Wong SS, Durie PR. Serum immunoreactive cationic trypsinogen: a useful indicator of severe exocrine dysfunction in the paediatric patient without cystic fibrosis. Gut, 1986; 27:1362–1368

1627. Aggett PJ, Cavanagh NPC, Matthew DJ, Pincott JR, Sutcliffe J, Harries JT. Shwachman's syndrome. A review of 21 cases. Arch Dis Child, 1980; 55:331–347

1628. Ginzberg H, Shin J, Ellis L et al. Shwachman syndrome: phenotypic manifestations of sibling sets and isolated cases in a large patient cohort are similar. J Pediatr, 1999; 135:81–88

1629. Masuno M, Imaizumi K, Nishimura G et al. Shwachman syndrome associated with de novo reciprocal translocation t(6;12)(q16.2;q21.2). J Mol Genet, 1995; 32:894–895

1630. Higashi O, Hayashi T, Ohara K, Honda Y, Doi S. Pancreatic insufficiency with bone marrow dysfunction (Shwachman-Diamond-Oski-Khaw's syndrome). Report of a case. Tohoku J Exp Med, 1967; 92:1–12

1631. Spycher MA, Giedion A, Shmerling DH, Ruttner JR. Electron microscopic examination of cartilage in the syndrome of exocrine pancreatic insufficiency, neutropenia, metaphyseal dysostosis and dwarfism. Helv Paediatr Acta, 1974; 29:471–479

1632. Brueton MJ, Mavromichalis J, Goodchild MC, Anderson CM. Hepatic dysfunction in association with pancreatic insufficiency and cyclical neutropenia. Shwachman-Diamond syndrome. Arch Dis Child, 1977; 52:76–78

1633. Liebman WM, Rosental E, Hirshberger M, Thaler MM. Shwachman-Diamond syndrome and chronic liver disease. Clin Pediatr (Phila), 1979; 18:695–698

1634. Wilschanski M, van der Hoeven E, Phillips J, Shuckett B, Durie P. Shwachman-Diamond syndrome presenting as hepatosplenomegaly. J Pediatr Gastroenterol Nutr, 1994; 19:111–113

1635. Ventura A, Dragovich D, Luxardo P, Zanazzo G. Human granulocyte colony-stimulating factor (rHuG-CSF) for treatment of neutropenia in Shwachman syndrome. Haematologica, 1995; 80:227–229

1636. Woods WG, Roloff JS, Lukens JN, Krivit W. The occurrence of leukemia in patients with the Shwachman syndrome. J Pediatr, 1981; 99:425–428

1637. Smith OP, Hann IM, Chessells JM, Reeves BR, Milla P. Haematological abnormalities in Shwachman-Diamond syndrome. Br J Haematol, 1996; 94:279–284

1638. Bunin N, Leahey A, Dunn S. Related donor liver transplant for veno-occlusive disease following T-depleted unrelated donor bone marrow transplantation. Transplantation, 1996; 61:664–666

1639. Okcu F, Roberts WM, Chan KW. Bone marrow transplantation in Shwachman-Diamond syndrome: report of two cases and review of the literature. Bone Marrow Transplant, 1998; 21:849–851

1640. Burke V, Colebatch JH, Anderson CM, Simon MJ. Association of pancreatic insufficiency and chronic neutropenia in childhood. Arch Dis Child, 1976; 42:147–157

1641. Graham AR, Walson PD, Paplanus SH, Payne CM. Testicular fibrosis and cardiomegaly in Shwachman's syndrome. Arch Pathol Lab Med, 1980; 104:242–244

1642. Struben VMD, Hespenheide EE, Caldwell SH. Nonalcoholic steatohepatitis and cryptogenic cirrhosis within kindreds. Am J Med, 2000; 108:9–13

1643. Maddrey WC, Iber FL. Familial cirrhosis: A clinical and pathologic study. Ann Intern Med, 1964; 61:667–679

1644. Caldwell SH, Oelsner DH, Iozzoni IC, Hespenheide EE, Battle EH, Driscoll CH. Cryptogenic cirrhosis: Clinical characterization and risk factors for underlying disease. Hepatology, 1999; 29:664–669

1645. Powell EE, Searle J, Mortimer R. Steatohepatitis associated with total lipodystrophy. Gastroenterology, 1989; 97:1022–1024

1646. Robertson DAF, Wright R. Cirrhosis in partial lipodystrophy. Postgrad Med, 1989; 65:318–320

1647. Awazu M, Tanaka T, Sato S et al. Hepatic dysfunction in two sibs with Alstrom syndrome: case report and review of the literature. Am J Med Genet, 1997; 69:13–16

1648. Quiros-Tejeira RE, Vargas J, Ament ME. Early-onset liver disease complicated with acute liver failure in Alstrom syndrome. Am J Med Genet, 2001; 101:9–11

1649. Satman I, Yilmaz MT, Gursoy N et al. Evaluation of insulin resistant diabetes mellitus in Alstrom syndrome: a long-term prospective follow-up of three siblings. Diabetes Res Clin Pract, 2002; 56:189–196

1650. Wang H, Cornford ME, German J, French SW. Sclerosing hyaline necrosis of the liver in Bloom syndrome. Arch Pathol Lab Med, 1999; 123:346–350

1651. Gurakan F, Kaymaz F, Kocak N, Ors U, Yuce A, Atakan N. A cause of fatty liver: Neural lipid storage disease with ichthyosis—electron microscopic findings. Dig Dis Sci, 1999; 44:2214–2217

1652. Mela D, Goretti R, Varagona G et al. Dorfman-Chenarin syndrome: a case with prevalent hepatic involvement. J Hepatol, 1996; 25:769–771

1653. Roberts EA. Steatohepatitis in children. Best Pract Res Clin Gastroenterol, 2002; 16:749–765

1654. Garg A. Acquired and inherited lipodystrophies. N Engl J Med, 2004; 350:1220–1234

1655. Garg A, Wilson R, Barnes R et al. A gene for congenital generalized lipodystrophy maps to human chromosome 9q34. J Clin Endocrinol Metab, 1999; 84:3390–3394

1656. Uzon O, Blackburn ME, Gibbs JL. Congenital lipodystrophy and peripheral pulmonary artery stenosis. Arch Dis Child, 1997; 76:456–457

1657. Berge T, Brum A, Hansing B, Kjellman B. Congenital generalized lipodystrophy. Acta Pathol Microbiol Scand Sect A, 1976; 84:47–54

1658. Case Records of the Massachusetts General H. Case, 1–1975. N Engl J Med, 1975; 292:35–41

1659. de Craemer D, Van Maldergem L, Roels F. Hepatic ultrastructure in congenital total lipodystrophy with special refinance to peroxisomes. Ultastruct Pathol, 1992; 16:307–316

1660. Harbour JR, Rosenthal P, Smuckler EA. Ultrastructural abnormalities of the liver in total lipodystrophy. Hum Pathol, 1981; 12:856–862

1661. Ipp MM, Howard NJ, Tervo RC, Gelfand EW. Sicca syndrome and total lipodystrophy. A case in a fifteen-year-old female patient. Ann Intern Med, 1975; 85:443–446

1662. Klar A, Livni N, Gross-Kieselstein E, Navon P, Shahin A, Branski D. Ultrastructural abnormalities of the liver in total lipodystrophy. Arch Pathol Lab Med, 1987; 111:197–199

1663. Ruvalcara RHA, Kelley VC. Lipoatrophic diabetes. II. Metabolic studies concerning the mechanism of lipemia. Am J Dis Child, 1965; 109:287–294

1664. Senior B, Gellis SS. The syndromes of total lipodystrophy and of partial lipodystrophy. Pediatrics, 1964; 33:593–612

1665. Forehand JR, Nauseef WM, Johnston RB Inherited disorders of phagocyte killing. In: The metabolic and molecular basis of inherited disease. C.R. Scriver, Editors. 1989, McGraw-Hill: New York. p. 2779–2801

1666. Buescher ES, Alling DW, Gallin JI. Use of an X-linked human neutrophil marker to estimate timing of lyonization and size of the dividing stem cell pool. J Clin Invest, 1985; 76:1581–1584

1667. Baehner RL, Kunkel LM, Monaco AP et al. DNA linkage analysis of X chromosome-linked chronic granulomatous disease. Proc Nat Acad Sci USA, 1986; 83:3398–3401

1668. Royer-Pokora B, Kunkel LM, Monaco AP et al. Cloning the gene for an inherited human disorder-chronic granulomatous disease-on the basis of its chromosomal location. Nature, 1986; 322:32–38

1669. Dinauer MC, Orkin SH. Chronic granulomatous disease: molecular genetics. Hematol Oncol Clin North Am, 1988; 2:225–240

1670. Rae J, Newburger PE, Dinauer MC et al. X-linked chronic granulomatous disease: mutations in the CYBB gene encoding the gp91-phox component of respiratory-burst oxidase. Am J Hum Genet, 1988; 62:1320–1331

1671. de Boer M, Bolscher BGJM, Sijmons RH, Scheffer H, Weening RS, Roos D. Prenatal diagnosis in a family with X-linked chronic granulomatous disease with the use of the polymerase chain reaction. Prenatal Diag, 1992; 12:773–777

1672. Wu YC, Huang YF, Lin CH, Shieh CC. Detection of defective granulocyte function with flow cytometry in newborn infants. J Microbiol Immunol Infect, 2005; 38:17–24

1673. Quie PG, White JG, Holmes B, Good RA. In vitro bactericidal capacity of human polymorphonuclear leukocytes: diminished activity in chronic granulomatous disease of childhood. J Clin Invest, 1967; 46:668–679

1674. Ezekowitz RAB, Dinauer MC, Jaffe HS, Orkin SH, Newburger PE. Partial correction of the phagocyte defect in patients with X-linked chronic granulomatous disease by subcutaneous interferon gamma. N Engl J Med, 1988; 319:146–151

1675. Chen LE, Minkes RK, Shackelford PG, Strasberg SM, Kuo EY, Langer JC. Cut it out: Managing hepatic abscesses in patients with chronic granulomatous disease. J Pediatr Surg, 2003; 38:709–713

1676. Ho CML, Vowels MR, Lockwood L, Ziegler JB. Successful bone marrow transplantation in a child with X-linked chronic granulomatous disease. Bone Marrow Transpl, 1996; 18:213–215

1677. Ikinciogullari A, Dogu F, Solaz N et al. Granulocyte transfusions in children with chronic granulomatous disease and invasive aspergillosis. Ther Apher Dial, 2005; 9:137–141

1678. Gungor T, Halter J, Klink A et al. Successful low toxicity hematopoietic stem cell transplantation for high-risk adult chronic granulomatous disease patients. Transplantation, 2005; 79:1596–1606

1679. Malech HL, Choi U, Brenner S. Progress toward effective gene therapy for chronic granulomatous disease. Jpn J Infect Dis, 2004; 57:S27–S28

1680. Goebel WS, Mark LA, Billings SD et al. Gene correction reduces cutaneous inflammation and granuloma formation in murine X-linked chronic granulomatous disease. J Invest Dermatol, 2005; 125:705–710

1681. Sadat MA, Pech N, Saulnier S et al. Long-term high-level reconstitution of NADPH oxidase activity in murine X-linked chronic granulomatous disease using a bicistronic vector expressing gp91phox and a Delta LNGFR cell surface marker. Hum Gene Ther, 2003; 14:651–666

1682. Ament ME, Ochs HD. Gastrointestinal manifestations of chronic granulomatous disease. N Engl J Med, 1973; 288:382–387

1683. Levine S, Smith VV, Malone M, Sebire NJ. Histopathological features of chronic granulomatous disease (CGD) in childhood. Histopathology, 2005; 47:508–516

1684. Lindahl JA, Williams FH, Newman SL. Small bowel obstruction in chronic granulomatous disease. J Pediatr Gastroenterol Nutr, 1984; 3:637–640

1685. Werlin SL, Chusid MJ, Caya J, Oechler HW. Colitis in chronic granulomatous disease. Gastroenterology, 1982; 82:328–331

1686. Bridges RA, Berendes H, Good RA. A fatal granulomatous disease of childhood. Am J Dis Child, 1959; 97:387–408

1687. Nakhleh RE, Glock M, Snover DC. Hepatic pathology of chronic granulomatous disease of childhood. Arch Pathol Lab Med, 1992; 116:71–75

1688. Tauber AI, Borregaard N, Simons E, Wright J. Chronic granulomatous disease. Medicine, 1983; 62:286–309

1689. Rodey DE, Landing BH. Chronic granulomatous disease of males. In: Birth defects atlas and compendium. D. Bergsma, Editor. 1973, Williams & Wilkins: Baltimore. p. 255–256

1690. Carson M, Chadwick DL, Brubaker CA, Cleland RS, Landing BH. Thirteen boys with progressive septic granulomatosis. Pediatrics, 1965; 35:405–412

1691. Levy J, Espanol-Boven T, Thomas C et al. Clinical spectrum of X-linked hyper-IgM syndrome. J Pediatr, 1997; 131:47–64

1692. Rodrigues F, Hadzic N, Davies G, Jones A, Veys P, Mieli-Vergani G. Liver disease in children with hyper IgM syndrome. J Hepatol, 2000; 32 (Suppl 2):127A

1693. Hayward AR, Levy J, Fachetti et al. Cholangiopathy and tumors of the pancreas, liver, and biliary tree in boys with X-linked immunodeficiency with hyper-IgM. J Immunol, 1997; 158:977–983

1694. Rodriguez C, Carrion F, Marinovic MA et al. [X-linked hyper-IGM syndrome associated to sclerosing cholangitis and gallbladder neoplasm: clinical case]. Rev Med Chil, 2003; 131:303–308

1695. Hadzic N. Liver disease in primary immunodeficiencies. J Hepatol, 2000; 32 (Suppl 2):9–10

1696. Tomizawa D, Imai K, Ito S et al. Allogeneic hematopoietic stem cell transplantation for seven children with X-linked hyper-IgM syndrome: a single center experience. Am J Hematol, 2004; 76:33–39

1697. Aarskog D. A familial syndrome of short stature associated with facial dysplasia and genital anomalies. J Pediatr, 1970; 77:856–861

1698. Grier RE, Farrington FH, Kendig R, Mamunes P. Autosomal dominant inheritance of the Aarskog syndrome. Am J Med Genet, 1983; 15:39–46

1699. Teebi AS, Rucquoi JK, Meyn MS. Aarskog syndrome: report of a family with review and discussion of nosology. Am J Med Genet, 1993; 46:501–509

1700. Welch JP. Elucidation of a 'new' pleiotropic connective tissue disorder. Birth Defects Orig Artic Ser, 1974; 10:138–146

1701. Escobar V, Weaver DD. Aarskog syndrome. New findings and genetic analysis. JAMA, 1978; 240:2638–2644

1702. Donohue WL, Uchida IA. Leprechaunism: a euphemism for a rare familial disorder. J Pediatr, 1954; 45:505–519

1703. Elsas LJ, Endo F, Strumlauf E, Elders J, Priest JH. Leprechaunism: an inherited defect in a high-affinity insulin receptor. Am J Hum Genet, 1985; 37:73–88

1704. Rosenberg AM, Howorth JC, Degroot GW, Trevenen CL, Rechler MM. A case of leprechaunism with severe hyperinsulinemia. Am J Dis Child, 1980; 134:170–175

1705. Evans PR. Leprechaunism. Arch Dis Child, 1955; 30:479–483

1706. Summitt RL, Favara BE. Leprechaunism (Donohue's syndrome): a case report. J Pediatr, 1960; 74:601–610

1707. Patterson JH, Watkins WL. Leprechaunism in a male infant. J Pediatr, 1962; 60:730–739

1708. Rogers DR. Leprechaunism (Donohue's syndrome): a possible case, with emphasis on changes in the adrenohypophysis. Am J Clin Pathol, 1966; 15:614–619

1709. Ordway NK, Stout LC. Intrauterine growth retardation, jaundice and hypoglycemia in a neonate. J Pediatr, 1973; 83:867–874

1710. Kritzler RA, Terner JY, Lindenbaum J et al. Chediak-Higashi syndrome: cytologic and serum lipid observations in a case and family. Am J Med, 1964; 36:583–594

1711. Spritz RA. Chediak-Higashi syndrome. In: Primary immunodeficiency diseases: a molecular and genetic approach. H.D. Ochs, C.I.E. Smith, and J.M. Puck, Editors. 1999, Oxford University Press: New York

1712. Barrat FJ, Le Deist F, Benkerrou M et al. Defective CTLA-4 cycling pathway in Chediak-Higashi syndrome: a possible mechanism for deregulation of T lymphocyte activation. Proc Natl Acad Sci, 1999; 96:8645–8650

1713. Hermansky F, Pudlak P. Albinism associated with hemorrhagic diathesis and unusual pigmented reticular cells in the bone marrow: report of two cases with histochemical studies. Blood, 1959; 14:162–169

1714. Weiss HJ, Witte LD, Kaplan KL et al. Heterogeneity in storage pool deficiency: studies in granule-bound substances in 18 patients including variants deficient in alpha-granules, platelet factor 4, beta-thromboglobin, and platelet-derived growth factor. Blood, 1979; 54:1296–1319

1715. Fukai K, Oh J, Frenk E, Almodovar C, Spritz RA. Linkage disequilibrium mapping of the gene for Hermansky-Pudlak syndrome to chromosome 10q23.1–q23.3. Hum Mol Genet, 1995; 4:1665–1669

1716. Oh J, Ho L, Ala-Mello S et al. Mutation analysis of patients with Hermansky-Pudlak syndrome: a frameshift hot spot in the HPS gene and apparent locus heterogeneity. Am J Hum Genet, 1998; 62:593–598

1717. Schallreuter KU, Frenk E, Wolfe LS, Witkop CJ, Wood JM. Hermansky-Pudlak syndrome in a Swiss population. Dermatology, 1993; 187:248–256

1718. Schinella PA, Greco MA, Garay SM, Lackner H, Wolman SR, Fazzini EP. Hermansky-Pudlak syndrome. A clinicopathologic study. Hum Pathol, 1985; 16:366–376

Alcoholic liver disease 6

Pauline de la M. Hall

Archaeological records of the earliest civilizations show that the history of alcohol dates back over 50 000 years.[1] Reuben gives a fascinating description of 'the love–hate relationship with alcohol that humankind has endured since the earliest recorded history'.[2] Alcohol-related diseases are recorded in Ayurveda, an ancient text of medicine from India, written around 567 BC. Many reviews of the epidemiology of alcoholic liver disease document a direct relationship between alcohol consumption per capita and mortality from alcoholic cirrhosis.[3–6] After heart disease and cancer, alcoholism and alcohol-related diseases constitute the third largest health problem in the USA, affecting over 10 million people, causing about 200 000 deaths each year and costing in the region of 60 billion dollars annually.[7] In the USA, and almost certainly in many other developed countries, alcohol is the leading cause of end-stage liver disease; alcohol causes 7.9 deaths/100 000 in the USA.[8] In addition alcohol, even when not causing overt alcoholic liver disease, can hasten the progression of other forms of chronic liver disease in terms of progression, risk of malignancy, and morbidity—this is particularly true of chronic hepatitis C.[9] Thus the true impact of alcohol on health and economic burden throughout the world is most certainly underestimated.

The spectrum of alcoholic liver disease which includes fatty change (steatosis), perivenular fibrosis alcoholic foamy degeneration (microvesicular steatosis), alcoholic hepatitis, occlusive venous lesions, cirrhosis and hepatocellular carcinoma is well recognized and described.[10–19] While there is no doubt that alcohol is a direct hepatotoxin, there is now an acceptance that both genetic and environmental factors influence the susceptibility of the individual to alcohol-associated liver injury.[20–23] The increased susceptibility of women to alcoholic liver injury does not appear to be explained by differences in the first-pass metabolism of alcohol.[24] It is possible that the susceptibility of women reported to be drinking as few as two drinks a day[25] may at least in some be related to other concomitant risk factors for non-alcoholic steatohepatitis (NASH; see Chapter 7).[26] Racial differences in alcohol metabolism, and possibly susceptibility, are associated with genetic polymorphisms of alcohol dehydrogenase and acetaldehyde dehydrogenase.[27]

The metabolism of alcohol

Alcohol metabolism and associated metabolic disturbances are comprehensively reviewed elsewhere[28–33] and will be discussed only briefly. Alcohol is readily absorbed from the gastrointestinal tract and is distributed throughout the body in proportion to the amount of fluid in the tissues. Less than 10% is eliminated through the lungs and kidneys, the remainder being oxidized in the body, predominantly in the liver; this probably explains the marked metabolic disturbances that occur in that organ. Furthermore, the liver has a limited capacity for safe disposal of large amounts of alcohol.

There are three pathways for alcohol metabolism in the liver.

1. Alcohol dehydrogenase (ADH) pathway

ADH catalyses the oxidative metabolism of alcohol to acetaldehyde.

$$CH_3CH_2OH + NAD^+$$
$$\downarrow ADH$$
$$CH_3CHO + NADH + H^+$$
Acetaldehyde

Hydrogen is transferred from alcohol to the cofactor nicotinamide adenine dinucleotide (NAD), converting it to the reduced form NADH, and acetaldehyde is produced. The generation of excess reducing equivalents (NADH) in the cytosol results in a marked shift in the redox potential, as indicated by the increased lactate : pyruvate ratio. Some of the hydrogen equivalents are transferred from the cytosol to the mitochondria via several shuttle systems.

The major rate-limiting factor in the ADH pathway is the ability of the liver to reoxidize NADH; the regeneration of NAD from NADH ultimately requires oxygen. Chronic alcohol consumption accelerates ADH-related alcohol metabolism to a limited extent. ADH activity, however, does not increase and a hypermetabolic state has been proposed as a possible mechanism for this acceleration.[34]

2. The microsomal ethanol-oxidizing system (MEOS)

This is a cytochrome P-450-dependent pathway and in particular involves the ethanol-inducible cytochrome P-450 2E1 (CYP2E1).[35,36] Until recently CYP2E1 was thought to be the only isoenzyme involved in ethanol metabolism but ethanol can also induce CYP1A1,[37] CYP3A,[38] and CYP4A.[39]

$$CH_3CH_2OH + NADPH + H^+ + O_2$$
$$\downarrow MEOS$$
$$CH_3CHO + NADP^+ + 2H_2O$$
Acetaldehyde

Increased CYP2E1 activity following chronic alcohol consumption is probably the major mechanism for the increased rates of clearance of alcohol from the blood and metabolic tolerance that develops in regular drinkers.[35] Animal studies have shown that the activity of this isoenzyme increases after relatively short-term alcohol consumption in doses that do not even cause fatty change.[40] The increased xenobiotic toxicity and carcinogenicity seen in association with chronic alcohol consumption, in both humans and various animal models, can be explained largely by the induction of CYP-450 2E1 which leads to enhanced metabolism of a wide variety of agents e.g. paracetamol (acetaminophen) that are metabolized by this isoenzyme.[31,41-44]

3. Catalase pathway

Catalase, located in peroxisomes, plays only a minor role in alcohol metabolism, although there is some evidence for increased metabolism of alcohol by peroxisomes in chronic drinkers.[45]

$$CH_3CH_2OH + H_2O_2 \xrightarrow{catalase} CH_3CHO + 2H_2O$$
Ethanol ... Acetaldehyde

Acetaldehyde metabolism

Acetaldehyde is oxidized to acetate; again, this occurs predominantly in the liver. Some of the acetaldehyde and most of the acetate are excreted by the liver into the blood stream and metabolized peripherally. Chronic alcoholics have accelerated alcohol metabolism and higher levels of blood acetaldehyde than non-drinkers.[44,46] The metabolism of acetaldehyde produces excess reducing equivalents (NADH) in liver mitochondria which in turn leads to a decrease in β-oxidation of long-chain fatty acids by inhibiting long-chain 3-hydroxyacyl CoA dehydrogenase (LCHAD) activity.

Chronic alcohol consumption results in high levels of acetaldehyde, which is highly toxic due to a variety of mechanisms including glutathione depletion, oxidative stress, lipid peroxidation, and the formation of adducts with proteins.[44]

In the last decade there have been major advances in the understanding of lipid metabolism in the liver as reviewed by You and Crabb.[47] The main regulatory molecules that control fatty acid oxidation and synthesis are peroxisome proliferator-activated receptor-α (PPAR-α) and sterol regulatory element binding protein 1 (SREBP-1).

Metabolic disturbances associated with alcohol metabolism (Fig. 6.1)

The increased NADH : NAD ratio which results from the oxidation of ethanol causes:

1. An increase in the lactate : pyruvate ratio, because of both decreased utilization and increased lactate production by the liver. There is lactic acidosis with a reduced renal capacity for uric acid excretion producing a secondary hyperuricaemia.
2. Impaired carbohydrate metabolism with reduced gluconeogenesis from amino acids; this may produce hypoglycaemia.
3. Impaired fat metabolism: H$^+$ ions replace two-carbon fragments derived from fatty acids as the main energy source in hepatocyte mitochondria and also depress the citric acid cycle. There is decreased fatty acid oxidation; an increase in α-glycerophosphate also occurs with a consequent increase in trapping of fatty acids, and an accompanying increased synthesis of triglycerides.[48] In long-standing alcohol abuse, protein synthesis is depressed and this, together with impaired liver-cell secretory function, causes retention of lipoproteins and contributes to the accumulation of fat in hepatocytes.
4. Impaired metabolism of serotonin, other amines and galactose.
5. Alterations in steroid metabolism; this may explain some of the hormonal disturbances in chronic alcoholism.

Pathology of alcoholic liver disease

Alcoholic steatosis (fatty change)

Steatosis, the earliest and the most common manifestation of alcoholic liver injury, is seen in up to 90% of patients presenting for treatment of chronic alcoholism.[49] The

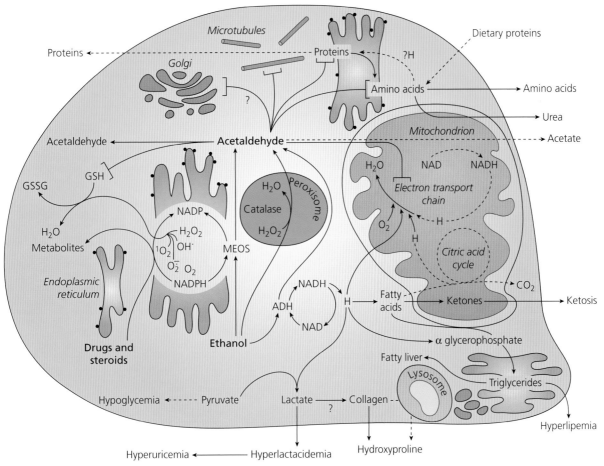

Fig. 6.1 • Metabolism of ethanol. Oxidation of ethanol in the hepatocyte and link of the two products (acetaldehyde and H⁺ ions) to disturbances in intermediary metabolism, including abnormalities of lipid, carbohydrate and protein metabolism. The broken lines indicate pathways that are depressed by ethanol. The symbol ─{ denotes interference or binding. NAD = nicotinamide adenine dinucleotide; NADH = reduced NAD; NADP = nicotinamide adenine dinucleotide phosphate; NADPH = reduced NADP; MEOS = microsomal ethanol oxidizing system; ADH = alcohol dehydrogenase. Redrawn from C.S. Lieber (ed.) Medical Disorders of Alcoholism: Pathogenesis and Treatment (1982) with permission from WB Saunders.

spectrum of clinical manifestations ranges from asymptomatic hepatomegaly, through non-specific digestive symptoms, to life-threatening hepatic failure.[6] Sudden death may occur in alcoholics and has been attributed to alcohol withdrawal.[50,51] At autopsy, the liver may show severe fatty change and a review of the illustrations of the pathology in these, and other similar case reports, suggests that these patients may have died from acute liver failure due to severe microvesicular steatosis; the possible role of other metabolic complications, e.g. hypoglycaemia, cannot be excluded.

Fatty change occurs predominantly in the perivenular zone and is seen initially in hepatocytes adjacent to the terminal hepatic venule. As the liver injury progresses, fatty change can be seen in hepatocytes in all zones. Fat disappears from the hepatocytes in 2–4 weeks following abstinence from alcohol but may persist in portal tract macrophages.

Initially, fat droplets appear to be membrane-bound, presumably by endoplasmic reticulum. As the droplets become larger they fuse, forming non-membrane-bound droplets. Fat droplets are seen as clear, intracytoplasmic vacuoles in haematoxylin and eosin-stained sections of processed tissue (Fig. 6.2(A)). To retain fat in tissue specimens, formalin-fixed liver material can be post-fixed in osmium tetroxide;

the osmicated fat is seen as black droplets in unstained sections. Haematoxylin and eosin and 'routine' special stains can still be performed (Fig. 6.2(B)).[52] The amount of fat in sections of osmicated tissue can be readily quantified, for example by video-assisted image analysis.[53] As the fat droplets enlarge they are seen predominantly as single, large vacuoles which displace the nuclei of the hepatocytes; this appearance is termed macrovesicular fatty change.

Hepatocyte necrosis and inflammation are not usually seen at the fatty liver stage other than in association with lipogranuloma formation. Rupture of distended hepatocytes leads to the release of fat and an inflammatory response comprising lymphocytes, macrophages and occasionally eosinophils (Fig. 6.3).[54] Rarely, true epithelioid granulomas are seen, and serial sectioning may be required to demonstrate the presence of fat droplets.[55] Lipogranulomas predominantly occur in the region of the terminal hepatic venules, and are seen most frequently in severe fatty change. Small amounts of fibrous tissue may be present. However, lipogranulomas usually disappear without sequelae.

Until quite recently, alcoholic steatosis without evidence of hepatocyte necrosis or fibrosis was thought to be a 'benign' condition with little risk of progression to cirrhosis. This has been questioned by Teli et al.[56] who followed 88

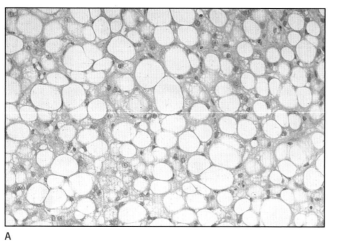
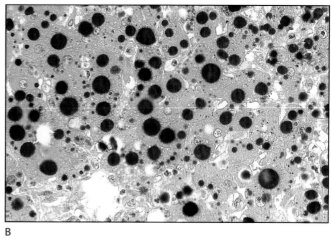

A   B

Fig. 6.2 • Macrovesicular fatty change. **(A)** Single, large fat droplets are seen in most of the hepatocytes; the liver-cell nuclei are situated peripherally. H&E. **(B)** Osmicated hepatic tissue. The osmicated fat is seen as black droplets of varying sizes. H&E.

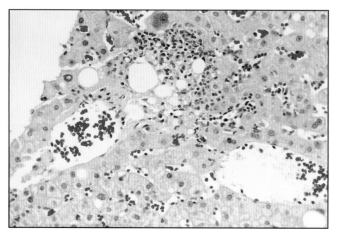

Fig. 6.3 • Lipogranuloma. Mildly fatty liver with a lipogranuloma in the region of a terminal hepatic venule. H&E.

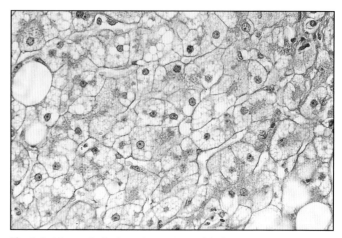

Fig. 6.4 • Microvesicular fatty change. Most of the hepatocytes are distended by large numbers of small fat droplets which surround centrally situated nuclei. Several cells contain slightly enlarged mitochondria, which are stained pink. Chromotrope-aniline blue.

patients with alcoholic steatosis for a mean of 10.5 years. Seven developed fibrosis, and another nine become cirrhotic; however, eight of the nine were known to have continued to drink at least 40 units of alcohol per week. The presence of mixed macrovesicular and microvesicular steatosis, and giant mitochondria, in the original biopsies were considered to be independent histological predictors of progression. Continued alcohol consumption by patients with these histological features on biopsy is associated with a 47–61% risk of progressive liver disease. Dam-Larsen et al. recently reported severity of steatosis on liver biopsy in alcoholic fatty liver disease to be a predictor of progression.[57]

Alcoholic foamy degeneration (microvesicular fatty change)

Alcoholic foamy degeneration was introduced as a term to described alcohol-induced microvesicular fatty change occurring at the fatty liver stage, in the absence of alcoholic hepatitis.[58] Uchida and co-workers described 20 patients with alcoholic foamy degeneration, all of whom recovered rapidly once alcohol was withdrawn. The authors considered alcoholic foamy degeneration to be a purely degenerative process since it occurred in the absence of inflammation. Jaundice and hepatomegaly are usually present in association with marked elevations of serum aminotransferases, alkaline phosphatase and bilirubin. The clinical and biochemical features are highly suggestive of extrahepatic biliary obstruction. The liver shows striking microvesicular fatty change which is maximal perivenularly but may extend into this mid-zone (Fig. 6.4). Some macrovesicular fat droplets may also be present. Bile is frequently seen in perivenular hepatocytes and canaliculi, while Mallory bodies, and an infiltrate of neutrophil polymorphs, are usually minimal or absent. Perivenular fibrosis is usually present, as is a small amount of perisinusoidal fibrosis. Enzyme histochemical studies revealed marked functional impairment of hepatocytes in the perivenular regions. Electron microscopy showed widespread damage or loss of organelles, particularly mitochondria and endoplasmic reticulum.[58]

Perivenular fibrosis

Baboons fed alcohol chronically have been observed to progress from the fatty liver stage to cirrhosis, without an intermediate stage of alcoholic hepatitis.[59] Perivenular fibrosis was present in the baboons' livers in association with alcoholic steatosis. A similar lesion occurs in humans[59,60] and it is now accepted as an intermediate stage in the development of alcoholic cirrhosis and distinct from alcoholic hepatitis.

Perivenular fibrosis has been defined as fibrosis extending around at least two-thirds of the perimeter of the terminal hepatic venule, the fibrous rim measuring over 4 mm in thickness (Fig. 6.5).[60] Serial liver biopsy studies have shown that patients with perivenular fibrosis at the fatty liver stage are likely to have progressive liver injury if drinking continues.[59,61] In the study of Worner & Lieber,[61] 13 of 15 patients with perivenular fibrosis in the first biopsy developed more severe disease within 4 years; nine had more extensive fibrosis, one incomplete cirrhosis and three established cirrhosis.[61] Morphometric studies of 'early alcoholic liver disease' failed to demonstrate fibrous thickening of the walls of the terminal hepatic venules.[62] Another study confirmed the presence of perivenular fibrosis as an early lesion in moderate to heavy drinkers;[63] 38.9% of males with a daily intake of 40–80 g alcohol for an average of 25 years had perivenular fibrosis and 44.4% had perivenular fibronectin deposition. Since only 20% of the heavy drinkers had cirrhosis, the authors suggest that factors in addition to the dose and duration of alcohol consumption must contribute to the progression from early perivenular fibrosis to cirrhosis.

Ultrastructural studies have shown myofibroblast proliferation around the terminal hepatic venule, occurring in association with perivenular fibrosis.[60] Perivenular fibrosis is thought to be the first lesion in a sequence of events which leads ultimately to the development of cirrhosis. The recognition of perivenular fibrosis at the fatty liver stage may permit the identification of patients who are likely to have progressive liver injury if they continue to drink.[61]

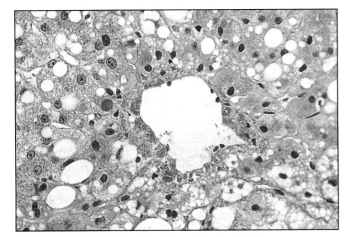

Fig. 6.5 • Perivenular fibrosis. Alcoholic fatty liver without evidence of alcoholic hepatitis. An abnormally thick rim of fibrous tissue surrounds the terminal hepatic venule; fibrous tissue also extends focally into the surrounding liver in a pericellular pattern. Several hepatocytes contain large mitochondria (discrete, pink globular masses). Chromotrope-aniline blue.

Alcoholic hepatitis

Beckett et al.[64] used the term 'acute alcoholic hepatitis' to describe a clinicopathological syndrome. Many subsequent studies have shown that a wide variety of clinical features and biochemical abnormalities may accompany the same morphological pattern of liver injury.[65-67] The term alcoholic steatonecrosis, used by some authors, is synonymous with alcoholic hepatitis.[68,69] Increasingly, the term alcoholic steatohepatitis (ASH) has been used as an alternative to alcoholic hepatitis.

Alcoholic hepatitis can only be reliably diagnosed morphologically, and the histological severity cannot be reliably predicted from the clinical features or the biochemistry. A liver biopsy study of patients presenting for treatment of alcoholism revealed alcoholic hepatitis in 17%.[70] Alcoholic hepatitis may be asymptomatic[71] but it is usually associated with non-specific digestive symptoms, hepatomegaly and raised liver enzymes.[65,67] About 25% of patients with severe liver injury show evidence of liver failure or hepatic encephalopathy.[65,67] Since alcoholic hepatitis may be asymptomatic, and up to 39% of patients have established cirrhosis at the time of first presentation,[72] the true incidence of alcoholic hepatitis remains to be determined. Alcoholic hepatitis is said to occur less commonly in Japan than in other parts of the world.[73]

The liver injury is characterized by fatty change, liver-cell necrosis and a neutrophil polymorph-rich infiltrate.[12,19,74] Mallory bodies (Chapter 2) are usually seen but their presence is not obligatory for the diagnosis. Unlike fat droplets, Mallory bodies persist in liver cells for many months (at least 8 months—personal observation) after alcohol consumption ceases. Giant mitochondria may be seen on light microscopy as eosinophilic, globular inclusions (Fig. 6.5) but occasionally they may be needle-shaped cytoplasmic inclusions. Where the liver injury is very mild, the presence of giant mitochondria may be a diagnostic hint of chronic alcohol consumption.[75]

When the liver injury is mild, only occasional foci of liver-cell necrosis are seen in the perivenular regions accompanied by a slight neutrophil polymorph infiltrate; occasional enlarged hepatocytes may contain Mallory bodies, and minimal pericellular fibrosis may also be present. However, on occasion liver biopsies from patients with a history of moderate to heavy alcohol consumption, show a non-specific pattern of injury characterized by mild to moderate hepatocyte injury—necrosis and/or apoptosis, with little or no ballooning degeneration, and accompanied by a mononuclear cell infiltrate with few or no polymorphs (Fig. 6.6). As discussed later this is the pattern of liver injury seen in most animal models of alcoholic liver disease,[76] and in steatohepatitis due to a wide variety of other causes (Chapter 7).

In fully developed alcoholic hepatitis, hepatocyte necrosis is more widespread and sometimes confluent; hepatocyte enlargement is a prominent feature and these ballooned hepatocytes frequently contain Mallory bodies (Fig. 6.7(A) and (C)). The neutrophil polymorph infiltrate is often concentrated around hepatocytes containing Mallory bodies

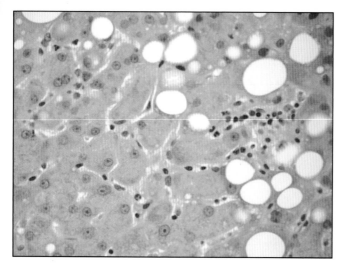

Fig. 6.6 • Nonspecific steatohepatitis. The liver shows moderate steatosis and a nonspecific pattern of injury in the form of small scattered areas on necroinflammation. Polymorphs, ballooning degeneration and Mallory bodies are not seen. H&E.

(Fig. 6.7(B))—so-called satellitosis. Monoclonal antibodies to hepatocyte cytokeratins, K8 and K18, anti-ubiquitin antibody (ubiquitin, a polypeptide, is present on intracytoplasmic aggregates of intermediate filament in a variety of cells) or anti-p62 antibody can be used to confirm the presence of Mallory bodies[77] (Fig. 6.7(D)). Immunohistochemical staining will also detect small Mallory bodies that are not readily apparent in routinely stained sections. A review of 700 articles on Mallory bodies found a mean prevalence of 65% in alcoholic hepatitis and 51% in alcoholic cirrhosis.[78]

Fatty change is usually present but is variable in severity and may be absent in patients who have been hospitalized for several weeks prior to the liver biopsy. Unlike NASH, the presence of steatosis is not a diagnostic requirement. Pericellular fibrosis is often present but may be limited to the perivenular zones in the early stages of alcoholic liver disease.

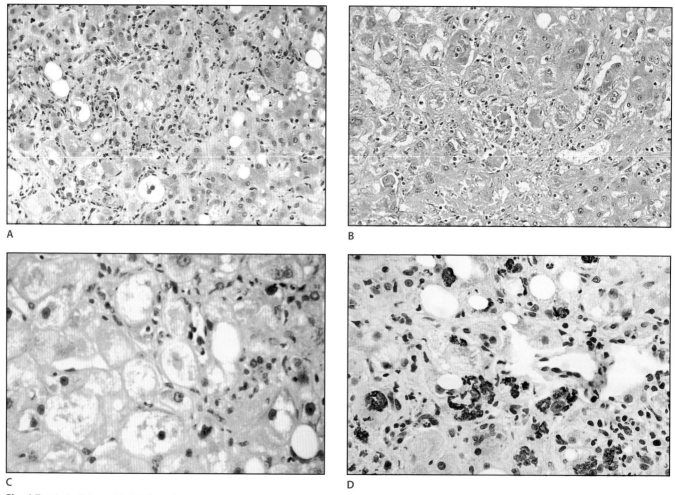

Fig. 6.7 • Alcoholic hepatitis. **(A)** The architecture is disturbed and there is a considerable liver-cell necrosis with an associated neutrophil polymorph infiltrate. Macrovesicular fat droplets are present in some hepatocytes. The patient, a woman aged 30 years, had a 12-year history of heavy drinking. H&E. **(B)** Numerous, slightly enlarged hepatocytes contain Mallory bodies and a heavy neutrophil polymorph infiltrate is seen in proximity to these cells. A marked degree of liver cell necrosis is apparent and a few large fat droplets are seen. H&E. **(C)** Hepatocytes showing marked ballooning degeneration. Most of the enlarged cells contain Mallory bodies. H&E. **(D)** Mallory bodies. A monoclonal antibody to ubiquitin reacts strongly with Mallory bodies. PAP.

Other features that may be seen include lipogranulomas, apoptosis[79] (previously described as acidophilic necrosis of hepatocytes), induced hepatocytes which have a 'ground-glass' appearance due to the proliferation of smooth endoplasmic reticulum, oncocytic hepatocytes, bile stasis, Kupffer cell proliferation, and enlargement due to ingested lipid and ceroid, 'microscopic cholangitis', a mild mononuclear cell infiltrate in the portal tracts, and variable degrees of perivenular fibrosis. Features indicating liver regeneration include mitotic figures in hepatocytes, microregenerative nodules and a ductular 'reaction'.

Sclerosing hyaline necrosis

Sclerosing hyaline necrosis, described by Edmondson et al.,[80] is not a separate pattern of alcohol-induced liver injury but rather forms part of the morphological spectrum of alcoholic hepatitis,[75] characterized by extensive perivenular liver-cell necrosis associated with the deposition of fibrous tissue (Fig. 6.8). The terminal hepatic venules may become occluded and portal hypertension can occur in the absence of cirrhosis.[81] Initially, fibrosis is seen only in the perivenular region and in association with foci of necrosis (Fig. 6.9(A)).

With progression, more extensive pericellular fibrosis is seen (Fig. 6.9(B)). More severe bridging necrosis between adjacent terminal hepatic venules or between terminal hepatic venules and portal tracts results in condensation of pericellular fibrosis tissue and the formation of septa.[82] Elastic fibres, which stain with orcein, can be seen in active fibrous septa, but not in areas of passive collapse of the reticulin framework.[83]

The anatomical pathologist is frequently asked to assess prognosis and the likelihood of the liver injury being reversible on the basis of the liver biopsy findings. Semiquantitative scoring systems have been described for assessing histological severity in steatohepatitis;[84,85] these are yet to be fully validated. The features which indicate a risk of progression to cirrhosis are: (i) the severity of the fatty change, particularly if it is microvesicular, and the extent of the hepatic fibrosis in livers seen at the fatty liver stage; (ii) the severity of hepatocyte necrosis and extent of pericellular and perivenular fibrosis[86]—the formation of fibrous septa with elastic fibre deposition[83] and architectural disturbance are bad prognostic indicators; (iii) diffuse parenchymal disease, which can also have an acute fulminant course; (iv) widespread obliteration of hepatic venules; and (v) widespread Mallory body formation.

Harinasuta & Zimmerman[68] and Christoffersen et al.[87] reviewed the significance of Mallory bodies in relation to the severity of liver injury and found that in non-cirrhotic livers parenchymal fibrosis appeared to be more marked when Mallory bodies were present. Bouchier et al.[88] reported a prospective study of 510 patients with a liver biopsy diagnosis of alcoholic liver disease who were followed for a 10-year period; 72% of those with simple fatty liver were alive at 10 years while only 37% of patients in whom alcoholic hepatitis was the predominant histological lesion survived. The highest mortality rate for patients with alcoholic

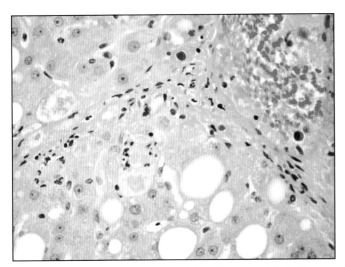

Fig. 6.8 • Sclerosing hyaline necrosis. Mild fatty change, mild alcoholic hepatitis and several Mallory bodies are apparent in the region of a hepatic venule. Increased amounts of fibrous tissue are seen in the parenchyma adjacent to the venule. H&E.

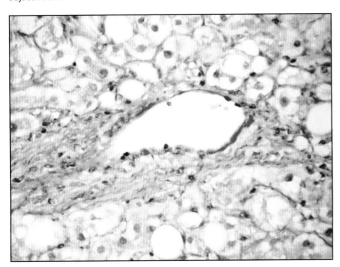

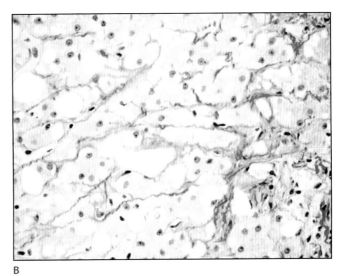

A   B

Fig. 6.9 • Hepatic fibrosis. **(A)** Mild perivenular fibrosis and mild pericellular fibrosis in zone 3. Sirius red. **(B)** More extensive pericellular fibrosis seen as thin re strands that are located in the perisinusoidal space of Disse and surround cords of hepatocytes. Sirius red.

hepatitis, both with and without cirrhosis, is in the first year after diagnosis.[89] The 30-day mortality rate for severe alcoholic hepatitis exceeds 40%.[90] Clinical scoring systems have been developed to predict mortality in acute alcoholic hepatitis.[91] Patients with alcoholic hepatitis are likely to have progressive injury leading to cirrhosis;[91] in one study 50% of patients with alcoholic hepatitis, who continued drinking, developed cirrhosis in 10–13 years.[92] Pares et al.[93] documented three variables that independently increase the risk of progression to cirrhosis: the severity of the initial histological injury, continuation of drinking, and female sex, while Morgan concludes that survival is significantly reduced in women, the elderly, and if drinking continues.[90]

Occlusive venous lesions in alcoholic liver disease

Goodman & Ishak[94] reviewed 200 autopsy cases of alcoholic liver disease, and described three types of venous lesions: (i) lymphocytic phlebitis; (ii) phlebosclerosis, due to perivenular fibrosis gradually obliterating vein lumens; and (iii) veno-occlusive lesions characterized by intimal proliferation, fibrosis of the vein wall and varying degrees of luminal obliteration.

Lymphocytic phlebitis was noted in 16% of patients with alcoholic hepatitis and in 4% of those with cirrhosis. Phlebosclerosis was found in all cases of alcoholic hepatitis and cirrhosis. Veno-occlusive lesions (Fig. 6.10) were found in 52% of cases of alcoholic hepatitis with portal hypertension, totally occluded veins were found in 47%, and partial occlusion of varying severity was found in 74% of cirrhotics. Portal hypertension correlated significantly with the degree of phlebosclerosis and veno-occlusive change. In biopsy material, Burt & MacSween[95] confirmed that phlebosclerosis was a universal finding in alcoholic hepatitis and cirrhosis but they found veno-occlusive lesions in only 10% of 256 biopsies and lymphocytic phlebitis in 4%. These occlusive venous lesions may contribute to the atrophy of hepatic parenchyma and functional impairment.

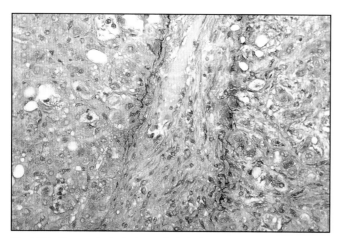

Fig. 6.10 • Veno-occlusive lesion in alcoholic liver disease: note the marked intimal proliferation producing considerable narrowing of the lumen of a hepatic vein branch. Verhoef-van Gieson.

Alcoholic cirrhosis

Alcohol is the most common cause of cirrhosis in Western countries.[5,25,96] In France, alcoholic liver disease-related mortality is 14.3 deaths per 100 000 population.[97] In the USA, in the 35–54 age group, cirrhosis, predominantly alcoholic, is the fourth commonest cause of death in men and the fifth commonest cause in women.[4]

A WHO group[98] defined cirrhosis as a diffuse process characterized by fibrosis and the conversion of the normal liver architecture into structurally abnormal nodules. Micronodular cirrhosis, which is the most common type of cirrhosis seen in association with alcohol,[99] is characterized by remarkably uniform-sized regenerative nodules, most of which are less than 3 mm in diameter. Bands of fibrous tissue completely surround the regenerative nodules; the terminal hepatic venules are not recognizable, but new vessel formation is apparent within the fibrous tissue (Fig. 6.11(A)).

Biopsies of cirrhotic livers may also show features of alcoholic hepatitis; the hepatocyte injury occurs

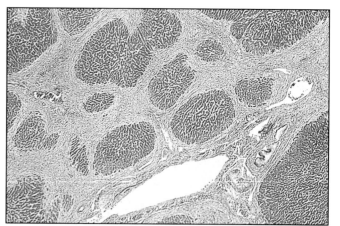

A

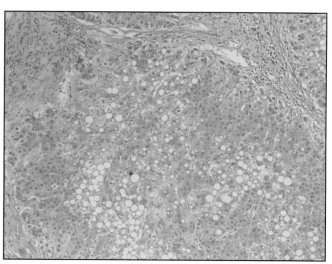

B

Fig. 6.11 • Alcoholic cirrhosis. **(A)** 'Inactive cirrhosis'. There is complete loss of the normal architecture and replacement by small regenerative nodules that are completely surrounded by broad bands of fibrous tissue. Masson's trichrome. **(B)** Steatosis superimposed on established micronodular cirrhosis. H&E.

predominantly at the periphery of the regenerative nodules. A variable mixture of neutrophil polymorphs, lymphocytes, plasma cells and macrophages is seen in the fibrous tissue. The presence of alcoholic hepatitis usually means continued drinking, even though there may be little or no fatty change. Autopsies sometimes reveal an unexpected finding of inactive cirrhosis in patients have been drinkers in the past (Fig. 6.11(A)) but, if drinking continues up until the time of death, steatosis, with or without the features of alcoholic hepatitis, may be seen (Fig. 6.11(B)).

In the past chronic (active) hepatitis has been described in alcoholic patients[100] because of the presence of interface hepatitis (piecemeal necrosis), but it now appears that superimposed hepatitis C virus, and to a lesser extent hepatitis B virus infection, explains many of the reported cases.[101,102] The liver may show features due both to alcohol-related liver injury and to chronic viral hepatitis (Fig. 6.12). It is not unusual for the predominant pattern of injury to be that of viral injury but with advanced fibrosis or even cirrhosis, often at a relatively young age, due to the potentiating effect of alcohol.[103] However, liver biopsies showing features of chronic hepatitis that resembles chronic viral hepatitis, are still being described in patients who are serologically negative for both hepatitis B and C virus, and it seems likely that other hepatitis viruses will be identified. Consequently, the role of alcohol per se as a cause of a chronic hepatitis-like injury remains controversial.[104]

A ductular 'reaction' is commonly seen in alcoholic liver disease; special stains and immunohistochemical studies have demonstrated glycogen, α_1-antitrypsin (α_1AT) and glucose 6-phosphatase in the ductular cells.[105] Immunohistochemical studies using a variety of monoclonal and polyclonal antibodies to cytokeratins have demonstrated the presence of the bile duct cytokeratins K7 and K19 in the ductular cells[106] (Fig. 6.13(A)). Until relatively recently the 'proliferating' ductules seen in the portal tracts and periportal regions, in alcoholic cirrhosis as well as cirrhosis due to other aetiologies, have been regarded as regenerating hepatocytes showing ductal metaplasia. An

alternative explanation is that these proliferating bile ductular cells are the progeny of 'proliferating' hepatic stem cells.[107-109] Small epithelial cells and 'proliferating' bile ductules often become particularly prominent in cirrhotic livers following abstinence from alcohol (Fig. 6.13(B)). The small epithelial cells seen in human livers closely resemble the oval cells that are seen in animal models of hepatocarcinogenesis. Oval cells from animal models, both in vivo and in culture, have been shown to differentiate into hepatocytes as well as biliary epithelial cells.[107-109] Immunohistochemical studies of a wide range of liver disease, including alcoholic liver disease, in humans have provided convincing evidence in support of the concept that these 'reactive' ductules are the progeny of hepatic, and possibly sometimes, bone marrow stem cells.[110]

Cirrhosis may become macronodular, particularly if drinking ceases.[99,111,112] The regenerative nodules then vary greatly in size, and many measure up to several centimetres in diameter; many such nodules contain portal tracts and terminal hepatic venules which are abnormally related to

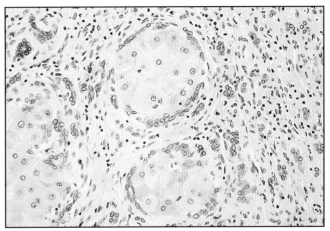

A

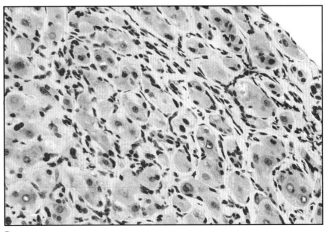

B

Fig.6.13 • Proliferation of ductules and small epithelial cells in alcoholic cirrhosis. **(A)** Explanted liver showing numerous small epithelial cells and ductules in the portal tracts and at the periphery of regenerative nodules. Reactivated with antibodies to bile-duct cytokeratins K7 and K19. PAP. **(B)** Small epithelial cells infiltrating between hepatocytes in a regenerative nodule. The liver biopsy was obtained from a patient with alcoholic cirrhosis who had been abstinent from alcohol for over 6 months prior to liver transplantation. H&E.

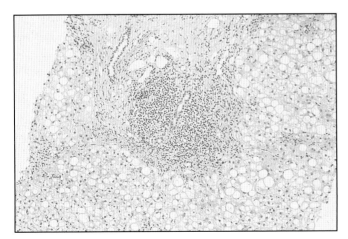

Fig. 6.12 • Chronic hepatitis C and alcoholic liver disease. A heavy infiltrate of mononuclear cells is seen in a portal tract, there is also evidence of interface hepatitis (piecemeal necrosis) and mild acinar hepatitis. The liver also shows moderate macrovesicular steatosis and elsewhere there was mild alcoholic hepatitis. H&E.

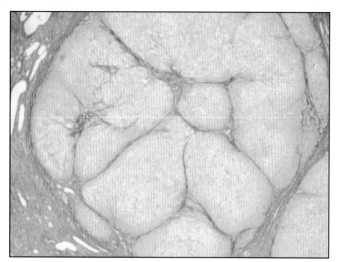

Fig. 6.14 • Macronodular cirrhosis. A large macroregenerative nodule contains several rudimentary portal areas. Sirius red.

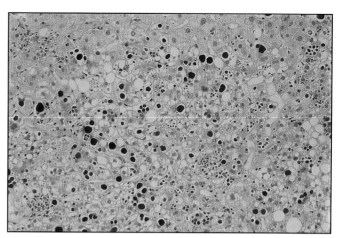

Fig. 6.15 • Alcoholic steatohepatitis and co-existing α_1AT deficiency. Many of the hepatocytes contain diastase resistant/PAS positive globules. In addition there is fatty change, hepatocyte necrosis and inflammation. D/PAS.

each other (Fig. 6.14). In some cases the architectural changes are best described as incomplete septal cirrhosis.[112a] A mixed micronodular and macronodular cirrhosis, with a variable proportion of micro- and macronodules, is not an uncommon finding at autopsy.

Large regenerative nodules may, on occasion, have clinical and radiological features suggestive of hepatocellular carcinoma. Nagasue et al.[113] reported several such cases and proposed the term hepatocellular 'pseudotumour' in the cirrhotic liver to describe these nodules. Focal nodular hyperplasia-like lesions are also described.[113a]

Steatosis and alcoholic hepatitis are reliably diagnosed by needle biopsy of the liver, but cirrhosis may be underdiagnosed because of sampling difficulty, particularly when an aspiration-type of needle is used.[114] Macronodular cirrhosis may be suspected, but cannot be confidently diagnosed by needle biopsy, because of the large size, by definition greater than 5 mm in diameter, of the nodules. Anthony et al.[98] and Scheuer & Lefkowitch[115] describe helpful criteria for the needle biopsy diagnosis of cirrhosis.

Globules of α_1AT are frequently seen in hepatocytes at the periphery of regenerative nodules; this accumulation is considered to be a consequence of impaired protein secretion.[116] However, recent studies in liver transplant units have revealed a higher than predicted prevalence of heterozygote α_1AT deficiency in patients undergoing transplantation for a variety of diseases, including alcoholic cirrhosis (8.2% Pi MZ in the transplant patients compared to 2–4% in the general population). This observation raises the possibility that α_1AT deficiency may potentiate other forms of liver disease including alcohol-related liver disease.[117] On rare occasions alcoholic liver disease and homozygous α_1AT deficiency may co-exist (Fig. 6.15). Again there is the possibility of an interaction between the two aetiological factors leading to cirrhosis at a relatively early age. Copper may also accumulate in hepatocytes in alcoholic liver disease. Copper bound to protein is seen as periodic acid-Schiff (PAS)-positive, diastase-resistant globules that stain positively with orcein,[118] and other more specific stains for copper such as rhodanine.

Oxyphilic granular hepatocytes, which have been termed hepatic oncocytes, are frequently seen at the periphery of regenerative nodules in alcoholic cirrhosis.[119,120] Oncocytes and induced hepatocytes can be differentiated from classic ground-glass hepatocytes which contain HBsAg, by orcein staining or immunohistochemistry.

Prognosis and reversibility of cirrhosis

A Veterans Administration Cooperative Study Group followed 281 alcoholic patients prospectively for 4 years to assess prognosis;[121] the worst prognosis, 35% survival at 48 months, was seen in patients with alcoholic hepatitis superimposed on cirrhosis. The most significant predictors of survival included age, grams of alcohol consumed, the ratio of serum (aspartate and alanine) aminotransferases (AST : ALT), and the histological and clinical severity of the disease.

Numerous studies have shown that abstinence can prolong survival in alcoholic cirrhosis.[65,122,123] In Powell & Klatskin's series,[122] 68% of cirrhotics who abstained survived 5 years, compared with 41% of those who continued to drink. Traditionally, cirrhosis has been thought to be an irreversible process; this concept is now being challenged. Cirrhosis in animal models is reversible, provided that the aetiological agent, e.g. carbon tetrachloride, is removed, and that sufficient time is allowed for the liver to return to its normal structure.[124] There are reports of reversal of established cirrhosis in humans;[125] this is a rare occurrence and reported instances are open to some doubt, particularly since micronodular cirrhosis can become macronodular, following the removal of the aetiological agent, in this case long-term abstinence from alcohol, and a follow-up needle biopsy—taken from within a macroregenerative nodule—may fail to detect the presence cirrhosis. Another possible explanation for some cases of apparently reversible cirrhosis could be overdiagnosis of cirrhosis in livers which in reality show widepread areas of confluent necrosis interspersed with groups of regenerating hepatocytes that are separated by bands of collapsed reticulin framework—an appearance that can resemble cirrhosis.

A recent review by Desmet & Roskams address the issues involved in the current controversies related to the possible reversibility of cirrhosis.[126] This is also discussed in Chapter 2.

Other morphological features of alcoholic liver injury

Cholestatic syndromes

Alcoholic liver disease may present with clinical and biochemical features that are strongly suggestive of extra-hepatic biliary obstruction.[49,127–129] The features include jaundice, right upper quadrant pain and tenderness, hepatomegaly, and marked elevation of serum bilirubin, serum alkaline phosphatase and serum cholesterol. Biliary obstruction, due to gallstones or alcoholic pancreatitis,[130] can be excluded by ultrasound, transhepatic cholangiography or endoscopic retrograde cholangiopancreatography (ERCP).

A high index of clinical suspicion of intrahepatic cholestasis is required in order to avoid unnecessary surgery in patients with alcoholic liver disease, as the risk of postoperative hepatic and/or renal failure is considerable. Severe cholestasis has been described in association with: (i) fatty liver[49,50,131] (Fig. 6.16); (ii) alcoholic foamy degeneration;[52] (iii) alcoholic hepatitis;[65,68,69,131] (iv) decompensated alcoholic cirrhosis; and (v) Zieve syndrome which comprises alcoholic steatosis, jaundice, hyperlipidaemia and haemolytic anaemia.[132]

A Veterans Administration Cooperative Study[133] showed a significant correlation between tissue cholestasis and mortality in alcoholic liver disease. The possibility that jaundice occurring in patients with a history of excess alcohol consumption may be due to non-alcoholic liver disease, such as viral hepatitis or drug-induced cholestasis, must also be considered.[134]

In patients with a severe fatty liver who develop a cholestatic syndrome, the liver biopsy may show portal tract changes with oedema, increased prominence of marginal bile ducts and a mild to moderate cholangitis with a neutrophil polymorph infiltrate—so-called microscopic cholangitis.[135]

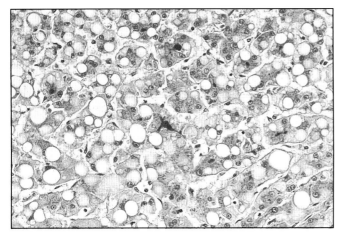

Fig. 6.16 • Fatty liver and cholestasis. The hepatocytes show fatty change and bile is present in some canaliculi. H&E.

Portal tract changes

Portal fibrosis has not classically been considered to occur as a result of alcohol injury per se. However, it may sometimes be a feature; Morgan et al.[136] found that the presence of portal fibrosis correlated with a previous history of viral hepatitis or episodes of acute pancreatitis. More recently, Michalak et al.[137] have suggested that portal fibrosis is part of progressive alcoholic liver disease. In their experience, portal and septal fibrosis was more frequent than perivenular fibrosis. Furthermore, it appeared to contribute to a greater proportion of overall fibrosis than did perivenular scarring. These intriguing findings merit further investigation.

Increased numbers of portal tract macrophages are seen frequently in alcoholic liver disease. A study by Karakucuk et al.[138] describes this feature at virtually all stages and has shown that the macrophages have markedly enhanced lysosomal enzyme release, compared with the resident macrophages in normal livers, suggesting that cytotoxic mediators released by these activated cells may be contributing to liver injury.

Hepatic siderosis

Excess stainable iron is found in both hepatocytes and Kupffer cells in many patients with alcoholic liver disease (Chapter 5). In one study, 57% of patients had mild siderosis while 7% had grade 3–4 siderosis.[139] The explanation for the excessive iron accumulation is still unclear but supports increased iron absorption, that has been attributed a variety of factors including the high iron content of some alcoholic beverages,[140] in particular home-brewed beer, which in sub-Saharan Africa is made in iron pots;[141] a direct effect of alcohol on the small intestine,[142] haemolysis associated with spur cell leading to increased iron absorption,[143] and upregulation of the transferrin receptor.[144] It is now generally accepted that only mild siderosis, grade 1–2, is alcohol-related—so-called alcoholic siderosis; patients with alcoholic liver disease in whom iron accumulation is massive (grade 3–4) are also suffering from hereditary haemochromatosis (Fig. 6.17(A),(B)).[146] Nevertheless, iron overload can be seen in extrahepatic tissues of patients with end-stage alcoholic liver disease in the absence of HFE mutations.[145]

In alcoholic siderosis, the iron-containing hepatocytes are distributed in a random fashion and the iron granules are often few in number; this contrasts with the zonal distribution of iron, with a periportal predominance, and often a pericanalicular distribution in the hepatocytes in hereditary haemochromatosis.

Porphyria cutanea tarda

Alcohol is thought to hasten the onset of the hepatic and cutaneous manifestations of porphyria cutanea tarda; alcohol withdrawal is followed by a dramatic clinical and biochemical improvement.[141] The hepatocytes may contain needle-shaped cytoplasmic inclusions of uroporphyrin which show brilliant-red autofluorescence under ultraviolet;

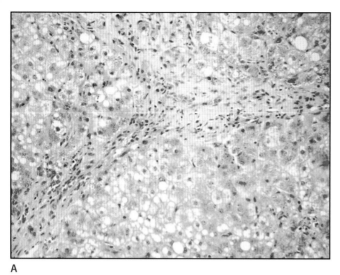

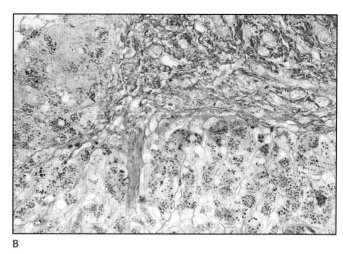

Fig. 6.17 • Hereditary haemochromatosis and alcoholic liver disease. **(A)** The liver shows the features of established micronodular cirrhosis, moderate fatty change. Also grade 4 siderosis with brown granules of iron being seen in the hepatocytes. Iron is also seen in bile-duct epithelium and portal tact macrophages. **(B)** Another area of the same liver—the iron is seen as blue granules and the fibrous tissue is stained red. Perls/Sirius red.

this is specific for porphyria cutanea tarda. Variable degrees of siderosis are usually present in the liver, and in addition there may be evidence of alcoholic liver disease.[141]

Hepatocellular carcinoma (HCC)

HCCs develop in 5–15% of patients with alcoholic cirrhosis, usually in association with macronodular cirrhosis[99] (Fig. 6.18). Studies from the USA and Italy suggest that in Western countries, alcohol may be the commonest cause of HCC accounting for 32–45% of cases.[147] Tumours are often seen in association with a combination of alcoholic and viral liver disease (hepatitis B and C viruses),[148] but are also described with negative markers for viral hepatitis.[149] There is now some evidence that alcohol may cause genetic alterations.[150] In addition, alcohol can act as a co-carcinogen because of its ability to induce the hepatic microsomal P-450-dependent biotransformation system, in particular the ethanol-inducible isoenzyme cytochrome P-450, leading to enhanced activation of a variety of pro-carcinogens that are present in food, tobacco smoke and alcoholic beverages.[18,44,151,152] A study of American patients with cirrhosis, with and without hepatocellular carcinomas, showed that alcohol, tobacco and obesity were independent, and synergistic, risk factors for hepatocellular carcinomas.[153] These authors suggest that increased oxidative stress plays a role in the pathogenesis of such tumours.

The role of alcohol and hepatitis B

The role of the hepatitis B virus (HBV) in the pathogenesis of hepatocellular carcinomas associated with alcoholic cirrhosis has been controversial, although clinical studies by Bellentani et al.[154] and molecular biological studies by Brechot et al.[155] support a role for the virus in the development of liver cancer. On the other hand, a study from Korea showed that alcohol, cigarette smoking and hepatitis B were

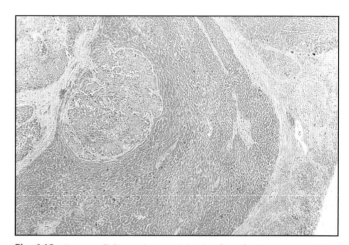

Fig. 6.18 • Hepatocellular carcinoma arising in a liver showing macronodular cirrhosis. The patient, a man aged 58 years, had a past history of heavy drinking but had abstained for several years. H&E.

independent risk factors for hepatocellular carcinoma but did not act synergisitically.[156]

The role of alcohol and hepatitis C

In contrast, alcohol is recognized as an important potentiating factor for hepatitis C virus (HCV)-associated hepatocellular carcinoma.[157–159] Yamauchi et al. reported a 10-year cumulative occurrence rate of hepatocellular carcinoma of 80.7% in patients with alcoholic cirrhosis who were anti-HCV-positive and drank more than 120 g alcohol per day; in contrast 18.5% of those with alcoholic cirrhosis alone developed hepatocellular carcinoma over 10 years while the 10-year rate for tumours in HCV-related cirrhosis in non-drinkers was 56.5%.[157] Another hospital-based, case-control study in the USA showed a significant synergy between heavy alcohol consumption, chronic hepatitis B or C virus infection as well as diabetes mellitus.[160] A review of alcohol and hepatocellular carcinoma reports that chronic alcohol consumption >80 g per day for >10 years increases the risk of hepatocellular almost five-fold, and that alcohol doubles the risk of this tumour in chronic hepatitis C compared to the risk with the virus alone.[147]

Autopsy studies in the past, as well as recent prospective studies of liver biopsies, have suggested that dysplastic nodules, which develop within cirrhotic nodules—especially macroregenerative nodules (>5 mm diameter)—may be the precursor lesion to hepatocellular carcinoma.[161–163] A prospective liver biopsy study of radiologically-identified hepatic nodules concluded that an increased ratio of nuclear density of >1.5, clear-cell change and small-cell dysplasia are features indicating a high risk for evolution to hepatocellular carcinoma.[162]

Lee et al.[164] evaluated large cell dysplasia, seen as foci of hepatocellular enlargement, nuclear pleomorphism, hyperchromasia and multinucleation, and concluded that this feature is an independent risk factor for hepatocellular carcinoma, with an estimated odds ratio of 3.3. However, large-cell dysplasia is not thought to be a direct precursor of hepatocellular carcinoma, but rather is an indicator of an increased risk of tumour development.[163,164] A comment about the presence, or absence, of both small-cell and large-cell dysplasia should always be included in reports of cirrhotic livers.

The role of liver biopsy in alcoholic liver disease

In a study by Levin et al. only 80% of patients with a heavy alcohol intake were found to have alcohol-associated liver injury.[134] The other 20% had various types of non-alcoholic liver disease including cholangitis, viral hepatitis, granulomatous hepatitis, passive venous congestion and non-specific changes; however, a more recent study showed that a clinical diagnosis of alcoholic liver disease was significantly associated with a histological diagnosis of alcoholic liver disease, with a 98% specificity and a 79% sensitivity.[165] Nevertheless, a liver biopsy is recommended under the following circumstances:

1. In patients suspected of having alcoholic liver disease since it allows the clinical diagnosis of alcoholic liver disease to be confirmed or refuted.
2. For assessment of the severity and stage and thus the prognosis of the liver injury. This information will sometimes be used in counselling patients to abstain from alcohol.
3. To determine whether there is any unsuspected co-existing, and sometimes treatable, liver disease such as an infection or some form of hepatic iron overload.
4. To monitor the effects of various therapeutic modalities, including anti-inflammatory agents such as prednisolone[166] and agents such as pentoxifylline,[167] and S-adenosyl-L-methionine[168,169] for the treatment of alcoholic hepatitis.

5. As part of the work-up of some patients being considered for orthotopic liver transplantation particularly if cofactors are suspected, e.g. iron overload which may require treatment prior to transplantation.

Differential diagnosis

Fatty liver diseases

The entire histopathological spectrum of alcohol-associated liver injury is non-specific—for example, macrovesicular fatty change is seen frequently in association with diabetes mellitus, obesity and drugs, e.g. corticosteroids; microvesicular fatty change is the lesion seen characteristically in Reye syndrome, fatty liver of pregnancy and in association with a variety of drugs e.g. sodium valproate, tetracycline and amiodarone.[170]

Both non-specific steatohepatitis and alcohol hepatitis-like patterns of injury can occur in non-drinkers when it is termed non-alcoholic fatty liver disease (NAFLD) or non-alcoholic steatohepatitis (NASH; see Chapter 7). The histological features of so-called type 3 and 4 NAFLD (NASH) are identical to those of alcoholic hepatitis (Fig. 6.7(A)–(C)) although the liver injury tends to be less severe in NAFLD/NASH and Mallory bodies may be sparse or absent.[171] In contrast, drugs such as perhexiline maleate[172] (Fig. 6.19) and amiodarone[173–176] can cause a severe, and sometimes fatal, alcoholic hepatitis-like injury; progression to cirrhosis is also well described with both drugs. Thus, the pathologist requires a reliable alcohol history in order to differentiate between alcoholic or 'non-alcoholic' liver disease.[177]

Some patients, especially obese women, in whom a there is a liver biopsy diagnosis of NASH, may actually have liver disease which is aetiologically and pathogenetically related to both the risk factors that are associated with NAFLD/NASH and to the small, so-called 'insignificant' amounts of alcohol that they are consuming. This suggestion is supported by a rodent nutritional model study of NAFLD in which liver injury was worsened by 'low-dose' alcohol.[178]

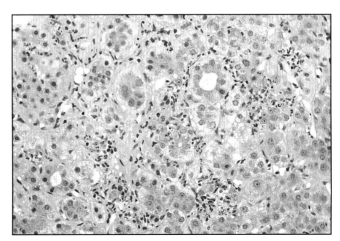

Fig. 6.19 • Perhexiline maleate-induced hepatitis. The liver shows severe alcoholic hepatitis-like injury. There is widespread focal necrosis of liver cells with a prominent infiltrate of neutrophils. Several regenerative acini are apparent. H&E.

Viral and drug hepatitis

It is now well recognized that heavy drinkers, as a result of an impaired immune response, have an increased risk of infection. Consequently, both acute and chronic viral hepatitis occur not infrequently in patients with a history of excess alcohol consumption.[100–102] The liver biopsy may show the features of viral hepatitis[100,101,134] without overt evidence of alcoholic liver disease, although the stage of chronic hepatitis may be advanced due to the potentiating effect of alcohol; this potentiation is, at least in part, due to enhanced viral replication.[200] Alternatively the liver may show the combined features of both viral and alcohol-related injury (Fig. 6.12).

Chronic alcohol ingestion also increases the risk of drug-induced liver injury due to the induction of the isoenzyme cytochrome CYP2E1 by alcohol.[41,42] Animal model studies also suggest that alcohol may selectively deplete mitochondrial glutathione and that this is an additional mechanism for the potentiating effect of alcohol on liver injury due to paracetamol (acetaminophen).[201] The pattern of liver injury may be purely that of drug-associated injury[170] but may also be superimposed on the various stages of alcohol-related injury.

Hereditary haemochromatosis

Prior to the identification of genetic abnormalities involved in iron metabolism, alcoholic siderosis and hereditary haemochromatosis were differentiated by biochemical measurement of the hepatic iron concentration and calculation of the hepatic iron index (HII) i.e. the hepatic iron concentration divided by the patient's age; an HII of greater than 2 is virtually diagnostic of hereditary haemochromatosis,[202] but calculation of the HII has been largely replaced by genotyping.[203] However, if genotyping is not available, and where marked iron overload is an unexpected finding in a liver biopsy specimen, the hepatic iron, demonstrated by the Perls method, can either be measured by computerized image analysis[204] or the remainder of the liver tissue can be removed from the paraffin block and the iron concentration can be measured biochemically in the de-waxed specimen.

The liver of chronic drinkers who are homozygous or heterozygous for the *HFE* (C282Y) mutation, or one of the less common mutations involved in iron overload, may show evidence of both hepatic iron overload and alcohol-related liver injury. A liver-biopsy-based study of 206 subjects with *HFE*-associated haemochromatosis showed that cirrhosis was almost nine times as common in those who drank >60 g of alcohol per day than in those who drank less than this amount.[205] In such patients, episodes of alcoholic hepatitis, in which iron is released from dead hepatocytes, can lead to an altered distribution of liver iron, with haemosiderin appearing in Kupffer cells and portal tract macrophages.[206]

Both primary and secondary hepatic iron overload appear to potentiate liver injury, due to a variety of causes including alcohol and chronic viral infections, in humans.[206] Similarly, dietary iron overload potentiated alcohol/hepatotoxin-mediated fibrosis and cirrhosis in an animal model.[207] Possible mechanisms for this potentiation of hepatic fibrosis included increased amounts of lipid peroxidation, iron-induced activation of hepatic stellate cells,[208] and iron-dependent activation of NF-κB in Kupffer cells leading to the production of proinflammatory cytokines.[209] The effect of alcohol on iron storage diseases of the liver have been reviewed recently by Fletcher et al.[210] and Tavill.[211]

Pathogenesis of alcoholic liver disease

Ultrastructural changes

The direct hepatotoxic effect of alcohol has been clearly demonstrated in numerous human[212,213] and animal studies.[212–216] Various forms of dietary manipulation have failed to prevent the hepatotoxic effects of alcohol.[213,217] Non-intoxicating doses of alcohol given to healthy non-alcoholic volunteers caused liver injury in only 2–4 days;[213] the ultrastructural changes included the accumulation of fat droplets, proliferation of smooth endoplasmic reticulum (SER) and mitochondrial damage. The mitochondria are enlarged and distorted in shape, with disrupted cristae and sometimes crystalline inclusions. Alterations in mitochondrial structure and function are due to the effects of alcohol metabolism, particularly acetaldehyde accumulation and the shift in redox potential.[28–31,218] Mitochondrial damage is always present at the fatty liver stage and persists as liver disease progresses. The presence of giant mitochondria, although non-specific (they can sometimes be seen in NASH), is highly suggestive of alcoholic liver disease (Fig. 6.20).[76] Giant mitochondria may be seen at all stages of alcoholic injury but are seen most frequently in association with alcoholic hepatitis.[219] They are often easily recognized in hepatocytes showing microvesicular steatosis; this is not unexpected since development of microvesicular steatosis can be directly attributed to mitochondrial dysfunction.[220] Mitochondrial DNA gene deletions have been described in

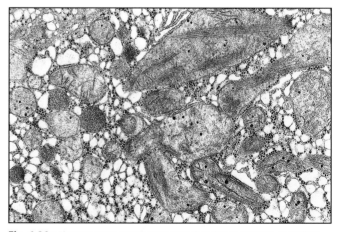

Fig. 6.20 • Electron microscopy: giant mitochondria containing crystalline inclusions; a number of normal-sized mitochondria are also seen, some with inclusions. ×17 500.

alcoholic liver disease.[221–223] Chronic ethanol consumption results in a generalized depression in hepatic mitochondrial energy metabolism which is one of the factors contributing to liver injury.

Proliferation of SER (Fig. 6.21) has been confirmed by the isolation and chemical measurement of microsomes.[212] The proliferation of SER is an adaptive response, the structural counterpart to ethanol-induction of CYP2E1, that accelerates alcohol metabolism and with a resultant increase in acetaldehyde production[35,224] The associated enhancement of vitamin metabolism can lead to a reduction in hepatic vitamin A and the appearance of multivesicular lysosomes in hepatocytes and macrophages (Fig. 6.22).[225] Enhanced metabolism of drugs, e.g. paracetamol (acet-aminophen),[226,227] and environmental chemicals, e.g. xylene[228] can cause severe acute liver injury which is sometimes fatal;[227] while chronic interactions between alcohol and vitamin A[229] or alcohol and carbon tetrachloride[230] can cause chronic injury with progressive hepatic fibrosis and eventually cirrhosis.

Mitochondrial and plasma membranes exhibit increased fluidity after acute ethanol ingestion, but become more rigid following chronic alcohol consumption.[218,231–233] The increased rigidity is thought to be due to changes in the lipid composition of the membranes.[234,235] Episodes of acute hepatocyte injury may occur in association with chronic alcohol consumption, because hepatocytes with membranes altered by alcohol are more susceptible to other membrane toxins such as products of intestinal bacteria, viruses and drugs; influx of calcium ions across damaged hepatocyte membranes has been proposed as a final common pathway for acute hepatocyte necrosis.[236,237] Hoek et al.[238] reviewed studies on the interaction of ethanol with biological membranes, in particular the actions of ethanol on hormonal signal transduction systems.

Lipid peroxidation (to be discussed later in more detail), which is peroxidative decomposition of membrane lipids initiated by reactive oxygen species (ROS), is now thought to be one of the important pathogenetic mechanisms for alcohol-related liver injury.[239–244]

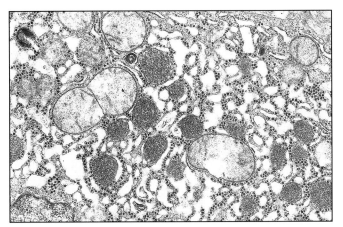

Fig. 6.21 • Proliferation of smooth endoplasmic reticulum (SER) in alcoholic liver disease: note the prominent, vesiculated SER, a number of mitochondria, and also a few dense bodies. ×24 000.

Perivenular hypoxia and enhanced oxygen requirements

Alcohol-induced liver injury selectively affects the perivenular region in the early stages. It has been postulated that a relatively lower oxygen tension in this zone may exaggerate the shift in redox potential that accompanies alcohol metabolism.[245] Hypoxia has been shown to induce perivenular liver-cell necrosis in chronic ethanol-fed rats.[246] Israel et al.[34] have likened the acceleration of alcohol metabolism with an associated enhancement of oxygen requirement to a hypermetabolic state and this has been the basis for animal and human studies of propylthiouracil.[247,248] Rats fed ethanol in the Lieber-De-Carli diet plus propylthiouracil, in doses that made the animals hypothyroid, did not show the hepatocyte ballooning that was seen in the alcohol alone group; they also had significantly less hepatic fibrosis.[249] CYP2E1 induction by alcohol,[250,251] and consequently the metabolism of alcohol occur maximally in the perivenular regions; Lieber et al.[252] suggested that impaired oxygen utilization rather than lack of oxygen supply, and enhanced alcohol metabolism in this zone, are factors in alcohol-associated liver injury. Fluctuations in blood flow have also been suggested as a mechanism for hypoxia-related injury in animal models for alcoholic liver disease; the role of hypoxia on liver injury has recently been comprehensively reviewed by French.[253]

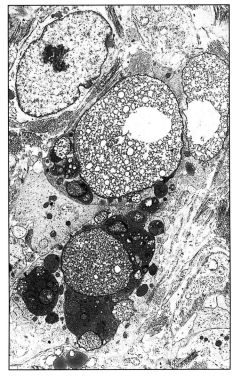

Fig. 6.22 • Multivesicular lysosomes. Portion of a cell containing several multivesicular lysosomes of the type also seen in vitamin A deficiency. ×4570.

Hepatocyte enlargement

Hepatomegaly, seen in association with chronic alcohol consumption, is at least in part due to the accumulation of both lipid and protein in hepatocytes (Fig. 6.7(C)).[254] Acetaldehyde and acetate impair microtubule-mediated protein secretion by hepatocytes;[255] water is retained in the cytoplasm of hepatocytes in proportion to protein retention, leading to hepatocyte enlargement, which may progress through ballooning degeneration to necrosis. Microtubules have a role in the maintenance of the shape of the hepatocytes, and a decrease in the number of microtubules may also contribute to the ballooning of hepatocytes.[256]

Some studies report a strong positive correlation between hepatocyte enlargement and intrahepatic pressure;[257–259] however, other studies in baboons[260] and humans[261] failed to demonstrate this relationship. Okanoue et al.[262] performed liver biopsies and measured the intrahepatic portal vein pressure in 12 patients immediately after abstinence from alcohol and repeated both investigations after the biochemistry improved; the reduction in intrahepatic pressure correlated with the reduction in size of swollen hepatocytes in patients with mild fibrosis, but in those with severe fibrosis the intrahepatic portal pressure remained high despite the reduction in hepatocyte size. It would seem that hepatocyte enlargement is only one of the mechanisms responsible for portal hypertension in pre-cirrhotic, alcoholic liver disease.

Mallory bodies

In 1911 Mallory[263] described the aggregates of amorphous, eosinophilic material in hepatocytes in alcoholic liver disease which today bear his name. The term Mallory body is favoured over alcoholic hyalin since the same material is seen in a wide variety of non-alcoholic liver diseases (Chapters 2 and 7). Mallory bodies are seen in NAFLD type 4 (NASH). Mallory bodies are also seen in association with prolonged cholestasis[264] which occurs in diseases such as primary biliary cirrhosis,[265] in Wilson disease,[266] Indian childhood cirrhosis,[267] focal nodular hyperplasia,[268] and

hepatocellular carcinoma.[269] Mallory bodies have been produced experimentally using griseofulvin,[270] diethylnitrosamine,[271] dieldrin[272], tautomycin[273] and 3,5-diethoxy carbonyl-1,4 dihydrocollidine (DDC).[274]

Three ultrastructurally distinct forms of Mallory bodies have been described:[275]

Type I	bundles of filaments in parallel arrays;
Type II	clusters of randomly oriented fibrils;
Type III	granular or amorphous substance containing only scattered fibrils.

The filament thickness varies from 5 to 20 nm, depending on the method of measurement. Type II Mallory bodies (Fig. 6.23(A),(B)) are the type seen most frequently in alcoholic liver disease. Isolation of Mallory bodies in a purified fraction has made chemical analysis possible.[276] Mallory bodies, purified from human liver, are composed predominantly of protein; five polypeptide bands have been detected by electrophoretic analysis, with molecular weights ranging from 32 kD to 56 kD.[277] Small amounts of carbohydrate have also been detected.[278,279] Mallory body formation is thought to result from derangement of the intermediate filament component of the cytoskeleton of the hepatocyte,[278,280] but they are not composed only of intermediate filament proteins; antibodies to Mallory bodies react with the cytoplasmic filament system of normal hepatocytes—cytokeratins 8 and 18[280–284]—but they also contain a number of unique antigenic determinants[280,285,286] together with cytokeratins 19 and 20. The cytokeratin molecules may be hyperphosphorylated[287] Mallory bodies from alcoholic and non-alcoholic liver disease have been shown to share a common antigenic determinant.[288]

Jenson & Gluud[289] reviewed previously published studies of Mallory bodies and concluded that Mallory bodies are stereotypical histological byproducts of diverse hepatic injuries (mostly alcohol-related), and of questionable pathogenic importance.[289] Previous hypotheses concerning the pathogenesis of Mallory body formation include those by

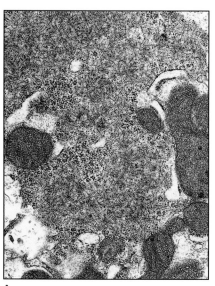

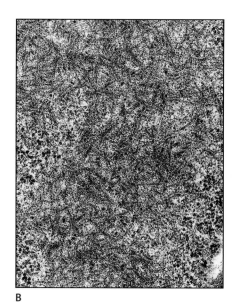

Fig. 6.23 • Mallory body, type II. **(A)** The Mallory body consists of a mass of randomly orientated filaments. Several mitochondria, of varying sizes and shapes, are also seen. ×25 100. **(B)** Higher magnification showing the randomly arranged filaments. ×57 000.

A

B

Janig et al.,[274] Denk et al.,[290] French,[282–284] French et al.,[291] and Worman.[292]

1. *Microtubular failure.* This theory is based on the observation that agents such as colchicine and alcohol cause microtubular disassembly and an increase in perinuclear intermediate filaments, which are thought to favour the development of Mallory bodies. Microtubules have been demonstrated in Mallory bodies.[293] However, other studies which used morphometry failed to show a relationship between microtubular abnormalities and Mallory body formation.

2. *Preneoplasia* with a structural phenotypic change. Hepatic carcinogens, such as griseofulvin and diethylnitrosamine, induce Mallory body formation and also the appearance of oncofetal markers in the same benign and malignant cells. It has therefore been postulated that Mallory body formation is part of the disorganization of the cytoskeleton caused by oncogenic transformation.[294] This hypothesis obviously does not explain the presence of Mallory bodies in non-neoplastic liver disease but would be consistent with the presence of Mallory bodies in hepatocellular carcinoma.

3. *Altered keratins and interaction with stress proteins.* Mallory body formation is considered to be pathological and a predominantly hepatocytic form of keratinization. This is based on the observation that vitamin A deficiency can induce Mallory body formation in mice and that serum vitamin A levels show a significant inverse correlation with the number of hepatocytes containing Mallory bodies.[295,296] Jenson & Gluud[289] favour the concept of defective protein systems in the pathogenesis of Mallory bodies. This concept is supported by the calcium antagonist properties of drugs such as amiodarone and perhexiline maleate that are associated with Mallory body formation, and the physiological characteristics of ubiquitin, the stress-response protein, that is seen in association with Mallory bodies. Recent studies have demonstrated that the stress proteins Hsp70, Hsp25 and p62 are also part of the complex of proteins in Mallory bodies.[274] The role of uncoordinated changes in hepatic oxygen delivery and consumption, and oxygen-derived free radicals are also under investigation, while Yuan et al.[273] suggest that activation of a protein kinase mechanism is involved. It would appear that the ubiquitin-proteosome pathway that is normally involved in protein degradation is blocked and as a consequence ubiquinated and misfolded proteins accumulate in aggregates giving rise to Mallory bodies.[274]

Irrespective of the mechanism of formation, all current data suggest that Mallory bodies form as a consequence of disruption of the normal intermediate filament network in the hepatocyte and that they are composed, at least in part, of the pre-existing intermediate filaments. Various cytokeratin antibodies[297,298] and anti-ubiquitin antibody[78,299] can be used to demonstrate the presence of Mallory bodies (Fig. 6.7(D)). The use of sensitive immunohistochemical techniques has confirmed the presence of Mallory bodies in a wide variety of non-alcoholic liver diseases; nevertheless, Mallory bodies are seen most frequently in alcoholic liver disease (71%) compared with non-alcoholic liver disease (40%).[297] Van Eyken et al.[106] demonstrated the presence of biliary cytokeratins K7 and K19 in Mallory bodies and suggested that hepatocytes that exhibit ductal metaplasia and express K7 and K19 may be showing pre-Mallory body changes. De Vos & Desmet,[300] in an electron microscopic study, described small epithelial cells, which are now recognized as hepatic stem cells; the relationship of these to cells showing pre-Mallory body changes remains to be elucidated.

Hepatic fibrogenesis

Hepatic fibrosis reflects an imbalance between the production and the degradation of extracellular matrix. A number of excellent review articles on hepatic fibrosis include those by Bataller and Brenner,[301] Friedman,[302] and Pinzani and Rombouts.[303]

Alcohol produces several highly characteristic, although not entirely specific, patterns of fibrosis. As discussed above, the early lesion may be that of perivenular fibrosis[58,60,304] (Fig. 6.9(A)), while the pericellular fibrosis, 'chicken-wire' pattern of fibrosis, may be seen in association with both perivenular fibrosis of central hyaline sclerosis and alcoholic hepatitis (Fig. 6.9(A),(B)). In Japan, progressive alcoholic fibrosis, apparently unrelated to alcoholic hepatitis, is has been described in the livers of heavy drinkers,[79,305,306] but the role of co-existent hepatitis C virus infection, and possibly other as yet unidentified hepatitis viruses, in this type of progressive hepatic fibrosis remains to be elucidated.

In the normal liver, the perisinusoidal extracellular matrix consists predominantly of a basement membrane-like matrix containing non-fibril-forming collagens—types IV and VI, and small amounts of collagen types I and III—while in alcoholic fibrosis and cirrhosis, as in cirrhosis of other aetiologies, fibronectin and laminin,[307] and type III collagen, with lesser amounts of type I collagen,[308] and also proteoglycans, tenascin, decorin and biglycan, are deposited in the space of Disse (Chapter 2).

Cells involved in collagen synthesis in the liver

It is now generally accepted that hepatic stellate cells, 'transitional' cells, myofibroblasts and fibroblasts belong to the same lineage and that these are the principal collagen-producing cells in the liver.[309] In contrast, the conversion of peribiliary fibrogenic cells is considered to be a separate process that is stimulated by platelet-derived growth factor (PDGF).[310]

Hepatic stellate cells

As described in Chapter 1, these cells are situated in the perisinusoidal space of Disse and are characterized by the presence of numerous vitamin A-containing fat droplets[311,312] (Fig. 6.24(A)). Stellate cells in culture have been shown to divide and to produce collagen type I, collagen type III and

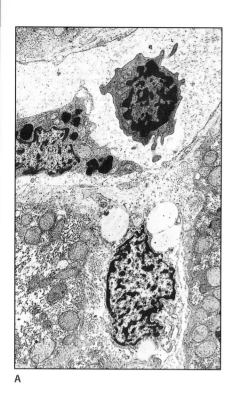
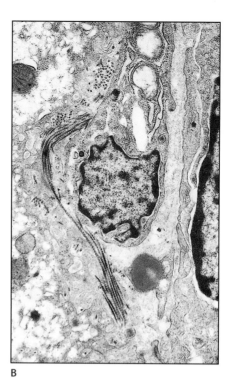

Fig. 6.24 • (A) A lipid-containing hepatic stellate cell and a small amount of collagen are situated in the space of Disse. Portion of a hepatocyte is seen on each side of the stellate cell. A sinusoid containing a lymphocyte and portion of a Kupffer cell are also shown (top). ×6160. **(B)** A transitional cell is situated in the space of Disse. Prominent rough endoplasmic reticulum is seen in the cell but fat droplets are absent. Bundles of collagen are seen in the space of Disse closely apposed to the outer surface of the cell. ×12 700.

laminin.[313] The presence of increased numbers of stellate cells in areas of hepatocyte necrosis in animal models can be demonstrated by anti-desmin antibodies.[314]

A very recent study has established human hepatic stellate cell culture lines, LX-1 and LX-2, that express key receptors reulating hepatic fibrosis.[315] These cell lines should prove invaluable in testing a range of antifibrotic drugs.

Transitional cells

In this context the term transitional cell is used to describe activated stellate cells, which show a morphological transition towards fibroblastic differentiation[316–321] (Fig. 6.24(B)). Studies in the chronic alcohol-fed baboon model, and in humans, suggest that this activation is associated with alcohol or, more likely, its metabolite acetaldehyde.[317,318,320,321] Less than 20% of the volume of transitional cells is composed of lipid droplets. The cells contain prominent rough endoplasmic reticulum (RER), microfilaments, dense bodies, pinocytotic vesicles and an oval or slightly irregular nucleus. Following chronic alcohol consumption, over 50% of stellate cells are seen to have the features of transitional cells,[319] and these cells are thought to increase in number. Stellate cells and transitional cells are closely related to collagen fibres in the space of Disse (Fig. 6.24(A),(B)).[317] There is a significant correlation between the percentage of transitional cells, the area of their RER and the amount of collagen in the space of Disse, suggesting that alcohol, or its metabolites, has a direct effect on collagen synthesis by stellate cells.[317,319]

Myofibroblasts

Myofibroblasts were first described in human livers in association with cirrhosis.[322] They are seen in the perivenular region in normal baboon liver; their number increases fol-

lowing alcohol ingestion and shows a correlation with the thickness of the rim of fibrous tissue around the terminal hepatic venules.[60,323] Myofibroblasts are characterized by prominent bundles of actin microfilaments, which usually run parallel to the long axis of the cell; microtubules are closely related to the microfilaments. Immunohistochemical studies have shown both desmin and vimentin intermediate filaments as well as contractile protein, actin, within myofibroblasts.[324] Myofibroblasts in the liver are considered to be activated stellate cells and to be responsible for the fibrosis that occurs in the perivenular region.[37,323] Both acetaldehyde and lactate have been shown to stimulate collagen production by baboon myofibroblasts in culture.[325] The contractile properties of myofibroblasts may contribute to scar contraction in cirrhosis and, by occluding hepatic venules, to the development of portal hypertension.[321,325]

Fibroblasts

Fibroblasts contain large amounts of RER with dilated cisternae filled with fluffy material thought to be procollagen. They contain intermediate filaments of the vimentin type. The number of fibroblasts in the perivenular region and the perisinusoidal space increases as fibrosis progresses.[60] Fibroblasts predominantly produce type I collagen and lesser amounts of type III, and also collagenase, fibronectin and glycosaminoglycans.[325] Acetaldehyde has been shown to stimulate the production of both collagen and non-collagenous proteins by human fibroblasts.[327]

Regulation of collagen synthesis in the liver

The pathogenesis of hepatic fibrosis involves a cascade of events in which inflammatory/immune mechanisms play a major role; current evidence suggests that a complex interplay of cytokines, with one another, and with the extracellular matrix of the liver modulates collagen synthesis in vivo. Friedman and colleagues[301,302,328] have proposed several models for stellate cell activation in hepatic fibrosis in which hepatocyte necrosis and apoptosis, both caused by and resulting in oxidative stress, accompanied by a variety of inflammatory/immunological changes that lead to a complex cascade of events that include: (i) paracrine stimuli e.g. Kupffer cell-derived cytokines such as transforming growth factor (TGF) β1, autocrine cytokines, lipid peroxidation, aldehyde adducts and NF-kB which all play a role in the initiation of stellate cell activation; and (ii) perpetuation of stellate cell activation, resulting in increased amounts of extracellular matrix, with a switch from type III to type I collagen production and deposition in the space of Disse.

A recent and novel suggestion is that stellate cells are 'hepatic neuroglia' that may be regulated by the sympathetic nervous system; mouse stellate cell culture studies have shown that cell growth can be increased by neurotransmitters such as catecholamines.[329] A recent morphological study of 87 human liver biopsies showing the features of alcoholic liver disease, with varying stages of fibrosis, is of particular interest.[330] Stellate cell activation, indicated by the expression of smooth muscle actin (SMA), was most intense in the perivenular regions in the 'earlier stages' and became diffuse as fibrosis progressed; Kupffer cell activation, as judged by the expression of CD68, was intense and diffuse, while the expression of CD34 by endothelial cells was seen in the periportal regions at all stages of fibrosis.

Factors involved in extracellular matrix degradation include matrix metalloproteinases (MMPs), as well as other enzymes such as plasmin. Membrane-type MMP can activate some latent metalloproteinases and gelatinases which can degrade basement membrane (type IV) collagen[331,332] in the space of Disse. Stellate cells express many of these components involved in matrix degradation.[302,331,332] During early activation, stellate cells release MMPs with the ability to degrade the matrix but when the cells are fully activated they show increased synthesis and release of tissue inhibitors of metalloproteinase (TIMP)-1 and -2, resulting in a net down-regulation of matrix degradation and consequently accumulation of extracellular matrix.[332]

Removal of activated stellate cells as a result of apoptosis is a key factor in the reversal of fibrosis and this requires downregulation of TIMP-1.[333] It is also noteworthy that leptin (the main hormone regulating metabolic rate and appetite) expression by activated stellate cells has recently been reported, thus giving the cell an endocrine function.[334]

'Capillarization of the sinusoids'

In 1963, Schaffner & Popper introduced the term capillarization of hepatic sinusoids;[335] today, this phenomenon is recognized as being due to disruption of the normal extracellular matrix in the space of Disse and replacement by mainly type I collagen, but also basal lamina-like material containing laminin and type IV collagen, all of which are produced by activated stellate cells. This process occurs in early alcoholic liver injury and is seen first in the perivenular zone;[336] capillarization occurs independently of parenchymal necrosis, alcoholic hepatitis or Mallory bodies in humans.[337]

Capillarization of the sinusoids results in a significant barrier between the blood and the hepatocyte which may provoke further activation of stellate cells and may also be a factor in hepatocyte dysfunction and injury, as well as reducing the transport of solutes from the sinusoidal blood to the hepatocyte via the space of Disse.

This phenomenon is often accompanied by structural changes in the sinusoidal endothelial cells. These unique endothelial cells have flattened processes perforated by small fenestrae about 0.1 mm in diameter; the fenestrae are arranged in groups termed the 'sieve plate'.[312] Since the normal sinusoidal lining does not have a basement membrane, the presence of the fenestrae permits a full exchange of fluid, solutes and particles between the blood and the space of Disse. The term 'defenestration' is used to describe changes in the fenestrae, which lessen the porosity of the sinusoidal lining. Scanning electron micrographic studies of needle biopsies from non-cirrhotic alcoholic patients have shown evidence of defenestration in the perivenular zone, occurring in both the presence and absence of collagenization of the space of Disse.[336] Morphometric studies of the sinusoidal barrier in alcoholic fatty liver without fibrosis showed changes in the porosity of the liver sieve due to dilatation of the fenestrae[338] but no difference in the volume and surface density of endothelial cells and stellate cells in control livers and alcoholic fatty livers.[339] The authors of these studies suggested that alteration of the sinusoidal barrier, which leads to impaired blood-hepatocyte exchange, may be a necessary and early step in the development of hepatic fibrosis. Horn et al.[340] demonstrated a positive correlation between defenestration and the occurrence and localization of subendothelial basal laminas, and between the presence of a basal lamina and the occurrence of collagen in the space of Disse, again suggesting that the phenomenon of defenestration is involved in the pathogenesis of hepatic fibrosis. The process of defenestration has been shown to be associated with increased vascular resistance in the sinusoidal bed, which suggests that alterations in the hepatic sinusoidal lining may be involved in the pathogenesis of portal hypertension.[341]

Clark et al.[342] made the interesting suggestion that defenestration of the hepatic sinusoids could be a cause of hyperlipoproteinaemia in chronic drinkers while Fraser et al.[338,343] suggested that defenestration could also contribute to hepatic steatosis.

Serum markers of hepatic fibrosis

Liver biopsy is still regarded as the 'gold standard' for assessing both the presence and type of necroinflammation, as well as the presence, distribution and severity of hepatic fibrosis. Nevertheless, the use of serial biochemical tests may provide a useful non-invasive method for objective assessment of progression of hepatic fibrosis and for monitoring antifibrotic therapy. Tsutsumi et al.[344] measured procollagen type III peptide, prolyl hydroxylase, the 7S domain (7S-IV) and the triple-helix domain of type IV (TH-IV) collagen, laminin and TIMP in serum and found that all but TIMP were elevated in patients with alcohol-related hepatic fibrosis; serum TH-IV collagen showed a good correlation with hepatic TH-IV collagen. Serum hyaluronate has been reported to correlate with the progression of alcoholic liver disease,[345] but further studies are required for validation. Panels of biochemical tests, for example the FibroTest for fibrosis,[346] and measurements of other serum markers for fibrosis such as aminoterminal peptide of type III, procollagen, laminin and hyaluronate, may ultimately provide a non-invasive ways to monitor therapy, but pretreatment liver biopsies will still be required.

The role of oxidative stress and lipid peroxidation

As discussed earlier in this chapter chronic ethanol ingestion results in induction of CYP2E1, in animal models and humans, which occurs predominantly in the perivenular regions of the liver. This CYP2E1 induction, usually 4–10 fold, results in enhanced lipid peroxidation and increased rates of ROS production.[240,243,244,347] Mitochondria are both the source of, and the target of, ROS.[348] Other sources of ROS include endotoxin-activated Kupffer cells and neutrophil polymorphs. Chronic ethanol ingestion simultaneously results in enhanced acetaldehyde production, due to CYP2E1 induction, and depletion of glutathione which impairs a major defence mechanism against oxidative stress.[240] Lipid peroxidation results in the formation of more free radicals which can further damage cell and organelle membranes causing more liver-cell injury. Depletion of mitochondrial glutathione sensitizes hepatocytes to the pro-oxidant effects of cytokines, in particular TNFα, and to the effects of ROS generated by the oxidative metabolism of alcohol.[347] Although the exact pathogenetic mechanism is unclear, the oxidative stress that develops during chronic ethanol administration by continuous intragastric infusion in rats appears to interfere with protease activities within the hepatocyte, leading to an accumulation of oxidized proteins which may contribute to liver injury in this model.[348,349]

A number of comprehensive review articles published in the last few years give a more detailed discussion of the role of oxidative stress.[350,351] Hoek et al.[352] discussed the effects of increased oxidative stress on mitochondrial structure and function; if damaged mitochondrial DNA is not repaired this can result in further oxidative stress and thus a vicious cycle develops with increasing hepatocyte injury. In addition, recent animal studies have shown that the change in mitochondrial function is, at least in part, dependent on the induction of inducible nitric oxide synthase (iNOS).[353]

Mitochondrial dysfunction can also promote both apoptosis and hepatocyte necrosis.[352] Apoptotic cells can be seen in liver biopsies from patients with alcoholic liver disease[79a] (Fig. 6.25), and DNA end-nick labelling has been used to confirm the presence of apoptotic bodies.[354,355] Apoptosis in

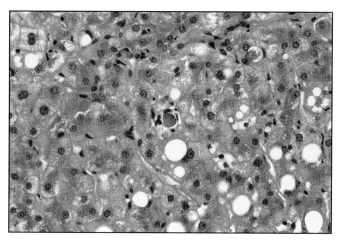

Fig. 6.25 • Alcoholic steatohepatitis. The hepatocytes show fatty change, and focal necrosis accompanied by a mixed inflammatory cell infiltrate. An apoptotic cell (centre) is also seen. H&E.

alcoholic liver disease is probably triggered by oxidative stress as well as by a variety of cytokines.[356] Recent studies suggest that antioxidant free radical scavengers are hepatoprotective; the use of such agents in alcoholic liver disease are under investigation as discussed in the review by Arteel.[350]

Endotoxaemia

Rao et al.[357] have recently reviewed the now considerable evidence supporting the concept that endotoxaemia, which results from alcohol-induced leakiness of the small intestine, plays an important role in the pathogenesis of alcoholic liver disease. Endotoxins, which consist of lipopolysaccharide derived from the walls of gram-negative bacteria, activate Kupffer cells and lead to cytokine production and the generation of ROS; destruction of Kupffer cells by gadolinium chloride prevents alcohol-induced steatohepatitis in the intragastric feeding model despite the 5- to 6-fold increase in CYP2E1.[358] Animal studies by Thurman and colleagues[359,360] have clearly demonstrated the increased susceptibility of female rats to alcohol/endotoxin-induced liver injury as judged by the severity of fatty change and neutrophil infiltrate in the liver, plasma endotoxin levels.

Immune mechanisms

The role of the immune system in the pathogenesis of alcoholic liver disease has been comprehensively reviewed by Leevy and Elbeshbeshly,[361] McFarlane[362] and Thiele et al.[363] Many immunological disturbances occur as a consequence of alcoholic liver injury and may be considered secondary events. Nevertheless, some of the morphological features raise the possibility that immunological mechanisms sometimes play a primary role in alcohol-related liver injury. These include the progression of liver disease that sometimes occurs despite abstinence from alcohol, and the recurrence of alcoholic liver disease following liver transplantation, which on rare occasions can have an accelerated progression to cirrhosis.[364]

Morphological pointers

The neutrophil polymorph infiltrate seen in and around hepatocytes, which contain Mallory bodies, could indicate a local Arthus reaction with humoral sensitization to Mallory bodies. An antibody to Mallory body antigen has been reported in alcoholic hepatitis, but was not demonstrated in patients with fatty liver or inactive cirrhosis.[365] However, subsequent studies by Kehl et al.[366] failed to detect either Mallory body antigen or antibody in the sera of patients with alcoholic hepatitis.

Several in vitro studies provided evidence of sensitization to Mallory body antigens and described the production of migration inhibition factor,[367] and a blastogenic factor.[368] Neutrophil polymorphs frequently surround hepatocytes which contain Mallory bodies (Fig. 6.7(b)); Mallory bodies per se do not appear to be chemotactic but peripheral mononuclear cells incubated with Mallory bodies secrete a chemotactic factor which may explain the accumulation of neutrophils seen around Mallory bodies in alcoholic hepatitis.[369]

As noted earlier a chronic hepatitis-like injury, with interface hepatitis, lobular hepatitis and a mononuclear cell infiltrate, is sometimes seen in association with chronic alcohol consumption and negative hepatitis B serology;[100,101,104] in some cases this pattern of injury has been shown to be associated with co-existent chronic hepatitis C virus infection (Fig. 6.12).[105,106] The suggestion that alcohol per se can cause chronic hepatitis remains controversial.[107] The presence of serum antibodies to liver-specific protein (LSP) in patients with active alcoholic cirrhosis correlates with the presence of a lymphocytic infiltrate in the portal tracts and interface hepatitis.[370,371] Antibody to LSP was not found in 'uncomplicated' alcoholic hepatitis, i.e. hepatitis without chronic hepatitis-like features, suggesting that sensitization to LSP may be causal in interface hepatitis.[372]

Other immunological features

Humoral immunity

Hypergammaglobulinaemia in alcoholic liver disease is characterized by a polyclonal increase in all classes of immunoglobulins, but with serum IgA levels being particularly increased and correlating closely with the severity of liver damage.[373–375] Perisinusoidal deposition of IgA has been reported in all forms of alcoholic liver disease, but it is not clear whether the antibody is present in immune complexes.[376] Van de Wiel et al.[377] suggest that the linear deposition of IgA along the sinusoids in alcoholic liver disease has such a high prevalence and specificity that this feature can be used as a reliable marker for the alcoholic aetiology of the liver disease.

Low titres of autoantibodies have been reported in alcoholic liver disease,[373,375] with anti-nuclear factor in 12–17% and anti-smooth muscle autoantibodies in 12–27% of patients with a slightly higher prevalence in women than men. A circulating IgA antibody against a 65 kD heat shock protein has been demonstrated in alcoholic hepatitis; the authors suggest this antibody may play a role in liver injury which continues after the cessation of alcohol.[378]

IgG and IgA antibodies to liver-cell membrane antigens (LMA) have been demonstrated in all stages of alcoholic liver injury.[379] The same group reported that IgG class antibodies reacting with ethanol-altered rabbit hepatocytes were detected in 74% of patients with fatty liver, 80% with alcoholic hepatitis and 70% with alcoholic cirrhosis but in only 25% with non-alcoholic liver disease.[380] A follow-up study of 39 patients with alcoholic liver disease, in whom LMA directed against alcohol-altered hepatocytes was detected, suggests that the presence of LMA is associated with a greater risk of progression to cirrhosis.[381]

Aldehyde-protein adducts

A number of studies have suggested that LMA is directed against acetaldehyde-protein adducts that are formed during the metabolism of alcohol.[382] Several different proteins have been detected in these adducts in hepatocytes. They include a 37 kD protein in the cytosol,[383] and CYP2E1 in microsomes.[384–386] Immunohistochemical studies have demonstrated the presence of protein-acetaldehyde adducts in perivenular hepatocytes at an early stage of alcoholic injury.[382,383] In addition, malondialdehyde and acetaldehyde can react together with proteins to form hybrid adducts termed malondialdehyde-acetaldehyde adducts (MAA).[387] A study in patients with alcoholic liver disease report that there is a T-cell response to these adducts and suggests that oxidative stress may play a role in the development of this cellular immune respone.[388] Similarly, products of lipid peroxidation 4-hydroxy-2'-nonenal (4-HNE) and 8-hydroxydeoxyguanosine (8-OHdG) can form adducts with proteins,[389] as can the free hydroxyethyl radicals that bind to hepatic proteins such as cytochrome P4502E1.[385,390]

In summary, there is growing evidence that a wide range of alcohol-induced neoantigens can be formed, in both human and animal livers, and that a T-cell mediated response can contribute to ongoing liver injury.

Cell-mediated immunity

Impaired delayed hypersensitivity is described in patients with alcoholic liver disease; this appears to be due to both nutritional deficiencies and a reduction in the number of circulating T-cells.[391] Circulating lymphocytes cytotoxic for autologous liver cells have been described in alcoholic hepatitis and active cirrhosis.[392,393] It is also of interest to note that natural killer cytotoxic activity is constantly depressed in patients with alcoholic cirrhosis,[394] explaining, at least in part, the impaired immunosurveillance in patients with alcoholic liver disease which results in increased susceptibility to various infections, including hepatitis B and C, and possibly also contributing to the increased incidence of some neoplasms. The lymphocytes that are recruited into the liver in alcoholic liver disease may have a regulatory role in the inflammatory process while others are cytotoxic.[388,395,396]

Cytokines and chemokines

Numerous human and animal studies of alcoholic liver disease have demonstrated an increased production of proinflammatory cytokines such as TNFα, which is produced primarily by Kupffer cells,[397-399] IL-1,[400] and IL-6.[400-402] The effects of TNFα, a mediator of many biological actions including the necroinflammatory response, is responsible for many of the clinical features seen in alcoholic hepatitis, for example fever, neutrophilia, and even hypotension that occurs in severe cases.[403] These effects are similar to those mediated by endotoxins.

Kupffer cells, which have been activated by endotoxin, also show enhanced production of macrophage inflammatory protein-2 (MIP-2), which is a potent chemotactic agent for polymorphs. Endotoxin also upregulates the expression of ICAM-1 on hepatocytes. The alcohol-related influx of endotoxin into the circulation is thought to lead to an enhanced interaction between adhesion molecules on neutrophils and intercellular adhesion molecule-1 (ICAM-1) on hepatocytes, thus contributing to liver injury and to the migration of polymorphs into the liver.[404] Furthermore, monocyte secretion of MIP-1 and MIP-1αI is increased in alcoholic hepatitis.[405]

Disturbances of IgA metabolism, with elevated total serum IgA and a characteristic linear deposition of IgA in the hepatic sinusoids, are well described in alcoholic liver disease;[376,377] IgA has also been shown to trigger the secretion of TNFα by monocytes and to synergistically enhance the endotoxin-induced secretion of this cytokine.[406]

There is now a growing interest in the part played by neutrophil polymorphs in generating the various cytokines that contribute to tissue injury.[407,408] The neutrophils are also a source hepatocyte growth factor (HGF), suggesting a role for these cell in liver regeneration.[409]

The compexities of the interactive role of cytokines and inflammatory mediators is discussed in the recent comprehensive review by Arteel et al.[410]

Nutritional factors

A number of reviews have addressed the interaction between nutritional factors, alcohol and liver disease in humans.[411-413] Primary malnutrition, due to poor diet, is well-recognized in the chronic drinker;[414] moreover, secondary malnutrition is now well-recognized in drinkers in whom the diet is adequate.[415]

A complete nutritional assessment of 666 patients showed evidence of protein calorie malnutrition in 62% of chronic drinkers who had clinical or laboratory evidence of early liver injury, while 100% of patients in whom liver injury was associated with jaundice had evidence of malnutrition.[415] Secondary malnutrition may be due to: (i) malabsorption with alcohol-related impairment of enterocyte function;[416] (ii) disturbed carbohydrate metabolism; (iii) impaired protein secretion by hepatocytes; (iv) impaired hepatic metabolism of vitamins; and (v) increased catabolic loss of zinc, magnesium and calcium.[417]

Vitamin A supplementation together with chronic alcohol administration has been shown to cause hepatic fibrosis in the rat;[418] it is consequently difficult to determine a safe dose of vitamin A supplementation for chronic alcoholics who are often deficient in vitamin A.

Mezey examined the role of dietary fat in alcoholic liver disease; the severity of alcoholic steatosis is clearly related to the amount of fat in the diet.[412] It is of note that patients with biopsy evidence of alcoholic liver disease have lower levels of polyunsaturated fatty acids in their livers than chronic drinkers who have morphologically normal livers.[419]

The recognition that metabolic/nutritional factors contribute to the pathogenesis of NASH[26,420] has stimulated a renewal of interest in the role of nutritional factors in the pathogenesis of alcoholic liver disease. There is now clear evidence that obesity potentiates the severity of alcohol-related hepatic injury although it is not yet clear whether the effect is additive or synergistic.[421] The liver injury of alcoholic hepatitis may well have the same, or at least a similar, pathogenesis as NASH. Factors involved in both alcoholic and non-alcoholic liver disease include nutritional deficiencies, metabolic disturbances, CYP2E1 induction and gut-derived endotoxins, and cytokine production.

In animal models, a high intake of polyunsaturated fat, particularly fish oil, is important for the development of necro-inflammation and fibrosis,[422] in contrast a diet containing beef fat appears to protect the liver from injury.[423] In various animal models manipulation of the type and amount of fat[424-426] and carbohydrate[37] in the diet can influence the development and severity of liver injury. Of considerable interest, and possibly with therapeutic implications, is the finding in the intra-gastric rat model for alcohol administration, that as the dietary unsaturated fat content increased oxidative stress and liver injury progressively decreased in a 'dose-response' fashion.[426] This effect appeared to be due to an increase in CYP4A-catalysed fatty acid oxidation and effects on lipid export.

Liver regeneration

The effect of alcohol on the liver includes not only direct and indirect injury to parenchymal and non-parenchymal cells but also impairment of hepatic regeneration.[427] Hepatic regeneration is controlled by a complex cell-to-cell interaction involving a wide variety of hormones and growth factors including HGF and epidermal growth factor (EGF); the responsiveness of hepatocytes is strongly influenced by their prior metabolic state[428] Chronic alcohol consumption impairs rat liver regeneration after partial hepatectomy; however, regenerative activity returns to normal after abstinence for one week.[429] Impaired liver regeneration associated with chronic alcohol ingestion could be an additional factor contributing to the severity and outcome of liver injury in humans.

Traditionally, liver regeneration has been attributed to division of mature hepatocytes but more recently hepatic stem (progenitor) cells have been recognized.[108,109] Hepatic stem cells, which are located in the region of the canals of Hering, were initially thought to proliferate only under extreme conditions such as fulminant hepatic failure and end-stage cirrhosis but as discussed earlier they are now recognized in many types of chronic liver disease, including alcoholic liver disease, in both humans (Fig. 6.13(A)) and animal models; they are seen first as small epithelial cells in the portal regions and have the capacity to differentiate into small bile ductules and hepatocytes. The microregenerative acini that are frequently seen in regenerating livers may have originated from stem cells which ultimately differented into hepatocytes. It is not uncommon to see ductular structures, a process that is now termed 'bile ductular reaction', which are lined by a mixture of cells some with a biliary phenotype and others showing hepatocellular features (see Fig. 3.30 in a chapter on alcoholic liver disease by Hall).[19] The small epithelial cells and bile ductules that are seen in alcoholic cirrhosis closely resemble the oval cells that are well described in many different experimental models of hepatocarcinogenesis.[430] More recently oval cells have been described in ethanol-fed mice.[431] The authors suggest 'that oval cell expansion is a component of the liver's adaptive response to oxidative stress'. Small epithelial cells are frequently seen in large numbers in alcoholic cirrhosis once the patient becomes abstinent (Fig. 6.13(B)). It now transpires that the requirement of the period of abstinence from alcohol, for 6 months or longer, in patients with alcoholic cirrhosis who are being considered for liver transplantation, is of great value in determining whether the liver can recover or not;[432] in many instances there will be sufficient regeneration, due to both improvement in hepatocyte regeneration and to hepatic stem cell proliferation and differentiation, to obviate the requirement for transplantation—at least in the short term.

Factors affecting individual susceptibility to alcoholic liver disease

Numerous studies since the 1960s[200,212–217] have established alcohol as a direct hepatotoxin and, until recently, alcoholic liver injury was thought to be purely dose-related.[25] The concept of genetic and acquired factors playing a role in the susceptibility of the individual to alcohol-associated liver disease is now widely accepted.[20–23]

Dose, duration and patterns of alcohol consumption

There are many ways of expressing the dose of alcohol but the simplest approach is to regard each standard drink, irrespective of whether it is beer, wine, spirit etc., as being equivalent to 10 g of alcohol. Lelbach[25] has clearly demonstrated a relationship between the risk of developing cirrhosis and the dose and duration of alcohol consumption; nevertheless, even with an intake as high as 226 g per day for a mean duration of 11.4 years, only 25% of drinkers develop cirrhosis. On the other hand, an intake as low as 20 g for women and 40 g for men per day has been claimed to be associated with the development of cirrhosis.[433,434] Indeed, an Australian case-control study has shown that the risk of cirrhosis development in both women and men increases significantly above the baseline when alcohol intake is greater than 40 g per day.[435] Sorensen et al.[92] performed serial liver biopsies over a 10–13-year period in 258 males, none of whom were cirrhotic at the beginning of the study; the average daily consumption of alcohol was over 50 g per day. Cirrhosis developed in 38, an overall risk of about 15%.

A study of the total lifetime alcohol intake (TLAL) in patients with biopsy-proven 'NAFLD' showed that 13% had a significantly higher alcohol intake than obtained in the original history suggesting that the alcohol intake may have been sufficient to have at least been contributing to the pathogenesis of the liver injury.[177] This type of study confirms the need for a reliable alcohol history to enable both the clinician and the pathologist to differentiate between alcohol and 'non-alcoholic' liver disease.

The pattern of drinking may also be important: an open population study in Italy of 6534 subjects, who did not have evidence of chronic viral hepatitis, suggested that drinking alcohol outside mealtimes and drinking multiple different types of alcoholic drinks each increased the risk of alcoholic liver disease.[436]

Analysis of the quantitative relationship between alcohol consumption and the occurrence of cirrhosis led Sorensen to consider whether alcohol abuse has a permissive rather than a dose-related effect.[22] Sorensen suggested that the risk of cirrhosis at a given level of alcohol consumption is higher or lower, depending on the action of other factors. Such cofactors could change the threshold for alcohol-associated liver injury as well as changing the level of risk with higher alcohol consumption. The group studied by Sorensen et al.[92] developed cirrhosis at a constant rate of 2% per year. This observation led the authors to suggest that other contributing factors affect approximately one in every 50 drinkers every year.

Genetic and ethnic factors

Female gender

The greater susceptibility of women to alcohol-associated liver injury is now widely accepted. A meta-analysis of 23 published liver biopsy studies of 5448 drinkers from many countries including Australia, England, France and the USA confirmed the greater susceptibility of women to the hepatotoxic effects of alcohol.[437] The increased susceptibility of women to alcoholic liver disease has a number of manifestations:

(i)   Women tend to present with more severe disease, often associated with a lower daily intake of alcohol for a shorter duration;[435,438]
(ii) Women, particularly those under 45 years, have a higher incidence of alcoholic hepatitis, and a worse long-term prognosis even if they abstain;[66,93]
(iii) American Negro women appear to be even more susceptible than Caucasian women to alcoholic hepatitis, and have a poor prognosis;[4]
(iv) Women with alcoholic cirrhosis have a higher mortality.[439]

It is not unusual to see liver biopsies from women in their 20s and 30s which show severe alcohol-related liver injury; progression to cirrhosis, liver failure and death can occur in 1 to 2 years if drinking continues (Fig. 6.26(A),(B)).

Gavaler & Arria suggest that the increased sensitivity of women to a given level of alcohol may be, at least in part, related to a gender-related differential in the mechanism(s) of the progression of initiated damage to the liver; they also speculate that the factors which are involved in susceptibility to alcoholic liver disease may be more prevalent in women than men.[437] In view of these suggestions it is of interest to note that obesity is a risk factor for alcoholic liver disease.[440,441] Similarly, the increased prevalence of NASH in women, which in turn is related to the increased prevalence of obesity and diabetes mellitus type 2 in women, may have some bearing on the increased susceptibility of women to alcoholic liver disease. Excess weight (BMI = or >23 in women and BMI = or >27 in men) has been reported as a risk factor for alcoholic liver disease.[441] Since similar pathogenic mechanisms are involved in alcohol-related liver injury and NASH and it seems likely that the 'insignificant'

amounts of alcohol that some patients with NASH consume may be contributing to liver injury which is currently being designated as NASH.[250,442]

The observations by Thurman's group that: (i) alcoholic liver injury involves the activation of Kupffer cells by endotoxin;[360] (ii) female rats are more sensitive than male rats to alcohol-induced injury, possibly due to increased levels of endotoxin in the serum and ICAM-1 expression in hepatic sinusoidal-lining cells;[443] and (iii) oestrogen increases the sensitivity of Kupffer cells to endotoxin,[359] provide further insights into factors that may contribute to the greater susceptibility of women to alcohol-induced liver injury.

Frezza et al.[24] suggested that the increased susceptibility of women could be linked to gender-related differences in first-pass metabolism. In non-alcoholic women first-pass metabolism of alcohol (i.e. oxidation in the stomach) and gastric alcohol dehydrogenase were considerably less, 23% and 59% respectively, than those in non-alcoholic men. These differences were even more pronounced in drinkers, where first-pass metabolism was virtually absent in women. The authors concluded that increased bioavailability of ethanol resulting from decreased gastric oxidation of ethanol may contribute to the enhanced vulnerability of women to acute and chronic complications of alcohol although this suggestion remains unproven.

Genetic polymorphisms of alcohol-metabolizing enzymes

Numerous studies have demonstrated racial differences in alcohol-metabolizing enzymes, raising the possibility that polymorphisms at the alcohol and aldehyde dehydrogenase loci play a role not only in genetic predisposition to alcoholism and alcoholic liver injury but could also act as protective factors against alcohol abuse[27,444-446] (also see reviews by Day & Bassendine,[447,448] Arnon et al.,[449] Agarwal[450] and Crabb et al.[451]). An atypical ALDH₂ isoenzyme (*ALDH2*1/*2*) is widely prevalent among Japanese,[445] Chinese[446] and other Orientals of Mongoloid origin; the 'deficiency' of ALDH2 results in a lower rate of elimination of alcohol and this is mainly responsible for their alcohol 'sensitivity' which manifests as facial flushing, sweating, headache and increased pulse rate. This sensitivity to alcohol generally acts as a deterrent against drinking, which no doubt accounts for the lower incidence of alcoholism and alcohol-related diseases in Oriental races. Enomoto et al.[452] investigated the relationship between the heterozygote ALDH2-deficient phenotype and the homozygous wild type and the severity of liver injury and found that patients who were homozygous for the normal gene had a lower incidence of alcoholic hepatitis/cirrhosis than those who were heterozygous for this gene. In contrast, Caucasians only show polymorphisms of ADH3 but in addition may show polymorphisms of CYP2E1; for example Grove et al.[453] in a study of Caucasians, which included 264 patients with alcoholic liver disease and 121 controls, examined the frequency of *RsaI* polymorphism of CYP2E1 and ADH3 genotype and found that male patients had a higher frequency of *ADH3*2/*2* genotype than controls (odds ratio 2.04). The rare *RsaI* polymorphism of

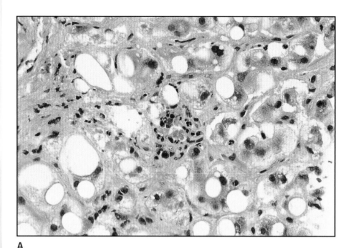

A

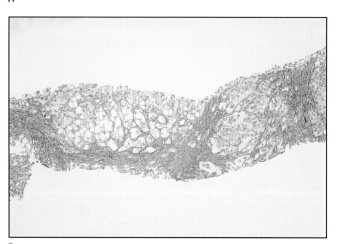

B

Fig. 6.26 • Alcoholic hepatitis and cirrhosis in a 32-year-old woman who continued to drink and died several months later from bleeding varices. **(A)** The liver shows steatosis and alcoholic hepatitis. H&E. **(B)** Established micronodular cirrhosis is apparent. Sirius red. A liver biopsy 2 years earlier showed only fatty change and mild pericellular fibrosis.

CYP2E1 (c2 CYP2E1) was not significantly increased in patients with advanced liver disease although those with the c2 allele presented at a younger age than those with the wild-type allele. It is of note that those patients with advanced liver disease who had the c2 allele had a significantly higher frequency of the ADH3*2/*2 genotype than those who were homozygous for the cl allele (odds ratio 3.71). The authors suggest that the mutant c2 allele of CYP2E1 is a risk factor for alcoholic liver disease particularly in the presence of the ADH3*2 allele; they also suggest that the ADH3 genotype, although not apparently a risk factor for advanced liver disease, may influence the risk of alcoholism, particularly in males.

Alcohol addiction is not necessarily associated with organ damage; for example, Wodak et al.[454] found alcoholic liver disease in only 18% of patients with severe alcohol dependence—an observation which is in keeping with Sorensen's hypothesis of the 'permissive' rather than dose-related role of alcohol in the pathogenesis of liver injury.[22] For a more detailed discussion about the correlation between genetic variants in alcohol metabolizing enzymes see recent reviews by Crabb et al.[451] and Lieber.[455]

Genetic polymorphisms of cytokines

Polymorphisms of genes ecoding for ADH, ALDH and CYP2E1 thus appear to play only a minor role in the susceptibility of Caucasians to alcoholic liver disease. Polymorphisms in cytokine genes may be more important. For example, polymorphisms in the promoter region of interleukin 10 (IL-10) have been described.[456] A clinical study of 287 heavy drinkers (>80 g alcohol per day for at least 10 years), compared to 212 controls, showed that the presence of the A allele at position −627 in the IL-10 promoter was associated with an increased risk of advanced alcoholic liver disease. The authors suggested that low expression of IL-10 inflammation and fibrogenesis. A Japanese study found that genetic polymorphisms of IL-1β was associated with the development of alcoholic liver disease.[457]

Histocompatibility antigens

A meta-analysis by List and Gluud[458] of 28 published studies, in which the distribution of HLA-antigens were reviewed, failed to show that any of the HLA-phenotypes that had been investigated in Caucasian patients with alcoholic disease were significantly more common than in controls, but the results of Japanese studies were less clear. McFarlane in a review of autoantibodies in alcoholic liver disease concluded that 'an association with various HLA phenotypes has not been confirmed by meta-analysis'.[362]

Chronic viral infections

Hepatitis B virus infection

Although in the past, studies of the association between chronic HBV infection and alcohol-induced liver injury have given conflicting results, a number of studies have shown an increased incidence of serological markers for hepatitis B in patients with alcoholic liver disease, suggesting increased susceptibility to infection. In addition, in some patients there appears to be an acceleration of the rate of progression to cirrhosis (Fig. 6.27(A)–(D)) due to the combined effects of chronic viral infection and alcohol, although this association is much less pronounced than with chronic HCV infection.[102,154,159,459–462] For example, Villa et al.[462] studied 296 HBsAg carriers prospectively for 3.5 years; one-third of the carriers developed raised liver enzymes while drinking less than 60 g alcohol per day. These researchers found that, for a given dose of alcohol, the risk of hepatic injury was much higher in the HBsAg carriers than in the age- and sex-matched HBsAg-negative controls. A study by Novick et al.[463] of alcoholic cirrhotics under 35 years of age also incriminated HBV in the development of cirrhosis at a relatively young age—98% had a history of heroin abuse, serological markers were detected in almost 94%, and 9.4% were carriers; while a study by Pereira et al.,[464] which examined the effect of ethanol intake on the development of HCCs, showed that the average age of tumour development in habitual drinkers who were HBsAg positive was significantly lower than in non-drinkers—44.3 ± 9.7 and 52.3 ± 15.7 years, respectively.

Hepatitis C virus infection

There is an increased prevalence of HCV infection in heavy drinkers.[101,102,157,465–467] In many, but not all, of the clinical studies, the liver injury was more severe in drinkers who were HCV positive;[102,465–467] in addition, chronic HCV infection accelerates the rate of progression to cirrhosis[467] and increases the risk of hepatocellular carcinoma developing in patients with alcohol-related liver disease.[157,158,468]

A variety of mechanisms are implicated for the potentiating effect of chronic alcohol consumption on chronic hepatitis C; these include immune dysfunction leading to persistence of the viral infection,[469] increased viral replication,[200,470,471] emergence of HCV quasi-species, apoptosis, and increased oxidative stress,[472] steatosis,[473] and hepatic iron overload. Interactions between alcohol and hepatitis C, including the increased risk of hepatocellular carcinoma, have recently been reviewed.[9,474]

HIV/AIDS

Alcohol consumption is a cofactor in the progression of HIV/AIDS;[475,476] in addition, patients who are coinfected with HIV and HCV, and who drink alcohol, are more likely to die of end-stage liver disease than those who do not drink.[477] Contributing factors include endotoxaemia and chemokine production by Kupffer cells,[478,479] impaired immune function—especially a decrease in proteosome—and immunoproteasome function in Kupffer cells.[480]

Drugs and toxins

The potentiation of acute drug-associated liver injury is well recognized,[41–43,226,227,229,230,481,482] e.g. the potential dangers

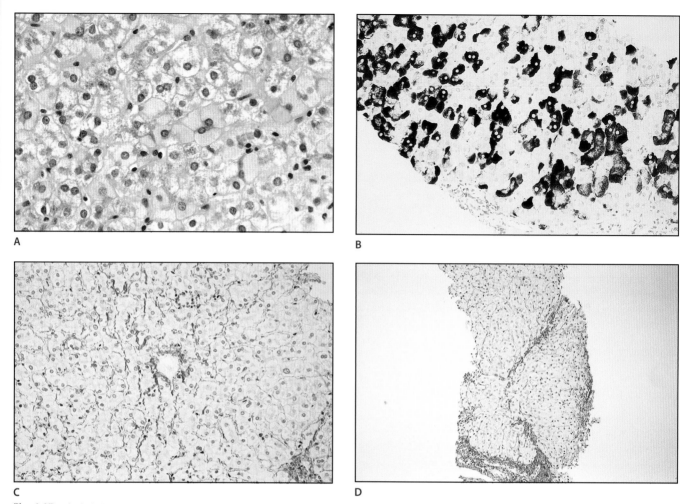

A

B

C

D

Fig. 6.27 • Alcoholic liver disease and chronic hepatitis B in a 19-year-old man who had been a heavy drinker since age 12. **(A)** Numerous 'ground-glass' hepatocytes are seen. Mild hepatitis (not shown) was also present. H&E. **(B)** The presence of HBsAg is confirmed immunohistochemically. PAP. **(C)** Perivenular and pericellular fibrosis is apparent. Sirius red. **(D)** The architecture is disturbed and the features are in keeping with developing cirrhosis. Sirius red.

of paracetamol (acetaminophen) ingestion, even in therapeutic doses, is now a well-recognized problem in chronic drinkers[227] but the idea of an alcohol–drug interaction causing chronic liver disease is a more recent concept.[230,483] Leo & Lieber[418] observed hepatic fibrosis in the rat following long-term administration of ethanol and a moderate dose of vitamin A, while Hall et al.[230] produced hepatic fibrosis and cirrhosis in rats by feeding ethanol in the Lieber–DeCarli diet together with exposure to low-dose CCl_4 vapour for 10 weeks. As discussed earlier, chronic alcohol ingestion induces the isoenzyme CYP2E1; this effect is seen maximally in perivenular hepatocytes[484] (Fig. 6.28). This enzyme induction, in turn, enhances the metabolism of a wide variety of drugs and toxins.[31,41–43] Relatively low doses of alcohol may well potentiate insidious liver injury by therapeutic doses of prescription drugs, non-prescription agents such as vitamin A, and environmental toxins.[230] This type of interaction may explain some cases of chronic liver injury seen in association with relatively low doses of alcohol and account for some cases of cryptogenic cirrhosis.

Chronic alcohol consumption is a risk factor in methotrexate-associated fibrosis and cirrhosis in patients

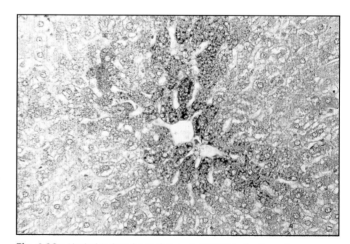

Fig. 6.28 • Alcohol-induced cytochrome P-450 2E1 in the liver of a young man. Increased amounts of the cytochrome P-450 2E1 (demonstrated immunohistochemically) are seen in perivenular hepatocytes that surround a terminal hepatic venule.

with psoriatic arthropathy[485-487] and is also thought to increase the risk of liver injury in rheumatoid patients receiving low doses of oral methotrexate.[488] The mechanism for this interaction has yet to be elucidated; however, one study reports increased risk factors for NAFLD/NASH in some psoriatic patients with progressive liver disease.[489]

Hepatic iron overload

As discussed earlier both primary (heriditary) and secondary iron overload can potentiate alcohol-related liver injury.[206-208,210,490] Activation of hepatic stellate cells by iron, and increased oxidative stress, are factors involved in the accelerated progression to cirrhosis in patients with homozygous haemochromatosis who are chronic drinkers.[491] It has been speculated that the death of Ludwig van Beethoven from end-stage liver disease was due to the combined effects of alcohol and iron overload.[492]

Treatment

Ideally, the goal should be prevention, rather than finding better ways to treat alcoholic liver disease. The recognition of inherited and acquired factors that increase the risk of development of alcohol-related liver injury has the potential to considerably reduce the prevalence of alcohol-related liver disease provided that the patients with risk factors e.g. medication such as methotrexate, chronic hepatitis C virus infection, can be persuaded to abstain from alcohol.[23]

Abstinence

Abstinence from alcohol remains the best way of preventing progression of liver injury, as well as prolonging survival of patients with established cirrhosis.[6] A more aggressive approach to liver biopsy in patients with suspected alcoholic liver disease, if accompanied by vigorous counselling about the need for abstinence, and explanation of the risk of progressive liver disease should drinking continue, could also significantly reduce the prevalence of alcoholic liver disease.

In addition, patients who as part of the work-up for liver transplantation are required to abstain from alcohol—usually for a minimum period of 6 months as a condition of eligibility for transplantation—may have sufficient return of function, due to cessation of alcohol-induced liver injury and liver regeneration, that transplantation can be delayed and/or avoided altogether.[432]

Medical management

The main purpose in mentioning drug therapy for alcohol-related liver disease in a chapter on liver pathology is for the insights into pathogenic mechanisms that the use of the various agents provide.[74,493,494] For example: *Prednisolone* which is used for severe alcoholic hepatitis,[166] modulates the immunological disturbances and downregulates cytokines such as TNFα and interleukin-8 production.

Pentoxifylline one of the newer agents that inhibit the synthesis and activity of TNF-α shows some promise in the treatment of alcoholic hepatitis.[167] *S-adenosyl-L-methionine*, glutathione precursor, can restore mitochondrial glutathione and significantly lessen hepatocyte injury.[168,169,244,347,495] *Propylthiouracil* can suppress the so-called hypermetabolic state as measured by increased liver oxygen consumption.[496] *Polyenylphosphatidylcholine*, which is a mixture of polyunsaturated fatty acids, is another agent that decreases alcohol-induced oxidative stress; its use, at least in baboons, has been shown to lessen hepatic fibrosis presumably by decreasing the amount of breakdown products of lipid peroxidation.[244,493,497]

The contribution of dietary deficiencies to the pathogenesis of alcoholic liver disease, and the effects of dietary modification in animal models, is well recognized.[414,415,417-419,423,426,498] Most of the studies involving dietary modification to enhance or lessen alcohol-induced liver injury have been in animal models; it is interesting to speculate about the possibility of dietary modification as a means of lessening the risk of alcoholic liver disease in humans. A diet of 'beefsteak and burgundy' has some appeal since it is known, at least in rats, that a diet high in beef fat lessens alcohol-related liver injury.[423] However, diets rich in saturated fatty acids,[423,424] fish oils[422] or cholesterol,[499] or a high carbohydrate diet are less acceptable.[37] Nevertheless, the dietary extremes used in models are unlikely to be palatable to humans and are therefore unlikely to provide protection from alcohol-related liver injury. For a detailed discussion of nutrition and alcoholic liver disease see a recent review by Halsted[413] and for a general review of on diagnosis and therapy see Levitsky & Mailliard.[494]

Liver transplantation

Although in the past the place of liver transplantation of alcoholic liver disease has been a controversial issue, today most transplant units, at least in developed countries, perform transplants on carefully selected patients.[500] A report on a workshop held jointly by the European Association for the Study of Liver (EASL) and the European Liver Transplant Registry (ELTR)[96] indicated that in Europe 5716 liver transplants were performed between January 1998 and June 2000 for alcoholic liver disease, making this condition the most common indication for liver transplantation in Europe.

The controversy related to liver transplantation for alcoholic liver disease has abated largely because of the growing acceptance of alcohol as a cofactor or 'permissive agent'[22] in a wide variety of inherited and acquired forms of liver disease.[23] As discussed earlier, excess alcohol consumption can hasten the progression of other liver diseases such as chronic hepatitis B or C virus infections, hereditary haemochromatosis with, or without, overt features of alcoholic liver disease in the liver. Thus, the belief that alcoholic liver disease is entirely self-inflicted and that transplantation cannot be justified has been modified in recent years.

The outcome of liver transplantation is similar to that in other forms of end-stage liver disease;[501,502] however, in one series the incidence of acute cellular rejection at 1 year was 29% compared to 48 ± 3% for other diseases such as primary biliary cirrhosis, autoimmune hepatitis and hepatitis C.[503] Much emphasis has been placed on the selection of patients for transplantation on the basis of likelihood of sobriety following transplantation, and a variety of prognostic models have been developed.[432,504] However, in 78 critically ill patients who had orthotopic liver transplants for alcoholic liver disease, at the Pittsburgh Medical Center, neither the preoperative length of sobriety nor alcohol rehabilitation predicted survival.[505] The study by Foster et al.[504] reached a similar conclusion about the period of pretransplant abstinence having little value as a predictor for post-transplant abstinence and suggests that other variables such as comorbid substance use and family history may have more predictive value.

Although some liver transplant units regard the consumption of any alcohol as a relapse,[506] others differentiate harmful drinking from other forms of drinking.[507] Some units now term the ingestion of low amounts of alcohol a 'slip', while a 'relapse' is more precisely defined in terms of consumption above a set amount e.g. 21 units/week for men and 14 units/week for women.[96]

Anecdotal reports of recurrent alcoholic liver disease abound but there are few published reports, some as letters[364] or abstracts.[508,509] Hepatic steatosis (Fig. 6.29) is the feature seen most frequently in the transplanted liver following resumption of drinking.[510] Two of the follow-up studies describe steatosis, without evidence of alcoholic hepatitis or cirrhosis, in post-transplant liver biopsies from patients who were consuming alcohol.[509,511] Burra et al. also describe fatty change, but with pericellular fibrosis, and suggest that these two features are 'the most relevant histological signs of heavy alcohol intake' post- transplant.[510] In contrast, Conjeevaram et al. reported severe alcoholic hepatitis in 50% of recidivists;[512] while Baddour et al.[508] reported steatosis in 20/23 patients and Mallory bodies in 23/23 patients, with four developing cirrhosis from day 177 to 711 post-transplant. An even more remarkable report is of a 45-year-old woman, who developed cirrhosis within 21 months of transplantation and was subsequently retransplanted.[364]

Animal models of alcohol-related liver disease

Animal models, initially rabbits in 1905, then dogs, rats, guinea-pigs, baboons, micropigs and mice, have been used to study the effects of alcohol on the liver (see the comprehensive review by French[513]). The use of animal models has yielded a wealth of information about pathogenetic mechanisms and factors that potentiate or protect against alcohol-related liver injury. Despite the variety of animal species, the innumerable dietary manipulations, and even the development of the intragastric tube feeding model in which a continuous high dose of alcohol is administered,[349,514,515] none of the animals have ever developed an alcoholic hepatitis-like pattern of injury.[64] It is therefore difficult to maintain the belief that alcohol per se causes alcoholic hepatitis.

Liver injury due to endotoxin, usually given as an injection of lipopolysaccharide, results in liver injury that shows a superficial resemblance to alcoholic hepatitis in as much as there is focal hepatocyte necrosis and a neutrophil polymorph infiltrate, but the hepatocyte necrosis is coagulative in type suggesting an ischaemic/hypoxic process, and hepatocyte enlargement and Mallory bodies are not seen (Fig. 6.30). As discussed earlier, endotoxin certainly contributes to alcohol-related liver injury but would not appear to be the factor that triggers alcoholic hepatitis.

Studies in ethanol-fed micropigs, with or without folate deficiency, have reported accelerated liver injury occurring in association with abnormal methionine metabolism that results in hyperhomocysteinaemia.[516,517] Ethanol-induced hyperhomocysteinaemia was also seen in the intragastric alcohol mouse model.[518] Ji and Kaplowitz have recently reviewed the possible clinical implications of hyperhomocysteinaemia.[519]

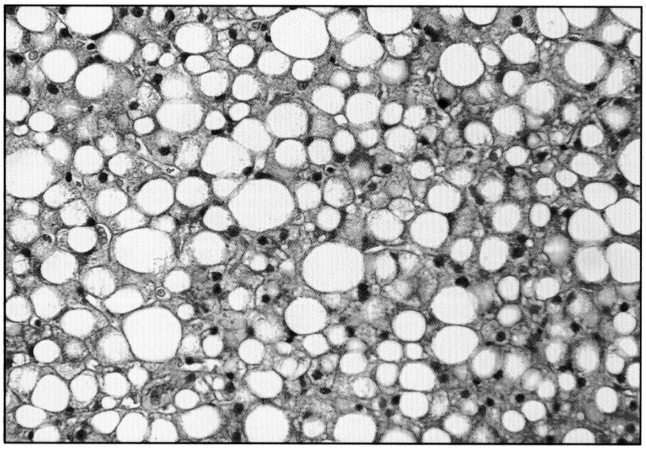

Fig 6.29 • Post-transplant liver biopsy from a 45-year-old man with presumed 'cryptogenic' cirrhosis who recommenced drinking following the transplant. The liver shows moderate macrovesicular fatty change without evidence of hepatitis or fibrosis. H&E.

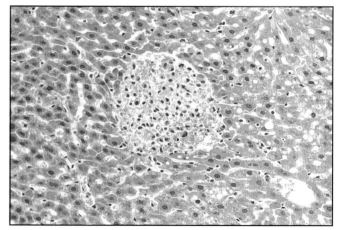

Fig. 6.30 • Alcohol/endotoxin-induced liver injury in a rat. The liver shows a large area of confluent hepatocyte necrosis and an associated heavy infiltrate of neutrophil polymorphs. H&E.

Currently one of the main values of animal models is in the evaluation of therapeutic agents, such as S-adenosyl-L-methionine and polyenylphosphatidylcholine,[126,244] S-adenosylmethionine (Ado-Met),[520] adiponectin,[521] pioglitazone,[522] and PPAR-α[523] prior to the commencement of clinical trials.

Conclusion

There is a paradoxical relationship between alcohol and an enjoyable lifestyle/culture and health on the one hand and disease/psychosocial problems on the other hand. This remains an unresolved issue for the medical profession, social workers and religious leaders. The media, with the assistance of breweries, wine makers, and distilleries, continue publicizing the beneficial effects of regular alcohol consumption on health. On the one hand 'moderate' alcohol consumption, up to 50 g per day, is associated with changes in the lipoprotein profile and a lower incidence of coronary artery disease,[524,525] but on the other hand relatively small doses of alcohol may be associated with liver disease.[433] In addition, alcohol can potentiate the hepatotoxicity of other agents.[229,230,483] Thus the concept that one or two drinks for women and up to four drinks per day for men is risk-free for everyone needs to be reconsidered. In particular, patients with chronic hepatitis should be counselled about the potentiating effects of alcohol and the increased risk of hepatocellular carcinoma.

In most countries, both developed and developing, the prevalence and mortality, and therefore the cost, of alcohol-related disease continues to rise.[8,526,527] Although financial constraints, as well as the lack of donor organs, severely limit the number of liver transplants that are performed each year, end-stage alcoholic liver is the most common reason for transplantation in Europe and the second most common in the USA.[96,527,500]

The growing understanding of the genetic and acquired factors that influence individual susceptibility to alcoholic liver disease has led to a progressively changing attitude towards the management of alcoholic liver disease. Consequently, at least in the more affluent countries, patients with end-stage alcohol-related liver disease may be offered intensive medical treatment and carefully selected patients are transplanted. In addition, the major advances in the understanding of pathogenic mechanisms involved in alcohol-related liver injury have major therapeutic implications not only for medical treatment, reversal of fibrosis/cirrhosis, but even offer the hope for prevention.

References

1. Keller M. A historical overview of alcohol and alcoholism. Cancer Res, 1979; 39:2822–2829
2. Reuben DB, Shekelle PG, Wenger NS. Quality of care for older persons at the dawn of the third millennium. J Am Geriatr Soc, 2003; 51:S346–S350
3. Saunders JB, Walters JR, Davies AP, Paton A. A 20-year prospective study of cirrhosis. Br Med J (Clin Res Ed), 1981; 282:263–266
4. Galambos JT. Epidemiology of alcoholic liver disease in the United States of America. In: Hall P de la M, ed. Alcoholic Liver Disease. London: Edward Arnold, 1985:230–249
5. Lelbach WK. The epidemiology of alcoholic liver disease in continental Europe. In: Hall P de la M, ed. Alcoholic liver disease. London: Edward Arnold, 1985, pp 130–166
6. Morgan MY. Epidemiology of alcoholic liver disease in the United Kingdom. In: Hall P de la M, ed. Alcoholic liver disease. London: Edward Arnold, 1985: pp 193–229
7. West LM. Alcoholism, In UCLA Conference, U.S.A, Ann Intern Med, 1984; 100:405–416
8. Roizen R, Kerr WC, Fillmore KM. Cirrhosis mortality and per capita consumption of distilled spirits, United States, 1949–94: trend analysis. BMJ, 1999; 319:666–670
9. Safdar K, Schiff ER. Alcohol and hepatitis C. Semin Liver Dis, 2004; 24:305–315
10. Orrego H, Israel Y, Blendis LM. Alcoholic liver disease: information in search of knowledge? Hepatology, 1981; 1:267–283
11. Popper H, Thung SN, Gerber MA. Pathology of alcoholic liver diseases. Semin Liver Dis, 1981; 1:203–216
12. MacSween RN, Burt AD. Histologic spectrum of alcoholic liver disease. Semin Liver Dis, 1986; 6:221–232
13. Diehl AM. Alcoholic liver disease. Med Clin North Am, 1989; 73:815–830
14. Maddrey WC. Alcoholic hepatitis: pathogenesis and approaches to treatment. Scand J Gastroenterol, 1990; 25 (suppl 175):118–130
15. Hall P de la M. Pathologic features of alcoholic liver disease. In: Okuda K, Benhamou J-P, ed. Portal hypertension: clinical and physiological aspects. Tokyo: Springer-Verlag, 1991: pp 41–68
16. Ishak KG, Zimmerman HJ, Ray MB. Alcoholic liver disease: pathologic, pathogenetic and clinical aspects. Alcohol Clin Exp Res, 1991; 15:45–66
17. French SW, Nash J, Shitabata P, Kachi K, Hara C, Chedid A, Mendenhall CL. Pathology of alcoholic liver disease. VA Cooperative Study Group 119. Semin Liver Dis, 1993; 13: 154–169
18. Lieber CS. Alcohol and the liver: 1994 update. Gastroenterology, 1994; 106:1085–1105
19. Hall P de la M. Pathology of pathogenesis of alcoholic liver disease. In: Hall P de la M, ed. Alcoholic Liver disease 2nd edition. London: Edward Arnold, 1995: pp 41–68
20. Saunders JB, Wodak AD, Williams R. What determines susceptibility to liver damage from alcohol?: discussion paper. J R Soc Med, 1984; 77:204–216
21. Johnson RD, Williams R. Genetic and environmental factors in the individual susceptibility to the development of alcoholic liver disease. Alcohol Alcohol, 1985; 20:137–160
22. Sorensen TI. Alcohol and liver injury: dose-related or permissive effect? Liver, 1989; 9:189–197
23. Hall P de la M. Genetic and acquired factors that influence individual susceptibility to alcohol-associated liver disease. J Gastroenterol Hepatol, 1992; 7:417–426
24. Frezza M, di Padova C, Pozzato G, Terpin M, Baraona E, Lieber CS. High blood alcohol levels in women. The role of decreased gastric alcohol dehydrogenase activity and first-pass metabolism. N Engl J Med, 1990; 322:95–99
25. Lelbach WK. Cirrhosis in the alcoholic and its relation to the volume of alcohol abuse. Ann N Y Acad Sci, 1975; 252:85–105
26. Ludwig J, Viggiano TR, McGill DB, Oh BJ. Nonalcoholic steatohepatitis: Mayo Clinic experiences with a hitherto unnamed disease. Mayo Clin Proc, 1980; 55:434–438
27. Day CP, Bashir R, James OF, Bassendine MF, Crabb DW, Thomasson HR, Li TK, Edenberg HJ. Investigation of the role of polymorphisms at the alcohol and aldehyde dehydrogenase loci in genetic predisposition to alcohol-related end-organ damage. Hepatology, 1991; 14:798–801
28. Lieber CS. Metabolism of alcohol. Clin Liver Dis, 2005; 9:1–35
29. Lieber CS. Alcohol metabolism. In: Hall P de la M, ed. Alcoholic liver disease. London: Edward Arnold, 1985: pp 3–40
30. Lieber CS. Mechanism of ethanol induced hepatic injury. Pharmacol Ther, 1990; 46:1–41
31. Lieber CS. Metabolism of ethanol and associated hepatotoxicity. Drug Alcohol Rev, 1991; 10:175–202
32. Mezey E. Metabolic effects of alcohol. Fed Proc, 1985; 44:134–138
33. French SW. Biochemical basis for alcohol-induced liver injury. Clin Biochem, 1989; 22:41–49
34. Israel Y, Videla L, Fernandez-Videla V, Bernstein J. Effects of chronic ethanol treatment and thyroxine administration on ethanol metabolism and liver oxidative capacity. J Pharmacol Exp Ther, 1975; 192:565–574
35. Lieber CS, DeCarli LM. Hepatic microsomal ethanol-oxidizing system. In vitro characteristics and adaptive properties in vivo. J Biol Chem, 1970; 245:2505–2512

36. Koop DR, Morgan ET, Tarr GE, Coon MJ. Purification and characterization of a unique isozyme of cytochrome P450 from liver microsomes of ethanol-treated rabbits. J Biol Chem, 1982; 257:8472–8480

37. Tsukada H, Wang PY, Kaneko T, Wang Y, Nakano M, Sato A. Dietary carbohydrate intake plays an important role in preventing alcoholic fatty liver in the rat. J Hepatol, 1998; 29:715–724

38. Kostrubsky VE, Szakacs JG, Jeffery EH et al. Role of CYP3A in ethanol-mediated increases in acetaminophen hepatotoxicity. Toxicol Appl Pharmacol, 1997; 143:315–323

39. Amet Y, Lucas D, Zhang-Gouillon ZQ, French SW. P-450-dependent metabolism of lauric acid in alcoholic liver disease: comparison between rat liver and kidney microsomes. Alcohol Clin Exp Res, 1998; 22:455–462

40. Lieber CS, Lasker JM, DeCarli LM, Saeli J, Wojtowicz T. Role of acetone, dietary fat and total energy intake in induction of hepatic microsomal ethanol oxidizing system. J Pharmacol Exp Ther, 1988; 247:791–795

41. Lieber CS, Lasker JM, Alderman J, Leo MA. The microsomal ethanol oxidizing system and its interaction with other drugs, carcinogens, and vitamins. Ann N Y Acad Sci, 1987; 492:11–24

42. Lieber CS. Metabolic effects of ethanol and its interaction with other drugs, hepatotoxic agents, vitamins, and carcinogens: a 1988 update. Semin Liver Dis, 1988; 8:47–68

43. Watkins PB. Role of cytochromes P450 in drug metabolism and hepatotoxicity. Semin Liver Dis, 1990; 10:235–250

44. Lieber CS. Ethanol metabolism, cirrhosis and alcoholism. Clin Chim Acta, 1997; 257:59–84

45. De Craemer D, Pauwels M, Van den Branden C. Morphometric characteristics of human hepatocellular peroxisomes in alcoholic liver disease. Alcohol Clin Exp Res, 1996; 20:908–913

46. Lindros KO, Stowell A, Pikkarainen P, Salaspuro M. Elevated blood acetaldehyde in alcoholics with accelerated ethanol elimination. Pharmacol Biochem Behav, 1980; 13 Suppl 1:119–124

47. You M, Crabb DW. Recent advances in alcoholic liver disease II. Minireview: molecular mechanisms of alcoholic fatty liver. Am J Physiol Gastrointest Liver Physiol, 2004; 287:G1–G6

48. Lieber CS, Savolainen M. Ethanol and lipids. Alcohol Clin Exp Res, 1984; 8:409–423

49. Edmondson HA, Peters RL, Frankel HH, Borowsky S. The early stage of liver injury in the alcoholic. Medicine, 1967; 46:119–129

50. Ballard H, Bernstein M, Farrar JT. Fatty liver presenting as obstructive jaundice. Am J Med, 1961; 30:196–201

51. Morgan MY, Sherlock S, Scheuer PJ. Acute cholestasis, hepatic failure, and fatty liver in the alcoholic. Scand J Gastroenterol, 1978; 13:299–303

52. Hall P, Smith RD, Gormley BM. 'Routine' stains on osmicated resin embedded hepatic tissue. Pathology, 1982; 14:73–74

53. Hall P, Gormley BM, Jarvis LR, Smith RD. A staining method for the detection and measurement of fat droplets in hepatic tissue. Pathology, 1980; 12:605–608

54. Christoffersen P, Braendstrup O, Juhl E, Poulsen H. Lipogranulomas in human liver biopsies with fatty change. A morphological, biochemical and clinical investigation. Acta Pathol Microbiol Scand [A], 1971; 79:150–158

55. Iversen K, Christoffersen P, Poulsen H. Epithelioid cell granulomas in liver biopsies. Scand J Gastroenterol,1970; 7(suppl):61–67

56. Teli MR, Day CP, Burt AD, Bennett MK, James OF. Determinants of progression to cirrhosis or fibrosis in pure alcoholic fatty liver. Lancet, 1995; 346:987–990

57. Dam-Larsen S, Franzmann MB, Christoffersen P et al., Histological characteristics and prognosis in patients with fatty liver Scand J Gastroenterol, 2005; 40:460–467

58. Uchida T, Kao H, Quispe-Sjogren M, Peters RL. Alcoholic foamy degeneration—a pattern of acute alcoholic injury of the liver. Gastroenterology, 1983; 84:683–692

59. Van Waes L, Lieber CS. Early perivenular sclerosis in alcoholic fatty liver: an index of progressive liver injury. Gastroenterology, 1977; 73:646–650

60. Nakano M, Worner TM, Lieber CS. Perivenular fibrosis in alcoholic liver injury: ultrastructure and histologic progression. Gastroenterology, 1982; 83:777–785

61. Worner TM, Lieber CS. Perivenular fibrosis as precursor lesion of cirrhosis. JAMA, 1985; 254:627–630

62. Junge J, Horn T, Vyberg M, Christoffersen P, Svendsen LB. The pattern of fibrosis in the acinar zone 3 areas in early alcoholic liver disease. J Hepatol, 1991; 12:83–86

63. Savolainen V, Perola M, Lalu K, Penttila A, Virtanen I, Karhunen PJ. Early perivenular fibrogenesis—precirrhotic lesions among moderate alcohol consumers and chronic alcoholics. J Hepatol, 1995; 23:524–531

64. Beckett AG, Livingstone AV, Hill KR. Acute alcoholic hepatitis. Br Med J, 1961; 5260:1113–1119

65. Brunt PW, Kew MC, Scheuer PJ, Sherlock S. Studies in alcoholic liver disease in Britain. I. Clinical and pathological patterns related to natural history. Gut, 1974; 15:52–58

66. Krasner N, Davis M, Portmann B, Williams R. Changing pattern of alcoholic liver disease in Great Britain: relation to sex and signs of autoimmunity. Br Med J, 1977; 1:1497–1500

67. Morgan MY, Sherlock S. Sex-related differences among 100 patients with alcoholic liver disease. Br Med J, 1977; 1:939–941

68. Harinasuta U, Zimmerman HJ. Alcoholic steatonecrosis. I. Relationship between severity of hepatic disease and presence of Mallory bodies in the liver. Gastroenterology, 1971; 60: 1036–1046

69. Birschbach HR, Harinasuta U, Zimmerman HJ. Alcoholic steatonecrosis. II. Prospective study of prevalence of Mallory bodies in biopsy speciemens and comparison of severity of hepatic disease in patients with and without this histological feature. Gastroenterology, 1974; 66:1195–1202

70. Bhathal PS, Wilkinson P, Clifton S, Rankin JG, Santamaria JN. The spectrum of liver diseases in alcoholism. Aust N Z J Med, 1975; 5:49–57

71. French SW, Burbridge EJ. Alcoholic hepatitus: clinical, morphological and therapeutic aspects. Prog Liver Dis., 1979; 6:557–580

72. Hislop WS, Bouchier IA, Allan JG, Brunt PW, Eastwood M, Finlayson ND, James O, Russell RI, Watkinson G. Alcoholic liver disease in Scotland and northeastern England: presenting features in 510 patients. Q J Med, 1983; 52:232–243

73. Karasawa T, Kushida T, Shikata T, Kaneda H. Morphologic spectrum of liver diseases among chronic alcoholics. A comparison between Tokyo, Japan and Cincinnati, U.S.A. Acta Pathol Jpn, 1980; 30:505–514

74. Baptista A. Alcoholic liver disease: morphological manifestations. Lancet, 1981; i:707–711

75. Bruguera M, Bertran A, Bombi JA, Rodes J. Giant mitochondria in hepatocytes: a diagnostic hint for alcoholic liver disease. Gastroenterology, 1977; 73:1383–1387

76. Hall P, Lieber CS, DeCarli L et al. Models of alcoholic liver disease in rodents: a critical evaluation. Alcohol Clin Exp Res, 2001; 25 (suppl):254–261

77. Vyberg M, Leth P. Ubiquitin: an immunohistochemical marker of Mallory bodies and alcoholic liver disease. APMIS (suppl), 1991; 23:46–52

78. Jensen K, Gluud C. The Mallory body: morphological, clinical and experimental studies (Part 1 of a literature survey). Hepatology, 1994; 20:1061–1077

79. Feldstein AE, Gores GJ. Apoptosis in alcoholic and nonalcoholic steatohepatitis. Front Biosci, 2005; 10:3093–3099

80. Edmondson HA, Peters RL, Reynolds TB, Kuzma OT. Sclerosing hyaline necrosis of the liver in the chronic alcoholic. A recognizable clinical syndrome. Ann Intern Med, 1963; 59:646–673

81. Reynolds TB, Hidemura R, Michel H, Peters R. Portal hypertension without cirrhosis in alcoholic liver disease. Ann Intern Med, 1969; 70:497–506

82. Gerber MA, Popper H. Relation between central canals and portal tracts in alcoholic hepatitis. A contribution to the pathogenesis of cirrhosis in alcoholics. Hum Pathol, 1972; 3:199–207

83. Scheuer PJ, Maggi G. Hepatic fibrosis and collapse: histological distinction by orcein staining. Histopathology, 1980; 4: 487–490

84. Brunt EM, Janney CG, Di Bisceglie AM, Neuschwander-Tetri BA, Bacon BR. Nonalcoholic steatohepatitis: a proposal for grading and staging the histological lesions. Am J Gastroenterol, 1999; 94:2467–2474

85. Matteoni CA, Younossi ZM, Gramlich T, Boparai N, Liu YC, McCullough AJ. Nonalcoholic fatty liver disease: a spectrum of clinical and pathological severity. Gastroenterology, 1999; 116:1413–1419

86. Nasrallah SM, Nassar VH, Galambos JT. Importance of terminal hepatic venule thickening. Arch Pathol Lab Med, 1980; 104:84–86

87. Christoffersen P, Eghoje K, Juhl E. Mallory bodies in liver biopsies from chronic alcoholics. A comparative morphological, biochemical, and clinical study of two groups of chronic alcoholics with and without Mallory bodies. Scand J Gastroenterol, 1973; 8:341–346

88. Bouchier IA, Hislop WS, Prescott RJ. A prospective study of alcoholic liver disease and mortality. J Hepatol, 1992; 16:290–297

89. Orrego H, Blake JE, Blendis LM, Medline A. Prognosis of alcoholic cirrhosis in the presence and absence of alcoholic hepatitis. Gastroenterology, 1987; 92:208–214

90. Morgan MY. The prognosis and outcome of alcoholic liver disease. Alcohol Alcohol (suppl) 1994; 2:335–343

91. Forrest EH, Evans CD, Stewart S et al. Analysis of factors predictive of mortality in alcoholic hepatitis and derivation and validation of the Glasgow alcoholic hepatitis score. Gut, 2005; 54:1174–1179

92. Sorensen TI, Orholm M, Bentsen KD, Hoybye G, Eghoje K, Christoffersen P. Prospective evaluation of alcohol abuse and alcoholic liver injury in men as predictors of development of cirrhosis. Lancet, 1984; ii:241–244

93. Pares A, Caballeria J, Bruguera M, Torres M, Rodes J. Histological course of alcoholic hepatitis. Influence of abstinence, sex and extent of hepatic damage. J Hepatol, 1986; 2:33–42

94. Goodman ZD, Ishak KG. Occlusive venous lesions in alcoholic liver disease. A study of 200 cases. Gastroenterology, 1982; 83:786–796

95. Burt AD, MacSween RN. Hepatic vein lesions in alcoholic liver disease: retrospective biopsy and necropsy study. J Clin Pathol, 1986; 39:63–67

96. Neuberger J, Schulz KH, Day C et al. Transplantation for alcoholic liver disease. J Hepatol, 2002; 36:130–137

97. Pageaux GP, Perney P, Larrey D. Liver transplantation for alcoholic liver disease. Addict Biol, 2001; 6:301–308

98. Anthony PP, Ishak KG, Nayak NC, Poulsen HE, Scheuer PJ, Sobin LH. The morphology of cirrhosis. Recommendations on definition, nomenclature, and classification by a working group sponsored by the World Health Organization. J Clin Pathol, 1978; 31:395–414

99. Lee FI. Cirrhosis and hepatoma in alcoholics. Gut, 1966; 7:77–85

100. Goldberg SJ, Mendenhall CL, Connell AM, Chedid A. 'Nonalcoholic' chronic hepatitis in the alcoholic. Gastroenterology, 1977; 72:598–604

101. Brillanti S, Barbara L, Miglioli M, Bonino F. Hepatitis C virus: a possible cause of chronic hepatitis in alcoholics. Lancet, 1989; 2:1390–1391

102. Mendenhall CL, Seeff L, Diehl AM et al. Antibodies to hepatitis B virus and hepatitis C virus in alcoholic hepatitis and cirrhosis: their prevalence and clinical relevance. The VA Cooperative Study Group No. 119. Hepatology, 1991; 14:581–589

103. Uchimura Y, Sata M, Kage M, Abe H, Tanikawa K. A histopathological study of alcoholics with chronic HCV infection: comparison with chronic hepatitis C and alcoholic liver disease. Liver, 1995; 15:300–306

104. Takase S, Takada N, Enomoto N, Yasuhara M, Takada A. Different types of chronic hepatitis in alcoholic patients: does chronic hepatitis induced by alcohol exist? Hepatology, 1991; 13:876–881

105. Uchida T, Peters RL. The nature and origin of proliferated bile ductules in alcoholic liver disease. Am J Clin Pathol, 1983; 79:326–333

106. Van Eyken P, Sciot R, Desmet VJ. A cytokeratin immunohistochemical study of alcoholic liver disease: evidence that hepatocytes can express 'bile duct-type' cytokeratins. Histopathology, 1988; 13:605–617

107. Van Eyken P. Progenitor ('stem cells') in alcoholic liver disease. In: Hall P de la M, ed. Alcoholic liver disease. London: Edward Arnold, 1995: pp 160–171

108. Haruna Y, Saito K, Spaulding S, Nalesnik MA, Gerber MA. Identification of bipotential progenitor cells in human liver development. Hepatology, 1996; 23:476–481

109. Smith PG, Tee LB, Yeoh GC. Appearance of oval cells in the liver of rats after long-term exposure to ethanol. Hepatology, 1996; 23:145–154

110. Tan J, Hytiroglou P, Wieczorek R, Park YN, Thung SN, Arias B, Theise ND. Immunohistochemical evidence for hepatic progenitor cells in liver diseases. Liver, 2002; 22:365–373

111. Rubin E, Krus S, Popper H. Pathogenesis of postnecrotic cirrhosis in alcoholics. Arch Pathol, 1962; 73:288–299

112. Fauerholdt L, Schlichting P, Christensen E, Poulsen H, Tygstrup N, Juhl E. Conversion of micronodular cirrhosis into macronodular cirrhosis. Hepatology, 1983; 3:928–931

112a. Schinoni MI, Andrade Z, de Frietas LA, Oliviera R, Parena R. Incomplete septal cirrhosis; an enigmatic disease. Liver Int, 2004; 24:452–456

113. Nagasue N, Akamizu H, Yukaya H, Yuuki I. Hepatocellular pseudotumor in the cirrhotic liver. Report of three cases. Cancer, 1984; 54:2487–2494

113b. Nakashima O, Kurogi M, Yamaguchi R et al. Unique hypervascular nodules in alcoholic liver cirrhosis; identical to focal nodular hyperplasia-like lesions. J Hepatol, 2004; 41:992–998

114. Abdi W, Millan JC, Mezey E. Sampling variability on percutaneous liver biopsy. Arch Intern Med, 1979; 139: 667–669

115. Scheuer P. Liver biopsy interpretation., 5th edn. WB Saunders, ed. London: Baillière Tindall, 1994

116. Pariente EA, Degott C, Martin JP, Feldmann G, Potet F, Benhamou JP. Hepatocytic PAS-positive diastase-resistant inclusions in the absence of alpha-1-antitrypsin deficiency—high prevalence in alcoholic cirrhosis. Am J Clin Pathol, 1981; 76:299–302

117. Graziadei IW, Joseph JJ, Wiesner RH, Therneau TM, Batts KP, Porayko MK. Increased risk of chronic liver failure in adults with heterozygous alpha1-antitrypsin deficiency. Hepatology, 1998; 28:1058–1063

118. Berresford PA, Sunter JP, Harrison V, Lesna M. Histological demonstration and frequency of intrahepatocytic copper in patients suffering from alcoholic liver disease. Histopathology, 1980; 4:637–643

119. Lefkowitch JH, Arborgh BA, Scheuer PJ. Oxyphilic granular hepatocytes. Mitochondrion-rich liver cells in hepatic disease. Am J Clin Pathol, 1980; 74:432–441

120. Gerber MA, Thung SN. Hepatic oncocytes. Incidence, staining characteristics, and ultrastructural features. Am J Clin Pathol, 1981; 75:498–503

121. Chedid A, Mendenhall CL, Gartside P, French SW, Chen T, Rabin L. Prognostic factors in alcoholic liver disease. VA Cooperative Study Group. Am J Gastroenterol, 1991; 86:210–216

122. Powell WJ, Jr., Klatskin G. Duration of survival in patients with Laennec's cirrhosis. Influence of alcohol withdrawal, and possible effects of recent changes in general management of the disease. Am J Med, 1968; 44:406–420

123. Borowsky SA, Strome S, Lott E. Continued heavy drinking and survival in alcoholic cirrhotics. Gastroenterology, 1981; 80:1405–1409

124. Pérez-Tamayo R. Cirrhosis of the liver: a reversible disease? Pathology Annual, 1979; 14 (part 2):183–213

125. Baker AL, Elson CO, Jaspan J, Boyer JL. Liver failure with steatonecrosis after jejunoileal bypass: recovery with parenteral nutriton and reanastomosis. Arch Intern Med, 1979; 139: 289–292

126. Desmet VJ, Roskams T. Cirrhosis reversal: a duel between dogma and myth. J Hepatol, 2004; 40:860–867

127. Phillips GB, Davidson CS. Liver disease of the chronic alcoholic simulating extrahepatic biliary obstruction. Gastroenterology, 1957; 33:236–244

128. Popper H, Szanto PB. Fatty liver with hepatic failure in alcoholics. J Mt Sinai Hosp N Y, 1957; 24:1121–1131

129. Perrillo RP, Griffin R, DeSchryver-Kecskemeti K, Lander JJ, Zuckerman GR. Alcoholic liver disease presenting with marked elevation of serum alkaline phosphatase. A combined clinical and pathological study. Am J Dig Dis, 1978; 23:1061–1066

130. Afroudakis A, Kaplowitz N. Liver histopathology in chronic common bile duct stenosis due to chronic alcoholic pancreatitis. Hepatology, 1981; 1:65–72

131. Glover SC, McPhie JL, Brunt PW. Cholestasis in acute alcoholic liver disease. Lancet, 1977; 2:1305–1307

132. Zieve L. Jaundice, hyperlipemia and hemolytic anemia: a heretofore unrecognized syndrome associated with alcoholic fatty liver and cirrhosis. Ann Intern Med, 1958; 48:471–496

133. Nissenbaum M, Chedid A, Mendenhall C, Gartside P and the VA Cooperative Study Group #119. Prognostic significance of cholestatic alcoholic hepatitis. Dig Dis Sci, 1990; 35:891–896

134. Levin DM, Baker AL, Riddell RH, Rochman H, Boyer JL. Nonalcoholic liver disease. Overlooked causes of liver injury in patients with heavy alcohol consumption. Am J Med, 1979; 66:429–434

135. Afshani P, Littenberg GD, Wollman J, Kaplowitz N. Significance of microscopic cholangitis in alcoholic liver disease. Gastroenterology, 1978; 75:1045–1050

136. Morgan MY, Sherlock S, Scheuer PJ. Portal fibrosis in the livers of alcoholic patients. Gut, 1978; 19:1015–1021

137. Michalak S, Rousselet MC, Bedossa P et al. Respective roles of porto-septal and centrilobular fibrosis in alcoholic liver disease. J Pathol, 2003; 201:55–62

138. Karakucuk I, Dilly SA, Maxwell JD. Portal tract macrophages are increased in alcoholic liver disease. Histopathology, 1989; 14:245–253

139. Jakobovits AW, Morgan MY, Sherlock S. Hepatic siderosis in alcoholics. Dig Dis Sci, 1979; 24:305–310

140. Macdonald R. Wine and iron in haemochromatosis. Lancet, 1963; i:727

141. Hift R. Alcohol and porphyria. In: Hall P de la M, ed. Alcoholic Liver disease 2nd edition. London: Edward Arnold, 1995: pp 219–231

142. Duane P RK, Simpson RJ, Peters TJ. Intestinal iron absorption in chronic alcoholics. Alcohol Alcohol, 1992; 27:539–544

143. Pascoe A, Kerlin P, Steadman C, Clouston A, Jones D, Powell L, Jazwinska E, Lynch S, Strong R. Spur cell anaemia and hepatic iron stores in patients with alcoholic liver disease undergoing orthotopic liver transplantation. Gut, 1999; 45:301–305

144. Suzuki Y, Saito H, Suzuki M, Hosoki Y, Sakurai S, Fujimoto Y, Kohgo Y. Up-regulation of transferrin receptor expression in hepatocytes by habitual alcohol drinking is implicated in hepatic iron overload in alcoholic liver disease. Alcohol Clin Exp Res, 2002; 26:26S–31S

145. LeSage GD, Baldus WP, Fairbanks VF, Baggenstoss AH, McCall JT, Moore SB, Taswell HF, Gordon H. Hemochromatosis: genetic or alcohol-induced? Gastroenterology, 1983; 84:1471–1477

146. Eng SC, Taylor SL, Reyes V, Raaka S, Bereger J, Kowdley KV. Hepatic iron overload in alcoholic end-stage liver disease is associated with iron deposition in other organs in the absence of HFE-1 hemochromatosis. Liver Int, 2005; 25:513–517

147. Morgan TR, Madayam S, Jamal MM. Alcohol and hepatocellular carcinoma. Gastroenterology, 2004; 127:587–596

148. Kuper H, Ye W, Broome U et al. The risk of liver and bile duct cancer in patients with chronic viral hepatitis, alcoholism, or cirrhosis. Hepatology, 2001; 34:714–718

149. Yamagishi Y, Horie Y, Kajihara M, Konishi M, Ebinuma H, Saito H, Kato S, Yokoyama A, Maruyama K, Ishii H. Hepatocellular carcinoma in heavy drinkers with negative markers for viral hepatitis. Hepatol Res, 2004; 28:177–183

150. Laurent-Puig P, Legoix P, Bluteau O et al. Genetic alterations associated with hepatocellular carcinomas define distinct pathways of hepatocarcinogenesis. Gastroenterology, 2001; 120:1763–7173

151. Faber E. Alcohol and other chemicals in the development of hepatocellular carcinoma. Clin Lab Med, 1996; 16:377–394

152. Sietz HK, Poschl G, Simanowski UA. Alcohol and Cancer. Recent Dev Alcohol, 1998; 14:67–95

153. Marrero JA, Fontana RJ, Fu S et al. Alcohol, tobacco and obesity are synergistic factors for hepatocellular carcinoma. J Hepatol, 2005; 42:218–224

154. Bellentani S, Tiribelli C, Saccoccio G, Sodde M, Fratti N, De Martin C, Cristianini G. Prevalence of chronic liver disease in the general population of northern Italy: the Dionysos Study. Hepatology, 1994; 20:1442–1449

155. Brechot C, Nalpas B, Courouce AM et al. Evidence that hepatitis B virus has a role in liver-cell carcinoma in alcoholic liver disease. N Engl J Med, 1982; 306:1384–1387

156. Jee SH, Ohrr H, Sull JW, Samet JM. Cigarette smoking, alcohol drinking, hepatitis B, and risk for hepatocellular carcinoma in Korea. J Natl Cancer Inst, 2004; 96:1851–1856

157. Yamauchi M, Nakahara M, Maezawa Y et al. Prevalence of hepatocellular carcinoma in patients with alcoholic cirrhosis and prior exposure to hepatitis C. Am J Gastroenterol, 1993; 88:39–43

158. Noda K, Yoshihara H, Suzuki K et al. Progression of type C chronic hepatitis to liver cirrhosis and hepatocellular carcinoma—its relationship to alcohol drinking and the age of transfusion. Alcohol Clin Exp Res, 1996; 20:95A–100A

159. Colombo M. The role of hepatitis C virus in hepatocellular carcinoma. Recent Results Cancer Res, 1998; 154:337–344

160. Hassan MM, Hwang LY, Hatten CJ, Swaim M, Li D, Abbruzzese JL, Beasley P, Patt YZ. Risk factors for hepatocellular carcinoma: synergism of alcohol with viral hepatitis and diabetes mellitus. Hepatology, 2002; 36:1206–1123

161. Arakawa M, Kage M, Sugihara S, Nakashima T, Suenaga M, Okuda K. Emergence of malignant lesions within an adenomatous hyperplastic nodule in a cirrhotic liver. Observations in five cases. Gastroenterology, 1986; 91:198–208

162. Terasaki S, Kaneko S, Kobayashi K, Nonomura A, Nakanuma Y. Histological features predicting malignant transformation of nonmalignant hepatocellular nodules: a prospective study. Gastroenterology, 1998; 115:1216–1222

163. Libbrecht LDV, Roskams T. Preneoplastic lesions in human hepatocarcinogenesis. Liver Int, 2005; 25:16–27

164. Lee RG, Tsamandas AC, Demetris AJ. Large cell change (liver cell dysplasia) and hepatocellular carcinoma in cirrhosis: matched case-control study, pathological analysis, and pathogenetic hypothesis. Hepatology, 1997; 26:1415–1422

165. Talley NJ, Roth A, Woods J, Hench V. Diagnostic value of liver biopsy in alcoholic liver disease. J Clin Gastroenterol, 1988; 10:647–650

166. Mathurin P, Duchatelle V, Ramond MJ, Degott C, Bedossa P, Erlinger S, Benhamou JP, Chaput JC, Rueff B, Poynard T. Survival and prognostic factors in patients with severe alcoholic hepatitis treated with prednisolone. Gastroenterology, 1996; 110:1847–1853

167. Akriviadis E, Botla R, Briggs W, Han S, Reynolds T, Shakil O. Pentoxifylline improves short-term survival in severe acute alcoholic hepatitis: a double-blind, placebo-controlled trial. Gastroenterology, 2000; 119:1637–1648

168. Mato JM, Camara J, Fernandez de Paz J et al. S-adenosylmethionine in alcoholic liver cirrhosis: a randomized, placebo-controlled, double-blind, multicenter clinical trial. J Hepatol, 1999; 30:1081–1089

169. Lieber CS. S-Adenosyl-L-methionine and alcoholic liver disease in animal models: implications for early intervention in human beings. Alcohol, 2002; 27:173–177

170. Hall P de la M. Histopathological spectrum of drug-induced liver injury. In: Farrell GC, ed. Drug-induced liver disease. Edinburgh: Churchill Livingstone, 1994: pp 115–151

171. Diehl AM, Goodman Z, Ishak KG. Alcohol-like liver disease in nonalcoholics. A clinical and histologic comparison with alcohol-induced liver injury. Gastroenterology, 1988; 95:1056–1062

172. Poupon R, Rosensztajn L, Prudhomme de S-M P, Lageron A, Gombeau T, Darnis F. Perhexiline maleate-associated hepatic injury prevalence and characteristics. Digestion, 1980; 20:145–150

173. Poucell S, Ireton J, Valencia-Mayoral P, Downar E, Larratt L, Patterson J, Blendis L, Phillips MJ. Amiodarone-associated phospholipidosis and fibrosis of the liver. Light, immunohistochemical, and electron microscopic studies. Gastroenterology, 1984; 86:926–936

174. Gilinsky NH, Briscoe GW, Kuo CS. Fatal amiodarone hepatoxicity. Am J Gastroenterol, 1988; 83:161–163

175. Bach N, Schultz BL, Cohen LB, Squire A, Gordon R, Thung SN, Schaffner F. Amiodarone hepatotoxicity: progression from steatosis to cirrhosis. Mt Sinai J Med, 1989; 56:293–296

176. Lewis JH, Ranard RC, Caruso A, Jackson LK, Mullick F, Ishak KG, Seeff LB, Zimmerman HJ. Amiodarone hepatotoxicity: prevalence and clinicopathologic correlations among 104 patients. Hepatology, 1989; 9:679–685

177. Hayashi PH, Harrison SA, Torgerson S, Perez TA, Nochajski T, Russell M. Cognitive lifetime drinking history in nonalcoholic fatty liver disease: some cases may be alcohol related. Am J Gastroenterol, 2004; 99:76–81

178. Clarkson VC, Hall P, Shepard E, Kirsch R, Marais D. Ethanol feeding increases CYP2E11 activity in the methionine choline deficient mouse model for NASH. Liver Int, 2004; 24:18

179. Adler M, Schaffner F. Fatty liver hepatitis and cirrhosis in obese patients. Am J Med, 1979; 67:811–816

180. Capron J-P. Fasting in obesity. Another cause of liver injury with alcoholic hyaline? Dig Dis Sci, 1982; 27:265–268

181. Silverman JF, O'Brien KF, Long S et al. Liver pathology in morbidly obese patients with and without diabetes. Am J Gastroenterol, 1990; 85:1349–1355

182. Thaler H. Relation of steatosis to cirrhosis. Clin Gastroenterol, 1975; 4:273–280

183. Falchuk KR, Fiske SC, Haggitt RC, Federman M, Trey C. Pericentral hepatic fibrosis and intracellular hyalin in diabetes mellitus. Gastroenterology, 1980; 78:535–541

184. Batman PA, Scheuer PJ. Diabetic hepatitis preceding the onset of glucose intolerance. Histopathology, 1985; 9:237–243

185. Peters RL, Gay T, Reynolds TB. Post-jejunoileal-bypass hepatic disease. Its similarity to alcoholic hepatic disease. Am J Clin Pathl, 1975; 63:318–331

186. Hamilton DL, Vest TK, Brown BS, Shah AN, Menguy RB, Chey WY. Liver injury with alcoholic-like hyalin after gastroplasty for morbid obesity. Gastroenterology, 1983; 85:722–726

187. Peura DA, Stromeyer FW, Johnson LF. Liver injury with alcoholic hyaline after intestinal resection. Gastroenterology, 1980; 79:128–130

188. Nakanuma Y, Ohta G, Konishi I, Shima Y. Liver injury with perivenular fibrosis and alcoholic hyalin after pancreatoduodenectomy for pancreatic carcinoma. Acta Pathol Jpn, 1987; 37:1953–1960

189. Powell EE, Searle J, Mortimer R. Steatohepatitis associated with limb lipodystrophy. Gastroenterology, 1989; 97:1022–1024

190. Nazim M, Stamp G, Hodgson HJ. Non-alcoholic steatohepatitis associated with small intestinal diverticulosis and bacterial overgrowth. Hepatogastroenterology, 1989; 36:349–351

191. Partin JS, Partin JC, Schubert WK, McAdams AJ. Liver ultrastructure in abetalipoproteinemia: Evolution of micronodular cirrhosis. Gastroenterology, 1974; 67:107–118

192. Kimura H, Kako M, Yo K, Oda T. Alcoholic hyalins (Mallory bodies) in a case of Weber–Christian disease: electron microscopic observations of liver involvement. Gastroenterology, 1980; 78:807–812

193. Paliard P, Vitrey D, Fournier G, Belhadjali J, Patricot L, Berger F. Perhexiline maleate-induced hepatitis. Digestion, 1978; 17:419–427

194. Pessayre D, Bichara M, Degott C, Potet F, Benhamou JP, Feldmann G. Perhexiline maleate-induced cirrhosis. Gastroenterology, 1979; 76:170–177

195. Itoh S, Igarashi M, Tsukada Y, Ichinoe A. Nonalcoholic fatty liver with alcoholic hyalin after long-term glucocorticoid therapy. Acta Hepatogastroenterol (Stuttg), 1977; 24:415–441

196. Seki K, Minami Y, Nishikawa M, Kawata S, Miyoshi S, Imai Y, Tarui S. 'Nonalcoholic steatohepatitis' induced by massive doses of synthetic estrogen. Gastroenterol Jpn, 1983; 18:197–203

197. Babany G, Uzzan F, Larrey D, Degott C, Bourgeois P, Rene E, Vissuzaine C, Erlinger S, Benhamou JP. Alcoholic-like liver lesions induced by nifedipine. J Hepatol, 1989; 9:252–255

198. Itoh S. Clinico-pathological and electron microscopical studies on a coronary dilating agent: 4,4'-diethylaminoethoxyhexestrol-induced liver injuries. Acta Hepatogastroenterol, 1973; 20:204–215

199. Wanless IR, Bargman JM, Oreopoulos DG, Vas SI. Subcapsular steatonecrosis in response to peritoneal insulin delivery: a clue to the pathogenesis of steatonecrosis in obesity. Mod Pathol, 1989; 2:69–74

200. Cromie SL, Jenkins PJ, Bowden DS, Dudley FJ. Chronic hepatitis C: effect of alcohol on hepatitic activity and viral titre. J Hepatol, 1996; 25:821–826

201. Zhao P, Kalhorn TF, Slattery JT. Selective mitochondrial glutathione depletion by ethanol enhances acetaminophen toxicity in rat liver. Hepatology, 2002; 36:326–335

202. Bassett ML, Halliday JW, Powell LW. Value of hepatic iron measurements in early hemochromatosis and determination of the critical iron level associated with fibrosis. Hepatology, 1986; 6:24–29

203. Feder JN, Gnirke A, Thomas W et al. A novel MHC class I-like gene is mutated in patients with hereditary haemochromatosis. Nat Genet, 1996; 13:399–408

204. Olynyk J, Hall P, Sallie R, Reed W, Shilkin K, Mackinnon M. Computerized measurement of iron in liver biopsies: a comparison with biochemical iron measurement. Hepatology, 1990; 12:26–30

205. Fletcher LM, Dixon JL, Purdie DM, Powell LW, Crawford DH. Excess alcohol greatly increases the prevalence of cirrhosis in hereditary hemochromatosis. Gastroenterology, 2002; 122:281–9

206. Powell LW. Distinction between haemochromatosis and alcoholic siderosis. In: Hall P de la M, ed. Alcoholic liver disease 2nd edition. London: Edward Arnold, 1995: pp 199–216

207. MacKinnon M, Clayton C, Plummer J, Ahern M, Cmielewski P, Ilsley A, Hall P. Iron overload facilitates hepatic fibrosis in the rat alcohol/low-dose carbon tetrachloride model. Hepatology, 1995; 21:1083–1088

208. Ramm GA, Crawford DH, Powell LW, Walker NI, Fletcher LM, Halliday JW. Hepatic stellate cell activation in genetic haemochromatosis. Lobular distribution, effect of increasing hepatic iron and response to phlebotomy. J Hepatol, 1997; 26:584–592

209. Xiong S, She H, Sung CK, Tsukamoto H. Iron-dependent activation of NF-kappaB in Kupffer cells: a priming mechanism for alcoholic liver disease. Alcohol, 2003; 30:107–113

210. Fletcher LM, Bridle KR, Crawford DH. Effect of alcohol on iron storage diseases of the liver. Best Pract Res Clin Gastroenterol, 2003; 17:663–677

211. Tavill AS, Qadri AM. Alcohol and iron. Semin Liver Dis, 2004; 24:317–325

212. Lane BP, Lieber CS. Ultrastructural alterations in human hepatocytes following ingestion of ethanol with adequate diets. Am J Pathol, 1966; 49:593–603

213. Rubin E, Lieber CS. Alcohol-induced hepatic injury in nonalcoholic volunteers. N Engl J Med, 1968; 278:869–876

214. Lieber CS, DeCarli LM. An experimental model of alcohol feeding and liver injury in the baboon. J Med Primatol, 1974; 3:153–163

215. Rubin E, Lieber CS. Fatty liver, alcoholic hepatitis and cirrhosis produced by alcohol in primates. N Engl J Med, 1974; 290:128–135

216. Lieber CS, DeCarli L, Rubin E. Sequential production of fatty liver, hepatitis, and cirrhosis in sub-human primates fed ethanol with adequate diets. Proc Natl Acad Sci USA, 1975; 72:437–441

217. Lieber CS, Leo MA, Mak KM, DeCarli LM, Sato S. Choline fails to prevent liver fibrosis in ethanol-fed baboons but causes toxicity. Hepatology, 1985; 5:561–572

218. Rubin E, Beattie DS, Lieber CS. Effects of ethanol on the biogenesis of mitochondrial membranes and associated mitochondrial functions. Lab Invest, 1970; 23:620–627

219. Inagaki T, Koike M, Ikuta K, Kobayashi S, Suzuki M, Kato K. Ultrastructural identification and clinical significance of light microscopic giant mitochondria in alcoholic liver injuries. Gastroenterol Jpn, 1989; 24:46–53

220. Fromenty B, Pessayre D. Impaired mitochondrial function in microvesicular steatosis. Effects of drugs, ethanol, hormones and cytokines. J Hepatol, 1997; 26 (suppl) 2:43–53

221. Caldwell SH, Swerdlow RH, Khan EM, Iezzoni JC, Hespenheide EE, Parks JK, Parker WD, Jr. Mitochondrial abnormalities in non-alcoholic steatohepatitis. J Hepatol, 1999; 31:430–434

222. Cahill A, Stabley GJ, Wang X, Hoek JB. Chronic ethanol consumption causes alterations in the structural integrity of mitochondrial DNA in aged rats. Hepatology, 1999; 30:881–888

223. Tsuchishima M, Tsutsumi M, Shiroeda H, Yano H, Ueshima Y, Shimanaka K, Takase S. Study of mitochondrial DNA deletion in alcoholics. Alcohol Clin Exp Res, 2000; 24:12S–15S

224. Lieber CS, DeCarli LM. Ethanol oxidation by hepatic microsomes: adaptive increase after ethanol feeding. Science, 1968; 162:917–918

225. Leo MA, Sato M, Lieber CS. Effect of hepatic vitamin A depletion on the liver in humans and rats. Gastroenterology, 1983; 84:562–572

226. McClain CJ, Kromhout JP, Peterson FJ, Holtzman JL. Potentiation of acetaminophen hepatotoxicity by alcohol. JAMA, 1980; 244:251–253

227. Seeff LB, Cuccherini BA, Zimmerman HJ, Adler E, Benjamin SB. Acetaminophen hepatotoxicity in alcoholics. A therapeutic misadventure. Ann Intern Med, 1986; 104:399–404

228. Riihimaki V, Savolainen K, Pfaffli P, Pekari K, Sippel HW, Laine A. Metabolic interaction between m-xylene and ethanol. Arch Toxicol, 1982; 49:253–263

229. Leo MA, Arai M, Sato M, Lieber CS. Hepatotoxicity of vitamin A and ethanol in the rat. Gastroenterology, 1982; 82:194–205

230. Hall P, Plummer JL, Ilsley AH, Cousins MJ. Hepatic fibrosis and cirrhosis after chronic administration of alcohol and 'low-dose' carbon tetrachloride vapor in the rat. Hepatology, 1991; 13:815–819

231. Waring AJ, Rottenberg H, Ohnishi T, Rubin E. Membranes and phospholipids of liver mitochondria from chronic alcoholic rats are resistant to membrane disordering by alcohol. Proc Natl Acad Sci USA, 1981; 78:2582–2586

232. Rubin E, Rottenberg H. Ethanol-induced injury and adaptation in biological membranes. Fed Proc, 1982; 41:2465–2471

233. Sun GY. Ethanol and membrane lipids. Alcoholism: Clin Exp Res, 1985; 9:164–180

234. Yamada S, Lieber CS. Decrease in microviscosity and cholesterol content of rat liver plasma membranes after chronic ethanol feeding. J Clin Invest, 1984; 74:2285–2289

235. Taraschi TF, Rubin E. Effects of ethanol on the chemical and structural properties of biologic membranes. Lab Invest, 1985; 52:120–131

236. Schanne FA, Kane AB, Young EE, Farber JL. Calcium dependence of toxic cell death: a final common pathway. Science, 1979; 206:700–702

237. Farber JL. Calcium and the mechanisms of liver necrosis. Prog Liver Dis, 1982; 7:347–460

238. Hoek JB, Taraschi TF, Rubin E. Functional implications of the interaction of ethanol with biologic membranes: actions of ethanol on hormonal signal transduction systems. Semin Liver Dis, 1988; 8:36–46

239. Shaw S, Rubin KP, Lieber CS. Depressed hepatic glutathione and increased diene conjugates in alcoholic liver disease. Evidence of lipid peroxidation. Dig Dis Sci, 1983; 28:585–589

240. Strubelt O, Younes M, Pentz R. Enhancement by glutathione depletion of ethanol-induced acute hepatotoxicity in vitro and in vivo. Toxicology, 1987; 45:213–223

241. Tribble DL, Aw TY, Jones DP. The pathophysiological significance of lipid peroxidation in oxidative cell injury. Hepatology, 1987; 7:377–386

242. Younes M, Strubelt O. Alcohol-induced hepatotoxicity: a role for oxygen free radicals. Free Radic Res Commun, 1987; 3:19–26

243. Shigesawa T, Sato C, Marumo F. Significance of plasma glutathione determination in patients with alcoholic and non-alcoholic liver disease. J Gastroenterol Hepatol, 1992; 7:7–11

244. Lieber CS. Role of oxidative stress and antioxidant therapy in alcoholic and nonalcoholic liver diseases. Adv Pharmacol, 1997; 38:601–628

245. Jauhonen P, Baraona E, Miyakawa H, Lieber CS. Mechanism for selective perivenular hepatotoxicity of ethanol. Alcohol Clin Exp Res, 1982; 6:350–357

246. French SW, Benson NC, Sun PS. Centrilobular liver necrosis induced by hypoxia in chronic ethanol-fed rats. Hepatology, 1984; 4:912–917

247. Yuki T, Israel Y, Thurman RG. The swift increase in alcohol metabolism. Inhibition by propylthiouracil. Biochem Pharmacol, 1982; 31:2403–2407

248. Orrego H, Blake JE, Blendis LM, Compton KV, Israel Y. Long-term treatment of alcoholic liver disease with propylthiouracil. N Engl J Med, 1987; 317:1421–1427

249. Gonzalez-Reimers E, Santolaria-Fernandez F, Perez-Labajos J et al. Relative and combined effects of propylthiouracil, ethanol and

protein deficiency on liver histology and hepatic iron, zinc, manganese and copper contents. Alcohol Alcohol, 1996; 31:535–545

250. Weltman MD, Farrell GC, Hall P, Ingelman-Sundberg M, Liddle C. Hepatic cytochrome P450 2E1 is increased in patients with nonalcoholic steatohepatitis. Hepatology, 1998; 27:128–133

251. Tsutsumi M, Lasker JM, Shimizu M, Rosman AS, Lieber CS. The intralobular distribution of ethanol-inducible P450IIE1 in rat and human liver. Hepatology, 1989; 10:437–446

252. Lieber CS, Baraona E, Hernandez-Munoz R, Kubota S, Sato N, Kawano S, Matsumura T, Inatomi N. Impaired oxygen utilization. A new mechanism for the hepatotoxicity of ethanol in sub-human primates. J Clin Invest, 1989; 83:1682–1690

253. French SW. The role of hypoxia in the pathogenesis of alcoholic liver disease. Hepatol Res, 2004; 29:69–74

254. Israel Y. Alcohol-induced hepatomegaly: pathogenesis and role in the production of portal hypertension. Fed Proc, 1982; 41:2472–2477

255. Matsuda Y, Takada A, Kanayama R, Takase S. Changes of hepatic microtubules and secretory proteins in human alcoholic liver disease. Pharmacol Biochem Behav, 1983; 18 (suppl) 1:479–482

256. Berman WJ, Gil J, Jennett RB, Tuma D, Sorrell MF, Rubin E. Ethanol, hepatocellular organelles, and microtubules. A morphometric study in vivo and in vitro. Lab Invest, 1983; 48:760–767

257. Orrego H, Blendis LM, Crossley IR, Medline A, Macdonald A, Ritchie S, Israel Y. Correlation of intrahepatic pressure with collagen in the Disse space and hepatomegaly in humans and in the rat. Gastroenterology, 1981; 80:546–556

258. Blendis LM, Orrego H, Crossley IR, Blake JE, Medline A, Isreal Y. The role of hepatocyte enlargement in hepatic pressure in cirrhotic and noncirrhotic alcoholic liver disease. Hepatology, 1982; 2:539–546

259. Grossman HJ, Grossman VL, Bhathal PS. The effect of hepatocyte enlargement on the hemodynamic characteristics of the isolated perfused rat liver preparation. Hepatology, 1998; 27:446–451

260. Miyakawa H, Iida S, Leo MA, Greenstein RJ, Zimmon DS, Lieber CS. Pathogenesis of precirrhotic portal hypertension in alcohol-fed baboons. Gastroenterology, 1985; 88:143–150

261. Krogsgaard K, Gluud C, Henriksen JH, Christoffersen P. Correlation between liver morphology and portal pressure in alcoholic liver disease. Hepatology, 1984; 4:699–703

262. Okanoue T. Clinical and experimental studies of the pathophysiology of portal hypertension. Hepatology, 1988; 8:677 (abstract)

263. Mallory FB. Cirrhosis of the liver. Five different types of lestions from which it may arise. Bull John Hopkins Hosp, 1911; 22:69–75

264. Gerber MA, Orr W, Denk H, Schaffner F, Popper H. Hepatocellular hyalin in cholestasis and cirrhosis: its diagnostic significance. Gastroenterology, 1973; 64:89–98

265. MacSween RN. Mallory's ('alcoholic') hyaline in primary biliary cirrhosis. J Clin Pathol, 1973; 26:340–342

266. Sternlieb I. Evolution of the hepatic lesion in Wilson's disease (hepatolenticular degeneration). Prog Liver Dis, 1972; 4:511–525

267. Nayak NC, Sagreiya K, Ramalingaswami V. Indian childhood cirrhosis. The nature and significance of cytoplasmic hyaline of hepatocytes. Arch Pathol, 1969; 88:631–637

268. Wetzel WJ, Alexander RW. Focal nodular hyperplasia of the liver with alcoholic hyalin bodies and cytologic atypia. Cancer, 1979; 44:1322–1326

269. Keeley AF, Iseri OA, Gottlieb LS. Ultrastructure of hyaline cytoplasmic inclusions in a human hepatoma: relationship to Mallory's alcoholic hyalin. Gastroenterology, 1972; 62:280–293

270. Denk H, Gschnait F, Wolff K. Hepatocellar hyalin (Mallory bodies) in long term griseofulvin-treated mice: a new experimental model for the study of hyalin formation. Lab Invest, 1975; 32:773–776

271. Borenfreund E, Bendich A. In vitro demonstration of Mallory body formation in liver cells from rats fed diethylnitrosamine. Lab Invest, 1978; 38:295–303

272. Meierhenry EF, Ruebner BH, Gershwin ME, Hsieh LS, French SW. Mallory body formation in hepatic nodules of mice ingesting dieldrin. Lab Invest, 1981; 44:392–396

273. Yuan Q. Tautomycin induces extensive Mallory body formation in drug primed mouse livers. Hepatology, 1998; 28:A376

274. Janig E, Strumptner C, Fuchsbichler A, Denk H, Zattonkar K. Interaction of stress proteins with misfolded keratins. Eur J Cell Biol, 2005; 84:329–339

275. Yokoo H, Minick OT, Batti F, Kent G. Morphologic variants of alcoholic hyalin. Am J Pathol, 1972; 69:25–40

276. French SW, Ihrig TJ, Norum ML. A method of isolation of Mallory bodies in a purified fraction. Lab Invest, 1972; 26:240–244

277. Tinberg HM, Regan RJ, Geier EA, Peterson GE, French SW. Mallory bodies: isolation of hepatocellular hyalin and electrophoretic

resolution of polypeptide components. Lab Invest, 1978; 39:483–490

278. Denk H, Franke WW, Eckerstorfer R, Schmid E. Kerjaschki D. Formation and involution of Mallory bodies ('alcoholic hyalin') in marine and human liver revealed in immunofluorescence microscopy with antibodies to prekeratin. Proc Natl Acad Sci USA, 1979; 76:4112–4116

279. Denk HF, Kerjaschi WWD. Mallory bodies: new facts and findings. In: Berk PDC, Chalmers TC, ed. Frontiers in liver disease. New York: Thieme-Stratton: 1981: pp 93–105

280. Schirmacher P, Dienes HP, Moll R. De novo expression of nonhepatocellular cytokeratins in Mallory body formation. Virchows Arch, 1998; 432:143–452

281. Denk H, Franke WW, Dragosics B, Zeiler I. Pathology of cytoskeleton of liver cells: demonstration of Mallory bodies (alcoholic hyalin) in murine and human hepatocytes by immunofluorescence microscopy using antibodies to cytokeratin polypeptides from hepatocytes. Hepatology, 1981; 1:9–20

282. French SW. The Mallory body: structure, composition, and pathogenesis. Hepatology, 1981; 1:76–83

283. French SW. Nature, pathogenesis and significance of the Mallory body. Semin Liver Dis, 1981; 1:217–231

284. French SW. Present understanding of the development of Mallory's body. Arch Pathol Lab Med, 1983; 107:445–450

285. Morton JA, Fleming KA, Trowell JM, McGee JO. Mallory bodies— immunohistochemical detection by antisera to unique non-prekeratin components. Gut, 1980; 21:727–733

286. Morton JA, Bastin J, Fleming KA, McMichael A, Burns J, McGee JO. Mallory bodies in alcoholic liver disease: identification of cytoplasmic filament/cell membrane and unique antigenic determinants by monoclonal antibodies. Gut, 1981; 22:1–7

287. Stumptner C, Omary MB, Fickert P, Denk H, Zatloukal K. Hepatocyte cytokeratins are hyperphosphorylated at multiple sites in human alcoholic hepatitis and in a mallory body mouse model. Am J Pathol, 2000; 156:77–90

288. Fleming KA, Morton JA, Barbatis C, Burns J, Canning S, McGee JO. Mallory bodies in alcoholic and non-alcoholic liver disease contain a common antigenic determinant. Gut, 1981; 22:341–344

289. Jensen K, Gluud C. The Mallory body: theories on development and pathological significance (Part 2 of a literature survey). Hepatology, 1994; 20:1330–1342

290. Denk H, Franke WW, Eckerstorfer R, Schmid E, Kerjaschki D. Formation and involution of Mallory bodies ('alcoholic hyalin') in murine and human liver revealed by immunofluorescence microscopy with antibodies to prekeratin. Proc Natl Acad Sci U S A, 1979; 76:4112–4116

291. French SW, Katsuma Y, Ray MB, Swierenga SH. Cytoskeletal pathology induced by ethanol. Ann N Y Acad Sci, 1987; 492:262–276

292. Worman HJ. Cellular intermediate filament networks and their derangement in alcoholic hepatitis. Alcohol Clin Exp Res, 1990; 14:789–804

293. Irie T, Koyama W, Ikeuchi Y, Kanaseki T. On the three-dimensional structure of quick-frozen hepatic Mallory bodies with special reference to the appearance of cytoplasmic vesicles. Cell Struct Funct, 1991; 16:1–16

294. Nakanuma Y, Ohta G. Is mallory body formation a preneoplastic change? A study of 181 cases of liver bearing hepatocellular carcinoma and 82 cases of cirrhosis. Cancer, 1985; 55:2400–2404

295. Akeda S, Fujita K, Kosaka Y, French SW. Mallory body formation and amyloid deposition in the liver of aged mice fed a vitamin A deficient diet for a prolonged period. Lab Invest, 1986; 54:228–233

296. Ray MB, Mendenhall CL, French SW, Gartside PS. Serum vitamin A deficiency and increased intrahepatic expression of cytokeratin antigen in alcoholic liver disease. Hepatology, 1988; 8:1019–1026

297. Ray MB. Distribution patterns of cytokeratin antigen determinants in alcoholic and nonalcoholic liver diseases. Hum Pathol, 1987; 18:61–66

298. Yoshioka K, Kakumu S, Tahara H, Arao M, Fuji A, Hirofuji H, Hayashi T, Kano H. Occurrence of immunohistochemically detected small Mallory bodies in liver disease. Am J Gastroenterol, 1989; 84:535–539

299. Ohta M, Marceau N, Perry G, Manetto V, Gambetti P, Autilio-Gambetti L, Metuzals J, Kawahara H, Cadrin M, French SW. Ubiquitin is present on the cytokeratin intermediate filaments and Mallory bodies of hepatocytes. Lab Invest, 1988; 59:848–856

300. De Vos R, Desmet V. Ultrastructural characteristics of novel epithelial cell types identified in human pathologic liver specimens with chronic ductular reaction. Am J Pathol, 1992; 140:1441–1450

301. Battaler R, Brenner DA. Liver fibrosis J Clin Invest, 2005; 115:209–218

302. Friedman SL. Mechanisms of Disease: mechanisms of hepatic fibrosis and therapeutic implications. Nature Clinical Practice: Gastroenterology & Hepatology, 2004; 1:98–105

303. Pinzani M, Rombouts K. Liver fibrosis: from the bench to clinical targets. Dig Liver Dis, 2004; 36:231–242

304. Karasawa T, Chedid A. Sclerosing hyaline necrosis in noncirrhotic chronic alcoholic hepatitis. Am J Clin Pathol, 1976; 66:802–809

305. Takada A, Nei J, Matsuda Y, Kanayama R. Clinicopathological study of alcoholic fibrosis. Am J Gastroenterol, 1982; 77:660–666

306. Ohnishi K. Epidemiology of alcholic liver desease in Japan. In: Hall P de la M , ed. Alcoholic liver disease. London: Edward Arnold, 1985: pp 167–183

307. Hahn E, Wick G, Pencev D, Timpl R. Distribution of basement membrane proteins in normal and fibrotic human liver: collagen type IV, laminin, and fibronectin. Gut, 1980; 21:63–71

308. Rojkind M. Collagen metabolism in the liver. In: Hall P de la M, ed. Alcoholic liver disease. London: Edward Arnold, 1985: pp 90–112

309. Cassiman D, Libbrecht L, Desmet V, Denef C, Roskams T. Hepatic stellate cell/myofibroblast subpopulations in fibrotic human and rat livers. J Hepatol, 2002; 36:200–209

310. Kinnman N, Francoz C, Barbu V et al. The myofibroblastic conversion of peribiliary fibrogenic cells distinct from hepatic stellate cells is stimulated by platelet-derived growth factor during liver fibrogenesis. Lab Invest, 2003; 83:163–173

311. Bioulac-Sage P. Perisinusoidal and pit cells in liver sinusoids. In: Bioulac-Sage P, Balabaud, C, eds. Sinusoids in human liver: health and disease. Rijswijk: Kupffer Cell Foundation, 1988: pp 39–62

312. Brouwer A. Sinusoidal endothelial cells and perisinusoidal fat-storing cells. In: Arias IM, Jakoby WB, Popper H, Schachter D, Shafritz DA, eds. The liver: biology and pathobiology 2nd edition. New York: Raven, 1988: pp 665–682

313. De Leeuw AM, McCarthy SP, Geerts A, Knook DL. Purified rat liver fat-storing cells in culture divide and contain collagen. Hepatology, 1984; 4:392–403

314. Burt AD, Robertson JL, Heir J, MacSween RN. Desmin-containing stellate cells in rat liver; distribution in normal animals and response to experimental acute liver injury. J Pathol, 1986; 150:29–35

315. Xu L, Hui AY, Albanis E, Arthur MJ et al. Human hepatic stellate cell lines, LX-1 and LX-2: new tools for analysis of hepatic fibrosis. Gut, 2005; 54:142–145

316. Kent G, Gay S, Inouye T, Bahu R, Minick OT, Popper H. Vitamin A-containing lipocytes and formation of type III collagen in liver injury. Proc Natl Acad Sci USA, 1976; 73:3719–3722

317. Minato Y, Hasumura Y, Takeuchi J. The role of fat-storing cells in Disse space fibrogenesis in alcoholic liver disease. Hepatology, 1983; 3:559–566

318. Okanoue T, Burbige EJ, French SW. The role of the Ito cell in perivenular and intralobular fibrosis in alcoholic hepatitis. Arch Pathol Lab Med, 1983; 107:459–463

319. Mak KM, Leo MA, Lieber CS. Alcoholic liver injury in baboons: transformation of lipocytes to transitional cells. Gastroenterology, 1984; 87:188–200

320. Horn T, Junge J, Christoffersen P. Early alcoholic liver injury. Activation of lipocytes in acinar zone 3 and correlation to degree of collagen formation in the Disse space. J Hepatol, 1986; 3:333–340

321. Mak KM, Lieber CS. Lipocytes and transitional cells in alcoholic liver disease: a morphometric study. Hepatology, 1988; 8:1027–1033

322. Bhathal PS. Presence of modified fibroblasts in cirrhotic livers in man. Pathology, 1972; 4:139–144

323. Nakano M, Lieber CS. Ultrastructure of initial stages of perivenular fibrosis in alcohol-fed baboons. Am J Pathol, 1982; 106:145–155

324. Skalli O, Schurch W, Seemayer T et al. Myofibroblasts from diverse pathologic settings are heterogeneous in their content of actin isoforms and intermediate filament proteins. Lab Invest, 1989; 60:275–285

325. Savolainen ER, Leo MA, Timpl R, Lieber CS. Acetaldehyde and lactate stimulate collagen synthesis of cultured baboon liver myofibroblasts. Gastroenterology, 1984; 87:777–787

326. Rudolph R, McClure WJ, Woodward M. Contractile fibroblasts in chronic alcoholic cirrhosis. Gastroenterology, 1979; 76:704–709

327. Friedman SL. Acetaldehyde and alcoholic fibrogenesis: fuel to the fire, but not the spark. Hepatology, 1990; 12:609–612

328. Olaso E, Friedman SL. Molecular regulation of hepatic fibrogenesis. J Hepatol, 1998; 29:836–847

329. Oben JA, Roskams T, Yang S et al. Hepatic fibrogenesis requires sympathetic neurotransmitters. Gut, 2004; 53:438–445

330. Chedid A, Arain S, Snyder A, Mathurin P, Capron F, Naveau S. The immunology of fibrogenesis in alcoholic liver disease. Arch Pathol Lab Med, 2004; 128:1230–1238

331. Arthur MJ. Collagenases and liver fibrosis. J Hepatol, 1995; 22:43–48

332. Arthur MJ, Mann DA, Iredale JP. Tissue inhibitors of metalloproteinases, hepatic stellate cells and liver fibrosis. J Gastroenterol Hepatol, 1998; 13 (suppl):S33–S38

333. Murphy FR, Issa R, Zhou X et al. Inhibition of apoptosis of activated hepatic stellate cells by tissue inhibitor of metalloproteinase-1 is mediated via effects on matrix metalloproteinase inhibition: implications for reversibility of liver fibrosis. J Biol Chem, 2002; 277:11069–1176

334. Potter JJ, Womack L, Mezey E, Anania FA. Transdifferentiation of rat hepatic stellate cells results in leptin expression. Biochem Biophys Res Commun, 1998; 244:178–182

335. Schaffner F. Capillarization of hepatic sinusoids in man. Gastroenterology, 1963; 44:239–242

336. Horn T, Junge J, Christoffersen P. Early alcoholic liver injury: changes of the Disse space in acinar zone 3. Liver, 1985; 5: 301–310

337. Horn T. Alcoholic liver injury: defenestration in non-cirrhotic livers. A scanning electron microscopic study. Hepatology, 1987; 7:77–82

338. Fraser R, Rogers WT, Dobbs BR. Alcohol and the 'liver sieve.' In: Hall de la M P, ed. Alcoholic Liver Disease. Volume 2nd edition. London: Edward Arnold, 1995: pp 248–259

339. Sztark F, Latry P, Quinton A, Balabaud C, Bioulac-Sage P. The sinusoidal barrier in alcoholic patients without liver fibrosis. A morphometric study. Virchows Arch A Pathol, Anat Histopathol, 1986; 409:385–393

340. Horn T. The 'blood-hepatocyte barrier'. A light microscopical transmission and scanning electron microscopic study. Liver, 1986; 6:233–245

341. Oda M, Azuma T, Nishizaki Y et al. Alterations of hepatic sinusoids in liver cirrhosis: their involvement in the pathogenesis of portal hypertension. J Gastroenterol Hepatol, 1989; 4 (suppl 1):111–113

342. Clark SA, Angus HB, Cook HB, George PM, Oxner RB, Fraser R. Defenestration of hepatic sinusoids as a cause of hyperlipoproteinaemia in alcoholics. Lancet, 1988; 2:1225–1227

343. Fraser R, Bowler LM, Day WA. Damage of rat liver sinusoidal endothelium by ethanol. Pathology, 1980; 12:371–376

344. Tsutsumi M, Takase S, Urashima S, Ueshima Y, Kawahara H, Takada A. Serum markers for hepatic fibrosis in alcoholic liver disease: which is the best marker, type III procollagen, type IV collagen, laminin, tissue inhibitor of metalloproteinase, or prolyl hydroxylase? Alcohol Clin Exp Res, 1996; 20:1512–1517

345. Stickel F, Poeschl G, Schuppan D, Conradt C, Strenge-Hesse A, Fuchs FS, Hofmann WJ, Seitz HK. Serum hyaluronate correlates with histological progression in alcoholic liver disease. Eur J Gastroenterol Hepatol, 2003; 15:945–950

346. Poynard T, Imbert-Bismut F, Munteanu M et al. Overview of the diagnostic value of biochemical markers of liver fibrosis (FibroTest, HCV FibroSure) and necrosis (ActiTest) in patients with chronic hepatitis C. Comp Hepatol, 2004; 3:8

347. Fernandez-Checa JC, Garcia-Ruiz C, Colell A et al. Oxidative stress: role of mitochondria and protection by glutathione. Biofactors, 1998; 8:7–11

348. Fataccioli V, Andraud E, Gentil M, French SW, Rouach H. Effects of chronic ethanol administration on rat liver proteasome activities: relationship with oxidative stress. Hepatology, 1999; 29:14–20

349. French SW. Intragastric ethanol infusion model for cellular and molecular studies of alcoholic liver disease. J Biomed Sci, 2001; 8:20–27

350. Arteel GE. Oxidants and antioxidants in alcohol-induced liver disease. Gastroenterology, 2003; 124:778–790

351. Loguercio C, Federico A. Oxidative stress in viral and alcoholic hepatitis. Free Radic Biol Med, 2003; 34:1–10

352. Hoek JB, Cahill A, Pastorino JG. Alcohol and mitochondria: a dysfunctional relationship. Gastroenterology, 2002; 122:2049–2063

353. Venkatraman A, Shiva S, Wigley A et al. The role of iNOS in alcohol-dependent hepatotoxicity and mitochondrial dysfunction in mice. Hepatology, 2004; 40:565–573

354. Zhao M, Laissue JA, Zimmermann A. TUNEL-positive hepatocytes in alcoholic liver disease. A retrospective biopsy study using DNA nick end-labelling. Virchows Arch, 1997; 431:337–444

355. Ziol M, Tepper M, Lohez M et al. Clinical and biological relevance of hepatocyte apoptosis in alcoholic hepatitis. J Hepatol, 2001; 34:254–260

356. Nanji AA. Apoptosis and alcoholic liver disease. Semin Liver Dis, 1998; 18:187–190

357. Rao RK, Seth A, Sheth P. Recent advances in alcoholic liver disease I. Role of intestinal permeability and endotoxemia in alcoholic liver disease. Am J Physiol Gastrointest Liver Physiol, 2004; 286: G881–G884

358. Koop DR, Klopfenstein B, Iimuro Y, Thurman RG. Gadolinium chloride blocks alcohol-dependent liver toxicity in rats treated chronically with intragastric alcohol despite the induction of CYP2E1. Mol Pharmacol, 1997; 51:944–950

359. Ijejima K. Estrogen increases sensitivty of hepatic Kupffer cells to endotoxin. Am J Physiol, 1998; 274:G669–G676

360. Thurman RG. Alcoholic liver injury involves activation of Kupffer cells by endotoxin. Am J Physiol, 1998; 275:G605–G611

361. Leevy CB, Elbeshbeshy HA. Immunology of alcoholic liver disease Clin Liver Dis, 2005; 9:55–66

362. McFarlane IG. Autoantibodies in alcoholic liver disease. Addict Bio, 2000; 5:141–151

363. Thiele GM FTL, Klaasen LW. Immunologic Mechanisms of Alcoholic Liver Injury. Seminars in Liver Disease, 2004; 24:273–287

364. Bernard PH. Liver retransplantation for alcoholic cirrhosis recurring within a 21 month period. Transpl Int, 1996; 9: 524–525

365. Kanagasundaram N, Kakumu S, Chen T, Leevy CM. Alcoholic hyalin antigen (AHAg) and antibody (AHAb) in alcoholic hepatitis. Gastroenterology, 1977; 73:1368–1367

366. Kehl A. Solid phase radioimmunoassay for detection of alcoholic hyaline antigen (AH Ag) and antibody (Anti-AH). Clin Exp Immunol, 1981; 43:214–221

367. Triggs SM, Mills PR, MacSween RN. Sensitisation to Mallory bodies (alcoholic hyalin) in alcoholic hepatitis. J Clin Pathol, 1981; 34:21–24

368. Zetterman RK, Sorrell MF. Immunologic aspects of alcoholic liver disease. Gastroenterology, 1981; 81:616–624

369. Peters M, Liebman HA, Tong MJ, Tinberg HM. Alcoholic hepatitis: granulocyte chemotactic factor from Mallory body-stimulated human peripheral blood mononuclear cells. Clin Immunol Immunopathol, 1983; 28:418–430

370. Manns M, Meyer zum Buschenfelde KH, Hess G. Autoantibodies against liver-specific membrane lipoprotein in acute and chronic liver diseases: studies on organ-, species-, and disease-specificity. Gut, 1980; 21:955–961

371. Perperas A, Tsantoulas D, Portmann B, Eddleston AL, Williams R. Autoimmunity to a liver membrane lipoprotein and liver damage in alcoholic liver disease. Gut, 1981; 22:149–152

372. Meliconi R, Perperas A, Jensen D, Alberti A, McFarlane IG, Eddleston AL, Williams R. Anti-LSP antibodies in acute liver disease. Gut, 1982; 23:603–607

373. Bailey RJ, Krasner N, Eddleston AL. Histocompatibility antigens, autoantibodies, and immunoglobulins in alcoholic liver disease. Br Med J, 1976; 2:727–729

374. Iturriaga H, Pereda T, Estevez A, Ugarte G. Serum immunoglobulin A changes in alcoholic patients. Ann Clin Res, 1977; 9:39–43

375. Morgan MY, Ross MG, Ng CM, Adams DM, Thomas HC, Sherlock S. HLA-B8, immunoglobulins, and antibody responses in alcohol-related liver disease. J Clin Pathol, 1980; 33:488–492

376. Swerdlow MA, Chowdhury LN. IgA deposition in liver in alcoholic liver disease. An index of progressive injury. Arch Pathol Lab Med, 1984; 108:416–419

377. Van De Wiel A. Characteristics of serum IgA and liver IgA deposits in alcoholic liver disease. Hepatology, 1987; 7:95–99

378. Winrow VR, Bird GL, Koskinas J, Blake DR, Williams R, Alexander GJ. Circulating IgA antibody against a 65 kDa heat shock protein in acute alcoholic hepatitis. J Hepatol, 1994; 20:359–363

379. Burt AD, Anthony RS, Hislop WS, Bouchier IA, MacSween RN. Liver membrane antibodies in alcoholic liver disease: 1. Prevalence and immunoglobulin class. Gut, 1982; 23:221–225

380. Anthony RS, Farquharson M, MacSween RN. Liver membrane antibodies in alcoholic liver disease. II. Antibodies to ethanol-altered hepatocytes. J Clin Pathol, 1983; 36:1302–1308

381. Takase S, Tsutsumi M, Kawahara H, Takada N, Takada A. The alcohol-altered liver membrane antibody and hepatitis C virus infection in the progression of alcoholic liver disease. Hepatology, 1993; 17:9–13

382. Tuma DJ, Sorrell MF. The role of acetaldehyde adducts in liver injury. In: Hall P de la M, ed. Alcoholic liver disease 2nd edition. London: Edward Arnold, 1995: pp 89–99

383. Li CJ, Nanji AA, Siakotos AN, Lin RC. Acetaldehyde-modified and 4-hydroxynonenal-modified proteins in the livers of rats with alcoholic liver disease. Hepatology, 1997; 26:650–657

384. Behrens UJ, Hoerner M, Lasker JM, Lieber CS. Formation of acetaldehyde adducts with ethanol-inducible P450IIE1 in vivo. Biochem Biophys Res Commun, 1988; 154:584–590

385. Clot P. Cytochrome P4502E1 hydroxyethyl radical adducts as the major antigen in antibody formation among alcoholics. Gastroenterology, 1996; 111:206–216

386. Niemela O, Parkkila S, Juvonen RO, Viitala K, Gelboin HV, Pasanen M. Cytochromes P450 2A6, 2E1, and 3A and production

387. of protein-aldehyde adducts in the liver of patients with alcoholic and non-alcoholic liver diseases. J Hepatol, 2000; 33:893–901

387. Xu D, Thiele GM, Beckenhauer JL, Klassen LW, Sorrell MF, Tuma DJ. Detection of circulating antibodies to malondialdehyde-acetaldehyde adducts in ethanol-fed rats. Gastroenterology, 1998; 115:686–692

388. Stewart SF, Vidali M, Day CP, Albano E, Jones DE. Oxidative stress as a trigger for cellular immune responses in patients with alcoholic liver disease. Hepatology, 2004; 39:197–203

389. Seki S, Kitada T, Sakaguchi H, Nakatani K, Wakasa K. Pathological significance of oxidative cellular damage in human alcoholic liver disease. Histopathology, 2003; 42:365–371

390. Albano E. Free radical mechanisms in immune reactions associated with alcoholic liver disease. Free Radic Biol Med, 2002; 32: 110–114

391. Muller C, Wolf H, Gottlicher J, Eibl MM. Helper-inducer and suppressor-inducer lymphocyte subsets in alcoholic cirrhosis. Scand J Gastroenterol, 1991; 26:295–301

392. Actis G, Mieli-Vergani G, Portmann B, Eddleston AL, Davis M, Williams R. Lymphocyte cytotoxicity to autologous hepatocytes in alcoholic liver disease. Liver, 1983; 3:8–12

393. Izumi N, Hasumura Y, Takeuchi J. Lymphocyte cytotoxicity for autologous human hepatocytes in alcoholic liver disease. Clin Exp Immunol, 1983; 54:219–224

394. Laso FJ, Madruga JI, Giron JA et al. Decreased natural killer cytotoxic activity in chronic alcoholism is associated with alcohol liver disease but not active ethanol consumption. Hepatology, 1997; 25:1096–1100

395. Batey RG, Cao Q, Gould B. Lymphocyte-mediated liver injury in alcohol-related hepatitis. Alcohol, 2002; 27:37–41

396. Haydon G, Lalor PF, Hubscher SG, Adams DH. Lymphocyte recruitment to the liver in alcoholic liver disease. Alcohol, 2002; 27:29–36

397. McClain CJ, Cohen DA. Increased tumor necrosis factor production by monocytes in alcoholic hepatitis. Hepatology, 1989; 9:349–351

398. Bird G, Sheron N, Goka AJK, Alexander GJ, Williams RS. Increased tumour necrosis factor in severe alcoholic hepatitis. Ann Intern Med, 1990; 112:917–920

399. Felver ME, Mezey E, McGuire M et al. Plasma tumor necrosis factor alpha predicts decreased long-term survival in severe alcoholic hepatitis. Alcohol Clin Exp Res, 1990; 14:255–259

400. Khoruts A, Stahnke L, McClain CJ, Logan G, Allen JI. Circulating tumor necrosis factor, interleukin-1 and interleukin-6 concentrations in chronic alcoholic patients. Hepatology, 1991; 13:267–276

401. Sheron N. Elevated plasma interleukin-6 and increased severity and mortality in alcoholic hepatitis. Clin Exp Immunol, 1991:449–453

402. Daniluk J, Szuster-Ciesielska A, Drabko J, Kandefer-Szerszen M. Serum cytokine levels in alcohol-related liver cirrhosis. Alcohol, 2001; 23:29–34

403. McClain CJ, Hill DB, Song Z, Deaciuc I, Barve S. Monocyte activation in alcoholic liver disease. Alcohol, 2002; 27:53–61

404. Bautista AP. Chronic alcohol intoxication induces hepatic injury through enhanced macrophage inflammatory protein-2 production and intercellular adhesion molecule-1 expression in the liver. Hepatology, 1997; 25:335–342

405. Fisher NC, Neil DA, Williams A, Adams DH. Serum concentrations and peripheral secretion of the beta chemokines monocyte chemoattractant protein 1 and macrophage inflammatory protein 1alpha in alcoholic liver disease. Gut, 1999; 45:416–420

406. Devière J, Vaerman JP, Content J et al. IgA triggers tumor necrosis factor alpha secretion by monocytes: a study in normal subjects and patients with alcoholic cirrhosis. Hepatology, 1991; 13:670–675

407. Bautista AP. Neutrophilic infiltration in alcoholic hepatitis. Alcohol, 2002; 27:17–21

408. Jaeschke H. Neutrophil-mediated tissue injury in alcoholic hepatitis. Alcohol, 2002; 27:23–27

409. Taieb J, Delarche C, Paradis V et al. Polymorphonuclear neutrophils are a source of hepatocyte growth factor in patients with severe alcoholic hepatitis. J Hepatol, 2002; 36:342–348

410. Arteel G, Marsano L, Mendez C, Bentley F, McClain CJ. Advances in alcoholic liver disease. Best Pract Res Clin Gastroenterol, 2003; 17:625–647

411. Marsano L, McClain CJ. Nutrition and alcoholic liver disease. JPEN J Parenter Enteral Nutr, 1991; 15:337–344

412. Mezey E. Dietary fat and alcoholic liver disease. Hepatology, 1998; 28:901–905

413. Halsted CH. Nutrition and alcoholic liver disease. Semin Liver Dis, 2004; 24:289–304

414. Mendenhall CL, Anderson S, Weesner RE, Goldberg SJ, Crolic KA. Protein-calorie malnutrition associated with alcoholic hepatitis.

Veterans Administration Cooperative Study Group on Alcoholic Hepatitis. Am J Med, 1984; 76:211–222

415. Mendenhall C, Roselle GA, Gartside P, Moritz T. Relationship of protein calorie malnutrition to alcoholic liver disease: a reexamination of data from two Veterans Administration Cooperative Studies. Alcohol Clin Exp Res, 1995; 19:635–641

416. Krasner N, Cochran KM, Russell RI, Carmichael HA, Thompson GG. Alcohol and absorption from the small intestine. 1. Impairment of absorption from the small intestine in alcoholics. Gut, 1976; 17:245–248

417. Patek AJ, Jr. Alcohol, malnutrition, and alcoholic cirrhosis. Am J Clin Nutr, 1979; 32:1304–1312

418. Leo MA, Lieber CS. Hepatic fibrosis after long-term administration of ethanol and moderate vitamin A supplementation in the rat. Hepatology, 1983; 3:1–11

419. de la Maza MP, Hirsch S, Nieto S, Petermann M, Bunout D. Fatty acid composition of liver total lipids in alcoholic patients with and without liver damage. Alcohol Clin Exp Res, 1996; 20:1418–1422

420. Ludwig J, McGill DB, Lindor KD. Review: nonalcoholic steatohepatitis. J Gastroenterol Hepatol, 1997; 12:398–403

421. Diehl AM. Obesity and alcoholic liver disease. Alcohol, Alcoholism 2004; 34:81–87

422. Polavarapu R, Spitz DR, Sim JE et al. Increased lipid peroxidation and impaired antioxidant enzyme function is associated with pathological liver injury in experimental alcoholic liver disease in rats fed diets high in corn oil and fish oil. Hepatology, 1998; 27:1317–1323

423. Bode C, Bode JC, Erhardt JG, French BA, French SW. Effect of the type of beverage and meat consumed by alcoholics with alcoholic liver disease. Alcohol Clin Exp Res, 1998; 22:1803–1805

424. Nanji AA, Mendenhall CL, French SW. Beef fat prevents alcoholic liver disease in the rat. Alcohol Clin Exp Res, 1989; 13:15–19

425. Nanji AA, Sadrzadeh SM, Yang EK, Fogt F, Meydani M, Dannenberg AJ. Dietary saturated fatty acids: a novel treatment for alcoholic liver disease. Gastroenterology, 1995; 109:547–554

426. Ronis MJ, Korourian S, Zipperman M, Hakkak R, Badger TM. Dietary saturated fat reduces alcoholic hepatotoxicity in rats by altering fatty acid metabolism and membrane composition. J Nutr, 2004; 134:904–912

427. Diehl AM. Recent events in alcoholic liver disease V. effects of ethanol on liver regeneration. Am J Physiol Gastrointest Liver Physiol, 2005; 288:G1–G6

428. Bucher NL. Liver regeneration: an overview. J Gastroenterol Hepatol, 1991; 6:615–624

429. Duguay L, Coutu D, Hetu C, Joly JG. Inhibition of liver regeneration by chronic alcohol administration. Gut, 1982; 23:8–13

430. Sell S. Comparison of liver progenitor cells in human atypical ductular reactions with those seen in experimental models of liver injury. Hepatology, 1998; 27:317–231

431. Roskams T, Yang SQ, Koteish A et al. Oxidative stress and oval cell accumulation in mice and humans with alcoholic and nonalcoholic fatty liver disease. Am J Pathol, 2003; 163:1301–1311

432. Neuberger J. Transplantation for alcoholic liver disease: a perspective from Europe. Liver Transpl Surg, 1998; 4:S51–S57

433. Péquignot G, Tuyns AJ, Berta JL. Ascitic cirrhosis in relation to alcohol consumption. Int J Epidemiol, 1978; 7:113–120

434. Tuyns AJ, Pequignot G. Greater risk of ascitic cirrhosis in females in relation to alcohol consumption. Int J Epidemiol, 1984; 13:53–57

435. Batey RG, Burns T, Benson RJ, Byth K. Alcohol consumption and the risk of cirrhosis. Med J Aust, 1992; 156:413–416

436. Bellentani S, Saccoccio G, Costa G et al. Drinking habits as cofactors of risk for alcohol induced liver damage. The Dionysos Study Group. Gut, 1997; 41:845–850

437. Gavaler J, Arria AM. Increased susceptibility of women to alcoholic liver disease: Artifactual or real? In: Hall P de la M, ed. Alcoholic liver disease 2nd edition. London: Edward Arnold, 1995: pp 123–133

438. Coates RA, Halliday ML, Rankin JG, Feinman SV, Fisher MM. Risk of fatty infiltration or cirrhosis of the liver in relation to ethanol consumption: a case-control study. Clin Invest Med, 1986; 9:26–33

439. Berglund M. Mortality in alcoholics related to clinical state at first admission. A study of 537 deaths. Acta Psychiatr Scand, 1984; 70:407–416

440. Bunout D, Munoz C, Lopez M et al. Interleukin 1 and tumor necrosis factor in obese alcoholics compared with normal-weight patients. Am J Clin Nutr, 1996; 63:373–376

441. Naveau S, Giraud V, Borotto E, Aubert A, Capron F, Chaput JC. Excess weight risk factor for alcoholic liver disease. Hepatology, 1997; 25:108–111

442. Zimmerman HJ, Ishak KG. Non-alcoholic steatohepatitis and other forms of pseudoalcoholic liver disease. In: Hall P de la M, ed. Alcoholic liver disease 2nd edition. London: Edward Arnold, 1995: pp 175–198

443. Iimuro Y, Frankenberg MV, Arteel GE, Bradford BU, Wall CA, Thurman RG. Female rats exhibit greater susceptibility to early alcohol-induced liver injury than males. Am J Physiol, 1997; 272: G1186–G1194

444. Bosron WF, Lumeng L, Li TK. Genetic polymorphism of enzymes of alcohol metabolism and susceptibility to alcoholic liver disease. Mol Aspects Med, 1988; 10:147–158

445. Tanaka F, Shiratori Y, Yokosuka O, Imazeki F, Tsukada Y, Omata M. Polymorphism of alcohol-metabolizing genes affects drinking behavior and alcoholic liver disease in Japanese men. Alcohol Clin Exp Res, 1997; 21:596–601

446. Chao YC, Young TH, Tang HS, Hsu CT. Alcoholism and alcoholic organ damage and genetic polymorphisms of alcohol metabolizing enzymes in Chinese patients. Hepatology, 1997; 25:112–117

447. Day CP, Bassendine MF. Genetic predisposition to alcoholic liver disease. Gut, 1992; 33:1444–1447

448. Bassendine MF, Day CP. The inheritance of alcoholic liver disease. Baillières Clin Gastroenterol, 1998; 12:317–335

449. Arnon R, Esposti SD, Zern MA. Molecular biological aspects of alcohol-induced liver disease. Alcohol Clin Exp Res, 1995; 19:247–256

450. Agarwal DP. Molecular genetic aspects of alcohol metabolism and alcoholism. Pharmacopsychiatry, 1997; 30:79–84

451. Crabb DW, Matsumoto M, Chang D, You M. Overview of the role of alcohol dehydrogenase and aldehyde dehydrogenase and their variants in the genesis of alcohol-related pathology. Proc Nutr Soc, 2004; 63:49–63

452. Enomoto N, Takase S, Takada N, Takada A. Alcoholic liver disease in heterozygotes of mutant and normal aldehyde dehydrogenase-2 genes. Hepatology, 1991; 13:1071–1075

453. Grove J, Brown AS, Daly AK, Bassendine MF, James OF, Day CP. The RsaI polymorphism of CYP2E1 and susceptibility to alcoholic liver disease in Caucasians: effect on age of presentation and dependence on alcohol dehydrogenase genotype. Pharmacogenetics, 1998; 8:335–342

454. Wodak AD, Saunders JB, Ewusi-Mensah I, Davis M, Williams R. Severity of alcohol dependence in patients with alcoholic liver disease. Br Med J (Clin Res Ed), 1983; 287:1420–1422

455. Lieber CS. CYP2E1: from ASH to NASH. Hepatol Res, 2004; 28:1–11

456. Grove J, Daly AK, Bassendine MF, Gilvarry E, Day CP. Interleukin 10 promoter region polymorphisms and susceptibility to advanced alcoholic liver disease. Gut, 2000; 46:540–545

457. Takamatsu M, Yamauchi M, Maezawa Y, Saito S, Maeyama S, Uchikoshi T. Genetic polymorphisms of interleukin-1beta in association with the development of alcoholic liver disease in Japanese patients. Am J Gastroenterol, 2000; 95:1305–1311

458. List S, Gluud C. A meta-analysis of HLA-antigen prevalences in alcoholics and alcoholic liver disease. Alcohol Alcohol, 1994; 29:757–764

459. Hislop WS, Follett EA, Bouchier IA, MacSween RN. Serological markers of hepatitis B in patients with alcoholic liver disease: a multi-centre survey. J Clin Pathol, 1981; 34:1017–1019

460. Mills PR, Follett EA, Urquhart GE, Clements G, Watkinson G, Macsween RN. Evidence for previous hepatitis B virus infection in alcoholic cirrhosis. Br Med J (Clin Res Ed), 1981; 282:437–438

461. Orholm M, Aldershvile J, Tage-Jensen U, Schlichting P, Nielsen JO, Hardt F, Christoffersen P. Prevalence of hepatitis B virus infection among alcoholic patients with liver disease. J Clin Pathol, 1981; 34:1378–1380

462. Villa E, Rubbiani L, Barchi T. Susceptibility of chronic symptomless HBsAg carriers to ethanol-induced hepatic damage. Lancet, 1982; 2:1243–1244

463. Novick DM, Enlow RW, Gelb AM, Stenger RJ, Fotino M, Winter JW, Yancovitz SR, Schoenberg MD, Kreek MJ. Hepatic cirrhosis in young adults: association with adolescent onset of alcohol and parenteral heroin abuse. Gut, 1985; 26:8–13

464. Pereira FE, Goncalves CS, Zago Mda P. The effect of ethanol intake on the development of hepatocellular carcinoma in HBsAg carriers. Arq Gastroenterol, 1994; 31:42–46

465. Nishiguchi S, Kuroki T, Yabusako T, Seki S, Kobayashi K, Monna T, Otani S, Sakurai M, Shikata T, Yamamoto S. Detection of hepatitis C virus antibodies and hepatitis C virus RNA in patients with alcoholic liver disease. Hepatology, 1991; 14:985–989

466. Shimizu S, Kiyosawa K, Sodeyama T, Tanaka E, Nakano M. High prevalence of antibody to hepatitis C virus in heavy drinkers with chronic liver diseases in Japan. J Gastroenterol Hepatol, 1992; 7:30–35

467. Mendenhall CL, Moritz T, Chedid A et al. Relevance of anti-HCV reactivity in patients with alcoholic hepatitis. VA cooperative Study Group #275. Gastroenterol Jpn, 1993; 28 Suppl 5:95–100

468. Tsutsumi M, Ishizaki M, Takada A. Relative risk for the development of hepatocellular carcinoma in alcoholic patients

with cirrhosis: a multiple logistic-regression coefficient analysis. Alcohol Clin Exp Res, 1996; 20:758–762

469. Encke J. Chronic ethanol consumption inhibits immune responses against hepatitis C virus nonstructural NS5 protein. Hepatology, 1998:A304, 565

470. Pessione F, Degos F, Marcellin P et al. Effect of alcohol consumption on serum hepatitis C virus RNA and histological lesions in chronic hepatitis C. Hepatology, 1998; 27:1717–1722

471. Zhang T, Li Y, Lai JP et al. Alcohol potentiates hepatitis C virus replicon expression. Hepatology, 2003; 38:57–65

472. Rigamonti C, Mottaran E, Reale E et al. Moderate alcohol consumption increases oxidative stress in patients with chronic hepatitis C. Hepatology, 2003; 38:42–49

473. Serfaty L, Poujol-Robert A, Carbonell N, Chazouilleres O, Poupon RE, Poupon R. Effect of the interaction between steatosis and alcohol intake on liver fibrosis progression in chronic hepatitis C. Am J Gastroenterol, 2002; 97:1807–1812

474. Jamal MM, Morgan TR. Liver disease in alcohol and hepatitis C. Best Pract Res Clin Gastroenterol, 2003; 17:649–662

475. Penkower L, Dew MA, Kingsley L et al. Alcohol consumption as a cofactor in the progression of HIV infection and AIDS. Alcohol, 1995; 12:547–552

476. Wang Y, Watson RR. Is alcohol consumption a cofactor in the development of acquired immunodeficiency syndrome? Alcohol, 1995; 12:105–109

477. Bica I, McGovern B, Dhar R et al. Increasing mortality due to end-stage liver disease in patients with human immunodeficiency virus infection. Clin Infect Dis, 2001; 32:492–497

478. Bautista AP. Acute alcohol intoxication and endotoxemia desensitize HIV-1 gp120-induced CC-chemokine production by Kupffer cells. Life Sci, 2001; 68:1939–1934

479. Bautista AP. Chronic alcohol intoxication primes Kupffer cells and endothelial cells for enhanced CC-chemokine production and concomitantly suppresses phagocytosis and chemotaxis. Front Biosci, 2002; 7:117–125

480. Haorah J, Heilman D, Diekmann C et al. Alcohol and HIV decrease proteasome and immunoproteasome function in macrophages: implications for impaired immune function during disease. Cell Immunol, 2004; 229:139–248

481. Strubelt O. Interactions between ethanol and other hepatotoxic agents. Biochem Pharmacol, 1980; 29:1445–1449

482. Zimmerman HJ. Effects of alcohol on other hepatotoxins. Alcohol Clin Exp Res, 1986; 10:3–15

483. Schenker S, Maddrey WC. Subliminal drug-drug interactions: users and their physicians take notice. Hepatology, 1991; 13:995–998

484. Buhler R, Lindros KO, Nordling A, Johansson I, Ingelman-Sundberg M. Zonation of cytochrome P450 isozyme expression and induction in rat liver. Eur J Biochem, 1992; 204:407–412

485. Nyfors A. Liver biopsies from psoriatics related to methotrexate therapy. 3. Findings in post-methotrexate liver biopsies from 160 psoriatics. Acta Pathol Microbiol Scand [A], 1977; 85:511–518

486. Weinstein G. Psoriasis-liver-methotrexate interactions: cooperative study. Arch Dermatol, 1977:36–42

487. Zachariae H, Kragballe K, Sogaard H. Methotrexate induced liver cirrhosis. Studies including serial liver biopsies during continued treatment. Br J Dermatol, 1980; 102:407–412

488. Whiting-O'Keefe QE, Fye KH, Sack KD. Methotrexate and histologic hepatic abnormalities: a meta-analysis. Am J Med, 1991; 90:711–716

489. Langman G, Hall PM, Todd G. Role of non-alcoholic steatohepatitis in methotrexate-induced liver injury. J Gastroenterol Hepatol, 2001; 16:1395–1401

490. Fletcher LM, Powell LW. Hemochromatosis and alcoholic liver disease. Alcohol, 2003; 30:131–136

491. Pietrangelo A. Iron-induced oxidant stress in alcoholic liver fibrogenesis. Alcohol, 2003; 30:121–129

492. Davies PJ. Was Beethoven's cirrhosis due to hemochromatosis? Renal Failure, 1995; 17:77–86

493. Lieber CS. New concepts of the pathogenesis of alcoholic liver disease lead to novel treatments. Curr Gastroenterol Rep, 2004; 6:60–65

494. Levitsky J, Mailliard ME. Diagnosis and therapy of alcoholic liver disease. Semin Liver Dis, 2004; 24:233–247

495. Colell A, Garcia-Ruiz C, Miranda M et al. Selective glutathione depletion of mitochondria by ethanol sensitizes hepatocytes to tumor necrosis factor. Gastroenterology, 1998; 115:1541–1551

496. Carmichael FJ, Orrego H, Saldivia V, Israel Y. Effect of propylthiouracil on the ethanol-induced increase in liver oxygen consumption in awake rats. Hepatology, 1993; 18:415–421

497. Lieber CS. The discovery of the microsomal ethanol oxidizing system and its physiologic and pathologic role. Drug Metab Rev, 2004; 36:511–529

498. Nanji AA, Zakim D, Rahemtulla A et al. Dietary saturated fatty acids down-regulate cyclooxygenase-2 and tumor necrosis factor alfa and reverse fibrosis in alcohol-induced liver disease in the rat. Hepatology, 1997; 26:1538–1545

499. Nanji AA, Rahemtulla A, Daly T, Khwaja S, Miao L, Zhao S, Tahan SR. Cholesterol supplementation prevents necrosis and inflammation but enhances fibrosis in alcoholic liver disease in the rat. Hepatology, 1997; 26:90–97

500. Watt KDS, McCashland TM. Transplantation in the alcoholic patient. Semin Liv Dis, 2004; 24:249–255

501. Lucey MR, Merion RM, Henley KS, Campbell DA, Jr., Turcotte JG, Nostrant TT, Blow FC, Beresford TP. Selection for and outcome of liver transplantation in alcoholic liver disease. Gastroenterology, 1992; 102:1736–1741

502. Tome S, Martinez-Rey C, Gonzalez-Quintela A. Influence of superimposed alcoholic hepatitis on the outcome of liver transplantation for end-stage alcoholic liver disease. J Hepatol, 2002; 36:793–798

503. Farges O, Saliba F, Farhamant H, Samuel D, Bismuth A, Reynes M, Bismuth H. Incidence of rejection and infection after liver transplantation as a function of the primary disease: possible influence of alcohol and polyclonal immunoglobulins. Hepatology, 1996; 23:240–248

504. Foster PF, Fabrega F, Karademir S, Sankary HN, Mital D, Williams JW. Prediction of abstinence from ethanol in alcoholic recipients following liver transplantation. Hepatology, 1997; 25:1469–1477

505. DiMartini A, Jain A, Irish W, Fitzgerald MG, Fung J. Outcome of liver transplantation in critically ill patients with alcoholic cirrhosis: survival according to medical variables and sobriety. Transplantation, 1998; 66:298–302

506. Howard L, Fahy T, Wong P, Sherman D, Gane E, Williams R. Psychiatric outcome in alcoholic liver transplant patients. Q J Med, 1994; 87:731–736

507. Berlakovich GA, Steininger R, Herbst F, Barlan M, Mittlbock M, Muhlbacher F. Efficacy of liver transplantation for alcoholic cirrhosis with respect to recidivism and compliance. Transplantation, 1994; 58:560–565

508. Baddour N. The prevalence, rate of onset and spectrum of histologic liver disease in alcohol abusing liver allograft recipients. Gastroenterology, 1992:A779

509. Pageaux GP. Alcoholism recurrence influences the clinical course of patients transplanted for alcoholism. J Hepatol, 1995; 23 (suppl):138

510. Burra P, Mioni D, Cecchetto A et al. Histological features after liver transplantation in alcoholic cirrhotics. J Hepatol, 2001; 34:716–722

511. Lucey MR, Carr K, Beresford TP et al. Alcohol use after liver transplantation in alcoholics: a clinical cohort follow-up study. Hepatology, 1997; 25:1223–1227

512. Conjeevaram HS, Hart J, Lissoos TW et al. Rapidly progressive liver injury and fatal alcoholic hepatitis occurring after liver transplantation in alcoholic patients. Transplantation, 1999; 67:1562–1568

513. French SW. Animal models of alcohol-associated liver injury. In: Hall P de la M, ed. Alcoholic liver disease 2nd edition. London: Edward Arnold, 1995: pp 279–296

514. Tsukamoto H, Reidelberger RD, French SW, Largman C. Long-term cannulation model for blood sampling and intragastric infusion in the rat. Am J Physiol, 1984; 247:R595–R599

515. Tsukamoto H, French SW, Benson N et al. Severe and progressive steatosis and focal necrosis in rat liver induced by continuous intragastric infusion of ethanol and low fat diet. Hepatology, 1985; 5:224–232

516. Halsted CH, Villanueva JA, Devlin AM. Folate deficiency disturbs hepatic methionine metabolism and promotes liver injury in the ethanol-fed micropig. Proc Natl Acad Sci USA, 2002; 99:10072–10077

517. Villanueva JA, Halsted CH. Hepatic transmethylation reactions in micropigs with alcoholic liver disease. Hepatology, 2004; 39:1303–1130

518. Ji C, Deng Q, Kaplowitz N. Role of TNF-alpha in ethanol-induced hyperhomocysteinemia and murine alcoholic liver injury. Hepatology, 2004; 40:442–451

519. Ji C, Kaplowitz N. Hyperhomocysteinemia, endoplasmic reticulum stress, and alcoholic liver injury. World J Gastroentero, 2004; 10:1699–1708

520. McClain CJ, Hill DB, Song Z et al. S-Adenosylmethionine, cytokines, and alcoholic liver disease. Alcohol, 2002; 27:185–192

521. Xu A, Wang Y, Keshaw H, Xu LY, Lam KS, Cooper GJ. The fat-derived hormone adiponectin alleviates alcoholic and nonalcoholic fatty liver diseases in mice. J Clin Invest, 2003; 112:91–100

522. Tomita K, Azuma T, Kitamura N et al. Pioglitazone prevents alcohol-induced fatty liver in rats through up-regulation of c-Met. Gastroenterology, 2004; 126:873–885

523. Nakajima T, Kamijo Y, Tanaka N et al. Peroxisome proliferator-activated receptor alpha protects against alcohol-induced liver damage. Hepatology, 2004; 40:972–980

524. Devenyi P, Robinson GM, Roncari DA. Alcohol and high-density lipoproteins. Can Med Assoc J, 1980; 123:981–984

525. Duhamel G, Nalpas B, Goldstein S, Laplaud PM, Berthelot P, Chapman MJ. Plasma lipoprotein and apolipoprotein profile in alcoholic patients with and without liver disease: on the relative roles of alcohol and liver injury. Hepatology, 1984; 4:577–585

526. Parry CDH. Alcohol policy and public health in South Africa, Cape Town: Oxford Press, 1998

527. Mandayam S, Jamal MM, Morgan TR. Epidemiology of alcoholic liver disease. Semin Liver Dis, 2004; 24:217–232

Non-alcoholic fatty liver disease

Elizabeth M. Brunt

Introduction

Over the 25 years following the seminal publication of Ludwig et al.'s[1] 'Nonalcoholic steatohepatitis: a hitherto unnamed disease', there has been increasing acceptance of the entity as a bona fide, significant and indeed common form of chronic liver disease. During the past 5 years non-alcoholic steatohepatitis (NASH) has been recognized as the hepatic manifestation of the metabolic syndrome, characterized by obesity, insulin resistance or diabetes, hyperlipidaemia and hypertension (Table 7.1).[2–5] There has been an exponential growth in investigations into epidemiology, clinical associations, pathophysiological pathways and early therapeutic intervention trials. Microscopic examination remains central for both diagnostic and research purposes.[6]

The increasing incidence of obesity, calculated to approach 40% of the US population by the year 2025[7] and the attendant rise in insulin resistance and type 2 diabetes in up to 10% of obese subjects,[3,8] are concerns for significant health and economic impacts of these disorders.[9] Disconcertingly, these statistics are neither exclusive to adults, nor to Western cultures.

Nomenclature

The descriptive term, non-alcoholic, is not ideal as it groups together divergent entities that result in steatosis.[6]

Additionally, no other liver disease currently is a 'non' disease. For known clinical associations of entities that relate to non-alcoholic fatty liver disease, some authors have recommended use of the terms that link to the aetiology,[9a] such as 'MSSH' (metabolic syndrome steatohepatitis)[2,10,11] or 'drug-induced' steatohepatitis, when appropriate.[12]

Just as the clinician cannot diagnose steato*hepatitis* with clinical tests, the pathologist cannot always discern *non-alcoholic* by microscopic evaluation.[13] Ludwig recommended the histological features be classified as 'steatohepatitis', regardless of aetiology.[14] A suggestion has been made to align histopathological diagnoses with currently accepted diagnostic terminology for other forms of chronic liver disease[15,16] such that the pathologists' diagnoses reflect presence of microscopic lesions and *pattern of injury* (i.e. steatohepatitis), and separately state a clinical association, if known and provided (i.e. obesity, diabetes, as examples).

However, in recognition of the widespread acceptance of the rubrics 'non-alcoholic steatohepatitis' (NASH) popularized by Ludwig et al.[1] and the broader term, 'non-alcoholic fatty liver disease', (NAFLD) these are the terms used in this chapter.

Background

NAFLD was recognized as a distinct, potentially progressive liver disease with histological similarities to alcoholic liver

Table 7.1	Metabolic syndrome[1]

1. Obesity: BMI ≥30 kg/m² or waist : hip ratio >0.9 (males), >0.85 (females)
2. Hypertension: blood pressure ≥140/90 mmHg
3. Dyslipidemia: low HDL <0.9 mmol/L and/or hypertriglyceridemia: >1.7 mmol/L
4. Microalbuminuria: urinary albumin excretion >20 μg/min

At least two of the above plus

5. Type 2 diabetes mellitus **OR** Insulin resistance **OR** impaired glucose tolerance

[1] Panel. Executive summary of the Third Report of the National Cholesterol Education Program (NCEP) expert panel on detection, evaluation, and treatment of high blood cholesterol in adults (Adult Treatment Panel III). JAMA 2001; 285:2486–2497. Copyright © (2001) American Medical Association. All rights reserved.

disease in obese subjects by pathologists decades ago. Rokitansky stated in 1839 that 'fat accumulation may be the primary affection upon which the granular shaped cirrhosis develops'; it was in the 1950s that studies documented and discussed the possible link(s) of fatty liver with morbid obesity,[17] nutritional disorders, diabetes and cirrhosis.[18] Thaler documented the presence of steatosis in 26.5% of his series of 10 900 liver biopsies in a 1975 review.[19] This insightful review discussed putative or known processes and associated culprits that may result in hepatic steatosis and included many discussed today: reduction of lipid export (malnutrition; certain medications), increased lipid delivery to the liver (weight reduction therapy, small-bowel bypass surgery, over-nutrition, hyperlipoproteinemia), increased hepatic lipid synthesis (over-nutrition; alcoholism; hyperlipoproteinemia), and reduced lipid oxidation (alcoholism). Thaler recognized the link of obesity and 'diabetic fatty liver'; although earlier studies had shown an increased prevalence of cirrhosis in diabetics,[20–23] he suggested the body of evidence did not support a cirrhotogenic role for fatty liver and suggested other unidentified 'factors' were important for that progression.

Histopathological studies in patients with clinically apparent liver disease related to obesity but not alcohol,[17,24–32] diabetes,[21,32–35] in patients who later developed glucose intolerance and/or diabetes,[36] and evaluation of liver biopsies from subjects undergoing surgical bypass procedures for morbid obesity[25,37–41] documented lesions already known in alcoholic fatty liver disease and that we now recognize as NAFLD and NASH. Previously, the entity was referred to by investigators that emphasized either the histological findings or presumed aetiology: non-alcoholic fatty liver with alcoholic hyaline,[42] non-alcoholic fatty hepatitis,[43] fatty liver hepatitis,[24,44] diabetic hepatitis,[35,36] steatofibrosis,[39] 'alcohol-like' liver disease,[45] non-alcoholic steatonecrosis,[46,47] pseudoalcoholic liver disease,[48] and idiopathic steatohepatitis.[49]

Prevalence of NAFLD and NASH

NAFLD is a global problem. In addition to Western countries, NASH is recognized in the Middle East,[50] in cultures that are strictly non-alcoholic,[51] and in Asia.[52,53] In the USA, adult[54–56] and paediatric subjects of Hispanic ethnicity[57–59] have higher prevalence of NASH. By contrast there is a lower prevalence of NASH (and cryptogenic cirrhosis presumed to be due to NASH) in African Americans, in spite of increased incidence of obesity and diabetes in this ethnic group.[54,60]

While histological confirmation is considered pivotal for an accurate diagnosis, liver biopsy is neither warranted nor ethical for population studies. The true prevalence of both NAFLD and NASH are elusive due to the lack of definitive laboratory tests. In studies done to date, ascertainment methods and both clinical and histopathological definitions have varied. Despite these difficulties, NAFLD is currently considered the most common cause of asymptomatic chronic liver test elevation.[7,55,61,62] Yu et al. have suggested that NAFLD is likely to be more common in the US population than hepatitis C (1.3–2.0%), alcoholic liver disease (1%), hepatitis B (0.3–0.4%), hereditary haemochromatosis (1 : 200–1 : 400 of northern European descent) and the chronic liver diseases with low prevalence autoimmune hepatitis, primary biliary cirrhosis, primary sclerosing cholangitis, A1AT deficiency and Wilson disease.[63]

Fundamental to all studies is the concept of 'non-alcoholic, yet the exact definition of 'insignificant alcohol use' is not uniform; values in published studies have ranged from <20 g/wk to <140 g/wk.[6,64] Furthermore, the difficulties of accuracy in self-reporting alcohol use and the utility of standardized questionnaires, confirmed in a group of clinically considered NAFLD subjects,[65] are recognized, but to date, standardized methods of assessment are not uniformly utilized. Intriguingly, the study of Dixon et al. of morbidly obese subjects showed that use of alcohol up to 210 g/week was 'protective' for developing NASH; the authors speculated this may be due to the effects of alcohol consumption on hyperinsulinemia.[66] In addition, gut-derived endogenously produced alcohol has been implicated in the complex of cellular events that may result in the hepatic manifestations of NASH.[67,68]

Table 7.2 shows historical studies of prevalence based on ultrasound detection of 'bright liver'[69–71] and in autopsy series.[44,72–74] The results of these early studies emphasize the relationship of steatosis and obesity. Other factors associated with hepatic steatosis are listed.

Population screening

Two recent studies utilized detailed anthropomorphic and biochemical data from the third US National Health and Nutrition Examination Survey (1988–1994) of over 15 000 American adult subjects and considered elevated liver biochemical tests (in the absence other documentable forms of chronic liver disease or reported alcohol use >2 drinks/day) as surrogate markers of NAFLD.[55,56,62] Ruhl et al.[55] excluded diabetics in analyses; of the 2.8% of non-diabetic adults

Table 7.2 Prevalence of fatty liver in adults*

Ultrasound series

Author	Database (n)	Prevalence of bright liver	Associated factors
Nomura, 1988[69]	Japanese population screening; n = 2574; all ages included	14%	Age: >19 yr–<49 yr Obesity, alcohol (in men), elevated serum triglycerides
Lonardo, 1997[70]	Diagnostic evaluation; n = 363 Italian adults	19.8%	Increased BMI Mean age 56 yr; controls 63 yr Elevated triglycerides, cholesterol, apoB
Bellentani, 2000[71]	Subpopulation of Dionysus Study Italian adults n = 257	16.4% (controls) 75.8% (obese) 46.4% (alcohol) 94.5% (obese + alcohol)	Obesity; alcohol When both present, obesity > alcohol

* Not exclusive of alcohol use

Autopsy series

Author	n	Subjects	Prevalence	Associated factors	Comments
Hilden, 1977[72]	503 adults	Consecutive victims of car accidents	24% overall 1% in <20 yr 18% in 20–40 yr 39% in >60 yr	Increased age Increased weight	Steatosis is 'normal' aging process
Hornboll, 1982[73]	678 adults	Consecutive, not selected	11% overall 25% in overweight subjects with short disease duration	Age up to 40 yr; not older Degree of overweight Diabetes	Diabetes not independent factor from weight
Underwood-Ground, 1984[74]	166 male adults	Accidental death, not related to alcohol	21%	Not assessed	
Wanless, 1990[44]	351 adults	Negative history for alcohol in all 207 obese 144 non-oebse	Steatosis: — Obese: 29.2% — Lean: 7.1% Steatohepatitis: — Obese: 18.5% — Lean: 2.7%	Steatosis: Degree of obesity Steatohepatitis: Additive effects of Type 2 DM, preterminal weight loss, amount of steatosis	Severe fibrosis in obese patients explained by higher prevalence of diabetes

that have elevated ALT (fasting level > 43 U/L), 65% were overweight (BMI ≥ 25 kg/m^2) or obese (BMI ≥ 30 kg/m^2). Other associations were younger age, male gender, and Mexican–American ethnicity (8.4% v 2.6% non-Hispanic Caucasians, and 1.9% non-Hispanic blacks). Impaired fasting glucose levels, higher BMI and waist : hip ratio (a measure of visceral adiposity), increased fasting serum leptin, triglycerides, and insulin levels, and criteria of metabolic syndrome were univariate factors associated with elevated ALT; >40% of subjects with elevated ALT had defined criteria for metabolic syndrome. Subjects with criteria for metabolic syndrome were 5 times more likely to have ele-

vated ALT compared with the remainder of the population. The investigators noted that if newer, lower values for 'normal' ALT had been applied (19 U/L for women, 30 U/L for men),[75] the results of elevated ALT would have risen to 12.4% for men and 13.9% for women.

Clark et al.[56] included diabetics and evaluated both AST and ALT. The cut-off values for ALT were lower than Ruhl et al.: AST > 37 IU/L, ALT > 40 IU/L for men, AST or ALT > 31 IU/L for women. 7.9% of the study population had elevated aminotransferases; of these, 69% were considered unexplained, and therefore considered as NAFLD. This results in a total of 5.5% adults in the NHANES population.

If newly recommended values for upper limits of ALT[75] were applied, there would be 26% incidence of elevated ALT, 81.7% of which were unexplained, for a total of 21.2% of the US NHANES study population with unexplained liver test elevations. Elevated ALT was associated with some features similar to that of Ruhl et al.,[55] but a notable difference was the increased prevalence of elevated ALT among non-Hispanic blacks (8.1%) compared with 1.9% in the study of Ruhl et al.[55]

Important and acknowledged difficulties with estimates derived from NHANES data include lack of histological confirmation,[55,56,62] a possible source of overestimation, and establishing 'normal' ALT values in the increasingly obese population.[75,76] On the other hand, two possible sources of underestimation include the use of frozen sera for ALT,[61] and the concept of screening with serological liver tests, as tests may be 'normal' in patients with chronic liver disease(s), including hepatitis C[76] and NAFLD.[77]

NAFLD in unusual patient settings

There are unusual patient settings for which the prevalence of NAFLD/NASH is not established. Biopsy-based studies introduced and confirmed that NASH may occur in non-obese individuals.[3,78] NAFLD and NASH have also been documented in subjects with normal ALT;[77,79,80] potential donors for living-related liver transplantation,[77] subjects undergoing obesity surgery,[79] and patients undergoing cholecystectomy.[80]

Other settings in which NASH has been reported, but for which prevalence is not known, include forms of lipodystrophy, conditions due to varying mutations of peroxisome proliferator activated receptor gamma, PPARγ, alleles that results in aberrant adipose tissue development and insulin resistance;[11] insulin resistance syndromes outside the setting of metabolic syndrome, such as polycystic ovary syndrome; metabolic diseases of childhood (see below); and hypothalamic or pituitary dysfunction, including craniopharyngioma and Prader–Willi syndrome.[81–83] Hypothyroidism, noted in 6%–15% of 33 and 174 subjects respectively with NASH[78,84] compared with 7.2% of 442 liver disease controls,[84] has been cautiously interpreted as an associated risk factor worth further exploration.[84] The inherent difficulties in discerning prevalence of NAFLD/NASH in cases of cryptogenic cirrhosis are discussed below.

Drugs, toxins and NAFLD

Table 7.3 shows a variety of medications, occupational toxins and illicit drugs that have been implicated in NASH[12,85–87] or associated with hepatic steatosis.[88] Farrell estimates, however, that <2% of NASH is attributable to drugs as there are few definitive histological studies.[12] Stravitz et al.[86] and Farrell[12] emphasize the concept that many of the drugs reported to cause NASH may be exacerbating the condition(s) in individuals with other manifestations of obesity and/or metabolic syndrome. Mechanisms postulated to be related to drug-induced phospholipidosis, steatosis and steatohepatitis[12,86] include: direct hepatoxicity

Table 7.3	Drugs, occupational exposures and toxins

Drugs implicated in NASH*

Nifedipine[a]
Diltiazem[b]
Tamoxifen[c,d]
Oestrogens[c,d]
Corticosteroids[e]
*Methotrexate[c,d,f]

Toxins implicated in NASH

Industrial solvent dimtethylformamide[g]
Paint thinners and solvents[c]
Petrochemical exposure[h]
Rapeseed cooking oil[i]
Cocaine[j]

* See text

References

a. Babany G, Uzzan F, Larrey D, et al. Alcohol-like liver lesions induced by nifedipine. Hepatology, 1989; 9:252–255

b. Itoh S, Tsukada Y. Clinico-pathological and electron microscopical studies on a coronary dilating agent: 4,4'-diethyl-aminoehtoxyhexestrol-induced liver injuries. Acta Hepato-Gastroenterology, 1973; 20:204–215

c. Farrell GC. Drugs and steatohepatitis. Seminars in Liver Disease, 2002; 22:185–194

d. Stravitz RT, Sanyal AJ. Drug-induced steatohepatitis. Clinics in Liver Disease, 2003; 7:435–451

e. Itoh S, Igarashi M, Tsukada Y, Ichinoe A. Nonalcoholic fatty liver with alcoholic hyalin after long-term glucocorticoid therapy. Acta Hepato-Gastroenterology, 1977; 24:415–418

f. Langman G, Hall PM, Todd G. Role of non-alcoholic steatohepatitis in methotrexate-induced liver injury. J Gastroenterol Hepatol, 2001; 16:1395–1401

g. Redlich CA, West AB, Fleming L, True LD, Cullen MR, Riely CA. Clinical and pathologic characteristics associated with occupational exposure to dimethylformamide. Gastroenterology 1990; 99:748–757

h. Cotrim HP, Andrade ZA, Parana R, Portugal M, Lyra LG, Freitas LA. Nonalcoholic steatohepatitis: a toxic liver disease in industrial workers. Liver, 1999; 19:299–304

i. Solis-Herruzo JA, Vidal JV, Colina F, Castellano G, Munoz-Yague MT, Morillas JD. Clinico-biochemical evolution and late hepatic lesions in the toxic oil syndrome. Gastroenterology, 1987; 93:558–568

j. Wanless IR, Dore S, Gopinath N et al. Histopathology of cocaine hepatotoxicity. Report of four patients. Gastroenterolgy, 1990; 98:497–501

and mitochondrial injury (coralgil, amiodarone, possibly tamoxifen); aggravation of underlying obesity-related conditions of hyperinsulinemia or hyperlipidemia (tamoxifen, oestrogens, corticosteroids), or exacerbation of pre-existing fibrosis (methotrexate). Finally, some reported cases may be spurious associations in which alcohol has not been adequately excluded, or circumstantial in patients with other conditions of metabolic syndrome (calcium channel blockers).[12]

Highly active antiretroviral therapy (HAART) for HIV has been associated with lipodystrophy and insulin resistance, but many of the histological lesions described in the related hepatoxicity of these agents, specifically cholestasis and hepatocellular injury, are not characteristic of NASH.[12]

Incidence of NASH in NAFLD

NAFLD is considered to be a spectrum that ranges from 'simple' steatosis on one end to steatohepatitis (NASH), fibrosis, and cirrhosis on the other.[89] By definition, therefore, studies quoted to estimate the prevalence of NASH, fibrosis and cirrhosis are based on individuals selected for histological evaluation by liver biopsy or transplantation; results of such studies are influenced by clinical findings and selection criteria. Published series include ranges from 2–5%[7,8,64] to 20–30% in subjects with metabolic syndrome,[3] obese individuals,[44] and morbidly obese patients undergoing surgical bypass procedures[66,90] to the highest value of 69.5% in a series of obese subjects.[91] A study reported from a single transplant centre[92] documented histological NASH in 2.6% of 1207 native hepatectomies of patients with end-stage liver disease undergoing liver transplant.

Value of liver biopsy in NAFLD

Liver biopsy remains the 'gold standard' for diagnosis in NASH as there are no imaging tests, serological or other laboratory tests that can replace liver tissue analysis for diagnosis, evaluation of the extent of active injury, the presence and character of fibrosis, and presence and degree of architectural remodeling.[6,15,16,93–95] Of equal importance is the value of biopsy for exclusion of other causes of liver disease in the clinical setting of marker-negative, unexplained liver enzyme elevations.[15,16,96] For example, liver test abnormalities in type 1 diabetics may be associated with histological findings of accumulation of glycogen in hepatocytes—hepatic glycogenosis,[97,98] or a recently described pattern of patchy dense perisinsoidal fibrosis, 'diabetic hepatosclerosis'[99] without steatosis (Chapter 17). Skelly et al.[100] showed in the study of 354 biopsies for unexplained abnormal liver function tests that while 34% had steatohepatitis, and 32% had steatosis, 9% remained unexplained and 6% were 'normal'; the remainder (13%) had features that led to subsequently confirmed, yet previously undiagnosed disease, including autoimmune hepatitis, haemochromatosis, primary biliary cirrhosis, sarcoid and drug-related injury.

As discussed in other forms of chronic liver disease, sampling 'error' in liver biopsy is a concern in NAFLD. Merriman et al.[101] studied 24 sets of paired right and left lobe liver biopsies from morbidly obese patients; there was 79% agreement in the amounts of steatosis, 61% in degree of lobular inflammation and 67% agreement in fibrosis score. Ratziu et al.[101a] studied 51 patients with NAFLD in whom two percutaneous samples were obtained. Discordance rates for the presence of ballooning were 18%. Furthermore there was discordance of 1 stage or more in 41%. Janiec et al.[101b] could detect no appreciable difference in grade between right and left lobes when they compared paired biopsies in patients undergoing bariatric surgery but again noted variation in staging. This heterogeneity of the degree of fibrosis was also noted by Goldstein et al.[101c] who stressed the importance of adequate biopsy length in assessing stage. Variability of this degree, particularly in fibrosis scores due

to sampling, has important implications in natural history studies as well as interpretation of results of treatment trials.[102]

Several clinico-pathological studies have emphasized the value of distinguishing the biopsy findings of NAFLD from those of NASH by showing significant differences in calculated indices or euglycemic clamp measures of insulin resistance, glucose homeostasis, laboratory values, metabolic syndrome features and natural history between the respective subject groups.[3,103–107] Interestingly, while this confirms the importance of utilization of specific criteria for diagnosis, there remain differences in 'required' lesions and injury pattern among experienced liver pathologists.[16]

Histopathological findings in NAFLD and NASH

Histopathological descriptions of NASH[1,13,14,24,30,32,38,39,44,45,48,104,108–113] have noted a spectrum of features similar to many known for alcoholic steatosis and steatohepatitis: specifically, macrovesicular steatosis, hepatocellular ballooning, lobular inflammation which includes a component of polymorphonuclear leukocytes, zone 3 perisinusoidal fibrosis and Mallory's hyaline (Mallory bodies). Clinical and laboratory studies have validated these lesions by demonstrating correlations with clinical features of metabolic syndrome[3,77,103,114] and with known pathogenetic processes[7,115–118] (see below).

Contrary to a commonly stated theme in the literature, however, NAFLD and NASH are not always histologically 'identical' to alcoholic liver disease; there are lesions of alcoholic hepatitis that are not described to date in NAFLD or NASH.[15,109,119] Specifically, sclerosing hyaline necrosis, the veno-occlusive lesion of alcoholic liver disease, ductular proliferation (ductular reaction), cholangiolitis, and acute cholestasis (Chapter 6) are not lesions described in NAFLD or NASH. A comparison of biopsies from non-alcoholic subjects, outpatient alcoholics and hospitalized alcoholics showed less necroinflammatory activity in the former two groups.[111] Ludwig et al.[14] and Burt[13] have commented that steatohepatitis with abundant Mallory's hyaline is more likely of alcoholic rather than non-alcoholic origin.

A review of the literature detailed the frequency of specific features noted in studies in adults and children.[15] Differences are present in requirements for, and quantitative analysis of, most of the lesions associated with NASH. A consideration not often discussed is that variances in histological lesions may actually reflect true variances in the specific metabolic status of the patient at the time of the biopsy. This area may receive further consideration as current studies in NASH are including more detailed studies of insulin resistance and related metabolic and inflammatory parameters.

An assessment of histological features of NASH and requirements for making the diagnosis among 10 international hepatopathologists who have published in NAFLD and NASH was included in a recent review.[16] A unifying

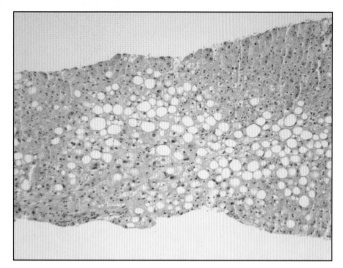

Fig. 7.1 • Non-cirrhotic non-alcoholic steatohepatitis is characterized by zone 3 accentuation of lesions, as shown in this low power view. H&E.

theme was that the diagnosis of NASH results from evaluation of a combination of lesions.

Non-cirrhotic steatohepatitis

In recognition that: (i) in cirrhosis, vascular landmarks and relationships are remodeled, and (ii) many or all of the active lesions of steatohepatitis may no longer exist in established cirrhosis, the lesions of non-cirrhotic and cirrhotic NASH will be discussed separately. As in other forms of liver disease, the overall pattern of injury is important in adult NASH (Fig. 7.1). Steatosis and necroinflammatory lesions in non-cirrhotic NASH are frequently noted as zone 3 predominant, rather than nonzonal.[15,119] This accentuation may not be as common in paediatric NASH,[120] as discussed below.

Steatosis

Processes that are reported to result in macrovesicular steatosis are listed in Table 7.4. Pathological conditions that result in predominantly or purely microvesicular steatosis, for example, Reye Syndrome, are clinically characterized by precipitous onset and markedly increased risk of short-term mortality. These conditions are not, therefore, included here but are referred to elsewhere (see Chapter 17).

Implied in discussions of NAFLD and NASH therefore is the presence of predominantly macrovesicular or large droplet steatosis. It is recognized that 'small amounts' of steatosis are common in liver biopsies,[13] and to date, amounts of steatosis to be considered 'pathological' are not known. This is a seemingly critical determination. A commonly accepted normal value for liver steatosis of 5% is based on lipid content measurements.[13] Steatosis is a minimum criterion for a diagnosis of NAFLD, and a hallmark of the spectrum of lesions considered in non-cirrhotic NAFLD and NASH. It was reported present in 100% of 433 cases of NASH from 13 series published between 1979 and 2000.[15] Studies that utilized oil red O stain for steatosis often report much greater amounts than those with standard H&E staining;

| Table 7.4 | Conditions associated with predominantly macrovesicular steatosis |

- **Alcoholic liver disease**

- **Non-alcoholic fatty liver disease and non-alcoholic steatohepatitis**
  - Obesity
  - Metabolic disorders of insulin resistance
    - Metabolic syndrome, syndrome X, insulin resistance syndrome
    - Type 2 diabetes
    - Alstrom syndrome, Bardet–Beidl syndrome
    - Polycystic ovary syndrome
    - Lipodystrophy syndromes; PPARγ mutations
  - Leptin deficiencies or resistance
    - Hypothalamic obesity; Prader–Willi syndrome

- **Drugs and toxins** (see Table 7.3)

- **Viral hepatitis**
  - HCV >>>> HBV
  - Labrea hepatitis (Hepatitis D)

- **Disorders of lipoprotein metabolism**
  - Abetalipoproteinemia
  - Familial hypobetalipoproteinemia
  - Dorfman–Chinarin syndrome
  - Pseudoneonatal adrenoleukodystrophy

- **Nutritional disorders other than obesity**
  - Total parenteral nutrition
  - Protein-calorie malnutrition (kwashiorkor)
  - Pancreatic insufficiency with bone marrow suppression, Shwachman syndrome
  - Obesity surgery: J-I bypass, gastric bypass, gastroplasty
  - Rapid weight loss
  - Post-surgical: bilio-pancreatic bypass, small bowel resections

- **Systemic disorders**
  - Cachexia, febrile illnesses, heatstroke
  - Inflammatory bowel disease
  - Weber–Christian disease
  - Cystic fibrosis
  - Pituitary dysfunction; craniopharyngioma

- **Non-insulin related metabolic or endocrine disorders**
  - Wilson disease
  - Galactosemia
  - Tyrosinemia
  - Hereditary fructose intolerance
  - Cystinuria
  - Sandhoff disease
  - Pituitary dysfunction
  - Hypothyroidism

- **Other**
  - Hepatic ischaemia
  - Small bowel diverticulosis with bacterial overgrowth
  - Age

most pathologists agree that special stains for fat are not required. In addition to the predominant large droplet steatosis there may be some hepatocytes with combinations of large single droplets and multiple small droplets, or clusters of hepatocytes with intracytoplasmic delicate septations due to microvesicular steatosis (Fig. 7.2).

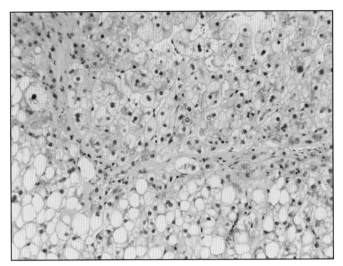

Fig. 7.2 • In the illustrated field, a portion of the parenchyma shows macrovesicular steatosis, while another area is predominantly microvesicular. H&E.

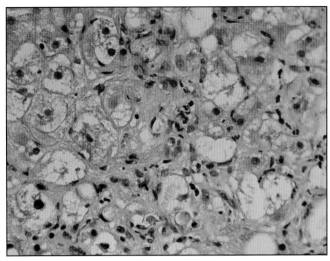

Fig. 7.4 • There is mixed acute and chronic inflammation in this field of steatosis and ballooned hepatocytes. H&E.

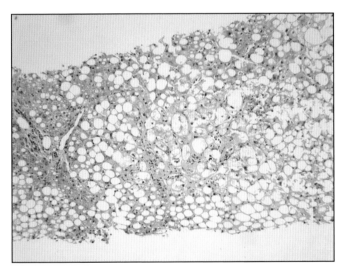

Fig. 7.3 • Ballooned hepatocytes are found in zone 3 admixed with steatosis; the involved hepatocytes are enlarged and swollen and may or may not contain Mallory's hyaline. H&E.

Common semi-quantitative assessments for steatosis are based on the percentage the surface area of a histological section involved and are usually considered as thirds or quartiles. By light microscopy, subdivisions of thirds is relatively straightforward as this incorporates the acinar divisions of the liver into zones 3, 2 and 1; thus the assessments are <33% (or 0–5%, 5–33%), 33–66%, >66%. Although a recent comparison of this approach with stereological point counting has suggested that semi-quantitative analysis overestimates the area/volume of fat content,[120a] it remains a useful means of assessing the degree of steatosis.

Ballooning

Hepatocyte ballooning (Fig. 7.3) is considered a manifestation of significant cell injury, and a required lesion of NASH in adults by many investigators.[16] Excluding the 2 paediatric studies,[49,121] a review of published series[15] found 82% of eleven reports described ballooning as a feature of NASH.

In the study of Matteoni et al. of clinical correlations with the spectrum of histology in NAFLD, ballooning was a distinct feature of progressive NAFLD (types 3 and 4).[104]

Ballooned hepatocytes are recognized most easily when they contain Mallory bodies; however, the two are not interchangeable as not all ballooned hepatocytes contain Mallory bodies. Furthermore, Mallory bodies are not restricted to ballooned hepatocytes. Hepatocyte ballooning is a structural manifestation of microtubular disruption;[13] this finding is likely a representation of cells undergoing lytic necrosis[122] and is not unique to alcoholic or non-alcoholic steatohepatitis.

An abstract of an ultrastructural examination of ballooned hepatocytes in 31 NAFLD biopsies challenges the dogma of ballooning as a degenerative change. Caldwell et al.[123] found little evidence of intracytoplasmic degenerative alterations; instead, varying amounts of lipid droplets were noted and these investigators concluded that the cells resembled mature brown fat of animals suggesting that it may represent an adaptive change.

Inflammation

Lobular inflammation in NASH is integral to the diagnosis, even though it is usually mild. 93% of the cases in series reviewed specifically noted lobular inflammation[15] (Fig. 7.4). Lobular inflammation is often mixed, in which polymorphonuclear leukocytes are a small but apparent component; in the early reported series of NASH, polymorphonuclear leukocytes were noted in 56–100% of cases in series in which the feature had been specifically examined.[15] The presence of polymorphs in NASH is, however, an area of divergence of opinion among pathologists. Other forms of lobular inflammation described include small lipogranulomas, some with associated eosinophils, Kupffer cell aggregates or single pigmented Kupffer cells. An immunohistochemical study corroborates the zone 3 accentuation of injury in NASH: the study showed Kupffer cell enlargement and aggregation in zone 3 in cases of steatohepatitis

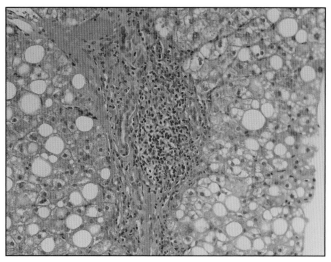

Fig. 7.5 • Portal inflammation in NASH is common, but usually mild. H&E.

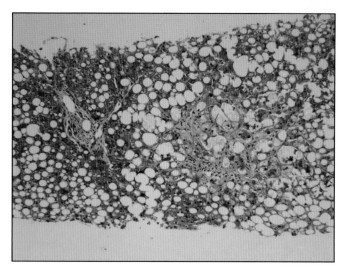

Fig. 7.6 • Collagen deposition can be appreciated in zone 3 in this low power photomicrograph. Masson trichrome.

(either alcoholic or non-alcoholic), whereas in steatosis and normal livers, CD68 Kupffer cells were diffusely present in the lobules.[124]

Mild portal chronic inflammation is an underappreciated yet relatively common lesion[15,113,125] (Fig. 7.5). However, as noted by Dixon et al.,[126] portal inflammation does not correspond with biochemical features of NASH and or metabolic syndrome. Portal inflammation that is more marked and out of keeping with the degree of lobular inflammation has been noted in resolving NASH;[127] in untreated subjects, this may represent concurrent liver injury of another origin, such as chronic viral hepatitis (see below).

Fibrosis

Whether fibrosis is a 'requirement' for the diagnosis or not is a matter of debate; the majority of pathologists, however, do not consider fibrosis obligatory for diagnosis.[16] The characteristic pattern of fibrosis that distinguishes non-cirrhotic steatohepatitis (alcoholic and non-alcoholic) from other forms of chronic liver disease is the presence of collagen in zone 3 perisinusoidal or pericellular spaces (Figs 7.6, 7.7). This pattern was noted in many of the early series of fatty liver disease.[31,113,128,129] When dense, the fibrosis may be observed by H&E, but when present is readily detected with specific histochemical stains for collagen, such as Masson's trichrome, Sweet's reticulin, picrosirius red and others. Just as lesions of activity and fibrosis are not always related in chronic viral hepatitis, zone 3 perisinusoidal fibrosis in the absence of active lesions may be an indication of prior episodes of steatohepatitis. A potential source of inconsistency in observations of fibrosis in published studies may be due to the use of different histochemical stains to detect collagen, such as Sweet's reticulin and picrosirius red stains. With progression of fibrosis, periportal fibrous spurs may be noted; bridging fibrous septa (central-central, central-portal, portal-portal) and cirrhosis may eventually develop (Fig. 7.8). With extensive bridging fibrosis or cirrhosis and

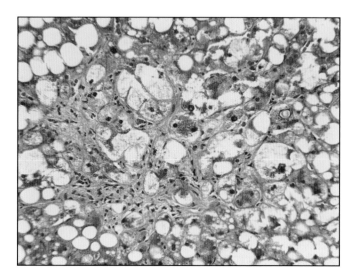

Fig. 7.7 • On this higher power view, the distinct pericellular, perisinusoidal location of collagen deposition can be seen. Masson trichrome.

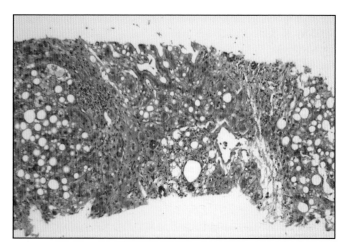

Fig. 7.8 • In this low power photomicrograph, there is evidence of zone 3 perisinusoidal fibrosis as well as portal expansion and bridging fibrosis. Terminal hepatic venule approximation suggests progressive architectural alteration. Masson trichrome.

Table 7.5	Clinical correlations of histologically significant fibrosis in liver biopsies					
Author	Biopsies (n) (% with fibrosis)	Correlations with fibrosis				
		Age	Obesity or increased BMI	Abnormal glucose or diabetes	ALT level or AST : ALT ratio >1	Other findings
Wanless, 1990[44]	207 (58%)	n/a	All were obese	+	n/a	Steatosis Diabetes explained differences of fibrosis in obese subjects
Bacon, 1994[78]	33 (39%)	n/a	+	+	n/a	Women > men Hyperlipidemia
Marceau, 1999[114]	551 (74%)	+	+	+	n/a	Steatosis
Angulo, 1999[261]	144 (27%)	+	+	+	Both	Serum albumin Serum Tf Saturation
Matteoni, 1999[104]	132 (16%)	No	No	No	AST : ALT >1	
Ratziu, 2000[130]	93 (30%)	+	+	+	*ALT*	Serum GGT Serum triglycerides
Garcia-Monzon, 2000[91]	46 (41%)	+	+	No	No	Steatosis Inflammation
Willner, 2001[296]	90 (49%)		+	+		
Crespo, 2001[295]	181 (10%)	+	All were obese	+	n/a	
Shimada, 2002[190]	81 (28%)	+	No	+	Lower ALT *AST : ALT >1*	Low platelet count, absence of hyperlipidemia, low ferritin; Mallory hyaline
Adams, 2003[199]	100 (17% cirrhosis)	+	+	+	ALT	Albumin, glucose, low platelet count
Marchesini, 2003[3]	163 (21%)	No	No	No	No	Criteria for metabolic syndrome
Beymer, 2003[90]	48 (12%)	No	All were obese	+	n/a	

Italic values: univariate and multivariate; nonbolded: univariate only

* BMI: body-mass index; for the table, BMI is used synonymously for results stated as weight or waist : hip (W : H) ratio

Tf: transferrin

architectural remodeling, perisinusoidal fibrosis may no longer be discerned.

Portal-based fibrosis in the absence of zone 3 perisinusoidal fibrosis has been reported in some studies of liver disease in obesity[113,130] and in paediatric NAFLD[49,58,59,120,121] but has not been considered common in adult NASH. A study comparing METAVIR portal-based scoring developed for chronic hepatitis C[131] with a published system for NASH[125] showed 47% agreement of fibrosis score; the differences were attributed to lack of detection of zone 3 perisinusoidal fibrosis by METAVIR.[103] Abrams et al.[131a] have, however, drawn attention to the existence of isolated portal fibrosis in patients with risk factors for NAFLD. The lesion was reported in 33.3% of their cohort of morbidly obese patients and they suggested that this histological change be considered within the spectrum of NAFLD. As the subjects whose biopsies had the lesion described also had clinical findings between NAFLD and NASH, it is possible the lesion may represent resolution from NASH rather than an interim lesion in progression.

Numerous clinico-pathological studies in recent years have examined clinical markers that correlate with hepatic fibrosis in patients with NASH; variability of findings may be related to different study designs, histochemical stains used and scoring systems, but common features are age, obesity, diabetes and ALT. Table 7.5 shows statistically significant clinical associations from representative series. Analysis of histological features associated with fibrosis have shown various combinations of steatosis, inflammation, and Mallory bodies as markers of fibrosis, or progression of disease. Results from studies are shown in Table 7.6.

Two groups have derived formulae from clinical and laboratory values to predict the presence of fibrosis,[130] or presence of NASH[106] in obese or morbidly obese subjects, respectively. The first is referred to by the acronym BAAT (BMI, Age, ALT, Triglycerides) and the second by HAIR (Hypertension, ALT, Insulin Resistance index). Hui et al.[107] have recently proposed a score based on adiponectin levels and insulin resistance calculations; this novel system closely

Table 7.6 Histologic features reported to correlate with fibrosis

Author (n = biopsies)	Steatosis	Lobular inflammation	Mallory hyaline	Other
Wanless, 1990[44] (n = 207)	+	n/a	n/a	n/a
Matteoni, 1999[104]* (n = 98)	+	+	+	
Angulo, 1999[261] (n = 144)	No	No	+	
George, 1998[151] (n = 51)	+	+		Stainable iron
Shimada, 2002[190] (n = 81)	+	No	+	
Ratziu, 2000[130] (n = 93)	+	+ with polymorphs	+	
Garcia-Monzon, 2000[91] (n = 46)	+	+		
Gramlich, 2004[95] (n = 107)	No	No	+	Ballooning

n/a: Not specifically discussed

* The combination of steatosis, inflammation, Mallory's hyaline, in the initial biopsy correlated with later development of cirrhosis in 21%; additional feature of fibrosis resulted in 28% with cirrhosis at follow-up

correlates with growing evidence of the significance of adiponectin and insulin resistance in pathogenesis of NAFLD and NASH.

Immunohistochemical studies of hepatic stellate cells (HSC) in human biopsies[133,134] have shown varying results. Washington et al.[133] found activated HSC in zone 3 in 97% of 76 cases of steatosis or NASH, compared to none in controls; in contrast, Cortez-Pinto et al.[134] found HSC reactivity in zone 3 in all liver biopsies examined, including 'normal' controls, but with greater numbers of activated cells in the 15 NASH biopsies. The association with fibrosis scores also varied: Washington et al. showed greater numbers of activated HSC in those with higher fibrosis scores,[133] while Cortez-Pinto did not.[134] Washington et al. showed a trend of increased HSC with increased steatosis, but no correlation with inflammatory grade,[133] while Cortez-Pinto noted a significant correlation with lobular and portal inflammation, but not with the degree of steatosis.[134] One group concluded that HSC activation in NASH is correlated with steatosis and is significant in fibrosis,[133] while the other group concluded that inflammation likely drives the fibrogenesis of NASH.[134] Larger studies may further clarify these considerations.

Paradis et al. showed elevated connective tissue growth factor with fibrosis in human NASH, in rodent models and in vitro hepatic stellate cells exposed to glucose and to insulin.[132] Experimental work with animals has demonstrated the necessity for leptin for hepatic fibrosis.[135]

Other lesions of non-cirrhotic NAFLD and NASH

Mallory's hyaline

Mallory's hyaline (MH) (also referred to as Mallory bodies—see Chapter 6) comprises intracellular, perinuclear ropy inclusion hepatocytes recognized in alcoholic hepatitis, NASH, a variety of chronic cholestatic liver diseases, in copper toxicity, in certain drugs (phospholipidosis-associated amiodarone toxicity), and in hepatocellular pro-

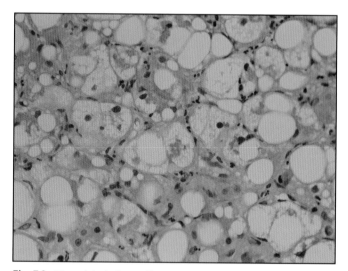

Fig. 7.9 • Most of the ballooned hepatocytes in this field contain intracytoplasmic ropy material consistent with Mallory's hyaline. Satellitosis can be seen. H&E.

liferative lesions such as focal nodular hyperplasia, adenomata and hepatocellular carcinoma.[13,136] (Chapters 2 and 6). In non-alcoholic steatohepatitis, MH is often described as 'poorly-formed' and is noted in ballooned hepatocytes, usually in zone 3.[1,137] MH is chemotactic; affected hepatocytes may be surrounded by polymorphs—so-called satellitosis (Fig. 7.9). Matteoni et al.[104] use MH as a lesion to delineate types 3 and 4 from types 1 and 2; other published studies of NASH have concurred that MH is more commonly found in higher necroinflammatory grades of steatohepatitis.[125] Abundant and well-formed MH is suggestive of alcoholic hepatitis.[13,137]

Detailed histological studies have reported MH in a range from none (primarily in paediatric cases) to 90% in one series.[15] In early studies that did not exclude alcoholics in descriptions of steatohepatitis, the presence of MH was interpreted as related to alcohol, and not obesity or diabetes.[28,129,138]

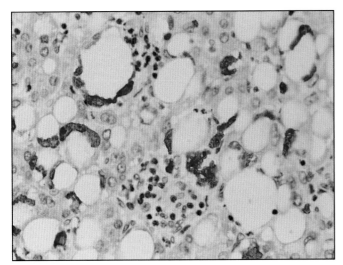

Fig. 7.10 • Immunohistochemical reactivity of Mallory's hyaline to p62 is illustrated (courtesy of Dr Cornelia Stumptner).

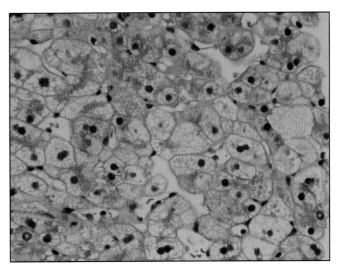

Fig. 7.11 • The frequency of megamitochondria in NAFLD and NASH has not been rigorously evaluated. This example shows round intracytoplasmic inclusions that are characteristic of megamitochondria. Needle-shaped inclusions may also be seen. H&E (reproduced with permission from Kliener DE et al. Hepatology 2005; 41: 1313–1321 with permission).

There is ongoing discussion of the requirement of MH for a diagnosis of NASH. Unquestionably the presence of MH is useful. Some pathologists use MH as a choice for any two of three lesions (along with steatosis and perisinusoidal fibrosis) necessary for a diagnosis.[16] However, others concur that MH are not required lesions, and the absence of MH does not mitigate against the diagnosis. There are immunohistochemical stains that aid in confirmation of MH: CK8, CK18, ubiquitin and p62, discussed below.

An extensive literature exists regarding the biology of MH.[136,139] Rather than reflecting a passive process of collapse of intracytoplasmic structures, MH are a result of concerted active metabolic pathways that include hyperphosphorylation, ubiquitination of abnormally-folded intermediate filaments CK 8 associated with heat shock proteins.[136] p62, a protein product of an early-response gene, associates with MH, and represents the hepatoprotective nature of sequestration of the abnormal proteins into biologically inert inclusions[139] (Fig. 7.10). One study has shown elevated serum levels of ubiquitin in NASH patients compared with controls and proposed this marker is an indication of cytoprotection against oxidative stress, rather than a marker of inflammation.[140]

Apoptosis and necrosis

Apoptotic hepatocytes (acidophil bodies) are either not mentioned or noted only in passing in most studies of NASH. However, a recent study in human biopsies[117] has highlighted their presence with use of assays specific for apoptosis (TUNEL and IHC for caspases 3 and 7). This study also showed upregulated FAS (death receptor) expression was present in human NASH; apoptotic bodies were more numerous than in cases of alcoholic hepatitis and non-alcoholic simple steatosis, and corresponded with biochemical and histological determinants (fibrosis) of severity.

The subacute necrosis with rapid liver failure reported in studies of obese patients undergoing gastric bypass is rare.[14] Seven non-surgical cases have been reported;[141,142,143] all

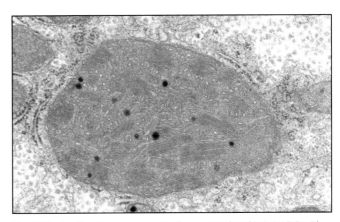

Fig. 7.12 • An ultrastructural example of megamitochondria in NAFLD with bundles of crystals noted. Studies of the significance of megamitochondria are discussed in the text. (Glutaraldehyde fixation, osmium tetroxide postfixed. Uranyl acetate. ×20 000, courtesy of Dr Steven Caldwell and Jan Redick).

were female. Two were patients who developed liver failure following prednisolone therapy for systemic lupus erythematosis;[141,142] neither had evidence of prior liver disease. Caldwell's series[143] documented NASH-related cirrhosis in liver explants or autopsies of 5 obese women with a clinical course of subacute liver failure; no other aetiology or prior diagnosis of liver disease had been made in these cases. Histological details are sparse in these cases, but they raise the awareness of the possibility of rapidly progressive disease in NASH.

Megamitochondria (Figs 7.11, 7.12)

Intrahepatocellular megamitochondria (giant mitochondria) observed in NASH are rounded or needle-shaped inclusions. Ultrastructural changes have been noted (Fig. 7.12).[105,144] Mitochondria are essential organelles involved in cellular energy production and lipid oxidation, but, in contrast with the association of progression in alcoholic liver disease,[145] the significance of megamitochondria in NAFLD is not clear. Le et al.[146] have recently showed non-zonal distribution of megamitochondria in an ultrastructural study of 31 human biopsies; there was no relationship with fibrosis stage, or degree of histochemically detectable products of oxidative stress. Unlike alcoholic liver disease, mitochondrial DNA deletion is uncommon in NASH.[144] Pessayre and Fromenty have recently drawn attention to functional abnormalities in hepatocytic mitochondria in NASH. They have also highlighted abnormalities in skeletal muscle mitochondria and have provocatively described NASH as a 'mitochondrial disease'.[144a] Caldwell's group has speculated that megamitochondria are a manifestation of either cell injury or hepatocellular adaptation.[11,144,146]

Iron deposition

The inconsistent evaluation of liver biopsies with iron stain may be one of the reasons iron deposition is not routinely discussed. When evaluated, granular iron pigment in hepatocytes is typically graded as mild (1+ to 2+); sinusoidal cell iron may also be present or there may be both parenchymal and non-parenchymal loading. Stainable iron has been reported in 10%,[147] to 95%[148] of cases. The variation in findings may be a manifestation of patient populations selected.[149]

In a study of 139 well-characterized subjects with insulin resistance, Turlin et al.[150] showed a predominantly non-parenchymal distribution, in contrast with hereditary haemochromatosis. When present, there was heterogeneity of staining reactivity in zone 1 hepatocytes. Another study showed a positive correlation between increased iron (either stainable or by biochemical determination) with increased portal fibrosis;[151] subsequent studies however have not corroborated this finding.[103,147,152–154] The significance of iron deposition, aberrant iron genetics and development of fibrosis are ongoing topics of debate, discussed below.[147,152,154]

Glycogenated nuclei

Glycogenated nuclei (GN) are well recognized in NAFLD and NASH; GN are common in paediatric liver tissue, Wilson disease, and diabetes.[35] In the literature review of NASH pathology,[15] this lesion was reported in 8 of 13 series and was found in 35–100% of cases. Two series reported 100% incidence: one was diabetics and the other paediatrics. A comparative study noted an incidence of 10–15% GN in alcoholic hepatitis compared with 75% in NASH biopsies; the lesion was associated with clinical evidence of diabetes and obesity.[111]

Histological resolution (Figs 7.13, 7.14, 7.15, 7.16)

Current therapeutic trials in NASH include histopathological evaluation at entry and post-treatment. The latter is of value as a measure of efficacy; further, post-treatment tissue provides an opportunity for characterization of lesions that resolve with therapy, providing validation of the histologi-

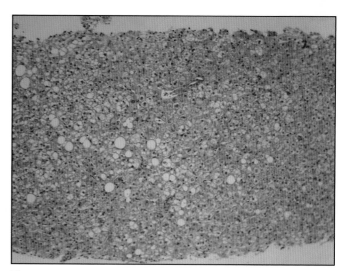

Fig. 7.13 • A pretreatment biopsy shows mild steatohepatitis. H&E.

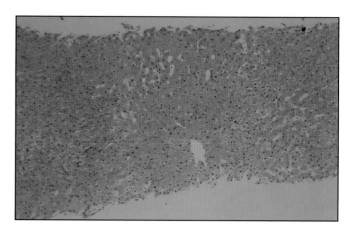

Fig. 7.14 • The same patient's post-treatment biopsy shows complete resolution with no steatosis, ballooning or inflammation. H&E.

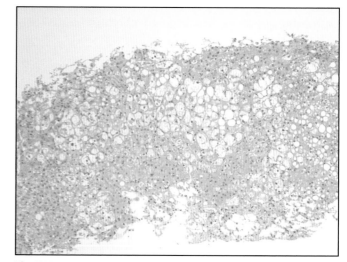

Fig. 7.15 • Nonalcoholic steatohepatitis with severe activity is illustrated. H&E.

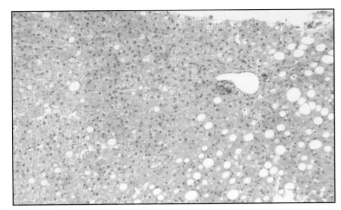

Fig. 7.16 • The same patient as Fig. 7.15 was rebiopsied two years later; there had been no interventional therapy in the interim but the loss of steatosis and lesions of steatohepatitis are apparent. H&E.

cal lesions of significance of NASH and metabolic syndrome.[126] Early studies utilized variable methods of analysis; results are included in reviews.[11,155,156]

Some recent trials have shown resolution in treated subjects[126,127,157] but in others there was no effect of treatment compared with placebo controls.[102] Tetri et al.[127] detailed clinico-pathological results of a 'proof of principle' treatment trial with the thiazolidinedione PPARγ agonist insulin-sensitizing agent, rosiglitazone, in 30 biopsy-proven NASH subjects. In addition to improvement of measures of insulin sensitivity, biochemical improvement and decreased CT-detected hepatic steatosis, 45% no longer met criteria for NASH. Histological features that improved on blinded biopsy review included decrease in global activity grade,[125] improvement (or no change) in the components of grade (steatosis, ballooning, lobular inflammation), loss of zone 3 accentuation of lesions, and two novel observations. The first was a qualitative shift in proportion of lobular and portal inflammation towards a relatively greater portal component. The second was a change in the qualitative nature of zone 3 perisinusoidal fibrosis from dense to delicate in 33% of cases; total fibrosis scores however did not change.

Promrat et al.[157] reported results of a pilot study of 18 nondiabetic NASH subjects following pioglitazone; the histological analysis separately scored individual components of steatohepatitis. In addition to improved insulin sensitivity, transaminase levels and decreased hepatic fat content by imaging, significant histological changes were noted in 66% of subjects and included lower sum histological score and values for steatosis, ballooning, parenchymal inflammation, presence of Mallory's hyaline and fibrosis, but no change in portal inflammation. Dixon et al.[126] showed significant improvement in weight, liver tests, insulin resistance and other features of metabolic syndrome in 36 obese patients after gastric banding; paired liver biopsies showed significant improvement in necroinflammatory grade and fibrosis stage[125] and zone 3 components of steatosis, lobular inflammation, Mallory's hyaline and perisinusoidal fibrosis. Follow-up biopsies showed complete resolution in 82% and improvement in 9%. No changes were seen in portal inflammation extent, intensity or fibrosis. The 4 subjects with no improvement had either insignificant weight loss, long standing insulin dependent diabetes or cirrhosis.

Reproducibility studies

Two histological studies of inter and intra-observer reproducibility have validated the significant lesions of NAFLD and NASH. In both, the pathologists met together prior to blinded reviews. The first[158] included 53 biopsies from adults with the full range of lesions of NAFLD. The second[159] included 30 adult biopsies and 18 paediatric biopsies submitted by the pathologists for the multicentre NIDDK-sponsored NASH Clinical Network Research and included the spectrum of biopsies submitted clinically for consideration of NAFLD or NASH. Both studies showed high kappa values for inter-observer correlations with extent of steatosis, hepatocellular ballooning, presence of perisinusoidal fibrosis and fibrosis grade. Mallory's hyaline had higher inter-observer correlation in one[159] and high agreement for intra-observer correlation in both. Lobular inflammation was the variable with least agreement in both studies.

Grading and staging in NASH

Pathologists are familiar with the evolution of semi-quantitative scoring systems for evaluation of necro-inflammatory activity (grade) and fibrosis architectural alterations (stage) in chronic viral hepatitis;[160] methods currently in use vary, but are based on assessments of portal inflammation and interface activity, lobular inflammation and necrosis, and portal fibrosis. One of the primary goals of standardized assessments in any histopathological scoring system is the assurance that across the spectrum of observers, the same lesions are being evaluated and given similar diagnostic weight; a system of grading and staging, therefore enhances reproducibility.

The lesions of steatohepatitis are sufficiently distinct from the portal-based lesions of chronic hepatitis of viral and autoimmune origin to warrant specific methods of evaluation. Matteoni et al.[104] categorized fatty liver on the presence of specific histological lesions, but did not include assessments of severity or acinar localization of lesions; the classification system was derived for clinical assessment rather than a morphological scoring system.

A novel grading and staging system was developed from evaluation of 51 biopsies from well-characterized adult patients with NASH.[125] The method was developed to score relevant histological lesions, to derive a semi-quantitative global 'activity' grade and to standardize reporting of the pattern of fibrosis progression in NASH.[125] This represents an alternative to prior methods that combined assessment of activity with those of fibrosis[24] and follows the accepted paradigm for chronic hepatitis in the recognition that processes that result in necroinflammatory lesion, grade, and fibrosis with architectural changes, stage, are separately evaluated and reported.[160]

Tables 7.7a and b describe the method. Determination of grades 1–3 is based on the constellation of features, steatosis, hepatocellular ballooning, lobular inflammation, and

Table 7.7a	Brunt system[125]: grade		
Grade	**Steatosis**	**Ballooning**	**Inflammation**
Mild, Grade 1	1–3 (up to 66%)	Minimal	L: 1–2 P: None-mild
Moderate, Grade 2	2–3 (>33%; may be >66%)	Present	L: 2 P: Mild–moderate
Severe, Grade 3	2–3	Marked	L: 3 P: Mild-moderate

Steatosis Grade 1: ≤33%; Grade 2: >33% <66%; Grade 3: ≥66%
L = lobular, P = portal

Lobular (0–3):
0: None
1: <2 foci/20x field
2: 2–4 foci/20x field
3: >4/20x field

Portal: (0–3):
0: None
1: Mild
2: Moderate
3: Marked

Table 7.7b	Brunt system[125]: stage		
Stage	**Zone 3, peri-sinusoidal**	**Portal-based**	**Bridging**	**Cirrhosis**
1	Focal or extensive	0	0	0
2	As above	Focal or extensive	0	0
3	Bridging septa	Bridging septa	+	0
4	+/−	+/−	Extensive	+

Fibrosis analysis is based on use of Masson's trichrome histochemical stain

Table 7.8	NASH CRN scoring system[159]

Component scores

Steatosis grade	Lobular inflammation	Hepatocellular ballooning
0: <5%	0: None	0: None
1: 5–33%	1: <2 foci/20x field	1: Mild, few
2: 34–66%	2: 2–4 foci/20x field	2: Moderate-marked, many
3: >66%	3: >4 foci/20x field	

NAFLD activity score (NAS): 0–8
Steatosis (0–3) + Lobular Inflammation (0–3) + Ballooning (0–2)

Fibrosis:*
0: None
1a: Mild zone 3 perisinusoidal fibrosis, requires trichrome stain to identify
1b: Moderate zone 3 perisinusoidal fibrosis, may be appreciated on H&E
1c: Portal fibrosis only
2: Zone 3 perisinusoidal fibrosis and periportal fibrosis
3: Bridging fibrosis
4: Cirrhosis

* based on the use of Masson's trichrome stain

portal inflammation; emphasis is placed on gradation of injury and inflammation rather than steatosis, as marked steatosis may occur without significant cell injury or inflammation. In addition, Mallory's hyaline, is neither required for diagnosis, nor considered as a feature of additive benefit for grade.

Fibrosis staging involves observation of the presence of zone 3 perisinusoidal and/or pericellular, chickenwire fibrosis either alone, or in conjunction with periportal or bridging fibrosis. Thus, stage 1 is perisinusoidal fibrosis (focal or extensive); stage 2 is stage 1 with additional periportal fibrosis; stage 3 is bridging fibrosis and stage 4 is cirrhosis (Fig. 7.17). During remodelling of the parenchyma, perisinusoidal fibrosis may or may not persist; caution is warranted in interpreting residual perisinusoidal fibrosis in cirrhosis, as evidence of steatohepatitis however.

Just as Ishak[161] and Scheuer[162] have discussed in grading viral hepatitis, the numerical values are not to be considered the equivalent of laboratory tests; rather, the system can serve as guideline for assessment of lesions of significance, a method to assure some uniformity of assessment of steatohepatitis among varying pathologists, as a useful method for comparisons of interval biopsies, and as a research instrument.

The NASH Clinical Research Network has recently developed and validated a further feature-based scoring system for the spectrum of lesions of NAFLD[159,163] (Table 7.8). The system is inclusive of the lower end of the histological spectrum of fatty liver disease, as represented by >5% steatosis for minimum criterion for NAFLD. The remaining lesions are graded as noted. The fibrosis score developed is a modification of the Brunt score[125] to separate delicate and dense zone 3 perisinusoidal fibrosis (1a and 1b), and to document non-bridging, portal-only fibrosis (1c) (Fig. 7.17). The results of the validation study[159] have been referred to above; this study further showed that of the 14 lesions evaluated, steatosis, lobular inflammation, hepatocellular ballooning and acidophil bodies independently correlated with the diagnostic categories of 'NASH', 'possible NASH' and 'not NASH' in univariate and multivariate analyses. Based on this, the NAFLD Activity Score (NAS) was created as a sum of scores for steatosis grade (0–3), lobular inflammation (0–3) and ballooning (0–2), thus the total NAS ranges from 0 to 8. An alternative system in which an overall activity score out of 12 and a three tier severity assessment has recently been described by Mendler et al.[163a]

Paediatric NAFLD and NASH

A population screening study from Japan in 1988 documented fatty liver in 2.8% of the 369 children less than 19 years of age.[69] However, recognition of paediatric NAFLD has lagged behind that of adults.

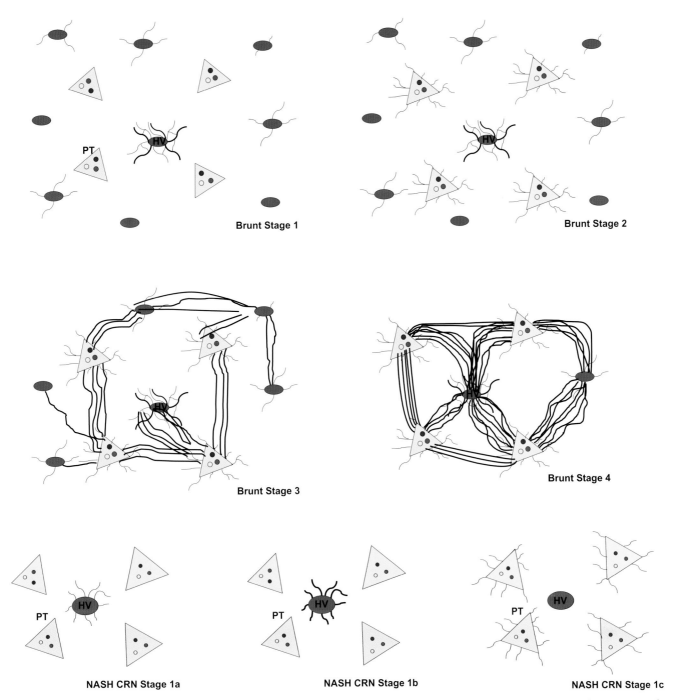

Brunt Stage 1

Brunt Stage 2

Brunt Stage 3

Brunt Stage 4

NASH CRN Stage 1a

NASH CRN Stage 1b

NASH CRN Stage 1c

Fig. 7.17 • Schematic representation of the proposed staging systems discussed in the text. The top four panels illustrate the Brunt method for assessment of fibrosis while the bottom three panels illustrate the modifications to Grade 1 in the NASH CRN system. HV—hepatic vein; PT—portal tract.

The rising incidence of NAFLD and NASH in children is not restricted to Western populations, and has paralleled that of the dramatic increase in obesity, type 2 diabetes mellitus in this age group.[52,57,59] Lifestyle changes including a shift to less physically-demanding pastimes and dietary exposure to high fats and refined sugars are all implicated.[59] Distinctive epidemiological findings reported in paediatric series are male predominance and strong association with

Hispanic ethnicity. An insulin-resistance associated cutaneous disorder, acanthosis nigricans, characterized by darkening in flexural areas, the posterior neck folds, axillae and groins, is a clinical feature described in 85% of 81 subjects in 3 series of paediatric NAFLD.[58] Weiss et al.[164] reported the increased incidence of metabolic syndrome with severity of obesity in a study of 490 children and adolescents, none of whom were diabetic or taking medications to lower blood pressure, lipids or glucose. All of the findings were independent of age or pubertal status, confirming that well-recognized features of metabolic syndrome in adults are present in children. In a 2 year follow-up of 77 patients, metabolic syndrome persisted in all affected subjects and 8 had progressed to type 2 diabetes.[164]

Reported inherited metabolic syndromes that are risk factors for NAFLD share the common features of obesity and either impaired glucose tolerance, insulin resistance or type 2 diabetes: Bardet–Biedl syndrome, Alstrom syndrome,[59,121] and Prader–Willi syndrome.[81] A recent report of a lean child with an inherited multisystem triglyceride breakdown and storage disorder, Dorfman–Chanarin syndrome[165] documented steatohepatitis and cirrhosis. Hypothalamic dysfunction with subsequent obesity is a recognized complication of many forms of treated childhood cancer;[166] a small percentage of cases in each series of reported paediatric NAFLD are in such children or adolescents.[49,58,121] The rare disorder, pseudoneonatal adrenoleukodystrophy, due to homozygous deficiency of acly-CoA-oxidase, an enzyme essential for fatty acid oxidation, is associated with hepatic steatosis.[167]

Imaging studies from Japan and Italy have confirmed that the presence of fatty liver in children is related to obesity;[168] interestingly, there has been disagreement about duration of obesity in relationship to NAFLD in children.[169] As examples, a Japanese study found greater incidence related to longer duration of obesity,[170] while an Italian study found the risk of fatty liver was associated with short duration.[171] Prevalence estimates in the obese paediatric population range from 16.2 % by elevated ALT assay[172] to as high as 83% by ultrasound detection.[170] As in adult prevalence studies, evaluation without biopsy are at risk of both over and under-estimation of steatosis in children.[169] Guzzaloni et al. studied 375 children and confirmed the value of hypertriglyceridemia in predicting steatosis, but questioned the value of GGT, and hyperinsulinemia for screening.[169] Literature reviews indicate that similar factors and markers of inflammation are present in paediatric NAFLD as in adults;[58,59] additionally, low serum levels of antioxidants have been seen in obese children. Schwimmer's recent study of 43 subjects with biopsy documentation noted relationships of significant histological findings with pertinent clinical parameters: steatosis was predicted by a combination of clinical features of insulin resistance calculated by QUICKI, age and ethnicity; portal inflammation was related to ALT and fasting insulin levels; portal fibrosis was related to calculated HOMA-IR and right upper quadrant pain and perisinusoidal fibrosis to AST, fasting insulin and BMI.[57]

Table 7.9 summarizes the histological lesions reported from published series or cases of 202 patients, 152 of whom had biopsies.[58,120,121,165,172–178] Of the 152, there were 8 (5%) with cirrhosis; bridging fibrosis was noted in an additional 27 (23%). These figures highlight the aggressive potential of NAFLD in children. Steatosis ranges from mild to severe; in the majority of these cases however the latter predominated. Differences noted in comparison to adult histology include: (i) greater severity of steatosis, (ii) little or no ballooning or Mallory's hyaline, (iii) less lobular inflamma-

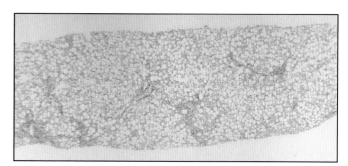

Fig. 7.18 • Paediatric NAFLD. A low power photomicrograph of a paediatric liver biopsy shows diffuse steatosis with prominent portal tracts. The latter is due to inflammation and slightly increased fibrosis. There was no ballooning or zone 3 perisinusoidal fibrosis. H&E. (Courtesy Dr Cynthia Behling)

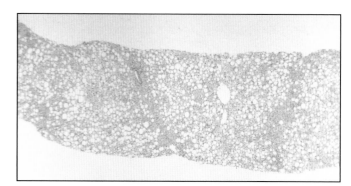

Fig. 7.19 • Paediatric NAFLD. In this example, there is centrizonal accentuation of steatosis; on higher power, there were occasional ballooned hepatocytes. There was no zone 3 or portal fibrosis. H&E. (Courtesy Dr Cynthia Behling)

tion, (iv) few or no polymorphonuclear leukocytes, and (v) more portal tract inflammation. Portal fibrosis without concomitant perisinusoidal fibrosis is commonly reported, however, this is not a universal observation (personal communications). A more subtle feature not often mentioned in paediatric series is the apparent lack of zone 3 predominance (Figs 7.18, 7.19). Anecdotal experience with paediatric NASH suggests that some cases may more closely resemble adult histology than in published reviews. Further documentation of paediatric NASH histology, as well as possible explanations for the differences will likely evolve from the increased research in this area.

Two paediatric treatment trials involving 11 and 31 subjects respectively have shown beneficial results with vitamin E[179] but no effect with ursodeoxycholic acid.[180]

Steatohepatitis-related cirrhosis and cryptogenic cirrhosis (Figs 7.20, 7.21 and 7.22)

The recognition that NAFLD may be a source of otherwise cryptogenic cirrhosis was suggested by: (i) a natural history study of 42 NASH patients,[181] (ii) a case report with repeat biopsy,[182] and (iii) subsequent clinical correlation studies.[54,183–185] Currently the association has evolved such that some investigators utilize the term 'cryptogenic' inter-

Table 7.9	Paediatric NAFLD					
Author	Country/ethnicity	n	M : F	Steatosis ballooning mallory	Inflammation	Portal fibrosis cirrhosis (n) Perisinusoidal fibrosis
Srinivasan, 2004[165]	UK: East Indian	n = 1 bx: 1	1F*	Diffuse, mixed N/A N/A	Present	Micronodular cirrhosis
Schwimmer, 2003[120]	USA: Hispanic 53%; Black: 5%; White: 25%; other: 17%	n = 43 bx: 43	30 : 13	Present in 74% 5% 2%	Portal: 58%; lobular: 2% portal > lobular	Portal: 46%; 70% had no psf Cirrhosis: 2% (n = 1) Perisinusoidal fibrosis: 19%
Molleston, 2002[178]	USA: Hispanic (1) Not Stated: (1)	n = 2 bx: 2	2M	100% N/A N/A	Portal: 100% Lobular: 50%	Cirrhosis: 50% (n = 1)
Sathya, 2002[174]	Montreal, Canada Not stated	n = 27 bx: 5	17 : 10	60% N/A N/A	Portal: 20% (n = 1)	Portal: 20% (n = 1)
Rashid, 2000[121]	Toronto, Canada Not stated	n = 36 bx: 24	21 : 15	100% N/A N/A	Not specified, present in 86%	Portal, Mild: 42% Portal Mod-Severe: 33% Cirrhosis: 4% (n = 1) Perisinusoidal fibrosis: N/A
Manton, 2000[177]	Australia Not stated	n = 17 bx: 17	11 : 6	100% N/A N/A	Present in 47% Portal: 41%	Portal: 35%; of these, 5 (71%) were bridging Cirrhosis: 6% (n = 1) 'evolving' Perisinusoidal fibrosis: 18%
Baldridge, 1995[49]	USA Not stated	n = 14 bx: 14	10 : 4	100% N/A N/A	Portal: 100% Lobular: present, unspecified %	Portal: 100% 90% exhibited bridging fibrosis and/or centrilobular and zone 3 perisinusoidal fibrosis
Vajro, 1994[173]	Italy	n = 9 bx: 1	6 : 3	Steatohepatitis, not otherwise described	N/A	N/A
Kinugasa, 1984[172]	Japan	n = 11 bx: 11	9 : 2	All N/A N/A	Portal: 100% Lobular: 64%	Portal: 91% Cirrhosis: 9% (n = 1) Perisinusoidal fibrosis: 55%
Moran, 1983[175]	USA White 100%	n = 3 bx: 3	2 : 1	100%	Foci of acute: 33% Portal, chronic: 33%	Portal: 66%; bridging fibrosis in 1
Squires, personal communication Roberts, 2003[58]	USA: Hispanic 51%; White 36%; Black 2.5%; Asian 10%*	n = 39 bx: 31	28 : 21		Steatohepatitis: 100%	Fibrosis (not specified): 68% Cirrhosis: 7% (n = 2)
Totals		**n = 202 bx: 152**	**M: 136 F: 76**			**Bridiging fibrosis: Cirrhosis: 5% (n = 8)**

* Dorfman–Chanarin syndrome. bx = biopsied

changeably with NASH-related cirrhosis.[54] The true prevalence of cryptogenic cirrhosis and/or the association with prior NASH is unknown. The study of Browning et al.[54] of 41 patients with cryptogenic cirrhosis highlighted differences in ethnic distribution that were similar to those reported in a separate study of ethnic differences in NASH:[60] greater incidence in Hispanic and Caucasian Americans of European descent compared with African Americans. Investigators have noted the paradox of this finding in view of the greater prevalence of metabolic syndrome in African Americans (and Hispanics) than European Americans.[55,62,186]

Abdelmalek et al.[182] and Powell et al.[181] documented histologically that cases with NASH had progressed to cirrhosis

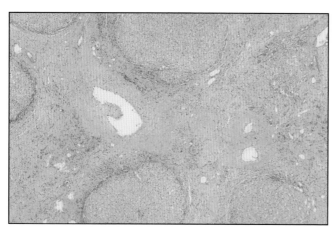

Fig. 7.20 • The biopsy findings and clinical studies fulfilled criteria for 'cryptogenic' cirrhosis. H&E.

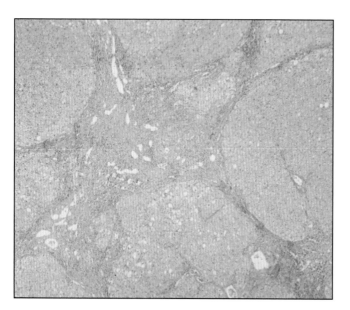

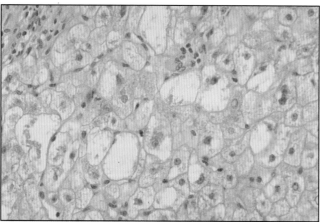

Figs 7.21 and 7.22 • A review of a biopsy obtained 11 years prior to that shown in Fig. 7.20 showed cirrhosis (Fig. 7.21) with evidence of active steatohepatitis (Fig. 7.22). This case illustrates that active lesions may persist in cirrhosis, that NASH may 'burn-out' and result in bland, non-steatotic cirrhosis. However, once the underlying aetiology is known, the label 'cryptogenic' is no longer appropriate.

on repeat biopsy and no longer retained diagnostic features of steatohepatitis. These reports provide evidence in support for the subsequently proposed concept that NASH may result in 'burned-out', otherwise cryptogenic, cirrhosis for which no histological hallmarks remain. Caldwell et al.[183] and Poonwala et al.[184] presented series of 70 and 65 cases respectively of cryptogenic cirrhosis; both studies showed the increased prevalence of clinical features such as diabetes and obesity, similar to patients with NAFLD,[183,184] but different from matched controls with other forms of chronic liver disease-related cirrhosis.[183] Other investigators have speculated that histological evidence of NAFLD and NASH in allograft livers of patients transplanted for cryptogenic cirrhosis may represent disease recurrence, and by definition, proof of NAFLD as the initial disease.[187–189]

It is increasingly common in the literature for cryptogenic cirrhosis, with or without biopsy, to be attributed to NAFLD or NASH, but this is an area in which definitional variances play a remarkable role in study results. For example, if prior biopsy-proven NASH were known, by definition the subsequent cirrhosis would not be cryptogenic. On the other hand, there may yet be undiscovered or undetected viral infections, autoimmune or metabolic diseases that may result in cirrhosis, but that currently are grouped under the rubric of cryptogenic.

NASH cirrhosis may in fact retain some or all of the characteristic histological features.[92,190,191] Shimada et al.[190] documented that all of the lesions of active steatohepatitis were present in each of 6 cirrhotic livers that also harboured hepatocellular carcinoma (HCC). Hui et al.[191] stressed the importance of histological criteria in categorizing cases of NASH cirrhosis. This group proposed criteria for pathological interpretation of cirrhotic livers with NASH: the categories were *definite* (steatosis with mixed lobular inflammation), *probable* (steatosis with only chronic inflammation), *possible* (with either steatosis only or mixed inflammation only) and *cryptogenic* (no steatosis or inflammation). In their 23 cases clinically consistent with NASH, 20 were definite and 3 were probable; ballooning was noted in 91% of cases and residual perisinusoidal fibrosis in 78%.

Determining the frequency and mechanisms of loss of each of the active lesions is challenging due to the requirement of follow-up tissue samples and are currently speculative.

Steatohepatitis in the allograft liver

Recurrence of NASH in allograft livers has been documented in case reports at 5.5 months[192] and 16 months post transplant[193] and in a series of 8 patients.[194] The latter included 3 patients with prior jenuno-ileal bypass; in the follow-up period, all of these patients and 3 other patients showed varying degrees of steatosis (3 weeks to 2.0 years), 3 of whom further progressed to NASH (6 weeks to 2.5 years). Zone 3 fibrosis was present in the latter group.[194] Of note, Czaja has discussed the challenges of discerning 'occurrence' from 'recurrence' of a steatohepatitis given the alterations of glucose and lipid metabolism, immune system

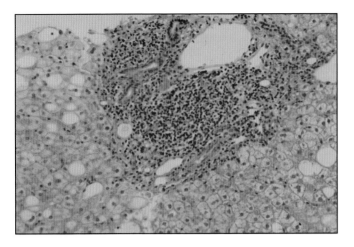

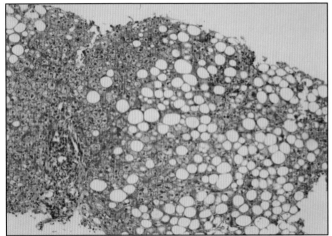

Figs 7.23 and 7.24 • An AMA positive case of primary biliary cirrhosis with nonalcoholic steatohepatitis. The PAS-D photomicrograph (Fig. 7.23) shows the portal inflammation and bile duct lesion while the trichrome (Fig. 7.24) highlights the zone 3 steatosis as well as fibrosis involving zone 3 and the portal tract.

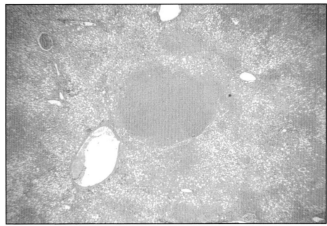

Fig. 7.25 • A microscopic focus of adenoma can be seen in this liver with background steatohepatitis. H&E.

function and cytokines that occur in the setting of liver transplantation.[195]

NAFLD and other liver disease

(Figs 7.23, 7.24)

Several clinico-pathological studies of NASH have shown the presence of ANA in small percentage of patients;[15,196,197] Loria et al.[197] specifically studied the prevalence of 'non-organ specific' antibodies in 84 subjects with NAFLD. This group documented positivity for ANA in 21%, ASMA in 5%, both in 6%, and AMA in 2%; three subjects with ANA showed overlapping histology of NASH and autoimmune hepatitis. Two recent abstracts have confirmed the prevalence of autoantibodies in subjects with NAFLD and NASH;[198,199] Kanji et al.[198] noted a lack of histological differences in 240 biopsy-proven subjects by auto-antibody status. In contrast, Adams et al.[199] reported higher stages of fibrosis in the nearly one-third of 225 biopsied NAFLD subjects who had autoantibodies.

Other groups have shown concurrence of histological (and clinical) features of NASH in patients with viral hepa-

titis C[200-203] and in subjects with non-viral serologically-diagnosed liver disease.[200] Numerous studies have documented the incidence and effects of hepatic steatosis and steatohepatitis in hepatitis C infection and response to therapy.[77,200,201,203-209] Currently, it is understood that with most genotypes of HCV, hepatic steatosis is related to underlying host predispositions (such as obesity); in genotype 3 however, steatosis is a direct viral cytopathic effect.[209,210] Recent work has further shown aberrations of insulin metabolism in animal models and non-cirrhotic patients by hepatitis C viral infection.[211-214] Hui et al. speculate the relationship is not spurious, as they demonstrated a relationship of insulin resistance and fibrosis stage in biopsies from patients with hepatitis C.[214]

Benign and malignant primary liver tumours in NAFLD

There is a rodent model of adenomatosis in steatohepatitis[215] but only a single report in a human of benign liver tumours in NASH[216] (Fig. 7.25).

The increased mortality from malignancies in multiple organ systems due to concurrent obesity is calculated as 14% for men and 20% for women.[217] A review of the United Organ Sharing (UNOS) Database of 19 271 explant hepatectomies found obesity to be an independent factor for the prevalence of HCC in cirrhosis due to alcoholic or cryptogenic cirrhosis, but not other known aetiologies of chronic liver disease and cirrhosis.[218] Hyperinsulinemia has been identified with an increased risk of HCC in a longitudinal survey of 6237 French men in the Paris Prospective Study.[219] In a case control study from Greece, Lagiou et al. documented a positive association of diabetes (presumed to be type 2) and HCC not confounded by other major risk factors for hepatic malignancy such as viral hepatitis, alcohol and tobacco.[220] By contrast in a case control study of 823 men with HCC, El-Serag et al. found that diabetes was not a risk for HCC independent of other forms of underlying chronic liver disease.[221] However, a more recent, larger cohort study of 173 643 American patients of the Veterans Administration Hospital followed for 15 years showed that the presence of type 2 diabetes in patients was associated with increased risk of both chronic liver disease and HCC compared with age and sex matched controls.[222] Clearly, these studies were not limited to the subset of patients within each group with NAFLD.

Hepatocellular carcinoma is now a recognized complication of cirrhosis in NASH patients. In the series of 42 patients by Powell et al., HCC was reported in one.[181] Ludwig et al. found 1 case of 7 explants with end-stage liver disease due to NASH cirrhosis during the 10 year period ending in 1995.[137] Cotrim et al. reported a case of fatal HCC 4 years following the diagnosis of NASH-cirrhosis.[223] Orikasa reported a case of lipid-rich clear cell HCC in a diabetic patient with NASH and early cirrhosis.[224] Zen et al. reported a NASH patient with multicentric hepatocellular lesions that developed 10 and 11 years after the initial diagnosis; two of the lesions were HCC and one was a dysplastic nodule.[225] Mori et al.[226] reported an elderly man who was diagnosed simultaneously with NASH cirrhosis and a 1.9 cm HCC. Shimada et al.[190] reported that from 82 cases of biopsy-proven NASH, 13 were cirrhotic and 6 of those 13 had HCC (7.3% of total cohort; 47% of cirrhotics). On the other hand, Hui et al. followed 23 patients with biopsy-proven NASH-related cirrhosis for 10 years; no cases of HCC occurred during the observation period, compared with 17% incidence of HCC in patients with hepatitis C-related cirrhosis.[191] Kudo has noted that greater length of follow-up may be necessary for determining prevalence of HCC; he further discussed the fact that Japanese patients are over-represented in reported cases of HCC secondary to NASH. Whether this may be a result of more vigilant screening for HCC in this patient population is not known. His review highlights the lower risk of NASH-related HCC (1.3–2.4 fold) compared with that of HCV cirrhosis (13–19 fold).[227]

Finally, three anecdotal cases of incidentally discovered HCC in non-cirrhotic livers of patients with clinico-pathological NASH have been observed (P. Bilouc-Sage, personal communication; Z. Goodman, personal communication personal observation). All three cases occurred in middle-aged men.

HCC and cryptogenic cirrhosis

In a survey of 641 cirrhosis-associated HCC, Bugianesi et al. found 44 cases arose in cryptogenic cirrhosis; compared with case-control for viral and alcoholic cirrhosis-associated HCC, the cases with cryptogenic cirrhosis showed higher prevalence of obesity, diabetes, indices of insulin resistance and elevated triglycerides. The authors concluded that the natural history of NASH should include cryptogenic cirrhosis and HCC.[185] Two additional studies of patients with cryptogenic cirrhosis found a range of 18%[228] to 27%[229] incidence of hepatocellular carcinoma; in the latter, only the obese cryptogenics showed increased risk of HCC. Both groups noted the incidence to be similar to that

of HCC in hepatitis C-related cirrhosis. In both studies, NAFLD was the inferred underlying pathogenesis of the cryptogenic cirrhosis, based on associated clinical features of metabolic syndrome.

Possible mechanisms for HCC in NAFLD include the known presence of insulin-like growth factor receptors in HCC, hyperinsulinemia of NAFLD,[218–220] increased susceptibility of the steatotic liver to lipid peroxidation, production of free radicals and subsequent DNA mutations,[218] increased susceptibility to carcinogens due to impairment of ATP production,[219] disordered energy and/or hormonal regulation in obesity,[230] the known metabolic derangements of 'metabolic syndrome' in NAFLD,[185] and aberrations in regenerative processes occurring in cirrhosis of any cause.

In ob/ob mice, an obesity animal model with genetic leptin deficiency, obesity-related hepatic steatosis and insulin resistance, hepatocyte hyperplasia and decreased apoptosis have been documented in enlarged fatty livers without fibrosis or cirrhosis.[231] The investigators speculated that these results support considerations that factors related to obesity and associated insulin resistance may promote hepatocyte proliferation even in the absence of cirrhosis, and further, that the changes may represent a pre-malignant condition. Subsequent studies have documented increased numbers of immunohistochemically-detected hepatocyte progenitor and intermediate hepatocyte-like cells in livers of ob/ob mice and humans with NAFLD.[232,233] Hepatic progenitor cells are a recent focus of investigation as precursors of hepatocellular carcinoma in animals and humans.[234]

Soga et al.[215] reported a non-obese inbred mouse model with spontaneous fatty liver that develops steatohepatitis; with time, many of the animals develop hepatocellular adenomas and hepatocellular carcinomas. These lesions show a gender predilection occurring in up to 40% of male mice but less than 10% of female mice. The investigators reviewed other reported animal models with the propensity for HCC development, and concluded that steatosis alone is not sufficient for tumour genesis, but inflammation may be a necessary component.

Finally, an additional potential mechanism for HCC includes the alterations of the peroxisome proliferators activated receptor α, (PPAR α) a nuclear receptor involved in fatty acid metabolism and resultant byproducts that lead to oxidative stress, potentially damaging to DNA and gene expression.[235,236] Animal models with genetic alterations of pathways involved in fatty acid metabolism have been reported to produce adenomas and HCC.[235,237] The role of PPARα activation in these models is an ongoing area of investigation.[167,238]

Hepatocellular regeneration in fatty liver

Studies have demonstrated decreased regeneration of mature hepatocytes with fatty livers in animals and humans after partial hepatectomy.[239,240] Severe macrovesicular steatosis (>60%) is a recognized cause of early allograft failure ('primary nonfunction') and patients with fatty liver have higher postoperative mortality compared with unaffected subjects.[240] Leclercq et al. showed the necessity of leptin and adipocyte-related cytokines TNFα and IL-6 in toxin-induced regenerative response in the leptin-deficient *ob/ob* mouse model.[241] Roskams et al.[232–234] documented that inhibition of replication of mature hepatocytes, or 'replicative senescence' is another manifestation of histologically proven oxidative stress in NAFLD. Immunohistochemical detection of increased numbers of cells positive for OV6 in mice and CK7 in humans was evidence of expansion of the putative hepatic progenitor cell compartment in this setting. The increased numbers of oval cells (in mice models of fatty liver) or progenitor cells (in human NAFLD tissue) as well as 'intermediate hepatocyte-like cells' correlated with the amount of fibrosis.[234] The authors conclude that expansion of the progenitor cell compartment represents an adaptive response to impaired regeneration caused by oxidative injury, and further speculate these immature cells may have survival advantage in conditions that are deleterious to mature hepatocytes, but also may serve as precursors for malignant tumours.

Natural history of NAFLD

Studies of the natural history of NAFLD are inherently challenging. Ideally, studies include biopsy series, but subjects that come to biopsy are already a highly selected group that may not be representative of an entire population with NAFLD. Furthermore, ideally natural history studies would include histological documentation in repeat biopsies to elucidate long-term outcome. Finally, it is difficult to document onset in a process such as NAFLD. To date, a spectrum of clinical outcomes has been reported; early case series reported a lack of progression in obesity-related steatosis/steatohepatitis in the absence of diabetes.[28,32,113] Calculations of fibrosis progression rates from recent studies has varied from 0.08 fibrosis stage/year[242] to 0.65 fibrosis stage/year.[243]

Angulo's recent literature review indicated that of 673 biopsies reported in the literature, fibrosis was documented in 66%, and cirrhosis in 14%; of the subset of patients that were rebiopsied in 3–11 years of follow-up, 28% had progressed, 13% had less fibrosis, and 59% were unchanged.[93] Falck-Ytter and co-workers' recent literature review also noted that advanced fibrosis and cirrhosis are documented in the initial biopsy in 15–19% of patients with presumed steatohepatitis.[64]

Massarrat et al. documented no progression to cirrhosis in 92 subjects with nonalcoholic fatty liver, 56 of whom had repeat biopsies in the 5 year follow-up.[244] Teli et al. confirmed the non-progressive nature of 'simple' steatosis: in a 10 year follow-up study of 40 patients with steatosis on index biopsy, only one had progressed to fibrosis, and none to cirrhosis.[245] Ratziu et al. confirmed the benign course of 'simple' steatosis in a study of 93 obese subjects; no progression of fibrosis was noted in 10/14 re-biopsied obese subjects with steatosis only on the index biopsy after 15 years follow-up. On the other hand, 2 of the remaining 4 with steatohepatitis on index biopsy did show progression.[130]

The concept of nonprogressive nature of steatosis proposed by Thaler in 1975[19] and reported in the studies of Massarrat et al.[244] and Teli et al.[245] has not been confirmed in all series. Itoh reported 5 patients with nonalcoholic 'diabetic cirrhosis'.[34] Watanabe and co-workers' series of 20 adults with fatty liver included 8 with fibrosis;[31] and in the study of Adler et al. of 20 adults, 7 had fibrosis and a further 7 cirrhosis.[24] The retrospective study of Matteoni et al. of 98 subjects with 10 year follow-up data documented cirrhosis and liver-related mortality increased according to the categorization based on histological lesions: hepatic steatosis defined type 1 and was a common denominator in the remainder; inflammation (type 2), ballooning (type 3), ballooning, and either Mallory's hyaline or fibrosis (type 4) further defined the groups. The study showed that prevalence of severe liver disease (cirrhosis) was greatest in types 3 (21%) and 4 (28%), but progression was also documented in those with 'simple steatosis' or NAFLD, type 1 (4%). Liver-related mortality was less than 2% in those with simple fatty liver, compared with 11% in types 3 and 4.[104] Saksena et al. have recently reported rates of progression to cirrhosis in an 8 year follow-up of 91 biopsied NAFLD patients: regardless of the diagnosis of NASH or simple steatosis on the index biopsy, progression rates were similar.[246] In addition, on rebiopsy, steatosis score increased in 61% (and decreased in 10%) in follow-up biopsies from subjects with initial NAFLD, in contrast with the 2% that increased or the 60% that decreased in steatohepatitis biopsies during the follow-up. No clinical findings were predictive of which patients remained stable or which progressed.

Powell et al.[181] showed progression to cirrhosis over a 5 year observation period in 3 of 42 subjects with biopsy-proven NASH. Evans et al. showed statistically insignificant progression of fibrosis in the 7 of 62 subjects who had repeat biopsies after mean follow-up of 8.2 years; the group calculated a rate of progression of 0.08 fibrosis units/year and projected the median years to cirrhosis as 45.[242] Harrison et al. studied 22 NAFLD subjects with follow-up biopsies after a mean of 5.7 years: 5% progressed and 18% improved.[247] Fassio et al.'s study of rebiopsy in 22 patients showed progression of fibrosis in 32%; none progressed to cirrhosis.[243] Adams et al. studied 100 untreated NAFLD patients with rebiopsy after a mean interval of 3.2 years. Progression of fibrosis occurred in 37%; fibrosis remained stable in 37% and spontaneously regressed in 29%. The rate of fibrosis progression ranged from −2.05 to 1.7 stage/year. The study showed that fibrosis progression rate positively correlated with a lower stage on the initial biopsy and with BMI and presence of diabetes.[248]

Adams et al.[249a] have recently reported on a population-based cohort study which may provide further insights into the natural history of NAFLD in the community. They compared 420 patients from a defined geographic region in the USA and compared overall survival with an age and sex-matched population. Survival was lower than that of the general population (standardized mortality ratio 1.34) and higher mortality was associated with age, fasting glucose and cirrhosis. Liver disease was the third leading cause of death, compared with thirteenth leading cause in the general population of that area.

Recent clinical treatment trials have provided further insight into natural history in well-characterized patients. A trial of rosiglitazone found histological improvement in 23% of subjects in the interval between initial biopsy and entry into the treatment trial; none had been actively treated in the interval.[103,127] An analysis by Lindor et al. of 107 subjects who completed a trial randomized for treatment with ursodeoxycholic acid or placebo and maintained stable body weight, showed biochemical improvement as well as biopsy-proven decrease in steatosis (in 40%) and fibrosis (in 20%) of subjects in both the placebo group and the treatment group. Fibrosis was stable in 52%, but progressed in 25%. While concerns of parenchymal 'sampling' were addressed, both studies confirm that the natural history of NASH may include spontaneous regression.[102]

Pathogenesis

The pathogenetic mechanisms that perpetuate the cycle of hepatocellular injury and fibrogenesis in NASH are not all understood, but some of the proposed pathways serve as a basis for therapeutic trials, i.e. weight loss, anti-oxidant treatments, insulin-sensitizing agents and hypolipidemic drugs.[11,155,156,156a,156b]

Mechanisms studied include interacting causes and manifestations of insulin resistance, hepatic steatosis, and aberrations in pathways of lipid oxidation and export; collectively, these mechanisms result in hepatocellular necrosis, apoptosis, inflammation and fibrosis.[7,8,85,115–117,250,251] In the original 'two-hit' hypothesis of Day and James[252] steatosis is the first 'hit' and the inflammatory and fibrogenic results of disordered metabolism of intracellular triglycerides, the second. Therapeutic intervention trials based on known and putative mechanisms have met with varying success, as reviewed elsewhere.[11,155]

Accumulation of triglycerides in the liver derives from cumulative imbalances of fatty acid delivery, and de novo production on the one hand, and disposal (oxidation or esterification and export) on the other (Figs 7.26, 7.27). A recent review discusses emerging understanding of the molecular basis of many of these inter-related pathways.[118] Broadly, these include: (i) aberrations in insulin-related lipolysis with resultant increased free fatty acid circulation and delivery to the liver and skeletal muscle; (ii) excess dietary carbohydrate with resultant de novo fatty acid synthesis in the liver, at least in part related to insulin-activation of sterol regulatory element-binding protein (SREBP-1c);[118] (iii) aberrations in the complex mechanisms of triglyceride assembly and export. Pathways of initiation and perpetuation of injury include impairment of mitochondrial β oxidation, with resultant production of reactive oxygen species; utilization of alternate pathways of peroxisomal and microsomal fatty acid oxidation;[85,253–255] lipid peroxidation and oxidative stress; impaired mitochondrial respiratory chain function and ATP depletion; depletion of intracellular anti-oxidants;

Hepatic Metabolism Free Fatty Acids

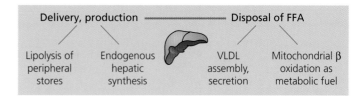

Nonalcoholic Fatty Liver Disease

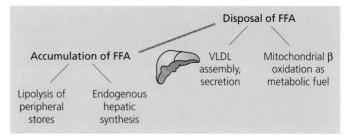

Fig. 7.26 and Fig. 7.27 • Schematic conception of the normal metabolic balance of fatty acid in the liver; when excess lipolysis and increased endogenous hepatic synthesis exceeds the capacity of the liver to synthesize and export VLDL particle or oxidize the free fatty acids, the imbalance results in steatosis.

mitochondrial DNA damage; production of the pro-inflammatory cytokines, including TNFα; induction of pro-apoptotic Fas ligand.[62,93,116,118,250,251,256] Self-perpetuating cycles of injury due to insulin resistance, hepatic and skeletal muscle fat accumulation, TNFα overexpression, chronic activation of inhibitor of kinase kappa beta (IKKβ), and interactions with nuclear transcription factor NF-κβ, have been inferred from animal models[62,115,250,256] (Figs 7.28, 7.29). Recently a tissue culture system has demonstrated a role of intracellular free fatty acids in lysosomal breakdown, induction of TNFα and lipotoxicity.[251]

Wanless proposed a '4 hit' hypothesis for initiation and perpetuation of progressive liver injury related to lipid accumulation and release based on histological observations: (i) insulin-induced steatosis; (ii) lipotoxicity and necrosis; (iii) inflammation secondary to released lipids; (iv) parenchymal extinction and fibrosis secondary to terminal hepatic venular obstruction.[257]

Iron

The role of iron overload as an underlying aetiology or as a promoter of progression and fibrosis in NAFLD and NASH, continues to be debated. Table 7.10 summarizes studies of the past 20 years; studies have shown increased *HFE* mutations[147,151,154] or increased iron stores[148,258,259] in subjects with NASH. The study of George et al. showed a positive correlation of increased hepatic iron stores with portal fibrosis;[151] this has not however been confirmed by others.[78,103,104,106,125,147,148,152–154,258,260,261]

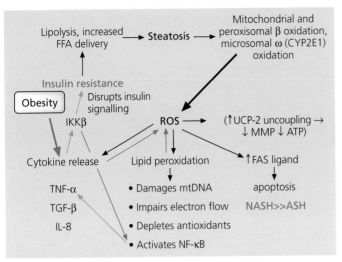

Fig. 7.28 • A simplified flow chart of the cyclic pathogenic events that both lead to and result in steatosis and steatohepatitis.

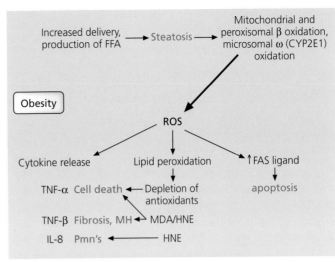

Fig. 7.29 • The same flow chart as Fig. 7.28 with emphasis on the concepts developed largely in animal models that the lesions associated with steatohepatitis are explained by pathogenetic models.

Table 7.10	Iron studies in NAFLD			
Author	No. pts or biopsies	% with stainable iron	Stainable iron: associated with histological fibrosis?	Serum iron studies or HFE mutations: associated with fibrosis?
Ludwig, 1980[1]	20	15	n/a	n/a
Bacon, 1994[78]	33	55	n/a	no
George, 1998[151]	51	41	yes	yes
Angulo, 1999[261]	144	n/a	n/a	no
Mendler, 1999[258]	161	21 H only, 79 H + RES	n/a	no
Bonkovsky, 1999[154]	57	n/a	n/a	no
Younossi, 1999[152]	65	n/a	n/a	no
Matteoni, 1999[164]	123	18	no	n/a
Brunt, 1999[125]	51	18 H	no	no
Ratziu, 2000[130]	93	26	no	no
Dixon, 2001[106]	105	0	no	n/a
Fargion, 2001[148]	40, hyperferritinemia	76 H; 35 H + RES	n/a	n/a
Fargion, 2001[148]	20, ultrasound	19	n/a	n/a
Chitturi, 2002[264]	93	10	no	no
Deguti, 2003[260]	32	10	no	no
Bugianesi, 2004[153]	263	n/a	n/a	no
Brunt, 2004[103]	30	30 H; 23 H + RES	no	no

H = hepatocellular iron
RES = reticulo-endothelial, includes sinusoidal lining cells, endothelia of portal and terminal hepatic venules
n/a: not stated

There are nevertheless studies that have demonstrated a relationship between insulin resistance and iron-overload; clinical manifestations include hyperferritinemia, normal transferrin saturation in most subjects, increased iron stores not related to hereditary haemochromatosis by HLA typing or *HFE* mutation.[148,258,262,263] Mendler et al.[258] studied 161 non-C282Y homozygous subjects from specialty clinic referrals with 'unexplained' iron overload; 94% had insulin resistance. Interestingly, 86% were men. Compound heterozygosity for *HFE* was related to increased iron stores, but also to lower incidence of histological NASH and steatosis, compared to subjects with no mutations or other genotypes.

Fargion et al.[148] found insulin resistance (69%), *HFE* mutations (65%), and biopsy-proven NASH (77%) respectively in 40 subjects with hyperferritinemia, all of whom had elevated liver iron. Of 90 patients with ultrasonograph evidence of steatosis, 27% had hyperferritinemia and normal transferrin saturation; 3 also had elevated serum glucose. In a study of 42 carbohydrate-intolerant non-obese patients without *HFE* mutations, Facchini et al.[263] documented NAFLD in 17 (40%); the diagnosis of NAFLD was made by a combination of clinical exclusions (alcohol, viral hepatitis studies, evaluation of copper and ceruloplasmin, α1AT levels and alkaline phosphatase, 'acute or chronic illness'), elevated ALT (>30 IU/L) and bright liver on ultrasound. All 42 subjects were phlebotomized to 'near-iron deficiency'; in the 17/42 patients with NAFLD, phlebotomy resulted in no change in body weight or medication use, but decrease in fasting insulin, glucose, AST, and ALT compared with the remaining 25/42 phlebotomized subjects without NAFLD. The possible relationship of venesection to improved insulin sensitivity is discussed in a recent review.[264]

Whether elevation of serum ferritin is a result of necrosis and inflammation[261,265] or truly a marker of metabolic syndrome[148,258,263] remains debated. Interestingly, as pointed out by Ferrannini[266] and Bugainesi et al.,[153] in vitro studies have shown that insulin binding causes simultaneous translocation of transferrin receptors, some glucose transporters and insulin-like growth factor II receptors from microsomal membranes to the cell membrane. Insulin may thus be linked to redistribution of transferrin receptors and cellular uptake of iron. These considerations are not exclusive of the concept of cytokine stimulation from inflammatory cascades in metabolic syndrome with resultant increased ferritin mRNA transcription.[266] Against the connection of iron and IR is the fact that, as noted by Bugianesi et al., iron overload is not associated with type 2 diabetes mellitus.[153]

The role of adipose tissue in NAFLD

Gut-derived peptides cholecystokinin, gherlin, PYY-36, glucagon-like peptide 1, and fat-derived protein leptin, interact with the central nervous system in the regulation of hunger and satiety; energy expenditure is regulated by thyroxine and T3 and the sympathetic nervous system;[267] for survival of the organism, these mechanisms are redundant and favour energy intake and accumulation.[268] Adipose tissue itself is no longer considered a simple excess energy storage depot, but rather a metabolically active endocrine organ that is the source of physiologically-active products, collectively referred to as adipokines or adipocytokines[269] that are involved in the metabolic linkage of glucose and lipid metabolism and the deleterious consequences of obesity[267] (Fig. 7.30). There is growing evidence that these mediators may play an important role in NAFLD.[269a] Adipogenesis and regulation of adipokine gene expression are regulated by the nuclear receptor, peroxisome proliferator activated receptor gamma (PPARγ); other members of this nuclear receptor superfamily, PPARα and PPARβ/δ are differentially expressed in liver, muscle and fat tissues and

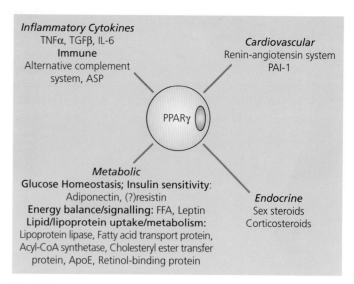

Fig. 7.30 • Visceral adipocyte endocrine products. This diagram illustrates the growing body of knowledge that identifies fat as a central effector organ in the multiple metabolic and cardiovascular manifestations of metabolic syndrome.[269,270,280]

play significant roles in lipid sensing and oxidation, glucose homeostasis and cellular metabolism, as reviewed.[267]

As stated by Arner,[270] 'not all fat is alike'. Visceral adipose tissue comprises 10–20% of total fat mass, and the proteins produced and fatty acids released in lipolysis drain directly into the liver via the portal system.[270] Animal studies have documented differences in adipose-related gene products (mRNA) in visceral vs subcutaneous depots[271] and cDNA levels[272] in cultured rodent white vs brown preadipocytes. Visceral adipose tissue is increasingly recognized as more significant than peripheral fat in the risk of cardiovascular disease related to metabolic syndrome.[256] The significance of truncal (visceral) obesity compared with overall body mass is also documented in NAFLD,[62,273,274] and may explain the recognized discrepancy of relatively lower BMI (body mass index) in Asians with the growing incidence of NAFLD.[52,53] A recent liposuction study[275] highlighted the differences: in spite of a 28–44% decrease in subcutaneous adipose tissue, no changes were noted in insulin-related effects of muscle glucose disposal, hepatic glucose production or adipose tissue lipolysis; in markers related to coronary artery disease risk (glucose, blood pressure and serum lipids); or in inflammatory markers, C-reactive protein, IL-6, TNFα, or adiponectin. Serum leptin levels, however, did decrease significantly.

PPARγ

PPARγ is a nuclear receptor central to regulation of adipogenesis and adipose tissue function; when bound by ligand, PPARγ codimerizes with retinoid X receptor and results in downstream regulation of a variety of key adipocyte-specific genes.[267,276] Two broad areas of active investigation are elucidating the essential role of this receptor in pathological conditions of insulin resistance, the known features of metabolic syndrome, and NASH: the beneficial effects of PPARγ ligands thiazolidinediones (TZDs) (troglitazone, rosiglitazone, pioglitazone) and the consequences of aberrant PPARγ gene expression or gene mutations in lipodystrophic conditions. Recent reviews[267,276] of a growing body of literature discuss differential tissue distribution of the three subclasses of PPARγ, and the molecular events and biological results of activation related to insulin sensitivity, adipocyte storage of fatty acids, and anti-inflammatory events following activation. Interestingly, endogenous ligands for the PPARγ receptors are yet to be discovered.[276]

Early studies with PPARγ agonists, thiazolidinediones (TZDs) in small numbers of patients with NASH, have shown biochemical and histological efficacy.[127,157,277,278] The multifactorial effects of TZDs are under study and include increased insulin sensitivity in liver and muscle, increased tissue glucose uptake, and decreased hepatic glucose output; decreased inflammation[279] and alteration of a variety of fat-derived biochemically active signalling molecules discussed below.[267]

Adipokines

Adipokines act variably in autocrine, endocrine and paracrine fashions and include proteins related to immune regulatory molecules and cytokines (TNF-α, IL-6, TGF-β, alternate complement proteins), proteins that affect vascular and endothelial function (angiotensinogen, other proteins of the renin-angiotensin system, and plasminogen-activator inhibitor), hormones being recognized in glucose homeostasis, insulin regulation and energy stores, (adiponectin, resistin, and leptin), lipid and lipoprotein metabolism (free fatty acids, lipoprotein lipase, fatty acid transport protein, cholesteryl ester transfer protein, apolipoprotein E, retinal-binding protein), and various endocrine and reproductive factors (corticosteroids and sex steroids).[269,280] Investigations have identified varying roles for these products in manifestations of metabolic syndrome.[256,281] Two adipokines studied in NASH are discussed briefly below.

Leptin

First recognized as the product of the 'obesity' gene,[282] the anorectic hormone leptin is an adipokine product of subcutaneous fat that plays a role in central (hypothalamic) signalling of energy status; absence or resistance to the signal correlates with starvation, even in the setting of obesity.[267] Leptin is functionally absent in the genetically obese *ob/ob* mouse model and the leptin receptor is absent or deficient in the *db/db* model. In humans, leptin levels are elevated in obesity, but may be in 'insufficient' amounts for the fat mass in subjects who develop NASH.[283] Chitturi et al. have shown elevated leptin levels and speculate NASH represents 'peripheral leptin resistance'.[284] Leptin has been shown to be: (i) involved in glucose metabolism,[284,285] (ii) profibrogenic,[135] (iii) an immune system modulator,[286] (iv) a mediator in hepatocyte regeneration in a steatotic mouse model[241] and, in animal models, is also postulated to be protective against lipotoxicity.[115]

Adiponectin

Adiponectin is the most abundant circulating hormone known in humans; intriguingly, there is an inverse relationship in concentrations of adiponectin in obesity, hypertriglyceridemia, type 2 diabetes and serum atherogenic markers, apo B and apo E.[287] A review of current work[287] indicates a growing focus on proposed central roles of adiponectin: (i) negative correlation with obesity and insulin resistance conditions is putatively through a negative feedback mechanism that may involve increased adipose-tissue derived TNFα; (ii) the globular domain of the protein is structurally similar to TNFα, and the two proteins have been shown to have locally antagonistic and opposite effects in arterial walls and in adipose tissue; (iii) hypoadiponectinemia has been demonstrated in conditions related to PPARγ mis-sense mutations or polymorphisms, suggesting this protein is a marker of PPARγ function; (iv) genetic regulation of adiponectin is not known, but mis-sense mutations in the globular domain have been identified in hypoadiponectinemia and type 2 diabetics; (v) thiazolidinedione (troglitazone, rosiglitazone, pioglitazone) treatments for diabetes have resulted in increased adiponectin levels.

In various animal models, adiponectin has been shown to decrease fibrosis in CCl_4-induced liver injury,[288] reverse insulin resistance in models of lipoatrophy and models of obesity,[289] and to protect against endotoxin-induced liver damage.[290] A study of steatohepatitis in both an obese mouse model and an alcoholic mouse model showed exogenously infused adiponectin improved hepatic steatosis, a variety of biochemical markers and insulin, and glucose and lipid metabolic parameters.[291] Hui et al.[107] documented hypoadiponectinemia in patients with biopsy-proven NASH, compared with those with simple steatosis; the reduced serum levels were related to inflammatory grades, but not serum ALT, in NASH. Leptin and TNFα levels did not show such correlations. The authors proposed a novel scoring system that utilizes serum adiponectin levels and insulin resistance calculations for differentiating subjects with NAFLD and NASH.[107]

The importance of perturbations in adiponectin regulation are reinforced by the study of Kaser et al.,[292a] who have recently demonstrated a reduction in hepatic expression of both adiponectin and its receptor adipo RII in biopsy tissue from patients with NASH.

Genetics

Just as not all patients who consume alcohol develop alcoholic liver disease,[292] not all subjects who are obese have insulin resistance, or metabolic syndrome will develop significant liver disease.[2,55,66,91,293–295] Furthermore, just as obesity is multifactorial, clearly NASH is also a complex process which may be influenced by environmental and genetic factors.

Two groups have documented kindreds with NAFLD and related cirrhosis,[296,297] in support of a role for a genetic predisposition. There is growing work utilizing newer technologies for DNA, RNA and protein analysis. For example, genetic variants in genes related to fatty acid mobilization (hormone specific lipase) and oxidation (adiponectin) have been shown in a preliminary study of 89 subjects with NASH.[298] Proteomic studies in mice and obese patients[299] showed various abnormalities in mitochondrial protein expression in steatohepatitis;[299] another group utilized proteomic analysis to identify distinct serum proteins in subjects with histologically confirmed NASH compared with NAFLD.[300] DNA microarray analysis of liver biopsies from patients with NASH- related cirrhosis provided evidence of altered expression in several genes related to insulin and mitochondrial function in patients with NASH.[301]

Day has reviewed other proposed genetic factors and polymorphisms in human or animal models focused on hepatic fat accumulation and progression of necroinflammatory damage. Broadly, these include predisposition for truncal pattern of obesity; factors that affect insulin sensitivity; lipolysis and secretion of free fatty acids; hepatic lipid storage and export; mitochondrial and peroxisomal oxidation; mechanisms that result in production of reactive oxygen species, lipid peroxidation, oxidative stress, and production of antioxidants, and various pro-inflammatory and fibrogenic cytokines.[115,250] Of particular interest is the recent identification of a polymorphism of the gene encoding phosphatidylethanomine N-methyltransferase which may confer susceptibility to NAFLD.[302] It is highly likely that further novel predisposing genetic factors will be identified in future studies.

Acknowledgement

The author appreciates the critical reading of the Pathogenesis section by Dr Brent A. Neuschwander Tetri.

References

1. Ludwig J, Viggiano TR, McGill DB, Oh BJ. Nonalcoholic steatohepatitis: Mayo Clinic experiences with a hitherto unnamed disease. Mayo Clin Proc, 1980; 55:434–438
2. Marchesini G, Brizi M, Bianchi G et al. Nonalcoholic fatty liver disease: a feature of the metabolic syndrome. Diabetes, 2001; 50:1844–1850
3. Marchesini G, Bugianesi E, Forlani G et al. Nonalcoholic fatty liver, steatohepatitis, and the metabolic syndrome. Hepatology, 2003; 37:917–923
4. Chitturi S, Abeygunasekera S, Farrell GC et al. NASH and insulin resistance: insulin hypersecretion and specific association with insulin resistance syndrome. Hepatology, 2002; 35:373–379
5. Adams LA, Angulo P. Recent concepts in non-alcoholic fatty liver disease. Diabet Med. 2005; 22:1129–1133
6. Clinical Practice Committee AGA. AGA Technical review on nonalcoholic fatty liver disease. Gastroenterology, 2002; 123:1705–1725
7. McCullough AJ. Update on nonalcoholic fatty liver disease. J Clin Gastroenterol, 2002; 34:255–262
8. Youssef WI, McCullough AJ. Diabetes mellitus, Obesity, and hepatic steatosis. Seminars in Gastrointestinal Disease, 2002; 13:17–30
9. O'Brien PE, Dixon JB. The extent of the problem of obesity. Am J Surg, 2002; 184:4S–8S
9a. Loria P, Lonardo A, Carulli N. Should nonalcoholic fatty liver disease be renamed? Dig Dis, 2005; 23:72–82
10. Dixon JB, O'Brien PE, Bhatal PS. A wider view on diagnostic criteria of nonalcoholic steatohepatitis (Reply). Gastroenterology, 2002; 122:841–842
11. Neuschwander-Tetri BA, Caldwell SH. Nonalcoholic steatohepatitis: Summary of an AASLD Single Topic Conference. Hepatology, 2003; 37:1202–1219
12. Farrell GC. Drugs and steatohepatitis. Semin Liv Dis, 2002; 22:185–194
13. Burt AD, Mutton A, Day CP. Diagnosis and interpretation of steatosis and steatohepatitis. Semin Diagn Pathol, 1998; 15:246–258
14. Ludwig J, McGill DB, Lindor KD. Review: nonalcoholic steatohepatitis. J Gastroenterol Hepatol, 1997; 12:398–403
15. Brunt EM. Nonalcoholic steatohepatitis: Definition and pathology. Semin Liv Dis, 2001; 21:3–16
16. Brunt EM. Nonalcoholic steatohepatitis. Semin Liver Dis, 2004; 24:3–20
17. Zelman S. The liver in obesity. Arch Int Med, 1958; 90:141–156
18. Thaler H. Die felleber und ihre pathogenethische Beziehung uzr libercirrhose. Virch Arch, 1962; 335:180–188
19. Thaler H. Relation of steatosis to cirrhosis. Clin Gastroenterol, 1975; 4:273–280
20. Connor CL. Fatty infiltration of liver and development of cirrhosis in diabetes and chronic alcoholism. Am J Pathol, 1938; 14:347–363
21. Reinberg MH, Lipson M. The association of Laennec's cirrhosis with diabetes mellitus. Ann Int Med, 1950; 33:1195–1202
22. Bloodworth JMB. Diabetes mellitus and cirrhosis of the liver. Arch Intern Med, 1961; 108:95–101
23. Jacques WE. The incidence of portal cirrhosis and fatty metamorphosis in patients dying with diabetes mellitus. N Engl J Med, 1953; 249:442–445
24. Adler M, Schaffner F. Fatty liver hepatitis and cirrhosis in obese patients. Am J Med, 1979; 67:811–816
25. Marubbio AT, Buchwald H, Schwartz MZ, Vargo R. Hepatic lesions of central pericellular fibrosis in morbid obesity and after jejunoileal bypass. Am J Clin Pathol, 1976; 66:684–691
26. Galambos JT, Wills CE. Relationship between 505 paired liver tests and biopsies to 242 obese patients. Gastroenterology, 1976; 74:1191–1195
27. Nasrallah SM, Wills CE, Galambos JT. Hepatic morphology in obesity. Dig Dis Sci, 1981; 26:325–327
28. Andersen T, Christoffersen P, Gluud C. The liver in consecutive patients with morbid obesity: a clinical, morphological and biochemical study. Int J Obes, 1984; 8:107–115
29. Eriksson S, Eriksson KF, Bondesson L. Nonalcoholic steatohepatitis in obesity: a reversible condition. Acta Medica Scand, 1986; 220:83–88
30. Klain J, Fraser D, Goldstein J et al. Liver histology abnormalities in the morbidly obese. Hepatology, 1989; 10:873–876
31. Watanabe A, Kobayashi M, Yoshitomi S, Nagashima H. Liver fibrosis in obese patients with fatty livers. J Med, 1989; 20:357–362
32. Silverman JF, O'Brien KF, Long S et al. Liver pathology in morbidly obese patients with and without diabetes. Am J Gastroenterol, 1990; 85:1349–1355
33. Zimmerman HJ, MacMurray FG, Rappaport H, Alpert LK. Studies of the liver in diabetes mellitus. J Lab Clin Med, 1950; 36:912–921
34. Itoh S, Tsukada N, Motomure Y, Ichinoe A. Five patients with nonalcoholic diabetic cirrhosis. Acta Hepato-Gastroenterol, 1979; 26:90–97
35. Nagore N, Scheuer PJ. The pathology of diabetic hepatitis. J Pathol, 1988; 156:155–160
36. Batman PA, Scheuer PJ. Diabetic hepatitis preceding the onset of glucose intolerance. Histopathology, 1985; 9:237–243
37. Peters RL. Hepatic morphologic changes after jejunoileal bypass. Progress in Liver Diseases, 1979; 6:581–594
38. Hamilton DL, Vest K, Brown BS, Shah AN, Menguy RB, Chey WY. Liver injury with alcoholic-like hyalin after gastroplasty for morbid obesity. Gastroenterology, 1983; 85:722–726
39. Vyberg M, Ravn V, Andersen B. Pattern of progression in liver injury following jejunoileal bypass for morbid obesity. Liver, 1987; 7:271–276
40. Peters RL, Gay T, Reynolds TB. Post-jejunoileal bypass hepatic disease. Am J Clin Pathol, 1975; 63:318–331
41. Silverman EM, Sapala JA, Appelman HD. Regression of hepatic steatosis in morbidly obese persons after gastric bypass. Am J Clin Pathol, 1995; 104:23–31
42. Itoh S, Igarashi M, Tsukada Y, Ichinoe A. Nonalcoholic fatty liver with alcoholic hyalin after long-term glucocorticoid therapy. Acta Hepato-Gastroenterol, 1977; 24:415–418

43. French SW, Eidus LB, Freeman J. Nonalcoholic fatty hepatitis: An important clinical condition. Can J Gastroenterol, 1989; 3:189–197

44. Wanless IR, Lentz JS. Fatty liver hepatitis (steatohepatitis) and obesity: an autopsy study with analysis of risk factors. Hepatology, 1990; 12:1106–1110

45. Diehl AM, Goodman Z, Ishak KG. Alcohollike liver disease in nonalcoholics. A clinical and histologic comparison with alcohol-induced liver injury. Gastroenterology, 1988; 95:1056–1062

46. Baker AL. Nonalcoholic steatonecrosis: A unique histopathologic lesion of the liver with multiple causes. Surv Dig Dis, 1985; 3:154–164

47. Wanless IR, Bargman J, Oreopoulos D, Vas S. Subcapsular steatonecrosis in response to peritoneal insulin deliver: A clue to the pathogenesis of steatonecrosis in obesity. Mod Pathol, 1989; 2

48. Deschamps D, DeBeco V, Fisch C et al. Inhibition by perhexiline of oxidative phosphorylation and the B-oxidation of fatty acids: possible role in pseudoalcoholic liver lesions. Hepatology, 1994; 19:948–961

49. Baldridge AD, Perezatayde AR, Graemecook F, Higgins L, Lavine JE. Idiopathic steatohepatitis in childhood—a multicenter retrospective study. J Pediatr, 1995; 127:700–704

50. Tankurt E, Biberoglu S, Ellidokuz E et al. Hyperinsulinemia and insulin resistance in non-alcoholic steatohepatitis. J Hepatol, 1999; 31:963

51. Bahrami H, Daryani NE, Mirmomen S, Kamangar F, Haghpanah B, Djalili M. Clinical and histological features of nonalcoholic steatohepatitis in Iranian patients. BMC Gastroenterology, 2003; 2003: http://www.biomedcentral.com/1471-230X/3/27

52. Chitturi S, Farrell GC, George J. Nonalcoholic steatohepatitis in the Asia-Pacific region: Future shock? J Gastroenterol Hepatol, 2004; 19:368–374

53. Farrell GC. Nonalcoholic steatohepatitis: What is it, and why is it important in the Asia-Pacific region? J Gastroenterol Hepatol, 2003; 18:124–138

54. Browning JD, Kumar KS, Saboorian H, Thiele DL. Ethnic differences in the prevalence of cryptogenic cirrhosis. Am J Gastroenterol, 2004; 99:292–298

55. Ruhl CE, Everhart JE. Determinants of the association of overweight with elevated serum alanine aminotrasferase activity in the United States. Gastroenterology, 2003; 124:71–79

56. Clark JM, Brancati FL, Diehl AM. The prevalence and etiology of elevated aminotransferase levels in the United States. Am J Gastroenterol, 2003; 98:960–967

57. Schwimmer JB, Deutsch R, Rauch J, Behling C, Newbury R, Lavine JE. Obesity, insulin resistance and other clinicopathological correlates of pediatric nonalcoholic fatty liver disease. J Pediatr, 2003; 143:500–505

58. Roberts EA. Nonalcoholic steatohepatitis in children. Current Gastroenterol Reports, 2003; 5:253–259

59. Roberts EA. Steatohepatitis in children. Best Practice & Research in Clinical Gastroenterology, 2002; 16:749–765

60. Caldwell SH, Harris DM, Patrie JT, Hespenheide EE. Is NASH underdiagnosed among African Americans? Am J Gastroenterol, 2002; 97:1496–1500

61. Clark JM, Diehl AM. Defining nonalcoholic fatty liver disease: implications for epidemiologic studies. Gastroenterology, 2003; 124:248–250

62. Clark JM, Brancati FL, Diehl AM. Nonalcoholic fatty liver disease. Gastroenterology, 2002; 122:1649–1657

63. Yu AS, Keefe EB. Elevated AST or ALT to nonalcoholic fatty liver disease: Accurate predictor of disease prevalence? (Editorial). Am J Gastroenterol, 2003; 98:955–956

64. Falck-Ytter Y, Younossi ZM, Marchesini G, McCullough AJ. Clinical features and natural history of nonalcoholic steatosis syndromes. Semin Liv Dis, 2001; 21:17–26

65. Hayashi PH, Harrison SA, Torgerson S, Perez TA, Nochajski T, Russell M. Cognitive lifetime drinking history in nonalcoholic fatty liver disease: some cases may be alcohol related. Am J Gastroenterol, 2004; 99:76–81

66. Dixon JB, Bhathal PS, O'Brien PE. Nonalcoholic fatty liver disease: Predictors of nonalcoholic steatohepatitis and liver fibrosis in the severely obese. Gastroenterology, 2001; 121:91–100

67. Wigg AJ, Roberts-Thomson IC, Dymock RB, McCarthy PJ, Grose RH, Cummins AG. The role of small intestinal bacterial overgrowth, intestinal permeability, endotoxaemia, and tumour necrosis factor alpha in the pathogenesis of non-alcoholic steatohepatitis. Gut, 2001; 48:206–211

68. Farrell GC. Is bacterial ash the flash that ignites NASH? Gut, 2001; 48:148–149

69. Nomura H, Kashigawai S, Hayashi J, Kaiyama W, Tani S, Goto M. Prevalence of fatty liver in a general population of Okinawa, Japan. Jap J Med, 1988; 27:142–149

70. Lonardo A, Bellini M, Tartoni P, Tondelli E. The bright liver syndrome—prevalence and determinants of a 'bright' liver echopattern. Ital J Gastroenterol Hepatol, 1997; 29:351–356

71. Bellentani S, Saccicio G, Masutti F, Croce LS, Cristanini G et al. Prevalence of and risk factors for hepatic steatosis in northern Italy. Ann Int Med, 2000; 132:112–117

72. Hilden M, Christoffersen P, Juhl E, Dalgaard JB. Liver histology in a 'normal' population-Examinations of 503 consecutive fatal traffic casualties. Scand J Gastroenterol, 1977; 12:593–597

73. Hornboll P, Olsen TS. Fatty changes in the liver. Acta Pathologia Microbiol Immunol Scand Sect A 1982; 90:199–205

74. Underwood Ground KE. Prevalence of fatty liver in healthy male adults accidently killed. Aviation, Space and Environmental Medicine, 1984; 55:59–61

75. Prati D, Taioli E, Zanella A et al. Updated definitions of healthy ranges for serum alanine aminotransferase levels. Ann Int Med, 2002; 137:1–9

76. Clinical Practice Committee AGA. AGA medical position statement: Evaluation of liver chemistry tests. Gastroenterology 2003; 123:1364–1366

77. Mofrad P, Contos MJ, Haque M et al. Clinical and histologic spectrum of nonalcoholic fatty liver disease associated with normal ALT values. Hepatology, 2003; 37:1286–1292

78. Bacon BR, Farahvash MJ, Janney CG, Neuschwandertetri BA. Nonalcoholic steatohepatitis—an expanded clinical entity. Gastroenterology, 1994; 107:1103–1109

79. Latham PS, Borum ML, Nsien EE. Nonalcoholic steatohepatitis (NASH) in patients with morbid obesity is commonly associated with normal liver enzymes. Hepatology, 2003; 38:233A

80. Weltman MD, Das A, Martin C, Wyatt JM, Cox M. Nonalcoholic fatty liver disase—A common disorder in patients presenting for laparascopic cholecystectomy. Hepatology, 2003; 38:234A

81. Adams LA, Feldstein AE, Lindor KD, Angulo P. Nonalcoholic fatty liver disease among patients with hypothalamic and pituitary dysfunction. Hepatology, 2004; 39:909–914

82. Altuntas B, Ozcakar B, Bideci A, Cinaz P. Cirrhotic outcome in patients with craniopharyngioma. J Pediatr Endocrinol Metabol 2002; 58:1057–1058

83. Basenau D, Stephani U, Fischer G. Development of complete liver cirrhosis in hyperphagia-induced fatty liver. (In German). Klin Padiatr, 1994; 206:62–64

84. Liangpunsakul S, Chalasani N. Is hypothyroidism a risk factor for nonalcoholic steatohepatitis? J Clin Gastroenterol, 2003; 37:340–343

85. Chitturi S, Farrell GC. Etiopathogenesis of nonalcoholic steatohepatitis. Semin Liv Dis, 2001; 21:27–41

86. Stravitz RT, Sanyal AJ. Drug-induced steatohepatitis. Clin Liv Dis, 2003; 7:435–451

87. Cotrim HP, Andrade ZA, Parana R, Portugal M, Lyra LG, Freitas LA. Nonalcoholic steatohepatitis: a toxic liver disease in industrial workers. Liver, 1999; 19:299–304

88. Wanless IR, Dore S, Gopinath N et al. Histopathology of cocaine hepatotoxicity. Report of four patients. Gastroenterology 1990; 98:497–501

89. Diehl AM. Nonalcoholic steatohepatitis. Semin Liv Dis, 1999; 19:221–229

90. Beymer C, Kowdley KV, Larson A, Edmonson P, Dellinger P, Flum DR. Prevalence and prdictors of asymptomatic liver disease in patients undergoing gastric bypass surgery. Arch Surg, 2003; 138:1240–1244

91. Garcia-Monzon C, Martin-Perez E, Lo Iacono O et al. Characterization of pathogenic and prognostic factors of nonalcoholic steatohepatitis associated with obesity. J Hepatol, 2000; 33:716–724

92. Charlton M, Kasparova P, Weston S et al. Frequency of nonalcoholic steatohepatitis as a cause of advanced liver disease. Liver Transpl, 2001; 7:608–614

93. Angulo P. Nonalcoholic fatty liver disease. N Engl J Med, 2002; 346:1221–1231

94. Neuschwander-Tetri BA. Nonalcoholic steatohepatitis: an evolving diagnosis. Can J Gastroenterol, 2000; 14:321–326

95. Gramlich T, Kleiner DE, McCullough AJ, Matteoni CA, Boparai N, Younossi ZM. Pathologic features associated with fibrosis in nonalcoholic fatty liver disease. Hum Pathol, 2004; 35:196–199

96. Neuschwander-Tetri BA. Evolving pathophysiologic concepts in nonalcoholic steatohepatitis. Current Gastroenterology Reports 2002; 4:31–36

97. Chatila R, West AB. Hepatomegaly and abnormal liver tests due to glycogenosis in adults with diabetes. Medicine, 1996; 75:327–333

98. Chen YY, Brunt EM, Jakate SM et al. Glycogenic hepatopathy: An under-recognized complication of diabetes mellitus. Mod Pathol, 2004; 17:297A

99. Harrison SA, Brunt EM, Goodman ZD, Di Bisceglie AM. Diabetic hepatosclerosis: perisinusoidal hepatic fibrosis without steatohepatitis among diabetics. Hepatology, 2003; 38:266A

100. Skelly MM, James PD, Ryder SD. Findings on liver biopsy to investigate abnormal liver function tests in the absence of diagnostic serology. J Hepatol, 2001; 35:195–199

101. Merriman RB, Ferrell LD, Patti MG et al. Histologic correlation of paired right lobe and left lobe liver biopsies in morbidly obese individuals with suspected nonalcoholic fatty liver disease. Hepatology, 2003; 39:232A

101a. Ratziu V, Charlotte F, Heurtier A et al. Sampling variability of liver biopsy in nonalcoholic fatty liver disease. Gastroenterology, 2005; 128:1898–1906

101b. Janiec DJ, Jacobson ER, Freeth A, Spaulding L, Blaszyk H Histologic variation of grade and stage of non-alcoholic fatty liver disease in liver biopsies. Obes Surg, 2005; 15:497–501

101c. Goldstein NS, Hastah F, Galan MV, Gordon SC. Fibrosis heterogeneity in nonalcoholic steatohepatitis and hepatitis C virus needle core biopsy specimens. Am J Clin Pathol, 2005; 123:382–387

102. Lindor KD, Kowdley KV, Heathcote EJ et al. Ursodeoxycholic acid for treatment of nonalcoholic steatohepatitis: results of a randomized trial. Hepatology, 2004; 39:770–778

103. Brunt EM, Neuschwander-Tetri BA, Oliver DA, Wehmeier KR, Bacon BR. Nonalcoholic steatohepatitis: histologic features and clinical correlations with 30 blinded biopsies. Hum Pathol, 2004; 35; 1070–1082

104. Matteoni CA, Younossi ZM, Gramlich T, Boparai N, Liu YC, McCullough AJ. Nonalcoholic fatty liver disease: A spectrum of clinical and pathological severity. Gastroenterology, 1999; 116:1413–1419

105. Sanyal AJ, Campbell-Sargent C, Mirshahi F et al. Nonalcoholic steatohepatitis: association of insulin resistance and mitochondrial abnormalities. Gastroenterology, 2001; 120:1183–1192

106. Dixon JB, Bhatal PS, O'Brien PE. Nonalcoholic fatty liver disease: predictors of nonalcoholic steatohepatitis and liver fibrosis in the severely obese. Gastroenterology, 2001; 121:91–100

107. Hui JM, Hodge A, Farrell GC, Kench JG, Kriketos A, George J. Beyond insulin resistance in NASH: TNF-a or adiponectin? Hepatology, 2004; 40:46–54

108. Lee RG. Nonalcoholic steatohepatitis: a study of 49 patients. Human Pathology, 1989; 20:594–598

109. Itoh S, Yougel T, Kawagoe K. Comparison between nonalcoholic steatohepatitis and alcoholic hepatitis. Am J Gastroenterol, 1987; 82:650–654

110. Contos MJ, Sanyal AJ. The clinicopathologic spectrum and management of nonalcoholic fatty liver disease. Adv Anatomic Pathol, 2002; 1:37–51

111. Cortez-Pinto H, Baptista A, Camilo ME, Valente A, Saragoca A, Demoura MC. Nonalcoholic steatohepatitis—clinicopathological comparison with alcoholic hepatitis in ambulatory and hospitalized patients. Dig Dis Sci 1996; 41:172–179

112. Crawford DH, Powell EE, Searle J, Powell LW. Steatohepatitis: comparison of alcoholic and non-alcoholic subjects with particular reference to portal hypertension and hepatic complications. J Gastroenterol Hepatol, 1989; 1:36–38

113. Andersen T, Gluud C. Liver morphology in morbid obesity: a literature study. Int J Obes, 1984; 8:97–106

114. Marceau P, Biron S, Hould FS et al. Liver pathology and the metabolic syndrome X in severe obesity. J Clin Endocrinol Metabol,1999; 84:1513–1517

115. Day CP. Pathogenesis of steatohepatitis. Best Practice & Research in Clinical Gastroenterology, 2002; 16:663–678

116. Pessayre D, Berson A, Fromenty B, Mansouri A. Mitochondria in steatohepatitis. Semin Liv Dis, 2001; 21:57–69

117. Feldstein AE, Canbay A, Angulo P et al. Hepatocyte apoptosis and fas expression are prominent features of human nonalcoholic steatohepatitis. Gastroenterology, 2003; 125:437–443

118. Browning JD, Horton JD. Molecular mediators of hepatic steatosis and liver injury. J Clin Invest 2004; 114:147–152

119. Brunt EM. Alcoholic and nonalcoholic steatohepatitis. Clin Liv Dis, 2002; 6:399–420

120. Schwimmer JB, Behling C, Newbury R et al. Histopathology of pediatric nonalcoholic fatty liver disease. Hepatology. 2005; 42:641–649

120a. Franzen LE, Ekstedt M, Kechagias S, Bodin L. Semiquantitative evaluation overestimates the degree of steatosis in liver biopsies: a comparison to stereological point counting. Mod Pathol, 2005; 18:912–916

121. Rashid M, Roberts EA. Nonalcoholic steatohepatitis in children. J Ped Gastroenterol Nutr, 2000; 30:48–53

122. Ishak KG. Light microscopic morphology of viral hepatitis. Am J Clin Pathol, 1976; 65:787–827

123. Caldwell SH, Chang C, Krugner-Higby LA, Redick JA, Davis CA, Al-Osaimi AMS. The ballooned hepatocyte in NAFLD: Denegerative or adaptive? J Hepatol, 2004; 40(suppl 1):168A

124. Lefkowitch JH, Haythe J, Regent N. Kupffer cell aggregation and perivenular distribution in steatohepatitis. Mod Pathol, 2002; 15:699–704

125. Brunt EM, Janney CG, Di Bisceglie AM, Neuschwander-Tetri BA, Bacon BR. Nonalcoholic steatohepatitis: a proposal for grading and staging the histological lesions. Am J Gastroenterol, 1999; 94:2467–2474

126. Dixon JB, Bhatal PS, Hughes NR, O'Brien PE. Nonalcoholic fatty liver disease: Improvement in liver histological analysis with weight loss. Hepatology, 2004; 39:1647–1654

127. Neuschwander-Tetri BA, Brunt EM, Wehmeier KR, Oliver D, Bacon BR. Improvement in nonoalcholic steatohepatitis following 48 weeks of treatment with the PPAR-g ligand rosiglitazone. Hepatology, 2003; 38:1008–1017

128. Marrubio AT, Buchwald H, Schwartz MZ, Varco R. Hepatic lesions of central pericellular fibrosis in morbid obesity and after jejunoileal bypass. Am J Clin Pathol, 1976; 66:684–691

129. Schaffner F, Thaler H. Nonalcoholic fatty liver disease. Progress in Liver Diseases, 1986; 8:283–298

130. Ratziu V, Giral P, Charlotte F et al. Liver fibrosis in overweight patients. Gastroenterology, 2000; 118:1117–1123

131. Group TFMCS. Intraobserver and interobserver variations in liver biopsy interpretation in patients with chronic hepatitis C. Hepatology, 1994; 20:15–20

131a. Abrams GA, Kunde SS, Lazenby AJ, Clements RH. Portal fibrosis and hepatic steatosis in morbidly obese subjects: a spectrum of nonalcoholic fatty liver disease. Hepatology, 2004; 40:475–483

132. Paradis V, Perlemuter G, Bonvoust F et al. High glucose and hyperinsulinemia stimulate connective tissue growth factor expression: a potential mechanism involved in progression to fibrosis in nonalcoholic steatohepatitis. Hepatology, 2001; 34:738–744

133. Washington K, Wright K, Shyr Y, Hunter EB, Olson S, Raiford DS. Hepatic stellate cell activation in nonalcoholic steatohepatitis and fatty liver. Hum Pathol, 2000; 31:822–828

134. Cortez-Pinto H, Baptista A, Camilo ME, de Moura MC. Hepatic stellate cell activation occurs in nonalcoholic steatohepatitis. Hepato-Gastroenterology, 2001; 48:87–90

135. Leclercq IA, Farrell GC, Schriemer R, Robertson GR. Leptin is essential for the hepatic fibrogenic response to chronic liver injury. J Hepatol, 2002; 37:206–213

136. Denk H, Stumptner C, Zatloukal K. Mallory bodies revisited. J Hepatol, 2000; 32:689–702

137. Ludwig J, McGill DB, Lindor KD. Nonalcoholic steatohepatitis. J Gastroenterol Hepatol, 1997; 12:398–403

138. Braillon A, Capron JP, Herve MA, Degott C, Quenum C. Liver in obesity. Gut, 1985; 26:133–139

139. Stumptner C, Fuchsbichler A, Heid H, Zatloukal K, Denk H. Mallory Body—A disease-associated type of sequestosome. Hepatology, 2002; 35:1053–1062

140. Savas MC, Koruk M, Pirim I et al. Serum ubiquitin levels in patients with nonalcoholic steatohepatitis. Hepato-Gastroenterology, 2003; 50:738–741

141. Nanki T, Koike R, Miyasaka N. Subacute severe steatohepatitis during prednisolone therapy for systemic lupus erythematosis (Letter to editor). Am J Gastroenterol, 1999; 94:3379

142. Dourakis SP, Sevastinaos VA, Kaliopi P. Acute severe steatohepatitis related to prednisolone therapy (Letter to editor). Am J Gastroenterol, 2002; 97:1074–1075

143. Caldwell SH, Hespenheide EE. Subacute liver failure in obese women. Am J Gastroenterol 2002; 97:2058–2062

144. Caldwell SH, Swerdlow RH, Khan EM et al. Mitochondrial abnormalities in non-alcoholic steatohepatitis. J Hepatol, 1999; 31:430–434

144a. Pessayre D, Fromenty B. NASH: a mitochodrial disease. J Hepatol, 2005; 928–940

145. Teli MR, Day CP, Burt AD, Bennett MJ, James OF. Determinants of progression to cirrhosis or fibrosis in pure alcoholic fatty liver. Lancet 1995; 346:987–990

146. Le TH, Caldwell SH, Redick JA et al. The zonal distribution of megamitochondria with crystalline inclusions in nonalcoholic steatohepatitis. Hepatology, 2004; 39:1423–1429

147. Chitturi S, Weltman M, Farrell GC et al. HFE Mutations, hepatic iron, and fibrosis: Ethnic-specific association of NASH with C282Y but not with fibrotic severity. Hepatology, 2002; 36:142–149

148. Fargion S, Mattioli M, Fracanzani AL et al. Hyperferritinemia, iron overload and multiple metabolic alterations identify patients at risk for nonalcoholic steatohepatitis. Am J Gastroenterol, 2001; 96:2448–2455

149. Bhattacharya R, Kowdley KV. Iron and *HFE* mutations in nonalcoholic steatohepatitis: innocent bystanders or accessories to the crime? Gastroenterology, 2003; 125:615–616

150. Turlin B, Mendler MH, Moirand R, Guyader D, Guillygomarc'h A, Deugnier Y. Histologic features of the liver in insulin resistance-associated iron overload. Am J Clin Pathol, 2001; 116:263–270

151. George DK, Goldwurm S, MacDonald GA et al. Increased hepatic iron concentration in nonalcoholic steatohepatitis is associated with increased fibrosis. Gastroenterology, 1998; 114:311–318

152. Younossi ZM, Gramlich T, Bacon BR et al. Hepatic iron and nonalcoholic fatty liver disease. Hepatology, 1999; 30:847–850

153. Bugianesi E, Manzini P, D'Antico S et al. Relative contribution of iron burden, HFE mutations, and insulin resistance to fibrosis in nonalcoholic fatty liver. Hepatology, 2004; 39:179–187

154. Bonkovsky HL, Jawaid Q, Tortorelli K et al. Non-alcoholic steatohepatitis and iron: increased prevalence of mutations of the HFE gene in non-alcoholic steatohepatitis. J Hepatol, 1999; 31:421–429

155. Angulo P, Lindor KD. Treatment of nonalcoholic fatty liver: Present and emerging therapies. Semin Liv Dis, 2001; 21:81–88

156. Harrison SA, Di Bisceglie AM. Advances in the understanding and treatment of nonalcoholic fatty liver disease. Drugs, 2003; 63:2379–2394

156a. Bugianesi E, McCullough AJ, Marchesini G. Insulin resistance: a metabolic pathway to chronic liver disease. Hepatology, 2005 Nov; 42(5):987–1000

156b. Sanyal AJ. Mechanisms of Disease: pathogenesis of nonalcoholic fatty liver disease. Nat Clin Pract Gastroenterol Hepatol., 2005 Jan; 2(1):46–53

157. Promrat K, Lutchman G, Uwaifo GI et al. A pilot study of pioglitazone treatment fo nonalcoholic steatohepatitis. Hepatology, 2004; 39:188–196

158. Younossi ZM, Gramlich T, Liu YC et al. Nonalcoholic fatty liver disease—assessment of variability in pathologic interpretations. Mod Pathol, 1998; 11:560–565

159. Kleiner DE, Brunt EM, Van Natta M et al. Nonalcoholic steatohepatitis Clinical Research Network: Design and validation of a histological scoring system for nonalcoholic fatty liver disease. Hepatology, 2005; 41:1313–1321

160. Brunt EM. Grading and staging the histopathologcial lesions of chronic hepatitis: The Knodell histology activity index and beyond. Hepatology, 2000; 31:241–246

161. Ishak KG, Baptista A, Bianchi L et al. Histological grading and staging of chronic hepatitis. J Hepatol, 1995; 22:696–699

162. Scheuer PJ. Scoring of liver biopsies: are we doing it right? European J Gastroenterol Hepatol, 1996; 8:1141–1142

163. Mendler MH, Kanel G, Govindarajan S. Proposal for a histological scoring and grading system for non-alcoholic fatty liver disease. Liver Int. 2005; 25:294–304

164. Weiss R, Dziura J, Burgert TS et al. Obesity and the metabolic syndrome in children and adolescents. N Engl J Med, 2004; 350

165. Srinivasan R, Hadzic N, Fischer J, Knisely AS. Steatohepatitis and unsuspected micronodular cirrhosis in Dorfman-Chanarin syndrome with documented *ABHD5* mutation. J Pediatr, 2004; 144:662–665

166. Lustig R. Hypothalamic obesity: the sixth cranial endocrinopathy. Endocrinologist, 2002; 12:210–217

167. Bass NM. Three for the price of one knockout—a mouse model of a congenital peroxisomal disorder, steatohepatitis, and hepatocarcinogenesis. Hepatology, 1999; 29:606–608

168. Tominaga K, Kurata JH, Chen YK et al. Prevalence of fatty liver in Japanese children and relationship to obesity. An epidemiological ultrasonographic survey. Dig Dis Sci, 1995; 40:2002–2009

169. Guzzaloni G, Grugni G, Minocci A, Moro D, Morabito F. Liver steatosis in juvenile obesity: correlations with lipid profile, hepatic biochemical parameters and glycemic and insulinemic responses to an oral glucose tolerance test. Int J Obes, 2000; 24:772–776

170. Tazawa Y, Noguchi H, Nishinomiya F, Takada G. Serum alanine aminotransferase activity in obese children. Acta Paediatrica, 1997; 86:238–241

171. Franzese A, Vajro P, Argenziano A et al. Liver involvement in obese children—ultrasonography and liver enzyme levels at diagnosis and during follow-up in an Italian population. Dig Dis Sci, 1997; 42:1428–1432

172. Kinugasa A, Tsunamoto K, Furukawa N, Sawada T, Kusunoki T, Shimada N. Fatty liver and its fibrous changes found in simple obesity of children. J Pediatr Gastroenterol Nutr, 1984; 3:408–414

173. Vajro P, Fontanella A, Perna C, Orso G, Tedesco M, De Vincenzo A. Persistent hypertransaminasemia resolving after weight reduction in obese children. J Pediatr, 1994; 125:239–241

174. Sathya P, Martin S, Alvarez F. Nonalcoholic fatty liver disease (NAFLD) in children. Curr Opin Pediatr, 2002; 14:593–600

175. Moran JR, Ghishan FK, Halter SA, Greene HL. Steatohepatitis in obese children: a cause of chronic liver dysfunction. Am J Gastroenterol, 1983; 78:374–377

176. Baldridge AD, Perez-Atayde AR, Graeme-Cook F, Higgins L, Lavine JE. Idiopathic steatohepatitis in childhood: a multicenter retrospective study. J Pediatr, 1995; 127:700–704

177. Manton ND, Lipsett J, Moore DJ, Davidson GP, Bourne AJ, Couper RT. Non-alcoholic steatohepatitis in children and adolescents. Med J Austr, 2000; 173:476–479

178. Molleston JP, White F, Teckman J, Fitzgerald JF. Obese children with steatohepatitis can develop cirrhosis in childhood. Am J Gastroenterol, 2002; 97:2460–2462

179. Lavine JE. Vitamin E treatment of nonalcoholic steatohepatitis in children: a pilot study. J Pediatr, 2000; 136:734–738

180. Vajro P, Franzese A, Valerio G, Iannucci MP, Aragione N. Lack of efficacy of ursodeoxycholic acid for the treatment of liver abnormalities in obese children. J Pediatr, 2000; 136:739–743

181. Powell EE, Cooksley WG, Hanson R, Searle J, Halliday JW, Powell LW. The natural history of nonalcoholic steatohepatitis: a follow-up study of forty-two patients for up to 21 years. Hepatology, 1990; 11:74–80

182. Abdelmalek M, Ludwig J, Lindor KD. Two cases from the spectrum of nonalcoholic steatohepatitis. J Clin Gastroenterol, 1995; 20:127–130

183. Caldwell SH, Oelsner DH, Iezzoni JC, Hespenheide EE, Battle EH, Driscoll CJ. Cryptogenic cirrhosis: Clinical characterization and risk factors for underlying disease. Hepatology, 1999; 29:664–669

184. Poonawala A, Nair SP, Thuluvath PJ. Prevalence of obesity and diabetes in patients with cryptogenic cirrhosis: A case-control study. Hepatology, 2000; 32:689–692

185. Bugianesi E, Leone N, Vanni E et al. Expanding the natural history of non-alcoholic steatohepatitis: from cryptogenic cirrhosis to hepatocellular carcinoma. Gastroenterology, 2002; 123:134–140

186. Mokdad AH, Bowman BA, Ford ES, Vinicor F, Marks JS, Koplan JP. The continuing epidemics of obesity and diabetes in the United States. JAMA, 2001; 286:1195–2000

187. Ong JP, Younossi ZM, Reddy V et al. Cryptogenic cirrhosis and posttransplantation nonalcoholic fatty liver disease. Liver Transpl, 2001; 7:797–801

188. Maor-Kendler Y, Batts KP, Burgart LJ et al. Comparative allograft histology after liver transplantation for cryptogenic cirrhosis, alcohol, hepatitis C, and cholestatic liver diseases. Transplantation, 2000; 70:292–297

189. Contos MJ, Cales W, Sterling RK et al. Development of nonalcoholic fatty liver disease after orthotopic liver transplantation for cryptogenic cirrhosis. Liver Transplantation, 2001; 7:363–373

190. Shimada M, Hashimoto E, Taniai M et al. Hepatocellular carcinoma in patients with non-alcoholic steatohepatitis. J Hepatol, 2002; 37:154–160

191. Hui JM, Kench JG, Chitturi S et al. Long-term outcomes of cirrhosis in nonalcoholic steatohepatitis compared with hepatitis C. Hepatology, 2003; 38:420–427

192. Molloy RM, Komorowski R, Varma RR. Recurrent nonalcoholic steatohepatitis and cirrhosis after liver transplantation. Liver Transpl Surg, 1997; 3:177–178

193. Carson K, Washington MK, Treem WR, Clavien PA, Hunt CM. Recurrence of nonalcoholic steatohepatitis in a liver transplant recipient. Liver Transpl Surg, 1997; 3:174–176

194. Kim WR, Poterucha JJ, Porayko MK, Dickson ER, Steers JL, Wiesner RH. Recurrence of nonalcoholic steatohepatitis following liver transplantation. Transplantation, 1996; 62:1802–1805

195. Czaja AJ. Recurrence of nonalcoholic steatohepatitis after liver transplantation. Liver Transpl Surg, 1997; 3:185–186

196. Shimada M, Hashimoto E, Kaneda H, Noguchi S, Hayashi N. Nonalcoholic steatohepatitis: risk factors for liver fibrosis. Hepatol Res, 2002; 24:429–438

197. Loria P, Lonardo A, Leonardi F et al. Non-organ-specific autoantibodies in nonalcoholic fatty liver disease: prevalence and correlates. Dig Dis Sci 2003; 48:2173–2181

198. Kanji K, Jakate S, Keshavarzian A, Jensen DM, Cotler SJ. Prevalence and clinical features associated with autoantibodies in nonalcoholic steatohepatitis (NASH). Hepatology, 2003; 34:506A

199. Adams LA, Keach JC, Lindor KD, Angulo P. Prevalence of autoantibodies and autoimmune hepatitis in nonalcoholic fatty liver disease. Hepatology, 2003; 34:503A

200. Brunt EM, Ramrakhiani S, Cordes BG et al. Concurrence of histologic features of steathepatitis with other forms of chronic liver disease. Mod Pathol, 2003; 16:49–56

201. Ong JP, Younossi ZM, Speer C, Olano A, Gramlich T, Boparai N. Chronic hepatitis C and superimposed nonalcoholic fatty liver disease. Liver, 2001; 21:266–271

202. Sanyal AJ, Contos MJ, Sterling RK et al. Nonalcoholic fatty liver disease in patients with hepatitis C is associated with features of the metabolic syndrome. Am J Gastroenterol, 2003; 98:2064–2071

203. Clouston AD, Powell EE. Interaction of non-alcoholic fatty liver disease with other liver diseases. Best Practice & Research in Clinical Gastroenterology, 2002; 16:767–781

204. Brunt EM, Tiniakos DG. Steatosis, steatohepatitis: review of effects on chronic hepatitis C. Current Hepatitis Reports, 2002; 1:38–44

205. Hourigan LF, Macdonald GA, Purdie D et al. Fibrosis in chronic hepatitis C correlates significantly with body mass index and steatosis. Hepatology, 1999; 29:1215–1219

206. Adinolfi LE, Utili R, Ruggiero G. Body composition and hepatic steatosis as precursors of fibrosis in chronic hepatitis C patients. Hepatology, 1999; 30:1530

207. Adinolfi LE, Utili R, Andreana A et al. Serum HCV RNA levels correlate with histological liver damage and concur with steatosis in progression of chronic hepatitis C. Dig Dis Sci 2001; 46

208. Adinolfi LE, Gambardella M, Andreana A, Tripodi MF, Utili R, Ruggiero G. Steatosis accelerates the progression of liver damage of chronic hepatitis C patients and correlates with specific HCV genotype and visceral obesity. Hepatology, 2001; 33:1358–1364

209. Lonardo A, Adinolfi LE, Loria P, Carulli N, Ruggiero G, Day CP. Steatosis and hepatitis C virus: Mechanisms and significance for hepatic and extrahepatic disease. Gastroenterology 2004; 126:586–597

210. Hui JM, Kench J, Farrell GC et al. Genotype-specific mechanisms for hepatic steatosis in chronic hepatitis C infection. J Gastroenterol Hepatol. 2002; 17:873–881

211. Maeno T, Okumura A, Ishikawa T et al. Mechanisms of increased insulin resistance in non-cirrhotic patients with chronic hepatitis C infection. J Gastroenterol Hepatol, 2003; 18:1358–1363

212. Shintani Y, Fujie H, Miyoshi H et al. Hepatitis C virus infection and diabetes: direct involvement of the virus in the development of insulin resistance. Gastroenterology, 2004; 126:840–848

213. Weinman SA, Belalcazar LM. Hepatitis C: A metabolic liver disease. Gastroenterology, 2004; 126:917–919

214. Hui JM, Sud A, Farrell GC et al. Insulin resistance is associated with chronic hepatitis C virus infection fibrosis progression. Gastroenterology, 2003; 125:1695–1704

215. Soga M, Kishimoto Y, Kawaguchi J et al. The FLS mouse: A new inbred strain with spontaneous fatty liver. Laboratory Animal Science, 1999; 49:269–275

216. Brunt EM, Wolverson MK, Di Bisceglie AM. Hepatic adenomatosis in nonalcoholic steatohepatitis: A case report. in preparation

217. Calle EE, Rodriguez C, Walker-Thurmond K, Thun MJ. Overweight, obesity, and mortality from cancer in a prospectively studied cohort of U.S. adults. N Engl J Med, 2003; 348:1625–1638

218. Nair S, Mason A, Eason J, Loss G, Perillo RP. Is obesity an independent risk factor for hepatocellular carcinoma in cirrhosis? Hepatology, 2002; 36:150–155

219. Balkau B, Kahn HS, Courbon D, Eschwege E, Ducimetiere P. Hyperinsulinemia predicts fatal liver cancer but is inversely associated with fatal cancer at some other sites. Diabetes Care, 2001; 24:843–849

220. Lagiou P, Kuper H, Stuver SO, Tzonou A, Trichopoulos D, Adami HO. Role of diabetes mellitus in the etiology of hepatocellular carcinoma. J N C I, 2000; 92:1096–1099

221. El-Serag HB, Richardson PA, Everhart JE. The role of diabetes in hepatocellular carcinoma: a case-control study among United States Veterans. Am J Gastroenterol, 2001; 96:2462–2467

222. El-Serag HB, Tran T, Everhart JE. Diabetes increases the risk of chronic liver disease and hepatocellular carcinoma. Gastroenterology, 2004; 126:460–468

223. Cotrim HP, Parana R, Braga E, Lyra L. Nonalcoholic steatohepatitis and hepatocellular carcinoma: natural history? Am J Gastroenterol, 2000; 95:3018–3019

224. Orikasa H, Ohyama R, Tsukada N, Eyden BP, Yamazaki K. Lipid-rich clear-cell carcinoma arising in nonalcoholic steatohepatitis in a patient with diabetes mellitus. J Submicrosc Cytol Pathol, 2001; 33:195–200

225. Zen Y, Katayanagi K, Tsuneyama K, Harada K, Araki I, Nakanuma Y. Hepatocellular carcinoma arising in non-alcoholic steatohepatitis. Path Int 2001; 51:127–131

226. Mori S, Yamasaki T, Sakaida I et al. Hepatocellular carcinoma with nonalcoholic steatohepatitis. J Gastroenterol, 2004; 39:391–396

227. Kudo M. Hepatocellular carcinoma and NASH. Editorial. J Gastroenterol, 2004; 39:409–411

228. Marrero JA, Fontana RJ, Su GL, Conjeevaram HS, Emick DM, Lok AS. NAFLD may be a common underlying liver disease in patients with hepatocellular carcinoma in the United States. Hepatology, 2002; 36:1349–1354

229. Ratziu V, Bonyhay L, Di Martino V et al. Survival, liver failure and hepatocellular carcinoma in obesity-related cryptogenic cirrhosis. Hepatology, 2002; 35:1485–1493

230. Adami HO, Trichopoulos D. Obesity and mortality from cancer. (Editorial). N Engl J Med, 2003; 348:1623–1624

231. Yang S, Lin HZ, Hwang J, Chacko VP, Diehl AM. Hepatic hyperplasia in noncirrhotic fatty livers: is obesity-related hepatic steatosis a premalignant condition? Cancer Res, 2001; 61:5016–5023

232. Yang S, Koteish A, Lin HZ et al. Oval cells compensate for damage and replicative senescence of mature hepatocytes in mice with fatty liver disease. Hepatology, 2004; 39:403–411

233. Roskams T, Yang SQ, Koteish A et al. Oxidative stress and oval cell accumulation in mice and humans with alcoholic and nonalcoholic fatty liver disease. Am J Pathol, 2003; 163:1301–1311

234. Roskams TA, Libbrecht L, Desmet VJ. Progenitor cells in diseased human liver. Semin Liv Dis, 2003; 23:385–396

235. Rao MS, Reddy JK. Hepatocarcinogensis of peroxisome proliferators. Ann NY Acad of Sci, 1996; 804:573–587

236. Ockner RK, Kaikus RM, Bass NM. Fatty-acid metabolism and the pathogenesis of hepatocellular carcinoma: Review and hypothesis. Hepatology, 1993; 18:669–676

237. Fan CY, Pan J, Usuda N, Yeldandi AV, Rao MS, Reddy JK. Steatohepatitis, spontaneous peroxisome proliferation and liver tumors in mice lacking peroxisomal fatty acyl-coa oxidase—implications for peroxisome proliferator-activated receptor alpha natural ligand metabolism. J Biol Chem, 1998; 273:15639–15645

238. Fan CY, Pan J, Usuda N, Yeldandi AV, Rao MS, Reddy JK. Steatohepatitis, spontaneous peroxisome proliferation and liver tumors in mice lacking peroxisomal fatty acyl-CoA oxidase. Implications for peroxisome proliferator-activated receptor alpha natural ligand metabolism. J Biol Chem, 1998; 273:15639–15645

239. Yang SQ, Lin HZ, Mandal AK, Huang J, Diehl AM. Disrupted signaling and inhibited regeneration in obese mice with fatty livers: implications for nonalcoholic fatty liver disease pathophysiology. Hepatology, 2001; 34:694–706

240. Selzner M, Clavien PA. Fatty liver in liver transplantation and surgery. Semin Liv Dis, 2001; 21:105–113

241. Leclercq I, Field J, Farrell G. Leptin-specific mechanisms for impaired liver regeneration in ob/ob mice after toxic injury. Gastroenterology, 2003; 124:1451–1464

242. Evans CDJ, Oien KA, MacSween RNM, Mills PR. Nonalcoholic steatohepatitis: a common cause of advanced liver injury? J Clin Pathol, 2002; 55:689–692

243. Fassio E, Alvarez E, Dominguez N, Landeira G, Longon C. Natural history of nonalcoholic steatohepatitis: A longitudinal study of repeat liver biopsies. Hepatology, 2004; 40:820–826

244. Massarrat S, Jordan G, Sahrhage G, Korb G, Bode JC, Dolle W. Five-year follow-up study of patients with nonalcoholic and nondiabetic fatty liver. Acta Hepato-Gastroenterol, 1974; 21:176–186

245. Teli MR, James OFW, Burt AD, Bennett MK, Day CP. The natural history of nonalcoholic fatty liver—a follow-up study. Hepatology, 1995; 22:1714–1719

246. Saksena S. Natural history and determinants of disease progression in nonalcoholic fatty liver disease: Good and bad news. Hepatology, 2003; 39:232A

247. Harrison SA, Torgerson S, Hayashi PH. The natural history of nonalcoholic fatty liver disease: a clinical histopathological study. Am J Gastroenterol, 2003; 98:2042–2047

248. Adams LA, Sanderson S, Lindor KD, Angulo P. The histological course of nonalcoholic fatty liver disease: a longitudinal study of 103 patient with sequential liver biopsies. Hepatology, 2005; 42:132–138

249. Adams LA, Lymp JF, St Sauver J et al. The natural history of nonalcoholic fatty liver disease: a population-based cohort study. Gastroenterology, 2005; 129:113–121

250. Day CP, Saksena S. Nonalcoholic steatohepatitis: Definitions and pathogenesis. J Gastroenterol Hepatol, 2002; 17:S377–S384

251. Feldstein AE, Werneburg NW, Canbay A et al. Free fatty acids promote hepatic lipotoxicity by stimulating TNFa expression via a lysosomal pathway. Hepatology, 2004; 40:185–194

252. Day CP, James OFW. Steatohepatitis—a tale of two hits. Gastroenterology, 1998; 114:842–845

253. Ip E, Farrell GC, Roberston G, Hall P, Kirsch R, Leclercq I. Central role of PPARa-dependent hepatic lipid turnover in dietary steatohepatitis in mice. Hepatology, 2003; 38:123–132

254. Leclercq IA, Field J, Enriquez A, Farrell GC, Robertson GR. Constitutive and inducible expression of hepatic CYP2E1 in leptin-deficient ob/ob mice. Biochem Biophys Res Comm, 2000; 268:337–344

255. Leclercq IA, Farrell GC, Field J, Bell DR, Gonzalez FJ, Robertson GR. CYP2E1 and CYP4A as microsomal catalysts of lipid peroxides

in murine nonalcoholic steatohepatitis. J Clin Invest, 2000; 105:1067–1075

256. Lebovitz HE. The relationship of obesity to the metabolic syndrome. Int J Clin Pract. Supplement, 2003; 134:18–27

257. Wanless IR, Shiota K. The pathogenesis of nonalcoholic steatohepatitis and other fatty liver diseases: A four-step model including the role of lipid release and hepatic venular obstruction in the progression to cirrhosis. Semin Liver Dis, 2004; 24:99–106

258. Mendler MH, Turlin B, Moirand R et al. Insulin resistance-associated hepatic iron overload. Gastroenterology, 1999; 117:1155–1163

259. Fargion S. Dysmetabolic iron overload syndrome. Haematologica 1999; 84:97–98

260. Deguti MM, Sipahi AM, Gayotto LCC et al. Lack of evidence for the pathogenic role of iron and HFE mutations in Brazilian patients with nonalcoholic steatohepatitis. Brazilian J Med Biol Res, 2003; 36:739–745

261. Angulo P, Keach JC, Batts KP, Lindor KD. Independent predictors of liver fibrosis in patients with nonalcoholic steatohepatitis. Hepatology, 1999; 30:1356–1362

262. Moirand R, Mortaji AM, Loreal O, Paillard F, Brissot P, Deugnier Y. A new syndrome of liver iron overload with normal transferrin saturation. Lancet, 1997; 349:95–97

263. Facchini FS, Hua NW, Stoohs RA. Effect of iron depletion in carbohydrate-intolerant patients with clinical evidence of nonalcoholic fatty liver disease. Gastroenterology, 2002; 122:931–939

264. Chitturi S, George J. Interaction of iron, insulin resistance, and nonalcoholic steatohepatitis. Current Gastroenterology Reports, 2003; 5:18–25

265. Bacon BR, Farahvash MJ, Janney CG, Neuschwander-Tetri BA. Nonalcoholic steatohepatitis: an expanded clinical entity. Gastroenterology, 1994; 107:1103–1109

266. Ferrannini E. Insulin resistance, iron, and the liver. Lancet, 2000; 355:2181–2182

267. Evans RM, Barish GD, Wang Y-X. PPARs and the complex journey to obesity. Nat Med, 2004; 10:1–7

268. Korner J, Leibel RL. To eat or not to eat—how the gut talks to the brain. N Engl J Med, 2003; 349:926–928

269. Prins JB. Adipose tissue as an endocrine organ. Best Practice and Research Clinical Endocrinology and Metabolism, 2002; 16:639–651

269a. Schaffler A, Scholmerich J, Buchler C. Mechanisms of disease: adipocytokines and visceral adipose tissue—emerging role in nonalcoholic fatty liver disease. Nat Clin Pract Gastroenterol Hepatol. 2005; 2:273–280

270. Arner P. Not all fat is alike. Lancet, 1998; 351:1301–1302

271. Atzmon G, Yang XM, Muzumdar R, Ma XH, Gabriely I, Barzilai N. Differential gene expression between visceral and subcutaneous fat depots. Hormone & Metabolic Research, 2002; 34:622–628

272. Boeuf S, Klingenspor M, Van Hal NLW, Schneider T, Keijer J, Klaus S. Differential gene expression in white and brown preadipocytes. Physiologic Genomics, 2001; 7:15–25

273. McCullough AJ, Falck-Ytter Y. Body composition and hepatic steatosis as precursors for fibrotic liver disease. Hepatology, 1999; 29:1328–1330

274. Reid AE. Nonalcoholic steatohepatitis. Gastroenterology, 2001; 121:710–723

275. Klein S, Fontana L, Young L et al. Absence of an effect of liposuction on insulin action and risk factors for coronary heart disease. New England Journal of Medicine, 2004; 350:2549–2557

276. Gurnell M, Savage DB, Chatterjee KK, O'Rahilly S. The metabolic syndrome: peroxisome proliferator-activated receptor γ and its therapeutic modulation. J Clin Endocrinol Metab, 2003; 88:2412–2421

277. Caldwell SH, Hespenheide EE, Redick JA, Iezzoni JC, Battle EH, Sheppard BL. A pilot study of a thiazolidinedione, troglitazone, in nonalcoholic steatohepatitis. Am J Gastroenterol, 2001; 96:519–525

278. Neuschwander-Tetri BA, Brunt EM, Wehmeier KR, Sponseller CA, Hampton K, Bacon BR. Interim results of a pilot study demonstrating the early effects of the PPAR-g ligand rosiglitazone on insulin sensitivity, aminotransferases, hepatic steatosis and body weight in patients with non-alcoholic steatohepatitis. J Hepatol, 2003; 38:434–440

279. Stumvoll M. Thiazolidinediones—some recent developments. Expert Opin Investig Drugs, 2003; 12:1179–1187

280. Arner P. The adipocyte in insulin resistance: key molecules and the impact of the thiazolidinediones. Trends in Endocrinology and Metabolism, 2003; 14:137–145

281. Das UN. Is metabolic syndrome X an inflammatory condition? Exp Biol Med, 2002; 227:989–997

282. Zhang Y, Proenca R, Maffei M, Barone M, Leopold L, Friedman JM. Positional cloning of the mouse obese gene and its human homologue. Nature, 1994; 372:425–432

283. Saibara T. 'Insufficient' leptin production for the fat mass: a risk factor for nonalcoholic steatohepatitis in obese patients? J Gastroenterol, 2003; 38:522–523

284. Chitturi S, Farrell G, Frost L et al. Serum leptin in NASH correlates with hepatic steatosis but not fibrosis: A manifestation of lipotoxicity? Hepatology, 2002; 36:403–409

285. Kamohara S, Burcelin R, Halaas JL, Friedman JM, Charron MJ. Acute stimulation of glucose metabolism in mice by leptin treatment. Nature, 1997; 389:374–377

286. Lord GM, Matarese G, Howard JK, Baker RJ, Bloom SR, Lechler RI. Leptin modulates the T-cell immune response and reverses starvation-induced immunosuppression. Nature, 1998; 394

287. Diez JJ, Iglesias P. The role of the novel adipocyte-derived hormone adiponectin in human disease. European Journal of Endocrinology, 2003; 148:293–300

288. Kamada Y, Tamura S, Kiso S et al. Enhanced carbon tetrachloride-induced liver fibrosis in mice lacking adiponectin. Gastroenterology 2003; 125:1796–1807

289. Yamauchi T, Kamon J, Waki H et al. The fat-derived hormone adiponectin reverses insulin resistance associated with both lipoatrophy and obesity. Nat Med, 2001; 7:941–946

290. Masaki T, Chiba S, Tatsukawa H et al. Adiponectin protects LPS-induced liver injury through modulation of TNF-a in KK-Ay obese mice. Hepatology, 2004; 40:177–184

291. Xu A, Wang Y, Keshaw H, Xu YL, Lam KSL, Cooper GJS. The fat-derived hormone adiponectin alleviates alcoholic and nonalcoholic fatty liver diseases in mice. J Clin Invest, 2003; 112:91–100

292. Day CP. Who gets alcoholic liver disease: nature or nurture? Journal of the Royal College of Physicians of London, 2000; 34:557–562

292a. Kaser S, Moschen A, Cayon A, Kaser A, Crespo J, Pons-Romero F, Ebenbichler CF, Patsch JR, Tilg H. Adiponectin and its receptors in non-alcoholic steatohepatitis. Gut, 2005; 54:117–121

293. Green RG. NASH-Hepatic metabolism and not simply the metabolic syndrome. (Editorial). Hepatology, 2003; 38:14–17

294. Spaulding L, Trainer T, Janiec D. Prevalence of nonalcoholic steatohepatitis in morbidly obese subjects undergoing gastric bypass. Obes Surg, 2003; 13:347–349

295. Crespo J, Fernandez-Gil P, Hernandez-Guerra M et al. Are there predictive factors of severe liver fibrosis in morbidly obese patients with non-alcoholic steatohepatitis? Obes Surg, 2001; 11:254–257

296. Wilner IR, Waters B, Patil R, Reuben A, Morelli J, Riely CA. Ninety patiens with nonalcoholic steatohepatitis: insulin resistance, familial tendency and severity of disease. Am J Gastroenterol, 2001; 96:2957–2961

297. Struben VM, Hespenheide EE, Caldwell SH. Nonalcoholic steatohepatitis and cryptogenic cirrhosis within kindreds. Am J Med, 2000; 108:9–13

298. Merriman RB, Aouizerat BE, Yankovich M et al. Variants of adipocyte genes affecting free fatty acid flux in patients with nonalcoholic fatty liver disease. Hepatology, 2003; 34:508A

299. Santamaria E, Avila MA, Latasa MU et al. Functional proteomics of nonalcoholic steatohepatitis: Mitochondrial proteins as targets of s-adenosylmethionine. Proceedings of the National Academy of Sciences of the United States of America, 2003; 100:3065–3070

300. Younossi ZM, Baranova A, Ziegler K, Del Giacco L, Schlauch K, Born TL, Elariny H, Gorreta F, VanMeter A, Younoszai A, Ong JP, Goodman Z, Chandhoke V. A genomic and proteomic study of the spectrum of nonalcoholic fatty liver disease. Hepatology. 2005; 42(3):665–674

301. Sreekumar R, Rosado B, Rasmussen D, Charlton M. Hepatic gene expression in histologically progressive nonalcoholic steatohepatitis. Hepatology, 2003; 38:244–251

302. Song J, da Costa KA, Fischer LM, Kohlmeier M, Kwock L, Wang S, Zeisel SH. Polymorphism of the PEMT gene and susceptibility to nonalcoholic fatty liver disease (NAFLD). FASEB J, 2005; 19:1266–1271

Acute and chronic viral hepatitis

Neil D. Theise   Henry C. Bodenheimer, Jr.   Linda D. Ferrell

8

The subject of this chapter is the pathological consequences of infection with hepatotropic viruses. These infections are responsible for viral hepatitis which is generally classified by viral type (Table 8.1). Distinction can also be made by the duration of infection and by the clinicopathological syndrome that develops (Table 8.2). Although some pathological features are unique to the type of virus responsible for infection, many aspects of the pathological injury and clinical progression are common to multiple types of hepatotropic viral infection.

Acute viral hepatitis

Clinical features

Acute viral hepatitis occurrence may be sporadic or epidemic. Transmission of disease is commonly via the faecal–oral route through contaminated food or water. Alternatively, transmission may be through parenteral exposure, such as by intravenous drug use, blood transfusion or occupational needle stick exposure.

The acute infection is often subclinical and anicteric. If symptoms are present, they may be non-specific and not readily identifiable as due to viral hepatitis. Typical symptoms include fatigue, anorexia and nausea in the early stages, followed by dark urine and jaundice. Right upper quadrant abdominal pain or discomfort, arthritis, urticaria, pruritus and low-grade fever may be present. In patients without jaundice, the symptoms may be mistaken for gastrointestinal viral infection or another non-specific viral syndrome.[1]

The severity of acute viral hepatitis may vary from a mild asymptomatic infection to fatal fulminant hepatic failure. The latter is characterized clinically by the development of hepatic encephalopathy within 8 weeks of the onset of clinical illness[2] and pathologically by massive or severe bridging hepatocyte necrosis. The terms 'subacute hepatitis' and 'subacute hepatic necrosis' are used to describe serious injury developing after 8 weeks of illness. In patients with acute viral hepatitis, the surviving parenchyma may be characterized by varying degrees of regeneration. Nodular hyperplasia, two-cell-thick hepatocyte plates between sinusoids, and mitotic figures within hepatocytes may indicate liver cell regeneration and a potential for recovery. Serum markers of hepatocyte regeneration, such as alpha-fetoprotein,[3] or measures of hepatic synthetic capacity such as factor VII,[4] have been used as prognostic indicators in acute hepatitis. Death may result from complications of infection or renal failure rather than from hepatic synthetic dysfunction directly.

Portal hypertension and ascites are typically associated with chronic liver disease and rarely develop in patients with acute liver injury. These complications, in acute disease, may be the result of hepatocyte loss and consequent collapse of the sinusoidal network.[5]

Acute viral hepatitis is typically characterized by injury to hepatocytes and is identified by a marked rise in aminotransferase activities. Rise in aminotransferase values precedes a rise in bilirubin and may peak prior to the development of jaundice. Jaundice, in the presence of significant elevation of aminotransferase values, indicates a severe degree of liver injury. A fall in hepatic synthesis of clotting factors may be reflected in a prolongation of protime and elevation of international normalized ratio (INR). This is another indication of severe hepatic injury.

Aminotransferase values generally rise over a period of weeks, and in those individuals who subsequently clear the virus, may normalize over weeks to months. Bilirubin elevation follows the aminotransferase rise. The onset of jaun-

Table 8.1	Clinical characteristics of human hepatotropic viral agents
Viral agents	**Characteristics**
Hepatitis A (HAV)	RNA picornavirus
	Sporadic or epidemic occurrence with faecal–oral transmission, resulting in acute disease only
Hepatitis B (HBV)	DNA hepadnavirus
	Sporadic or endemic occurrence through sexual, perinatal and parenteral transmission
	Chronic disease persists in 5% of adults and in up to 90% of infants
	Chronic infection is associated with hepatocellular carcinoma
Hepatitis C (HCV)	RNA flavi-like virus
	Sporadic occurrence with parenteral transmission
	Perinatal and sexual spread is less common
	Chronic disease develops in 60–80% of persons infected and cirrhosis is associated with hepatocellular carcinoma
Hepatitis D (HDV)	RNA defective virus
	Sporadic or endemic disease occurs as coinfection with HBV
	Transmission is parenteral and sexual
	Chronic disease is seen in patients with chronic HBV
	HDV worsens the clinical severity of HBV infection
Hepatitis E (HEV)	RNA virus
	Sporadic or epidemic occurrence
	Transmission is faecal–oral, resulting in acute disease only
	Mortality rate is 25% in pregnant women

Table 8.2	Clinical–pathological syndromes of viral hepatitis
Acute	Subclinical/anicteric
	Symptomatic/icteric
	Fulminant
	Cholestatic
	Atypical presentation in immunosuppressed patients (including fibrosing cholestatic hepatitis)
Chronic	Asymptomatic without hepatocyte necrosis
	Chronic infection with hepatic injury
	Chronic hepatitis compensated with cirrhosis
	Decompensated chronic hepatitis with cirrhosis
	Chronic post-transplant

dice is clinically recognized when bilirubin levels rise above approximately 2.5 mg/dl. Jaundice or icterus may persist at lower levels of serum bilirubin during recovery due to bilirubin that is conjugated to albumin in tissue, particularly if hyperbilirubinaemia has been prolonged. This bilirubin and albumin complex has been termed delta bilirubin.[6]

Cholestatic hepatitis is a clinical variant of acute viral hepatitis in which biliary dysfunction predominates. This syndrome is characterized by elevation of alkaline phosphatase and bilirubin values with proportionately less elevation of aminotransferase activities. The cholestatic biochemical abnormalities may persist for weeks to months. The prognosis of this pattern of hepatic injury is generally favourable when not associated with prominent hepatocellular necrosis. Cholestatic hepatitis must be distinguished clinically from biliary obstruction by biliary imaging studies (Table 8.2).

Pathological features

Acute viral hepatitis is characterized morphologically by a combination of inflammatory-cell infiltration, macrophage activity, hepatocellular damage and regeneration. The proportion and detailed nature of these components vary widely according to the particular virus responsible, the host response and the passage of time. The pathological features are considerably different from those of classic acute inflammation, because they primarily represent a response of the patient's immune system to viral antigens displayed on cells, rather than a vascular and cellular response to injury. Some features of acute inflammation are nevertheless present to a limited extent; thus, for instance, the liver in acute viral hepatitis is swollen and tender, its capsule is tense and blood vessels are engorged. In addition, polymorphonuclear leukocytes may be seen as a secondary response to epithelial injury, and are often seen associated with bile ductular proliferation.

Macroscopic appearances

Information on the macroscopic appearances of the liver in non-fatal acute hepatitis is mainly derived from laparoscopy[7] and from liver transplantation. Initially the liver is swollen and red, its capsule oedematous and tense; exuded tissue fluid may be seen on the capsular surface. Focal depressions are the result of localized subcapsular necrosis and collapse. In patients with severe cholestasis, the colour of the liver is bright yellow or green. In fulminant hepatitis, the organ shrinks and softens as a result of extensive necrosis, and the capsule becomes wrinkled. The left lobe may be more severely affected than the right. If the patient survives for weeks or months, tan to yellow-green nodules of regenerating parenchyma may be seen protruding from the capsular surface or deep within the liver (Fig. 8.1), separated or surrounded by more haemorrhagic, or redder, necrotic areas. In other examples, necrosis is uniform throughout the organ.

In patients dying of fulminant hepatitis, there is often damage to organs other than the liver and this may significantly contribute to the immediate cause of death.[8] Findings at autopsy include pneumonia, septicaemia, cerebral oedema, gastrointestinal haemorrhage and pancreatitis. Such lesions help to explain death when liver-cell damage is limited in extent or when there has already been substantial regeneration.

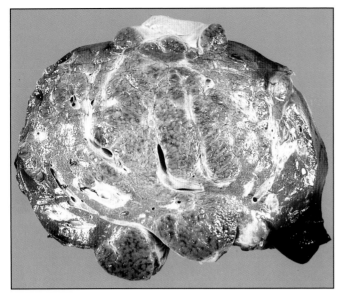

Fig. 8.1 • Massive necrosis with regenerative foci in severe hepatitis that progressed to liver failure over a time period of several weeks. The tan nodular zones represent regenerative foci, and the red zones represent massive necrosis with no residual hepatocytes.

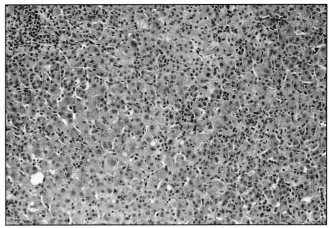

Fig. 8.2 • Classic acute hepatitis. Hepatocyte swelling and lymphocytic infiltrates are seen in the lobule. H&E.

Light-microscopic appearances: types of necrosis

The histological classification of acute hepatitis given in this chapter is based on different patterns of hepatocellular necrosis. These patterns will therefore be briefly discussed before the microscopic changes of acute hepatitis are described in detail. More than one of the patterns of necrosis described below may be seen in different parts of the same liver, and even within a single biopsy specimen.

Spotty (focal) necrosis and apoptosis. In this form of necrosis, which represents the fundamental lesion of acute viral hepatitis, individual hepatocytes within otherwise intact parenchyma die and are removed. The mode of death of hepatocytes probably includes both lytic necrosis and apoptosis (Chapter 2), but the relative contribution of each is uncertain. In the case of apoptosis (or formation of acidophilic or Councilman bodies in older terminology), it is likely that T-lymphocytes play a role. The remnants of cells affected by either process are rapidly removed from the site by blood flow or phagocytosis.

Confluent and bridging necrosis. This type of necrosis comprises groups of adjacent dead hepatocytes or the site where a group of hepatocytes has undergone previous necrosis and removal, so that areas of confluent necrosis are formed. These are often perivenular (centrilobular) in location. Confluent necrosis linking vascular structures and portal zones is known as bridging necrosis. Bridging at the periphery of complex acini links terminal hepatic venules (central veins) to each other, but does not involve portal tracts. This is called 'central–central' bridging in the lobular nomenclature. The other form of bridging necrosis links terminal hepatic venules to portal tracts ('central–portal' bridging in the lobular nomenclature). This form is best explained as

necrosis of zone 3 of the simple acinus, as described by Rappaport,[9] because this zone touches both terminal hepatic venule and portal tract. Zone 3 bridges are sometimes curved, in keeping with the shape of the zone. When confluent necrosis is more extensive, involving zones 2 and 1 in addition to zone 3 so that entire acini are destroyed, the process is described as panacinar or panlobular necrosis.

Interface hepatitis. Interface hepatitis, formerly known as piecemeal necrosis, can be defined as death of hepatocytes at the interface of parenchyma and the connective tissue of the portal zone, accompanied by a variable degree of inflammation and fibrosis. The older term 'piecemeal necrosis' is now considered inappropriate in part because the pathogenetic process involved is almost certainly apoptosis rather than necrosis.[10] In the acinar concept, interface hepatitis typically involves zone 1 and leads to apparent widening of portal tracts. These are therefore more likely to be cut longitudinally by a microtome knife, and this is seen in two-dimensional sections as linking of adjacent portal tracts, that is to say portal–portal bridging. Interface hepatitis was a defining feature of the formerly used category of chronic active hepatitis,[11] but very similar periportal necrosis is found in some cases of acute hepatitis.

Light microscopic appearance: patterns of acute hepatitis

Classic acute hepatitis

Features seen in the parenchyma in this form of acute hepatitis include liver-cell damage and cell death, liver-cell regeneration, cholestasis, infiltration with inflammatory cells and prominence of sinusoidal cells (Fig. 8.2). The necrosis may be spotty or confluent. The histological changes, especially confluent necrosis, are often most severe near the terminal hepatic venule. The reason for this zonal distribution has not been established, but possible explanations include metabolic and functional differences between hepatocytes in different zones, and the lower oxygen content of the blood in perivenular areas. There is a variable degree of condensation of the reticulin framework but, in the classic form of hepatitis, this does not amount to substantial alteration of structure and vascular relationships. Portal tracts are inflamed and bile ducts may be damaged. Macrovesicular steatosis is relatively uncommon in the fully developed stage of hepatitis.

Little is known about the earliest changes of acute viral hepatitis in man. Available information suggests that Kupffer cells are prominent and may show mitotic activity, and that hepatocellular necrosis occurs early in the course of the disease.[12] In the setting of acquired hepatitis after liver transplantation, necrosis is seen as an early indicator of hepatitis.[13]

Hepatocyte swelling is a common feature in acute hepatitis, and results mainly from dilatation of the endoplasmic reticulum. The swollen cells are pale-staining as a result of intracellular oedema (Fig. 8.3). Because of the combination of swelling and rounding of the affected cells, the term 'ballooning degeneration' is sometimes applied. It should be noted, however, that such ballooning degeneration is not a diagnostic feature of viral hepatitis, since it may also be seen in other circumstances, for example in alcoholic or drug-induced hepatitis, and following liver transplantation as part of the spectrum of ischaemia and/or preservation injury. The nuclei of the affected cells are also swollen, because of the accumulation of proteins.[14] Nucleoli of hepatocytes may be more prominent than usual, mitotic figures are occasionally seen, and multinucleation may be increased.

In addition to swollen cells, there are hepatocytes with deeply acidophilic cytoplasm, in which the nucleus is sometimes seen to be undergoing pyknosis, or apoptosis. Such acidophilic hepatocytes are small in comparison with ballooned cells, but may occasionally be larger than normal hepatocytes. This suggests that the two types of cell change, ballooning and acidophilic change, could represent stages of cell degeneration rather than fundamentally different responses to injury. Acidophilic cells have round or irregular outlines, sometimes assuming rhomboid, angular shapes, apparently determined by the pressure from adjacent swollen hepatocytes. The formation of acidophil

(Councilman) bodies (Fig. 8.4) is probably a later stage of this process. Acidophil bodies are generally rounded hepatocyte remnants, but some may be ovoid or have other irregular forms, may or may not contain nuclear remnants and may appear thick and refractile. Affected cells eventually undergo fragmentation, the whole process representing an example of apoptosis.[10] Some acidophil bodies are in close contact with lymphocytes or Kupffer cells, while others appear to lie free within liver-cell plates or sinusoids, with no other cells in close proximity. Like ballooned hepatocytes, acidophil bodies are not specific for acute viral hepatitis, although they often constitute a striking histological feature of the disease.

Loss of individual hepatocytes leads to localized defects in the liver-cell plates, with consequent distortion and condensation of the supporting reticulin framework, especially when the necrosis is confluent. While an overall increase in connective tissue fibres is probably slight in acute hepatitis and therefore difficult to detect by light microscopy (with conventional staining methods), immunocytochemical and ultrastructural evidence indicates synthesis of collagen

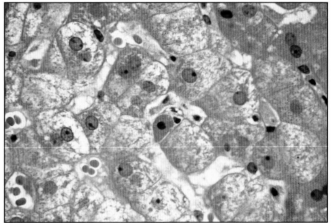

A

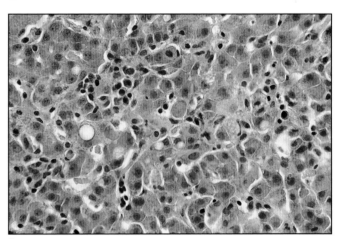

B

Fig. 8.4 • **(A)** Classic acute hepatitis. Focal apoptosis of hepatocyte with nuclear remnant present. Inflammatory cells are present next to the apoptotic cell within the sinusoid. Hepatocyte swelling is also present. H&E. **(B)** Classic acute hepatitis. Focal apoptosis of hepatocytes is present (rounded acidophil body) as well as inflammation of the lobule and disarray of the plate architecture. H&E.

Fig. 8.3 • Classic acute hepatitis. Swollen hepatocytes are present, together with a mononuclear infiltrate in the sinusoids. Disarray of the plate architecture is present due to loss of hepatocytes. H&E.

fibres[15] and associated proteins such as fibronectin, as well as increased prominence of stellate cells. There may also be degradation of these components, so that there is presumably a dynamic balance which determines the degree of fibrosis in an individual case. The distortion of cell plates is accentuated by regeneration of hepatocytes. This is recognized by the appearance of mitotic figures, rare in normal liver, and by a change in the structure of the cell plates; these become more than one cell thick, or assume the structure of short cylinders known as liver-cell rosettes. The end result of focal necrosis, reticulin condensation and regeneration is a diagnostically helpful disarray of the liver-cell plates (Fig. 8.3).

Cholestasis is common in acute hepatitis. It varies from the presence of scanty, small bile plugs in perivenular canaliculi to extensive bile plug formation with canalicular dilatation. Intracellular bile is more difficult to recognize because bile is easily confused with lipofuscin pigment. For this reason cholestasis should only rarely be diagnosed on the basis of routine stains in the absence of canalicular bile plugs. Morphological cholestasis may be accompanied by clinical and biochemical features of cholestasis, but this is variable.

The inflammatory infiltrate of acute viral hepatitis is mainly composed of lymphocytes, plasma cells and macrophages in varying proportions (Figs 8.2 and 8.4). Within the parenchyma, the infiltrate is most abundant where liver-cell damage is greatest, usually in the perivenular zones. Lymphocytes are often attached to endothelial cells of the central and portal venules.[16] Mononuclear phagocytes, either activated Kupffer cells or circulating phagocytes, are seen as large irregular cells in areas of liver-cell drop-out (Fig. 8.5). They often show brown pigmentation, due to phagocytosis of bile or to the accumulation of lipid-rich ceroid (also known as lipochrome) pigment. Iron is also abundant in some cases. The iron-containing phagocytes are sometimes found in the form of small clumps composed of several cells.[17] Whatever the pigment, the periodic acid-Schiff (PAS) reaction after diastase digestion is usually strongly positive (Fig. 8.5).

Most portal tracts in acute viral hepatitis are infiltrated with inflammatory cells to a greater or lesser extent and, in the classic form, lymphoid cells predominate. Cytotoxic T-cells (CD45RO+) typically are more prominent than B-cells (CD20+).[18] Plasma cells are common, the majority containing IgG.[19] Perls-positive, iron-rich macrophages may be present. Portal infiltration may be diffuse or focal. Mild bile-duct damage is common, and is seen as minor irregularities of shape, size and arrangement of the epithelial nuclei of the small, interlobular ducts. Less commonly, the ductal epithelium becomes vacuolated and disrupted; such lesions are seen most often near or within lymphoid follicles, but granulomas are not associated with the duct lesion as in primary biliary cirrhosis. Irregular dilatation of ductules is not typical but has been described in type A hepatitis.[20] In general, however, a finding of dilated, bile-containing ductules or canals of Hering should arouse a suspicion of sepsis, a complication of severe acute hepatitis in some patients. Bile-duct damage in acute hepatitis does not usually correlate with a prolonged cholestatic clinical course, probably because there is not the widespread and progressive destruction of the duct system found in disorders such as primary biliary cirrhosis.

The outlines of the portal tracts may remain intact and sharply delineated in classic acute hepatitis with spotty necrosis. More often, infiltration by lymphoid cells and accompanying disruption of the limiting plate of hepatocytes leads to an irregular outline (or interface hepatitis). Severe periportal necrosis and inflammation in acute hepatitis is discussed below.

All the above features of classic acute hepatitis with spotty (focal) necrosis vary in extent. There is therefore a wide range of appearances, from a mild hepatitis with little cell damage or inflammatory-cell infiltration, to one with widespread changes throughout the parenchyma. In the latter case the diagnosis presents no great difficulty, but in the former the distinction from non-specific reactive changes or from non-hepatitic cholestasis may be difficult or even impossible. These characteristics of classic acute hepatitis with spotty (focal) necrosis also form the basis of the other three forms of acute hepatitis, which may be regarded as exaggerations of one or other component of the classic form.

Variants of classic acute viral hepatitis. Multinucleation may be very prominent with the formation of giant hepatocytes (Fig. 8.6).[21] When this change is widespread the appearances resemble those of neonatal giant-cell hepatitis. In addition, cholestatic variants have been described, especially in association with hepatitis A and E. In these cases, the degree of necrosis may be minimal and the cholestasis quite prominent, mimicking biliary obstruction.

Acute hepatitis with confluent (bridging) necrosis

In this form of acute hepatitis, the features described under classic acute hepatitis with spotty (focal) necrosis are seen but, in addition, bridging in the form of confluent necrosis linking central venules to portal tracts ('central–portal' bridging) or linking central venules to each other ('central–central' bridging) can also be present.

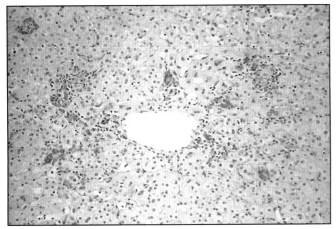

Fig. 8.5 • Classic acute hepatitis. Clumps of hypertrophied Kupffer cells are most prominently seen near the centrizonal region and stain strongly with PAS–diastase. PASD.

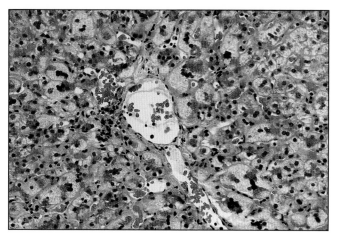

Fig. 8.6 • Giant-cell change of hepatocytes in an adult. Many of the hepatocytes in the centrizonal area contain large numbers of nuclei. H&E.

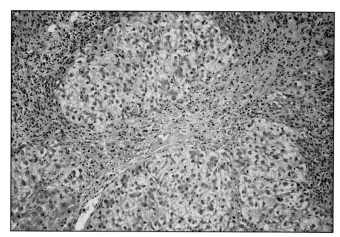

Fig. 8.7 • Acute hepatitis with bridging necrosis. Curving bridges are formed as a result of confluent necrosis linking central and portal zones. H&E.

Of these two forms of confluent necrosis, central–portal bridging has been considered to be possibly more significant for the progression of the lesion than the central–central necrosis. For example, in patients who develop chronic liver disease, central–portal confluent necrosis may hasten the onset of cirrhosis by creating early disruption of the normal architectural relationships upon conversion of the bridges into fibrous septa, which undergo contraction. In patients who do not develop chronic hepatitis, bridging necrosis of central to portal type may lead to a certain degree of scarring and distortion, sometimes seen in biopsy specimens taken many months after the acute attack. The prognostic significance of central–portal bridging necrosis remains somewhat controversial. Boyer & Klatskin[22] considered that patients with this type of bridging necrosis were more likely to develop chronic hepatitis, a conclusion later supported by another study.[23] However, both groups of authors included not only central–portal bridging as described above, but also bridges linking portal tracts, probably representing periportal necrosis. Others have not considered bridging as a good predictor of chronicity.[24,25] It must nevertheless be regarded as an important histological feature seen in the more severe forms of acute hepatitis.

The appearance of the necrosis varies according to the stage of the illness. In the early stages of bridge formation, there is death of substantial numbers of hepatocytes. This is followed by disappearance of the affected cells, leaving a loose connective tissue stroma infiltrated with lymphocytes and macrophages (Fig. 8.7). With time, the stroma collapses to form more or less dense 'passive' septa, which intersect the liver tissue. Confluent/bridging necrosis can develop in the early weeks of acute hepatitis, but its absence on a biopsy sample does not exclude the possibility that it will develop later.

The combination of necrosis, collapse and hepatocellular regeneration leads to architectural distortion which, in turn, can easily be mistaken for that of chronic hepatitis or cirrhosis. Helpful differentiating features include the presence of other lesions of acute viral hepatitis and staining properties of the septa; recently formed passive septa are virtually devoid of elastic fibres (Fig. 8.8) whereas the older

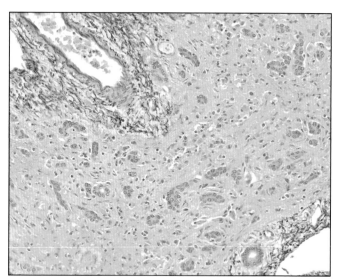

Fig. 8.8 • Acute hepatitis with bridging necrosis. Deeply stained elastic fibres are present in the portal tract. Adjacent areas of collapse have no elastic tissue. Orcein.

septa of chronic hepatitis and cirrhosis contain increasing numbers of these fibres.[26] In addition, the stroma in zones of recent necrosis will tend to show the residual structure of the cell plates on reticulin stain (Fig. 8.9); this is not readily seen in chronic hepatitis and cirrhosis. The stroma is often more haemorrhagic or contains more macrophages than in typical chronic hepatitis (Fig. 8.10). Trichrome stain may also show a two-tone appearance, with darker staining of established areas of scar due to thicker collagen bundles (comparable to the normal residual portal tract collagen), as compared to lighter staining of areas of recent collapse, where the residual framework and lack of hepatocytes account for the staining. Extensive liver cell destruction in acute hepatitis with confluent necrosis may also lead to a significant ductular reaction within the periportal areas, which mimics bile-duct obstruction, and a more florid portal inflammatory reaction than is normally found in classic acute hepatitis. Neutrophils may be more abundant, and often seen adjacent to the ductular structures.

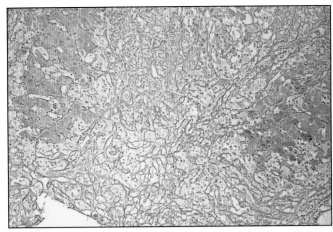

Fig. 8.9 • Acute hepatitis with bridging necrosis. The reticulin framework remains intact and has not significantly collapsed at this time point. Reticulin.

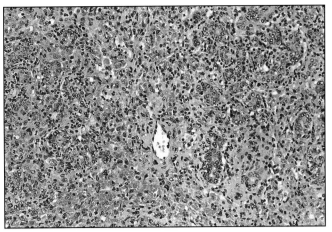

Fig. 8.11 • Acute hepatitis with massive necrosis. The hepatocytes have been destroyed, and the collapsed stroma is haemorrhagic. Ductular structures (ductular metaplasia) are prominent. H&E.

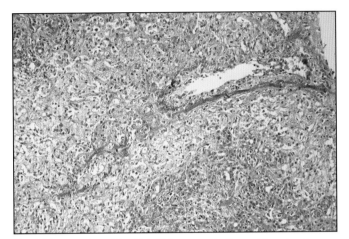

Fig. 8.10 • Acute hepatitis with bridging necrosis. The centrizonal region shows large numbers of macrophages that stain light blue to grey. The wall of the vein, in contrast, is bright blue and lined by dense collagen bundles. Trichrome.

Acute hepatitis with panlobular (panacinar) necrosis

This form of acute hepatitis represents the most severe degree of necrosis, with complete or near-complete destruction of hepatocytes in entire lobules. When several adjacent lobules undergo necrosis, the term 'multilobular' is applicable. The term massive hepatic necrosis generally is used when the liver shows extensive, diffuse panlobular (panacinar) and multilobular necrosis. This lesion is typically the morphological counterpart of the clinical condition of fulminant hepatitis (Table 8.2), or fulminant liver failure, which is often fatal. The term submassive necrosis is used generally for lesions that involve necrosis of perivenular zones with sparing of the periportal zone.

For reasons as yet unknown, panlobular necrosis may spare large areas of the liver (Fig. 8.1), though the more viable zones usually show lesser degrees of damage, including bridging necrosis. Thus, determination of the degree of total loss of liver parenchyma based on needle biopsy alone is not recommended owing to the patchy nature of the necrosis that can occur in acute viral hepatitis.[27] Panlobular necrosis on a smaller scale is not necessarily accompanied by severe disease clinically, and may be seen particularly in

a subcapsular location (or rarely at other sites), adjacent to less severely damaged liver tissue. It is even likely that panlobular necrosis can occur in the entire absence of severe symptoms, because areas of old necrosis and collapse may be found incidentally in the livers of patients with no history of acute hepatitis. Conversely, some patients have severe clinical hepatitis in the absence of panlobular necrosis, and it must then be assumed that a large proportion of hepatocytes has sustained sublethal damage.

The macroscopic appearances in this form of acute hepatitis have been described above. Microscopically, acute hepatitis with panlobular necrosis is characterized by extensive liver-cell loss, proliferation of ductular-like structures around portal tracts, inflammatory-cell infiltration and collapse (Figs 8.11 and 8.12). The degree of collapse may be judged by the extent of approximation of adjacent portal tracts, which increases with time, and by the density of the collapsed reticulin framework. As in the case of confluent/bridging necrosis, areas of recent collapse contain few if any elastic fibres whereas staining for these fibres becomes positive later.[28] Haemorrhage in the collapsing zone may be prominent in some cases (Fig. 8.11). Inflammatory-cell infiltration is mixed and variable in degree. The main infiltrating cells are often macrophages (Fig. 8.12), which usually contain ceroid pigment and should not be mistaken for residual hepatocytes. Mononuclear infiltrates in areas of surviving parenchyma are sometimes surprisingly mild in comparison with classic acute hepatitis.[29] Many of the ductule-like structures contain both liver-cell and bile-duct elements, and these have been designated as zones of ductular metaplasia, ductular reaction or neocholangioles.[30] They may reflect proliferation of a hepatic stem cell/progenitor cell population[31] or transformation of hepatocytes into ductular-like structures. These structures generally are most prominent in the periportal zone, and their location would correspond to the former canals of Hering now transformed into complex arborizing networks of proliferating cells.[31] Venulitis of central veins can be seen (Fig. 8.13). Evidence of significant parenchymal cell regeneration is present even in fatal cases.[32]

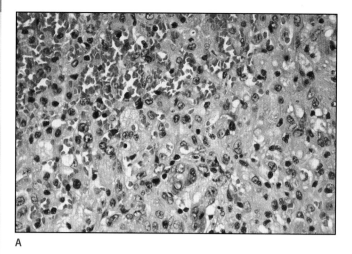

A

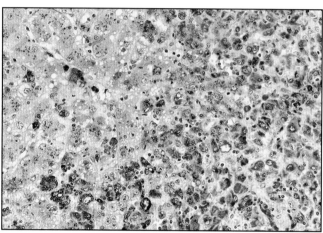

B

Fig. 8.12 • **(A)** Acute hepatitis with submassive necrosis. The necrotic zone is filled with macrophages. H&E. **(B)** Acute hepatitis with submassive necrosis. The macrophages as seen in Fig. 8.12A stain intensely for CD68. A few residual hepatocytes are present in upper left. Immunoperoxidase for CD68.

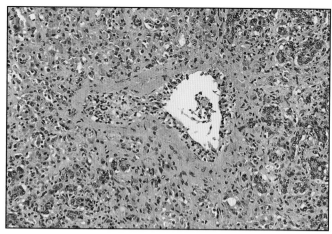

Fig. 8.13 • Acute hepatitis with submassive necrosis and central venulitis. H&E.

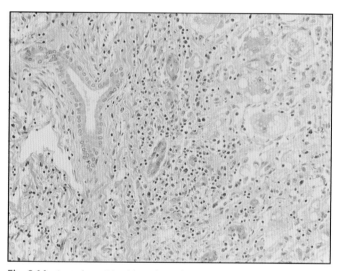

Fig. 8.14 • Acute hepatitis with periportal necrosis. In this example of type A hepatitis, extensive inflammation and necrosis are seen at the edge of a portal tract. H&E.

The common hepatotropic viruses can cause panlobular necrosis, but the mechanisms responsible for development of massive necrosis, instead of the more typical pattern of spotty necrosis, are unknown. Possibilities include overwhelming viral infection, superinfection with a second virus[33] and microcirculatory failure.[29] In some instances, mutants of the hepatitis B virus have been implicated.[34,35]

Acute hepatitis with periportal necrosis

In this pattern of hepatitis, the usual changes of classic acute hepatitis are seen to a greater or lesser extent, but there is additionally a substantial degree of necrosis in the periportal zones, accompanied by significant periportal inflammatory infiltration (Fig. 8.14). Lymphocytes and plasma cells usually predominate in the portal and periportal infiltrate. Ductular proliferation/reaction may be present. One effect of the periportal necrosis is to cause apparent widening of the portal tracts, and linking of tracts as seen in two-dimensional sections. Changes in other parts of the parenchyma may be mild or severe. In some examples of hepatitis A, for instance, the portal and periportal changes may be accompanied by very little perivenular necrosis. In contrast, there are patients in whom biopsy shows a combination of periportal necrosis with central–portal bridging.

In contrast to the periportal necrosis (interface hepatitis) of chronic hepatitis, trapped periportal hepatocytes are usually absent or scant in number in the necrotic zone. There is, nevertheless, a close resemblance between these two kinds of necrosis; biopsies from patients with acute hepatitis may thus be wrongly diagnosed as chronic hepatitis, an error usually avoidable if the patient's history is both unequivocal and available to the pathologist, and if an examination is carried out for the typical parenchymal changes of acute hepatitis.

Evolution of the lesion

As already noted, little is known about the early stages of acute hepatitis in man. The descriptions given in this chapter refer to the fully developed acute lesion, but the time over which this lesion develops varies widely from patient to patient. In some, the lesion begins to regress after a few weeks, while in others the course is one of many months. There is international agreement that the term 'chronic hepatitis' should be used for inflammation of the liver continuing without improvement for more than 6 months[37] but there is overlap between acute and chronic disease: the former may last for more than 6 months in some instances, regressing slowly thereafter, while the latter possibly becomes established in the first few weeks or months of the disease.[38]

Following the fully developed stage of acute hepatitis, there is a stage of regressing and finally residual hepatitis. During regression, necrosis diminishes or ceases and phagocytic activity predominates. Portal inflammation is still seen, and in severe hepatitis there may be ductular proliferation/reaction. In patients with marked cholestasis, bile stasis can persist after much of the inflammatory activity and necrosis has subsided, often in association with a cholestatic clinical course. Condensation of the reticulin framework marks zones of liver-cell loss, and necrotic bridges undergo collapse to form passive septa. The risk of confusion with chronic liver disease and/or cirrhosis thus increases. In this regressing stage, however, the lesion can still be recognized as acute hepatitis on the basis of hepatocellular changes, parenchymal inflammation and phagocytic activity. In severe forms of acute hepatitis with collapsing stroma, the absence of established scarring, as evidenced by lack of dense bundles of collagen and elastic fibres, can help distinguish acute from chronic disease.

The stage of regression passes imperceptibly into a residual stage, which is much less characteristic and easily mistaken for a non-specific reaction unconnected with viral hepatitis. Changes include slight alterations of architecture, minor degrees of septum formation, focal liver-cell regeneration as shown by variation in liver-cell size and appearance from one area to another, inflammatory infiltration and Kupffer-cell activation. Clumps of Kupffer cells containing iron or ceroid pigment are often present. Cholestasis, if still present, is mild. Gradually these residual changes fade and the liver returns to normal. Minor degrees of inflammation and phagocytic activity may be seen as long as a year or more after onset.

Differential diagnosis of acute hepatitis

Acute viral hepatitis is only one cause of the acute hepatitis syndrome and the typical clinical question upon presentation is the aetiology of new-onset hepatic injury. This challenge is generally a clinical question rather than a pathological differential because diagnostic liver biopsy is usually not pursued in the acute setting. If a biopsy is done, the lesions of acute hepatitis are sufficiently diffuse within the liver to be diagnosed with confidence on small specimens.[39] This may not hold true for some examples of panlobular necrosis, but this exception rarely presents real diagnostic problems when clinical data are taken into account. It should be noted, however, that it is very difficult to distinguish a cause for acute hepatitis by morphological means alone, so clinical information and correlation are imperative.

The most common causes of acute hepatitis syndrome include hepatotropic viral infection, drug toxicity, toxin or alcohol exposure and hepatic hypoperfusion. Other aetiologies may present as an acute hepatitis syndrome but be the presenting feature of a chronic underlying disorder such as autoimmune hepatitis, hepatic lymphoma or Wilson disease.

In general, acute viral hepatitis should be considered in any presentation of acute hepatitis and appropriate history obtained to assess possible exposure to each of the hepatotropic viruses. The aetiology of acute viral hepatitis is appropriately evaluated by assessing the presence of antibody to the respective viral types (see sections below on specific viral types for more details). Acute hepatitis A infection is indicated by the presence of IgM anti-HAV antibody. Acute hepatitis B infection is identified by the presence of hepatitis B surface antigen (HbsAg) with coexisting IgM antihepatitis B core antibody (IgM anti-HBc). Acute hepatitis C infection is defined earliest by the presence of hepatitis C RNA but current assays for hepatitis C antibody (anti-HCV) are sensitive and able to detect anti-HCV after several weeks of infection.[40] Acute infection with hepatitis D (HDV) is defined by Delta antigen in the serum. HDV always exists in the context of hepatitis B coinfection as the Delta agent requires the metabolic capability of the hepatitis B virus to survive. The assay for IgM anti-HD indicates acute delta infection, but is not generally available. Hepatitis E infection can be detected by the presence of an antibody to the virus (anti-HEV).

Other viral infections, such as Epstein–Barr or cytomegalovirus may also be responsible for acute liver injury. Histological clues may be present to suggest these viral infections. In infectious mononucleosis (EBV-related), for example, liver-cell damage is usually absent or mild, and atypical lymphocytes are seen in sinusoids and portal tracts. In the other herpes-type viral infections, for example herpes simplex and cytomegalovirus, the necrosis is often confluent rather than single-cell, spotty type, and a minimal associated lymphoid infiltrate is present in the sinusoids. The typical viral inclusions can often be seen. The histological findings of these viral infections are discussed in Chapter 9. Other infectious agents including syphilis, dengue fever or yellow fever may be considered as the clinical history suggests.

Acute cholestatic hepatitis may be induced by hepatotropic viral infection, but must be distinguished from acute large bile-duct obstruction, which can present with prominent aminotransferase elevation during the first days of presentation. This pattern is generally followed by a rise in alkaline phosphatase and bilirubin values, especially when obstruction is high-grade and unremitting. The presentation is usually accompanied by right upper quadrant or abdominal pain but may be occult, particularly in patients with diabetes or in the elderly. Biliary imaging studies, such as ultrasound or magnetic resonance cholangiograms, are sensitive in defining this pathology.

Other relatively common cholestatic hepatitis syndromes include drug or toxin injury and alcoholic hepatitis. Less commonly this syndrome may be simulated by cholestasis of pregnancy, benign recurrent cholestasis or the exacerbation of a chronic underlying cholestatic disorder such as primary sclerosing cholangitis or primary biliary cirrhosis.

The bile-duct lesion of acute hepatitis can usually be distinguished from that of biliary tract diseases, such as primary biliary cirrhosis, by the presence of the parenchymal features of acute hepatitis, lack of granulomatous duct lesions, ductopenia and other clinical and biochemical findings. Granulomas associated with bile-duct lesions are almost never seen in acute hepatitis. The presence of lobular changes also helps to distinguish hepatitis from primary biliary cirrhosis; however, sinusoidal lymphocytic infiltrates are relatively common and even spotty necrosis has been noted in primary biliary cirrhosis,[41] so clinical correlation is always advised if the histological changes are equivocal. In addition, bile ductular reaction tends to be less in hepatitis (except in more severe forms of hepatitis), and the periportal hepatocytes do not retain copper as in the chronic cholestatic diseases. Overall, the key features for separation of these two entities lie in the examination for granulomatous duct lesions or loss of the interlobular bile ducts in primary biliary cirrhosis.

In cholestasis from any cause, secondary changes in hepatocytes and accompanying inflammation may cause confusion with acute hepatitis. In cholestasis, the changes are generally confined to the cholestatic areas, and liver-cell plates show little or no disruption, although some regenerative changes can be present. The presence of spotty hepatocellular necrosis can be a key histological feature to differentiate a cholestatic hepatitis such as hepatitis A from bile duct obstruction. Furthermore, bile retention is almost never seen in early stages of primary biliary cirrhosis, so, in the absence of ductopenia, the presence of canalicular cholestasis would favour a hepatitis or obstruction. Portal changes vary according to the cause of the cholestasis, and may also help to establish a correct diagnosis, but both hepatitis and biliary diseases may show varying degrees of portal mononuclear infiltrates and interface hepatitis.

Drugs and toxic agents should always be suspected as a possible cause of acute hepatitis syndrome (see Chapter 14). Correlation of the temporal relationship of liver disease to the usage of the drug is essential in any type of possible drug reaction, either idiosyncratic or toxic. Hepatic injury is generally recognized at least 5 days after initiating drug exposure but may become evident during the first year or later of administration.[42] The pattern of liver test abnormalities may be hepatocellular with prominent aminotransferase elevation, although some agents such as chlorpromazine generate a predominant cholestatic pattern of liver test results.[43] Mixed patterns are also possible. Drugs, environmental toxins, 'health' supplements, vitamin preparations and over-the-counter therapies all need to be considered as possible causes when evaluating acute hepatic injury. Most recently, the growing use of alternative medicine has focused attention on the potential hepatotoxicity of 'natural' products, or herbal agents. Although systemic evidence of hypersensitivity, such as rash or eosinophilia, may support drug hepatotoxicity, these findings are not necessary for the diagnosis. Histopathological findings included injury of varying severity from bridging necrosis to massive necrosis.[44] Features that should arouse a greater than average degree of suspicion for an idiosyncratic type of drug hepatitis include

a poorly developed or absent portal inflammatory reaction, abundant neutrophils or eosinophils, granuloma formation, sharply defined perivenular necrosis with little inflammation, or a mixed pattern of hepatitic and cholestatic features with duct damage; the latter may be a prominent feature. Direct toxic reactions such as paracetamol (acetaminophen) toxicity will tend to have a uniform pattern of perivenular necrosis with a minimal inflammatory component.

Acute alcoholic hepatitis is usually an exacerbation of a chronic condition. The degree of elevation of aminotransferase values is generally modest and does not reflect the severity of injury. Typically, AST levels are greater than ALT values and prominent elevation of GGT is typical.[45] GGT activity is a reflection of enzyme induction rather than the severity of hepatotoxicity. Alkaline phosphatase and bilirubin values commonly rise as aminotransferase values improve following abstinence.

In alcoholic hepatitis, ballooning of hepatocytes is usually seen in perivenular (central) zones, often accompanied by a predominantly neutrophilic infiltrate with or without the presence of new collagen fibres around affected hepatocytes; fatty change and Mallory bodies are often present (see Chapter 6). In contrast, non-alcoholic steatohepatitis (NASH, see Chapter 7) may have a more intense lymphocytic infiltrate and absent or less prominent Mallory bodies but this entity is not typically in the clinical differential diagnosis owing to the lack of jaundice and the milder, more chronic nature of the aminotransferase abnormalities.

Autoimmune hepatitis can present as an acute hepatitis syndrome as well (see Chapter 10), with aminotransferase values more than five times the upper limit of normal. When this occurs, histological changes are similar to those of acute viral hepatitis with extensive hepatocyte necrosis and inflammatory infiltrates, especially in the perivenular (central) zone. Plasma cells are likely to be prominent in autoimmune hepatitis, but they may be variable in number in viral hepatitis, and have been noted to be a common component of the inflammatory infiltrate in acute hepatitis A, so the presence of these cells cannot be used as a definitive distinguishing feature. Serum markers for autoimmune antibodies as well as elevated gamma globulin levels above 2 gm/dl are typically present to distinguish these lesions.[46]

Wilson disease (see Chapter 5) can also rarely present as fulminant liver failure, and, in these instances, the histology can be similar to acute viral hepatitis. However, some of these patients may have underlying evidence of chronic injury such as established scarring, demonstrated by densely staining collagen bands in the form of septa and/or increased elastic fibre deposition in septa. Tissue from Wilson disease patients may also show copper deposits by histochemical stains (see Chapter 5).

Additional causes of acute liver injury are multiple and are pursued according to evidence supplied within the medical history. Liver pathology evaluation may be of value in focusing consideration on unanticipated results and assessing the severity of injury. As many as 15–20% of patients with fulminant liver failure may have no known case for the hepatitis. The histology of these cases is often similar to the types of changes described in this chapter for severe hepatitis with panlobular necrosis.

Lastly, areas of collapse in acute hepatitis must be distinguished from the fibrous septa of chronic liver disease, as discussed above.

Sequelae of acute hepatitis

The morphological consequences of acute viral hepatitis are shown in Table 8.3. Restitution to normal liver occurs in the classic forms of acute viral hepatitis, and the results of fulminant hepatitis are described under acute hepatitis with panlobular necrosis. The spectrum of lesions of chronic hepatitis is discussed later in this chapter. A viral carrier state without significant histological changes (other than ground-glass hepatocytes in hepatitis B virus carriers) may possibly develop in both hepatitis B and C as a temporary state,[47] but some question remains whether a permanent, non-progressive infection by these two viruses exists.

It is likely that cirrhosis may develop following acute hepatitis due to ongoing hepatitic changes or chronic hepatitis. The idea that cirrhosis can develop directly from massive hepatic necrosis, without the intervention of chronic hepatitis, is expressed in the old term 'post-necrotic cirrhosis'. Karvountzis et al.[47] followed 22 patients surviving acute hepatitis with coma, and concluded that such patients rarely if ever developed chronic hepatitis. On the other hand, Horney & Galambos[29] reported that chronic hepatitis had developed in three of nine patients having follow-up biopsies 6 to 60 months after fulminant hepatitis. Certainly, nodular regeneration of surviving parenchyma is seen in patients dying some weeks or months after the acute attack, but this should not be considered as cirrhosis as the septa are formed by collapse of pre-existing fibres rather than by true new collagen deposition (fibrosis); in addition, the nodularity is not usually uniform or diffuse. It is possible that in a small number of patients who recover from the acute attack, there is sufficient nodularity, portal–systemic shunting, fibrosis and portal hypertension to warrant a diagnosis of inactive cirrhosis even in the absence of chronic hepatitis,[25,48] but this is probably the exception rather than the rule.

A role for vascular occlusion in the pathogenesis of chronic liver disease and cirrhosis has been proposed,[49] and one could also speculate that similar lesions play a role in postnecrotic scarring following acute hepatitis. The mechanism for the injury would probably start with phlebitis of the hepatic venules (Fig. 8.13) or portal veins, with resultant vascular sclerosis. Occlusion of these veins, in turn, would lead to ischaemia or outflow obstruction in these areas, a process which would impair regeneration and enhance the formation of scar tissue in those zones with severe hepatocyte necrosis and dropout.

Hepatocellular carcinoma (see Chapter 15) is a long-term complication of hepatitis B and C; it is usually (but not always) seen in end-stage disease associated with cirrhosis.

Chronic viral hepatitis

Clinical features

Chronic viral hepatitis is a syndrome of persisting hepatotropic viral infection usually associated with chronic inflammation, hepatocyte injury and progressive fibrosis. By convention, infection for more than 6 months is considered evidence that spontaneous resolution of infection is unlikely and hepatitis is no longer acute. A clinical diagnosis of chronic viral hepatitis may be made on an initial clinical evaluation when clinical history or pathological findings suggest chronic infection even in the absence of earlier laboratory data. Chronic viral hepatitis is typically classified by the responsible infecting virus and modified by the extent of pathological injury and clinical compensation. Hepatotropic viruses responsible for this syndrome include hepatitis B, C and D. The injury from hepatitis A and E viruses may be severe and relapsing but represents acute injury rather than chronic hepatitis. The epidemiologies of the various forms of viral hepatitis share modes of transmission and thus a small, but significant, number of individuals may have chronic coinfection with multiple viruses. In addition to hepatotropic viruses, HIV also shares epidemiological features with the hepatitis viruses. Individuals with HIV coinfection may experience accelerated injury and progression of disease (Chapter 9).[50]

The hepatotropic viruses form a group of diverse agents which utilize liver tissue as a site of replication and major pathological injury. The liver, usually, is the predominant focus of injury but the course of disease may vary considerably from patient to patient. Many patients are asymptomatic and most are anicteric. Infection with hepatitis B or C may be discovered through screening, which is most fruitful in populations at high risk of exposure (Table 8.4).[51,52]

Symptoms of chronic hepatitis may be non-specific with fatigability being the most common. Patients may have mild discomfort in the right upper quadrant, pruritus, joint pain or anorexia. As liver disease progresses, muscle atrophy, jaundice, fluid retention and loss of mental acuity may develop.

The characteristic biochemical abnormality associated with chronic viral hepatitis is an elevation of aminotransferase values. Typically, aminotransferase activities range from normal to less than 10 times the upper limit of normal. On occasion, patients may have flares of hepatitic activity

Table 8.3	Sequelae of acute hepatitis
Restitution to normal morphology	
Death from severe liver damage or its complications	
Posthepatitic scarring	
Viral carrier state	
Chronic hepatitis and cirrhosis	
Hepatocellular carcinoma	

Table 8.4	Populations at risk of exposure to hepatitis B or C[51,52]

Populations at risk for exposure to Hepatitis B
  Persons born in high endemic areas
  Men who have sex with men
  Injection drug users
  Dialysis patients
  Persons with HIV infections
  Family/household and sexual contacts of HBV-infected patients

Populations at risk for exposure to Hepatitis C
  Injection-drug users
  Persons with HIV infection
  Haemophiliacs who received clotting factors before 1987
  Dialysis patients
  Persons who received a transfusion of blood or blood products
    before 1992
  Persons who received an organ transplant before 1992
  Children born to HCV-infected mothers
  Health care workers with needle-stick injury or mucosal exposure
    to HCV-positive persons

with enzyme activities more than 20 times the upper limit of normal. In patients with hepatitis C, this hectic course of aminotransferase values is more commonly seen early in infection, and in patients with hepatitis B infection, a rise in aminotransferase value may be associated with seroconversion of HBe antigen positive to HBe antibody reactivity or delta superinfection.

In many patients with chronic viral hepatitis, aminotransferase values are normal. Although the correlation with aminotransferase values and the degree of liver injury is not precise, generally asymptomatic individuals with consistently normal aminotransferase values have a more favourable prognosis than individuals with elevated test results.[53] Patients however can have significant pathological abnormality, even cirrhosis, in spite of normal alanine aminotransferase (ALT) values. In one study, 16% of patients with persistently normal ALT values had significant necroinflammation or fibrosis.[54] Disease progression has been demonstrated in patients with hepatitis C and persistently normal aminotransferase values.[55]

As chronic hepatitis progresses, evidence of hepatic synthetic dysfunction is demonstrated by a fall in serum albumin and rise of INR and serum bilirubin. The presence of cirrhosis may be suspected by the presence of signs of portal hypertension such as splenomegaly and laboratory results may show a fall in platelet count. The AST/platelet ratio has recently been shown to correlate with the presence of cirrhosis.[56]

Once a patient is defined as having chronic viral hepatitis due to a specific hepatotropic virus, it is important to assess the severity of illness and the presence or absence of complications such as portal hypertension or hepatocellular carcinoma. Liver biopsy is particularly useful in this assessment and currently forms the basis for the most secure assessment of the stage of disease and the urgency of initiating antiviral therapy.

Pathological features

Chronic viral hepatitis is characterized by a combination of inflammatory cell infiltration, hepatocyte death, atrophy and regeneration, and fibrosis. These components, while all present in acute viral hepatitis to some degree, have a different relative proportion and distribution in chronic viral infection. The proportion and distribution may also differ between one viral infection and another, as well as in the same patient with the same infection, over time. Patterns of inflammation and scarring will be discussed first, followed by descriptions of the types of scarring that may be seen, if and when the disease is progressive. The possible mechanisms of injury and repair responsible for these gross and light microscopic changes will then be summarized. Finally, grading and staging of chronic hepatitis will be discussed along with consideration of the impact of tissue sampling on such assessments.

Macroscopic appearances

The macroscopic appearances of livers with chronic viral hepatitis in advance of cirrhosis have not been systematically described. However, anecdotal observations of such livers obtained at autopsy or in partial hepatectomy for tumours indicate that they may appear normal, have focal areas of fibrosis with a somewhat gritty texture, or have a diffuse or focally lobulated appearance indicative of fibrous septa and local regeneration (Fig. 8.15). The colour of the liver at these early stages is generally the normal beefy red as these patients are rarely cholestatic. Some yellow colour will indicate steatosis, particularly to be expected in hepatitis C infection.

As cirrhosis develops, there is increasingly diffuse nodularity and obvious fibrous scarring. Classically, cirrhosis associated with chronic viral hepatitis appears either macronodular or mixed micro- and macronodular. However, a diffusely micronodular cirrhosis does not exclude the diagnosis. A predominantly macronodular cirrhosis seems to be most often present in patients younger than 40 years old, while strictly micronodular cirrhosis in chronic hepatitis should raise the question of concomitant alcoholic liver disease. Nodules may vary in colour, ranging from beefy red to dark green, signifying cholestasis, to yellow, if there is focal fat. Some nodules may appear necrotic, presumably because they have either outgrown their blood supply or because their blood supply has become compromised by mechanical distortions and/or thrombosis. Examination of the larger branches of the portal vein often demonstrates thrombotic occlusion.

Light microscopic appearances: patterns of necrosis, inflammation, and fibrosis

Hepatocyte injury and inflammation in chronic hepatitis is now generally referred to as 'activity', which is 'graded' (see below). Distribution of inflammatory cells may vary from case to case or even in sequential biopsies from the same patient. However, all cases of chronic viral hepatitis are

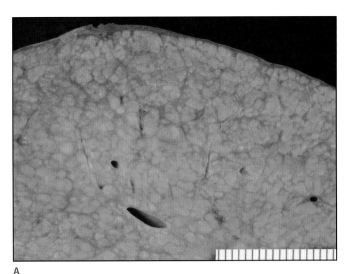

A

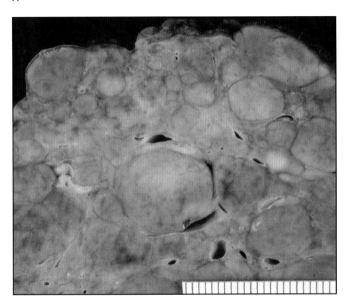

B

Fig. 8.15 • **(A)** Micronodular cirrhosis due to chronic hepatitis C. Nodules of regenerating hepatic parenchyma separated by fibrous bands are rarely greater than 3 mm in greatest dimension. The two green nodules are foci of hepatocellular carcinoma. Courtesy of Dr I Wanless. **(B)** Macronodular cirrhosis in chronic hepatitis B. Nodules vary greatly in size, though most are greater than 3 mm in greatest dimension. Courtesy of Dr I Wanless.

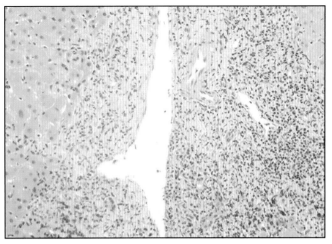

Fig. 8.16 • Phlebitis of a portal vein in a liver with chronic hepatitis C. The portal tract is expanded by a dense mononuclear cell infiltrate which focally encroaches on the vein. Damage to the endothelium is evidenced by focal lifting of the endothelium from its basement membrane and adherent inflammatory cells. Such damage has been hypothesized to lead to thrombosis of veins with subsequent ischaemia and extinction of dependent regions of parenchyma. H&E. Courtesy of Dr I Wanless.

distinguished by a relatively dense monocytic infiltration of the portal tracts. If nearly all the inflammation is confined within the portal tracts and if hepatocyte injury is scant or absent, the pattern corresponds to what was originally classified as 'chronic persistent hepatitis' by the International Working Group.[57] This phrase, however, is no longer in use. When there is more obvious inflammation and apoptosis of hepatocytes involving the limiting plate and lobular hepatocytes, the hepatitis may be termed active, though the phrase 'chronic active hepatitis' should also be avoided.

Portal inflammation

Mononuclear infiltration of portal tracts is the defining lesion of chronic hepatitis of any cause. Some or all portal tracts may be involved and the portal infiltrates are usually much more dense than those seen in acute viral hepatitis. The portal tracts may be of normal size or appear widened by the influx of mononuclear cells. The infiltrate includes predominantly CD4+helper/inducer T-lymphocytes with an admixture of plasma cells.[58-60] Some portal macrophages may also be seen to contain periodic acid–Schiff (PAS)-positive, diastase-resistant material and iron pigment, representing the removal of hepatocyte debris.

Portal inflammation will often fill and expand the portal fibrous stroma, pushing structures aside without obvious injury. Lymphoid aggregates or fully formed follicles may be seen; while most common in hepatitis C, they are also seen in other forms of hepatitis. However, inflammation with damage or even destruction of bile ducts may be seen, particularly in hepatitis C.[61-63] Inflammation may also encroach on the portal blood vessels, in particular the portal veins (Fig. 8.16), endophlebitis may be present, and there may be associated fresh or organizing venous thrombosis; such lesions may be particularly evident with trichrome-stained sections.[64]

Interface hepatitis

The region of liver tissue where the hepatic parenchyma comes into contact with the mesenchymal stroma of the intact or scarred portal tract may be referred to as an interface region. Thus, hepatocyte apoptosis and inflammation of this area are generally referred to as 'interface hepatitis,' this being the currently favoured term. Previously, this classical histological feature of active chronic hepatitis was called 'piecemeal necrosis', referring to the way in which the limiting plate of hepatocytes was eroded in a piecemeal, that is focal, fashion (Fig. 8.17).[65]

In regions of interface hepatitis, there is a predominantly mononuclear infiltration, though in these regions, Fas-ligand positive CD8+ suppressor/cytotoxic T-cells predominate.[66] Close contact of hepatocytes with these lymphocytes, and with macrophages and plasma cells, is seen.[67-72] Emperipolesis, the invagination of lymphocytes into hepa-

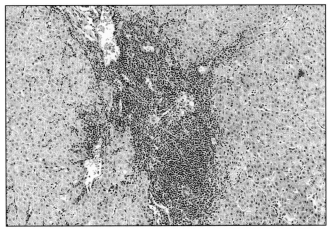

A

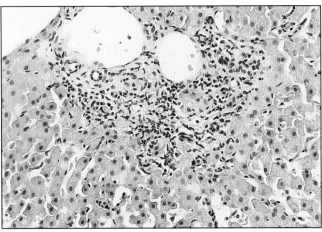

B

Fig. 8.17 • (A) Interface hepatitis in chronic viral hepatitis. Previously referred to as 'piecemeal necrosis,' this lesion can often be observed at low power, evidenced by irregular contours of a portal tract containing a dense mononuclear cell infiltrate eroding the limiting plate of hepatocytes in a piecemeal fashion. H&E. (B) Higher-power view of an inflamed portal tract in hepatitis C shows mononuclear cells extending beyond the limiting plate, surrounding individual or small clusters of hepatocytes. H&E.

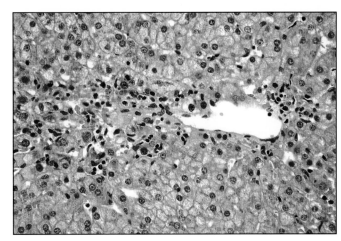

Fig. 8.18 • Lobular hepatitis in chronic hepatitis C. Foci of inflammation and parenchymal necrosis located in the hepatic parenchyma near the hepatic venule are a form of activity in chronic hepatitis. Another term for this lesion is spotty necrosis. H&E.

tocytes, has been described.[70] While the inflammation interweaving amongst hepatocytes at the interface is sufficient by itself for describing the lesion as interface hepatitis, dead or dying hepatocytes may also be seen in these areas. These hepatocytes will show the typical features of cells undergoing apoptosis, including nuclear hyperchromasia and disintegration, cytoplasmic eosinophilia and fragmentation, and a pulling away from adjacent cells with rounding of the cell surface.[71,72]

Lobular hepatitis and confluent necrosis

Another form of activity in chronic viral hepatitis is that found within the hepatic lobule away from the portal areas or septal scars. Such lesions may be referred to as 'lobular hepatitis' or 'spotty necrosis'. Cases in which such lesions predominate have historically been referred to as 'chronic lobular hepatitis', though, like the terms chronic persistent and chronic active hepatitis, this classification is no longer in favour (Fig. 8.18).[73–77] The inflammatory infiltrates in these areas of activity are the same as those seen in interface hepatitis, but their relative importance to the development of scarring and progression in chronic viral hepatitis remains uncertain.

Some foci of lobular hepatitis are relatively devoid of mononuclear cells. In these areas there may be rare or numerous acidophil bodies, macrophages containing PAS-positive, diastase-resistant material indicating prior cell death, or simply cellular debris and loosely aggregated collagen and reticulin fibres. Such lesions are similar to the lobular damage found in acute viral hepatitis and tend to focus on the hepatic venules. If large areas are involved, one may refer to the lesion as 'confluent necrosis' and, if such areas span from central vein to central vein or from central vein to portal tract, then the term 'bridging necrosis' is used. Such bridging necrosis is considered the most ominous finding in terms of progression toward scarring and cirrhosis.[76,77] In some cases, when one or more entire lobule has been destroyed, it may be referred to as panlobular or multilobular collapse. In these areas, portal tracts will be in abnormally close proximity, separated only by regions filled with necrotic debris, macrophages, loose or more mature collagen, and elastic fibres.[78] A ductular reaction, which is now recognized as activation of a hepatic stem cell compartment, is also present (Fig. 8.19).[78,79]

Fibrosis and hepatocyte regeneration

While some patients with chronic viral hepatitis do not show fibrous scarring, most will have some. Increasing fibrosis is now assessed as advancing 'stages' of disease. The scarring will usually develop as an extension of the portal stroma, though perivenular and pericellular fibrosis may also be seen. The perivenular fibrosis usually develops following collapse and condensation of the reticulin meshwork in an area of confluent or bridging necrosis. The resulting scars are bland and generally acellular, and often lack an extensive accompanying interface hepatitis. These septa will either link central veins to neighbouring portal tracts or to other hepatic veins and, in these cases, probably represent an area of healed bridging necrosis. If these scars

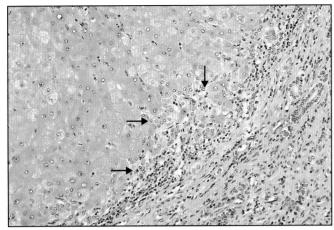

Fig. 8.19 • A ductular reaction, consisting of a disorganized array of cholangiocyte-like cells (arrows), is present at the margin of a fibrous septum in hepatitis B cirrhosis. Such cells can also be seen focally within the fibrous tissue. H&E.

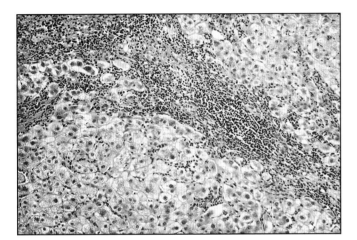

Fig. 8.20 • A fibrous septum in hepatitis C cirrhosis with a dense mononuclear cell infiltrate and extensive interface hepatitis. H&E.

persist, mature forms of collagen will deposit, as will elastin fibres demonstrated by orcein or Victoria blue stains. Thus, deposition of elastic fibres suggests increasing age of the scar.[78]

Fibrous expansion of the portal tract probably results from a more active process of injury and repair. There is as yet little agreement on the use of the terms periportal fibrosis and portal fibrosis. Whichever term is used, it refers to fibrous stroma extending from the portal tract beyond its usual boundaries. This fibrosis is usually conceptualized as following Rappaport's acinus zone 1 and, thus, eventually leads to linking of one portal tract to another. These septa usually contain mononuclear inflammatory cells as described above and may be associated with interface hepatitis (Fig. 8.20). The fibrosis is usually mature, darkly staining with trichrome stains, and containing abundant type I collagen in addition to type III collagen (Fig. 8.21A) and reticulin fibres (Fig 8.21B).[80] Again, elastic fibres are easily demonstrated, indicating that the scars are of at least several months duration. Immunohistochemical staining for α-smooth muscle actin highlights numerous activated stellate

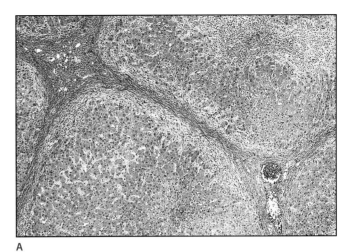

A

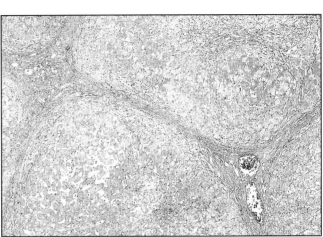

B

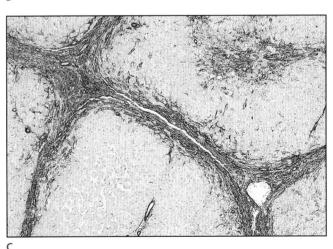

C

Fig. 8.21 • **(A)** Trichrome stain of a fibrous septum in hepatitis C cirrhosis, lining two portal tracts, shows dark blue staining of a mature scar, abundant in type I and type III collagen. Gomori's trichrome. **(B)** Reticulin stain of the same scar demonstrates collapse of the reticulin meshwork in the scar and highlights the regenerative thickening of liver cell plates in adjacent nodules of parenchyma. Gomori's reticulin. **(C)** Immunohistochemistry for smooth-muscle actin demonstrates actin fibres depositing in the scar, but also highlights individual activated stellate cells within the scar and in adjacent sinusoids. These cells are the resident myofibroblasts in the liver and are primarily responsible for deposition of matrix proteins which make up the scar. Immunoperoxidase, DAB.

cells in these regions and these cells are thought to be largely responsible for most of the scarring (Fig. 8.21C).[81]

Regeneration of hepatocytes becomes increasingly evident in parallel with the formation of fibrous septa and advancing stages of disease. The thickening of liver cell plates to two or three cells thick evidences this regeneration. Haematoxylin and eosin (H & E) or silver stains for reticulin can demonstrate these changes. An incomplete periportal nodular transformation may thus be noted around portal tracts that are becoming fibrotic. However, in the later stages of developing cirrhosis, hepatocyte regeneration markedly diminishes in parallel with an increasingly proliferative ductular reaction at the mesenchymal/parenchymal interface.[79] The implication is that as hepatocytes reach replicative senescence there is activation of the intrahepatic facultative stem cell compartment.

Regression of fibrosis and cirrhosis

Development of scarring in a chronically diseased liver is actually the result of a balance in favour of matrix deposition in a liver dynamically producing and degrading matrix at all time points. That fibrosis can regress with elimination of viral activity and infection has now been demonstrated in all forms of chronic viral hepatitis.[82-87] Cirrhosis itself, however, has generally been thought to be an 'end stage' of chronic liver disease and therefore not reversible. However, exceptions to this concept have been noted in many liver diseases over the years.[83,85]

In 2000, Ian Wanless and colleagues examined sequential biopsies from a patient with chronic hepatitis B infection who, with successful antiviral treatment and elimination of viral infection, apparently reversed the scarring and re-established some degree of functional, non-cirrhotic parenchyma.[85] These changes were documented on biopsy. Wanless's suggestion that cirrhosis was reversible when the impetus to hepatic injury ceases was exceedingly controversial at the time. The formal paper was finally published in a particularly interesting fashion: all in the same volume of the journal there appeared his paper, responses/critiques written by each of the reviewers,[88-91] and then his response to their comments.[92] Despite the controversial nature of the proposal, however, the concept rapidly entered the realm of general knowledge as clinical papers exploring the impact of successful eradication of HCV infection on stage of disease in patients with paired pre- and post-eradication biopsy specimens demonstrated the possibility of regression of fibrosis and, in some cases, regression of cirrhosis.

Wanless and colleagues described eight histological features of regression as the 'hepatic repair complex' which can be grouped into features evincing three regenerative phenomena: fragmentation and regression of scar (e.g. delicate, perforated septa; isolated thick collagen fibres; delicate, periportal fibrous spikes; hepatocytes within or splitting septa), evidence of prior, now resolving, vascular derangements (e.g. portal tract remnants, hepatic vein remnants with prolapsed hepatocytes, aberrant parenchymal veins) and parenchymal regeneration in the form of hepatocyte 'buds'. These hepatocyte buds are small clusters of hepatocytes, usually emerging from within portal/septal stroma;

the interpretation that these represented a regenerative phenomenon rather than entrapment of parenchyma by active scarring was supported by Falkowski et al.[79]

Pathogenetic mechanisms

There appear to be general mechanisms of injury and repair common to all hepatotropic viral infections. Some mechanisms of disease involve viral determinants whereas others are defined by the host response. It is the complex interplay of these viral determinants with the host immune system that determines the outcome of viral hepatitis.[93] Most importantly, the continued testing and development of antiviral drugs and immunomodulators is allowing clinicians increasingly to influence the balance and, therefore, the outcome of these infections.

Viral determinants include gene products that cause or inhibit apoptosis of infected or reacting cell populations.[94-96] Direct cytotoxicity of the hepatotropic viruses is probably a smaller contributor. The viruses may produce gene products that interfere with cell-mediated immunity and cytokine actions.[97] Mutations of the viruses may lead to escape from both humoral and cell-mediated immune responses.[98,99] Infection of extrahepatic, immunologically tolerant or privileged sites may encourage viral persistence.[100] On the other hand, the host has a wide range of possible responses to prevent infection or to clear virus from the liver or at least inhibit viral activity. Non-immunological responses include apoptosis of an infected cell.[101] Immune responses include those of humoral- and cell-mediated immunity as well as a range of cytokines released by immune cells plus parenchymal and non-parenchymal liver cells. These responses may be viral specific or non-specific.[93]

In acute hepatitis, the most appropriate response is one where the immune system can outpace the spread of the infection and eliminate viral replication from all infected cells, or eliminate the infected cells directly. With efficient regeneration of hepatocytes, either from mature hepatocyte division or from activation of a stem/progenitor-cell compartment, the liver can then recover, re-establishing normal architecture and function. If the viral infection is not kept in check by an active immune response, however, then progressive immune destruction of the liver results in fulminant hepatic failure.

Alternatively, the immune system may be generally or selectively impaired in response to the specific viral infection. Patients with a generalized immunosuppression, such as those coinfected with HIV or patients receiving immunosuppressive therapy for unrelated diseases, are at increased risk for developing chronic infection following acute exposure to a hepatitis virus.[102,103] Selective immune system defects may also occur, either pre-existent (perhaps genetically determined) or influenced or induced by viral factors.[104,105]

Regardless of the specific mechanisms involved, the virus is able to infect hepatocytes beyond the ability of the immune system to kill the infected cells or to induce suppression of the viral replication. Outpacing the immune system, the viral infections maintain a chronic presence in the liver and provoke, to variable degrees in different individuals, ongoing immune-mediated damage to the liver and its sequelae. In many patients, the outcome of this damage is development of scarring, sometimes leading to cirrhosis. There is also likely to be an increased risk for development of hepatocellular carcinoma related, at least in part, to increased hepatocellular turnover.[106,107]

The role of humoral immunity

Virus-specific antibodies play a relatively limited role in the development of viral hepatitis. Specific antiviral antibodies can protect against infection in the first place; thus, vaccine-induced anti-HAV and anti-HBV antibodies can prevent these infections.[108,109] Humoral immunity against hepatitis C, however, appears very limited.[110] Once infection has occurred, the humoral response serves primarily to help clear virus from the body, preventing its spread to uninfected cells. However, humoral responses to the viruses can lead to immune complex diseases such as glomerulonephritis, vasculitis and cryoglobulinaemia.[111–113] Autoantibody production can also be induced, perhaps leading to an autoimmune component of the hepatitis or autoimmune diseases affecting other organs.[113]

The role of cellular immunity

Cell-mediated immunity, particularly the cytotoxic T lymphocyte (CTL) response, is thought to be central to elimination of viral infections of the liver (Chapter 2). Through specific cell-to-cell recognition of host (major histocompatibility complex, MHC class I) and viral antigens on the surface of infected cells, CTL-induced cell death eliminates infected hepatocytes. Activation of CD4+ T-helper cells throughout the MHC class II pathway is also important for viral clearance, whether by stimulating CTL responses, inducing different patterns of cytokine production, or perhaps through some direct, Fas-mediated cytotoxic activity.[114–116] However, the number of potentially infected cells in the liver can far outweigh the available, though proliferating, virus-directed lymphocytes. Thus, though direct cell–cell interactions are probably important, diffusible cytokines produced or induced by these lymphocytes may be a more important factor in viral clearance.[117] Most recently, CD1d-reactive T cells, variants of natural killer cells, are seen to play important roles in production of these diverse cytokines as well, mediating via both Th1 and Th2 pathways.[118]

The role of cytokines

Cytokines may have direct antiviral activity and thus be important in modulation of the immune system. For example, the interferons have been shown to inhibit all viral infective/replicative processes, from entry into the cell, through uncoating, to viral gene translation and protein synthesis. Through these activities viral clearance from infected cells, even in the absence of cell death, can occur, extending the antiviral capabilities beyond the limits of cell-mediated immunity. They also induce production of host-cell proteins, including HLA class I and class II antigens. Macrophages, natural killer cells, and cytotoxic T-cells are also stimulated by these cytokines. Tumour necrosis factor (TNF), produced by macrophages and T-cells, stimulates chemotaxis, activation of macrophages, induction of class I and class II antigens and T-cell activation, and modulates acute-phase protein transcription, amongst other functions. IL-1 is produced by multiple cell types, including epithelial cells, macrophages, dendritic cells, endothelial cells and B-cells. Actions include enhancement of lymphocyte and fibroblast proliferation and activation, and induction of acute-phase reactants. IL-6, produced by monocytes, fibroblasts and endothelial cells, induces B-cell differentiation and acute phase proteins and is a growth factor for T-cells. Profibrotic cytokines, including IL-4 and IL-13, may also play a role in fibrosis. Thus, these cytokines have overlapping as well as distinct effects.[119–121]

The role of vascular injury

While hepatocyte injury often precedes cirrhosis, it is insufficient per se for its development. Even after significant hepatocyte necrosis, the liver can regenerate to a normal architecture without permanent fibrosis. Moreover, despite distribution of significant hepatocyte injury evenly throughout the hepatic lobule in chronic hepatitis, the formation of fibrous septa only occurs in limited regions. Some fibrous septa probably develop as scar tissue to replace bridging necrosis due to direct hepatocyte injury. However, some septa form in response to regions of parenchymal extinction following injury and thrombosis of intrahepatic arteries and veins with resultant parenchymal atrophy. In chronic hepatitis this injury is probably a 'bystander' phenomenon, resulting from the inflammatory response directed against, but not limited to, the infected parenchymal cell. Once cirrhosis is established, stasis leads to further thrombosis of portal and hepatic veins and secondary parenchymal loss that is independent of the activity of the original disease.[64]

Mechanisms of fibrogenesis and fibrotic regression

As noted above, scarring during chronic liver disease represents a balance between new deposition of matrix and its resorption. As long as the disease persists, the balance favours deposition and scar formation. If the disease is inhibited or eliminated, then fibrosis and even cirrhosis can regress.

The principal cell responsible for collagen deposition and scar formation in the liver is the hepatic stellate cell, though it is becoming clear that this class of cells is markedly heterogeneous.[122] Many factors probably initiate stellate cell activation.[122] Oxidant stress is one influence. For example, in vitro lipid peroxidation products, such as malondialdehyde, can stimulate stellate cell activation, inducing collagen synthesis.[123] Interestingly, such products have been identified in the regions of hepatocyte injury and fibrous septum formation in chronic hepatitis.[124] Once activated, stellate cells respond to a variety of cytokines that up-regulate collagen synthesis and deposition, including TGF-β, IL-1 and IL-4, many of which are primarily or secondarily produced in inflammatory responses typical of chronic viral hepatitis. Fibrogenic cytokines may derive from autocrine, paracrine and matrix-bound sources.[125]

Certainly, regression of fibrosis requires breaking up and digestion of collagen and elastin fibres which make up the principal components of the scar. Various metalloproteinases accomplish some, if not all, of these tasks and may be produced by hepatocytes as well as non-parenchymal cells, particularly those of macrophage lineages. However, the appearance of fractured, 'perforated' septa with hepatocytes within or completely interrupting the septa, usually in the absence of inflammation or activated macrophages, suggests that hepatocytes themselves may play a major role. Expression of various metalloproteinases by hepatocytes supports this concept.[126,127]

Multiple chronic viral infections

Coinfection by multiple hepatotropic viruses

Since hepatitis B, C and D viruses are all parenterally spread, it is not surprising that dual or triple infection of these viruses occurs.[128] Viral interference appears to be most common in coinfections. Experimentally, in chimpanzees, non-A non-B hepatitis (presumably HCV) interfered with both acute hepatitis A and chronic hepatitis B.[129] Interference has also been demonstrated in clinical settings, usually HCV interfering with HBV replication,[130] though the reverse has also been reported when HBV infection followed HCV infection.[131] The clinical course, however, does not seem to be consistently altered by such coinfections.[128,132]

Histopathologically, there are no specific findings to suggest the possibility of multiple infections and the diagnosis usually depend on serological investigations. However, immunohistochemical investigations have revealed some important features. In particular, it seems that there is suppression of HBV core antigen by simultaneous HCV infection. It may be reasonable to suggest that, in a patient serologically positive for hepatitis B surface antigen (HBsAg), the absence of demonstrable tissue staining for HBV antigens indicates that clinical suspicion of coinfection not only with HDV, but also with HCV, should be raised.[133]

Coinfection by hepatotropic viruses and HIV

Since HBV, HCV, HDV and the human immunodeficiency virus (HIV) are all parenterally acquired, and HBV and HIV are also frequently transmitted sexually, coinfection of these hepatitis viruses and HIV is often seen clinically.[128] Additionally, coinfection between HIV and HAV has been identified, though this does not seem to lead to a difference in HAV's clinical course.[134,135] HIV coinfection with HEV has been reported and transmission to the fetus and maternal mortality may be increased in this setting.[136]

Though acute hepatitis B is less commonly icteric in the setting of HIV infection, viral persistence and development of chronic infection is more common.[128] Most studies indicate a diminished histological activity of chronic hepatitis B, though greater activity has also been reported. Reactivation of hepatitis B has also been reported with HIV coinfection.[128] Rarely, the fibrosing cholestatic variant of hepatitis B is seen, as it is in hepatitis C.[137–139] As far as HDV is concerned, coinfection with HIV seems to worsen liver damage as evidenced by increased serum aminotransferase levels and worsened histological severity.[140] Replication of both HBV by itself and together with HDV is increased and may be demonstrated by more diffuse staining for hepatitis B and delta antigens in tissue specimens.[128]

Coinfection of HCV and HIV is also common.[141] As HIV-infected individuals are surviving longer with new antiviral therapies, the importance of HCV infection in these patients increases. Acute hepatitis C seems to be more often symptomatic and much more likely to result in liver failure when HIV is simultaneously acquired. Many studies indicate that untreated HIV with significant immunosuppression increases the severity and accelerates the course of chronic hepatitis C, though successful anti-HIV treatment accompanied by immune reconstitution seems to lead, generally, to a more typical HCV course. However, it has been reported that even with minimal or absent immunosuppression in such treated patients, fibrosis is still more prevalent and more rapid, though the mechanism is uncertain.[142] Conversely, it has also been suggested that HCV is a poor prognostic indicator for HIV disease and patients with coinfection, even with successful immune reconstitution, have increased mortality and morbidity due to viral interactions directly or to interactions between the large battery of medications required to treat both infections.[141,143]

Differential diagnosis of chronic hepatitis

Many disease states can mimic chronic viral hepatitis and other, non-viral conditions can cause the same chronic hepatitic patterns of injury. To evaluate this fully in a biopsy or resection specimen, clinical history must be considered. In all cases, if a diagnosis of chronic viral hepatitis is contemplated, serological tests for hepatitis B, C and D must be obtained. In the absence of positive viral serology, the following diseases must be considered.

Other causes of chronic hepatitis

Infecting viruses are not the only aetiology of the typical histological features of chronic hepatitis. Autoimmune hepatitis is characterized by autoantibodies such as antinuclear antibodies or antiliver kidney microsome (LKM) antibodies (see Chapter 10). Histologically, abundant plasma cells in the inflammatory infiltrate and widespread parenchymal collapse are hints that an autoimmune process rather than a viral infection is present. Serological studies demonstrating autoantibodies, in the absence of those confirming viral infection, should establish the diagnosis. However, one caveat is that in chronic hepatitis C and less commonly in chronic hepatitis B, serological studies may indicate the presence of circulating autoantibodies. In the case of hepatitis C, false-positive results of the early antibody tests in patients with hypergamma globulinaemia and antinuclear antibodies accounted for some of these cases. It is also clear, however, that in chronic infection with HBV, HCV or HDV there may be breakdown of self tolerance and induction of autoantibodies.[144] For example, chronic hepatitis B infection may stimulate the formation of circulating immune complexes of viral antigens and reactive antibody. These complexes may fix complement and induce tissue damage such as vasculitis, arthritis and glomerulonephritis.[145] Chronic hepatitis C is also associated with autoimmune phenomena. HCV and less frequently HBV are associated with mixed cryoglobulinaemia.[146,147] Autoantibodies, including antinuclear antibodies, may be seen in chronic hepatitis C but are generally of low titre.

Metabolic diseases may also have chronic hepatitic patterns of injury. α_1-Antitrypsin deficiency can have the same necroinflammatory lesions and pattern of scarring, but histological demonstration of α_1-antitrypsin globules by H & E, PAS staining after diastase digestion, or immunohistochemistry will confirm the diagnosis. Typically, liver disease is seen in individuals with ZZ phenotype. Phenotypes such as SS or a heterozygous pattern are not predictably related to chronic liver disease. Care must be taken, however, to exclude concomitant viral infection serologically, as it appears that most chronic hepatitides in the setting of metabolic diseases are due to a superimposed viral infection.[148]

Similarly, Wilson disease can cause the same pattern of injury, but histological confirmation, while suggested by abundant Mallory bodies, fatty change, or even some copper accumulation in periportal hepatocytes, can be achieved only in combination with clinical and biochemical findings.[149] The diagnostic tests are complex but attempt to establish abnormalities of copper metabolism by documenting low levels of serum ceruloplasmin or by finding evidence of increased tissue stores of copper. Provocative testing with urine copper measurements before and after penicillamine administration has been most extensively validated in children.[150] However, none of the test results is pathognomonic for Wilson disease and may be abnormal in patients with other causes of abnormal copper retention as is seen in patients with primary biliary cirrhosis or primary sclerosing cholangitis. Wilson disease should be remembered as a confounding impostor and considered in the differential diagnosis of non-viral chronic hepatitis irrespective of age.

Hereditary haemochromatosis (HH) is a common, inherited disorder that also results in chronic liver disease, but not typically in individuals under the age of 40 years.[151] HH typically does not have any significant chronic inflammatory response, so in a clinical setting suspicious for HH, but with chronic hepatitis-like changes seen on biopsy, one should investigate other aetiologies.

Some drugs can also cause chronic hepatitis, including: α-methyldopa, isoniazid, oxyphenasatin, nitrofurantoin and diclofenac (see Chapter 14). Some of these drugs may actually induce autoantibodies, suggesting induction of an autoimmune hepatitis.[152] Again, the absence of serological markers of viral infection will help diagnostic accuracy and careful history taking will often reveal the offending toxin.

Diseases that mimic chronic viral hepatitis

Any disease leading to dense lymphoplasmacytic infiltrate in the portal tracts may mimic chronic viral hepatitis. For example, primary biliary cirrhosis (PBC) not only often has a dense portal infiltrate, but may also have extensive interface and lobular hepatitis. A diagnostic biopsy for this disease demonstrating granulomatous destruction of bile ducts is unlikely to cause this confusion. A later-stage lesion, with ductular proliferation and features of chronic cholestasis adjacent to fibrotic septa, is also unlikely to cause confusion. However, non-diagnostic early lesions of PBC may be difficult to distinguish from chronic viral hepatitis, particularly type C, as the latter may have marked bile-duct damage and even loss.[61] In these instances, clinical correlation is important, as PBC predominantly affects women and is characterized by elevation of alkaline phosphatase and gamma-glutamyl transpeptidase associated with elevated IgM and the presence of mitochondrial antibody. Aminotransferase values are generally less than five times the upper limit of normal but may fluctuate to higher levels. Similar confusion may be encountered, although less frequently, with a non-diagnostic biopsy specimen for primary sclerosing cholangitis. Again, clinical correlation for possible chronic inflammatory bowel disease (usually ulcerative colitis) and characteristic bile-duct abnormalities on imaging studies are very helpful.

Lymphoma or leukaemic infiltrates may also mimic the inflammatory infiltrate of chronic viral hepatitis, particularly when the infiltrate is most prominently located in the portal tracts with overflow into neighbouring sinusoids. In such cases, careful inspection of the lesion will reveal an absence of true interface hepatitis at the margins of portal tracts where the malignant cells extend past hepatocytes that are atrophic, but not truly apoptotic. Similarly, parenchymal hepatocytes may appear atrophic, but acidophil bodies are generally absent. The typical scarring of progressive chronic hepatitis is also not usually present in such specimens. Most important, of course, is that the infiltrating cells will have features suggesting a lymphoproliferative disorder, including monomorphism or marked atypia.

Semiquantitative scoring in chronic hepatitis

Adequacy of biopsy sampling for grading and staging

Though one might argue that this section should follow those that describe the history and use of the varied schemata for grading and staging chronic viral hepatitis, the importance of the topic and the lack of consistent application of well-documented principles warrants its being highlighted at the start. As summarized by Guido and Rugge,[153] there are two basic issues which bear on the adequacy of tissue acquisition for grading and staging: (i) can a small random sample adequately reflect the overall state of a diffuse liver disease, such as chronic hepatitis? and (ii) can sample size affect the accuracy of histological assessments?[153]

The answer to both questions is a clear 'yes'. *If* sufficient tissue is obtained, *then* the little needle biopsy core of tissue, estimated to be 1/50 000 of the total liver parenchyma, can reflect the status of disease in the organ as a whole. However, it would seem that, indeed, there is little attention paid to what is 'sufficient' in routine hepatology and hepatopathology practice. Recent studies suggest a simple and clear answer: a total of 2.0 cm of liver tissue, containing 11 to 15 portal tracts, is necessary to avoid underscoring of grade and stage of disease. Less than that and there are likely to be significant inaccuracies in assessment.[154–159]

An additional sampling problem concerns small biopsy specimens obtained from the subcapsular region. For perhaps as much as 1 cm below the capsule, increased stroma, including septum formation and perhaps focal nodularity, may be within the spectrum of normal. Thus, such biopsy specimens may overestimate the stage of disease.[153]

It cannot be overemphasized, therefore, that the pathologist must assess samples of tissue provided either by hepatologists or radiologists for *adequacy* before supplying an assessment of grade (necroinflammatory activity) and stage (scarring) to the clinician and the patient. It behoves the pathologists to educate their clinical colleagues to supply adequate samples, either by obtaining one long needle core or through repeat passes. It should particularly be made clear to radiologists that they should eschew the easier approach, into the left lobe, for the more traditional right lobe sampling, thus making it more likely to avoid sampling the subcapsular region alone.

Development and application of scoring systems

The first scoring system specifically designed for the study of chronic hepatitis was that of Knodell and colleagues.[160] The purpose of their histical activity index (HAI) was to follow the course of chronic hepatitis in asymptomatic patients, in whom conventionally used clinical events, such as jaundice, ascites and encephalopathy, could not be evaluated. The HAI was based on four components: periportal and bridging necrosis; intralobular degeneration and focal necrosis; portal inflammation; and fibrosis. The scores allotted to these components were respectively 0–10, 0–4, 0–4 and 0–4, giving a maximum possible total of 22. The system and its components were used extensively after its publication for the evaluation of therapy and for correlation of histological changes with other factors such as viral load, viral genotype and liver function tests, principally in chronic hepatitis B and C.

Several other scoring systems followed. Of these, the most notable are those of Batts and Ludwig[161] (Table 8.5) and the METAVIR group (a co-operative group of French investigators) (Fig. 8.22).[162] An important feature of these

Table 8.5	A simple scoring system (after Batts and Ludwig[161])	

Portal/periportal activity		*Lobular activity*	
None or minimal	0	None	0
Portal inflammation only	1	Inflammatory cells but no hepatocellular death	1
Mild interface hepatitis	2	Focal cell death	2
Moderate interface hepatitis	3	Severe focal cell death, +/– confluent necrosis without bridging	3
Severe interface hepatitis	4	Damage includes bridging necrosis	4

Fibrosis	
None	0
Enlarged, fibrotic portal tracts	1
Periportal or portal–portal septa but intact architecture	2
Fibrosis with architectural distortion but no obvious cirrhosis	3
Probable or definite cirrhosis	4

Note: separate scores are generated for portal/periportal and lobular activity

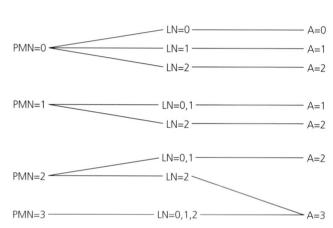

Fig. 8.22 • Algorithm for the evaluation of histological activity: PMN, piecemeal necrosis; 0, none; 1, mild; 2, moderate; 3, severe; LN, lobular necrosis; 0, none or mild; 1, moderate; 2, severe; A, histological activity; 0, none; 1, mild; 2, moderate; 3, severe. (After Bedossa et al.[162])

systems recognized that grading of necroinflammatory activity should be separated from staging (i.e. the extent of fibrosis, structural distortion, development of cirrhosis).[163] In recognition of this, the 'Knodell scoring system' was modified by Ishak and colleagues in 1995 (Tables 8.6 and 8.7).[164]

An alternative approach to the problem of assessing the extent of pathological change, in particular of fibrosis, has been the use of morphometry.[165,166] Additionally, there is currently an active hunt for the 'holy grail' of non-invasive approaches to grading and, particularly, staging. However, none of these non-invasive approaches, using serological assessments or radiological/ultrasonagraphic measurements, have yet reached appropriate levels of sensitivity and specificity to make them clinically reliable.[167] Liver biopsy remains, therefore, a very important diagnostic tool in the management of most patients with chronic basal hepatitis.[168]

Table 8.6	A complex grading system (after Ishak et al.[164])

A. Periportal or periseptal interface hepatitis (piecemeal necrosis)

Absent	0
Mild (focal, few portal areas)	1
Mild/moderate (focal, most portal areas)	2
Moderate (continuous around <50% of tracts or septa)	3
Severe (continuous around >50% of tracts or septa)	4

B. Confluent necrosis

Absent	0
Focal confluent necrosis	1
Zone 3 necrosis in some areas	2
Zone 3 necrosis in most areas	3
Zone 3 necrosis + occasional portal–central (P–C) bridging	4
Zone 3 necrosis + multiple P–C bridging	5
Panacinar or multiacinar necrosis	6

*C. Focal (spotty) lytic necrosis, apoptosis and focal inflammation**

Absent	0
1 focus or less per 10 × objective	1
2 to 4 foci per 10 × objective	2
5 to 10 foci per 10 × objective	3
More than 10 foci per 10 × objective	4

D. Portal inflammation

None	0
Mild, some or all portal areas	1
Moderate, some or all portal areas	2
Moderate/marked, all portal areas	3
Marked, all portal areas	4

* Does not include diffuse sinusoidal infiltration by inflammatory cells
Note: other features such as bile-duct damage should be noted but not scored

Table 8.7	Example of staging system (after Ishak et al.[164])

Architectural changes, fibrosis and cirrhosis

No fibrosis	0
Fibrous expansion of some portal areas, with or without short fibrous septa	1
Fibrous expansion of some portal areas, with or without short fibrous septa	2
Fibrous expansion of most portal areas with occasional portal to portal (P–P) bridging	3
Fibrous expansion of portal areas with marked bridging (portal to portal (P–P) as well as portal to central (P–C))	4
Marked bridging (P–P and/or P–C) with occasional nodules (incomplete cirrhosis)	5
Cirrhosis, probable or definite	6

Intra- and interobserver variation

Histological evaluation of liver biopsies includes a subjective element and is therefore liable to both inter- and intra-observer variation; this must be taken into account when interpreting numbers generated by different pathologists or

Table 8.8	Accuracy and reproducibility of scoring: helpful precautions

Two simultaneous observers if possible
Agreement on criteria before starting study
Only adequate biopsy specimens evaluated
Biopsies from same patient scored within a short period of time
Test of intra- and interobserver variation at end of study

by the same pathologist at different times.[169] Staging appears to be less subject to variation than grading.[170,171] Moreover a simple scoring system proved more reliable than a complex one when intra- and interobserver variation were investigated.[171] Variation was reduced in a study by the METAVIR group when biopsies were evaluated simultaneously by two observers. The precautions listed in Table 8.8 are recommended for the achievement of maximal reliability in scoring.

Handling data from semiquantitative analysis

When semiquantitative scoring data are evaluated, it is important to bear in mind the nature of the generated numbers. The numbers represent categories rather than measurements, and cannot therefore be used as real numbers in statistical analyses.[172,173] Even adding the numbers representing different grading components (e.g. interface hepatitis, confluent necrosis, lobular activity and portal inflammation) together to create a total grading score can lead to inaccuracies, because the scales for these components are linear, and differ from each other. At best, a total grading score serves only to give an approximate idea of the severity of a chronic hepatitis; it usually gives no information on the types of liver damage and inflammation involved. It follows that statistical evaluation must be appropriate for categories rather than measurements, and that correlations should be made with individual grading components rather than with grading totals.

Uses and choice of scoring methods

Simple scoring methods not requiring much time may be used routinely, but like all methods involving subjective assessment of categories they are prone to intra- and inter-observer variation. Scoring should not be undertaken unless pathologist and clinician agree that it is likely to be helpful for patient management. The METAVIR group's algorithm is an example of a simple, carefully evaluated method easily applicable to routine use.[162] In some centres, scores form part of the evaluation of patients for possible antiviral therapy. There is then merit in using the same system for pre- and post-treatment evaluation. In general, the more complex schemes are likely to enable smaller therapeutic effects to be recognized. Whichever system is chosen for a particular purpose, the user should ensure that the features evaluated and the numbers generated are appropriate for the particular purpose. If necessary, an existing system can be modified for an individual project. Features not included in the scoring system, such as bile-duct damage and immuno-histochemical findings, can be separately recorded. In inter-preting the results of any scoring system, it is relevant to note that grading scores greater than zero can sometimes be generated in biopsies from patients without liver disease.[174]

In addition to the role of scoring in routine reporting and in the evaluation of therapies, it plays an important part in clinical research. Among the many examples using a variety of scoring methods are the observations that patients infected with different HCV serotypes show relatively little difference in histological activity,[175] that cirrhosis com-monly develops during long-term follow-up in chronic hepatitis C,[176] and that progression of fibrosis in this disease is related to age at infection, male sex and alcohol intake.[177] Indeed, biopsy-based evaluation of outcomes is central for determining efficacy of antiviral clinical interventions and requires detailed quantitative grading and staging of disease activity.[178]

Individual types of viral hepatitis

There are more histological similarities than differences between the various viral hepatitides (Table 8.1). All share the same basic features of liver-cell damage and inflamma-tion, and the principal histological patterns of acute hepa-titis may all be found in association with any of the viruses, with the possible exception of panlobular necrosis, which is rarely, if ever, due to HCV infection. Likewise, the histo-logical features of chronic hepatitis overlap for hepatitis B and C; thus, it is not currently possible to differentiate reli-ably between the viruses on histological grounds alone. However, there are different, sometimes characteristic, pat-terns associated with some of the agents, and these will now be described. They represent tendencies rather than defini-tive differential diagnostic criteria.

Type A hepatitis

Viral particles of hepatitis A (HAV) were first demonstrated in faeces of infected volunteers by Feinstone and coworkers in the early 1970s.[179] The infective agent is a small, un-enveloped RNA hepatovirus approximately 27 nm in dia-meter. The genome is a linear, single-stranded plus-sense RNA. Viral antigen can be demonstrated in the cytoplasm of Kupffer cells and hepatocytes[180,181] and in situ hybridiza-tion has been used to detect viral RNA.[182] In practice, however, diagnosis rests on demonstration of antibody to the virus in serum rather than on tissue-based methods. Current infection is shown by the presence of the IgM form of the antibody, and past infection by the corresponding IgG antibody.

Spread is by the faecal–oral route, either directly from person to person or by contaminated food or water.[183] Improving hygiene in many countries has led to later and less frequent infection of the population, so that the preva-lence of immunity to the virus is falling. This, together with the commonly greater severity of infection in older subjects, has determined a need for the development of vaccines, some of which are now in use.

The hepatitis is characteristically mild in the young, although protracted or relapsing hepatitis (also known as polyphasic hepatitis)[184] is not uncommon and a very small number of patients develop fulminant, potentially fatal disease[185] that may require liver transplantation. A rare case of recurrent hepatitis A after transplantation for acute liver failure has been reported.[186] At the other end of the spec-trum, asymptomatic attacks are probably very common. Chronic type A hepatitis, if it occurs at all, is extremely rare.[187,188] McDonald and colleagues[188] reported a patient in whom chronic disease developed over a period of 4 years, with persistence of IgM anti-HAV for an unusually long period. Of particular interest is the possibility that HAV might be one of several viruses capable of triggering the onset of autoimmune hepatitis. In a prospective study of healthy relatives of patients with autoimmune hepatitis, three out of 58 developed subclinical HAV infection over a period of 4 years, and two of these developed autoimmune hepatitis shortly thereafter.[189]

Histopathology of hepatitis A

The histological features of HAV infection are those of acute hepatitis in general, but two features are especially common. One is a periportal pattern of inflammation and necrosis (interface hepatitis), with little or no perivenular necro-sis.[190] Plasma cells are prominent, and so the lesion may be mistaken for that of autoimmune hepatitis. The other feature is perivenular cholestasis with little or no associated hepato-cellular necrosis (Fig. 8.23), so-called cholestatic hepatitis, that can be mistaken for obstructive liver disease. The peri-portal hepatitis and cholestasis are sometimes found in the same biopsy, and it is possible that the cholestasis is then the result of interruption of bile drainage by the periportal damage.[20] In other patients there is classic perivenular hepa-titis with hepatocellular ballooning, multinucleation and

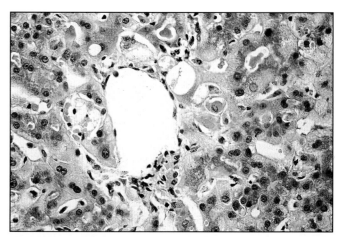

Fig. 8.23 • Type A hepatitis. There is severe cholestasis in the form of bile plugs in dilated canaliculi and bile-laden Kupffer cells. Inflammation and liver-cell loss are relatively slight. H&E.

necrosis.[191,192] In the rare fulminant form of hepatitis A, the histological features are those of panlobular necrosis, with microvesicular fatty change in surviving hepatocytes noted in some cases (Fig. 8.24).[185] Fibrin-ring granulomas have been reported in hepatitis A.[193–195]

Pathogenetic mechanisms of hepatitis A

The mechanism whereby HAV produces liver disease has been the subject of several studies. T-lymphocytes of CD8 type derived from the livers of patients with hepatitis A were shown to exhibit specific anti-HAV activity, and killed skin fibroblasts infected with the virus.[196] Immunocytochemical staining of lymphoid cells in liver biopsy sections of 10 patients showed a predominance of T-memory cells (CD45RO+) with lesser numbers of B-cells.[18] This finding, in addition to the more prominent plasma cell infiltrates in HAV, may support the concept of a mixed cell-mediated and humoral immune response. In peripheral blood, the most striking early change is an increase in the number of natural killer lymphocytes, consistent with the view that non-MHC-restricted cellular cytotoxicity is involved in the control of viral infection.[197] A substantial direct cytopathic effect of the virus on hepatocytes seems unlikely.

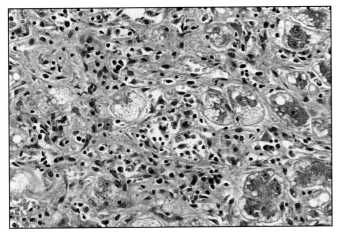

Fig. 8.24 • Fulminant type A hepatitis. Many of the surviving hepatocytes are swollen and finely vacuolated. H&E.

Type B hepatitis

It has been estimated that up to 350 million people are infected by hepatitis B virus (HBV) world-wide. It is particularly prominent in China, Southeast Asia and sub-Saharan Africa, where as many as 15% of the population are infected. These regions and the overall global spread of HBV make it the probable leading cause of chronic liver disease and hepatocellular carcinoma world-wide.[198,199]

HBV is a blood-borne virus, spread primarily through parenteral contact, in adults particularly through intravenous drug use with needle sharing or through blood transfusions, or perinatally from mother to neonate (transplacental spread is rare).[198,199] HBV is also found in other bodily fluids, such as semen and saliva, and is therefore also spread by close personal contact, including sexually.[200] Vertical transmission appears to be common in China and Taiwan. In other countries with endemic HBV, particularly in Africa, horizontal transmission between children in the first few years of life also appears to be a common, if not the predominant mode of spread. Similarly, horizontal spread is also very common amongst institutionalized children. Much of this epidemiology should change in the future as vaccination programmes become more widely implemented.[198,199] Screening for viral protein, where implemented rigorously, has virtually eliminated post-transfusional hepatitis B.[198,201]

Molecular virology

The complete virion, known as the Dane particle, measures 42 nm and consists of a 27-nm core containing circular, incompletely double stranded DNA, surrounded by an envelope of surface material (Fig. 8.25).[202] HBV is a prototype member of the Hepadnaviridae. Based on nucleotide diversity, eight major genotypes (A to H) have been identified which have a distinct global distribution.[203]

The virus was first identified following the discovery of the surface antigen (HBsAg) by Blumberg and colleagues in the serum of an infected patient.[204] It was termed the 'Australian antigen' as this first patient was Australian Aborigine. This antigen and the antibodies directed against

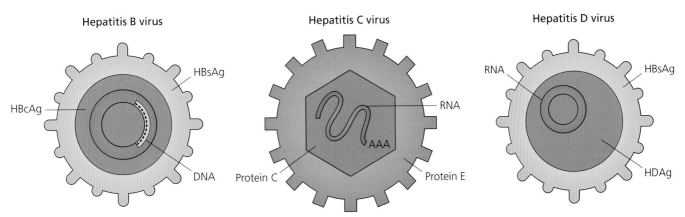

Fig. 8.25 • Schematic structure of hepatitis B, C, and delta viruses, the predominant causes of chronic viral hepatitis. HbsAg = hepatitis B surface antigen; HbcAg = hepatitis B core antigen; HDAg = hepatitis delta antigen.

it remain the most important serological markers for HBV infection. HbsAg appears in the blood as part of the virion, but also as part of incomplete viral forms.

The 3.2-kb genome of HBV has been sequenced and contains four open reading frames coding for the two non-structural antigens Pol and X, for HBsAg (including pre-S1 and pre-S2), and for HBcAg (Fig. 8.26). These latter two reading frames also have multiple initiation sites leading to production of proteins of different length with different biological functions.[203] Two important antigens are located within the core, associated with the viral DNA: core protein (HBcAg) and e antigen (HBeAg). Other important antigens include pre-S1, considered important for attachment of the virus to hepatocyte membranes, pre-S2, X antigen, and the Pol (i.e. polymerase) protein. X antigen, a transactivating protein, interacts with a variety of inhibitors and promoters of cell growth and may be important not only in the development of chronic infection, but in hepatocarcinogenesis. X antigen may be found in tumour cells in the absence of other viral proteins.[203,205]

Viral replication takes place following viral attachment and entry into the hepatocyte; this is mediated by pre-S1 protein on the viral surface. The virus uncoats during this process and the viral DNA travels to the nucleus where it is converted to a covalently closed circular (ccc) viral DNA by modifications to both plus and minus strands of DNA. This cccDNA serves as the template for transcription and formation of viral messenger RNA in a long form and a short form. The long form of viral mRNA serves as the template for minus-strand DNA synthesis and is packaged, in the cytoplasm, with viral DNA polymerase (reverse transcriptase) and a priming protein into a viral capsid composed of HBcAg. Within this core particle, minus-strand DNA is then synthesized, which, in turn, serves a template for synthesis of the shorter plus-strand DNA. The mRNA template is disintegrated during this process. Such a reverse transcriptase mechanism is very rare in DNA viruses, but shares many features with retrovirus replication.[206,207]

The core particles thus formed, containing the double stranded viral DNA, are then assembled into complete virions with HBsAg and cell membrane lipid containing envelope. Apparently, assembly of virions and release from the cell can happen at any point in this replicative process, as HBV particles containing DNA–RNA hybrid molecules can be found in the serum. Some capsids also move back into the nucleus where their newly synthesized viral DNA becomes an additional template for viral mRNA transcription, feeding back into the replicative system. Meanwhile, at some point in the nuclear DNA transcription, integration of segments of viral DNA to the host cell genome takes

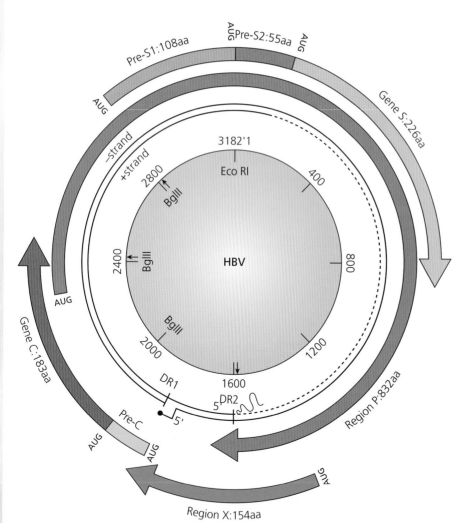

Fig. 8.26 • Structure and genetic organization of the HBV genome. The partially double-stranded DNA genome has four open reading frames: the *pre-S1/pre-S2/S* gene encoding for HBsAg, the *pre-core/core* gene encoding the structural HBcAg and hepatitis B e antigen (HBeAg), the polymerase gene *P* encoding the viral DNA polymerase/reverse transcriptase, and the *X* gene encoding the hepatitis B ¥ protein. In addition, the viral genome contains several cis-acting regulatory elements (promoters, enhancers, and others), as well as regions involved in viral replication, such as the direct repeats *DR1* and *DR2*.

place. This has been seen in both the normal hepatocytes of HBV-infected patients and in hepatocellular carcinoma cells.[206,207]

Clinical course

In the course of acute self-limited infection, a standard pattern of serological changes can be charted (Fig. 8.27). The most commonly followed serological tests include those for HBsAg, anti-HBs (HBsAb), IgM or IgG anti HBc, HBeAg and anti-HBe. In patients with acute hepatitis B, there is almost always an antibody response to HBcAg and usually an antibody response to HBsAg. HbsAg appears in the serum between 4 and 28 weeks after infection (average = 8 weeks). Serum titres of the antigen may disappear before the onset of symptoms, or persist into the symptomatic phase of disease or even somewhat after symptoms have abated. After HBsAg disappears from the serum there is a window of several weeks before HbsAb appears. With the appearance of HBsAb, the patient becomes immune to a new HBV infection; indeed, it is by induction of HBsAb that HBV vaccination is successful. HBsAb may persist for the entire life of the patient, or may decline over years and eventually disappear.[207,208]

Shortly after the appearance of HBsAg in the serum, HBeAg also appears and an IgM anti-HBcAg response becomes detectable. Within a few weeks of the onset of acute self-limited HBV infection, HbeAg disappears and anti-HBe titres develop, which may persist for years. A few months to over a year later, IgG anti-HBc comes to dominate the serological response to the infection. It is this response that becomes the serological hallmark of either prior exposure or ongoing HBV infection.[207–209]

A different pattern of serological test results is found in chronic HBV infection (Fig. 8.28). HBsAg appears in the serum in a similar time course, but does not abate, and HBsAb fails to develop. HBsAg is thus the hallmark of active current HBV, whether acute or chronic. IgM anti-HBc arises and is followed, as in the acute self-limited infection, by IgG anti-HBcAg and HBeAg which persist for years, HBsAg usually lasts for the life of the patient, while HBeAg abates to varying degrees. When serum HBeAg declines and anti-HBe appears, there is often a clinical flare-up of hepatitis activity marked by elevated serum liver enzymes and, in some, acute symptomatology. Anti-HBe then persists for years or the lifetime of the patient. PCR-detectable HBV-DNA can also be found in the serum of chronically infected patients, although in some it may decline to undetectable levels, often at the time of seroconversion to anti-HBe. Following this seroconversion, disease activity (as indicated by serum aminotransferase levels or symptoms) generally declines, although progression to cirrhosis may still occur.[207–209]

Of the patients who are acutely infected by HBV, approximately 65% are asymptomatic. Typical symptoms exhibited by the remaining 35% range from mild flu-like syndromes to nausea, vomiting and jaundice. Less than 1% of individuals develop fulminant failure leading to either death or liver transplantation. Less than 5% of patients acutely infected, whether symptomatic or not, develop chronic infection in which virus is not cleared from the body. Some of these will become so-called healthy carriers who remain infectious, but have no symptoms of liver disease. Others will go on to develop progressive scarring of the liver, eventually leading to cirrhosis; some will also develop hepatocellular carcinoma. While it is tempting to think of healthy carriers as distinct from those with the disease activity of chronic hep-

Fig. 8.27 • Acute HBV infection with recovery: typical serological course.

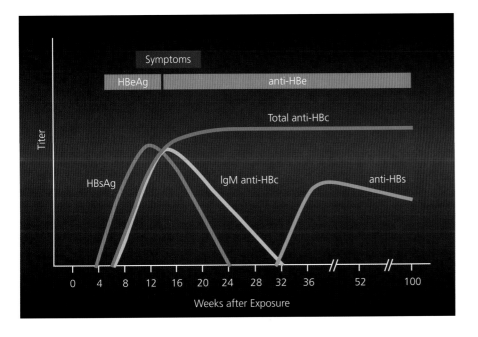

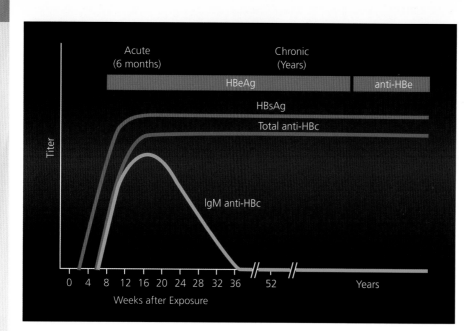

Fig. 8.28 • Chronic HBV infection: typical serological course.

atitis, these two categories are, in fact, relatively labile; patients move from one category to the other, depending on various factors including immune function, coinfections or age. It is estimated that 30% of chronically infected patients will eventually develop cirrhosis at a rate of approximately 2% each year.[209–211]

HBV mutants

Several mutant strains of HBV have been identified. These mutant viruses can result in a variety of atypical serological patterns in acute and chronic infection. Moreover, many of these mutant strains have an impact on clinical outcome, with an increased likelihood of chronicity and increased severity of disease.[203,212] Emergence of such mutants arises both from viral and host factors, but now, increasingly, from exogenous factors such as treatment with nucleoside and nucleotide analogues, hepatitis B immunoglobulin, and vaccination.[203,213] The ease with which these mutants arise is, in some measure, due to the error-prone nature of viral reverse transcriptase, though other mechanisms are also probably involved. This leads to extensive development of quasispecies in infected patients.[213,214]

For example, mutations of the pre-S region have been detected, this region of the genome exhibiting the highest heterogeneity.[215] These result in escape from vaccine-induced viral clearance in already-infected patients as well as an ability to infect despite prior vaccination.[216] Such mutations result in changes in the antigenic properties of HBsAg, thereby decreasing their affinity for neutralizing antibodies. They probably arise via immune pressure generated by vaccination and only rarely seem to arise naturally.

Introduction of antiviral therapies utilizing nucleoside analogues has resulted in the emergence of HBV DNA poly-merase mutants that are resistant to treatment.[203] These probably do not occur naturally, and are only seen in response to prolonged treatment. Interestingly, they also seem to lead to defects in viral replication and, therefore, following cessation of treatment, they appear to be overtaken by wild-type HBV.[217] Moreover, since the DNA polymerase domain overlaps the HBsAg domain in the genome, drug-resistant strains are often also vaccine escape mutants.[203]

Core/precore mutants have been described that generally lead to increased viral replication and disease activity, and respond poorly to interferon therapy. Some of these mutations result in diminished HBeAg and continued anti-HBe in serum despite relatively high levels of replication of the virus.[203,214] X-gene mutants have also been described, many of which also lead to decreased production of HBeAg and greater disease activity.[214]

Histopathology of hepatitis B

Histologically, acute hepatitis B infection appears essentially similar to other forms of acute hepatitis. There are varying numbers of apoptotic bodies scattered through the lobule, perivenular confluent necrosis and, in the most severe cases, bridging necrosis and parenchymal collapse. Similarly, chronic hepatitis B can have all the typical hallmarks of chronic hepatitis from any cause: interface hepatitis, lobular activity and lymphoplasmacytic infiltrates in portal tracts and focally in the lobules. One other major clinicopathological variation of hepatitis B occurring following orthotopic liver transplant and, more rarely, in other settings of immune compromise is called 'fibrosing cholestatic hepatitis' (Fig. 8.29). This variant is rapidly progressive, has a poor prognosis and a distinctive histopathology:

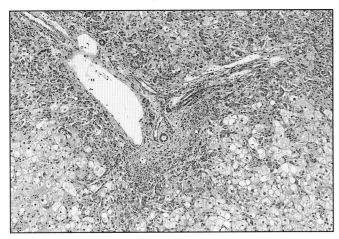

Fig. 8.29 • Fibrosing cholestatic variant of hepatitis B following orthotopic liver transplantation. This severe variant of viral hepatitis is usually seen in the immunocompromised patient. The lesion shows less dense portal mononuclear infiltrates than typically seen in chronic viral hepatitis, but portal areas are more fibrotic and ductular reactions associated with parenchymal cholestasis are prominent. H&E.

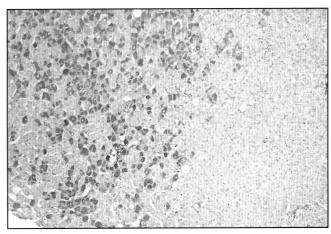

Fig. 8.31 • Histochemical staining of hepatitis B surface antigen with orcein (seen here) or Victoria blue stains can highlight the presence of ground glass hepatocytes in chronic hepatitis B.

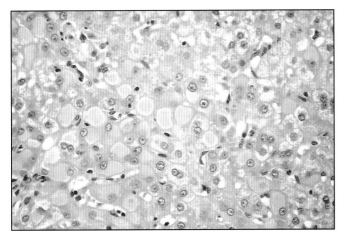

Fig. 8.30 • Ground glass hepatocytes in chronic hepatitis B infection can be identified by the homogeneous pink cytoplasmic inclusions, which can be surrounded by a clear halo. The inclusion pushes the cytoplasmic contents and the nucleus to the sides of the cell. The inclusion represents endoplasmic reticulum filled with hepatitis B surface antigen. H&E.

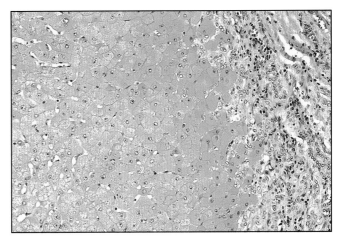

Fig. 8.32 • Oncocytic hepatocytes, seen in a wide range of chronic liver diseases, are seen in this section from a chronic hepatitis C cirrhosis. These cells have abundant mitochondria filling the cytoplasm and, while superficially easy to mistake for ground-glass cells in hepatitis B, they are more eosinophilic and granular, and lack the halo and consistent displacement of cytoplasmic contents to the cell margin. H&E.

fibrous expansion of portal tracts, extensive ductular reaction often with ductular cholestasis, and marked bilirubinostasis in hepatocytes.[218,219]

The most distinctive histological feature that readily distinguishes chronic HBV infection is the so-called ground-glass hepatocyte. These cells have a finely granular cytoplasmic inclusion which consists of proliferated endoplasmic reticulum containing abundant HBsAg that pushes the cell contents, including the nucleus, to the side, usually leaving a visible halo separating the inclusion from the cell membrane (Fig. 8.30). Ground-glass cells can be highlighted by histochemical stains such as Shikata's orcein (Fig. 8.31) and Victoria blue stains as well as by immunohistochemical staining.[220] Such hepatocytes are usually scattered singly and often non-uniformly throughout the liver. In cirrhosis, some nodules may contain abundant ground-glass cells, while other nodules are totally devoid of them. The differ-

ential diagnosis suggested by these cells includes oncocytic hepatocytes (Fig. 8.32), cyanamide toxicity, Lafora disease, and fibrinogen storage disease.[221] Nuclear inclusions may also be seen on routine H & E stained biopsy specimens of chronic hepatitis B. These pale pink, very finely granular inclusions are referred to as 'sanded nuclei' and contain abundant core material (Fig. 8.33).[222] Confirmation can be obtained with immunohistochemical staining for HBcAg.

Detection of HBV in tissue sections

Immunohistochemical staining of various viral antigens is straightforward and widely applied. The patterns of staining in a given specimen can confirm the presence of HBV infection and can also provide information regarding viral replication.

HBcAg. Immunohistochemical staining for core antigen shows a predominant localization in hepatocyte nuclei and, less prominently, in the cytoplasm or associated with the

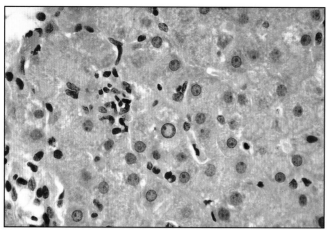

Fig. 8.33 • The hepatocyte in the centre of the field from a hepatitis B infected liver has a pale pink, finely granular intranuclear inclusion. This 'sanded nucleus' is evidence of hepatitis B core antigen accumulating in the nucleus of an infected cell. H&E.

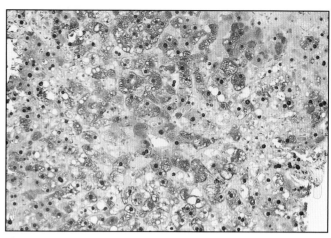

Fig. 8.35 • Diffuse immunohistochemical staining for hepatitis B core antigen of most of the hepatocytes in this biopsy specimen is related to the spread of HBV in an immunocompromised host, in this case a post-liver transplant patient. Immunoperoxidase, DAB.

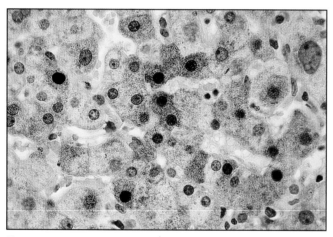

Fig. 8.34 • Immunohistochemical staining for hepatitis B core antigen is prominent in nuclei and slightly less so in the cytoplasm of some hepatocytes, confirming the presence of viral infection and replication. Immunoperoxidase, DAB.

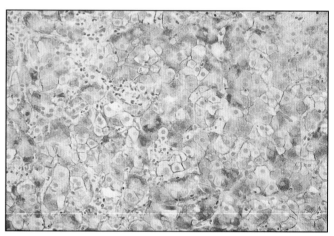

Fig. 8.36 • Extensive membranous immunohistochemical staining for hepatitis B surface antigen is associated with high rates of viral replication. Staining of parallel sections for core antigen will usually show many positive cells as well. Immunohistochemistry, DAB.

cell membrane (Fig. 8.34).[223,224] The presence of nuclear staining correlates well with active viral replication as indicated by HBV DNA, DNA polymerase and HBeAg in the liver and serum.[225,226] On the other hand, cytoplasmic staining for core antigen correlates best with hepatocyte regenerative activity.[227]

Immunostaining for HBcAg is an important clinical adjunct to histochemical assessment of biopsy specimens from HBV-infected patients for particular reasons. First, while absence of staining for core antigen in a biopsy specimen may simply be due to sampling error, as expression can be variable in different parenchymal regions, coinfection with other hepatotropic viruses may suppress HBV replication and, thus, core antigen expression. Therefore, in the absence of core immunostaining, clinical investigation of possible coinfection is important.[228] On the other hand, diffuse staining of nuclei throughout a specimen generally suggests unbridled viral replication in the setting of immune compromise, such as following organ transplantation or in

HIV infection. Likewise, in this setting, the pattern of core antigen detection warrants additional clinical investigation, to rule out perhaps unsuspected causes of immunosuppression (Fig. 8.35).[229]

HBsAg. While immunohistochemical demonstration of HBV surface antigens in the presence of ground-glass cells can readily confirm the diagnosis of chronic HBV, such staining can also give information about the replicative state of the virus. On the one hand, there may be extensive membranous staining for surface antigen, which is usually associated with core antigen staining (Fig. 8.36); such a pattern would indicate a high replicative state for the virus. Alternatively, there may be intracytoplasmic staining for surface antigen, not only in ground-glass cells, but also in many more cells without apparent inclusions. Such staining may range from a faint perinuclear blush to a dense signal throughout the cytoplasm corresponding to the ground-glass cells (Fig. 8.37). This pattern of staining indicates an inability of the hepatocytes to secrete fully-formed viruses

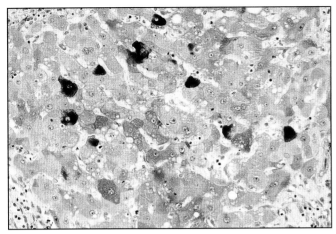

Fig. 8.37 • Immunohistochemical staining for hepatitis B surface antigen can often highlight ground-glass hepatocytes (darkly staining intracytoplasmic inclusions), but also demonstrates surface antigen in hepatocytes without obvious inclusions. Such widespread cytoplasmic staining is usually associated with relatively low viral replication rates and immunostaining for core antigen in parallel sections would demonstrate few positive cells. Immunoperoxidase, DAB.

and, if these cells are numerous, one may expect a relatively low level of viral replication.[230]

HBeAg. Immunohistochemical staining for e antigen in chronic hepatitis B generally follows that for core antigen. When the core antigen is present in the cytoplasm, e antigen colocalizes to the same cells. Similarly, e antigen is generally only seen in cells with nuclear core staining, though staining for core antigen is often more widespread. Staining for e antigen is therefore thought to be an indicator of viral replication, particularly when nuclear.[223]

HBXAg. Immunohistochemical staining demonstrates that X antigen is more widely present in hepatocytes of patients with chronic hepatitis B than either surface or core antigens and may therefore represent a more sensitive immunohistochemical test for HBV infection. This finding also suggests that X antigen, being expressed independently of other viral antigens, indicates integration of this segment of the viral genome into the host genome.[231] Moreover, its presence in hepatocellular carcinoma cells from chronic hepatitis B patients, in the absence of the other HBV antigens, also supports the concept that it is involved in hepatocarcinogenesis.[232]

Pathogenetic mechanisms of hepatitis B

It would appear that in most hepatitis B infections the virus is not directly cytopathic; rather, damage to liver tissue results from immunological attempts to eradicate the virus. For example, the relatively common 'healthy carrier state' in humans, in which the immune system is essentially minimally reactive or non-reactive to HBV antigens, demonstrates that the virus itself may cause little, if any, damage.[233] Furthermore, with the interesting exception of fibrosing cholestatic hepatitis in immunocompromised patients, HBV-related liver disease demonstrates active inflammation within tissue specimens. In fact, with the possible exception

of the POL protein, viral antigens produced in HBV transgenic mice show little evidence of T-lymphocyte-mediated, directly cytotoxic liver disease.[234–236] Indeed, suppression of viral replication in these models appears to be through induction of interferons which lead to suppression of activity through non-cytotoxic pathways.[235]

Multiple arms of the immune system are involved in acute, self-limited HBV infection.[237–239] Simultaneously with the rise of serum liver enzymes following an incubation period of several weeks, antiviral antibodies appear, beginning with IgM anti-HBc. The acute phase of the illness comes with the subsequent production of anti-HBs, a neutralizing antibody. Production of this antibody through vaccination can successfully induce viral clearance in children who are infected perinatally.[240] In addition to the antibody response, there is a type-1 helper T-lymphocyte response against HBc, HBe and HBs, which helps to activate CTL and B-cell responses through cytokine release and, to a seeming much lesser extent, a direct cytotoxic effect.[203,239,241] Supporting this concept, it has been demonstrated that transgenic mice expressing HBV antigens or actively replicating virus develop necroinflammatory lesions only after adoptive transfer of HBsAg-specific CTL lines and clones.[242] On the other hand, the CTL response, although thought to be the most significant for viral clearance in these acute infections, may not actually be the central player, as it has been demonstrated experimentally that viral clearance occurs before full T-cell infiltration of the liver, and so presumably occurs via cytokine activity.[243] Even in individuals who recover from the acute infection and fail to develop chronic hepatitis B, there is long-term persistence of HBV-specific CTLs displaying recent activation markers, suggesting that an exceedingly low-level infection persists, with new virions restimulating the CTL response over time.[239,244]

In a minority of patients, this combined immune attack fails to terminate clinically apparent infection and the infected individual goes on to chronic disease. Age at acquisition of infection influences the likelihood of this event, with earlier (particularly perinatal) infection more likely to result in chronicity.[198,209] Men are also at greater risk for chronic disease, although the reasons are uncertain, as are immunocompromised individuals.[245,246]

In contrast to individuals who clear the infection in the acute phase, individuals progressing to chronic hepatitis B seem to have diminished CD4+ and CD8+ cellular responses in the peripheral blood.[203,239,247] Weak CTL responses due to immune tolerance to the virus are likely to be responsible for viral persistence in neonatal hepatitis B transmission, the most common setting of chronic HBV infection. The mechanism for the development of such tolerance in adults, however, is not well understood.[203,247] Infection of privileged sites, selective immune suppression and down-regulation of viral gene expression, are all proposed mechanisms. A very large viral load that overwhelms the T-cell response might be responsible and induction of peripheral tolerance might also contribute. Viral mutants that escape surveillance by the immune system are also likely contributors to the development of tolerance.[203,214]

Type C hepatitis

The hepatitis C virus (HCV) was first identified in 1989 by molecular cloning and was found to be the agent responsible for a majority of sporadic and post-transfusion hepatitides, previously referred to as non-A non-B hepatitis. Since its identification, it has become evident that HCV is a globally widespread infectious agent which has been present for more than five decades. It has been calculated that there are more than 170 million chronic carriers world-wide, that is approximately 3% of the world's population. With its high rates of chronic infection, progression to cirrhosis and end-stage liver disease, and development of hepatocellular carcinoma, it represents a formidable public health challenge world-wide.[248,249]

Molecular virology

HCV is a small (30–38 nm) single-stranded RNA virus with a lipoid envelope (Fig. 8.25). It is classified as a subgenus of the Flaviviridae family. Consisting of a large open reading frame, the genome contains approximately 9400 nucleotides (Fig. 8.38).[249] At the 5' end is a highly conserved region with significant homology between different subtypes of HCV that is thus useful for amplification in polymerase chain reaction assays. The polyprotein produced from translation of this open reading frame yields 10 mature proteins which have been identified as: core (C) and envelope glycoproteins (E1, E2/NS1), p7 (possibly an ion channel), non-structural regions involved in viral replication (NS2, 3, 4A, 4B, 5A, 5B) that code for proteases, a helicase, membrane anchoring proteins and an RNA-dependent RNA polymerase.[248] In plasma, HCV virus particles appear to be associated with lipoproteins; lipoprotein receptors on hepatocytes may facilitate infection of cells.[250]

Variations in genomic sequences in viral isolates from around the world have allowed for phylogenetic classification of six viral genotypes which, in turn, contain many subtypes.[251] There are clear differences in genotype prevalences in different geographic regions (Fig. 8.39), as well as differences between genotypes and their subtypes in terms of treatment responses, but confirmation of any association between different genotypes and severity or progression of disease is still lacking. Whether this is due to cohort study design or a true lack of difference remains unclear.[251,252]

Epidemiology and clinical course

Parenteral spread is the most efficient means of viral transmission, which results in the high prevalence rates in intra-venous drug users. Also, prior to identification of the virus and the resultant screening of donated blood products patients receiving such therapies (such as persons with haemophilia), were at high risk of infection. Other percutaneous modes of transmission are suspected including needle-stick injuries in health-care workers, tattoos, piercings, scarification, and intranasal cocaine use.[253] Though sexual promiscuity is associated with increased risk of HCV infection, sexual activity is an inefficient means of disease transmission in monogamous couples. Sexual transmission probably occurs only rarely, but is significantly increased in the setting of concomitant immunosuppresion.[253–256] Household contact transmission and maternal–infant transmission is also rare. Finally, poor socioeconomic status is a risk factor for HCV infection.[257] Altogether, in many surveys, approximately 60% of hepatitis C infections can be accounted for by these various modes of transmission, but in approximately 40% of cases the means of infection are uncertain and such cases are often referred to as 'sporadic' or 'community acquired'.[253]

However HCV is acquired, its acute phase is usually asymptomatic and is therefore rarely diagnosed. Additionally, with virus identification and awareness of the dangers of parenteral exposure highlighted by the HIV epidemic, there has been a dramatic decline in the number of new infections of HCV, particularly in the United States and Europe. Rare cases of fulminant hepatitis due to HCV have been documented. Elevation of aminotransferases is usually seen from 2 to 4 weeks after infection. The first viral marker found in the serum is HCV RNA between 1 and 3 weeks. Antibodies to specific viral proteins are seen from 2 weeks to 6 months after infection.[258]

As many as 90% of acutely infected individuals go on to some degree of chronic infection, most of whom have some degree of liver damage.[259,260] As with acute hepatitis C infection, chronic hepatitis C is commonly asymptomatic or only mildly symptomatic for most of the course of the disease. When symptoms do occur, they are usually non-specific, such as fatigue, and do not specifically suggest viral hepatitis. Thus, diagnosis is often made when patients are incidentally discovered to have elevated serum liver enzymes on routine testing with serological follow-up studies revealing anti-HCV antibodies or HCV RNA. Of those individuals who are chronically infected, approximately one-quarter will go on to develop cirrhosis with liver-related mortality ranging from 1 to 11.7% in various studies.[248,261] Risk factors for progression of chronic hepatitis C include male gender, 40 years of age or older at the time of infection, an alcohol intake of greater than 50 g per day, and increased activity or fibrosis identified in the biopsy specimen.[253,254] The inci-

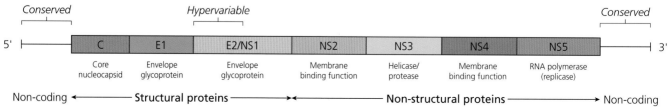

Fig. 8.38 • Structure of the hepatitis C viral genome and encoded proteins.

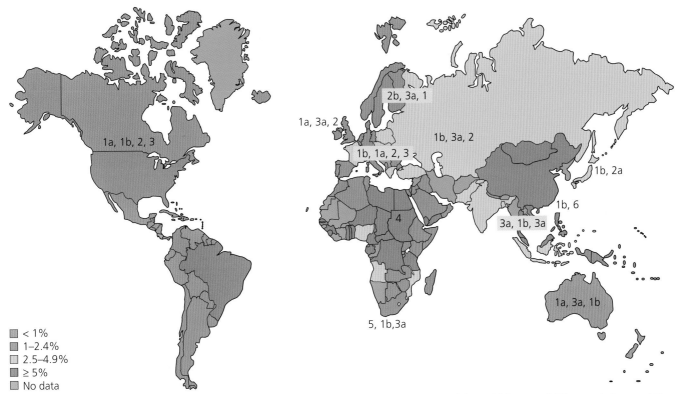

Fig. 8.39 • The hepatitis C prevalences and distribution of predominant hepatitis C virus genotypes around the world. Because of differences in the population groups studied, in methods of data collection and in interpretation between countries, and because data from several countries are limited, the prevalence shown does not necessarily represent the true prevalence in the country.

dence of hepatocellular carcinoma is also dramatically increased in chronic hepatitis C, probably taking 20 to 40 years to develop and usually (though not invariably) doing so in the presence of cirrhosis as a related development.[261,262]

Histopathology of hepatitis C

The histopathology of acute hepatitis C is similar to that of acute hepatitis related to other viral or toxic agents, namely scattered acidophil bodies, predominantly near the central vein and a variable, though mild to moderate, lymphoplasmacytic infiltrate in portal tracts and in the lobule (Fig. 8.40). As will be seen for chronic HCV infection, steatosis and bile-duct damage may also be found.[263] In more severe injury, confluent necrosis around terminal hepatic venules may be seen. Very rarely, bridging necrosis or parenchymal collapse, associated with clinically severe hepatitis, may also be seen.[264] Furthermore, in a similar fashion to recurrent hepatitis B arising following orthotopic liver transplant, there is a progressive variant of recurrent HCV infection referred to as fibrosing cholestatic hepatitis (or severe cholestatic hepatitis) (Fig. 8.41).[265,266]

The histopathology of chronic infection is variably active and progressive, with all the features of any chronic viral hepatitis as described above. The severity of changes in the biopsy does not correlate well with symptoms or with the serum liver enzymes at the time of biopsy and therefore the biopsy may provide information independent of serum tests. In fact, asymptomatic patients, even those without

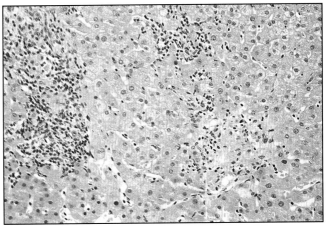

Fig. 8.40 • Acute type C hepatitis. A portal tract (left) and sinusoids are infiltrated by lymphocytes. Liver-cell damage is slight in this example. The hepatitis followed a needle-stick injury. H&E.

serum aminotransferase elevations, may have significantly abnormal histology.[267,268]

While not specific, some histological features may be considered characteristic of HCV infection, when seen in the otherwise typical chronic hepatitis biopsy. These changes include prominent lymphoid aggregates or even fully developed lymphoid follicles with germinal centres (Fig. 8.42), prominent bile-duct damage (Fig. 8.43), and steatosis (Fig. 8.44).[269–271] The lymphoid aggregates, with or without germinal centres, are not restricted to chronic hepatitis C, as they may also be seen in autoimmune hepatitis and chronic

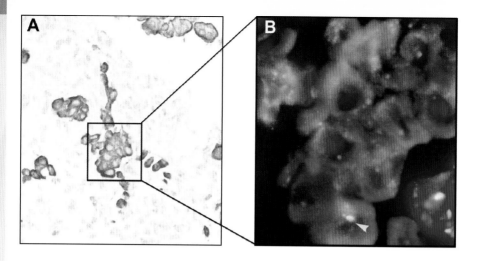

Fig. 8.41 • **(A)** A region of the ductular reaction in aggressive/fibrosing cholestatic recurrent hepatitis C, highlighted by immunohistochemical staining for cytokeratins. Immunoperoxidase, DAB. **(B)** Fluorescence in situ hybridization for X and Y chromosomes shows X chromosomes (red) in many cholangiocyte nuclei but the cholangiocyte at the bottom (yellow arrow) also contains a Y chromosome (turquoise), indicating origin from the male recipient rather than from the female donor, and indicating derivation from an extrahepatic source of hepatic progenitor cells, probably from the donor's bone marrow. Y-positive nuclei in the lower right belong to inflammatory cells. DAB, FITC, rhodamine, DAPI counterstain.

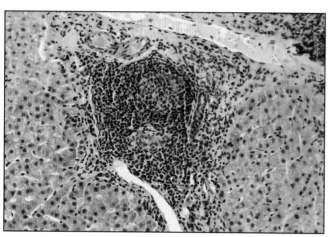

Fig. 8.42 • Portal lymphoid follicle in chronic hepatitis C. While not pathognomonic for hepatitis C (they may occasionally be seen in hepatitis B or autoimmune hepatitis), they are most frequently seen with HCV and should suggest this aetiology if it is not clinically suspected. Complete follicles are not always seen; instead, only lymphoid aggregates may be identified, but these also are highly suggestive of HCV infection. Also note the reactive ductal changes (present below the follicle). H&E.

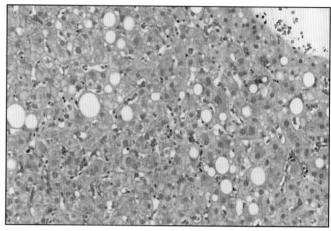

Fig. 8.44 • Steatosis in chronic hepatitis C. Mild, small and large droplet fat within hepatocytes is often seen in HCV infection, in a patchy distribution in biopsy specimens. Diffuse steatosis is more suggestive of fatty liver disease of other causes. The presence of steatohepatitis or steatofibrosis would favour other aetiologies rather than HCV infection as the primary cause of the steatosis. H&E.

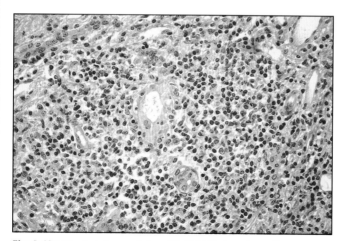

Fig. 8.43 • Bile-duct damage in hepatitis C. A bile duct shows disruption, intraepithelial mononuclear cells, and regenerative changes. Such bile-duct damage is commonly seen in chronic hepatitis C infection. H&E. Courtesy of Dr S N Thung.

hepatitis B.[269,271] However, they are far more common with HCV infection and their identification should raise the possibility of HCV infection. When present, they contain activated B-cells, surrounded by follicular dendritic cells and a B-cell mantle zone, and are surrounded by an outer T-cell zone suggesting that they are fully functioning lymphoid follicles.[272] The lymphocytic infiltration of the liver is otherwise similar to that seen with other causes of chronic hepatitis, though a striking bead-like appearance of intrasinusoidal lymphocytes reminiscent of infectious mononucleosis can sometimes be seen.[273]

The fatty change seen in hepatitis C is usually a mixed micro- and macrovesicular steatosis of mild to moderate degree. Such steatosis may relate to increased body mass index (particularly in genotype 1) and insulin resistance,[274] though direct viral effects also seem to be involved (genotype 3).[275] More severe degrees of steatosis, particularly if associated with Mallory bodies, neutrophilic infiltration and other histological features of fatty liver disease, suggest concomitant injury by any of the aetiologies of such disease, including alcohol, obesity, diabetes mellitus, and hyperlipidaemia syndromes.[277] Interestingly, steatosis is less common in patients coinfected with HIV than those with HCV alone.[276]

The bile-duct injury seen in hepatitis C may be relatively mild with focal reactive changes in epithelium, with vacuolation, stratification and crowding. More severe injury, however, with pyknosis of cholangiocytes and lymphocytic infiltration is frequently identified. Bile-duct loss may also occur. Confusion with early stages of primary biliary cirrhosis must therefore be guarded against, though clinical information should establish the diagnosis.[269,270] HCV has been detected in bile-duct epithelium.[278]

Hepatic iron stores are frequently increased in chronic hepatitis C. Reticuloendothelial iron deposition is likely to be secondary to necroinflammatory activity and is associated with a poorer response to interferon treatment.[279,280] When hepatocytic iron is also seen, particularly in advance of cirrhosis, it may be associated with concomitant genetic haemochromatosis, porphyria cutanea tarda, increased oral uptake, previous treatment with Ribavirin for the HCV infection, and alcohol use.[281,282] In cirrhosis, parenchymal iron is often related to the cirrhosis itself.[283]

Detection of HCV in tissue sections

Clinically useful and reliable methods for detection of virus in tissue sections have been hampered by the paucity of viral particles and proteins in infected tissue.[284,285] In situ hybridization for viral RNA[286] and in situ RT-PCR[287] are of variable specificity and sensitivity depending on the probes being used. Immunohistochemical staining has been successfully performed, but still remains a research tool rather than demonstrating utility for diagnostic or prognostic purposes.[288,289]

Pathogenetic mechanisms of hepatitis C

Information regarding pathogenetic mechanisms of acute hepatitis C infection is limited. Though antibodies to a range of HCV antigens are produced in acute infection, a significant role for humoral immunity in the injury in acute infection has not been demonstrated. There is a strong CD4+ proliferation and cytokine response to the HCV NS3 protein that correlates with viral clearance in the acute phase of disease. CD8+CTL responses may also be important and, as has been shown in chimpanzees, chronic infection follows an undetectable or minimal CTL response, whereas early, durable, multispecific CTL responses result in viral clearance.[258]

It is not known if the virus is directly cytotoxic in the acute phase. Studies of such direct cytotoxicity have been made difficult by the absence of a high-titre in vitro tissue culture system. The fibrosing cholestatic variant of recurrent hepatitis C may, however, be a clinical example of such direct cytotoxicity. Given the relative paucity of lymphocytes in tissue sections from such specimens and the depressed cell-mediated immunity post-transplant, it has been suggested that the severe damage is primarily virus-mediated.[290]

On the other hand, cytopathic viruses rarely lead to persistent viral infections, chronic infection is marked by lymphocytic infiltration, and there are individuals with persistent viraemia in the absence of elevated serum liver enzymes or tissue damage. Thus, it seems that the damage in chronic infection is primarily immune-mediated. Furthermore, transgenic mice expressing structural proteins of HCV have been studied and in none of these is there any evidence of liver cell injury.[291] It may be possible, however, that viral proteins enhance the reactivity of hepatocytes to inflammatory cytokines. For example, in vitro studies show that HCV core protein increases sensitivity to Fas-ligand binding without increasing Fas expression on the cell surface.[292] Further insights into HCV–host interactions are likely to lead from the recent development of a robust in vitro system[293,294] and an in vivo animal model harbouring a functional liver cell xenograft utilizing uPA-SCID mouse chimeras.[295]

Once chronic infection is established, HCV-specific CD4+ responses compartmentalize within the liver. HCV-specific CTL responses have been identified in the livers of patients with chronic hepatitis C as well as in peripheral blood mononuclear cells in the same population.[237,256] Circumstantial evidence that cellular immune responses actually limit viral replication includes the increased viral titres seen in individuals with depressed cellular immunity, such as following liver transplantation or those with HIV infection, and the flare-up of viral activity in non-A, non-B hepatitis patients following treatment with steroids and their subsequent withdrawal, with significantly grater subsequent progression.[237,249,256] Experimentally, there is also evidence that CTL should be able to recognize and kill infected cells.[248] Hepatitis C, however, is obviously capable of escaping from immune-mediated inhibition of replication, which may relate to the ease with which this RNA virus produces an ever-changing array of quasispecies during infection, with compartmentalization of these quasispecies in different regions of the liver.[296] A direct suppressive effect on intrahepatic dendritic cell function may play a role in the tolerogenic mechanisms.[297] Of course, while these cell-mediated mechanisms may serve to limit ideas to some extent, they are also responsible for the damage seen in chronic hepatitis C. The number of CD8+ cells correlates with aminotransferase levels, suggesting a prominent role of T-cell mediated damage in the disease.[260,298] Increased Fas antigen expression in HCV-infected livers, particularly on hepatocytes adjacent to infiltrating lymphocytes, further supports this mechanism of injury.[299]

Extrahepatic manifestations of HCV infection

A number of extrahepatic complications have been associated with hepatitis C infection, including mixed cryoglobulinaemia, glomerulonephritis, porphyria cutanea tarda, polyarteritis nodosa, Sjögren's syndrome and lichen planus.[300,301] While the pathogenetic mechanisms of the manifestations are not clear, it has also been observed that various autoantibodies are commonly detected in patients with hepatitis C, including anti-LKM, anti-smooth muscle, antithyroid, and anti-GOR antibodies. These findings suggest a B-cell response to HCV, which could contribute to the autoimmune effects associated with the disease.[301] In particular, more than half of HCV-infected individuals have a marked expansion of CD5+ B lymphocytes peripherally. Activation of this B-cell subset has been linked to auto-immune diseases.[302] Selective clonal B-cell activation may also be related to the development of B-cell lymphomas in patients with hepatitis C.[303]

Hepatitis C and alcoholic liver injury

It is well recognized that, in many populations, alcoholic liver disease and chronic hepatitis C often coexist. Alcoholics with alcohol-related liver disease are at significantly increased risk for developing chronic HCV infection, while those without alcohol-related liver disease are not. In fact, several studies report an increase in the frequency of HCV markers as the histological severity of alcoholic liver disease increases. These findings suggest that HCV infection enhances the injury induced by alcohol or, conversely, that alcoholic liver disease increases the risk of HCV infection or progression of HCV infection to chronicity.[304–306]

From the diagnostic point of view, if biopsy specimens taken for documentation of alcoholic liver disease contain features more typical of chronic hepatitis, a significant proportion will be hepatitis C positive.[307] When histological features of both diseases are identified, the speed of progression is greater. Survival for individuals with both diseases is significantly lower than for those with only one disease or the other.[308] The precise mechanisms for these effects are not known, but are hypothesized to include: enhancement of immune-mediated antiviral damage to alcohol-altered hepatocyte membranes; alcohol inhibition of liver regeneration; enhancement by alcohol of viral replication; and concomitant immune suppression.[304,306]

As noted above, mild to moderate steatosis is often identified in association with hepatitis C and, by itself, neither suggests nor excludes the possibility of concomitant alcoholic liver disease. However, more severe fatty change, involving entire lobules, should raise the possibility of concomitant alcoholic liver injury, particularly if associated with steatohepatitis (in the form of ballooning degeneration of hepatocytes or neutrophilic infiltration) or perivenular/pericellular fibrosis. In fact, scarring with this distribution in the absence of fatty change may suggest alcohol injury in the past and should be noted as such in chronic hepatitis C biopsy specimens.[275,309]

Type D (delta) hepatitis

Hepatitis D virus (HDV) was first discovered by Rizzetto and colleagues as a nuclear antigen in the hepatocytes of HBV-infected patients.[310] HDV was originally thought to be an antigenic variant of HBV, and referred to as the delta antigen. It was subsequently recognized as a separate infectious viral agent, but a highly unusual one in that is defective in terms of replicative ability and requires coinfection with HBV for propagation.[311–313] It shares some functional and structural similarities with infectious agents in plants, but seems to be the only viral agent of its type in animals. Despite these similarities, however, it shares no sequence homologies with these plant viruses and occupies its own separate genus and family, *Deltaviridae*.[314]

HDV has three components, two of which are provided by HDV itself, and one of which comes from HBV. The 36-nm particle contains a negative-stranded RNA genome, two forms of the delta antigen (HDAg), and an envelope consisting of hepatitis B surface antigen (HBsAg) (Fig. 8.25). The genome is a 1.7-kb single-stranded circular RNA. Because of intramolecular base-pairing it is capable of collapsing into an unbranched rod with 70% of the nucleotides being paired. The genome replicates via a double rolling circle with transcription by a host RNA polymerase II, a DNA-dependent enzyme. Both the genome and its transcript contain autocatalytic sites, ribozymes that process the linear transcripts into circular structures. Because these ribozyme activities are unique to the virus they make good potential targets for antiviral therapies.[311–313,315–317]

The delta antigen is produced from the antisense mRNA transcript and has multiple biological roles. In the viral particle, HDAg is bound with HDV RNA into a spherical 18-nm nucleocapsid structure. The protein exists in two species, large and small, the larger having a 19 amino acid extension. Despite the identity of the proteins beside that extension, the two forms have different conformations yielding different functions. The small HDAg is required for RNA replication and thus predominates in the early replicative cycle. Only large HDAg is present in the virion, bound to the viral RNA, and it therefore predominates later in the cycle. How and where large HDAg, localized to the nucleus, interacts with the cytoplasmically localized HBsAg remains unclear.[318]

Spread of HDV follows that of HBV, primarily through parenteral exposure, although sexual transmission also occurs. It can either be acquired at the same time as a primary HBV infection or later, superimposed on a pre-existent chronic hepatitis B.[311] HDV is rare in the USA and other countries with a relatively low HBV incidence and is most often found amongst intravenous drug abusers. In regions where HBV is moderately endemic, as in southern Europe and the Middle East, 15 to 50% of individuals with chronic hepatitis B also had HDV infection in the late 1980s; however, this has diminished dramatically to where predictions of its disappearance are now made.[319] In areas where the incidence of HBV infections is relatively high, the incidence of HDV coinfections varies widely and is likely to change as advances in vaccination for hepatitis B proceed.[312]

The clinical course of hepatitis D depends somewhat on whether HDV is acquired as a coinfection simultaneously with HBV or as a superinfection in a person who already has chronic hepatitis B.[320] In coinfection, HDV viraemia typically appears after HBsAg has appeared in the serum, reflecting the dependence of HDV propagation on HBsAg production. In most cases the acute infection is self-limiting and the individual will clear HDV with the clearance of its obligatory companion, HBV. The antibody response to HDV, usually IgM to HDAg, is often weak and transitory in the case of acute self-limited infection.[321] The humoral response is neither protective nor involved in clearance since HDAg is only present internally within the virus.[318] Though the majority of individuals with coinfection have acute self-limited infection, there is an increased risk of fulminant hepatic failure (up to 20%).[320] Progression of the coinfection to chronicity remains infrequent.[320]

With superinfected HDV, several different outcomes are possible. Though some of these superinfections will be asymptomatic, an exacerbation of hepatitis occurs in this setting more often than with simultaneous primary infections. Furthermore, those patients who have symptomatic or fulminant HDV superinfections will go on to also develop chronic hepatitis D.[322] These patients will have HDV viraemia and an antibody response to HDAg of both IgM and IgG classes.[322] If the prior HBV infection was unsuspected, the patient may appear to have an acute HBV infection rather than a superimposed acute hepatitis D.[323] Similarly, a patient with known chronic hepatitis B might be thought to have an acute exacerbation of that disease, rather than a new HDV infection; a full panel of HBV and HDV serology should clarify the situation. Chronic HDV infection does not necessarily follow from superinfection on chronic hepatitis B though most patients will not resolve the acute HDV infection and clear the virus.[322]

Histopathology of hepatitis D

Histologically, acute and chronic hepatitis D infections look like any other acute or chronic hepatitis, with the same range of necroinflammatory lesions and patterns of scarring. Activity in chronic hepatitis D is usually fairly high with widespread interface and lobular hepatitis. The single distinguishing feature is the sanded nucleus, similar to that seen occasionally in hepatitis B (Fig. 8.33). In hepatitis D this feature is due to HDAg accumulating in the nucleus of infected cells.[324]

Detection of hepatitis D in tissue sections

Immunohistochemistry for HDAg demonstrates intense nuclear staining in infected hepatocytes; cytoplasmic staining is weak or absent (Fig. 8.45).[311] The more time that has passed from the time of the acute HDV infection, the less likely is it that stainable antigen will be found, probably reflecting diminished replication over time. Sampling error may be significant then, and a negative biopsy specimen should not be considered definitive in ruling out chronic hepatitis D. In situ hybridization for HDV RNA has also been described and may be more sensitive than immunohistochemical staining for HDAg.[311]

Pathogenetic mechanisms of hepatitis D

Whether or not HDV is directly cytopathic remains unclear, though differences in outcome may relate to issues of antigen/viral load or viral subtype. Against direct cytotoxicity are the findings that transgenic mice expressing HDAg

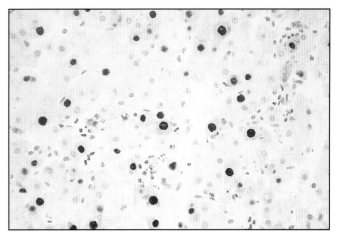

Fig. 8.45 • Hepatitis D virus (delta virus) infection. Positive staining is seen in many hepatocyte nuclei and there is weak cytoplasmic positivity. Polyclonal anti-HDV antibody; immunoperoxidase. Courtesy of Dr S N Thung.

do not display liver damage,[325,326] neither do mice infected with the virus, despite the ability to maintain viral replication.[327] Furthermore, there have been many studies of stable infection of cultured cell lines without evident cell injury.[318] On the other hand, the expression of a small amount of HDAg, inducibly driven by a metallothionein promoter, led to cell death.[328] Another possible mechanism of cytotoxicity might relate to the virus utilizing host RNA polymerase II, thereby competing with host gene transcription and viral replication are inhibited.[318] Clinically, there is also a description of microvesicular steatosis, suggesting mitochondrial injury, in epidemics of severe hepatitis D in regions of South America, although this may specifically relate to a particular subtype of the virus.[329]

As in hepatitis B and C, the immune response is probably important in causing hepatocellular injury, though the details of immunopathogenesis are poorly understood. It is known that disease activity in acute hepatitis D is associated temporally with increased immune response and diminished HDV replication.[318] However, separating this from the immune response triggered against HBV directly is clearly difficult.

Type E hepatitis

Hepatitis E virus (HEV), formerly classified as one of the forms of non-A, non-B hepatitis viruses,[330] is an unenveloped, single-stranded RNA virus. Viral particles measure approximately 27 to 34 nm in diameter, and have spiky outlines. These can be found in faeces of infected patients and have also been demonstrated within bile ductules and hepatic sinusoidal cells of a patient with fatal cholestatic hepatitis E,[331] as well as in the hepatocytes in infected monkeys. The virus can be transmitted to a number of primates,[332–334] and the viral genome has been cloned after isolation from gallbladder bile of infected cynomolgus monkeys.[335] In these animals, close contact between lymphocytes and damaged hepatocytes suggests that immunological mechanisms are involved in the pathogenesis of the disease.[336] The serological finding of IgM and IgG antibody to HEV is generally the means of identifying currently and previously infected patients. Detection of the HEV RNA and genotypes of the virus can be made by RT-PCR techniques.[337] A fluorescent antibody assay that can identify HEV proteins in liver tissue has also been used.[338]

The virus can cause a spectrum of disease from mild hepatitis to fulminant disease. The hepatitis resembles that of hepatitis A in that it is spread by the faecal–oral route and can have a cholestatic pattern.[339] However, unlike hepatitis A, there is little infection from secondary contacts (through family members or other close contacts); rather, most patients become infected through the primary source.[340] It is common in Asia, where the virus gives rise to water-borne epidemics[341] as well as to sporadic disease. The infection has also been identified in Africa and Latin America,[342] and occasional cases are reported in industrialized nations following travel to endemic areas[343,344] or exposure to contaminated sewage.[345] Infection can be more severe in pregnancy,[346] and with the combination of hepatitis A and E in young children.[340] In addition, some have reported a rare association of past exposure to hepatitis E and the occurrence of autoimmune hepatitis[347] or primary biliary cirrhosis,[348,349] suggesting a possible role in the development of autoimmune liver disease, again similar to that seen in hepatitis A.

Histopathology of hepatitis E

Compared to the other viral types of hepatitis, there is less information on detailed histological appearances in hepatitis E. However, the injury has been reported to include classical as well as cholestatic types of acute viral hepatitis.[339,350] The classic types showed the focal hepatocyte necrosis including frequent acidophil bodies, swollen (or ballooned) hepatocytes, and lymphocytic parenchymal and portal infiltrates (Fig. 8.46A, B). Cholestatic forms have features of canalicular cholestasis and gland-like transformation of hepatocytes, while degenerative hepatocytic changes and necrosis were less prominent than in the classical types. Neutrophils were also found in larger numbers in the lobules and portal tracts, although the lymphocyte was still the predominant inflammatory cell type present. These histological features of cholestatic hepatitis E have been noted to be similar to those of hepatitis A.[351] In the fatal case cited above,[331] extensive necrosis and collapse of the parenchyma was present. Surviving hepatocytes were swollen and foamy, and sometimes formed gland-like structures around bile-filled canaliculi. Other features included bile ductular proliferation and phlebitis involving both portal and hepatic venules and Kupffer-cell hyperplasia. Portal inflammation was mild. A lymphocytic destructive cholangitis has been reported in one case of acute hepatitis E.[352]

Other forms of viral hepatitis

Various other viruses have been implicated in acute or chronic hepatitis in the recent past. Some have been described as hepatitis F,[353,354] but none of these have been

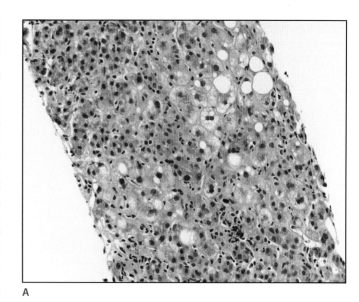

A

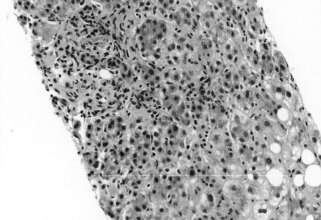

B

Fig. 8.46 • Hepatitis E infection. Acute hepatitis with mild portal inflammation and reactive bile ductular changes. **(A)** There are changes of acute hepatitis including some focal hepatocyte swelling, regenerative hepatocellular changes, acinar formation, cholestasis, and mononuclear infiltrates. Minimal fat is also present. **(B)** The portal infiltrate is predominantly mononuclear, composed of lymphocytes, but some neutrophils are present as well, especially in the vicinity of the reactive ductular structures. H&E.

accepted by the virological and hepatological communities as valid hepatotropic agents. The GBV-C virus,[356,357] designated as hepatitis G by some, was also considered a potential additional cause of viral hepatitis, but most now consider this a passenger virus with minimal contribution to liver damage. Of some interest, however, is the possibility that this agent may inhibit HIV replication leading to a better course in patients coinfected compared to those with HIV alone, although this remains controversial.[358] More recently, the TT[359,360] and the SEN viruses,[361] were also investigated as potential causes of viral hepatitis, including possible modulatory effects on HBV[346] and HCV[362] infection, but as with GBV-C, the significance of these viruses in the aetiology of acute or chronic liver disease remains unproven at this time.

References

1. Regev A, Schiff ER. Viral hepatitis A, B, and C. Clin Liver Dis, 2000; 4:47–63
2. Sass DA, Shakil AO. Fulminant hepatic failure. Gastroenterol Clin, 2003; 4:1195–1211
3. Sakurai T, Marusawa H, Santomura S, et al. Lens culinaris agglutinin-A reactive alpha-fetoprotein as a marker for liver atrophy in fulminant hepatic failure. Hepatol Res, 2003; 26:98–105
4. Gazzard BG, Henderson JM, Williams R. Factor VII levels as a guide to prognosis in fulminant hepatic failure. Gut, 1976; 17:489–491
5. Valla D, Flejou JF, Lebrec D, et al. Portal hypertension and ascites in acute hepatitis: clinical, hemodynamic and histological correlations. Hepatology, 1989; 10:482–487
6. Lauff, JJ, Kasper ME, Wu TW, Ambrose RT. Isolation and preliminary characterization of a fraction of bilirubin in serum that is firmly bound to protein. Clin Chem, 1982; 28:629–637
7. Bruguera M, Bordas J, Rodes J. Atlas of laparoscopy and biopsy of the liver. Philadelphia: WB Saunders, 1979
8. Gazzard BG, Portmann B, Murray-Lyon IM, Williams R. Causes of death in fulminant hepatic failure and relationship to quantitative histological assessment of parenchymal damage. Q J Med, 1975; 44:615–626
9. Rappaport AM. The microcirculatory acinar concept of normal and pathological hepatic structure. Beitr Pathol, 1976; 157:215–243
10. Lau JY, Xie X, Lai MM, Wu PC. Apoptosis and viral hepatitis. Semin Liver Dis, 1998; 18:169–176
11. De Groote J, Desmet V, Gedigk P, et al. A classification of chronic hepatitis. Lancet, 1968; ii:626–628
12. Thaler H. Die Virushepatitis. In: Thaler H, ed., Leberbiopsie. Berlin: Springer, 1969; p. 51
13. Ferrell L, Wright T, Roberts J, Ascher N, Lake J. Pathology of hepatitis C viral infection in liver transplant recipients. Hepatology, 1992; 16:865–876
14. Ranek L. Cytophotometric studies of the DNA, nucleic acid and protein content of human liver cell nuclei. Acta Cytol, 1976; 20:151–157
15. Inuzuka S, Ueno T, Torimura T, Sata M, Abe H, Tanikawa K. Immunohistochemistry of the hepatic extracellular matrix in acute viral hepatitis. Hepatology, 1990; 12:249–256
16. Nonomura A, Mizukami Y, Matsubara F, Kobayashi K. Clinicopathological study of lymphocyte attachment to endothelial cells (endothelialitis) in various liver diseases. Liver, 1991; 11:78–88
17. Hengeveld P, Zuyderhoudt FM, Jobsis AC, van Gool J. Some aspects of iron metabolism during acute viral hepatitis. Hepatogastroenterology, 1982; 29:138–141
18. Hashimoto E, Kojimahara N, Noguchi S, Taniai M, Ishiguro N, Hayashi N. Immunohistochemical characterization of hepatic lymphocytes in acute hepatitis A, B, and C. J Clin Gastroenterol, 1996; 23:199–202
19. Mietkiewski JM, Scheuer PJ. Immunoglobulin-containing plasma cells in acute hepatitis. Liver, 1985; 5:84–88
20. Sciot R, Van Damme B, Desmet VJ. Cholestatic features in hepatitis A. J Hepatol, 1986; 3:172–181
21. Tordjmann T, Grimbert S, Genestie C, et al. Hépatite à cellules multinuclées de l'adulte: étude chez 17 malades. Gastroenterol Clin Biol, 1998; 22:305–310
22. Boyer JL, Klatskin G. Pattern of necrosis in acute viral hepatitis. Prognostic value of bridging (subacute hepatic necrosis). N Engl J Med, 1970; 283:1063–1071
23. Ware AJ, Eigenbrodt EH, Combes B. Prognostic significance of subacute hepatic necrosis in acute hepatitis. Gastroenterology, 1975; 68:519–524
24. Spitz RD, Keren DF, Boitnott JK, Maddrey WC. Bridging hepatic necrosis. Etiology and prognosis. Am J Dig Dis, 1978; 23:1076–1078
25. Nisman RM, Ganderson AP, Vlahcevic ZR, Gregory DH. Acute viral hepatitis with bridging hepatic necrosis. An overview. Arch Intern Med, 1979; 139:1289–1291
26. Scheuer PJ, Maggi G. Hepatic fibrosis and collapse: histological distinction by orcein staining. Histopathology, 1980; 4:487–490
27. Hanau C, Munoz SJ, Rubin R. Histopathological heterogeneity in fulminant hepatic failure. Hepatology, 1995; 21:345–351
28. Thung SN, Gerber MA. The formation of elastic fibers in livers with massive hepatic necrosis. Arch Pathol Lab Med, 1982; 106:468–469
29. Horney JT, Galambos JT. The liver during and after fulminant hepatitis. Gastroenterology, 1977; 73:639–645
30. Phillips MJ, Poucell S. Modern aspects of the morphology of viral hepatitis. Hum Pathol, 1981; 12:1060–1084
31. Theise ND, Saxena R, Portmann BC, et al. The canals of Hering and hepatic stem cells in humans. Hepatology, 1999; 30:1425–1430
32. Milandri M, Gaub J, Ranek L. Evidence for liver cell proliferation during fatal acute liver failure. Gut, 1980; 21:423–427
33. Smedile A, Farci P, Verme G, et al. Influence of delta infection on severity of hepatitis B. Lancet, 1982; 2:945–947
34. Omata M, Ehata T, Yokosuka O, Hosoda K, Ohto M. Mutations in the precore region of hepatitis B virus DNA in patients with fulminant and severe hepatitis. N Engl J Med, 1991; 324:1699–1704
35. Liang TJ, Hasegawa K, Rimon N, Wands JR, Ben-Porath E. A hepatitis B virus mutant associated with an epidemic of fulminant hepatitis. N Engl J Med, 1991; 324:1705–1709
36. Fagan EA, Ellis DS, Tovey GM et al. Toga virus-like particles in acute liver failure attributed to sporadic non-A, non-B hepatitis and recurrence after liver transplantation. J Med Virol, 1992; 38:71–77
37. Leevy C, Sherlock S, Tygstrup N, Zetterman R, eds. Diseases of the liver and biliary tract. Standardization of nomenclature, diagnostic criteria, and prognosis. New York: Raven Press, 1994
38. Shikata T, Karasawa T, Abe K. Two distinct types of hepatitis in experimental hepatitis B virus infection. Am J Pathol, 1980; 99:353–367
39. Hølund B, Poulsen H, Schlichting P. Reproducibility of liver biopsy diagnosis in relation to the size of the specimen. Scand J Gastroenterol, 1980; 15:329–335
40. Pawlotsky JM. Use and interpretation of virological tests for hepatitis C. Hepatology, 2002; 36:s65–s73
41. Nakanuma Y. Necroinflammatory changes in hepatic lobules in primary biliary cirrhosis with less well-defined cholestatic changes. Hum Pathol, 1993; 24:378–383
42. Danan G, Benichou C. Causality assessment of adverse reactions to drug. I. A novel method based on the conclusions of international consensus meetings: application to drug-induced liver injuries. J Clin Epidemiol, 1993; 46:1323–1330
43. Derby L, Gutthann SP, Jick H, Dean A. Liver disorders in receiving chlorpromazine or isoniazid. Pharmacotherapy, 1993; 13:354–358
44. Estes JD, Stoplman D, Olyaei A, et al. High prevalence of potentially hepatotoxic herbal supplement use in patients with fulminant hepatic failure. Arch Surg, 2003; 138:852–858
45. Levitsky J, Mailliard ME. Diagnosis and therapy of alcoholic liver disease. Sem Liver Dis, 2004; 24:233–247
46. Czaja AJ, Freese DK. Diagnosis and treatment of autoimmune hepatitis. Hepatology, 2002; 36:479–497
47. Karvountzis GG, Redeker AG, Peters RL. Long term follow-up studies of patients surviving fulminant viral hepatitis. Gastroenterology, 1974; 67:870–877
48. Thaler H. Hepatitis and cirrhosis. Dtsch Med Wochenschr, 1975; 100:1018–1025
49. Wanless I, Wong F, Blendis L, Greig P, Heathcote E, Levy G. Hepatic and portal vein thrombosis in cirrhosis: possible role in development of parenchymal extinction and portal hypertension. Hepatology, 1995; 21:1238–1247
50. Rockstroh JK, Spengler U. HIV and hepatitis C virus co-infection. Lancet Infectious Dis, 2004; 4:437–444
51. Strader DB, Wright T, Thomas DI, Seeff LB. Diagnosis, management, and treatment of hepatitis C. J Hepatol, 2004; 39:1147–1171
52. Lok ASF, McMahon BJ, Chronic hepatitis B. Hepatology, 2001; 34:1225–1241
53. Alberti A, Noventa F, Benvegnu L, Boccato S, Gatta A. Prevalence of liver disease in population of asymptomatic persons with hepatitis C virus infection. Ann Int Med, 2000; 137:961–965
54. Kyrlagitsis I, Portmann B, Smith H, O'Grady J, Cramp ME. Liver histology and progression of fibrosis in individuals with chronic hepatitis C and persistently normal ALT. Am J Gastroenterol, 2003; 98:1588–1593
55. Hui CK, Belaye T, Montegrande K, Wright TL. A comparison in the progression of liver fibrosis in chronic hepatitis C between persistently normal and elevated transaminase. J Hepatol, 2003; 38:511–517
56. Wai CT, Greenson JK, Fontana RJ, et al. A simple noninvasive index can predict both significant fibrosis and cirrhosis in patients with chronic hepatitis C. J Hepatol, 2003; 38:518–526
57. Groote JD, Desmet V, Gedigk P, et al. A classification of chronic hepatitis. Lancet, 1968; ii:626–628
58. Amaraa R, Mareckova H, Urbanek P, Fucikova T. T helper, cytotoxic T lymphocyte, NK cell and NK-T cell subpopulations in patients with chronic hepatitis C. Folia Microbiol (Praha) 2002; 47:717–722

59. Kakumu S, Yoshioka K, Wakita T, Ishikawa T, et al. Comparisons of peripheral blood and hepatic lymphocyte subpopulations and interferon production in chronic viral hepatitis. J Clin Lab Immunol, 1990; 33:1–6

60. Torres B, Martin JL, Caballero A, Villalobos M, Olea N. HCV in serum, peripheral blood mononuclear cells and lymphocyte subpopulations in C-hepatitis patients. Hepatol Res, 2000; 18:141–151

61. Bach N, Thung SN, Schaffner F. The histological features of chronic hepatitis C and autoimmune chronic hepatitis: a comparative analysis. Hepatology, 1992; 15:572–577

62. Danque PO, Bach N, Schaffner F, Gerber MA, Thung SN. HLA-DR expression in bile duct damage in hepatitis C. Mod Pathol, 1993; 6:327–332

63. Scheuer PJ, Ashrafzadeh P, Sherlock S, Brown D, Dusheiko GM. The pathology of hepatitis C. Hepatology, 1992; 15:567–571

64. Wanless IR, Wong F, Blendis LM, Greig P, Heathcote EJ, Levy G. Hepatic and portal vein thrombosis in cirrhosis: possible role in development of parenchymal extinction and portal hypertension. Hepatology, 1995; 21:1238–1247

65. Popper H, Paronetto F, Schaffner F. Immune processes in the pathogenesis of liver disease. Ann NY Acad Sci, 1965; 124:781–799

66. Ibuki N, Yamamoto K, Yabushita K, et al. In situ expression of granzyme B and Fas-ligand in the liver of viral hepatitis. Liver, 2002; 22:198–204

67. Eddleston AL, Mondelli M. Immunopathological mechanisms of liver cell injury in chronic hepatitis B virus infection. J Hepatol, 1986; 3 Suppl. 2:S17–23

68. Antonaci S, Schiraldi O. Costimulatory molecules and cytotoxic T cells in chronic hepatitis C: defence mechanisms devoted to host integrity or harmful events favouring liver injury progression? A review. Immunopharmacol Immunotoxicol, 1998; 20:455–472

69. Pianko S, Patella S, Ostapowicz G, Desmond P, Sievert W. Fas-mediated hepatocyte apoptosis is increased by hepatitis C virus infection and alcohol consumption, and may be associated with hepatic fibrosis: mechanisms of liver cell injury in chronic hepatitis C virus infection. J Viral Hepat, 2001; 8:406–413

70. Kerr JF, Cooksley WG, Searle J, et al. The nature of piecemeal necrosis in chronic active hepatitis. Lancet, 1979; 2:827–828

71. Chen NL, Bai L, Li L, et al. Apoptosis pathway of liver cells in chronic hepatitis. World J Gastroenterol, 2004; 10:3201–3204

72. Calabrese F, Pontisso P, Pettenazzo E, Benvegnu L, Vario A, Chemello L, Alberti A, Valente M. Liver cell apoptosis in chronic hepatitis C correlates with histological but not biochemical activity or serum HCV-RNA levels. Hepatology, 2000; 31:1153–1159

73. Popper H, Schaffner F. Chronic hepatitis: taxonomic, etiologic, and therapeutic problems. Prog Liver Dis, 1976; 5:531–558

74. Popper H. Changing concepts of the evolution of chronic hepatitis and the role of piecemeal necrosis. Hepatology, 1983; 3:758–762

75. Liaw YF, Chu CM, Chen TJ, Lin DY, Chang-Chien CS, Wu CS. Chronic lobular hepatitis: a clinicopathological and prognostic study. Hepatology, 1982; 2:258–262

76. Cooksley WG, Bradbear RA, Robinson W, et al. The prognosis of chronic active hepatitis without cirrhosis in relation to bridging necrosis. Hepatology, 1986; 6:345–348

77. Chen TJ, Liaw YF. The prognostic significance of bridging hepatic necrosis in chronic type B hepatitis: a histopathologic study. Liver, 1988; 8:10–16

78. Scheuer PJ, Maggi G. Hepatic fibrosis and collapse: histological distinction by orcein staining. Histopathology, 1980; 4:487–490

79. Falkowski O, An HJ, Ianus IA, et al. Regeneration of hepatocyte 'buds' in cirrhosis from intrabiliary stem cells. J Hepatol, 2003; 39:357–364

80. Bedossa P. [Fibrosis in chronic hepatitis C infection: mechanisms and cofactors]. Gastroenterol Clin Biol, 2002; 26 Spec No 2: B163–167

81. Guido M, Rugge M, Chemello L, et al. Liver stellate cells in chronic viral hepatitis: the effect of interferon therapy. J Hepatol, 1996; 24:301–307

82. Arif A, Levine RA, Sanderson SO, et al. Regression of fibrosis in chronic hepatitis C after therapy with interferon and ribavirin. Dig Dis Sci, 2003; 48:1425–1430

83. Farci P, Roskams T, Chessa L, et al. Long-term benefit of interferon alpha therapy of chronic hepatitis D: regression of advanced hepatic fibrosis. Gastroenterology, 2004; 126:1740–1749

84. Poynard T, McHutchison J, Manns M, et al. Impact of pegylated interferon alfa-2b and ribavirin on liver fibrosis in patients with chronic hepatitis C. Gastroenterology, 2002; 122:1303–1313

85. Wanless IR, Nakashima E, Sherman M. Regression of human cirrhosis. Morphologic features and the genesis of incomplete septal cirrhosis. Arch Pathol Lab Med, 2000; 124:1599–1607

86. Dufour JF, DeLellis R, Kaplan MM. Regression of hepatic fibrosis in hepatitis C with long-term interferon treatment. Dig Dis Sci, 1998; 43:2573–2576

87. Poynard T, McHutchison J, Davis GL, et al. Impact of interferon alfa-2b and ribavirin on progression of liver fibrosis in patients with chronic hepatitis C. Hepatology, 2000; 32:1131–1137

88. Ray MB. Regression of cirrhosis. A timely topic. Arch Pathol Lab Med, 2000; 124:1589–1590; discussion 1592–1593

89. Geller SA. Coming or going? What is cirrhosis? Arch Pathol Lab Med, 2000; 124:1587–1588; discussion 1592–1593

90. Chejfec G. Controversies in pathology. Is cirrhosis of the liver a reversible disease? Arch Pathol Lab Med, 2000; 124:1585–1586; discussion 1592–1593

91. Chedid A. Regression of human cirrhosis. Arch Pathol Lab Med, 2000; 124:1591; discussion 1592–1593

92. Wanless IR. In reply. Arch Pathol Lab Med, 2000; 124:1592–1593

93. Koziel MJ. Immunology of viral hepatitis. Am J Med, 1996; 100:98–109

94. Pawlotsky JM. Pathophysiology of hepatitis C virus infection and related liver disease. Trends Microbiol, 2004; 12:96–102

95. Kidd-Ljunggren K, Miyakawa Y, Kidd AH. Genetic variability in hepatitis B viruses. J Gen Virol, 2002; 83:1267–1280

96. Taylor JM. Replication of human hepatitis delta virus: recent developments. Trends Microbiol, 2003; 11:185–190

97. Francois C, Duverlie G, Rebouillat D, et al. Expression of hepatitis C virus proteins interferes with the antiviral action of interferon independently of PKR-mediated control of protein synthesis. J Virol, 2000; 74:5587–5596

98. Blum HE. Hepatitis viruses: genetic variants and clinical significance. Int J Clin Lab Res, 1997; 27:213–224

99. Kantzanou M, Lucas M, Barnes E, et al. Viral escape and T cell exhaustion in hepatitis C virus infection analysed using Class I peptide tetramers. Immunol Lett, 2003; 85:165–171

100. Rosenberg W. Mechanisms of immune escape in viral hepatitis. Gut, 1999; 44:759–764

101. Kiyici M, Gurel S, Budak F, et al. Fas antigen (CD95) expression and apoptosis in hepatocytes of patients with chronic viral hepatitis. Eur J Gastroenterol Hepatol, 2003; 15:1079–1084

102. Gitnick G. Hepatitis infection in immunocompromised patients. Gastroenterol Clin North Am, 1994; 23:515–521

103. Garcia G, Terrault N, Wright TL. Hepatitis C virus infection in the immunocompromised patient. Semin Gastrointest Dis, 1995; 6:35–45

104. Thimme R, Bukh J, Spangenberg HC, et al. Viral and immunological determinants of hepatitis C virus clearance, persistence, and disease. Proc Natl Acad Sci USA, 2002; 99:15661–15668

105. Wieland S, Thimme R, Purcell RH, Chisari FV. Genomic analysis of the host response to hepatitis B virus infection. Proc Natl Acad Sci USA, 2004; 101:6669–6674

106. Schaff Z, Kovalszky I, Nagy P, Zalatnai A, Jeney A, Lapis K. Human and experimental hepatocarcinogenesis. Scand J Gastroenterol, 1998; 228 Suppl.:90–97

107. Theise ND. Cirrhosis and hepatocellular neoplasia: more like cousins than like parent and child. Gastroenterology, 1996; 111:526–528

108. Franco E, Giambi C, Ialacci R, Maurici M. Prevention of hepatitis A by vaccination. Expert Opin Biol Ther, 2003; 3:965–974

109. Mele A. Progress in prevention and control of hepatitis B: a congress reviewing the first ten years since the introduction of mass vaccination in Italy. J Med Virol, 2002; 67:432

110. Chen M, Sallberg M, Sonnerborg A, et al. Limited humoral immunity in hepatitis C virus infection. Gastroenterology, 1999; 116:135–143

111. Nityanand S, Holm G, Lefvert AK. Immune complex mediated vasculitis in hepatitis B and C infections and the effect of antiviral therapy. Clin Immunol Immunopathol, 1997; 82:250–257

112. Stokes MB, Chawla H, Brody RI, et al. Immune complex glomerulonephritis in patients coinfected with human immunodeficiency virus and hepatitis C virus. Am J Kidney Dis, 1997; 29:514–525

113. Chattopodhyay D, Sen MR. Circulating immune complex in murine autoimmune hepatitis. Indian J Exp Biol, 1999; 37:308–310

114. Bertoletti A, Maini M, Williams R. Role of hepatitis B virus specific cytotoxic T cells in liver damage and viral control. Antiviral Res, 2003; 60:61–66

115. Gremion C, Grabscheid B, Wolk B, et al. Cytotoxic T lymphocytes derived from patients with chronic hepatitis C virus infection kill bystander cells via Fas-FasL interaction. J Virol, 2004; 78:2152–2157

116. Guidotti LG. The role of cytotoxic T cells and cytokines in the control of hepatitis B virus infection. Vaccine, 2002; 20 Suppl 4: A80–82

117. Chisari FV. Cytotoxic T cells and viral hepatitis. J Clin Invest, 1997; 99:1472–1477

118. Exley MA, Koziel MJ. To be or not to be NKT: natural killer T cells in the liver. Hepatology, 2004; 40:1033–1040

119. Peters M. Actions of cytokines on the immune response and viral interactions: an overview. Hepatology, 1996; 23:909–916

120. Koziel MJ. Cytokines in viral hepatitis. Semin Liver Dis, 1999; 19:157–169

121. de Lalla C, Galli G, Aldrighetti L, et al. Production of profibrotic cytokines by invariant NKT cells characterizes cirrhosis progression in chronic viral hepatitis. J Immunol, 2004; 173:1417–1425

122. Friedman SL. Stellate cells: A moving target in hepatic fibrogenesis. Hepatology, 2004; 40:1041–1043

123. Casini A, Ceni E, Salzano R, et al. Neutrophil-derived superoxide anion induces lipid peroxidation and stimulates collagen synthesis in human hepatic stellate cells: role of nitric oxide. Hepatology, 1997; 25:361–367

124. Paradis V, Kollinger M, Fabre M, Holstege A, Poynard T, Bedossa P. In situ detection of lipid peroxidation by-products in chronic liver diseases. Hepatology, 1997; 26:135–142

125. Friedman SL. Cytokines and fibrogenesis. Semin Liver Dis, 1999; 19:129–140

126. Haruyama T, Ajioka I, Akaike T, Watanabe Y. Regulation and significance of hepatocyte-derived matrix metalloproteinases in liver remodeling. Biochem Biophys Res Commun, 2000; 272:681–686

127. Lee HS, Huang GT, Miau LH, Chiou LL, Chen CH, Sheu JC. Expression of matrix metalloproteinases in spontaneous regression of liver fibrosis. Hepatogastroenterology, 2001; 48:1114–1117

128. Shukla NB, Poles MA. Hepatitis B virus infection: co-infection with hepatitis C virus, hepatitis D virus, and human immunodeficiency virus. Clin Liver Dis, 2004; 8:445–460

129. Bradley DW, Maynard JE, McCaustland KA, Murphy BL, Cook EH, Ebert JW. Non-A, non-B hepatitis in chimpanzees: interference with acute hepatitis A virus and chronic hepatitis B virus infections. J Med Virol, 1983; 11:207–213

130. Pontisso P, Gerotto M, Ruvoletto MG, et al. Hepatitis C genotypes in patients with dual hepatitis B and C virus infection. J Med Virol, 1996; 48:157–160

131. Guido M, Rugge M, Colombari R, Cecchetto A, Scarpa A, Cadrobbi P. Prompt hepatitis C virus suppression following hepatitis B virus superinfection in chronic untreated hepatitis C. Ital J Gastroenterol Hepatol, 1998; 30:414–417

132. Colombari R, Dhillon AP, Piazzola E, et al. Chronic hepatitis in multiple virus infection: histopathological evaluation. Histopathology, 1993; 22:319–325

133. Guido M, Thung SN, Fattovich G, et al. Intrahepatic expression of hepatitis B virus antigens: effect of hepatitis C virus infection. Mod Pathol, 1999; 12:599–603

134. Lefkowitch JH. The liver in AIDS. Semin Liver Dis, 1997; 17:335–344

135. Newell A, Francis N, Nelson M. Hepatitis and HIV: interrelationship and interactions. Br J Clin Pract, 1995; 49:247–251

136. Singh S, Mohanty A, Joshi YK, Deka D, Mohanty S, Panda SK. Mother-to-child transmission of hepatitis E virus infection. Indian J Pediatr, 2003; 70:37–39

137. Rosenberg PM, Farrell JJ, Abraczinskas DR, Graeme-Cook FM, Dienstag JL, Chung RT. Rapidly progressive fibrosing cholestatic hepatitis—hepatitis C virus in HIV coinfection. Am J Gastroenterol, 2002; 97:478–483

138. Tolan DJ, Davies MH, Millson CE. Fibrosing cholestatic hepatitis after liver transplantation in a patient with hepatitis C and HIV infection. N Engl J Med, 2001; 345:1781

139. Fang JW, Wright TL, Lau JY. Fibrosing cholestatic hepatitis in patient with HIV and hepatitis B. Lancet, 1993; 342:1175

140. Housset C, Pol S, Carnot F, et al. Interactions between human immunodeficiency virus-1, hepatitis delta virus and hepatitis B virus infections in 260 chronic carriers of hepatitis B virus. Hepatology, 1992; 15:578–583

141. Sabin CA, Walker AS, Dunn D. HIV/HCV coinfection, HAART, and liver-related mortality. Lancet, 2004; 364:757–758; author reply 758

142. Rullier A, Trimoulet P, Neau D, et al. Fibrosis is worse in HIV-HCV patients with low-level immunodepression referred for HCV treatment than in HCV-matched patients. Hum Pathol, 2004; 35:1088–1094

143. Nunez M, Soriano V. New hopes for HIV and HCV coinfection in 2004. HIV Clin Trials, 2004; 5:232–251

144. Hansen KE, Arnason J, Bridges AJ. Autoantibodies and common viral illnesses. Semin Arthritis Rheum, 1998; 27:263–271

145. Trepo C, Guillevin L. Polyarteritis nodosa and extrahepatic manifestations of HBV infection: The case against autoimmune intervention in pathogenesis. J Autoimmunity, 2001; 16:269–274

146. Kayali Z, Buckwold VE, Zimmerman B, Schmidt WN. Hepatitis C, cryoglobulinemia and cirrhosis a meta-analysis. Hepatology, 2002; 36:978–985

147. Cesur S, Akin K, Kurt H. The significance of cryoglobulinemia in patients with chronic hepatitis B and C virus infection. Hepatogastroenterology, 2003; 50:1487–1489

148. Propst T, Propst A, Dietze O, Judmaier G, Braunsteiner H, Vogel W. High prevalence of viral infection in adults with homozygous and heterozygous alpha 1-antitrypsin deficiency and chronic liver disease. Ann Intern Med, 1992; 117:641–645

149. Loudianos G, Gitlin JD. Wilson's disease. Semin Liver Dis, 2000; 20:353–364

150. Martins Da Coasta C, Baldwin D, Portmann B, Lolin Y, Mowat AP, Meili Vergani G. Value of urinary copper excretion after penicillamine challenge diagnosis of Wilson's disease. Hepatology, 1992; 15:609–615

151. Tavill AS. Diagnosis and management of hemochromatosis. Hepatology, 2001; 33:1321–1328

152. Dansette PM, Bonierbale E, Minoletti C, Beaune PH, Pessayre D, Mansuy D. Drug-induced immunotoxicity. Eur J Drug Metab Pharmacokinet, 1998; 23:443–451

153. Guido M, Rugge M. Liver biopsy sampling in chronic viral hepatitis. Semin Liver Dis, 2004; 24:89–97

154. Fanning L, Loane J, Kenny-Walsh E, et al. Tissue viral load variability in chronic hepatitis C. Am J Gastroenterol, 2001; 96:3384–3389

155. Regev A, Berho M, Jeffers LJ, et al. Sampling error and intraobserver variation in liver biopsy in patients with chronic HCV infection. Am J Gastroenterol, 2002; 97:2614–2618

156. Persico M, Palmentieri B, Vecchione R, Torella R, de Sio I. Diagnosis of chronic liver disease: reproducibility and validation of liver biopsy. Am J Gastroenterol, 2002; 97:491–492

157. Siddique I, El-Naga HA, Madda JP, Memon A, Hasan F. Sampling variability on percutaneous liver biopsy in patients with chronic hepatitis C virus infection. Scand J Gastroenterol, 2003; 38:427–432

158. Bedossa P, Dargere D, Paradis V. Sampling variability of liver fibrosis in chronic hepatitis C. Hepatology, 2003; 38:1449–1457

159. Goldstein NS, Hastah F, Galan MV, Gordon SC. Fibrosis heterogeneity in nonalcoholic steatohepatitis and hepatitis C virus needle core biopsy specimens Am J Clin Pathol, 2005; 123:382–387

160. Knodell RG, Ishak KG, Black WC, et al. Formulation and application of a numerical scoring system for assessing histological activity in asymptomatic chronic active hepatitis. Hepatology, 1981; 1:431–435

161. Batts KP, Ludwig J. Chronic hepatitis. An update on terminology and reporting. Am J Surg Pathol, 1995; 19:1409–1417

162. Bedossa P, Poynard T. An algorithm for the grading of activity in chronic hepatitis C. The METAVIR Cooperative Study Group. Hepatology, 1996; 24:289–293

163. Desmet VJ, Gerber M, Hoofnagle JH, Manns M, Scheuer PJ. Classification of chronic hepatitis: diagnosis, grading and staging. Hepatology, 1994; 19:1513–1520

164. Ishak K, Baptista A, Bianchi L, et al. Histological grading and staging of chronic hepatitis. J Hepatol, 1995; 22:696–699

165. Maduli E, Andorno S, Rigamonti C, et al. Evaluation of liver fibrosis in chronic hepatitis C with a computer-assisted morphometric method. Ann Ital Med Int, 2002; 17:242–247

166. Zaitoun AM, Al Mardini H, Awad S, Ukabam S, Makadisi S, Record CO. Quantitative assessment of fibrosis and steatosis in liver biopsies from patients with chronic hepatitis C. J Clin Pathol, 2001; 54:461–465

167. Di Sario A, Feliciangeli G, Bendia E, Benedetti A. Diagnosis of liver fibrosis. Eur Rev Med Pharmacol Sci, 2004; 8:11–18

168. Almasio PL, Niero M, Angioli D, et al. Experts' opinions on the role of liver biopsy in HCV infection: a Delphi survey by the Italian Association of Hospital Gastroenterologists (A.I.G.O.) J Hepatol, 2005; 43:381–387

169. Winkfield B, Aube C, Burtin P, Cales P. Inter-observer and intra-observer variability in hepatology. Eur J Gastroenterol Hepatol, 2003; 15:959–966

170. The French METAVIR Cooperative Study Group. Intraobserver and interobserver variations in liver biopsy interpretation in patients with chronic hepatitis C. Hepatology, 1994; 20:15–20

171. Goldin RD, Goldin JG, Burt AD, et al. Intra-observer and inter-observer variation in the histopathological assessment of chronic viral hepatitis. J Hepatol, 1996; 25:649–654

172. Cross SS. Grading and scoring in histopathology. Histopathology, 1998; 33:99–106

173. Macnaughton RJ. Numbers, scales, and qualitative research. Lancet, 1996; 347:1099–1100
174. Kay EW, O'Dowd J, Thomas R, et al. Mild abnormalities in liver histology associated with chronic hepatitis: distinction from normal liver histology. J Clin Pathol, 1997; 50:929–931
175. Guido M, Rugge M, Thung SN, et al. Hepatitis C virus serotypes and liver pathology. Liver, 1996; 16:353–357
176. Yano M, Kumada H, Kage M, et al. The long-term pathological evolution of chronic hepatitis C. Hepatology, 1996; 23:1334–1340
177. Poynard T, Bedossa P, Opolon P. Natural history of liver fibrosis progression in patients with chronic hepatitis C. The OBSVIRC, METAVIR, CLINIVIR, and DOSVIRC groups. Lancet, 1997; 349:825–832
178. Scheuer PJ, Standish RA, Dhillon AP. Scoring of chronic hepatitis. Clin Liver Dis, 2002; 6:335–347
179. Feinstone S, Kapikian A, Purcell R. Hepatitis A: detection by immune electron microscopy of a virus-like antigen associated with acute illness. Science, 1973; 182:1026–1028
180. Mathiesen LR, Fauerholdt L, Moller AM et al. Immunofluorescence studies for hepatitis A virus and hepatitis B surface and core antigen in liver biopsies from patients with acute viral hepatitis. Gastroenterology, 1979; 77:623–628
181. Shimizu YK, Shikata T, Beninger PR et al. Detection of hepatitis A antigen in human liver. Infect Immun, 1982; 36:320–324
182. Fagan E, Yousef G, Brahm J et al. Persistence of hepatitis A virus in fulminant hepatitis and after liver transplantation. J Med Virol, 1990; 30:131–136
183. Tilzey AJ, Banatvala JE. Hepatitis A (editorial). Brit Med J, 1991; 302:1552–1553
184. Villari D, Raimondo G, Attard L et al. Polyphasic type A hepatitis: histological features. Infection, 1993; 21:46–48
185. Masada CT, Shaw BW, Jr, Zetterman RK, Kaufman SS, Markin RS. Fulminant hepatic failure with massive necrosis as a result of hepatitis A infection. J Clin Gastroenterol, 1993; 17:158–162
186. Gane E, Sallie R, Saleh M, Portmann B, Williams R. Clinical recurrence of hepatitis A following liver transplantation for acute liver failure. J Med Virol, 1995; 45:35–39
187. Inoue K, Yoshida M, Yotsuyanagi H, Otsuka T, Sekiyama K, Fujita R. Chronic hepatitis A with persistent viral replication. J Med Virol, 1996; 50:322–324
188. McDonald GS, Courtney MG, Shattock AG, Weir DG. Prolonged IgM antibodies and histopathological evidence of chronicity in hepatitis A. Liver, 1989; 9:223–228
189. Vento S, Garofano T, Di Perri G, Dolci L, Concia E, Bassetti D. Identification of hepatitis A virus as a trigger for autoimmune chronic hepatitis type 1 in susceptible individuals. Lancet, 1991; 337:183–187
190. Abe H, Beninger PR, Ikejiri N, Setoyama H, Sata M, Tanikawa K. Light microscopic findings of liver biopsy specimens from patients with hepatitis type A and comparison with type B. Gastroenterology, 1982; 82:938–947
191. Teixeira MR, Jr., Weller IV, Murray A et al. The pathology of hepatitis A in man. Liver, 1982; 2:53–60
192. Okuno T, Sano A, Deguchi T et al. Pathology of acute hepatitis A in humans. Comparison with acute hepatitis B. Am J Clin Pathol, 1984; 81:162–169
193. Ponz E, Garcia-Pagan JC, Bruguera M, Bruix J, Rodes J. Hepatic fibrin-ring granulomas in a patient with hepatitis A. Gastroenterology, 1991; 100:268–270
194. Yamamoto T, Ishii M, Nagura H et al. Transient hepatic fibrin-ring granulomas in a patient with acute hepatitis A. Liver, 1995; 15:276–279
195. Ruel M, Sevestre H, Henry-Biabaud E, Courouce AM, Capron JP, Erlinger S. Fibrin ring granulomas in hepatitis A. Dig Dis Sci, 1992; 37:1915–1917
196. Vallbracht A, Maier K, Stierhof YD, Wiedmann KH, Flehmig B, Fleischer B. Liver-derived cytotoxic T cells in hepatitis A virus infection. J Infect Dis, 1989; 160:209–217
197. Muller C, Godl I, Gottlicher J, Wolf HM, Eibel MM. Phenotypes of peripheral blood lymphocytes during acute hepatitis A. Acta Paediatr Scand, 1991; 80:931–937
198. Lavanchy D. Hepatitis B virus epidemiology, disease burden, treatment, and current and emerging prevention and control measures. J Viral Hepat, 2004; 11:97–107
199. Lai CL, Ratziu V, Yuen MF, Poynard T. Viral hepatitis B. Lancet, 2003; 362:2089–2094
200. Davison F, Alexander GJ, Trowbridge R, Fagan EA, Williams R. Detection of hepatitis B virus DNA in spermatozoa, urine, saliva and leucocytes, of chronic HBsAg carriers. A lack of relationship with serum markers of replication. J Hepatol, 1987; 4:37–44
201. Seeff LB. Transfusion-associated hepatitis B: past and present. Transfus Med Rev, 1988; 2:204–214
202. Dane DS, Cameron CH, Briggs M. Virus-like particles in serum of patients with Australia-antigen-associated hepatitis. Lancet, 1970; 1:695–698
203. Locarnini S. Molecular virology of hepatitis B virus. Semin Liver Dis, 2004; 24 Suppl. 1:3–10
204. Blumberg BS, Alter HJ, Visnich S. A 'new' antigen in leukemia sera. JAMA, 1965; 191:541–546
205. Wen YM. Structural and functional analysis of full-length hepatitis B virus genomes in patients: implications in pathogenesis. J Gastroenterol Hepatol, 2004; 19:485–489
206. Lee JY, Locarnini S. Hepatitis B virus: pathogenesis, viral intermediates, and viral replication. Clin Liver Dis, 2004; 8:301–320
207. Servoss JC, Friedman LS. Serologic and molecular diagnosis of hepatitis B virus. Clin Liver Dis, 2004; 8:267–281
208. Nair S, Perrillo RP. Hepatitis B and D. In: Zakim D and Boyer TD, eds. Hepatology: A textbook of liver disease, Vol 2, 4th edn. Philadelphia, PA: WB Saunders, 2003:959–1017
209. McMahon BJ. The natural history of chronic hepatitis B virus infection. Semin Liver Dis, 2004; 24 Suppl. 1:17–21
210. Liaw YF, Tai DI, Chu CM, Chen TJ. The development of cirrhosis in patients with chronic type B hepatitis: a prospective study. Hepatology, 1988; 8:493–496
211. McMahon BJ, Alberts SR, Wainwright RB, Bulkow L, Lanier AP. Hepatitis B-related sequelae. Prospective study in 1400 hepatitis B surface antigen-positive Alaska native carriers. Arch Intern Med, 1990; 150:1051–1054
212. Chen WN, Oon CJ. Human hepatitis B virus mutants: significance of molecular changes. FEBS Lett, 1999; 453:237–242
213. Torresi J. The virological and clinical significance of mutations in the overlapping envelope and polymerase genes of hepatitis B virus. J Clin Virol, 2002; 25:97–106
214. Ngui SL, Hallet R, Teo CG. Natural and iatrogenic variation in hepatitis B virus. Rev Med Virol, 1999; 9:183–209
215. Gunther S, Fischer L, Pult I, Sterneck M, Will H. Naturally occurring variants of hepatitis B virus. Adv Virus Res, 1999; 52:25–137
216. Shields PL, Owsianka A, Carman WF, et al. Selection of hepatitis B surface 'escape' mutants during passive immune prophylaxis following liver transplantation: potential impact of genetic changes on polymerase protein function. Gut, 1999; 45:306–309
217. Chayama K, Suzuki Y, Kobayashi M, et al. Emergence and takeover of YMDD motif mutant hepatitis B virus during long-term lamivudine therapy and re-takeover by wild type after cessation of therapy. Hepatology, 1998; 27:1711–1716
218. Fang JW, Wright TL, Lau JY. Fibrosing cholestatic hepatitis in patient with HIV and hepatitis B. Lancet, 1993; 342:1175
219. Harrison RF, Davies MH, Goldin RD, Hubscher SG. Recurrent hepatitis B in liver allografts: a distinctive form of rapidly developing cirrhosis. Histopathology, 1993; 23:21–28
220. Nayak NC, Sachdeva R. Localization of hepatitis B surface antigen in conventional paraffin sections of the liver. Comparison of immunofluorescence, immunoperoxidase, and orcein staining methods with regard to their specificity and reliability as antigen marker. Am J Pathol, 1975; 81:479–492
221. Callea F, de Vos R, Togni R, Tardanico R, Vanstapel MJ, Desmet VJ. Fibrinogen inclusions in liver cells: a new type of ground-glass hepatocyte. Immune light and electron microscopic characterization. Histopathology, 1986; 10:65–73
222. Bianchi L, Gudat F. Sanded nuclei in hepatitis B: eosinophilic inclusions in liver cell nuclei due to excess in hepatitis B core antigen formation. Lab Invest, 1976; 35:1–5
223. Chu CM, Liaw YF. Immunohistological study of intrahepatic expression of hepatitis B core and E antigens in chronic type B hepatitis. J Clin Pathol, 1992; 45:791–795
224. Trevisan A, Gudat F, Busachi C, Stocklin E, Bianchi L. An improved method for HBcAg demonstration in paraffin-embedded liver tissue. Liver, 1982; 2:331–339
225. Chu CM, Yeh CT, Chien RN, Sheen IS, Liaw YF. The degrees of hepatocyte nuclear but not cytoplasmic expression of hepatitis B core antigen reflect the level of viral replication in chronic hepatitis B virus infection. J Clin Microbiol, 1997; 35:102–105
226. Ballare M, Lavarini C, Brunetto MR, et al. Relationship between the intrahepatic expression of 'e' and 'c' epitopes of the nucleocapsid protein of hepatitis B virus and viraemia. Clin Exp Immunol, 1989; 75:64–69
227. Park YN, Han KH, Kim KS, Chung JP, Kim S, Park C. Cytoplasmic expression of hepatitis B core antigen in chronic hepatitis B virus infection: role of precore stop mutants. Liver, 1999; 19:199–205
228. Guido M, Thung SN, Fattovich G, et al. Intrahepatic expression of hepatitis B virus antigens: effect of hepatitis C virus infection. Mod Pathol, 1999; 12:599–603

229. McDonald JA, Harris S, Waters JA, Thomas HC. Effect of human immunodeficiency virus (HIV) infection on chronic hepatitis B hepatic viral antigen display. J Hepatol, 1987; 4:337–342

230. Callea F. Immunohistochemical techniques for the demonstration of viral antigens in liver tissue. Ric Clin Lab, 1988; 18:223–231

231. Wang WL, London WT, Lega L, Feitelson MA. HBxAg in the liver from carrier patients with chronic hepatitis and cirrhosis. Hepatology, 1991; 14:29–37

232. Wang WL, London WT, Feitelson MA. Hepatitis B x antigen in hepatitis B virus carrier patients with liver cancer. Cancer Res, 1991; 51:4971–4977

233. Hoofnagle JH, Shafritz DA, Popper H. Chronic type B hepatitis and the 'healthy' HBsAg carrier state. Hepatology, 1987; 7:758–763

234. Kakimi K, Isogawa M, Chung J, Sette A, Chisari FV. Immunogenicity and tolerogenicity of hepatitis B virus structural and nonstructural proteins: implications for immunotherapy of persistent viral infections. J Virol, 2002; 76:8609–8620

235. Guidotti LG. The role of cytotoxic T cells and cytokines in the control of hepatitis B virus infection. Vaccine, 2002; 20 Suppl. 4: A80–82

236. Akbar SK, Onji M. Hepatitis B virus (HBV)–transgenic mice as an investigative tool to study immunopathology during HBV infection. Int J Exp Pathol, 1998; 79:279–291

237. Koziel MJ. Immunology of viral hepatitis. Am J Med, 1996; 100:98–109

238. Koziel MJ. Cytokines in viral hepatitis. Semin Liver Dis, 1999; 19:157–169

239. Koziel MJ. The immunopathogenesis of HBV infection. Antivir Ther, 1998; 3:13–24

240. Bracebridge S, Irwin D, Millership S. Prevention of perinatal hepatitis B transmission in a health authority area: an audit. Commun Dis Public Health, 2004; 7:138–141

241. Guidotti LG, Chisari FV. Noncytolytic control of viral infections by the innate and adaptive immune response. Annu Rev Immunol, 2001; 19:65–91

242. Guidotti LG, Morris A, Mendez H, et al. Interferon-regulated pathways that control hepatitis B virus replication in transgenic mice. J Virol, 2002; 76:2617–2621

243. Guidotti LG, Rochford R, Chung J, Shapiro M, Purcell R, Chisari FV. Viral clearance without destruction of infected cells during acute HBV infection. Science, 1999; 284:825–829

244. Rehermann B, Ferrari C, Pasquinelli C, Chisari FV. The hepatitis B virus persists for decades after patients' recovery from acute viral hepatitis despite active maintenance of a cytotoxic T-lymphocyte response. Nat Med, 1996; 2:1104–1108

245. London WT, Drew JS, Lustbader ED, Werner BG, Blumberg BS. Host responses to hepatitis B infection in patients in a chronic hemodialysis unit. Kidney Int, 1977; 12:51–58

246. McCarron B, Main J, Thomas HC. HIV and hepatotropic viruses: interactions and treatments. Int J STD AIDS, 1997; 8:739–45; quiz 745–746

247. Jung MC, Pape GR. Immunology of hepatitis B infection. Lancet Infect Dis, 2002; 2:43–50

248. Pawlotsky JM. Pathophysiology of hepatitis C virus infection and related liver disease. Trends Microbiol, 2004; 12:96–102

249. Penin F, Dubuisson J, Rey FA, Moradpour D, Pawlotsky JM. Structural biology of hepatitis C virus. Hepatology, 2004; 39:5–19

250. Andre P, Perlemuter G, Budkowska A, Brechot C, Lotteau V. Hepatitis C virus particles and lipoprotein metabolism. Semin Liver Dis, 2005; 25:93–104

251. Simmonds P. Genetic diversity and evolution of hepatitis C virus—15 years on. J Gen Virol, 2004; 85:3173–3188

252. Davidson F, Simmonds P, Ferguson JC, et al. Survey of major genotypes and subtypes of hepatitis C virus using RFLP of sequences amplified from the 5′ non-coding region. J Gen Virol, 1995; 76:1197–1204

253. Feitelson MA. Hepatitis C Virus: From laboratory to clinic. Cambridge University Press, 2002

254. Thomas DL, Seeff LB. Natural history of hepatitis C. Clin Liver Dis, 2005; 9:383–398, vi

255. Eyster ME, Alter HJ, Aledort LM, Quan S, Hatzakis A, Goedert JJ. Heterosexual co-transmission of hepatitis C virus (HCV) and human immunodeficiency virus (HIV). Ann Intern Med, 1991; 115:764–768

256. Einav S, Koziel MJ. Immunopathogenesis of hepatitis C virus in the immunosuppressed host. Transpl Infect Dis, 2002; 4:85–92

257. Alter MJ, Kruszon-Moran D, Nainan OV, et al. The prevalence of hepatitis C virus infection in the United States, 1988 through 1994. N Engl J Med, 1999; 341:556–562

258. Orland JR, Wright TL, Cooper S. Acute hepatitis C. Hepatology, 2001; 33:321–327

259. Hoofnagle JH. Hepatitis C: the clinical spectrum of disease. Hepatology, 1997; 26:15S–20S

260. Bowen DG, Walker CM. Adaptive immune responses in acute and chronic hepatitis C virus infection. Nature, 2005; 436:946–952

261. El-Serag HB. Hepatocellular carcinoma and hepatitis C in the United States. Hepatology, 2002; 36:S74–83

262. Theise ND. Cirrhosis and hepatocellular neoplasia: more like cousins than like parent and child. Gastroenterology, 1996; 111:526–528

263. Kobayashi K, Hashimoto E, Ludwig J, Hisamitsu T, Obata H. Liver biopsy features of acute hepatitis C compared with hepatitis A, and non-A, non-B, non-C. Liver, 1993; 13:69–72

264. Chu CM, Sheen IS, Liaw YF. The role of hepatitis C virus in fulminant viral hepatitis in an area with endemic hepatitis A and B. Gastroenterology, 1994; 107:189–195

265. Theise ND, Nimmakayalu M, Gardner R, et al. Liver from bone marrow in humans. Hepatology, 2000; 32:11–16

266. Rosenberg PM, Farrell JJ, Abraczinskas DR, Graeme-Cook FM, Dienstag JL, Chung RT. Rapidly progressive fibrosing cholestatic hepatitis—hepatitis C virus in HIV coinfection. Am J Gastroenterol, 2002; 97:478–483

267. Haber MM, West AB, Haber AD, Reuben A. Relationship of aminotransferases to liver histological status in chronic hepatitis C. Am J Gastroenterol, 1995; 90:1250–1257

268. Kyrlagkitsis I, Portmann B, Smith H, O'Grady J, Cramp ME. Liver histology and progression of fibrosis in individuals with chronic hepatitis C and persistently normal ALT. Am J Gastroenterol, 2003; 98:1588–1593

269. Bach N, Thung SN, Schaffner F. The histological features of chronic hepatitis C and autoimmune chronic hepatitis: a comparative analysis. Hepatology, 1992; 15:572–577

270. Kaji K, Nakanuma Y, Sasaki M, et al. Hepatitic bile duct injuries in chronic hepatitis C: histopathologic and immunohistochemical studies. Mod Pathol, 1994; 7:937–945

271. Lefkowitch JH, Schiff ER, Davis GL, et al. Pathological diagnosis of chronic hepatitis C: a multicenter comparative study with chronic hepatitis B. The Hepatitis Interventional Therapy Group. Gastroenterology, 1993; 104:595–603

272. Mosnier JF, Degott C, Marcellin P, Henin D, Erlinger S, Benhamou JP. The intraportal lymphoid nodule and its environment in chronic active hepatitis C: an immunohistochemical study. Hepatology, 1993; 17:366–371

273. Khakoo SI, Soni PN, Savage K, et al. Lymphocyte and macrophage phenotypes in chronic hepatitis C infection. Correlation with disease activity. Am J Pathol, 1997; 150:963–970

274. Fartoux L, Poujol-Robert A, Guechot J, Wendum D, Poupon R, Serfaty L. Insulin resistance is a cause of steatosis and fibrosis progression in chronic hepatitis C. Gut, 2005; 54:1003–1008

275. Hezode C, Roudot-Thoraval F, Zafrani ES, Dhumeaux D, Pawlotsky JM. Different mechanisms of steatosis in hepatitis C virus genotypes 1 and 3 infections. J Viral Hepat, 2004; 11:455–458

276. Monto A, Dove LM, Bostrom A, Kakar S, Tien PC, Wright TL. Hepatic steatosis in HIV/hepatitis C coinfection: prevalence and significance compared with hepatitis C monoinfection. Hepatology, 2005; 42:310–316

277. Dev A, Patel K, McHutchison JG. Hepatitis C and steatosis. Clin Liver Dis, 2004; 8:881–892, ix

278. Fillipowicz EA, Xiao S, Sower LE, Weems J, Payne DA. Detection of HCV in bile duct epithelium by laser capture microdissection (LCM). In Vivo, 2005; 19:737–739

279. Kaji K, Nakanuma Y, Harada K, Sakai A, Kaneko S, Kobayashi K. Hemosiderin deposition in portal endothelial cells is a histologic marker predicting poor response to interferon-alpha therapy in chronic hepatitis C. Pathol Int, 1997; 47:347–352

280. Boucher E, Bourienne A, Adams P, Turlin B, Brissot P, Deugnier Y. Liver iron concentration and distribution in chronic hepatitis C before and after interferon treatment. Gut, 1997; 41:115–120

281. Chiaverini C, Halimi G, Ouzan D, Halfon P, Ortonne JP, Lacour JP. Porphyria cutanea tarda, C282Y, H63D and S65C HFE gene mutations and hepatitis C infection: a study from southern France. Dermatology, 2003; 206:212–216

282. Fiel MI, Schiano TD, Guido M, et al. Increased hepatic iron deposition resulting from treatment of chronic hepatitis C with ribavirin. Am J Clin Pathol, 2000; 113:35–39

283. Deugnier Y, Turlin B, le Quilleuc D, et al. A reappraisal of hepatic siderosis in patients with end-stage cirrhosis: practical implications for the diagnosis of hemochromatosis. Am J Surg Pathol, 1997; 21:669–675

284. Scheuer PJ, Krawczynski K, Dhillon AP. Histopathology and detection of hepatitis C virus in liver. Springer Semin Immunopathol, 1997; 19:27–45

285. De Vos R, Verslype C, Depla E, et al. Ultrastructural visualization of hepatitis C virus components in human and primate liver biopsies. J Hepatol, 2002; 37:370–379

286. Qian X, Guerrero RB, Plummer TB, Alves VF, Lloyd RV. Detection of hepatitis C virus RNA in formalin-fixed paraffin-embedded sections with digoxigenin-labeled cRNA probes. Diagn Mol Pathol, 2004; 13:9–14

287. Biagini P, Benkoel L, Dodero F, de Lamballerie X, et al. Hepatitis C virus RNA detection by in situ RT-PCR in formalin-fixed paraffin-embedded liver tissue. Comparison with serum and tissue results. Cell Mol Biol (Noisy-le-grand), 2001; 47 Online Pub: OL167–171

288. Benkoel L, Biagini P, Dodero F, De Lamballerie X, De Micco P, Chamlian A. Immunohistochemical detection of C-100 hepatitis C virus antigen in formaldehyde-fixed paraffin-embedded liver tissue. Correlation with serum, tissue and in situ RT-PCR results. Eur J Histochem, 2004; 48:185–90

289. Verslype C, Nevens F, Sinelli N, et al. Hepatic immunohistochemical staining with a monoclonal antibody against HCV-E2 to evaluate antiviral therapy and reinfection of liver grafts in hepatitis C viral infection. J Hepatol, 2003; 38:208–214

290. Schluger LK, Sheiner PA, Thung SN, et al. Severe recurrent cholestatic hepatitis C following orthotopic liver transplantation. Hepatology, 1996; 23:971–976

291. Rosenberg S. Recent advances in the molecular biology of hepatitis C virus. J Mol Biol, 2001; 313:451–464

292. Ruggieri A, Harada T, Matsuura Y, Miyamura T. Sensitization to Fas-mediated apoptosis by hepatitis C virus core protein. Virology, 1997; 229:68–76

293. Chisari FV. Unscrambling hepatitis C virus–host interactions. Nature, 2005; 436:930–932

294. Wakita T, Pietschmann T, Kato T, et al. Production of infectious hepatitis C virus in tissue culture from a cloned viral genome. Nat Med, 2005; 11:791–796

295. Meuleman P, Libbrecht L, De Vos R, et al. Morphological and biochemical characterization of a human liver in a uPA-SCID mouse chimera. Hepatology, 2005; 41:847–856

296. Sakai A, Kaneko S, Honda M, Matsushita E, Kobayashi K. Quasispecies of hepatitis C virus in serum and in three different parts of the liver of patients with chronic hepatitis. Hepatology, 1999; 30:556–561

297. Pachiadakis I, Pollara G, Chain BM, Naoumov NV. Is hepatitis C virus infection of dendritic cells a mechanism facilitating viral persistence? Lancet Infect Dis, 2005; 5:296–304

298. Ballardini G, Groff P, Pontisso P, et al. Hepatitis C virus (HCV) genotype, tissue HCV antigens, hepatocellular expression of HLA-A,B,C, and intercellular adhesion-1 molecules. Clues to pathogenesis of hepatocellular damage and response to interferon treatment in patients with chronic hepatitis C. J Clin Invest, 1995; 95:2067–2075

299. Hayashi N, Mita E. Involvement of Fas system-mediated apoptosis in pathogenesis of viral hepatitis. J Viral Hepat, 1999; 6:357–365

300. Sene D, Limal N, Cacoub P. Hepatitis C virus-associated extrahepatic manifestations: a review. Metab Brain Dis, 2004; 19:357–381

301. Cacoub P, Poynard T, Ghillani P, et al. Extrahepatic manifestations of chronic hepatitis C. MULTIVIRC Group. Multidepartment Virus C. Arthritis Rheum, 1999; 42:2204–2212

302. Vassilopoulos D, Younossi ZM, Hadziyannis E, et al. Study of host and virological factors of patients with chronic HCV infection and associated laboratory or clinical autoimmune manifestations. Clin Exp Rheumatol, 2003; 21:S101–111

303. Roboz GJ. Hepatitis C and B-cell lymphoma. AIDS Patient Care STDS, 1998; 12:605–609

304. Safdar K, Schiff ER. Alcohol and hepatitis C. Semin Liver Dis, 2004; 24:305–315

305. Schiff ER, Ozden N. Hepatitis C and alcohol. Alcohol Res Health, 2003; 27:232–239

306. Jerrells TR. Association of alcohol consumption and exaggerated immunopathologic effects in the liver induced by infectious organism. Front Biosci, 2002; 7:d1487–1493

307. Anderson S, Nevins CL, Green LK, El-Zimaity H, Anand BS. Assessment of liver histology in chronic alcoholics with and without hepatitis C virus infection. Dig Dis Sci, 2001; 46:1393–1398

308. Shiomi S, Kuroki T, Minamitani S, et al. Effect of drinking on the outcome of cirrhosis in patients with hepatitis B or C. J Gastroenterol Hepatol, 1992; 7:274–276

309. Hourigan LF, Macdonald GA, Purdie D, et al. Fibrosis in chronic hepatitis C correlates significantly with body mass index and steatosis. Hepatology, 1999; 29:1215–1219

310. Rizzetto M, Canese MG, Arico S, et al. Immunofluorescence detection of new antigen-antibody system (delta/anti-delta) associated to hepatitis B virus in liver and in serum of HBsAg carriers. Gut, 1977; 18:997–1003

311. Bean P. Latest discoveries on the infection and coinfection with hepatitis D virus. Am Clin Lab, 2002; 21:25–27

312. Karayiannis P. Hepatitis D virus. Rev Med Virol, 1998; 8:13–24

313. Taylor JM. Replication of human hepatitis delta virus: recent developments. Trends Microbiol, 2003; 11:185–190

314. Diener TO. Hepatitis delta virus-like agents: an overview. Prog Clin Biol Res, 1993; 382:109–115

315. Chen PJ, Wu HL, Wang CJ, Chia JH, Chen DS. Molecular biology of hepatitis D virus: research and potential for application. J Gastroenterol Hepatol, 1997; 12:S188–192

316. Macnaughton TB, Lai MM. Hepatitis delta virus RNA transfection for the cell culture model. Methods Mol Med, 2004; 96:351–357

317. Macnaughton TB, Li YI, Doughty AL, Lai MM. Hepatitis delta virus RNA encoding the large delta antigen cannot sustain replication due to rapid accumulation of mutations associated with RNA editing. J Virol, 2003; 77:12048–12056

318. Lai MM. Molecular biologic and pathogenetic analysis of hepatitis delta virus. J Hepatol, 1995; 22:127–131

319. Gaeta GB, Stroffolini T, Chiaramonte M, et al. Chronic hepatitis D: a vanishing Disease? An Italian multicenter study. Hepatology, 2000; 32:824–827

320. Caredda F, Rossi E, d'Arminio Monforte A, et al. Hepatitis B virus-associated coinfection and superinfection with delta agent: indistinguishable disease with different outcome. J Infect Dis, 1985; 151:925–928

321. Negro F, Rizzetto M. Diagnosis of hepatitis delta virus infection. J Hepatol, 1995; 22:136–139

322. Smedile A, Farci P, Verme G, et al. Influence of delta infection on severity of hepatitis B. Lancet, 1982; 2:945–947

323. Farci P, Smedile A, Lavarini C, et al. Delta hepatitis in inapparent carriers of hepatitis B surface antigen. A disease simulating acute hepatitis B progressive to chronicity. Gastroenterology, 1983; 85:669–673

324. Moreno A, Ramon y Cajal S, Marazuela M, et al. Sanded nuclei in delta patients. Liver, 1989; 9:367–371

325. Polo JM, Jeng KS, Lim B, et al. Transgenic mice support replication of hepatitis delta virus RNA in multiple tissues, particularly in skeletal muscle. J Virol, 1995; 69:4880–4887

326. Guilhot S, Huang SN, Xia YP, La Monica N, Lai MM, Chisari FV. Expression of the hepatitis delta virus large and small antigens in transgenic mice. J Virol, 1994; 68:1052–1058

327. Netter HJ, Kajino K, Taylor JM. Experimental transmission of human hepatitis delta virus to the laboratory mouse. J Virol, 1993; 67:3357–3362

328. Cole SM, Gowans EJ, Macnaughton TB, Hall PD, Burrell CJ. Direct evidence for cytotoxicity associated with expression of hepatitis delta virus antigen. Hepatology, 1991; 13:845–851

329. Popper H, Thung SN, Gerber MA, et al. Histologic studies of severe delta agent infection in Venezuelan Indians. Hepatology, 1983; 3:906–912

330. Khuroo MS. Study of an epidemic of non-A, non-B hepatitis. Possibility of another human hepatitis virus distinct from post-transfusion non-A, non-B type. Am J Med, 1980; 68:818–824

331. Asher LV, Innis BL, Shrestha MP, Ticehurst J, Baze WB. Virus-like particles in the liver of a patient with fulminant hepatitis and antibody to hepatitis E virus. J Med Virol, 1990; 31:229–233

332. Arankalle VA, Ticehurst J, Sreenivasan MA et al. Aetiological association of a virus-like particle with enterically transmitted non-A, non-B hepatitis. Lancet, 1988; i:550–554

333. Panda SK, Datta R, Kaur J, Zuckerman AJ, Nayak NC. Enterically transmitted non-A, non-B hepatitis: recovery of virus-like particles from an epidemic in south Delhi and transmission studies in rhesus monkeys. Hepatology, 1989; 10:466–472

334. Zuckerman AJ. Hepatitis E virus. The main cause of enterically transmitted non-A, non-B hepatitis. Br Med J, 1990; 300:1475–1476

335. Reyes G, Purdy M, Kim J et al. Isolation of a cDNA from the virus responsible for enterically transmitted non-A, non-B hepatitis. Science, 1990; 247:1335–1339

336. Soe S, Uchida T, Suzuki K et al. Enterically transmitted non-A, non-B hepatitis in cynomolgus monkeys: morphology and probable mechanism of hepatocellular necrosis. Liver, 1989; 9:135–145

337. Takahashi K, Kang JH, Ohnishi S, et al. Full-length sequences of six hepatitis E virus isolates of genotypes III and IV from patients with sporadic acute or fulminant hepatitis in Japan. Intervirology, 2003; 46:308–318

338. Purdy MA, Carson D, McCaustland KA, Bradley DW, Beach MJ, Krawczynski K. Viral specificity of hepatitis E virus antigens identified by fluorescent antibody assay using recombinant HEV proteins. J Med Virol, 1994; 44:212–214

339. Krawczynski K. Hepatitis E. Hepatology, 1993; 17:932–941

340. Harrison T. Hepatitis E virus—an update. Liver, 1999; 19:171–176

341. Ramalingaswami V, Purcell RH. Waterborne non-A, non-B hepatitis. Lancet, 1988; 1:571–573

342. Velazquez O, Stetler HC, Avila C et al. Epidemic transmission of enterically transmitted non-A, non-B hepatitis in Mexico, 1986–1987. JAMA, 1990; 263:3281–3285

343. Skidmore SJ, Yarbough PO, Gabor KA, Tam AW, Reyes GR, Flower AJ. Imported hepatitis E in UK. Lancet, 1991; 337:1541

344. Johansson PJ, Mushahwar IK, Norkrans G, Weiland O, Nordenfelt E. Hepatitis E virus infections in patients with acute hepatitis non-A-D in Sweden. Scand J Infect Dis, 1995; 27:543–546

345. Clemente-Casares P, Pina S, Buti M, Jardi R, Martin M, Bofill-Mas S, Girones R. Hepatitis E virus epidemiology in industrialized countries. Emerg Infect Dis, 2003; 9:448–454

346. Khuroo MS, Teli MR, Skidmore S, Sofi MA, Khuroo MI. Incidence and severity of viral hepatitis in pregnancy. Am J Med, 1981; 70:252–255

347. Le Cann P, Tong MJ, Werneke J, Coursaget P. Detection of antibodies to hepatitis E virus in patients with autoimmune chronic active hepatitis and primary biliary cirrhosis. Scand J Gastroenterol, 1997; 32:387–389

348. Wang CH, Tschen SY. Hepatitis E virus and primary biliary cirrhosis. Q J Med, 1997; 90:154–155

349. Sylvan SP, Hellstrom UB, Hampl H, Kapprell HP, Troonen H. Hepatitis E in patients with chronic autoimmune liver disease. JAMA, 1995; 273:377–378

350. Gupta D, Smetana H. The histopathology of viral hepatitis as seen in the Delhi epidemics (1955–56). Indian J Med Res, 1957; 45(suppl):101–113

351. Uchida T. Hepatitis E: review. Gastroenterol Jpn, 1992; 27:687–696

352. Wendum D, Nachury M, Yver M, et al. Acute hepatitis E: a cause of lymphocytic destructive cholangitis. Hum Pathol, 2005; 36:436–438

353. Fagan EA, Ellis DS, Tovey GM et al. Toga virus-like particles in acute liver failure attributed to sporadic non-A, non-B hepatitis and recurrence after liver transplantation. J Med Virol, 1992; 38:71–77

354. Deka N, Sharma M, Mukerjee R. Isolation of the novel agent from human stool samples that is associated with sporadic non-A, non-B hepatitis. J Virol, 1994; 68:7810–7815

355. Kasirga E, Sanlidag T, Akcali S, et al. Clinical significance of TT virus infection in children with chronic hepatitis B. Pediatr Int, 2005; 47:300–304

356. Simons J, Leary T, Dawson G et al. Isolation of novel virus-like sequences associated with human hepatitis. Nature Med, 1995; 1:564–569

357. Kao JH, Chen PJ, Lai MY et al. GB virus-C/hepatitis G virus infection in an area endemic for viral hepatitis, chronic liver disease, and liver cancer. Gastroenterology, 1997; 112:1265–1270

358. Kaiser T, Tillmann HL. GB virus C infection: is there a clinical relevance with the human immunodeficiency virus? AIDS Rev, 2005; 7:3–12

359. Nishizawa T, Okamoto H, Konishi K, Yoshizawa H, Miyakawa Y, Mayumi M. A novel DNA virus (TTV) associated with elevated transaminase levels in posttransfusion hepatitis of unknown etiology. Biochem Biophys Res Commun, 1997; 241:92–97

360. Poovorawan Y, Tangkijvanich P, Theamboonlers A, Hirsch P. Transfusion transmissible virus TTV and its putative role in the etiology of liver disease. Hepatogastroenterology, 2001; 48:256–260

361. Umemura T, Tanaka E, Ostapowicz G, et al. Investigation of SEN virus infection in patients with cryptogenic acute liver failure, hepatitis-associated aplastic anemia, or acute and chronic non-A-E hepatitis. J Infect Dis, 2003; 188:1545–1552

362. Moriyama M, Mikuni M, Matsumura H, et al. SEN virus infection influences the pathological findings in liver but does not affect the incidence of hepatocellular carcinoma in patients with chronic hepatitis C and liver cirrhosis, Liver Int, 2005; 25:226–235

Other viral and infectious diseases and HIV-related liver disease

9

Sebastian B. Lucas

As a major blood-filtering organ, the liver is affected in many infections, be they systemic or arriving via the portal venous system. The large component of phagocytic Kupffer cells, which engulf blood-borne bacteria, fungi and protozoa, ensures that hepatomegaly is almost as frequent as fever. In addition, several viral infections are solely hepatotropic; the commonest viral hepatitides are described in Chapter 8, and the remainder here.

The infections are described in taxonomic groupings. The final section discusses the hepatic manifestations of human immunodeficiency virus (HIV) infection and AIDS. Parasite life cycles are not detailed in this chapter, and the reader is referred to standard texts.[1] Covering dozens of different infectious agents, this chapter cannot detail all the appearances that aid differential diagnosis. The pathology of protozoal and helminthic diseases of the liver and other organs is illustrated and discussed by Gutierrez,[2] and the AFIP volumes cover the pathology of most infections.[3] An encyclopaedic description of the clinical and pathogenetic aspects of infectious diseases can be found in the textbook by Mandell et al.[4]

Viral infections

A comprehensive account of the pathology and pathogenesis of human viral infections is given by Craighead.[5]

Viral haemorrhagic fevers

These viral infections share several epidemiological and clinico-pathological features,[4] and their liver pathologies are similar. The diseases caused by these agents and their geographical distribution are listed in Table 9.1. Although much attention has been paid to the hepatic pathology of the viral haemorrhagic fevers, and abnormal liver function tests are common, clinically significant liver disease and death from liver failure are rare except in yellow fever. The viruses cause small vessel damage in multiple organs, which is often associated with haemorrhage. The clinico-pathological correlations of the viral haemorrhagic fevers were reviewed by Ishak et al.[6]

Yellow fever

Despite the existence of a safe and effective vaccine against yellow fever for over 50 years, the disease is still endemic in Africa and South America. This flavivirus is transmitted by several *Aedes* species of mosquito. Young adult males are predominantly affected. During an epidemic in rural West Africa, the clinical attack rate was estimated to be 5% and the mortality was nearly 3% of the local population.[7] The presenting features are an acute illness of sudden onset with fever, myalgia and headache, followed by jaundice after a few days; death occurs in the second week after onset, and is preceded by coma. The diagnosis is usually confirmed by the serological demonstration of specific IgM by an ELISA method, or by virus isolation from blood.

The histopathological appearances depend on the stage of the disease, and the classic features are seen only in the acute stage. At autopsy the liver is yellow and soft. Microscopically, there is confluent focal necrosis with a predominantly mid-zonal distribution. Some hepatocytes undergo acidophilic degeneration and lose their nuclei, forming the classic (but non-specific) Councilman bodies (Fig. 9.1). Rarely, eosinophilic intranuclear inclusions

Table 9.1	The viral haemorrhagic fevers	
Disease	**Virus group**	**Geography**
Yellow fever	Flaviviridae	Africa, South America
Dengue	Flaviviridae	Africa, Asia, tropical America
Lassa fever	Arenaviridae	West Africa
Argentine haemorrhagic fever (Junin virus)	Arenaviridae	Argentina
Ebola fever	Filoviridae	Central Africa
Marburg fever	Filoviridae	Central and southern Africa
Rift valley fever	Bunyaviridae	East and central Africa
Haemorrhagic fever with renal syndrome (Hantaan virus)	Bunyaviridae	Northern Eurasia
Congo–Crimea haemorrhagic fever	Bunyaviridae	Former Soviet Union, central-west Asia, Africa

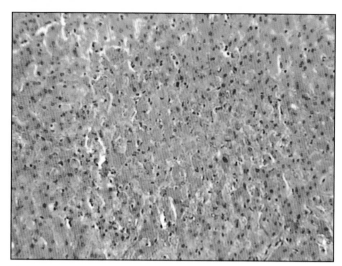

Fig. 9.2 • Dengue haemorrhagic fever: necrosis of the hepatocytes with no associated inflammation. H&E. Photograph courtesy of the Wellcome Trust International Health Image Collection.

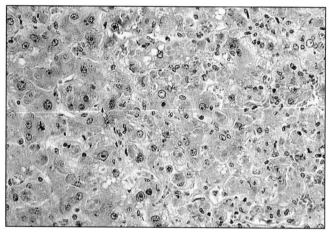

Fig. 9.1 • Yellow fever. Mid-zonal liver necrosis with minimal inflammation. Note the acidophilic (Councilman) bodies. H&E.

(Torres bodies) are present. Fatty change may be prominent. The surviving liver shows ballooned hepatocytes and regenerative hyperplasia; multinucleate hepatocytes are common. Cholestasis is unusual. Some portal lymphocytic infiltration may be seen. Biopsies taken from survivors up to 2 months after the acute illness show a non-specific intraacinar hepatitis.[8]

Dengue

Dengue is also transmitted by *Aedes* mosquitoes. The initial disease is influenza-like with a rash—dengue fever, which is unlikely to be biopsied. The clinically more severe diseases[9]—dengue haemorrhagic fever (DHF) and dengue shock syndrome (DSS)—follow from reinfection by dengue virus but with a different serotype of the virus. In DHF there are widespread petechial haemorrhages and multiple organ damage; in DSS there is widespread capillary leakage and fluid depletion. Untreated, the mortality approaches 50%. In DHF the liver is enlarged, pale from steatosis and blotchy from multifocal haemorrhages. Microscopically, there are focal necroses or more coalescent perivenular or mid-zonal necrosis, with little or no inflammation (Fig. 9.2).[10,11] Pathogenetically, there is dengue virus within hepatocytes and cell death is from apoptosis.[11]

Lassa fever

The natural reservoir of Lassa virus is the multimammate rat *Mastomys natalensis*. Man is infected directly from its urine. Following the alarming emergence of the disease in the early 1970s, serological surveys have shown that the infection is widespread in West Africa, but clinical disease occurs in 5–10% and the case fatality rate is less than 25%. The features include abdominal pain, pharyngitis and fever, but not jaundice.

The liver is mottled in appearance (Fig. 9.3(A)). Histologically, there is necrosis without inflammation. Individual hepatocytes or groups of cells throughout the acini are acidophilic (Fig. 9.3(B)). There is no cholestasis, or steatosis, but lipofuscin deposition is evident.[12] Arenaviruses are present in large numbers under electron microscopy, but there are no light-microscopic viral inclusions.

Lassa virus is readily transmitted by inoculation of infected blood. The pathologist who performed the early autopsies (1970s) in West Africa died of the disease following an accident. In the UK, autopsies on patients with known or suspected viral haemorrhagic fever should only be performed in specialist centres;[13] post-mortem needle sampling may be done. In a British case of imported Lassa fever, such a needle sample showed only changes of shock, two weeks of therapeutic ribavirin having eliminated the virus (personal observations).

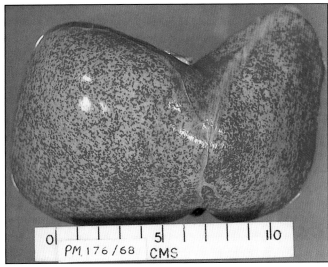

A

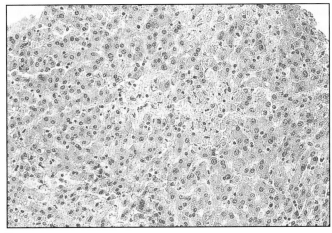

B

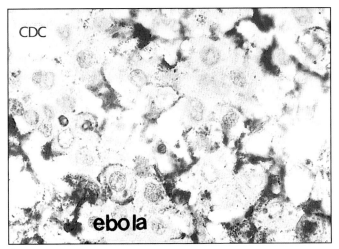

C

Fig. 9.3 • Haemorrhagic fevers. **(A)** Autopsy liver from Lassa fever patient showing foci of haemorrhagic necrosis under the capsule. **(B)** Lassa fever: focal liver-cell necrosis without associated inflammation. H&E. **(C)** Ebola virus infection: immunocytochemical stain showing vast quantities of filovirus in the sinusoids of the liver. Photograph courtesy of Dr S Zaki, CDC, Atlanta.

Ebola and Marburg fevers

The natural reservoirs of these viruses are still unknown. Between 1976 and 1979, three epidemics of Ebola disease occurred in Zaire and Sudan with a rapid course and 70% mortality. Marburg disease first occurred in 1967 in people who had been in contact with African green monkeys imported from Uganda. The mortality was 25%; subsequently there were isolated cases in Kenya and South Africa up to 1982. Clinically, patients had fever and widespread haemorrhages, shock and disseminated intravascular coagulation. The hepatic pathology is similar to that in Lassa fever: hepatocyte necrosis that ranges from spotty to widespread, no cholestasis, and minimal inflammation.[14] Experimental studies[15] show that the Ebloa filovirus is present in large quantities free in the blood, throughout the mononuclear phagocyte system, in endothelial cells and hepatocytes (Fig. 9.3(C)); the reticular network of lymph nodes is also heavily infected and damaged.

These infections are still relevant. In 1989, monkeys imported into the USA from the Philippines were found to be dying of Ebola virus infection. Transmission to some laboratory staff occurred although no clinical disease developed. In 1995, an epidemic of Ebola infection occurred in Zaire, with many deaths.[16] Outbreaks still occur in West Africa, and the possibility of undiagnosed patients arriving in industrialized countries is real. Epidemiological and clinical information on these ongoing outbreaks is available on the WHO website: www.who.int/topics/haemorrhagic_fevers_viral/en/.

Congo Crimea haemorrhagic fever

A review of this infection in southern Africa shows that the pathology is similar to that of the other viral haemorrhagic fevers.[17]

Herpes virus group

The five members of this group of DNA viruses that may directly affect the liver are herpes simplex, herpes zoster, cytomegalovirus, the Epstein–Barr virus, and human herpes virus-6 (HHV6). The Kaposi sarcoma virus (HHV8) is considered in the section on HIV/AIDS. In most societies, infection is near universal for most of the herpes viruses (except HHV8), and occurs in childhood or adolescence. Once infected with a herpes virus, infection is life-long, hence its tendency to reactivate and induce aggressive lesions in immunosuppressed persons.

Herpes simplex

Primary herpes simplex infection produces oral or genital lesions, and latent infection lasts for life. There are two strains of this virus: type 1 is responsible for generalized infections in older children and adults, and type 2 affects the genital tract in the neonate. In the latter, dissemination may occur, with necrotizing hepatitis. The liver is also involved in the severe fulminant systemic herpes infection that immunocompromised patients may suffer. Organ transplantation and treatment for haematological malignancy are the most frequent underlying predispositions[18] but HIV infection is increasingly important. Fatal herpetic hepatitis also occurs in apparently immunocompetent adults.[19] The clinical features resemble those of septic endotoxic shock; jaundice is not always present.

At autopsy the liver is enlarged and mottled with yellow or white foci surrounded by congestion (Fig. 9.4(A)). Microscopically, there is little inflammation but irregular coagulative necrosis of the parenchyma is present. At the margins, hepatocytes show purple nuclear inclusions with a clear surrounding halo, and some hepatocytes are multinucleate (Fig. 9.4(B)).

Herpes zoster

Herpes zoster causes chicken pox and—as a reactivation of latent infection—shingles. After infection, there is a primary viraemia with viral replication in the epithelium of the gut, respiratory tract, liver, pancreas and adrena. A secondary viraemia leads to skin infection with the usual rash. Liver

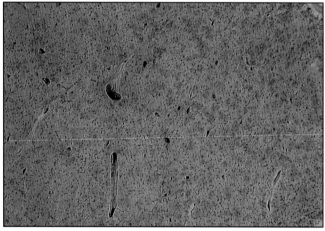

A

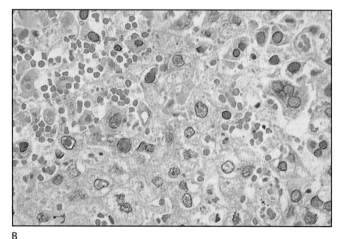

B

Fig. 9.4 • Herpes simplex. (A) Autopsy liver (fixed) of an HIV-positive child with disseminated herpes. The extensive, paler areas are necrotic, with adjacent congested liver. **(B)** At the edge of a necrotic zone, some hepatocytes are multinucleate and many nuclei contain eosinophilic viral inclusions. H&E.

disease is restricted to those patients who are immunocompromised, most often from cancer treated with chemotherapy. Rarely, steroid therapy given during the phases of viral dissemination may precipitate severe zoster.[20] In these severe infections there is focal or massive liver necrosis without much inflammation, similar to the lesions of herpes simplex infection. Intranuclear inclusions may be plentiful or scanty.

In herpetic lesions, electron microscopy shows abundant herpes virions. Immunocytochemistry is useful for confirming the presence of a herpes virus although, depending on the specificity of the antibodies used, it may not identify which one is present. Polymerase chain reaction analysis, even on formalin-fixed paraffin-embedded material, is highly sensitive and specific.

Cytomegalovirus

Most adult populations have a prevalence of latent, asymptomatic cytomegalovirus infection greater than 50%, as judged by serological surveys. Primary infection with clinical disease does occur in immunocompetent adults, but most significant cytomegalovirus disease occurs in the newborn or in the immunocompromised host. In renal transplant recipients, it is the commonest specific cause of hepatitis and, in liver transplant recipients, cytomegalovirus hepatitis needs to be distinguished from graft rejection.

In immunocompetent individuals, cytomegalovirus produces an infectious mononucleosis-like syndrome. Liver biopsy shows focal hepatocyte and bile duct damage with lymphocytic infiltration of sinusoids. In some cases, there are non-caseating epithelioid cell granulomas, but neither viral inclusions nor immunocytochemically demonstrable antigen are seen.[21,22]

Cytomegalovirus is a cause of neonatal hepatitis with giant cell transformation, cholestasis, inflammation and viral inclusions. The characteristic finding is an enlarged cell (endothelial, hepatocyte, or bile-duct epithelium) that contains basophilic granules in the cytoplasm and a swollen nucleus. An amphophilic intranuclear inclusion is surrounded by a clear halo, so that it resembles an owl's eye. Both the nuclear and cytoplasmic inclusions represent closely packed virions[23] (Fig. 9.5). Immunocytochemical staining for cytomegalovirus will highlight evident and ambiguous inclusions, but usually does not provide a positive signal if inclusions are absent on ordinary stains.

In immunocompromised hosts, cytomegalovirus inclusions are often seen without necrosis or inflammation—a 'passenger infection'—but when tissue damage is evident, the virus is presumed to be pathogenic. In the fetal liver, cytomegalovirus disease has been associated with obliteration of bile ducts.[24] The commonest predisposition to cytomegalovirus hepatitis at present is HIV infection.

Epstein–Barr virus

In the tropics, the Epstein–Barr virus is transmitted early in childhood and is aetiologically associated with Burkitt

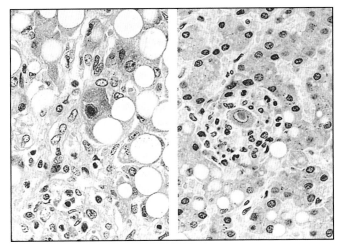

Fig. 9.5 • Cytomegalovirus infection. Two cytomegalovirus lesions with intranuclear inclusions, and no or little associated inflammation in the adjacent parenchyma. The basophilic material within the cytoplasm is also viral. H&E.

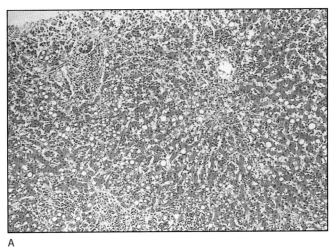

A

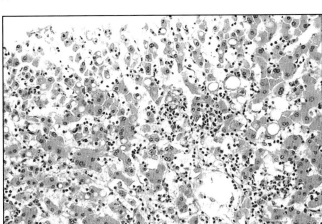

B

Fig. 9.6 • Epstein–Barr virus infection. (A) There is a diffuse portal tract and intra-acinar mononuclear cell infiltrate of the fatty liver; at a higher power (B) there is perivenular focal liver-cell necrosis and an intense intra-sinusoidal mononuclear cell infiltrate. H&E.

lymphoma. In industrialized countries, infection usually occurs in adolescence and causes infectious mononucleosis. Abnormal liver function tests indicate frequent hepatic involvement, but jaundice is rare.

The usual liver histopathology in infectious mononucleosis is of a diffuse lymphocytic infiltrate in the sinusoids.[25] When this is marked, focal apoptotic hepatocytes are seen.[26] The infiltrate—which is composed of infected B-lymphocytes, activated T-lymphocytes and natural killer cells—can be atypical and suggest leukaemia/lymphoma. Any part of the liver acinus is affected. Steatosis may occur but cholestasis is not a feature (Fig. 9.6). Non-necrotic tuberculoid granulomas are occasionally found in infectious mononucleosis.[27]

Immunosuppressed patients suffer from poly- and oligoclonal lymphoproliferative disease caused by EBV, the underlying predispositions including inherited, iatrogenic (post-transplantation) and HIV infection.[28] Patients with the X-linked lymphoproliferative syndrome are especially vulnerable to Epstein–Barr virus infection[29] and may suffer severe liver necrosis. In a fatal case, herpes-like viral intranuclear inclusions were seen.[30] Rarely, EBV causes the virus-associated haemophagocytic syndrome,[5] with macrophages in the sinusoids engulfing red blood cells. Apart from acute EBV infection per se, underlying causes include X-linked lymphoproliferative syndrome and T-cell lymphoma.

Human herpes virus-6 (HHV6)

This virus infects T-cells. Primary infection in children usually causes transient fever and skin rash (erythema subitum). Occasionally severe visceral infection, including hepatitis and haemophagocytic syndrome, can result. This can occur in transplant recipients and other immunosuppressed patients (including those with HIV/AIDS), and occasionally in normal persons. The histopathology is of a non-specific lobular hepatitis. In a heart transplant recipient, syncitial giant cell transformation of bile ductular epithelium is described.[31]

Other viruses

The adenovirus group

These DNA viruses usually affect the respiratory tract and conjunctiva. In children and in adults immunosuppressed because of HIV infection, severe combined immunodeficiency, haematological malignancy or organ transplantation, adenovirus may cause a severe hepatitis and liver failure.[32–34] The pathology is similar to that seen in herpes simplex infection. There are extensive areas of liver cell necrosis with little inflammation; intranuclear inclusions may be frequent (Fig. 9.7).

Enteroviruses

Group B Coxsackie virus infections can produce multisystem disease in neonates, including liver involvement, but in adults they are a rare cause of hepatitis.[35] The histopathology in neonates is of haemorrhagic necrosis. In adults, there is perivenular bile stasis and hydropic swelling of hepatocytes, accompanied by infiltration of mononuclear cells and polymorphs in sinusoids and portal tracts.

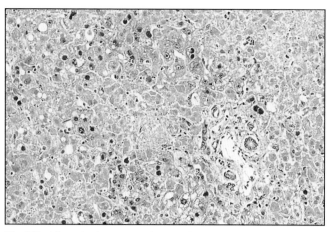

Fig. 9.7 • Adenovirus hepatitis. Widespread liver cell necrosis; irregular dark viral inclusions are seen in the nuclei of some surviving hepatocytes. H&E.

Measles (rubeola)

In children dying of measles, the liver usually shows non-specific features. There is frequently steatosis (especially when associated with malnutrition in the tropics), portal inflammation and focal necroses.[36] Viral inclusions and giant cells are rarely seen, but have been reported in a patient with immunoglobulin deficiency.[37] Inclusions are not present in the liver when measles is associated with HIV infection. Measles can also cause an acute hepatitis syndrome in adults.[38]

Rubella

Childhood rubella is not associated with liver disease. However, this virus can be associated with giant cell transformation in neonatal hepatitis. In mild cases, focal necroses, cholestasis and a lymphocytic infiltrate occur.[39] Rarely, there is massive necrosis.

Parvovirus

Human parvovirus (B19 virus) is the cause of erythema infectiosum in childhood. If a pregnant woman acquires the infection, it can be transmitted to the fetus and cause hydrops fetalis. Many fetal organs, including the liver, are damaged. There is excessive erythropoietic activity; erythroblasts and hepatocytes have eosinophilic nuclear inclusions as well as swollen hydropic nuclei.[40] In children, B19 virus is associated with acute hepatitis,[41] and also with fulminant liver failure at the time of liver transplantation.[42]

Coronavirus: severe acute respiratory syndrome (SARS)

Severe acute respiratory syndrome is caused by a novel coronavirus which mainly affects the lung and gastrointestinal system.[43] It emerged as a 'new' disease in 2002 and to date has caused the death of some 1000 patients in the Far East and Canada. The virus is detectable in the intestines and in over one-quarter of affected individuals there is derange-

ment of liver function tests.[44] Histopathological examination of the livers of such patients has shown marked apoptosis of hepatocytes and (presumably compensatory) mitotic activity.[45] There was also ballooning of hepatocytes and a lobular hepatitis. There is some evidence that co-infection with HBV infection may be associated with more severe respiratory disease[46] but this is disputed.[47]

Rickettsial and chlamydial infections

Rickettsiae are obligate intracellular parasites that contain both DNA and RNA. They are coccobacilli, 0.3 μm in size, and in human infection they are found in endothelial cells. Although mild derangement of liver function tests may occur in any of the rickettsial fevers, including typhus, clinical liver disease is seen in Q fever, Boutonneuse fever, Rocky Mountain spotted fever, and bacillary angiomatosis.

Q fever

Q fever, caused by *Coxiella burnettii*, exists as a zoonosis in domestic and other animals. Transmission to man is probably via inhalation, with a resulting rickettsaemia. Clinical presentations include pneumonia, hepatitis and fever of unknown origin. Liver function tests are usually abnormal. The typical microscopic hepatic lesions are intra-acinar granulomas.[48] These have a central fat vacuole, an intermediate ring of fibrin, and a peripheral rim of activated macrophages (Fig. 9.8). Non-vacuolated granulomas and tuberculoid granulomas with giant cells and central necrosis may also occur. Thus, the differential diagnosis on histology includes brucellosis and tuberculosis.

The fibrin-ring granuloma itself is not a lesion specific for Q fever. It is also seen in patients with lymphoma, staphylococcal bacteraemia, Epstein–Barr virus infection, cytomegalovirus infection, leishmaniasis, and allopurinol hypersensitivity.[49,50]

Boutonneuse fever

The tick-borne infection, *Rickettsia conorii*, occurs around the Mediterranean, in East and South Africa, and in India. Although it usually takes the form of a mild febrile disease, there is a fatality rate of up to 5%. The liver lesions have been described as granulomatous.[51] However, a series of biopsies taken from Boutonneuse fever patients without clinical hepatitis showed focal hepatocyte necrosis without granulomas, and a local lymphocytic infiltrate; the portal tracts were normal.[52] Immunocytochemical staining may reveal rickettsial antigen in endothelial cells lining the sinusoids.

Rocky Mountain spotted fever

The causative tick-borne infection, *Rickettsia rickettsii*, occurs in the Americas. Hepatitis is part of the Rocky Mountain spotted fever syndrome. As with *R. conorii* infection, the

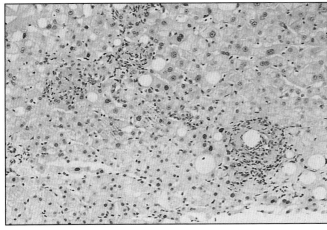

A

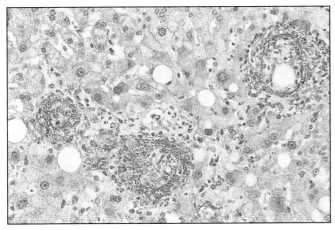

B

Fig. 9.8 • Liver biopsy from a patient with proven Q fever. **(A)** The granulomas have a central fatty vacuole and the surrounding macrophages are trapped in a mesh of fibrin, H&E; this is better seen on an MSB stain **(B)**.

primary target of infection is the endothelial cell. The portal tracts are inflamed, with mononuclear and polymorph perivascular inflammation, and vasculitis (predominantly mononuclear). Fibrin thrombi may form over damaged portal endothelial cells. Erythrophagocytosis by Kupffer cells may be prominent, but there is no significant hepatocyte necrosis or cholestasis.[53,54] Immunostaining demonstrates the rickettsial antigen within endothelial cells.

Chlamydia infection

Chlamydiae are obligate intracellular parasites that contain both RNA and DNA and have a characteristic life cycle with inclusion bodies. The liver is involved in two chlamydial diseases—psittacosis and genital infection.

Infection with *Chlamydia psittaci* causes pneumonia and systemic illness with hepatomegaly and sometimes jaundice. Focal hepatocyte necrosis and Kupffer cell hypertrophy have been described in autopsy material.[3] The intracellular inclusion bodies are difficult to identify even with a Giemsa stain. Genital tract infection with *Chlamydia trachomatis* causes salpingitis and may produce the Fitz–Hugh–Curtis syndrome of perihepatitis.[55]

Ehrlichiosis

Ehrlichiosis is a tick-borne zoonosis caused most frequently by *E.chaffeensis*, which is related to *Rickettsia*. Most cases are reported from the USA. The syndrome of human monocytic ehrlichiosis is a mild to severe febrile multi-system illness. The liver pathology has been described:[56] there is lobular hepatitis with variable hepatocyte injury and death, Kupffer cell hyperplasia, and cholestasis. With immunocytochemistry, the intracytoplasmic inclusion bodies may be seen in lobular or portal mononuclear cells, and in the peripheral blood monocytes.

Bacterial infections

Septicaemia and pyogenic liver abscess

Hepatomegaly and jaundice are commonly associated with septicaemia, i.e. bacteriaemia with clinical shock.[57] Various histological features may be seen depending on the aetiology and severity of the condition. Canalicular cholestasis is frequent, sometimes with inspissated bile in cholangioles ('ductular cholestasis'). This has been referred to as cholangitis lenta. Steatosis and perivenular ischaemic necrosis are non-specific but common. Microabscesses may occur in the parenchyma and contain visible bacteria.

Bacterial infection may reach the liver via the portal vein, the hepatic artery and the biliary tree. The first route is less common now in industrialized countries; the sources of sepsis are the appendix, colon and pancreas. This results in septic portal thrombophlebitis and hepatic abscesses. In some developing countries, a significant proportion of idiopathic splenomegaly has been attributed to a late complication of neonatal portal pyaemia and secondary splenic vein occlusion that originated from umbilical sepsis.[58]

Hepatic arterial spread of infection is common, but patients often succumb before visible abscesses can develop. One of the more frequent identifiable lesions is seen in staphylococcal sepsis: clusters of Gram-positive cocci are surrounded by necrosis and polymorphs. In chronic granulomatous disease (see Chapter 5), disseminated bacterial infection (commonly staphylococcal) also involves the liver;[59] portal macrophages with lipofuscin pigment, parenchymal necrotizing granulomas, and portal fibrosis are seen. In septicaemia due to *Neisseria gonorrhoeae*, jaundice is a common complication with focal necrosis and neutrophil infiltration in the liver. Liver tenderness described as perihepatitis can complicate pelvic infection by gonococci and *Chlamydia trachomatis* (the Fitz–Hugh–Curtis syndrome); it may simulate acute cholecystitis.[60,61] The liver parenchyma is normal in this condition, but the organisms can be isolated from the capsule.

Septicaemic plague, caused by *Yersinia pestis* (Gram-negative coccobacillus) is occasionally encountered at autopsy in developing countries; it is a highly virulent infection and stringent safety measures must be employed to ensure that material is not inhaled or inoculated accidentally into skin. The liver shows multiple necrotic foci with little inflammatory response, but they are packed with short Gram-negative rods.[62] *Yersinia enterocolitica* infection is more common, a global per-oral infection. It causes an enteritis and mesenteric adenitis with characteristic purulent granulomas, and can occasionally affect the liver. This is usually via a bacteriaemia. The liver lesions include granulomas[63] and large pyogenic abscesses. One point to note is the growth-potentiating role of iron for *Yersinia*: multiple liver abscesses have led to the diagnosis of underlying haemochromatosis.[64]

Spread of infection within the liver via the biliary tree follows an acute ascending cholangitis (see Fig. 9.62(a)). This often complicates large duct obstruction due to stones, but may follow suppurative cholecystitis, postoperative biliary strictures, acute or chronic pancreatitis, and tumours in the biliary tree or pancreas.

In many cases of pyogenic abscess, the origin of the infection is not obvious. Underlying causes include diabetes mellitus, perforated duodenal ulcer or diverticular disease. The commonest aetiological agents are *E. coli* and other coliforms, but anaerobes are reported with increasing frequency.[4,65] *Streptococcus milleri* is also common. The differential diagnosis of pyogenic liver abscess includes amoebiasis and several worm infections of the biliary tree that predispose to bacterial cholangitis (ascariasis, clonorchiasis and fascioliasis).

Typhoid fever, brucellosis, melioidosis and listeriosis

This group of infections has common clinicopathological features. They are intracellular parasites of macrophages, and all may cause granulomatous hepatitis.

Typhoid fever

Salmonella typhi is a Gram-negative bacillus. The classic clinicopathological phases of typhoid disease are incubation, active invasion (dissemination throughout the lymphoreticular system), fastigium, and lysis. During the phase of invasion, the liver shows a range of non-specific histological lesions: sinusoidal and portal lymphocytosis, focal parenchymal necrosis, and Kupffer cell hypertrophy, sometimes with erythrophagocytosis. Small macrophage clusters, which evolve into non-necrotizing epithelioid cell granulomas, are often seen. Microvesicular steatosis in hepatocytes is common. In the symptomatic phase of fastigium, there is hepatomegaly and sometimes jaundice. The granulomas in the liver enlarge and become necrotic, as they do in the lymph nodes of the bowel and mesentery (Fig. 9.9). There are no Langhans giant cells, and bacilli are very hard to detect with standard methods such as Gram stains. Although typhoid bacilli multiply readily in the bile and gallbladder, ascending cholangitis is rare.

Brucellosis

Brucellosis is a zoonosis of ruminants. Man may be infected by the Gram-negative bacilli *Brucella melitensis*, *B. abortus*, or

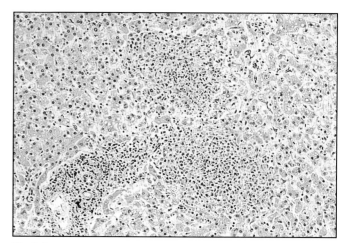

Fig. 9.9 • Typhoid fever. Autopsy liver showing portal and parenchymal granulomas. H&E.

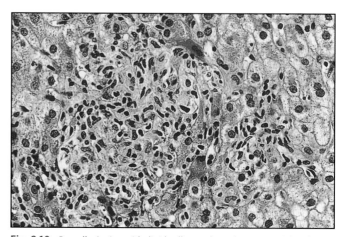

Fig. 9.10 • Brucellosis. An epithelioid cell granuloma (non-necrotic) within the liver parenchyma. In addition to tuberculosis and sarcoidosis, the presence of such granulomas should also prompt a suspicion of brucellosis. H&E.

B. suis, and infection comes through occupational exposure or ingestion of milk products. The clinical manifestations are protean—brucellosis is a great mimic. Three main patterns occur, all including fever and weakness: acute, recurrent, and chronic. In all, there is haematogenous dissemination of bacteria to all lymphoreticular organs, including the liver. Hepatomegaly and altered liver function tests are common. Histological examination shows a non-specific reactive hepatitis, microgranulomas, or epithelioid cell granulomas (Fig. 9.10). The latter may have giant cells and, in the chronic pattern of brucellosis, there may be fibrinoid necrosis, rendering the histological appearances indistinguishable from tuberculosis or histoplasmosis. Patients with large caseous granulomas (coin lesions) in the liver have been reported.[66] When granulomatous hepatitis without evident cause is encountered in biopsy material, brucellosis should always be considered.[67] Serology is the means of establishing the diagnosis.

Melioidosis

Disease due to the Gram-negative bacillus *Burkholderia (ex-Pseudomonas) pseudomallei* is endemic in South-East Asia and the Indian sub-continent, and sporadic cases occur in other parts of the tropics and sub-tropics (although not in Africa).[68] The organism is a saprophyte of soil and water. Clinically, it presents as acute pulmonary, septicaemic, or chronic suppurative disease. The acute infections are rapid and have high mortality. Hepatomegaly and jaundice are complications. The histopathology of the liver in acute melioidosis includes small and large abscesses, in which the rods may be seen on a Gram or Giemsa stain. In the chronic form of the disease, there are necrotic granulomas. These may mimic tuberculosis, or be stellate in form, resembling cat-scratch disease. Bacteria are rarely seen.[69]

Listeriosis

Listeria monocytogenes is a Gram-positive bacillus that is saprophytic in soil and water. It may be transmitted to man through soft cheeses. Disease occurs in pregnant women and their infants via the transplacental route, in immunosuppressed patients and, less commonly, in immunocompetent individuals. HIV infection does not play a predisposing role. The clinical disease in neonates is septicaemia with multiple organ lesions. The liver shows miliary microabscesses that contain abundant Gram-positive rods (Fig. 9.11). In routine sections, this may resemble acute neonatal syphilis. In adults with listeriosis, the clinical picture can mimic viral hepatitis, though microabscesses with bacilli are common and some patients have a granulomatous hepatitis.[70]

Cat-scratch disease and peliosis (Bartonella infection)

Advances in bacterial taxonomy have clarified and unified a complex group of unusual diseases. *Bartonella henselae* and, less commonly, *B. quintana* are the agents causing cat-scratch disease, bacillary peliosis (including peliosis), and bacillary angiomatosis, as well as trench foot and some cases of endocarditis.[71]

Although most cases of cat-scratch disease manifest only as a skin lesion and local lymphadenopathy, dissemination to the viscera, including the liver, occurs in a small proportion.[72] Occasionally this can occur without lymphadenopathy.[73] Clinically, disseminated cat-scratch disease is an illness presenting in children as fever with tender hepatosplenomegaly. The liver lesions have the same histological features as the typical lymph node: stellate microabscesses with a granulomatous border. With a Warthin–Starry stain, extracellular clumps of short Gram-negative bacilli may be demonstrated at the edges of the necrosis.

Peliosis hepatis (see below, Fig. 9.56) occurs mainly in immunocompromised patients (e.g. HIV/AIDS) and in many cases is due to *Bartonella* infection. It also may develop in transplant patients on immunosuppressive drugs.[74]

Actinomycete infections

Most cases of actinomycosis in man are caused by *Actinomyces israelii*, a globally distributed soil organism. Actinomycosis

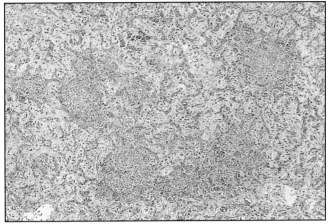

A

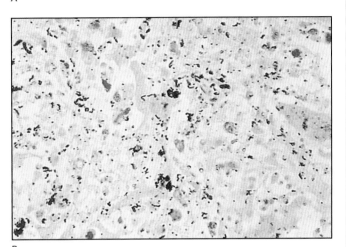

B

Fig. 9.11 • Listeriosis. **(A)** Necrotic granulomas in the parenchyma. H&E. **(B)** Gram stain shows abundant Gram-positive bacilli.

of the liver is usually secondary to intra-abdominal or thoracic infection, the bacilli reaching the liver by direct extension or via the portal vein.[75] The latter follows caecal or appendiceal infection. Occasionally an apparently primary hepatic lesion is seen,[76] which presents clinically as other liver abscesses. Grossly, there is usually a honeycomb of confluent small abscesses, containing greenish pus. Microscopically, amidst the acute inflammation there are grains (colonies) of *Actinomyces*, which are basophilic in H&E-stained sections. These are composed of closely packed, radiating, Gram-positive bacilli, 1 μm across, which can be impregnated with silver by the Grocott method (Fig. 9.12). There is often a fibrinoid Hoeppli–Splendore reaction at the perimeter. These abscesses may rupture, forming sinuses into the retroperitoneum.

A related infection, *Nocardia brasiliensis* or *asteroides*, may also spread to the liver as part of haematogenous dissemination. *N. asteroides* is usually an opportunistic infection in immunosuppressed individuals (due to transplantation or HIV infection). The bacilli within the abscess may form grain-like colonies or be more diffusely spread (Fig. 9.13). They are also Gram-positive and beaded, and are silver-positive on Grocott stains but, unlike *Actinomyces*, they are weakly acid-fast, staining well with a Wade–Fite method.[77]

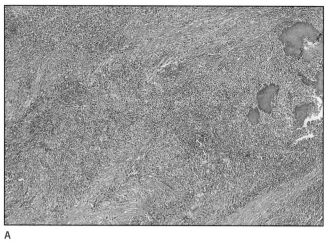

A

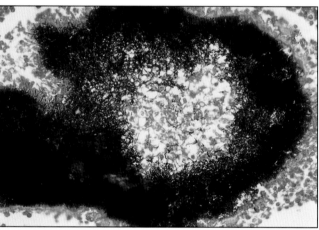

B

Fig. 9.12 • Actinomycosis. **(A)** Liver abscess with bacterial colonies in the purulent inflammation. H&E. **(B)** Silver stain shows fine brancing bacilli within the colony.

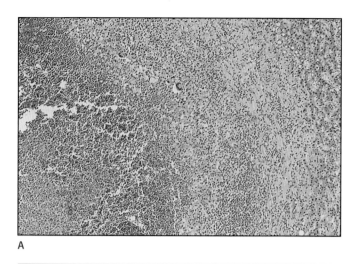

A

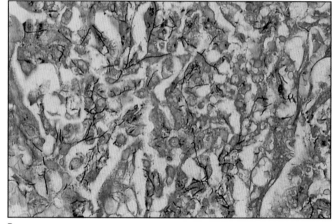

B

Fig. 9.13 • Nocardiosis. **(A)** Edge of a liver abscess with a purulent centre and a granulomatous border. Note the giant cell. H&E. **(B)** Clusters of thin branching filaments of *N. asteroides* within the abscess. Grocott stain.

Spirochaete infections

Syphilis (Treponema pallidum)

Congenital syphilis often manifests early as intra-uterine death or infantile disease, both with hepatosplenomegaly. In the earlier phases there may be miliary necroses, portal inflammation and hepatocyte giant cell transformation. In neonatal deaths, the degree of persistent haemopoiesis is excessive for gestational age. The Warthin–Starry stain demonstrates large numbers of spirochaetes, particularly when there is necrosis. Later, the liver shows a characteristic progressive pericellular fibrosis with apparent withering of the liver-cell plates (Fig. 9.14).[78]

Primary syphilis has no notable liver histology, but in the secondary phase there is focal hepatocyte necrosis, portal inflammation with numerous polymorphs around bile ductules, and sometimes granulomas. The portal vessels may show vasculitis.[79,80] Spirochaetes are less often seen compared with congenital lesions. The lesion of tertiary disease is the gumma. In the liver these are single or multiple, ranging in size from millimetres to centimetres. They are tuberculoid giant cell granulomas with amorphous pale

necrotic centres, mimicking caseation, although the classic description emphasizes the preservation of cellular architecture within the necrotic zone. Accompanying this are plasma cells and endarteritis obliterans. Healing is by fibrosis and broad bands of scarring which may distort the liver to produce 'hepar lobatum'.

Relapsing fever (borreliosis)

Relapsing fever may be louse- or tick-borne and is caused by many *Borrelia* spp. The louse-borne infection is due to *B. recurrentis*. Most infections occur in East Africa. As the name suggests, it presents as periodic fever lasting a week and recurring another week or so later. The diagnosis is made by finding the spirochaetes in peripheral blood smears.

In severe infections, jaundice and hepatosplenomegaly occur. In fatal cases an enlarged, congested liver is seen. There are foci of hepatocyte necrosis with surrounding haemorrhage in acinar zones 2 and 3. The sinusoids are infiltrated by lymphocytes and polymorphs, which are associated with Kupffer cell hypertrophy and erythrophagocytosis.[81] Warthin–Starry or Dieterle stains may reveal the 10–20 μm long spirochaetes lying free in the sinusoids.

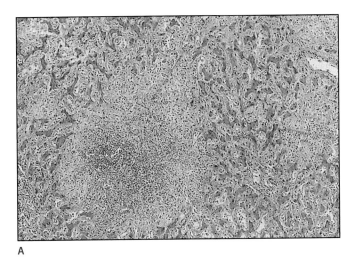

A

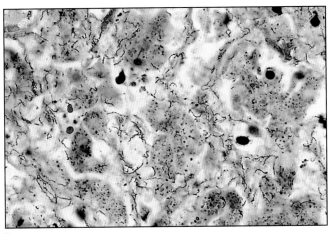

B

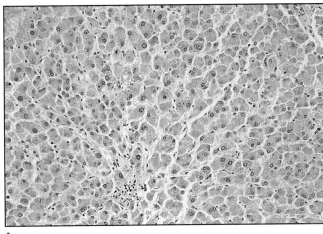

A

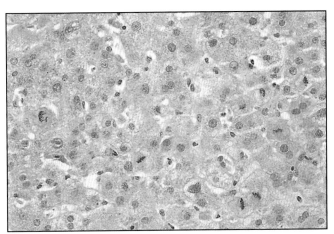

B

Fig. 9.14 • Congenital syphilis. **(A)** Liver showing both a focal necrotic and inflammatory lesion, and the typical diffuse sinusoidal fibrosis with attenuation of the liver plates. H&E. **(B)** The focal lesion contains abundant silver-positive spirochaetes. Warthin–Starry stain.

Leptospirosis (Weil disease)

Leptospirosis is a zoonosis of rats, dogs and pigs. The agent, *Leptospira icterohaemorrhagica*, is ubiquitous in wet environments, and man acquires the infection via water contaminated with animal urine. The clinical features are fever with jaundice and renal failure, and bleeding into conjunctiva, skin and viscera. Hepatomegaly is often present. The haemorrhagic phenomena are not due to liver failure, but to direct damage to small vessels by leptospirae. With appropriate therapy, mortality is now low.

At autopsy the liver may be normal or enlarged and icteric. The major histological features are individual hepatocyte damage, regeneration, canalicular cholestasis, and only slight portal or sinusoidal lymphocytosis. Ballooning and hydropic change of hepatocytes is less marked than that seen in viral hepatitis; apoptotic bodies are the more prominent evidence of liver damage. Many liver cells are binucleate and show mitoses; variation in size is a further indication of regenerative activity. Autopsy material shows dissociation and separation of liver-cell plates, but biopsy samples have intact plates, so the separation is probably a post-mortem artefact (Fig. 9.15). Kupffer cells are hyper-

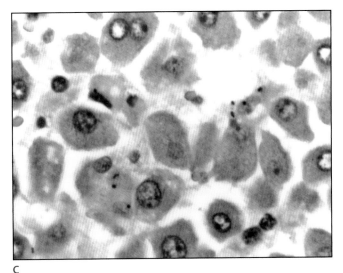

C

Fig. 9.15 • Leptospirosis. **(A)** Autopsy liver: the liver cells appear dissociated and there is cholestasis. H&E. Slide courtesy of Dr C Corbett, Brazil. **(B)** Liver biopsy: no dissociation of liver cells is seen but there are numerous mitoses. H&E. **(C)** Immununocytochemical stain showing scanty leptospiral antigen in Kupfer cells. Photograph courtesy of Dr S Zaki, CDC, Atlanta.

trophied and contain erythrocytes. In a proportion of cases, a Warthin–Starry stain shows the spirochaetes, which are 10–20 μm long. Immunocytochemical staining with specific polyclonal antibodies can demonstrate leptospiral antigen in Kupffer cells, portal tracts and endothelium.[82,83]

Lyme disease

Lyme disease is a multisystem infection caused by *Borrelia burgdorferi*. It is tick-borne and occurs throughout the world. It has acute and chronic clinical patterns, and the liver may be involved in both. Hepatomegaly and abnormal liver function tests, associated with portal tract inflammation on biopsy, are noted in the acute disease. Recurrent Lyme disease may cause a more marked hepatitis, with ballooned hepatocytes, mitotic activity, microvesicular steatosis, Kupffer cell hyperplasia, and sinusoidal infiltration by lymphocytes and polymorphs. On Warthin–Starry or Dieterle silver stains, the spirochaetes can be seen in the sinusoids and in liver cells.[84,85]

Mycobacterial infections

Of the 50-odd mycobacterial species, *M. tuberculosis* and *M. leprae* are the most frequent causes of disease in man. However, the advent of the HIV pandemic has highlighted the predisposition of immunosuppressed people to develop other mycobacterioses, particularly of the *M. avium* complex.

Tuberculosis

One third of the global population are infected with *M. tuberculosis*, generating more than 8 million cases per annum and about 2 million deaths (current data from the WHO website: www.who.org). Factors leading to the present re-emergence of tuberculosis as a global medical problem include HIV infection, poor case management and relapse, migration and refugees, and drug resistance. Since this organism is a parasite of macrophages, the liver is frequently involved. There are broadly four patterns of hepatic tuberculosis as outlined below.

Primary tuberculosis

During the primary infection, whether it be in lung or intestine, the liver is involved if there is haematogenous dissemination leading to miliary tuberculosis. Hepatomegaly is common but jaundice is unusual. In rare cases of congenital tuberculosis, the infection is transmitted via the umbilical vein and the liver is the most severely affected organ. At autopsy or on liver biopsy, there is a range of histological appearances. The classic pattern is of miliary portal and parenchymal tubercles composed of epithelioid cells and a Langhans giant cell. There may or may not be central fibrinoid necrosis, and acid-fast bacilli are often scanty or absent on Ziehl–Neelsen stain. In severe cases, the tubercles are of the 'soft' type. These are immature granulomas with much central fibrinoid necrosis, no giant cells and numerous acid-fast bacilli.[86] Rarely, a tuberculoma may form; this is a solitary caseating mass measuring up to several centimetres in size. Microscopy shows the classic giant cell granuloma pattern at the border, with scanty acid-fast bacilli.

Congenital tuberculosis

This is the rarest form of tuberculosis. The liver is the first organ infected as organisms come from the infected placenta via the umbilical vein. The appearance is of miliary tuberculosis and the necrotic lesions are generally 'soft' and anergic and contain abundant acid-fast bacilli.[87] This may be found as a cause of hydrops fetalis and intra-uterine death at autopsy.

Post-primary tuberculosis

This, the commonest manifestation of tuberculosis, is a pulmonary disease and is usually considered to arise from reactivation of previous infection. Bacilli (or antigen) are shed into the blood stream, and in many organs including the liver, granulomas are found. These are usually of the 'hard' non-necrotic type, with epithelioid and giant cells. Acid-fast bacilli are demonstrated infrequently.[86]

Anergic (immunosuppressed, non-reactive) tuberculosis

Patients with primary or reactivated tuberculosis who are immunocompromised often manifest a non-specific disease with wasting, termed 'cryptic tuberculosis'.[88] The underlying causes range from old age and immunosuppressive chemotherapy to leukaemia and HIV infection. Multiple organs, including the liver, show miliary necrotic lesions 1–2 mm in diameter (see Fig. 9.53). Histological examination shows a rim of unactivated macrophages with clear cytoplasm (hydropic swelling) surrounding a necrotic centre with much haematoxyphilic debris. Enormous numbers of acid-fast bacilli are characteristic in these lesions (Fig. 9.16).

Leprosy (Hansen disease)

Leprosy as a clinical disease affects some 10 million people, mainly in the tropics and subtropics. However, significant involvement of the liver is uncommon and is mainly due to drug reactions and amyloidosis.

Systematic studies of large numbers of leprosy patients show that about 20% of those with paucibacillary (tuberculoid) disease have liver lesions, rising to about 60% of those with multibacillary (lepromatous) disease.[89] Abnormalities of liver function tests are mild. Histological examination reveals good correlation between the patterns of skin and liver lesions. In the liver of paucibacillary leprosy patients, there are tuberculoid granulomas with few or no acid-fast bacilli. Conversely, lepromatous patients have foamy macrophage aggregates (Virchow cells) with acid-fast bacilli, distributed randomly within the acinus or near the portal tracts (Fig. 9.17). Such patients may also have acid-fast bacilli in Kupffer cells: this is a result of mycobacteraemia that may reach 10^5 bacilli per ml of blood.[90] It is possible that the liver is a source of bacilli in cases of relapse.

Occasionally, multibacillary patients undergoing the leprosy reaction of erythema nodosum leprosum are jaundiced and have hepatomegaly. These lepromatous hepatic

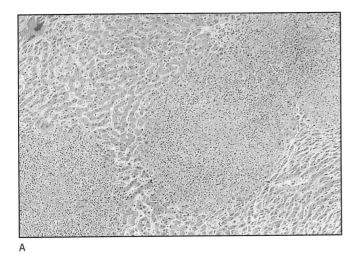

A

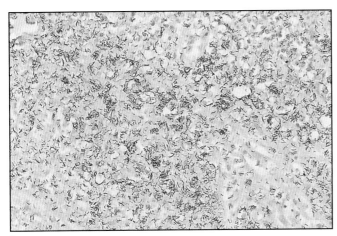

B

Fig. 9.16 • Tuberculosis (anergic). **(A)** Multiple necrotic lesions within the parenchyma; these are not true granulomas, being composed of 'non-activated' hydropic and dead macrophages. H&E. **(B)** Ziehl–Neelsen stain of same liver, showing vast numbers of extra cellular acid-fast bacilli.

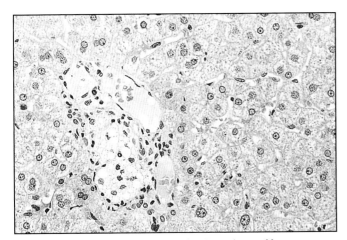

Fig. 9.17 • Lepromatous leprosy. Biopsy showing a cluster of foamy macrophages. On Wade–Fite stain, these contained degenerate acid-fast bacilli. H&E.

lesions are accompanied by neutrophil polymorph infiltrates, as in the skin lesions of such patients.[91]

The incidence of systemic amyloidosis in leprosy varies widely, depending on geography, and thus host factors.[92] The liver is usually affected.[93] Drug reactions may occur

Table 9.2	Liver disease caused by non-tuberculosis, non-leprosy mycobacterial infections
Species	**Reference**
BCG	94
M. avium complex	95, 96
M. bovis	97
M. chelonei	98
M. fortuitum	99–101
M. gordonae	102
M. kansasii	100–105
M. scrofulaceum	104, 106
M. simiae	107
M. terrae	108
M. xenopi	109, 110

with rifampicin (see Chapter 14), the main potentially hepatotoxic drug that patients with leprosy receive.

Other mycobacterioses

Many other mycobacteria cause disease in man, especially when the subject is immunocompromised: the predispositions include congenital immunodeficiency states, chronic granulomatous disease, HIV infection, myeloid and hairy cell leukaemias, pancytopenia, steroid and cytotoxic therapy, alcoholism and old age.[87] Systemic infection often involves the liver as a lymphoreticular organ, and unexplained hepatomegaly may be a presenting feature. The mycobacteria known to cause hepatic lesions are listed in Table 9.2.[94–110]

The pathologies of these mycobacterioses vary widely according to the species of infection and the underlying state of the host. At one end of a spectrum, immunological responses result in epithelioid cell granulomas with or without giant cells, with few or no acid-fast bacilli evident on Ziehl–Neelsen stains, and necrosis (caseating or often admixed with a neutrophil infiltrate). At the anergic end of the spectrum, the more virulent mycobacteria (e.g. *M. kansasii*) produce parenchymal necrosis with no granulomatous reaction and numerous acid-fast bacilli, whilst the less virulent infections (e.g. *M. avium* and BCG) result in nodules of histiocytic cells in the sinusoids and parenchyma. Here, the macrophages are stuffed with acid-fast bacilli (see Fig. 9.55).

Mycotic infections

The liver is involved in many fungal infections as part of haematogenous dissemination. With the exception of candidiasis and zygomycosis, these organisms enter the body by inhalation. They produce a primary lesion in the lung, with contemporary or later spread to other organs: the sequence is similar to that of tuberculosis. Significant visceral disease, including liver involvement, is often precipitated by immunosuppression.

Identification of the fungus on histological examination alone is usually possible from the size and morphology of the yeasts or the hyphae. Some fungi—the commonest of which is Candida—manifest both forms within a lesion. The special stains of Grocott or PAS are helpful in clarifying the morphology of fungi in tissues. Sometimes (particularly with yeast forms), this is misleadingly atypical in size or shape. Culture of tissue or blood, serological techniques and detection of specific fungal antigenaemia are aids to speciation. Immunocytochemical techniques using antibodies and lectins can identify fungi in sections, but are of limited availability. A comprehensive atlas of the clinical pathology of mycoses has been produced by Chandler et al.[77]

Aspergillosis

Aspergilli are abundant in the environment and cause a wide range of diseases. Disseminated infection that involves the liver is opportunistic and the host is debilitated by malignancy (typically leukaemia), immunosuppressive therapy, steroids and antibiotics. Hepatic failure is also a predisposing cause.[111] The commonest agents are *Aspergillus fumigatus* and *flavus*. The liver is affected in about one-fifth of such cases. Macroscopically, in severe cases there are multiple foci of haemorrhagic necrosis. Microscopically, the hyphae are seen to penetrate blood vessel walls and produce thrombosis and infarction. The hyphae are basophilic, 3–6 μm in diameter, septate, and branch regularly at a 45° angle. In less fulminant cases, there are chronic inflammatory lesions of granulomas with purulent centres (as with candidiasis): the hyphae are more scanty, may appear less regular, and may not branch (Fig. 9.18).

Candidiasis

Candida infection is global. *C. albicans* is the most frequent species, being a commensal organism in the mouth and intestine of most healthy individuals. Liver infection is usually encountered in neonates and in the immunocompromised host, such as leukaemic patients with low blood neutrophil counts. Occasionally it occurs in pregnant women and as a result of hyperalimentation. Multiple portal and periportal chronic abscesses form, sometimes with granulomas. The yeasts and hyphae may be plentiful or scanty (Fig. 9.19). This infection is very hard to eliminate, and persistent lesions can induce considerable scarring.

Cryptococcosis

Cryptococcus neoformans is also distributed globally. Clinical disease is usually a meningo-encephalitis or pneumonia, and the liver is involved during dissemination in an immunosuppressed host. Previously the usual association was

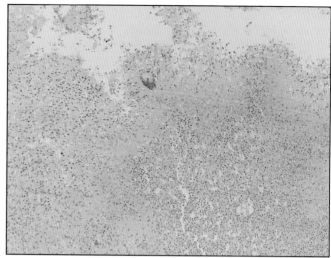

A

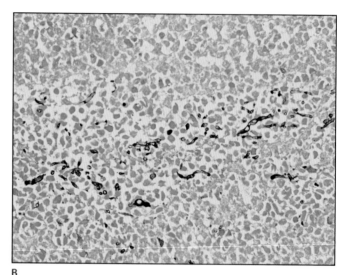

B

Fig. 9.18 • Aspergillosis. **(A)** Mixed acute and granulomatous inflammation with necrosis. The fungi are not visible. H&E. **(B)** distorted fungal hyphae of *Aspergillus*. Grocott silver stain.

chemotherapy for lymphoma, but HIV-associated opportunism is now more important. Macroscopically, liver cryptococcosis is usually unremarkable. Rarely, there are multiple foci of necrosis,[112] and occasionally the extrahepatic biliary tree is involved, mimicking sclerosing cholangitis.[113] The fungal yeasts have a wide range of size, from 5 to 20 μm, relatively thin walls, and are usually encapsulated. This characteristic thick mucoid capsule appears as an empty space on H&E, PAS and Grocott stains, and is best shown with a mucicarmine stain (or by dark-ground illumination in cerebrospinal fluid). Sometimes the yeasts are small and non-encapsulated, in which case the distinction from histoplasmosis can be made only on culture or by specific immunostaining. The usual host reaction is single or multiple budding yeasts engulfed by Kupffer cells in the sinusoids or by portal macrophages, with minimal accompanying lymphocytic inflammation (Fig. 9.20).

Sometimes, epithelioid cell granulomas develop and large multinucleate giant cells may be seen containing many yeasts.

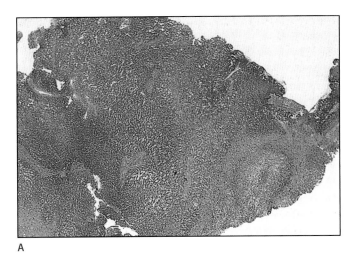

A

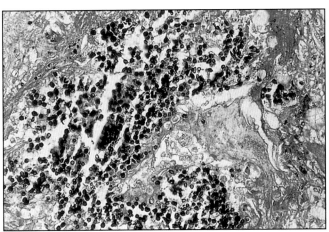

B

Fig. 9.19 • Candidiasis associated with leukaemia. **(A)** Low-power view of liver with a focal inflammatory lesion surrounded by fibrosis. H&E. **(B)** Multiple small budding yeasts within the inflammation. Grocott stain.

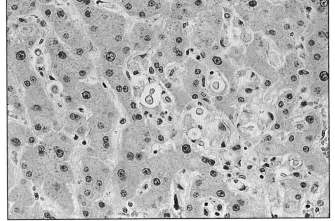

Fig. 9.20 • Cryptococcosis. Sinusoids infiltrated by yeasts. The central one is budding. They have thick walls and all show an apparently empty rim which is the mucoid capsule. H&E.

Histoplasmosis

There are two organisms causing histoplasmosis. *Histoplasma capsulatum* is found in most parts of the world; *H. duboisii* is restricted to Africa. In some zones endemic for *H. capsulatum*, such as the southern USA, infection is almost

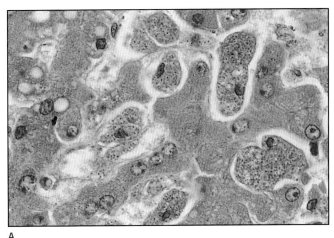

A

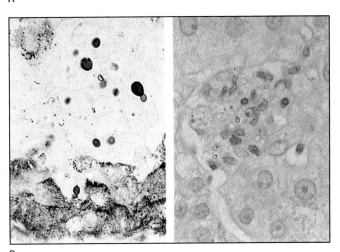

B

Fig. 9.21 • Histoplasmosis capsulatum. **(A)** Kupffer cells contain abundant yeasts, with purple nuclei. The yeasts are about the same size as *Leishmania amastigotes*, but the latter have a smaller nucleus. H&E. **(B)** In a case with granulomas and fewer organisms, special stains highlight the *H. capsulatum*: right—PAS stain emphasizes the cell membrane and the nucleus; left—Grocott silver stain shows a budding yeast.

universal. The various clinico-pathological patterns of histoplasmosis (analogous to tuberculosis) have been described.[114] Disseminated infection is usually associated with deficient cell-mediated immunity, of which the commonest cause is now HIV infection, or with age over 50 years.[115] Histoplasmosis is a classic example of an infection that may lie latent in the body for decades after primary infection, becoming manifest if host defences decline, and causing diagnostic confusion in non-endemic countries if a travel history is not sought.

The liver in histoplasmosis is usually enlarged. The yeast forms are 3–4 µm across and parasitize Kupffer cells and portal macrophages (Figs 9.21 and 9.57). They may be seen budding and in chains, and are best visualized with a Grocott silver stain. Various histological patterns are seen: diffuse or focal parasitization of sinusoidal Kupffer cells or the formation of small tuberculoid granulomas with fewer yeasts. Rarely, a large 'histoplasmoma' forms, consisting of a central fibronecrotic mass, often calcified and containing variable numbers of yeasts, which is surrounded by a granulomatous rim. The yeasts are refractile and have an amphophilic central nucleus, yet can resemble amastigotes of leishmaniasis on H&E stains. However, the latter possess a kinetoplast and are negative with fungal special stains. On Grocott silver stains, the fungi may also resemble cysts of *Pneumocystis carinii*, but the latter appear as an extracellular honeycomb agglomeration, the cysts do not bud, and they often appear crenated.

H. duboisii rarely involves the liver. The yeasts are larger, 10–15 µm in diameter, and similar to *Blastomyces*. They are usually contained within macrophages of giant cell granulomas.

Blastomycosis (North American)

Blastomyces dermatitidis infection occurs in the Americas, Africa and Israel. Liver lesions are incidental to widespread dissemination and take the form of miliary nodules. The histological reaction shows a range from purulent abscesses to chronic granulomas, or a mixture of the two. Yeasts may be seen surrounded by polymorphs; in the granulomatous pattern they may be inside or outside epithelioid cells and giant cells. The fungi are 6–15 µm diameter yeasts with a thick refractile cell wall (Fig. 9.22). They bud with a distinctively broad base, but in histological sections they may resemble *Cryptococcus* or *H. duboisii*.

Paracoccidioidomycosis (South American blastomycosis)

In rural areas of South America, infection with *Paracoccidioides brasiliensis* is endemic. Systemic infection follows from pulmonary disease. In the liver there are miliary nodules related to portal tracts.[116] The host cell reaction is similar to that of blastomycosis. A variable amount of portal fibrosis is seen. The morphology is characteristic: the round to oval amphophilic yeasts are 5–60 µm in diameter and show small peripheral buds that resemble a ship's steering wheel.

Coccidioidomycosis

The agent *Coccidioides immitis* is restricted to the southern USA and Central and South America. Pulmonary disease is

the commonest manifestation but, like tuberculosis, it may disseminate to viscera, including the liver. The pleomorphic host reaction is like that in blastomycosis. The fungi are large spherules ranging in size from 20 to 200 µm in diameter and contain endospores.[3,77]

Penicilliosis

Infection with *Penicillium marneffei* is endemic in South-East Asia. Clinically it presents much like disseminated tuberculosis. All parts of the lymphoreticular system are involved, including the liver and spleen.[117] The host inflammatory reaction varies from tuberculoid granulomas, with or without suppuration, to a diffuse histiocytosis. Like *H. capsulatum*, which it closely resembles, *P. marneffei* is an intracellular macrophage infection. The yeasts are ovoid, 5 × 2 µm in size, do not bud but multiply by schizogony, and have a prominent septum which distinguishes them from histoplasmosis. Tubular forms are also seen (Fig. 9.23).

Zygomycosis

This group of diseases, which includes mucormycosis and phycomycosis, is caused by several fungal genera such as

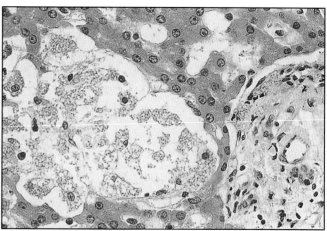

A

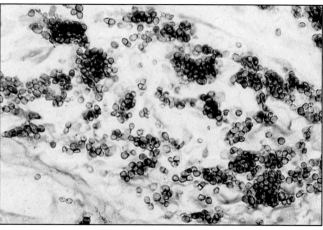

B

Fig. 9.23 • Penicilliosis. **(A)** Small yeasts filling the Kupffer cells and expanding the sinusoids. H&E. **(B)** Grocott silver stain shows the yeasts: they are similar in size to *H. capsulatum*, but some show characteristic transverse septae. Slides courtesy of Dr W Tsui, Hong Kong.

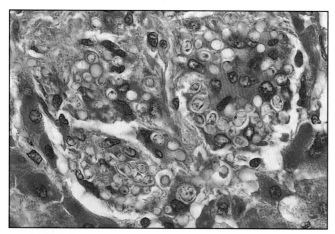

Fig. 9.22 • Blastomycosis. A giant cell granuloma containing abundant large yeasts with prominent nuclear material. H&E.

Rhizopus, Mucor and *Absidia*. They share a characteristic morphology: broad, branching hyphae, 6–25 μm in diameter with few or no septae. The fungi are ubiquitous and cause opportunistic, disseminated disease when the host is immunocompromised, usually from haematological malignancy or transplantation.[118] Liver involvement, as seen at autopsy, may show multiple, necrotic, 1 cm diameter nodules. Histologically, there is coagulative necrosis infiltrated by hyphae. This pattern of widespread vascular invasion with ischaemic necrosis is similar to that seen in aspergillosis, but the hyphae in the latter infection are narrower and septate.

Protozoal infections

Malaria

Clinical and epidemiological features
The *P. falciparum* parasite—clinically the most important malarial species—continues to infect more than 1 billion people in Africa, Asia and South America, and in many African countries it is a major cause of childhood mortality. Chronologically, there are three phases to malaria in endemic areas:

1. Up to three months of age, children are protected by maternal antibodies.
2. Thereafter, repeated attacks of acute malaria occur, which may be fatal, until immunity is acquired in survivors by late childhood.
3. Adults maintain immunity by repeated clinically silent infections. This immunity may be broken in women by pregnancy, and in anyone who leaves an endemic zone. A few adults go on to develop the 'tropical splenomegaly syndrome'.

Thus, clinical malaria is encountered in children and pregnant women; in adults who have lost acquired immunity by emigration and have been reinfected; and in non-immune travellers to endemic malarial areas. HIV infection does not influence the prevalence or severity of falciparum malaria.[119] In malaria, death from hepatic failure that is directly due to plasmodial infection does not occur. Nonetheless, many liver-related phenomena may develop: jaundice, hepatomegaly, hypoglycaemia, low serum albumin, prolonged prothrombin time, and mildly elevated transaminases.[120]

Pathology
The initial phase of infection after a mosquito bite requires multiplication in the liver. Schizonts develop within hepatocytes and then seed into the blood. There are no clinical sequelae until the erythrocytic part of the life cycle with consequent haemolysis commences.

The gross appearance of the liver at autopsy in severe malaria is of an enlarged, congested dark brown or grey organ, the colour being due to pigment deposition (Fig. 9.24). This colour may be mimicked by severe acute schis-

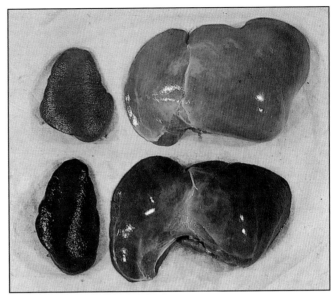

Fig. 9.24 • Malaria. Pairs of liver and spleen from autopsied young children, one of whom died of malaria. The lower set is dark brown owing to the haemozoin pigment of malaria.

tosomiasis and by dissemination of gas-producing Gram-negative bacilli after death.

Microscopically, in the liver as in other organs of the mononuclear phagocyte system, the striking feature is the accumulation of malarial pigment, *haemozoin*. It is seen as small dark-brown dots in parasitized erythrocytes and as larger lumps within macrophages. In acute attacks, the pigment accumulates in Kupffer cells, which are increased in number and size. When parasitaemia subsides, the pigment shifts to portal tract macrophages and is eventually cleared. The sinusoids are usually distended by erythrocytes. Parasites are visible in them as faint, clear rings with a haematoxyphilic dot, the nucleus (Fig. 9.25), but they are often obscured by the pigment. The hepatocytes may show steatosis (a non-specific product of anaemia and infection) but in most cases are otherwise unaffected. A mild portal lymphocytosis and plasmacytosis are often present.[121]

The old-fashioned clinical entity 'malarial hepatitis' does not exist. Significant clinico-biochemical liver damage is associated with shock in severe malaria; histopathologically there is perivenular ischaemic necrosis and sometimes cholestasis.[122] The hypoglycaemic state—mainly seen in African children and adult pregnant women[120]—has its histological counterpart in a complete absence of glycogen in hepatocytes. Electron microscopic studies of the liver in malaria have shown mitochondrial damage, and swelling and loss of microvilli: these are secondary non-specific effects of shock.[123]

Pathogenesis
Haemozoin is an iron porphyrin proteinoid complex formed by the parasite from the breakdown of haemoglobin. It does not react with Prussian blue stain and can be removed from tissue sections by a saturated alcoholic solution of picric acid. Haemozoin is birefringent under polarized light in a

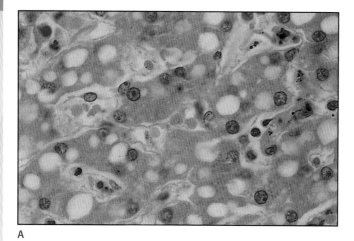

A

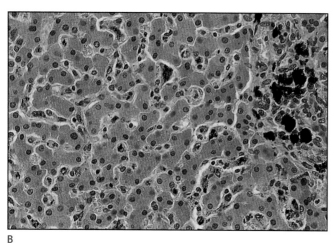

B

Fig. 9.25 • Malaria. **(A)** Acute falciparum malaria with some fatty change; haemozoin pigment is in Kupffer cells, and two erythrocytes (centre, top) contain falciparum ring forms. H&E. **(B)** Acute falciparum malaria showing large clumps of haemozoin in portal tract macrophages and Kupffer cells. H&E.

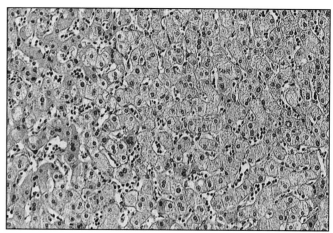

Fig. 9.26 • 'Tropical splenomegaly syndrome'. Liver sinusoids contain numerous reactive T-lymphocytes. Note the absence of haemozoin pigment. H&E.

red–yellow colour. It is to be distinguished from porphyria pigment, which is darker red in polarized light and is seen in hepatocytes and ductules. It is ordinarily indistinguishable from schistosomal haemozoin pigment, but differences are revealed by electron microscopy and biochemical methods.[124] There is evidence that the haemozoin in macrophages compromises their functions of phagocytosis and cell-mediated immunity.[125]

The jaundice of malaria is mainly haemolytic, as erythrocytes rupture and the merozoites are released. The mechanisms causing the shock state of severe malaria and the uncommon hepatic necrosis and cholestasis are uncertain.[120] They include sequestration of parasitized erythrocytes in the splanchnic vasculature with subsequent hypoperfusion, endotoxaemia, and elevated production of tumour necrosis factor.

'Tropical splenomegaly syndrome'

In malarial areas, chronic splenomegaly has many causes, but a syndrome of 'big spleen disease' in adults, without evident cause, has long been recognized. In such cases the spleen may weigh 2–4 kg. The splenic morphology is a non-specific hyperplasia, whilst the liver, which is only slightly enlarged, shows a characteristic lymphocytic infiltrate—'hepatic sinusoidal lymphocytosis'—morphologically resembling that seen in Felty syndrome (Fig. 9.26). The lymphocytes are T-cells, and may form fairly dense clusters. The Kupffer cells are hypertrophied and contain phagocytosed immune complexes; there is no haemozoin pigment.

The evidence that the underlying pathogenesis of tropical splenomegaly syndrome is an idiosyncratic immune response to *P. falciparum* infection comes from several sources. The geographical epidemiology, its rarity in people with sickle-cell trait, the good response to antimalarial chemotherapy, and serological abnormalities with raised IgM levels all implicate a low-grade chronic *P. falciparum* infection. The entity has been renamed 'hyper-reactive malarial splenomegaly'.[126]

Other malaria infections

The clinically mild *P. vivax*, *P. ovale* and *P. malariae* infections cause less haemolysis than *P. falciparum*, and jaundice is rare. Grossly the liver may be grey, but as death seldom occurs, it is rarely encountered at autopsy. The histological findings are similar to those in falciparum malaria though less marked.

Babesiosis

Babesia species are transmitted by ticks, and the disease is a zoonotic infection. In Europe, people who have had splenectomy may occasionally become infected by the cattle babesia parasite *B. divergens*. The clinical course is similar to falciparum malaria with fever, renal failure and haemolysis, but jaundice is more severe.[127] Mortality is high. At autopsy, the liver is enlarged and congested. Microscopically, there is focal ischaemic necrosis, hypertrophied Kupffer cells, and erythrocytes containing parasites morphologically similar to *P. falciparum*. However, there is no production of haemozoin pigment.

Visceral leishmaniasis

Clinical and epidemiological features

Visceral leishmaniasis (kala azar) is endemic in southern Europe, the Middle East, Asia, China, South America and Africa. In recent years, epidemics have occurred in Italy, India and Sudan. *Leishmania donovani* is the agent except in Europe, where its variant, *L. infantum*, is responsible, and in South America where it is the related *L. donovani chagasi.* Infection follows the bite of an infected sandfly. Apart from India, where leishmaniasis is an anthroponotic infection, visceral leishmaniasis is a zoonosis and canines are the reservoir.

The ratio of those infected to those who develop disease is between 10 and 30 to one.[128] The clinical spectrum of manifestations is protean. It ranges from mild malaise, through growth retardation in children, to the classic picture of hepatosplenomegaly, lymphadenopathy, fever, pancytopenia and hypergammaglobulinaemia.[129] Liver function tests are little altered, apart from a low albumin, and jaundice is uncommon. Untreated clinical visceral leishmaniasis is usually fatal; treated leishmaniasis has a mortality range of 2–17%. Children suffer a more acute form of the disease than adults, with a higher mortality.

Pathology

The liver is enlarged, sometimes massively, up to 4 kg, with no specific macroscopic appearance. Accounts of the histopathology are confusing. Liver biopsies taken during an epidemic in Italy showed that infected but asymptomatic patients (with positive anti-leishmanial serology) had epithelioid cell granulomas scattered throughout the parenchyma. These only rarely contained the parasite.[130]

In patients with acute overt leishmaniasis, the liver generally shows two overlapping histopathological patterns. The classic type consists of Kupffer cell hypertrophy and hyperplasia, portal inflammation and a diffuse sinusoidal chronic inflammatory infiltrate with conspicuous plasma cells. The parasites are present in Kupffer cells and portal macrophages, but the numbers vary widely (Fig. 9.27). They are seen as 2–3 μm diameter, ovoid or round, clear blobs of cytoplasm with a basophilic nucleus (the amastigote form); the characteristic paranuclear rod-shaped kinetoplast is not always evident in sections. Rarely, parasites are seen in hepatocytes also.[131] In the second pattern, the macrophages are seen within the acinus as small nodules with scanty parasites.[132] Sometimes epithelioid cell granulomas are found. Fatty change is common, but non-specific, and cholestasis is seen in some fatal cases. Occasionally, fibrin-ring granulomas form within the nodules, similar to those seen in Q fever.[133]

Necrosis is not normally a feature of the liver in leishmaniasis but it occurs in some acute fatal cases. The granulomas may show central necrosis and resemble those of tuberculosis and brucellosis, but amastigotes are usually visible. Hepatic necrosis around granulomas with bile-duct proliferation has been described and sometimes haemorrhagic necrosis is seen.[134,135] The extent to which terminal

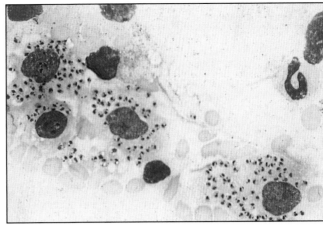

A

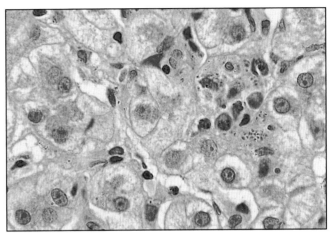

B

Fig. 9.27 • Visceral leishmaniasis. **(A)** Splenic aspirate: macrophages contain amastigotes that have a nucleus and an eccentric bar of DNA, the kinetoplast. Giemsa. **(B)** Liver biopsy showing Kupffer cells with amastigotes and associated plasma cells. H&E.

shock or other processes contribute to these more severe lesions is unclear.

In chronic adult cases of visceral leishmaniasis, a diffuse panacinar fibrosis may develop, similar to that seen in congenital syphilis. Amastigotes are scanty in this phase.[136] A denser form of fibrosis, leaving the portal structures intact but dividing the parenchyma into small groups of hepatocytes, was described as 'Rogers' cirrhosis'.[137] It is not a true cirrhosis and is now uncommon (Fig. 9.28).

Liver biopsy is not the most sensitive diagnostic technique for leishmaniasis, but a liver aspirate can demonstrate parasites in 75% or more of cases.[138,139] The main treatment for visceral leishmaniasis is liposomal amphotericin.

Many cases of leishmaniasis in HIV-1-positive patients are now reported although it is not an AIDS-defining disease.

Pathogenesis

Resistance to leishmaniasis depends on cell-mediated immunity. In the mouse, a single autosomal gene controls the persistence or elimination of the infection.[140] In patients with clinical leishmaniasis, interleukin-2 and α-interferon

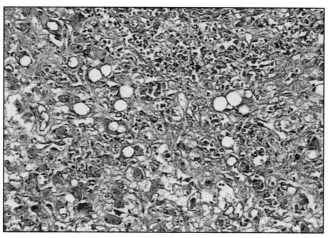

Fig. 9.28 • Chronic leishmaniasis: 'Roger cirrhosis'. Progressive sinusoidal fibrosis separating the liver plates. Trichrome stain. Photograph courtesy of Dr C Corbett, Brazil.

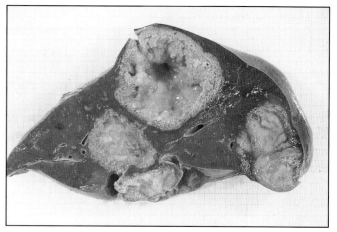

Fig. 9.29 • Amoebiasis. Liver with four large amoebic abscesses.

production are poor, resulting in a lack of macrophage activation to eliminate the parasites. Macrophages throughout the body are also parasitized. A major contribution to the morbidity and mortality is the immune paralysis consequent upon macrophage malfunction, and secondary bacterial infections are common. Conversely, the granulomatous lesions in asymptomatic, infected cases reflect parasite elimination.

Amoebiasis

Epidemiology and clinical features

Entamoeba histolytica-related infections are globally distributed, with about 10% of the world's population being infected. Whilst most of these reside in tropical and subtropical areas, no country is exempt. However, only 10% overall of people infected develop amoebiasis—either colorectal or extra-intestinal. The remaining 90% are asymptomatic carriers of amoebic trophozoites in the gut. Infection is via the faecal–oral route and results from ingestion of cysts. An invasive lesion in the large bowel is a prerequisite for the parasite to pass into the portal vein circulation, but only one-third of patients with amoebic liver abscess have a history of bowel symptoms.

Amoebic liver abscess presents with an enlarged, tender liver, fever and leucocytosis. Ultrasound is now the usual mode of diagnosis in hospital practice, supported by serology, which is positive in nearly all cases. Aspiration of an abscess is usually performed as a therapeutic measure to prevent rupture rather than as a diagnostic procedure, but amoebae may be identified in the aspirate.

The major differential diagnoses are hepatocellular carcinoma and pyogenic abscess. Jaundice is more common in pyogenic than in amoebic liver abscess. However, in a large series studied in India, cholestasis was present in nearly 30% of patients. This was associated with large, inferior abscesses and compression of the hepatic ducts. The mortality is increased (up to 43%, despite treatment) in such patients.[141]

Pathology

Most amoebic abscesses are in the right lobe, reflecting its greater portal venous drainage compared with the left lobe, and are often multiple (Fig. 9.29). The earliest macroscopic lesion, which is rarely encountered, is one or more small nodules of pale necrotic liver tissue. Fully developed abscesses have a ragged margin without a fibrous rim, and liquid contents. These have been likened to anchovy sauce, being brown-red and often paste-like in consistency. The size of an abscess varies greatly, but most are between 5 and 20 cm in diameter. Old lesions can develop a fibrotic capsule up to a centimetre thick.

The earliest histological finding is the presence of amoebic trophozoties in the sinusoids, associated with coagulative necrosis between the portal tract and terminal venule of an acinus.[142] There is a mild polymorph reaction with oedema. Trophozoites are 20–50 μm in diameter. They have a cytoplasm that ranges from nearly clear to purple and granular, depending on fixation and quality of staining (Fig. 9.30(A)). Phagocytosed erythrocytes are often present. The round nucleus is the size of a red cell with a sharp nuclear membrane and a prominent central karyosome. The usual confusion is with macrophages; the latter are smaller, have more basophilic nuclei and less granular cytoplasm. Amoebae are intensely PAS positive due to glycogen in the cytoplasm. Immunocytochemical stains (human anti-amoeba serum works well) also highlight amoebae (Fig. 9.30(B)), even in tissues stored for over a century.

As the lesion enlarges, amoebae cluster at the advancing edge of the abscess, leaving behind haemorrhagic granular necrotic material with much nuclear debris. Oedema is prominent around the abscess, associated with lymphocytes and plasma cells, but polymorphs are scanty—hence it is technically not a true 'abscess'. Older lesions generate peripheral granulation tissue and, eventually, dense fibrosis.

Amoebic abscesses may rupture through the liver capsule. Sub-diaphragmatic lesions may penetrate into the pleural cavity and the lung tissue. A sinus may drain through the abdominal wall and progressively digest away the surrounding skin. Rupture into the peritoneal cavity has a par-

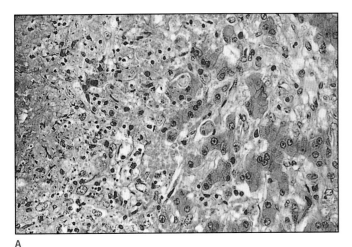

A

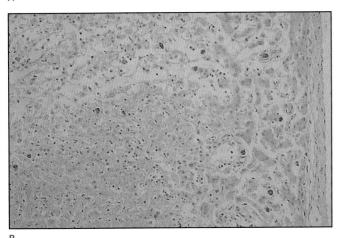

B

Fig. 9.30 • Amoebiasis. **(A)** Edge of an established amoebic abscess: necrotic liver on left; several purple-staining trophozoities in the centre and between hepatocytes. H&E. **(B)** Early stage of invasive amoebiasis in liver: single trophozoites visible in sinusoids and around a focus of necrosis. Anti-Entamoeba immunoperoxidase stain.

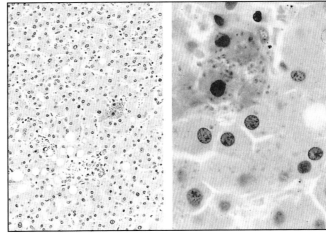

Fig. 9.31 • Toxoplasmosis. A small cluster of degenerating hepatocytes containing small haematoxyphilic zoites of *T. gondii*. H&E.

ticularly high mortality from the resulting amoebic peritonitis.

Pathogenesis

The majority of people with *E. histolytica* in the bowel harbour strains that are non-pathogenic but morphologically identical to the potentially invasive and disease-associated virulent strains. After decades of controversy, it is now established that the pathogenic and non-pathogenic strains, originally described by enzyme electrophoresis, are distinct genotypic entities.[143] Thus there is the potentially invasive species *Entamoeba histolytica*, and the non-invasive species *Entamoeba dispar*.[144]

The pathogenicity of *E. histolytica* depends on direct contact with the target cell. The process has five stages: binding, cytolysis of target cells, dissolution of tissue, phagocytosis, and spread of amoebae. Binding involves a 170 kD galactose/*N*-acetyl galactosamine-inhibitable lectin, which is expressed on the surface of the parasite. The mechanisms of amoebic cytotoxicity are still unclear.[145] Under investigation are contact-dependent calcium influx into the target cell, a phospholipase associated with the plasma membrane, and an ionophore secreted by the amoeba. This 'amoebapore' is a 77 amino acid peptide, which produces large pores in the target cell membrane, followed by lethal leak of ions.[146] Evidence for apoptotic death of cells has been presented, but this does not utilize a Fas-dependent or tumour necrosis factor (TNF-α) dependent pathway.[147] Tissue dissolution may be mediated by secretion of collagenase and cysteine proteinases by trophozoites.[148] The amoeba phagocytoses the injured cell, and continues its motion through the tissue by pseudopodial action.

Balantidiasis

Balantidium coli, a rare cause of enteritis, may occasionally pass via the portal vein and produce a liver abscess.[2] This parasite is the largest protozoon that infects man, the trophozoites measuring 50–100 μm.

Toxoplasmosis

Infection with *Toxoplasma gondii*, whose definitive host phase is in the enterocytes of cats, is ubiquitous. Man is infected from cat faeces or, more usually, from consuming undercooked meat. Most infections in adults are asymptomatic and toxoplasmosis is a latent, lifelong infection. The prevalence depends on climate, contact with pets, and culinary habits. In France and West Africa, adult seroprevalence rates are over 80%, but in dry, hot countries only 10% of adults may have serological evidence of infection.

A giant cell hepatitis may occur in congenital toxoplasmosis, but more frequently there are focal necroses associated with parasitized sinusoidal cells. Toxoplasmosis acquired after birth is only rarely associated with liver problems in normal hosts. Immunocompromised individuals, however, can have a marked toxoplasmic hepatitis with focal necroses and cholestasis.[149] The parasites are seen as cysts containing many zoites or as free tachyzoites (Fig. 9.31). The commonest clinical association is now HIV infection. Toxoplasmosis is also a cause of granulomatous hepatitis with non-necrotic epithelioid and giant cell lesions.[150]

Helminth infections

Nematodes

Ascariasis

In the tropics and subtropics, more than one billion people are infected with *Ascaris lumbricoides*—it is the commonest helminth infection of man. These 25 cm long roundworms inhabit the small bowel, but the liver is involved as a phase in the life cycle and by adult worms causing biliary obstruction. Infection occurs via the faecal–oral route by ingesting eggs and, when heavy, it may cause hepatomegaly during larval migration. If the liver is biopsied, an eosinophilic granulomatous reaction may be seen around degenerate small larvae. Ascaris worms migrate, and as they move into and out of the biliary tree and pancreatic duct, complications may arise. These include acalculous cholecystitis, biliary colic, acute bacterial cholangitis and hepatic abscess.[151] The diagnosis may be made by ERCP and ultrasound, in addition to finding the ova in the faeces. The organisms causing secondary cholangitis are usually *E.coli*, *Klebsiella* spp., and *Pseudomonas aeruginosa*. These complications usually resolve with appropriate chemotherapy and removal or spontaneous migration of the worms. Once a hepatic abscess has developed it may perforate the liver capsule or lead to septicaemia.

The worms may be seen obstructing and distending the bile ducts (Fig. 9.32). If they are trapped and die within the biliary tree, the remnants can form nidi for biliary calculi to form. Such remnants may adhere to the biliary epithelium, and cause glandular proliferation and intestinal metaplasia.[152] Eggs deposited by adult worms may also be seen within necrotic peribiliary foci, where they induce a mixed suppurative and granulomatous reaction around the characteristic brown-shelled and mamillated eggs.

Enterobiasis

Enterobius (Oxyuris) vermicularis, or the pinworm, is endemic in temperate zones, but less so in the tropics. Normally the only clinical sequel is pruritus from the eggs that the gravid female worm deposits around the anus. Occasionally the worm migrates up the female genital tract and into the peritoneal cavity. There, a florid inflammatory reaction occurs around the adult worm and eggs to produce a mass which causes abdominal pain and is associated with blood eosinophilia. Several cases of such nodules in the liver ('enterobioma') have been reported.[153,154] These join the list of non-neoplastic lesions that can mimic a benign tumour or a deposit of metastatic carcinoma in the liver.

Macroscopically, the lesions are about 1 cm in diameter and white or greenish in colour. Histologically, there is usually a fibrous and granulomatous rim surrounding a bland eosinophilic necrotic centre. This contains the degenerate worm, which may be seen to have characteristic triangular, pointed alae along the cuticle. The eggs are 25 × 50 μm in size, and one lateral aspect is flattened; they are seen within and outside the worm (Fig. 9.33).

Strongyloidiasis

Strongyloides stercoralis is endemic in tropical and subtropical areas around the world, including the southern USA. It is almost unique in that, once a person is infected, the auto-infection cycle perpetuates the infection indefinitely in many instances. Thus, decades after leaving an endemic zone, an infected but previously asymptomatic patient may present with unsuspected strongyloidiasis.

The liver is involved, like other visceral organs, when immunosuppression precipitates a hyperinfection syndrome. In this situation, the autoinfection process is acceler-

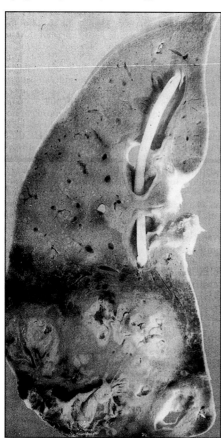

Fig. 9.32 • Ascariasis. Ascarid worm within a dilated bile duct, associated with several cholangitic abscesses in the lower half. Photograph courtesy of the Wellcome Trust International Health Image Collection.

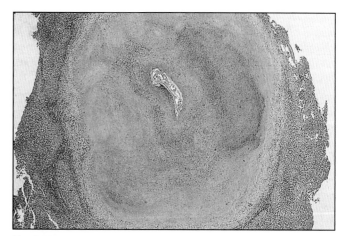

Fig. 9.33 • Enterobiasis. Necrotic nodule with a central female *E. vermicularis* worm. The extensive surrounding eosinophilic necrosis is typical. H&E.

ated and the infection load in the intestine augments rapidly. Predisposing events include malnutrition, high-dose steroid therapy and cytotoxic drugs for organ transplantation and cancer.[155] Human T-cell leukaemia virus type 1 (HTLV-1) infection has a particularly high risk of promoting the hyperinfection syndrome. This may occur before or after the HTLV-1-associated adult T-cell leukaemia/lymphoma has developed, and may be a presenting feature of leukaemia.[156] HIV infection, however, is not epidemiologically associated with strongyloidiasis.

The filariform larvae disseminate haematogenously and there is often an associated Gram-negative septicaemia. The larvae are $600 \times 16\,\mu m$, but they are rarely seen in a complete longitudinal section. In the liver, they are present in small portal vessels and sinusoids without any inflammation; or they may be surrounded by a chronic inflammatory infiltrate, often with giant cells but usually not many eosinophils (Fig. 9.34).[157]

Capillariasis

Infection with *Capillaria hepatica* is a worldwide zoonosis of small mammals, and human disease is rare. Man is infected by ingesting eggs in foodstuffs contaminated with soil. Clinically, there is fever, hepatomegaly and eosinophilia, and mortality is high.[158] Macroscopically, the liver is enlarged, sometimes fibrotic, and shows numerous small white foci of necrosis. Histologically, there are many eosinophils and a granulomatous reaction to adult worms ($20 \times 0.1\,mm$) and abundant eggs ($60 \times 30\,\mu m$). The eggs have characteristic striated shells and bipolar plugs (Fig. 9.35).

Visceral larva migrans (toxocariasis)

Certain ascarid intestinal worms of dogs (*Toxocara canis*) and cats (*T. cati*) are able to parasitize virtually any host paratenically: that is, larvae migrate through the body for years but they do not develop or mature. The term 'visceral larva migrans', when used unqualified, is taken to indicate infection with *T. canis* larvae.

Visceral larva migrans is a disease of children, who ingest the larvae from faeces of infected dogs. Seroprevalence surveys have shown that many infections are asymptomatic. Hepatomegaly and blood eosinophilia are part of the syndromes of both mild ('covert') and overt visceral larva migrans disease.[159,160] Histologically, the liver may show small foci of necrosis, many degranulating eosinophils and some giant cells. This is the track lesion of a migrating larva (Fig. 9.36). Rarely, part of a larva, which is $300 \times 20\,\mu m$ in size, is seen within the granuloma.

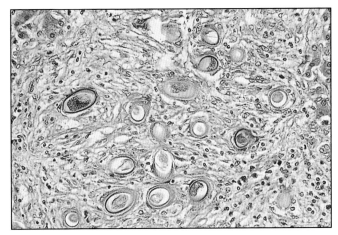

Fig. 9.35 • Capillariasis. Intrahepatic granuloma around numerous eggs. H&E.

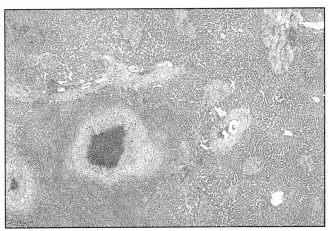

A

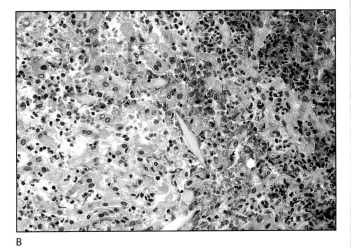

B

Fig. 9.36 • Visceral larva migrans. **(A)** miliary-type abscesses within the liver, locating the site of a migrating larva. H&E. **(B)** Trichrome stain shows the Charcot–Leyden crystals formed from degranulated eosinophils.

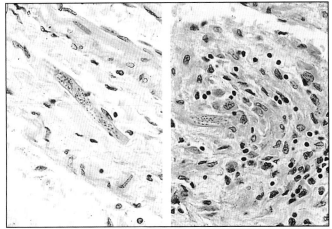

Fig. 9.34 • Strongyloidiasis. Two views of *Strongyloides* filariform larvae invading a portal tract; they contain many small nuclei. On the right, the larva has evoked a granulomatous reaction with eosinophilis. H&E.

Other hepatic larval helminthic diseases

The life cycles of many anthroponotic worm infections involve the liver, so larvae and an attendant inflammatory reaction may occasionally be encountered in liver biopsy or autopsy material as an incidental finding. These infections include not only *Ascaris lumbricoides*, the hookworms, and *Stronglyoides stercoralis*, but also certain zoonotic infections. These include *Baylisascaris*, *Gnathostoma*, and *Sparganum*.[2,3]

Cestodes

Hydatid disease is caused by the larval forms of *Echinococcus* tapeworms. *E. granulosus* is the most frequent parasite, the adults being found in dogs and jackals in all continents including Europe. Many mammals can serve as intermediate hosts, but sheep are the most frequent. *E. multilocularis* is less common but causes a more aggressive clinical disease. The definitive host is the fox and the infection occurs in eastern Europe, Turkey, the southern Russian states and the northern states of the USA and Canada. Intermediate hosts are usually rodents.

Unilocular hydatidosis

This is the classic hydatid cyst, caused by *E. granulosus*. After ingestion, the eggs hatch and the larval oncospheres pass to the liver by the portal vein. About 75% of infected individuals develop one or more cysts in the liver. These grow slowly, about 1 cm a year. The right lobe of the liver is affected more often than the left. Many hepatic hydatid cysts are asymptomatic and are discovered incidentally on X-ray. Clinical symptoms arise from large cysts as space-occupying lesions, when they compress the biliary tree, become bacterially infected (and cause septic shock) or, rarely, press on the portal vein and produce portal hypertension. A small proportion of liver cysts rupture into the peritoneal cavity, resulting in secondary dissemination of infection there. Rupture into the biliary tree and across the diaphagm into the pleural cavity are other complications. *E.granulosus* cysts may also develop in the lung, kidneys, spleen, brain and musculo-skeletal system.

The typical hydatid cyst is spherical, up to 30 cm or more in diameter, and has a fibrous rim. It may be single and unilocular or, more frequently, contain several daughter cysts which have developed by growth and invagination of the germinal membrane (Fig. 9.37). The wall has three structural components: (i) an outer acellular laminated membrane, which is 1 mm thick, ivory white, friable, and rather slippery to touch; (ii) the germinal membrane, a transparent nucleated lining; and (iii) the protoscolices, which are attached to the membrane and budding from it. These are about 100 μm across, ovoid in shape, and contain two circles of hooklets, and a sucker (Figs 9.38 and 9.39). Many cysts are partly or wholly degenerate. Collapsed daughter cysts have closely rolled laminated membranes. Histologically, these are anucleate and devoid of viable protoscolices. They may contain many shed hooklets, which have a characteristic scimitar shape, and small calcareous bodies.

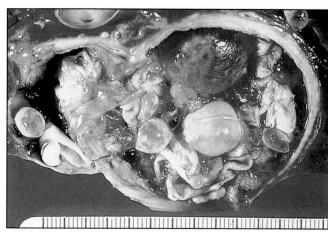

Fig. 9.37 • Hydatid cyst. A single cyst within the liver, containing numerous daughter cysts. The white laminated membranes are seen and also the thin fibrous rim around the cyst.

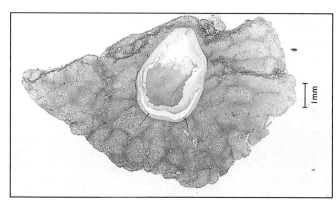

Fig. 9.38 • Hydatid cyst. A liver resection containing a small apparently dead cyst. There is a fibrous rim, a detached laminated membrane, and granular or fluid contents. H&E.

The host reaction to unilocular hydatid cyst is slight: there is some granulation tissue and a relatively thin fibrous wall. Eosinophils are not conspicuous but if a cyst has died or ruptured, they may be more evident, along with giant cell granulomas.

The diagnosis is usually made by ultrasound or CT scan, supported by positive hydatid serology. Leakage of antigen-laden hydatid cyst fluid into the circulation may result in anaphylactic shock, which can be fatal. Thus, liver biopsy is not encouraged if a hydatid cyst is suspected. Fine needle aspiration, however, is a safe diagnostic procedure.[161] The fluid obtained should be spun down and searched for protoscolices or hooklets. The latter are acid-fast on Ziehl-Neelsen stain and also stain well with trichrome methods.

Current chemotherapy is with long-term albendazole (a benzimidazole carbamate), but although this kills the larval stage it is not well absorbed and has limited diffusion across the cyst wall, and so is not definitive therapy. Modern surgical treatment avoids hepatectomy if possible: the laminated membrane and contents are sucked out, taking care not to disseminate germinal membrane or protoscolices. More recently, percutaneous treatment appears satisfactory for non-complicated cysts: puncture–aspiration–injection–re-aspiration (PAIR).[162] Covered by a short course of alben-

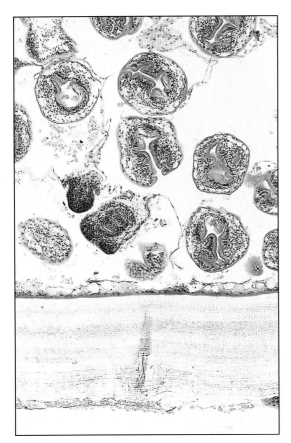

Fig. 9.39 • Hydatid cyst. From bottom to top: non-staining laminated membrane, the thin nucleated germinal membrane, and several protoscolices with sucker and refractile hooklets. H&E.

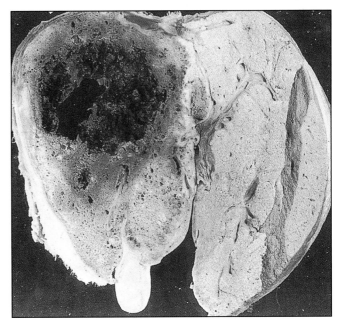

Fig. 9.40 • Alveolar hydatid cyst. Autopsy liver with a large irregular necrotic and invasive mass on the left. Photograph courtesy of the Wellcome Trust International Health Image Collection.

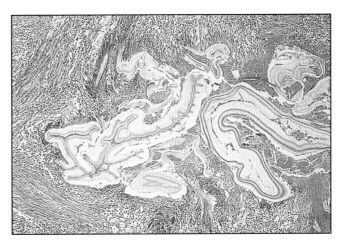

Fig. 9.41 • Alveolar hydatid cyst. Necrotic and fibrotic liver tissue infiltrated by irregular membranes that have no apparent nuclei. Protoscolices are not seen in human infection. H&E.

dazole, a 12–20 gauge needle is used to aspirate about 50% of the cyst fluid, inject hypertonic saline (to kill the scolices) and re-aspirate after 15 minutes.

The histopathologist is often asked whether resected or aspirated cysts are sterile, searching for an endpoint to therapy. This is impossible to answer. The presence of germinal membrane with nuclei or of protoscolices indicates that the cyst is potentially viable; however, retained remnants of hydatid cysts, even in the absence of apparent nucleated membrane or protoscolices, are capable of continued growth and dissemination.

Alveolar (multilocular) hydatidosis

The liver is also the primary site of infection with *E. multilocularis*. Patients present with hepatomegaly, jaundice and ascites.[163] Untreated, this infection is usually fatal (80%), for spontaneous resolution rarely occurs. Surgery and chemotherapy have improved this dismal outlook.[164]

The liver lesions appear as multilocular, necrotic, cystic cavities, containing thick pasty material. A fibrous rim is absent (Fig. 9.40). Rupture into the abdominal cavity or biliary tree and distant spread to other organs may occur. Histologically, the irregular cysts have a laminated membrane, but no nucleated germinal membrane or protoscolices are seen. The laminated membrane is often fragmented and is highlighted by PAS stain. These structures invade necrotic liver tissue much like a malignant tumour. The host

response is variable. There may be a granulomatous reaction with polymorphs and eosinophils, or an extensive peripheral rim of necrosis, fibrosis and focal calcification (Fig. 9.41). Fine needle aspiration can make the diagnosis, as with classical hydatid disease.[165]

Trematodes

The four major genera of trematode flatworms or flukes that affect man are *Schistosoma*, *Clonorchis*, *Opisthorchis* and *Fasciola*, and all cause liver damage. Trematodes require specific aquatic snail intermediate hosts for their life cycles.

Schistosomiasis

Epidemiology and clinical features

Schistosomiasis (bilharzia) is one of the great tropical diseases, with more than 200 million people infected. However, only 10% of those infected have clinically evident disease. Hepatosplenic schistosomiasis is the commonest cause of portal hypertension in the world. It results from infection with *Schistosoma mansoni*, *S. japonicum* and *S. mekongi*. *S. mansoni* is endemic in Africa, the Caribbean and South America; *S. japonicum* is prevalent in several countries in South-East Asia including the Philippines, China, Indonesia and Thailand; *S. mekongi* occurs in Laos and Cambodia.[166,167] Of the other species, *S. haematobium* and *S. intercalatum* mainly involve the bladder or bowel respectively, and cause minor non-symptomatic hepatic lesions.[168,169]

After infection by schistosome cercariae, there is a latent period before the worms settle in the veins of their preferred visceral sites. For *S. mansoni*, *S. japonicum* and *S. mekongi* these are the mesenteric and portal veins. Adult worms are 10–20 mm long and up to 1 mm in diameter. About 4 weeks after infection, female worms commence egg-laying. Eggs not retained in the intestinal wall or excreted in the faeces are carried to the liver; about 50% of all eggs laid are retained in the body. An acute infection syndrome called 'Katayama fever' may occur at this time, with fever, systemic upset, eosinophilia and transient hepatosplenomegaly.[170] The histopathology of Katayama in the liver is an infiltrate of eosinophils and young schistosome eggs in the portal tracts, surrounded by eosinophil microabscess.

Clinical hepatosplenic schistosomiasis presents with splenomegaly and gastrointestinal bleeding from oesophageal varices. Young adults are the main age group affected. Liver metabolic function is generally well preserved, and encephalopathy is rare after variceal haemorrhage. Ascites is found in up to one-third of patients presenting with haemorrhage,[171] but is more frequent in advanced decompensated cases.[172]

Pathology

The typical macroscopic features of advanced hepatosplenic schistosomiasis are a firm, enlarged liver with a bosselated thickened capsule, and a characteristic portal fibrosis termed Symmers clay-pipe stem fibrosis.[173] On cut section, there are thick, white tracts of collagen around major portal tracts, in rounded or stellate shapes (Fig. 9.42). Liver acinar architecture is preserved and there is no cirrhosis.

The microscopic features depend on duration of infection.[174] Eggs arriving in the liver are trapped in portal vein radicles of about 50 μm diameter. In early lesions the live eggs are surrounded by eosinophils and an eosinophil abscess may form with fibrinoid material surrounding the egg, a Hoeppli–Splendore reaction. Later an epithelioid granuloma with or without giant cells develops around the egg, the eosinophils being distributed round the periphery (Fig. 9.43). Schistosomal haemozoin pigment, which is indistinguishable from malarial pigment on light microscopy, is phagocytosed by macrophages in granulomas and in the portal tracts and sinusoids. This pigment is a product of haemoglobin catabolism by adult worms. Fibrous scar tissue forms around the granulomas and it eventually replaces them. The eggs live for about 3 weeks then gradually degenerate into empty shells which may be seen in long-standing lesions (Figs 9.43 and 9.44). Within the thick

clay-pipe stem fibrous lesions, one sees variable numbers of dead eggs, healing granulomas, fibroblasts, myofibroblasts, dense collagen, hypertrophied elastic fibres, tortuous arterioles and venules, and entrapped bile ducts.[170] Electron microscopic studies reveal deposition of collagen in the

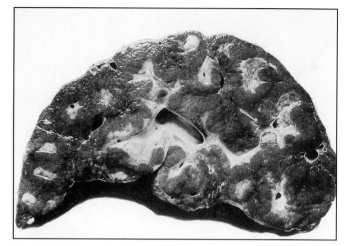

Fig. 9.42 • Schistosomiasis. Autopsy liver showing the thick periportal fibrosis ('Symmers clay-pipe stem fibrosis').

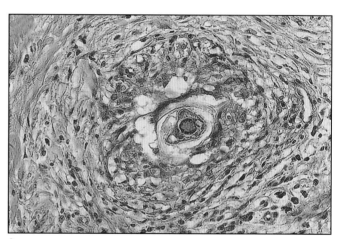

A

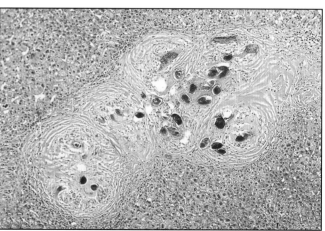

B

Fig. 9.43 • Schistosomiasis. (A) Acute infection: within the granuloma is a live egg with brown shell and spine, and the circular ring of nuclei. H&E. (B) Chronic infection: numerous dead calcified eggs with minor residual granulomatous reaction, surrounded by fibrosis. H&E.

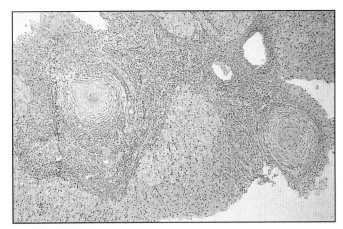

Fig. 9.44 • Schistosomiasis. Portal fibrosis associated with two periportal granulomas, each with concentric fibrosis. Van Gieson.

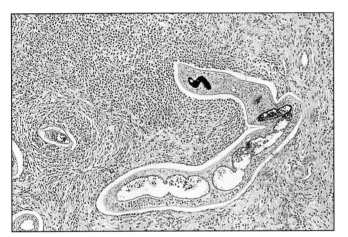

Fig. 9.45 • Schistosomiasis. Wedge liver biopsy: the adult worm within a portal vein has haemozoin pigment within its intestine, and is causing no host inflammatory reaction; the egg (left) is surrounded by eosinophils. H&E.

space of Disse, resulting in obstruction of sinusoidal fenestrations.[171]

S. mansoni eggs are $60 \times 140\,\mu m$ in size and bear a lateral spine; *S. japonicum* eggs measure $60 \times 85\,\mu m$, *S. mekongi* eggs are $50 \times 60\,\mu m$ and both have a small lateral knob. The shells of these eggs are characteristically brown in colour, and they are acid-fast with Ziehl–Neelsen stain. Occasionally in biopsy material and more often at autopsy, a pair of adult worms, eliciting no inflammatory reaction, may be seen within a portal vein (Fig. 9.45).

Where schistosomiasis is common so is cirrhosis, thus a proportion of patients will have incidental schistosome eggs in a liver biopsy specimen showing cirrhosis. The distinction between cirrhosis and schistosomal fibrosis is usually straightforward on wedge biopsies, but there may be problems with needle biopsies. If schistosome eggs are seen in a fibrotic liver, features in favour of cirrhosis as the main disease are small liver nodules, hyperplastic liver-cell plates, interface hepatitis, fibrotic bands of uniform thickness around the nodules, and the absence of granulomas and eosinophilia. If a biopsy of liver from a patient in an endemic area shows a portal lymphocytic infiltrate, non-necrotic tuberculoid granulomas and eosinophils, this is evidence

that the process is due to schistosomiasis even in the absence of eggs.

Pathogenesis

The portal hypertension of hepatosplenic schistosomiasis is pre-sinusoidal in type. It results from fibrosis due to the host's cell-mediated granulomatous reaction to secreted egg antigens.[172–179] The major determinants of liver disease are the intensity and duration of infection. Autopsy studies of *S. mansoni* show that clinically significant hepatic fibrosis does not usually develop until there has been chronic infection from more than 160 worms.[180] However, the degree of fibrosis does not correlate closely with infection load. Individuals vary in their fibrogenic potential to given stimuli. Hepatosplenic schistosomiasis is associated with various HLA types which may influence the degree of fibrosis. Linkage disequilibrium has been demonstrated with HLA-A1, -A2, -B5 and -B12, according to the population studied. T-lymphocyte responses to schistosomal antigens show a correlation with the degree of fibrosis. Blood mononuclear cells from patients with hepatic fibrosis show a higher blastogenic response to antigen than from schistosomiasis patients without fibrosis; the latter also have a lower blood CD4 : CD8 T-cell ratio than fibrotic patients and uninfected controls.[181,182] *S. japonicum* is considered to cause more severe liver disease than *S. mansoni* since adult females lay more than 1000 eggs/day, in comparison with 300/day from *S. mansoni* females. It is also possible that, within species, different strains of the parasite vary in their propensity to cause fibrosis.

It is not clear why the typical localized clay-pipe stem pattern develops rather than a more diffuse peri-acinar portal fibrosis. Morphological and haemodynamic studies of portal veins and hepatic arteries in schistosomiasis are conflicting. In schistosomal fibrosis, total hepatic blood flow is normal. Impregnation of vessels in autopsy material suggests an augmented arterial network and arterio-portal venous shunting.[183] However, radiographic studies during life indicate amputation of the large portal veins, proliferation of smaller vein branches around them, diminished hepatic arterial diameters, and shunting of hepatic arterial blood towards the spleen.[172] It is possible that once portal fibrosis has developed, with the accompanying distortion of vascular architecture, incoming eggs are swept into the smaller veins proliferating around the large portal veins, and via the granuloma/fibrosis sequence this results in progressively expanding tracts of collagen that characterize the clay-pipe stem pattern. The mechanisms of pre-sinusoidal portal hypertension in hepatosplenic schistosomiasis are thus multifactorial. In addition, since schistosomiasis is an intravascular infection, reactive lymphoid hyperplasia contributes to splenomegaly.

Clinically decompensated hepatosplenic schistosomiasis is characterized by wasting, low serum albumin, prolonged prothrombin time, ascites and hepatic encephalopathy. Its pathogenesis is disputed but the factors proposed include malnutrition, severe deposition of collagen in the space of Disse, ischaemic damage from repeated variceal bleeding, and severely distorted arterio-venous relationships in the portal tracts. Alcohol abuse and viral hepatitis types B and C will produce additional effects.[184]

Hepatitis B virus (HBV) infection is common in areas where schistosomiasis is endemic. However, there is no epidemiological association between the prevalences of hepatitis B virus and *S. mansoni* or *S. japonicum* infections.[185-187] HBV coinfection may be important in determining the prognosis of individual patients with hepatosplenic schistosomiasis. Thus, mortality from acute viral hepatitis is increased, and splenomegaly and HBsAg carriage are prolonged after acute B viral hepatitis in patients with schistosomiasis. Cross-sectional studies have also indicated that the chronic sequelae of HBV infection—chronic hepatitis and cirrhosis—are more likely to develop.[186,188] An explanation for these associations may lie in the interactions of cytokines, T-lymphocytes and macrophage responses to both infections. Epidemiological studies have not shown that schistosomiasis per se is a risk factor for hepatocellular carcinoma.

More recently, the impact of co-infection of schistosomiasis and hepatitis C infection (HCV) has been assessed. The extraordinarily high prevalence of HCV infection in Egypt is attributable to the mass parenteral chemotherapy campaigns against schistosomiasis that ended in the 1980s,[189] which has rendered HCV infection as the single predominant cause of chronic disease in that country.[190] In more than three-quarters of Egyptian patients with chronic liver disease both infections are present, whilst only 12% have HBV infection.[191] The progression of HCV-related liver disease appears not to be affected by co-schistosomal infection.[192] However, in schistosomal patients, co-infection with HCV leads to earlier decompensation of liver function due to chronic hepatitis and cirrhosis.[189,193,194] The contribution of schistosomiasis to the development of hepatocellular carcinoma in HCV-infected patients is debated,[195] although improbable; careful analysis of HCV, HBV and liver schistosomal infection are required.

Ultrasound studies

Most clinicopathological studies of hepatosplenic schistosomiasis have relied on hospitalized patients studied clinically, parasitologically, and histopathologically by biopsy and autopsy. Ultrasonography has changed this perspective. It provides a non-invasive means of assessing hepatic fibrosis and can be correlated with morphological studies.[196] The technology is suitable for epidemiological studies of schistosomal liver disease in the community (Fig. 9.46). In rural Zimbabwe, ultrasonography showed that an overall 10% of the population studied had schistosomiasis-related portal fibrosis, rising to 19% in those over 50 years of age, but severe fibrosis was rare.[197] Ultrasound studies in Egypt also suggest that a mild degree of fine portal fibrosis accompanies mild hepatosplenomegaly in children infected only with *S. haematobium*.[169]

Therapy

The fibrosis of advanced hepatosplenic schistosomiasis is not reversible on anti-schistosomal therapy with praziquantel. Biochemical studies of patients treated before variceal

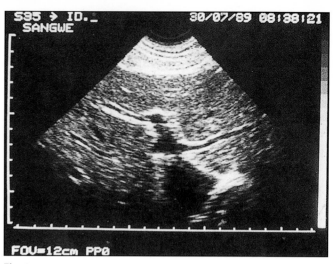

Fig. 9.46 • Schistosomiasis. Liver ultrasound shows thick white bands of fibrous tissue around major portal tracts. Photograph courtesy of Dr S Houston, Canada.

haemorrhage has occurred show a reduction in fibrogenesis and a diminution of the obstruction to portal vein blood flow.[198] Ultrasound evaluation of patients with *S. japonicum* has indicated that moderate but not severe hepatic fibrosis diminishes on praziquantel with a reduction in spleen size, and that serum total bile acid levels can predict which patients are more likely to improve with chemotherapy.[199]

Comprehensive reviews of the clinical pathology of the schistosomiases have been provided by Chen & Mott.[178,179,200,201]

Clonorchiasis and opisthorchiasis

Epidemiology and clinical features

Infection with the human liver flukes *Clonorchis* and *Opisthorchis* mainly occurs in the Far East. *C. sinensis* is prevalent in China, Taiwan, Hong Kong, Korea, and Vietnam. *O. viverrini* is frequent in the adult population of north-east Thailand. There are foci of *O. felineus* infection in eastern Europe, and apparently many cases in the former Soviet Union. The infection is acquired by ingesting cercariae in uncooked freshwater fish. Immature worms ascend and settle in the biliary tract, and occasionally the pancreatic duct.

Clonorchiasis and opisthorchiasis are clinically and pathologically similar and will be described together. Adult *C. sinensis* flukes are 8–25 mm long, 2–5 mm wide and 1 mm thick; *O. viverrini* is smaller, 11–20 mm long and 3 mm wide. They usually live less than 10 but occasionally up to 25 years. They excrete their eggs into the bile. The diagnosis is usually made by identifying eggs in the faeces, but ultrasonography is increasingly important.

One-third of chronically infected people are asymptomatic. Surveys in Thailand found a prevalence of 5–10% of symptomatic cases in the population. Symptoms and pathology broadly correlate with the intensity of infection. The clinical disease is usually insidious. Blood eosinophilia is usual. Patients may present with abdominal pain, hepatomegaly and, less commonly, jaundice.[202] Portal hypertension and splenomegaly do not develop. Specific complications of the infection include biliary obstruction from the worms themselves, stricture and calculus formation, secondary ascending cholangitis and liver abscess, and occasionally cholecystitis. An important sequel in adults is cholangiocarcinoma. In endemic areas clonorchiasis and opisthorchiasis increase the incidence of this carcinoma by a factor of 20–40.[203] In some areas, the incidence reaches 87 per 100 000 per annum, approaching the frequency of hepatocellular carcinoma. One large hospital-based autopsy study in Thailand found that 55% of cadavers with opisthorchiasis had liver cancer, of which 44% were cholangiocarcinoma.[204]

Pathology

In light infections, worms are mainly found in the distal bile ducts, but with heavier loads the proximal ducts and the gallbladder are parasitized (Fig. 9.47). Worms in the gallbladder are usually dead. The left lobe of the liver is more commonly affected than the right because the left intrahepatic bile duct is straighter and wider, allowing more ready access to worms. The largest number of *Clonorchis* worms found in a liver was 27 000.

The pathology of heavy *Clonorchis* infection is detailed in the classic description by Hou.[205] The liver is enlarged but not cirrhotic. The commonest macroscopic feature is focal dilatation of segments of smaller bile ducts to a diameter of 3–6 mm. The walls are thickened and worms are visible in the lumen (Fig. 9.48). Generalized bile-duct dilatation is uncommon and signifies a proximal stricture, stone or tumour.

Histologically, the bile-duct lining adjacent to the worms is hyperplastic, with infoldings of the epithelium ('adenomatous hyperplasia'). There is fibrosis and variable eosinophilia. Eggs are not seen in the tissues. Ascending cholangitis, usually due to *E. coli* infection, produces a purulent exudate in the dilated ducts and sometimes liver abscesses may form. Stones in the ducts often have dead worms as their nidus.

The cholangiocarcinoma associated with clonorchiasis is usually intrahepatic, multicentric and mucin-secreting. The pathogenesis is not certain. Malnutrition and carcinogens—either ingested or formed in the bile—are factors proposed. The fluke itself may be only weakly carcinogenic, but constant irritation of biliary epithelium by the worms could act as a promoting agent.[206] This subject is discussed further in Chapter 15.

For a comprehensive review of the literature on the clinical pathology of clonorchiasis, see Chen et al.[207]

Fascioliasis

Fasciola hepatica is a common zoonotic infection of sheep, goats and cattle. Man is only occasionally affected although many infections may be subclinical. Human infections are distributed globally but most cases occur in Europe. Eating watercress contaminated by metacercariae is the mode of infection. The immature fluke penetrates the liver capsule and migrates through the parenchyma to reside in the large bile ducts and the gallbladder. The leaf-like worm is up to 30 mm long and 13 mm wide, and lives for about 9 years. It adheres to and irritates the biliary epithelium via its suckers.

The clinical features are fever, upper abdominal pain and hepatomegaly during the phase of invasion and, in the chronic phase, ascending bacterial cholangitis with obstructive jaundice. Severe bleeding may occur from the biliary tract. A marked blood eosinophilia, reaching 30% or more of the total white cell count, is typical. The diagnosis is made at laparotomy, on ERCP, or by finding eggs in the faeces. Fatalities due to fascioliasis are uncommon.

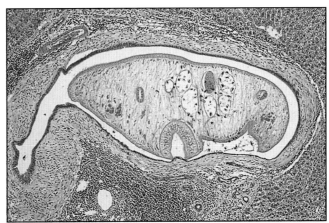

A

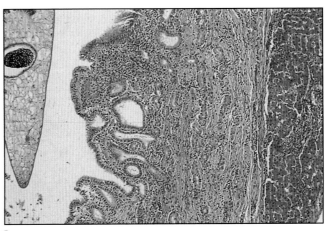

B

Fig. 9.48 • Opisthorchiasis. **(A)** Fluke in bile duct, attached to the epithelium via its sucker. H&E. **(B)** Biliary epithelial proliferation associated with a fluke. H&E.

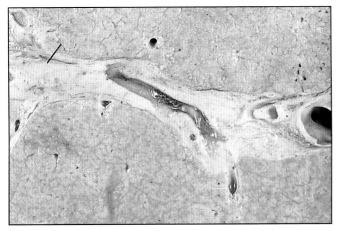

Fig. 9.47 • Clonorchiasis. Fluke within a bile duct.

Because the parasite migrates through the parenchyma, the liver may show yellow surface nodules 5–20 mm across. As in enterobiasis, these may be mistaken for metastatic carcinoma. Histologically, tracks are seen with much necrosis and eosinophilia around the worm. Subsequently, scars develop under the capsule.

Up to 40 worms may be found in an infected liver. Focal bile-duct dilatation is associated with a worm and there may be an acute cholangitis. Histologically, the bile epithelium is eroded, inflamed, and hyperplastic, and the surrounding portal tract is thickened and fibrotic (Fig. 9.49). Large necrotic granulomas can develop around trapped eggs. Tissue eosinophilia is typical in all these lesions. Adult flukes are often seen, along with gallstones, in the gallbladder, which shows a hypertrophied muscle coat and hyperplastic inflamed mucosal epithelium.[208]

Fascioliasis is not associated with cholangiocarcinoma. A comprehensive review of the clinical pathology of this infection has been provided.[209]

Pentastomiasis

Pentastomes are worm-like organisms that share morphological features of helminths and arthropods. In Africa, most cases of visceral infection are caused by *Armillifer (Porocephalus) armillatus*. In Asia, other species are prevalent. Occasional cases of pentastomiasis with hepatic lesions have been reported in the USA.[210] The adult pentastomes live in snakes, and man is infected from ingesting either eggs in contaminated drinking water or larvae in raw snake meat. The larval nymphs migrate within the abdominal organs, including the liver; they do not mature to adults but die and degenerate. Most hepatic pentastomiasis is encountered as calcified nodules enclosing dead parasites. Autopsy and radiological surveys have produced remarkably high prevalences of healed pentastomiasis, such as 25% in West Africans[211] and 45% among certain groups of Malaysians.[212] In Africa, it is said to be the commonest cause of calcification in the liver.

The calcified lesions are 5–10 mm in diameter and histologically are often non-specific; there is old necrotic tissue and surrounding fibrosis. Earlier lesions show an identifiable or even viable parasite. It is folded in a C shape, has a thick crenellated cuticle, and contains an intestinal canal and striated muscle (Fig. 9.50).

HIV infection and AIDS

Infection by the human immunodeficiency viruses type 1 (HIV-1) and type 2 (HIV-2) causes the acquired immunodeficiency syndrome, AIDS, which represents advanced HIV disease. First observed in the USA in the early 1980s, the epidemic of HIV-1 infection is now global and some 40 million adults and children are living with HIV/AIDS. The worldwide prevalence of HIV infection varies greatly, with 95% of people affected residing in resource-poor developing countries—see Table 9.3.

In many capital cities of Africa, particularly east and southern Africa, HIV-1 seroprevalence rates in sentinel groups such as women of child-bearing age reach 25% or more. HIV-2 infection is mainly restricted to West Africa,

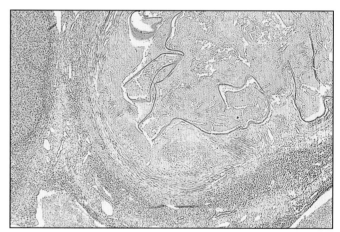

Fig. 9.50 • Pentastomiasis. Typical appearance of a dead pentastome in liver. The irregular cuticle is surrounded by fibrous and granulomatous reaction. H&E.

Table 9.3	Global data on HIV/AIDS (numbers in millions). Current information is accessed from the UNAIDS website: www.unaids.org/wad2004/report.html	
Living with HIV/AIDS at end-2004	37 m adults	2.2 m children
New HIV infections in 2004	4.3 m adults	0.64 m children
HIV/AIDS deaths in 2004	2.6 m adults	0.51 m children
Persons with HIV/AIDS by region:	Sub-Saharan Africa	25.4 m
	South & south-east Asia	7.1 m
	East Asia	1.1 m
	Latin America	1.7 m
	North America	1.0 m
	Western Europe	0.61 m
	Eastern Europe & central Asia	1.4 m
	Caribbean	0.44 m
	Oceania	0.035 m

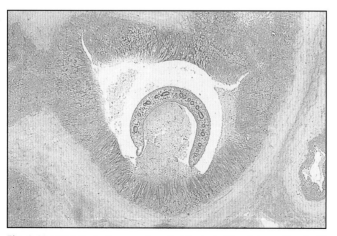

Fig. 9.49 • Fascioliasis. Cross-section of a bile duct with a fluke exciting florid epithelial proliferation. H&E.

although cases are occasionally seen elsewhere in immigrants or their sexual partners. Within two decades, HIV-related disease has come totally to dominate hospital medicine and pathology in many countries in Africa.

Transmission of the HIVs is through sexual intercourse (vaginal and anal), transfusion of blood and blood products, needle sharing among intravenous drug users, and from mother to fetus. Among HIV-positive people in European countries, homosexual males and immigrants from Africa predominate. In Eastern Europe, intravenous drug use is a major driver of infection. However, heterosexual transmission is the dominant mode in resource-poor countries, where the prevalence of infection is similar among males and females.

Pathogenesis

The essential pathogenesis of the disease is the initial HIV infection and immune response, followed by the progressive destruction of CD4+ T-lymphocytes (T-helper cells) by the virus and, ultimately, AIDS.[213] The course runs from the time of infection, when there may be a seroconversion illness, through the latent asymptomatic phase, to the development of certain diseases that constitute AIDS. The latter are indicative of severely compromised cellular immunity, the most commonly used marker of which is the blood CD4+ T-lymphocyte count. These diseases include, according to the surveillance criteria for cases of AIDS: (i) specific opportunistic infections and tumours, (ii) clinically defined states such as wasting and dementia.[214,215] Once AIDS has developed, death is inevitable sooner or later. The survival period with HIV infection and disease varies widely according to geographical location and the availability of medical treatment; in industrialized countries, 10 to 20 or more years is now common (Fig. 9.51). The advent of highly active anti-retroviral therapy (HAART) since 1996 has resulted in a dramatic fall in deaths due to HIV/AIDS even whilst the incidence and prevalence of new HIV infection has increased (see UK data on the Health Protection Agency website: *www.hpa.org.uk*/infections/topics_az/hiv_and_sti/hiv/hiv.htm). This survival has come with cost in terms of treatment side effects—see 'Drug toxicity in HIV disease', p. 483.

General pathological features in the liver

The liver and the biliary tree are commonly affected by HIV-associated opportunistic infections and tumours, and liver biopsy is a means of establishing such diagnoses (Table 9.4).[216] However, HIV disease rarely produces liver failure unless there is drug toxicity or coinfection with hepatitis C. There is no evidence of a direct 'HIV-hepatitis' although other viral hepatitides are modified by HIV infection. HIV-positive people consume numerous drugs as prophylaxis and therapy, some of which are hepatotoxic. As the pandemic spreads and seroprevalence rates augment, any disease may be encountered in the liver of an HIV-infected person by chance. The HIV-associated diseases are those whose prevalences are significantly increased in HIV-positive people compared with the HIV-negative population, and/or whose clinico-pathological features are distinctly worsened by HIV infection.

The following account is primarily of HIV-1 disease, the major infection (see below for HIV-2 infection). There are autopsy and many biopsy series documenting the

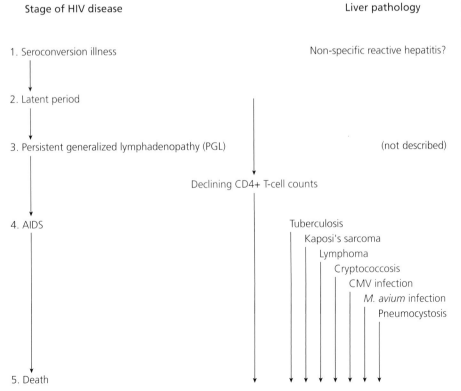

Stage of HIV disease	Liver pathology
1. Seroconversion illness	Non-specific reactive hepatitis?
2. Latent period	
3. Persistent generalized lymphadenopathy (PGL)	(not described)
	Declining CD4+ T-cell counts
4. AIDS	Tuberculosis / Kaposi's sarcoma / Lymphoma / Cryptococcosis / CMV infection / *M. avium* infection / Pneumocystosis
5. Death	

Fig. 9.51 • The time course of HIV disease and liver pathology, indicating some of the diseases found and their relative presentation over time.

Table 9.4	The main HIV-associated opportunistic diseases found in the liver of HIV-infected patients. Those marked* are AIDS-defining conditions for surveillance purposes

1. Non-specific: peliosis hepatis; sclerosing cholangitis (some cases are pathogen negative).

2. Specific infections:
   a. viral: cytomegalovirus*, herpes simplex virus*, Epstein–Barr virus, adenovirus, hepatitis B and C viruses.
   b. bacterial: *Bartonella henselae* (bacillary angiomatosis, peliosis); Gram-negative bacillus sepsis*.
   c. mycobacterial; *Mycobacterium tuberculosis*, *M. avium** complex and other.
   d. fungal: *Candida**, *Cryptococcus neoformans**, *Histoplasma capsulatum**, *Penicillium marneffei*, *Pneumocystis jiroveci**, *Coccidioides immitis.**
   e. protozoal: *Toxoplasma gondii**, *Cryptosporidium parvum**, microsporidia, *Leishmania* spp.

3. Tumours: Kaposi sarcoma*, high-grade B-cell lymphoma*, B-cell lymphoproliferative disease.

hepatic pathology in HIV disease,[221] and reviews of the same.[100,217–224] Most emanate from industrialized countries. However, the patterns of infections and tumours in AIDS depend both on the mode of HIV transmission and where the infected person lives. Many of the most significant opportunistic infections in AIDS are reactivations of latent asymptomatic infections acquired since birth, and these are often regionally restricted. Autopsy studies from Africa[225] and India[221] have emphasized the overwhelming importance of tuberculosis in HIV-associated liver disease, paralleling that infection's importance in all organ pathologies in those continents. In industrialized countries, tuberculosis is much less common, with the exception of those patients immigrating from developing countries. Thus the hepatic pathology is not uniform around the world. Moreover, it is changing as therapy (HAART) alters the clinical pathology and cadence of HIV disease.

HIV seroconversion illness

Up to 50% of HIV-infected people experience a seroconversion illness resembling infectious mononucleosis between 3 weeks and 6 months after infection. A small proportion of these develop an acute hepatitis syndrome with vomiting, upper abdominal pain and hepatomegaly. The serum transaminases are raised but there is no jaundice nor elevated serum alkaline phosphatase.[226,227] Serological evidence is against co-infection by other hepatitis viruses in these patients, and the liver disease resolves. No histopathological reports of liver biopsies are available, and the pathogenesis of this 'HIV-associated hepatitis' is uncertain.

Other general features

At some time during HIV disease, hepatomegaly is seen in 60% of patients in industrialized countries, and at autopsy

the liver weight is more than 1800 g in 72% of cases.[224] This may not be universal: in a West African autopsy study, the mean liver weight (approximately 1550 g) was no different in HIV-negative and HIV-positive patients, nor different between those dying with or without an AIDS-defining condition (personal observations).

Mild to moderate degrees of macrovesicular steatosis are common in liver biopsy and autopsy material in HIV-positive patients, particularly those with AIDS. Moderate chronic lymphocytic inflammation of portal tracts is common as a non-specific reactive hepatitis. These are regarded as the non-specific consequences of a chronic wasting disease. Haemosiderin deposits in Kupffer cells are common in those to whom blood transfusions have been given to maintain haemoglobin levels. There is a close correlation between the amount of blood transfused and the degree of iron overload. Progressive fibrosis can occur, as documented from repeat liver biopsies.[228]

If there is bone marrow failure, haemopoiesis may be seen in the sinusoids. Rarely, massive and sometimes fatal macrovesicular steatosos occurs, with the liver at autopsy weighing 5 kg or more.[229] In the cases reported, such patients have not had terminal AIDS (their CD4 counts were more than $100/mm^3$). Anti-retroviral therapy has been implicated as the cause in many cases.

Granulomas are found in liver biopsy and autopsy material in up to one-third of HIV-positive patients.[214,215,230] The main causes are *M. avium* complex infection, tuberculosis, and mycoses. In patients with AIDS, HIV-1 can usually be demonstrated in the liver by in situ hybridization probes and by immunocytochemistry against p24 antigen.[231,232] Kupffer cells and endothelial cells contain more virus than hepatocytes, and the liver is probably a site of active replication of the virus.

Veno-occlusive disease

Hepatic veno-occlusive disease is associated with HIV infection, with the typical pathological features of sinusoidal congestion, fibrosis, perivenular hepatocyte degeneration, central vein obliteration and sclerosis. From a large USA study, the condition is associated with IV drug use and presents before the development of AIDS defining conditions.[233]

Amyloidosis

Amyloidosis is reported in HIV patients without other predisposing conditions, and the liver may be affected.[234,235] In Africa, despite the high frequency of tuberculosis associated with HIV infection, amyloidosis is only occasionally seen.

Nodular regenerative hyperplasia

Diffuse nodular regenerative hyperplasia has been observed in association with visceral leishmaniasis (see below);[236] and also at autopsy in an HIV-infected patient without this infection or a viral hepatitis (personal observations).

Infections of the liver in HIV disease

Viral infections

Cytomegalovirus

Reactivation of cytomegalovirus (CMV) is frequent in HIV disease but significant pathology is unusual until CD4+ T-lymphocyte counts are very low (less than 50/mm^3). Hepatic disease due to parenchymal cytomegalovirus infection is minor.[222] In up to 10% of patients, microscopic examination shows scanty cytomegalovirus inclusions in hepatocytes, Kupffer cells and endothelial cells. This is usually associated with only a small zone of necrosis and inflammation (microabscess). However, cytomegalovirus infection can occasionally be a cause of severe bile-duct necrosis (Fig. 9.52), and it is also associated with sclerosing cholangitis.

Herpes simplex virus

Disseminated Herpes simplex virus infection is uncommon in HIV disease. However, it can present with liver failure. At autopsy, the enlarged liver shows hepatic necrosis affecting zones 2 and 3 of the acini, multinucleate hepatocytes, ground-glass nuclear inclusions, and minimal inflammation[237] (Fig. 7.3).

Epstein–Barr virus

An Epstein–Barr-virus-associated lymphoproliferative disorder affecting many lymphoreticular organs is associated with HIV infection. Histologically, the liver shows an infiltrate of immunoblasts in sinusoids but no necrosis.[238] An EBV-associated haemophagocytic syndrome is also reported.[239]

Adenovirus

Adenovirus hepatitis in HIV-positive patients appears to be restricted to children and, occasionally, to young adults.[33,34] As well as fever and hepatomegaly, it presents with a bleeding diathesis. Histologically, there is extensive zone 3 hepatocyte necrosis, little inflammation, and abundant intranuclear viral inclusions.

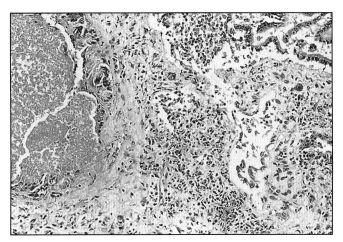

Fig. 9.52 • CMV infection. Large, inflamed portal tract with two CMV inclusions and necrotic bile duct (at left). H&E. See also Fig. 9.5.

Viral hepatitides—HAV, HBV, HCV, HDV

Risk factors that greatly increase the likelihood of hepatotropic virus infections are intravenous drug use (HBV, HCV and HDV), homosexual activity (HBV), and being African (HBV). There is no evidence of an association between HIV and hepatitis A virus infections.

Hepatitis B HIV-positive men infected with HBV are at an increased risk of becoming chronic carriers as CD4+ T-lymphocyte counts fall.[240] Moreover, HIV infection seems to permit the reactivation of, or reinfection by, HBV infection in those who had earlier become HBsAg-seronegative.[241] In terms of clinical manifestations, HIV-positive patients are less likely to be icteric following HBV infection than HIV-negative individuals.[242] Liver biopsy studies have also demonstrated that HIV-positive patients have less active chronic HBV disease and less scarring, and HBV-associated cirrhosis is less frequent. Further, expression of HBeAg and HBV-DNA polymerase is greater, indicating that HBV viral replication is more active in HIV-positives.[242] Within HIV-positive cohorts, acute hepatitis (HBV, and 'non-A, non-B') and chronic hepatitis are found more often in those who have not developed AIDS, and therefore have better cell-mediated immunity than those with AIDS.[243] Occasionally HIV may cause so-called fibrosing cholestatic hepatitis in HBeAg positive individuals (p. 416).

Concerning the effect of HBV infection on the biology of HIV disease, one European study has suggested that, among HIV-positive men, those who are HBcAg-seropositive progress to AIDS faster than those without evidence of active HBV infection,[244] but this association may be spurious, confounded by other behaviour and infection co-factors.

Hepatitis C HCV and HIV co-infection are common given the large number of intravenous drug users globally (5 million in industrialized countries alone). Acute HCV infection is generally as asymptomatic in HIV-infected persons as in those not infected.[245]

The long-term biological sequelae of co-infection are complex. Initial studies indicated that the cadence of HCV disease is unchanged or milder in HIV-positive patients.[246] Longer follow-up reveals that HCV behaves as an opportunistic infection, particularly in the later stages of HIV disease. Whereas 20–30% of immunocompetent individuals with HCV will progress to cirrhosis over an average of 15–30 years, controlled studies show that HCV-infected persons with HIV have faster progression to end stage liver disease: faster fibrosis, more interface hepatitis, higher rates of cirrhosis, higher HCV-RNA loads, and a greater likelihood to go into liver failure.[247–251] One study found a median time to cirrhosis of 23 years in co-infected persons compared with 32 years in HCV-only infected. These effects correlate with the severity of HIV-related immunosuppression. The development of hepatocellular carcinoma is also accelerated by HIV co-infection.[252]

There has been debate whether the progression of HIV disease is affected by HCV (or HBV, HDV) status.[253] Most data indicate that HCV coinfection does accelerate progression to AIDS and HIV-related death, and that this may be HCV genotype-dependent.[254,255]

As a result of the increasing number of HIV/HCV co-infected persons and the decline of many other classic HIV-related diseases because of anti-retroviral therapy, the significance of HCV-related liver disease has increased significantly, particularly in Europe. A large study in France noted that half of deaths in HIV-infected persons were not from classic HIV-related diseases and, within that category, liver disease was the single commonest cause of death.[256]

Updated information about, and treatment guidelines for, HIV/HCV co-infected persons is available on the BHIVA website: www.bhiva.org (HIV and chronic hepatitis C virus infection).

Hepatitis D Although HDV is dependent on HBV infection, it is not known whether its pathogenicity is modified by HIV co-infection.[222,253]

Bacterial infections

Tuberculosis

From being rare initially, the prevalence of tuberculosis in HIV-positive patients in industrialized countries is increasing, and it is high in Africa and India.[257] An autopsy study in West Africa found that 50% of adults dying of AIDS had active tuberculosis and in 85% of them the liver was involved (Fig. 9.53). Tuberculosis was, in fact, the commonest specific hepatic HIV-associated lesion.[225] In India, 41% of a cadaveric series had tuberculosis of the liver.[258]

The macroscopic features include single or multiple mass lesions, and miliary tuberculosis which is the commonest pattern in AIDS patients. Depending on the cellular immune status of the patient, the pathology of the lesions varies. Granulomas with Langhans giant cells and caseation may be seen, or non-giant cell epithelioid cell granulomas. Acid-fast bacilli are usually scanty in these cases. However, at the extreme of immune deficiency commonly seen in terminal AIDS patients with tuberculosis, the histological pattern is that of non-reactive (anergic) tuberculosis. Foci of granular necrosis are surrounded by degenerate swollen macro-

phages, and large numbers of acid-fast bacilli are present[259] (Fig. 9.16(b)).

Other mycobacterioses

The prevalence of *M. avium* complex infection in HIV-positive patients depends on geography, being rare in developing countries, and on survival. Some 25% of those with *M. avium* bacillaemia have liver infection on biopsy or at autopsy.[260] However, the prevalence is inversely correlated with CD4+ T-lymphocyte count, rising to 40% when it is less than 10/mm³. *M. avium* may eventually infect most patients who do not die earlier from another HIV-related event.[261]

M. avium complex infection is frequently associated with raised serum alkaline phosphatase as enlarged lymph nodes compress the bile duct, or intrahepatic *M. avium* granulomas obstruct terminal ductules. Abscesses may develop and contain numerous bacilli on Ziehl–Neelsen stain.[96] More frequently, there are miliary nodules of non-necrotic epithelioid cell granulomas throughout the parenchyma, and acid-fast bacilli are scanty (Fig. 9.54). When immune deficiency is extreme, clusters of histiocytes are seen with bluish and even striated cytoplasm due to the vast numbers of acid-fast bacilli (Fig. 9.55).[95]

Disseminated infections with many other species of mycobacteria are recorded in HIV-positive patients and often involve the liver. The histopathological appearances are not distinct from tuberculosis and culture is required to identify them. Against expectations, leprosy is not more frequent or more severe in HIV-positive people.[262]

Bartonellosis: peliosis, bacillary angiomatosis and cat-scratch disease

Peliosis hepatitis is a condition with many underlying aetiologies. It is the presence of multiple blood-filled cystic spaces in the liver, previously associated with tuberculosis, cancer cachexia and androgen therapy. In HIV infection, the main cause is *Bartonella henselae* bacterial infection,[71] which also causes bacillary angiomatosis and cat-scratch disease.

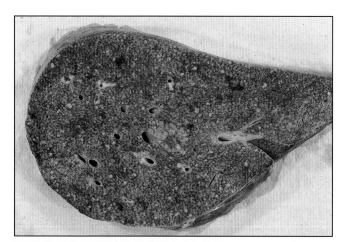

Fig. 9.53 • Miliary tuberculosis of the liver in an HIV-positive adult. Slice of liver with numerous small white spots of necrosis.

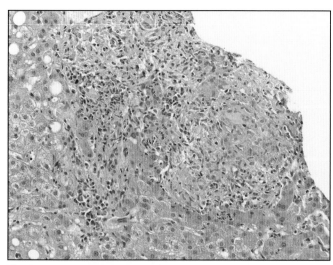

Fig. 9.54 • *M. avium* complex infection. Non-necrotic granuloma near the portal tract. Acid-fast bacilli were not seen. H&E.

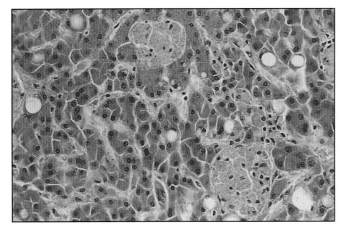

A

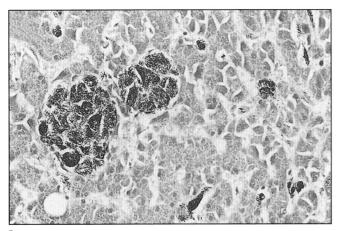

B

Fig. 9.55 • *M. avium* complex infection. **(A)** Discrete, non-necrotic aggregates of unactivated macrophages in the sinusoids. The blue haematoxyphilic cytoplasm results from the tightly packed mycobacteria. H&E. **(B)** Ziehl–Neelsen stain of same liver, showing large numbers of intracellular acid-fast bacilli.

Peliosis is infrequently seen in patients with AIDS.[263] The lesions are visible as red spots beneath the capsule of the liver, which may be greatly enlarged. Histologically, they appear as 1–4 mm cysts within the parenchyma, containing blood. A partial endothelial lining may be present and adjacent sinusoids are ectatic.

In the livers of some patients with HIV-associated peliosis hepatis, lesions resembling bacillary angiomatosis of the skin are also found. Macroscopically these are greyish or haemorrhagic nodules, and microscopically show fibrovascular and vascular proliferation accompanied by neutrophils.[264] Between liver-cell plates and the blood vessels, there is a myxoid stroma that contains clumps of granular material.[265] On Warthin–Starry stain (Fig. 9.56), these are masses of bacilli that are morphologically similar to those seen in the lesions of cutaneous bacillary angiomatosis.

Rarely, cat-scratch disease also affects the liver in HIV-positive patients, with pathology similar to that in non-HIV-infected individuals.[266]

Q fever

Serological evidence suggests that infection with *Coxiella burnetii* is three times more frequent among HIV-positive individuals than in HIV-negative controls, and cases of disease are 12 times more frequent. However, the course of the disease with treatment is unaffected by HIV status. There is fever and sometimes hepatomegaly. Liver biopsy shows a granulomatous hepatitis.[267]

Gram-positive and Gram-negative sepsis

Septicaemia due to Gram-positive cocci (staphylococci and streptococci) and Gram-negative bacilli (particularly non-typhoid salmonellae) is strongly associated with HIV infection.[268,269] These infections may produce hepatic abscesses.

Fungal infections

Many disseminated fungal infections involving the liver have been reported. The most important infections are by *Candida albicans*, *Cryptococcus neoformans*, *Histoplasma capsulatum*, *Penicillium marneffei*, *Coccidioides immitis*, and *Pneumocystis jiroveci*. *Histoplasmosis duboisii*, blastomycosis and aspergillosis have also been encountered occasionally.[270–273] Liver biopsy may detect these diseases, but the most sensitive techniques for identifying them (except pneumocystosis) are blood culture or blood antigenaemia tests.[224]

Candidiasis and cryptococcosis

Candidiasis and cryptococcosis are ubiquitous infections and are documented in the liver in 2–14% of HIV-positive patients in industrialized countries.[230] Candidiasis often presents as small purulent abscesses containing the yeasts and hyphae. Cryptococcosis may cause hepatomegaly. It was found in 5% of a cadaveric series in India.[258] There is a diffuse intracellular infection of Kupffer cells and portal macrophages (Fig. 9.20). Foreign-body-type giant cells may also be seen containing many yeasts.

Histoplasmosis

The prevalence of histoplasmosis in HIV disease depends on geography since the infection is rare in Europe or Australasia. A 1–4% prevalence of hepatic histoplasmosis in the USA has been quoted.[224,229] Histologically, small non-giant cell granulomas may be seen throughout the parenchyma or portal tracts, containing budding yeasts 3–5 μm in diameter (Figs 9.21 and 9.57). In heavy infections, Kupffer cells may be filled with yeasts.

Penicilliosis

Although infection with *Penicillium marneffei* is not currently an AIDS-defining condition, it is strikingly frequent in patients with HIV infection in Thailand and Hong Kong. Histologically, a diffuse infiltrate of yeast-laden macrophages replaces the liver parenchyma (Fig. 9.23).[274,275] The 3–4 μm diameter yeasts closely resemble *H. capsulatum* in size, but also show the characteristic features of forming tubes and elongated, septate spores.[216]

Coccidioidomycosis

This mycosis is endemic in the Americas only, and is found in the liver as part of disseminated disease in AIDS patients.

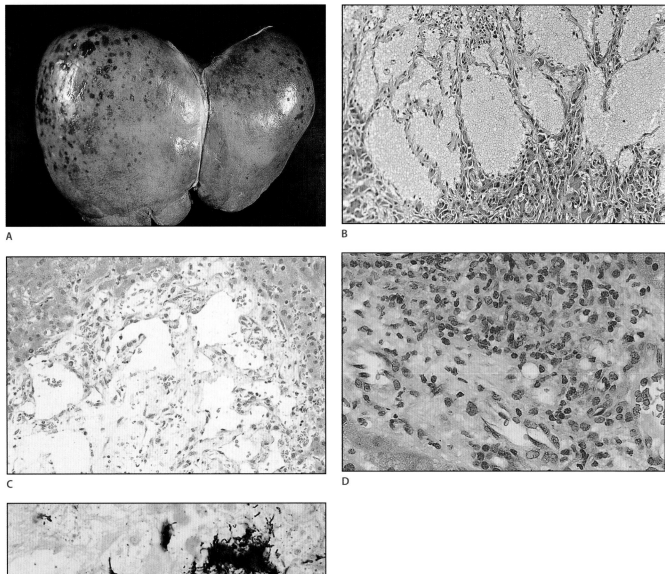

A

B

C

D

E

Fig. 9.56 • Peliosis hepatis and bacillary angiomatosis. **(A)** Peliosis hepatis. Liver showing multiple sub-capsular blood filled spaces. **(B)** dilated vascular spaces within the parenchyma; endothelial cells are mostly absent and the liver cells are attenuated. H&E. **(C)** Bacillary angiomatosis. Dilated vascular components with surrounding myxoid stroma. **(D)** Portal tract with chronic inflammatory cells around blood vessels, and granular greyish stroma which contains abundant bacteria. **(E)** Warthin–Starry stain of the same liver showing clumps of silver-positive bacilli. Slides courtesy of Dr T J Stephenson, Sheffield.

Histologically there are multiple granulomas containing the characteristic 20–200 μm diameter spherules.[218,276]

Nocardiosis

Nocardiosis (mainly *N. asteroides*) is uncommon but is seen with HIV infection.[277] Hepatic lesions occur as part of disseminated disease. Macroscopically, they resemble miliary tuberculosis. Histologically the lesions are small or large purulent abscesses, sometimes with a granulomatous edge, containing branching and beaded bacilli. These are invisible in H&E-stained sections but are clearly demonstrated by Grocott silver stain; they are also Gram-positive and are weakly acid-fast by the Wade–Fite method (Fig. 9.13).

Pneumocystis jiroveci (ex-carinii)

Previously considered to be a protozoon, *P. jiroveci* is now classed as a fungus on the basis of studies of ribosomal RNA homology. It is probably ubiquitous in soil or air, and, globally, most children manifest a subclinical antibody response to infection before the age of 10 years.[278] Immunodepression from malnutrition, steroid therapy and HIV infection predisposes to *Pneumocystis* pneumonia. Before systematic

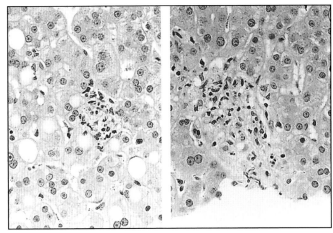

Fig. 9.57 • Histoplasmosis. Liver biopsy of an HIV-positive man with fever revealed small non-necrotic granulomas. The yeasts are difficult to see, but can be highlighted by special stains. H&E. See also Fig. 7.18b.

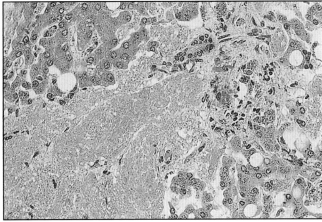

A

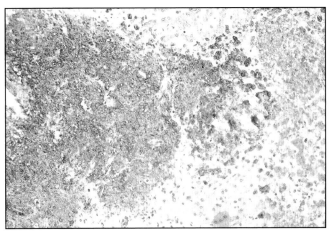

B

Fig. 9.58 • *Pneumocystis jiroveci* infection. **(A)** Post-mortem liver: eosinophilic granular material composed of cysts has infiltrated the sinusoids and replaced the liver cells. H&E. Slide courtesy of Dr R Goldin, London. **(B)** Immunocytochemical stain to demonstrate pneumocystosis (monoclonal anti-Peumocystis).

anti-pneumocystis prophylaxis was instituted, more than 85% of patients with AIDS in industrialized countries developed pneumocystis pneumonia some time before death. Spread of the infection outside the lungs is common in HIV-positive patients with CD4+ T-lymphocyte counts less than 50/mm³, often associated with use of nebulized (inhaled) pentamidine therapy for pneumocystosis. The liver may then be involved in up to 40% of such cases.[219,279,280] Extra-pulmonary pneumocystosis has not yet been seen in HIV disease in Africa.

There is no notable macroscopic appearance. Microscopically there are focal areas where the sinuses are widened and the liver cells are necrotic, being replaced by extracellular frothy pink material on H&E stain. On high power, pale cysts containing a haematoxyphilic dot are seen amongst the eosinophilic material (Fig. 9.58). With a Grocott stain, the characteristic cysts are more evident, their membranes often folded over and bearing a solid dark spot.

Protozoal infections

The protozoa that are more frequent in the liver in HIV-positive patients are *Leishmania* spp., *Toxoplasma gondii*, *Cryptosporidium parvum*, and microsporidia. The last two primarily affect the biliary tree and are considered below.

Toxoplasmosis

Disseminated toxoplasmosis (i.e. outside the usual location of the brain) is uncommon in AIDS patients. Hepatic lesions are occasionally encountered in autopsy material, with microscopic lesions composed of one or more parasitized parenchymal cells which contain zoites and are surrounded by a few lymphocytes or polymorphs (Fig. 9.31). Occasionally large necrotic lesions are seen.[281,282]

Leishmaniasis

The prevalence of leishmaniasis in the liver in HIV-positive patients depends on geography, since the species and strains of *Leishmania* that cause visceral infection are restricted to southern Europe, South America and Africa. Like *H. capsulatum* and *M. tuberculosis*, leishmanial parasites can remain latent in the body for years, only to reactivate as immune competence declines.

The majority of HIV-positive patients with visceral leishmaniasis are intravenous drug users in Europe, and the agent is *L. infantum*.[283] Three-quarters present with leishmaniasis when they already have AIDS and the CD4+ T-lymphocyte counts are about 150/mm³. This infection is not currently an AIDS-defining condition for surveillance purposes, although HIV-positive people are more likely to develop disease than HIV-negative individuals.[284] The potential magnitude of this co-infection is illustrated by a 17% prevalence of leishmanial infection in one Spanish series of HIV-positive people with a fever of unknown origin.[285]

The presentation in HIV-positive people may be atypical, a smaller proportion having hepatosplenomegaly or positive anti-leishmanial serology. The response to chemotherapy is more variable and there is a greater likelihood of relapse.[286] About one-quarter of patients die within one month of presentation.[287] The liver pathology is similar to that in symptomatic non-HIV-infected people: numerous amastigotes within Kupffer cells and portal macrophages, and sometimes within endothelial cells and vessel lumina (Fig. 9.27).[219,288,289] Given the number of intravenous drug users with leishmaniasis, it is not surprising that triple co-infection of HIV, leishmania and HCV is frequent; liver biopsies may show chronic hepatitis or cirrhosis and leishmaniasis. Unusual forms of HIV/leishmania pathology include significant liver necrosis[290] and nodular regenerative hyperplasia.[236]

Amoebiasis

Amoebiasis (infection with *Entamoeba histolytica*) was expected to be an opportunistic infection in HIV-infected patients, but there is no epidemiological evidence for this association.[291] In regions where amoebiasis is common, incidental co-infection may occur. A series from Taiwan documented a protracted course of amoebic liver absess in patients who were co-infected with HIV.[292]

Helminthic infections

Helminthic infections are not more virulent in immuno-compromised patients since few of them proliferate in the host. Common infections (e.g. schistosomiasis) and rarities (e.g. dicrocoeliasis) have been reported in the livers of HIV-positive patients, but their effects are not modified by HIV infection.[293,294] Disseminated infection by *Strongyloides stercoralis*—a worm which does multiply in the host—was initially expected to occur with increased frequency in HIV-positive patients and to be an AIDS-defining disease.[291] Although a few cases have been reported with hepatic involvement,[295] epidemiological studies have not found a significant association between strongyloidiasis and HIV infection.

Tumours

The established HIV-associated tumours are Kaposi sarcoma and non-Hodgkin lymphoma. Spindle cell tumours are recorded in children with AIDS (see below).

Kaposi sarcoma

In 1994 it was established that Kaposi sarcoma is associated with a herpes virus, HHV8 (human herpes virus 8).[296] There are monoclonal antibodies for immunocytochemical demonstration of HHV8 in the nuclei of infected endothelial cells and lymphoid cells, that work well on formalin-fixed tissue. The virus is transmitted by blood and sexual contact, and probably vertically from mother to child.

Kaposi sarcoma involves the liver in up to one fifth of autopsied AIDS patients in industrialized countries, though its prevalence elsewhere is less. This frequency has declined in countries that use anti-retroviral therapy widely, along with the general reduction of classic HIV-associated opportunistic diseases. Only rarely is hepatic Kaposi sarcoma the first presentation of AIDS since the liver is usually involved as part of cutaneous and visceral disseminated disease.[297]

Macroscopically, there may be capsular deposits of tumour, 5–10 mm in diameter, appearing as dark-red blebs. On cut section, Kaposi sarcoma radiates out from the portal tracts and follows the bile ducts.[298] It also causes multiple dark-red spots in the parenchyma (Fig. 9.59). Histologically, the typical lesion is a bland spindle-cell tumour arising around bile ducts and forming a mesh that contains erythrocytes (Fig. 9.60). Early lesions may be difficult to diagnose. They consist of irregular thin-walled dilated vessels which separate the collagen fibres of capsular and portal connective tissue. Clues to the diagnosis of Kaposi sarcoma include the diffuse presence of plasma cells, infrequent and normal mitoses, and clusters of intracytoplasmic eosinophilic inclusions which resemble erythrocytes but are smaller. Immunocytochemistry against HHV8 can assist diagnosis in suspicious cases. Although it is called a sarcoma, it is likely that Kaposi 'disease' is probably a benign reactive vascular hyperplasia.[299]

Lymphomas

HIV-infected people are at high risk of developing non-Hodgkin lymphoma. It is nearly always a high-grade B-cell

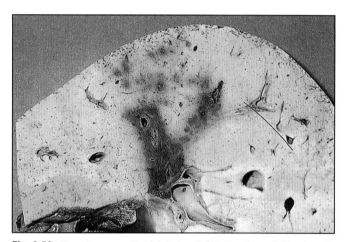

Fig. 9.59 • Kaposi sarcoma. Purplish lesions infiltrating the portal tracts and spreading into the parenchyma. Fixed liver.

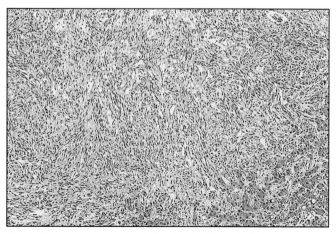

Fig. 9.60 • Kaposi sarcoma. Interlacing bands of Kaposi spindle cells infiltrating a portal tract and extending into the parenchyma. H&E.

lymphoma and the proportion having extra-nodal disease is greater than among HIV-negative patients. Typically, B-cell lymphoma develops when the CD4+ T-lymphocyte counts are below 100/mm³. As treatment of complications prolongs the survival of HIV-infected patients, it is expected that the proportion with lymphoma will increase, perhaps to one-third or more of those who survive more than 3 years with AIDS.[300] In Africa, HIV-associated lymphoma is relatively common compared with the non-HIV population, but less common than in HIV patients in industrialized countries.[301]

The liver is involved in over a quarter of HIV-positive patients with lymphoma and it may be primary there.[302] Infiltration is often diffuse but mass lesions also occur, with multifocal pale tumours several centimetres in diameter. These are often necrotic and can mimic tuberculosis or *M. avium* complex infection. Primary bile-duct lymphoma, clinically and radiologically mimicking sclerosing cholangitis, has also been reported.[303] Histologically, the lymphoma cells are centroblastic or immunoblastic, often with bizarre polylobated nuclei (Fig. 9.61).

The pathogenesis of HIV-associated lymphoma is complicated, with many different histomorphologies and genetic events described.[304,305] Overall, Epstein–Barr virus infection is important. Development in understanding of HHV8 (the Kaposi sarcoma virus) indicates that it is involved in body-cavity lymphomas in HIV patients and in solid organ lymphoma also.[306] Diffuse liver sinusoidal involvement with HHV8-infected B-cells is part of the HHV8-associated lymphoproliferative disease spectrum in HIV.

Although Hodgkin disease has been reported in AIDS patients, it is not clear whether it is aetiologically associated with HIV infection.[307] However, it tends to pursue a more rapidly progressive clinical course.

Other tumours

There is no evidence for an increased frequency of visceral carcinomas but there is an impression that such tumours are more aggressive in HIV-positive patients. Whilst earlier studies in the USA suggested that hepatocellular carcinoma was associated with HIV infection, subsequent larger series have not confirmed this.[308] Nonetheless, the more frequent persistence of HBV envelope protein in HIV-positive people suggests the potential for an association. The more rapid progression of HCV disease in co-infected persons will probably result in more hepatocellular carcinoma.

Inflammatory pseudotumour

Inflammatory pseudotumour simulating liver carcinoma has been described.[309] The histology was of dense fibrous tissue, spindle cells, foamy histiocytes, lymphocytes and plasma cells.

Cholangitis

Two types of cholangitis are seen in HIV-positive patients: ascending bacterial cholangitis and HIV-associated sclerosing cholangitis. The frequency of bacterial cholangitis is not known; the organisms are usually Gram-negative bacilli. The disease resembles that seen in non-HIV-infected people, with dilated biliary tracts and parenchymal abscesses (Fig. 9.62(A)).

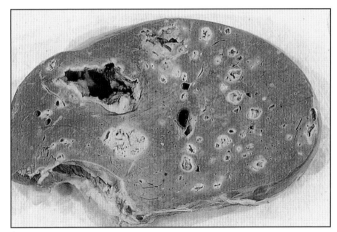

A

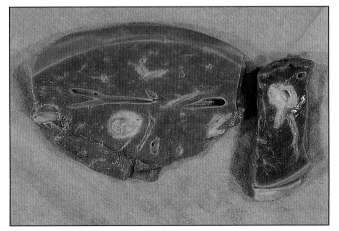

B

Fig. 9.62 • Cholangitis in HIV-positive patients. **(A)** Slice of liver with bacterial ascending cholangitis and several associated hepatic abscesses. **(B)** Sclerosing cholangitis with fibrotic portal tracts.

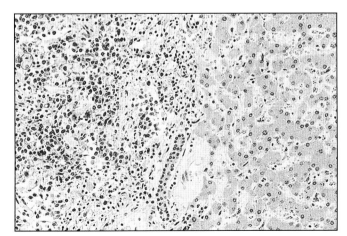

Fig. 9.61 • HIV-associated non-Hodgkin lymphoma. Autopsy liver showing malignant lymphoid cells infiltrating a portal tract. H&E.

Sclerosing cholangitis

HIV-associated sclerosing cholangitis is increasingly recognized as a complication of advanced immune depression: the median CD4+ T-lymphocyte count of patients at diagnosis was 24/mm³.[310] It is characterized by chronic abdominal pain, fever, and cholestasis with dilatation and irregularities of the bile ducts, both intra- and extrahepatic (Fig 9.62(B)). The diagnosis is usually made by ERCP; some cases are virtually identical to primary sclerosing cholangitis (see Chapter 11).

The role of infectious agents

Cryptosporidiosis

Cryptosporidiosis (C. parvum) and cytomegalovirus infections are the most frequently documented. Two-thirds of patients with cholangitis are infected with one or both agents.[310] In a study of HIV-positive men with cryptosporidial diarrhoea, 26% had sclerosing cholangitis.[311] The extrahepatic biliary mucosa is inflamed, often fibrotic, and the epithelium is hyperplastic. The cryptosporidia are seen adhering to the surface of biliary epithelial cells (Fig. 9.63), although electron microscopy shows them to be intracellular, covered by brush-border membrane. Intrahepatic portal tracts are frequently normal but may show mild inflammation, periductal fibrosis or ductal obliteration. Uncommonly, one sees the cryptosporidia attached to small intrahepatic bile ducts in liver biopsies. Similarly, cytomegalovirus inclusions are more often seen in the extrahepatic than in the intrahepatic ducts. Currently, it is thought that C. parvum is the major aetiological agent in HIV-associated sclerosing cholangitis, and that cytomegalovirus is usually a passenger infection.

Analysis of MHC class I and II antigens in the liver in HIV disease has shown that HLA-DR II expression is only found in biliary epithelium, but this does not correlate with biliary pathology.[312] Whether HIV itself causes cholangitis is not clear. Since a similar association with cryptosporidiosis is seen in congenitally immuno-deficient children without HIV infection,[313] it is considered that C. parvum is a sufficient cause of sclerosing cholangitis. However, the pathogenetic mechanisms are unknown.

Microsporidiosis

Microsporidiosis is being diagnosed in an increasing number of the 'pathogen-negative' cases of HIV-associated sclerosing cholangitis. Microsporidia are small oval obligate intracellular protozoan parasites that live and multiply in the cytoplasm of host cells. In man, two genera are important, Enterocytozoon and Encephalitozoon.[314,315] They are recognizable with some difficulty on H&E-stained sections in the supranuclear cytoplasm as clusters of pale refractile spores with a tiny haematoxyphilic nucleus. More sensitive is toluidine blue stain on semi-thin resin sections, or electron microscopy, which is needed to determine the genus and species (Fig. 9.64). A characteristic feature of microsporidia is an electron-dense coiled polar tube.

Enterocytozoon bieneusi is a parasite of small bowel enterocytes found in a proportion of HIV-positive patients with diarrhoea. It has also been observed in the bile of patients with HIV-associated sclerosing cholangitis, and within the cytoplasm of biliary epithelial cells of liver, extrahepatic ducts and gallbladder. There is usually an associated mild mononuclear inflammation of the lamina propria. Cases of co-infection of the biliary tree involving microsporidia, cytomegalovirus, Cryptosporidium and M. avium infection are being reported.[316–319]

Another species, Encephalitozoon intestinalis, is known to disseminate widely among the viscera (in macrophages as well as epithelial cells)[320,321] and has been noted within hepatocytes in a patient with a necrotizing granulomatous and suppurative hepatitis.[316] The same organism has also been seen in sinusoidal lining cells and lying free in clusters in the portal vein.[316]

A study of cholecystitis in HIV/AIDS patients documents both microsporidial species, cytomegalovirus and Cryptosporidium as frequent infections of the gallbladder, and single examples of Pneumocystis jiroveci and Isospora belli.[322]

Paediatric HIV-associated liver disease

At end-2004, UNAIDS estimates that there are 2.2 million living HIV-infected children, >85% of them residing in sub-Saharan Africa. 90% are infected by their mothers, perinatally or through breast milk. The course of HIV disease in children is bimodal: a proportion infected earliest become ill and die within 1–2 years of birth; those infected later, present when some years older.[323] A comprehensive account is given by Moran & Mullick in an AFIP fascicle on paediatric HIV/AIDS pathology.[28]

The liver is often enlarged and shows non-specific features of steatosis and mild portal inflammation. Whilst cytomegalovirus and M. avium complex infections, tuberculosis, Kaposi sarcoma and lymphoma occur in HIV-positive children, they are less frequent than in adults. Hepatic granulomas are uncommon, and hepatic pneumocystosis has not been reported; neither has HIV-associated cholangitis,

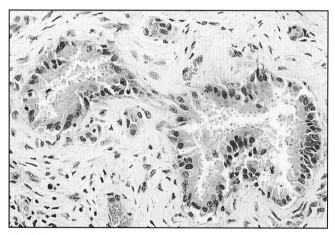

Fig. 9.63 • Cryptosporidial cholangitis. Medium-sized bile duct with numerous Cryptosporidium bodies at the luminal surface of epithelial cells. With electron microscopy, these are seen to reside just within the plasma membrane. H&E.

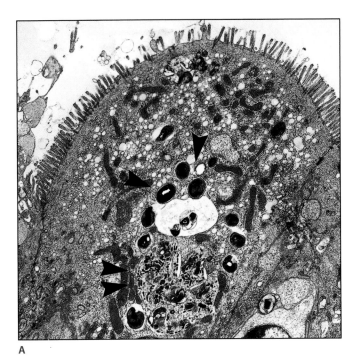

A

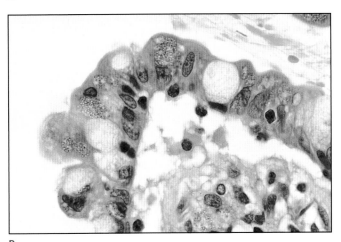

B

Fig. 9.64 • Microsporidiosis. **(A)** Electron micrograph of *Enterocytozoon bieneusi* forms within an epithelial cell: spores (single arrowheads); proliferating plasmodia (double arrowheads). Photograph courtesy of Mr G Tovey, London. **(B)** *Encephalitozoon intestinalis* infection of the duodenum, which also infected the biliary tree. The parasites are seen in the supranuclear portions of enterocytes and in the lamina propria macrophages. H&E.

Table 9.5	Potentially hepatotoxic (non-antiretroviral) drugs commonly used in HIV-positive
Drug	**Indication**
Co-trimoxazole	*Pneumocystis* infection
Pentamidine	*Pneumocystis* and *Toxoplasma* infections
Ketoconazole	Anti-fungal
Fluconazole	Anti-fungal
Rifampicin	Anti-mycobacterial
Isoniazid	Anti-mycobacterial
Ganciclovir	Anti-cytomegalovirus

not more prevalent in HIV-positive children than in controls.[119] This, and unusual infection such as aggressive alveolar hydatid disease,[165] suggest that HIV may influence disease cadence in unpredictable ways.

Spindle-cell tumours that are not Kaposi sarcoma are reported involving the liver of children with HIV, along with gastro-intestinal and tracheopulmonary systems.[327-329] They include fibrosarcoma and smooth muscle tumours of benign, malignant and undetermined potential type.

Drug toxicity in HIV disease

The polypharmacy of HIV-positive patients in industrialized countries is such that drug reactions are an important concern, and a major indication for liver biopsy. The potential for significant interactions between the many drugs that HIV patients take is considerable and complicated.[330] Table 9.5 lists the anti-infection drugs commonly given to HIV/AIDS patients which are potentially hepatotoxic.

Of greater significance are the increasing range of anti-retroviral drugs that inhibit the replication of HIV within cells. These have dramatic effects in prolonging the life of HIV patients and reversing many associated opportunistic diseases[331] but are also associated with significant toxicity, often centred on the liver. Table 9.6 lists the main agents by class and indicates the hepatotoxic pathologies. These drugs are used in combinations (highly active anti-retroviral therapy, HAART), the standard backbone in UK therapy being two NRTIs and one NNRTI, or two NRTIs and a ritonavir-boosted PI. The development and use of anti-HIV drugs is a moving field, and the current status of treatment options and issues, including drug side effects, can be seen on the website of the British HIV Association (BHVIA): www.bhiva.org (HIV treatment guidelines update).

The nucleoside analogue reverse transcriptase inhibitor (NRTI)-associated hepatotoxicity is the most important. The steatosis may be macrovesicular or microvesicular. Like the lactic acidosis syndrome, it is thought to follow from mitochondrial toxicity.[333] In addition to abnormal liver function tests, which become evident a few weeks after commencing the treatments, severe liver damage with failure and death are well documented.[332,338] The histopa-

despite the fact that intestinal cryptosporidiosis is common in children.

Conversely, two hepatic lesions are restricted to children: *giant cell transformation* and a *nodular lympho-plasmacytic portal infiltrate*. It has been suggested that these changes represent abnormal responses to Epstein–Barr virus.[324,325] Some children with hepatomegaly have chronic hepatitis and bile-duct damage.[326] Unlike in hepatitis B virus infection and autoimmune liver disease, these HIV-positive children have predominantly CD8+ T-lymphocytes in the portal tracts. Adenovirus hepatitis is also usually confined to children.

In African children dying with HIV infection, specific hepatic lesions are uncommon although cytomegalovirus, necrotizing herpes simplex, miliary tuberculosis and toxoplasmosis have all been noted. Severe malaria infection is

Table 9.6	Anti-retroviral drugs used in treating HIV-infected patients, and their hepato-toxicities

A. Nucleoside analogue reverse transcriptase inhibitors (NRTI): zidovudine (AZT); zalcitabine; didanosine (ddI); stavudine (d4T) associated with lactic acidosis, steatosis and pancreatitis[332–334] lamivudine (3TC); abacavir; tenofovir (TDF); entricitabine (FTC) not (yet) associated with significant hepatotoxicity

B. Non-nucleoside reverse transcriptase inhibitors (NNRTI): nevirapine; efavirenz; nevirapine has been associated with hepatitis[335]

C. Protease inhibitor (PI): Saquinavir; ritonavir; indinavir; nelfinavir; lopinavir; fosamprenavir associated with lipodystrophy, hyperglycaemia, hyperlipidaemia, and hepatitis[336]

D. Hydroxyurea associated with hepatitis[337]

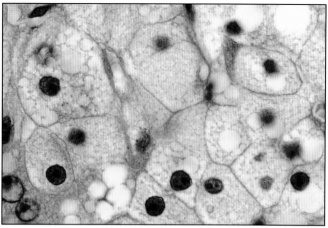

A

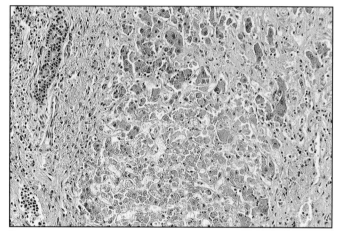

B

Fig. 9.65 • Drug toxicity in HIV disease. **(A)** microvesicular steatosis due to NRTI ddI treatment: the patient died of liver failure. H&E. **(B)** fatal massive liver necrosis due to protease inhibitor therapy. H&E.

thology of acute failure includes microvesicular steatosis, confluent hepatocellular necrosis, inflammation and cholestasis (Fig. 9.65). Severe hepatitis has also been rarely documented in health care workers given short-course HAART as post-exposure prophylaxis following needlestick injury.[339] Didanosine, as well as causing steatosis,[334] has been noted to induce Mallory body formation in hepatocytes.[340]

HCV infection appears to render the liver more liable to toxic damage from antiretroviral therapy,[341] but not such that therapy is precluded. Further, HAART that includes the NNRTI nevirapine appears to accelerate the development of liver fibrosis in HCV/HIVco-infected persons.[342] This contrasts with the overall beneficial effect of HAART on slowing the rate of fibrosis due to HCV when therapy is commenced early.[343]

HIV-2 and liver disease

HIV-2 infection is mainly confined to West Africa, although patients with this infection, with or without HIV-1 co-infection, are also encountered in Europe. HIV-2 causes AIDS, although the progression of disease may be slower than with HIV-1. The same range of pathological manifestations is seen in the liver of such patients, including tuberculosis, sclerosing cholangitis and leishmaniasis.[344,345] An African autopsy study noted more cholangitis, from all causes, in HIV-2 patients compared with HIV-1.[225]

The role of liver biopsy in HIV disease

Many studies of HIV-positive patients with fever, hepatomegaly and abnormal liver function tests of unknown aetiology have been published, and diagnostic strategies involving liver biopsy proposed.[224,346,347] Diagnostic yields of 30–90% are quoted, higher than in the investigation of fever of unknown origin in non-HIV patients,[348] and related to the local prevalence of infectious diseases such as tuberculosis, leishmaniasis, and mycoses.[216] In centres that

Table 9.7	Indications for liver biopsy in HIV infected patients

- Fever of unknown origin

- Suspicion of specific infection: mycobacteria, mycoses, leishmaniasis

- Suspicion of sclerosing cholangitis (see Chapter 11)

- Suspicion of drug toxicity

- Suspicion of lymphoproliferative disease

manage HIV patients intensively, biopsy studies show that jaundice is more likely due to drugs than opportunistic infections.[349] In paediatric patients, liver biopsy is useful in identifying mycobacterial and viral infections, haemophagocytosis, and evaluating jaundice.[350]

The diagnostic sensitivity of liver histology for disseminated infections such as mycobacterioses and mycoses is lower than other techniques such as blood culture, marrow and lymph node examination, and the detection of fungal antigenaemia. Liver biopsy is most useful in evaluation of liver masses, drug hepatotoxicity versus infections, suspected lymphoproliferative disease, biliary tree abnormalities, and undiagnosed fever and hepatosplenomegaly (Table 9.7).

It is essential to examine liver biopsies from all HIV-positive patients with Grocott silver stain for fungi and nocardiosis, Ziehl–Neelsen for mycobacteria and, if bacillary angiomatosis is suspected, a Warthin–Starry stain.

Liver biopsy in AIDS patients is not risk-free. A multicentre study in London found a 1.6% mortality from haemorrhage (4/248) following percutaneous biopsy; this is related to thrombocytopaenia and clotting abnormalities.[351]

References

1. Lucas SB. Pathology of Tropical Infections. In McGee JO, Isaacson PG, Wright NA, eds. Oxford Textbook of Pathology, pp 2187–266. Oxford: OUP, 1992
2. Gutierrez Y. Diagnostic Pathology of Parasitic Infections with Clinical Correlations. Oxford: Oxford University Press, 2000
3. Connor DH, Chandler FW, Manz HJ, Schwartz DA, Lack EE. Pathology of Infectious Diseases. Stanford: Appleton & Lange, 1997
4. Mandell GL, Bennett JE, Dolin R. Principles and Practice of Infectious Diseases. Philadelphia: Churchill Livingstone, 2005
5. Craighead JE. Pathology and Pathogenesis of Human Viral Disease. San Diego: Academic Press, 2000
6. Ishak KG, Walker DH, Coetzer JAW, Gardner JJ, Gorelkin L. Viral hemorrhagic fevers with hepatic involvement: pathologic aspects with clinical correlations. In Popper H, Schaffner F, eds. Progress in Liver Diseases, vol VII, pp 495–515. New York: Grune & Stratton, 1982
7. De Cock KM, Nasidi A, Enriquez J et al. Epidemic yellow fever in Eastern Nigeria, 1986. Lancet, 1989; 1:630–633
8. Francis TI, Moore DL, Edington GM, Smith JA. A clinicopathological study of human yellow fever. Bull WHO, 1972; 46:659–667
9. Wahid SF, Sanusi S, Zawawi MM, Ali RA. A comparison of the pattern of liver involvement in dengue hemorrhagic fever with classic dengue fever. Southeast Asian J Trop Med Public Health, 2000; 31:259–263
10. Bhamarapravati N, Tuchida P, Boonyapaknavik V. Pathology of Thailand haemorrhagic fever: a study of 100 autopsy cases. Ann Trop Med Parasit, 1967; 61:500–510
11. Huerre M, Lan NT, Marianneau P et al. Liver histopathology and biological correlates in 5 cases of fatal dengue fever in Vietnamese children. Virchows Arch[A], 2001; 438:107–115
12. Edington GM, White HA. The pathology of Lassa fever. Trans R Soc Trop Med Hyg, 1972; 66:381–389
13. Health Services Advisory Committee. Safe working and the prevention of infection in the mortuary and post-mortem room. London: HSE Books, 2003
14. Rippey JJ, Schepers NJ, Gear JHS. The pathology of Marburg virus disease. S Afr Med J, 1984; 66:50–54
15. Davis KJ, Anderson AO, Geisbert TW et al. Pathology of experimental Ebola virus infection in African green monkeys. Arch Pathol Lab Med, 1997; 121:805–819
16. Zaki SR, Greer PW, Goldsmith CS et al. Ebola virus hemorrhagic fever: pathologic, immunopathologic and ultrastructural studies. Lab Invest, 1996; 74:133A
17. Burt FJ, Swanepoel R, Shieh WJ et al. Immunohistochemical and in situ localisation of Crimean–Congo Hemorrhagic Fever (CCHF) virus in human tissues and implications for CCHF pathogenesis. Arch Pathol Lab Med, 1997; 121:839–846
18. Walker DP, Longson M, Lawler W, Mallick NP, Davies JS, Jphnson RWG. Disseminated herpes simplex virus infection with hepatitis in an adult renal transplant recipient. J Clin Pathol, 1981; 34:1044–1046
19. Goodman ZD, Ishak KG, Sesterhenn IA. Herpes simplex hepatitis in apparently immunocompetent adults. Am J Clin Pathol, 1986; 85:694–699
20. Kasper WJ, Howe PM. Fatal varicella after a single course of corticosteroids. Pediatr Infect Dis J, 1990; 9:729–732
21. Clarke J, Craig RM, Saffro R, Murphy P, Yokoo H. Cytomegalovirus granulomatous hepatitis. Am J Med, 1979; 66:264–269
22. Snover DC, Horwitz CA. Liver disease in cytomegalovirus mononucleosis: a light microscopical and immunoperoxidase study of six cases. Hepatolology, 1984; 4:408–412
23. Vanstapel M-J, Desmet VJ. Cytomegalovirus hepatitis: a histological and immunohistochemical study. Appl Pathol, 1983; 1:41–49
24. Finegold MJ, Carpenter RJ. Obliterative cholangitis due to cytomegalovirus: a possible precursor of paucity of intrahepatic bile ducts. Hum Pathol, 1982; 13:662–665
25. Purtilo DT, Sakamoto K. Epstein–Barr virus and human disease: immune response determines the clinical and pathologic expression. Hum Pathol, 1981; 12:677–679
26. Kilpatrick ZM. Structural and functional abnormalities of liver in infectious mononucleosis. Arch Intern Med, 1966; 117:47–53
27. Ishak KG. Granulomas of the liver. In Ioachim HL, ed. Pathology of Granulomas, p 309. New York: Raven Press, 1983
28. Moran C, Mullick FG. Systemic Pathology of HIV infection and AIDS in Children. Washington DC: AFIP, 1997
29. Purtilo DT, DeFlorio D, Hutt LM et al. Variable phenotypic expression of an X-linked recessive lymphoproliferative syndrome. N Engl J Med, 1977; 297:1077–1080
30. Chang MY, Campbell WG. Fatal infectious mononucleosis. Association with liver necrosis and herpes-like virus particles. Arch Pathol Lab Med, 1975; 99:185–191
31. Randhawa PS, Jenkins FJ, Nalesnik MA et al. Herpesvirus 6 variant A infection after heart transplantation with giant cell transformation on the bile ductluar and gastroduodenal epithelium. Am J Surg Pathol, 1997; 21:847–853
32. Carmichael GP, Zahradnik JM, Moyer GH, Porter DD. Adenovirus hepatitis in an immunosuppressed adult patient. Am J Clin Pathol, 1979; 71:352–355
33. Janner D, Petru AM, Belchis D, Azimi PH. Fatal adenovirus infection in a child with acquired immunodefiency syndrome. Pediatr Infect Dis J, 1990; 9:434–436
34. Krilov LR, Rubin LG, Frogel M, Gloster E, Ni K, Kaplan M et al. Disseminated adenovirus infection with hepatic necrosis in patients with human immunodeficiency virus infection and other immunodefiency states. Rev Infect Dis, 1990; 12:303–307
35. Sun NC, Smith VC. Hepatitis associated with myocarditis: unusual manifestations of infection with coxsackiie Group B, type 3. N Engl J Med, 1966; 274:190–193
36. Williams AO. Autopsy study of measles in Ibadan, Nigeria. Ghana Med J, 1970; 9:23–27
37. Scully RE, Mark EJ, McNeely WF, McNeely BU. Case records of the Massachusetts General Hospital [measles hepatitis]. N Engl J Med, 1988; 319:495–509
38. McLellan RK, Gleiner JA. Acute hepatitis in an adult with rubeola. JAMA, 1982; 247:2000–2001
39. Heathcote J, Deodhar KP, Scheuer PJ, Sherlock S. Intrahepatic cholestatis in childhood. N Engl J Med, 1976; 295:801–805
40. Anand A, Gray ES, Brown T, Clewley JP, Cohen BJ. Human parvovirus infection in pregnancy and hydrops fetalis. N Engl J Med, 1987; 316:183–186
41. Yoto Y, Kudoh T, Haseyama K, Suzuki N, Chiba S. Human parvovirus B19 infection associated with acute hepatitis. Lancet, 1996; 347:868–869
42. Langnas AN, Markin RS, Cattral MS, Naides SJ. Parvovirus B19 as a possible causative agent of fulminant liver failure and associated applastic anaemia. Hepatolology, 1995; 22:1661–1665
43. Ksiazek TG, Erdman D, Goldsmith CS et al. A novel coronavirus in patients with severe acute respiratory syndrome. N Engl J Med, 2003; 348:1953–1966
44. Lee N, Hui D, Wu A et al. A major outbreak of severe acute respiratory syndrome in Hong Kong. N Engl J Med, 2003; 348:1986–1994
45. Chau TN, Lee KC, Yao H et al. SARS-associated viral hepatitis caused by a novel coronavirus: report of three cases Hepatology, 2004; 39:302–310
46. Wong WM, Ho JC, Hung IF et al. Temporal patterns of hepatic dysfunction and disease activity in patients with SARS. JAMA, 2003; 290:2663–2665
47. Chan HLY, Kwan ACP, To KF et al. Clinical significance of hepatic derangement in severe acute respiratory syndrome. World J Gastroenterol, 2005; 11:2148–2153
48. Pellegrin M, Delsol G, Auvergant JC, Familiades J, Faure H, Guiu M et al. Granulomatous hepatitis in Q fever. Hum Pathol, 1980; 11:51–57
49. Lobdell DH. 'Ring' granulomas in cytomegaloviral hepatitis. Arch Pathol Lab Med, 1987; 111:881–882
50. Murphy E, Griffiths MR, Hunter JA, Burt AD. Fibrin-ring granulomas: a non-specific reaction to liver injury? Histopathol, 1991; 19:91–93
51. Guardia J, Martinez-Vazquez JM, Moragas A. The liver in boutonneuse fever. Gut, 1974; 15:549–551

52. Walker DH, Staiti A, Mansueto G, Tringali G. Frequent occurrence of hepatic lesions in boutonneuse fever. Acta Trop, 1986; 43:175–181

53. Adams JS, Walker DH. The liver in Rocky Mountain spotted fever. Am J Clin Pathol, 1981; 75:156–161

54. Jackson MD, Kirkman C, Bradford WD, Walker DH. Rocky Mountain spotted fever. Hepatic lesions in childhood cases. Pediatr Pathol, 1986; 5:379–388

55. Wollner-Hanssen P, Weström L, Mårdh P-A. Perihepatitis and chlamydial salpingitis. Lancet, 1980; 1:901–904

56. Sehdev AE, Dumler JS. Hepatic pathology in human monocytic ehrlichiosis. Ehrlichia chaffeensis infection. Am J Clin Pathol, 2003; 119:859–865

57. Rackow EC, Astiz ME. Pathophysiology and treatment of septic shock. JAMA, 1991; 266:548–554

58. Bagshawe A, Miller JRM. The aetiology of portal hypertension associated with gross haemorrhage in Kenya. East Afr Med J, 1970; 47:185–187

59. Nakhleh RE, Glock M, Snover DC. Hepatic pathology of chronic granulomatous disease in childhood. Arch Pathol Lab Med, 1992; 116:71–75

60. Kimball MW, Knee S. Gonococcal perihepatitis in a male. N Engl J Med, 1970; 282:1082–1083

61. Lopez-Zeno JA, Keith LG, Berger GS. The Fitz–Hugh–Curtis syndrome revisted: changing perspectives after half a century. J Reprod Med, 1985; 30:567–582

62. Butler T. Plague and other *Yersinia* infections. New York: Plenum, 1983

63. Stjernberg U, Silseth C, Rifland S. Granulomatous hepatitis in Yersinia enterocolitica infection. Hepatoology-Gastroenterol, 1987; 34:56–57

64. Vadillo M, Corbella X, Pac V, Fernandez-Viladrich P, Pujol R. Multiple liver abscesses due to Yersinia enterocolitica discloses primay hemochromatosis. Clin Infect Dis, 1994; 18:938–941

65. Greenstein AJ, Lowenthal BA, Hammer GFS, Schaffner F, Aufses AH. Continuing patterns of disease in pyogenic liver abscess: a study of 38 cases. Am J Gastroenterol, 1984; 79:217–226

66. Cervantes F, Carbonell J, Bruguera M, Force L, Webb S. Liver disease in brucellosis. A clinical and pathologic study of 40 cases. Postgrad Med J, 1982; 58:346–350

67. Christou LG, Dalekos GN, Barbati K, Tsianos EV. A 54-year old stockbreeder with ascites. Lancet, 1997; 349:994

68. Dance DAB. Melioidosis as an emerging global problem. Acta Trop, 2000; 74:115–119

69. Piggot JA, Hochholzer L. Human melioidosis. A histopathologic study of acute and chronic melioidosis. Arch Pathol Lab Med, 1970; 90:101–111

70. Yu VL, Miller WP, Wing EJ, Romano JM, Ruiz CA, Bruns FJ. Disseminated listeriosis presenting as acute hepatitis. Am J Med, 1982; 73:773–777

71. Spach DH, Koehler JE. Bartonella-associated infections. Infect Dis Clinic N Amer, 1998; 12:137–155

72. Rizkallah MF, Meyer L, Ayoub EM. Hepatic and splenic abscesses in cat-scratch disease. Pediatr Infect Dis J, 1988; 7:191–195

73. Delbeke D, Sandler MP, Shaff MI, Miller SF. Cat-scratch disease: report of a case with liver lesions and no lymphadenopathy. J Nucl Med, 1988; 29:1454–1456

74. Ahsan N, Holman MJ, Riley TR, Abendroth CS, Langhoff EG, Yang HC. Peliosis hepatis due to Bartonella henselae in transplantation: a hemato-hepato-renal syndrome. Transplant, 1998; 65:1003–1007

75. Putman HC, Dockerty MB, Waugh JM. Abdominal actinomycosis: an analysis of 122 cases. Surgery, 1993; 28:781–790

76. Kazmi KA, Rab SM. Primary hepatic actinomycosis: a diagnostic problem. Am J Trop Med Hyg, 1989; 40:310–311

77. Chandler FW, Kaplan W, Ajello L. A Color Atlas and Text of the Histopathology of Mycotic Diseases. London: Wolfe Medical Publications Ltd, 1980

78. Brooks SEH, Audretsch JJ. Hepatic ultrastructure in congenital syphilis. Arch Pathol Lab Med, 1978; 102:502–505

79. Sobel HJ, Wolf EH. Liver involvement in early syphilis. Arch Pathol Lab Med, 1972; 93:565–568

80. Romeu J, Rybak B, Dave P, Coven R. Spirochetal vasculitis and bile ductular damage in early hepatic syphilis. Am J Gastroenterol, 1980; 74:352–354

81. Judge DM, Samuel I, Perine PL, Vukotic D. Louse-born relapsing fever in man. Arch Pathol Lab Med, 1974; 97:136–140

82. Ferreira VA, Vianna MR, Yasuda PH, de Brito T. Detection of leptospiral antigen in the human liver and kidney using an immunoperoxidase staining procedure. J Pathol, 1987; 151:125–131

83. Zaki SR, Shieh WJ. Leptospirosis associated with an outbreak of acute febrile illness and pulmonary haemorrhage, Nicaragua 1995. Lancet, 1996; 347:535–536

84. Goellner MH, Agger WA, Burgess JH, Duray PH. Hepatitis due to recurrent Lyme disease. Ann Intern Med, 1988; 108:707–708

85. Duray PH. Clinical pathologic correlations of Lyme disease. Rev Infect Dis, 1989; 11(suppl 6):S1487–S1493

86. Rich AR. The Pathogenesis of Tuberculosis. Springfield: C.C.Thomas, 1951

87. Siegel M. Pathological findings and pathogenesis of congenital tuberculosis. Am Rev Tuberc, 1934; 29:297–309

88. O'Brien JR. Non-reactive tuberculosis. J Clin Pathol, 1954; 7:216–225

89. Karat ABA, Job CK, Rao PSS. Liver in leprosy: histological and biochemical findings. Br.Med.J. 1971; 1:307–310

90. Chen TSN, Drutz DJ, Whelan GE. Hepatic granulomas in leprosy. Arch Pathol Lab Med, 1976; 100:182–185

91. Kramarsky B, Edmondson HA, Peters RL, Reynolds TB. Lepromatous leprosy in reaction. Arch Pathol Lab Med, 1968; 85:516–531

92. Lucas SB. Mycobacteria and the tissues of man. In Ratledge C, Stanford J, eds. The biology of the mycobacteria, vol 3, pp 107–76. London: Academic Press, 1988

93. Desikan KV, Job CK. A review of post mortem findings in 37 cases of leprosy. Int J Lepr, 1968; 36:32–44

94. MacKay A, Alcorn MJ, MacLeod IM, Stack BHR, MacLeod T, Laidlaw M et al. Fatal disseminated BCG infection in an 16-year old boy. Lancet, 1980; 2:1332–1334

95. Sohn CC, Schroff RW, Kliewer KE, Lebel DM, Fligiel S. Disseminated Mycobacterium avium-intracellulare infection in homosexual men with acquired cell-mediated immunodeficiency: a histological and immunologic study of two cases. Am J Clin Pathol, 1983; 79:247–252

96. Maasenkeil G, Opravil M, Salfinger M, Von Graevenitz A, Lüthy R. Disseminated coinfection with Mycobacterium avium complex and Mycobacterium kansasii in a patient with AIDS and liver abscess. Clin Infect Dis, 1992; 14:618–619

97. Simor AE, Patterson C. Disseminated Mycobacterium bovis infection in an elderly patient. Diag Microbiol Infect Dis, 1987; 7:149–153

98. Ausina V, Gurgui M, Verger G, Prats G. Iatrogenic disseminated Mycobacterium chelonei infection. Tubercle, 1984; 65:53–57

99. Dreisin RB, Scoggin C, Davidson PT. The pathogenicity of Mycobacterium fortuitum and Mycobacterium chelonei in man: a report of seven cases. Tubercle, 1976; 57:49–57

100. Bültmann BD, Flad HD, Kaiserling E, Müller-Hermelink HK, Kratzch G, Galle J et al. Disseminated mycobacterial histiocytosis due to M.fortuitum associated with helper T-lymphocyte immune deficiency. Virchows Arch[A], 1982; 395:217–225

101. Razon-Veronesi S, Visconti A, Boeri R, Casiraghi G, Canova G. Linfogranulomatosi disseminata da Mycobacterium fortuitum in eta pediatrica. Minerv Pediatr, 1983; 35:775–783

102. Kurnik PB, Padmanabh U, Bonatsos C, Cynamon MH. Mycobacterium gordonae as a human hepato-peritoneal pathogen, with a review of the literature. Am J Med Sci, 1983; 285:45–48

103. Stewart C, Jackson L. Spleno-hepatic tuberculosis due to Mycobacterium kansasii. Med J Aust, 1976; 2:99–101

104. Zamorano J, Tompsett R. Disseminated atypical mycobacterial infection and pancytopenia. Arch Intern Med, 1968; 121:424–427

105. Bach N, Thung SN, Berk PD. The liver in acquired immunodeficiency syndrome (AIDS). In Bianchi L, Gerok W, Maier KP, Deinhardt FJ, eds. Infectious diseases of the liver, pp 333–351. Dordrecht: Kluwer Academic, 1990

106. Patel KM. Granulomatous hepatitis due to Mycobacterium scrofulaceum: report of a case. Gastroenterol, 1981; 81:156–158

107. Torres RA, Nord J, Feldman R, LaBombardi V, Barr M. Disseminated mixed Mycobacterium simiae-Mycobacterium avium complex infection in acquired immunodeficiency syndrome. J Infect Dis, 1991; 164:432–433

108. Cianculli FD. The radish bacillus (Mycobacterium terrae): saprophyte or pathogen? Am Rev Respir Dis, 1974; 109:138–141

109. Weinberg JR, Gertner D, Dootson G, Chambers ST, Smith H. Disseminated Mycobacterium xenopi infection. Lancet, 1985; 1:1033–1034

110. Tecson-Tumang FT, Bright JL. Mycobacterium xenopi and the acquired immunodeficiency syndrome. Ann Intern Med, 1984; 100:461–462

111. Walsh TJ, Hamilton SR. Disseminated aspergillosis complicating hepatic failure. Arch Intern Med, 1983; 143:1189–1191

112. Sabesin SM, Fallon HJ, Andriole VT. Hepatic failure as a manifestation of cryptococcosis. Arch Intern Med, 1963; 111:661–669

113. Buculvalas JC, Bove KE, Kaufman RA, Gilchrist MJR, Oldham KT, Balistreri WF. Cholangitis associated with Cryptococcus neoformans. Gastroenterology, 1985; 88:1055–1059

114. Goodwin RA, Shapiro JL, Thurman GH, Thurman SS, Des Prez RM. Disseminated histoplasmosis: clinical and pathologic correlations. Medicine, 1980; 59:1–33

115. Wheat LJ, Slama TG, Norton JA, Kohler RB, Eitzen HE, French MLV et al. Risk factors for disseminated or fatal histoplasmosis. Ann Intern Med, 1982; 96:159–163

116. Teixeira F, Gayotto LCdaC, de Brito T. Morphological patterns of the liver in South American blastomycosis. Histopathology, 1978; 2:231–237

117. Jayanetra P, Nitiyanant P, Ajello L et al. Penicilliosis marneffei in Thailand: report of five human cases. Am J Trop Med Hyg, 1984; 33:637–644

118. Meyer RD, Rosen P, Armstrong D. Phycomycosis complicating leukaemia and lymphoma. Ann Intern Med, 1972; 77:871–879

119. Butcher GA. HIV and malaria: a lesson in immunology. Parasitology Today 1992; 8:307–311

120. Warrell DA, Molyneux ME, Beales PF. Severe and complicated malaria. Trans R Soc Trop Med Hyg, 1990; 84(suppl 2):S1–S65

121. Deller JJ, Cifarelli PS, Berque S, Buchanan R. Malaria hepatitis. Milit Med, 1967; 132:614–620

122. Joshi YK, Tandon SK, Acharya SK, Babu S, Tandon M. Acute hepatic failure due to Plasmodium falciparum liver injury. Liver, 1986; 6:357–360

123. de Brito T, Barone AA, Faria RM. Human liver biopsy in P. falciparum and P. vivax malaria: a light and electron microscopy study. Virchows Arch.[A], 1969; 348:220–229

124. Moore G, Homewood CA, Gilles HM. A comparison of pigment from S. mansoni and P. berghei. Ann Trop Med Parasit, 1975; 69:373–374

125. Turrini F, Schwarzer E, Arese P. The involvement of hemozoin toxicity in depression of cellular immunity. Parasitology Today, 1993; 9:297–300

126. Crane GG. Hyperreactive malarious splenomegaly (tropical splenomegaly syndrome). Parasitology Today, 1986; 2:4–9

127. Enrtrican JH, Williams H, Cook IA et al. Babesiosis in man: report of a case from Scotland with observations on the infecting strain. J Infect, 1979; 1:227–1234

128. Bryceson ADM. The liver in leishmaniasis. In Bianchi L, Maier K-P, Gerok W, Deinhardt F, eds. Infectious Diseases of the Liver, pp 215–23. Dordrecht: Kluwer Academic Press, 1989

129. Badaró R, Jones TC, Carvalho EM, et al. New perspectives on a subclinical form of visceral leishmaniasis. J Infect Dis, 1986; 154:1003–1011

130. Pampiglione S, Manson-Bahr PEC, Giungi F, Giunti G, Parenti A, Trotti GC. Studies in Mediterranean leishmaniasis 2. Asymptomatic cases of visceral leishmaniasis. Trans R Soc Trop Med Hyg, 1974; 68:447–453

131. Duarte MIS, Mariano ON, Corbett CEP. Liver parenchymal cell parasitism in human visceral leishmaniasis. Virchows Arch.[A], 1989; 415:1–6

132. Khaldi F, Bennaceur B, Othman HB, Achouri E, Ayachi R, Regaieg R. Les formes sévères d'atteinte hépatique au cours de la leishmaniose viscérale. A propos de 7 cas. Arch Fr Pediatr, 1990; 47:257–260

133. Moreno A, Marazuela M, Yerba M et al. Hepatic fibrin ring granulomas in visceral leishmaniasis. Gastroenterology, 1988; 95:1123–1126

134. Pampiglione S, La Placa M, Schlick G. Studies on Mediterranean leishmaniasis. 1. an outbreak of visceral leishmaniasis in Northern Italy. Trans R Soc Trop Med Hyg, 1974; 68:349–359

135. Daneshbod K. Visceral leishmaniasis (kala azar) in Iran: a pathologic and electron microscopic study. Am J Clin Pathol, 1972; 57:156–166

136. Duarte MIS, Corbett CEP. Histopathological patterns of the liver involvement in visceral leishmaniasis. Rev Inst Med Trop Sao Paulo, 1987; 29:131–136

137. Rogers L. A peculiar intralobular cirrhosis of the liver produced by the protozoal parasite of kala-azar. Ann Trop Med Parasit, 1908; 2:147–152

138. Kumar PV, Omrani GH, Saberfirouzi M, Arshadi C, Arjmand F, Parhizgar A. Kala-azar: liver fine needle aspiration in 23 cases presenting with fever of unknown origin. Acta Cytol, 1996; 40:263–268

139. Ho EA, Suong T-H, Li Y. Comparative merits of sternum, spleen and liver puncture in the study of human visceral leishmaniasis. Trans R Soc Trop Med Hyg, 1948; 41:315–320

140. Bradley DJ, Taylor BA, Blackwell JA et al. Regulation of Leishmania populations within the host: III. Mapping of the locus controlling susceptibility to visceral leishmaniasis in the mouse. Clin Exp Immunol, 1979; 37:7–14

141. Nigam P, Gupta AK, Kapoor KK, Sharan GR, Goyal BM, Joshi LD. Cholestasis in amoebic liver abscess. Gut, 1985; 26:140–145

142. Palmer RB. Changes in the liver in amebic dysentery. With special reference to the origin of amebic abscess. Arch Pathol Lab Med, 1938; 25:327–335

143. Spice WM, Cruz-Reyes JA, Ackers JP. Entamoeba histolytica. In Myint S, Cann A, eds. Molecular and Cell Biology of Opportunistic Infections in AIDS, pp 95–137. London: Chapman & Hall, 1993

144. Clark CG. Entamoeba dispar, an organism reborn. Trans R Soc Trop Med Hyg, 1998; 92:361–364

145. Berninghausen O, Leippe M. Necrosis versus apoptosis as the mechanism of target cell death induced by Entamoeba histolytica. Infect Immun, 1997; 65:3615–3621

146. Young JD, Young TM, Lu LP, Unkless JC, Cohn ZA. Characterization of a membrane pore-forming protein from Entamoeba histolytica. J Exp Med, 1982; 156:1677–1690

147. Seydel KB, Stanley SL. Entamoeba histolytica induces host-cell death in amebic liver abscess by a non-Fas-dependent, non-tumour necrosis alpha-dependent pathway of apoptosis. Infect Immun, 1998; 66:2980–2981

148. Tannich E. Amoebic disease. Entamoeba histolytica and E. dispar: comparison of molecules considered important for host tissue destruction. Trans R Soc Trop Med Hyg, 1998; 92:593–596

149. Tiwari I, Rolland CF, Popple AW. Cholestatic jaundice due to toxoplasma hepatitis. Postgrad Med J, 1982; 58:299–300

150. Weitberg AB, Alper JC, Diamond I, Fligiel Z. Acute granulomatous hepatitis in the course of acquired toxoplasmosis. N Engl J Med, 1979; 300:1093–1096

151. Khuroo MS, Zargar SA, Mahajan R. Hepatobiliary and pancreatic ascariasis in India. Lancet, 1990; 335:1503–1506

152. Gayotto LCdaC, Muszkat RML, Souza IV. Hepatobiliary alterations in massive biliary ascariasis. Histopathological aspects of an autopsy case. Rev Inst Med Trop Sao Paulo, 1990; 32:91–95

153. Daly JJ, Baker GF. Pinworm granuloma of the liver. Am J Trop Med Hyg, 1984; 33:62–64

154. Mondou EN, Gnepp DR. Hepatic granuloma resulting from Enterobius vermicularis. Am J Clin Pathol, 1989; 91:97–100

155. Genta RM. Global prevalence of strongyloidiasis: critical review and epidemiologic insights into the prevention of disseminated disease. Rev Infect Dis, 1989; 11:755–767

156. Nakada K, Yamaguchi K, Furgen S et al. Monoclonal integration of HTLV-1 proviral DNA in patients with strongylodiasis. Int J Cancer, 1987; 40:145–148

157. Poltera AA, Katsimbura N. Granulomatous hepatitis due to Strongyloides stercoralis. J Pathol, 1974; 113:241–246

158. Choe G, Lee HS, Seo JK et al. Hepatic capillariasis: first case report in the Republic of Korea. Am J Trop Med Hyg, 1993; 48:610–625

159. Taylor MRH, Keane CT, O'Connor P, Mulvihill E, Holland C. The expanded spectrum of toxocaral disease. Lancet, 1988; 1:692–695

160. Schantz PM. Toxocara larva migrans now. Am J Trop Med Hyg, 1989; 41(suppl):21–34

161. Hira PR, Lindberg LG, Francis I et al. Diagnosis of cystic hydatid disease: role of aspiration cytology. Lancet, 1988; 2:655–657

162. Pelaez V, Kugler C, Correa D et al. PAIR as percutaneous treatment of hydatid liver cysts. Acta Trop, 2000; 75:197–202

163. Akinoglu A, Demiryurek H, Guzel C. Alveolar hydatid disease of the liver: a report on thirty-nine surgical cases in eastern Anatolia. Am J Trop Med Hyg, 1991; 45:182–189

164. Wilson JF, Rausch RL, Wilson FR. Alveolar hydatid disease. Review of the surgical experience in 42 cases of active disease among Alaskan Eskimos. Ann Surg, 2000; 221:315–323

165. Ciftcioglu MA, Yildirgan MI, Akcay MN, Reis A, Safali M, Aktas E. Fine needled aspiration biopsy in hepatic Echinococcus multilocularis. Acta Cytol, 1997; 41:649–652

166. WHO. The Control of Schistosomiasis. Second report of the WHO expert committee. Geneva: WHO, 1993

167. Wittes R, MacLean JD, Law C, Lough JO. Three cases of schistosomiasis mekongi from northern Laos. Am J Trop Med Hyg, 1984; 33:1159–1163

168. Van Wijk HB, Elias EA. Hepatic and rectal pathology in Schistosoma intercalatum infection. Trop Geog Med, 1975; 27:237–248

169. Nafeh MA, Medhat A, Swifae Y et al. Ultrasonographic changes of the liver in Schistosoma haematobium infection. Am J Trop Med Hyg, 1992; 47:225–230

170. Hiatt RA, Sotomayor ZR, Sanchez G, Zambrana M, Knight WB. Factors in the pathogenesis of acute schistosomiasis mansoni. J Infect Dis, 1979; 139:659–666

171. De Cock KM, Awadh S, Raja RS, Wankya BM, Lucas SB. Eosophageal varices in Nairobi, Kenya: a study of 68 cases. Am J Trop Med Hyg, 1982; 31:579–588

172. Da Silva LC, Carrilho FJ. Hepatosplenic schistosomiasis. Pathophysiology and treatment. Gastroenterol Clin N Am, 1992; 21:163–177

173. Symmers WStC. Note on a new form of liver cirrhosis due to the presence of the ova of Bilharzia haematobia. J Path Bact, 1903; 9:237–239

174. Bhagwandeen SB. The histopathology of early hepatic schistosomiasis. Afr J Med Sci, 1976; 5:125–130

175. Andrade ZA, Peixoto E, Guerret S, Grimaud J-E. Hepatic connective tissue changes in hepatosplenic schistosomiasis. Hum Pathol, 1992; 23:566–573

176. Grimaud JA, Borojevic R. Chronic human schistosomiasis mansoni: pathology of the Disse's space. Lab Invest, 1977; 36:268–273

177. Dunn MA, Kamel R. Hepatic schistosomiasis. Hepatology, 1981; 1:653–661

178. Chen MG, Mott KE. Progress in assessment of morbidity due to Schistosoma japonicum infection. A review of recent literature. Trop Dis Bull, 1988; 85:R1–R45

179. Chen MG, Mott KE. Progress in assessment of morbidity due to Schistosoma mansoni infection. A review of recent literature. Trop Dis Bull, 1988; 85:R1–R56

180. Cheever AW. A quantitative post-mortem study of schistosomiasis mansoni in man. Am J Trop Med Hyg, 1968; 17:38–64

181. Colley DG, Garcia AA, Lambertucci JR, Parra JC, Katz N, Rocha RS et al. Immune responses during human schistosomiasis. XII. Differential responsiveness in patients with hepatosplenic disease. Am J Trop Med Hyg, 1986; 35:793–802

182. Hafez M, Hassan SA, El-Tahan H et al. Immunogenetic susceptibility for post-schistosomal hepatic fibrosis. Am J Trop Med Hyg, 1991; 44:424–433

183. Andrade ZA, Cheever AW. Alterations of the intrahepatic vasculature in hepatosplenic schistosomiasis mansoni. Am J Trop Med Hyg, 1971; 20:425–432

184. Watt G, Padre L, Tuazon M, Wotherspoon A, Adapon B. Hepatic parenchymal dysfunction in Schistosoma japonicum infection. J Infect Dis, 1991; 164:186–192

185. Ye XP, Anderson RM, Nokes DJ. Absense of relationship between Schistosoma japonicum and hepatitis B virus infection in the Dongting lake region, China Epidemiol Infect 1998; 121:193–195

186. Conceicao MJ, Argento CA, Chagas VL et al. Prognosis of schistosomiasis mansoni patients infected with hepatitis B virus. Mem Inst Osw Cruz, 1998; 93:255–288

187. Serufo JC, Antunes CM, Pinto-Silva RA et al. Chronic carriers of hepatitis B surface antigen in an endemic area for schistosomiasis mansoni in Brazil. Mem Inst Osw Cruz, 1998; 93:249–253

188. Ghaffar YA, Fatah SA, Kamel M, Badr RM, Mahomed FF, Strickland GT. The impact of endemic schistosomiasis on acute viral hepatitis. Am J Trop Med Hyg, 1991; 45:743–750

189. Frank C, Mohammed MK, Strickland GT. The role of parenteral antischistosomal therapy in the spread of hepatitic C virus in Egypt. Lancet, 2000; 355:887–891

190. Strickland GT, Elhefni H, Salman T et al. Role of hepatitis C infection in chronic liver disease in Egypt. Am J Trop Med Hyg, 2002; 67:436–442

191. Halim A-B, Garry RF, Dash S, Gerber MA. Effect of schistosomiasis and hepatitis on liver disease. Am J Trop Med Hyg, 1999; 60:915–920

192. Helal TE, Danial MF, Ahmed HF. The relationship between HCV and schistosomiasis: histopathologic evaluation of liver biopsy specimens. Hum Pathol, 1998; 29:743–749

193. Mohamed A, Elsheikh A, Ghandour Z, Al Karawi M. Impact of hepatitis C virus on schistosomal liver disease. Hepato-Gastroenterology, 1998; 45:1492–1496

194. Gad A, Tanaka E, Orii K et al. Relationship between hepatitis C virus infection and schistosomal liver disease: not simply an additive effect. J Gastroenterol, 2001; 36:753–758

195. Mabrouk GM. Prevalence of HCV infection and schistosomiasis in Egyptian patients with hepatocellular carcinoma. Dis Markers, 2000; 13:177–182

196. Homeida M, Abdel GAF, Cheever AW, Bennett JL. Diagnosis of pathologically confirmed Symmers' periportal fibrosis by ultrasonography: a prospective blinded study. Am J Trop Med Hyg, 1988; 38:86–91

197. Houston S, Munjoma M, Kanyimo K, Davidson RN, Flowerdew G. Use of ultrasound in a study of schistosomal periportal fibrosis in rural Zimbabwe. Acta Trop, 1993; 53:51–58

198. Zwingenberger K, Richter J, Vergetti JGS, Feldmeier H. Praziquantel in the treatment of hepatosplenic schistosomiasis: biochemical disease markers indicate deceleration of fibrogenesis and diminution of portal flow obstruction. Trans R Soc Trop Med Hyg, 1990; 84:252–526

199. Ohmae H, Tanaka M, Hayashi M et al. Improvement of ultrasonographic and serologic changes in Schistosoma japonicum-infected patients after treatment with praziquantel. Am J Trop Med Hyg, 1992; 46:99–104

200. Chen MG, Mott KE. Progress in assessment of morbidity due to Schistosoma intercalatum infection: a review of recent literature. Trop Dis Bull, 1989; 86(no 8):R1–R18

201. Chen MG, Mott KE. Progress in assessment of morbidity due to Schistosoma haematobium infection. A review of recent literature. Trop Dis Bull, 1989; 86(no 4):R1–R36

202. Upatham ES, Viyanant V, Kurathong S et al. Relationship between prevalence an intensity of Opisthorcis viverrini infection, and clinical symptoms and signs in a rural community in north-east Thailand. Bull WHO, 1984; 62:451–461

203. Vatanasapt V, Uttaravichien T, Mairiang E-O, Pairojkul C, Chartbanchachai W, Haswell EM. Cholangiocarcinoma in north-east Thailand. Lancet, 1990; 335:117–118

204. Koompirochana C, Sonakul D, Chinda K, Stitnimankarn T. Opisthorcis: a clinicopathologic study of 154 autopsy cases. Southeast Asian J Trop Med Public Health, 1978; 9:60–64

205. Hou PC. The pathology of Clonorchis sinensis infestation of the liver. J Pathol, 1955; 70:53–64

206. Flavell DJ. Liver-fluke infection as an aetiological factor in bile-duct carcinoma of man. Trans R Soc Trop Med Hyg, 1981; 75:814–824

207. Chen MG, Lu WP, Hua XJ, Mott KE. Progress in assessment of morbidity due to Clonorchis sinensis infection: a review of recent literature. Trop Dis Bull, 1994; 91:R7–R65

208. Acosta-Ferreira W, Vercelli-Hetta J, Falconi LM. Fasciola hepatica human infection. Histopathological study of 16 cases. Virchows Arch.[A], 1979; 383:319–327

209. Chen MG, Mott KE. Progress in assessment of morbidity due to Fasciola hepatica infection: a review of recent literature. Trop Dis Bull, 1990; 87:R1–R37

210. Gardiner CH, Dyke JW, Shirley SF. Hepatic granuloma due to a nymph of Linguatula serrata in a woman from Michigan. A case report and review of the literature. Am J Trop Med Hyg, 1984; 33:187–189

211. Self JT, Hopps HC, Williams AO. Pentastomiasis in Africans. Trop Geog Med, 1975; 27:1–13

212. Prathap K, Lau KS, Bolton JM. Pentastomiasis: a common finding at autopsy in Malaysian aborigines. Am J Trop Med Hyg, 1969; 18:20–27

213. Feinberg MB. Changing the natural history of HIV disease. Lancet, 1996; 348:239–246

214. Centers for Disease Control and Prevention. Revision of the CDC surveillance case definition for AIDS. MMWR 1987; 36:1S–15S

215. Buehler JW, Ward JW. A new case definition for AIDS surveillance. Ann Intern Med, 1993; 118:390–392

216. Piratvisuth T, Siripaitoon P, Sriplug H, Ovartlarnporn B. Findings and benefit of liver biopsies in 46 patients infected with HIV. J Gastroenterol Hepatol, 1999; 14:146–149

217. Nakanuma Y, Liew CI, Peters RL, Govindarajan S. Pathologic features of the liver in AIDS. Liver 1986; 6:158–166

218. Schneiderman DJ, Arenson DM, Cello JP, Margaretten W, Weber TE. Hepatic disease in patients with the acquired immunodeficiency syndrome (AIDS). Hepatology, 1987; 7:925–930

219. Wilkins MJ, Lindley R, Doukaris SP, Goldin RD. Surgical pathology of the liver in HIV infection. Histopathology, 1991; 18:459–464

220. Cello JP. Acquired immunodeficiency syndrome cholangiopathy: spectrum of disease. Am J Med, 1989; 86:539–546

221. Rathi PM, Amrapurkar DN, Borges NE, Koppikar GV, Kalro RH. Spectrum of liver diseases in HIV infection. Ind J Gastroenterol, 1997; 16:94–95

222. Palmer M, Braly LF, Schaffner F. The liver in AIDS disease. Semin Liv Dis, 1987; 7:192–202

223. Dowsett JF, Miller R, Davidson R, Vaira D, Polydorou A, Cairns SR et al. Sclerosing cholangitis in acquired immunodeficiency syndrome. Case reports and a review of the literature. Scand J Gastroenterol, 1988; 23:1267–1274

224. Bonacini M. Hepatobiliary complications in patients with human immunodeficiency virus infection. Am J Med, 1992; 92:404–411

225. Lucas SB, Hounnou A, Peacock CS et al. The mortality and pathology of HIV disease in a West African city. AIDS, 1993; 7:1569–1579

226. Boag FC, Dean R, Hawkins DA, Lawrence AG, Gazzard BG. Abnormalities of liver function during HIV seroconversion illness. Int J STD AIDS, 1992; 3:46–48

227. Molina JM, Welker Y, Ferchal F, Decazes JM, Shenmetzler C, Modaï J. Hepatitis associated with primary HIV infection. Gastroenterology, 1992; 102:739

228. Goldin R, Wilkins M, Dourakis S, Parkin J, Lindley R. Iron overload in multiply transfused patients who are HIV seropositive. J Clin Pathol, 1993; 46:1036–1038

229. Freiman JP, Helfert KE, Hamrell MR, Stein DS. Hepatomegaly with severe steatosis in HIV-seropositive patients. AIDS, 1993; 7:379–385

230. Klatt EC. Practical AIDS Pathology. Chicago: ASCP Press, 1992

231. Housset C, Bouchier O, Girard PM et al. Immunohistochemical evidence for human immunodeficiency virus-1 infection of liver Kupffer cells. Hum Pathol, 1990; 21:404–408

232. Cao Y, Dieterich D, Thomas PA, Huang Y, Mirabile M, Ho DD. Identification and quantification of HIV-1 in the liver of patients with AIDS. AIDS, 1992; 6:65–70

233. Buckley JC, Hutchins GM. Association of hepatic veno-occlusive disease with AIDS. Mod Pathol, 2000; 8:398–401

234. Welch K, Finkbeiner W, Alpers CE, Blumenfeld W, Davis RL, Smuckler EA et al. Autopsy findings in the acquired immune deficiency syndrome. JAMA, 1984; 252:1152–1159

235. Cozzi PJ, Abu-Jawdeh GM, Green RM, Green D. Amyloidosis in association with human immunodeficiency virus infection. Clin Infect Dis, 1992; 14:189–191

236. Fernandez-Miranda C, Colina F, Delgado JM, Lopez-Carreira M. Diffuse nodular regenerative hyperplasia of the liver associated with HIV and visceral leishmaniasis. Am J Gastroenterol, 1993; 88:433–435

237. Zimmerli W, Bianchi L, Gudat F et al. Disseminated herpes simplex type 2 and systemic Candida infection in a patient with previous asymptomatic HIV infection. J Infect Dis, 1988; 157:597–598

238. Beissner RS, Rappaport ES, Diaz JA. Fatal case of Epstein–Barr virus-induced lymphoproliferative disorder associated with a human immunodeficiency virus infection. Arch Pathol Lab Med, 1987; 111:250–253

239. Albrecht H, Schafer H, Stellbrink H-J, Greten H. Epstein–Barr-virus-associated hemophagocytic syndrome. A cause of fever of unknown origin in HIV infection. Arch Pathol Lab Med, 1997; 121:853–858

240. Bodsworth NJ, Cooper DA, Donovan B. The influence of human immunodeficiency virus type 1 infection on the development of hepatitis B virus carrier state. J Infect Dis, 1991; 163:1138–1140

241. Waite J, Gilson RJC, Weller IVD, Lacey CJN, Hambling MH, Hawkins A et al. Hepatitis B virus reactivation or reinfection associated with HIV-1 infection. AIDS, 1988; 2:443–448

242. Goldin RD, Fish DE, Hay A, Waters JA, McGarvey MJ, Main J et al. Histological and immunohistochemical study of hepatitis B virus in human immunodeficiency virus infection. J Clin Pathol, 1990; 43:203–205

243. Prufer-Kramer L, Kramer A, Weigel R et al. Hepatic involvement in patients with human immunodeficiency virus infection: discrepancies between AIDS patients and those with earlier stages of infection. J Infect Dis, 1991; 163:866–869

244. Eskild A, Magnus P, Petersen G et al. Hepatitis B antibodies in HIV-infected homosexual men are associated with more rapid progression to AIDS. AIDS, 1992; 6:571–574

245. Ghosn J, Pierre-Francois S, Thibault V et al. Acute hepatitis C in HIV-infected men who have sex with men. HIV Med, 2004; 5:303–306

246. Vento S, Cruciani M, Di Perri G et al. Hepatitis C virus with normal liver histology in symptomless HIV-1 infection. Lancet, 1992; 340:1161

247. García-Samaniego J, Soriano V, Castilla J et al. Influence of hepatitis C virus genotypes and HIV infection on histological severity of chronic hepatitis C. The Hepatitis/HIV Spanish Study Group. Am J Gastroenterol, 1997; 92:1130–1134

248. Bierhoff E, Fischer HP, Willsch E et al. Liver histopathology in patients with concurrent chronic hepatitis C and HIV infection. Virchows Arch.[A], 1997; 430:271–277

249. Dragoni F, Cafolla A, Gentile G et al. HIV-HCV RNA loads and liver failure in coinfected patients with coagulopathy. Haematologica, 1999; 84:525–529

250. Lesens O, Deschenes M, Steben M, Belanger G, Tsoukas CM. Hepatitis C virus is related to progressive liver disease in HIV+ve haemophiliacs and should be treated as an opportunistic infection. J Infect Dis, 1999; 179:1254–1258

251. Ghany MG, Leissinger C, Lagier R, Sanchez-Pescador R, Lok AS. Effect of HIV infection on hepatitis C virus infection in hemophiliacs. Dig Dis Sci, 1996; 41:1265–1272

252. Garcia-Samaniego J, Rodriguez M, Berenguer J et al. Hepatocellular carcinoma in HIV-infected patients with chronic hepatitis C. Am J Gastroenterol, 2001; 96:179–183

253. Macias J, Pineda JA, Leal M et al. Influence of hepatitis C virus on the mortality of antiretroviral-treted patients with HIV disease. Eur J Clin Microbiol Infect Dis, 1998; 17:167–170

254. Sabin CA, Telfer P, Phillips AN, Bhagani S, Lee CA. The association between hepatitis C virus genotype and HIV disease progression in a cohort of hemophiliac men. J Infect Dis, 1997; 175:164–168

255. Piroth L, Duong M, Quantin C et al. Does hepatitis C virus co-infection accelerate the clinical and immunological evolution of HIV-infected patients? AIDS, 1999; 12:381–388

256. Bonnet F, Morlat P, Chene G et al. Causes of death among HIV-infected patients in the era of highly active antiretroviral therapy, Bordeaux, France, 1998–99. HIV Med, 2002; 3:195–199

257. De Cock KM, Soro B, Coulibaly I-M, Lucas SB. Tuberculosis and HIV infection in sub-Saharan Africa. JAMA, 1992; 268:1581–1587

258. Lanjewar DN, Rao RJ, Kulkarni S, Hira SK. Hepatic pathology in AIDS: a pathological study from Mumbai, India. HIV Med, 2004; 5:253–257

259. Nambuya A, Sewankambo NK, Mugerwa J, Goodgame RW, Lucas SB. Tuberculous lymphadenitis associated with human immunodeficiency virus (HIV) in Uganda. J Clin Pathol, 1988; 41:93–96

260. Wallace JM, Hannah JB. Mycobacterium avium complex infection in patients with the acquired immunodeficiency syndrome. A clinicopathologic study. Chest, 1988; 93:926–932

261. Nightingale SD, Byrd LT, Southern PM, Jockusch JD, Cal SX, Wynne BA. Incidence of Mycobacterium avium-intracellulare complex bacteremia in human immunodeficiency virus-positive patients. J Infect Dis, 1992; 165:1082–1085

262. Lucas SB. HIV and leprosy (editorial). Lepr Rev, 1993; 64:97–103

263. Czapar CA, Weldon-Linne CM, Moore DM, Rhone DP. Peliosis hepatis in acquired immunodeficiency syndrome. Arch Pathol Lab Med, 1986; 110:611–613

264. Steeper TA, Rosenstein H, Weiser J, Inampudi S, Snover DC. Bacillary epithelioid angiomatosis involving the liver, spleen, and skin in an AIDS patient with concurrent Kaposi's sarcoma. Am J Clin Pathol, 1992; 97:713–718

265. Perkocha LA, Geaghan SM, Yen TSB et al. Clinical and pathological features of bacillary peliosis hepatitis in association with human immunodeficiency virus infection. N Engl J Med, 1990; 323:1581–1586

266. Schlossberg D, Morad Y, Krouse TB, Wear DJ, English CK. Culture-proven disseminated cat-scratch disease in acquired immunodeficiency syndrome. Arch Intern Med, 1989; 149:1437–1439

267. Raoult D, Levy P-Y, Dupont HT et al. Q fever and HIV infection. AIDS, 1993; 7:81–86

268. Nichols L, Balogh K, Silverman M. Bacterial infections in the acquired immunodeficiency syndrome. Clinicopathologic correlations in a series of autopsy cases. Am J Clin Pathol, 1989; 92:787–790

269. Gilks CF, Ojoo SA, Brindle RJ. Non-opportunistic bacterial infections in HIV-seropositive adults in Nairobi, Kenya. AIDS, 1991; 5(suppl 1):S113–S116

270. Filce C, Brunetti E, Carnevale G, Dughetti S, Pirola F, Rondanelli EG. Ultrasonographic and microbiological diagnosis of mycotic liver abscess in patients with AIDS. Microbiologica, 1989; 12:101–104

271. Pursell KJ, Telzak EE, Armstrong D. Aspergillus species colonization and invasive disease in patients with AIDS. Clin Infect Dis, 1992; 14:141–148

272. Harding CV. Blastomycosis and opportunistic infections in patients with acquired immunodeficiency syndrome. An autopsy study. Arch Pathol Lab Med, 1992; 115:1133–1136

273. Carme B, Ngaporo AI, Ngolet A, Ibara JR, Ebikili B. Disseminated African histoplasmosis in a Congolese patient with AIDS. J Med Vet Mycol, 1992; 30:245–248

274. Tsui WMS, Ma KF, Tsang DNC. Disseminated Penicillium marneffei infection in HIV-infected subject. Histopathology, 1992; 20:287–291

275. Cooper CR, McGinnis MR. Pathology of Penicillium marneffei. An emerging AIDS-related pathogen. Arch Pathol Lab Med, 1997; 121:798–804

276. Bronnimann DA, Adam RD, Galgiani JN, Habib MP, Petersen EA, Porter B et al. Coccidioidomycosis in the acquired immunodeficiency syndrome. Ann Intern Med, 1987; 106:372–379

277. Lucas SB, Hounnou A, Peacock CS, Beaumel A, Kadio A, De Cock KM. Nocardiosis in HIV-positive patients: an autopsy study in West Africa. Tuberc Lung Dis, 1994; 75:301–307

278. Wakefield AE, Stewart TJ, Moxon ER, Marsh K, Hopkin JM. Infection with Pneumocystis carinii is prevalent in healthy Gambian children. Trans R Soc Trop Med Hyg, 1990; 84:800–802

279. Telzak EE, Cote RJ, Gold JWM, Campbell SW, Armstrong D. Extrapulmonary Pneumocystis carinii infection. Rev Infect Dis, 1990; 12:380–386

280. Coker RJ, Clark D, Claydon EL, Gompels M, Ainsworth JG, Lucas SB et al. Disseminated Pneumocystis carinii infection in AIDS. J Clin Pathol, 1991; 44:820–833

281. Mastroianni CM, Coronado O, Scarani P, Manfredi R, Chiodi F. Liver toxoplasmosis and AIDS. Recenti Prog Med, 1996; 87:353–355

282. Artigas J, Grosse G, Niedobitek F. Anergic disseminated toxoplasmosis in a patient with the acquired immunodeficiency syndrome. Arch Pathol Lab Med, 1993; 117:540–541

283. Albrecht H, Sobottka I, Emminger C et al. Visceral leishmaniasis emerging as an important opportunistic infection in HIV-infected persons living in areas non-endemic for Leishmania donovani. Arch Pathol Lab Med, 1997; 121:189–198

284. Altes J, Salas A, Riera M et al. Visceral leishmaniasis: another HIV-associated opportunistic infection? Report of eight cases and review of the literature. AIDS, 1991; 5:201–207

285. Alvar J, Gutierrez-Solar B, Molina R et al. Prevalence of Leishmania infection among AIDS patients. Lancet, 1992; 339:1427

286. Peters BS, Fish D, Goldin R, Evans DA, Bryceson ADM, Pinching AJ. Visceral leishmaniasis in HIV infection and AIDS: clinical features and response to therapy. Q J Med, 1990; 77:1101–1111

287. Lopez-Velez R, Perez-Molina JA, Guerrero A et al. Clinicorepidemiologic characteristics, prognostic factors, and survival analysis of patients co-infected with HIV and Leishmania in an area of Madrid, Spain. Am J Trop Med Hyg, 1998; 58:436–443

288. Hofman V, Marty P, Perrin C, Saint-Paul M-C et al. The histological spectrum of visceral leishmaniasis caused by Leishmania infantum MON-1 in AIDS. Hum Pathol, 2000; 31:75–84

289. Falk S, Helm EB, Hübner K, Stutte HJ. Disseminated visceral leishmaniasis (kala azar) in acquired immunodeficiency syndrome (AIDS). Path Res Pract, 1989; 183:253–255

290. Angarano G, Maggi P, Rollo MA et al. Diffuse necrotic hepatic lesions due to visceral leishmaniasis in AIDS. J Infect, 1998; 36:167–169

291. Lucas SB. Missing infections in AIDS. Trans R Soc Trop Med Hyg, 1990; 84(Suppl 1):34–38

292. Liu CJ, Hung CC, Chen MY et al. Amebic liver abscess and HIV infection: a report of three cases. J Clin Gastroenterol, 2001; 33:64–68

293. Tuur SM, Macher AM, De Vinatea ML, Baird JK, Neafie RC, McGivney RK et al. Case for diagnosis. Milit Med, 1987; 152: M10–M16

294. Drabick JJ, Egan JE, Brown SL, Vick RG, Sandman BM, Neafie RC. Dicroceliasis (lancet fluke disease) in an HIV seropositive man. JAMA, 1988; 259:567–568

295. Harcourt-Webster JN, Scaravilli F, Darwish AH. Strongyloides stercoralis hyperinfection in an HIV positive patient. J Clin Pathol, 1991; 44:346–348

296. Chang Y, Cesarman E, Pessin MS et al. Identification of herpes virus like sequences in AIDS-associated Kaposi's sarcomas. Science, 1994; 266:1865–1869

297. Hasan FA, Jeffers LJ, Welsh SW, Reddy KR, Schiff ER. Hepatic involvement as the primary manifestation of Kaposi' sarcoma in the acquired immune deficiency syndrome. Am J Gastroenterol, 1989; 84:1449–1451

298. Glasgow BJ, Anders K, Layfield LJ, Steinsapir KD, Gitnick GL, Lewin KJ. Clinical and pathologic findings of the liver in acquired immune deficiency syndrome (AIDS). Am J Clin Pathol, 1985; 83:582–588

299. Bayley AC, Lucas SB. Kaposi's sarcoma or Kaposi's disease? A personal reappraisal. In Fletcher CDM, McKee PM, eds. Pathobiology of soft tissue tumours, pp 141–64. Edinburgh: Churchill Livingstone, 1990

300. Pluda JM, Yarchoan R, Jaffe ES et al. Development of non-Hodgkin lymphoma in a cohort of patients with severe human immunodeficiency virus (HIV) infection on long-term antiretroviral therapy. Ann Intern Med, 1990; 113:276–282

301. Lucas SB, Diomandé M, Hounnou A et al. HIV-associated lymphoma in Africa: an autopsy study in Côte d'Ivoire. Int J Cancer, 1994; 59:20–24

302. Caccamo D, Pervez NK, Marchevsky A. Primary lymphoma of the liver in the acquired immunodeficiency syndrome. Arch Pathol Lab Med, 1986; 110:553–555

303. Kaplan LD, Kahn J, Jacobson M, Bottles K, Cello J. Primary bile duct lymphoma in the acquired immunodeficiency syndrome (AIDS). Ann Intern Med, 1989; 110:161–162

304. Knowles DM. Immunodeficiency-associated lymphoproliferative disorders. Mod Pathol, 1999; 12:200–217

305. Knowles DM. Molecular pathology of AIDS-related non-Hodgkin's lymphoma. Semin Diag Pathol, 1997; 14:67–82

306. Cesarman E, Knowles DM. The role of Kaposi's sarcoma-associated herpesvirus (KSHV/HHV8) in lymphoproliferative diseases. Semin Canc Biol, 1999; 9:165–174

307. Ioachim HL, Dorsett B, Cronin W, Maya M, Wahl S. Acquired immunodeficiency syndrome-associated lymphomas: clinical, pathologic, immunologic, and viral characteristics of 111 cases. Hum Pathol, 1991; 22:659–673

308. Rabkin CS, Blattner WA. HIV infection and cancers other than non-Hodgkin lymphoma and Kaposi's sarcoma. In Beral V, Jaffe HW, Weiss RA, eds. Cancer, HIV and AIDS, pp 151–60. New York: Cold Spring Harbour Laboratory Press, 1991

309. Tai YS, Lin PW, Chen SG, Chang KC. Inflammatory pseudotumour of the liver in a patient with HIV infection. Hepato-Gastroenterology, 2005; 45:1760–1763

310. Forbes A, Blanshard C, Gazzard BG. Natural history of AIDS sclerosing cholangitis: a study of 20 cases. Gut, 1993; 34:116–121

311. McGowan I, Hawkins AS, Weller IVD. The natural history of cryptosporidial diarrhoea in HIV-infected patients. AIDS, 1993; 7:349–354

312. Sieratzki J, Thung SN, Gerber MA, Ferrone S, Schaffner F. Major histocompatibility antigen expression in the liver in acquired immunodeficiency syndrome. Arch Pathol Lab Med, 1987; 111:1045–1049

313. David JJ, Heyman MB, Ferrell L, Kerner J, Kerlan R, Tahler MM. Sclerosing cholangitis associated with chronic cryptosporidiosis in a child with a congenital immunodeficiency disorder. Am J Gastroenterol, 1987; 82:1196–1202

314. Shadduck JA, Orenstein JM. Comparative pathology of microsporidiosis. Arch Pathol Lab Med, 1993; 117:1215–1219

315. Schwartz DA, Sobottka I, Leitch GJ, Cali A, Visvesvara GS. Pathology of microsporidiosis. Arch Pathol Lab Med, 1996; 120:173–188

316. Orenstein JM, Dieterich DT, Kotler DP. Systemic dissemination by a newly recognised intestinal microsporidia species in AIDS. AIDS, 1992; 6:1143–1150

317. Beaugerie L, Teilhac MF, Deluol A-M, Fritsch J, Girard P-M, Rozenbaum W et al. Cholangiopathy associated with Microsporidia infection of the common bile duct mucosa in a patient with HIV infection. Ann Intern Med, 1992; 117:401–402

318. Pol S, Romana C, Richard S, Carnot F, Dumont J-L, Bouche H et al. Enterocytozoon bieneusi infection in acquired immunodeficiency syndrome-related sclerosing cholangitis. Gastroenterology, 1992; 102:1778–1781

319. Pol S, Romana C, Richard S, Amouyal P, Desportes-Livage I, Carnot F et al. Microsporidia infection in patients with the human immunodeficiency virus and unexplained cholangitis. N Engl J Med, 1993; 328:95–99

320. Cowley GP, Miller RF, Papadaki L, Canning EU, Lucas SB. Disseminated microsporidiosis (Encephalitozoon intestinalis) in a patient with AIDS. Histopathology, 1997; 30:386–389

321. Terada S, Reddy KR, Jeffers LJ, Cali A, Schiff ER. Microsporidian hepatitis in the acquired immunodeficiency syndrome. Ann Intern Med, 1987; 107:61–62

322. French AL, Beaudet LM, Benator DA, Levy CS, Kass M, Orenstein JM. Cholecystectomy in patients with AIDS: clinicopathological correlations in 107 cases. Clin Infect Dis, 1995; 21:852–858

323. Blanche S, Tardieu M, Duliege A-M et al. Longitudinal study of 94 symptomatic infants with perinatally acquired human immunodeficiency virus infection. Am J Dis Child, 1990; 144:1210–1205

324. Kahn E, Greco MA, Daum F et al. Hepatic pathology in pediatric acquired immunodeficiency syndrome. Hum Pathol, 1991; 22:1111–1119

325. Jonas MM, Roldan EO, Lyons HJ, Fojaco RM, Reddy RK. Histopathologic features of the liver in pediatric acquired immunodeficiency syndrome. J Pediatr Gastroenterol Nutr, 1989; 9:73–81

326. Duffy LF, Daum F, Kahn E et al. Hepatitis in children with acquired immune deficiency syndrome. Gastroenterology, 1986; 90:173–181

327. Ninane J, Moulin D, Latinne D et al. AIDS in two African children: one with fibrosarcoma of the liver. Eur J Pediatr, 1985; 144:385–390

328. Ross JS, Varin F, Mayaux MJ et al. Primary hepatic leiomyosarcoma in a child with AIDS. Hum Pathol, 1992; 23:69–72

329. van Hoeven KH, Factor SM, Kress Y, Woodruff JM. Visceral myogenic tumours. A manifestation of HIV infection in children. Am J Surg Pathol, 1993; 17:1176–1181

330. Piscitelli SC, Flexner C, Minor JR, Polis MA, Masur H. Drug interactions in patients infected with HIV. Clin Infect Dis, 1996; 23:685–693

331. BHIVA Writing Committee. BHIVA guidelines for the treatment of HIV-infected adults with antiretroviral therapy. HIV Med. 2000; 1:76–101

332. Sundar K, Suarez M, Banogon PE, Shapiro JM. Zidovudine-induced fatal lactic acidosis and hepatic failure in patients with AIDS: report of two patients and review of the literature. Crit Care Med, 1997; 25:1425–1430

333. Chariot P, Drogou I, de Lacroix-Szmania I et al. Zidovudine-induced mitochondrial disorder with massive liver steatosis, myopathy, lactic acidosis, and mitochondrial DNA depletion. J Hepatol, 1999; 30:156–160

334. Lai KK, Gang DL, Zawacki JK, Cooley TP. Fulminant hepatic failure associated with 2′,3′-dideoxyinosine (ddI). Ann Intern Med, 1991; 115:283–284

335. Leitze Z, Nadeem A, Saul Z, Roberts IMCA. Nevaripine-induced hepatitis treated with corticosteroids. AIDS, 1998; 12:1115–1117

336. Brau N, Leaf HL, Wieczorek RL, Margolis DM. Severe hepatitis in three AIDS patients treated with indinavir. Lancet, 1997; 349:924–925

337. Wiessmann SB, Sinclair GI, Green CL, Fissell WH. Hydroxyurea-induced hepatitis in HIV+ve patients. Clin Infect Dis, 1999; 29:223–224

338. Clark SJ, Creighton S, Portmann B, Taylor C, Wendon JA, Cramp M. Acute liver failure associated with antiretroviral treatment for HIV: a report of six cases. J Hepatol, 2002; 36:295–301

339. Struble KA, Platt RD, Gitterman SR. Toxicity of antiretroviral agents. Am J Med, 1997; 102:65–67

340. Hu B, French SW. 2′,3′-Dideoxyinosine-induced Mallory bodies in patients with HIV. Am J Clin Pathol, 1997; 108:280–283

341. Sulkowski MS, Thomas DL, Chaisson RE, Moore RD. Hepatotoxicity associated with antiretroviral therapy in adults infected with HIV and the role of hepatitis C or B virus infection. JAMA, 2000; 283:74–80

342. Marcias J, Castellano V, Merchante N et al. Effect of antiretroviral drugs on liver fibrosis in HIV-infected patients with chronic hepatitis C: harmful impact of nevirapine. AIDS 2004; 18:767–774

343. Marine-Barajon E, Saint-Paul MC, Pradier C et al. Impact of antiretroviral treatment on progression of hepatic fibrosis in HIV/hepatitis C virus co-infected patients. AIDS, 2004; 18:2163–2170

344. Roulot D, Valla D, Brun-Vézinet F et al. Cholangitis in the acquired immunodeficiency syndrome: report of two cases and review of the literature. Gut, 1987; 28:1653–1660

345. Sabbatani S, Isulerdo Calzado A, Ferro A et al. Atypical leishmaniasis in an HIV-2 seropositive patient from Guinea-Bissau. AIDS 1991; 5:899–901

346. Taillan B, Garnier G, Fuzibet J-G, Pesce A, Vinti H, Hoffman P et al. Liver biopsy in patients with serum antibodies to HIV. Am J Med, 1990; 89:694

347. Garcia-Ordonez MA, Colmenero JD, Jiminez-Onate F, Martos F, Martinez J, Juarez C. Diagnostic usefulness of percutaneous liver biopsy in HIV-infected patients with fever of unknown origin. J Infect, 1999; 38:94–98

348. Mitchell DP, Hanes TE, Hoyumpa AM, Schenker S. Fever of unknown origin: assessment of the value of percutaneous liver biopsy. Arch Intern Med, 1977; 137:1001–1004

349. Chalasani N, Wilcox CM. Etiology, evaluation, and outcome of jaundice in patients with AIDS. Hepatology, 1996; 23:728–733

350. Lacaille F, Founet JC, Blanche S. Clinical utility of liver biopsy in children with AIDS. Pediatr Infect Dis J, 2000; 18:143–147

351. Churchill DR, Mann D, Coker RJ et al. Fatal haemorrhage following liver biopsy in patients with HIV infection. Genitourin Med, 1996; 72:62–64

Autoimmune hepatitis 10

Albert J. Czaja   Herschel A. Carpenter

Autoimmune hepatitis is a non-resolving hepatocyte-directed inflammation of the liver with characteristic but non-specific histological findings, hypergammaglobulinaemia, and liver-related autoantibodies.[1] Lymphocytic, often lymphoplasmacytic, inflammatory infiltrates extend from portal tracts into parenchymal tissue where they are associated with hepatocyte injury.[2] Parenchymal inflammation may be limited to periportal areas (interface hepatitis) or it may involve the entire acinus. The diagnosis requires a characteristic histological pattern and appropriate clinical features.

The clinical criteria for diagnosis have been codified by the International Autoimmune Hepatitis Group.[3,4] A definite diagnosis requires absence of viral markers, abstinence from alcohol, denial of blood transfusion, no recent exposures to hepatotoxic medication or chemicals, and a compatible histological pattern of injury (Table 10.1) Atypical or less pronounced findings and/or inability to satisfy the inclusion criteria support an alternative diagnosis (Table 10.1).[5,6]

An acute, even fulminant presentation, has been recognized[7-14] and the requirement for 6 months of disease activity to establish chronicity has been waived.[3,4] The histological patterns that characterize acute onset autoimmune hepatitis are a panacinar hepatitis that resembles an acute viral or drug-induced hepatitis and a perivenular (zone 3) hepatitis that resembles an acute toxic injury.[12-16] Earlier reports that virtually all patients with acute onset disease had portal lymphoplasmacytic infiltrates, bridging (septal) fibrosis, or cirrhosis focused on individuals who likely had an exacerbation of previously unrecognized chronic disease.[10,11] Transitions from perivenular (zone 3) hepatitis to interface hepatitis have been demonstrated in successive biopsy specimens from patients with acute onset disease, and the perivenular (zone 3) pattern of injury may be an early histological manifestation of autoimmune hepatitis that is unrecognized in specimens obtained later in the course.[12,13] It also may be a clue to triggering agents, such as drugs or toxins. The long lag time between the onset of autoimmune hepatitis and its clinical recognition limits the ability to identify aetiologic factors.

There are no disease-specific clinical or histological features. The diagnosis of autoimmune hepatitis requires the confident exclusion of other similar disorders including Wilson disease, genetic haemochromatosis, α-1 antitrypsin deficiency, chronic viral hepatitis, drug-related chronic liver disease, primary biliary cirrhosis (PBC), and primary sclerosing cholangitis (PSC) (Table 10.1).[1,3,4] Minocycline is the drug that has been most commonly implicated as a cause of the syndrome.[17-19]

A combined clinical and histopathological scoring system designed to standardize the evaluation and enhance the accuracy and strength of the clinical diagnosis was originally proposed in 1993[3] and revised in 1999[4] (Table 10.2). The diagnoses of definite, probable, and inconclusive autoimmune hepatitis are based on the aggregate score before and after corticosteroid treatment (Table 10.2). The scoring system was developed as a research tool to ensure comparability between patient populations in clinical trials, and this application is still its intent. The virtues of the scoring system are that it quantifies the diagnosis, facilitates objective comparisons between patient populations, accommodates individuals with atypical manifestations, and assesses the degree of resemblance of variant disorders to the classical disease. Its drawbacks are its complexity, and its failure to consistently distinguish cholestatic syndromes from autoimmune hepatitis.[20,21] The sensitivity of the scoring system for autoimmune hepatitis ranges from 97% to 100%,

Table 10.1 Diagnostic criteria for autoimmune hepatitis

Diagnostic requirement	Diagnosis of autoimmune hepatitis	
	Probable	**Definite**
Exclusion of genetic disease	Partial (heterozygous) α1-antitrypsin deficiency Non-diagnostic serum copper or ceruloplasmin abnormality Non-diagnostic serum iron and/or ferritin abnormalities	Normal α-antitrypsin phenotype Normal ceruloplasmin level Normal serum iron and/or ferritin level
Exclusion of viral infection	Previous blood transfusion but not implicated in liver disease False positive anti-HCV Past HBV infection	No blood transfusion No anti-HCV (or HCV RNA) Negative HBsAg, IgM anti-HBc, IgM anti-HAV, Epstein-Barr and CMV tests
Exclusion of toxic injury	Exposure to drugs or chemicals but unrelated to liver injury Moderate daily alcohol (35–50 g in men; 25–40 g in women)	No exposures to drugs or chemicals Limited daily alcohol (<35 g in men; <25 g in women)
Inflammatory indices	Predominant serum aminotransferase abnormalities	Predominant serum aminotransferase abnormalities
Immunoglobulins	Hypergammaglobulinaemia of any degree	Total globulin, γ-globulin or IgG level ≥1.5 × normal
Autoantibodies	ANA, SMA or anti-LKM1 titres ≥1 : 40 in adults and ≥1 : 10 in children Other autoantibodies	ANA, SMA, or anti-LKM1 titres ≥1 : 80 in adults and ≥1 : 20 in children
Histological features	Portal, portal/periportal interface and/or panacinar lymphoplasmacytic hepatitis Absence of significant biliary injury or particular features of other diseases	Portal, portal/periportal interface and/or panacinar lymphoplasmacytic hepatitis with numerous plasma cells. Absence of significant biliary injury or particular features of other diseases

ANA = antinuclear antibodies; anti-HAV = antibodies to hepatitis A virus; anti-HBc = antibodies to hepatitis B core antigen; CMV = cytomegalovirus; HBsAg = hepatitis B surface antigen; HBV = hepatitis B virus; HCV = hepatitis C virus; IgM = serum immunoglobulin M level; IgG = serum immunoglobulin G level; SMA = smooth muscle antibodies; anti-LKM1 = antibodies to liver/kidney microsome type 1.

and its specificity for excluding autoimmune hepatitis in patients with chronic hepatitis C ranges from 66% to 92%.[3]

The histological findings are important components of the scoring system. Lymphoplasmacytic inflammatory infiltrates in portal areas, the portal/periportal interface, and acinar tissue with evidence of hepatocyte injury (necrosis) and repair (rosette formation) are graded heavily in support of the diagnosis. In contrast, the presence of biliary changes, granulomas, extensive steatosis, copper deposition, or iron overload greatly reduces the score (Table 10.2). The scoring system is not a discriminative diagnostic index, and it should not be used to distinguish autoimmune hepatitis from other classical liver diseases. The components of the scoring system are not unique to autoimmune hepatitis, nor has the scoring system been developed by head-to-head comparisons with other liver disorders.[22]

Classification of autoimmune hepatitis

Three types of autoimmune hepatitis have been proposed, but only two types have distinctive serological profiles (Table 10.3).[23] None has been ascribed a unique cause, individual management strategy, or special behaviour, and they have not been endorsed as separate entities by the International Autoimmune Hepatitis Group.[3,4] All types are diagnosed by the same criteria, and they have similar histological manifestations and identical treatment strategies. The designations are used mainly as clinical descriptors.

Type 1 autoimmune hepatitis

This is the most common form of the disease worldwide, constituting at least 80% of cases in adults (Table 10.3).[23] It is characterized by the presence of smooth muscle antibodies (SMA) and/or antinuclear antibodies (ANA), hypergammaglobulinaemia, and concurrent immune disease. Human leucocyte antigen (HLA) DR3 and/or DR4 are commonly present (85%) in white northern European and North American patients. The specificity of SMA for the diagnosis can be enhanced if antiactin antibodies are sought.[24–26]

Type 1 disease affects mainly women (71%) of age 40 years or less (48%), and an acute onset of illness occurs in 40%.[23] In the latter instance, the presence of hypoalbuminaemia, hypergammaglobulinaemia, or features of portal hypertension, such as thrombocytopenia, ascites or oesophageal varices, commonly suggest the presence of chronic liver disease.[11,27] The possibility of autoimmune hepatitis

Category	Factor	Score
Gender	Female	+2
Alk phos: AST (or ALT) ratio	<1.5	+2
	1.5–3.0	0
	>3.0	−2
γ-globulin or IgG levels above normal	>2.0	+3
	1.5–2.0	+2
	1.0–1.5	+1
	<1.0	0
ANA, SMA, or anti-LKM1 titres	>1 : 80	+3
	1 : 80	+2
	1 : 40	+1
	<1 : 40	0
AMA	Positive	−4
Viral markers	Positive	−3
	Negative	+3
Drugs	Yes	−4
	No	+1
Alcohol	<25 g/day	+2
	>60 g/day	−2
HLA	DR3 or DR4	+1

Table 10.2 Scoring system for the diagnosis of autoimmune hepatitis

Category	Factor	Score
Immune disease	Thyroiditis, colitis, synovitis, others	+2
Other liver-defined autoantibody	Anti-SLA/LP, anti-actin, anti-LC1, pANCA	+2
Histological features	Interface hepatitis	+3
	Plasma cells	+1
	Rosettes	+1
	None of above	−5
	Biliary changes	−3
	Other features	−3
Treatment response	Complete	+2
	Relapse	+3
Pretreatment score		
Definite diagnosis	>15	
Probable diagnosis	10–15	
Posttreatment score		
Definite diagnosis	>17	
Probable diagnosis	12–17	

Alk phos = serum alkaline phosphatase level; AST = serum aspartate aminotransferase level; ALT = serum alanine aminotransferase level; IgG = serum immunoglobulin G level; ANA = antinuclear antibodies; SMA = smooth muscle antibodies; anti-LKM1 = antibodies to liver/kidney microsome type 1; AMA = antimitochondrial antibodies; anti-SLA/LP = antibodies to soluble liver antigen/liver-pancreas; anti-LC1 = antibodies to liver cytosol type 1; pANCA = perinuclear anti-neutrophil cytoplasmic antibodies

should always be considered in individuals with an acute or fulminant presentation,[7–14] and the histological findings of panacinar hepatitis or perivenular (zone 3) hepatitis should not dissuade the diagnosis.[12–16] Twenty-five per cent of patients with type 1 autoimmune hepatitis have cirrhosis at presentation, indicating the presence of an indolent, clinically unsuspected, aggressive stage.[28–30]

HLA DR3 and DR4 are independent risk factors for type 1 autoimmune hepatitis,[31] and they influence the clinical features, disease severity, and treatment response.[32–39] Eighty-five percent of white North American and northern European patients with type 1 autoimmune hepatitis have HLA DR3, DR4, or both DR3 and DR4. Patients with HLA DR3 are younger than patients with other phenotypes, and they have greater degrees of inflammatory activity at presentation and a poorer response to corticosteroid therapy.[33,34,36–40] In contrast, patients with HLA DR4 are older and more commonly female than patients with HLA DR3.[33,36,41] They also have higher serum levels of γ-globulin and immunoglobulin G (IgG), higher titres of ANA, and a greater frequency of concurrent immune diseases. Most

importantly, they enter remission more commonly and fail treatment less frequently than counterparts with HLA DR3.[33,36] High resolution DNA-based techniques have indicated that the alleles associated with susceptibility, clinical expression and outcome in caucasoid northern European and North American patients with type 1 autoimmune hepatitis are *DRB1*0301* and *DRB1*0401*.[34,35] These findings implicate the *DRB1* locus as the principal susceptibility region of the major histocompatibility complex (MHC).[34,35,38,39]

The risk of type 1 autoimmune hepatitis may relate to amino acid sequences in the antigen binding groove of the class II MHC molecule, and multiple alleles may encode the same or similar sequence.[37–39] The critical shared motif in white North Americans and Northern Europeans with type 1 autoimmune hepatitis is a six-amino-acid sequence represented by the code LLEQKR.[34] This sequence is located between positions 67 and 72 of the DRβ polypeptide chain of the class II MHC molecule, and lysine (K) in position 71 is the critical determinant of susceptibility. *DRB1*0301* and *DRB1*0401* encode identical amino acid sequences in the

Table 10.3 Distinctive types of autoimmune hepatitis

Clinical features	Type 1	Type 2
Signature autoantibodies	Smooth muscle Antinuclear	Liver/kidney microsome type 1
Age (years)	Infancy–elderly	2–14
Female (%)	78	89
Associated immune diseases (%)	41	34
Common types of immune diseases	Immune thyroiditis Graves' disease Ulcerative colitis	Vitiligo Type 1 diabetes Immune thyroiditis APECED
Concurrent autoantibodies	Anti-actin Anti-SLA/LP Anti-ASGPR pANCA	Anti-LC 1 Anti-ASGPR
γ-globulin elevation	Marked	Mild
Low IgA	No	Occasional
HLA	B8, DR3, DR4 A1-B8-DR3	B14, DR3, C4A-QO DR7
Allelic risk factors	DRB1 *0301 DRB1 *0401 DRB3 *0101 DRB4 *0103	DRB1 *07
Steroid response	Excellent	Good
Development of cirrhosis (%)	45	82

APECED = autoimmune polyendocrinopathy candidiasis ectodermal dystrophy; anti-LC1 = antibodies to liver cytosol type 1; AMA = antimitochondrial antibodies; anti-SLA/LP = antibodies to soluble liver antigen/liver pancreas; anti-ASGPR = antibodies to asialoglycoprotein receptor; SMA = smooth muscle antibodies; ANA = antinuclear antibodies; pANCA = perinuclear anti-neutrophil cytoplasmic antibodies

DRβ 67–72 region, and they affect susceptibility similarly. DRB1*0404 and DRB1*0405, which also encode similar six amino acid sequences in this region, are the susceptibility alleles in Mexican,[42] Japanese,[43,44] and Argentinian adults.[45,46] In contrast, DRB1*1301, which encodes a dissimilar amino acid sequence in this region, is associated with type 1 autoimmune hepatitis in Argentinian children[45,46] and Brazilian patients.[47–49] DRB1*1501 protects against type 1 autoimmune hepatitis in white North Americans and Northern Europeans, and it encodes another different sequence in this region.[34] Other non-disease-specific autoimmune promoters, such as polymorphisms of genes encoding immune regulatory cytokines[50–52] or region-specific genetic factors that favour susceptibility to indigenous aetiological agents,[53] may also contribute to the occurrence and phenotype of the disease.

Type 2 autoimmune hepatitis

This is characterized by the presence of antibodies to liver/kidney microsome type 1 (anti-LKM1) (Table 10.3).[54] These antibodies strongly react by indirect immunofluorescence with the proximal tubules of mouse kidney and the hepatocytes of mouse liver.[54–57] Exuberant immunofluorescence of the proximal tubules can render an indeterminate result or be mistaken for the reaction of antimitochondrial antibodies (AMA).[55] Enzyme-linked immunosorbent assays (ELISA) based on recombinant antigens have largely replaced indirect immunofluorescence for the detection of anti-LKM1 and AMA in clinical laboratories, and discrimination between these reactivities can now be made with confidence.[58]

Sera from patients with type 2 autoimmune hepatitis react on Western blots with a 50 kDa microsomal protein, and the major antigen of anti-LKM1 is the cytochrome mono-oxygenase, CYP2D6.[59–61] Five antigenic sites located between peptides 193–212, 257–269, 321–351, 373–389, and 410–429 are recognized by anti-LKM1. The amino acid sequence spanning 193–212 of the cytochrome mono-oxygenase CYP2D6 molecule is the target of anti-LKM1 in 93% of patients with type 2 autoimmune hepatitis.[61–63]

Homologies have been recognized between epitopes on the CYP2D6 molecule and the genome of the hepatitis C virus,[61–64] and the detection of anti-LKM1 in occasional patients with chronic hepatitis C (≤10%) probably reflects molecular mimicry and antibody cross-reactivity.[64–66] The hexameric amino acid sequence, RLLDLA, spanning 193–212 of the CYP2D6 molecule is homologous to the sequence, RLLDLS, spanning region 2985–2990 of the hepatitis C virus (HCV) genome and identical to the sequence spanning region 130–135 of the cytomegalovirus (CMV) genome.[63] These homologies, which can generate cross-reactivities between antibodies against the antigenic target of one form of autoimmune hepatitis and two unrelated viruses, suggest that multiple exposures to viruses mimicking self may be a mechanism by which to break self-tolerance.[63,67]

Antibodies to LKM1 are extremely rare in North American patients with chronic hepatitis C,[55,68] and this rarity may reflect differences in the indigeneous virus or the genetic susceptibility of the host.[56] Studies in Germany and Italy have not found an association between structural changes within the viral genome and the presence of anti-LKM1, and a host factor for anti-LKM1 expression has been implicated.[69,70]

Patients with type 2 autoimmune hepatitis are predominantly children (ages 2 to 14 years), but adults can be affected (Table 10.3).[54] In the USA, the disease occurs in only 4% of adults with autoimmune hepatitis[55] whereas in western Europe (France and Germany) as many as 20% of patients with type 2 autoimmune hepatitis are adults.[54] Regional variations in the occurrence of type 2 disease may reflect differences in genetic risk factors. Patients with type 2 autoimmune hepatitis from Germany have DRB1*03 and DRB1*04 less commonly and DRB1*07 more frequently than white North American patients with type 1 autoimmune hepatitis and normal control subjects.[71] In Brazil, type 2 autoimmune hepatitis is also associated with DRB1*07.[47] Ten per cent of normal caucasoid adults lack CYP2D6[72] and absence of this target autoantigen may also affect prevalence of the disease in certain regions. HLA B14, HLA DR3 and C4A-QO have also been incriminated as genetic risk factors.[73]

Associated immunological disorders are common (40%), including vitiligo, autoimmune thyroiditis, insulin-dependent diabetes, autoimmune haemolytic anaemia, idiopathic thrombocytopenic purpura, pernicious anaemia, rheumatoid arthritis and ulcerative colitis (Table 10.3).[54] Hypergammaglobulinaemia is less pronounced than in type 1 disease and serum immunoglobulin A (IgA) levels may be low. Non-organ-specific autoantibodies are rare whereas organ-specific antibodies are common (30%), including antibodies against thyroid microsomes, thyroglobulin, islets of Langerhans and gastric parietal cells.[54] Early experiences suggested that type 2 autoimmune hepatitis progressed more rapidly to cirrhosis than type 1 disease (82% versus 43% within 3 years).[54] These observations have not been corroborated, and outcomes are now considered to be similar between both types.[70,71] As in type 1 autoimmune hepatitis, an acute, even fulminant, presentation is possible.[9]

A distinct form of anti–LKM1-positive autoimmune hepatitis occurs in association with the syndrome of autoimmune polyendocrinopathy-candidiasis-ectodermal dystrophy (APECED).[76] APECED consists of multiple endocrine organ failure (parathyroids, adrenals, ovaries), mucocutaneous candidiasis, and ectodermal dysplasia in various syndromic combinations that may include autoimmune hepatitis in 15% of instances. The syndrome is caused by a single-gene mutation located on chromosome 21q22.3 which affects the generation of the autoimmune regulator (AIRE). AIRE is a transcription factor that is expressed in epithelial and dendritic cells within the thymus, and it regulates clonal deletion of autoreactive T cells (negative selection). APECED has an autosomal recessive pattern of inheritance, complete penetrance of the gene, no HLA-DR associations, and no female predominance. The autoantigens associated with APECED are CYP1A2 and CYP2A6.

Type 3 autoimmune hepatitis

This is the least established form of autoimmune hepatitis, and it has been characterized by the presence of antibodies to soluble liver antigen/liver pancreas (anti-SLA/LP).[77,78] These antibodies are directed against a 50 kDa cytosolic protein[79] which may be a transfer RNA complex (tRNP$^{(ser)sec}$) involved in the incorporation of selenocysteine into polypeptide chains.[80] Patients with type 3 disease are mostly women (91%) with a mean age of 37 years (range: 17 to 67 years).[77] They may have ANA, SMA (35%), anti-LKM1, antibodies to liver membrane antigen (26%), and AMA (22%), including antibodies to the M2 antigens of primary biliary cirrhosis (PBC). Recent studies have not distinguished patients with anti-SLA/LP from patients with type 1 autoimmune hepatitis by clinical or laboratory features, HLA

phenotype, or response to corticosteroids.[81,82] Currently, there is no justification for a type 3 autoimmune hepatitis.

Associated autoantibodies

Antibodies to SLA/LP, which had been used to designate a type 3 autoimmune hepatitis, may have important diagnostic and prognostic implications that warrant continued investigation (Table 10.4). Patients who have anti-SLA/LP have more severe disease than seronegative patients,[83] and they invariably relapse after corticosteroid withdrawal.[84-86] Furthermore, the expression of anti-SLA/LP is closely associated with HLA DR3.[83,84] This association may explain the low frequency of anti-SLA/LP in Japan (7%) where HLA DR3 is rare[87,88] and the refractory nature of the disease in many patients with anti-SLA/LP.[83-86] Antibodies to SLA/LP have a 100% specificity and positive predictability for relapse after corticosteroid withdrawal,[84-86] and they have a worldwide occurrence.[87] They are found in 16%–20% of white North American patients with type 1 autoimmune hepatitis, and they occur in 17% of patients from Brazil and 19% from Germany. Antibodies to SLA/LP have high specificity for autoimmune hepatitis (99%), and they can be present in both type 1 and type 2 disease. Testing for anti-SLA/LP may also be useful in reclassifying patients with cryptogenic chronic hepatitis.[87]

Other autoantibodies that are found in autoimmune hepatitis are antibodies to asialoglycoprotein receptor (anti-ASGPR),[89-94] actin (anti-actin),[24-26,86] chromatin (anti-chromatin),[95,96] liver cytosol type 1 (anti-LC1),[97-100] double-stranded DNA (anti-ds DNA),[101,102] histones (anti-histones),[103,104] neutrophil cytoplasm (pANCA),[105-108] Saccharomyces cerevisiae,[109,110] lactoferrin,[111] endomysium,[112] and tissue transglutaminase[110] (Table 10.4). These autoantibodies do not define clinically distinct subpopulations,[113] but some have promise as prognostic indices or ancillary diagnostic tools.[26,56-58,86,90,94,96,102]

Immunoglobulin A (IgA) endomysial antibodies (EMA) have a sensitivity of 94% and specificity of 99% for coeliac disease, and antibodies to tissue transglutaminase (anti-tTG), which is the target antigen of coeliac disease within the endomysium, have similar performance parameters (Table 10.4).[58] Assays for these antibodies should be incorporated into diagnostic algorithms for autoimmune hepatitis and cryptogenic chronic hepatitis since coeliac disease can cause liver dysfunction[114-119] or occur coincidentally with autoimmune liver disease.[112,117,119,120] Furthermore, gluten restriction can improve the liver test abnormalities.[116,118] The liver dysfunction associated with coeliac disease is diverse (acute, chronic, fulminant, cholestatic), and the histological patterns resemble those of autoimmune hepatitis, fulminant hepatitis, nonalcoholic fatty liver disease, and primary biliary cirrhosis.[116-119] IgA EMA may have greater specificity for coeliac disease in patients with autoimmune hepatitis than anti-tTG since tissue transglutaminase activity can be upregulated during fibrogenesis and result in a falsely positive test.[110,121,122]

Table 10.4 Autoantibodies of autoimmune hepatitis

Autoantibody	Target antigen (s)	Clinical utility
Smooth muscle	Microfilaments (actin, myosin) Microtubules (tubulin) Intermediate filaments (vimentin)	Type 1 AIH Standard repertoire
Antinuclear	Ribonucleoproteins Ribonucleoprotein complexes Centromere	Type 1 AIH Standard repertoire
Liver/kidney microsome type 1	CYP2D6	Type 2 AIH Standard repertoire Mistaken for AMA by IF

Perinuclear antineutrophil cytoplasm	Uncertain	Type 1 AIH (not in type 2 AIH);
		Standard repertoire
		  Ulcerative colitis
		  PSC

Endomysium (IgA)	Tissue transglutaminase	Coeliac disease
		Standard repertoire
		  Cryptogenic hepatitis
		  Cholestatic hepatitis

Tissue transglutaminase (IgA)	Calcium-dependent enzyme
	Tissue transglutaminase
		Coeliac disease
		Standard repertoire
		  Target antigen within endomysium
		  Can be falsely increased in liver disease

Histones	H3 core nuclear protein Histone-DNA complex (nucleosome)	Type 1 AIH with ANA Nonstandard repertoire Severe inflammation

ds DNA	Nuclear DNA	Type 1 AIH with ANA
		Nonstandard repertoire
		  Poor response
		  Assay dependent

Actin	Actin microfilaments Polymerized F-actin	Type 1 AIH Nonstandard repertoire Poor long-term outcome

Liver cytosol type 1	Formimino-transferase cyclodeaminase	Type 2 AIH
		Nonstandard repertoire
		  Young patients
		  Aggressive disease

Soluble liver antigen/liver pancreas	Transfer RNP$^{(ser)sec}$ complex
	50 kilodalton cytosolic protein
		Type 3 AIH (unestablished type)
		Nonstandard repertoire
		  Predicts relapse
		  Present in all types

Asialoglycoprotein receptor	Asialoglycoprotein receptor	Not generally available
		Generic marker of AIH
		  Associated with histologic activity
		  Predicts relapse

Chromatin	Octameric macromolecule Chromatin fibre	Under investigation Type 1 AIH Predicts relapse
Saccharomyces cerevisiae	Brewer's yeast	Under investigation Unproven value Type 1 AIH
Lactoferrin	Iron binding protein Granulocyte granules	Under investigation Unproven value Type 1 AIH

AIH = autoimmune hepatitis; ANA = antinuclear antibodies; ds DNA = double-stranded deoxyribonucleic acid; CYP2D6 = cytochrome 2D6; AMA = antimitochondrial antibodies; IF = indirect immunofluorescence; RNP = ribonucleoprotein; PSC = primary sclerosing cholangitis

Assays based on indirect immunofluoresence have been endorsed by the International Autoimmune Hepatitis Group as the gold standards of serological diagnosis.[123] These assays have been validated as markers of autoimmune hepatitis and correlated with the clinical phenotype and course of the disease. In contrast, kit-based, semi-automated, commercial assays commonly lack validation in autoimmune hepatitis and concordance with the classical detection techniques and their clinical applications. The International Autoimmune Hepatitis Group has also emphasized the importance of establishing standardized methods of testing. Serum exchange workshops with calibrated reference sera containing known autoantibodies were proposed as an essential mechanism to standardize testing and to minimize discrepancies between laboratories and clinical experiences. A similar exchange workshop has been in place since 1986 for the autoantibodies of type 1 diabetes mellitus, and the publication requirements in the major journals of diabetes now require validation of the serological assays under international workshop conditions.

Histological diagnosis

Interface hepatitis (hepatitis at the portal-parenchymal interface) is a constant but non-discriminating feature of autoimmune hepatitis.[1–4] In addition to interface hepatitis, autoimmune hepatitis is characterized by periportal lymphocytic or lymphoplasmacytic inflammation, hepatocyte swelling and/or pyknotic necroses (Fig. 10.1).[124–126] Interface hepatitis is not disease-specific and patients with drug-related, viral, other immune-mediated, and cryptogenic forms of acute and chronic hepatitis may show this feature.[2,127,128] Hepatic mesenchymal cells containing γ-globulin are invariably demonstrated in regions of interface hepatitis.[129,130] Lymphocytes, plasma cells and histiocytes typically accompany these cells. They surround and engulf individual dying hepatocytes at the portal/parenchymal interface or elsewhere in the acinus (spotty necrosis).

Panacinar hepatitis is present less commonly, but it is part of the histological spectrum[3,4] and may occur in acute

onset disease[10–14] or in autoimmune hepatitis that has relapsed after corticosteroid withdrawal (Fig. 10.2).[2,131] Severe inflammatory activity may be manifest by panacinar hepatitis and bridging necrosis (Fig. 10.3) or multiacinar necrosis (Fig. 10.4).[132,133] In contrast, fibrous or granulomatous cholangitis and changes such as granulomas, siderosis, copper deposits, and extensive macrovesicular steatosis, are incompatible with the definite diagnosis of autoimmune hepatitis.[3,4] These changes suggest other diagnoses or variant syndromes of autoimmune hepatitis.

Plasma cells are typically abundant at the interface and throughout the acinus (Fig. 10.5), but their sparsity or absence in the inflammatory infiltrate does not preclude the diagnosis.[1,2] The intensity of the plasma cell infiltration can be useful in discriminating autoimmune hepatitis from viral hepatitis.[2,134–136] Only 66% of patients with autoimmune hepatitis have plasma cells in groups or sheets in the portal tracts, but this finding, in conjunction with moderate-to-severe interface hepatitis and/or panacinar hepatitis, has an 81% specificity and 68% positive predictability for the disease. In contrast, 34% of patients with autoimmune hepatitis have few or no portal or acinar plasma cells.[2]

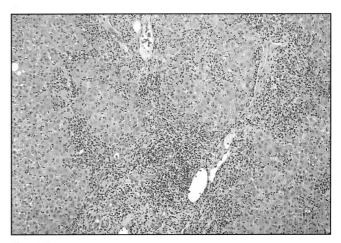

Fig. 10.2 • Panacinar hepatitis. Portal and acinar lymphoplasmacytic infiltrates with early bridging between portal tracts and terminal hepatic venules. Hepatocyte swelling and active regeneration with hepatic plate thickening and distortion are present. H&E.

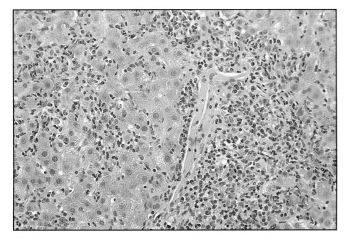

Fig. 10.1 • Autoimmune hepatitis. Lymphoplasmacytic portal and periportal infiltrates with active interface hepatitis. Hepatocyte swelling, architectural distortion, pyknotic necroses and acinar inflammation are present. H&E.

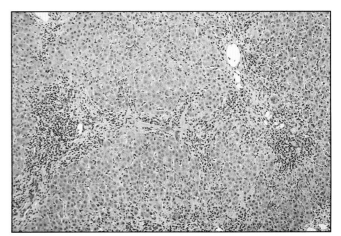

Fig. 10.3 • Bridging necrosis. Panacinar hepatitis with well-developed bridging necrosis and inflammation link portal tracts and terminal hepatic venules. Hepatic plate disorganization and rosette formation indicate regeneration. H&E.

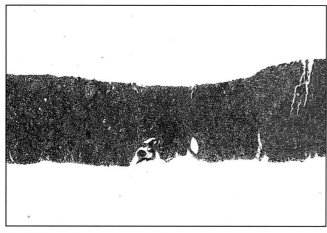

Fig. 10.4 • Massive necrosis. Massive hepatocyte necrosis, dropout and stromal collapse are present. Trichrome.

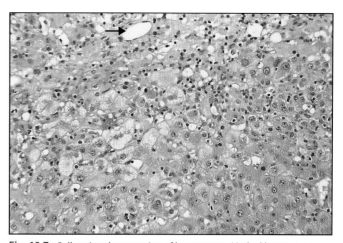

Fig. 10.7 • Ballooning degeneration of hepatocytes. Marked hepatocyte swelling, architectural disruption, and cell dropout near the terminal hepatic venule (arrow) are present. Double nucleated hepatocytes and disorganized plate architecture indicate regeneration. H&E.

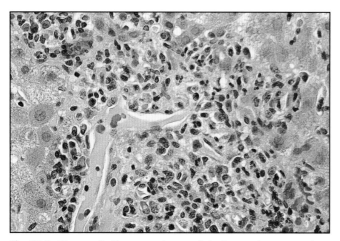

Fig. 10.5 • Plasma cells. Numerous plasma cells in the portal tract extend into the parenchyma (interface hepatitis). H&E.

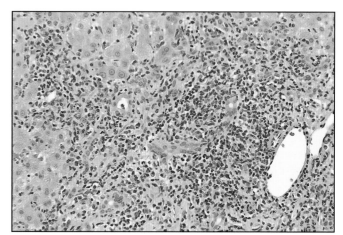

Fig. 10.8 • Lymphocytic cholangitis. Lymphocytes infiltrate the epithelium of an interlobular bile duct but significant damage to the biliary epithelium is not evident. H&E.

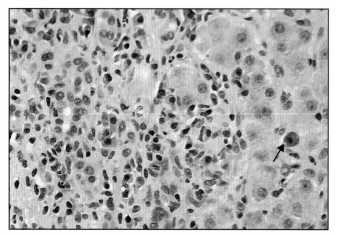

Fig. 10.6 • Pyknotic cell necrosis. A pyknotic hepatocyte is extruded into the sinusoid (arrow). Plasma cells and lymphocytes extend across the limiting plate to encircle damaged hepatocytes. H&E.

Pyknotic cell necroses (Fig. 10.6) and ballooning degeneration of hepatocytes (Fig. 10.7) are present in 39% of all patients with autoimmune hepatitis.[2] The presence of lymphoid aggregates surrounding and infiltrating a bile duct—lymphocytic cholangitis (Fig. 10.8)—and/or a pleomorphic

or mixed inflammatory infiltrate encircling and infiltrating a bile duct—pleomorphic cholangitis (Fig. 10.9)—constitute an exuberant inflammatory reaction within the portal tracts and do not preclude the diagnosis of autoimmune hepatitis.[137–139] These findings, however, occur in only 9% and 7% of biopsy specimens, respectively.[137]

Extensive interface hepatitis, panacinar hepatitis, bridging or massive necrosis and collapse are all features of increasing disease severity which may lead to fibrosis and loss of hepatocyte function.[132,140–142] Milder injury is followed by regeneration in the form of thickening of the hepatic plates and hepatic rosette formation (multiple hepatocytes surrounding bile canaliculi) (Fig. 10.10). The formation of new ductal structures (neocholangioles) may be exuberant following extensive bridging or massive necrosis and is a manifestation of a more severe injury (Fig. 10.11).

The histological patterns at presentation not only reflect severity but also predict prognosis if the disease is untreated.[132,140–141] Interface hepatitis (Fig. 10.1) progresses to cirrhosis in 17% of patients within 5 years and untreated individuals with this histological feature have a normal

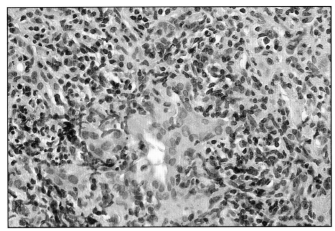

Fig. 10.9 • Pleomorphic cholangitis. Lymphocytes and histiocytes surround, infiltrate and damage an interlobular bile duct. Reactive changes are present in the biliary epithelium and there is loss of the normal orderly appearance of the epithelial cells. Furthermore, these cells are enlarged; they have abundant eosinophilic cytoplasm; and they have lost the normal nuclear orientation. H&E.

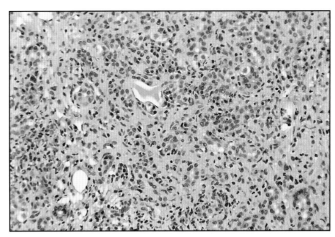

Fig. 10.11 • Neocholangioles in massive necrosis. Liver tissue is replaced by a proliferation of cholangioles, collapsed stroma and fibrous tissue. The cholangioles are uniformly distributed throughout the areas of necrosis. H&E.

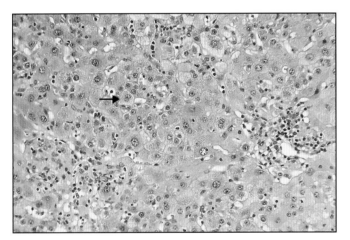

Fig. 10.10 • Hepatic rosette formation. Liver plates are thickened by hepatocyte swelling and proliferation. A cluster of hepatocytes surround a single canaliculus (rosette) in the centre of the field (arrow), indicating regeneration. H&E.

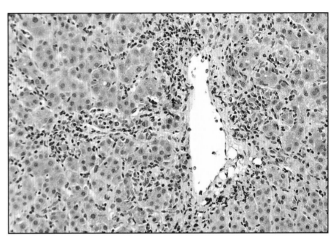

Fig. 10.12 • Perivenular necrosis with rosettes. Inflammation and hepatocyte drop out are present around a terminal hepatic venule. Mild diffuse inflammation, hepatic plate thickening, and disorganization of the hepatic plate architecture with rosette formation are also present. H&E.

5-year life expectancy.[140] In contrast, bridging necrosis (Fig. 10.3) is associated with an 82% frequency of cirrhosis and a 5-year mortality of 45%.[132,140,141] Similar consequences occur in patients with massive necrosis at presentation (Fig. 10.4) and cirrhosis with active inflammation.[132,140,142,143] Importantly, patients with cirrhosis respond as well to corticosteroid therapy as patients with other findings, and they should be treated as vigorously.[29,30]

Sampling variation is common with needle biopsy of the liver, especially in patients with cirrhosis, and the application of uniform diagnostic criteria for this finding is especially important.[144–147] Whereas intra-observer consistency in grading the type and degree of inflammatory activity is 90% and the sampling error for inflammatory changes is trivial, the diagnosis of cirrhosis by needle biopsy is highly variable.[145] Multiple biopsies from the same liver show cirrhosis in each specimen in only 33% of instances,[145] and the reproducibility of an interpretation of cirrhosis by the same observer is 78%.[145,148] The presence of a complete

regenerative nodule in the biopsy specimen would decrease the frequency of a false positive result, but biopsy cores obtained by intermediate gauge needles may not consistently afford this reassurance.[145]

Other histological manifestations of autoimmune hepatitis include (i) perivenular (zone 3) necrosis with or without inflammation of the portal tracts (Fig. 10.12)[12–15] and (ii) giant syncytial multinucleated hepatocytes (Fig. 10.13).[149–152] Perivenular (zone 3) necrosis occurs in viral hepatitis and drug-induced liver disease, and its presence raises a broad differential diagnosis (Fig. 10.12). Perivenular (zone 3) necrosis has not been formally included within the histological spectrum of autoimmune hepatitis, but patients with this finding can respond to corticosteroid therapy. The presence of perivenular (zone 3) necrosis with clinical features of autoimmune hepatitis and no other explanation for the disease warrants treatment as autoimmune hepatitis.[12–15] Fifty per cent of reported patients with perivenular (zone 3) necrosis lack autoantibodies and hypergammaglobulinaemia, and they are best categorized as having cryptogenic chronic hepatitis.

Giant syncytial multinucleated hepatocytes are non-specific reactions to injury that are associated most commonly with drug exposure, viral infection (especially with paramyxovirus), and autoimmune diseases (Fig. 10.13). Multiple other associations have been described.[149-152] These changes are most commonly found in the neonatal period, but giant syncytial multinucleated hepatocytes have been described after infancy (ages 2–80 years), and many patients have concurrent immune manifestations (ANA, direct Coombs reaction, concurrent immune disease) and corticosteroid responsiveness. The designation of these patients as cryptogenic chronic hepatitis is appropriate since infection with an unconventional hepatotropic virus cannot be excluded and the histological changes are not included within the spectrum of classical autoimmune hepatitis.

Variant syndromes

Codification of the clinical criteria for the diagnosis of autoimmune hepatitis[1,3,4] has facilitated recognition of variant syndromes.[5,6] These syndromes include patients with autoimmune hepatitis and another type of chronic liver disease (overlap syndrome) or findings suggestive but non-diagnostic of autoimmune hepatitis (outlier syndrome) (Table 10.5).[5,6] Overlap syndromes include patients with mixed features of autoimmune hepatitis and PBC, PSC or true chronic viral infection, and outlier syndromes include patients with autoimmune cholangitis (or AMA-negative PBC) and cryptogenic chronic hepatitis (Table 10.5).[5,6,153-156] These variant conditions currently lack an established identity, official designation and treatment strategy. Their occurrences, however, must be recognized,

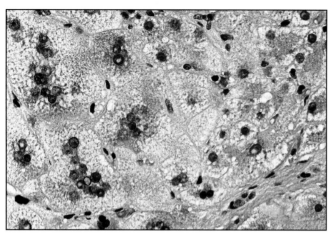

Fig. 10.13 • Multinucleated syncytial giant cells. Giant hepatocytes have numerous nuclei. H&E.

Table 10.5	Variant forms of autoimmune hepatitis	
Variant Form	**Disease component**	**Salient features**
Overlap	Primary biliary cirrhosis	Disproportionate alkaline phosphatase elevation
		Antimitochondrial antibodies
		Cholangitis (lymphoid, granulomatous)
		Hepatic copper deposition
		Improvement during corticosteroid trial common unless serum alkaline phosphatase level > ×2 normal
	Primary sclerosing cholangitis	Cholestatic laboratory features
		Cholangitis (lymphoid, fibrous obliterative)
		Hepatic copper deposition
		Abnormal cholangiogram (except interlobular ducts only/'small duct disease')
		Inflammatory bowel disease
		Recalcitrance to corticosteroids
	Chronic hepatitis C-immune predominant	SMA and/or ANA ≥1 : 320
		Moderate–severe interface hepatitis, lobular hepatitis, and/or portal plasma cell infiltrate
	Chronic hepatitis C-viral predominant	SMA or ANA <1 : 320
		Steatosis, bile-duct injury, and/or portal lymphoid aggregates
Outlier	Autoimmune cholangitis	ANA and/or SMA present
		Cholestatic laboratory features
		Cholangitis (lymphoid, granulomatous) or ductopenia
		No antimitochondrial antibodies
		Variable response to corticosteroids/ursodeoxycholic acid
		No histological improvement with therapy
	'Autoantibody-negative autoimmune hepatitis' (cryptogenic chronic hepatitis)	No ANA, SMA or anti-LKM1
		Late appearance of ANA, SMA or anti-LKM1 or seropositivity to anti-SLA/LP or pANCA
		Corticosteroid responsive

SMA = smooth muscle antibodies; ANA = antinuclear antibodies; anti-LKM1 = antibodies to liver/kidney microsome type 1; anti-SLA/LP = antibodies to soluble liver antigen/liver pancreas; pANCA = perinuclear anti-neutrophil cytoplasmic antibodies

and they should not be assimilated into diagnoses that hide their individuality or imperil the homogeneity of the classical diseases.

Autoimmune hepatitis-PBC overlap variant

The overlap syndrome of autoimmune hepatitis and PBC is characterized by the clinical features of autoimmune hepatitis, including marked serum aspartate aminotransferase elevation, hypergammaglobulinaemia, and SMA and/or ANA seropositivity (Table 10.5).[153-155] There is also a blend of PBC-like clinical features, including seropositivity for AMA and cholestatic biochemical findings. The histological features include a variable combination of inflammatory cell infiltrates directed at bile ducts and hepatocytes; portal and periportal lymphoplasmacytic infiltrates associated with pleomorphic or granulomatous destructive cholangitis and/or bile-duct loss; and interface or diffuse inflammatory cell infiltrates associated with hepatocyte swelling or acidophilic necroses (Fig. 10.14).[156,157] Patients who have predominantly hepatocellular rather than cholestatic clinical and histological features frequently respond to corticosteroid therapy.[153,154,158,159] Patients with predominantly cholestatic features, including serum alkaline phosphatase levels more than four-fold the upper limit of normal and/or florid duct lesions on histological examination, can be treated with ursodeoxycholic acid or a combination of prednisone and ursodeoxycholic acid.[160]

Separation of autoimmune hepatitis from stage 2 PBC may be impossible by histological examination if the portal inflammation and interface hepatitis are not accompanied by obvious diffuse hepatitis (autoimmune hepatitis) or ductopenia (PBC) (Fig. 10.15).[157] Both conditions have a similar inflammatory infiltrate, including the lymphoplasmacytic component.

Differentiation requires analysis of the laboratory and serological manifestations. Predominant cholestatic features (mainly disproportionate increase in the serum alkaline phosphatase level) and seropositivity for AMA justify classification as PBC. Predominant hepatocellular features (mainly disproportionate increase in serum aminotransferase levels), seropositivity for ANA, SMA or anti-LKM1, and seronegativity for AMA warrant classification as autoimmune hepatitis. Mixed cholestatic and hepatocellular features and autoantibody profiles support classification as an overlap syndrome. Patients with the overlap variant of autoimmune hepatitis and PBC (Figs 10.14 and 10.15) have high scores for autoimmune hepatitis by the modified scoring system of the International Autoimmune Hepatitis Group (Table 10.2).[153,154]

Useful histological findings that discriminate 'ordinary' PBC from 'ordinary' autoimmune hepatitis are bile-duct destruction (granulomatous or otherwise), bile-duct loss, isolated granulomas and copper accumulation. Lymphocytic infiltration of bile ducts is a non-specific feature which may be seen in autoimmune hepatitis, PBC, viral hepatitis and drug-induced liver disease (Fig. 10.8).[137,157] In up to 20% of normal portal tracts, bile ducts may not be seen due to the plane of section, and inspection of multiple sections is necessary to secure the diagnosis of ductopenia. The absence of a bile duct adjacent to a portal arteriole signifies bile-duct loss (Fig. 10.15).[157]

Ductular reaction occurs whenever the flow of bile from the canaliculus to the bile duct is interrupted, and it can be present in autoimmune hepatitis or PBC.[157] In PBC, hepatocytes at the portal-parenchymal interface may be swollen as a result of cholate stasis but hepatocytes elsewhere are normal. The hepatic plate architecture also remains normal in PBC despite the frequent and sometimes confusing increase in the number of mononuclear cells in the sinusoids. Hepatocyte swelling, pyknosis and regenerative rosette formation are all indications of a process in which hepatocyte injury is the primary pathological mechanism (Figs 10.6, 10.7 and 10.10).

Some patients (12%) with clinical and laboratory features that are typical of autoimmune hepatitis have isolated florid duct lesions (granulomatous destructive cholangitis) or ductopenia in biopsy specimens (Fig. 10.14).[138,139] These

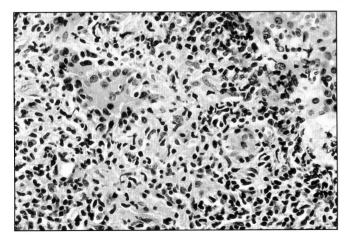

Fig. 10.14 • Florid duct lesion in PBC-autoimmune hepatitis overlap syndrome. Histiocytes and a mixture of lymphocytes and plasma cells produce an ill-defined granuloma which distorts and disorganizes the residual biliary epithelia. The damaged biliary cells have an eosinophilic cytoplasm. H&E.

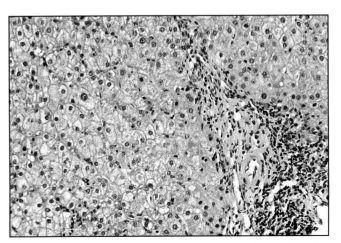

Fig. 10.15 • Ductopenia in PBC-autoimmune hepatitis overlap syndrome. A portal arteriole is not accompanied by an interlobular bile duct. Inflammatory cells are clustered toward the periphery of the portal tract at the interface; hepatocytes are swollen; and the plate architecture is disorganized. H&E.

sparse background changes are present in the clinical and histological context of typical autoimmune hepatitis, and they should not alter the primary diagnosis or change the treatment strategy. Patients with the incidental bile duct changes do not have a cholestatic clinical or laboratory phenotype; they are clinically indistinguishable from patients who lack these histological findings; and they respond as well to corticosteroid therapy as patients with classical features of autoimmune hepatitis.[138,139] The changes may reflect collateral bile duct injury during an exuberant and promiscuous immune mediated response, or they may be weak expressions of a variant cholestatic syndrome. Serological assessments for PBC-specific AMA, antibodies to nuclear pore complex antigen gp210, and nuclear antigen Sp100 have been negative in these patients.[139] Theoretically, the bile-duct destruction may remain clinically inapparent and biologically unimportant, or it could progress later to a cholestatic syndrome affecting prognosis.

Autoimmune hepatitis-PSC overlap variant

The overlap syndrome of autoimmune hepatitis and PSC (Table 10.5) is characterized by SMA and/or ANA seropositivity, interface hepatitis, and hypergammaglobulinaemia in conjunction with cholestatic biochemical changes (mainly serum alkaline phosphatase elevation greater than two-fold the upper limits of normal), frequent concurrence of inflammatory bowel disease, and histological features of fibrous obliterative cholangitis, ductopenia, portal tract oedema and/or bile stasis (Fig. 10.16).[6,21,153–155,161,162] The diagnosis is supported by cholangiographic changes of intrahepatic and/or extrahepatic PSC. These changes are not requisites for the diagnosis since only the interlobular bile ducts may be involved (small duct PSC).[163,164] The overlap form of autoimmune hepatitis and PSC is commonly resistant to corticosteroid therapy,[153,164] and empirical treatments include short-term trials with ursodeoxycholic acid that are often of limited or no benefit.[165]

An autoimmune sclerosing cholangitis has been described in children with autoimmune hepatitis, and it may be different from the overlap syndrome of autoimmune hepatitis and PSC described in adults. The term 'autoimmune sclerosing cholangitis' rather than primary sclerosing cholangitis has been applied mainly because these children improve during immunosuppressive treatment.[74,75] Therapy with prednisone, azathioprine and ursodeoxycholic acid induces laboratory remission in 89% of patients during a median follow-up of 4 years, and this response is similar to that of children with classical autoimmune hepatitis. Cirrhosis does not develop; vanishing bile ducts are rare; cholangiograms are unchanged in most patients; and 10-year survivals are similar to those with classical autoimmune hepatitis. Only a lower transplant-free survival time distinguishes them from children with classical disease. As in adults with autoimmune hepatitis and PSC, children with autoimmune sclerosing cholangitis have a higher frequency of concurrent inflammatory bowel disease, lower serum aminotransferase levels at presentation, and greater frequency of bile duct changes on initial histological examination than children with normal cholangiograms. These group differences do not distinguish individual patients, and the presence of autoimmune sclerosing cholangitis can be excluded only by cholangiography.

Autoimmune hepatitis-chronic hepatitis C overlap variant

The overlap syndrome of autoimmune hepatitis and chronic hepatitis C implies the co-existence of autoimmune hepatitis with high titre (serum titres, ≥1 : 320) SMA or ANA and hypergammaglobulinaemia with a true hepatitis C infection (Table 10.5).[136,166–169] Since corticosteroid therapy of chronic hepatitis C can enhance viral replication[170] and interferon therapy of autoimmune hepatitis can intensify immune reactivity,[171–173] there is no single drug strategy that accommodates all contingencies. The histological examination is often the basis for determining the predominant (viral versus autoimmune) manifestations of this rare mixed form and directing treatment.[134–136,166,169]

Biopsy specimens from patients with chronic hepatitis C may show the following histological patterns: (i) portal lymphocytic infiltrates, nodular aggregates and mild macrovesicular steatosis which is typical of hepatitis C infection (Fig. 10.17); (ii) diffuse portal, interface or panacinar hepatitis with a significant plasma cell infiltration (usually less than 10%) that resembles autoimmune hepatitis (Figs 10.18 and 10.19); (iii) co-dominant mixtures of patterns 1 and 2; and (iv) diffuse portal, interface or panacinar hepatitis without plasma cells or features typical of chronic hepatitis C or autoimmune hepatitis (non-discriminative pattern).[134–136,174] The non-discriminative pattern is most common (40%) but the other composites are also frequent (20% each).[136]

Patients with portal, interface and acinar hepatitis in conjunction with portal or acinar plasma cell infiltrates (Figs 10.18 and 10.19) have more laboratory manifestations of immune reactivity (higher serum immunoglobulin levels, notably IgG, and a greater frequency of autoantibodies) than patients with portal lymphoid aggregates and steato-

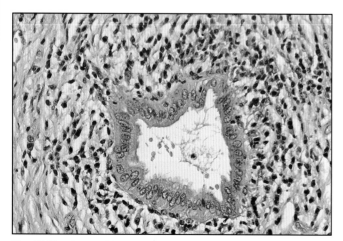

Fig. 10.16 • Fibrous obliterative cholangitis in autoimmune hepatitis-PSC overlap syndrome. Oedema and a mild inflammatory infiltrate are present in the wall of a septal bile duct. The bile duct lumen is compressed and encircling stromal cells are in a characteristic laminar pattern. H&E.

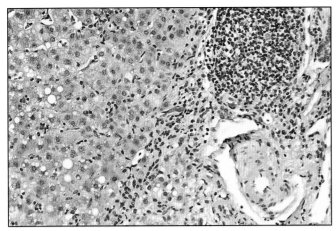

Fig. 10.17 • Classic chronic hepatitis C. The portal lymphoid aggregate, mild diffuse portal lymphocytic inflammation, minimal parenchymal inflammation and mild steatosis are characteristic of relatively quiescent disease. H&E.

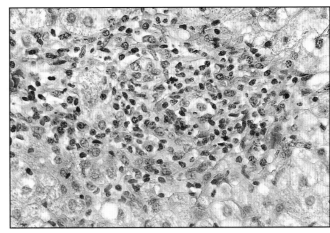

Fig. 10.19 • Chronic hepatitis C with portal plasma cells resembling autoimmune hepatitis. The diffuse portal inflammation consists mainly of lymphocytes and plasma cells and it extends across the limiting plate—interface hepatitis. H&E.

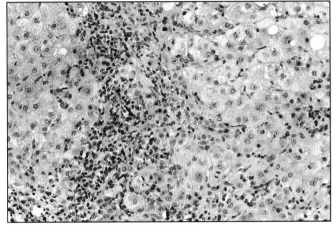

Fig. 10.18 • Chronic hepatitis C with interface and acinar hepatitis resembling autoimmune hepatitis. The diffuse portal lymphoplasmacytic inflammation with interface hepatitis and mild acinar hepatitis is indistinguishable from autoimmune hepatitis. H&E.

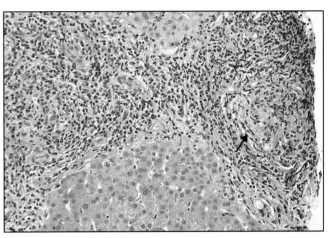

Fig. 10.20 • Autoimmune cholangitis. The portal tracts are expanded by a mixed, mainly lymphoplasmacytic inflammatory infiltrate and an interlobular bile duct (arrow) is being destroyed (pleomorphic or granulomatous destructive cholangitis or florid duct lesion). The hepatocytes and plate architecture are relatively normal and the sinusoids are open. H&E.

sis.[136,166–169] They also have higher total Knodell scores and modified scores for inflammatory activity and fibrosis than patients with portal lymphoid aggregates and steatosis (Fig. 10.17).[136,169] Although these features may reflect differences in the degree of inflammatory activity, they suggest an immune-predominant pathogenic process in one condition (Figs 10.18 and 10.19) and a viral-predominant process in the other (Fig. 10.17).[136,166–169] By defining these various histological patterns, the principal nature of the overlap syndrome can be deduced and properly weighted within the clinical context to develop an appropriate treatment strategy (Table 10.5).[169,175–177] Mixed and non-discriminative patterns are common in chronic hepatitis C, and these histological findings do not characterize the principal nature of the syndrome or indicate the most appropriate therapeutic action.[136,169]

The nature of concurrent immune diseases can also help differentiate autoimmune hepatitis with incidental hepatitis C virus infection from chronic hepatitis C with incidental immune features.[167–169,178] The concurrent immune diseases of autoimmune hepatitis are mainly autoantigen-driven, cell-mediated disorders such as autoimmune thyroiditis, Graves' disease, ulcerative colitis, and rheumatoid arthritis, whereas the concurrent immune diseases of chronic hepatitis C (with the exception of Sjögren syndrome and autoimmune thyroiditis) are mainly viral antigen-driven, humoral responses such as vasculitis, glomerulonephritis, and symptomatic cryoglobulinemia.

Autoimmune cholangitis

Autoimmune cholangitis is an outlier syndrome that is characterized by seropositivity for ANA and/or SMA, histological evidence of bile-duct injury, and absence of AMA (Table 10.5).[179–184] The cholestatic features preclude classification as autoimmune hepatitis and the lack of AMA restricts categorization as PBC.[3,4] The histological findings may be indistinguishable from PBC (Fig. 10.20),[182,184] and the diagnosis is based on the absence of AMA and a normal cholangiogram (Table 10.5).[184]

Patients with autoimmune cholangitis have been distinguished from patients with PBC by having higher serum levels of aspartate aminotransferase and lower serum concentrations of immunoglobulin M.[179] They also have been characterized by the presence of antibodies to carbonic anhydrase;[185,186] HLA risk factors that are different from PBC;[187] and clonal expansion of liver-infiltrating lymphocytes that express Vβ5.1 T cell receptors.[188] These findings have suggested that autoimmune cholangitis is an entity distinct from PBC. Its cholestatic features and failure to respond consistently to corticosteroid therapy have also distanced it from autoimmune hepatitis.

Patients with autoimmune cholangitis have low scores for autoimmune hepatitis by the system of the International Autoimmune Hepatitis Group,[153] and they respond variably to empirical therapies with corticosteroids or ursodeoxycholic acid.[153,179–181,183,184] Clinical and laboratory improvements during treatment may not be accompanied by histological resolution.[153,179,180] These features suggest a kinship that is closer to PBC or PSC than autoimmune hepatitis.[153,182,189,190]

AMA-negative PBC is a diagnostic entity, but it is unclear if all cases of autoimmune cholangitis can be classified in this fashion. Patients previously diagnosed as having AMA-negative PBC have been compared retrospectively to patients with AMA-positive PBC, and the conditions have been indistinguishable.[182,183,189,190] Histological features were similar;[182,183] clinical phenotype and treatment outcomes were comparable;[183,189,190] antibodies to carbonic anhydrase did not differentiate the conditions;[191] histochemical analyses demonstrated pyruvate dehydrogenase complex on the biliary epithelia of AMA-negative patients;[192] and antibodies to the PBC-specific 2-oxo-acid dehydrogenase complex were found in each disorder.[192,193] These findings confirmed the similarity of AMA-negative and AMA-positive PBC, but they did not define the essential nature of autoimmune cholangitis. Most studies have been biased by their largely retrospective nature and their use of pre-selected patient populations as discovery fields for autoimmune cholangitis. Under such circumstances, similarities between autoimmune cholangitis and its parent population can be anticipated. Similar biases in favour of an association between autoimmune cholangitis and autoimmune hepatitis can be anticipated if examples of autoimmune cholangitis are sought only from within this group.

Prospective studies have indicated that autoimmune cholangitis is a generic term that encompasses patients with diverse histological features of bile duct injury or loss and varying degrees of inflammatory activity.[184] Histological findings may resemble PBC, PSC, or a mixed condition of autoimmune hepatitis (interface hepatitis) and PBC (destructive cholangitis) or PSC (ductopenia, portal tract oedema). The morphological findings that suggest PBC are portal lymphocytic or lymphoplasmacytic infiltration, destructive cholangitis, ductopenia, and isolated granulomas. The morphological features that suggest PSC are ductular reaction, mild mixed inflammation with little or no portal lymphocytic or lymphoplasmacytic infiltration, portal tract oedema or fibrosis, ductopenia, and fibrous

obliterative cholangitis. These observations suggest that autoimmune cholangitis that is discovered prospectively is a heterogeneous group that includes patients with atypical PBC, small duct PSC, concurrent diseases of autoimmune hepatitis and AMA-negative PBC, transition stages in the early development of a classical syndrome, or a separate and distinct entity with variable histological manifestations.[184] The possibility of a drug reaction must also be excluded. As diagnostic criteria are codified, pathogenic mechanisms are clarified, and the natural history is described, individual entities may be split from the designation of autoimmune cholangitis and the generic term eliminated.

'Autoantibody-negative autoimmune hepatitis'

In a small percentage (less than 15%) of adult patients with clinical, laboratory and histological features of autoimmune hepatitis, conventional liver-related autoantibodies (ANA, SMA and anti-LKM1) are undetectable.[5,6,194–196] These patients with 'autoantibody-negative autoimmune hepatitis' constitute an outlier syndrome that is commonly included under the designation of cryptogenic chronic hepatitis (Table 10.5).[5,6] Marked serum aminotransferase abnormalities, hypergammaglobulinaemia, increased serum IgG levels, and histological features of portal, interface and acinar hepatitis in any combination with and without portal or acinar plasma cell infiltration typify the syndrome (Fig. 10.1).[194,195] The HLA susceptibility factors for classical autoimmune hepatitis (DR3 and DR4) occur as commonly in this condition as in autoantibody-positive disease, and patients respond as well to corticosteroid treatment.[194] These patients probably have an autoimmune hepatitis that has escaped detection by conventional serological testing. Late expression of SMA and/or ANA[113] or seropositivity for novel autoantibodies such as anti-SLA/LP[81,82,87] (Table 10.4) may ultimately define an autoimmune nature. All patients should be tested repeatedly for the late expression of the conventional autoantibodies,[113] and assessments for the presence of pANCA[106,108] and IgA EMA[58,112,114,116] are appropriate during the initial evaluation. 'Autoantibody-negative autoimmune hepatitis' must be distinguished from cryptogenic cirrhosis which is typically an advanced inactive disease of indeterminate nature.[197]

Modified appearances following therapy

Immunosuppressive agents are the mainstays of therapy for autoimmune hepatitis. Corticosteroids and azathioprine (either alone or in combination) are most frequently used but several new front line therapies are currently being assessed.[198] It has recently been suggested that patients with asymptomatic autoimmune hepatitis may not require immunosuppression.[199]

While the majority of cases respond rapidly with resolution of histological changes, some will subsequently relapse after therapy is discontinued. In others there is no initial response and in some there may be a shift in the phenotype of the disease. For those in whom therapy is ineffective, transplantation remains an option.[200] Autoimmune hepatitis may recur in the graft, but recurrence is typically mild and successfully treated.

Remission

Prednisone alone or in combination with azathioprine induces resolution of the histological features of autoimmune hepatitis in 65% of patients within 18 months.[1,198–201] Improvements in the biopsy appearances lag behind clinical and laboratory improvements by 3 to 8 months, and histological remission cannot be established by clinical and laboratory indices.[202,203] The absence of symptoms and normal laboratory tests during corticosteroid therapy are associated with histological evidence of activity in the majority of cases that are biopsied immediately at biochemical resolution.[203] Liver biopsy evaluation is the only way to confirm remission of the disease during treatment, and it should be undertaken in all patients prior to drug withdrawal. Premature discontinuation of medication is the most common cause of relapse. Twenty-one per cent of patients treated with conventional regimens of prednisone alone or in combination with azathioprine sustain their remission for a median of 76 months after drug withdrawal, and an effort should be made to withdraw all patients from initial therapy after criteria for remission have been satisfied.[204]

Histological remission of autoimmune hepatitis is defined as the absence of interface hepatitis.[205] The liver tissue can be normal, fibrotic, cirrhotic (Fig. 10.21) or non-cirrhotic with mild portal inflammation (Fig. 10.22). The histological findings prior to drug withdrawal predict the likelihood of a sustained remission. Reversion of the liver architecture to normal during therapy is associated with a 20% frequency of clinical relapse after drug withdrawal;[148] improvement to portal inflammation (Fig. 10.22) during therapy is associated with a 50% frequency of clinical relapse within 6 months;[148,205] interface hepatitis at the time of drug withdrawal is associated with an 80% frequency of clinical relapse;[148] and progression to cirrhosis during therapy is nearly always associated with relapse.[148,206] The presence of portal plasma cells is predictive of relapse after drug withdrawal in tissue specimens otherwise satisfying criteria for remission (Fig. 10.22).[131] The positive predictability of portal plasma cell infiltration for relapse is 92%, but its occurrence in individuals who relapse is only 31%. Portal plasma cell infiltration may be indicative of an active antibody-dependent pathogenic mechanism that perpetuates inflammatory activity after drug withdrawal, but the low sensitivity of this histological finding for relapse indicates the need for other complementary predictors of outcome.[131,206]

Unexpected histological evidence of active inflammation (interface hepatitis or active cirrhosis) during corticosteroid treatment in an otherwise asymptomatic individual with normal laboratory tests justifies continuation of therapy for an additional 3 to 8 months. Reduction or elimination of inflammatory activity inhibits fibrogenesis, and it may facilitate fibrolytic activity, especially in early stage fibrosis (Fig. 10.23(A), 10.23(B)).[207–211]

Cirrhosis develops in 40% of patients within 10 years.[29,30] It is a consequence of the severity of inflammatory activity and the difficulty in achieving a permanently inactive disease. Typically, cirrhosis develops early during the most active stages of inflammatory activity. Thereafter, the frequency of cirrhosis increases by only 1% to 2% per year regardless of subsequent relapse and retreatment.[29] Histologically confirmed cirrhosis at presentation or subsequently does not affect responsiveness to corticosteroid therapy or the 5- and 10-year survival expectations. The clinical stage of the disease (Child–Pugh classification) and the degree of associated inflammatory activity are probably the most important determinants of long-term outcome after therapy has been instituted.[29,30] Recent studies have suggested that fibrosis can decrease during corticosteroid therapy, and there have been isolated reports suggesting

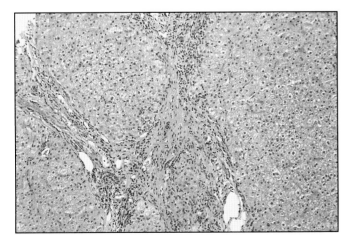

Fig. 10.21 • Treated cirrhosis with minimal activity. Regenerative nodules separated by fibrous septa establish the presence of cirrhosis. The mild portal and septal inflammation and focal minimal interface hepatitis are consistent with histological remission of autoimmune hepatitis during corticosteroid treatment. H&E.

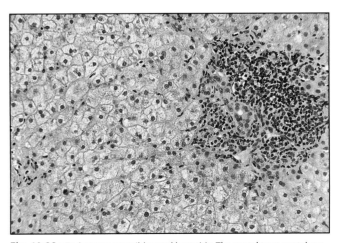

Fig. 10.22 • End-treatment mild portal hepatitis. The portal tract contains a mild mixed, mainly lymphoplasmacytic, infiltrate in the absence of significant interface or acinar hepatitis. These findings satisfy histological criteria for remission of autoimmune hepatitis during corticosteroid treatment. H&E.

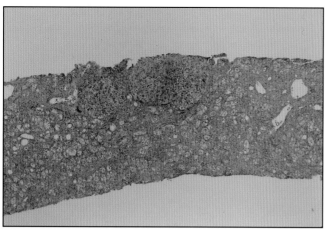

A

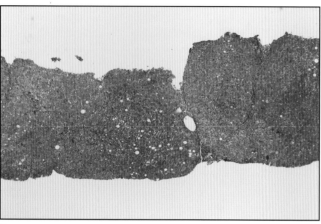

B

Fig. 10.23 • **(A)** Dense fibrous bands crisscross the sample isolating nodules of hepatic parenchyma. Trichrome stain. **(B)** Delicate fibrous septae interesect hepatic parenchyma after 4 years of treatment. Trichrome stain. Mild steatosis is probably related to corticosteroid therapy.

reversal of cirrhosis during treatment.[207–210] These possibilities may affect long-term outcome and in part explain the excellent long-term prognosis of patients with histological cirrhosis.

Relapse

Relapse is common after corticosteroid withdrawal and implies recurrence of interface hepatitis usually in conjunction with symptoms of easy fatigability, arthralgias and myalgias.[202,204,205,212,213] The serum aspartate aminotransferase level typically exceeds three-fold normal and hypergammaglobulinaemia reappears or worsens. The histological appearance resembles that of the pretreatment tissue specimen (Fig. 10.1) or there can be more extensive inflammatory activity with bridging necrosis (Fig. 10.3) or massive necrosis (Fig. 10.4). Active cirrhosis may be present or a diffuse panacinar hepatitis may reflect the abruptness of the recurrence and its severity (Fig. 10.2). In each instance, alternative and/or superimposed infectious, toxic or drug-related aetiologies must be excluded. Liver biopsy examination is usually not necessary to document relapse since the clinical and biochemical changes accurately reflect the

histological findings, and they are sufficient indications for the resumption of treatment.[203]

The frequency of treatment-related complications increases to 70% after two relapses and repeat treatments, and the probability of a sustained long-term remission decreases.[213] The diminishing benefit-to-risk ratio of further treatment after relapse justifies the use of long-term maintenance schedules. Prednisone administered alone in the lowest dose possible to control symptoms and laboratory findings,[214] or indefinite azathioprine therapy (2 mg per kg daily), are each effective as long-term management strategies.[215,216] Reversion of the liver architecture to normal is not the objective of treatment during maintenance therapy, and liver biopsy tissue may show mild focal interface hepatitis or mildly active cirrhosis. Liver biopsy evaluation is seldom necessary during long-term maintenance therapy since histological activity is usually absent or mild, asymptomatic, and non-progressive.[203,214–216]

Treatment after relapse need not be indefinite. Twenty-eight per cent of patients who are re-treated after relapse can enter a sustained long-term remission without medication, and the probability of achieving this outcome after initial or repeated treatments is 47% after 10 years.[204] The frequency of ultimately inducing a sustained remission and the ready ability to diagnose and treat relapse effectively support the effort to withdraw treatment in all patients with stable inactive disease even after repeated earlier relapses.

Treatment failure

Clinical, laboratory, and/or histological deterioration despite compliance with conventional corticosteroid regimens occur in 9% of patients.[1] Treatment failure justifies reassessment of the original diagnosis and exclusion of superimposed factors, such as viral infection, steatohepatitis, or alcohol injury.[157] Reclassification of the disease as an overlap or outlier syndrome may be warranted (Table 10.5) or a concurrent viral or drug-induced disease may be found. Histological examination, appropriate laboratory tests, and cholangiography may be necessary to establish the diagnosis. In most instances, there is no alternative basis for the deterioration.

Transformations

The classical syndrome of autoimmune hepatitis can undergo apparent transformation to another disease in rare instances. Liver biopsy assessment is essential to recognize this transition, and the histological findings can affect management.[157] PSC is one condition that can emerge from autoimmune hepatitis.[161,162,164] Its presence is typically heralded by the development of resistance to corticosteroid treatment and the appearance of cholestatic features. Cholangiography and liver tissue examination are required for the diagnosis. The histological findings are compatible with PSC (Fig. 10.16); the cholangiographic findings are usually characteristic; and ulcerative colitis is commonly present.[164] The two diseases could be independent and coincidental conditions or reflective of a phenotype affected by cross-reacting autoantibodies and tissue infiltrating cytotoxic lymphocytes associated with an emerging ulcerative colitis. Autoimmune hepatitis and PSC are each associated with HLA DR3, and a similar genetic predisposition may contribute to the metamorphosis.[187,217,218]

Patients with clinical, laboratory and histological features of classical autoimmune hepatitis at presentation can develop AMA later and isolated florid duct lesions (Fig. 10.14).[219] These serological and histological transformations in the absence of cholestatic laboratory findings do not alter the clinical manifestations of the disease or its responsiveness to corticosteroid treatment. The PBC-like manifestations may be transient, intermittent or permanent; they may represent changing or cross-reacting immune reactivities which are insufficient to affect clinical expression or treatment outcome. The emergence of autoimmune hepatitis from PBC has also been described,[220] and this experience further emphasizes the phenotypic transitions that can occur between the classical disorders.

Steatosis is present in 7% of patients with corticosteroid-treated autoimmune hepatitis,[2,174] and in rare instances, it may be associated with perpetuation, intensification, or recrudescence of inflammatory activity (Fig. 10.24). Typically, patients who have undergone transition from autoimmune hepatitis to nonalcoholic fatty liver disease (NAFLD) have had the recognized risk factors for NAFLD, including obesity, hyperlipidemia, glucose intolerance, or protracted corticosteroid treatment.[174] They may be misclassified as having treatment failure or relapse of their autoimmune hepatitis, and corticosteroid treatment may be intensified or re-introduced. Liver biopsy assessment is essential in these patients to direct the appropriate strategy of corticosteroid withdrawal, exercise and weight reduction. Autoantibodies, mainly ANA, occur in 23–36% of patients with NAFLD and hypergammaglobulinemia is present in 50%.[221–223] ANA in patients with NAFLD has been associated with insulin resistance,[222] and it may indicate a more severe disease.[223] Patients with NAFLD and autoantibodies commonly (88%) satisfy the international scoring criteria for autoimmune hepatitis, and liver biopsy examination is essential to distinguish NAFLD from autoimmune hepati-

tis.[223] Rare patients may have histological features of NAFLD and autoimmune hepatitis, and these patients may benefit from low calorie diet, exercise, weight reduction and corticosteroid therapy.[222]

Successive liver biopsy examinations have shown that corticosteroid therapy decreases fibrosis in autoimmune hepatitis, and there may be an inability to re-document histological cirrhosis (Fig. 10.23(a), 10.23(b)). Fibrosis scores improved in 56% of patients followed for 55 ± 9 months and did not progress in 33% of patients followed for 62 ± 14 months.[210] Histological activity indices decreased concurrently, and patients in whom the histological activity indices improved had a higher frequency of improvement in the fibrosis scores (80% versus 25%, $p = 0.002$). These findings suggested that improvement in hepatic fibrosis occurred in conjunction with reductions in liver inflammation and that corticosteroids could facilitate the disappearance of fibrosis by suppressing inflammatory activity. Small case studies have also suggested that cirrhosis can disappear during treatment, but this possibility must await confirmation by assays more reliably reflective of cirrhosis than conventional needle biopsy of the liver.[207–209]

The assessment of fibrosis in liver biopsy tissue is compromised by intra-observer interpretative variation, sampling error, and specimen size.[145–147,224–226] The anatomical changes of cirrhosis are more complex than those of fibrosis,[227,228] and they may not be apparent on needle biopsy specimens. Reductions in fibrosis score by 1 or 2 points may be insufficient to conclude that there has been significant improvement in fibrosis or disappearance of cirrhosis.[229] These factors justify wariness when speculating about changes in fibrosis in sequential liver tissue specimens.

Changes in fibrosis are best assessed by applying a standardized scoring system, interpreting all specimens in batch under code by a single experienced liver pathologist, and focusing on changes in fibrosis rather than the complex histological requirements for cirrhosis.[230–233] The Ishak system[126] may be better able to evaluate the mild changes of fibrosis that are unevenly distributed in autoimmune hepatitis than the system developed specifically for chronic hepatitis C.[232,233] Furthermore, its reproducibility and validity for staging chronic hepatitis are recognized.[232,233] Reductions in the length of the tissue core erroneously decrease the grade and stage of the disease,[224] but there has been no consensus about the optimal length, diameter, and number of portal tracts per specimen to assess histological change.[226] Recent studies recommend that tissue cores be at least 2.5 cm long,[225] 1.4 mm wide,[224] and possess 6–8 portal tracts.[226,234] These idealized criteria may have set the standard too high for consistent satisfaction by current needle biopsy techniques.

Liver transplantation

Liver transplantation is effective in the management of patients with decompensated autoimmune hepatitis.[235] There are no features at presentation that predict prognosis, and projections of outcome require assessments of response

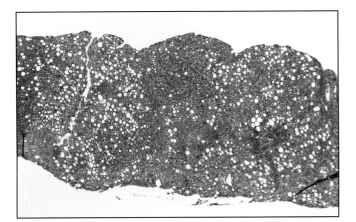

Fig. 10.24 • Macrovesicular steatosis is the predominant histological feature after corticosteroid treatment and disappearance of interface hepatitis and portal lymphoplasmacytic infiltrate. Trichrome stain.

to corticosteroids. Patients with massive necrosis in whom the hyperbilirubinaemia fails to improve after two weeks of treatment invariably die without liver transplantation,[142] and patients who fail to enter remission after 4 years of continuous treatment should be considered for transplantation when ascites first develops.[235]

The 5-year survival of patient and graft ranges from 83% to 92%, and the actuarial 10-year survival after transplantation is 75%.[236] Autoimmune hepatitis recurs in at least 17%,[237-240] and it develops de novo in 3%–5% of patients transplanted for non-autoimmune liver disease.[241-244] Acute rejection, steroid resistant rejection, and chronic rejection occur more commonly in patients transplanted for autoimmune hepatitis than for other conditions, and patients with autoimmune hepatitis are more difficult to withdraw from glucocorticoids.[245,246]

The histological features of recurrence include portal and interface hepatitis, portal lymphoplasmacytic infiltration and/or panacinar hepatitis (Fig. 10.25).[157,237-240] Panacinar hepatitis due to viral hepatitis, especially infection with hepatitis C virus, or a drug toxicity must be distinguished from allograft rejection.[157,239,242] The time interval between transplantation and disease occurrence, the laboratory and serological findings, the character of the inflammatory infiltrate (especially if plasmacytic), the sparsity of activated lymphocytes, and the absence of significant lymphocytic cholangitis and endothelitis are distinguishing features. Adjustments in the immunosuppressive regimen are usually sufficient to control the process.[237-240] Progression to cirrhosis and graft failure are possible.[247] Patients with autoimmune hepatitis who undergo liver transplantation also have a higher frequency of acute allograft rejection, corticosteroid-resistant acute rejection, and chronic rejection than counterparts without immune-mediated chronic liver disease,[245] and they should be followed closely for these manifestations.[246]

De novo autoimmune hepatitis is a clinical syndrome that affects mainly children who undergo transplantation for non-autoimmune liver disease.[241,242] Its occurrence is rare (3%–5% of liver transplant recipients), but its consequences can be severe if unrecognized and untreated. Immunosuppression with cyclosporine is a common feature, and treatment with prednisone and azathioprine is typically effective. Those patients with de novo autoimmune hepatitis who fail corticosteroid therapy have worsening fibrosis and possible graft loss, and those who do not receive corticosteroids progress to cirrhosis, require retransplantation, or die of liver failure.[243] De novo autoimmune hepatitis can occur in adults,[243,244] and in these patients, it has been associated with severe perivenular (zone 3) necrosis and an atypical anti-liver/kidney cytosolic antibody of uncertain pathogenic significance.[243] Antibodies to cytokeratin 8/18 have also been described.[248]

Immunosuppressive therapy may have the paradoxical effect of enhancing autoreactivity and promoting de novo autoimmune hepatitis after transplantation, especially in individuals with an immature immune system.[242] Cyclosporine inhibits the calcineurin-mediated pathway in the signalling of apoptosis, and it may also have a direct toxic effect on the thymic stroma.[249,250] These actions may alter the editing of T lymphocytes within the thymus and impair the negative selection of autoreactive cells. Tacrolimus can affect the thymic microenvironment in a similar fashion. An immature T cell antigen receptor repertoire, drug-induced injury of the thymic stroma, impaired apoptosis of autoreactive immunocytes, and repeated exposure to multiple infectious and/or drug-related antigens that are homologous to self antigens may be sufficient to induce de novo autoimmune hepatitis. The emergence of autoimmune hepatitis should be considered in all liver biopsy specimens obtained after transplantation that show acute panacinar hepatitis, interface hepatitis, and portal or acinar plasma cell infiltration.

References

1. Czaja AJ, Freese DK. Diagnosis and treatment of autoimmune hepatitis. Hepatology, 2002; 36:479–497
2. Czaja AJ, Carpenter HA. Sensitivity, specificity and predictability of biopsy interpretations in chronic hepatitis. Gastroenterology, 1993; 105:1824–1832
3. Johnson PJ, McFarlane IG, Alvarez F et al. Meeting report. International Autoimmune Hepatitis Group. Hepatology, 1993; 18:998–1005
4. Alvarez F, Berg PA, Biandin FB et al. International Autoimmune Hepatitis Group Report: review of criteria for diagnosis of autoimmune hepatitis. J Hepatol, 1999; 31:929–938
5. Czaja AJ. Chronic active hepatitis: the challenge for a new nomenclature. Ann Int Med, 1993; 119:510–517
6. Czaja AJ. The variant forms of autoimmune hepatitis. Ann Intern Med, 1996; 125:588–598
7. Crapper RM, Bhathal PS, Mackay IR et al. 'Acute' autoimmune hepatitis. Digestion, 1986; 34:216–325
8. Amontree JS, Stuart TD, Bredfeldt JE. Autoimmune chronic active hepatitis masquerading as acute hepatitis. J Clin Gastroenterol, 1989; 11:303–307
9. Porta G, Da Costa Gayotto LC, Alvarez F. Anti-liver-kidney microsome antibody-positive autoimmune hepatitis presenting as fulminant liver failure. J Pediatric Gastroenterol Nutr, 1990; 11:138–140
10. Nikias GA, Batts KP, Czaja AJ. The nature and prognostic implications of autoimmune hepatitis with an acute presentation. J Hepatol, 1994; 21:866–871
11. Burgart LJ, Batts KP, Ludwig J et al. Recent onset autoimmune hepatitis: biopsy findings and clinical correlations. Am J Surg Pathol, 1995; 19:699–708

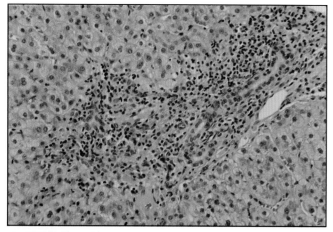

Fig. 10.25 • Recurrent autoimmune hepatitis after liver transplantation. Mononuclear infiltrate with plasma cells involve portal area; interface hepatitis is mild; bile ducts are present and unaffected. H&E.

12. Singh R, Nair S, Farr G et al. Acute autoimmune hepatitis presenting with centrizonal liver disease: case report and review of the literature. Am J Gastroenterol, 2002; 97:2670–2673

13. Okano N, Yamamotos K, Sakaguchi K et al. Clinicopathological features of acute-onset autoimmune hepatitis. Hepatol Res, 2003; 25:263–270

14. Kessler WR, Cummings OW, Eckert G et al. Fulminant hepatic liver failure as the initial presentation of acute autoimmune hepatitis. Clin Gastroenterol Hepatol, 2004; 2:625–631

15. Te HS, Konkoulis G, Ganger DR. Autoimmune hepatitis: a histological variant associated with prominent centrilobular necrosis. Gut, 1997; 41:269–271

16. Pratt DS, Fawaz KA, Rabson A et al. A novel histological lesion in glucocorticoid-responsive chronic hepatitis. Gastroenterology, 1997; 113:664–668

17. Teitelbaum JE, Perez-Atayde AR, Cohen M et al. Minocycline-related autoimmune hepatitis: case series and literature review. Arch Pediatr Adolesc Med, 1998; 152:1132–1136

18. Goldstein NS, Bayati N, Silverman AL et al. Minocycline as a cause of drug-induced autoimmune hepatitis. Report of four cases and comparison with autoimmune hepatitis. Am J Clin Pathol, 2000; 114:591–598

19. Abe M, Furukawa S, Takayama S et al. Drug-induced hepatitis with autoimmune features during minocycline therapy. Intern Med, 2003; 42:48–52

20. Czaja AJ, Carpenter HA. Validation of a scoring system for the diagnosis of autoimmune hepatitis. Dig Dis Sci, 1996; 41:305–314

21. Boberg KM, Fausa O, Haaland T et al. Features of autoimmune hepatitis in primary sclerosing cholangitis: an evaluation of 114 primary sclerosing cholangitis patients according to a scoring system for the diagnosis of autoimmune hepatitis. Hepatology, 1996; 23:1369–1376

22. Talwalkar JA, Keach JC, Angulo P et al. Overlap of autoimmune hepatitis and primary biliary cirrhosis: an evaluation of a modified scoring system. Am J Gastroenterol, 2002; 97:1191–1197

23. Czaja AJ, Manns MP. The validity and importance of subtypes of autoimmune hepatitis: a point of view. Am J Gastroenterol, 1995; 90:1206–1211

24. Lidman K, Biberfield G, Fagraeus A et al. Anti-actin specificity of human smooth muscle antibodies in chronic active hepatitis. Clin Exp Immunol, 1976; 24:266–272

25. Fusconi M, Cassani F, Zauli D et al. Anti-actin antibodies: a new test for an old problem. J Immunol Methods, 1990; 130:1–8

26. Czaja AJ, Cassani F, Cataleta M et al. Frequency and significance of antibodies to actin in type 1 autoimmune hepatitis. Hepatology, 1996; 24:1068–1073

27. Davis GL, Czaja AJ, Baggenstoss AH et al. Prognostic and therapeutic implications of extreme serum aminotransferase elevation in chronic active hepatitis. Mayo Clin Proc, 1982; 57:303–309

28. Czaja AJ, Davis GL, Ludwig J et al. Autoimmune features as determinants of prognosis in steriod-treated chronic active hepatitis of uncertain etiology. Gastroenterology, 1983; 85:713–717

29. Davis GL, Czaja AJ, Ludwig J. Development and prognosis of histologic cirrhosis in corticosteroid-treated HBsAg-negative chronic active hepatitis. Gastroenterology, 1984; 87:1222–1227

30. Roberts SK, Therneau T, Czaja AJ. Prognosis of histological cirrhosis in type 1 autoimmune hepatitis. Gastroenterology, 1996; 110:848–857

31. Donaldson PT, Doherty DG, Hayllar KM et al. Susceptibility to autoimmune chronic active hepatitis human leukocyte antigens DR4 and A1-B8-DR3 are independent risk factors. Hepatology, 1991; 13:701–706

32. Czaja AJ, Carpenter HA, Santrach PJ, Moore SB. Genetic predispositions for the immunological features of chronic active hepatitis. Hepatology, 1993; 18:816–822

33. Czaja AJ, Carpenter HA, Santrach PJ et al. Significance of HLA DR4 in type 1 autoimmune hepatitis. Gastroenterology, 1993; 105:1502–1507

34. Doherty DG, Donaldson PT, Underhill JA et al. Allelic sequence variation in the HLA class II genes and proteins in patients with autoimmune hepatitis. Hepatology, 1994; 19:609–615

35. Strettell MDJ, Donaldson PT, Thomson LJ et al. Allelic basis for HLA-encoded susceptibility to type 1 autoimmune hepatitis. Gastroenterology, 1997; 112:2028–2035

36. Czaja AJ, Strettell MDJ, Thomson LJ et al. Associations between the alleles of the major histocompatibility complex and type 1 autoimmune hepatitis. Hepatology, 1997; 25:317–323

37. Czaja AJ, Donaldson PT. Genetic susceptability for immune expression and liver cell injury in autoimmune hepatitis. Immunol Rev, 2000; 174:250–259

38. Czaja AJ, Doherty DG, Donaldson PT. Genetic bases of autoimmune hepatitis. Dig Dis Sci, 2002; 47:2139–2150

39. Donaldson PT, Czaja AJ. Genetic effects on susceptibility, clinical expression, and treatment outcome of type 1 autoimmune hepatitis. Clin Liver Dis, 2002; 6:799–824

40. Czaja AJ, Rakela J, Hay JE et al. Clinical and prognostic implications of human leukocyte antigen B8 in corticosteroid-treated severe autoimmune chronic active hepatitis. Gastroenterology, 1990; 98:1587–1593

41. Czaja AJ, Donaldson PT. Gender effects and synergisms with histocompatibility leukocyte antigens in type 1 autoimmune hepatitis. Am J Gastroenterol, 2002; 97:2051–2057

42. Vazquez-Garcia MN, Alaez C et al. MHC class II sequences of susceptibility and protection in Mexicans with autoimmune hepatitis. J Hepatol, 1998; 28:985–990

43. Seki T, Kiyosawa K, Inoko H et al. Association of autoimmune hepatitis with HLA-Bw54 and DR4 in Japanese patients. Hepatology, 1990; 12:1300–1304

44. Seki T, Ota M, Furuta S et al. HLA class II molecules and autoimmune hepatitis susceptibility in Japanese patients. Gastroenterology, 1992; 103:1041–1047

45. Fainboim L, Marcos Y, Pando M et al. Chronic active autoimmune hepatitis in children. Strong association with a particular HLA DR6 (DRB1*1301) haplotype. Hum Immunol, 1994; 41:146–150

46. Pando M, Larriba J, Fernandez GC et al. Pediatric and adult forms of type 1 autoimmune hepatitis in Argentina: evidence for differential genetic predisposition. Hepatology, 1999; 30:1374–1380

47. Bittencourt PL, Goldberg AC, Cancado ELR. Genetic heterogeneity in susceptibility to autoimmune hepatitis types 1 and 2. Am J Gastroenterol, 1999; 94:1906–1913

48. Goldberg AC, Bittencourt PL, Mougin B et al. Analysis of HLA haplotypes in autoimmune hepatitis type 1: identifying the major susceptibility locus. Hum Immunol, 2001; 62:165–169

49. Czaja AJ, Souto EO, Bittencourt PL et al. Clinical distinctions and pathogenic implications of type 1 autoimmune hepatitis in Brazil and the United States. J Hepatol, 2002; 37:302–308

50. Czaja AJ, Cookson S, Constantini PK et al. Cytokine polymorphisms associated with clinical features and treatment outcome in type 1 autoimmune hepatitis. Gastroenterology, 1999; 117:645–652

51. Cookson S, Constantini PK, Clare M et al. Frequency and nature of cytokine gene polymorphisms in type 1 autoimmune hepatitis. Hepatology, 1999; 30:851–856

52. Agarwal K, Czaja AJ, Jones DEJ et al. CTLA-4 gene polymorphism and susceptibility to type 1 autoimmune hepatitis. Hepatology, 2000; 31:49–53

53. Fainboim L, Velasco VCC, Marcos CY et al. Protracted, but not acute, hepatitis A virus infection is strongly associated with HLA-DRB1*1301, a marker for pediatric autoimmune hepatitis. Hepatology, 2001; 33:1512–1517

54. Homberg J-C, Abuaf N, Bernard O et al. Chronic active hepatitis associated with antiliver/kidney microsome antibody type 1: a second type of 'autoimmune' hepatitis. Hepatology, 1987; 7:1333–1339

55. Czaja AJ, Manns MP, Homburger HA. Frequency and significance of antibodies to liver/kidney microsome type 1 in adults with chronic active hepatitis. Gastroenterology, 1992; 103:1290–1295

56. Czaja AJ. Autoantibodies. Baillieres Clin Gastroenterol, 1995; 9:723–744

57. Czaja AJ, Homburger HA. Autoantibodies in liver disease. Gastroenterology, 2001; 120:239–249

58. Czaja AJ, Norman GL. Autoantibodies in the diagnosis and management of liver disease. J Clin Gastroenterol, 2003; 37:315–329

59. Gueguen M, Meunier-Rotival M, Bernard O, Alvarez F. Anti-liver kidney microsome antibody recognizes a cytochrome P450 from the IID subfamily. J Exp Med, 1988; 168:801–806

60. Zanger UM, Hauri H-P, Loeper J, Homberg J-C, Meyer UA. Antibodies against human cytochrome P-450db1 in autoimmune hepatitis type II. Proc Natl Acad Sci USA, 1988; 85:8256–8260

61. Manns MP, Griffin KJ, Sullivan KF et al. LKM-1 autoantibodies recognize a short linear sequence in P450IID6, a cytochrome P-450 monooxygenase. J Clin Invest, 1991; 88:1370–1378

62. Yamamoto AM, Cresteil D, Homberg JC et al. Characterization of the anti-liver-kidney microsome antibody (anti-LKM1) from hepatitis C virus-positive and -negative sera. Gastroenterology, 1993; 104:1762–1767

63. Kerkar N, Choudhuri K, Ma Y et al. Cytochrome P4502D6$_{193-212}$: a new immunodominant epitope and target of virus/self cross-reactivity in liver kidney microsomal autoantibody type 1-positive liver disease. J Immunol, 2003;170:1481–1489

64. Klein R, Zanger UM, Berg T et al. Overlapping but distinct specificities of anti-liver-kidney microsome antibodies in autoimmune hepatitis type II and hepatitis C revealed by recombinant native CYP2D6 and novel peptide epitopes. Clin Exp Immunol, 1999; 118:290–297

65. Mackie FD, Peakman M, Yun M et al. Primary and secondary liver/kidney microsomal autoantibody response following infection with hepatitis C virus. Gastroenterology, 1994; 106:1672–1675

66. Giostra F, Manzin A, Lenzi M et al. Low hepatitis C viremia in patients with anti-liver/kidney microsomal antibody type 1 positive chronic hepatitis. J Hepatol, 1996; 25:433–438

67. Vergani D, Choudhuri K, Bogdanos DP et al. Pathogenesis of autoimmune hepatitis. Clin Liver Dis, 2002; 6:727–737

68. Reddy RK, Krawitt EL, Homberg JC et al. Absence of anti-LKM1 in hepatitis C viral infection in the United States. J Viral Hepat, 1995; 2:175–179

69. Durazzo M, Philipp T, van Pelt FNAM et al. Heterogeneity of microsomal autoantibodies (LKM) in chronic hepatitis C and D virus infection. Gastroenterology, 1995; 108:455–462

70. Gerotto M, Pontisso P, Giostra F et al. Analysis of the hepatitis C virus genome in patients with anti-LKM-1 autoantibodies. J Hepatol, 1994; 21:273–276

71. Czaja AJ, Kruger M, Santrach PJ et al. Genetic distinctions between types 1 and 2 autoimmune hepatitis. Am Gastroenterol, 1997; 92:2197–2200

72. Manns MP. Cytoplasmic autoantigens in autoimmune hepatitis: molecular analysis and clinical relevance. Semin Liver Dis, 1991; 11:205–214

73. Manns MP, Kruger M. Immunogenetics of chronic liver diseases. Gastroenterology, 1994; 106:1676–1697

74. Gregorio GV, Portmann B, Reid F et al. Autoimmune hepatitis in childhood. A 20 year survey. Hepatology, 1997; 25:541–547

75. Gregorio GV, Portmann B, Karani J et al. Autoimmune hepatitis/sclerosing cholangitis overlap syndrome in childhood: a 16-year prospective study. Hepatology, 2001; 33:544–553

76. Clemente MG, Obermayer-Straub P, Meloni A et al. Cytochrome P450 1A2 is a hepatic autoantigen in autoimmune polyglandular syndrome type 1. J Clin Endocrinol Metab, 1997; 82:1353–1361

77. Manns MP, Gerken G, Kyriatsoulis A et al. Characterization of a new subgroup of autoimmune chronic active hepatitis by autoantibodies against a soluble liver antigen. Lancet, 1987; i:292–294

78. Stechemesser E, Klein R, Berg PA. Characterization and clinical relevance of liver-pancreas antibodies in autoimmune hepatitis. Hepatology, 1993; 18:1–9

79. Wies I, Brunner S, Henniger J et al. Identification of target antigen for SLA/LD autoantibodies in autoimmune hepatitis. Lancet, 2000; 355:1510–1515

80. Costa M, Rodriques-Sanchez JL, Czaja AJ et al. Isolation and characterization of cDNA encoding the antigenic protein of the human tRNA(Ser)Sec complex recognized by autoantibodies from patients with type 1 autoimmune hepatitis. Clin Exp Immunol, 2000; 121:364–374

81. Czaja AJ, Carpenter HA, Manns MP. Antibodies to soluble liver antigen, P450IID6, and mitochondrial complexes in chronic hepatitis. Gastroenterology, 1993; 105:1522–1528

82. Kanzler S, Weidemann C, Gerken G et al. Clinical significance of autoantibodies to soluble liver antigen in autoimmune hepatitis. J Hepatol, 1999; 31:635–640

83. Ma Y, Okamoto M, Thomas MG et al. Antibodies to conformational epitopes of soluble liver antigen define a severe form of autoimmune liver disease. Hepatology, 2002; 35:658–664

84. Czaja AJ, Donaldson PT, Lohse AW. Antibodies to soluble liver antigen/liver pancreas and HLA risk factors in type 1 autoimmune hepatitis. Am J Gastroenterol, 2002; 97:413–419

85. Czaja AJ, Shums Z, Norman GL. Frequency and significance of antibodies to soluble liver antigen/liver pancreas in variant autoimmune hepatitis. Autoimmunity, 2002; 35:475–483

86. Czaja AJ, Shums Z, Norman GL. Nonstandard antibodies as prognostic markers in autoimmune hepatitis. Autoimmunity, 2004; 35:475–483

87. Baeres M, Herkel J, Czaja AJ et al. Establishment of standardized SLA/LP immunoassays: specificity for autoimmune hepatitis, worldwide occurrence, and clinical characteristics. Gut, 2002; 51:259–264

88. Miyakawa H, Kawashima Y, Kitazawa E et al. Low frequency of anti-SLA/LP autoantibody in Japanese adult patients with autoimmune liver disease: analysis with recombinant antigen assay. J Autoimmun, 2003; 21:77–82

89. McFarlane IG, McFarlane BM, Major GN et al. Identification of the hepatic asialoglycoprotein receptor (hepatic lectin) as a component of liver specific membrane lipoprotein (LSP). Clin Exp Immunol, 1984; 5:347–354

90. McFarlane IG, Hegarty JE, McSorley CG et al. Antibodies to liver-specific protein predict outcome of treatment withdrawal in autoimmune chronic active hepatitis. Lancet, 1984; 2:954–956

91. McFarlane BM, McSorley CG, McFarlane IG et al. Serum autoantibodies reacting with the hepatic asialoglycoprotein receptor (hepatic lectin) in acute and chronic liver disorders. J Hepatol, 1986; 3:196–205

92. Treichel U, Poralla T, Hess G et al. Autoantibodies to human asialoglycoprotein receptor in autoimmune-type chronic hepatitis. Hepatology, 1990; 11:606–612

93. Poralla T, Treichel U, Lohr H et al. The asialoglycoprotein receptor as target structure in autoimmune liver diseases. Semin Liver Dis, 1991; 11:215–222

94. Czaja AJ, Pfeifer KD, Decker RH et al. Frequency and significance of antibodies to asialoglycoprotein receptor in type 1 autoimmune hepatitis. Dig Dis Sci, 1996; 41:1733–1740

95. Li L, Chen M, Huang DY et al. Frequency and significance of antibodies to chromatin in autoimmune hepatitis type 1. J Gastroenterol Hepatol, 2000; 15:1176–1782

96. Czaja AJ, Shums Z, Binder WL et al. Frequency and significance of antibodies to chromatin in autoimmune hepatitis. Dig Dis Sci, 2003; 48:1658–1664

97. Martini E, Abuaf N, Cavalli F et al. Antibody to liver cytosol (anti-LC1) in patients with autoimmune chronic active hepatitis type 2. Hepatology, 1988; 8:1662–1666

98. Abuaf N, Johanet C, Chretien P et al. Characterization of the liver cytosol antigen type 1 reacting with autoantibodies in chronic active hepatitis. Hepatology, 1992; 16:892–898

99. Han S, Tredger M, Gregorio GV et al. Anti-liver cytosolic antigen type 1 (LC1) antibodies in childhood autoimmune liver disease. Hepatology, 1995; 21:58–62.

100. Muratori L, Cataleta M, Muratori P et al. Liver/kidney microsomal antibody type 1 and liver cytosol antibody type 1 concentrations in type 2 autoimmune hepatitis. Gut, 1998; 42:721–726

101. Wood JR, Czaja AJ, Beaver SJ et al. Frequency and significance of antibody to double stranded DNA in chronic active hepatitis. Hepatology, 1986; 6:976–980

102. Czaja AJ, Morshed SA, Darveen S et al. Antibodies to single stranded and double stranded DNA in antinuclear antibody positive type 1 autoimmune hepatitis. Hepatology, 1997; 26:567–572

103. Czaja AJ, Ming C, Shirai M et al. Frequency and significance of antibodies to histones in autoimmune hepatitis. J Hepatol, 1995; 23:32–38

104. Chen M, Shirai M, Czaja AJ et al. Characterization of anti-histone antibodies in patients with type 1 autoimmune hepatitis. J Gastroenterol Hepatol, 1998; 13:483–489

105. Mulder AHL, Horst G, Haagsma EB et al. Prevalence and characterization of neutrophil cytoplasmic antibodies in autoimmune liver diseases. Hepatology, 1993; 17:411–417

106. Targan SR, Landers C, Vidrich A et al. High-titer antineutrophil cytoplasmic antibodies in type 1 autoimmune hepatitis. Gastroenterology, 1995; 108:1159–1166.

107. Bansi D, Chapman R, Fleming K. Antineutrophil cytoplasmic antibodies in chronic liver diseases: prevalence, titre, specificity and IgG subclass. J Hepatol, 1996; 24:581–586

108. Zauli D, Ghetti S, Grassi A et al. Anti-neutrophil cytoplasmic antibodies in type 1 and type 2 autoimmune hepatitis. Hepatology, 1997; 25:1105–1107

109. Muratori P, Muratori L, Guidi M et al. Anti-Saccharomyces cerevisiae antibosies (ASCA) and autoimmune liver diseases. Clin Exp Immunol, 2003; 132:473–476

110. Czaja AJ, Shums Z, Donaldson PT et al. Frequency and significance of antibodies to Saccharomyces cerevisiae in autoimmune hepatitis. Dig Dis Sci, 2004; 49:611–618

111. Ohana M, Okazaki K, Hajiro K et al. Antilactoferrin antibodies in autoimmune liver diseases. Am J Gastroenterol, 1998; 93:1334–1339

112. Volta U, De Franceschi L, Molinaro N et al. Frequency and significance of anti-gliadin and anti-endomysial antibodies in autoimmune hepatitis. Dig Dis Sci, 1998; 43:2190–2195

113. Czaja AJ. Behavior and significance of autoantibodies in type 1 autoimmune hepatitis. J Hepatol, 1999; 30:394–401

114. Bardella MT, Fraquelli M, Quatrini M et al. Prevalence of hypertransaminasemia in adult celiac patients and effect of gluten-free diet. Hepatology, 1995; 22:833–836

115. Volta U, Granito A, De Franceschi L et al. Anti tissue transglutaminase antibodies as predictors of silent coeliac disease in patients with hypertransaminasaemia of unknown origin. Dig Liver Dis, 2001; 33:420–425

116. Kaukinen K, Halme L, Collin P et al. Celiac disease in patients with severe liver disease: gluten-free diet may reverse hepatic failure. Gastroenterology, 2002; 122:881–888

117. Volta U, Rodrigo L, Granito A et al. Celiac disease in autoimmune cholestatic liver disorders. Am J Gastroenterol, 2002; 97:2609–2613

118. Sedlack RE, Smyrk TC, Czaja AJ et al. Celiac-disease-associated autoimmune cholangitis. Am J Gastroenterol, 2002; 97:3196–3198

119. Abdo A, Meddings J, Swain M. Liver abnormalities in celiac disease. Clin Gastroenterol Hepatol, 2004; 2:107–112

120. Biecker E, Stieger M, Zimmerman A, Reichen J. Autoimmune hepatitis, cryoglobulinaemia and untreated coeliac disease: a case report. Eur J Gastroenterol Hepatol, 2003; 15:423–427

121. Leon F, Camarero C, Pena R et al. Anti-transglutaminase IgA ELISA: clinical potential and drawbacks in celiac disease diagnosis. Scand J Gastroenterol, 2001; 36:849–853

122. Carroccio A, Giannitrapani L, Soresi M et al. Guinea pig transglutaminase immunolinked assay does not predict coeliac disease in patients with chronic liver disease. Gut, 2001; 49:506–511

123. Vergani D, Alvarez F, Bianchi FB et al. Liver autoimmune serology: a consensus statement from the committee for autoimmune serology of the International Hepatitis Group. J Hepatol, 2004; 41:677–683

124. Desmet VJ, Gerber M, Hoofnagle JH et al. Classification of chronic hepatitis: diagnosis, grading and staging. Hepatology, 1994; 19:1513–1520

125. International Working Party. Terminology of chronic hepatitis Am J Gastroenterol, 1995; 90:181–189

126. Ishak K, Baptista A, Bianchi L et al. Histological grading and staging of chronic hepatitis. J Hepatol, 1995; 22:696–699

127. Boyer JL. Chronic hepatitis. A perspective on classification and determinants of prognosis. Gastroenterology, 1976; 70:1161–1171

128. Czaja AJ. Autoimmune chronic active hepatitis-a specific entity? The negative argument. J Gastroenterol Hepatol, 1990; 5:343–351

129. Cohen S, Ohta G, Singer EJ et al. Immunocytochemical study of gamma globulin in liver in hepatitis and postnecrotic cirrhosis. J Exp Med, 1960; 11:285–293

130. Paronetto F, Rubin E, Popper H. Local formation of gamma-globulin in the diseased liver and its relation to hepatic necrosis. Lab Invest, 1962; 11:150–158

131. Czaja AJ, Carpenter HA. Histological features associated with relapse after corticosteroid withdrawal in type 1 autoimmune hepatitis. Liver International, 2003; 23:116–123

132. Baggenstoss AH, Soloway RD, Summerskill WHJ et al. Chronic active liver disease. The range of histologic lesions, their response to treatment, and evolution. Hum Pathol, 1972; 3:183–198

133. Dienes HP, Popper H, Manns M et al. Histologic features in autoimmune hepatitis. Z Gastroenterol, 1989; 27:325–330

134. Bach N, Thung SN, Schaffner F. The histological features of chronic hepatitis C and autoimmune chronic hepatitis: a comparative analysis. Hepatology, 1992; 15:572–577

135. Scheuer PJ, Ashrafzadeh P, Sherlock S, Brown D, Dusheiko GM. The pathology of hepatitis C. Hepatology, 1992; 15:567–571

136. Czaja AJ, Carpenter HA. Histological findings in chronic hepatitis C with autoimmune features. Hepatology, 1997; 26:459–466

137. Ludwig J, Czaja AJ, Dickson ER et al. Manifestations of nonsuppurative cholangitis in chronic hepatobiliary disease: morphologic spectrum, clinical correlations and terminology. Liver, 1984; 4:105–116

138. Czaja AJ, Carpenter HA. Autoimmune hepatitis with incidental histologic features of bile duct injury. Hepatology, 2001; 34:659–665

139. Czaja AJ, Muratori P, Muratori L et al. Diagnostic and therapeutic implications of bile duct injury in autoimmune hepatitis. Liver Int, 2004; 24:1–8

140. Schalm SW, Korman MG, Summerskill WHJ et al. Severe chronic active liver disease. Prognostic significance of initial morphologic patterns. Am J Dig Dis, 1977; 22:973–980

141. Cooksley WGE, Bradbear RA, Robinson W et al. The prognosis of chronic active hepatitis without cirrhosis in relation to bridging necrosis. Hepatology, 1986; 6:345–348

142. Czaja AJ, Rakela J, Ludwig J. Features reflective of early prognosis in corticosteroid-treated severe autoimmune chronic active hepatitis. Gastroenterology, 1988; 95:448–453

143. Murray-Lyon IM, Stern RB, Williams R. Controlled trial of prednisone and azathioprine in active chronic hepatitis. Lancet, 1973; i:735–737

144. Czaja AJ, Steinberg AS, Saldana M, Marin GA. Peritoneoscopy: its value in the diagnosis of liver disease. Gastrointest Endosc, 1973; 20:23–25

145. Soloway RD, Baggenstoss AH, Schoenfield LJ et al. Observer error and sampling variability tested in evaluation of hepatitis and cirrhosis by liver biopsy. Am J Dig Dis, 1975; 20:1087–1090

146. Theodossi A, Skene AM, Portmann B et al. Observer variation in assessment of liver biopsies including analysis by kappa statistics. Gastroenterology, 1980; 79:232–241

147. Bedossa P, Bioulac-Sage P, Callard P et al. Intraobserver and interobserver variations in liver biopsy interpretation in patients with chronic hepatitis C. Hepatology, 1994; 20:15–20

148. Czaja AJ, Davis GL, Ludwig J et al. Complete resolution of inflammatory activity following corticosteroid treatment of HBsAg-negative chronic active hepatitis. Hepatology, 1984; 4:622–627

149. Phillips MJ, Blendis LM, Poucell S et al. Syncytial giant-cell hepatitis. Sporadic hepatitis with distinctive pathological features, a severe clinical course, and paramyxoviral features. N Engl J Med, 1991; 324:455–460

150. Devaney K, Goodman ZD, Ishak KG. Postinfantile giant-cell transformation in hepatitis. Hepatology, 1992; 16:327–333

151. Lau JYN, Koukoulis G, Mieli-Vergani G et al. Syncytial giant-cell hepatitis—a specific disease entity? J Hepatol, 1992; 15:216–219

152. Rabinovitz M, Demetris AJ. Postinfantile giant cell hepatitis associated with anti-M2 mitochondrial antibodies. Gastroenterology, 1994; 107:1162–1164

153. Czaja AJ. The frequency and nature of the variant syndromes of autoimmune hepatitis. Hepatology, 1998; 28:360–365

154. Czaja AJ. Variant forms of autoimmune hepatitis. Curr Gastroenterol Rep, 1999; 1:63–90

155. Ben-Ari Z, Czaja AJ. Autoimmune hepatitis and its variant syndromes. Gut, 2001; 49:589–594

156. Kloppel G, Seifert G, Lindner H et al. Histopathological features in mixed types of chronic aggressive hepatitis and primary biliary cirrhosis. Correlations of liver histology with mitochondrial antibodies of different specificity. Virchows Arch Pathol Anat Histol, 1977; 373:143–160

157. Carpenter HA, Czaja AJ. The role of histologic evaluation in the diagnosis and management of autoimmune hepatitis and its variants. Clin Liver Dis, 2002; 6:685–705

158. Kenny RP, Czaja AJ, Ludwig J et al. Frequency and significance of antimitochondrial antibodies in severe chronic active hepatitis. Dig Dis Sci, 1986; 31:705–711

159. Lohse AW, Meyer zum Buschenfelde KH, Kanzler FB et al. Characterization of the overlap syndrome of primary biliary cirrhosis (PBC) and autoimmune hepatitis: evidence for it being a hepatitic form of PBC in genetically susceptible individuals. Hepatology, 1999; 29:1078–1084

160. Chazouilleres O, Wendum D, Serfaty L et al. Primary biliary cirrhosis-autoimmune hepatitis overlap syndrome: clinical features and response to therapy. Hepatology, 1998; 28:296–301

161. Rabinovitz M, Demetris AJ, Bou-Abboud CF et al. Simultaneous occurrence of primary sclerosing cholangitis and autoimmune chronic active hepatitis in a patient with ulcerative colitis. Dig Dis Sci, 1992; 37:1606–1611

162. McNair ANB, Moloney M, Portmann BC et al. Autoimmune hepatitis overlapping with primary sclerosing cholangitis in 5 cases. Am J Gastroenterol, 1998; 93:777–784

163. Wee A, Ludwig J. Pericholangitis in chronic ulcerative colitis: primary sclerosing cholangitis of the small bile ducts? Ann Intern Med, 1985; 102:581–587

164. Perdigoto R, Carpenter HA, Czaja AJ. Frequency and significance of chronic ulcerative colitis in severe corticosteroid-treated autoimmune hepatitis. J Hepatol, 1992; 14:325–331

165. Lindor KD. Ursodiol for primary sclerosing cholangitis. N Engl J Med, 1997; 336:691–695

166. Czaja AJ. Autoimmune hepatitis and viral infection. Gastroenterol Clin North Am, 1994; 23:547–566

167. Czaja AJ, Carpenter HA, Santrach PJ et al. Immunologic features and HLA associations in chronic viral hepatitis. Gastroenterology, 1995; 108:157–164

168. Czaja AJ, Carpenter HA, Santrach PJ et al. Significance of human leukocyte antigens DR3 and DR4 in chronic viral hepatitis. Dig Dis Sci, 1995; 40:2098–2106

169. Czaja AJ. The autoimmune hepatitis/hepatitis C overlap syndrome. Does it exist? In: Leueschner U, Broome U, Stiehl A, eds. Cholestatic liver diseases: therapeutic options and perspectives. Falk Symposium No. 136. Lancaster: Lancaster Publishing, 2004; 132–146

170. Magrin S, Craxi A, Fabiano C et al. Hepatitis C viremia in chronic liver disease: relationship to interferon-alpha or corticosteroid therapy. Hepatology, 1994; 19:273–279

171. Vento S, DiPerri G, Garofano T et al. Hazards of interferon therapy for HBV-seronegative chronic hepatitis. Lancet, 1989; ii:926

172. Conlon KC, Urba WJ, Smith JW et al. Exacerbation of symptoms of autoimmune disease in patients receiving alpha-interferon therapy. Cancer, 1990; 65:2237–2242

173. Papo T, Marcellin P, Bernuau J et al. Autoimmune chronic hepatitis exacerbated by alpha-interferon. Ann Intern Med, 1992; 116:51–53

174. Czaja AJ, Carpenter HA, Santrach PJ et al. Host- and disease-specific factors affecting steatosis in chronic hepatitis C. J Hepatol, 1998; 29:198–206

175. Czaja AJ, Magrin S, Fabiano C et al. Hepatitis C virus infection as a determinant of behavior in type 1 autoimmune hepatitis. Dig Dis Sci, 1995; 40:33–40

176. Bellary S, Schiano T, Hartman G et al. Chronic hepatitis with combined features of autoimmune chronic hepatitis and chronic hepatitis C: favorable response to prednisone and azathioprine. Ann Int Med, 1995; 123:32–34

177. Tran A, Benzaken S, Yang G et al. Chronic hepatitis C and autoimmunity: good response to immunosuppressive treatment. Dig Dis Sci, 1997; 42:778–780

178. Czaja AJ. Extrahepatic immunologic features of chronic viral hepatitis. Dig Dis, 1997; 15:125–144

179. Michieletti P, Wanless IR, Katz A et al. Antimitochondrial antibody negative primary biliary cirrhosis: a distinct syndrome of autoimmune cholangitis. Gut, 1994; 35:260–265

180. Taylor SL, Dean PJ, Riely CA. Primary autoimmune cholangitis: an alternative to antimitochondrial antibody-negative primary biliary cirrhosis. Am J Clin Pathol, 1994; 18:91–99

181. Ben-Ari Z, Dhillon AP, Sherlock S. Autoimmune cholangiopathy: part of the spectrum of autoimmune chronic active hepatitis. Hepatology, 1993; 18:10–15

182. Goodman ZD, McNally PR, Davis DR et al. Autoimmune cholangitis: a variant of primary biliary cirrhosis. Clinicopathologic and serologic correlations in 200 cases. Dig Dis Sci, 1995; 40:1232–1242

183. Lacerda MA, Ludwig J, Dickson ER et al. Antimitochondrial antibody-negative primary biliary cirrhosis. Am J Gastroenterol, 1995; 90:247–249

184. Czaja AJ, Carpenter HA, Santrach PJ et al. Autoimmune cholangitis within the spectrum of autoimmune liver disease. Hepatology, 2000; 31:1231–1238

185. Gordon SC, Quattrociocchi-Longe TM, Khan BA et al. Antibodies to carbonic anhydrase in patients with immune cholangiopathies. Gastroenterology, 1995; 108:1802–1809

186. Akisawa N, Nishimori I, Miyaji E et al. The ability of anti-carbonic anhydrase II antibody to distinguish autoimmune cholangitis from primary biliary cirrhosis in Japanese patients. J Gastroenterol, 1999; 34:366–371

187. Czaja AJ, Santrach PJ, Moore SB. Shared genetic risk factors in autoimmune liver disease. Dig Dis Sci, 2001; 46:140–147

188. Shimizu Y, Higuchi K, Kashii Y et al. Clonal accumulation of Vβ5.1-positive cells in the liver of a patient with autoimmune cholangiopathy. Liver, 1997; 17:7–12

189. Nakanuma Y, Harada K, Kaji K et al. Clinicopathological study of primary biliary cirrhosis negative for antimitochondrial antibodies. Liver, 1997; 17:281–287

190. Omagari K, Ikuno N, Matsuo I et al. Autoimmune cholangitis syndrome with a bias towards primary biliary cirrhosis. Pathology, 1996; 28:255–258

191. Muratori P, Muratori L, Lenzi M et al. Antibodies to carbonic anhydrase in autoimmune cholangiopathy. Gastroenterology, 1997; 112:1053–1059

192. Tsuneyama K, Van de Water J, Van Thiel D et al. Abnormal expression of PDC-E2 on the apical surface of biliary epithelial cells in patients with antimitochondrial antibody-negative primary biliary cirrhosis. Hepatology, 1995; 22:1440–1446

193. Kinoshita H, Omagari K, Whittingham S et al. Autoimmune cholangitis and primary biliary cirrhosis—an autoimmune enigma. Liver, 1999; 19:122–128

194. Czaja AJ, Carpenter HA, Santrach PJ et al. The nature and prognosis of severe cryptogenic chronic active hepatitis. Gastroenterology, 1993; 104:1755–1761

195. Czaja AJ, Hay JE, Rakela J. Clinical features and prognostic implications of severe corticosteroid-treated cryptogenic chronic active hepatitis. Mayo Clin Proc, 1990; 65:23–30

196. Kaymakoglu S, Cakaloglu Y, Demir K et al. Is severe cryptogenic chronic hepatitis similar to autoimmune hepatitis? J Hepatol, 1998; 28:78–83

197. Greeve M, Ferrell L, Kim M et al. Cirrhosis of undefined pathogenesis: absence of evidence for unknown viruses or autoimmune processes. Hepatology, 1993; 17:593–598

198. Czaja AJ, Bianchi FB, Carpenter HA et al. Treatment challenges and investigational opportunities in autoimmune hepatitis. Hepatology, 2005; 41:207–215

199. Feld JJ, Dinh H, Arenovich T et al. Autoimmune hepatitis: effect of symptoms and cirrhosis on natural history and outcome. Hepatology, 2005; 42:53–62

200. Tan P, Marotta P, Ghent C, Adams P. Early treatment response predicts the need for liver transplantation in autoimmune hepatitis. Liver Int, 2005; 25:728–733

201. Czaja AJ. Treatment of autoimmune hepatitis. Semin Liver Dis, 2002; 22:365–377

202. Czaja AJ, Ammon HV, Summerskill WHJ. Clinical features and prognosis of severe chronic active liver disease (CALD) after corticosteroid-induced remission. Gastroenterology, 1980; 78:518–523

203. Czaja AJ, Wolf AM, Baggenstoss AH. Laboratory assessment of severe chronic active liver disease (CALD): correlation of serum transaminase and gamma globulin levels with histologic features. Gastroenterology, 1981; 80:687–692

204. Czaja AJ, Menon KVN, Carpenter HA. Sustained remission after corticosteroid therapy for type 1 autoimmune hepatitis: a retrospective analysis. Hepatology, 2002; 35:890–897

205. Czaja AJ, Ludwig J, Baggenstoss AH et al. Corticosteroid-treated chronic active hepatitis in remission. Uncertain prognosis of chronic persistent hepatitis. N Engl J Med, 1981; 304:5–9

206. Verma S, Gunuwan B, Mendler M et al. Factors predicting relapse and poor outcome in type 1 autoimmune hepatitis: role of cirrhosis development, patterns of transaminases during remission, and plasma cell activity in the liver biopsy. Am J Gastroenterol, 2004; 99:1510–1516

207. Schvarcz R, Glaumann H, Weiland O. Survival and histological resolution of fibrosis in patients with autoimmune chronic active hepatitis. J Hepatol, 1993; 18:15–23

208. Dufour J-F, DeLellis R, Kaplan MM. Reversibility of hepatic fibrosis in autoimmune hepatitis. Ann Inter Med, 1997; 127:981–985

209. Cotler SJ, Jakate S, Jensen DM. Resolution of cirrhosis in autoimmune hepatitis with corticosteroid therapy. J Clin Gastroenterol, 2001; 32:428–430

210. Czaja AJ, Carpenter HA. Decreased fibrosis during corticosteroid therapy of autoimmune hepatitis. J Hepatol, 2004; 40:644–650

211. Czaja AJ, Carpenter HA. Progressive fibrosis during corticosteroid therapy of autoimmune hepatitis. Hepatology, 2004; 39:1631–1638

212. Hegarty JE, Nouri-Aria KT, Portmann B et al. Relapse following treatment withdrawal in patients with autoimmune chronic active hepatitis. Hepatology, 1983; 3:685–689

213. Czaja AJ, Beaver SJ, Shiels MT. Sustained remission following corticosteroid therapy of severe HBsAg-negative chronic active hepatitis. Gastroenterology, 1987; 92:215–219

214. Czaja AJ. Low dose corticosteroid therapy after multiple relapses of severe HBsAg-negative chronic active hepatitis. Hepatology, 1990; 11:1044–1049

215. Stellon AJ, Keating JJ, Johnson PJ et al. Maintenance of remission in autoimmune chronic active hepatitis with azathioprine after corticosteroid withdrawal. Hepatology, 1988; 8:781–784

216. Johnson PJ, McFarlane IG, Williams R. Azathioprine for long-term maintenance of remission in autoimmune hepatitis. N Engl J Med, 1995; 333:958–963

217. Mieli-Vergani G, Lobo-Yeo A, McFarlane BM et al. Different immune mechanisms leading to autoimmunity in primary sclerosing cholangitis and autoimmune chronic active hepatitis of childhood. Hepatology, 1989; 9:198–203

218. Farrant JM, Doherty DG, Donaldson PT et al. Amino acid substitutions at position 38 of the DRβ polypeptide confer susceptibility to and protection from primary sclerosing cholangitis. Hepatology, 1992; 16:390–395

219. Horsmans Y, Piret A, Brenard R et al. Autoimmune chronic active hepatitis responsive to immunosuppressive therapy evolving into a typical primary biliary cirrhosis syndrome: a case report. J Hepatol, 1994; 21:194–198

220. Angulo P, El-Amin O, Carpenter HA et al. Development of autoimmune hepatitis in the setting of long-standing primary biliary cirrhosis. Am J Gastroenterol, 2001; 96:3021–3027

221. Czaja AJ, Carpenter HA, Santrach PJ, Moore SB. Genetic predispositions for immunological features in chronic liver diseases other than autoimmune hepatitis. J Hepatol, 1996; 24:52–59

222. Loria P, Lonardo A, Leonardi F et al. Non-organ-specific autoantibodies in nonalcoholic fatty liver disease: prevalence and correlates. Dig Dis Sci, 2003; 48:2173–2181

223. Adams LA, Lindor KD, Angulo P. The prevalence of autoantibodies and autoimmune hepatitis in patients with nonalcoholic fatty liver disease. Am J Gastroenterol, 2004; 99:1316–1320

224. Colloredo G, Guido M, Sonzogni A et al. Impact of liver biopsy size on the histological evaluation of chronic hepatitis: the smaller the sample, the milder the disease. J Hepatol, 2003; 39:239–244

225. Bedossa P, Dargere D, Pardis V. Sampling variability of liver fibrosis in chronic hepatitis C. Hepatology, 2003; 38:1449–1457

226. Scheuer PJ. Liver biopsy size matters in chronic hepatitis: bigger is better. Hepatology, 2003; 38:1356–1358

227. Wanless IR, Nakashima E, Sherman M. Regression of human cirrhosis: morphologic features and the genesis of incomplete septal fibrosis. Arch Pathol Lab Med, 2000; 124:1599–1607

228. Wanless IR. Use of corticosteroid therapy in autoimmune hepatitis resulting in resolution of cirrhosis (editorial) J Clin Gastroenterol, 2001; 32:371–372

229. Desmet VJ, Roskams T. Cirrhosis reversal: a duel between dogma and myth (editorial). J Hepatol, 2004; 40:860–867

230. Arthur MJP. Reversibility of liver fibrosis and cirrhosis following treatment for hepatitis C (editorial). Gastroenterology, 2002; 122:1525–1528

231. French METAVIR Cooperative Study Group. Intraobserver and interobserver variations in liver biopsies in patients with chronic hepatitis C. Hepatology, 1994; 20:15–20

232. Westin J, Lagging LM, Wejstal R et al. Interobserver study of liver histopathology using the Ishak score in patients with chronic hepatitis C virus infection. Liver, 1999; 19:183–187

233. Brunt EM. Grading and staging the histopathological lesions of chronic hepatitis: the Knodell histology activity index and beyond. Hepatology, 2000; 31; 241–246

234. Kaserer K, Fiedler R, Steindl P et al. Liver biopsy is a useful predictor of response to interferon therapy in chronic hepatitis C. Histopathology, 1998; 32:454–461

235. Sanchez-Urdazpal L, Czaja AJ, van Hoek B et al. Prognostic features and role of liver transplantation in severe corticosteroid-treated autoimmune chronic active hepatitis. Hepatology, 1992; 15:215–221

236. Seaberg EC, Belle SH, Beringer KC et al. Liver transplantation in the United States from 1987–1998: updated results from the Pitt-UNOS liver transplant registry. In: Cecka JM, Terasaki PI, eds. Clinical Transplants 1998. Los Angeles: UCLA Tissue Typing Laboratories, 1999; 17–37

237. Neuberger J, Portmann B, Calne R, Williams R. Recurrence of autoimmune chronic active hepatitis following orthotopic liver grafting. Transplantation, 1984; 37:363–365

238. Devlin J, Donaldson P, Portmann B, Heaton N, Tan K-C, Williams R. Recurrence of autoimmune hepatitis following liver transplantation. Liver Transplantation and Surgery, 1995; 1:162–165

239. Sempoux C, Horsmans Y, Lerut J et al. Acute lobular hepatitis as the first manifestation of recurrent autoimmune hepatitis after orthotopic liver transplantation. Liver, 1997; 17:311–315

240. Gonzalez-Koch A, Czaja AJ, Carpenter HA et al. Recurrent autoimmune hepatitis after orthotopic liver transplantation. Liver Transplantation, 2001; 7:302–310

241. Kerkar N, Hadzic N, Davies ET et al. De-novo autoimmune hepatitis after liver transplantation. Lancet, 1998; 353:409–413

242. Czaja AJ. Autoimmune hepatitis after liver transplantation and other lessons of self-intolerance. Liver Transplantation, 2002; 8:505–513

243. Salcedo M, Vaquero J, Banares R et al. Response to steroids in de novo autoimmune hepatitis after transplantation. Hepatology, 2002; 35:349–356

244. Heneghan MA, Portmann BC, Norris SM et al. Graft dysfunction mimicking autoimmune hepatitis following liver transplantation in adults. Hepatology, 2001; 34:464–470

245. Hayashi M, Keefe EB, Krams SM et al. Allograft rejection after liver transplantation for autoimmune liver disease. Liver Transplant Surg, 1998; 4:208–214

246. Neuberger J. Transplantation for autoimmune hepatitis. Semin Liver Dis, 2002; 22:379–385

247. Ratziu V, Samuel D, Sebagh M et al. Long-term follow-up after liver transplantation for autoimmune hepatitis: evidence of recurrence of primary disease. J Hepatol, 1999; 30:131–141

248. Inui A, Sogo T, Komatsu H et al. Antibodies against cytokeratin 8/18 in a patient with de novo autoimmune hepatitis after living donor liver transplantation. Liver Transpl, 2005; 11:504–507

249. Beschorner WE, Namnoum JD, Hess AD et al. Thymic immunopathology after cyclosporin: effect of irradiation and age on medullary involution and recovery. Transplant Proc, 1988; 20:1072–1078

250. Hess AD, Fischer AC, Horwitz LR et al. Cyclosporine-induced autoimmunity: critical role of autoregulation in the prevention of major histocompatibility class II-dependent autoaggression. Transplant Proc, 1993; 25:2811–2813

Diseases of the bile ducts 11

Bernard C. Portmann   Yasuni Nakanuma

This chapter covers the different diseases in which there is injury to the intrahepatic and/or extrahepatic bile ducts; these are summarized in Table 11.1. The disorders are varied; some, although selectively affecting the bile ducts, are discussed in more detail elsewhere in this volume and appropriate cross-references are given. We shall emphasize those histological features that characterize the early stages of the disease in which there are distinctive bile-duct lesions that may be identified in liver biopsies. In some of these conditions, especially primary biliary cirrhosis (PBC), chronic liver allograft rejection and graft-versus-host disease (GVHD), the interlobular bile ducts up to a diameter of 100 µm are damaged and progressively disappear from the liver—the so-called vanishing or disappearing bile-duct disorders. These are characterized histologically by ductopenia, of which the number of recognized aetiologies or associations has been steadily growing. In others, these structures may be affected together with larger intrahepatic and extrahepatic bile ducts; this is especially true in primary sclerosing cholangitis (PSC). Progressive destruction and loss of the intrahepatic bile ducts lead to portal–portal bridging fibrosis and eventual development of a biliary cirrhosis. Thus, in their later stages, the various diseases have many pathological features in common. These, in turn, closely resemble the changes observed with secondary biliary cirrhosis that are reviewed at the end of this chapter. The term cholangiopathy is collectively applied to the diseases in which cholangiocytes or biliary epithelial cells are the primary target of the disease process.[1]

In contrast to extrahepatic biliary obstruction, chronic intrahepatic bile-duct lesions may evolve over many years without obvious morphological cholestasis or bilirubinostasis. This period of evolution is characterized by profound and characteristic changes at the interface between portal tracts and parenchyma—cholate stasis or biliary interface activity, previously known as biliary piecemeal necrosis. It seems pertinent to review them in depth as, in the absence of characteristic bile-duct lesions, their recognition is essential to distinguish biliary from other forms of chronic liver disease. As biliary disorders selectively affect different segments of the biliary tree, the first section outlines the anatomical features relevant to the classification and nomenclature of the biliary disorders (see Chapter 1 for the development and a more detailed morphological account of the biliary tree). It is followed by an account of basic pathogenetic mechanisms that are shared by many of the distinct entities discussed later in the chapter.[2]

The normal morphology of the biliary tree and peribiliary glands

The intrahepatic branching of the bile ducts is best visualized on a biliary injection cast (Fig. 11.1). There is no sharp delineation of the various segments, but from a practical point of view the ducts proximal to the confluence of the hepatic duct can be classified into two main categories:

Table 11.1	Diseases of the intra- and/or extrahepatic bile ducts

Neonates and children

Ductal plate malformation (infantile polycystic disease, congenital hepatic fibrosis, Caroli disease) (Ch. 4)

Extrahepatic biliary atresia (Ch. 4)*

Paucity of the interlobular bile ducts (syndromic and non-syndromic) (Ch. 4)

α_1-Antitrypsin deficiency (Ch. 5)

Cystic fibrosis (Ch. 5)

Primary sclerosing cholangitis* with or without ulcerative colitis with autoimmune features ('autoimmune sclerosing cholangitis') perinatal onset

Acquired sclerosing cholangitis (immunodeficiency, Langerhans cell histiocytosis)

Adults

1. Destruction and progressive loss of bile ducts

   Primary biliary cirrhosis

   Primary sclerosing cholangitis with or without ulcerative colitis*

   Acquired sclerosing cholangitis:

      Opportunistic (primary or secondary immunodeficiency—AIDS)*

      Ischaemic (arterial cytotoxic infusion, liver allograft)* (Ch. 16)

      Toxic (treated hydatid cyst)

      Associated with sclerosing pancreatitis

   Idiopathic adulthood ductopenia

   Hepatic allograft rejection (Ch. 16)

   Graft-versus-host disease (Ch. 16)

   Suppurative cholangitis usually with biliary obstruction

   Sarcoidosis (Ch. 17)

   Hodgkin disease (Ch. 17)

   Drug reactions (Ch. 14)

2. Usually reversible injury to bile ducts

   Extrahepatic obstruction*

   Viral hepatitis, especially HCV, cytomegalovirus (Chs 8 and 9)

   Drug reactions (Ch. 14)

   Septicaemia, endotoxic shock and toxic shock syndrome

   Parasitic infestation (Ch. 9)*

   Recurrent pyogenic cholangitis/hepatolithiasis

* Extrahepatic bile ducts additionally and/or preferentially affected

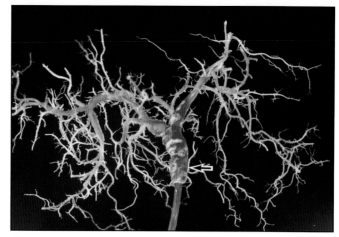

Fig. 11.1 • Normal biliary tree. Biliary cast of the normal adult liver prepared at autopsy. Note that branching does not show an exact dichotomy. Arrow: Common bile duct.

1. *Large intrahepatic bile ducts.* These consist of the right and left hepatic ducts, the segmental (large perihilar) ducts, and the first and second branches of the large area ducts, all of which are grossly visible.[3]

2. *Small intrahepatic bile ducts.* These are the septal and interlobular bile ducts which are visible only under the microscope, the former being inconsistently sampled by biopsy needles.

Like the large intrahepatic ducts, the septal ducts (>100 µm in diameter) are lined by tall columnar cells with basal nuclei and are surrounded by a layer of hypocellular collagen, the duct wall. In contrast, the interlobular bile ducts are lined by cuboidal cells resting on a thin basement membrane. The interlobular bile ducts are connected to the bile canicular network by ductules or cholangioles (<20 µm diameter) similarly lined by cuboidal cells and the canals of Hering, which are lined partly by biliary epithelium and partly by hepatocytes. Neither ductules nor canals of Hering are clearly identifiable in haematoxylin- and eosin-(H & E) stained sections of normal liver, but they become obvious in various pathological conditions and by immunostaining of biliary cytokeratin.[4]

Peribiliary glands are present within the fibromuscular walls of extrahepatic bile ducts and neck of gallbladder, and also along the large intrahepatic bile ducts[5] (Fig. 11.2A–C). Glandular acini arise from ductal plates and their density decreases progressively through infancy and childhood.[6] Around the large intrahepatic bile ducts, peribiliary glands are subdivided into intramural, non-branching tubular glands and extramural ramified glands. The latter lie in the periductal connective tissue and, in a three-dimensional model, have a linear distribution along two opposite sides of the bile ducts (Fig. 11.2A–C); they indirectly drain into the bile-duct lumen via their own conduit (Fig. 11.3A). The extramural glands show anastomosing bridges and consist of serous and mucous acini (Fig. 11.3B, C).[5] Pancreatic acini without Langerhans islets are found intermingled with peribiliary glandular acini in some 4% of autopsy livers and are probably an intrinsic component of these glands (Fig. 11.3D).[7,8] The glands are thought to have absorptive and secretory activities and may be a site of biliary epithelial regeneration.[5] Von Meyenburg complexes or ductular reaction in the hepatic parenchyma near hepatic hilar and peri-hilar regions can be differentiated from the extramural type of peribiliary glands, which are located in the connective tissue around large intrahepatic bile ducts.

Immune-related molecules involved in self-defence system of the bile ducts

The human bile ducts, particularly the intrahepatic ones, and bile are sterile under normal conditions, yet bacterial components such as lipopolysaccharide (LPS) and bacterial DNA are detectable in normal bile,[9–11] and bacteria are also detectable in bile and biliary epithelial cells in chronic

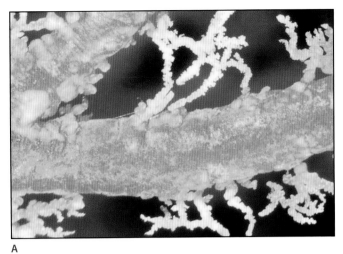

A

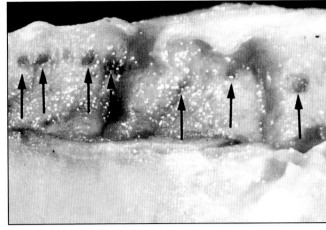

B

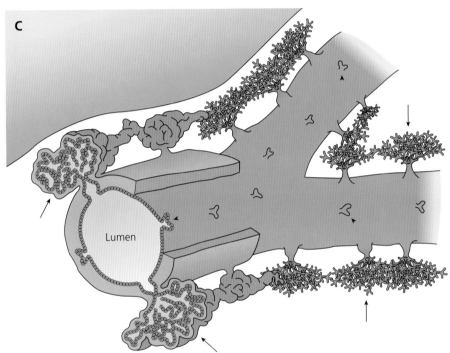

C

Lumen

Fig. 11.2 • Intrahepatic peribiliary glands in normal human liver. **(A)** Extramural peribiliary glands regularly distributed on either side of left lateral segment ducts with anastomotic bridges near the duct bifurcation. Biliary cast. **(B)** Extramural peribiliary glands outlets appear as small depressions (arrowed) with a linear distribution on the luminal surface of the bile duct. Biliary cast. **(C)** Schematic representation of the intramural (arrowheads) and extramural (thin arrows) peribiliary glands. Redrawn from Nakanuma et al. with permission from Blackwell Publishing Ltd.[5]

inflammatory biliary diseases.[9,12,13] The biliary tract is equipped with defence mechanisms, which are physical (bile flow and biliary mucus), chemical (bile salts), and immunological, such as secretory IgA and biliary intra-epithelial lymphocytes (bIEL).[14–16]

Non-specific bactericidal enzymes (lactoferrin and lyso-zyme) have been demonstrated in intrahepatic biliary tree, peribiliary glands and bile.[15] Human β-defensins (hBDs), an important group of antimicrobial peptides contributing to innate immunity at mucosal surfaces, is expressed in the biliary tree;[17] hBD-1 is constitutively expressed in epithelial tissues[18] including intrahepatic biliary epithelium,[17] while hBD-2 expression is induced following exposure to bacteria or cytokines.[19] hBD-2 is not found in normal livers, but is expressed in large intrahepatic bile ducts in extrahepatic biliary obstruction, hepatolithiasis and to a lesser degree in PBC and PSC[17] (Fig.11.4A), suggesting a response to local infection and/or active inflammation. Trefoil factor family

(TFF)-1,2,3 peptides expressed at the apical surface of the epithelium play a major role in mucosal repair.[20] TFF1 and TFF3 may secure non-specifically biliary epithelial repair in intrahepatic large bile ducts.[21] Toll-like receptor(s), which are involved in the recognition of bacterial components, are expressed in biliary epithelia of normal and pathologic bile ducts (Fig.11.4B).[22]

IgA, which is known to be secreted into bile by binding with the secretory component, is likely to be part of the natural immune defence.[14,15] bIEL are occasionally encountered in normal intrahepatic bile ducts and markedly increased in bile-duct injuries, particularly in immune-mediated cholangitis. Their number in normal livers is a tenth of that in the intestinal epithelium, and most of them are positive for CD8, while some are CD57 +ve; these cells may participate in the biliary innate immunity. The distri-bution of these molecules and bIEL along the intrahepatic biliary tree is schematically shown in Fig.11.4C.

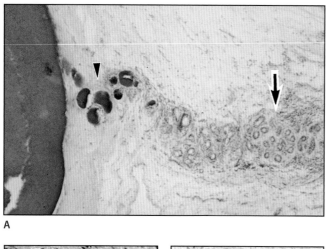

A

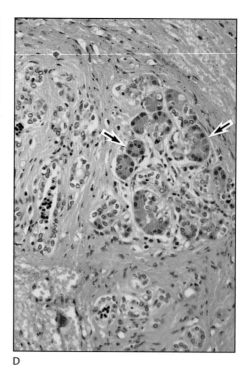

D

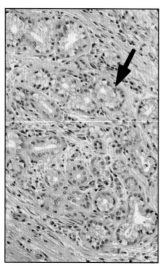

B

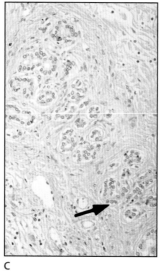

C

Fig. 11.3 • Peribiliary glands. **(A)** The glands (arrow) are arranged as lobules and drain into the intrahepatic large bile duct (*) via their own conduit (arrowhead), the latter being filled with contrast medium. H & E. **(B)** and **(C)** At higher magnification, extramural glands are arranged as lobules surrounded by fibrous tissue. The lobules (arrowed) consist of mucinous (B) and serous (C) acini, which are usually mixed in individual lobules. H & E. **(D)** Admixed with extramural peribiliary glands, there are acini resembling pancreatic exocrine acini (arrows). H & E.

Biliary epithelium injury

Pathological changes in response to injury

Biliary epithelium may undergo a range of histopathological changes that often lack specificity and differ according to the size of the affected ducts. They are summarized in this section; more characteristic histopathological alterations are considered and illustrated later in relation to individual disorders.

In the large bile ducts, biliary epithelial swelling and atrophy, disordered nuclear polarity and sloughing around the circumference are encountered in both inflammatory and neoplastic conditions. This may lead to ulceration with a granulomatous or xanthomatous reaction induced by extravasated bile products. In the interlobular bile ducts, cytoplasmic vacuolation, eosinophilic change, nuclear pleomorphism and hyperchromasia are common degenerative changes. Nuclear 'piling up' suggests regeneration which may be substantiated by immunostaining for proliferative marker antigens, although mitoses are rarely seen. Proliferation of biliary epithelium is associated with subsequent luminal enlargement and may lead to an overestimation of the actual size of the affected ducts.[23] Nuclear pyknosis, apoptosis, fading and uneven spacing anticipate

duct loss.[24] Mucin may become detectable histochemically in the supranuclear cytoplasm and on the luminal surface as a non-specific response to various injuries. This is occasionally marked, leading to the formation of mucus lakes lined by pleomorphic epithelium which may be misinterpreted as carcinomatous transformation (Fig. 11.5A,B). Injured ducts can be variably distorted with an irregularly shaped lumen. Rupture of the duct basement membrane is followed by dilatation which, as in the case of early PBC, may lead to an overestimation of the actual size of the affected duct; small diverticula may rarely form. Damaged bile ducts can show 'inappropriate' or aberrant expression of immune molecules such as cytokines, chemokines and other antigens (see below).

Impacted erythrocytes are encountered in bile-duct lumens in cases of haemobilia (Fig. 11.5C) or within the epithelium of the interlobular bile ducts in liver biopsy specimens taken after recent endoscopic or surgical biliary manipulation[25] (Fig. 11.5D) or in association with primary or secondary malignancy.

Metaplasia of biliary epithelia can be observed as follows. *Hepatocytic metaplasia* of biliary epithelium occurs in interlobular bile ducts and bile ductules in various pathological situations but remains of uncertain significance (Fig. 11.6A).[26] The cells have a clear or weakly eosinophilic,

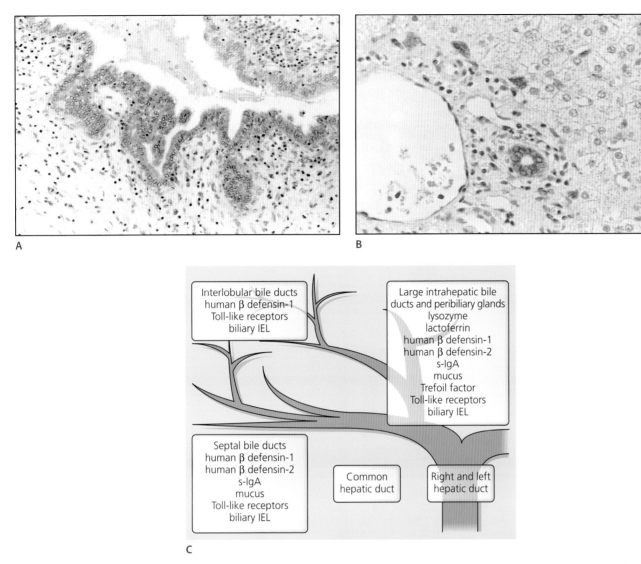

Fig. 11.4 • Expression of innate immunity related molecules and distribution of intraepithelial lymphocytes along the intrahepatic bile ducts. **(A)** Chronic inflammation of a large intrahepatic bile duct (hepatolithiasis) showing an aberrant expression of human β-defensin 2 in the cytoplasm of biliary epithelial cells and also several inflammatory cells. **(B)** Toll-like receptor 4 is constitutively expressed on interlobular bile duct, Kupffer cells and endothelial cells. **(C)** Schematic presentation of molecules related to self-defence and intraepithelial lymphocytes at different anatomical levels of the intrahepatic biliary tree. S-IgA, secretory IgA.

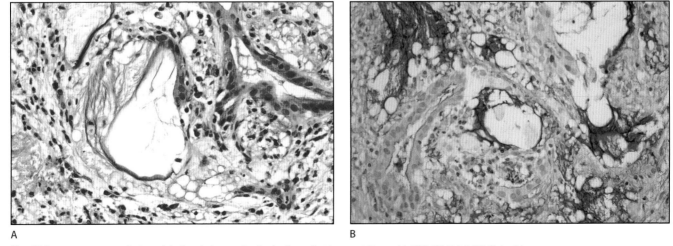

Fig. 11.5 • Secretory metaplasia and cholangiodestruction in the liver of a 10-year-old boy with PSC. **(A)** H & E. **(B)** Alcian blue.

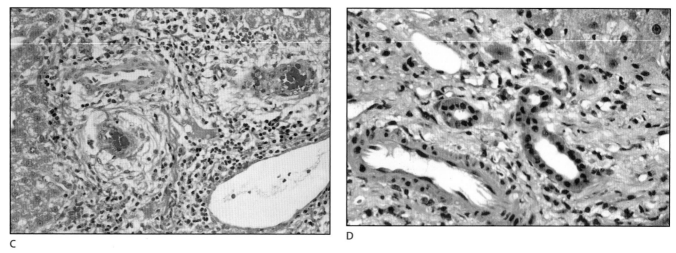

C

Fig. 11.5 • cont'd (C) Haematobilia following rupture of a hepatic arterial aneurysm with cast of red cells in the lumen of two interlobular bile ducts. H & E. **(D)** Red cells are impacted within epithelial lining of interlobular bile ducts in a biopsy taken shortly after ERCP. H & E. Courtesy of Dr L. Ferrell.

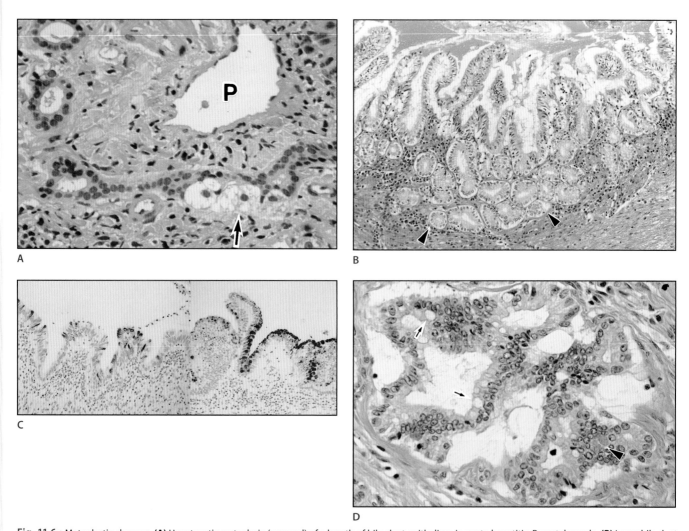

Fig. 11.6 • Metaplastic changes. (A) Hepatocytic metaplasia (arrowed) of a length of bile-duct epithelium in acute hepatitis. P, portal venule. **(B)** Large bile duct in hepatolithiasis showing an increased number of glands (arrowheads) which resemble pyloric glands. The surface epithelium is also hyperplastic. **(C)** Gastrointestinal metaplasia demonstrated by immunostaining for mucus core protein (MUC). MUC 2 protein, colonic mucin, (left) and MUC 5AC protein, gastric mucin (right), are aberrantly expressed on the biliary epithelium, particularly goblet cells. **(D)** Goblet cell metaplasia (arrows) with Paneth cell (arrowhead) within hyperplastic peribiliary glands in hepatolithiasis. H & E.

glycogen-rich cytoplasm with a distinct border and rest on a basement membrane alongside normal biliary cells. They are identical to hepatocytes, although some may express a mixed hepatocytic and bile-duct phenotype.[26] They may be newly formed hepatocytes derived from facultative hepatic stem cells in the canals of Hering (intrabiliary stem cells).[27] *Gastrointestinal metaplasia* resembling pyloric glands, goblet cells or intestinal metaplasia is seen in chronically inflamed large bile ducts, peribiliary glands and the gallbladder (Fig. 11.6B). The change is associated with gastric type mucus core protein (MUC) 5AC (Fig. 11.6C left) and MUC6 expression and with intestinal type MUC2 (Fig. 11.6C right).[28-30] This MUC expression pattern differs from the normal constitutive MUC3.[31] Invagination of the biliary epithelium seems in part responsible for this lesion, which manifests as an increased number of intramural glands. *Goblet cells* are frequently seen amongst the bile-duct lining cells, but infrequently in pathological peribiliary glands where *intestinal metaplasia* may include Paneth cells (Fig. 11.6D). Expression of other molecules at the intrahepatic large bile ducts, such as REG I and trefoil factors, appears to be related to intestinal or gastric metaplasia.[32,33] *Squamous metaplasia* is rarely encountered in longstanding inflammation of large bile ducts[34] or in the lining of developmental biliary cysts.

Hyperplasia of septal and large bile ducts manifests as micropapillary projections or as a stratification of the epithelium with or without dilatation of the duct lumen. Intramural and extramural peribiliary glands participate in the process with variable luminal dilatation, a change associated with an increased content of neutral, carboxylated and sulphated mucins. When prominent, in particular with *Clonorchis sinensis* infection, the term adenomatous hyperplasia has been used.[35]

Biliary epithelial dysplasia is characterized by atypical, enlarged and hyperchromatic nuclei, an increased nucleo-cytoplasmic ratio, and a loss of polarity (Fig. 11.7). It is either micropapillary or flat with a portion of the duct circumference being replaced by a single- or multilayered dysplastic epithelium. Low-grade and high-grade dysplasia are seen in association with chronic inflammation, clonorchiasis or deposition of thorotrast, within both large bile ducts and peribiliary glands, and are considered steps in the neoplastic transformation of the biliary epithelium.[36]

Biliary epithelial cell renewal

Homeostasis of the biliary epithelium operates through a balance between apoptotic cell death and cell renewal. This is mainly regulated by the *bcl-2* family of proteins.[37] *Bcl-2*, which prolongs cell survival by counteracting apoptosis, is diffusely expressed by cells of the interlobular bile ducts and ductules, while *bax*, a promoter of apoptosis, is expressed throughout the biliary tree.[38] It has been proposed that a liver stem cell or bipotential progenitor cell residing in the canal of Hering[39] is continuously feeding the biliary tree with new cells (see Chapter 1). The offspring may migrate toward larger branches of the bile ducts and then toward the hepatic hilum. However, this streaming theory[40] remains

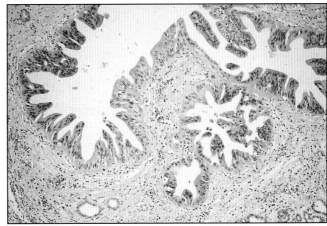

A

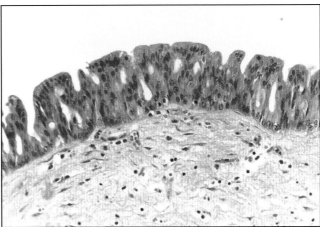

B

Fig. 11.7 • Biliary epithelial dysplasia associated with hepatolithiasis. **(A)** Lining epithelium of a large intrahepatic bile duct shows micropapillary hyperplasia with cellular dysplasia. H & E. **(B)** Close-up of micropapillary hyperplasia with mild dysplasia illustrating nuclear pseudostratification. H & E.

speculative and, in biliary disorders, the contribution of a stem cell compartment to replenish the epithelium of the injured bile ducts remains to be demonstrated. As already mentioned, the conduits of the peribiliary glands may be an additional site of biliary epithelium regeneration. Ductular reaction, a common process associated with intra- and extrahepatic cholestasis, has been re-evaluated recently;[4] it is discussed later on p. 532.

Cholangitis

Cholangitis, or inflammation of the bile ducts with biliary epithelial damage, can be histologically classified into a suppurative and a non-suppurative form.[41] These terms are descriptive and not necessarily related to a specific aetiology.

Suppurative cholangitis implies the presence of numerous polymorphonuclear cells around and within the wall as well as within the lumen of the ducts. This may involve ducts of any size and is occasionally associated with abscess formation—cholangitic abscess (Fig. 11.8A). Microbial infection is often responsible, but the change also occurs in the presence of a sterile bile, in particular after bile extrava-

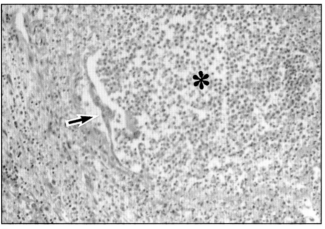

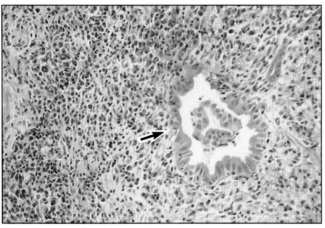

Fig. 11.8 • (A) Suppurative cholangitis with cholangitic abscess (*) and remnants of the bile-duct epithelium (arrow) in a case of bacterial cholangitis. **(B)** Non-suppurative cholangitis showing epithelial damage (arrow) and periductal infiltration of lymphocytes and plasma cells in primary biliary cirrhosis. H & E.

sation where the detergent effect of the bile salts may produce a chemical cholangitis, and in the acutely rejected liver graft (rejection cholangitis) where the release of cytokines is the likely cause.

Non-suppurative cholangitis includes a spectrum of bile-duct inflammation (Fig. 11.8B) which may be granulomatous, lymphoid, or sclerosing according to the predominant type of inflammatory reaction present.

Granulomatous cholangitis of the interlobular bile ducts is usually destructive and constitutes the hallmark of PBC. Similar cholangitis is found in drug-induced liver disease and in sarcoidosis. Non-specific biliary damage with a granulomatous reaction and lymph follicle formation rarely occurs in livers with non-specific biliary strictures and other longstanding biliary disease, in particular PSC.[42] PBC-type granulomatous cholangitis with epithelioid cells forming a mantle around the injured bile duct has to be distinguished from the giant-cell reaction to extravasated bile seen near ruptured ducts, for example in PSC and extrahepatic biliary atresia.[42]

Lymphoid cholangitis refers to a close association between duct branches and lymphocytic aggregates, which may show a follicular arrangement. This is found in PBC and PSC with

concomitant bile-duct destruction, or in non-biliary disorders, in particular autoimmune and viral hepatitis C where progressive bile-duct destruction is generally not a feature.[43,44]

Sclerosing cholangitis (bile-duct fibrosis) develops as a consequence of longstanding bile-duct inflammatory or ischaemic injury; it can be obliterative or non-obliterative. The former is characteristic of PSC, though, in our experience, it may be seen in secondary forms of sclerosing cholangitis. In the fibrotic ducts, there is an aberrant expression of stem cell factor, a ligand for c-kit receptor expressed on mast cells.[45] The bile-duct wall in longstanding sclerosing cholangitis shows a marked increase in the number of mast cells which secrete histamine, basic fibroblast growth factor (bFGF) and/or tumour necrosis factor-alpha (TNFα), all known fibrogenic factors.[45] In the fibrosis which surrounds the interlobular bile ducts and ductules, the biliary epithelium itself produces and secretes fibrogenic substances such as epidermal growth factor (EGF), bFGF, transforming growth factor-beta (TGFβ) and platelet-derived growth factor (PDGF), as well as basement membrane proteins and extracellular matrix proteins laminin and collagen.[46–49] The biliary epithelium also has receptors for EGF, leading to autocrine growth stimulation, and for hepatocyte growth factor (HGF), which is released from the activated portal fibroblasts or adjacent hepatic stellate cells.[50,51]

Biliary apoptosis

The role of apoptosis in bile-duct injury may be underestimated as apoptotic cells are rapidly eliminated from the biliary tree and probably shed into bile.[52] Apoptosis is difficult to identify and quantify accurately in H&E stained sections, but shrunken slender cells with pyknotic nuclei and fragmented and condensed nuclei in the biliary epithelial layer and bile-duct lumen are regarded as apoptotic bodies[52] (Fig. 11.9A). This can be confirmed using in situ nick-end labelling which detects DNA fragmentation[53] (Fig. 11.9B). Ultrastructurally, there is a reduction of cell volume, increased density, and aggregation of cytoplasmic organelles.[53,54]

Biliary apoptosis has been considered as an important pathogenetic process in several cholangiopathies.[55,56] An excessive apoptotic activity that exceeds the proliferative response of bile-duct cells will result in ductopenia. In contrast, inhibition of the apoptotic process may cause hyperplasia of bile-duct epithelium[56] with an increased risk of neoplastic transformation.[57]

Bile-duct loss or ductopenia

Ductopenia is defined as an absence of identifiable bile ducts from the portal tract. When severe inflammation is present, the duct may be obscured by numerous inflammatory cells and immunostaining for cytokeratins 19 or 7 may assist their identification.

Within portal tracts, hepatic arterial branches and interlobular bile ducts of similar size run parallel. This parallelism is useful to appreciate the size of affected ducts and the

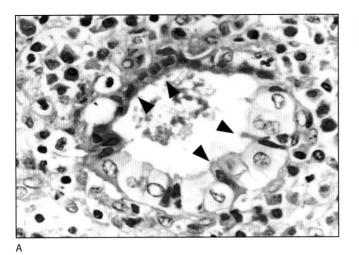

A

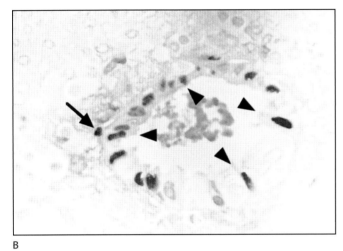

B

Fig. 11.9 • Apoptosis of interlobular bile-duct cells (arrowheads) in florid lesion of primary biliary cirrhosis shown in consecutive sections stained with H & E **(A)** and TUNEL method **(B).** Note TUNEL-positive lymphocytes around the bile duct (arrow).

Table 11.2	Diseases associated with ductopenia (vanishing bile duct syndrome)
Primary biliary cirrhosis	
Primary sclerosing cholangitis	
Severe acute and chronic hepatic allograft rejection	
Chronic graft-versus-host disease (GVHD)	
Secondary sclerosing cholangitis (ischaemic cholangitis)	

Infantile and childhood diseases (Chs 4 and 5)
    Syndromatic paucity of interlobular bile ducts
    Non-syndromatic paucity of interlobular bile ducts
    Progressive familial intrahepatic cholestasis (some cases)
    Extrahepatic biliary atresia (extension to intrahepatic ducts)	

Drug or toxin-induced biliary injury[61]	
Idiopathic adulthood ductopenia[60]	
Hepatic sarcoidosis[62]	
Hodgkin disease (usually post-treatment)[63]	

degree of bile-duct loss.[23,58] The proportion of portal tracts without identifiable bile ducts is of practical use to estimate bile-duct loss. Ten or more portal tracts in a liver specimen are usually considered adequate and ductopenia is typically defined as the absence of interlobular bile ducts in at least 50% of the portal tracts.[59]

Vanishing bile-duct syndrome (VBDS)

Vanishing bile-duct syndrome defines a clinicopathological complex in which chronic cholestasis is associated with a progressive loss of the intrahepatic bile ducts or ductopenia.[60] A heterogeneous group of conditions have been, to a variable extent, associated with the VBDS.[61–63] They are summarized in Table 11.2, and will be discussed in detail later in the chapter. Immune processes, infections, drugs and/or ischaemia have been incriminated as causes of the bile-duct destruction which may be achieved within months or develop over many years. In this respect one can distinguish an acute or subacute form evolving over months, in which ductular reaction and portal fibrosis are inconspicuous, and features of acute rather than chronic cholestasis dominate the picture; this is exemplified by the ductopenia

observed in allograft rejection,[64] severe graft-versus-host disease (GVHD),[65] with some drugs[66] and in treated Hodgkin disease.[63] In contrast, progressive disappearance of the bile ducts may evolve over one or two decades accompanied by the changes of chronic cholestasis, portoseptal fibrosis and eventually a biliary cirrhosis; this is the pattern characteristic of PBC, sclerosing cholangitides, and occasionally sarcoidosis[62] and drugs. The interlobular bile ducts and bile ductules are mainly affected in PBC, GVHD, hepatic allograft rejection and drug-induced ductopenia, whereas ductopenia generally follows the involvement of septal and large intrahepatic bile ducts in PSC and in extrahepatic biliary atresia in children.

Recovery from VBDS has been observed, in particular in the liver allograft or after drug toxicity. In that situation regrowth of the bile ducts is preceded by marginal ductular reaction. Hepatic stem cells or progenitor cells presumably migrating from the periportal areas into the biliary channels may be involved in the process.[67]

Immune-mediated cholangitis

Primary biliary cirrhosis, PSC, GVHD, and hepatic allograft rejection are examples of autoimmune or alloimmune mediated cholangiopathy.[2] The level and extent of the biliary tree affected differs across and within individual diseases. The peribiliary glands are involved in PSC[68] and in GVHD.[69] Immunologically mediated events are evidenced by the accumulation of activated auto- or alloreactive T-lymphocytes at the site of bile-duct destruction.[70] There is a mixture of immunocompetent cells, particularly CD3+, CD4+ and CD8+ T-cells that bear the T-cell receptor α/β.[70,71] This supports T-cell cytotoxicity and/or cytokine release in the pathogenesis of the bile-duct lesion; but a humoral immune mechanism may also contribute. The proportion of CD4+

and CD8+ T-cells does, however, differ according to individual diseases or stage of development.[72,73]

Target antigens

The immune process is targeted against allo- or autoantigens that may be normally or aberrantly expressed in the biliary epithelium, or absorbed from the bile. Some may be related to major histocompatibility complex (MHC) substances, while others may be exogenous substances such as bacteria or viruses, which bear a molecular mimicry for biliary epithelial cell components.[74,75]

The alloimmune response preferentially affects the small interlobular bile ducts.[76] In hepatic rejection, the recipient's immune response is directed against allogeneic antigens (peptide antigens presented by allogeneic MHC or allogeneic MHC themselves) on the donor bile ducts.[2] In GVHD, MHC related antigens induced on the biliary epithelial cells by locally released cytokines or viral infections are targeted by grafted lymphoid cells.[2] Antimitochondrial antibodies (AMA) are detected against antigens such as pyruvate dehydrogenase E2-subunit (PDC-E2),[77,78] and biliary epithelial antigen in PBC.[79] In PSC, cross-reactive peptides shared by biliary and colonic epithelium have been proposed as possible targets.[80]

Additional antigens that may initiate or aggravate the immune reaction include heat shock protein,[81,82] and bacterial antigens.[83,84] Increased expression of both heat shock protein-60[85] and lipid A, a constituent of endotoxin,[84] have been demonstrated in the biliary epithelium in PBC and PSC, but heat shock protein expression may be a nonspecific feature of chronic cholestasis.[85] In addition, the biliary epithelial cells contain many antigenic substances such as blood-group related antigens and carbonic anhydrase II, against which autoantibodies have been detected in sera of patients with immune-mediated cholangitis.[86,87]

Antigen presentation and recognition

Two kinds of antigen presenting cells (APC), professional APC and biliary epithelial cells, are potentially involved in immune-mediated cholangitis.[88] Professional APC, especially dendritic cells and to a lesser degree macrophages, are the most important regulators of initial T-cell activation.[89,90] Dendritic cells that express B7, human lymphocyte antigen (HLA)-class II and S100 molecules are observed around and occasionally within the epithelial layer of damaged bile ducts[89–91] (Fig. 11.10). At least two molecules, B7–1 and B7–2, work as costimulatory ligands for CD28 expressed on surrounding T-cells.[92,93] Focal staining for B7–2[90,92] on bile-duct cells that aberrantly express MCH-class II[94,95] suggests that the biliary epithelium may present self antigens to surrounding helper T-cells.[88,94,96]

T helper 1 (Th1) and T helper 2 (Th2) balance and cytokine networks

Along with the breakdown of self-tolerance, the relative strength of Th1 and Th2 responses and the resultant cyto-

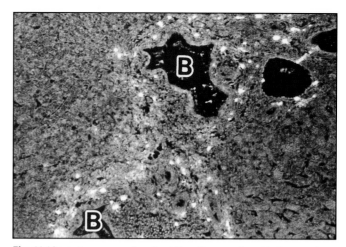

Fig. 11.10 • Antigen-presenting dendritic cells are scattered in the portal area with some accentuation in the vicinity of the bile ducts in primary biliary cirrhosis. Immunostaining for costimulatory factor B7–2 demonstrated with confocal laser microscopy. B = bile duct; white spots indicate positive staining.

kine milieu are determinants for the continuation of bile-duct damage.[76,97–100] In PBC, PSC and liver allograft rejection, there is a predominance of Th1 subsets which produce interleukin (IL)-2 and interferon-gamma (INFγ), and stimulate both the proliferation of cytotoxic T-lymphocytes,[98] and the local production of INFγ and TNFα. The latter are known to induce and up-regulate expression of MHC class I, MHC class II and adhesion molecules on biliary epithelial cells.[76,99] The detection of mRNA for IL-5, IL-6 and transforming growth factor-β (TGFβ) in the majority of cases of immune-mediated cholangitis,[99] and of Th2 type (IL-10) cytokine, particularly in PBC,[100] suggest that antibody production by B-lymphocytes is also involved.

Altered portal microenvironments and expression of immune molecules on bile ducts

The inflammatory microenvironment associated with T-cell activation and proliferation, and the secretion of cytokines, particularly INFγ, TNFα and chemokines, induce and up-regulate the bile-duct expression of MHC class II (HLA-DR, DP, DQ) (Fig. 11.11A, B),[2,101–103] intercellular adhesion molecule-1 (ICAM-1), lymphocyte-associated antigen (LFA)-3, and vascular adhesion molecule-1 (VCAM)-1 (Fig. 11.11C, D). In addition, constitutive surface immune-molecules such as MHC class I and very late antigen (VLA)-2, -3 and -6 are expressed on biliary epithelial cells.[76,102] Induction and up-regulation of immune molecules also occurs on the nearby microvasculature which leads to recruitment of more inflammatory cells. Immune molecules serve as ligands or receptors for inflammatory cells and matrix proteins. These changes facilitate various aspects of the immune reaction around the bile ducts, such as cell positioning or adhesion, antigen presentation, costimulatory signalling and the activation of antigen-specific CD4+ T-cells.

Cytokines, chemokines, and their receptors, which are produced and expressed by multiple cell types around the damaged bile ducts as well as by biliary cells themselves, are central to the progression of the bile-duct lesion in

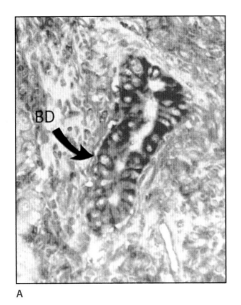

A

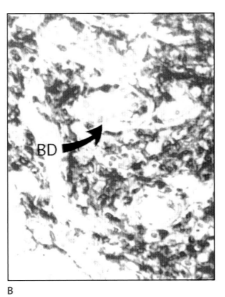

B

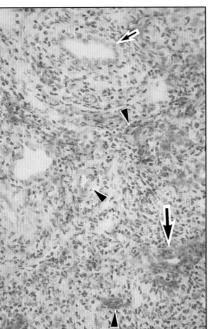

C

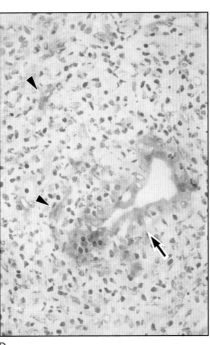

D

Fig. 11.11 • **(A)** Strong HLA-DR staining on an injured bile duct (curved arrow) in primary biliary cirrhosis. **(B)** Absence of HLA-DR expression on injured bile duct (curved arrow) in chronic hepatitis C; the surrounding lymphoid cells are positive. **(C)** Primary biliary cirrhosis; intercellular adhesion molecule-1 (ICAM-1) is expressed on some bile ducts (large arrow) and also small vessels (arrowheads), while another duct is negative (small arrow). **(D)** Same case as (C) showing expression of vascular adhesion molecule-1 (VCAM-1) on an injured interlobular bile duct (arrow) and also on small vessels (arrowheads). Immunostaining with appropriate antibody, (A) and (B) coloured with Vecta-Red.

immune cholangitides,[104] but a triggering event that damages biliary epithelial cells or changes the inflammatory micro-environments of the portal tract is required to start the process in genetically susceptible individuals.[22,105,106]

Recruitment of inflammatory cells and epitheliotropism

The leukocytes, which accumulate around the bile ducts, migrate from the peribiliary vascular plexus[107] whose constituent capillaries strongly express chemokine-induced adhesion molecules—ICAM-1, VCAM-1, and ELAM-1 (E-selectin).[108] These are involved in the extravasation and localization of inflammatory cells.[109,110] The latter express integrins, LFA-1 and VLA-4 which are essential for their migration out of the blood vessels.[111,112] Angiogenesis may contribute to the vascular network around bile ducts follow-

ing injury, driven by enhanced expression of vascular endo-thelial growth factor (VEGF) and angiopoietins 1 and 2.[113]

Following migration, the immunocompetent cells have to penetrate into the bile duct epithelium—*epitheliotropism* (Fig. 11.12A). The presence on duct basement membranes of binding sites for lymphocyte receptors,[108] and the up-regulation of integrins and other adhesion molecules, facilitate the process.[114,115] Surface expression of ICAM-1, LFA-3, and VCAM-1 on bile-duct cells[76,98] suggests linkages between damaged bile ducts and lymphocytes which secure antigen presentation to periductal lymphocytes and trigger effector mechanisms. Point and broad contacts between infiltrating lymphocytes and both biliary epithelial cells and extracel-lular matrix are demonstrated ultrastructurally.[54] Such interactions appear to involve binding of CX3CR1 to frac-talkine, the latter being up-regulated in injured bile-duct epithelium.[116]

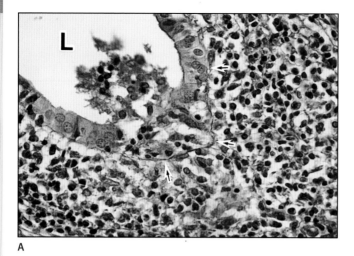

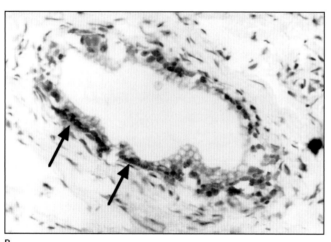

Fig. 11.12 • (A) Lymphoid cells penetrating the biliary epithelial layer through the basement membrane (arrows). Note also biliary epithelial and lymphoid cells sloughing into the bile duct lumen (L). PAS after diastase. **(B)** Membranous expression of Fas receptor (arrows) on the bile duct in primary biliary cirrhosis. Immunostaining for FasR.

Effector mechanisms

Several effector mechanisms have been proposed for the immune-mediated bile-duct damage, but autoreactive or alloreactive T-cells, particularly cytotoxic T-lymphocytes, probably play the major role in causing epithelial cell death.[99,117-120]

Apoptosis and T-cell mediated cytotoxicity

Apoptosis is considered a major mode of cell death.[55,118] In PBC and allograft rejection, a relatively insufficient proliferative response will result in the progressive loss of bile ducts due to apoptosis.[121,122] The initiation of apoptosis may occur through different, yet interrelated mechanisms:

(a) Direct cytotoxicity by CD4+ and CD8+ T-cells,[76] the former mainly dependent on the Fas/Fas ligand (FasL) interaction[123,124] while the latter rely on the perforin–granzyme exocytosis pathway.[99,125] Most cytotoxic lymphocytes in allograft rejection are MHC class I-restricted CD8+ T-cells,[76] while CD4+ cells belonging mainly to the Th1-subset predominate in PBC and PSC.[125-128]

(b) Activation of the Fas receptor (FasR)/FasL system is the best-studied model of apoptosis.[127] In PBC, PSC and allograft rejection, FasR is strongly expressed on the damaged bile-duct cells (Fig. 11.12B) which are surrounded or infiltrated by FasL-expressing cytotoxic T-cells of Th1 subset.[122,124] The exact stimuli for FasR expression on the bile-duct epithelium may vary with individual diseases.

(c) Induction of cytokines TNFα and INFγ. The occurrence of apoptotic cell death through this system is supported by expression of both mRNA and protein for the TNFα and TNFα receptor on damaged biliary epithelial cells.[55,104]

Autoantibody-mediated injury

Serum autoantibodies are detected in PBC and PSC, but there is only weak evidence that AMA or centromere type antinuclear antibodies (ANA) in PBC and ANA or p-antineutrophil cytoplasmic antibodies (pANCA) in PSC have a pathogenic role. IgA- and IgM-class AMA which are secreted through the biliary epithelial cytoplasm via the secretory component (SC)-mediated transport could injure mitochondria.[129] A majority of the plasma cells infiltrating the portal tracts in PBC secrete AMA of IgG, IgA and IgM classes,[130,131] and these antibodies may be involved in antibody-dependent cell-mediated cytotoxicity. The CD20+ B-cells and immunoglobulin-positive cells which are detected in the portal areas may result from a proliferation of auto-reactive B-cells stimulated by CD4+ T cells of Th2 subset.[132,133] Immunoglobulins and complement components on the surface of biliary epithelial may recognize antigens on the biliary epithelium, and provoke an antibody-mediated attack by IgA and IgG antibodies present in bile.[134] The recent demonstration of selective caspase activation by dimeric IgA with specificity for the PDC-E2 component of AMA in an in vitro cell line transfected with human polymeric immunoglobulin receptor adds strong support to a pathogenetic role of AMA in bile-duct injury of PBC.[135]

In liver allograft rejection and GVHD, preformed anti-donor MHC class I antibodies and antibodies directed against major ABO blood group antigens, which are normally expressed on the biliary epithelium, may be responsible for antibody binding and complement fixing damage.[136]

Other mechanisms

In acute liver allograft and to a lesser degree in PBC and PSC at early stages, there is a marked eosinophil infiltration of portal tracts with widespread deposition of eosinophil cationic protein granules that are known to be cytotoxic for bile ducts.[137-139] Blood eosinophilia may be associated with this infiltrate. Eosinophils are correlated with an up-regulation of eosinophil chemotactic factor IL-5.[140]

Oxidative stress generated in biliary epithelial cells themselves and also by inflammatory cells around and within the bile-duct epithelium may be responsible for biliary epithelial apoptosis in PBC and allograft rejection.[141,142] In PBC and allograft rejection, the interlobular bile ducts frequently show cytoplasmic eosinophilia, cellular and nuclear enlargement, and irregular arrangement with uneven nuclear spacing (Fig. 11.13A). Some biliary epithelial cells are multinucleated and frequently express senescence-associated-β-galactosidase, suggesting the occurrence of senescence and impaired regeneration of bile-duct cells (Fig.11.13B).[24,143]

Predisposing and augmenting factors

Genetic background
There is good evidence that genetically determined abnormalities of immunoregulation play a role in the development of bile-duct damage in PBC and PSC, although an association with certain HLA haplotype(s) is not always evident.[144] Genetic factors in addition to HLA disparity are also likely determinants of whether individuals will be strong or weak rejectors after liver grafting, but none have been specifically identified except for non-Caucasian recipients being at an increased risk for graft rejection.[2]

Infections
Bacterial or viral infections may play a primary or secondary role in the progression of immune-mediated bile-duct injury. Bacteria, particularly enterobacteria, may be involved in the progression of PBC, PSC and hepatolithiasis.[12,145-149] Bacterial or viral infections may aggravate or initiate the alloimmune-mediated bile-duct lesions in GVHD[150] and hepatic allograft rejection.[151] Cytomegalovirus (CMV) infection has been shown to increase the risk of ductopenic rejection,[151,152] although there remains doubt as to the pathogenetic role of CMV.[153] Hepatitis C infection and treatment with INFα may predispose to the development of ductopenic rejection after orthotopic liver transplantation.[154]

Hydrophobic bile acids
Normally, the biliary epithelium is protected against the detergent effects of bile acids by phospholipids, resulting from the incorporation of the bile acids into mixed micelles with phospholipids and cholesterol. The detergent power of bile acids increases with increasing relative hydrophobicity of bile acids.[155] Endogenous hydrophobic bile acids may enhance the bile-duct lesion by dissolving membrane lipids or stripping key hydrophobic proteins off the outer layer of the apical membrane of biliary epithelial cells and by promoting apoptosis.[156,157]

Ischaemic bile-duct injury

The peribiliary vascular plexus is essentially supplied by branches of the hepatic artery which makes the bile ducts, unlike the parenchyma, particularly vulnerable to any interference with arterial flow. The small constituent vessels are well demonstrated by immunostaining for CD34 or factor VIII-related substance (Fig. 11.14A). They form a three-layer plexus around the extrahepatic, large intrahepatic and septal bile-ducts,[107] the small portal vein branches

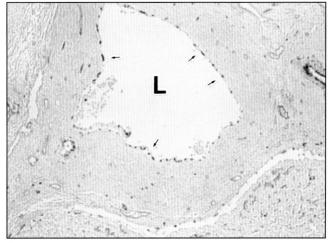

A

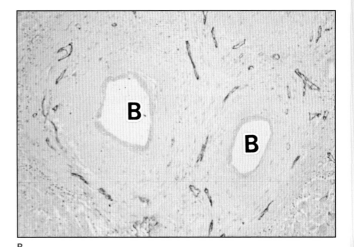

B

Fig. 11.14 • Peribiliary vascular plexus around normal and diseased bile duct. **(A)** Normal septal bile duct (L, lumen) showing a chain-like capillary network (inner layer) (arrows) beneath the lining epithelium and several small vessels within and around the wall (middle and outer layer). **(B)** Autopsy liver after transarterial embolization therapy. The inner layer of the plexus is lost, while the vessels around the bile duct (B) (outer layer) remain. Immunohistochemistry for *Ulex europaeus* agglutinin (UEA-1).

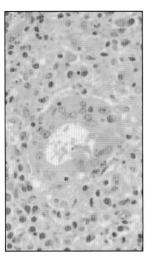

A

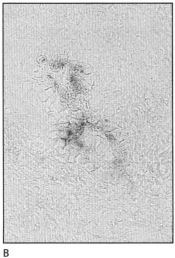

B

Fig. 11.13 • Primary biliary cirrhosis. **(A)** Biliary epithelial cells of an interlobular bile duct show cytoplasmic eosinophilia, ansocytosis and uneven spacing of focally crowded nuclei. H & E. **(B)** Senescence-associated-β-galactosidase activity is detected as a blue reaction using the senescence detection kit (BioVision, Mountain View, CA).

and small arteries around the bile ducts (peribiliary arteries), being included in the outer layer. This organization becomes less evident around the interlobular bile duct and ductules[107] which nevertheless remain entirely dependent on arterial blood.

Primary and secondary damage to the hepatic arterial branches or to the plexus itself, whether due to thrombotic occlusion, foam cell arteriopathy and/or vasculitis, may lead to ischaemic cholangitis.[158,159] This may take the form of biliary epithelial damage, cholangitis without necrosis and bile-duct fibrosis. Erosion, focal necrosis or infarction of bile ducts and extravasation of bile (biloma) may ensue.[160] Ductopenia, biliary stricture and cholangiectasis are common complications with infection often developing in the devascularized tissue. The biliary tree in allografts is particularly susceptible to ischaemia because of a lack of vascular collaterals in the early post-transplant period.[158] In this situation, both thrombotic occlusion and rejection-related arteriopathy may contribute to ischaemic bile-duct damage and loss (see also Chapter 16).

Transcatheter arterial embolization and intra-arterial infusion chemotherapy have been followed by a form of sclerosing cholangitis, often associated with thrombotic occlusion and/or considerable reduction or even absence of the peribiliary plexus (Fig. 11.14B). Irradiation-induced bile-duct injury is also associated with sclerosing and obliterative arterial changes;[161] a sclerosing cholangitis with stricture may follow.[162,163]

In all forms of sclerosing cholangitis, a marked attenuation of the peribiliary vascular plexus is seen within the sclerotic duct wall, but it remains uncertain whether these changes are secondary to, or responsible for, the bile-duct fibrosis.[164] Necrotizing arteritis (polyarteritis nodosa) of hepatic arterial branches is a rare cause of ischaemic bile-duct injury.[165]

Pathological features secondary to impaired bile flow

Cholestasis

The complex mechanisms of bile secretion have been described in detail in Chapters 1 and 2. Cholestasis denotes a defect in bile secretory mechanisms leading to an accumulation in the blood of substances normally excreted in the bile—*biochemical cholestasis*. This is often, but not invariably, associated with deposition of bile in the biliary passages which can be visualized microscopically—*morphological cholestasis*.[166] Mechanical or obstructive cholestasis usually refers to lesions of the extrahepatic biliary tract (extrahepatic cholestasis), but is occasionally produced by intrahepatic processes which cause jaundice only when the flow is compromised in the majority of the intrahepatic biliary passages, as for instance in the late stage of PBC. Although mechanical obstruction thus clearly contributes to cholestasis originating within the anatomical confines of the liver, that is intrahepatic, the term 'intrahepatic cholestasis' is used by most authors to indicate cholestatic syndromes

without demonstrable mechanical obstruction. Such functional intrahepatic cholestasis is common to a number of parenchymal injuries of various aetiologies when complex metabolic alterations at the level of the hepatocyte produce an abnormally thick bile which becomes inspissated in the canaliculi, first and predominantly in the perivenular region.

There may be a striking discrepancy between morphological and clinical cholestasis. Conditions which are clinically cholestatic and considered as primarily biliary diseases may progress without evident bilirubinostasis on biopsy. This is mainly the case in partial obstruction of the biliary passages, for instance, obstruction of one hepatic duct or narrowing of several duct segments in the early stages of PBC and PSC. In this situation, the patient experiences pruritus and there are biochemical signs of cholestasis, such as raised serum alkaline phosphatase, γ-glutamyl transpeptidase (γ-GT), cholesterol and bile acids, whereas the level of conjugated bilirubin remains normal or is only marginally raised and remains so until the disease is very advanced. Morphologically, this pre-icteric phase is characterized by profound changes at the portal or portoseptal interface: *biliary interface activity*, which is discussed in the second part of this section.

Morphology of cholestasis

Microscopically, cholestasis of any aetiology is characterized by an exclusively or predominantly perivenular localization of bilirubin deposition in hepatocytes, inspissated bile in dilated canaliculi and a variable degree of bile regurgitation into the perisinusoidal space with phagocytosis by Kupffer cells (Fig. 11.15A, B) (see also Chapter 2); it may be more correctly described as 'bilirubinostasis', though products other than the bilirubin are concomitantly retained, yet not readily visualized microscopically. In severe cholestasis or in cholestasis of longer duration, such pigment deposition may extend to the periportal region and cholestatic or biliary liver-cell rosettes may develop. These are particularly common in children and consist of dilated canaliculi surrounded by more than two hepatocytes in a pseudotubular arrangement (Fig. 11.16A). The rosettes express some biliary cytokeratins (Fig 11.16B) and by three-dimensional reconstruction they are found to communicate with bile ducts and ductules.[167] The predominantly perivenular localization of bilirubinostasis may be explained by both the lower oxygen tension in the perivenular region and the fact that bile acid secretion and corresponding bile water flow are assured by mechanisms different from those responsible for bilirubin secretion.[168] Since the periportal zone is the main contributor to 'bile-acid-dependent' bile flow, the canaliculi of the perivenular zones are perfused with a smaller amount of fluid which is generated by mechanisms progressively independent of bile acids as one approaches the hepatic venule. Such zonal differences predispose to a primarily perivenular distribution of canalicular precipitates during cholestasis of any cause.[168]

In addition to bilirubinostasis, cholestasis is associated with changes in staining patterns of various enzymes. In

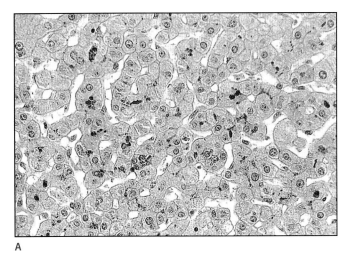

A

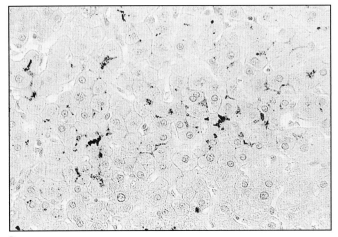

B

Fig. 11.15 • Perivenular cholestasis in early large-duct obstruction. There is marked bilirubinostasis with bile plugging of dilated canaliculi. **(A)** H & E. **(B)** Hall's bilirubin stain.

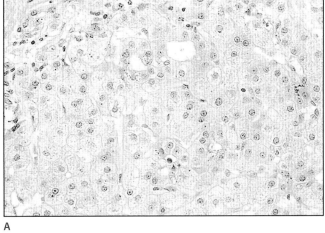

A

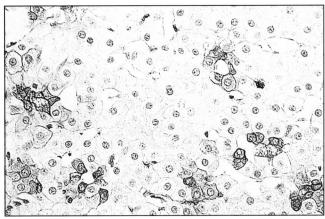

B

Fig. 11.16 • Liver parenchyma in chronic bile-duct obstruction, revealing tubular arrangement of hepatocytes (cholestatic liver-cell rosettes). **(A)** H & E. **(B)** Cytokeratin 7 immunostaining.

particular, the basolateral membrane of the hepatocyte acquires microvilli that show a positive reaction for Mg^{++}-ATPase whereas this has disappeared in the canalicular membrane. The pattern suggests a reverse secretory polarity which has been confirmed by the demonstration of the canalicular bile-salt export carrier on the basolateral membrane. The latter also shows a striking increase in histochemically demonstrable serum alkaline phosphatase and γ-GT,[169] possibly due to a high local concentration in detergent bile acids causing release of these enzymes from the liver cell membrane.[166]

Electron microscopically (Figs 11.17 and 11.18)[166] cholestasis is recognized by a typical pattern of changes in and around the canaliculi, even in the absence of any visible bile pigment accumulation on light microscopy. The canaliculi are variably dilated with a loss of microvilli and their lumen may be filled with electron-dense material representing bile concretions, but the tight junctions are preserved; the pericanalicular ectoplasm is thickened and the hepatocytes show dilated endoplasmic reticulum with the presence of vacuoles containing whorled membranous material and lipofuscin inclusions. Mitochondria exhibit curled or circular cristae.

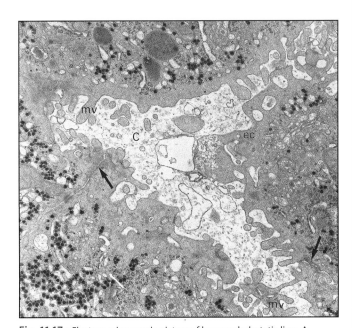

Fig. 11.17 • Electron microscopic picture of human cholestatic liver. A canaliculus (C) is dilated and shows loss of microvilli as well as irregular and plump microvilli (mv); the pericanalicular ectoplasm (ec) is thickened; tight junctions are preserved (arrow). Original magnification: ×23 000. Courtesy of Professor R. de Vos.

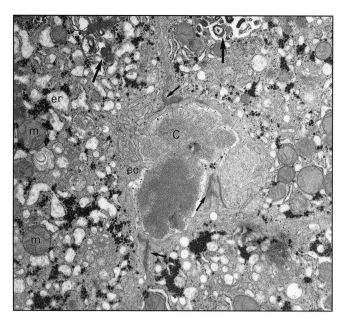

Fig. 11.18 • Electron microscopy picture of human cholestatic liver. In the centre of the picture, a dilated canaliculus (c) is seen filled with variably electron-dense material (bile concretion). Microvilli have largely disappeared. The pericanalicular ectoplasm (ec) is thickened; tight junctions (small arrow) are preserved. The hepatocytes show dilatation of the endoplasmic reticulum (er), focal cytoplasmic degeneration and bile pigment (arrow) and mitochondria with curled cristae (m). Original magnification: ×18 400. Courtesy of Professor R de Vos.

Biliary interface activity

Biliary interface activity, previously known as biliary piece-meal necrosis,[170] refers to a disruption of the parenchymal limiting plates by a complex process which includes cholate stasis, ductular reaction and fibroplasia in variable combinations (Figs 11.19A–D and 11.20A–C). The recognition of biliary interface activity is important as, in the absence of cholestasis and of characteristic bile-duct injury, it is the main clue to diagnosing a primarily biliary disorder. The two main components—cholate stasis and ductular reaction—are discussed separately as either of them may dominate the picture and evolve distinctively, which may reflect the severity and duration of interference with bile flow, or at times maybe for no obvious reason. Fibrosis invariably develops when cholate stasis and ductular reaction persist.

Cholate stasis

The term cholate stasis acknowledges the fact that the cytological alterations are thought to be caused by the intracellular detergent action of retained bile acids[171] (see also Chapter 2). Periportal hepatocytes are preferentially affected as they are the site of maximal bile acid transport in the normal liver.[171] The hepatocytes are swollen and rounded with a distinct border and a clear cytoplasm which may contain web-like membranous and perinuclear granular remnants (Fig. 11.19A). They often contain copper and its binding protein, a polymerized form of metallothionein, which accumulates in lysosomes where it is readily demonstrated as black/brown granules by Shikata orcein stain.[172] This indirect method, unlike the rhodanine stain for copper,

is not influenced by fixation;[173] it is therefore a useful diagnostic tool since, at an early stage, in the absence of bilirubinostasis, the demonstration of orcein-positive granules in the periportal regions is a good indicator of a chronic biliary process (Fig. 11.19B).[174] Similarly, expression by periportal hepatocytes of biliary cytokeratin 7 and 19 is an early marker of cholate stasis.[175] As the lesion progresses, the thread-like reticular cytoplasm—*feathery degeneration*—acquires a greenish-brown tinge from impregnation with bilirubin, and bile pigment may later accumulate (Fig. 11.19C). During the process, there is cytoskeletal injury, which often results in the formation of Mallory bodies (Fig. 11.19D).[176] This is thought to be due to a toxic effect of bile acids, and possibly copper, on the microtubules with consequent aggregation of intermediate microfilament proteins. Mallory bodies in chronic cholestasis are identical morphologically and chemically to those observed in alcoholic liver disease,[177] but differ in their perilobular rather than centrilobular location.

Ductular reaction and fibroplasia

The small intralobular bile ducts, ductules and canals of Hering have the property of increasing in number in many forms of liver disease, especially in cholestasis. The ductules are accompanied by an inflammatory infiltrate and by fibrosis, the composite picture referred to as ductular reaction (Fig. 11.20).[4] Their origin is still a matter of debate. The neoductules, lined by cuboidal or flattened cells, seem, in longstanding cholestasis, to arise from 'ductular metaplasia' of periportal hepatocytes[4,56] and to a lesser extent from a proliferation of pre-existing ductules, although the relative role of these two mechanisms may vary depending on the degree of biliary obstruction[178] or the duration of cholestasis.[179] A shift from the hepatocellular to the biliary cell phenotype can be demonstrated for cytokeratins[4,180] (Fig. 11.20D), blood group antigens,[181] chromogranin[182] and 'bile-duct type' integrins VLA-2, -3 and -6.[183] The mechanism inducing ductular metaplasia of periportal hepatocytes appears to be complex, involving pericellular matrix components,[184,185] possibly bile salts,[186] hepatic stellate cells[56] and various humoral and neural factors.[187,188] A contribution of bone marrow-derived progenitor or stem cells to the ductular reaction remains speculative in the human liver.

Reactive ductular cells contain dense-core neuroendocrine-type granules and express chromogranin, neural cell adhesion molecule (NCAM)[189] and parathyroid hormone-like peptide,[190] a factor which modulates cellular growth and differentiation. These findings led to speculation that reactive ductular cells may produce a substance that exerts an autocrine or paracrine regulatory role on the growth of ductules or in the ductular metaplasia of periportal hepatocytes.[171,191] In the setting of primary cholangiopathies, reactive ductules coexpress NCAM and bcl-2, suggesting a histogenesis which recapitulates the early stages of biliary ontogenesis.[192]

The role of the ductular reaction is incompletely understood. The ductules may provide abortive bypass mechanisms for the drainage of bile in diseases associated with

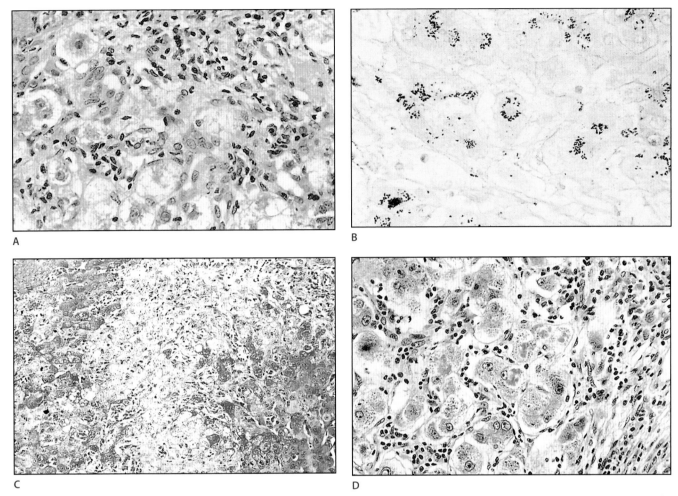

Fig. 11.19 • Biliary interface activity in primary biliary cirrhosis. **(A)** Cholate stasis: distended and rounded hepatocytes with a clear cytoplasm containing web-like eosinophilic remnants are intermingled with ductular epithelium. H & E. **(B)** The hepatocytes contain orcein-positive copper-associated protein. Shikata orcein. **(C)** Later stage with an extensive accumulation of feathery cells, some of which are hepatocytes and others macrophages. PAS. **(D)** Cholestatic phase with accumulation of bilirubin pigment and formation of Mallory bodies. H & E.

destruction of interlobular bile ducts, such as PBC.[193] The ductular cells reabsorb bile acids[194] and may thus protect the hepatocytes from the deleterious effect of bile acid overload. Reabsorption with leakage of bile components leads to a marked inflammatory reaction, which consists mainly of polymorphonuclear leukocytes closely associated with the reactive ductules in the oedematous fibrous matrix at the portal periphery (Fig. 11.20C). These morphological features of acute cholangiolitis represent a tissue reaction to irritant chemical stimuli rather than a true bacterial infection.[195]

Ductular reaction and the accompanying inflammatory reaction play an important role in portal and periportal fibroplasia.[196] The ductules produce and secrete a variety of biologically active materials such as cytokines and chemokines including TNF-α, IL-6, IL-8, monocyte chemotactic protein-1 (MCP-1) and nitric oxide (NO), and also express aberrant NCAM,[192] which underpin their potential role in the inflammatory reaction and concomitant fibrogenesis. Surrounded by a PAS-positive basement membrane the neoductules are invariably set in a loose connective tissue matrix deposition which contains type IV collagen and laminin, in part synthesized by the ductular cells them-

selves.[47] Fibroplasia is also due to stimulation of mesenchymal cells. Reactive ductules express growth factors, such as human growth factor (HGF), connective tissue growth factor (CTGF), transforming growth factor-β2 (TGF-β2) and platelet-derived growth factor (PDGF),[47,197,198] which activate mesenchymal cells and matrix production. Intimately associated with the ductules are myofibroblasts and transitional cells between hepatic stellate cells and myofibroblasts expressing smooth muscle actin and desmin.[56,199,200] They are responsible for the production of tenascin in the early stage of ductular reaction,[201,202] followed later on by deposition of type VI collagen,[203] matrix components, and interstitial collagen types I, III and V.[204]

In this way, the ductular reaction is a pacemaker for the development of progressive fibrosis in chronic cholestatic liver disease, eventually resulting in biliary cirrhosis and the associated haemodynamic alterations.[191] It is of interest that in the two chronic cholestatic disorders, paucity of the intrahepatic bile ducts (Alagille syndrome) and chronic liver allograft rejection, in which ductular reaction is essentially absent, periportal fibrosis is similarly inconspicuous. The ductular reaction and periductular fibrosis is reversible in the early stage. Following removal of the proliferative

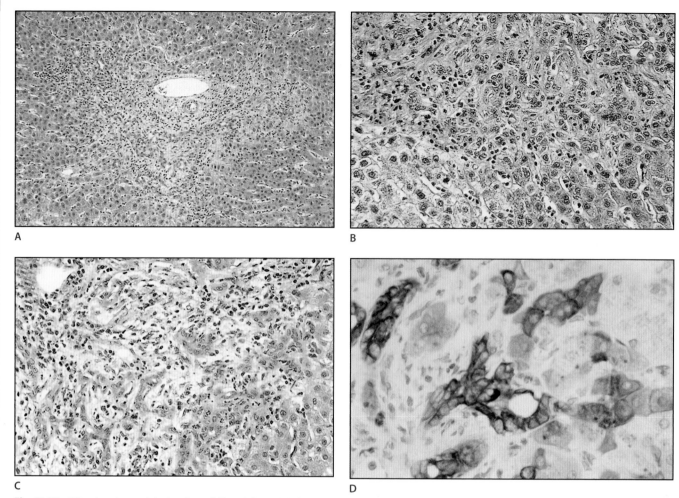

Fig. 11.20 • Biliary interface activity in primary biliary cirrhosis. **(A)** There is no bile duct in the portal tract; the periportal parenchyma is disturbed due to loose connective tissue containing a mixed inflammatory cell infiltrate in the liver cell plates **(B)**, some of which show a tubular transformation. (A) H & E; (B) Masson trichrome. **(C)** Ductular proliferation is more marked in this case and closely associated with a predominantly neutrophil infiltrate. H & E. **(D)** Both ductules and periportal hepatocytes express bile duct cytokeratin 7. Immunostaining for cytokeratin 7.

stimulus (e.g. after relief of bile-duct obstruction) the excess ductular cells are deleted by apoptosis.[205] Regression of the ductular reaction is accompanied by regression of the periductular fibrosis.[206]

Biliary fibrosis/cirrhosis

In chronic large-duct obstruction and intrahepatic bile-duct loss, biliary interface activity and fibroplasia steadily progress. The limiting plates become irregular with separation of hepatocytes by deposition of loose fibrous tissue which contrasts sharply with the compact collagen of the original portal tract or, later, of the central core of the fibrous septa (Fig. 11.21A). Hepatocytes manifesting cholate stasis become intermingled with smaller hepatocytes having a darker staining cytoplasm which acquire phenotypic characteristics of duct cells, in particular the expression of cytokeratin 7 and 19;[175] these merge imperceptibly with the reactive neoductules. The associated inflammatory infiltrate is usually less dense and of different cellular composition from that observed at the interface in autoimmune hepatitis (see Chapter 10);[170] neutrophils predominate and there is a variable accumulation of cholesterol/lipid-laden macro-

phages with a foamy or microvesicular appearance—xanthomatous cells (Fig. 11.19C). They may at times be difficult to distinguish from hepatocytes showing cholate stasis on H & E stained sections.

Progressive fibrosis in the periportal zone produces gradual enlargement of the portal tracts followed by the formation of fibrous septa bridging adjacent portal tracts and eventually the development of a micronodular cirrhosis with parenchymal regeneration and distortion. Until very advanced, the basic architecture is preserved with hepatic venules and portal tracts maintaining an almost normal anatomical relationship; hence the term *monolobular cirrhosis*. This provides a hint as to the biliary aetiology of the lesion but may lead to difficulty in deciding morphologically when a true cirrhosis has been established (Fig. 11.21B). The features of cholate stasis and the deposition of oedematous collagen matrix produce a striking 'halo' at the interface between hepatocytes and septa, a further pointer to the biliary nature of the lesion (Fig. 11.21B–D).

Much of the cellular and tissue damage is due to retention of hydrophobic, cytotoxic bile acids. Ursodeoxycholic acid (UDCA) appears to protect rat hepatocytes in vitro and in vivo against such cytotoxic damage.[207] UDCA inhibits, at

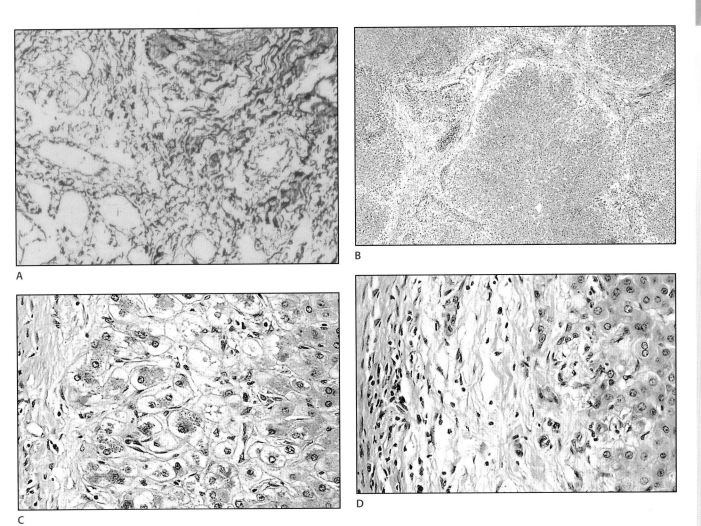

Fig. 11.21 • Biliary fibrosis and cirrhosis. **(A)** Fibrous portal-tract expansion. The original portal area can be recognized by the denser appearance of coarse collagen (golden-brown), whereas newly added fibrosis appears black as condensed reticulin. Gordon & Sweets' silver method for reticulin. **(B)** Irregularly shaped parenchymal areas, some having a normally positioned hepatic venule, are delineated by oedematous bands of connective tissue with centrally located inflammation and a marginal 'halo'. H & E. **(C)** and **(D)** The 'halo' may be predominantly cellular as in (C) or fibrous as in (D). H & E.

least in part, the biological and toxic effects of the endogenous bile acids by reducing their concentration within and around the liver cells, while UDCA itself is devoid of toxicity.[208] This explains the wide use of this drug in the treatment of chronic cholestatic disorders in both adults[209] and children.

Diseases affecting primarily the intrahepatic bile ducts

Primary biliary cirrhosis

Primary biliary cirrhosis (PBC) is an autoimmune liver disease of unknown aetiology which selectively affects the small intrahepatic bile ducts (Fig. 11.22A–C) and variably the hepatocytes. Along with the progressive bile-duct damage, chronic cholestasis, biliary fibrosis and then cirrhosis develop. The term PBC was established by Ahrens et al.[210] in 1950, but it is inaccurate, for only in the later stages is a true cirrhosis established, and a presymptomatic, or symptomatic but precirrhotic, stage may last for many

years. The term chronic non-suppurative destructive cholangitis (CNSDC)[211] more accurately describes the initial lesions. Nevertheless, the term PBC is almost invariably used to describe the entire spectrum of this disease.

Clinical features

Familiarity with the clinical and laboratory aspects of the disease is essential in establishing a diagnosis as pathognomonic histological features tend to be found only in the early stages and, even then, the biopsy needle may fail to sample the duct lesions owing to their focal distribution within the liver.[212] The presence of AMA in the serum is the major marker of the disease. PBC usually affects middle-aged to elderly women with a peak incidence in the 40–60 age group. It is rare under 30 years of age and, unlike PSC, has only exceptionally been reported in the paediatric age group.[213] There is a female preponderance of 9–10 to 1. This could be related to the increased expression of oestrogen receptor found in bile-duct cells and hepatocytes in PBC.[81] The disease is generally similar in both sexes, except that males were found to have less pruritus and skin pigmenta-

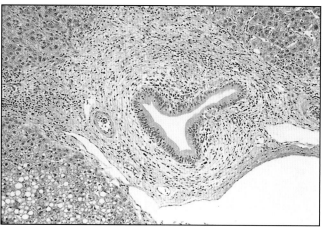

A

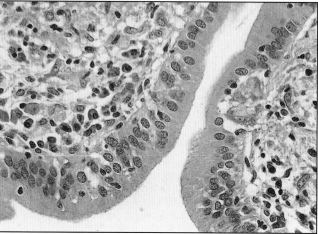

B

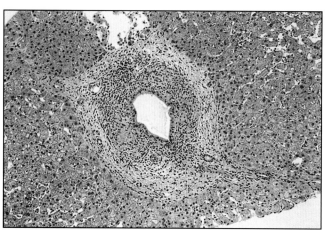

C

Fig. 11.22 • Primary biliary cirrhosis. **(A)** A mixed chronic inflammatory cell and granulomatous infiltrate surrounds this intermediate-sized bile duct and there is focal disruption of the basement membrane. H & E. **(B)** At a higher magnification note that the inflammatory cell infiltrate extends into hyperplastic biliary epithelium and there is focal dissolution of the epithelium. H & E. **(C)** In this case note the bile duct is completely surrounded by an epithelioid cell granulomatous reaction and there is focal disruption of the epithelium. H & E.

tion, and a higher incidence of hepatocellular carcinoma.[214] Although PBC occurs world-wide and has been found in all races, there is some geographical variation in incidence[215] with few cases reported from the Indian and African continents. In a combined European study[216] the overall prevalence was 23 per million, but with regional variations ranging from <10 to >60 per million. An increased awareness of the condition and the diagnosis of asymptomatic patients seem to account for the apparent rise in incidence and prevalence of PBC noted in the late 1980s.[217]

Insidious in onset, the presenting features are usually intense pruritus and lethargy with increasing skin pigmentation and eventually cholestatic jaundice, although icterus may not develop for years after the initial symptoms. Some patients first present with jaundice, particularly during pregnancy[218] or following drug intake, and in a very few instances hepatic decompensation may bring the patient to clinical notice. Portal hypertension may become manifest before a true cirrhosis is established.[219] Xanthomas/xanthelasma occur in 30% of patients.

The incidental finding of hepatomegaly (sometimes massive), a raised serum alkaline phosphatase or of serum AMA may result in the recognition of patients who are asymptomatic. They may remain asymptomatic for some years and experience a normal life expectancy,[220] although an increased mortality is shown for those in whom symptoms subsequently develop.[221,222]

PBC eventually progresses in most cases. Its natural history is presumed to be about 20 years, and the onset of jaundice, usually in the last 5 to 7 years, heralds clinical deterioration.[223] Death is usually due to hepatocellular failure, with bleeding from oesophageal varices in approximately 30% of cases;[224] non-hepatic causes of death are found in less than 20% of the patients.[225] Predicting the prognosis is a major issue, with the use of liver transplantation as the only treatment option in patients with advanced disease. Several models based on multiple regression analysis of clinical, biochemical and histopathological variables have been proposed, and in these the serum bilirubin levels and the presence of bridging fibrosis/cirrhosis are the most significant risk factors. These statistical models have proved useful in determining the optimal timing and in assessing the efficacy of liver transplantation in PBC.[226,227]

Associated conditions

The coexistence of PBC with other diseases which are themselves associated with immunological abnormalities is not uncommon. Features of Sjögren syndrome or the 'sicca complex' of dry eyes and dry mouth may be found in more than half the patients;[228] this led to the hypothesis that a common mechanism may be responsible for damaging epithelium-lined ducts in lacrimal and salivary glands and in the liver.[229] PBC may be associated with all or some of the features of the CREST syndrome: Calcinosis, Raynaud phenomenon, oEsophageal dysfunction, Sclerodactyly and Telangiectasis,[230] to which the presence of anticentromere antibodies and keratoconjunctivitis sicca were later added. CREST association may represent a distinct subgroup of patients with a high prevalence of HLA DR9.[231] Other reported associations include seropositive and seronegative arthritis,[232] autoimmune thyroiditis,[233] renal tubular acidosis,[234] coeliac disease,[235,236] systemic lupus erythematosus[237] and vasculitis.[238,239] Rare, possibly coincidental, associations include interstitial pulmonary fibrosis,[240] pulmonary haemorrhage and glomerulonephritis,[241] rapidly progressive glomerulonephritis,[242] multiple sclerosis,[243] idiopathic myelofibrosis, [244] ulcerative colitis,[245] tubulointerstitial nephritis and Fanconi syndrome,[246] systemic amyloidosis,[247] fibrinogen storage disease,[248] and a single case of autoimmune haemolysis.[249] Patients with PBC, in common with other chronic cholestatic syndromes, develop progressive bone loss in the course of the disease leading to severe osteoporosis.[250]

Laboratory tests

Liver function tests show a mild elevation of bilirubin (34–68 µmol/l; 2–4 mg/dl), accompanied by a striking and disproportionate elevation of serum alkaline phosphatase to levels three to five times normal, although a normal value does not preclude the diagnosis.[251] There is a moderate elevation of serum aminotransferase levels (100–150 iu/l). Serum immunoglobulins of all three major classes may be raised, but markedly elevated IgM in excess of 150% of normal is most consistent and is a distinctive feature of PBC.[252]

The most helpful diagnostic test is the demonstration of AMA, which are found in more than 95% of patients' sera.[253] Following antigen cloning and better definition, the major autoantigens which AMA recognize are now identified as components of the 2-oxo-acid dehydrogenase complex (2-OADC), an enzyme complex which is located on the mammalian inner mitochondrial membranes.[254-256] AMA of more than 95% of PBC patients are strongly reactive with epitopes in the E2 components of the pyruvate dehydrogenase complex (PDC-E2) and also with components of other 2-OADC;[257,258] AMA of about a half of PBC patients are known to react with BCOAD-E2 (E2 component of branched chain 2-oxo-acid dehydrogenase complex, 52 kD), AMA of 40 to 88% of PBC patients with OGDC-E2 (E2 component of 2-oxoglutarate dehydrogenase complex, 48 kD), and AMA of 95% of PBC patients with protein X (dihydrolipoamide dehydrogenase-binding protein, 55 kDa). Occurrence of ANA of centromere type is also characteristic for PBC.[259] In addition, autoantibodies against nuclear pore protein (gp210), and antibodies against inner membrane protein lamin B receptor (LBR) are characteristically detected in PBC, while their incidence is low compared to AMA.[260,261]

Aetiology and pathogenesis

PBC is characterized by a breakdown in self-tolerance of T and B cells to the conserved mitochondrial self-antigen E2-component of 2-OADC, particularly a major self-antigen PDC-E2, and then occurrence of autoreactive T and B cells against PDC-E2. The key pathologic process is damage to the interlobular bile ducts with apoptotic loss of biliary

epithelial cells.[53,55] However, the aetiology and precise pathogenesis of PBC remain obscure.[262,263] A clear association with class I HLA antigens has not been demonstrated and genetic associations with chromosomes 6p21.3 and 2q, which include HLA DRBI*08 haplotypes, CTLA4* G, IL1RN-IL1B haplotypes, CASP8, and nramp1, remain to be confirmed in independent series.[264] Genetic factors are suggested by a familial predisposition, an increased prevalence of autoantibodies in relatives of PBC patients,[265] and the recent suggestion of a high rate of monosomy X in women;[266] while geographical clustering of cases may militate in favour of either a genetic susceptibility or an environmental factor triggering bile-duct destruction in genetically predisposed hosts.[267] Also, a high concordance rate of PBC in monozygotic twins has been described, but the identification of three discordant pairs out of eight monozygotic pairs emphasizes that either epigenetic and/or environment factors play a critical role.[268]

Expression of potential target antigen(s) on bile ducts

The major AMA-related antigen, PDC-E2, is aberrantly expressed on the small intrahepatic bile ducts in PBC,[269-272] either diffusely[269] or on the luminal or supranuclear regions[270,272] (Fig. 11.23), a staining pattern which does not parallel the distribution of mitochondria.[273] In situ hybridization for the mRNA encoding these proteins is negative in biliary epithelial cells[274] which suggests that the molecules reacting with PDC-E2 may have been taken up, possibly from the bile, rather than synthesized, by bile-duct cells.[98] Aberrant expression of PDC-E2 has been shown to recur on biliary epithelium after transplantation for PBC in one study,[275] but this was not confirmed by other investigators.[276]

Molecular mimicry and autoantibodies

The events provoking initial activation of AMA- and PDC-E2-recognizing T-cells remain unknown; the hypothesis of molecular mimicry implies that foreign pathogens with homology to self-protein or modified self-protein can break tolerance.[277] Several reports have suggested the association

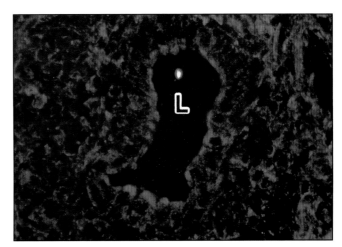

Fig. 11.23 • Expression of pyruvate dehydrogenase complex (PDC-E2) on the luminal border of an interlobular bile duct (L, lumen). PDC-E2 immunofluorescent staining.

of PBC with environmental factors such as microbes, drugs and chemicals.

Bacterial infections or mycobacteria have long been incriminated.[278,279] PDC-E2 are intracellular enzymes highly conserved during evolution and there is cross-reactivity between AMA and subcellular constituents of microbes, in particular *Escherichia coli* and mycobacteria. Sera from patients with PBC react with a variety of prokaryotes, including *E. coli*. Cloned T-cells from PBC livers are known to react with PDC-E2 elements of *E. coli*.[279] A strong correlation between anti-sp100 reactivity and AMA seropositivity in women with recurrent urinary tract infection, with or without evidence of primary biliary cirrhosis, further supports an involvement of *E. coli* infection in the induction of PBC-specific autoimmunity[260] and the large number of *E. coli* immunogenic mimics may account for the dominance of the major PDC-E2 autoepitope.[280] Recent evidence suggests that patients with PBC may exhibit a hypersensitive innate immune system to pathogen-associated stimuli which may facilitate loss of tolerance.[281]

Granuloma formation, a well-known product of mycobacterial infection, is part of the early bile-duct injury in PBC. A high prevalence of AMA has been demonstrated in the serum of patients with tuberculosis[282] and a PBC lesion has been produced experimentally in the mouse by mycoplasma-like organism.[283] To date, positive bacterial culture from liver tissue with PBC has not been obtained, but CD1—a family of four distinct non-polymorphic HLA class I-like molecules—which can present microbial antigens to T-cells is expressed in epithelioid granulomas and epithelial cells of the small bile ducts in early stages of PBC and may be involved in presenting microbial lipid antigen(s) to surrounding T-cells.[278] Disease-specific cross-reactivity between mimicking peptides of heat shock protein of *Mycobacterium gordonae* and dominant epitope of E2 subunit of pyruvate dehydrogenase seems to have a geographical distribution, being common in Spanish but not British patients with PBC.[284] Harada et al.[285] have identified several indigenous bacteria, and among them *Propionibacterium acnes* (*P. acnes*) DNA as a major clone in granulomas of PBC, suggesting that *P. acnes* and other enteric bacteria are involved in the pathogenesis of granuloma.

Chlamydia pneumoniae (*C. pneumoniae*) antigens have been universally found in all liver tissue samples of patients with PBC (but in only 8.5% of control livers) and the eight tested for *C. pneumoniae* 16S RNA by in situ hybridization were positive.[286] Another study detected *C. pneumoniae*-specific antibodies, but not *C. pneumoniae* rRNA gene and *C. pneumoniae* antigens, suggesting that *Chlamydia* infection is unlikely to be involved in PBC.[287] Recently, IgG3 antibodies which react both to PDC-E2 and beta-galatosidase of *Lactobacillus delbrueckii* have been identified in the serum of PBC patients.[288]

Viral particles have been identified by electron microscopy and exogenous retroviral nucleotide sequences cloned from biliary epithelium of patients with primary biliary cirrhosis.[289] The virus referred to as human betaretrovirus virus was found to have a high nucleotide homology with mouse mammary tumour virus (MMTV) and with retroviral sequences derived from human breast cancer samples. Evidence of infection in PBC patients led Mason et al.[290] to conduct a limited clinical trial with an apparent beneficial effect of antiviral therapy with Combivir in the short term. Conversely, Selmi et al.[291] failed to detect immunohistochemical or molecular evidence for MMTV in either liver specimens or peripheral blood lymphocytes of PBC patients.

In addition to foreign pathogens, which can break tolerance through molecular homology to cell components, it has been proposed that halogenated xenobiotics actively metabolized in the liver can modify self-molecules to render them immunogenic and result in the development of PBC in genetically susceptible hosts.[292]

AMA and bile-duct lesion

The above data suggest that AMA may be pathogenetic, but their precise role remains uncertain. It must be noted that the 2-OADC which is recognized by AMA is not restricted to the small intrahepatic bile ducts, but distributed throughout the body. Furthermore, AMA do not seem to be correlated with disease activity, particularly with the degree of bile-duct injury.

IgA, which is both produced by biliary cells and derived from the portal blood and then bound to the secretory component, is transported to the luminal surface of biliary epithelial cells.[293] Bile from PBC patients contains IgG and secretory IgA in similar amounts,[293,294] and has been shown to contain IgG and IgA anti-PDC-E2 antibodies.[134] IgA-PDC-E2 antibody may bind to PDC-E2 within the cytoplasm,[129,131] preventing uptake of PDC-E2 into the inner membrane of, and leading to deficient PDC-E2 transport into, the mitochondria. This will, in turn, cause mitochondrial dysfunction and damage or induction of apoptosis, both followed by cell death.[131,132] In PBC, colocalization of IgA and PDC-E2, both within the cytoplasm and at the apical surface of bile-duct cells, suggests a direct effect of IgA-class AMA on the mitochondrial function of biliary cells which have IgA receptors.[134]

Autoreactive T cells

Growing evidence has implicated the involvement of autoreactive T cells, recognizing PDC-E2 component, in the pathogenesis of bile-duct injuries. In patients with autoimmune diseases, the organ damage reportedly is caused by CD4+CD28− T cells, which express high levels of IFNγa and possess cytolytic activity. In PBC, CD4+ T cells have been shown to recognize amino acids 163–176 of PDC-E2 and there is a corresponding marked increase of CD4+ CD28− T cells in PBC livers.[119] Furthermore, CD8+ cytotoxic T lymphocytes that recognize components of amino acids 159–167 of PDC-E2 have an effector role in the bile-duct injury.[130]

Pathological features

The early lesion of PBC is characterized by portal inflammation with destructive injury to the small intrahepatic bile ducts (Fig. 11.24A–C). The majority of lymphocytes in the portal tracts are CD4+ and CD8+ T cells, although B cells

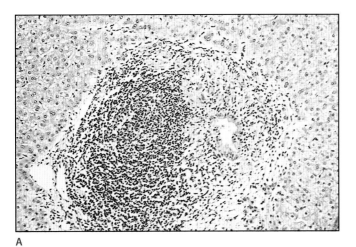

A

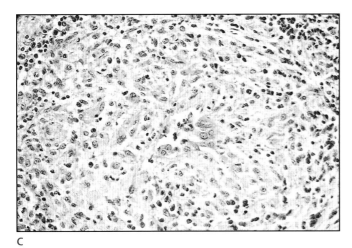

B

C

Fig. 11.24 • Primary biliary cirrhosis. Variations which may characterize the bile-duct lesions. **(A)** A lymphocytic aggregate with a germinal centre is present beside a damaged duct surrounded by an epithelioid granulomatous reaction. H & E. **(B)** Focally dense, chronic inflammatory cell infiltrates are closely associated with hyperplastic bile ducts, the number of which appears to be excessive. H & E. **(C)** Degenerate bile-duct epithelium surrounded by an epithelioid granulomatous reaction with some plasma cells. H & E.

are occasionally dense around the bile ducts and may form lymph follicles.[132,133,295] In addition, plasma cells and eosinophils can be conspicuous. Aggregates of epithelioid cells are common and well-defined non-caseating granulomas are characteristically seen in the early stages.

The initial injury affects interlobular bile ducts 40–80 μm in diameter; the smaller are the first to disappear,[296] and to a lesser degree septal bile ducts.[23] Epithelial cells of the bile ducts are variably swollen with a vacuolated cytoplasm and an irregular luminal border, or show an eosinophilic shrunken appearance with pyknotic nuclei. The epithelium also shows proliferative changes with stratification. This, together with some duct ectasia following the rupture of its basement membrane, leads to an overestimation of the actual size of the duct affected.[297] CD8+ and/or CD4+ T cells (Th1 subset) are the predominant cells infiltrating the ducts.[119] In the early stages, bile-duct damage and portal inflammation are distributed heterogeneously within the liver, and might not be sampled by liver biopsy needles. Non-specific portal inflammation can therefore be found in early liver biopsies from patients with a clinical diagnosis of PBC. Epithelioid cell granulomas, particularly when they are intimately associated with damaged bile ducts, are a characteristic finding of PBC (Figs 11.22C and 11.24C). Epithelioid cells may form a mantle around or be loosely arranged in the vicinity of the bile ducts.[298] There may be an admixture of foamy macrophages, suggesting phagocytosis of phospholipid substances, probably released from the injured duct.[170,298] Hyaline deposits may also be seen in the portal areas, at times within lymphocytic aggregates.[170] Around some ducts, polymorphonuclear neutrophils and/or oedema may be prominent.

These bile-duct lesions have been called chronic non-suppurative destructive cholangitis (by Rubin et al.[211]) or florid duct lesions. Serial sections disclose the segmental disappearance of interlobular bile ducts associated with a variable degree of granulomatous and lymphocytic reaction (Fig. 11.25A–D). Necrotic or ruptured bile ducts are variably surrounded by lymphocytes, plasma cells, epithelioid cells (Fig. 11.26A) and also foamy macrophages (Fig. 11.26B). Later, only remnants of duct epithelium will be identifiable as isolated cytokeratin 7-positive cells or small amorphous deposits of PAS-positive material amongst the inflammatory cell infiltrate. Finally, even such vestigial remnants are absent and only some focal condensation of the portal fibrous tissue or a lymphocytic aggregate remain to identify the site from which a bile duct has disappeared (Fig. 11.27A–B). The presence of arteries unaccompanied by ducts is used as a useful, yet rough, marker of bile-duct loss or ductopenia (Fig. 11.27A,B).[23] In contrast, the septal and large intrahepatic ducts, although they may show some inflammation in their wall, are preserved even at an advanced stage of the disease.

Changes in the lobular parenchyma are initially mild and may variably include single-cell necrosis, acidophilic bodies, Kupffer-cell hyperplasia and sinusoidal infiltration with lymphocytes and lipid-laden macrophages. Rarely, a more intense perivenular inflammation with cell loss may be seen (Fig. 11.28A). Well-formed epithelioid granulomas may also be found outside the portal areas (Fig. 11.28B). As discussed below, the activity at the interface may simulate an autoimmune hepatitis (Fig. 11.28C). Hepatocyte hyperplasia with twin-cell and pseudoglandular plates may be prominent from an early stage (Fig. 11.29A, B); this has been

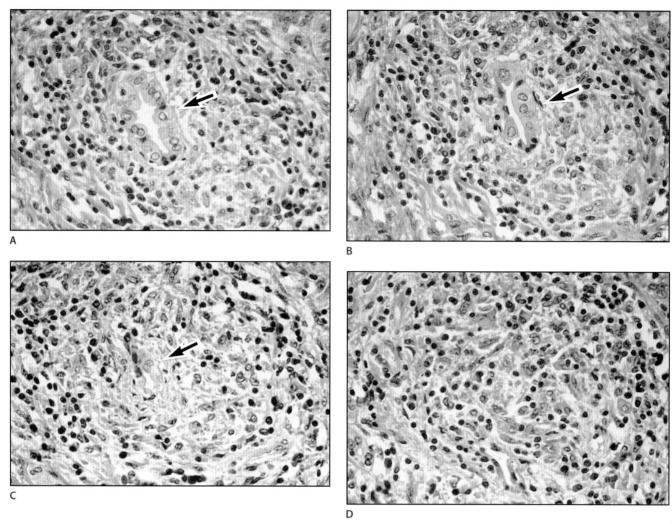

Fig. 11.25 • Primary biliary cirrhosis. Serial transverse sections of a disappearing interlobular bile duct. **(A)** A damaged interlobular bile duct (arrow) with several apoptotic biliary cells is surrounded by epithelioid and lymphoid cells. H & E. **(B)** and **(C)** The bile duct is gradually attenuated. H & E. **(D)** The bile duct has disappeared leaving a granulomatous focus. H & E.

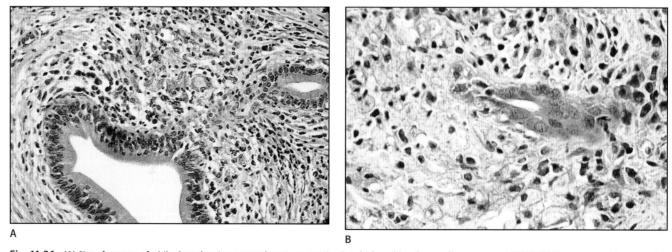

Fig. 11.26 • **(A)** Site of rupture of a bile duct showing a granulomatous reaction in which multinucleate cells are present. H & E. **(B)** Foamy macrophages and a few plasma cells have accumulated near a damaged bile duct. H & E.

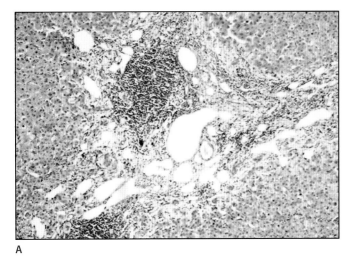

A

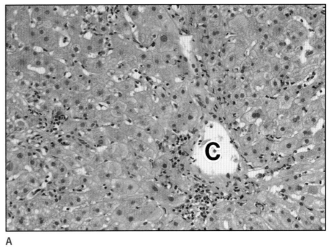

A

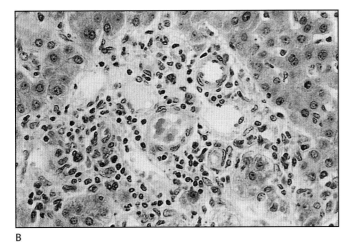

B

Fig. 11.27 • Evidence of ductopenia in primary biliary cirrhosis. **(A)** In this portal tract a lymphocytic aggregate is present at the presumed site of a disappeared bile duct. There are dilated lymphatics and small vessels. **(B)** Small chronically inflamed portal tract in which a number of hepatic arterioles are present, but no bile ducts. H & E.

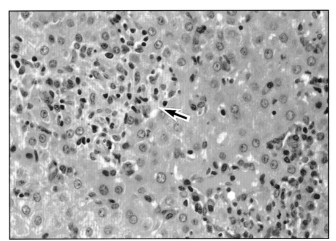

B

C

Fig. 11.28 • Hepatic parenchymal changes in primary biliary cirrhosis. **(A)** There are foci of cell necrosis and loss accentuated in the perivenular region (C, hepatic venule). Kupffer cells are prominent. H & E. **(B)** Small epithelioid granulomas are also seen (arrow). H & E. **(C)** Lymphocytic interface hepatitis (lymphocytic piecemeal necrosis) may be prominent with hepatocytes entrapped within the lymphocytic infiltrate. H & E.

confirmed by increased uptake of bromodeoxyuridine[299] and enhanced proliferating cell nuclear antigen (PCNA) immunostaining.[300] Sometimes, the change is prominent with nodule formation and atrophy of the intervening parenchyma similar to nodular regenerative hyperplasia (Fig. 11.29C).[301,302] It is probably an important factor both in the hepatomegaly of PBC and in the development of portal hypertension, which may be clinically significant before cirrhosis has set in.[219]

Progression of the liver injury

In the early stage, the bile-duct injury and associated inflammation described in the preceding paragraphs remain confined within the portal tract boundaries. The subsequent progression of the disease is characterized by an extension of the necroinflammatory process to the periportal parenchyma—interface activity. This may take two different forms which are often present in variable combination:[170]

1. *Lymphocytic interface activity* (Fig. 11.28C) resembles the lesion seen in autoimmune hepatitis (AIH) and suggests an extension to adjacent hepatocytes of the same immunological process as that affecting the duct system.[170] Lymphocytic interface activity is present in a substantial number of cases, generally early in conjunction with florid bile-duct damage and inflammation. In less than 10% of cases, it may even

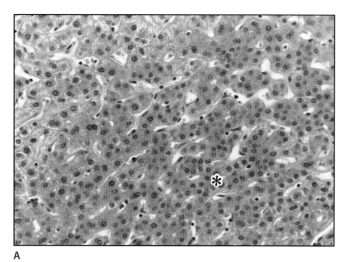

A

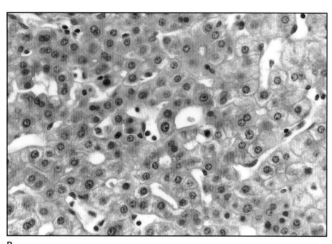

B

C

Fig. 11.29 • Primary biliary cirrhosis, parenchymal hyperplasia. **(A)** Foci of small hepatocytes (*) form two-cell-thick plates in some part of the liver lobule. H & E. **(B)** Some regenerating cells form pseudoglandular structures. H & E. **(C)** Regenerative hyperplasia with twin-cell plates producing some compression of the adjacent parenchyma. Gordon & Sweets' silver method for reticulin.

dominate the picture and be associated with clinical features of AIH, so-called PBC and AIH overlap syndrome.[303]

2. *Biliary interface activity* is superimposed or, as the duct loss advances, becomes the main feature. In common with other chronic cholestatic disorders, it results from the 'toxic' effect of hydrophobic bile acids and other retained bile products. There is cholate stasis (Figs 11.19A and 11.30A) and deposition of copper or copper-associated protein granules (Figs 11.19B and 11.30B).[304] The degree of copper deposition generally correlates with biochemical markers of cholestasis and stages of PBC.[305] Xanthoma cells, often in aggregates, may be present (Fig. 11.30C). Ductular reaction may be a striking feature, although the ductular elements often disappear in the advanced stages of the disease when pericellular fibrosis (Fig. 11.31A, B), Mallory bodies and intracellular or canalicular bile pigment dominate the picture at the interface (Fig. 11.19D).

In time, the necroinflammatory process accompanied by fibrosis extends along the terminal distribution of the portal tracts leading to portal–portal bridging septa.[306] Dilated lymphatics and venules forming a microcavernous structure (Fig. 11.27A) are frequently seen in the enlarged portal tracts. Periseptal changes are usually continuous with, and similar to, the periportal changes. There is a close association between the ductular reaction, activation of the surrounding mesenchyme, particularly hepatic stellate cells, and deposition of extracellular substances. The biliary type fibrosis is dense and scar-like in the deeper portions of the septa, but oedematous at the periphery where it gives rise to a 'halo' effect (Figs 11.21B, 11.30A and 11.31A, B).

Macroscopically, the cirrhotic liver is of a larger size than that of post-hepatitic type cirrhosis following viral or autoimmune hepatitis. The cirrhotic pattern is predominantly micronodular, of a regular appearance and there is variable bile staining (Fig. 11.32). Rarely a shrunken, macronodular liver is observed.

The histological changes may be difficult to distinguish from those of cirrhosis of other aetiology. Primary biliary cirrhosis should be suspected, however, on the following features: (i) virtual absence of medium- and small-sized bile ducts; (ii) focal lymphocytic aggregates in portal areas; (iii) peripheral cholate stasis or cholestasis with Mallory bodies and copper deposition regularly highlighting the parenchymal limiting plates; (iv) a biliary or monolobular pattern of fibrosis; and (v) partial or focal preservation of the normal architecture. In a few instances the diagnostic bile-duct lesions may persist at the cirrhotic stage and granulomas may also be seen.

The histological distinction between PBC and primary sclerosing cholangitis is discussed later. The main clinicopathological features of the two conditions are compared in Table 11.3.

Hepatocellular carcinoma has been reported as a terminal complication in a small number of PBC patients,[307] a low risk thought to reflect the female preponderance of PBC and the relatively short duration of the truly cirrhotic stage. This assumption is confirmed in a study of 667 patients which recorded an overall incidence of 5.9% in patients

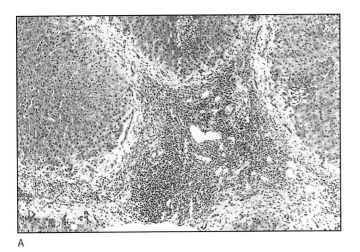

A

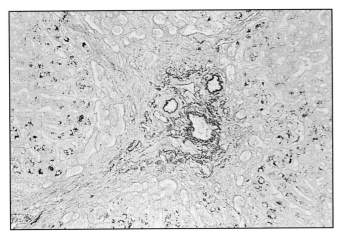

B

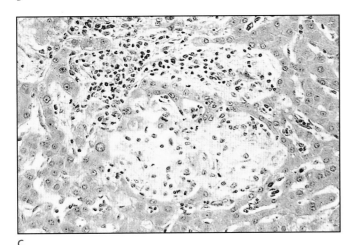

C

Fig. 11.30 • Primary biliary cirrhosis, stage 3. **(A)** Characteristic portal–septal fibrous expansion in which, centrally, there is chronic inflammation and fibrosis while there are clear margins ('halo' effect) indicating continuing biliary interface activity. H & E. **(B)** Orcein staining highlights the original boundaries of the portal tract with its abundant elastic content and copper-associated granules within what is now the parenchymal limiting plate. Shikata orcein. **(C)** Periportal aggregates of xanthoma cells. Masson trichrome.

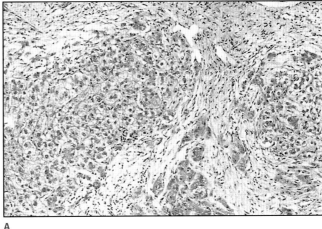

A

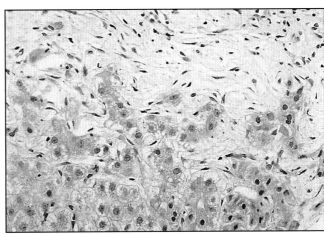

B

Fig. 11.31 • Primary biliary cirrhosis, fibrous interface in stage 4. **(A)** Inflammation is now minimal and the margins of the septa mostly comprise loose fibrous tissue which extends between the disrupted liver-cell plates. H & E. **(B)** The peripheral liver-cell plates seem to end blindly in the fibrous matrix of the septum. H & E.

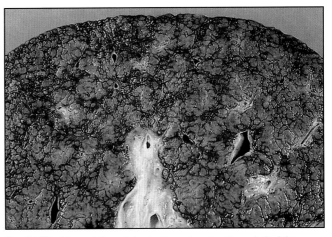

Fig. 11.32 • Primary biliary cirrhosis. Coronal section through the hilar region of a liver with PBC. The cirrhosis is of a regular micronodular pattern with marked bile staining at the periphery of the nodules.

with stage 3–4 disease, with a male incidence of 20% vs. 4.1% in female patients.[308] The true increased risk in males may be accounted for by a higher DNA synthetic activity than in female cirrhotic liver.[309] Hepatocellular carcinoma typically develops several years after the onset of cirrhosis

and carries a poor prognosis similar to that in cirrhosis of other aetiology.[308] An autopsy series suggested that the tumour cells in PBC are more likely to accumulate fat, copper and its binding protein and also Mallory bodies, particularly at an early stage.[310] There are reports also of an increased incidence of extrahepatic malignancies, notably breast cancer, the incidence of which was found to be 4.4 times that predicted for the general population.[311]

Histological staging of PBC

As early as 1965, Rubin et al.[211] proposed to divide the histological changes of PBC into four successive stages, a staging system which has been subsequently modified by other workers,[312–314] as shown in Table 11.4. The versions of Scheuer et al.[312] or Ludwig et al.[314] are used by most pathologists. Although these authors have given different names to the four stages, the systems overlap and can be summari-zed as follows: *Stage 1* refers to inflammation and non-suppurative destructive cholangitis (florid bile-duct lesion) confined within the portal boundaries; *Stage 2* denotes a destruction of the parenchymal limiting plates (interface activity) with variable degrees of ductular proliferation and early short radiating septa; *Stage 3* implies an extension of the portal-septal fibrosis to include portal–portal bridging septa (biliary fibrosis) (Fig. 11.30A); *Stage 4* is a fully developed cirrhosis (Fig. 11.31A).

The value of staging needle biopsy specimens has been somewhat downgraded owing to the uneven distribution of the lesion within the liver as a whole. Several stages, and occasionally all four, may be seen in a single liver removed at transplantation. In addition, there is a marked individual variation in the rate of progression of the disease. As a consequence, the histological staging is of little assistance in assessing the likely prognosis, except for the demonstration of severe bridging fibrosis or an established cirrhosis (stages 3–4) which, combined with the clinical development of jaundice, indicate a poor prognosis. Evaluation of a large series of yearly biopsies repeated for the purpose of a therapy trial[170] has been unable to confirm an earlier report that the presence of granulomas, irrespective of the stage, indicated a more favourable outlook.[315]

Treatment

The treatment of choice is ursodeoxycholic acid (UDCA), a hydrophilic bile acid which reduces the intrahepatic more hydrophobic bile-salt concentration, and competitively inhibits their reabsorption in the gut, thereby reducing the overall bile-acid pool size.[156] UCDA may also exert immunological effects:[316] in particular UDCA therapy is associated with a reduction of HLA molecule expression within the liver.[317] Clinically, UCDA often improves or even normalizes serum levels of cholestatic enzymes.[318] Results of the studies assessing the beneficial effect of UCDA on liver histology diverge, a discrepancy which can be expected given the known sampling variation and the small number of paired biopsies reviewed in the various studies.[319–321] Immunosuppressive therapy has been disappointing in PBC,[322,323] although anecdotal cases and observations made after liver transplantation suggest that corticosteroids could

Table 11.3	Comparison of clinicopathological features in primary biliary cirrhosis and primary sclerosing cholangitis	
Feature	**Primary biliary cirrhosis**	**Primary sclerosing cholangitis**
Clinical		
Sex, M/F	1/9	2/1
Symptomatic	>65%	>80%
Pruritus	>70%	>70%
Cholangitis	Absent	<15%
Hyperpigmentation	>50%	<25%
Xanthelasma	<20%	<5%
Laboratory tests		
Alkaline phosphatase	++++	++++
Bilirubin	+ to +++	+/++
Raised immunoglobulin M	++++	++
AMA	>95%	Absent or low titre
Other autoantibodies	<30%	Children > adults
HLA association	Not certain	B8; DR3, DR2, DRw52a
Associated diseases		
Inflammatory bowel disease	<4%	>65%
Sicca syndrome	>65%	<2%
Arthritis	>15%	<10%
Thyroid disease	>15%	<2%
Cholangiography	Often normal	Diagnostic
Histological features (needle biopsy)		
Granulomatous cholangitis	30–50%	Very rarely
Fibro-obliterative cholangitis	Absent	>10%
Cholestasis	Late	Variable
Copper-associated granules	>80%	>70%

Table 11.4	Histological staging of primary biliary cirrhosis			
Author	**Stage 1**	**Stage 2**	**Stage 3**	**Stage 4**
Rubin et al.[211]	Damage to intrahepatic bile ducts	Ductular proliferation	Ductular proliferation	Cirrhosis
Scheuer[312]	Florid duct lesion	Ductular proliferation	Scarring	Cirrhosis
Popper & Schaffner[313]	Cholangitis	Ductular proliferation and destruction	Precirrhotic stage	Cirrhosis
Ludwig et al.[314]	Portal hepatitis	Periportal hepatitis	Bridging necrosis or fibrosis or both	Cirrhosis

be beneficial if administered before ductopenia is too advanced. Studies using combined UCDA/steroid therapy are not large enough to appropriately evaluate the results.[324] Other agents have been used including methotrexate but a recent multicentre study of combined methotrexate with UDCA showed no additional benefit over UDCA alone.[325]

Variants of PBC

Primary biliary cirrhosis and AIH (see Chapter 10), the two main autoimmune liver diseases, differ in their clinical, biochemical, serological and histological features and, in most instances, a diagnosis of PBC or AIH can be achieved using accepted criteria. However, in some 18% of cases problems arise because PBC patients lack serum AMA antibody on standard indirect immunofluorescence (AMA negative PBC) or because features of both conditions in various combinations co-exist in a single patient.[326] At the present time these autoimmune variants can be grouped into three main categories:[327] (i) AMA-negative PBC (autoimmune cholangitis);[328] (ii) PBC–AIH overlap syndrome, both of which are discussed in this section and (3) PSC-AIH-overlap ('autoimmune sclerosing cholangitis') which is considered on p. 557.

AMA-negative PBC (autoimmune cholangitis)

The term 'immunocholangitis' was first introduced by Brunner & Klinge[329] to describe three women (two were mother and daughter) who had liver disease which clinically, biochemically and histologically was typical of PBC, except that AMA testing was negative and all three were ANA-positive in high titre. Ben-Ari et al.[330] later reported four similar patients with clinical and histological features of PBC, all four testing negative for AMA, but positive for both ANA and anti-alpha smooth-muscle actin (ASMA). The beneficial effect of prednisolone alone[330] or with azathioprine[329] recorded in these early studies has not been confirmed in subsequent studies dealing with larger numbers of patients.[328,331–333] IgM levels were lower and high-titre ANA positivity was more frequent in AMA-negative than AMA-positive PBC cases in one study.[331] Serum antibodies to carbonic anhydrase, a zinc metal enzyme abundant in biliary epithelium, has been detected in higher frequency in AMA-negative than AMA-positive PBC and AIH patients,[86] but these results could not be confirmed by others.[334] Based on sequential study in a single patient, accumulation of Vβ5.1-positive cells in the liver was put forward as a distinctive feature of autoimmune cholangitis.[335]

In all other aspects the two groups are identical.[333,334,336] There is also immunophenotypic similarity of the infiltrating inflammatory cells in both.[337,338] In both AMA-positive and AMA-negative PBC, ANA are reactive with a 210 kD glycoprotein of the nuclear membrane (gp 210), nuclear pore complex proteins and/or Sp100 nucleoprotein. In addition, the majority of AMA-negative PBC cases are found positive for recombinant elements of either of the two OADC-E2.[339] Thus, the general view is that autoimmune cholangitis can be considered as synonymous with AMA-negative PBC.[336] The sole distinctive feature between these

patients is the autoantibody profile (AMA, ANA),[340] which in itself should not lead to a diagnosis of overlap syndrome.[341]

PBC–AIH overlap syndrome

This PBC–AIH overlap syndrome is defined by the association of PBC and AIH in a single patient, either simultaneously or consecutively.[303,342] The frequency is about 20% of patients with autoimmune liver disease,[343] but the incidence varies at the grace of broader or narrower definitions, and long-term follow-up with frequent histological examinations may considerably reduce the number of cases initially considered as AIH–PBC overlap.[344]

Chazouillere et al.[303] have proposed diagnostic criteria for PBC–AIH overlap syndrome, namely the presence in an individual patient of at least two out of three accepted features for PBC (positive AMA, florid bile-duct lesion on histology and raised alkaline phosphatase × 5) and AIH (raised ALT levels × 5, serum IgG levels × 2 or a positive ASMA and moderate or severe lymphocytic interface activity on histology). Using these criteria, they found 9.2% of PBC patients having an overlap syndrome.[303] It must be stressed that the histological finding of PBC-like bile-duct injury in an otherwise classical AIH[345] or of lymphocytic interface hepatitis in an otherwise classical PBC[170] is in itself not sufficient for a diagnosis of overlap. The consecutive occurrence of PBC–AIH, with flare-up of AIH, either spontaneously or during treatment with UDCA, has been documented;[342] in two patients clinicopathological features of AIH occurred after transplantation for PBC.[346] Classical AIH evolving into a typical PBC has also been reported.[347]

Already in 1976, Geubel et al.[348] highlighted that response to therapy can differentiate overlap PBC–AIH from classical PBC. The combination of corticosteroids and UCDA, and in some cases azathioprine, may be required to achieved biochemical remission in patients with PBC–AIH overlap syndromes.[303]

PBC and sarcoidosis

Liver involvement in sarcoidosis is discussed in detail in Chapter 17. However, it must be mentioned here that in a few cases of sarcoidosis, a granulomatous cholangitis with progressive ductopenia leads to a cholestatic syndrome which raises the differential diagnosis of a PBC.[349] In that respect sarcoidosis can be considered as a cause of vanishing bile-duct syndrome.[60] Very few patients will have convincing features of both PBC and sarcoidosis[350-352] and these could be regarded as overlap syndromes.

Idiopathic adulthood ductopenia

Several authors[60,353] have identified patients who present in young adult life with a chronic cholestatic syndrome and a loss of the interlobular bile ducts leading to biliary fibrosis/cirrhosis, but in whom the clinical, radiological and immunological features did not satisfy the criteria for any of the recognized causes of vanishing bile-duct syndrome. Ludwig et al.[60] first used the term 'idiopathic adulthood ductopenia' for this condition. The patients show a male preponderance, are AMA-negative, have an essentially normal cholangiogram, a negative drug history and no evidence of chronic inflammatory bowel disease nor sarcoidosis.[354] Most reported cases present with pruritus or jaundice, in one case mimicking benign recurrent intrahepatic cholestasis,[355] and show a progressive course resulting in death or liver transplantation.[356] The diagnosis is one of exclusion.

Idiopathic adulthood ductopenia may constitute a heterogeneous group waiting for further characterization.[357,358] Most of the patients reported were younger than the lower age limit encountered in PBC, making a diagnosis of AMA-negative PBC unlikely; some may represent small-duct PSC without associated ulcerative colitis, while others may be a late onset of infantile non-syndromatic paucity of interlobular bile ducts.[359] A number of patients have been related.[353,356] Genetic studies might help in solving such cases which may represent forms of progressive familial intrahepatic cholestasis. Hereditary or acquired dysfunction of the canalicular membrane transporters bile-salt export pump (BSEP, ABCB11) and multidrug resistance protein type 3 (MDR3, ABCB4) seem not to play a role in the pathogenesis of PBC and PSC, but this remain to be evaluated in patients with idiopathic adulthood ductopenia.[360] Recently, asymptomatic cases of idiopathic adulthood ductopenia have been reported, possibly the result of a partial genetic defect.[361] These have apparently shown a good response to UDCA.

Bile-duct injury in the liver allograft and graft-versus-host disease

The interlobular bile ducts are the main targets of the immune attack during liver allograft rejection and graft-versus-host disease (GVHD), and so these lesions are of significant relevance to the discussion of biliary injury in the liver. These changes are discussed in Chapter 16, and so will not be presented here.

Other disorders associated with intrahepatic bile-duct injury

Acute and chronic hepatitis

A hepatitis-associated bile-duct lesion was first reported by Poulsen & Christoffersen[362] and subsequent studies by these and other workers have shown that this lesion occurs most commonly in chronic hepatitis C[44,363] and also in AIH.[41,364,365] The reported prevalence of bile-duct lesions varies markedly in different series; this probably reflects uncertainty about the aetiology of the underlying acute or chronic hepatitis in early series and variations in the criteria used to diagnose bile-duct lesions. The approximate frequency is 10–15% in acute viral hepatitis,[44,362] 20–35% in chronic viral hepatitis overall[44] and 25–30% in AIH.[41,364]

The distinctive lesions (Fig. 11.33A,B) are characterized by prominent swelling and vacuolation of the small bile-duct epithelium with piling up of irregularly spaced and hyperchromatic nuclei. The surrounding inflammatory cell infiltrate often includes lymphocytic aggregates with or without a follicular arrangement. The lumen may be con-

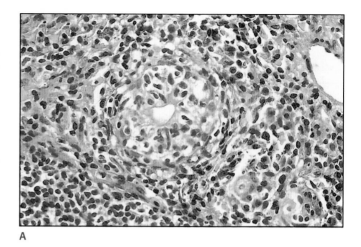

A

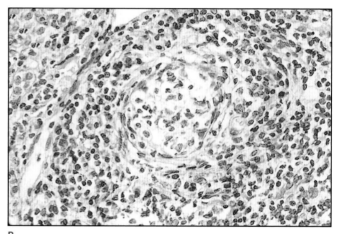

B

Fig. 11.33 • Hepatitis-associated bile-duct lesion. **(A)** There is an intense chronic inflammatory cell infiltrate in the portal tract; the bile-duct epithelium is swollen and stratified producing reduction of the luminal diameter; the epithelial cell cytoplasm is vacuolated and intraepithelial inflammatory mononuclear cells are present. H & E. **(B)** Serial section from the same case showing virtual obliteration of the lumen; there appears to be some reduplication of the basement membrane. PAS. Courtesy of Professor H Poulsen.

siderably narrowed and there may be reduplication of the epithelial basement membrane (Fig. 11.33B). The lesions involve only a segment of the duct circumference. Vyberg,[365] using serial three-dimensional studies, described a diverticular variant of this hepatitis-associated bile-duct injury. While a blinded, multiobserver assessment of trimmed bile ducts showed that histological differentiation of hepatitis associated bile-duct lesions from PBC is possible in most instances, bile-duct injury indistinguishable from the PBC lesion can be encountered in a significant number of chronic viral hepatitis cases.[366]

The lesion is common in chronic hepatitis C with a reported incidence ranging from 35 to 90%.[44,363,367,368] While granulomas are occasionally seen in portal tracts,[369] granulomatous cholangitis with duct loss is not a feature.[44] A single report claims loss of bile ducts in chronic hepatitis C, particularly at an advanced stage.[370] This must be viewed with caution as ductopenia may be difficult to quantify in cirrhosis owing to concomitant arteriolar hyperplasia. In addition, the changes of chronic cholestasis are not part of chronic hepatitis C in the non-immunocompromised host.

Viral infection of biliary epithelium[371] may be responsible for the bile-duct lesion observed in hepatitis C, and this is supported by the similarity to the benign lymphoepithelial lesion of Sjögren syndrome in which an association with chronic hepatitis C has been reported.[372] The bile-duct injury differs from that seen in immune-mediated cholangitis in that ectopic expression of HLA-DR (Fig. 11.11A,B) and enhanced expression of HLA-A,B,C are generally absent or mild in hepatitis-associated lesions.[44,373] Expression levels of ICAM-1 and LFA-3 on the bile ducts correlate with the severity of bile-duct damage,[374] and dendritic cells are frequently encountered in associated lymphoid follicles.[44,373] Lymphocytic cholangitis has also been recently described in hepatitis E.[375]

Reversible injury to bile-duct epithelium is not unusual in CMV hepatitis. In the neonate, viral inclusions of biliary epithelium are seen as a feature of CMV hepatitis (Fig. 11.34). In adults, mostly in immunocompromised hosts, CMV can occasionally be a cause of severe bile-duct necrosis.[376] It has been suggested that the paucity of interlobular bile ducts of neonates may be a sequela of CMV infection, but this is not supported by hard data.[377]

Drug and toxin-induced injury

Although biliary epithelial cells have a low metabolic activity compared with hepatocytes, bile-duct injury, cholangitis and ductopenia are occasionally reported in drug-induced reactions.[378] These are reviewed in Chapter 14. Following jaundice of acute onset, there may be extensive duct loss leading to prolonged cholestasis.[60,66,379]

The most commonly implicated drugs are neuroleptics (e.g. chlorpromazine),[380] tricyclic antidepressants, anticonvulsants (e.g. phenytoin), ajmaline, antibiotics (e.g. clindamycin, flucloxacillin, erythromycin, thiabendazole, amoxicillin/clavulanic acid[381,382]), and non-steroidal anti-inflammatory drugs (e.g. ibuprofen[66]). In many instances the severe and prolonged jaundice eventually disappears, leaving a biochemical cholestasis which may persist for months. In this form extensive ductular reaction and some

fibrosis precede restoration of the interlobular bile ducts whose numbers, however, may remain reduced after clinical recovery.[383] The prognosis has been reported as favourable with ultimate resolution in most cases.[384,385] However, a few cases show a rapid progression, even in children,[382] and development of cirrhosis is well recorded.[380] Some patients present a syndrome which closely resembles the clinical course and serum abnormalities of PBC, and when AMA is found in the serum, one can anticipate that the drug has unmasked or triggered a genuine PBC.

Morphologically, perivenular bilirubinostasis is a constant finding. The epithelium of the small bile ducts shows variable vacuolation or eosinophilic degeneration with nuclear pleomorphism, pyknosis and signs of regeneration with nuclear crowding and mitotic activity (Fig. 11.35A). The portal tract is oedematous with a mild to moderate inflammatory cell infiltrate. This may show a periductal reinforcement with a predominance of eosinophils and neutrophils (Fig. 11.35A), but granulomatous destructive cholangitis indistinguishable from PBC is exceptionally recorded.[386] A granulomatous reaction with eosinophils may be seen in patients presenting signs of hypersensitivity (Fig. 11.35B,C). Rarely, ductopenia occurs without significant portal tract inflammation. In longstanding cases, progressive ductopenia leads to portal fibrosis and signs of chronic cholestasis with copper accumulation in periportal hepatocytes.

Similar bile-duct injury has been produced experimentally or accidentally by toxic substances such as α-naphthylisothiocyanate or 4,4'-diaminodiphenylmethane.[387] The latter, which is an aromatic amine contained in bread, was the cause of so-called Epping jaundice in the UK; liver biopsy specimens from the patients showed cholangitic inflammation with many eosinophils, bile-duct necrosis and bilirubinostasis.[388] In paraquat poisoning, eosinophilic shrinkage of duct epithelium, nuclear pyknosis and epithelial detachment from the basement membrane have been noted (see Fig. 14.15) but with a very scanty inflammatory reaction.[389,390]

The *Stevens–Johnson syndrome*,[391] a drug hypersensitivity reaction with severe mucocutaneous manifestations, has been associated with a vanishing bile-duct syndrome.[392,393] The association occurs more often in patients with an abnormal immune status.[394] Stevens–Johnson syndrome is accompanied by immune complex deposition, followed by cytokine release and/or cell-mediated response. Several drugs have been linked with both vanishing bile-duct syndrome and Stevens–Johnson syndrome which provides evidence for immune pathogenetic mechanisms being common to both syndromes. Chamuleau et al.[395] reported a case of *toxic epidermal necrolysis* of unknown origin and vanishing bile-duct syndrome; both eventually improved after a year, leaving a mild elevation of alkaline phosphatase and γ-GT as the only sequelae.

Hodgkin lymphoma

Prolonged intrahepatic cholestasis has been observed in some patients with non-Hodgkin and Hodgkin lym-

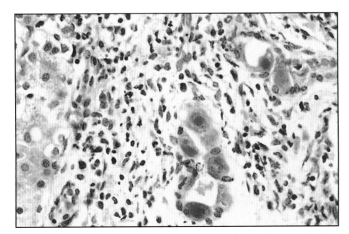

Fig. 11.34 • Neonatal hepatitis. Cytomegalovirus inclusions in the epithelial lining of a small bile duct. H & E.

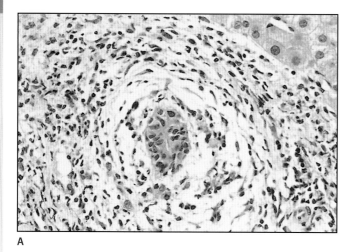

A

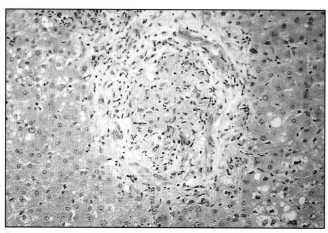

B

C

Fig. 11.35 • Drug-induced bile-duct injury. **(A)** Imipiramine-induced jaundice: the small bile duct shows epithelial atypia with nuclear pleomorphism and crowding; there is marked periductal oedema with a light mixed inflammatory cell infiltrate. H & E. **(B)** Carbamazepine (Tegretol): there is a granulomatous reaction in the portal tract with marked oedema and a neutrophil polymorph reaction; the damaged bile duct shows epithelial degeneration and a surrounding and infiltrative neutrophil polymorph reaction. H & E. **(C)** Chronic jaundice due to chlorpromazine: there is a continuing inflammatory reaction of the portal tract with a periportal ductular reaction; there is some periductal fibrosis, the epithelium shows degenerative change and there is a related neutrophil polymorph reaction. H & E.

phoma,[396,397] including vanishing bile-duct syndrome in the latter.[63] This is further discussed in Chapter 17.

Septicaemia, endotoxic and toxic shock syndrome

Septicaemia and severe bacterial infection may result in marked cholestatic jaundice.[398] Histological changes may be non-specific, comprising mild perivenular bilirubinostasis and portal inflammatory infiltration.[399] At times septicaemia of any cause may produce a suppurative cholangitis. In one female patient with *E. coli* septicaemia and severe cholestasis, liver histology showed reversible bile-duct damage characterized by epithelial swelling with nuclear pleomorphism, hyperchromasia or pyknosis; some ducts were ectatic, and there were polymorphonuclear cells within and around the damaged bile ducts.[399]

In severe *septic/endotoxic shock*, jaundice is frequently present. The mechanisms are complex with impairment of both bile salt-dependent and bile salt-independent bile formation.[400] Experimentally, there is release of cytokines secondary to increased bacterial lipopolysaccharides in the circulation with consequent down-regulation of bile acid transporters and reduced bile secretion.[401]

Biopsy specimens show a marked cholangiolitis, so called cholangitis lenta.[402] The portal tracts are surrounded by dilated ductules and canals of Hering which extend into the periportal zone; their lumens contain PAS-positive, bilirubin-stained casts with neutrophil polymorphs present within and around the ductules (Fig. 11.36A).[402,403] This is an important lesion to recognize, in that the picture of an acute cholangiolitis without a suppurative cholangitis suggests septicaemia rather than duct obstruction.[402] In long-standing cases of septicaemia or at autopsy[403] the portal tracts are ringed by the bile-containing dilated cholangioles (Fig. 11.36B). Similar, striking cholangiolar bile retention may often also be seen at autopsy after submassive liver-cell necrosis of viral or drug aetiology, and in decompensated cirrhosis. In these situations, the change may reflect septic complications associated with spontaneous bacterial peritonitis. This is also a somewhat common finding in biopsy specimens from liver allografts, and, in this setting, may also represent ischaemia to the biliary tree.

The *toxic shock syndrome*[404] is thought to be due to an exotoxin produced by *S. aureus* and in some cases was associated with the use of vaginal tampons; in other cases skin infection was present, but in many patients no source of infection could be identified. The syndrome is associated with a high mortality rate. Patients present with multisystem involvement; vomiting and diarrhoea, impaired renal function, thrombocytopenia, mental deterioration and jaundice with elevated serum aminotransaminases. Jaundice was a feature in 50% of patients. Histologically, there is a severe cholangitis and cholangiolitis with intense mural, luminal and periductal infiltration of neutrophil polymorphs (Fig. 11.37). The lesions were attributed to chemical irritation, probably resulting from exotoxin excretion in the bile, combined with liver hypoperfusion.

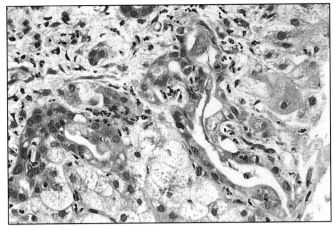

A

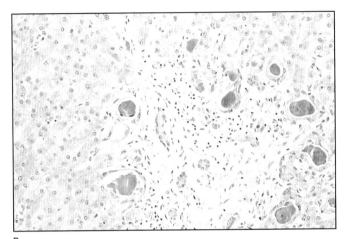

B

Fig. 11.36 • Cholangiolar cholestasis associated with septicaemia. **(A)** Biopsy 14 days postoperative showing prominence and swelling of cholangioles, the presence of a bile concretion and an intense acute cholangiolitis. H & E. **(B)** Autopsy case showing dilated periportal cholangioles with numerous bile concretions. H & E.

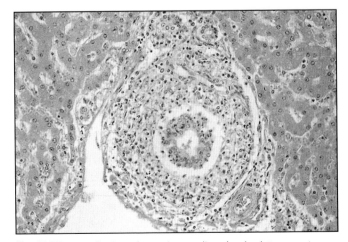

Fig. 11.37 • Toxic shock syndrome. Autopsy liver showing intense acute inflammatory cell infiltrate of the portal tract with a cholangitis. H & E.

Diseases affecting the extra- and intrahepatic biliary tree

Primary sclerosing cholangitis

Primary sclerosing cholangitis (PSC) is a chronic cholestatic disorder characterized by non-specific inflammatory fibrosis in the wall of the biliary tree leading to unevenly distributed stenosis and ectasia. The lesion usually affects the extrahepatic and large intrahepatic bile ducts, but the small intrahepatic bile ducts are often involved and in some 5% of the cases are affected exclusively—so-called *small-duct primary sclerosing cholangitis*.[405] The disease has to be distinguished from the secondary sclerosing cholangitis which may follow biliary surgery, cholelithiasis, congenital biliary abnormalities or infectious, ischaemic or iatrogenic cholangiopathy, as well as from sclerosing bile-duct carcinoma which may produce similar clinicopathological features. In that respect, the classic diagnostic criteria for PSC included: (i) absence of previous biliary tract surgery; (ii) absence of choledocholithiasis; (iii) diffuse involvement of the extrahepatic biliary tract; and (iv) exclusion of cholangiocarcinoma. However, with the recognition of small-duct disease, diffuse involvement of the extrahepatic biliary tract is no longer a prerequisite, and there is mounting evidence that a strict adherence to the first two criteria would underestimate the frequency and clinicopathological spectrum of the disease. In reality, a proportion of patients who underwent recurrent biliary surgery had PSC, and cholelithiasis and/or choledocholithiasis develops in a third of otherwise classic PSC cases.[406] Exclusion of a cholangiocarcinoma is not simple; cholangiographic appearances may be difficult to interpret against the background of a markedly distorted biliary tree.[407] Furthermore, a reasonably long follow-up does not exclude malignancy as cholangiocarcinoma may develop de novo, after years, in 10 to 20% of patients with PSC.[408]

As previously mentioned, there is a tendency to separate sclerosing cholangitis into a *primary* or *idiopathic* form, of which around 70% of cases are associated with ulcerative colitis, and an *acquired* or *secondary* form, of which infectious, toxic or ischaemic causes are recognized. Although this distinction might prove useful for further studies on pathogenesis and for the development of specific treatments, it must be stressed that the two subgroups are often indistinguishable clinically and radiologically,[409] as well as morphologically. In our experience, fibro-obliterative bile-duct lesions are more commonly, but far from exclusively, observed in the primary form.

Clinical features

Seventy-five per cent of patients are less than 50 years old at the time of diagnosis, but the disease can affect any age group.[410] Unlike PBC, it is well recognized in infancy[411] and in childhood.[412,413] There is a male preponderance of 2–3 to 1. Patients asymptomatic with respect to their hepatobiliary disease (5–25% in some series[414]) are discovered because of an isolated rise in alkaline phosphatase found as part of regular screening of patients with chronic inflammatory bowel disease.[415]

The classic presentation is with fatigue,[416] vague upper abdominal pain, intermittent or progressive jaundice and, less commonly, with recurrent attacks of cholangitis.[417,418] In the majority of patients, including those who are asymptomatic at the time of diagnosis,[419] the disease will progress and biliary cirrhosis develops with progressive liver failure, deepening jaundice and death within 5–17 years of diagnosis. However, follow-up studies show a considerable variation in clinical course[408,419–422] with survival in one patient of up to 30 years.[422]

As with PBC, a number of studies using multivariate analysis have been carried out to identify prognostic factors which might indicate the need to proceed to liver transplantation;[423,424] increasing age and serum bilirubin levels usually indicate a poor prognosis. Pretransplant prediction of prognosis after liver transplantation has also been determined using a Cox regression model where univariate analysis showed high serum creatinine, high serum bilirubin, biliary tree malignancy, previous upper abdominal surgery, hepatic encephalopathy, ascites and Crohn disease to be associated with a decreased post-transplant survival, whereas ulcerative colitis was associated with a better survival.[424] Unfortunately, there are no means of identifying the 10% or more of patients who are at risk of developing a cholangiocarcinoma.[425]

Associated disorders

Primary sclerosing cholangitis may occur alone, but in 54–75% of patients[426] or more it is associated with chronic inflammatory bowel disease, mainly ulcerative colitis. Conversely, PSC may occur in approximately 2.5–7.5% of patients with ulcerative colitis.[426,427] These figures vary considerably in different series, probably reflecting patient selection and differences in the diagnostic criteria applied.[428] A recent survey of 388 PSC cases in Japan identified two peaks of age distribution: the younger, including the 39% associated with ulcerative colitis, had characteristics similar to those in the West, whereas the older group appears specific to Japan;[429] this group included a proportion of patients with presumed autoimmune pancreatitis.[430,431] Primary sclerosing cholangitis may also be associated with Crohn disease.[432] The prevalence may be similar to that in ulcerative colitis, and the colon is usually involved in affected patients.[432,433] The term pericholangitis was previously synonymous both, clinically and histologically, with the liver involvement in chronic inflammatory bowel disease. The term covered a range of portal and biliary tract changes but, with the advent of cholangiography, it was applied to other patients with abnormal liver function tests and a normal endoscopic retrograde cholangiopancreatography (ERCP). The term small-duct PSC is now used for this subgroup.[405]

The pancreatic duct may be involved, causing chronic pancreatitis[434,435] which may dominate the clinical picture,[436] and in some instances may be associated with autoimmune

features.[430,431,437] Pancreatic involvement has also been associated with Sjögren syndrome.[438,439]

Recently, an apparently distinct disorder has been recognized in Japan.[440,441] The condition is characterized by variable degree and extent of fibrous thickening in the wall of the extrahepatic, hilar and/or perihilar bile ducts. Histologically, there is a dense fibrosis with obliterative phlebitis, many eosinophils, and heavy lymphoplasmacytic infiltrates (Fig. 11.38A,B,C), which, on immunohistochemistry, show a predominance of IgG4-positive cells (Fig. 11.38B). This accounts for the term 'IgG4-associated sclerosing cholangitis' tentatively applied to the condition.[441] Similar changes are characteristically found in the pancreas (sclerosing or autoimmune pancreatitis).[437,441] In contrast, IgG4-plasma cells are generally not prominent in classical PSC.[441] Interestingly, the cholangitis associated with inflammatory pseudotumours shows a similar predominance of both IgG4-positive plasma cells and obliterative phlebitis.[442,443] A case of pancreatic pseudotumour with sclerosing pancreatocholangitis reported in the West[444] shares many of the features recorded in Japanese patients, but IgG4 is not mentioned in the report. Additional cases are needed to further characterize what appears to be a new entity.

Less commonly reported clinical associations include multifocal fibrosclerosis and/or Riedel thyroiditis,[445–447] coeliac disease[448] (with ulcerative colitis in 2 sisters[449]) and hypereosinophilic syndrome.[450,451] There are isolated reports of associated Peyronie disease,[452] systemic lupus erythematosus,[453] lupus anticoagulant,[454] Budd–Chiari syndrome,[455] autoimmune haemolytic anaemia with hyperthyroidism,[456] Graves hyperthyroidism,[457] ulcerative lesions on skin and soft palate,[458] erythrocyte hyperaggregation,[459] and idiopathic thrombocytopenic purpura,[460] the majority of these reported associations appearing coincidental. One patient presented with acute pancreatitis with autoimmune haemolytic anaemia and subsequently developed ankylosing spondylitis in the absence of ulcerative colitis.[461] There are a few reports of associated extrahepatic sarcoidosis,[462,463] whereas others describe features of sclerosing cholangitis due to sarcoidosis diffusely affecting the intrahepatic bile ducts—a form of acquired sclerosing cholangitis.[464] A predisposition to osteopenia may be severe in advanced PSC, in a few cases below the fractures threshold.[465]

The high incidence of a complicating cholangiocarcinoma has already been mentioned. Approximately 7% of PSC patients develop cholangiocarcinoma over a mean follow-up of 11.5 years, which is markedly higher than the rates in the general population.[466] There are also reports of hepatocellular carcinoma in PSC,[467] in one case the fibrolamellar variant,[468] and of mixed hepatocholangiocellular carcinoma.[469] Inflammatory pseudotumour,[441,442] and an incidental focal nodular hyperplasia[470] may occasionally enter the differential diagnosis.

Laboratory tests

Liver function tests show cholestasis with a pattern similar to that seen in PBC except that the alkaline phosphatase levels are usually higher and there is no marked increase in

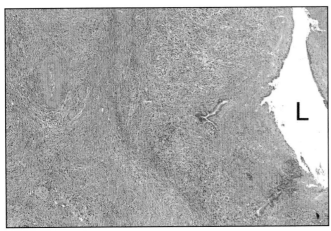

A

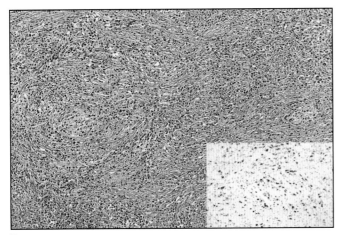

B

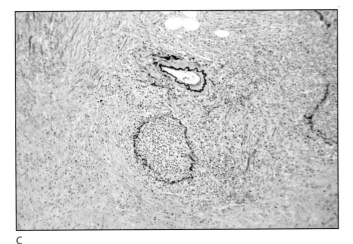

C

Fig. 11.38 • IgG4 sclerosing cholangitis associated with sclerosing pancreatitis (autoimmune pancreatitis). **(A)** The common bile duct shows a markedly thickened wall due to cellular fibroplasia with heavy inflammatory cell infiltration extending into the surrounding tissue. L, bile-duct lumen. H & E. **(B)** Prominent lymphoplasmacytic infiltration and myofibroblastic proliferation. The inset shows the majority of infiltrating plasma cells to react with IgG4 antibodies. H & E and immunostaining for IgG4. **(C)** An obliterated veins is demonstrated with elastic van Gieson stain.

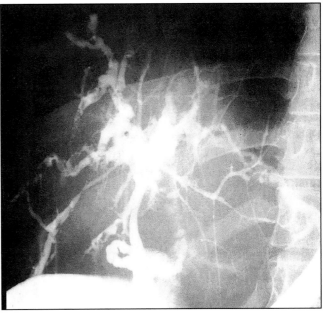

Fig. 11.39 • ERCP film in primary sclerosing cholangitis. Note the markedly distorted extra- and intrahepatic biliary tree with variable beading, stenosis and thinning of the bile ducts.

found as often in AIH and, to a lesser extent in PBC, and defining antigen specificity—catalase, alpha-enolase and lactoferrin—does not increase their clinical significance.[472] Low-titre anti-nuclear and anti-smooth muscle antibodies are found in one-third of the patients;[410] these were mainly of IgM class in one series.[473] The prevalence of antibodies is higher in children, in whom serum IgG is also often elevated.[412] In a survey of serum autoantibodies in 73 untreated patients anticardiolipins were the single group of autoantibodies that had a significant correlation with prognostic factors and histological stage.[474]

Radiological features

Imaging of the biliary tree is an extremely important diagnostic test in PSC. Either ERCP[475] or Chiba skinny-needle percutaneous transhepatic cholangiography (PTC) demonstrates irregular areas of stricture and beading of the bile ducts which, in 80% of patients, involve both intra- and extrahepatic bile ducts (Fig. 11.39).[476] Diverticular outpouchings and webs may be seen[477] and, in a few cases, cholangiectasis may mimic the changes seen in Caroli disease.[478] Later, decreased intrahepatic branching produces a 'pruned tree' appearance which may resemble the attenuated pattern seen in PBC and other forms of cirrhosis.[479] Magnetic resonance cholangiopancreatography (MRCP) has now been shown to be a sensitive and non-invasive technique to diagnose PSC although different bile-duct abnormalities leading to the diagnosis are depicted by MRCP and ERCP; more bile-duct stenoses and pruning are seen with ERCP and more skip dilatation with MRCP.[480,481]

Localized, high-grade stricture with marked progression in sequential cholangiograms, excessive duct dilatation proximal to strictures, and polypoid lesions suggest the development of cholangiocarcinoma, but the diagnosis of

serum IgM levels in PSC.[418] As in PBC, a normal alkaline phosphatase does not preclude the diagnosis.[471] AMA is not present in PSC, but circulating antibodies against cytoplasmic constituents of neutrophils (ANCA) are frequently present; however, they lack sensitivity and specificity, being

tumour is difficult and is often only made at autopsy or when the liver is removed at transplantation.[482] The value of brush cytology has been poor[483] although recent evidence suggests that sensitivity and specificity are improved if brush cytology is combined with measurement of serum CA19-9 levels.[484] Positron emission tomography (PET) using [18F]fluoro-2-deoxy-D-glucose, a glucose analogue that accumulates in various malignant tumours, has allowed the detection of small cholangiocarcinomas in PSC.[485]

Aetiology and pathogenesis

The various factors responsible for the acquired forms of sclerosing cholangitis (see Table 11.5) have all been considered as potential causes of PSC, but none has yet been convincingly implicated. As in PBC, deficiency in bile salt export pump and MDR3 do not appear to play a role.[360] The existence of a localized renin–angiotensin system within the liver has been proposed and an aberrant production of angiotensin II hypothesized as the critical event contributing to the pathogenesis of PSC, but this is supported only by the fact that biliary tract ischaemia can produce morphological changes identical to PSC.[486] In view of the frequent association with ulcerative colitis, chronic portal endotoxaemia and bacteraemia from the diseased colon have been proposed, but are not supported by appropriate data.[487] An increased expression of lipid A, a constituent of endotoxins, in bile-duct epithelium of PBC and PSC seems likely to be a secondary change.[84] Furthermore, chronic inflammatory bowel disease does not cause PSC; the two diseases occur independently. No differences have been demonstrated between PSC occurring in association with chronic inflammatory bowel disease and that occurring in its absence.[415] The interval between the onset of the bowel disease and the onset of biliary tract disease varies widely; the chronic inflammatory bowel disease may become symptomatic some years after PSC has been diagnosed and, conversely, PSC may become symptomatic years after colectomy. However, their frequent association strongly suggests that chronic inflammatory bowel disease and PSC have some aetiopathogenetic factor in common, and this is further supported by the demonstration that T cells activated in the gut can be recruited to an extraintestinal site of disease.[488]

Evidence of a genetic predisposition is provided by reports of familial cases,[489–491] and of a close association of PSC with HLA-B8 and DR3, to a lesser extent DR2 phenotypes,[492,493] and polymorphism of immune-related molecules.[494,495] A close association between HLA-DRW52 and PSC has been demonstrated.[496] Both DRW52 and DR2 encode a leucine residue at position 38 of the DRβ chain and it has been postulated that it is this feature of the DR molecule which confers susceptibility to PSC.[497] A genetic study of 256 PSC patients from five European countries has shown that three HLA class II haplotypes are associated with susceptibility to, and one with protection from PSC, in all five patients' groups when compared with 764 ethnically matched controls.[498] Subsequent studies have reaffirmed increased and decreased frequencies of haplotypes in the HLA-DRB3, DRB1, DQA1 and DQB1 regions suggesting that specific amino acids may determine the susceptibility/resistance to PSC encoded by these haplotypes.[499,500] A recent study demonstrated mutations/variants in the *CFTR* (cystic fibrosis) gene in PSC patients,[501] but *CFTR* alteration was not detected in Italian PSC patients.[500]

Humoral immune abnormalities recorded in PSC include: hypergammaglobulinaemia;[502] antineutrophil cytoplasmic and non-organ specific antibodies[428,503] (the latter more prevalent in children[412,504]); increased levels of soluble CD23[505] and of circulating immune complexes[506] (of which clearance by fixed macrophages could be impaired[507]); and activation of the complement system.[508] Cellular abnormalities include lymphocyte sensitization to biliary antigens,[509] an increased CD4 : CD8 ratio of circulating T cells,[510,511] and a predominance of T lymphocytes in the portal tract infiltrate, which in one study appeared to consist mainly of non-activated memory T lymphocytes expressing CD3-CD45RO markers.[512] Although some of these abnormalities may be secondary, they suggest that immune mechanisms play a role in perpetuating the bile-duct lesion, as further suggested by the overlapping features between PSC and AIH that are discussed below.[513] Increased expression of ICAM-1[514] and of heat-shock protein[82] by biliary epithelial cells has been documented in PSC. Autoantibodies against the specific epitope of tropomyosin(s) were suggested as putative antigenic peptide involved in the immunopathogenesis of ulcerative colitis and, perhaps, PSC.[515] Aberrant expression of HLA-DR antigens on the surface membrane of bile-duct epithelium is seen in PSC as in PBC;[516] it may enable the biliary epithelial cells to present antigens to sensitized T lymphocytes. CD44 is also expressed in bile-duct cells of both PBC and PSC livers and may play a role early in promoting lymphoepithelial interactions, whereas HLA-DR may be involved in the subsequent progression of the lesions.[517] Some of the infiltrating lymphocytes within the liver in PSC are mucosal T cells recruited through aberrant expression of the gut-specific chemokine CCL25 in hepatic endothelial cells.[518]

Thus, in PSC as in PBC, genetically predisposed individuals appear to become sensitized to triggering antigens, the nature of which remains unknown. There has been speculation on the role of viruses, in that PSC exhibits many morphological resemblances to biliary atresia which may be induced in weanling mice, but less often in humans, by infection with Reovirus type 3.[519] However, only a minority of patients with PSC had significantly elevated titres of serum antibody to Reovirus type 3 and the virus could not be detected in liver tissue.[520] An association with CMV, frequent in AIDS-related sclerosing cholangitis (p. 48), has not been found in PSC.[521] *Helicobacter pylori* and other helicobacter species were detected by PCR, hybridization and partial DNA sequencing in 20 out of 24 PBC and PSC livers with a weak association with ulcerative colitis in the PSC group. This was found in only one of the 13 patients of the non-cholestatic disease group, a boy who on subsequent examination showed histological changes of PSC, and in none of the 10 normal controls.[522]

Pathological features

The distinctive bile-duct lesion in PSC is a fibro-obliterative one, characterized by an 'onion-skin' type of periductal fibrosis around medium-sized or larger bile ducts, with degeneration and atrophy of the epithelial lining and eventual replacement of the bile duct by fibrous cords (Fig. 11.40A–C). These lesions, accompanied by reduced numbers of interlobular bile ducts, are virtually diagnostic of PSC. However, owing to the large size of the ducts involved, the lesions may be present in less than 40% of biopsy specimens. The small interlobular bile ducts may also be affected and replaced by fibrous scars (Fig. 11.40D), either in addition to the involvement of larger ducts or alone in the small-duct variant.[405] Thus, examination of the peripheral parenchyma obtained in needle biopsies may reveal portal tract changes which are either non-specific, but suggestive of a pathological process involving the major bile ducts, or are characteristic of small-duct PSC,[405] which may not invariably be associated with involvement of the extrahepatic bile ducts.

By analogy with PBC, the histological changes may be divided into four stages. In stage 1 the changes are confined within the boundaries of portal tracts. These contain a diffuse mixed inflammatory cell infiltrate of lymphocytes, plasma cells and neutrophils, and this tends to be more intense around the bile ducts (Fig. 11.41A). Lymphoid follicles or aggregates may be present (Fig. 11.41B), but granulomas are only very occasionally found in needle biopsy specimens,[410] perhaps less so in tissue blocks from livers removed at transplantation.[42] Small bile ducts may show degenerative epithelial changes (Fig. 11.41A,B). There may be increased portal fibrosis with some condensation around the bile ducts and also portal oedema.

In stage 2, portal tracts are swollen with variable degrees of disruption of the parenchymal limiting plates (Figs 11.41A,B and 11.42A). The histological picture varies, presumably depending on the severity of biliary obstruction,[523] the degree of superimposed cholangitis and the activity of the immune-mediated processes. Biliary interface activity with focal ductular reaction may predominate. These small ductules may be surrounded by typically mild neutrophilic

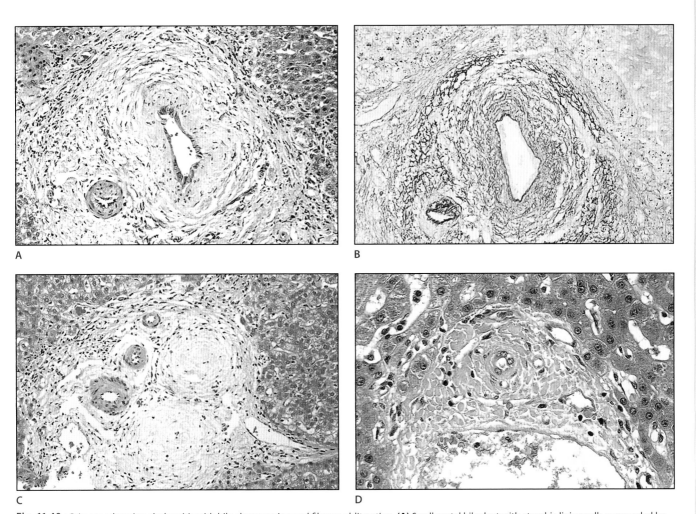

A

B

C

D

Fig. 11.40 • Primary sclerosing cholangitis with bile-duct scarring and fibrous obliteration. **(A)** Small septal bile duct with atrophic lining cells surrounded by dense hyaline collagen. H & E. **(B)** Same field as (A) to show the elastic content of the periductal collagen; note granular copper-associated protein deposits within periportal hepatocytes. Orcein. **(C)** Complete obliteration of bile ducts which are replaced by dense fibrous whorls; note the prominence of adjacent arterial branches. H & E. **(D)** In this patient with ulcerative colitis who had a negative ERCP, the liver biopsy shows fibro-obliterative lesions of the small bile ducts. H & E.

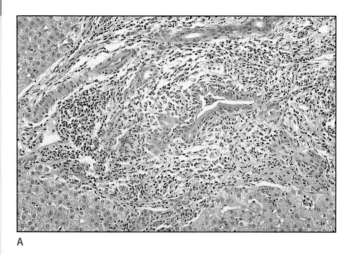

A

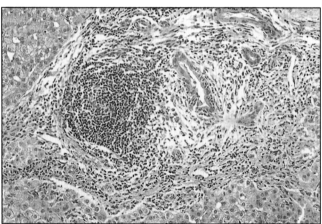

B

Fig. 11.41 • Primary sclerosing cholangitis. Ductal lesions and portal inflammation. **(A)** and **(B)** Two portal areas from the same biopsy specimen. A dense chronic inflammatory cell infiltrate surrounds the bile duct and inflammatory cells extend into the bile-duct epithelium raising the differential diagnosis of primary biliary cirrhosis; note a lymphoid follicle in (B). H & E.

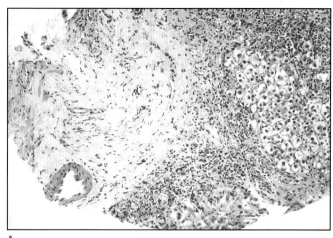

A

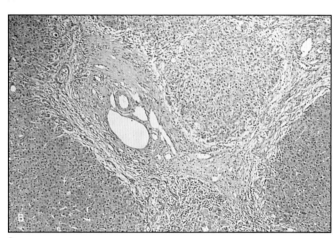

B

Fig. 11.42 • **(A)** Primary sclerosing cholangitis with lymphocytic interface activity raising the differential diagnosis of autoimmune hepatitis. Note, however, the collagenous scar in the portal tract which highlights the site of an obliterated duct. **(B)** Cirrhotic stage. A portal–portal fibrous septum is devoid of a bile duct and there is an unaccompanied hepatic artery branch; note the hyaline scar and the periseptal biliary interface activity with a 'halo' effect. H & E.

cell infiltrates. Less commonly, dense portal tract inflammation is present and can be associated with lymphocytic interface activity, with the appearance mimicking that of autoimmune hepatitis (Fig. 11.42A). This may cause diagnostic problems when hyperglobulinaemia and autoantibodies are present. In many instances, the inflammation seems to have subsided, the mildly fibrotic portal tracts have a stellate shape due to short and thin radiating septa and there is a slight excess of ductules and a few granules of copper-associated protein. Unless periductal fibrosis, cholangitis and focal ductopenia are present, the changes are not diagnostic, but suggestive enough to confirm a clinical and radiological diagnosis of PSC, or to indicate ERCP examination when this has not been already performed.

Further progression of the disease is characterized by increasing portal fibrosis with the formation of portal–portal linking septa (stage 3) and eventual development of cirrhosis—stage 4 (Fig. 11.42B). As the disease advances, the inflammation has a tendency to subside, leaving a combination of portal–septal fibrosis and oedema, focal ductular reaction, periseptal biliary interface activity with copper accumulation, Mallory bodies, 'halo' formation and pro-

gressive reduction in the number of bile ducts as described for PBC.[524] Bile ducts disappear, and their former site is often indicated by either small aggregates of lymphocytes or macrophages, as in PBC, or rounded scars which are much more common in PSC (Figs 11.40C and 11.42B). As in PBC, the presence of an unaccompanied hepatic artery branch is an indication of bile-duct loss (Figs 11.40C and 11.42A,B). Occasionally, the portal tract contains unusually prominent hepatic artery branches (Fig. 11.40C), which may reflect either an increased number of vessels or increased tortuosity of the peribiliary plexus as a result of the disappearance of the bile ducts and shrinkage of the scarred portal tract.

The distinction between PSC and PBC on histological appearances alone may be difficult; it was reliable in only 28% of a series of 318 patients who had one of these two syndromes.[418] The distinction is even more difficult on the basis of a single biopsy and where the size of the portal tracts contained in the biopsy specimen may determine the pattern of the histological lesions seen. Cholestasis can be an earlier and more frequent finding in PSC than in PBC.[420]

Periductal fibrosis or duct replacement by fibrous cords, with or without superimposed acute cholangitis, favours PSC, whereas granulomas are mostly found in PBC (Table 11.3).

Livers obtained at transplantation have allowed more detailed examination of the large intrahepatic and extrahepatic bile ducts and have highlighted the uneven distribution of the changes in the liver as a whole. This closely reflects the changes seen radiologically[525] and explains the high degree of sampling variability experienced in needle and even wedge liver biopsy evaluation.[526,527] On gross examination of explanted livers, one may see annular scars or fibrous cords which alternate with tubular or saccular cholangiectases, including luminal fibrous webs (Fig. 11.43A,B), ulceration of large ducts with or without cholangitic abscesses, and intrahepatic bile sludge or stones. It is important to mention that broad areas of confluent parenchymal collapse may be present (Fig. 11.43A), secondary to duct obliteration and/or vascular block, in particular portal venous occlusion, due to associated phlebitis. Large perihilar scars with yellow discoloration due to xanthomatous change may be seen. At times, these changes simulate a desmoplastic tumour and can radiographically mimic chol-

angiocarcinoma. In general, the pattern of cirrhosis is more irregular than that of PBC, reflecting the larger calibre of the ducts involved and possibly associated portal vein occlusion (Fig. 11.43C). Obliteration of segmental or main left or right hepatic ducts may occasionally lead to a segmental[528] or 'hemicirrhosis' respectively (Fig. 11.43C,D).

Histological examination of these livers may confirm ulceration of large bile ducts with bile impregnation and a xanthogranulomatous reaction in the surrounding tissue (Fig. 11.44A). There may also be distortion of bile-duct architecture and irregular periductal scarring (Fig. 11.44B,C,D), and obliteration of large intrahepatic bile ducts by fibrous scars (Fig. 11.45A–D); remnants of peribiliary glands may mark the site at which a large bile duct was present (Fig.11.45D). Areas of diffuse parenchymal collapse (Fig. 11.43A) may resemble posthepatitic collapse. Such areas, when sampled by a biopsy needle, may lead to an erroneous diagnosis of severe hepatitis. Acute inflammatory infiltrates as well as dense lymphoplasmacytic infiltrates are often seen around large intrahepatic bile ducts, while smaller portal tracts show the changes secondary to interference with bile flow with little inflammation only. This may account for the unusually mild inflammation sometimes

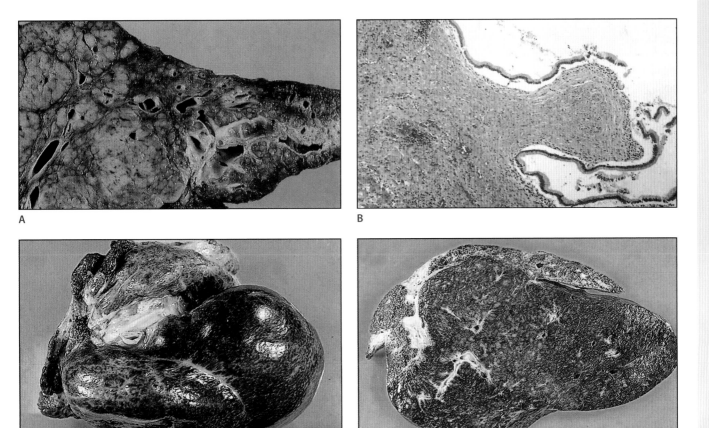

A

B

C

D

Fig. 11.43 • Primary sclerosing cholangitis with cirrhosis. **(A)** This liver shows a markedly and irregularly dilated duct almost reaching the capsular surface of an atrophic left lobe. Note intraductal fibrous webs and the prominent areas of confluent parenchymal collapse (dark staining) in the upper subcapsular portion of the lobe. **(B)** Histological illustration of an intraluminal fibrous web as seen in (A). H & E. **(C)** Inferior aspect of a grossly deformed liver showing massive expansion of left and caudate lobes contrasting with the markedly atrophic, cirrhotic right lobe. **(D)** Coronal section of the liver shown in (C); the cirrhotic right lobe is stretched at the periphery of the massively expanded caudate and left lobes which histologically showed stage 2 disease with marked features of regeneration and cholestasis.

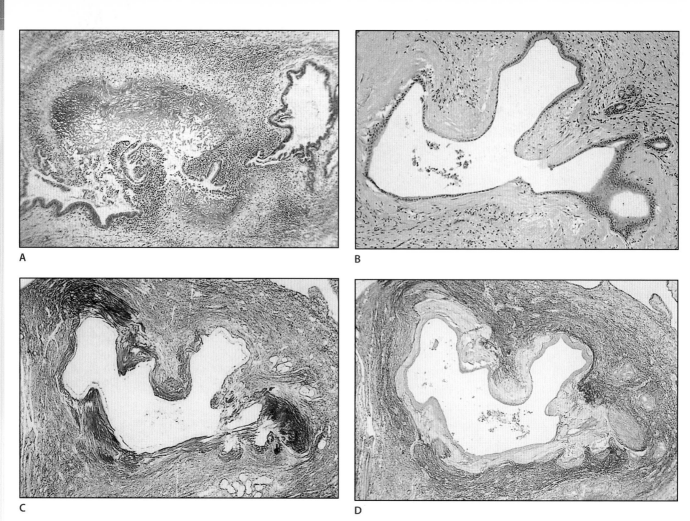

Fig. 11.44 • Primary sclerosing cholangitis. **(A)** Ulceration with bilirubin impregnation and inflammatory reaction in the wall of a large septal bile duct. H & E. A distorted septal duct with variably atrophic epithelial lining is stained with H & E in **(B)**, Gordon & Sweets reticulin in **(C),** and Shikata orcein in **(D)** to illustrate the uneven distribution and composition of the periductal scarring.

observed in the needle biopsy specimens of patients in whom clinical and laboratory features suggest an active autoimmune process. Occasionally, xanthogranulatous cholangitis, a lesion consisting of exuberant granulation tissue with prominent foamy macrophages, acute and chronic inflammation, fibrosis and foreign-body giant cells, can be found at the liver hilum. This lesion is similar to that found in the common bile duct and gallbladder and can be histologically similar to inflammatory pseudotumour. Bile extravasation into the tissue surrounding the damaged bile ducts is the likely cause. The change is said to carry an adverse effect on outcome after transplantation.[529]

In a few cases of undisputed PSC on cholangiography the changes are unexpectedly mild on liver biopsy. Conversely, there is a subgroup of patients with ulcerative colitis in whom histological features of PSC may be present or even advanced, but in whom ERCP examination is normal.[530] The apparent discrepancy between radiological and histological appearances at either end of the lesion spectrum emphasizes the heterogeneity of PSC, and the necessity for performing both cholangiography and liver biopsy to fully evaluate and stage the disease; indeed, each of the techniques provides information on essentially different segments of the biliary system.[531,532]

Treatment

Although immunosuppressive therapy added to ursodeoxycholic acid may alter the course of sclerosing cholangitis, particularly in children with autoimmune features,[533] in the majority of patients, it is of limited benefit and no specific treatment can arrest the progression of the disease. Sooner or later hepatic failure and complications of portal hypertension will develop and transplantation provides the only potential cure;[534] patients with PSC have a higher retransplantation rate and lower survival when compared to PBC.[535] The disease has been shown to recur with a prevalence, in various series, which ranges from 8.6 to 27% (see Chapter 16).[536,537] In that respect some controversy has arisen due to the difficulty in differentiating recurrent from acquired sclerosing cholangitis, especially from ischaemic cholangitis,[536] which in the liver graft may mimic the changes of PSC, but usually occurs at an early stage after transplantation.[537]

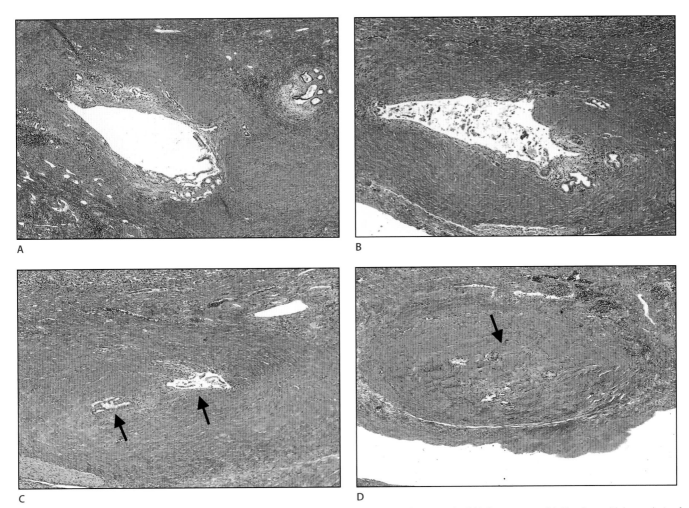

Fig. 11.45 • Semiserial sections of a large intrahepatic bile duct in PSC. **(A)** and **(B)** Periductal fibrosis and mild inflammatory cell infiltrations with hyperplasia of the peribiliary glands (intramural and extramural). **(C)** and **(D)** Fibrous narrowing and obliteration (arrows) of the lumen with few remnants of intramural glands. H & E.

Variant of primary sclerosing cholangitis

Primary sclerosing cholangitis—overlap autoimmune hepatitis ('autoimmune sclerosing cholangitis')

Autoimmune features are well recognized in both children[412,413,533] and adults with primary sclerosing cholangitis.[538-540] The most comprehensive study[513] evaluated 114 patients with PSC according to the scoring system proposed by the International Autoimmune Hepatitis Group for diagnosis of AIH.[541] Two of the patients scored above 15, satisfying the criterion for 'definite' AIH, whereas 33% of the patients scored between 10 and 15, falling into the category of 'probable' AIH. In these patients, bile-duct damage was indistinguishable from that seen in PSC without AIH features, but almost always involved the intrahepatic biliary tree. Another study recorded postinfantile giant cells in four adult cases.[542] PSC–AIH overlap in adults[538-540,542-544] is often associated with ulcerative colitis, and some patients showed a marked improvement once immunosuppressive therapy was combined with ursodeoxycholic acid treatment. These overlaps with AIH can occur simultaneously or sequentially[543-544] As with Mutatori et al.,[545] our experience is that an overlap AIH with PSC is more frequent than with

PBC, but the contrary is found in one study;[546] a difference possibly reflecting different patient selection or criteria used, particularly in the borderline AIH–PBC and AMA-negative ANA-positive PBC.

Autoimmune features seem more common in children.[412,413,547,548] In a prospective study of 55 consecutive children with clinical, serological and histological manifestations typical of AIH, 50% had bile-duct abnormalities diagnostic of sclerosing cholangitis on cholangiography performed at presentation.[548] Histologically, cholangitic changes and biliary interface activity was more frequent among, though not exclusive to, those with bile-duct damage on ERCP and one patient progressed from a normal ERCP to one typical of sclerosing cholangitis over an 8-year period. Histopathologists should be aware of this overlap between the two conditions, particularly in the young patient, when subtle biliary features, especially copper-associated protein deposition, may be an indication to perform an ERCP. Autoimmune phenomena have been described in at least one case of sclerosing cholangitis with a perinatal onset;[549] other such cases may be familial,[550] possibly a type of progressive intrahepatic cholestasis waiting for enzymatic and genetic characterization.

Acquired sclerosing cholangitis

The acquired forms of sclerosing cholangitis in which the radiological findings are similar to those of PSC are summarized in Table 11.5.

The condition may occur in patients with primary or acquired immunodeficiency syndromes and in whom chronic biliary infection is involved in the pathogenesis. In patients with AIDS, acalculous cholecystitis, sclerosing cholangitis and/or papillary stenosis (AIDS cholangiopathy) are well recognized,[551–554] and cryptosporidiosis and/or CMV infection coexist in up to 80% of patients (see Chapter 9). One study of patients with AIDS-related sclerosing cholangitis described, in 25% of patients, intraluminal polypoidal defects at ERCP, which microscopically consisted of exuberant granulation tissue.[553] In one patient with HIV infection but no previous AIDS-defining illness, ERCP features of sclerosing cholangitis were related to disseminated B-cell lymphoma and improved following chemotherapy.[555]

A few cases have been reported in children with congenital immunodeficiency syndromes (see Chapters 5 and 17), particularly boys suffering from X-linked immunodeficiency with hyper-IgM,[556] often in conjunction with chronic *Cryptosporidium* infection of the gastrointestinal tract.[557,558] Sclerosing cholangitis has been shown to relapse in transplanted immunodeficient children owing to reinfection of the biliary tree,[559] but one patient has been successfully treated with combined liver and non-myeloablative bone marrow transplantation, the latter allowing restoration of the immune system while avoiding the hepatotoxicity of the conditioning regimen.[560] The lesion has been reproduced by infecting immunodeficient mice with *Cryptosporidium*.[561] *Cryptosporidium parvum* is shown in vitro to trigger host cell apoptosis in bystander uninfected biliary epithelial cells,

which may limit spread of the infection, while it directly activates the NF-κB/I(κ)B system in infected biliary epithelia, thus protecting infected cells from death and facilitating parasite survival and propagation.[562] Cholangiocellular, hepatocellular and pancreatic carcinomas have complicated sclerosing cholangitis and cirrhosis in a few immunodeficient patients.[563]

Sclerosing cholangitis has occurred following rupture of hydatid cysts into the biliary tree,[564] more often as a complication of surgical treatment in which the cysts had been injected with scolicidal solutions, such as 2% formaldehyde or 20% sodium chloride.[565] In these patients, leakage through a cystic–biliary connection is supposed to produce a caustic sclerosing cholangitis similar to that induced experimentally.[566]

Sclerosing cholangitis has also been observed in up to 56% of patients receiving intra-arterial infusion of fluorodeoxyuridine (FUDR) for palliative treatment of liver metastases from colorectal adenocarcinoma (see also Chapter 14).[159,567–569] The cholangitis was assumed to be caused by the toxic effect of FUDR;[567,568] an ischaemic aetiology was later considered,[569] and was supported by the demonstration of obliterative changes in the periductal arteries in these livers.[159] Bile-duct scarring has also been produced experimentally by ethanol embolization of the hepatic artery in monkeys.[570] Ischaemic cholangitis is a well-documented complication of arterial occlusion in the liver allograft leading to changes that closely resemble those of sclerosing cholangitis (Chapter 16).

Langerhans cell histiocytosis (histiocytosis X) may produce a picture of sclerosing cholangitis, both in children[571] and adults.[572] This seems to follow infiltration of the bile ducts by Langerhans cell granulomatous tissue (Chapter 4). Langerhans cell histiocytosis with sclerosing cholangitis has been associated with a low rate of recurrence after liver transplantation,[573] but an apparently high incidence of post-transplant lymphoproliferative disease.[574] Increased immunosuppression due to the high incidence of refractory rejection in these children might have been partly responsible.[574]

Finally, mention should be made of a radiological and clinical syndrome identical to PSC which may develop secondary to extrahepatic portal vein obstruction.[575] The change is thought to be the result of choledochal varices, part of the collateral system bypassing the portal venous block, but these have yet to be demonstrated morphologically.[575,576]

Pathology of the peribiliary glands

Because of their location, most observations on the pathology of the peribiliary glands have been made at autopsy,[5,8,577] or in livers removed at transplantation. Accordingly, clinicopathological correlation studies are few and mainly deal with cystic and hyperplastic changes.[577–580] Thus, the clinical significance is uncertain and a role for these structures as the primary site of the necroinflammatory process in chronic cholangiopathy affecting the major bile ducts remains speculative.

Table 11.5	Disorders leading to secondary sclerosing cholangitis

Infectious
  Cryptosporidiosis and/or CMV infection
  Primary immunodeficiency (CD40 ligand, combined immunodeficiency)
  Secondary immunodeficiency (AIDS cholangiopathy)
  Hydatid cysts (rupture)

Ischaemic
  Liver allograft: thrombotic or foam cell arteriopathy
  Intra-arterial infusion chemotherapy
  Radiation injury
  Recurrent pyogenic cholangitis

Toxic (caustic)
  Scolicidal hydatic cyst injection

Neoplastic
  Langerhans cell histiocytosis
  Malignant infiltration (rare)

Mechanical
  Choledochal varices (portal vein block, cavernous transformation)

Necroinflammatory and degenerative changes

Necroinflammatory changes (peribiliary adenitis) usually include lymphoplasmacytic cell infiltration and variable glandular epithelial swelling, vacuolation or eosinophilic necrosis (Fig. 11.46A,B).[580] Suppurative peribiliary adenitis and fibroplasia is a common accompaniment of hepatolithiasis as well as of various liver conditions, including cirrhosis, submassive hepatocellular necrosis and ascending cholangitis.[580] In GVHD, bizarre nuclei and acidophilic cytoplasm[69] resemble the characteristic changes seen in small interlobular bile ducts and ductules (see Chapter 16) (Fig. 11.46B). Peribiliary glands are also involved in PSC as an extension of the inflammatory process.[68] In biliary atresia, the peribiliary glands are thought to undergo necroinflammatory destruction[581] as well as hyperplastic changes, which may reflect a transient attempt at bile drainage through paraductal anastomosing channels after occlusion of the main duct lumen. It seems plausible that severe adenitis will be followed by extensive loss of peribiliary glands, although the clinical and pathological consequences of this remains undetermined. The glands may be also affected in systemic amyloidosis (Fig. 11.46C).[582]

Peribiliary cysts (multiple hilar cysts)

Peribiliary cysts involving the hilar and perihilar regions are not uncommon.[583] They are located around, and are thought to arise from, the peribiliary glands of the large intrahepatic bile ducts. The cysts are usually multiple, ranging in size from a few millimetres to 1 cm, rarely up to 3 cm (Fig. 11.47A–C). Similar peribiliary cysts have been detected grossly and radiologically within the extrahepatic biliary tree in a few cases. On cholangiography, the cysts appear non-communicating with the lumen of the large bile ducts.[584] Peribilary cysts appear to have at least two pathogeneses.[583] Some appear acquired, as suggested by their preferential occurrence in cirrhotic livers, in portal vein thrombosis, or in idiopathic portal hypertension;[584–587] in this context, they may be used as markers of disease progression as their number and size increase in parallel with the advancing liver disease. Others seem of developmental origin given their detection on CT scan in 73% of polycystic livers associated with autosomal dominant polycystic kidney disease (ADPKD) and also in association with solitary simple cysts.[588]

The content of the cysts is mainly serous; their walls are thin, occasionally transparent. Histologically, the grossly visible cysts are usually associated with variably dilated peribiliary glands, suggesting developmental stages in the process. There may be associated inflammation and hyperplasia of the epithelial lining, which expresses c-MET protein, the HGF receptor.[585] Although the cysts are incidentally found during radiological examination or on livers removed at transplantation or autopsy, they occasionally cause compression of the biliary tree with intrahepatic biliary dilatation, bile stasis or cholangitis, and jaundice or cholangitis may be presenting symptoms.[589]

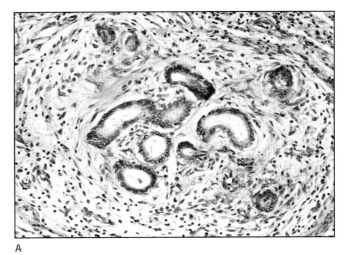

A

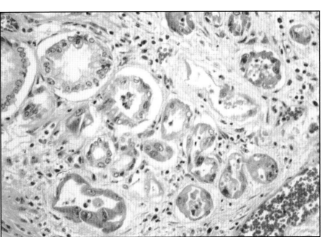

B

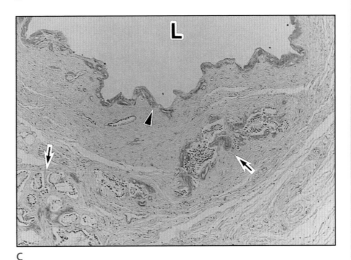

C

Fig. 11.46 • Necroinflammatory and degenerative changes of peribiliary glands. **(A)** There are focal cytopathic changes of acinar cells with interstitial oedema and sparse lymphoid cells. Case of ascending bacterial cholangitis. H & E. **(B)** Acinar cells show acidophilic cytoplasmic change, nuclear pleomorphism and sloughing into the acinar lumen. Graft-versus-host disease. H & E. **(C)** Deposition of amlyoid underneath the epithelial lining (arrowhead) and around the intramural and extramural peribiliary glands (arrows) of a large bile duct (L, lumen). Direct fast scarlet for amyloid.

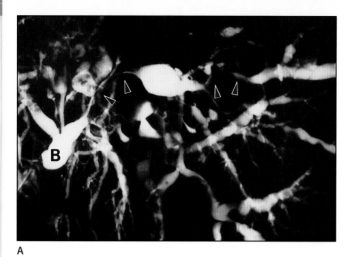

A

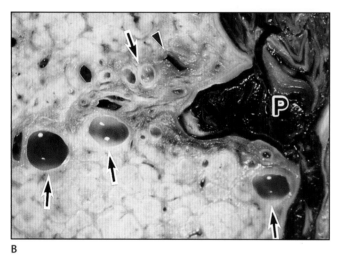

B

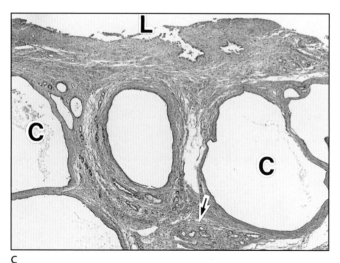

C

Fig. 11.47 • Peribiliary cysts. **(A)** Post-mortem cholangiogram in a case of alcoholic cirrhosis. The intrahepatic bile ducts show focal dilatation and compression, the latter due to peribiliary cysts (arrowheads) (B, common bile duct). **(B)** Cut section through the hilar region of a cirrhotic liver due to chronic hepatitis B. There are several peribiliary cysts (arrows) (arrowhead, intrahepatic bile duct). The portal vein (P) is occluded by fresh thrombus. **(C)** Histologically, the cysts (C) are intimately associated with peribiliary glands (arrow) in the large bile-duct wall (L, bile-duct lumen). H & E.

The cysts are radiologically visible and small cysts along the portal veins correspond to the periportal collar and abnormal signal intensity seen on CT and on MR scan respectively.[584] Ultrasound shows round or tubular anechoic lesions around the large portal tracts which mimic dilatation of the bile ducts. In about half of the cirrhotic cases the peribiliary cysts gradually increase in size and number. Peribiliary cysts must be differentiated from dilatation of bile ducts or oedema of portal tracts. Ahmadi et al.[590] reported that enlarged peribiliary cysts presented a central dot sign on contrasted CT such as is seen in Caroli disease. PSC and papillary tumour of the bile ducts also enter the differential diagnoses of peribiliary cysts.

Hilar peribiliary cysts have been reported as a rare post-transplant biliary tract complication,[578] occurring in 2.6% of 493 consecutive liver transplants; three patients had obstructive jaundice while the other 10 were identified by systematic search in the hepatic hilum. Two types were identified: (i) blind unilocular cavities, ranging between 0.5 and 5.5 cm in diameter, with viscid mucous content (mucoceles), located adjacent to the biliary tract anastomoses and thought to have arisen from sequestered remnants of the cystic duct; and (ii) cystically dilated peribiliary glands with multilocular, occasionally multiple cavities ranging from 0.5 to 2 cm in diameter; these were located adjacent to the left, right or common hepatic duct.

Hyperplasia of peribiliary glands

Hyperplasia of the peribiliary glands may be observed in association with a variety of hepatobiliary disorders, especially hepatolithiasis (Fig. 11.48A,B) or in apparently normal livers.[5,8,577] It may be multifocal or less often diffuse and involve intramural glands and/or extramural serous and mucinous acini in various combinations. Unfamiliarity with this pathology can lead to an erroneous diagnosis of well-differentiated cholangiocarcinoma.

Multifocal hyperplasia is characterized by both an increased number of glands and epithelial hyperplasia. Hyperplasia of extramural serous acini is more commonly associated with intrahepatic cholangitis and submassive hepatic necrosis, while hyperplasia of extramural mucous acini with increased mucus secretion is observed in cirrhosis, submassive hepatic necrosis, cholangitis, systemic infection and extrahepatic biliary obstruction. The change may resemble the pseudopyloric gland metaplasia observed in chronic cholecystitis.

Exceptionally, the lesion is focal and may simulate a tumour, with nodules up to 4 cm recorded. It may lead to stenosis of the biliary lumen and occasionally the lesion appears as an intraductal papillary neoplasm covered by non-neoplastic epithelium. A variant of hyperplasia with florid proliferative changes and intense inflammation of intramural glands—*glandularis proliferans*—may affect both intrahepatic and extrahepatic bile ducts.[591] It resembles changes seen in PSC, but usually affects women and is not associated with chronic inflammatory bowel disease.

Proliferation of intramural glands—*adenomatous hyperplasia*—with active secretion of mucin is also seen around

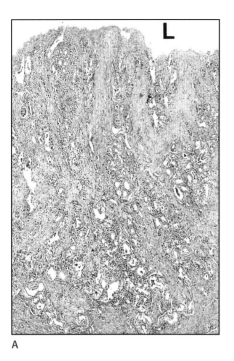 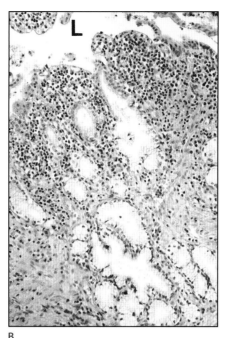

Fig. 11.48 • Hyperplasia of peribiliary glands in hepatolithiasis. **(A)** The bile-duct wall is fibrous and contains hyperplastic extramural as well as intramural glands (L, bile-duct lumen). H & E. **(B)** The intramural mucinous glands are prominent and surrounded by lymphoid cells (L, bile-duct lumen). H & E.

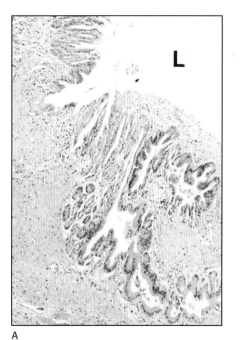 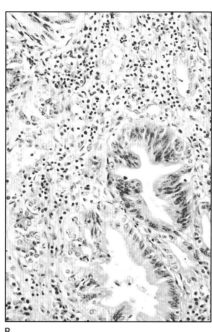

Fig. 11.49 • Dysplasia of peribiliary glands in hepatolithiasis. **(A)** Hyperplastic peribiliary glands with foci of mild dysplasia (L, bile-duct lumen). H & E. **(B)** There is nuclear hyperchromasia and stratification. H & E.

intrahepatic bile ducts containing calculi (see Hepatolithiasis below), or homing adult worms of *Clonorchis sinensis*.[592]

Diffuse peribiliary gland hyperplasia with a variable degree of cystic dilatation around intrahepatic and extrahepatic bile ducts[579] occurs in apparently normal liver or in liver with massive necrosis. One case of a 54-year-old man with obstructive jaundice due to compression of the extrahepatic bile ducts by diffuse periductal glandular hyperplasia with profuse mucinous secretion has been reported.[593]

Dysplasia and neoplasia of peribiliary glands

It has been suggested that some cholangiocarcinomas (especially those associated with PSC and hepatolithiasis) and other neoplasms may arise from peribiliary glands. Hyperplastic and dysplastic changes are frequent in these structures (Fig. 11.49A,B),[36,594,595] and a multistep manner of proliferation through hyperplasia, dysplasia, non-invasive adenocarcinoma and invasive adenocarcinoma is well recognized in the biliary tree.[36,596]

The rare hepatobiliary cystadenoma and cystadenocarcinoma harbour chromogranin-positive cells, which are otherwise exclusively located in the normal or proliferating intrahepatic peribiliary glands.[596] Dilated peribiliary glands containing endocrine cells were closely associated in three-quarters of the cases examined.[597]

The so-called bile-duct adenoma was shown to share the same two antigens expressed by intramural mucous glands and extramural tubuloalveolar seromucinous glands, suggesting that this lesion may represent a hamartoma derived from peribiliary glands.[598]

Isolated idiopathic bile ductular hyperplasia

An isolated ductular reaction in the absence of other histopathological changes is occasionally encountered in liver biopsies. This change was noted in 70 of 1235 patients studied by Sonzogni et al.[599] Of these, 16 had no identifiable aetiology. These patients had a mean age of 38 and were asymptomatic but had persistent low-grade abnormalities in LFTs including elevations of ALT and γGT. Histologically, the ductular reaction in these cases lacked accompanying inflammatory change and the epithelium comprised mature EMA-positive/NCAM-negative ductules. The long-term significance of this 'condition' remains to be determined.

Hepatolithiasis and recurrent pyogenic cholangitis

These two diseases are seen predominantly in the Far East and, to a lesser extent in Asian immigrants to the West, while they are rare among Caucasians.[600,601] The reasons for this geographical or racial prevalence remain unclear. In Japan and Taiwan, hepatolithiasis is decreasing, but it is still prevalent in Korea.[602] Many of their clinical and pathological features overlap and in many instances a clear distinction between the two conditions is difficult as recurrent pyogenic cholangitis can both cause and complicate hepatolithiasis.

Primary hepatolithiasis

Hepatolithiasis is characterized by the presence of calculi, usually multiple, in dilated intrahepatic bile ducts. Two types of intrahepatic stones have been identified: (i) brown pigment (calcium bilirubinate) and black-coloured mixed stones, by far the more common; and (ii) pure cholesterol stones.[603] Primary intrahepatic stones are formed de novo within the liver and, on the basis of distinctive pathogenesis, chemical composition and clinical course, they should be distinguished from stones which have migrated from the extrahepatic biliary tree[604,605] (see Chapter 12).

Calcium bilirubinate stones (brown pigment stones)
Hepatolithiasis commonly affects middle-aged and elderly people, but only occasional teenagers, in East Asian countries. Classically, hepatolithiasis is a progressive illness presenting with bouts of fever, abdominal pain, and ultimately death from acute bacterial cholangitis and sepsis. Recently, probably owing to improvement in hygiene and better control of bacterial infection, the incidence of the disease has decreased in Japan, including rural areas and islands.[604] Asymptomatic cases in whom stones are incidentally detected are occasionally encountered in these areas. Interventional radiology and minimal surgical treatment has been successfully applied, but there is still a significant number of patients who either remain undetected or have

a long clinical course which will eventually be complicated by the development of cholangiocarcinoma.[595,606]

Grossly, the intrahepatic bile ducts show irregular dilatations of their lumen which alternate with areas of relative stenosis (Fig. 11.50A). Calcium-bilirubinate stones and biliary sludge (Fig. 11.50B) are impacted in the dilated portions of the ducts which have thickened walls due to inflammation and fibrosis extending into the surrounding tissue. These changes are absent in the unaffected segment(s) or lobe. Biliary abscesses are associated in some cases.

Histologically, the bile ducts show marked fibrosis and a variable degree of multifocal hyperplasia of the peribiliary glands[607] which contain large amounts of acid and neutral mucin.[31] There is a variable lymphoplasmacytic cell infiltration which may include the formation of lymphoid follicles. Mast cells are also found and thought to contribute to the fibrosing process. The term *'chronic proliferative cholangitis'* is used collectively for these bile-duct lesions.

The aetiology of hepatolithiasis is as yet unknown and, in the majority of cases, no predisposing disease is identified. Bacterial infection,[9,145,146] bile stasis and hypersecretion of mucus are the common denominators of the disorder, in

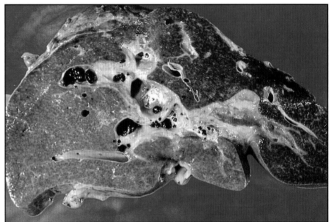

A

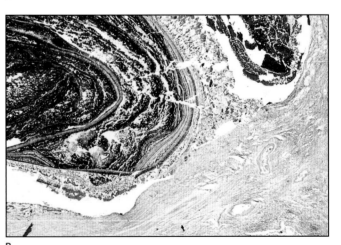

B

Fig. 11.50 • Hepatolithiasis with calcium bilirubinate stones. **(A)** The cut surface of an autopsy liver shows irregularly dilated and thick-walled bile ducts with some black stones remaining in their lumen. **(B)** The cut surface of the stones show lamellar pigment layers, characteristic of calcium bilirubinate stones. H & E.

which the mucus profile differs from that present in other hepatobiliary diseases.[31] In particular, gastric phenotypes of apomucin are important because these molecules form gel, and thus may contribute to stone formation, whereas MUC3, the constitutive mucin of the biliary tree, lacks this property. Calcium bilirubinate stones form in bile with a high cholesterol saturation and have significantly more cholesterol, and less calcium bilirubinate and bile acid, than the stones found in the extrahepatic bile ducts.[604,605] In primary hepatolithiasis, hepatic hyposecretion of phospholipids due to decreased multidrug resistance P-glycoprotein 3 (MDR3) expression levels may contribute to the formation of aggressive bile-duct lesions through a decreased formation of mixed micelles,[608] but the decreased transcription levels of MDR3 in the liver are not due to mutations detected in the *ABCB4* coding region of the gene.[609]

Pure cholesterol stones

Pure cholesterol stones are less common. Cholangitis or fever is the usual presentation, but the clinical symptoms are mild.[610] Like the calcium bilirubinate stones, they are mainly encountered in the Asian population.[611] The patients show excellent clinical outcome despite impaired bilioenteric drainage. Grossly, the cholesterol stones are impacted in (Fig. 11.51A) and easily removed from the lumen of the intrahepatic biliary tree. In comparison with calcium-bilirubinate stones, bile-duct inflammation, fibrous wall thickening, bile sludging and glandular hyperplasia are significantly less.[612] Foreign body reaction against cholesterol crystals may be seen at the periphery of the cholesterol stones. Cholesterol deposits are also present in both small bile ducts (Fig. 11.51B) and peribiliary glands.

Secondary hepatolithiasis

It must be mentioned that hepatolithiasis occurs in developmental disorders such as Caroli disease,[613] solitary cystic dilatation of the biliary tree and hepatobiliary malfunctions, usually in association with ulceration and infection of the cyst walls. Intrahepatic bile sludging and stone formation is also a known complication in various conditions where there is cholangiodestruction and/or biliary abscess formation, for example extrahepatic biliary atresia and ischaemic and/or suppurative cholangitis, in particular in the liver allograft (see Chapter 16). In these situations, cavities containing bile concretions are lined partly by biliary epithelium and partly by inflamed and sclerosing granulation tissue, so-called pseudo-Caroli cysts. Bile sludges reveal a collagen skeleton, suggesting their origin from sloughed-off portions of the necrotic bile-duct wall which may have acted as a nidus for subsequent bile precipitation.[614]

Recurrent pyogenic cholangitis

Recurrent pyogenic cholangitis is also a disease of the Far East,[615] but an increasing number of cases are reported in the West, mainly in Asian immigrants.[616]

Clinically, recurrent pyogenic cholangitis is characterized by abdominal pain, fever, chills and jaundice due to

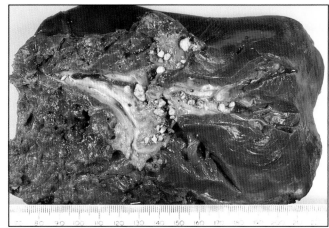

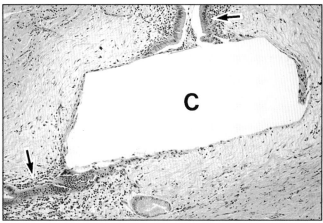

Fig. 11.51 • Hepatolithiasis with cholesterol stones. **(A)** Surgically resected liver whose dilated bile ducts have been cut open to show impacted cholesterol stones in the dilated intrahepatic biliary tree. **(B)** Segmental dilatation of a septal bile duct with a rectangular shaped lumen previously occupied by a cholesterol crystal (C). Arrows show normal bile duct on both sides.

recurrent attacks of suppurative cholangitis. *Clonorchis sinensis* or other parasites used to be detected in 30–40% of autopsy livers.[617] A recent case–control study shows that helminthiasis including ascariasis or clonorchiasis is a possible risk factor for hepatolithiasis in a small number of cases, and the patients with helminthiasis tend to have a history of an asymptomatic interval between the periods of recurrent abdominal pain in their childhood and the diagnosis of hepatolithiasis in their adulthood.[618] Enteric organisms, chiefly *E. coli*, can be cultured from bile in 95% of patients and from the portal blood during acute attacks.[619] Bacteria are believed to be in part responsible for the formation of stones as a result of bilirubin glucuronide deconjugation by bacterial E1-glucuronidase.[146]A low-protein oriental diet contributes to decreased bile levels of glucaro-1 : 4-lactone that normally inhibits E1-glucuronidase.[620] The role of diet and of nutritional deficiency can account for the higher prevalence in rural areas of Japan.[620]

Cholangiographic findings[615] include bile-duct stones, disproportionately severe dilatation of the extrahepatic ducts and straightening, rigidity, decreased arborization and an increased branching angle of the intrahepatic bile ducts. Sonography and CT scanning show intra- or extrahepatic duct stones, prominent dilatation of the extrahepatic ducts, localized dilatation of the segmental bile ducts, and segmental hepatic atrophy.

Morphologically, extrahepatic and large intrahepatic bile ducts show chronic and acute cholangitis with fibrosis and hyperplasia of the peribiliary glands. Both intra- and extrahepatic bile ducts contain soft, pigmented stones and pus. Liver abscesses are variably seen.[616]

The distinction between hepatolithiasis and recurrent pyogenic cholangitis is not always clear as they share many clinicopathological features and the latter can variably appear as a cause or a complication of hepatolithiasis.

Chronic cholangitis and cholangiocarcinoma

In PSC, hepatolithiasis, recurrent pyogenic cholangitis and infestation with liver flukes and longstanding inflammation and destruction of the intra- and/or extrahepatic bile ducts promote hyperplastic and dysplastic changes in the biliary epithelium and peribiliary glands.[36,595] This ultimately leads to the development of cholangiocarcinoma.[55,596] The concomitant or sequential demonstration of dysplasia, carcinoma in situ and foci of microinvasive carcinoma in various parts of the biliary tree suggest a multicentric and multistep carcinogenesis (Fig. 11.7A,B).[594] The dysregulation of apoptosis and increased cell proliferation during cholangiocellular carcinogenesis have been shown to be a multistep process;[55,57] shift of proto-oncogenes to oncogenes and deletion, mutation or functional inactivation of tumour suppressor genes or their products have been particularly well studied in the preneoplastic and neoplastic biliary epithelium.[55,57,594–596,621] Epidemiological and clinicopathological aspects of cholangiocarcinoma are presented in Chapter 15.

Diseases affecting mainly the extrahepatic bile ducts

Large duct obstruction (extrahepatic cholestasis)

The large bile ducts outside the liver or within the porta hepatis may be primarily affected by miscellaneous disorders which have in common the production of mechanical obstruction of the duct lumen—extrahepatic or 'surgical' cholestasis as opposed to intrahepatic or 'medical' cholestasis. This distinction has now been rendered somewhat artificial as the transplant surgeons correct certain causes of 'medical' jaundice and interventional gastroenterologists and radiologists now correct certain causes of 'surgical' jaundice.[622] In addition, the distinction between extra- and intrahepatic obstruction is not always a watertight one, especially when hilar ducts are involved.

The main diseases producing large duct obstruction are listed in Table 11.6.[623–634] Some of the diseases have already been discussed in this chapter, in particular PSC, acquired sclerosing cholangitis and recurrent pyogenic cholangitis,

Table 11.6	Causes of large bile-duct obstruction

Adults (+/– children)

Choledocholithiasis mostly originated from the gallbladder (Ch. 12) (+/– Suppurative cholangitis)

Recurrent pyogenic cholangitis (Far East) (see previous section)

Primary sclerosing cholangitis (localized strictures)

Acquired sclerosing cholangitis
Langerhans cell histiocytosis (Ch. 4)
Cryptosporidiosis (primary and secondary immunodeficiency) (p. 558 and Ch. 9)

Biliary stricture (postbiliary tract surgery)

Inflammatory stricture of the CHD secondary to cholelithiasis and cholecystitis (Mirizzi syndrome)[623]

Inflammatory polyps

Blunt (rare) or penetrating trauma

Parasitic invasion: *Clonorchis sinensis*, *Ascariasis lumbricoides*, *Fasciola hepatica*, *Strongyloides stercoralis* (Ch. 9)

Aneurysm of the hepatic or gastroduodenal artery

Pancreatitis, pancreatic pseudocyst

Penetrating duodenal ulcer

Annular pancreas (after positive exclusion of other causes)[624]

Amyloid deposition[625]

In liver allograft (Ch. 16) anastomotic strictures, ischaemic cholangitis, amputation neuroma[626]

Neoplasms (Ch. 15)
Papillary adenoma (single, multiple); simple adenoma
Rare benign neoplasm: granular cell tumour, leiomyoma, lipoma
Ampullary adenocarcinoma (lower end of CBD, pancreas, rarely duodenal mucosa)
Bile-duct carcinoma (papillary and/or scirrhous adenocarcinoma)
High-duct carcinoma (Klatskin tumour)[627]
Hepatocellular carcinoma invading bile ducts[628]
Carcinoid tumour[629]
Primary and metastatic tumours of the head of pancreas

Children (Ch. 4)
Extrahepatic biliary atresia
Choledochal cysts, choledococele
Inspissated bile plug syndrome[630]
Benign biliary strictures (common channel, idiopathic, radiotherapy)[639]
Spontaneous perforation of the bile ducts[631]
Extramural compression (Ladd bands in malrotation of the mid-gut)[632]
Gastric heterotopy in common bile duct[633]
Embryonal rhabdomyosarcoma of the bile duct[634]

Abbreviations: CBD, common bile duct; CHD, common hepatic duct; HCC, hepatocellular carcinoma

but they are listed here as they may predominantly affect the extrahepatic biliary tree and produce localized strictures. As the various conditions leading to extrahepatic biliary obstruction include developmental, necroinflammatory and neoplastic disorders in both children and adults, several are discussed in detail in other chapters and appropriate cross-references are given in Table 11.6.

Clinical features and diagnosis

Persistent jaundice with a predominant elevation of alkaline phosphatase and a prothrombin time that is normal or normalizes with vitamin K administration always raises the possibility of extrahepatic biliary obstruction. Abdominal pain, fever, rigors, prior biliary surgery and older age are features that favour a biliary obstruction. Colicky pain will suggest cholelithiasis, whereas severe painless jaundice in adults makes a malignant obstruction likely until proven otherwise. This is particularly true if there are no gallstones and the gallbladder is markedly dilated (Courvoisier sign), a sign which is obviously lacking when dealing with hilar tumours. An early diagnosis is important as surgery or interventional radiology can relieve the obstruction before septic complications or irreversible liver damage develop.

As a rule, ultrasonography is the first investigation which, in about a quarter of patients, will detect dilated intra- or extrahepatic bile ducts. Such a finding indicates the need for ERCP or percutaneous cholangiography, techniques which have the advantage over a liver biopsy of providing information on the level, if not the cause, of a biliary obstruction. Thus, liver biopsy is now only rarely performed. Nevertheless, with early, incomplete and/or proximal duct obstruction, bile ducts may fail to dilate, and a needle biopsy can be taken and occasionally provides the first hint that a patient may have extrahepatic biliary tract obstruction. Histopathologists should therefore be aware of the early changes which point to an obstructive cholangiopathy.

Pathology of large-duct obstruction

Our knowledge comes from earlier studies dealing with large numbers of biopsy specimens[635,636] as well as from animal experiments. The precise chronology of the changes is indeed difficult to evaluate in man where sequential specimens cannot be obtained. In addition, the changes in the liver depend not only on the duration and degree of obstruction, but also on superimposed infection, and the respective part played by mechanical duct obstruction per se. The histological changes are grouped into early and later manifestations.

Early lesions (first 2 weeks)
The earliest changes usually consist of perivenular bilirubinostasis, followed by portal tract oedema and inflammation. The presence of bilirubinostasis alone in some patients with early obstruction causes problems of differentiation from other conditions causing 'bland' or 'pure' cholestasis,

such as benign recurrent, drug-induced, infection-associated, or postoperative cholestasis.

Bilirubinostasis starts in the perivenular regions. It is characterized by the appearance of fine bilirubin granules in the cytoplasm of hepatocytes and bile plugs or concretions within variably dilated and shaped intercellular spaces (see Fig. 11.15). Some are located in cholestatic liver-cell rosettes, i.e. they are surrounded by three or more liver cells (see Fig. 11.16). Some bile concretions are PAS-positive; these are probably older. Calcium can be detected in bile plugs.[637] Single liver-cell necroses and acidophil bodies may be found, but cellular pleomorphism with the ballooning characteristic of a viral hepatitis is not a feature.[171] Kupffer cells often become prominent.

Portal tract oedema develops early[636] and is more pronounced in the smaller terminal ramifications. In medium-sized portal tracts the oedema causes a concentric periductal lamellar arrangement of the collagen fibres.[638] Biliolymphatic reflux[639] is held responsible for the portal oedema, activation of fibroblasts and infiltration of inflammatory cells[635,636] with a predominance of histiocytes and neutrophil leukocytes.

Ductular reaction occurs early and can be better visualized by immunostaining for bile-duct cytokeratins 7 or 19.[175] The reactive ductules have a recognizable lumen lined by cuboidal cells and surrounded by a PAS-D positive basement membrane.[635] The reactive ductules are almost always accompanied by a neutrophil polymorphonuclear infiltration in close relationship to, and even within, their basement membrane, so-called cholangiolitis, a pattern which is also seen, though generally less extensive, in diseases of the intrahepatic bile ducts, such as PBC (see Fig. 11.20C). This marginal bile ductular reaction has been reported to be present in 82% of portal areas in biopsy specimens with extrahepatic obstruction.[640]

Later lesions (several weeks to months)
With continuing obstruction, the parenchymal and portal changes become more pronounced and biliary periportal interface activity with cholate stasis develops, similar to that seen in chronic cholangitis affecting the intrahepatic bile ducts. However, in extrahepatic obstruction, bilirubinostasis is consistently more prominent. Intercellular bile plugs increase in number and size and some inspissated concrements may become very large and, with time, cholestasis extends to the periportal zone. There is an increasing number of 'cholestatic liver-cell rosettes'[167] of which lumens of variable size may appear empty, or may contain a precipitate of lightly bile-stained material or densely inspissated bile concrements.

Isolated (or groups of) hepatocytes, adjacent to plugs or concrements, or with no topographical relationship to biliary deposits, are enlarged and show a rarefaction of their cytoplasm which is reduced to a fine reticular net, sometimes impregnated with bilirubin, so-called feathery degeneration (Fig. 11.52A).[641] The changes may be difficult to differentiate from groups of histiocytes with foamy lipid-laden cytoplasm which are variably present (Fig. 11.52B). Lytic or acidophilic necrosis of liver cells leads to rupture of

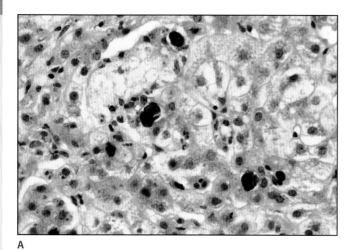

Fig. 11.52 • Large duct obstruction. **(A)** Hepatocytes adjacent to large bile concrements show a rarefied and reticular appearance of their cytoplasm with a light pigmentation—feathery degeneration. H & E. **(B)** Parenchymal accumulation of foamy histiocytes (xanthomatous cells). H & E.

canaliculi and release of bile plugs and concrements, which become surrounded by macrophages. Single (or groups of) large bulky macrophages may be found, with a voluminous cytoplasm, containing recognizable bile plugs and large amounts of PAS-positive ceroid pigment derived from phagocytosed cell debris.

Feathery degeneration of confluent liver-cell groups near portal tracts and their subsequent lytic necrosis are termed bile infarcts (Fig. 11.53A).[641] Large bile infarcts are diagnostic of extrahepatic cholestasis, although smaller areas of such biliary necrosis can occur in intrahepatic forms of cholestasis.[641] Large bile infarcts (Fig. 11.53B) show extensive lytic necrosis with irregular empty spaces and loosely arranged, bile-impregnated, reticulin fibres and necrobiotic cells; they are surrounded by a zone of hepatocytes showing feathery degeneration.[166] Bile infarcts appear to be caused by the toxic action of retained bile constituents, especially bile salts, combined with the injurious effect of increased biliary pressure.[642,643] Necrotic areas of bile infarcts are gradually replaced by fibrous scarring (Fig. 11.53C). Large concrements in bile ducts may lead to necrosis of the lining epithelium and extravasation of bile. Such biliary extravasates elicit a phagocytic reaction, often including

multinucleated foreign-body giant cells (Fig. 11.53D). Large bile infarcts and bile extravasates are rarely seen, as they are rather late changes and currently an early diagnosis generally leads to curative surgery or relief of the obstruction by insertion of a stent.

With incomplete relief or partial obstruction, subsequent changes at the interface recapitulate those observed in disorders of the intrahepatic bile ducts and in PSC. These findings include biliary interface activity with progressive ductular reaction, cholate stasis, copper accumulation, Mallory bodies and fibroplasia. The neoductules extend beyond the limits of the portal tract towards neighbouring portal tracts and invade the parenchyma, and are accompanied by fibroblastic proliferation. In large-duct obstruction the lumens of the ducts and ductules may be irregularly dilated and their lining cells may show various degenerative changes including anisocytosis, cytoplasmic vacuolation, nuclear pyknosis and epithelial sloughing (Fig. 11.54).

Larger interlobular bile ducts may show tortuosity and branching, and occasionally signs of damage to their lining cells or sloughing of the epithelium. The lumen appears variably empty or filled with mucoid material or biliary precipitate with or without neutrophilic polymorphs. Larger inspissated biliary concrements may lead to ulceration of the epithelial lining, whereas other areas may show epithelial hyperplasia with micropapillary projections. Periductal fibrosis interferes with the ductal blood supply from the periductal capillary plexus, resulting in progressive atrophy and even disappearance of the duct (secondary ischaemic cholangitis),[643] although the process is generally less extensive than in small intrahepatic bile-duct diseases such as PBC and PSC.

Superimposed infection: suppurative cholangitis

Ascending infection is suspected when dense collections of neutrophilic polymorphs obscure ducts and ductules and aggregate within their lumens. Pus in the lumen is sometimes associated with damage to the lining epithelium and, in severe infection, abscesses form (see Fig. 11.8A). Severe suppurative cholangitis is more often encountered in association with recurrent obstructive cholangiopathy such as recurrent pyogenic cholangitis, in choledocho- or hepatolithiasis, and in the liver allograft. In the last, there is often an ischaemic component that facilitates infection in creating protected sites where bacteria can grow freely away from the reach of antibiotics.[614] Cavitations and biliary abscesses (biloma) may follow.

Reversibility of changes

Relief of bile-duct obstruction leads to regression of the parenchymal and portal changes with varying speed.[644] Extensive periportal fibrosis and secondary biliary cirrhosis are largely irreversible, although considerable resolution is occasionally seen after relief of obstruction in children. Reversibility of the lesions after relief of obstruction has been well demonstrated in experimental animals.[206,645–649] Degenerate and necrotic hepatocytes are replaced within a few days by a process of rapid regeneration. Foci of feathery degeneration, perivenular bile plugs and macrophage pig-

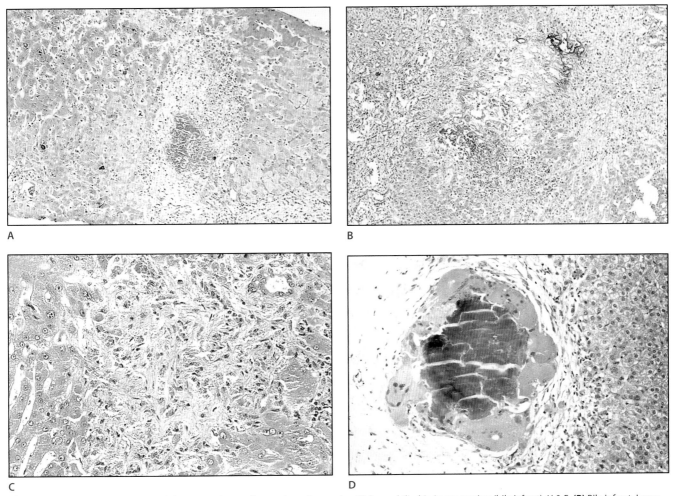

Fig. 11.53 • Large-duct obstruction. **(A)** Paraportal area of parenchymal necrosis with heavy bilirubin impregnation (bile infarct). H & E. **(B)** Bile infarct. Large area of necrosis of which the centre shows loss of liver cells and bilirubin impregnation of reticulin fibres and cellular debris. H & E. **(C)** Organizing paraportal bile infarct, containing scattered bilirubin-laden macrophages in the scar tissue. H & E. **(D)** Oedematous and fibrotic portal area with a bile extravasate surrounded by multinucleated giant macrophages which show a lightly pigmented cytoplasm.

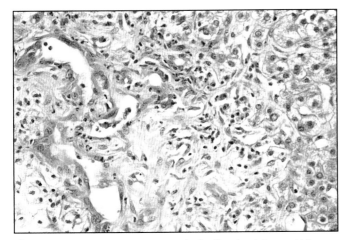

Fig. 11.54 • Large duct obstruction. Markedly dilated and distorted bile ductules with degenerative epithelial changes set in oedematous and mildly inflamed fibrous tissue. H & E.

mentation may persist for several weeks. The neoductules may disappear by apoptosis.[205] Inflammatory changes in the portal tracts will remain for some time, and eventually hyalinized collagen is deposited, resulting in a more permanent, slight enlargement of the tracts. Fully functional recovery of the liver may take considerable time following relief of bile-duct obstruction.[647–649]

Secondary biliary cirrhosis

Pathogenesis and morphogenesis

Secondary biliary cirrhosis is a relatively uncommon complication of extrahepatic biliary obstruction. It has been reported in 8.6% of a large series in the past,[650] a figure which would now certainly be lower owing to early imaging diagnosis, improvement in surgical or interventional radiology techniques and a greater use of broad-spectrum antibiotics. The pathogenesis of secondary biliary cirrhosis is controversial with respect to the relative roles of obstruction per se and the commonly accompanying cholangitis. In addition, portal occlusive phlebitis may play a role in the development of parenchymal collapse seen in some livers with advanced biliary cirrhosis.

That obstruction alone can cause secondary biliary cirrhosis is established in experimental animals subjected to aseptic ligation of the common bile duct,[651] and in the human by its occurrence in infants with extrahepatic biliary atresia, although in that model ongoing destruction of the intrahepatic bile ducts is probably related to other factors than mechanical obstruction per se. The time required for cirrhosis of the liver to develop in unrelieved extrahepatic obstruction is variable, and depends on the cause of the obstruction, associated infection and criteria used to diagnose cirrhosis. In infants with extrahepatic biliary atresia, cirrhosis develops after 5–6 months.[652]

In a series of 60 adults, Scobie & Summerskill[650] found a range of mean intervals between the onset of biliary obstruction and the confirmation of biliary cirrhosis: 7.1 years in patients with common bile-duct stricture, 4.6 years in those with common bile-duct stones, and 0.8 years in patients with malignant obstruction. Biliary cirrhosis developed less rapidly in patients with symptoms of cholangitis (fever, chills and intermittent jaundice) than in those without. This led to the postulation that cholangitis reflected partial or intermittent obstruction, with consequently slower development of cirrhosis, and that the earlier onset of cirrhosis in patients with carcinoma might be due to more complete obstruction.[652] Indeed patients who present with acute malignant obstruction may have had a subclinical cholangiopathy which may have evolved for months and explains the advanced biliary fibrosis seen in the liver.

A true secondary biliary cirrhosis due to extrahepatic mechanical obstruction has become rare. Benign obstructions are generally relieved surgically and, in the presence of inoperable malignancy, stenting of the obstructed duct will allow transient bile drainage and death generally occurs too early from cachexia, metastases and/or septic complications for cirrhosis to develop. Biliary cirrhosis is most frequently seen as a sequel to chronic obstructive cholangiopathies, in particular primary or acquired sclerosing cholangitis, which are generally not amenable to surgery or interventional radiology. In this situation, the morphogenesis of the cirrhosis is therefore identical to that described in relation to chronic cholestasis.

The ductular reaction with concomitant disappearance of periportal hepatocytes and the accompanying fibroplasia play the key role in the portoseptal fibrous expansion creating mesenchymal edges growing towards and eventually linking adjacent portal tracts together. Both the ductular cells and activated hepatic stellate cells contribute to lay down loose and cellular connective tissue which is rich in type IV collagen and laminin.[203] Connective tissue growth factor and periductal mast cells may be important in this process.[197,653] There then follows the deposition of type III fibres with a persistently active degrading activity (increased collagen turnover and reversible fibrosis), and later a progressive deposition of type I fibres with exhaustion of the breakdown system (irreversible fibrosis).[166]

As with the progression observed with chronic intrahepatic cholestasis, portal–portal fibrous linkages at first preserve intrahepatic vascular relationships (so-called biliary fibrosis) and it may be difficult to determine when a true cirrhosis sets in. Diffuse regeneration, suggested by thickened liver-cell plates, is common and may, together with fibrosis, contribute to portal hypertension even in the absence of cirrhosis.[654] Damage to periportal/periseptal hepatocytes is reflected in an impairment of the maximal

biosynthetic activity, as demonstrated experimentally at an early stage after obstruction.[655] More extensive loss of hepatocytes, possibly related to portal blood deprivation, leads to the formation of the bridging septa with the intrahepatic vascular shunts and ultimate nodular regeneration found in cirrhosis.

Pathology

The liver is increased in size, only to shrink to subnormal proportions in the final stages of the disease.[656] The surface is smooth, finely granular or nodular. Consistency and granularity vary with the stage of the cirrhosis: the liver feels firm, hard or even wooden. On slicing, the cut surface is yellow, greenish-grey or deep green, stippled with small grey or white areas corresponding to enlarged portal tracts. Small haemorrhages, grey or yellow necrotic patches and even small infarcts may be seen. Bile ducts may sometimes be considerably distended, with light or dark, occasionally inspissated, bile. In some cases the intrahepatic ducts are filled with white, glairy bile under pressure.[656] The large ducts near the hilum are accompanied by an increased amount of connective tissue.

Histologically, the picture also varies with the stage of the disease; it can be summarized as biliary fibrosis and later cirrhosis, with features of extrahepatic cholestasis. Bile stasis may be diffuse or predominantly periseptal, highlighting the periphery of irregularly shaped nodules. Microscopic bilirubinostasis may be associated with feathery degeneration of liver cells, bile infarcts and bile lakes; the latter are a characteristic sign of an obstructive cause of cirrhosis, but are seldom seen in needle biopsy specimens.

Within the oedematous fibrous septa, there is dense connective tissue, composed of coarse, hyalinized collagen bundles which are doubly refractile under polarized light with a paucity of mesenchymal and inflammatory cells. They constitute the original portal connective tissue and the old deep-seated portions of the septa and are made of irreversible type I collagen. This contrasts with a marginal expanding and potentially reversible zone of loosely woven reticulin fibres containing the reactive ductules and accompanying mesenchymal and inflammatory cells.

The inflammatory exudate usually continues to include neutrophil leukocytes. Significant from a diagnostic point of view is the number of ductular structures, especially well-formed ductules with recognizable lumens. Biliary casts may be present in these structures and in the ducts, particularly when there is associated sepsis. In the late stages of secondary biliary cirrhosis, both ducts and ductules may disappear.[635] Remaining ducts are often characterized by concentric periductal fibrosis.

Regenerative nodules are formed from single and multiple lobules, often resembling pieces of a jigsaw puzzle (Fig. 11.55).[641] The nodules are separated by broad serpiginous bands of connective tissue with parallel fibres and a typical zone of oedema and ductular proliferation, or 'halo', at the interface with the parenchyma. The liver cells in this area show cholate stasis and bilirubinostasis and contain orcein-positive deposits of copper-binding protein, rhodanine-

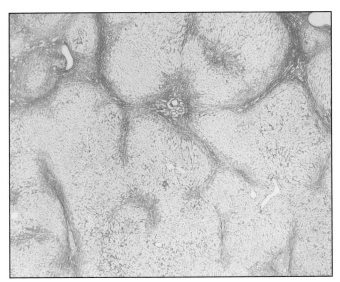

Fig. 11.55 • Biliary cirrhosis. Serpiginous fibrous septa delineate variably shaped parenchymal areas, which have been compared to the pieces of a jigsaw puzzle. Gordon & Sweets silver method for reticulin.

positive granules of copper and Mallory bodies. As already mentioned, secondary biliary cirrhosis may be complicated by bacterial infection. When infection is severe, pylephlebitis and cholangitic, often bile-stained, abscesses may result.

References

1. Lazaridis KN, Strazzabosco M, Larusso NF. The cholangiopathies: disorders of biliary epithelia. Gastroenterology, 2004; 127:1565–1577
2. Demetris AJ. Immunopathology of the human biliary tree. In: Sirica AE, Longnecker DS, eds, Biliary and pancreatic epithelia. Pathobiology and pathophysiology. New York: Marcel Dekker, 1997; pp 127–180
3. Nakanuma Y, Hoso M, Sanzen T, Sasaki M. Microstructure and development of the normal and pathologic biliary tract in humans, including blood supply. Microsc Res Tech, 1997; 38:552–570
4. Roskams TA, Theise ND, Balabaud C et al. Nomenclature of the finer branches of the biliary tree: canals, ductules, and ductular reactions in human livers. Hepatology, 2004; 39:1739–1745
5. Nakanuma Y, Katayanagi K, Terada T, Saito K. Intrahepatic peribiliary glands of humans. I. Anatomy, development and presumed function. J Gastroenterol Hepatol, 1994; 9:75–79
6. Terada T, Nakanuma Y. Expression of pancreatic enzymes (alpha-amylase, trypsinogen, and lipase) during human liver development and maturation. Gastroenterology, 1995; 108:1236–1245
7. Terada T, Nakanuma Y. Development of human intrahepatic peribiliary glands. Histological, keratin immunohistochemical, and mucus histochemical analyses. Lab Invest, 1993; 68:261–269
8. Terada T, Nakanuma Y, Kakita A. Pathologic observations of intrahepatic peribiliary glands in 1000 consecutive autopsy livers. Heterotopic pancreas in the liver. Gastroenterology, 1990; 98:1333–1337
9. Sheen-Chen S, Chen W, Eng H, Sheen C, Chou F, Cheng Y, Lee T. Bacteriology and antimicrobial choice in hepatolithiasis. Am J Infect Control, 2000; 28:298–301
10. Hiramatsu K, Harada K, Tsuneyama K et al. Amplification and sequence analysis of partial bacterial 16S ribosomal RNA gene in gallbladder bile from patients with primary biliary cirrhosis. J Hepatol, 2000; 33:9–18
11. Sasatomi K, Noguchi K, Sakisaka S, Sata M, Tanikawa K. Abnormal accumulation of endotoxin in biliary epithelial cells in primary biliary cirrhosis and primary sclerosing cholangitis. J Hepatol, 1998; 29:409–416
12. Harada K, Ozaki S, Kono N et al. Frequent molecular identification of Campylobacter but not Helicobacter genus in bile and biliary epithelium in hepatolithiasis. J Pathol, 2001; 193:218–223
13. Nilsson HO, Taneera J, Castedal M, Glatz E, Olsson R, Wadstrom T. Identification of Helicobacter pylori and other Helicobacter species by PCR, hybridization, and partial DNA sequencing in human liver samples from patients with primary sclerosing cholangitis or primary biliary cirrhosis. J Clin Microbiol 2000; 38:1072–1076
14. Sugiura H, Nakanuma Y. Secretory component and immunoglobulins in the intrahepatic biliary tree and peribiliary gland in normal livers and hepatolithiasis. Gastroenterol Jpn, 1989; 24:308–314
15. Saito K, Nakanuma Y. Lactoferrin and lysozyme in the intrahepatic bile duct of normal livers and hepatolithiasis. An immunohistochemical study. J Hepatol, 1992; 15:147–153
16. Fava G, Glaser S, Frances H, Alpini G. The immunophysiology of biliary epithelium. Semin Liver Dis, 2005; 25:251–264
17. Harada K, Ohba K, Ozaki S et al. Peptide antibiotic human beta-defensin-1 and -2 contribute to antimicrobial defense of the intrahepatic biliary tree. Hepatology, 2004; 40:925–932
18. Fellermann K, Stange EF. Defensins—innate immunity at the epithelial frontier. Eur J Gastroenterol Hepatol, 2001; 13:771–776
19. Schroder JM, Harder J. Human beta-defensin-2. Int J Biochem Cell Biol, 1999; 31:645–651
20. Podolsky D. Mucosal Immunity and Inflammation V. Innate mechanisms of mucosal defense and repair: the best offence is a good defense. Am J Physiol, 1999; 277:G495–G499
21. Sasaki M, Tsuneyama K, Saito T et al. Site-characteristic expression and induction of trefoil factor family 1, 2 and 3 and malignant brain tumor–1 in normal and diseased intrahepatic bile ducts relates to biliary pathophysiology. Liver Int, 2004; 24:29–37
22. Harada K, Ohira S, Isse K, Ozaki S, Zen Y, Sato Y, Nakanuma Y. Lipopolysaccharide activates nuclear factor-kappaB through toll-like receptors and related molecules in cultured biliary epithelial cells. Lab Invest, 2003; 83:1657–1667
23. Nakanuma Y, Ohta G. Histometric and serial section observations of the intrahepatic bile ducts in primary biliary cirrhosis. Gastroenterology, 1979; 76:1326–1332
24. Lunz JG 3rd, Contrucci S, Ruppert K et al. Replicative senescence of biliary epithelial cells precedes bile duct loss in chronic liver allograft rejection: increased expression of p21(WAF1/Cip1) as a disease marker and the influence of immunosuppressive drugs. Am J Pathol, 2001; 158:1379–1390
25. Hartshorne N, Hartman G, Markin RS, Demetris AJ, Ferrell L. Bile duct hemorrhage: a biopsy finding after cholangiography or biliary tree manipulation. Liver, 1992; 12:137–139
26. Nomoto M, Uchikosi Y, Kajikazawa N, Tanaka Y, Asakura H. Appearance of hepatocyte-like cells in the interlobular bile ducts of human liver in various liver disease states. Hepatology, 1992; 16:1199–1205
27. Falkowski O, An HJ, Ianus IA, Chiriboga L, Yee H, West AB, Theise ND. Regeneration of hepatocyte 'buds' in cirrhosis from intrabiliary stem cells. J Hepatol, 2003; 39:357–364
28. Zen Y, Harada K, Sasaki M, Tsuneyama K, Katayanagi K, Yamamoto Y, Nakanuma Y. Lipopolysaccharide induces overexpression of MUC2 and MUC5AC in cultured biliary epithelial cells: possible key phenomenon of hepatolithiasis. Am J Pathol, 2002; 161:1475–1484
29. Ishikawa A, Sasaki M, Ohira S et al. Aberrant expression of CDX2 is closely related to the intestinal metaplasia and MUC2 expression in intraductal papillary neoplasm of the liver in hepatolithiasis. Lab Invest, 2004; 84:629–638
30. Takao S, Uchikura K, Yonezawa S, Shinchi H, Aikou T. Mucin core protein expression in extrahepatic bile duct carcinoma is associated with metastases to the liver and poor prognosis. Cancer, 1999; 86:1966–1975
31. Sasaki M, Nakanuma Y, Kim YS. Expression of apomucins in the intrahepatic biliary tree in hepatolithiasis differs from that in normal liver and extrahepatic biliary obstruction. Hepatology, 1998; 27:54–61
32. Harada K, Zen Y, Kanemori Y et al. Human REG I gene is up-regulated in intrahepatic cholangiocarcinoma and its precursor lesions. Hepatology, 2001; 33:1036–1042
33. Sasaki M, Ikeda H, Ohira S, Ishikawa A, Nakanuma Y. Expression of trefoil factor family 1, 2, and 3 peptide is augmented in hepatolithiasis. Peptides, 2004; 25:763–770
34. Hoang MP, Murakata LA, Padilla-Rodriguez AL, Albores-Saavedra J. Metaplastic lesions of the extrahepatic bile ducts: a morphologic and immunohistochemical study. Mod Pathol, 2001; 14:1119–1125
35. Kim YI, Yu ES, Kim ST. Intraductal variant of peripheral cholangiocarcinoma of the liver with Clonorchis sinensis infection. Cancer, 1989; 63:1562–1566
36. Ludwig J, Wahlstrom HE, Batts KP, Wiesner RH. Papillary bile duct dysplasia in primary sclerosing cholangitis. Gastroenterology, 1992; 102:2134–2138

37. LeBrun DP, Warnke RA, Cleary ML. Expression of bcl-2 in fetal tissue suggests a role in morphogenesis. Am J Pathol, 1993; 142:743–753

38. Charlotte F, L'Hermine A, Martin N, Geleyen Y, Nollet M, Gaulard P, Zafrani ES. Immunohistochemical detection of bcl-2 in normal and pathologic human liver. Am J Pathol, 1994; 144:460–465

39. Gerber MA, Thung SN. Liver stem cells and development (editorial). Lab Invest, 1993; 68:261–263

40. Aber N, Zajicek G. Streaming liver VI. Streaming intra-hepatic bile ducts. Liver, 1990; 10:205–208

41. Ludwig J, Czaja AJ, Dickson ER, LaRusso NF, Wiesner RH. Manifestations of nonsuppurative cholangitis in chronic hepatobiliary diseases: morphologic spectrum, clinical correlations and terminology. Liver, 1984; 4:105–116

42. Ludwig J, Colina F, Poterucha JJ. Granulomas in primary sclerosing cholangitis. Liver, 1995; 15:307–312

43. Vyberg M. The hepatitis-associated bile duct lesion. Liver, 1993; 13:289–301

44. Kaji K, Nakanuma Y, Sasaki M et al. Hepatitic bile duct injuries in chronic hepatitis C: histopathologic and immunohistochemical studies. Mod Pathol, 1994; 7:937–945

45. Tsuneyama K, Kono N, Yamashiro M et al. Aberrant expression of stem cell factor on biliary epithelial cells and peribiliary infiltration of c-kit-expressing mast cells in hepatolithiasis and primary sclerosing cholangitis: a possible contribution to bile duct fibrosis. J Pathol, 1999; 189:609–614

46. Milani S, Herbst H, Schuppan D, Surrenti C, Riccken EO, Stein H. Cellular localization of type I, III and IV procollagen gene transcripts in normal and fibrotic human liver. Am J Pathol, 1990; 137:59–70

47. Milani S, Herbst H, Schuppan D, Riecken EO, Stein H. Cellular localization of laminin gene transcripts in normal and fibrotic human liver. Am J Pathol, 1989; 134:1175–1182

48. Milani S, Herbst H, Schuppan D, Stein H, Surrenti C. Transforming growth factor beta 1 and beta 2 are differently expressed in fibrotic liver diseases. Am J Pathol, 1991; 139:1221–1229

49. Napoli J, Prentice D, Niihami C, Bishop GA, Desmond P, McCaughan GW. Sequential increases in the intrahepatic expression of epidermal growth factor, basic fibroblast growth factor, and transforming growth factor β in a bile duct ligated rat model of cirrhosis. Hepatology, 1997; 26:624–633

50. Joplin R, Hishida T, Tsubouchi H et al. Human intrahepatic biliary epithelial cells proliferate in vitro in response to human hepatocyte growth factor. J Clin Invest, 1992; 90:1284–1290

51. Schuppan D, Schmid M, Somasundaran R et al. Collagens in the liver extracellular matrix bind hepatocyte growth factor. Gastroenterology, 1998; 114:139–152

52. Patel T, Tores GJ. Apoptosis and hepatobiliary disease. Hepatology, 1995; 21:1725–1741

53. Harada K, Ozaki S, Gershwin ME, Nakanuma Y. Enhanced apoptosis relates to bile duct loss in primary biliary cirrhosis. Hepatology, 1997; 26:1399–1405

54. Bernuau D, Feldmann G, Degott C, Gisselbrecht C. Ultrastructural lesions of bile ducts in primary biliary cirrhosis. A comparison with the lesions observed in graft versus host disease. Hum Pathol, 1981; 12:782–793

55. Celli A, Que FG. Dysregulation of apoptosis in the cholangiopathies and cholangiocarcinoma. Semin Liver Dis, 1998; 18:177–185

56. Harada K, Kono N, Tsuneyama K, Nakanuma Y. Cell-kinetic study of proliferating bile ductules in various hepatobiliary diseases. Liver, 1998; 18:277–284

57. Harnois DM, Que FG, Celli A, LaRusso NF, Gores GG. Bcl-2 is overexpressed and alters the threshold for apoptosis in a cholangiocarcinoma cell line. Hepatology, 1997; 26:884–890

58. Crawford AR, Lin XZ, Crawford JM. The normal adult human liver biopsy: a quantitative reference standard. Hepatology, 1998; 28:323–331

59. Ludwig J, Wiesner RH, LaRusso NF. Idiopathic adulthood ductopenia. A cause of chronic cholestatic liver disease and biliary cirrhosis. J Hepatol, 1988; 17:193–199

60. Ludwig J. New concepts in biliary cirrhosis. Semin Liver Dis, 1987; 7:293–310

61. Desmet VJ. Vanishing bile duct syndrome in drug-induced liver disease. J Hepatol, 1997; 26(suppl 1):31–35

62. Murphy JR, Sjögren MH, Kikendall JW, Peura DA, Goodman Z. Small bile duct abnormalities in sarcoidosis. J Clin Gastroenterol, 1990; 12:555–561

63. Hübscher SG, Lumley MA, Elias E. Vanishing bile duct syndrome: a possible mechanism for intrahepatic cholestasis in Hodgkin's lymphoma. Hepatology, 1993; 7:70–77

64. Ludwig J, Wiesner RH, Batts KP, Perkins JD, Krom RA. Vanishing bile duct syndrome (acute irreversible) after orthotopic liver transplantation. Hepatology, 1987; 7:476–483

65. Yeh KH, Hsieh HC, Tang JL, Lin MT, Yang CH, Chen YC. Severe isolated acute graft-versus-host disease with vanishing bile duct syndrome. Bone Marrow Transplant, 1994; 14:319–321

66. Alam I, Ferrell LD, Bass NM. Vanishing bile duct syndrome temporally associated with ibuprofen use. Am J Gastroenterol, 1996; 91:1626–1630

67. Sirica AE, Mathis GA, Sano N, Elmore LW. Isolation, culture, and transplantation of intrahepatic biliary epithelial cells and oval cells. Pathobiology, 1990; 58:44–64

68. Terasaki S, Nakanuma Y, Unoura M, Kaneko S, Kobayashi K. Involvement of peribiliary glands in primary sclerosing cholangitis: A histopathologic study. Int Med, 1997; 36:766–770

69. Nakanuma Y, Terada T, Ohtake S, Govindarajan S. Intrahepatic periductal glands in graft-versus-host disease. Acta Pathol Jpn, 1988; 38:281–289

70. McCaughan GW, Davis JS, Waugh JA et al. A quantitative analysis of T-lymphocyte populations in human liver allografts undergoing rejection: the use of monoclonal antibody and double immunolabelling. Hepatology, 1990; 12:1305–1313

71. Whiteside TL, Lasky S, Si L, Van Thiel DH. Immunologic analysis of mononuclear cells in liver tissue and blood of patients with primary sclerosing cholangitis. Hepatology, 1985; 5:468–474

72. Yamada G, Hyodo I, Tobe K et al. Ultrastructural immunocytochemical analysis of lymphocytes infiltrating bile duct epithelia in primary biliary cirrhosis. Hepatology, 1986; 6:385–391

73. Ibrahim S, Dawson DV, Killerberg PG, Sanfilippo F. The pattern and phenotype of T-cell infiltration associated with human liver allograft rejection. Hum Pathol, 1993; 24:1365–1370

74. Burroughs AK, Butler P, Sternberg MJE, Baum H. Molecular mimicry in liver disease. Nature, 1992; 358:377–378

75. Van de Water J, Ishibashi H, Coppel RL, Gershwin ME. Molecular mimicry and primary biliary cirrhosis: premises not promises. Hepatology, 2001; 33:771–775

76. Vierling JM. Immunology of acute and chronic hepatic allograft rejection. Liver Transpl Surg, 1999; 4:S1–S20

77. Fussey SP, Guest JR, James OF, Bassendine MF, Yeaman SJ. Identification and analysis of the major M2 autoantigen in primary biliary cirrhosis. Proc Natl Acad Sci USA, 1988; 85:8654–8658

78. Kita H, Matsumura S, He XS, Ansari AA, Lian ZX, Van de Water J, Coppel RL, Kaplan MM, Gershwin ME. Quantitative and functional analysis of PDC-E2-specific autoreactive cytotoxic T lymphocytes in primary biliary cirrhosis. J Clin Invest, 2002; 109:1231–1240

79. Miyamoto T, Maeda T, Ohnishi S, Yamatomo Y. T cell autoreactivity against a 28 kD biliary protein (B1-p28) in primary biliary cirrhosis. J Hepatol, 1995; 22:423–430

80. Mandel A, Dasgupta A, Jeffers L et al. Autoantibodies in sclerosing cholangitis against a shared peptide in biliary and colonic epithelium. Gastroenterology, 1994; 106:185–192

81. Jorge AD, Stati AO, Roig LV, Ponce G, Jorge OA, Ciocca DR. Steroid receptors and heat-shock proteins in patients with primary biliary cirrhosis. Hepatology, 1993; 18:1108–1114

82. Broome U, Scheynius A, Hulcrantz R. Induced expression of heat-shock protein on biliary epithelium in patients with primary sclerosing cholangitis and primary biliary cirrhosis. Hepatology, 1993; 18:298–303

83. Hopf U, Miller B, Stemerowicz R et al. Escherichia coli rough R mutants in the gut and lipid A in the liver from patients with primary biliary cirrhosis (PBC). Lancet, 1998; 2:1419–1422

84. Sasatomi K, Noguchi K, Sakisaka S, Sata M, Tanikawa K. Abnormal accumulation of endotoxin in biliary epithelial cells in primary biliary cirrhosis and primary sclerosing cholangitis. J Hepatol, 1998; 29:409–416

85. Martins EB, Chapman RW, Marron K, Fleming KA. Biliary expression of heat shock protein: a non-specific feature of chronic cholestatic liver diseases. J Clin Pathol, 1996; 49:53–56

86. Gordon SC, Quattrociocchi-Longe TM, Khan BA, Koali VP, Chen J, Silverman AL. Antibodies to carbonic anhydrase in patients with immune cholangiopathies. Gastroenterology, 1995; 108:1802–1809

87. Invernizzi P, Battezzati PM, Crosignani A et al. Antibody to carbonic anhydrase II is present in primary biliary cirrhosis (PBC) irrespective of antimitochondrial status. Clin Exp Immunol, 1998; 114:448–454

88. Kita H, Mackay IR, Van De Water J, Gershwin ME. The lymphoid liver: considerations on pathways to autoimmune injury. Gastroenterology, 2001; 120:1485–1501

89. Hart DNJ. Dendritic cells: unique leukocyte populations which control the primary immune response. Blood, 1997; 90:3245–3287

90. Tsuneyama K, Harada K, Yososhima M, Kaji K, Gershwin ME, Nakanuma Y. Expression of co-stimulatory factor B7-2 on the intrahepatic bile ducts in primary biliary cirrhosis and primary sclerosing cholangitis: an immunohistochemical study. J Pathol, 1998; 186:126–130

91. Demetris AJ, Sever C, Kakizoe S, Oguma S, Starzl TE, Jaffe R. S100 protein positive dendritic cells in primary biliary cirrhosis and other chronic inflammatory liver diseases. Relevance to pathogenesis? Am J Pathol, 1989; 134:741–747

92. Leon MP, Kirby JA, Gibbs P, Burt AD, Bassendine MF. Immunogenicity of biliary epithelial cells: study of the expression of B7 molecules. J Hepatol, 1995; 22:591–595

93. Leon MP, Bassendine MF, Wilson JL, Ali S, Thick M, Kirby JA. Immunogenicity of biliary epithelium: investigation of antigen presentation to CD4+T cells. Hepatology, 1996; 24:561–567

94. Van den Oord JJ, Sciot R, Desmet VJ. Expression of MHC products by normal and abnormal bile duct epithelium. J Hepatol, 1986; 3:310–317

95. Nakanuma Y, Kono K. Expression of HLA-DR antigens on interlobular bile ducts in primary biliary cirrhosis and other hepatobiliary diseases: an immunohistochemical study. Hum Pathol, 1991; 22:431–436

96. Donaldson P, Underhill J, Doherty D et al. Influence of human leukocyte antigen matching on liver graft survival and rejection: 'the dualistic effect'. Hepatology, 1993; 17:1008–1015

97. Harada K, Tsuneyama K, Yasoshima M et al. Type1 and type2 memory T cells imbalance shown by expression of intrahepatic chemokine receptors relates to pathogenesis of primary biliary cirrhosis. Hepatol Res, 2002; 24:290

98. Harada K, Van de Water J, Leung PS et al. In situ nucleic acid hybridization of cytokines in primary biliary cirrhosis: predominance of the Th1 subset. Hepatology, 1997; 25:791–796

99. Martinez OM, Villanueva JC, Gershwin ME, Krams SM. Cytokine patterns and cytotoxic mediators in primary biliary cirrhosis. Hepatology, 1995; 21:113–119

100. Nakanuma Y, Yasoshima M, Tsuneyama K, Harada K. Histopathology of primary biliary cirrhosis with emphasis on expression of adhesion molecules. Semin Liver Dis, 1997; 17:35–47

101. Hübscher SG, Adams DH, Elias E. Changes in the expression of major histocompatibility class II antigens in liver allograft rejection. J Pathol, 1990; 162:165–171

102. Dienes HP, Lohse AW, Gerken G et al. Bile duct epithelia as target cells in primary biliary cirrhosis and primary sclerosing cholangitis. Virchow Arch, 1997; 431:119–124

103. Broome U, Glaumann H, Hultcrantz R, Forsum U. Distribution of HLA-DR, HLA-DP, and HLA-DQ antigens in liver tissue from patients with primary sclerosing cholangitis. Scand J Gastroenterol, 1990; 25:54–58

104. Yasoshima M, Kono N, Sugawara H, Katayanagi K, Harada K, Nakanuma Y. Increased expression of interleukin-6 and tumor necrosis factor-alpha in pathologic biliary epithelial cells: in situ and culture study. Lab Invest, 1998; 78:89–100

105. D'Amico E, Paroli M, Fratelli V et al. Primary biliary cirrhosis induced by interferon-alpha therapy for hepatitis C virus infection. Dig Dis Sci, 1995; 40:2113–2116

106. Moradpour D, Altorfer J, Flury R et al. Chlorpromazin-induced vanishing bile duct syndrome leading to biliary cirrhosis. Hepatology, 1994; 20:1437–1441

107. Kono N, Nakanuma Y. Ultrastructural and immunohistochemical studies of the intrahepatic peribiliary capillary plexus in normal livers and extrahepatic biliary obstruction in human beings. Hepatology, 1992; 15:411–418

108. Adams DH, Hübscher SG, Fisher NC, Williams A, Robinson M. Expression of E-selectin and E-selectin ligands in human liver inflammation. Hepatology, 1996; 24:533–538

109. Steinhoff G, Behrend M, Schrader B, Pichlmayr R. Intercellular immune adhesion molecules in human liver transplants: overview on expression pattern of leukocyte ligand molecules. Hepatology, 1993; 18:440–453

110. Morland CM, Fear J, McNab G, Joplin R, Adams DH. Promotion of leukocyte transendothelial cell migration by chemokines derives from human biliary epithelial cells in vitro. Proc Assoc Am Physicians, 1997; 109:372–382

111. Baron JL, Madri JA, Ruddle NH, Hashim G, Janeway Jr CA. Surface expression of α-4-integrin by CD4 T cells is required for their entry into brain parenchyma. J Exp Med, 1993; 177:57–58

112. Lobb RR, Abraham WM, Burkly LC et al. Pathophysiologic role of alpha-4 integrins in the lung. Ann NY Sci, 1996; 796:113–123

113. Medina J, Sanz-Cameno P, Garcia-Buey L et al. Evidence of angiogenesis in primary biliary cirrhosis: an immunohistochemical descriptive study. J Hepatol, 2005; 42:124–131

114. Yasoshima M, Nakanuma Y, Tsuneyama K, Van de Water J, Gershwin ME. Immunohistochemical analysis of adhesion molecules in the micro-environment of portal tracts in relation to aberrant expression of PDC-E2 and HLA-DR on the bile ducts in primary biliary cirrhosis. J Pathol, 1995; 175:319–325

115. Jaspars LH, Beljaards RC, Bonnet P, Willemze R, Meijer CJLM. Distinctive adhesion pathways are involved in epitheliotropic processes at different sites. J Pathol, 1996; 178:385–392

116. Isse K, Harada K, Zen Y et al. Fractalkine and CX3CR1 are involved in recruitment of intraepithelial lymphocytes of intrahepatic bile ducts. Hepatology, 2005; 41:506–516

117. Krams SM, Martinez O. Apoptosis as a mechanism of tissue injury in liver allograft rejection. Semin Liver Dis, 1998; 18:153–167

118. Que FG, Gores GJ. Cell death by apoptosis: Basic concepts and disease relevance for the gastroenterologist. Gastroenterology, 1996; 110:1238–1243

119. Kamihira T, Shimoda S, Harada K et al. Distinct costimulation dependent and independent autoreactive T-cell clones in primary biliary cirrhosis. Gastroenterology, 2003; 125:1379–1387

120. Matsumura S, Kita H, He XS et al. Comprehensive mapping of HLA-A*0201-restricted CD8 T-cell epitopes on PDC-E2 in primary biliary cirrhosis. Hepatology, 2002; 36:1125–1134

121. Gapany C, Zhao M, Zimmermann A. The apoptosis protector, bcl-2 protein, is downregulated in bile duct epithelial cells of human liver allografts. J Hepatol, 1997; 26:535–542

122. Kuroki T, Seki S, Kawakita N, Nakatani K, Hisa T. Expression of antigens related to apoptosis and cell proliferation in chronic nonsuppurative destructive cholangitis in primary biliary cirrhosis. Virchows Arch, 1996; 429:119–129

123. Lowin B, Hahne M, Mattmann C, Tschopp J. Cytolytic T-cell cytotoxicity is mediated through perforin and Fas lytic pathways. Nature, 1994; 370:650–652

124. Kagi D, Vignaux F, Ledermann B et al. Fas and perforin pathways as major mechanisms of T-cell mediated cytotoxicity. Science, 1994; 265:528–530

125. Apasov S, Redegeld F, Sitkovsky M. Cell-mediated cytotoxicity: contact and secreted factors. Curr Opin Immunol, 1993; 5:404–410

126. Lohr H, Schlaak JF, Gerken F, Fleischer B, Dienes HP, Meyer zum Buschenfelde KH. Phenotypical analysis and cytokine release of liver-infiltrating and peripheral blood T lymphocytes from patients with chronic hepatitis of different etiology. Liver, 1994; 14:161–166

127. Nagata S. Apoptosis by death factor. Cell, 1997; 88:355–365

128. Shimoda S, Nakamura M, Ishibashi H et al. Molecular mimicry of mitochondrial and nuclear autoantigens in primary biliary cirrhosis. Gastroenterology, 2003; 124:1915–1925

129. Malmborg AC, Shultz DB, Luton F et al. Penetration and co-localization in MDCK cell mitochondria of IgA derived from patients with primary biliary cirrhosis. J Autoimmun, 1998; 1:573–580

130. Bjorkland A, Loof L, Mendel-Hartvig I, Totterman TH. Primary biliary cirrhosis. High proportions of B cells in blood and liver tissue produce anti-mitochondrial antibodies of several Ig classes. J Immunol, 1994; 153:2750–2757

131. Matsuda J, Omagari K, Ohba K et al. Correlation between histopathological findings of the liver and IgA class antibodies to 2-oxo-acid dehydrogenase complex in primary biliary cirrhosis. Dig Dis Sci, 2003; 48:932–938

132. Krams SM, Van de Water J, Coppel RL et al. Analysis of hepatic T lymphocytes and immunoglobulin deposits in patients with primary biliary cirrhosis. Hepatology, 1990; 12:306–313

133. Nakanuma Y. Distribution of B lymphocytes in nonsuppurative destructive cholangitis in primary biliary cirrhosis. Hepatology, 1993; 18:570–575

134. Nishio A, Van de Water J, Leung PSC et al. Comparative studies of antimitochondrial autoantibodies in sera and bile in primary biliary cirrhosis. Hepatology, 1997; 25:1085–1089

135. Matsumura S, Van De Water J, Leung P et al. Caspase induction by IgA antimitochondrial antibody: IgA-mediated biliary injury in primary biliary cirrhosis. Hepatology, 2004; 39:1415–1422

136. Demetris AJ, Murase N, Nakamura K et al. Immunopathology of antibodies as effectors of orthotopic liver allograft rejection. Semin Liver Dis, 1992; 12:51–59

137. Terasaki T, Nakanuma Y, Yamazaki M, Unoura M. Eosinophilic infiltration of the liver in primary biliary cirrhosis: A morphologic study. Hepatology, 1993; 17:206–212

138. De Groen PC, Kephart GM, Gleich GJ, Ludwig J. Eosinophil cationic protein's role in human hepatic allograft rejection. Hepatology, 1994; 20:654–662

139. Foster PF, Sankary HN, Williams JW, Bhattacharyya A, Coleman J, Ashmann M. Morphometric inflammatory cell analysis of human liver allograft biopsies. Transplantation, 1991; 51:873–876

140. Martinez OM, Ascher NL, Ferrell L et al. Evidence for a nonclassical pathway of graft rejection involving interleukin 5 and eosinophils. Transplantation, 1993; 55:909–918

141. Wu CT, Eiserich JP, Ansari AA et al. Myeloperoxidase-positive inflammatory cells participate in bile duct damage in primary biliary cirrhosis through nitric oxide-mediated reactions. Hepatology, 2003; 38:1018–1025

142. Tsuneyama K, Harada K, Kono N et al. Damaged interlobular bile ducts in primary biliary cirrhosis show reduced expression of glutathione-S-transferase-pi and aberrant expression of 4-hydroxynonenal. J Hepatol, 2002; 37:176–183

143. Sasaki M, Ikeda H, Haga H, Manabe T, Nakanuma Y. Frequent cellular senescence in small bile ducts in primary biliary cirrhosis: a possible role for bile duct loss. J Pathol, 2005; 205:451–459

144. Jones DE, Donaldson PT. Genetic factors in the pathogenesis of primary biliary cirrhosis. Clin Liver Dis, 2003; 7:841–864

145. Cetta FM. Bile infection documented as the initial event in the pathogenesis of brown pigment biliary stones. Hepatology, 1986; 6:482–489

146. Maki T. Pathogenesis of calcium bilirubinate gallstone. Role of E. coli beta-glucuronidase and coagulation by inorganic ions, polyelectrolytes and agitation. Ann Surg, 1966; 164:90–100

147. Hiramatsu K, Harada K, Tsuneyama K et al. Amplification and sequence analysis of partial bacterial 16S ribosomal RNA gene in gallbladder bile from patients with primary biliary cirrhosis. J Hepatol, 2000; 33:9–18

148. Nilsson HO, Taneera J, Castedal M, Glatz E, Olsson R, Wadstrom T. Identification of Helicobacter pylori and other Helicobacter species by PCR, hybridization, and partial DNA sequencing in human liver samples from patients with primary sclerosing cholangitis or primary biliary cirrhosis. J Clin Microbiol, 2000; 38:1072–1076

149. Olsson R, Bjornsson E, Backman L et al. Bile duct bacterial isolates in primary sclerosing cholangitis: a study of explanted livers. J Hepatol, 1998; 28:426–432

150. Beschorner WE, Pino J, Boitnott JK, Tuschka PJ, Santos GW. Pathology of the liver with bone marrow transplantation. Effects of busulfan, carmustine, acute graft-versus-host disease and cytomegalovirus infection. Am J Pathol, 1980; 99:369–385

151. O'Grady JG, Alexander GJM, Sutherland S et al. Cytomegalovirus infection and donor/recipient HLA antigens: interdependent cofactors in the pathogenesis of vanishing bile duct syndrome after liver transplantation. Lancet, 1988; ii:301–305

152. Arnold JC, Nouri-Aria KT, O'Grady JG, Portmann BC, Alexander GJ, Williams R. Hepatic alpha-interferon expression in cytomegalovirus-infected liver allograft recipients with and without vanishing bile duct syndrome. Clin Invest, 1993; 1:191–196

153. Wright TL. Cytomegalovirus infection and the vanishing bile duct syndrome. Culprit or innocent bystander? Hepatology, 1992; 16:285–292

154. Hoffmann RM, Gunther C, Diepolder HM et al. Hepatitis C virus infection as a possible risk factor for ductopenic rejection (vanishing bile duct syndrome) after liver transplantation. Transpl Int, 1995; 8:353–359

155. Deleuze JF, Jacquemin E, Dubuisson C et al. Defect of multidrug-resistance 3 gene expression in a subtype of progressive familial intrahepatic cholestasis. Hepatology, 1996; 23:904–908

156. Paumgartner G, Beuers U. Ursodeoxycholic acid in cholestatic liver disease: mechanisms of action and therapeutic use revisited. Hepatology, 2002; 36:525–531

157. Komichi D, Tazuma S, Nishioka T, Hyogo H, Une M, Chayama K. Unique inhibition of bile salt-induced apoptosis by lecithins and cytoprotective bile salts in immortalized mouse cholangiocytes. Dig Dis Sci, 2003; 48:2315–2322

158. Ludwig J. Ischemic cholangitis in hepatic allografts. Mayo Clin Proc, 1992; 67:519–526

159. Ludwig J, Kim CH, Wiesner RH, Krom RA. Floxuridine-induced sclerosing cholangitis: an ischemic cholangiopathy? Hepatology, 1989; 9:215–218

160. Kobayashi S, Nakanuma Y, Terada T, Matsui O. Postmortem survey of bile duct necrosis and biloma in hepatocellular carcinoma after transcatheter arterial chemoembolization therapy: relevance to microvascular damages of peribiliary capillary plexus. Am J Gastroenterol, 1993; 88:1410–1415

161. Martensen JA, Gundersen LL, Buskirk SJ et al. Hepatic duct stricture after radiation therapy for biliary cancer: recurrence or fibrosis? Mayo Clin Proc, 1986; 61:530–536

162. Cherqui D, Plazzo L, Piedbois P et al. Common bile duct stricture as a late complication of upper abdominal radiotherapy. J Hepatol, 1994; 20:693–697

163. Geubel AP. Radiation-induced bile duct injury: a vanishing cause of obstructive jaundice. J Hepatol, 1994; 20:687–688

164. Kobayashi S, Nakanuma Y, Matsui O. Intrahepatic peribiliary vascular plexus in various hepatobiliary diseases: a histological survey. Hum Pathol, 1994; 25:940–946

165. Goritsas CP, Repanti M, Papadaki E, Lazarous N, Andonopoulos AP. Intrahepatic bile duct injury and nodular regenerative hyperplasia of the liver in a patient with polyarteritis nodosa. J Hepatol, 1997; 26:727–730

166. Desmet VJ. Cholestasis: extrahepatic obstruction and secondary biliary cirrhosis. In: MacSween RNM, Anthony PP, Scheuer PJ, Burt AD, Portmann BC, eds, Pathology of the liver, 3rd edn. Edinburgh: Churchill Livingstone, 1994, pp 425–476

167. Nagore N, Howe S, Boxer L, Scheuer PJ. Liver cell rosettes: structural differences in cholestasis and hepatitis. Liver, 1989; 9:43–51

168. Fevery J, Blanchaert N. Hyperbilirubinemia. In: McIntyre N, Benhamou JP, Bircher J, Rizzetto M, Rodes J, eds, Oxford textbook of clinical hepatology, vol 2. Oxford: Oxford University Press, 1991: pp 985–991

169. Meier-Abt PJ. Cellular mechanisms of intrahepatic cholestasis. Drugs, 1990; 40(suppl 3):84–97

170. Portmann B, Popper H, Neuberger J, Williams R. Sequential and diagnostic features in primary biliary cirrhosis, based on serial histologic study in 209 patients. Gastroenterology, 1985; 88:1777–1790

171. Popper H, Schaffner F. The pathophysiology of cholestasis. Hum Pathol, 1970; 1:1–24

172. Salaspuro M, Sipponen P. Demonstration of an intracellular copper-binding protein by orcein staining in long-standing cholestatic liver diseases. Gut, 1976; 17:787–790

173. Portmann BC. Histochemistry in diagnostic assessment of liver biopsy. In: Filipe MI, Lake BD, eds, Histochemistry in pathology, 2nd edn. Edinburgh: Churchill Livingstone, 1990: pp 221–234

174. Guarascio P, Yentis F, Cevikbas U, Portmann B, Williams R. Value of copper-associated protein in diagnostic assessment of liver biopsy. J Clin Pathol, 1983; 36:18–23

175. Van Eyken P, Sciot R, Desmet VJ. A cytokeratin immunohistochemical study of cholestatic liver disease: evidence that hepatocytes can express 'bile duct-type' cytokeratin. Histopathology, 1989; 15:125–136

176. Gerber MA, Orr W, Denk H, Schaffner F, Popper H. Hepatocellular hyalin in cholestasis and cirrhosis: its diagnostic significance. Gastroenterology, 1973; 64:89–98

177. Denk H, Lackinger E. Cytoskeleton in liver diseases. Semin Liver Dis, 1986; 6:199–211

178. Slott PA, Liu MH, Tavoloni N. Origin, pattern and mechanism of bile duct proliferation following biliary obstruction in the rat. Gastroenterology, 1990; 99:466–477

179. Burt AD, MacSween RNM. Bile duct proliferation—its true significance. Histopathology, 1993; 23:590–596

180. Nakanuma Y, Ohta G. Immunohistochemical study on bile ductular proliferation in various hepatobiliary diseases. Liver, 1986; 6:205–211

181. Nakanuma Y, Sasaki M. Expression of blood group-related antigens in the intrahepatic biliary tree and hepatocytes in normal livers and various hepatobiliary diseases. Hepatology, 1989; 10:174–178

182. Roskams T, Van den Oord JJ, De Vos R, Desmet VJ. Neuroendocrine features of reactive bile ductules in cholestatic liver disease. Am J Pathol, 1990; 137:1019–1025

183. Volpes R, Van den Oord JJ, Desmet VJ. Distribution of the VLA family of integrins in normal and pathological human liver tissue. Gastroenterology, 1991; 101:200–206

184. Hahn EG, Kirchner J, Schuppan D. Perisinusoidal fibrogenesis and ductular metaplasia of hepatocytes in focal nodular hyperplasia of the liver. J Hepatol, 1987; 5:S32

185. Bucher NLR, Robinson GS, Farmer SR. Effects of extracellular matrix on hepatocyte growth and gene expression: implications for hepatic regeneration and the repair of liver injury. Semin Liver Dis, 1990; 10:11–19

186. Lamireau T, Zoltowska M, Levy E, Yousef I, Rosenbaum J, Tuchweber B, Desmouliere A. Effects of bile acids on biliary epithelial cells: proliferation, cytoxicity, and cytokine secretion. Life Sci, 2003; 72:1401–1411

187. Hillan KJ, Burt AD, George WD, MacSween RNM, Griffiths MR, Bradley JA. Intrasplenic hepatocyte transplantation in rats with experimental liver injury: morphological and morphometric studies. J Pathol, 1989; 159:67–73

188. Cassiman D, Libbrecht L, Sinelli N, Desmet V, Denef C, Roskams T. The vagal nerve stimulates activation of the hepatic progenitor cell compartment via muscarinic acetylcholine receptor type 3. Am J Pathol, 2002; 161:521–530

189. Roskams T, De Vos R, Van den Oord JJ, Desmet V. Cells with neuroendocrine features in regenerating human liver. APMIS, 1991; (suppl 23):32–39

190. Roskams T, Campos RV, Drucker DJ, Desmet VJ. Reactive human bile ductules express parathyroid hormone-like peptide. Histopathology, 1993; 23:11–19

191. Shibayama Y, Nakata K. Haemodynamic alterations and their morphological basis in biliary obstruction. Liver, 1992; 12:175–178

192. Fabris L, Strazzabosco M, Crosby HA et al. Characterization and isolation of ductular cells coexpressing neural cell adhesion molecule and Bcl-2 from primary cholangiopathies and ductal plate malformations. Am J Pathol, 2000; 156:1599–1612

193. Yamada S, Howe S, Scheuer PJ. Three-dimensional reconstruction of biliary pathways in primary biliary cirrhosis: a computer-assisted study. J Pathol, 1987; 152:317–323

194. Buscher H-P, Miltenberger C, MacNelly G, Gerok W. The histoautoradiographic localization of taurocholate in rat liver after bile duct ligation. J Hepatol, 1989; 8:181–191

195. Carlson E, Zukoski CF, Campbell J, Chvapil M. Morphologic, biophysical, and biochemical consequences of ligation of the common biliary duct in the dog. Am J Pathol, 1977; 86:301–320

196. Aronson DC, De Haan J, James J et al. Quantitative aspects of the parenchyma–stroma relationship in experimentally induced cholestasis. Liver, 1988; 8:116–126

197. Sedlaczek N, Jia JD, Bauer M, Herbst H, Ruehl M, Hahn EG, Schuppan D. Proliferating bile duct epithelial cells are a major source of connective tissue growth factor in rat biliary fibrosis. Am J Pathol, 2001; 158:1239–1244

198. Grappone C, Pinzani M, Parola M et al. Expression of platelet-derived growth factor in newly formed cholangiocytes during experimental biliary fibrosis in rats. J Hepatol, 1999; 31:100–109

199. Cassiman D, Libbrecht L, Desmet V, Denef C, Roskams T. Hepatic stellate cell/myofibroblast subpopulations in fibrotic human and rat livers. J Hepatol, 2002; 36:200–209

200. Schmitt-Gräff A, Krüger S, Bochard F, Gabbiani G, Denk H. Modulation of alpha smooth muscle actin and desmin expression in perisinusoidal cells of normal and diseased human livers. Am J Pathol, 1991; 138:1233–1242

201. Van Eyken P, Greets A, Bleser PD et al. Localization and cellular source of the extracellular matrix protein tenascin in normal and fibrotic rat liver. Hepatology, 1992; 15:909–916

202. Miyazaki H, Van Eyken P, Roskams T, De Vos R, Desmet VJ. Transient expression of tenascin in experimentally induced cholestatic fibrosis in rat liver. An immunohistochemical study. J Hepatol, 1993; 19:353–366

203. Griffiths MR, Shepherd M, Ferrier R, Schuppan D, James OFW, Burt AD. Light microscopic and ultrastructural distribution of type VI collagen in human liver: alterations in chronic biliary disease. Histopathology, 1992; 21:335–344

204. Pinzani M, Milani S, Grappone C. Cholestasis and fibrogenesis. In: Gentilini P, Arias IM, McIntyre N, Rodes J, eds, Cholestasis. Amsterdam: Excerpta Medica, 1994: pp 129–139

205. Bhathal PS, Gall JAM. Deletion of hyperplastic biliary epithelial cells by apoptosis following removal of the proliferative stimulus. Liver, 1985; 5:311–325

206. Abdel-Aziz G, Lebeau G, Rescan PY et al. Reversibility of hepatic fibrosis in experimentally induced cholestasis in rat. Am J Pathol, 1990; 137:1333–1342

207. Heuman DM, Pandak WM, Hylemon PB, Vlahcevic ZR. Conjugates of ursodeoxycholate protect against cytotoxicity of more hydrophobic bile salts: in vitro studies in rat hepatocytes and human erythrocytes. Hepatology, 1991; 14:920–926

208. Paumgartner G, Beuers U. Mechanisms of action and therapeutic efficacy of ursodeoxycholic acid in cholestatic liver disease. Clin Liver Dis, 2004; 8:67–81

209. Poupon RE, Lindor KD, Pares A, Chazouilleres O, Poupon R, Heathcote EJ. Combined analysis of the effect of treatment with ursodeoxycholic acid on histologic progression in primary biliary cirrhosis. J Hepatol, 2003; 39:12–16

210. Ahrens T, Payne MA, Kunkel HG. Eisenmenger WJ, Blondheim SH. Primary biliary cirrhosis. Medicine, 1950; 29:299–364

211. Rubin E, Schaffner F, Popper H. Primary biliary cirrhosis. Chronic nonsuppurative destructive cholangitis. Am J Pathol, 1965; 46:387–407

212. Kaplan MM, Gershwin ME. Primary biliary cirrhosis. N Engl J Med, 2005; 353:1261–1275

213. Dahlan Y, Smith L, Simmonds D, Jewell LD, Wanless I, Heathcote EJ, Bain VG. Pediatric-onset primary biliary cirrhosis. Gastroenterology, 2003; 125:1476–1479

214. Lucey MR, Neuberger JM, Williams R. Primary biliary cirrhosis in men. Gut, 1986; 27:1373–1376

215. Selmi C, Invernizzi P, Zuin M et al. Genetica and geoepidemiology of primary biliary cirrhosis; following the footprints to disease aetiology. Semin Liver Dis, 2005; 25:265–280

216. Triger DR, Berg PA, Rodes J. Epidemiology of primary biliary cirrhosis. Liver, 1984; 4:195–200

217. Prince MI, James OF. The epidemiology of primary biliary cirrhosis. Clin Liver Dis, 2003; 7:795–819

218. Rabinovitz M, Appasamy R, Finkelstein S. Primary biliary cirrhosis diagnosed during pregnancy. Does it have a different cause? Dig Dis Sci, 1995; 40:571–574

219. Navasa M, Parés A, Bruguera M, Caballería J, Bosch J. Rodés J. Portal hypertension in primary biliary cirrhosis. Relationship with histological features. J Hepatol, 1987; 5:292–298

220. Prince MI, Chetwynd A, Craig WL, Metcalf JV, James OF. Asymptomatic primary biliary cirrhosis: clinical features, prognosis, and symptom progression in a large population based cohort. Gut, 2004; 53:865–870

221. Mitchison HC, Lucey MR, Kelly PJ, Neuberger JM, Williams R, James OFW. Symptom development and prognosis in primary biliary cirrhosis: a study in two centers. Gastroenterology, 1990; 99:778–784

222. Balasubramaniam K, Grambsch PM, Wiesner RH, Lindor KD, Dickson ER. Diminished survival in asymptomatic primary biliary cirrhosis: a prospective study. Gastroenterology, 1990; 98:1567–1571

223. Mahl TC, Schockcor W, Boyer JL. Primary biliary cirrhosis: survival of a large cohort of symptomatic and asymptomatic patients followed for 24 years. J Hepatol, 1994; 20:707–713

224. Takeshita E, Kumagi T, Matsui H et al. Esophagogastric varices as a prognostic factor for the determination of clinical stage in patients with primary biliary cirrhosis. J Gastroenterol, 2003; 38:1060–1065

225. Goudie BM, Burt AD, Macfarlane GJ et al. Risk factors and prognosis in primary biliary cirrhosis. Am J Gastroenterol, 1989; 84:713–716

226. Neuberger J, Altman D, Christensen E, Tygstrup N, Williams R. Use of a prognostic index in evaluation of liver transplantation for primary biliary cirrhosis. Transplantation, 1986; 41:713–716

227. Markus B, Dickson ER, Grambsch P et al. Efficacy of liver transplantation in patients with primary biliary cirrhosis. N Engl J Med, 1989; 320:1709–1713

228. Uddenfeldt A, Danielsson A, Forssell A, Holm M, Östberg Y. Features of Sjögren's syndrome in patients with primary biliary cirrhosis. J Int Med, 1991; 230:443–448

229. Epstein O, Thomas HC, Sherlock S. Primary biliary cirrhosis is a dry gland syndrome with features of chronic graft-versus-host (GVH) disease. Lancet, 1980; i:1166–1168

230. Powell FC, Shroeter AL, Dickson ER. Primary biliary cirrhosis and the CREST syndrome: a report of 22 cases. Quart J Med, 1987; 62:75–82

231. Tojo J, Ohira H, Suzuki T et al. Clinicolaboratory characteristics of patients with primary biliary cirrhosis associated with CREST symptoms. Hepatol Res, 2002; 22:187–195

232. Modena V, Marengo C, Amoroso A et al. Primary biliary cirrhosis and rheumatic diseases. A clinical, immunological and immunogenetical study. Clin Exp Immunol, 1986; 4:129–134

233. Crowe JP, Christensen E, Butler J et al. Primary biliary cirrhosis: The prevalence of hypothyroidism and its relationship to thyroid auto-antibodies and sicca syndrome. Gastroenterology, 1980; 78:1437–1441

234. Pares A, Rimola A, Bruguera M, Mas E, Rodes J. Renal tubular acidosis in primary biliary cirrhosis. Gastroenterology, 1981; 80:681–686

235. Floreani A, Betterle C, Baragiotta A et al. Prevalence of coeliac disease in primary biliary cirrhosis and of antimitochondrial antibodies in adult coeliac disease patients in Italy. Dig Liver Dis, 2002; 34:258–261

236. Fracchia M, Galatola G, Corradi F, Dall'Omo AM, Rovera L, Pera A, Vitale C, Bertero MT. Coeliac disease associated with Sjogren's syndrome, renal tubular acidosis, primary biliary cirrhosis and autoimmune hyperthyroidism. Dig Liver Dis, 2004; 36:489–491

237. Hall S, Axelsen PH, Larson DE, Bunch TW. Systemic lupus erythematosus developing in patients with primary biliary cirrhosis. Ann Int Med, 1984; 100:388–389

238. Mutimer DJ, Bassendine MF, Crook P, James OFW. Vasculitis in primary biliary cirrhosis—response to prednisolone. Q J Med, 1990; 75:509–514

239. Iannone F, Falappone P, Pannarale G et al. Microscopic polyangiitis associated with primary biliary cirrhosis. J Rheumatol, 2003; 30:2710–2712

240. Weissman E, Becker NH. Interstitial lung disease in primary biliary cirrhosis. Am J Med Sci, 1983; 285:21–27

241. Bissuel F, Bizollon T, Dijoud F et al. Pulmonary hemorrhage and glomerulonephritis in primary biliary cirrhosis. Hepatology, 1992; 16:1357–1361

242. Nakamura T, Kawagoe Y, Ueda Y, Koide H. Antineutrophil cytoplasmic autoantibody-associated rapidly progressive glomerulonephritis in a patient with primary biliary cirrhosis. Am J Med Sci, 2004; 328:176–179

243. Pontecorvo MJ, Levinson JD, Roth JA. A patient with primary biliary cirrhosis and multiple sclerosis. Am J Med, 1992; 92:433–436

244. Hernandez-Boluda JC, Jimenez M, Rosinol L, Cervantes F. Idiopathic myelofibrosis associated with primary biliary cirrhosis. Leuk Lymphoma, 2002; 43:673–674

245. Xiao WB, Liu YL. Primary biliary cirrhosis and ulcerative colitis: a case report and review of literature. World J Gastroenterol, 2003; 9:878–880

246. Lino M, Binaut R, Noel LH et al. Tubulointerstitial nephritis and Fanconi syndrome in primary biliary cirrhosis. Am J Kidney Dis, 2005; e41–e46

247. Rodriguez-Luna H, Vargas HE, Williams J et al. Primary biliary cirrhosis and systemic amyloidosis. Dig Dis Sci, 2004; 49:1196–1200

248. Mitsui H, Miyauchi E, Miyahara J et al. A case of primary biliary cirrhosis accompanied with fibrinogen storage disease. Path Res Pract, 2005; 201:341–345

249. Fuller SJ, Kumar P, Weltman M, Wiley JS. Autoimmune hemolysis associated with primary biliary cirrhosis responding to ursodeoxycholic acid as sole treatment. Am J Hematol, 2003; 72:31–33

250. Eastell R, Dickson ER, Hodgson SF, Wiesner RH et al. Rates of vertebral bone loss before and after liver transplantation in women with primary biliary cirrhosis. Hepatology, 1991; 14:296–300

251. Mitchison HC, Bassendine MF, Hendrick A. Positive antimitochondrial antibody but normal alkaline phosphatase: Is this primary biliary cirrhosis? Hepatology, 1986; 6:1279–1284

252. MacSween RNM, Horne CHW, Moffat AJ, Hughes HM. Serum protein levels in primary biliary cirrhosis. J Clin Pathol, 1972; 25:789–792

253. Walker JG, Doniach D, Roitt IM, Sherlock S. Serological tests in diagnosis of primary biliary cirrhosis. Lancet, 1965; i:827–831

254. Yeaman SJ. The mammalian 2-oxoacid dehydrogenases: a complex family. Trends Biochem Sci, 1986; 11:293–297

255. Gershwin ME, Mackay IR, Sturgess A, Coppel RL. Identification and specificity of a cDNA encoding the 74kD mitochondrial antigen recognized in primary biliary cirrhosis. J Immunol, 1987; 138:3525–3531

256. Nishio A, Coppel R, Ishibashi H, Gershwin ME. The pyruvate dehydrogenase complex as a target autoantigen in primary biliary cirrhosis. Baillière's Best Pract Res Clin Gastroenterol, 2000; 14:535–547

257. Cha S, Leung PSC, Van de Water J et al. Random phage mimotopes recognized by monoclonal antibodies against the pyruvate dehydrogenase complex-E2 (PDC-E2). Proc Natl Acad Sci USA, 1996; 93:10949–10954

258. Van de Water J, Gershwin ME, Leung P, Ansari A, Coppel RL. The autoepitopes of the 74-kD mitochondrial autoantigen of primary biliary cirrhosis corresponds to the functional site of dihydrolipoamide acetyltransferase. J Exp Med, 1988; 167:1791–1799

259. Marasini B, Gagetta M, Rossi V, Ferrari P. Rheumatic disorders and primary biliary cirrhosis: an appraisal of 170 Italian patients. Ann Rheum Dis, 2001; 60:1046–1049

260. Bogdanos DP, Baum H, Butler P et al. Association between the primary biliary cirrhosis specific anti-sp100 antibodies and recurrent urinary tract infection. Dig Liver Dis, 2003; 35:801–805

261. Lin F, Noyer CM, Ye Q, Courvalin JC, Worman HJ. Autoantibodies from patients with primary biliary cirrhosis recognize a region within the nucleoplasmic domain of inner nuclear membrane protein LBR. Hepatology, 1996; 23:57–61

262. Gershwin ME, Ansari AA, Mackay IR et al. Primary biliary cirrhosis: an orchestrated immune response against epithelial cells. Immunol Rev, 2000; 174:210–225

263. Leung PS, Coppel RL, Gershwin MF. Etiology of primary biliary cirrhosis; the search for the culprit. Semin Liver Dis, 2005; 25:327–336

264. Jones DE, Donaldson PT. Genetic factors in the pathogenesis of primary biliary cirrhosis. Clin Liver Dis, 2003; 7:841–864

265. Watt FE, James OF, Jones DE. Patterns of autoimmunity in primary biliary cirrhosis patients and their families: a population-based cohort study. Q J Med, 2004; 97:397–406

266. Invernizzi P, Miozzo M, Battezzati PM et al. Frequency of monosomy X in women with primary biliary cirrhosis. Lancet, 2004; 363:533–535

267. Abu-Mouch S, Selmi C, Benson GD et al. Geographic clusters of primary biliary cirrhosis. Clin Dev Immunol, 2003; 10:127–131

268. Selmi C, Mayo MJ, Bach N et al. Primary biliary cirrhosis in monozygotic and dizygotic twins: genetics, epigenetics, and environment. Gastroenterology, 2004; 127:485–492

269. Migliaccio C, Nishio A, Van de Water J et al. Monoclonal antibodies to mitochondrial E2 components define autoepitopes in primary biliary cirrhosis. J Immunol, 1998; 161:5157–5163

270. Tsuneyama K, Van de Water J, Van Thiel D et al. Abnormal expression of PDC-E2 on the apical surface of biliary epithelial cells in patients with antimitochondrial antibody-negative primary biliary cirrhosis. Hepatology, 1995; 22:1440–1446

271. Joplin R, Lindsay JG, Hübscher SG et al. Distribution of dihydrolipoamide acetyltransferase (E2) in the liver and portal lymph nodes of patients with primary biliary cirrhosis: an immunohistochemical study. Hepatology, 1991; 14:442–447

272. Van de Water J, Turchany J, Leung PS et al. Molecular mimicry in primary biliary cirrhosis. Evidence for biliary epithelial expression of a molecule cross-reactive with pyruvate dehydrogenase complex-E2. J Clin Invest, 1993; 91:2653–2664

273. Nakanuma Y, Tsuneyama K, Kono N, Hoso M, Van de Water J, Gershwin ME. Biliary epithelial expression of pyruvate dehydrogenase complex in primary biliary cirrhosis: an immunohistochemical and immunoelectron microscopic study. Hum Pathol, 1995; 26:92–98

274. Harada K, Van de Water J, Leung PSC, Coppel R, Nakanuma Y, Gershwin ME. In situ nucleic acid hybridization of pyruvate dehydrogenase complex-E2 in primary biliary cirrhosis: pyruvate dehydrogenase complex-E2 messenger RNA is expressed in hepatocytes but not in biliary epithelial cells. Hepatology, 1997; 25:27–32

275. Van de Water J, Gerson LB, Ferrell LD et al. Immunohistochemical evidence of disease recurrence after liver retransplantation for primary biliary cirrhosis. Hepatology, 1996; 24:1074–1084

276. Neuberger J, Wallace L, Joplin R, Hübscher S. Hepatic distribution of E2-component of pyruvate dehydrogenase complex after liver transplantation. Hepatology, 1995; 22:798–801

277. Amano K, Leung PS, Xu Q et al. Xenobiotic-induced loss of tolerance in rabbits to the mitochondrial autoantigen of primary biliary cirrhosis is reversible. J Immunol, 2004; 172:6444–6452

278. Tsuneyama K, Yasoshima M, Harada K, Hiramatsu K, Gershwin ME, Nakanuma Y. Increased CD1d expression on small bile duct epithelium and epithelioid granuloma in livers in primary biliary cirrhosis. Hepatology, 1998; 28:620–623

279. Hopf U, Moller B, Stemerowicz R et al. Relation between Escherichia coli R (rough)-forms in gut, lipid A in liver, and primary biliary cirrhosis. Lancet, 1989; ii:1419–1422

280. Bogdanos DP, Baum H, Grasso A et al. Microbial mimics are major targets of crossreactivity with human pyruvate dehydrogenase in primary biliary cirrhosis. J Hepatol, 2004; 40:31–39

281. Mao TK, Lian ZX, Selmi C et al. Altered monocyte responses to defined TLR ligands in patients with primary biliary cirrhosis. Hepatology, 2005; 42:802–808

282. Klein R, Berg PA. Demonstration of antibodies against the pyruvate dehydrogenase complex (M2) in sera from patients with tuberculosis. Hepatology, 1992; 16:556

283. Johnson L, Wirostko E, Wirostko W. Primary biliary cirrhosis in the mouse: induction by human mycoplasma-like organism. Int J Exp Pathol, 1990; 71:701–712

284. Bogdanos DP, Pares A, Baum H et al. Disease-specific cross-reactivity between mimicking peptides of heat shock protein of mycobacterium gordonae and dominant epitope of E2 subunit of pyruvate dehydrogenase is common in Spanish but not British patients with primary biliary cirrhosis. J Autoimmun, 2004; 22:353–362

285. Harada K, Tsuneyama K, Sudo Y, Masuda S, Nakanuma Y. Molecular identification of bacterial 16S ribosomal RNA gene in liver tissue of primary biliary cirrhosis: is Propionibacterium acnes involved in granuloma formation? Hepatology, 2001; 33:530–536

286. Abdulkarim AS, Petrovic LM, Kim WR, Angulo P, Lloyd RV, Lindor KD. Primary biliary cirrhosis: an infectious disease caused by Chlamydia pneumoniae? J Hepatol, 2004; 40:380–384

287. Leung PS, Park O, Matsumura S, Ansari AA, Coppel RL, Gershwin ME. Is there a relation between Chlamydia infection and primary biliary cirrhosis? Clin Dev Immunol, 2003; 10:227–233

288. Bogdanos DP, Baum H, Okamoto M et al. Primary biliary cirrhosis is characterised by IgG3 antibodies cross-reactive with the major mitochondrial auto-epitope and its Lactobacillus mimics. Hepatology, 2005; 42:458–465

289. Xu L, Sakalian M, Shen Z, Loss G, Neuberger J, Mason A. Cloning the human betaretrovirus proviral genome from patients with primary biliary cirrhosis. Hepatology, 2004; 39:151–156

290. Mason AL, Farr GH, Xu L, Hubscher SG, Neuberger JM. Pilot studies of single and combination antiretroviral therapy in patients with primary biliary cirrhosis. Am J Gastroenterol, 2004; 99:2348–2355

291. Selmi C, Ross SR, Ansari AA, Invernizzi P, Podda M, Coppel RL, Gershwin ME Lack of immunological or molecular evidence for a role of mouse mammary tumor retrovirus in primary biliary cirrhosis. Gastroenterology, 2004; 127:493–501

292. Kita H, He XS, Gershwin ME. Autoimmunity and environmental factors in the pathogenesis of primary biliary cirrhosis. Ann Med, 2004; 36:72–80

293. Nagura H, Smith PD, Nakane PK, Brown WR. IgA in human bile and liver. J Immunol, 1981; 126:587–595

294. Brown WR, Kloppel TM. The liver and IgA: immunological, cell biological, and clinical implications. Hepatology, 1989; 9:763–784

295. Hashimoto E, Lindor KD, Homburger HA et al. Immunohistochemical characterization of hepatic lymphocytes in primary biliary cirrhosis in comparison with primary sclerosing cholangitis and autoimmune chronic active hepatitis. Mayo Clin Proc, 1993; 68:1049–1055

296. Yamada S, Howe S, Scheuer PJ. Three-dimensional reconstruction of biliary pathways in primary biliary cirrhosis: a computer-assisted study. J Pathol, 1987; 152:317–323

297. Nakanuma Y, Harada K. Florid duct lesion in primary biliary cirrhosis shows highly proliferative activities. J Hepatol, 1993; 19:216–221

298. Nakanuma Y, Ohta G. Quantitation of hepatic granulomas and epithelioid cells in primary biliary cirrhosis. Hepatology, 1983; 3:423–427

299. Tarao K, Shimizu A, Ohkawa S et al. Increased uptake of bromodeoxyuridine by hepatocytes from early stage of primary biliary cirrhosis. Gastroenterology, 1991; 100:725–730

300. Shibata M, Watanabe M, Ueno Y et al. Clinicopathological study of proliferating cell nuclear antigen (PCNA) of hepatocytes in primary biliary cirrhosis. J Gastroenterol, 1994; 29:56–60

301. Nakanuma Y, Ohta G. Nodular hyperplasia of the liver in primary biliary cirrhosis of early histological stages. Am J Gastroenterol, 1987; 82:8–10

302. Colina F, Pinedo F, Solis JA, Moreno D, Nevado M. Nodular regenerative hyperplasia of the liver in early histologic stages of primary biliary cirrhosis. Gastroenterology, 1992; 102:1319–1324

303. Chazouilleres O, Wendum D, Serfaty L, Montembault S, Rosmorduc O, Poupon R. Primary biliary cirrhosis-autoimmune hepatitis overlap syndrome: clinical features and response to therapy. Hepatology, 1998; 28:296–301

304. Nakanuma Y, Karino T, Ohta G. Orcein positive granules in the hepatocytes in chronic intrahepatic cholestasis. Morphological, histochemical and electron X-ray microanalytical examination. Virchows Arch A Pathol Anat, 1979; 382:21–30

305. Kowdley KV, Knox TA, Kaplan MM. Hepatic copper content is normal in early primary biliary cirrhosis and primary sclerosing cholangitis. Dig Dis Sci, 1994; 39:2416–2420

306. Nakanuma Y. Pathology of septum formation in primary biliary cirrhosis: a histological study in the non-cirrhotic stages. Virchows Arch A Pathol Anat, 1991; 419:381–387

307. Shibuya A, Tanaka K, Miyakawa H et al. Hepatocellular carcinoma and survival in patients with primary biliary cirrhosis. Hepatology, 2002; 35:1172–1178

308. Jones DE, Metcalf JV, Collier JD, Bassendine MF, James OF. Hepatocellular carcinoma in primary biliary cirrhosis and its impact on outcomes. Hepatology, 1997; 26:1138–1142

309. Tarao K, Ohkawa S, Shimizu A et al. The male preponderance in incidence of hepatocellular carcinoma in cirrhotic patients may depend on the higher DNA synthetic activity of cirrhotic liver in men. Cancer, 1993; 72:369–374

310. Nakanuma Y, Terada T, Doishita K, Miwa A. Hepatocellular carcinoma in primary biliary cirrhosis: an autopsy study. Hepatology, 1990; 11:1010–1016

311. Wolke AM, Schaffner F, Kapelman B, Sacks HS. Malignancy in primary biliary cirrhosis. High incidence of breast cancer in affected women. Am J Med, 1984; 76:1075–1078

312. Scheuer PJ. Primary biliary cirrhosis. Proc Roy Soc Med, 1967; 60:1257–1260

313. Popper H, Schaffner F. Non-suppurative destructive chronic cholangitis and chronic hepatitis. In: Popper H, Schaffner F, eds, Progress in liver diseases, vol. 3. New York: Grune & Stratton, 1970: pp 336–354

314. Ludwig J, Dickson ER, McDonald GS. Staging of chronic nonsuppurative destructive cholangitis (syndrome of primary biliary cirrhosis). Virchows Arch A, 1978; 379:103–112

315. Lee RG, Epstein O, Jauregui H, Sherlock S, Scheuer PJ. Granulomas in primary biliary cirrhosis: a prognostic feature. Gastroenterology, 1981; 81:983–986

316. Yoshikawa M, Tsujii T, Matsumura K et al. Immunomodulatory effects of ursodeoxycholic acid on immune responses. Hepatology, 1992; 16:358–364

317. Calmus Y, Gane P, Rougier P, Poupon P. Hepatic expression of class I and class II major histocompatibility complex molecule in primary biliary cirrhosis: effect of ursodeoxycholic acid. Hepatology, 1990; 11:12–15

318. Jorgensen R, Angulo P, Dickson ER, Lindor KD. Results of long-term ursodiol treatment for patients with primary biliary cirrhosis. Am J Gastroenterol, 2002; 97:2647–2650

319. Paumgartner G. Ursodeoxycholic acid treatment of primary biliary cirrhosis: potential mechanisms of action. In: Lindon KD, Heathcote EJ, Poupon R eds, Primary biliary cirrhosis: from pathogenesis to clinical treatment. Dordrecht: Kluwer Academic Pub., 1997: pp 138–146

320. Batts KP, Jorgensen RA, Dickson ER, Lindor KD. Effects of ursodeoxycholic acid on hepatic inflammation and histological stage in patients with primary biliary cirrhosis. Am J Gastroenterol, 1996; 91:2314–2317

321. Poupon RE, Lindor KD, Pares A, Chazouilleres O, Poupon R, Heathcote EJ. Combined analysis of the effect of treatment with ursodeoxycholic acid on histologic progression in primary biliary cirrhosis. J Hepatol, 2003; 39:12–16

322. Lombard M, Portmann B, Neuberger J et al. Cyclosporin A treatment in primary biliary cirrhosis. Results of a long-term placebo controlled trial. Gastroenterology, 1993; 104:519–526

323. Mitchison HC, Palmer JM, Bassendine MF, Watson AJ, Record CO, James OFW. A controlled trial of prednisolone treatment in primary biliary cirrhosis. Three-year results. J Hepatol, 1992; 15:336–344

324. Heathcote EJ. Evidence based therapy of primary biliary cirrhosis. Eur J Gastroenterol Nutr, 1999; 11:607–615

325. Combes B, Emerson SS, Flye NL. Methotrexate (MTX) plus ursodeoxycholic acid (UDCA) in the treatment of primary biliary cirrhosis. Hepatology, 2005; 42:1184–1193

326. Poupon R. Autoimmune overlapping syndromes. Clin Liver Dis, 2003; 7:865–878

327. Beuers U, Rust C. Overlap syndromes. Semin Liver Dis, 2005; 25:311–320

328. Heathcote J. Autoimmune cholangitis. Gut, 1997; 40:440–442

329. Brunner G, Klinge O. Ein der chronisch-destruierenden nichteitrigen Cholangitis ähnliches Krankheitsbild mit antinukleären Antikörpern (immunocholangitis). Dsch Med Wochenschr, 1987; 112:1454–1458

330. Ben-Ari Z, Dhillon AP, Sherlock S. Autoimmune cholangiopathy: part of the spectrum of autoimmune chronic active hepatitis. Hepatology, 1993; 18:10–15

331. Michieletti P, Wanless IR, Katz A et al. Antimitochondrial antibody negative primary biliary cirrhosis: a distinctive syndrome of autoimmune cholangitis. Gut, 1994; 35:260–265

332. Taylor SL, Dean PJ, Riely CA. Primary autoimmune cholangitis. An alternative to antimitochondrial antibody-negative primary biliary cirrhosis. Am J Surg Pathol, 1994; 18:91–99

333. Lacerda MA, Ludwig J, Dickson ER, Jorgensen RA, Lindor KD. Antimitochondrial antibody-negative primary biliary cirrhosis. Am J Gastroenterol, 1995; 90:247–249

334. Akisawa N, Nishimori I, Miyaji E et al. The ability of anti-carbonic anhydrase II antibody to distinguish autoimmune cholangitis from primary biliary cirrhosis in Japanese patients. J Gastroenterol, 1999; 34:366–371

335. Shimizu Y, Higuchi K, Kashii Y et al. Clonal accumulation of Vβ5.1-positive cells in the liver of a patient with autoimmune cholangiopathy. Liver, 1997; 17:7–12

336. Goodman ZD, McNally PR, Davis DR, Ishak KG. Autoimmune cholangitis; a variant of primary biliary cirrhosis. Dig Dis Sci, 1995; 40:1232–1242

337. Kaserer K, Exner M, Mosberger I, Penner E, Wrab F. Characterization of the inflammatory infiltrates in autoimmune cholangitis. A morphologic and immunohistochemical study. Virchows Arch, 1998; 432:217–222

338. O'Donohue J, Wong T, Portmann B, Williams R. Immunohistochemical differences in the portal tract and acinar infiltrates between primary biliary cirrhosis and autoimmune cholangitis. Eur J Gastroenterol Hepatol, 2002; 14:1143–1150

339. Nakanuma Y, Harada K, Kaji K et al. Clinicopathological study of primary biliary cirrhosis negative for antimitochondrial antibodies. Liver, 1997; 17:281–287

340. Czaja AJ, Carpenter HA, Santrach PJ et al. Autoimmune cholangitis within the spectrum of autoimmune liver disease. Hepatology, 2000; 31:1231–1238

341. Muratori P, Muratori L, Gershwin ME et al. 'True' antimitochondrial antibody-negative primary biliary cirrhosis, low

sensitivity of the routine assays, or both? Clin Exp Immunol, 2004; 135:154–158

342. Lohse AW, Meyer zum Buschenfelde KH, Kanzler FB et al. Characterization of the overlap syndrome of primary biliary cirrhosis (PBC) and autoimmune hepatitis: evidence for it being a hepatitic form of PBC in genetically susceptible individuals. Hepatology, 1999; 29:1078–1084

343. Dienes HP, Erberich H, Dries V, Schirmacher P, Lohse A. Autoimmune hepatitis and overlap syndromes. Clin Liver Dis, 2002; 6:349–362

344. Suzuki Y, Arase Y, Ikeda K et al. Clinical and pathological characteristics of the autoimmune hepatitis and primary biliary cirrhosis overlap syndrome. J Gastroenterol Hepatol, 2004; 19:699–706

345. Sato Y, Harada K, Sudo Y et al. Autoimmune hepatitis associated with bile duct injury resembling chronic non-suppurative destructive cholangitis. Pathol Int, 2002; 52:478–482

346. Jones DEJ, James OFW, Portmann B, Burt AD, Williams R, Hudson M. Development of autoimmune hepatitis following liver transplantation for primary biliary cirrhosis. Hepatology, 1999; 30:53–57

347. Horsmans Y, Piret A, Brenard R, Rahier J, Geubel AP. Autoimmune chronic active hepatitis responsive to immunosuppressive therapy evolving into a typical primary biliary cirrhosis syndrome: a case report. J Hepatol, 1994; 21:194–198

348. Geubel AP, Baggenstoss AH, Summerskill WHJ. Response to treatment can differentiate chronic active liver disease with cholangitic features from the primary biliary cirrhosis syndrome. Gastroenterology, 1976; 71:444–449

349. Pereira-Lina J, Schaffner F. Chronic cholestasis in hepatic sarcoidosis with clinical features resembling primary biliary cirrhosis. Am J Med, 1987; 83:144–148

350. Sherman S, Nieland NS, Van Thiel DH. Sarcoidosis and primary biliary cirrhosis. Coexistence in a single patient. Dig Dis Sci, 1988; 33:368–374

351. Fagan EA, Moore-Gillon JC, Turner-Warwick M. Multi-organ granulomas and mitochondrial antibodies. N Engl J Med, 1983; 308:572–575

352. Spiteri MA, Clarke SW. The nature of latent pulmonary involvement in primary biliary cirrhosis. Sarcoidosis, 1989; 6:107–110

353. Zafrani ES, Metreau J-M, Douvin C et al. Idiopathic biliary ductopenia in adults: a report of five cases. Gastroenterology, 1990; 99:1823–1828

354. Ludwig J. Idiopathic adulthood ductopenia: an update. Mayo Clin Proc, 1998; 73:285–291

355. Faa G, van Eyken P, Demelia L, Vallebona E, Costa V, Desmet VJ. Idiopathic adulthood ductopenia presenting with chronic recurrent cholestasis. A case report. J Hepatol, 1991; 12:14–20

356. Burak KW, Pearson DC, Swain MG, Kelly J, Urbanski SJ, Bridge RJ. Familial idiopathic adulthood ductopenia: a report of five cases in three generations. J Hepatol, 2000; 32:159–163

357. Dominguez-Antonaya M, Coba-Ceballos JM, Gomez-Rubio M, de Cuenca B, Ortega-Munoz P, Garcia J. Idiopathic adulthood ductopenia: a diagnosis: two clinicopathologic courses. J Clin Gastroenterol, 2000; 30:210–212

358. Perez-Atayde AR. Idiopathic biliary ductopenia. N Engl J Med, 1997; 337:280–281

359. Bruguera M, Llach J, Rodés J. Nonsyndromic paucity of intrahepatic bile ducts in infancy and idiopathic ductopenia in adulthood: the same syndrome? Hepatology, 1992; 15:830–834

360. Pauli-Magnus C, Kerb R, Fattinger K, Lang T, Anwald B, Kullak-Ublick GA, Beuers U, Meier PJ. BSEP and MDR3 haplotype structure in healthy Caucasians, primary biliary cirrhosis and primary sclerosing cholangitis. Hepatology, 2004; 39:779–791

361. Moreno A, Carreno V, Cano A, Gonzalez C. Idiopathic biliary ductopenia in adult without symptoms of liver disease. N Engl J Med, 1997; 336:835–838

362. Poulsen H, Christoffersen P. Abnormal bile duct epithelium in liver biopsies with histological signs of viral hepatitis. Acta Path Microbiol Scand, 1969; 76:383–390

363. Scheuer PJ, Ashrafzadeh P, Sherlock S, Brown D, Dusheiko GM. The pathology of hepatitis C. Hepatology, 1992; 15:567–571

364. Christoffersen P, Poulsen N, Scheuer PJ. Abnormal bile duct epithelium in chronic aggressive hepatitis and primary biliary cirrhosis. Hum Pathol, 1972; 3:227–235

365. Vyberg M. Diverticular bile duct lesion in chronic active hepatitis. Hepatology, 1989; 10:774–778

366. Zen Y, Harada K, Sasaki M et al. Are bile duct lesions of primary biliary cirrhosis distinguishable from those of autoimmune hepatitis and chronic viral hepatitis?—interobserver histological agreement on trimmed bile ducts. J Gastroenterol, 2005; 40:164–170

367. Bach N, Thung SN, Schaffner F. The histological features of chronic hepatitis C and autoimmune chronic hepatitis: a comparative analysis. Hepatology, 1992; 15:572–577

368. Lefkowitch JH, Schiff ER, Davis GL et al. Pathological diagnosis of chronic hepatitis C: a multicenter comparative study with chronic hepatitis B. Gastroenterology, 1993; 104:595–603

369. Harada K, Minato H, Hiramatsu K, Nakanuma Y. Epithelioid cell granulomas in chronic hepatitis C: immunohistochemical character and histological marker of favourable response to interferon-alpha therapy. Histopathology, 1998; 33:216–221

370. Golding RD, Patel NK, Thomas HC. Hepatitis C and bile duct loss. J Clin Pathol, 1996; 49:836–838

371. Nouri Aria KT, Sallie R, Sangar F et al. Detection of hepatitis C virus genome in liver tissue by in situ hybridisation. J Clin Invest, 1993; 91:2226–2234

372. Haddad J, Deny P, Munz-Gotheil C et al. Lymphocytic sialoadenitis of Sjögren syndrome associated with chronic hepatitis C virus liver disease. Lancet, 1992; 339:321–323

373. Kaji K, Tsuneyama K, Nakanuma Y et al. B7-2 positive cells around interlobular bile ducts in primary biliary cirrhosis and chronic hepatitis C. J Gastroenterol Hepatol, 1997; 12:507–512

374. Mosnier JF, Scoazec JY, Marcellin P, Degott C, Benhamou JP, Feldmann G. Expression of cytokine-dependent immune adhesion molecules by hepatocytes and bile duct cells in chronic hepatitis C. Gastroenterology, 1994; 107:1457–1468

375. Wendrum D, Nachury M, Yver M et al. Acute hepatitis E: a cause of lymphocytic destructive cholangitis. Hum Pathol, 2005; 36:436–438

376. Lucas SB. Other viral and infectious diseases and HIV-related liver disease. In: MacSween RNM, Burt AD, Portmann BC, Scheuer PJ, Anthony PP, eds, Pathology of the liver, 4th edn. Edinburgh: Churchill Livingstone, 2002: pp 397

377. Kage M, Kosai K, Kojiro M, Nakamura Y, Fukuda S. Infantile cholestasis due to cytomegalovirus infection of the liver. A possible cause of paucity of interlobular bile ducts. Arch Pathol Lab Med, 1993; 117:942–944

378. Degott C, Feldmann G, Larvey D et al. Drug-induced prolonged cholestasis in adults: a histologic semiquantitation study demonstrating progressive ductopenia. Hepatology, 1992; 15:244–251

379. Forbes GM, Jeffrey GP, Shilkin KB, Reed WD. Carbamazepine hepatotoxicity: another cause of the vanishing bile duct syndrome. Gastroenterology, 1992; 102:1385–1388

380. Walker CO, Combes B. Biliary cirrhosis induced by chlorpromazine. Gastroenterology, 1985; 511:631–640

381. Richardet JP, Mallat A, Zafrani ES, Blazquez M, Bognel JC, Campillo B. Prolonged cholestasis with ductopenia after administration of amoxicillin/clavulanic acid. Dig Dis Sci, 1999; 44:1997–2000

382. Chawla A, Kahn E, Yunis EJ, Daum F. Rapidly progressive cholestasis: An unusual reaction to amoxicillin/clavulanic acid therapy in a child. J Pediatr, 2000; 136:121–123

383. Trak-Smayra V, Cazals-Hatem D, Asselah T, Duchatelle V, Degott C. Prolonged cholestasis and ductopenia associated with tenoxicam. J Hepatol, 2003; 39:125–128

384. Horsmans Y, Rahier J, Geubel AP. Reversible cholestasis with bile duct injury following azathioprine therapy. A case report. Liver, 1991; 11:89–93

385. Basile G, Villari D, Gangemi S, Ferrara T, Accetta MG, Nicita-Mauro V. Candesartan cilexetil-induced severe hepatotoxicity. J Clin Gastroenterol, 2003; 273–275

386. McMaster KR, Henniger GR. Drug induced granulomatous hepatitis. Lab Investigation, 1981; 44:61–73

387. Petersen BE, Zajac VF, Michalopoulos GK. Bile ductular damage induced by methylene dianiline inhibits oval cell activation. Am J Pathol, 1997; 151:905–909

388. Kopelman H, Scheuer PJ, Williams R. The liver lesion in the Epping jaundice. Quart J Med, 1966; 35:553–564

389. Matsumoto T, Matumori H, Kuwabara N, Fukuda Y, Ariwa R. A histopathological study of the liver in paraquat poisoning. An analysis of fourteen autopsy cases with emphasis on bile duct injury. Acta Pathol Japan, 1980; 30:859–870

390. Mullick FG, Ishak KG, Mahabir R, Stromeyer FW. Hepatic injury associated with paraquat toxicity in humans. Liver, 1981; 1:209–211

391. Wolkenstein P, Revuz J. Drug-induced severe skin reactions. Incidence, management and prevention. Drug Saf, 1995; 13:56–58

392. Srivastava M, Perez-Atayde A, Jonas MM. Drug-associated acute-onset vanishing bile duct syndrome and Stevens-Johnson syndrome in a child. Gastroenterology, 1998; 115:743–746

393. Cavanzo FJ, Garcia CF, Botero RC. Chronic cholestasis, paucity of bile ducts, red cell aplasia and the Stevens-Johnson syndrome. An ampicillin-associated case. Gastroenterology, 1990; 99:854–856

394. Revuz JE, Roujeau JC. Advances in toxic epidermal necrolysis. Semin Cutan Med Surg, 1996; 15:258–266

395. Chamuleau RA, Diekman MJ, Bos PJ, Smitt JH, Bosma A, Schellekens PT. Reappearance of vanished bile ducts. Hepatogastroenterology, 1992; 39:523–524

396. Lieberman DA. Intrahepatic cholestasis due to Hodgkin's disease: an elusive diagnosis. J Clin Gastroenterol, 1986; 8:304–307

397. Birrer MJ, Young RC. Differential diagnosis of jaundice in lymphoma patients. Semin Liver Dis, 1987; 3:269–277

398. Miller DJ, Keeton GR, Webber BL, Saunders SJ. Jaundice in severe bacterial infection. Gastroenterology, 1976; 71:94–97

399. Vyberg M, Poulsen H. Abnormal bile duct epithelium accompanying septicaemia. Virchows Arch (A), 1984; 71:1075–1078

400. Kullak-Ublick GA, Beuers U, Paumgartner G. Liver Disease 2000 and beyond. Hepatobiliary transport. J Hepatol, 2000; 32(suppl 1):3–18

401. Moseley RH. Sepsis-associated cholestasis. Gastroenterology, 1997; 112:302–306

402. Lefkowitch JH. Bile ductular cholestasis: an ominous histological sign related to sepsis and 'cholangitis lenta'. Hum Pathol, 1982; 13:19–24

403. Banks JG, Foulis AK, Ledingham IMA, MacSween RNM. Liver function in septic shock. J Clin Pathol, 1982; 35:1249–1252

404. Ishak KG, Rogers WA. Cryptogenic acute cholangitis—association with toxic shock syndrome. Am J Clin Pathol, 1981; 76:619–626

405. Ludwig J. Small-duct primary sclerosing cholangitis. Semin Liver Dis, 1991; 11:11–17

406. Kaw M, Silverman WB, Rabinovitz M, Shade RR. Biliary calculi in primary sclerosing cholangitis. Am J Gastroenterol, 1995; 90:72–75

407. Van Leeuwen DJ, Reeders JW. Primary sclerosing cholangitis and cholangiocarcinoma as a diagnostic and therapeutic dilemma. Ann Oncol, 1999; 10(suppl 4):89–93

408. Bergquist A, Glaumann H, Persson B, Broome U. Risk factors and clinical presentation of hepatobiliary carcinoma in patients with primary sclerosing cholangitis: a case-control study. Hepatology, 1998; 27:311–316

409. Sherlock S. Pathogenesis of sclerosing cholangitis: the role of immune factors. Semin Liver Dis, 1991; 11:5–10

410. Chapman RWG, Arborgh BAM, Rhodes JM et al. Primary sclerosing cholangitis: a review of its clinical features, cholangiography and hepatic histology. Gut, 1980; 21:870–877

411. Amedee-Manesme O, Bernard O, Brunelle F et al. Sclerosing cholangitis with neonatal onset. J Paediatr, 1987; 111:225–229

412. El-Shabrawi M, Wilkinson ML, Portmann B et al. Primary sclerosing cholangitis in childhood. Gastroenterology, 1987; 92:1226–1235

413. Wilschanski M, Chait P, Wade JA et al. Primary sclerosing cholangitis in 32 children: Clinical, laboratory, and radiographic features, with survival analysis. Hepatology, 1995; 22:1415–1422

414. Helzberg JH, Petersen JM, Boyer JL. Improved survival with primary sclerosing cholangitis. A review of clinicopathologic features and comparison of symptomatic and asymptomatic patients. Gastroenterology, 1987; 92:1869–1875

415. Rabinovitz M, Gavaler JS, Schade RR, Dindzans VJ, Chien M-C, van Thiel DH. Does primary sclerosing cholangitis occurring in association with inflammatory bowel disease differ from that occurring in the absence of inflammatory bowel disease? a study of sixty-six subjects. Hepatology, 1990; 11:7–11

416. Bjornsson E, Simren M, Olsson R, Chapman RW. Fatigue in patients with primary sclerosing cholangitis. Scand J Gastroenterol, 2004; 39:961–968

417. Schrumpf E, Fausa O, Kolmannskog F, Elgjo K, Ritland S, Gjone E. Sclerosing cholangitis in ulcerative colitis, a follow-up study. Scand J Gastroenterol, 1982; 17:33–39

418. Wiesner RH, LaRusso NF, Ludwig J, Dickson ER. Comparison of the clinicopathologic features of primary sclerosing cholangitis and primary biliary cirrhosis. Gastroenterology, 1985; 88:108–114

419 Porayko MK, Wiesner RH, LaRusso NF et al. Patients with asymptomatic primary sclerosing cholangitis frequently have progressive disease. Gastroenterology, 1990; 98:1595–1602

420. Farrant JM, Hayllar KM, Wilkinson ML, Karani J, Portmann BC, Westaby D, Williams R. Natural history and prognostic variables in primary sclerosing cholangitis. Gastroenterology, 1991; 100:1710–1717

421. Broome U, Olsson R, Loof L et al. Natural history and prognostic factors in 305 Swedish patients with primary sclerosing cholangitis. Gut, 1996; 38:610–615

422. Goudie BM, Birnie GG, Watkinson G, MacSween RNM. A case of long-standing primary sclerosing cholangitis. J Clin Pathol, 1983; 36:1298–1301

423. Kim WR, Therneau TM, Wiesner RH et al. A revised natural history model for primary sclerosing cholangitis. Mayo Clin Proc, 2000; 75:688–694

424. Neuberger J, Gunson B, Komolmit P, Davies MH, Christensen E. Pretransplant prediction of prognosis after liver transplantation in primary sclerosing cholangitis using a Cox regression model. Hepatology, 1999; 29:1375–1379

425. Harrison PM. Prevention of bile duct cancer in primary sclerosing cholangitis. Ann Oncol, 1999; 10(suppl 4):208–211

426. Olsson R, Danielsson A, Jarnerot G et al. Prevalence of primary sclerosing cholangitis in patients with ulcerative colitis. Gastroenterology, 1991; 100:1319–1323

427. Rasmussen HH, Fallingborg J, Mortensen PB et al. Primary sclerosing cholangitis in patients with ulcerative colitis. Scand J Gastroenterol, 1992; 27:732–736

428. Fausa O, Schrumpf E, Elgjo K. Relationship of inflammatory bowel disease and primary sclerosing cholangitis. Semin Liver Dis, 1991; 11:31–39

429. Takikawa H, Takamori Y, Tanaka A, Kurihara H, Nakanuma Y. Analysis of 388 cases of primary sclerosing cholangitis in Japan; Presence of a subgroup without pancreatic involvement in older patients. Hepatol Res, 2004; 29:153–159

430. Okazaki K, Chiba T. Autoimmune related pancreatitis. Gut, 2002; 51:1–4

431. Klöppel G, Luttges J, Lohr M, Zamboni G, Longnecker D. Autoimmune pancreatitis: pathological, clinical, and immunological features. Pancreas, 2003; 27:14–19

432. McGarity B, Bansi DS, Robertson DAF, Millward-Sadler GH, Shepherd HA. Primary sclerosing cholangitis: an important and prevalent complication of Crohn's disease. Eur J Gastroenterol Hepatol, 1991; 3:361–364

433. Rasmussen HH, Fallingborg JF, Mortensen PB, Vyberg M, Tage-Jensen U, Rasmussen SN. Hepatobiliary dysfunction and primary sclerosing cholangitis in patients with Crohn's disease. Scand J Gastroenterol, 1997; 32:604–610

434. Børkje B, Vetvik K, Odegaard S, Schrumpf E, Larssen TB, Kolmannskog F. Chronic pancreatitis in patients with sclerosing cholangitis and ulcerative colitis. Scand J Gastroenterol, 1985; 20:539–542

435. Imrie CW, Bombacher GD. Sclerosing cholangitis: a rare etiology for acute pancreatitis. Int J Pancreatol, 1998; 23:71–75

436. Kawaguchi K, Koike M, Tsuruta K, Tabata I, Fujita N. Lymphoplasmacytic sclerosing pancreatitis with cholangitis: A variant of primary sclerosing cholangitis extensively involving the pancreas. Hum Pathol, 1991; 22:387–395

437. Kojima E, Kimura K, Noda Y, Kobayashi G, Itoh K, Fujita N. Autoimmune pancreatitis and multiple bile duct strictures treated effectively with steroid. J Gastroenterol, 2003; 38:603–607

438. Montefulso PP, Geiss AC, Bronzo RL et al. Sclerosing cholangitis, chronic pancreatitis, and Sjögren's syndrome: A syndrome complex. Am J Surg, 1984; 147:822–826

439. Nieminen U, Koivisto T, Kahri A, Farkkila M. Sjögren's syndrome with chronic pancreatitis, sclerosing cholangitis, and pulmonary infiltrations. Am J Gastroenterol, 1997; 92:139–142

440. Kamisawa T, Funata N, Hayashi Y et al. A new clinicopathological entity of IgG4-related autoimmune disease. J Gastroenterol, 2003; 38:982–984

441. Zen Y, Harada K, Sasaki M et al. IgG4-related sclerosing cholangitis with and without hepatic inflammatory pseudotumor, and sclerosing pancreatitis-associated sclerosing cholangitis: do they belong to a spectrum of sclerosing pancreatitis? Am J Surg Pathol, 2004; 28:1193–1203

442. Nakanuma Y, Tsuneyama K, Masuda S, Tomioka T. Hepatic inflammatory pseudotumor associated with chronic cholangitis: report of three cases. Hum Pathol, 1994; 25:86–91

443. Toda K, Yasuda I, Nishigaki Y et al. Inflammatory pseudotumor of the liver with primary sclerosing cholangitis. J Gastroenterol, 2000; 35:304–309

444. Toosi MN, Heathcote J. Pancreatic pseudotumor with sclerosing pancreato-cholangitis: is this a systemic disease? Am J Gastroenterol, 2004; 99:377–382

445. Bartholomew LG, Cain JC, Woolner LB, Utz DC. Sclerosing cholangitis. Its possible association with Riedel's thyroiditis and fibrous retroperitonitis. N Engl J Med, 1963; 267:8–12

446. Comings DE, Skubi KB, van Eyes J, Motulsky AG. Familial multifocal fibrosclerosis. Findings suggesting that retroperitoneal fibrosis, mediastinal fibrosis, sclerosing cholangitis, Riedel's thyroiditis, and pseudotumor of the orbit may be different manifestations of a single disease. Ann Intern Med, 1967; 66:884–892

447. Oguz KK, Kiratli H, Oguz O, Cila A, Oto A, Gokoz A. Multifocal fibrosclerosis: a new case report and review of the literature. Eur Radiol, 2002; 12:1134–1138

448. Wurm P, Dixon AD, Rathbone BJ. Ulcerative colitis, primary sclerosing cholangitis and coeliac disease: two cases and review of the literature. Eur J Gastroenterol Hepatol, 2003; 15:815–817

449. Habior A, Rawa T, Orlowska J et al. Association of primary sclerosing cholangitis, ulcerative colitis and coeliac disease in female siblings. Eur J Gastroenterol Hepatol, 2002; 14:787–791

450. Delevaux I, Andre M, Chipponi J, Milesi-Lecat AM, Dechelotte P, Aumaitre O. A rare manifestation of idiopathic hypereosinophilic syndrome: sclerosing cholangitis. Dig Dis Sci, 2002; 47:148–151

451. Thurlow PJ, Marshall AW. Extreme hypereosinophilia in sclerosing cholangitis. Intern Med J, 2003; 33:134–136

452. Viteri AL, Hardin WJ, Dyck WP. Peyronie's disease and sclerosing cholangitis in a patient with ulcerative colitis. Dig Dis Sci, 1979; 24:490–491

453. Audan A, Bruley Des Varannes S, Georgelin T. Primary sclerosing cholangitis and systemic lupus erythematosus. Gastroenterol Clin Biol, 1995; 19:123–126

454. Kirby DF, Blei AT, Rosen ST et al. Primary sclerosing cholangitis in the presence of lupus anticoagulant. Am J Med, 1986; 83:1077–1080

455. Karatapanis T, McCormich PA, Burroughs AK. Ulcerative colitis complicated by Budd-Chiari syndrome and primary sclerosing cholangitis. Eur J Gastroenterol Hepatol, 1992; 4:683–686

456. Moeller DD. Sclerosing cholangitis associated with autoimmune hemolytic anaemia and hyperthyroidism. Am J Gastroenterol, 1985; 80:122–125

457. Janssen HL, Smelt AH, van Hoek B. Graves' hyperthyroidism in a patient with primary sclerosing cholangitis. Coincidence or combined pathogenesis? Eur J Gastroenterol Hepatol, 1998; 10:269–271

458. Fishman G, DeRowe A, Wasserman D, Leider-Trejo L, Reif S. Inflammatory bowel disease and sclerosing cholangitis with ulcerative lesions on skin and soft palate. Int J Pediatr Otorhinolaryngol, 2004; 68:1349–1352

459. Anwar MA, Rampling MW. Erythrocyte hyper-aggregation in a patient undergoing orthotopic transplantation for primary sclerosing cholangitis complicated by biliary stricture. Clin Hemorheol Microcirc, 2004; 31:169–172

460. Sakai M, Egawa N, Sakamaki H et al. Primary sclerosing cholangitis complicated with idiopathic thrombocytopenic purpura. Intern Med, 2001; 40:1209–1214

461. Pineau BC, Pattee LP, McGuire S, Sekar A, Scully LJ. Unusual presentation of primary sclerosing cholangitis. Can J Gastroenterol, 1997; 11:45–48

462. Schep GN, Scully LJ. Primary sclerosing cholangitis and sarcoidosis: An unusual combination. Case report and review of the literature. Can J Gastroenterol, 1990; 4:489–494

463. Keller K, Hofmann WJ, Kayser K et al. Coincidence of primary sclerosing cholangitis and sarcoidosis—case report and review of the literature. Z Gastroenterol, 1997; 35:33–39

464. Alam I, Levenson SD, Ferrell LD, Bass NM. Diffuse intrahepatic biliary strictures in sarcoidosis resembling sclerosing cholangitis. Case report and review of the literature. Dig Dis Sci, 1997; 42:1295–1301

465. Angulo P, Therneau TM, Jorgensen RA et al. Bone disease in patients with primary sclerosing cholangitis: prevalence, severity and prediction of progression. J Hepatol, 1998; 29:729–735

466. Burak K, Angulo P, Pasha TM, Egan K, Petz J, Lindor KD. Incidence and risk factors for cholangiocarcinoma in primary sclerosing cholangitis. Am J Gastroenterol, 2004; 99:523–526

467. Ismail T, Angrisani L, Hübscher S, McMaster P. Hepatocellular carcinoma complicating primary sclerosing cholangitis. Br J Surg, 1991; 78:360–361

468. Snook JA, Kelly P, Chapman RW, Jewell DP. Fibrolamellar hepatocellular carcinoma complicating ulcerative colitis with primary sclerosing cholangitis. Gut, 1989; 30:243–245

469. Wee A, Ludwig J, Coffey RJ, LaRusso NF, Wiesner RH. Hepatobiliary carcinoma associated with primary sclerosing cholangitis and chronic ulcerative colitis. Hum Pathol, 1985; 16:719–726

470. Gow PJ, Chapman RW. Simultaneous occurrence of focal nodular hyperplasia and primary sclerosing cholangitis in a young female. Eur J Gastroenterol Hepatol, 2000; 12:565–567

471. Balasubramaniam K, Wiesner RH, LaRusso NR. Primary sclerosing cholangitis with normal serum alkaline phosphatase activity. Gastroenterology, 1988; 95:1395–1398

472. Roozendaal C, de Jong MA, van den Berg AP, van Wijk RT, Limburg PC, Kallenberg CG. Clinical significance of anti-neutrophil cytoplasmic antibodies (ANCA) in autoimmune liver diseases. J Hepatol, 2000; 32:734–741

473. Zauli D, Schrumpf E, Crespi C, Cassani F, Fausa O, Aadland E. An autoantibody profile in primary sclerosing cholangitis. J Hepatol, 1987; 5:14–18

474. Angulo P, Peter JB, Gershwin E et al. Serum autoantibodies in patients with primary sclerosing cholangitis. J Hepatol, 2000; 32:182–187

475. Elias E, Summerfield JD, Dick R, Sherlock S. Endoscopic retrograde cholangiopancreatography in the diagnosis of jaundice associated with ulcerative colitis. Gastroenterology, 1974; 67:907–911

476. MacCarty RL, LaRusso NF, Wiesner RH, Ludwig J. Primary sclerosing cholangitis: Findings on cholangiography and pancreatography. Radiology, 1983; 149:39–44

477. Gulliver DJ, Baker ME, Putnam W, Baillie J, Rice R, Cotton PB. Bile duct diverticula and webs: nonspecific cholangiographic features of primary sclerosing cholangitis. Am J Roentgenol, 1991; 157:281–285

478. Geneve J, Dubuc N, Mathieu D, Zafrani ES, Dhumeaux D, Métreau JM. Cystic dilatation of intrahepatic bile ducts in primary sclerosing cholangitis. J Hepatol, 1990; 11:196–199

479. Chen V, Goldberg HI. Sclerosing cholangitis: Broad spectrum of radiographic features. Gastrointest Radiol, 1984; 9:39–47

480. Vitellas KM, Keogan MT, Freed KS et al. Radiologic manifestations of sclerosing cholangitis with emphasis on MR cholangiopancreatography. Radiographics, 2000; 20:959–975

481. Textor HJ, Flacke S, Pauleit D et al. Three-dimensional magnetic resonance cholangiopancreatography with respiratory triggering in the diagnosis of primary sclerosing cholangitis: comparison with endoscopic retrograde cholangiography. Endoscopy, 2002; 34:984–990

482. Rosen CB, Nagorney DM. Cholangiocarcinoma complicating primary sclerosing cholangitis. Semin Liver Dis, 1991; 11:26–30

483. Ponsioen CY, Vrouenraets SM, van Milligen de Wit AW et al. Value of brush cytology for dominant strictures in primary sclerosing cholangitis. Endoscopy, 1999; 31:305–309

484. Furmanczyk PS, Grieco VS, Agoff SN et al. Biliary brush cytology and the detection of cholangiocarcinoma in primary sclerosing cholangitis: evaluation of specific cytomorphological features and CA19-9 levels. Am J Clin Pathol, 2005; 124:355–360

485. Keiding S, Hansen SB, Rasmussen HH et al. Detection of cholangiocarcinoma in primary sclerosing cholangitis by positron emission tomography. Hepatology, 1998; 28:700–706

486. Patel T. Aberrant local renin-angiotensin II responses in the pathogenesis of primary sclerosing cholangitis. Med Hypotheses, 2003; 61:64–67

487. Narayanan Menon KV, Wiesner RH. Etiology and natural history of primary sclerosing cholangitis. J Hepatobiliary Pancreat Surg, 1999; 6:343–351

488. Eksteen B, Grant AJ, Miles A et al. Hepatic endothelial CCL25 mediates the recruitment of CCR9+ gut-homing lymphocytes to the liver in primary sclerosing cholangitis. J Exp Med, 2004; 200:1511–1517

489. Quigley EMM, LaRusso NF, Ludwig J, MacSween RNM, Birnie GG, Watkinson G. Familial occurrence of primary sclerosing cholangitis and ulcerative colitis. Gastroenterology, 1983; 85:1160–1165

490. Silber GH, Finegold MJ, Wagner ML, Klish WJ. Sclerosing cholangitis and ulcerative colitis in a mother and her son. J Pediatr Gastroenterol Nutr, 1987; 6:147–152

491. Bergquist A, Lundberg G, Saarinen S, Broome U. Increased prevalence of primary sclerosing cholangitis among first degree relatives. J Hepatol, 2005; 42:252–256

492. Schrumpf E, Fausa O, Forre O, Dobloug JH, Ritland S, Thorsby E. HLA antigens and immunoregulatory T cells in ulcerative colitis associated with hepatobiliary disease. Scand J Gastroenterol, 1982; 17:187–191

493. Donaldson PT, Farrant JM, Wilkinson ML, Hayllar K, Portmann B, Williams R. Dual association of HLA DR2 and DR3 with primary sclerosing cholangitis. Hepatology, 1991; 13:129–133

494. Yang X, Cullen SN, Li JH, Chapman RW, Jewell DP. Susceptibility to primary sclerosing cholangitis is associated with polymorphisms of intercellular adhesion molecule-1. J Hepatol, 2004; 40:375–379

495. Eri R, Jonsson JR, Pandeya N et al. CCR5-Delta32 mutation is strongly associated with primary sclerosing cholangitis. Genes Immun, 2004; 5:444–450

496. Prochazka EJ, Terasaki PI, Park MS, Goldstein LI, Busuttil RW. Association of primary sclerosing cholangitis with HLA-DRw52a. N Engl J Med, 1990; 322:1842–1844

497. Farrant JM, Doherty DG, Donaldson PT et al. Amino acid substitutions at position 38 of the DR beta polypeptide confer susceptibility to and protection from primary sclerosing cholangitis. Hepatology, 1992; 16:390–395

498. Spurkland A, Saarinen S, Boberg KM et al. HLA class II haplotypes in primary sclerosing cholangitis patients from five European populations. Tissue Antigens, 1999; 53:459–469

499. Donaldson PT, Norris S. Evaluation of the role of MHC class II alleles, haplotypes and selected amino acid sequences in primary sclerosing cholangitis. Autoimmunity, 2002; 35:555–564

500. Neri TM, Cavestro GM, Seghini P et al. Novel association of HLA-haplotypes with primary sclerosing cholangitis (PSC) in a southern European population. Dig Liver Dis, 2003; 35:571–576

501. Sheth S, Shea JC, Bishop MD et al. Increased prevalence of CFTR mutations and variants and decreased chloride secretion in primary sclerosing cholangitis. Hum Genet, 2003; 113:286–292

502. Aadland E, Schrumpf E, Fausa O et al. Primary sclerosing cholangitis: A long-term follow-up study. Scand J Gastroenterol, 1987; 22:655–664

503. Chapman RW, Cottone M, Selby WS, Shepherd HA, Sherlock S, Jewell DP. Serum autoantibodies, ulcerative colitis and primary sclerosing cholangitis. Gut, 1986; 27:86–91

504. Mieli-Vergani G, Lobo-Yeo A, McFarlane BM, McFarlane IG, Mowat AP, Vergani D. Different immune mechanism leading to autoimmunity in primary sclerosing cholangitis and autoimmune chronic active hepatitis of childhood. Hepatology, 1989; 9:198–203

505. Bansal AS, Thomson A, Steadman C et al. Serum levels of interleukins 8 and 10, interferon gamma, granulocyte-macrophage colony stimulating factor and soluble CD23 in patients with primary sclerosing cholangitis. Autoimmunity, 1997; 26:223–229

506. Bodenheimer HC, LaRusso NF, Thayer WP Jr et al. Elevated circulating immune complexes in primary sclerosing cholangitis. Hepatology, 1983; 3:150–154

507. Minuk GY, Angus M, Brickman CM et al. Abnormal clearance of immune complexes from the circulation of patients with primary sclerosing cholangitis and ulcerative colitis. Gastroenterology, 1985; 88:166–170

508. Senaldi G, Donaldson P, Magrin S et al. Activation of the complement system in primary sclerosing cholangitis. Gastroenterology, 1989; 97:1430–1434

509. McFarlane IG, Wojcicka BM, Tsantoulas DC, Portmann B, Eddleston ALWF, Williams R. Leucocyte migration inhibition in response to biliary antigens in primary biliary cirrhosis, sclerosing cholangitis, and other chronic liver disease. Gastroenterology, 1979; 76:1333–1340

510. Lindor KD, Wiesner RH, Katzmann JA et al. Lymphocyte subsets in primary sclerosing cholangitis. Dig Dis Sci, 1987; 32:720–725

511. Snook JA, Chapman RW, Sachdev GK et al. Peripheral blood and portal tract lymphocyte populations in primary sclerosing cholangitis. J Hepatol, 1989; 9:36–40

512. Ponsioen CY, Kuiper H, Ten Kate FJ, van Milligen de Wit M, van Deventer SJ, Tytgat GN. Immunohistochemical analysis of inflammation in primary sclerosing cholangitis. Eur J Gastroenterol Hepatol, 1999; 11:769–774

513. Boberg KM, Fausa O, Haaland T et al. Features of autoimmune hepatitis in primary sclerosing cholangitis: an evaluation of 114 primary sclerosing cholangitis patients according to a scoring system for the diagnostic of autoimmune hepatitis. Hepatology, 1996; 23:1369–1376

514. Adams DH, Hübscher SG, Shaw J et al. Increased expression of intercellular adhesion molecule 1 on bile ducts in primary biliary cirrhosis and primary sclerosing cholangitis. Hepatology, 1991; 14:426–431

515. Sakamaki S, Takayanagi N, Yoshizaki N et al. Autoantibodies against the specific epitope of human tropomyosin(s) detected by a peptide based enzyme immunoassay in sera of patients with ulcerative colitis show antibody dependent cell mediated cytotoxicity against HLA-DPw9 transfected L cells. Gut, 2000; 47:236–241

516. Chapman RW, Kelly PMA, Heryet A, Jewell DP, Fleming KA. Expression of HLA-DR antigens on bile duct epithelium in primary sclerosing cholangitis. Gut, 1988; 29:870–877

517. Cruickshank SM, Southgate J, Wyatt JI, Selby PJ, Trejdosiewicz LK. Expression of CD44 on bile ducts in primary sclerosing cholangitis and primary biliary cirrhosis. J Clin Pathol, 1999; 52:730–734

518. Eksteen B, Grant AJ, Miles A et al. Hepatic endothelial CCL25 mediates the recruitment of CCR9+ gut homing lymphocytes to the liver in primary sclerosing cholangitis. J Exp Med, 2004; 200:1511–1517

519. Glaser JH, Morecki R. Reovirus type 3 and neonatal cholestasis. Semin Liver Dis, 1987; 7:100–107

520. Minuk GY, Rascanin N, Paul RW, Lee PWK, Buchan K, Kelly JK. Reovirus type 3 infection in patients with primary sclerosing cholangitis. J Hepatol, 1987; 5:8–13

521. Mehal WZ, Hattersley AT, Chapman RW, Fleming KA. A survey of cytomegalovirus (CMV) DNA in primary sclerosing cholangitis (PSC) liver tissue using a sensitive polymerase chain reaction (PCR) based assay. J Hepatol, 1992; 15:396–399

522. Nilsson HO, Taneera J, Castedal M, Glatz E, Olsson R, Wadstrom T. Identification of Helicobacter pylori and other Helicobacter species by PCR, hybridization, and partial DNA sequencing in human liver samples from patients with primary sclerosing cholangitis or primary biliary cirrhosis. J Clin Microbiol, 2000; 38:1072–1076

523. Lefkowitch JH. Primary sclerosing cholangitis. Arch Intern Med, 1982; 142:1157–1160

524. Casali AM, Carbone G, Cavalli G. Intrahepatic bile duct loss in primary sclerosing cholangitis: a quantitative study. Histopathology, 1998; 32:449–453

525. Harrison RF, Hübscher SG. The spectrum of bile duct lesions in end-stage primary sclerosing cholangitis. Histopathology, 1991; 19:321–327

526. Angulo P, Larson DR, Therneau TM, LaRusso NF, Batts KP, Lindor KD. Time course of histological progression in primary sclerosing cholangitis. Am J Gastroenterol, 1999; 94:3310–3313

527. Burak KW, Angulo P, Lindor KD. Is there a role for liver biopsy in primary sclerosing cholangitis? Am J Gastroenterol, 2003; 98:1155–1158

528. Ito H, Imada T, Rino Y, Kondo J. A case of segmental primary sclerosing cholangitis. Hepatogastroenterology, 2000; 47:128–131

529. Keaveny AP, Gordon FD, Goldar-Najafi A et al. Native liver xanthogranulomatous cholangiopathy in primary sclerosing cholangitis: impact on posttransplant outcome. Liver Transpl, 2004; 10:115–122

530. Ludwig J, Barham SS, LaRusso NF, Elveback LR, Wiesner RH, McCall JT. Morphologic features of chronic hepatitis associated with primary sclerosing cholangitis and ulcerative colitis. Hepatology, 1981; 1:632–640

531. Harrison PM. Diagnosis of primary sclerosing cholangitis. J Hepatobiliary Pancreat Surg, 1999; 6:356–360

532. Sapey T, Turlin B, Canva-Delcambre V et al. Importance of liver puncture biopsy and endoscopic retrograde cholangiography in patients with chronic anicteric unexplained cholestasis. A retrospective study in 79 patients. Gastroenterol Clin Biol, 1999; 23:178–185

533. Feldstein AE, Perrault J, El-Youssif M, Lindor KD, Freese DK, Angulo P. Primary sclerosing cholangitis in children: a long-term follow-up study. Hepatology, 2003; 38:210–217

534. Narumi S, Roberts JP, Emond JC, Lake J, Asher NL. Liver transplantation for sclerosing cholangitis. Hepatology, 1995; 22:451–457

535. Maheshwari A, Yoo HY, Thuluvath PJ. Long-term outcome of liver transplantation in patients with PSC: a comparative analysis with PBC. Am J Gastroenterol, 2004; 99:538–542

536. Brandsaeter B, Schrumpf E, Clausen OP, Abildgaard A, Hafsahl G, Bjoro K. Recurrent sclerosing cholangitis or ischemic bile duct lesions—a diagnostic challenge? Liver Transpl, 2004; 10:1073–1074

537. Graziadei IW, Wiesner RH, Batts KP et al. Recurrence of primary sclerosing cholangitis following liver transplantation. Hepatology, 1999; 29:1050–1056

538. Gohlke F, Loshse AW, Dienes HP et al. Evidence for an overlap syndrome of autoimmune hepatitis and primary sclerosing cholangitis. J Hepatol, 1996; 24:699–705

539. McNair ANB, Molonay M, Portmann BC, Williams R, McFarlane IG. Autoimmune hepatitis overlapping with primary sclerosing cholangitis in five cases. Am J Gastroenterol, 1998; 93:777–784

540. Hong-Curtis J, Yeh MM, Jain D, Lee JH. Rapid progression of autoimmune hepatitis in the background of primary sclerosing cholangitis. J Clin Gastroenterol, 2004; 38:906–909

541. International Autoimmune Hepatitis Group Report. Review of criteria for the diagnosis of autoimmune hepatitis. J Hepatol, 1999; 31:929–938

542. Protzer U, Dienes HP, Bianchi L et al. Post infantile giant cell hepatitis in patients with primary sclerosing cholangitis and autoimmune hepatitis. Liver, 1996; 16:274–282

543. Rabinowitz M, Demetris AJ, Bou-Abboud CG, Van Thiel DH. Simultaneous occurrence of primary sclerosing cholangitis and autoimmune chronic active hepatitis in a patient with ulcerative colitis. Dig Dis Sci, 1992; 37:1606–1611

544. Abdo AA, Bain VG, Kichian K, Lee SS. Evolution of autoimmune hepatitis to primary sclerosing cholangitis: A sequential syndrome. Hepatology, 2002; 36:1393–1399

545. Muratori L, Cassani F, Pappas G et al. The hepatitic/cholestatic 'overlap' syndrome: an Italian experience. Autoimmunity, 2002; 35:565–568

546. Gheorghe L, Iacob S, Gheorghe C et al. Frequency and predictive factors for overlap syndrome between autoimmune hepatitis and primary cholestatic liver disease. Eur J Gastroenterol Hepatol, 2004; 16:585–592

547. Debray D, Pariente D, Urvoas E, Hadchouel M, Bernard O. Sclerosing cholangitis in children. J Pediatr, 1994; 124:49–56

548. Gregorio GV, Portmann B, Karani J et al. Autoimmune hepatitis/sclerosing cholangitis overlap syndrome in childhood: A 16-year prospective study. Hepatology, 2001; 33:543–544

549. Bar Meir M, Hadas-Halperin I, Fisher D et al. Neonatal sclerosing cholangitis associated with autoimmune phenomena. J Pediatr Gastroenterol Nutr, 2000; 30:332–334

550. Baker AJ, Portmann B, Westaby D, Wilkinson M, Karani J, Mowat AP. Neonatal sclerosing cholangitis in two siblings: a category of progressive intrahepatic cholestasis. J Ped Gastroenterol Nutr, 1993; 17:317–322

551. Bouche H, Housset C, Dumount JL et al. AIDS-related cholangitis; diagnostic features and course in 15 patients. J Hepatol, 1993; 17:34–39

552. Forbes A, Blanshard C, Gazzard B. Natural history of AIDS related sclerosing cholangitis: A study of 20 cases. Gut, 1993; 34:116–121

553. Collins CD, Forbes A, Harcourt-Webster JN, Francis ND, Gleeson JA, Gazzard BG. Radiological and pathological features of AIDS-related polypoid cholangitis. Clin Radiol, 1993; 48:307–310

554. Chen XM, LaRusso NF. Cryptosporidiosis and the pathogenesis of AIDS-cholangiopathy. Semin Liver Dis, 2002; 22:277–289

555. Teare JP, Price DA, Foster GR, McBride M, Goldin RD, Main J. Reversible AIDS-related sclerosing cholangitis. J Hepatol, 1995; 23:209–211

556. DiPalma JA, Strobel CT, Farrow JG. Primary sclerosing cholangitis associated with hyperimmunoglobulin M immunodeficiency (dysgammaglobulinemia). Gastroenterology, 1986; 91:464–446

557. Rodrigues F, Davies EG, Harrison P, McLauchlin J, Karani J, Portmann B, Jones A, Veys P, Mieli-Vergani G, Hadzic N. Liver disease in children with primary immunodeficiencies. J Pediatr, 2004; 145:333–339

558. Winkelstein JA, Marino MC, Ochs H, Fuleihan R, Scholl PR, Geha R, Stiehm ER, Conley ME. The X-linked hyper-IgM syndrome: clinical and immunologic features of 79 patients. Medicine, 2003; 82:373–384

559. Martinez Ibanez V, Espanol T, Matamoros N et al. Relapse of sclerosing cholangitis after liver transplant in patients with hyper-IgM syndrome. Transpl Proc, 1997; 29:432–433

560. Hadzic N, Pagliuca A, Rela M et al. Correction of hyper IgM after liver and bone marrow transplantation. N Engl J Med, 2000; 342:320–321

561. Stephens J, Cosyns M, Jones M, Hayward A. Liver and bile duct pathology following *Cryptosporidium parvum* infection of immunodeficient mice. Hepatology, 1999; 30:27–35

562. Chen XM, Levine SA, Splinter PL, Tietz PS, Ganong AL, Jobin C, Gores GJ, Paya CV, LaRusso NF. Cryptosporidium parvum activates nuclear factor kappaB in biliary epithelia preventing epithelial cell apoptosis. Gastroenterology, 2001; 120:1774–1783

563. Hayward AR, Levy J, Facchetti F et al. Cholangiopathy and tumors of the pancreas, liver, and biliary tree in boys with X-linked immunodeficiency with hyper IgM. J Immunol, 1997; 15:977–983

564. Van Steenbergen W, Fevery J, Broeckaert L et al. Hepatic echinococcosis ruptured into the biliary tract. J Hepatol, 1987; 4:133–139

565. Terés J, Gomez-Moll J, Bruguera M, Visa J, Bordas JM, Pera C. Sclerosing cholangitis after surgical treatment of hepatic echinococcal cyst. Report of three cases. Am J Surg, 1984; 148:694–697

566. Houry S, Languille O, Hugier M, Benhamou J-P, Belghiti J, Msika S. Sclerosing cholangitis induced by formaldehyde solution injected into the biliary tree of rats. Arch Surg, 1990; 125:1059–1061

567. Herrmann G, Lorenz M, Kirkowa-Reiman M et al. Morphological changes after intra-arterial chemotherapy of the liver. Hepatogastroenterology, 1987; 34:5–9

568. Shea WJ, Demas BE, Goldberg HI et al. Sclerosing cholangitis associated with hepatic arterial FUDR chemotherapy: radiographic-histologic correlation. Am J Roentgenol, 1986; 146:717–721

569. Dikengil A, Siskind BN, Morse SS, Swedlund A, Bober-Sorcinelli KE, Burrell MI. Sclerosing cholangitis from intra-arterial floxuridine. J Clin Gastroenterol, 1986; 8:690–693

570. Doppman JL, Girton ME. Bile duct scarring following ethanol embolization in the hepatic artery: An experimental study in monkeys. Radiology, 1984; 152:621–626

571. Jaffe R. Liver involvement in the histiocytic disorders of childhood. Pediatr Dev Pathol, 2004; 7:214–225

572. Gey T, Bergoin C, Just N, Paupard T, Cazals-Hatem D, Xuan KH, Tavernier JY, Wallaert B. Langerhans cell histiocytosis and sclerosing cholangitis in adults. Rev Mal Respir, 2004; 21:997–1000

573. Caputo R, Marzano AV, Passoni E, Fassati LR, Agnelli F. Sclerosing cholangitis and liver transplantation in Langerhans cell histiocytosis: a 14-year follow-up. Dermatology, 2004; 209:335–337

574. Newell KA, Alonso EM, Kelly SM et al. Association between liver transplantation for Langerhans cell histiocytosis, rejection, and development of posttransplant lymphoproliferative disease in children. J Pediatr, 1997; 131:98–104

575. Dilawari JB, Chawla YK. Pseudosclerosing cholangitis in extrahepatic portal vein obstruction. Gut, 1992; 33:272–276

576. Akaki S, Kobayashi H, Sasai N, Tsunoda M, Kuroda M, Kanazawa S, Togami I, Hiraki Y. Bile duct stenosis due to portal cavernomas: MR portography and MR cholangiopancreatography demonstration. Abdom Imaging, 2002; 27:58–60

577. Nakanuma Y, Sasaki M, Terada T, Harada K. Intrahepatic peribiliary glands of humans. II. Pathological spectrum. J Gastroenterol Hepatol, 1994; 9:80–86

578. Colina F, Castellano VM, Gonzalez-Pinto I et al. Hilar biliary cysts in hepatic transplantation. Report of three symptomatic cases and occurrence in resected liver grafts. Trans Int, 1998; 11:110–116

579. Dumas A, Thung SN, Lin CS. Diffuse hyperplasia of the peribiliary glands. Arch Pathol Lab Med, 1998; 122:87–89

580. Terada T, Nakanuma Y. Pathological observations of intrahepatic peribiliary glands in 1,000 consecutive autopsy livers. III. Survey of necroinflammation and cystic dilatation. Hepatology, 1990; 5:1229–1233

581. Gautier M, Jehan P, Odièvre M. Histologic study of biliary fibrous remnants in 48 cases of extrahepatic biliary atresia: correlation with postoperative bile flow restoration. J Pediatr, 1976; 89:704–709

582. Sasaki M, Nakanuma Y, Terada T et al. Amyloid deposition in intrahepatic large bile ducts and peribiliary glands in systemic amyloidosis. Hepatology, 1990; 12:743–746

583. Nakanuma Y, Kurumaya H, Ohta G. Multiple cysts in the hepatic hilum and their pathogenesis. A suggestion of periductal gland origin. Virchows Arch, 1984; 404:341–350

584. Hoshiba K, Matsui O, Kadoya M et al. Peribiliary cysts in cirrhotic liver: observation on computed tomography. Abdom Imaging, 1996; 21:228–232

585. Fujioka Y, Kawamura N, Tanaka S, Fujita M, Suzuki H, Nagashima K. Multiple hilar cysts of the liver in patients with alcoholic cirrhosis: report of three cases. J Gastroenterol Hepatol, 1997; 12:137–143

586. Nakanuma Y. Peribiliary cysts have at least two different pathogeneses. J Gastroenterol, 2004; 39:407–408

587. Seguchi T, Akiyama Y, Itoh H et al. Multiple hepatic peribiliary cysts with cirrhosis. J Gastroenterol, 2004; 39:384–390

588. Qian Q, Li A, King BF et al. Clinical profile of autosomal dominant polycystic liver disease. Hepatology, 2003; 37:164–171

589. Stevens W, Harford W, Lee E. Obstructive jaundice due to multiple hepatic peribiliary cysts. Am Coll Gastroenterol, 1996; 91:155–157

590. Ahmadi T, Itai Y, Minami M. Central dot sign in entities other than Caroli disease. Radiat Med, 1997; 15:381–384

591. Graham SM, Barwick K, Cahow CE, Baker CC. Cholangitis glandularis proliferans. A histologic variant of primary sclerosing cholangitis with distinctive clinical and pathologic features. J Clin Gastroenterol, 1988; 10:579–583

592. Chot TK, Wong KP, Wong J. Cholangiographic appearance in clonorchiasis. Br J Radiol, 1984; 57:681–684

593. Chin NW, Chapman I, Jimenez FA. Mucinous hamartoma of the biliary duct system causing obstructive jaundice. Hum Pathol, 1988; 19:1112–1114

594. Wee A, Ludwig J, Coffey RJ Jr, LaRusso NF, Wiesner RH. Hepatobiliary carcinoma associated with primary sclerosing cholangitis and chronic ulcerative colitis. Hum Pathol, 1985; 16:719–726

595. Nakanuma Y, Terada T, Tanaka M, Ohta G. Are hepatolithiasis and cholangiocarcinoma aetiologically related? A morphological study of 12 cases of hepatolithiasis associated with cholangiocarcinoma. Virchows Arch, 1985; 406:45–58

596. Terada T, Nakanuma Y. Pathological observations of intrahepatic peribiliary glands in 1,000 consecutive autopsy livers. II. A possible source of cholangiocarcinoma. Hepatology, 1996; 429:119–129

597. Terada T, Kitamura Y, Ohta T, Nakanuma Y. Endocrine cells in hepatobiliary cystadenomas and cystadenocarcinomas. Virchows Arch, 1997; 430:37–40

598. Bhathal PS, Hughes NR, Goodman ZD. The so-called bile duct adenoma is a peribiliary gland hamartoma. Am J Surg Pathol, 1996; 20:858–864

599. Sonzogni A, Colloredo G, Fabris L et al. Isolated idiopathic bile ductular hyperplasia in patients with persistently abnormal liver function tests. J Hepatol, 2004; 40:592–598

600. Kim MH, Sekijima J, Lee SP. Primary intrahepatic stones. Am J Gastroenterol, 1995; 90:540–548

601. Nakayama F, Koga A, Ichimiya H et al. Hepatolithiasis in East Asia: comparison between Japan and China. J Gastroenterol Hepatol, 1991; 6:155–158

602. Park YH, Park SJ, Jang JY, Ahn YJ, Park YC, Yoon YB, Kim SW. Changing patterns of gallstone disease in Korea. World J Surg, 2004; 28:206–210

603. Kim MH, Sekijima J, Park HZ, Lee SP. Structure and composition of primary intrahepatic stones in Korean patients. Dig Dis Sci, 1995; 40:2143–2151

604. Shoda J, Tanaka N, He BF, Matsuzaki Y, Osuga T, Miyazaki H. Alterations of bile acid composition in gallstones, bile, and liver of patients with hepatolithiasis, and their etiological significance. Dig Dis Sci, 1993; 38:2130–2141

605. Shoda J, He BF, Tanaka N, Matsuzaki Y, Yamamori S, Osuga T. Primary dual defect of cholesterol and bile acid metabolism in liver of patients with intrahepatic calculi. Gastroenterology, 1995; 108:1534–1546

606. Kim YT, Byun JS, Kim J et al. Factors predicting concurrent cholangiocarcinomas associated with hepatolithiasis. Hepatogastroenterology, 2003; 50:8–12

607. Nakanuma Y, Yamaguchi K, Ohta G, Terada T. Pathologic features of hepatolithiasis in Japan. Hum Pathol, 1988; 19:1181–1186

608. Shoda J, Oda K, Suzuki H et al. Etiologic significance of defects in cholesterol, phospholipid, and bile acid metabolism in the liver of patients with intrahepatic calculi. Hepatology, 2001; 33:1194–1205

609. Kano M, Shoda J, Sumazaki R, Oda K, Nimura Y, Tanaka N. Mutations identified in the human multidrug resistance P-glycoprotein 3 (ABCB4) gene in patients with primary hepatolithiasis. Hepatol Res, 2004; 29:160–166

610. Kondo S, Nimura Y, Hayakawa N et al. A clinicopathologic study of primary cholesterol hepatolithiasis. Hepatogastroenterology, 1995; 42:478–486

611. Ohta T, Nagakawa T, Takeda T et al. Histological evaluation of the intrahepatic biliary tree in intrahepatic cholesterol stones, including immunohistochemical staining against apolipoprotein A-1. Hepatology, 1993; 17:531–537

612. Saito K, Nakanuma Y, Ohta T et al. Morphological study of cholesterol hepatolithiasis. Report of three cases. J Clin Gastroenterol, 1990; 12:585–590

613. Ros E, Navarro S, Bru C, Gilabert R, Bianchi L, Bruguera M. Ursodeoxycholic acid treatment of primary hepatolithiasis in Caroli's syndrome. Lancet, 1993; 342:404–406

614. Portmann B, Koukoulis G. Pathology of the liver allograft. In: Berry CL, ed., Current topics in pathology, vol. 92. Transplantation pathology. Berlin Heidelberg: Springer-Verlag, 1999: pp 61–105

615. Lim JH. Oriental cholangiohepatitis: pathologic, clinical, and radiological features. Am J Roentgenol, 1991; 157:1–8

616. Sperling RM, Koch J, Sandhu JS, Cello HP. Recurrent pyogenic cholangitis in Asian immigrants to the United States. Natural history and role of therapeutic ERCP. Dig Dis Sci, 1997; 42:865–871

617. Chou ST, Chan CW. Recurrent pyogenic cholangitis: a necropsy study. Pathology, 1980; 12:415–428

618. Huang MH, Chen CH, Yen CM et al. Relation of hepatolithiasis to helminthic infestation. J Gastroenterol Hepatol, 2005; 20:141–146

619. Ong GB. A study of recurrent pyogenic cholangitis. Arch Surg, 1962; 84:199–225

620. Matsushiro T, Suzuki N, Sato T, Maki T. Effects of diet on glutaric acid concentration in bile and the formation of calcium bilirubinate gallstones. Gastroenterology, 1977; 72:630–633

621. Kokuryo T, Yamamoto T, Oda K et al. Profiling of gene expression associated with hepatolithiasis by complementary DNA expression array. Int J Oncol, 2003; 22:175–179

622. Lidosfsky SD. Jaundice. In: Bacon BR, O'Grady JG, Di Bisceglie AM, Lake JR, eds, Comprehensive clinical hepatology. Mosby Elsevier 2006: pp 83–99

623. Kadrademir S, Astarcioglu H, Sokmen S et al. Mirizzi's syndrome: diagnostic and surgical considerations in 25 patients. J Hepatobiliary Pancreat Surg, 2000; 7:72–77

624. Benger JR, Thompson MH. Annular pancreas and obstructive jaundice. Am J Gastroenterol, 1997; 92:713–714

625. Terada T, Hirata K, Hisada Y, Hoshii Y, Nakanuma Y. Obstructive jaundice caused by the deposition of amyloid-like substance in the extrahepatic bile ducts in patient with multiple myeloma. Histopathology, 1994; 24:485–487

626. Colina F, Garcia-Prats MD, Moreno E et al. Amputation neuroma of the hepatic hilum after orthotopic liver transplantation. Histopathology, 1994; 25:151–157

627. Gerhards MF, van Gulik TM, Bosma A et al. Long-term survival after resection of proximal bile duct carcinoma (Klatskin tumors). World J Surg, 1999; 23:91–96

628. Tanoue K, Kanematsu T, Matsumata T, Shirabe K, Sugimachi K, Yasunaga C. Successful surgical treatment of hepatocellular carcinoma invading into biliary tree. HPB Surg, 1991; 4:237–244

629. Chan C, Medina-Franco H, Bell W, Lazenby A, Vickers S. Carcinoid tumor of the hepatic duct presenting as a Klatskin tumor in an adolescent and review of the literature. Hepatogastroenterology, 2000; 47:519–521

630. Howard ER, Heaton N. Benign extrahepatic bile duct obstruction. In: Howard ER, ed., Surgery of liver disease in children. Oxford: Butterworth-Heinemann, 1991: pp 94–101

631. Davenport M, Howard ER. Spontaneous perforation of the bile ducts in infancy. In: Howard ER, ed., Surgery of liver disease in children. Oxford: Butterworth-Heinemann, 1991: pp 91–93

632. Spitz L, Orr JD, Harries JT. Obstructive jaundice secondary to chronic mid-gut volvulus. Arch Dis Child, 1983; 58:383–385

633. Martinez-Urrutia MJ, Vasquez-Estevez J, Larrauri J, Diez Pardo JA. Gastric heterotopy of the biliary tract. J Ped Surg, 1990; 25:356–357

634. Ruymann FB, Raney RB, Crist WM, Lawrence W, Lindberg RD, Soule EH. Rhabdomyosarcoma of the biliary tree in childhood. A report from the intergroup rhabdomyosarcoma. Cancer, 1985; 56:575–581

635. Shorter RG, Baggenstoss AH. Extrahepatic cholestasis. III. Chronology of histologic changes in the liver. Am J Clin Pathol, 1959; 32:10–17

636. Christoffersen P, Poulsen H. Histological changes in human liver biopsies following extrahepatic biliary obstruction. Acta Pathol Microbiol Scand (suppl), 1970; 212:150–157

637. Itoh S, Inomata R, Matsuyama Y, Matsuo S, Gohara S. Calcium staining in diseased liver. J Hepatol, 1992; 15:414–415

638. Bianchi L, Meinecke R. Histologie des Leberpunktates und Ikterus. In: Beck K, ed., Ikterus. Stuttgart: Schattauer Verlag, 1968: pp 351–356

639. Serrao D, Cardoso V. Histodynamic interpretation of biliary epithelio-mesenchymatous reactions in experimental cholestasis. Pathol Eur, 1973; 8:219–234

640. Matzen P, Junge J, Christoffersen P, Poulsen H. Reproducibility and accuracy of liver biopsy findings suggestive of an obstructive cause of jaundice. In: Brunner H, Thaler H, eds, Hepatology, a Festschrift for Hans Popper. New York: Raven Press, 1985: pp 285–293

641. Desmet VJ. Morphologic and histochemical aspects of cholestasis. In: Popper H, Schaffner F, eds, Progress in liver diseases, vol. 4, ch 7. New York: Grune & Stratton, 1972: pp 97–132

642. Heimann R. Factors producing liver cell necrosis in experimental obstruction of the common bile duct. J Pathol Bacteriol, 1965; 90:479–485

643. Gall EA, Dobrogorski O. Hepatic alterations in obstructive jaundice. Am J Clin Pathol, 1964; 41:126–139

644. Bunton GL, Cameron R. Regeneration of liver after biliary cirrhosis. Ann NY Acad Sci, 1963; 111:412–421

645. Yokoi H. Morphologic changes of the liver in obstructive jaundice and its reversibility—with special reference to morphometric analysis of ultrastructure of the liver in dogs. Acta Hepatol Jpn, 1983; 24:1381–1391

646. So SU, Bondar GF. Effect of transient biliary obstruction on liver function and morphology. Can J Surg, 1974; 17:49–58

647. Jalink D, Urbanski SJ, Lee SS. Bilioenteric anastomosis reverses hyperkinetic circulation in bile duct-ligated cirrhotic rats. J Hepatol, 1996; 25:924–931

648. Younes RN, Vydelingum NA, De Rooij P et al. Metabolic alterations in obstructive jaundice: effect of duration of jaundice and bile-duct decompression. HPB Surg, 1991; 5:35–48

649. Melzer E, Krepel Z, Ronen I, Bar-Meir S. Recovery of hepatic clearance and extraction following a release of common bile duct obstruction in the rat. Res Exp Med, 1992; 192:35–40

650. Scobie BA, Summerskill WHJ. Hepatic cirrhosis secondary to obstruction of the biliary system. Am J Dig Dis, 1965; 10:135–146

651. Kountouras J, Billing BH, Scheuer PJ. Prolonged bile duct obstruction: a new experimental model for cirrhosis in the rat. Br J Exp Pathol, 1984; 65:305–311

652. Desmet VJ, Callea F. Cholestatic syndromes of infancy and childhood. In: Zakim D, Boyer TD, eds, Hepatology. A textbook of liver disease, vol 2, 2nd edn. Philadelphia: Saunders, 1990: pp 1355–1395

653. Koda W, Harada K, Tsuneyama K et al. Evidence of the participation of peribiliary mast cells in regulation of the peribiliary vascular plexus along the intrahepatic biliary tree. Lab Invest, 2000; 80:1007–1017

654. Weinbren K, Hadjis NS, Blumgart LH. Structural aspects of the liver in patients with biliary disease and portal hypertension. J Clin Pathol, 1985; 38:1013–1020

655. Lee E, Ross BD, Haines JR. Effect of experimental bile-duct obstruction on critical biosynthetic functions of the liver. Br J Surg, 1972; 59:564–568

656. Cameron SR, Hou PC. Biliary cirrhosis. Edinburgh: Oliver & Boyd, 1962

Diseases of the gallbladder

Jose Jessurun   Jorge Albores-Saavedra

Normal gallbladder

Macroanatomy

Located in a depression on the inferior surface of the right and quadrate hepatic lobes, the gallbladder is attached to the liver by loose connective tissue containing blood vessels, lymphatics, and occasionally bile ducts; and to the duodenum by a peritoneal fold known as the cholecystoduodenal ligament. A blind-ending segment known as the fundus projects beyond the anterior liver margin. The central body, or corpus, has a portion that bulges forward toward the upper margin of the first portion of the duodenum forming the infundibulum or Hartmann pouch. A short neck is continuous with the cystic duct.

The gallbladder's blood supply is via the cystic artery, which in most cases originates from the right hepatic artery. Its venous blood is carried through small veins that traverse the gallbladder bed and drain into the liver. Lymph drains to one or more lymph nodes at the gallbladder neck, which connect with lymph nodes located near the hepatic hilum and at the hepatoduodenal ligament. From the anterior and posterior hepatic plexuses, the gallbladder and extrahepatic bile ducts receive sympathetic and parasympathetic nerve fibres.[1]

The cystic duct is a 3 cm tubular structure located in the right free edge of the lesser omentum. At the junction with the gallbladder neck several mucosal folds, forming the spiral valve of Heister, project into the lumen. These valvular infoldings regulate the filling and emptying of the gallbladder in response to pressure changes within the biliary system.

Microanatomy

The gallbladder is composed of three layers: mucosa, muscularis and adventitia. The mucosa, which consists of surface epithelium and lamina propria, projects into the lumen as branching folds that become more prominent when the gallbladder contracts and less so when distended. A single layer of columnar cells with basally orientated nuclei make up the surface epithelium. The predominant cell has a lightly eosinophilic cytoplasm and a few small, periodic acid-Schiff- (PAS) positive apical vacuoles. On electron microscopy these cells are coated with microvilli and display other characteristics of absorptive cells, including basolateral spaces and digitations, and are tightly joined together by apical junctional complexes.[2] Another type of cell occasionally seen in the surface epithelium is a narrow columnar cell with dark eosinophilic cytoplasm referred to as a 'pencil-like' cell. It appears to be more than a compressed common columnar cell since, ultrastructurally, it contains more organelles and shows basal cytoplasmic extensions that penetrate the basement membrane.[3] The basal cell is a rarely-observed type of epithelial cell found in contact with, and parallel to, the basement membrane. In addition to the epithelial cells a few T-lymphocytes are normally present between the surface columnar cells. Endocrine cells and melanocytes are absent.

Present exclusively at the neck of the gallbladder are tubuloalveolar glands composed of mucin-producing cuboidal cells with a clear cytoplasm. These glands are similar to those found in the extrahepatic ducts. Their presence in the body or fundus of the gallbladder is abnormal and represents antral (or gastric) metaplasia. The denomination

Rokitansky–Aschoff sinuses should be used to refer to pathological herniations of the mucosa into and/or through the muscularis. In this sense, they are analogous to intestinal diverticula (pseudodiverticula).

The lamina propria is composed of loose connective tissue, nerve fibres, blood vessels and lymphatics. Small numbers of lymphocytes, IgA-containing plasma cells, mast cells and macrophages may be seen.

The muscular layer is a slightly thickened version of the muscularis mucosa of the intestine, composed of bundles of loosely arranged smooth muscle separated by fibrovascular connective tissue. Fusiform cells with elongated bipolar or dendritic cytoplasmic projections located very close to, or in intimate contact with, the smooth muscle cells of the muscular layer have recently been recognized in the gallbladder. These cells, which are immunoreactive for CD117 and have been interpreted as interstitial cells of Cajal, may play a role in muscle contraction or may act as mediators of neurotransmission.[4]

The adventitia is composed of loose connective tissue, blood vessels, lymphatics, nerves and fatty tissue. Rare paraganglia may be seen adjacent to the vessels. The abdominal side of the adventitia is covered by a serosa. On the hepatic bed, solitary or multiple small bile ducts known as canals of Luschka may be present. The hepatic adventitia may also contain larger accessory biliary ducts. Leakage of bile into the peritoneum may occur if these ducts are left patent after a cholecystectomy.

The normal gallbladder epithelium has a low rate of cell renewal; however, the mitotic activity of the epithelium may be stimulated in certain conditions, such as with mechanical distension following ligation of the common bile duct, or with neoplastic obstruction. In addition, high DNA synthesis may be stimulated with hormones such as cholecystokinin (CCK), a diet rich in cholesterol or cholic acid, or by the presence of gallstones.[5]

Embryology

The gallbladder, bile ducts, liver and primitive ventral pancreas originate from a diverticulum that appears on the ventral surface of the primitive foregut near the yolk stalk. At 4 weeks of gestation, three separate buds can be recognized: the cranial bud penetrates the splanchnic mesenchyme of the septum transversum and develops into the liver; the caudal bud becomes the gallbladder; and a smaller basal bud gives rise to the ventral pancreas. Their centrifugal migration causes elongation of those segments originally attached to the foregut, which then become the hepatic, cystic and common bile ducts, respectively. Proliferation of epithelial cells transforms these hollow structures into solid cords that re-acquire a lumen by cellular vacuolization around the seventh week of gestation. The extrahepatic segments of the right and left hepatic ducts are recognizable from 12 weeks of gestation. The common hepatic duct and distal parts of both hepatic ducts connect to several ductules in the hilar region. Variations in the remodelling process of these ducts explain the various branching patterns that have been recognized.[6] The lumen of the common bile duct progressively widens during infancy and early childhood, reaching its definitive diameter in adulthood.

Physiology

The liver secretes approximately 1000 ml of bile each day. Bile flow is a consequence of the reciprocal activity of smooth muscle in the gallbladder and the sphincter of Oddi. The ingestion of food induces contraction of the gallbladder and relaxation of the sphincter of Oddi, allowing the release of bile into the duodenum. Fatty meals and, to a lesser degree, proteins stimulate contraction of the gallbladder smooth muscle mainly through the action of cholecystokinin, a polypeptide hormone secreted by the proximal small intestine.[1] Contraction of the gallbladder during the interdigestive period is most likely mediated by motilin, another polypeptide hormone found in the epithelium of the duodenum and jejunum. By contrast, somatostatin, a hormone secreted from the intestine and pancreas after the ingestion of a fatty meal, inhibits gallbladder contraction. Because cholecystokinin and somatostatin are released by the same stimuli, their opposing actions suggest that these hormones act as physiological 'balances' for each other.[7] During fasting, contraction of the sphincter of Oddi causes the progressive accumulation of bile in the common bile duct. When the pressure in this system exceeds the resting pressure of the gallbladder (approximately 10 mmHg), bile flows into the latter. Although the capacity of the gallbladder is small (40 to 70 ml), a larger quantity of bile constituents is effectively stored through concentration. Water is absorbed by the epithelial cells through an osmotic gradient generated by a Na^+ K^+-ATPase mediated sodium-coupled transport of chloride.[8]

In addition to storing bile, the gallbladder secretes mucin via the surface epithelial cells and neck mucous glands. Most of the mucus is neutral, heavily sulphated, and contains a few sialic residues.[9] Recent attention has been focused on these mucosubstances as researchers are discovering the role they play in the formation of gallstones.

Gallbladder bile is sterile in most individuals. Among the factors that contribute to its sterility are the antibacterial action of bile acids[10] and cholangiocyte secretion of immunoglobulin A and defensins.[11]

Congenital and developmental abnormalities

Even though congenital anomalies of the gallbladder are rare, they may represent a challenging group of disorders for the diagnostic radiologist and for the surgeon while performing a cholecystectomy.

Congenital malformations include anomalies in shape, number and position. The most common abnormality in shape is an angulation of the fundus called a *Phrygian cap* because of its resemblance to the folded hats worn in the ancient country of Phrygia in Asia Minor. Microscopically, a mucosal fold with some disorientation of the underlying muscle bundles characterizes this abnormality. Although clinically unimportant, it may be mistaken on radiological examination for a stone or a pathological septum.[12]

Congenital diverticula of the gallbladder are very rare, and consist of saccular outpouchings of the gallbladder wall. Diverticula are most often single, but may occasionally be multiple. They may involve any aspect of the gallbladder and generally come to clinical attention as an incidental finding, or when they become infected.

Septation of the gallbladder is characterized by the presence of one or multiple septa dividing the gallbladder lumen into several chambers.[13] This anomaly predominantly occurs in adults[13] and probably results from incomplete fusion of the vacuoles, which gives rise to the lumen after the solid stage (see embryology). In some cases the septa may contain muscle fibres that are continuous with those of the outer wall, a finding which has been used as an argument to support a developmental aetiology.[14] It is worth noting, however, that inflammatory diseases of the gallbladder can produce internal compartmentalization mimicking congenital septation. The inflammatory septa are usually thicker and made of inflamed fibrous tissue. In some cases, particularly those associated with gallstones, the distinction between inflamed congenital septa and acquired compartmentalization is impossible. Septation of the gallbladder has been associated with intermittent abdominal pain in young adults.[15] Stones are usually, but not invariably, absent. The term *hourglass gallbladder* has been used to describe those cases with a transverse septum that divides the lumen into a proximal and distal cavity. Inflammatory changes and stone formation tend to occur more frequently in the distal cavity.

Cystic malformations of the gallbladder may be analogous to the more common choledochal cysts or may arise by occlusion of a diverticulum.[16] In addition, dilatation of Luschka ducts may give rise to multilocular cysts around the gallbladder.

Failure of development of the caudal foregut diverticulum results in *agenesis* of the gallbladder. This developmental abnormality can either occur as an isolated phenomenon or be associated with other anomalies, the most common one being choledocholithiasis. Other abnormalities associated with gallbladder agenesis include absence of ascending colon, polycystic kidneys, tracheo-oesophageal fistulas, cardiac defects, imperforate anus, annular pancreas, the Klippel–Feil syndrome and horseshoe kidney combined with malrotation of the gut.[17] Clinical symptoms of gallbladder agenesis usually present in adults, mimic the symptoms of cholecystitis or cholangitis, and are frequently associated with jaundice.

A *hypoplastic gallbladder* may occur when the caudal bud undergoes incomplete development or when the solid stage of the bud is not recanalized. It may be found in association with congenital biliary atresia and in cystic fibrosis. This condition should be differentiated from acquired post-inflammatory fibrotic contraction of the gallbladder.[17]

At the opposite end of the spectrum from gallbladder agenesis and hypoplasia is *gallbladder duplication*, which occurs when there is excessive budding of the caudal diverticulum. The duplicated cystic ducts most commonly enter the common bile duct separately (so-called 'H-type' configuration) or unite to form a common cystic duct in such cases ('Y-type' configuration). Less frequently, they drain independently into the hepatic ducts. Stones, inflammatory conditions and tumours may preferentially involve one of the gallbladders.[17] A duplicate gallbladder may be an uncommon cause of recurrent acute right upper quadrant abdominal pain after cholecystectomy.[18]

The gallbladder may be *located in abnormal sites*. It may be found on the left side as the only malpositioned organ or, more commonly, as a part of *situs inversus*. The surgeon should be aware of possible anatomic anomalies associated with a left-sided gallbladder, such as right-sided round ligament associated with abnormal intrahepatic portal branching or ectopic gallbladder attached to the left lobe of the liver that connects to the left hepatic duct via the cystic duct or the accessory bile duct.[19] In other instances, the gallbladder is placed within the falciform ligament or abdominal wall, or totally surrounded by liver parenchyma (intrahepatic gallbladder). Another abnormality that may be clinically relevant is the wandering or *'floating' gallbladder*, so called because it lacks a firm connection to the hepatic parenchyma, and is instead completely surrounded by peritoneum. The extreme mobility of this floating gallbladder predisposes to kinking of the cystic duct with subsequent compromise of bile flow, or to twisting of the nutrient vessels resulting in haemorrhagic infarction.[20] A floating gallbladder may also result from agenesis or hypoplasia of the right hepatic lobe.[21]

Heterotopias

Ectopic tissues are rarely found in the wall of the gallbladder. More common in young adults than in children, ectopic gastric mucosa is usually symptomatic and in some cases may lead to perforation and haemorrhage.[22] Microscopically, fundic and antral mucosa are identified in most cases (Fig. 12.1(A),(B)). In contrast, ectopic pancreatic tissue is usually an incidental finding in cholecystectomy specimens (Fig. 12.1(C)). Rarely, however, it has given rise to clinical symptoms of acute pancreatitis.[23] Ectopic liver, adrenal cortex, and thyroid tissue are incidental microscopic findings.[24]

Gallstones

General comments

Historical perspective

Since antiquity, gallstones have been of interest to physicians. Surprisingly, no mention of gallstone disease in humans is encountered in ancient Greek writings. The first discussion of gallstones as 'dried up humours concreted like stones' and their relation to obstruction of the liver is ascribed to the Greek physician Alexander of Tralles (5th century AD). The 14th-century physician Gentile da Foligno

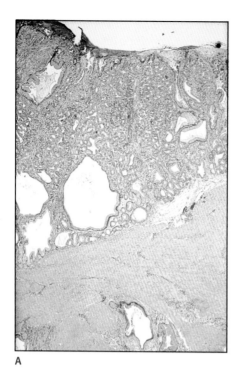

A

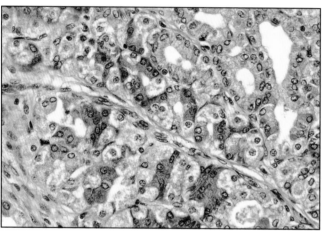

B

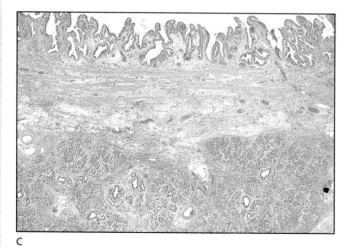

C

Fig. 12.1 • Heterotopias of the gallbladder. **(A)** Gastric mucosa. The thickened gastric mucosa is composed of small and dilated tubular glands that lie on a muscle coat and **(B)** are lined by parietal and chief cells. **(C)** Pancreas. A nodule of pancreatic tissue is seen in the perimuscular connective tissue of the gallbladder. H&E.

suggested for the first time the association of cholecystitis and gallstones, based on autopsy findings. Antonio Benivieni succeeded in predicting the presence of gallstones in a patient that was experiencing abdominal pain. His clinical impression was confirmed at autopsy. However, it was Jean Fernel (1581), physician to the King of France, who provided the most accurate clinical description of the symptoms associated with cholelithiasis.

Gallstones were removed from a living patient for the first time in 1618 by the German surgeon Wilhem Fabry. Two and a half centuries later, another German physician, Carl Langenbuch, performed the first cholecystectomy.

The composition of gallstones was unknown until the end of the 17th and 18th centuries. It was through the work of researchers such as Antonio Vallisneri, Pouilletier de la Salle and Vicq d'Azyr that the chemical composition of gallstones was determined and the fact that there are differences among them was realized.[25]

Because gallstones are a very common cause of morbidity throughout the world, they can be considered among the most expensive digestive tract disorders. More than 20 million Americans have gallbladder disease,[26] with an estimated annual direct and indirect cost in 2000 of $6.5 billion.[27] Recent technical advances such as shock-wave lithotripsy and pharmacological dissolution of gallstones have become increasingly popular therapeutic alternatives to open or laparoscopic cholecystectomy. Undoubtedly, further improvements in therapy and perhaps even mechanisms for prevention will derive from a better understanding of the epidemiology and pathophysiology of gallstone formation.

Classification of gallstones

Gallstones are composed predominantly of cholesterol, bilirubin and calcium salts with lesser amounts of other constituents. The most popular classification system is based on the relative amount of cholesterol in the stones, with two primary categories: cholesterol or non-cholesterol (Fig. 12.2). The latter are further classified as black or brown pigment stones.[28,29] Cholesterol gallstones constitute more than 80% of stones in the Western world and are composed predominantly of cholesterol crystals agglomerated by a mucin glycoprotein matrix. Non-cholesterol gallstones, in contrast, are much more common in other parts of the world, such as Asia. Black pigment stones are formed from calcium salts of unconjugated bilirubin in a polymerized matrix. Brown pigment stones may form within bile ducts and contain bacterial degradation products of biliary lipids, calcium salts of fatty acids, unconjugated bilirubin and precipitated cholesterol. Since the pathogenesis and epidemiology of these types of stones are considerably different, they will be discussed separately.

Cholesterol gallstones

Pathogenesis

The major lipid components of bile are bile salts, phospholipids and cholesterol. Since cholesterol is virtually

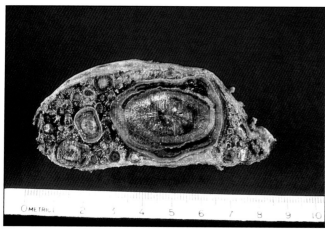

A

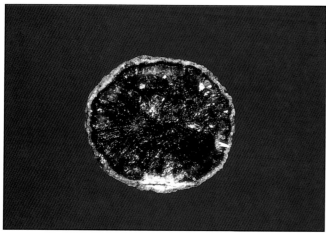

B

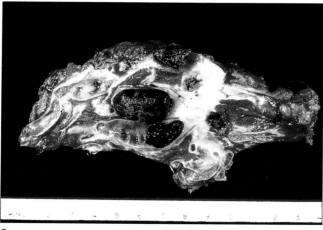

C

Fig. 12.2 • Gallstones. **(A)** Cholesterol gallstones. These are commonly numerous; the high concentration of calcium bilirubinate at the centre of the stone imparts a dark brown appearance which is surrounded by concentric layers of yellow concretions. **(B)** Black pigmented gallstones. Compared to cholesterol stones, they are usually smaller and on section exhibit a homogeneous black appearance. **(C)** Brown pigmented gallstones have a soft consistency and frequently form in situ within the extrahepatic bile ducts.

insoluble in water, it requires a solubilizing system, which is provided by its association with phospholipids and bile salts. After being co-secreted by hepatocytes, cholesterol and phospholipids form spherical structures or vesicles, made of a double layer of phospholipids, of which lecithin

(diacylphosphatidylcholine) is the main type. Vesicles are soluble by virtue of the outward orientation of the hydrophilic ('water loving') choline groups, allowing cholesterol to be inserted into the hydrophobic ('water fearing') milieu provided by the fatty acid chains.[30-32]

Bile acids are secreted by the hepatocytes through a different transport mechanism. Although soluble in water, bile salt monomers self-aggregate into simple micelles once they surpass the so-called critical micellar concentration (= 0.5 to 5 mM). The amphiphilic properties of bile acids render an extremely water-soluble structure due to the orientation of the hydrophobic portions away from water and the exposure of the hydrophilic surfaces to the aqueous environment. As detergents, bile acids can dissolve portions of vesicles and incorporate them as mixed micelles. The resulting structures are essentially discs composed of cholesterol and phospholipids surrounded by bile acids.[31-33]

As the concentration of cholesterol increases, more of it is carried in vesicles. In addition, increasing cholesterol concentration causes increased cholesterol transfer from vesicles to micelles during the micellation process. The resulting cholesterol-enriched unilamellar vesicles are unstable and fuse into large multilamellar vesicles. When the cholesterol-to-phospholipid ratio exceeds 1, cholesterol crystallizes at their surface. Enhancement of crystallization is influenced by the concentration of solutes in bile since aggregation occurs more efficiently when cholesterol carriers are close to each other.[31,32,34]

Cholesterol is most soluble in a mixture of lipids containing at least 50% bile acids and smaller amounts of phospholipids. Supersaturation occurs when a solution contains more cholesterol molecules than can be incorporated into mixed micelles. Theoretically, bile supersaturation may be due to hypersecretion of cholesterol, hyposecretion of bile acids or a combination of both. An increase in biliary cholesterol output—either due to increased synthesis or increased uptake—is the most common cause of supersaturation and subsequent stone formation. Increased uptake by hepatocytes may involve either endogenous cholesterol (transported via low density lipoprotein-LDL) or exogenous cholesterol (transported via chylomicrons).

As noted above, cholesterol supersaturation may also arise as a consequence of bile acid hyposecretion. However, this is much less common: in fact, most patients with gallstones have normal bile acid secretion. Adequate bile acid secretion depends on the integrity of the enterohepatic circulation. In a cycle that occurs 3–12 times per day, 90% of the bile acids are reabsorbed from the terminal ileum and returned to the liver via the portal system. There, the bile acids are re-utilized by the hepatocytes following passive and active re-uptake. Any interference with this recycling mechanism will contribute to bile acid hyposecretion and subsequent cholesterol supersaturation.[31-33]

Supersaturation of cholesterol is necessary but not sufficient for the formation of cholesterol gallstones. For any given degree of cholesterol saturation, patients with gallstones form cholesterol crystals more rapidly than individuals without gallstones. This observation led to the idea that stone formation may involve a nucleation process, and subsequent studies have confirmed this hypothesis. It has become apparent that the tendency of bile to nucleate its cholesterol depends on the balance between substances that promote and prevent nucleation. Pronucleating substances include N-aminopeptidase, haptoglobin, mucin, acidic glycoproteins, immunoglobulins, phospholipase C, fibronectin and orosomucoid. Antinucleating substances include apolipoproteins A-1 and A-2 (biliary glycoproteins belonging to the cytokeratin family of proteins), and certain immunoglobulins.[35-39] Although biliary proteins are abnormal in lithogenic biles, specificic alterations in pronucleating or antinucleating proteins have not been demonstrated to be the primary initiating event in gallstone pathogenesis.[40]

Biliary sludge is a viscous gel composed of mucin and microscopic precipitates of multilamellar vesicles, cholesterol monohydrate and calcium bilirubinate. Since mucin is present at the centre of almost all gallstones, it has been suggested that the formation of biliary sludge precedes the formation of macroscopic cholesterol gallstones.[40] Previous studies have suggested that infections do not play a significant role in the formation of pure cholesterol gallstones. However, DNA homology to bacterial rRNA has been found in cholsterol gallstones.[41] Recent studies have revealed the presence of bile-resistant *Helicobacter* species in bile samples and gallbladder mucosa.[42] Experimentally, it has been shown that infection of a gallstone-susceptible strain of mice with specific strains of *Helicobacter* promotes the development of cholesterol gallstones when fed with a lithogenic diet.[43]

Epidemiology

The prevalence of cholesterol gallstones varies greatly by age, sex, country and ethnic group. Geographical differences are most likely related to the interaction of genetic and environmental factors. In the USA it has been estimated that more than 20 million people have gallstones. The prevalence is higher and increases with age. An increased risk for gallstones is associated with multiparity, oestrogen-replacement therapy, oral-contraceptive use, obesity and rapid weight loss.[32] Obese patients have an increased incidence of gallbladder diseases and the relative risk appears to be correlated with the level of increase in the body mass index.[44] Most likely, gallbladder disorders will dramatically increase in incidence considering the general rise in obesity observed during the last decade. Whether diabetes predisposes to gallstone formation is still controversial. Interestingly, there is substantial evidence that suggests that alcohol intake protects against gallstones.[45]

In the USA, the highest prevalence of gallstones is observed among native Americans, with progressively lower risk among whites, blacks and some Asian groups. Mexican American women also have a higher prevalence of gallstones than other Hispanic women.[26,46-48] In other parts of the world, gallstones are extremely common in areas such as Chile and the Scandinavian countries, while they have a much lower incidence in areas such as Asia and Africa.[49,50]

The epidemiological data from North America suggest that populations with a high prevalence of gallstones carry dominant Amerindian lithogenic genes transmitted by common ancestral human groups of Asian origin that colonized the USA more than 20 000 years ago. In support of this hypothesis a recent epidemiological study from Chile found a positive correlation between native American genes (measured via ABO blood group distribution and determination of mitochondrial DNA polymorphisms) and the prevalence of gallstones in women younger than 35 years.[51] In this study, the highest prevalence of gallstone disease was found among native Mapuche Indians (35.2%), followed by residents of urban Santiago (27.5%) and Maoris of Easter Island (20.9%).[51] The high prevalence in native-American and Mexican-American women would also support this hypothesis. Most likely, specific genes associated with gallstone susceptibility will be identified in the future; at that time the influence of environmental factors may be further elucidated.

Pigment gallstones

Pathogenesis

There are two types of pigment stones: black and brown. The distinction is important since they differ in their aetiology, associated clinical conditions, morphology and chemical composition. *Black stones* are composed of calcium bilirubinate, phosphate and carbonate embedded in a glycoprotein matrix, and have a very low cholesterol concentration. *Brown stones* contain calcium salts of bilirubin and fatty acids (palmitate) in a glycoprotein matrix and have a higher concentration of cholesterol. Calcium carbonate and phosphate are usually not present.[34,52]

Because it is a precursor for calcium bilirubinate, unconjugated bilirubin plays a central role in the formation of both brown and black pigment stones. Unconjugated bilirubin is solubilized by bile salts in mixed micelles, and then combines with calcium to form calcium bilirubinate. Any condition resulting in elevated levels of unconjugated bilirubin can therefore predispose to stone formation. Thus, biliary infections contributing to bile stasis are a common cause of brown stones, as bacterial overgrowth generates hydrolases that can then form free bile acids from conjugated bile salts. In addition, bacteria elaborate phospholipase A, which cleaves phospholipids to form lysolecithin and free fatty acids. These free fatty acids (mainly palmitic and stearic) combine with the free bile salts generated by the bacterial hydrolases and precipate as calcium salts. It is not surprising, therefore, that bacteria are present within the matrix of most brown stones.[30,52]

Black pigment stone disease is not associated with bacterial infection. An increased concentration of unconjugated bilirubin originates from an increment in the secretion of bilirubin conjugates as occurs in haemolysis and chronic alcoholism, followed by non-bacterial enzymatic or non-enzymatic hydrolysis. An analogous effect may occur if there is a decrease in the secretion of bile salts, as occurs in cirrhosis, since these compounds are required to solubilize unconjugated bilirubin and buffer ionized calcium.[34,40] Phospholipids also play an important role in pigment sludge formation. Calcium bilirubinate sludge contains an increased amount of phospholipids and these compounds are present in the core of pigment gallstones. Carbohydrate-rich diets stimulate enzymes which are important in the synthesis of phospholipids, such as fatty acid synthetase. The increased activity of these enzymes may explain the higher hepatic bile phospholipid concentrations found in clinical situations such as total parenteral nutrition.

Interestingly, the gallbladder itself plays a role in lithogenesis. Biliary epithelium functions to acidify bile, thereby increasing the solubility of calcium carbonate. Mucosal inflammation interferes with the ability of the epithelium to perform this acidifying role, resulting in an increased biliary pH and subsequent calcium carbonate precipitation. In addition, reparative metaplastic changes in the mucosa cause an increased concentration of biliary glycoproteins, which in turn promotes gallstone formation.[40]

Epidemiology

Pigment gallstones occur in all countries. Although they account for only 20 to 25% of stones in the USA, they are the most common type worldwide. As with cholesterol gallstones, pigment stones develop more frequently in females and their incidence increases with age; however, at variance with the former, race does not appear to be a factor.

Clinical conditions associated with black gallstones include haemolytic anaemia, cirrhosis, alcoholism, malaria, pancreatitis, total parenteral nutrition and advanced age. In addition, black pigment stones develop more frequently in patients with Crohn disease, particularly those with extensive ileitis or who have undergone ileal resection. The predilection for stone formation in this last group of patients stems from the decreased or absent functionality of the terminal ileum, which, as discussed earlier, is the site of 90% of bile salt reabsorption in the normal individual. Any unconjugated bilirubin in normal patients then precipitates in the colon as calcium bilirubinate or other bilirubinates. By contrast, impaired or absent resorptive function in the ileum in patients with Crohn disease leads to increased levels of bile salts in the colon, where the salts solubilize unconjugated bilirubin.[53] Subsequent increased colonic resorption of this unconjugated bilirubin then leads to supersaturation of bile (up to three times normal levels) and stone formation.

Cholecystitis

Inflammatory diseases of the gallbladder are a frequent cause of morbidity in Western countries. It has been calculated that the cost to the US public to treat these disorders is more than 1.5 billion dollars per year.[54] The term cholecystitis encompasses a group of disorders that differ in their pathological, pathogenetic and clinical characteristics. As in other organs of the gastrointestinal tract, most inflammatory diseases of the gallbladder show non-specific histological features because they elicit non-distinctive types of cellular infiltrates. However, characterization of inflammatory patterns helps to establish a pathological diagnosis and provides insight into the pathogenesis of a disease. In addition, it is through the recognition of differences in the inflammatory patterns that clinically useful histological diagnoses are rendered.

Acute cholecystitis

Acute cholecystitis is clinically defined as an episode of acute biliary pain accompanied by fever, right upper quadrant tenderness, guarding, persistence of the symptoms beyond 24 hours, and leukocytosis.[55] Approximately 90% of cases are associated with gallstones. Ultrasonography demonstrates a thickened gallbladder wall or pericholecystic fluid. The diagnosis is also supported by failure to visualize the gallbladder during a hepatobiliary scintigram.[56] Because of their unique clinical and/or pathological characteristics, the following three types of acute cholecystitis will be discussed separately: acute calculous cholecystitis, acute acalculous cholecystitis and emphysematous cholecystitis.

Acute calculous cholecystitis

The precipitating event for the development of acute calculous cholecystitis appears to be occlusion of the neck of the gallbladder or cystic duct by a gallstone. The subsequent increased intraluminal pressure causes dilatation of the gallbladder and oedema of its wall. However, outflow obstruction does not always cause acute cholecystitis: indeed, animal models in whom the cystic duct has been ligated or obliterated experience only shrinkage of the gallbladder, not acute cholecystitis.[57] Other factors contributing to acute cholecystitis may therefore be mucosal ischaemia secondary to visceral distension or external compression of the nearby cystic artery by the impacted stone. Formation of inflammatory mediators such as lysolecithin and prostaglandins, and mucosal injury by concentrated bile, cholesterol or gallstones may also contribute to mucosal injury.[58] It has been postulated that trauma to the mucosa caused by stones releases phospholipase from lysosomes residing in mucosal epithelial cells. This enzyme converts lecithin to lysolecithin, which is an active detergent known to be toxic to the mucosa.[59] In addition, phospholipids can damage the biliary epithelial cells. It has been shown that the bile from patients with gallstones contains lysophosphatidylcholine, which induces mucosal necrosis and inflammation of the gallbladder wall.[60]

When bile cultures are obtained early enough (within 48 hours of onset) bacteria can be isolated in 42 to 72% of the cases. The predominant organisms are intestinal: *Escherichia coli*, other Gram-negative aerobic rods, enterococci and, in 20% of the cases, anaerobes.[61-63] Most authorities agree that the infection is secondary and does not contribute to the onset of acute cholecystitis.

Pathology

The surgeon identifies acute cholecystitis at the time of laparoscopy or laparotomy by signs of acute inflammation such as omental adhesions to the gallbladder wall, oedema, friability, pericholecystic fluid, and frank gangrene. The

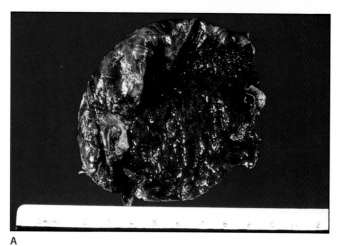

Fig. 12.3 • Acute cholecystitis. **(A)** Numerous cholesterol gallstones were present. The mucosal surface exhibits haemorrhagic necrosis, which microscopically **(B)** demonstrates coagulative necrosis of the epithelium, extensive transmural neutrophilic inflammation and haemorrhage. H&E. **(C)** Another case showing a combination of acute inflammation and ischaemia with the formation of fibrin-rich pseudomembranes. H&E.

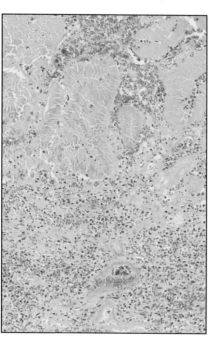

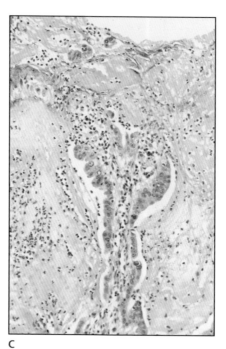

gallbladder is usually enlarged with a wall thickened by oedema, vascular congestion and haemorrhage. The serosa is dull and covered with patches of fibrinopurulent exudate (Fig. 12.3(A)). As mentioned previously, a gallstone is frequently found obstructing the outflow pathway. Thick, cloudy bile admixed with blood and pus fills the lumen. Depending on the severity of the inflammatory response, the mucosal changes range from oedema and congestion to widespread ulcers and necrosis. Histologically, an acute inflammatory reaction characterized by oedema, vascular congestion, haemorrhage, neutrophilic infiltration, and mucosal necrosis predominates in specimens obtained early in the course of the disease (Fig. 12.3(B)).

As the pathological process evolves, transmural inflammation, secondary acute vasculitis and mural necrosis follows. The type of inflammatory cells at this stage include lymphocytes, plasma cells, macrophages and abundant eoinsophils. Fibrinous pseudomembranes (pseudomembranous cholecystitis) may develop over necrotic-appearing mucosa (Fig. 12.3(C)). Granulation tissue and collagen deposition replace previously ulcerated or necrotic tissue.

A cholecystectomy for acute cholecystitis should preferably be performed within 2–3 days of the onset of symptoms, a time frame that has been referred to as the 'golden period'.[63,64] After inflammation has been present for >72 hours, the increasing fibrous adhesions and transmural inflammation make cholecystectomy far more laborious and prone to complications such as acute calculous cholecystitis, empyema, gangrene and perforation. The latter complication is usually sealed off by the omentum leading to the formation of pericholecystic adhesions and/or an abscess. In the less fortunate, however, life-threatening bacteraemia and septic complications may ensue.[55]

Clinical correlation

Most patients are women with a peak age incidence of 50 to 70 years. The typical symptoms are right upper quadrant pain of recent onset accompanied by abdominal guarding and local tenderness. These symptoms may be deceptively mild, or even absent in the elderly. Sometimes, the enlarged gallbladder may be palpated and/or pain may be elicited while palpating the right upper quadrant when the patient inhales deeply (Murphy's sign). Some patients are febrile and jaundiced and most show leukocytosis. Since the clinical features are not entirely specific, imaging techniques such as ultrasonography or cholescintigraphy are used to confirm the diagnosis. Preoperative clinical findings of acute cholecystitis are highly reliable for predicting intraoperative gross findings. However, intraoperative findings of acute cholecystitis are commonly found in the absence of preoperative clinical signs. For reasons that are not clear, the correlation between pathological diagnosis and intraoperative findings is poor.[56]

Acute acalculous cholecystitis

This infrequent but clinically serious disease is found in approximately 5% of all patients undergoing cholecystectomy.[65] It predominantly affects individuals with other clinicopathological conditions including trauma, non-biliary surgical procedures, sepsis, burns, parenteral nutrition, mechanical ventilation, numerous blood transfusions and use of narcotics or antibiotics. Its exact pathogenesis is not fully understood although it appears to be multifactorial.[66] Increased bile viscosity from stasis with subsequent obstruction of the cystic duct has been suggested as a contributing factor; this may explain the association of acalculous cholecystitis with a history of fasting, narcotic use, dehydration or anaesthesia, all of which may result in bile stasis. Undoubtedly, mucosal ischaemia plays a major role in patients with underlying cardiovascular diseases or those that develop acute acalculous cholecystitis following trauma, sepsis or surgical procedures.

Prostanoids and bile salts also appear to play an important role in the development of acalculous cholecystitis. Prostaglandins are involved in gallbladder contraction, water absorption, inflammation and pain associated with gallbladder disease. Different types of prostaglandins have various roles in acute inflammatory conditions of the gallbladder. Prostaglandin E (PGE) levels are increased as inflammation increases. In normal gallbladders the PGE/PGF ratio is 4 : 1. PGE levels are increased seven-fold in patients with acute acalculous cholecystitis. Tissue anoxia secondary to shock, bacterial contamination and invasion, stasis and changes in bile salt concentration also contribute to in the injury to the gallbladder mucosa. As a consequence, inflammation, distention, atonicity and pain develops.[67]

In animal models, platelet-activating factor (PAF) has been show to play a role in the induction of acute acalculous cholecystitis. This cytokine is released by basophils, eosinophils, neutrophils, macrophages, monocytes, mast cells, vascular endothelial cells and smooth muscle cells. It increases vascular permeability, and induces neutrophil aggregation and degranulation. Indirectly, PAF may cause acalculous cholecystitis by stimulating and releasing interleukin-1, tumour necrosis factor (TNF), and interleukin-6. PAF may also be associated with the development of arteriolar thrombosis and ischaemia.[68]

There are no specific clinical or histological differences between acute calculous and acalculous cholecystitis. However, in acalculous cases, there is a male preponderance, an increased rate of complications and a higher overall mortality. Patients at risk of developing severe complications from this condition are older and have high white blood cell counts. In these patients, earlier surgical intervention should be considered if the sonographic findings support the diagnosis of acute acalculous cholecystitis.[69]

Acute emphysematous cholecystitis

Acute emphysematous cholecystitis is an uncommon variant of acute cholecystitis in which the infecting bacteria produce gas. Clinically, this condition is indistinguishable from simple acute cholecystitis, and the distinction is more often made with radiographic studies, although abdominal radiographs are relatively insensitive in the diagnosis of emphysematous cholecystitis. As a result of the regular use of ultrasonography in suspected hepatobiliary disease, emphysematous cholecystitis is being diagnosed with increased frequency.[70] A delay in diagnosis results in a high incidence of complications such as gangrene and perforation, which explains the high overall mortality rate (15% vs 4.1% for acute calculous cholecystitis). About 50% of bile cultures are positive for clostridial organisms, the most common being *Clostridra welchii*. Vascular occlusion of the cystic artery or its branches by atherosclerosis and small vessel disease (both frequent complications of diabetes mellitus) are major contributory factors for emphysematous cholecystitis.[71,72]

Pathology
During cholecystectomy, the gallbladder may appear distended, tense and encased by the omentum, fibrous adhesions and/or an abscess. A necrotic, friable wall frequently leads to fragmentation of the gallbladder during removal. Upon opening, gas and foul-smelling purulent exudate escape from the lumen. Gallstones, frequently of the pigment type, are found in 70% of cases. The mucosa appears necrotic, congested and haemorrhagic. Microscopically, the necrotic and acutely inflamed mucosa often contains colonies of gram-positive bacilli. Gas bubbles are occasionally seen within the wall or in the subserosal connective tissue.

Chronic cholecystitis

Chronic cholecystitis is almost always associated with gallstones. The pathogenesis of this common disorder is poorly understood. It has been suggested that chronic cholecystitis develops as a result of recurrent attacks of mild acute cholecystitis. However, only a minority of patients provide a clinical history supportive of this hypothesis. The inflammatory and reparative changes may be in part explained by repetitive mucosal trauma produced by gallstones, although other factors also play a role. Because there is a poor correlation between the severity of the inflammatory response and the number and size of stones, it is possible that the intensity of the inflammatory response of the mucosa to gallstones in different populations is genetically determined. A potential and currently unproved hypothesis is that a florid inflammatory response in the gallbladder could be a residue of what may have been a 'protective effect' for those populations whose ancestors resided in geographical areas with a high incidence of parasitic biliary infections. This energetic inflammatory response of the gallbladder mucosa may at one time have been protective against parasites, but has evolved into a detrimental mechanism in the pathology of gallstone disease. Other scientists have postulated that both cholelithiasis and chronic cholecystitis are caused by an abnormal composition of the bile leading to stone formation and chemical injury to the mucosa.

In contrast to the high percentage of positive bile cultures in patients with acute cholecystitis, bacteria-mostly *E. coli* and enterococci-are cultured in less than a third of the cases of chronic cholecystitis.[73] A recent study has identified DNA from *Helicobacter* species in biliary tract specimens from a group of Chilean patients with gallbladder disease.[74] Whether this finding has pathogenetic significance or not awaits the results of future studies.

Pathology

The variable appearance of the gallbladder in chronic cholecystitis is a reflection of differences in the degree of inflammation and fibrosis. The gallbladder may be distended or shrunken. Fibrous serosal adhesions suggest previous episodes of acute cholecystitis. On macroscopic examination, the wall is usually thickened but it may be thin. The mucosa may be intact with preservation or accentuation of its folds, or it may be flattened in cases with outflow obstruction. Mucosal erosions or ulcers are frequently found in association with impacted stones (Fig. 12.4). The mere presence of gallstones is neither necessary nor sufficient for the diagnosis of chronic cholecystitis, which is based instead on the histological features of: (i) a predominantly mononuclear inflammatory cell infiltrate; (ii) fibrosis; and/or (iii) metaplastic changes.

The degree of the inflammatory reaction is variable. In some cases, the infiltrate is exclusively located in the mucosa while in others it extends into the muscularis and serosa. The distribution of the infiltrate varies from focal to patchy to diffuse. Commonly, lymphocytes predominate over plasma cells and histiocytes. It is important to recall that sparse, focally distributed lymphoid cells may be present in normal gallbladders obtained from healthy individuals who died of traumatic causes and whose livers were used for transplantation.[75] Occasional lymphoid follicles arise in a background of chronic inflammation. Most of the lymphoid follicles are located in the lamina propria but may infiltrate the full thickness of the gallbladder wall. When diffuse, the term *follicular cholecystitis* (Fig. 12.5(A)) is used to describe this condition.[76] A minor component of eosinophils and neutrophils may be also seen. When neutrophils are pre-

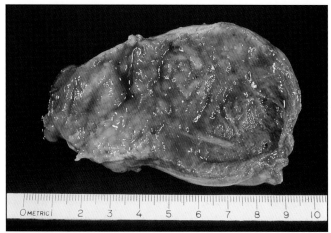

A

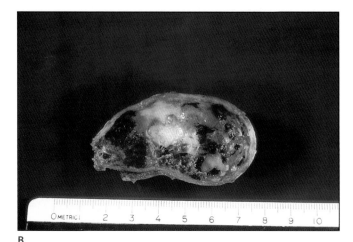

B

Fig. 12.4 • Chronic cholecystitis. **(A)** Numerous cholesterol stones were present. Areas of mucosal prominence alternate with areas showing an atrophic appearance. **(B)** This small, scarred, non-functioning gallbladder contained a single large gallstone.

dominantly found within the epithelium in a setting of chronic cholecystitis, it is preferable to view them as evidence of 'activity' of the inflammatory process rather than as a mixed acute and chronic or subacute condition. We believe that the term chronic active cholecystitis better defines these cases (Fig. 12.5(B)).[15]

When bile penetrates into the subepithelial layers through mucosal ulcers or fissures, it frequently elicits an inflammatory reaction composed of closely packed histiocytes with pale cytoplasm and containing abundant brown granular pigment. In addition to its colour, this pigment, referred to as ceroid, is characterized histochemically by its acid fastness and PAS positivity (diastase-resistant). A sparse lymphocytic reaction usually accompanies the histiocytes.[77,78] Most importantly, ceroid granulomas trigger a reparative response leading to the deposition of dense collagen. Fibrosis eventually replaces those areas previously involved by the inflammatory process and may, with time, replace the entire gallbladder. Dystrophic calcification is often associated with this fibrous tissue, and when diffuse, gives rise to the so-called porcelain gallbladder (Fig. 12.6).[79,80] For unknown reasons, carcinoma of the gallbladder is more frequently

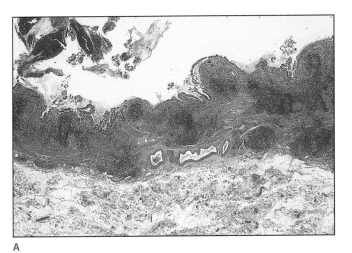

A

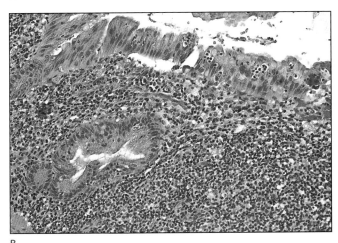

B

Fig. 12.5 • **(A)** Chronic follicular cholecystitis. Diffuse lymphoid hyperplasia with germinal centre formation characterizes this condition. **(B)** Chronic active cholecystitis. A dense lymphoplasmacytic infiltrate ('chronic') distends the lamina propria; intra-epithelial neutrophils ('active') are focally present. H&E.

associated with this condition than with other forms of chronic cholecystitis.[81,82]

In addition to ceroid granulomas, foreign body type granulomas characterized by aggregates of multinucleated giant cells and foamy histiocytes may be seen around clefts containing cholesterol crystals or concretions of bile. Foamy histiocytes are also the predominant cells in xanthogranulomas, usually in association with plasma cells and occasionally with giant cells or ceroid-containing histiocytes. These cells may form tumour-like aggregates that are sometimes confused with neoplasms.[83-86]

As with many other organ systems, chronic injury to the gallbladder mucosa can cause metaplastic changes.[87,88] The most common type of metaplasia is of the antral (or pyloric) type, characterized by tubular glands in the lamina propria formed by clear cells with abundant mucin vacuoles (Fig. 12.7(A)). The cells are similar to those found in the gastric antrum. The surface epithelium frequently undergoes metaplasia of superficial gastric type. This change is characterized by focal or diffuse replacement of the normal columnar epithelium by taller, mucin rich, PAS-positive, columnar cells. When the metaplastic pyloric glands proliferate and permeate smooth muscle fibres, their histological appear-

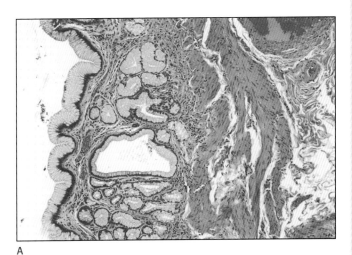

A

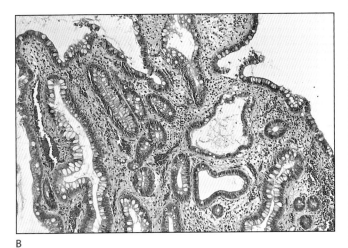

B

Fig. 12.7 • Metaplasia of gallbladder mucosa in chronic cholecystitis. **(A)** A lobule of pyloric glands is seen in the lamina propria. The surface epithelium is of gastric foveolar type. **(B)** Intestinal metaplasia with columnar and goblet cells; endocrine cells were identified by immunohistochemistry. H&E.

Fig. 12.6 • Porcelain gallbladder. Radiograph of a cholecystectomy specimen showing diffuse plaque-like calcifications in the wall of the gallbladder.

ance may be confused with an adenocarcinoma. Rarely, florid pyloric gland metaplasia may show perineural and intraneural 'invasion'. The lobular arrangement of the glands and the bland cytological features should prevent misinterpretation as adenocarcinoma.[89,90] Less frequently, intestinal metaplasia may occur. It is identified by the appearance of cells with intestinal phenotypes, such as goblet cells, absorptive columnar cells, Paneth cells, and endocrine cells (Fig. 12.7(B)). The aberrant expression of CDX2 protein, a marker for intestine-specific transcription factor, in areas of intestinal metaplasia within the gallbladder has been recently demonstrated by immunohistochemistry.[91] Very infrequently, squamous metaplasia may also be found.

Clinical correlation

Chronic cholecystitis is more easily defined by its macroscopic and histological features than by clinical characteristics. Uncertainty still prevails as to the precise symptom(s) associated with gallstone disease and chronic cholecystitis. Most persons with gallstones never experience pain attacks. The only symptom proven to be related to gallstones is episodic upper abdominal pain.[92] Dyspeptic symptoms, belching, bloating, abdominal discomfort, heartburn and food intolerances are frequently attributed to cholelithiasis and chronic cholecystitis, both by the patients and their physicians. However, most of these symptoms are probably unrelated to these conditions and frequently persist after cholecystectomy.

In the USA, laparoscopic cholecystectomy has become the preferred treatment for patients with cholelithiasis.[93,94] This minimally invasive surgical procedure offers the advantages of shorter hospitalization, limited postoperative pain, diminished disability and a better cosmetic result. In most instances, the gallbladder is easily removed through the umbilical puncture wound, although difficulties may arise when bile and/or gallstones distend the gallbladder, or when inflammation and fibrosis give rise to a thick, non-collapsible wall. This problem is usually solved by extending the umbilical incision or by removing the bile and stones after the neck of the gallbladder has been pulled through the skin and amputated. Large stones can be pulverized by mechanical devices, ultrasound or laser energy.[95] When examining a gallbladder the pathologist should differentiate the numerous artifacts produced by these procedures from the pathological changes due to disease.

Chronic acalculous cholecystitis

About 12 to 13% of patients with chronic cholecystitis do not have gallstones.[96] It has been suggested that postinflammatory stenosis or anatomic abnormalities of the cystic duct might impede normal emptying of the gallbladder. Such patients may pose diagnostic difficulties since ultrasound scans and oral cholecystograms are often normal. Patients with 'biliary dyskinesia' who may benefit from cholecystectomy are identified by a CCK provocation test. A positive test consists of reproduction of pain within 5 to 10 minutes after an intravenous injection of CCK.[97] Furthermore,

incomplete emptying of the gallbladder can be documented when this test is performed at the same time as oral cholecystography.[98]

Pathology

At the time of surgery, a normal, distended or thickened gallbladder may be found. Microscopic examination may show an unremarkable appearance or demonstrate changes consistent with outflow obstruction, inflammation or both. Thickening of the muscularis propria and the presence of Rokitansky–Aschoff sinuses identify outflow obstruction (Fig. 12.8(A)). Gallbladders excised from patients with biliary dyskinesia may show abundant Rokitansky–Aschoff sinuses in the absence of inflammation, a condition that has been referred to as microdiverticulosis or 'Rokitansky–Aschoff sinusosis' (Fig. 12.8(B)).[75] Other patients with this condition may have a normal appearing gallbladder or non-specific chronic cholecystitis. When present, the inflammatory pattern in patients with chronic acalculous cholecystitis is non-specific.

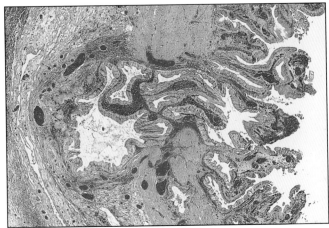

A

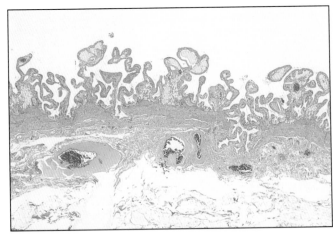

B

Fig. 12.8 • (A) Rokitansky–Aschoff sinuses. These 'sinuses' are mucosal pseudodiverticula. They are a morphological hallmark of increased intraluminal pressure. **(B)** Small intramural and transmural Rokitansky–Aschoff sinuses were present in this patient with biliary dyskinesia; note the absence of inflammation. H&E.

Inflammatory cell infiltrates in patients with acalculous cholecystitis contain a higher percentage of eosinophils than those seen in patients with gallstones. Referred to as 'lympho-eosinophilic cholecystitis', this type of cholecystitis is diagnosed when eosinophils comprise 50 to 75% of the total number of inflammatory cells. It has been hypothesized that abnormal biliary contents or certain hepatic metabolites may evoke a hypersensitivity reaction recruiting a large number of eosinophils that cause mucosal damage and gallbladder dysmotility.[99] In contradistinction, true *eosinophilic cholecystitis* is very rare, and is characterized histologically by an inflammatory infiltrate composed almost exclusively of eosinophils. The massive eosinophilic infiltrate commonly involves the extrahepatic bile ducts in addition to the gallbladder. Clinically, these patients may present with obstructive jaundice that mimics a neoplasm.[100]

A further type of chronic cholecystitis recently identified is characterized by diffuse lymphoplasmacytic infiltrates confined to the lamina propria with or without active lesions (intraepithelial neutrophilic infiltrates) (Fig. 12.9). In the absence of gallstones, this form of chronic cholecystitis was first thought to be found almost exclusively in patients with primary sclerosing cholangitis.[101] However, it has recently been shown this is not the case, and this inflammatory pattern is instead highly specific for extrahepatic biliary tract disease in general.[102]

Xanthogranulomatous cholecystitis

This uncommon form of chronic cholecystitis is nearly always associated with stones and frequently accompanied by fibrosis of variable extent. Its incidence ranges from 0.7% to 1.8% of excised gallbladders, although a recent report demonstrated an incidence of 9.0% in Japan and India.[103–105] The pathogenesis of this condition is uncertain: it has been proposed, however, that xanthogranulomas form as a reaction to the penetration of bile into the gallbladder wall from mucosal ulcers or ruptured Rokitansky–Aschoff sinuses in conjunction with outflow obstruction by stones and infection.[83–86] Positive bile cultures, mostly for enterobacteria, are found in about 50% of the patients.

Pathology

The areas involved by the xanthogranulomatous process may appear as firm yellow masses (Fig. 12.10(A)) that resemble carcinoma clinically and macroscopically.[84] Histological examination shows rounded to spindle shaped lipid laden macrophages, plasma cells and fibrosis (Fig. 12.10(B)). Cholesterol clefts, foreign-body and Touton-type giant cells, and other inflammatory cells (lymphocytes, eosinophils and neutrophils) are commonly found. Frequently, the xanthogranulomatous reaction occupies a limited area of the gallbladder and the remainder shows typical chronic cholecystitis, often with lymphoid follicles.

Xanthogranulomatous inflammation should be differentiated from *malakoplakia* of the gallbladder.[106] The characteristic microscopic findings of malakoplakia consist of a diffuse proliferation of histiocytes with abundant eosinophilic granular cytoplasm, some of which contain spherules

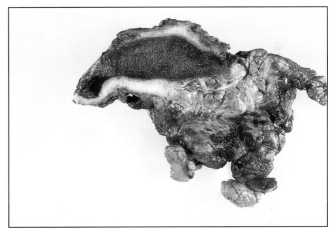

A

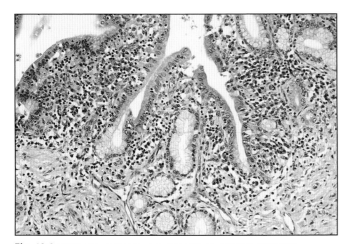

Fig. 12.9 • Diffuse lymphoplasmacytic acalculous cholecystitis. This condition is characterized by a diffuse lymphoplasmacytic infiltrate which mimics the superficial and diffuse distribution of the inflammatory infiltrate in colonic mucosa in ulcerative colitis. H&E.

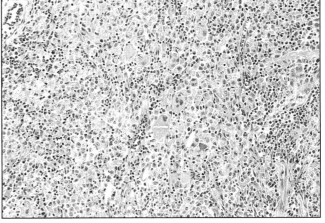

B

Fig. 12.10 • Xanthogranulomatous cholecystitis. **(A)** The gallbladder wall is irregularly thickened. Multiple yellow nodules involve the fundus and extend into adjacent soft tissues. **(B)** Sheets of histiocytes admixed with lymphocytes and multinucleated giant cells are seen. Bile pigment is also present. H&E.

(Michaelis–Guttman bodies) positive with PAS and von Kossa (calcium) stains.

Clinical correlation

Xanthogranulomatous cholecystitis may be difficult to distinguish from other forms of cholecystitis. However, in contrast to chronic cholecystitis, a history of at least one previous episode of acute cholecystitis is obtained from most patients. Some patients present with a clinical picture suggestive of an acute cholecystitis. Imaging studies demonstrate a thickened wall, and gallstones are found in almost all patients. An increased risk of adenocarcinoma of the gallbladder in patients with xanthogranulomatous cholecystitis was reported;[107] however, recent studies have not confirmed this association.[104] In cases where xanthogranulomatous cholecystitis resembles adenocarcinoma, intraoperative histologic examination is essential to ensure optimal surgical treatment.[105]

Cholecystitis in patients with AIDS

Acalculous cholecystitis has been cited in several reports as a complication of HIV infection.[108–111] *Cryptosporidium* is the most commonly identified cause of AIDS-related infection of the extrahepatic bile ducts and gallbladder. This organism has been identified in the bile ducts or stools in 20 to 62% of patients with symptoms of AIDS-related cholangitis (p. 482). *Cryptosporidia* organisms colonize the biliary cells and elicit an inflammatory response of variable intensity, being mild in those cases not associated with other organisms. Cytomegalovirus (CMV) infection is the second most common infection in AIDS-related cholecystitis. It has been estimated that 10% of AIDS patients with CMV develop biliary involvement.[112] Mucosal ulcers and a mixed inflammatory infiltrate are present. Intranuclear and intracytoplasmic inclusions are found in endothelial and epithelial cells. Occasionally, CMV and cryptosporidium infections co-exist in the same gallbladder (Fig. 12.11). Rare instances of infection by *Mycobacterium avium* have been reported. The diffuse histiocytic proliferation induced by this organism

may mimic xanthogranulomatous cholecystitis and malakoplakia. Other organisms that have been identified in the gallbladder include *Microsporidia*, particularly *Enterocytozoon bieneusi* and *Isospora*.[111,113]

Other miscellaneous diseases of the gallbladder

Helminth infestation

Infestation of the gallbladder with *Fasciola hepatica* and *Clonorchis sinensis* induces an inflammatory response rich in lymphocytes and eosinophils, usually accompanied by hyperplasia of metaplastic pyloric-type glands. Granulomatous cholecystitis has been described in association with the ova of *Schistosoma mansoni*, *Paragonimus westermani* and *Ascaris lumbricoides*.[114]

Polyarteritis nodosa and other vasculitis

Histological changes of classic polyarteritis nodosa are seen in the gallbladder in two clinical settings (Fig. 12.12), patients with isolated gallbladder involvement and patients with systemic disease including scleroderma and systemic lupus erythematosus.[115–117] The localized form of polyarteritis nodosa may rarely progress to systemic disease, especially in patients with serum autoantibodies (rheumatoid factor, antinuclear antibodies).[117] Other forms of vasculitis include granulomatous vasculitis as described in the gallbladder of patients with the Churg–Strauss syndrome or temporal giant-cell arteritis.

Cholesterolosis

Cholesterolosis is characterized by aggregates of lipid-containing macrophages in the lamina propria of the gallbladder. Autopsy and surgical studies have demonstrated a prevalence of 12% and 26%, respectively.[118–120] The

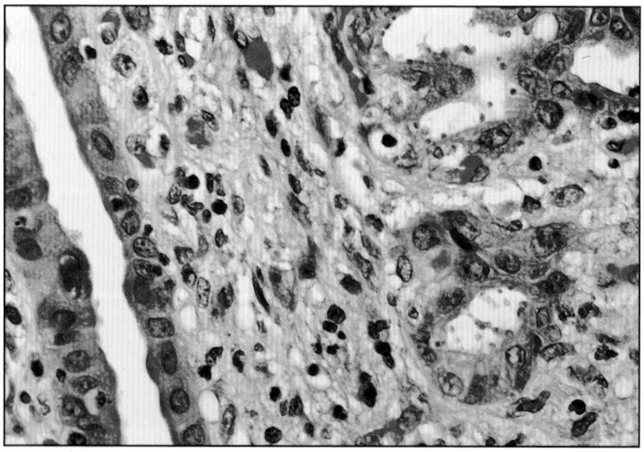

Fig. 12.11 • Cytomegalovirus and cryptosporidium infection. An epithelial cell of an invagination shows the characteristic nuclear CMV inclusions. *Cryptosporidia* are attached to the apical cells lining two metaplastic glands. H&E.

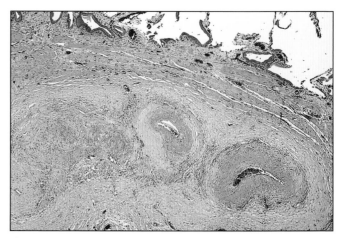

Fig. 12.12 • Polyarteritis nodosa. Medium-sized arteries with fibrinoid necrosis and an inflammatory infiltrate that involves their walls are seen in the muscular coat of the gallbladder. H&E.

aetiology and pathogenesis of cholesterolosis are poorly understood. Accumulation of cholesterol esters and triglycerides may reflect an increased hepatic synthesis of these lipids and/or an increased absorption and esterification by the gallbladder. The normal gallbladder can absorb free and non-esterified cholesterol from the bile. Cholesterol is esterified in the endoplasmic reticulum and forms lipid droplets that are released into the intercellular space, where they are phagocytosed by macrophages.[120] Patients with cholesterolosis, as those with cholesterol stones, have supersaturated bile; as expected, both conditions frequently co-exist. It is therefore probable that cholesterolosis results from increased cholesterol uptake from supersaturated bile. Another theory postulates the existence of a defect in macrophages with failure to metabolize or excrete the cholesterol absorbed from the bile.[119]

Pathology

On macroscopic examination, the lipid deposits appear as yellow flecks against a dark-green background, earning the sobriquet 'strawberry gallbladder'. When extensive, these deposits may form polypoid excrescences that project into the lumen. Commonly referred to as 'cholesterol polyps' but more properly called cholesterolosis polyps, these lesions are generally small but may be large enough to be detected by imaging techniques. Cholesterol gallstones are associated with cholesterolosis in half of the surgical cases, and in 10% of autopsy series.

Microscopically, the diagnostic feature of cholesterolosis is the accumulation of foamy macrophages within an expanded lamina propria resulting in thickened folds and/or polyps (Fig. 12.13). The adjacent mucosa may be normal or inflamed; however, inflammation occurs almost exclusively in those patients with co-existent stones.

Clinical correlation

Ninety years after the first description of this entity its clinical relevance is still debated. Some studies have suggested that cholesterolosis is associated with symptoms in patients having acalculous biliary disease, with colicky abdominal pain and selective food intolerance as the most common complaints. Cholesterolosis is present in some patients with biliary dyskinesia, in which case the resolution of symptoms following surgery is more likely due to eradication of the dyskinesia rather than removal of the cholesterolosis. Recent evidence suggests a possible relationship between cholesterolosis and acute pancreatitis. Temporary impaction of cholesterolosis polyps at the sphincter of Oddi may produce recurrent attacks of acute pancreatitis.[121] If the prevalence of cholesterolosis as derived from autopsy studies reflects the actual frequency in the general population, it is clear that most individuals with cholesterolosis do not develop severe symptoms.

Papillary hyperplasia

This is a proliferative lesion composed of tall, exaggerated epithelial folds lined by normal-appearing biliary epithelium. It is classified as of primary and secondary types.[122]

Secondary papillary hyperplasia is much more common and is usually seen in association with chronic cholecystitis or other inflammatory diseases such as ulcerative colitis and primary sclerosing cholangitis. Secondary papillary hyperplasia is focal or segmental in distribution and frequently accompanied by intestinal metaplasia. *Primary papillary hyperplasia* is uncommon and not associated with chronic inflammation. Primary papillary hyperplasia may be focal, segmental or involve the entire mucosa of the biliary tract. There is no intestinal metaplasia in primary papillary hyperplasia. Epithelial dysplasia develops in secondary but not in primary papillary hyperplasia.

Hydrops and mucocele

Gallbladders distended by clear watery fluid (hydrops) or mucus (mucocele) account for 3% of cholecystectomy specimens in adults.[17] In this age group, the most common cause is an impacted stone in the neck of the gallbladder or cystic duct. Less frequent causes include cystic fibrosis, tumours, fibrosis or kinking of the cystic duct, or external compression by inflammatory or neoplastic masses. In children, these conditions are usually acute processes associated with infectious diseases or inflammatory disorders of unknown aetiology, such as streptococcal infections, mesenteric adenitis, typhoid, leptospirosis, viral hepatitis, familial Mediterranean fever and Kawasaki syndrome. Symptoms may resolve with conservative treatment.[17,123]

Pathology

The gallbladder is considerably distended and may contain over 1500 ml of fluid or be filled by a mass of inspissated mucin. When associated with numerous stones, the wall is usually thickened. By contrast, a thin wall is the rule when a single stone obstructs the cystic duct or in acute cases in childhood. Microscopic examination usually reveals a flattened mucosa lined by low columnar or cuboidal cells (Fig. 12.14). As a result of increased intraluminal pressure,

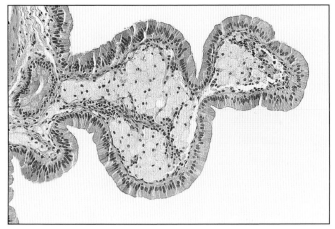

Fig. 12.13 • Cholesterolosis. Clusters of foamy macrophages expand the lamina propria. In contrast to xanthogranulomatous cholecystitis, these histiocytic aggregates do not elicit a fibrosing reaction. H&E.

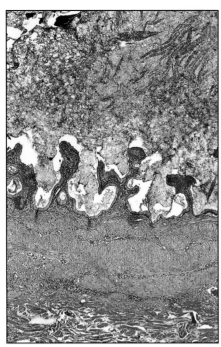

Fig. 12.14 • Mucocele. The lumen of the gallbladder contains abundant extracellular mucin but the lining epithelium is normal. H&E.

Rokitansky–Aschoff sinuses may be plentiful. In some cases the mucin may reach the peritoneal cavity and simulate mucinous adenocarcinoma. The amount of inflammatory cells varies from sparse to abundant. Acute cholecystitis with oedema of the lamina propria and abundant neutrophils occurs in some patients with Kawasaki syndrome.[123]

Diverticular disease

Congenital and traction diverticula are the two types of true diverticula that occur in the gallbladder. The congenital lesions have been discussed previously. They are differentiated from the more common acquired pseudodiverticula by the constituents of their wall: true diverticula have all the elements of the normal wall while the pseudodiverticula have little or no smooth muscle.

Traction diverticula are caused by the pulling action of post-inflammatory fibrous adhesions anchoring the serosa of the gallbladder to adjacent structures. Erosion by stones, healing fistulas, widespread peritonitis of any cause, or previous intra-abdominal surgery precede their formation. Traction diverticula are distinguished from congenital outpouchings principally by their relationship with intra-abdominal lesions in the vicinity of the gallbladder, and by the predominance of the serosal (rather than mucosal) inflammation and fibrosis. In some cases, however, this distinction may be impossible.

Acquired pseudodiverticula are mucosal herniations among the smooth muscle bundles of the wall and should be regarded as prominent Rokitansky–Aschoff sinuses. Almost invariably, these pulsion diverticula are associated with stones and chronic cholecystitis or with outflow obstruction. Analogous to diverticular disease of the colon, the intervening smooth muscle is usually hypertrophied. The mucosal outpouchings and the prominent muscle may form a localized tumour-like lesion that has been referred to as an *adenomyoma/localized adenomyomatous hyperplasia,* or may diffusely thicken the gallbladder wall—*diffuse adenomyomatous hyperplasia.*[124,125] The epithelium lining the mucosal herniations is usually normal but may rarely show gastric foveolar metaplasia, dysplastic or neoplastic changes. Perineural invasion has rarely been observed in adenomyomatous hyperplasia and should not be confused with adenocarcinoma.[89]

Ischaemic diseases

Deprivation of arterial blood flow or obstruction to venous drainage may result in infarction of the gallbladder. As mentioned previously, the blood supply of the gallbladder comes from the cystic artery, which usually originates from the right hepatic artery. The latter is a branch of the coeliac artery. Venous blood is carried though small veins that drain into the liver. Atherosclerosis and its common complication, thrombosis, are the usual causes of obliteration of the arterial blood flow. Embolic occlusion may occur as a complication of valvular heart disease or bacterial endocarditis. Another cause of ischaemia may be a dissecting aneurysm extending into the coeliac artery with occlusion of the origin of the hepatic artery. External compression of the arteries and/or interference with venous drainage may result from impingement on these vessels by stones, or tumours, or occlusion by surgical iatrogenic ligation.[126]

Gallbladders with a greater degree of mobility ('floating gallbladders') may twist on their pedicle, a condition known as torsion or volvulus. As mentioned previously the floating gallbladder lacks a firm attachment to the liver and is completely surrounded by peritoneum. Torsion in developmentally normal gallbladders may also result from loosening of the suspensory connective tissue, as seen in ageing, or from shrinkage of the liver (as in cirrhosis) leading to detachment of the gallbladder from its bed and visceroptosis.[17]

Uncommonly, ischaemic lesions result from vasculitis. Among the primary vascular diseases that may involve the gallbladder, polyarteritis nodosa appears to be the most frequent.[127–128] Other forms of vasculitis that affect this organ include allergic granulomatosis (Churg–Strauss), rheumatoid vasculitis, and a form of small vessel vasculitis restricted to the gallbladder known as localized or focal visceral angiitis. As in other locations, lymphocytic venulitis may be a manifestation of Behçet disease.[129,130] Secondary vasculitis frequently occurs in patients with calculous cholecystitis.

Pathology

The gallbladder wall is thickened and the mucosa is congested or haemorrhagic. Microscopic examination reveals partial or complete loss of the epithelium, oedema and/or haemorrhage in the lamina propria. When occlusion to venous outflow predominates, there is extensive, often transmural, haemorrhagic infarction. Ischaemic lesions associated with primary vasculitis are often focal and

confined to the mucosa. In patients with calculous cholecystitis, superimposed ischaemic damage caused by secondary vasculitis or small vessel thrombosis is frequently found.
Healed ischaemic lesions are at least partially responsible
for the deposition of fibrous tissue in so-called sclerosing
cholecystitis.

Clinical correlation

Most of the cases occur in patients older than 60 years. The
preoperative clinical diagnosis is rarely made since the
symptoms mimic those of acute cholecystitis.

Traumatic conditions and 'chemical' cholecystitis

The gallbladder is seldom damaged from abdominal trauma
since it is partially protected by the ribs and liver. On occasion, however, blunt abdominal trauma can disrupt a distended gallbladder causing contusion, laceration, torsion,
avulsion and intraluminal haemorrhage.[131] Penetrating
wounds may damage the gallbladder, usually in association
with injury to the adjacent organs. Iatrogenic injury can
result from liver biopsy or percutaneous transhepatic cholangiography. An acute cholecystitis with mucosal necrosis
followed by fibrosis may occur as a result of repeated infusion of chemotherapeutic agents through a catheter placed
in the hepatic artery.[132]

Biliary fistulas

In most cases, fistulas between the biliary tract and adjacent
organs are a consequence of gallstone-associated necrosis
with inflammation of the gallbladder and/or bile ducts.

Inflammatory adhesions precede their formation; these
lesions may form masses that could be confused with a fixed
inoperable tumour. A classical cholecystectomy in the presence of fistulas carries a high risk of injury to the bile ducts.
The most common fistulas are cholecystoduodenal, followed by cholecystocolic and choledochoduodenal fistulas.[17] Bilio-biliary fistulas form between the gallbladder and
the common bile duct. This complication should be suspected in patients with cholelithiasis and jaundice.[133]

Metachromatic leucodystrophy

Metachromatic leucodystrophy (MLD) is an inborn error of
metabolism associated with a deficiency in aryl sulphatase.[134] The disease is characterized by diffuse breakdown
of myelin in both the central nervous system and peripheral
nervous system. The microscopic changes in the gallbladder
consist of papillary hyperplasia (papillomatosis) and expansion of the lamina propria by macrophages containing the
abnormal metachromatic material (sulphatides). The metachromatic material is also found within the epithelial cells
and may be responsible for the hyperplastic epithelial
changes.[134]

Tumours

Despite its simple histological structure, the gallbladder
gives rise to a wide variety of neoplasms. The majority of
such tumours are carcinomas, and a small proportion are
adenomas, carcinoid and stromal tumours.[3] The histological classification of tumours of the gallbladder is shown in
Table 12.1. This classification is essentially similar to the
WHO classification published in 1991[135] and to the classification adopted by the Armed Forces Institute of Pathology
(AFIP) fascicle published in 1999.[3]

Epithelial tumours
Adenomas

Adenomas of the gallbladder are uncommon benign neoplasms of glandular epithelium that are typically polypoid,
single and well-demarcated (Fig. 12.15(A)). According to
their pattern of growth, adenomas of the extrahepatic
biliary tree are divided into three types: tubular, papillary
and tubulopapillary. Cytologically they are classified into:
pyloric gland type, intestinal type and biliary type.[136] Pyloric

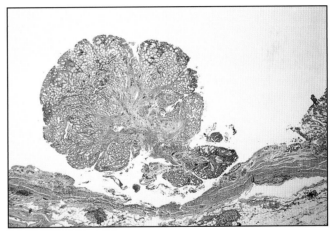

A

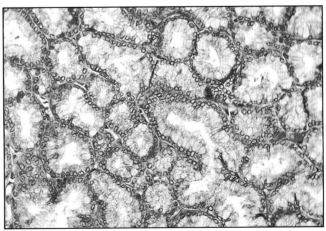

B

Fig. 12.15 • Tubular adenoma, pyloric gland type. **(A)** A small, well-
demarcated polypoid and pedunculated tumour projects into the lumen of
the gallbladder. **(B)** Closely packed tubular glands are lined by columnar cells
with vesicular basally placed nuclei. H&E.

Table 12.1 Histological classification of tumours of the gallbladder

Epithelial tumours		Non-epithelial tumours	
Benign	*Malignant*	*Benign*	*Malignant*
Adenoma	Adenocarcinoma	Leiomyoma	Malignant mesenchymal tumours
Tubular	Papillary adenocarcinoma	Stromal tumour with interstitial	Rhabdomyosarcoma
Papillary	Adenocarcinoma, intestinal type	cells of Cajal phenotype	Malignant fibrous histiocytoma
Tubulopapillary	Adenocarcinoma, gastric	Lipoma	Angiosarcoma
	foveolar type	Haemangioma	Leiomyosarcoma
	Clear-cell adenocarcinoma	Lymphangioma	Kaposi sarcoma
Cystadenoma	Mucinous carcinoma	Osteoma	
Papillomatosis	Signet-ring cell carcinoma	Granular cell tumour	
	Adenosquamous carcinoma	Neurogenic tumours	
		Neurofibroma	
Premalignant lesions	Squamous-cell carcinoma	Neurofibromatosis	
Dysplasia	Small-cell carcinoma (oat-cell	Ganglioneuromatosis	
	carcinoma)		
Carcinoma in situ	Large-cell neuroendocrine	**Miscellaneous tumours**	
	carcinoma	Carcinosarcoma	
	Undifferentiated carcinoma	Malignant melanoma	
	Spindle- and giant-cell type	Malignant lymphoma	
	Small-cell type	Yolk-sac tumour	
	With a nodular growth pattern	Secondary tumours	
	With osteoclast-like giant cells		
	Cystadenocarcinoma	**Tumour-like lesions**	
		Regenerative epithelial atypia	Mucocele
Endocrine tumours		Papillary hyperplasia	Heterotopia
Carcinoid tumour		Adenomyomatous hyperplasia	Cholesterol polyp
Adenocarcinoid		Rokitansky–Aschoff sinuses	Inflammatory polyp
(goblet-cell carcinoid)		Intestinal metaplasia	Fibrous polyp
Tubular carcinoid		Pyloric gland metaplasia	Xanthogranulomatous
Mixed carcinoid-adenocarcinoma			cholecystitis
		Squamous metaplasia	Cholecystitis with lymphoid
Tumours of paraganglia			hyperplasia
Paraganglioma		Luschka ducts	Malakoplakia
		Myofibroblastic proliferations	Myoproliferative proliferations

gland adenoma is the most common type followed by the intestinal and biliary types. A small proportion of adenomas progress to carcinoma.[136–138]

Clinical features

Adenomas are found in 0.3 to 0.5% of gallbladders removed for cholelithiasis or chronic cholecystitis and are more common in women than in men. In the largest series of 37 patients, 26 were females (70%).[135] The age of the patients ranged from 17 to 79 years with a mean of 58 years. Rarely, gallbladder adenomas occur in children.[139,140] Adenomas are often small, asymptomatic, and usually discovered incidentally during cholecystectomy; they can, however, be large, multiple, fill the lumen of the gallbladder and be symptomatic. Occasionally adenomas of the gallbladder occur in association with the Peutz–Jeghers syndrome[141] or with Gardner syndrome.[142,143] Tubular adenomas of pyloric gland type are more common in the gallbladder while intestinal type adenomas are more common in the extrahepatic bile ducts.[136]

Tubular adenoma, pyloric-gland type

This is a benign tumour composed of closely packed short tubular glands that are similar to pyloric glands and lined by mild to moderately dysplastic epithelium (Fig. 12.15). In their early phase of development pyloric gland type tubular adenomas appear as well-demarcated nodules embedded in the lamina propria and covered with normal biliary epithelium. Although most of the pyloric-type glands are small and short, some may be cystically dilated. The glands are lined by columnar or cuboidal cells with vesicular or hyperchromatic nuclei and small nucleoli. A variable amount of cytoplasmic mucin is present. Squamoid morules characterized by nodular aggregates of spindle cells with eosinophilic cytoplasm, but without intercellular bridges or keratinization are identified in approximately 10% of cases.[144,145] True squamous metaplasia, however, is exceedingly rare. Approximately 20% of the tumours contain Paneth cells as well as endocrine cells. By immunohistochemistry, serotonin and a variety of peptide hormones including somatostatin, pancreatic polypeptide and gastrin, have been detected in the cytoplasm of these cells. Dysplastic changes are more pronounced in the larger adenomas. Foci of carcinoma in situ and invasive carcinoma are seen in a small proportion of adenomas. As they enlarge, most adenomas develop a pedicle and project into the lumen. Rarely, they extend into or arise from Rokitansky–Aschoff sinuses, a finding that should not be mistaken for carcinoma.[136]

Tubular adenoma, intestinal type

This benign tumour is composed of tubular glands lined by cells with an intestinal phenotype. The lining cells characteristically show moderate to severe dysplastic changes. This type of adenoma closely resembles colonic adenomas: it consists of tubular glands lined by pseudostratified columnar cells with elongated hyperchromatic nuclei. The glands lack invasive properties and focally are arranged in well-defined lobules. The adenomatous epithelium may extend into the Rokitansky–Aschoff sinuses, a finding which should not be confused with stromal invasion. Clusters of goblet, Paneth and endocrine cells are usually admixed with the columnar cells. Serotonin and, less frequently, peptide hormones have been identified in the endocrine cells by immunohistochemistry. Hyperplasia of metaplastic pyloric type glands is often seen at the base of the adenomas.

Papillary adenoma, intestinal type

This benign tumour consists predominantly of papillary structures lined by dysplastic cells with an intestinal phenotype[1] (Fig. 12.16). The predominant cell is columnar with elongated hyperchromatic nuclei and little or no cytoplasmic mucin. The cells are pseudostratified, mitotically active

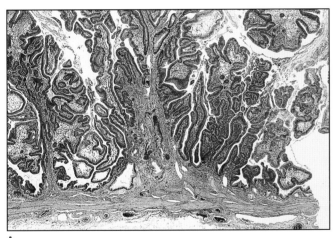

A

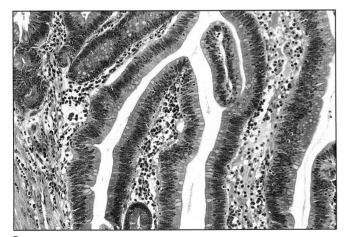

B

Fig. 12.16 • Papillary adenoma, intestinal type. **(A)** Low power view of a papillary neoplasm that projects into the lumen of the gallbladder. **(B)** The papillary structures are lined by pseudostratified columnar cells admixed with goblet and Paneth cells. H&E.

and indistinguishable from those of papillary adenomas arising in the large intestine. Tubular glands lined by the same type of epithelium but representing less than 20% of the tumour may also be found. Dysplastic changes are more extensive than in pyloric-gland type adenomas. Also present are goblet, Paneth and serotonin-containing cells (Fig. 12.16(B)). Some of the endocrine cells are immunoreactive for peptide hormones. These adenomas, which usually arise on a background of pyloric gland metaplasia, may occur in the gallbladder or the extrahepatic bile ducts. In a series of five intestinal type papillary adenomas of the gallbladder, one progressed to invasive carcinoma.[136]

Papillary adenoma, biliary type

This type of adenoma is well demarcated and consists of papillary structures lined by tall columnar cells, which, except for the presence of more cytoplasmic mucin, show minimal variation from normal gallbladder epithelium. Endocrine or Paneth cells are not found in these adenomas. Only mild dysplastic changes are noted and in situ or invasive carcinoma has not been reported.

This is the rarest form of adenoma of the gallbladder. In fact, we have seen only one case. Most papillary lesions composed of normal-appearing gallbladder epithelium are examples of hyperplasia secondary to chronic cholecystitis.

Tubulopapillary adenoma

When tubular glands and papillary structures each comprise more than 20% of the tumour, the term tubulopapillary adenoma is applied. Two subtypes are recognized: one is composed of tubular glands and papillary structures similar to those of mixed intestinal adenomas; the other subtype consists of tubular glands similar to pyloric glands and papillary structures often lined by foveolar epithelium. Paneth and endocrine cells are seen in some adenomas. Dysplastic changes are usually present. Rarely, tubulopapillary adenomas arise from the epithelial invaginations of adenomyomatous hyperplasia.

Molecular pathology

The molecular pathology of adenomas of the gallbladder differs from that of carcinomas. Of 16 adenomas (12 pyloric type and 2 intestinal type), subjected to genetic analysis, none showed p53 and p16 Ink4/CDKN2a gene mutations, which are the most common and sometimes the only molecular abnormalities detected in carcinomas.[140] Four adenomas (25%) had K-ras mutations (two in codon 12 and two in codon 61), which are considered rare and late events in the pathogenesis of carcinomas of the gallbladder. Only one adenoma of intestinal type showed loss of heterozygosity at 5q22.[130]

Cystadenoma

Cystadenomas are seen predominantly among adult females and are usually symptomatic. Some of the tumours may measure up to 20 cm in diameter, leading to obstructive jaundice or cholecystitis-like symptoms. More common in the extrahepatic bile ducts than in the gallbladder, cystadenomas are multiloculated neoplasms that contain mucinous or serous fluid and are lined by columnar epithelium reminiscent of bile duct or foveolar gastric epithelium.[146] Occasionally endocrine cells are present. The cellular subepithelial stroma resembles ovarian stroma and shows immunoreactivity for oestrogen and progesterone receptors.[147] The stroma also shows fibrosis of variable extent. Malignant transformation (cystadenocarcinoma) can occur.[146]

Papillomatosis (adenomatosis)

Papillomatosis is a clinicopathological condition characterized by multiple recurring papillary adenomas that may involve extensive areas of the extrahepatic bile ducts and even extend into the gallbladder and intrahepatic bile ducts. The disease affects both sexes equally. Most patients are adults between 50 and 60 years. Complete excision of the multicentric lesions is difficult and local recurrence is common.[148]

The lesion consists of numerous papillary structures as well as complex glandular formations. Because severe dysplasia is often present, papillomatosis is difficult to distinguish from papillary carcinoma. Some regard this lesion as a form of low-grade multicentric intraductal papillary carcinoma. Papillomatosis has a greater potential for malignant transformation than solitary adenomas.

Dysplasia and carcinoma in situ of the gallbladder

The rate of dysplasia and carcinoma in situ of the gallbladder reflects that of invasive carcinoma. The prevalence of dysplasia and carcinoma in situ is higher in countries in which carcinoma of the gallbladder is endemic than in countries in which this tumour is sporadic. Studies from different countries have shown that the incidence of high-grade dysplasia or carcinoma in situ in gallbladders with lithiasis has varied from 0.5 to 3%.[3] This variation in the incidence of dysplasia and carcinoma in situ may also be attributable to other factors, such as lack of uniformity in morphological criteria, sampling methods, etc.

Dysplasia and carcinoma in situ are usually not recognized on macroscopic examination because they often occur in association with chronic cholecystitis. Macroscopically, no distinctive features alert the pathologist to the presence of these two lesions. The mucosa may appear granular, nodular, plaque-like or trabeculated. The papillary type of dysplasia or carcinoma in situ usually appears as a small, cauliflower-like excrescence that projects into the lumen and can be recognized on close inspection. However, in most cases of dysplasia and carcinoma in situ, the gallbladder shows only a thickened and indurated wall, resulting from chronic inflammation and fibrosis.

Microscopic features

Microscopically, two types of dysplasia and carcinoma in situ are recognized: papillary and flat, the latter being more common. The papillary type is characterized by short fibro-

vascular stalks that are covered by dysplastic or neoplastic cells.[149,150]

Dysplasia and carcinoma in situ usually begin on the surface epithelium and subsequently extend downward into the Rokitansky–Aschoff sinuses and into metaplastic pyloric glands. Columnar, cuboidal and elongated cells with variable degrees of nuclear atypia, loss of polarity and occasional mitotic figures characterize dysplasia. The dysplastic cells are usually arranged in a single layer. However, because of cellular proliferation and nuclear crowding, pseudostratification often occurs. As the disease progresses, dysplastic cells extend into epithelial invaginations and even into metaplastic pyloric-type glands or may grow outward and cover small fibrovascular stalks that protrude into the lumen. The large nuclei of dysplastic cells may be round, oval or fusiform, with one or two nucleoli that are more prominent than those of normal cells. The cytoplasm usually stains eosinophilic and contains non-sulphated acid and neutral mucin. Goblet cells are found in one third of cases (Fig. 12.17). An abrupt transition between normal-appearing columnar cells and dysplastic epithelium is seen in nearly all cases, which is an important clue in the diagnosis of dysplasia. In general, the cell population of dysplasia is homogeneous, unlike the heterogeneous cell population of the epithelial atypia of repair. In many cases, the dysplastic lesions are continuous with areas of carcinoma in situ, although normal appearing epithelium may separate the two. Widespread involvement of the mucosa by dysplasia and in situ carcinoma often occurs. For this reason, we have suggested that some, if not most, invasive carcinomas of the gallbladder arise from a field change within the epithelium.

Cells from carcinoma in situ have all the cytological features of malignancy. Because of the excessive cellular proliferation, mitotic figures are more common and nuclear crowding and pseudostratification are more prominent in cases of carcinoma in situ than in cases of dysplasia. Neoplastic cells first appear along the surface epithelium and later spread into the epithelial invaginations and antral-type metaplastic glands. In the late stages of carcinoma in situ, the histological picture is that of back-to-back glands located in the lamina propria but often connected with the

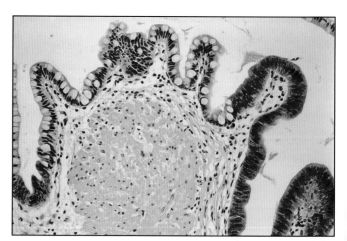

Fig. 12.17 • Dysplasia. High-grade dysplasia adjacent to intestinal metaplasia.

surface epithelium. However, not all in situ carcinomas exhibit this type of growth pattern. Some show distinctive papillary features with small fibrovascular stalks lined by neoplastic cells. Not infrequently, a combination of these growth patterns is seen.

Unusual histological variants of carcinoma in situ

An in situ carcinoma composed of goblet cells, columnar cells, Paneth cells and endocrine cells has been described, and is thought to represent the in situ phase of the tumour designated 'intestinal-type adenocarcinoma' because both the infiltrating and the intraepithelial forms have the same cell population.[3,151] In addition to the endocrine cells which are argyrophil and chromogranin-positive, this type of in situ carcinoma may contain goblet cells. Their presence in the conventional type of in situ carcinoma is regarded as an example of intestinal differentiation occurring within the neoplastic epithelium.

Another type of in situ intestinal type carcinoma is composed of cells closely resembling those of colonic carcinomas at the light and electron microscopic levels. The neoplastic columnar cells extend into the epithelial invaginations and the antral-type glands. Formation of cribriform structures in the lamina propria occurs. This tumour also has scattered endocrine cells, most of which are immunoreactive for serotonin.

Two examples of signet-ring cell carcinoma confined to the surface epithelium and to the epithelial invaginations of the gallbladder have been reported.[152] These in situ signet-ring cell carcinomas represented incidental findings in cholecystectomy specimens and were cytologically similar to those reported in the stomach. The signet-ring cells showed reactivity for cytokeratin and carcinoembryonic antigen (CEA). Despite multiple sections stromal invasion was not found. This unusual form of carcinoma in situ should be distinguished from epithelial cells, which acquire signet-ring cell morphology when desquamated within the lumen of dilated metaplastic pyloric glands in cases of chronic cholecystitis. These CEA-negative cells are often poorly preserved, lack nuclear atypia and appear floating with other degenerating epithelial and inflammatory cells.[3] Likewise, mucin-containing histiocytes (muciphages) that are occasionally seen in mucoceles of the gallbladder may simulate signet-ring cell carcinoma in situ. These muciphages however, are cytokeratin and CEA negative.

The mucosa adjacent to pure squamous-cell carcinomas of the gallbladder often shows areas of squamous metaplasia, dysplasia and carcinoma in situ. It seems, therefore, that squamous-cell carcinomas, which are unusual in the gallbladder, undergo the same pathological changes in their development as those arising in other sites.[3]

It is worth noting that the morphological type of in situ carcinoma does not always correspond with that of the invasive carcinoma. For example, we have seen conventional adenocarcinoma in situ in the mucosa adjacent to various invasive carcinomas including squamous-, small-cell and undifferentiated spindle- and giant-cell type.

The wall of the gallbladder with dysplasia or carcinoma in situ usually shows variable inflammatory changes. As expected, the most common type of inflammatory response is chronic, with a predominance of lymphocytes and plasma cells, although xanthogranulomatous inflammation or even an acute inflammatory reaction may be present. In some cases, lymphoid follicles with germinal centres may be seen in the lamina propria and muscle layer. Reactive epithelial atypia is discussed under differential diagnosis.

If dysplasia or carcinoma in situ is found, multiple sections should be taken to exclude invasive cancer. Cholecystectomy is a curative surgical procedure for patients with in situ carcinoma or with carcinoma extending into the lamina propria.[3]

Differential diagnosis

The differential diagnosis between severe dysplasia and carcinoma in situ is difficult and often impossible in many cases. This is not important because the two lesions, which vary only in degree histologically, are closely related biologically. However, differentiation of dysplasia or carcinoma in situ from the epithelial atypia of repair is of great clinical significance because the last lesion does not progress to carcinoma. The atypia of repair consists of a heterogeneous cell population in which columnar mucus-secreting cells, low cuboidal cells, atrophic-appearing epithelium and pencil-like cells are present. In addition, there is a gradual transition of the cellular abnormalities, in contrast with the abrupt transition seen in dysplasia and carcinoma in situ. The extent of nuclear atypia is less pronounced in the epithelial atypia of repair than in dysplasia or in carcinoma in situ. In contrast to dysplasia and carcinoma in situ, reactive atypia is usually CEA negative and does not express p53 protein.

Immunohistochemistry and molecular pathology

Immunohistochemically, dysplasia and carcinoma in situ are immunoreactive for CEA with polyclonal and monoclonal antibody and for the carbohydrate antigen CA 19-9.[3] The reactivity is usually focal and displays a linear pattern along the apical cytoplasmic border. However, faint cytoplasmic staining is also seen mainly for CEA. Although this oncofetal antigen can be detected in both the bile and in the serum, an elevated CEA level is not diagnostic of dysplasia or carcinoma because extrahepatic bile-duct obstruction from any cause results in high levels. The lack of specificity of CEA limits its use in the diagnosis of early carcinoma of the gallbladder.[143]

Recent studies have shown a crucial role of p53 gene mutations in the early pathogenesis of gallbladder carcinoma. By immunohistochemistry p53 nuclear staining was found in 32% of cases of dysplasia and in 44% of in situ carcinomas.[154] Genetic analysis has shown a high incidence of loss of heterozygosity of the p53 gene, in both dysplasia (58%) and carcinoma in situ (85%). Other molecular abnormalities include loss of heterozygosity at 9p and 8p loci and of the 18q gene. These molecular abnormalities are also early events and most likely contributing factors in the pathogenesis of gallbladder carcinoma. However, K-ras mutations were not detected in dysplasia or carcinoma in situ.[154]

Carcinoma

Epidemiology

The incidence of carcinoma of the gallbladder varies in different parts of the world and also differs among different ethnic groups within the same country. In the USA, for example, carcinoma of the gallbladder is more common in native Americans than in Caucasians or in African Americans; the rate among female American Indians is 21 per 100 000 compared with 1.4 per 100 000 among Caucasian females. In Latin American countries, the highest rates are found in Chile, Mexico and Bolivia. In other countries, such as Japan, the incidence rates are intermediate between those of American Indians and those of Caucasians. In the general population of the USA cancer of the gallbladder accounts for 0.17% of all cancers in males and 0.49% of cancers in females.[3]

Despite having certain features in common, carcinomas of the gallbladder and carcinomas of the extrahepatic bile ducts show a number of differences. Gallbladder carcinomas are usually associated with cholelithiasis and have a female preponderance. In contrast, extrahepatic bile-duct carcinomas occur more frequently in males and are usually not associated with choledocholithiasis. In addition extrahepatic bile-duct carcinomas typically produce early biliary obstruction, and are better differentiated histologically as a group, while gallbladder carcinomas tend to present late. Finally, extrahepatic bile-duct carcinomas are associated with primary sclerosing cholangitis and ulcerative colitis but gallbladder carcinomas show no significant association with these two disorders.[155]

Aetiology

The four most important factors associated with the development of gallbladder carcinoma are genetic abnormalities, gallstones, congenital abnormal choledochopancreatic junction and porcelain gallbladder.

Genetic factors

As discussed above, cancer of the gallbladder is concentrated in certain racial and ethnic groups. Unusually high rates are found among native Americans and Hispanic Americans, especially those living in Arizona and in California, and among South and Central American Indians. The Hispanic Americans, it should be recalled, are descendants of the early Spanish settlers and have an ethnic background of both native American and Spanish. Familial aggregation of gallbladder cancer has been recorded in the USA and in other countries.[3]

The high incidence of carcinoma of the gallbladder in Hispanic Americans seems to be the result of racial intermixture, since the Iberian Spaniards, the historical source of New Mexico's original settlers, do not have high rates of gallbladder cancer—2.7 per 100 000 for females and 1.8 per 100 000 for males. Studies of Hispanics in Colorado indicate that the Indian contribution to the gene pool is as high as 40%. It is possible, therefore, that the high rates observed in some countries in Latin America may also be the result of racial intermixture between the Spanish immigrants and the native Americans.

Gallstones

The association of carcinoma of the gallbladder with gallstones has been known since 1861. Found in more than 80% of cases, this association is cited by many as indicating a causal relationship and is the reason for the view that elective cholecystectomy for cholelithiasis is a preventive measure for carcinoma of the gallbladder.

Gallstones should be considered a risk factor for carcinoma of the gallbladder. The incidence of gallbladder cancer is higher in patients with gallstones than in patients without stones.[3] There is a higher incidence of carcinoma in females, which parallels the higher incidence of gallstones in this sex. Similarly, gallstones are more common in the gallbladder than in the bile ducts, and gallbladder cancer is more common than bile-duct cancer. The incidence of gallbladder cancer is higher in some ethnic groups, such as native Americans, who have a higher incidence of stones, and is lower in other ethnic groups, such as African Americans, who have a low incidence of stones. While some authors have reported a correlation between gallstone size and the risk of cancer, others have not found such a correlation.[3]

While gallstones are considered a risk factor, the overall incidence of carcinoma of the gallbladder in patients with cholelithiasis is less than 0.2%. This percentage, however, varies with race, sex and length of exposure to the stones.[3] Choledocholithiasis does not seem to play a role in the pathogenesis of carcinomas of the extrahepatic bile ducts.

Abnormal choledochopancreatic junction

Data largely reported from Japan indicates an association between gallbladder cancer and an abnormal junction of the pancreatic and common bile ducts.[156,157] The abnormal junction is defined as the union of the pancreatic and common bile ducts outside the wall of the duodenum proximal to the sphincter of Oddi. Normally, the main pancreatic duct and the common bile duct unite within the sphincter to form the pancreaticobiliary duct. The pancreaticobiliary duct and the junction are governed by the sphincter, but in the anomaly described the pancreaticobiliary duct is unusually long and no longer under control of the sphincter. As a result pancreatic juice can reflux into the common bile duct. The mixture of pancreatic juice and bile leads to chronic inflammation of the gallbladder with subsequent metaplasia, dysplasia and carcinoma.

Porcelain gallbladder

Diffuse calcification of the gallbladder wall (porcelain gallbladder) is another condition predisposing to carcinoma. Porcelain gallbladder is associated with carcinoma in 10–25% of cases.

Clinical features

Carcinoma of the gallbladder is a disease of older age groups. Most patients are female and in the sixth or seventh decade of life. Depending upon the series, the female to male ratio varies from 2 or 3 to 1. Cancer of the gallbladder usually presents late in its course. The signs and symptoms are not specific, often resembling those of chronic cholecystitis. Pain, usually the initial complaint, occurs in 75% of patients. It may be intermittent or persistent, severe and, for the most part, localized in the right upper quadrant. A small proportion of patients develop systemic manifestations.

Adenocarcinoma

Microscopic features

Well to moderately differentiated adenocarcinomas are the most common malignant epithelial tumours of the gallbladder. They are composed of short or long tubular glands lined by cells that vary in height from low cuboidal to tall columnar and superficially resemble biliary epithelium. Mucin is frequently present in the cells and glands. Rarely, the extracellular mucin may become calcified.[158,159] About one-third of the well-differentiated tumours show focal intestinal differentiation and contain goblet and endocrine cells.[160,161] The endocrine cells may be numerous and show immunoreactivity for serotonin and peptide hormones, but a diagnosis of carcinoid is not warranted. Paneth cells may rarely be seen. Adenocarcinomas may show cribriform or angiosarcomatous patterns. They may also contain cyto- and syncytiotrophoblast cells.

Grading

Adenocarcinomas can be divided into well, moderately or poorly differentiated types. The diagnosis of well-differentiated adenocarcinoma requires that 95% of the tumour contains glands (Fig. 12.18). For moderately differentiated adenocarcinoma, 40 to 94% of the tumour should

be composed of glands, and for poorly differentiated adenocarcinomas 5 to 39% of the tumour should contain glands. Undifferentiated carcinomas display less than 5% of glandular structures. Cystadenocarcinoma refers to a uni- or multilocular glandular tumour which may be the result of malignant transformation of a cystadenoma.

Papillary adenocarcinoma

This malignant tumour is composed predominantly of papillary structures lined by cuboidal or columnar epithelial cells often containing variable amounts of mucin.

Some tumours show intestinal differentiation with collections of goblet, endocrine and Paneth cells. Papillary adenocarcinomas may fill the lumen before invading the wall. Non-invasive papillary carcinomas are associated with a better prognosis than other types of invasive carcinomas.

Adenocarcinoma, intestinal type

This unusual variant of adenocarcinoma is composed of tubular glands or papillary structures lined predominantly by cells with an intestinal phenotype, namely goblet cells or colonic-type epithelium or both, with or without a variable number of endocrine and Paneth cells.[151]

Mucinous adenocarcinoma

Mucinous adenocarcinomas of the biliary tree are similar to those that arise in other anatomical sites. Characteristically, more than 50% of the tumour contains extracellular mucin.[135] There are two histological variants of mucinous adenocarcinomas of the gallbladder; one variant is characterized by neoplastic glands distended with mucin and lined by columnar cells with mild to moderate nuclear atypia, and the second variant is characterized by small groups or clusters of cells surrounded by abundant mucin. Some tumours show both growth patterns. The abundant mucin makes the tumour appear hypocellular.

Clear-cell adenocarcinoma

This rare malignant tumour is composed predominantly of glycogen-rich clear cells having well-defined cytoplasmic borders and hyperchromatic nuclei. In addition to clear cells, a variable number of cells contain eosinophilic granular cytoplasm. The clear cells line glands or are arranged in nests, sheets, cords, trabecula or papillary structures.[152,162,163] Foci of conventional adenocarcinoma with focal mucin production are usually found and are useful in separating primary from metastatic clear cell carcinomas. In some clear-cell adenocarcinomas of the biliary tree the columnar cells contain subnuclear and supranuclear vacuoles similar to those seen in secretory endometrium. Focal hepatoid differentiation with production of α-fetoprotein has been documented in clear cell carcinomas of the gallbladder.[164]

Signet-ring cell carcinoma

Signet-ring cell carcinoma of the gallbladder is histologically similar to its counterpart in other organs, and is characterized by cells with intracytoplasmic mucin that displaces the nuclei toward the cell. A variable amount of extracellu-

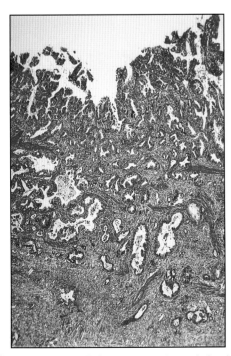

Fig. 12.18 • Well-differentiated adenocarcinoma. Long tubular glands infiltrate the full thickness of the gallbladder wall. The superficial portion of the tumour shows a papillary architecture. H&E.

lar mucin is usually present. Lateral spread through the lamina propria is a common feature. A diffusely infiltrating linear pattern resembling 'linitis plastica' of the stomach is observed in some cases.

Adenosquamous carcinoma

This tumour consists of two malignant components, one glandular and the other squamous. The extent of differentiation of the two components varies, but in general they tend to be moderately differentiated.[165,166] Keratin pearls are present in the well-differentiated squamous component, and mucin is usually demonstrable in the neoplastic glands, regardless of the degree of differentiation. Gastric foveolar epithelium is rarely observed in the neoplastic glands.[167] A small proportion of adenosquamous carcinomas contain endocrine cells.

Squamous cell carcinoma

This malignant epithelial tumour is composed entirely of squamous cells. The extent of differentiation varies considerably. Keratinizing and non-keratinizing types exist. Squamous cell carcinomas composed predominantly of clear cells have been described.[163] Spindle cells predominate in some poorly differentiated tumours which may be confused with sarcomas, especially malignant fibrous histiocytomas or carcinosarcomas. Immunocytochemical stains for cytokeratin may clarify the diagnosis in these spindle-cell cases. The tumour may arise from areas of squamous metaplasia. Dysplastic and in situ carcinomatous changes can be found in the metaplastic squamous mucosa.

Small-cell carcinoma (oat-cell carcinoma)

The cell population and growth patterns of this tumour are similar to those of small-cell carcinomas of the lung.[152,153,168,169] Most tumours are composed of round or fusiform cells arranged in sheets, nests, cords and festoons. Rosette-like structures and tubules are occasionally present. Extensive necrosis and subepithelial growth are constant features. In necrotic areas, intense basophilic staining of the blood vessels occurs. Membrane-bound, round, dense core granules are seen by electron microscopy. Neuron-specific enolase and less frequently chromogranin and synaptophysin reactivity are demonstrated by immunocytochemistry. Cushing syndrome has rarely been reported in association with small-cell carcinomas. About 30% of these tumours contain a minor adenocarcinomatous component (Fig. 12.19).[152,153] Foci of squamous differentiation are seen in 6% of the tumours.[152,170–173] Small-cell carcinomas appear to be more common in the gallbladder than in the extra-hepatic bile ducts. Some small-cell carcinomas simulate carcinoid tumours.

Undifferentiated carcinoma

A malignant epithelial tumour in which glandular structures are typically absent, undifferentiated carcinomas are

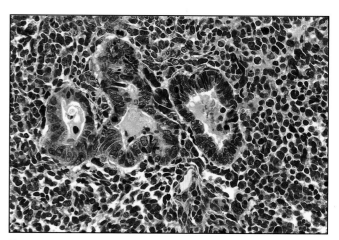

Fig. 12.19 • Combined small cell carcinoma and adenocarcinoma of gallbladder. Neoplastic glands are surrounded by cells characteristic of small-cell carcinoma. H&E.

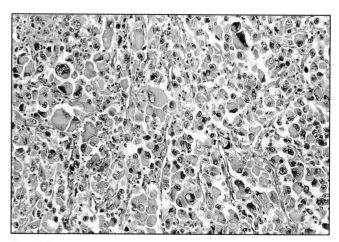

Fig. 12.20 • Spindle- and giant-cell carcinoma. Many large and multinucleated giant cells show abundant eosinophilic cytoplasm. H&E.

more common in the gallbladder than in the extrahepatic bile ducts. There are four histological variants: (i) *spindle- and giant-cell type*; (ii) *with osteoclast-like giant cell*; (iii) *small-cell type*; and (iv) *nodular or lobular type*.[152,171–173] The spindle and giant-cell type is the most common and resembles a sarcoma. These tumours have been referred to as pleomorphic spindle and giant-cell adenocarcinomas or sarcomatoid carcinomas (Fig. 12.20). They consist of variable proportions of spindle, giant and polygonal cells but foci of well-differentiated neoplastic glands are usually found in some, after extensive sampling. Areas of squamoid differentiation may also be seen. Rarely, foci of osteoclast-like multinucleated giant cells are present. The presence of cytokeratin in the spindle cells may help to distinguish this tumour from carcinosarcoma. The second variant of undifferentiated carcinoma contains mononuclear cells and numerous evenly spaced osteoclast-like giant cells resembling giant-cell tumour of bone. The mononuclear cells show immunoreactivity for cytokeratin and epithelial membrane antigen while the osteoclast-like giant cells are positive for histiocytic markers such as CD68. The third variant is composed of sheets of round cells with vesicular nuclei and prominent nucleoli that occasionally contain cytoplasmic mucin. The fourth variant consists of well-defined nodules or lobules of neoplastic cells superficially resembling breast carcinoma.

Molecular pathology

The immunohistochemical demonstration of a high incidence of p53 immunoreactivity in gallbladder carcinoma suggested that molecular abnormalities of this tumour suppressor gene are important in the pathogenesis of gallbladder cancer.[154,156] Subsequent studies showed loss of heterozygosity and mutations of the p53 gene in the vast majority of invasive carcinomas.[175,176] Moreover, loss of heterozygosity of the p53 gene was the only molecular abnormality detected in 27% of carcinomas. Likewise, loss of heterozygosity at 8p loci (44%) and 9p (50%) and the 18q gene (31%) were also detected in gallbladder carcinomas.[176,177] These molecular abnormalities were considered frequent and early events, while *ras* mutations and loss of heterozygous, at 3p, rb, and 5q occurred less frequently and were considered late events, probably related to tumour progression. The c-*erb*β-2 gene, a glycoprotein structurally similar to the epidermal growth factor receptor and related to cell growth has recently been investigated in gallbladder carcinoma.[178] Amplification of the c-*erb*β-2 gene was detected in 30 of 43 (69.8%) invasive carcinomas. However, no correlation between c-*erb*β-2 gene amplification and prognosis was found.

Although the frequency of K-*ras* mutations in gallbladder carcinomas has ranged from 0% to 34% in different studies most investigators have found these mutations to be significantly higher in extrahepatic bile duct tumours than in gallbladder carcinomas.[179] However, the incidence of K-*ras* mutations is greater in gallbladder carcinomas associated with an anomalous junction of the pancreatico-biliary duct.[180] These molecular pathology findings support the concept that gallbladder carcinogenesis requires a number of genetic alterations involving activation of oncogenes or inactivation of tumour suppressor genes.

In contrast to gallbladder carcinomas, K-*ras* mutations appear to be a common and early molecular event in the pathway of extrahepatic bile-duct carcinomas. Depending on the study, the incidence of K-*ras* mutations in extrahepatic bile-duct carcinomas has varied from 0 to 100%,[181] but the true incidence is most likely around 56%.[179] In contrast, the incidence of p53 mutations is lower and appears to be a late molecular event.

Endocrine tumours

Carcinoid tumour

Carcinoid tumours of the gallbladder and extrahepatic bile ducts are rare neoplasms of the diffuse endocrine cell system that usually exhibit trabecular, insular or nesting growth patterns with occasional tubule formation. The cell population includes different neuroendocrine cell types.

Carcinoid tumours of the gallbladder and extrahepatic bile ducts represent less than 1% of all digestive tract carcinoids. Patients are usually young or middle-aged adults.

There is no clear sex predominance. Small carcinoids (<1 cm) of the gallbladder are usually incidental findings in cholecystectomy specimens. Carcinoids of the gallbladder and extrahepatic bile ducts have been rarely associated with the Zollinger–Ellison, multiple endocrine neoplasia or the carcinoid syndromes.[182] Carcinoid tumours larger than 2 cm often extend into the liver or metastasize. Complete excision of small tumours is usually a curative procedure. The five-year survival rate of 18 patients with symptomatic carcinoid tumours of the gallbladder from the SEER programme of the National Cancer Institute was 41.3%.[183]

Pathological features

These tumours appear as grey to yellow intramural nodules measuring from a few milimetres to 4 cm. Submucosal growth is a common feature. Carcinoid tumours are composed of uniform relatively small cells with eosinophilic granular cytoplasm and round nuclei with finely stippled chromatin. The cells are arranged in nests, cords and trabeculae with occasional tubule formation. Peripheral palisading is common. The stroma is usually desmoplastic.

Most carcinoid tumours of the gallbladder are argyrophilic. Some show immunoreactivity for only the general neuroendocrine markers. Others are immunoreactive for serotonin and somatostatin, gastrin or pancreatic polypeptide. Rarely, reactivity for a single peptide hormone is demonstrated and the designation of somatostatinoma or gastrinoma has been employed. However, somatostatin-producing tumours are non-functioning tumours.

Mixed carcinoid-adenocarcinoma

This malignant tumour exhibits variable proportions of adenocarcinoma and carcinoid. The tumours behave as adenocarcinomas and, therefore, are clinically more aggressive than carcinoids. Adenocarcinoma with endocrine cells should not be included in this category.

Paraganglioma

This benign tumour is composed of chief cells and sustentacular cells arranged in a nesting or zellballen pattern. The chief cells are argyrophilic and stain for neuron-specific enolase and chromogranin. The sustentacular cells are S-100 protein positive. The tumour is located in either the subserosa or muscular wall of the gallbladder and apparently arises from normal paraganglia. This rare and small tumour is usually an incidental finding in cholecystectomy specimens. Paragangliomas also occur in the extrahepatic bile ducts, where they may be symptomatic.

Non-epithelial tumours

A number of non-epithelial tumours occur in the gallbladder. Among the benign lesions are granular cell tumour, leiomyoma, lipoma, haemangioma, lymphangioma, neurofibroma, ganglioneuromatosis and ganglioneurofibromatosis. A benign stromal tumour of the gallbladder with interstitial cells of Cajal phenotype has been reported.[4]

Among the malignant non-epithelial tumours are rhabdomyosarcoma, Kaposi sarcoma, leiomyosarcoma, malignant fibrous histiocytoma and angiosarcoma. Because of their clinicopathological significance several are discussed below.

Granular cell tumour

This is the most common benign non-epithelial tumour of the extrahepatic biliary tract.[184,185] It is more common in the bile ducts than in the gallbladder. Although usually single, granular cell tumours may be multicentric or may co-exist with one or more granular cell tumours in other sites, especially the skin. Granular cell tumours are poorly circumscribed, firm, yellow-tan nodules usually less than 2 cm in diameter. They are composed of sheets or clusters of large, ovoid or round cells separated by connective tissue bands. The cells have abundant granular eosinophilic cytoplasm and small hyperchromatic nuclei. The cytoplasm is PAS positive, diastase resistant and contains lysosomes when examined electron microscopically. Most tumour cells show S-100 protein reactivity. Though benign, this tumour may extend beyond the gallbladder wall. Reactive atypia of the overlying epithelium and of metaplastic pyloric glands occurs, in some cases mimicking carcinoma.

Ganglioneuromatosis

Ganglioneuromatosis of the gallbladder is a component of the type IIb multiple endocrine neoplasia syndrome. The histological changes consist of Schwann-cell and ganglion-cell proliferation in the lamina propria as well as enlarged and distorted nerves in the muscle layer and subserosa. Neurofibromatosis is exceedingly rare in the gallbladder but has been reported in association with multiple neurofibromatosis.

Leiomyosarcoma

Both conventional and epithelioid leiomyosarcomas have been described in the gallbladder and extrahepatic bile ducts. Dense cellularity, cytological atypia, mitotic activity and necrosis are useful criteria for the diagnosis of leiomyosarcomas. These tumours are immunoreactive for smooth muscle actin and muscle specific actin. Less frequently, they express desmin and cytokeratin.

Rhabdomyosarcoma

Embryonal rhabdomyosarcoma (sarcoma botryoides) is the most common malignant neoplasm of the biliary tract in childhood.[186] It occurs more frequently in the bile ducts than in the gallbladder. Embryonal rhabdomyosarcoma forms soft polypoid structures with a characteristic grape-like appearance that project into the lumen. Microscopically, the polypoid structures are covered with normal biliary epithelial cells. Immediately beneath the epithelium is a concentration of primitive mesenchymal cells, some of which contain abundant eosinophilic cytoplasm (rhabdomyoblasts). About one-third of the tumours show rhabdomyoblasts with cross-striations. Myxoid areas contain undifferentiated stellate cells. Desmin and muscle-specific actin are the most reliable immunohistochemical markers for the diagnosis of embryonal rhabdomyosarcoma.

Kaposi sarcoma

Foci of Kaposi sarcoma involving the gallbladder are incidental autopsy findings in the acquired immune deficiency syndrome. The haemorrhagic lesions are usually located in the subserosa or muscular wall of the gallbladder or in the periductal connective tissue of the bile ducts. The tumours show the characteristic spindle cells and vascular slits.

Miscellaneous tumours

Carcinosarcoma

This malignant tumour consists of a mixture of two components: carcinomatous and sarcomatous. The epithelial elements usually predominate in the form of glands but may be arranged in cords or sheets. Foci of malignant squamous cells are occasionally seen. The mesenchymal component includes foci of heterologous elements such as chondrosarcoma, osteosarcoma and rhabdomyosarcoma. Cytokeratin and carcinoembryonic antigen are absent from the mesenchymal component, which helps to distinguish carcinosarcomas from spindle- and giant-cell carcinomas.

Malignant melanoma

Primary malignant melanoma is exceedingly rare in the gallbladder.[187] Junctional activity in the epithelium overlying the tumour, absence of a primary melanoma elsewhere in the body and long-term survival are important features to distinguish primary from the more commonly occurring metastatic melanoma. It is important to keep in mind, however, that junctional activity has been reported in metastatic melanoma in the gallbladder.

Lymphomas

Malignant lymphomas of the gallbladder are usually part of a systemic process. The exceedingly rare primary lymphomas of the gallbladder are of small lymphocytic (MALToma) type and seem to arise on a background of lymphoid hyperplasia. Intravascular lymphomas have also been documented in the gallbladder.

Secondary tumours

Metastatic tumours in the gallbladder and extrahepatic bile ducts are not common and are generally discovered at autopsy. The majority result from transcoelomic spread and are associated with peritoneal carcinomatosis. Blood-borne metastases may be symptomatic and simulate primary tumours. The more common metastatic lesions include malignant melanoma and carcinomas of the kidney, lung,

Table 12.2	Summary of staging of tumours of the gallbladder[191]				
T1	Gallbladder wall	Stage 0	Tis	N0	M0
T1a	Lamina propria	Stage IA	T1	N0	M0
T1b	Muscle	Stage IB	T2	N0	M0
T2	Perimuscular connective tissue	Stage IIA	T3	N0	M0
T3	Serosa and/or one organ, liver, 2 cm	Stage IIB	T1–3	N1	M0
T4	Two or more organs, or liver >2 cm	Stage III	T4	Any N	M0
N1	Regional	Stage IV	Any T	Any N	M1

breast, ovary and oesophagus.[6,188,189] The gallbladder may be involved by direct extension from carcinomas of the pancreas, stomach, colon and liver.

Staging of tumours

The prognosis of tumours of the gallbladder depends primarily on the extent of disease.[190] For example, tumours that only extend into the lamina propria have a much better prognosis than those that infiltrate the serosa or invade the liver. The tumour, node, metastasis (TNM) system (Table 12.2) provides a uniform classification for the extent of disease.[191] In cholecystectomy specimens, pathological staging should be included in the pathologist's report.

References

1. Frierson HF Jr. The gross anatomy and histology of the gallbladder, extrahepatic bile ducts, Vaterian system, and minor papilla. Am J Surg Pathol, 1989; 13:146–162
2. Gilloteaux J. Introduction to the biliary tract, the gallbladder, and gallstones. Microsc Res Tech, 1997; 38:547–551
3. Albores-Saavedra J, Henson DE, Klimstra D. Tumors of the gallbladder, extrahepatic bile ducts and ampulla of Vater, 3rd edn, Fascicle 27. Washington DC: Armed Forces Institute of Pathology, 2001
4. Ortiz-Hidalgo C, deLeon B, Albores-Saavedra J. Stromal tumor of the gallbladder with phenotype of interstitial cells of Cajal. A previously unrecognized neoplasm. Amer J Surg Path, 2000; 24:1420–1423
5. Lamonte J, Willems G. DNA synthesis, cell proliferation index in normal and abnormal gallbladder epithelium. Microsc Res Tech, 1997; 38:609–615
6. MacSween RNM, Scothorne RJ. Developmental anatomy and normal structure. In: MacSween RNM, Anthony PP, Scheuer PJ, Burt AD, Portmann BC, eds. Pathology of the liver, 3rd edn. Edinburgh: Churchill Livingstone, 2001
7. Fisher RS, Rock E, Levin G et al. Effects of somatostatin on gallbladder emptying. Gastroenterology, 1987; 92:885–890
8. Frizzell RA, Heintze K. Transport functions of the gallbladder. In: Javitt NB, ed. Liver and biliary tract physiology. vol. 21, International review of physiology. Baltimore: University Park Press, 1980
9. Madrid JF, Hernandez F, Ballesta J. Characterization of glycoproteins in the epithelial cells of human and other mammalian gallbladders. Microsc Res Tech, 1997; 38:616–630
10. Lorenzo-Zuniga V, Bartoli R, Planas R et al. Oral bile acids reduce bacterial overgrowth, bacterial translocation and endotoxemia in cirrhotic rats. Hepatology, 2003; 37:551–557
11. Harada K, Ohba K, Ozaki S et al. Peptide antibiotic human beta-defensin-1 and -2 contribute to antimicrobial defense of the intrahepatic biliary tree. Hepatology, 2004; 40:925–932
12. Williams I, Slavin G, Cox A et al. Diverticular disease (adenomyomatosis) of the gallbladder: a radiological-pathological survey. Br J Radiol, 1986; 59:29–34
13. Esper E, Kaufman DB, Crary GS et al. Septate gallbladder with cholelithiasis: A cause of chronic abdominal pain in a 6-year-old child. J Pediatr Surg, 1992; 27:1560–1562
14. Haslam RH, Gayler BW, Ebert PA. Multiseptate gallbladder. a cause of recurrent abdominal pain in childhood. Am J Dis Child, 1966; 112:600–603
15. Bhagavan BS, Amin PB, Land AS et al. Multiseptate gallbladder. Embryogenetic hypotheses. Arch Pathol, 1970; 89:382–385
16. Lobe TE, Hayden CK, Merkel M. Giant congenital cystic malformation of the gallbladder. Pediatr Surg, 1986; 21:447–448
17. Weedon D. Pathology of the gallbladder. New York: Masson, 1984
18. Shapiro T, Rennie W. Duplicate gallbladder cholecystitis after open cholecystectomy. Ann Emerg Med, 1999; 33:584–587
19. Noritomi T, Watanabe K, Yamashita Y et al. Left-sided gallbladder associated with congenital hypoplasia of the left lobe of the liver: a case report and review of literature. Int Surg, 2004; 89:105
20. Chiavarini RL, Chang SF, Westerfield JD. The wandering gallbladder. Radiology, 1975; 115:47–48
21. Maeda N, Horie Y, Shiota G et al. Hypoplasia of the left hepatic lobe associated with floating gallbladder. A case report. Hepatogastroenterology, 1998; 45:1100–1103
22. Boyle L, Gallivan MVE, Chun B et al. Heterotopia of gastric mucosa and liver involving the gallbladder. Report of two cases with literature review. Arch Pathol Lab Med, 1992; 116:138–142
23. Qizilbash AH. Acute pancreatitis occurring in heterotopic pancreatic tissue in the gallbladder. Can J Surg, 1976; 19: 413–414
24. Busuttil A. Ectopic adrenal within the gallbladder wall. J Pathol, 1974; 113:231–233
25. Hendry A, O'Leary JP. The history of cholelithiasis. Am Surg, 1998; 64:801–802
26. Everhart JE, Khare M, Hill M, Maurer KR. Prevalence and ethnic differences in gallbladder disease in the United States. Gastroenterology 1999; 117:623–639
27. Sandler RS, Everhart JE, Donowitz M et al. The burden of selected digestive diseases in the United States. Gastroenterology, 2002; 122:1500–1511.
28. Cooper AD. Epidemiology, pathogenesis, natural history and medical therapy of gallstones. In: Sleisenger MH, Fordtran JS, eds. Sleisenger and Fordtran gastrointestinal disease. Philadelphia: Saunders, 1990; pp 1788–1804
29. Ostrow JD. The etiology of pigment gallstones. Hepatology, 1984; 4:215S–222S
30. Moser AJ, Abedin MZ, Roslyn JJ. The pathogenesis of gallstone formation. Adv Surg, 1993; 26:357–386
31. Bowen JC, Brenner HI, Ferrante WA et al. Gallstone disease. Pathophysiology, epidemiology, natural history, and treatment options. Med Clin North Am, 1992; 76:1143–1157
32. Everson GT. Gallbladder function in gallstone disease. Gastroenterol Clin North Am, 1991; 20:85–110
33. Paumgartner G, Sauerbruch T. Gallstones: pathogenesis. Lancet, 1991; 338:1117–1121
34. Donovan JM, Carey MC. Physical-chemical basis of gallstone formation. Gastroenterol Clin North Am, 1991; 20:47–66
35. Bennion LJ, Grundy SM. Effects of obesity and caloric intake on biliary lipid metabolism in man. J Clin Invest, 1975; 56:996–1011

36. Holan KR, Holzbach RT, Hermann RE et al. Nucleation time: a key factor in the pathogenesis of cholesterol gallstone disease. Gastroenterology, 1979; 77:611–617

37. Harvey PR, Strasberg SM. Will the real cholesterol-nucleating and -antinucleating proteins please stand up? Gastroenterology, 1993; 104(2):646–650

38. Ohya T, Schwarzendrube J, Busch N et al. Isolation of a human biliary glycoprotein inhibitor of cholesterol crystallization. Gastroenterology, 1993; 104:527–538

39. Abei M, Kawczak P, Nuutinen H et al. Isolation and characterization of a cholesterol crystallization promoter from human bile. Gastroenterology, 1993; 104:539–548

40. Donovan JM. Physical and metabolic factors in gallstone pathogenesis. Gastroesterol Clin North Amer, 1999; 28:75–97

41. Swidsinski A, Ludwig W, Pahlig H et al. Molecular genetic evidence of bacterial colonization of cholesterol gallstones. Gastroenterology, 1995; 108:860–864

42. Kawaguchi M, Saito T, Ohno H et al. Bacteria closely resembing *Helicobacter pylori* detected immunohistologically and genetically on resected gallbladder mucosa. J Gastroenterology, 1996; 31:294–298

43. Maurer KJ, Ihrig MM, Robers AB et al. Identification of cholelithogenic enterohepatic *Helicobacter* species and their role in murine cholesterol gallstone formation. Gastroenterology, 2005; 128:1023–1033

44. Dittrick GW, Thompson JS, Campos D et al. Gallbladder pathology in morbid obesity. Obes Surg, 2005; 15:238–242

45. Maclure KM, Hayes KC, Colditz GA et al. Dietary predictors of symptom-associated gallstones in middle-aged women. Am J Clin Nutr, 1990; 52:916–922

46. Weiss KM, Ferrell RE, Hanis CL et al. Genetics and epidemiology of gallbladder disease in New World native peoples. Am J Hum Genet, 1984; 36:1259–1278

47. Maurer KR, Everhart JE, Ezzati TM et al. Prevalence of gallstone disease in Hispanic populations in the United States. Gastroenterology, 1989; 96(2 Pt 1):487–492

48. Maurer KR, Everhart JE, Knowler WC et al. Risk factors for gallstone disease in the Hispanic populations of the United States. Am J Epidemiol, 1990; 131:836–844

49. Mendez-Sanchez N, Jessurun J, Ponciano-Rodriguez G et al. Prevalence of gallstone disease in Mexico. A necropsy study. Dig Dis Sci, 1993; 38:680–683

50. Simonovis NJ, Wells CK, Feinstein AR. In-vivo and post-mortem gallstones: support for validity of the 'epidemiologic necropsy' screening technique. Am J Epidemiol, 1991; 133:922–931

51. Miquel JF, Covarrubias C, Villaroel L et al. Genetic epidemiology of cholesterol cholelithiasis among Chilean Hispanics, Amerindians, and Maoris. Gastroenterology, 1998; 115:937–946

52. Trotman BW. Pigment gallstone disease. Gastroenterol Clin North Am, 1991; 20:111–126

53. Fevery J. Pigment gallstones in Crohn's disease. Gastroenterology, 1999; 116:1492–1494

54. Dudley SL, Starin RB. Cholelithiasis: diagnosis and current therapeutic options. Nurse Pract, 1991; 16:12–18

55. Sen M, Williamson RCN. Acute cholecystitis: surgical management. Baillières Clin Gastroenterol, 1991; 5:817–840

56. Fitzgibbons RJ Jr, Tseng A, Wang H et al. Acute cholecystitis. Does the clinical diagnosis correlate with the pathological diagnosis? Surg Endosc, 1996; 10:1180–1184

57. Salomonowitz E, Frick MP, Simmons RL et al. Obliteration of the gallbladder without formal cholecystectomy. A feasibility study. Arch Surg, 1984; 119:725–729

58. Sjodahl R, Wetterfors J. Lysolecithin and lecithin in the gallbladder wall and bile; their possible roles in the pathogenesis of acute cholecystitis. Scand J Gastroenterol, 1974; 9:519–555

59. Pellegrini CA, Way LW. Acute cholecystitis. In: Way LW, Pellegrini CA, eds. Surgery of the gallbladder and bile ducts. Philadelphia: Saunders, 1987

60. Neiderhiser DH. Acute acalculous cholecystitis induced by lysophosphotidylcholine. Am J Pathol, 1986; 124:559–563

61. Claesson BE, Holmlund DE, Matzsch TW. Microflora of the gallbladder related to duration of acute cholecystitis. Surg Gynecol Obstet, 1986; 162:531–535

62. Adam A, Roddie ME. Acute cholecystitis: radiological management. Baillières Clin Gastroenterol, 1991; 5:787–816

63. Hawasli A. Timing of laparoscopic cholecystectomy in acute cholecystitis. J Laparoendosc Surg, 1994; 4:9–16

64. Rattner DW, Ferguson C, Warshaw AL. Factors associated with successful laparoscopic cholecystectomy for acute cholecystitis. Ann Surg, 1993; 217:233–236

65. Babb RR. Acute acalculous cholecystitis: a review. J Clin Gastroenterol, 1992; 15:238–241

66. Frazee RC, Nagorney DM, Mucha P Jr. Acute acalculous cholecystitis. Mayo Clin Proc, 1989; 64:163–167

67. Sjodahl R, Tagesson C. Wetterfors J. On the pathogenesis of acute cholecystitis. Surg Gynecol Obstet, 1978; 146:199–202

68. Kaminski DL, Andrus CH, German D et al. The role of prostanoids in the production of acute acalculous cholecystitis by platelet-activating factor. Ann Surg, 1990; 212:455–461

69. Wang AJ, Wang TE, Lin CC et al. Clinical predictors of severe gallbladder complications in acute acalculous cholecystitis. World J Gastroenterol 2004; 9:2821–2823

70. Gill KS, Chapman AH, Weston MJ. The changing face of emphysematous cholecystitis. Br J Radiol, 1997; 70:986–991

71. Mentzer RM Jr, Golden GT, Chandler JG et al. A comparative appraisal of emphysematous cholecystitis. Am J Surg, 1975; 129:10–15

72. Lee BY, Morilla CV. Acute emphysematous cholecystitis: a case report and review of the literature. N Y State J Med, 1992; 92:406–407

73. Bergan T, Dobloug I, Liavag I. Bacterial isolates in cholecystitis and cholelithiasis. Scand J Gastroenterol, 1979; 14(5):625–631

74. Fox JG, Dewhirst FE, Shen Z et al. Hepatic Helicobacter species identified in bile and gallbladder tissue from Chileans with chronic cholecystitis. Gastroenterology, 1998; 114:755–763

75. Coad JE, Carlon J, Jessurun J. Microdiverticulosis (Rokitansky–Aschoff 'sinusosis') in patients with biliary dyskinesia (BD). Mod Pathol, 1999; 12:73A

76. Albores-Saavedra J, Gould E, Manivel-Rodriguez C et al. Chronic cholecystitis with lymphoid hyperplasia. Rev Invest Clin (Mex), 1989; 41:159–164

77. Hanada M, Tujimura T, Kimura M. Cholecystic granulomas in gallstone disease. A clinicopathologic study of 17 cases. Acta Pathol Jpn, 1981; 31:221–231

78. Amazon K, Rywlin AM. Ceroid granulomas of the gallbladder. Am J Clin Pathol, 1980; 73:123–127

79. Ashur H, Siegal B, Oland Y et al. Calcified gallbladder (porcelain gallbladder). Arch Surg, 1978; 113:594–596

80. Weiner PL, Lawson TL. The radiology corner. Porcelain gallbladder. Am J Gastroenterol, 1975; 64:224–227

81. Berk RN, Armbuster TG, Saltzstein SL. Carcinoma in the porcelain gallbladder. Radiology, 1973; 106:29–31

82. Polk HC Jr. Carcinoma and the calcified gall bladder. Gastroenterology, 1966; 50:582–585

83. Roberts KM, Parson MA. Xanthogranulomatous cholecystitis: clinicopathological study of 13 cases. J Clin Pathol, 1987; 40:412–417

84. Howard TJ, Bennion RS, Thompson JE Jr. Xanthogranulomatous cholecystitis: a chronic inflammatory pseudotumor of the gallbladder. Am Surg, 1991; 57:821–824

85. Goodman ZD, Ishak KG. Xanthogranulomatous cholecystitis. Am J Surg Pathol, 1981; 5:653–659

86. Dao AH, Wong SW, Adkins RB Jr. Xanthogranulomatous cholecystitis. A clinical and pathologic study of twelve cases. Am Surg, 1989; 55:32–35

87. Kozuka S, Hachisuka K. Incidence by age and sex of intestinal metaplasia in the gallbladder. Hum Pathol, 1984; 15:779–784

88. Albores-Saavedra J, Nadji M, Henson DE et al. Intestinal metaplasia of the gallbladder: a morphologic and immunocytochemical study. Hum Pathol, 1986; 17:614–620

89. Albores-Saavedra J, Henson DE. Adenomyomatous hyperplasia of the gallbladder with perineural invasion. Arch Pathol Lab Med, 1995; 199:117–176

90. Albores-Saavedra J, Henson DE. Pyloric gland metaplasia with perineural invasion of the gallbladder. A lesion that can be confused with adenocarcinoma. Cancer, 1999; 86:2625–2631

91. Osawa H, Kita H. Satoh K et al. Aberrant expression of CDX2 in the metaplastic epithelium and inflammatory mucosa of the gallbladder. Am J Surg Pathol, 2004; 28:1253–1254

92. Diehl AK. Symptoms of gallstone disease. Baillières Clin Gastroenterol, 1992; 6:635–657

93. Soper NJ, Flye MW, Brunt LM et al. Diagnosis and management of biliary complications of laparoscopic cholecystectomy. Am J Surg, 1993; 165:663–669

94. Deziel DJ, Millikan KW, Economou SG et al. Complications of laparoscopic cholecystectomy: a national survey of 4292 hospitals and an analysis of 77 604 cases. Am J Surg, 1993; 165:9–14

95. Fitzgibbons RJ Jr, Annibali R, Litke BS. Gallbladder and gallstone removal, open versus closed laparoscopy, and pneumoperitoneum. Am J Surg, 1993; 165:497–504

96. Raptopoulos V, Compton CC, Doherty P et al. Chronic acalculous gallbladder disease: multiimaging evaluation with clinical-pathologic correlation. AJR Am J Roentgenol, 1986; 147:721–724

97. Sykes D. The use of cholecystokinin in diagnosing biliary pain. Ann R Coll Surg Engl, 1982; 64:114–116

98. Griffen WO Jr, Bivins BA et al. Cholecystokinin cholecystography in the diagnosis of gallbladder disease. Ann Surg, 1980; 191:636–640

99. Dabbs DJ. Eosinophilic and lymphoeosinophilic cholecystitis. Am J Surg Pathol, 1993; 17:497–501

100. Rosengart TK, Rotterdam H, Ranson JH. Eosinophilic cholangitis: a self-limited cause of extrahepatic biliary obstruction. Am J Gastroenterol, 1990; 85:582–585

101. Jessurun J, Bolio-Solis A, Manivel JC. Diffuse lymphoplasmacytic acalculous cholecystitis: a distinctive form of chronic cholecystitis associated with primary sclerosing cholangitis. Hum Pathol, 1998; 28:512–517

102. Abraham SC, Cruz-Correa M, Argani P et al. Diffuse lymphoplasmacytic chronic cholecystitis is highly specific for extrahepatic biliary tract disease but does not distinguish between primary and secondary sclerosing cholangiopathy. Am J Surg Pathol, 2003; 27:1313–1320

103. Hanada K, Nakata H, Nakayama T et al. Radiologic findings in xanthogranulomatous cholecystitis. Am J Radiol, 1987; 148:727–730

104. Dixit VK, Prakash An Gupta A et al. Xanthogranulomatous cholecystitis. Dig Dis Sci, 1998; 43:940–942

105. Guzman-Valdivia G. Xanthogranulomatous cholecystitis: 15 years experience. World Surg, 2004; 28:254–257

106. Charpentier P, Prade M, Bognel C et al. Malacoplakia of the gallbladder. Hum Pathol, 1983; 14:827–828

107. Gockel HP. Xanthogranulomatous cholecystitis. Fortschr Roentgenstr, 1994; 140:223–224

108. Kavin H, Jonas RB, Chowdhury L et al. Acalculous cholecystitis and cytomegalovirus infection in the acquired immunodeficiency syndrome. Ann Intern Med, 1986; 104:53–54

109. Blumberg RS, Kelsey P, Perrone T et al. Cytomegalovirus- and Cryptosporidium-associated acalculous gangrenous cholecystitis. Am J Med, 1984; 76:1118–1123

110. Lebovics E, Dworkin BM, Heier SK et al. The hepatobiliary manifestations of human immunodeficiency virus infection. Am J Gastroenterol, 1988; 83:1–7

111. Nash JA, Cohen SA. Gallbladder and biliary tract disease in AIDS. Gastroenterol Clin North Am, 1997; 26:323–335

112. Forbes A, Blanshard C, Gazzard B. Natural history of AIDS-related sclerosing cholangitis: A study of 20 cases. Gut, 1993; 34:116–121

113. Garcia GR, Meza H, Sadowinski-Pine S. Colecistitis acalculosa por Microsporidium en un paciente con SIDA. Patologia (Mex), 1993; 31:37–39

114. Yellin AE, Donovan AJ. Biliary lithiasis and helminthiasis. Am J Surg, 1981; 142:128–134

115. Nohr M, Lausstsen J, Falk E. Isolated necrotizing panarteritis of the gallbladder. Case report. Acta Chir Scand, 1989; 155:485–587

116. Ito M, Sano K, Inaba H et al. Localized necrotizing arteritis. A report of two cases involving the gallbladder and pancreas. Arch Pathol Lab Med, 1991; 115:780–783

117. Burke AP, Sobin LH, Virmani R. Localized vasculitis of the gastrointestinal tract. Am J Surg Pathol, 1995; 19:338–349

118. Salmenkivi K. Cholesterosis of the gallbladder. Surgical considerations. Int Surg, 1966; 45:304–309

119. Jacyna MR, Bouchier IAD. Cholesterolosis: a physical cause of 'functional' disorder. Br Med J, 1987; 295:619–620

120. Satoh H, Koga A. Fine structure of cholesterolosis in the human gallbladder and the mechanism of lipid accumulation. Microsc Res Tech, 1997; 39:14–21

121. Parrilla-Paricio P, Garcia-Olmo D, Pellicer-Franco E et al. Gallbladder cholesterolosis: an etiological factor in acute pancreatitis of uncertain origin. Br J Surg, 1990; 77:735–736

122. Albores-Saavedra J, Defortuna SM, Smothermon WE. Primary papillary hyperplasia of the gallbladder and cystic and common bile ducts. Hum Pathol, 1990; 21:228–231

123. Suddleson EA, Reid B, Woolley MM, Takahashi M. Hydrops of the gallbladder associated with Kawasaki syndrome. J Pediatr Surg, 1987; 22:956–959

124. Williams I, Slavin G, Cox A et al. Diverticular disease (adenomyomatosis) of the gallbladder: a radiological-pathological survey. Br J Radiol, 1986; 59:29–34

125. Berk RN, van der Vegt JH, Lichtenstein JE. The hyperplastic cholecystoses: cholesterolosis and adenomyomatosis. Radiology, 1983; 146:593–601

126. Matz LR, Lawrence-Brown MM. Ischaemic cholecystitis and infarction of the gallbladder. Aust NZ J Surg, 1982; 52:466–471

127. Chen KT. Gallbladder vasculitis. J Clin Gastroenterol, 1989; 11:537–540

128. Dillard BM, Black WC. Polyarteritis nodosa of the gallbladder and bile ducts. Am Surg, 1970; 36:423–427

129. Puica-Sarage E, Costa J. Idiopathic entero-colic lymphocytic phlebitis. Am J Surg Pathol, 1989; 13:303–308

130. Bailey M, Chapin W, Licht H, Reynolds JC. The effects of vasculitis on the gastrointestinal tract and liver. Gastroenterol Clin North Am, 1998; 27:747–782

131. Salman AB, Yildirgan MI, Celebi F. Posttraumatic gallbladder torsion in a child. J Pediatr Surg, 1996; 31:1586

132. Carrasco CH, Freeny PC, Chuang VP et al. Chemical cholecystitis associated with hepatic artery infusion chemotherapy. Am J Roentgenol, 1983; 141:703–706

133. Rao PS, Tandon RK, Kapur BM. Biliobiliary fistula: review of nine cases. Am J Gastroenterol, 1988; 83:652–657

134. Burgess JH, Kalfayan B, Slungaard RK, Gilbert E. Papillomatosis of the gallbladder associated with metachromatic leukodystrophy. Arch Pathol Lab Med, 1982; 106:79–81

135. Albores-Saavedra J, Henson DE, Sobin LH. WHO histological typing of tumors of the gallbladder and extrahepatic bile ducts. Berlin: Springer-Verlag, 1991

136. Albores-Saavedra J, Vardaman C, Vuitch F. Non-neoplastic polypoid lesions and adenomas of the gallbladder. Pathol Ann, 1993; 28:145–177

137. Kijima H, Watanabe H, Iwafuchi M et al. Histogenesis of gallbladder carcinoma from investigation of early carcinoma and microcarcinoma. Acta Pathol Jpn, 1989; 39:235–244

138. Kosuka S, Tsubone M, Yasui A et al. Relation of adenoma to carcinoma in the gallbladder. Cancer, 1982; 50:2226–2234

139. Mogilner JG, Dharan M, Siplovich L. Adenoma of the gallbladder in childhood. J Pediatr Surg, 1991; 26:223–224

140. Wistuba I, Miquel AF, Gazdar AF et al. Gallbladder adenomas have molecular abnormalities different from those present in gallbladder carcinomas. Hum Pathol 1999; 30:21–25

141. Foster DR, Foster DBE. Gallbladder polyps in Peutz–Jeghers syndrome. Postgrad Med J, 1980; 56:373–376

142. Tantachamrun T, Borvonsombat S, Theetranont C. Gardner's syndrome associated with adenomatous polyp of the gallbladder. J Med Assoc Thai, 1979; 62:441–447

143. Walsh N, Qizilbash A, Banerjee R et al. Biliary neoplasia in Gardner's syndrome. Arch Pathol Lab Med, 1987; 111:76–77

144. Kushima R, Remmele W, Stolte M et al. Pyloric gland type adenoma of the gallbladder with squamoid spindle cell metaplasia. Pathol Res Pract, 1996; 192:963–969

145. Nishihara K, Yamaguchi K, Hashimoto H et al. Tubular adenoma of the gallbladder with squamoid spindle cell metaplasia. Acta Pathol Jpn, 1991; 41:41–45

146. Devaney K, Goodman ZD, Ishak KG. Hepatobiliary cystadenoma and cystadenocarcinoma. A light microscopic and immunohistochemical study of 70 patients. Am J Surg Pathol, 1994; 18:1078–1091

147. Vuitch F, Battifora H, Albores-Saavedra J. Demonstration of steroid hormone receptors in pancreato-biliary mucinous cystic neoplasms. Lab Invest, 1993; 68:114A

148. Hubens G, Delvaux G, Willems G et al. Papillomatosis of the intra- and extrahepatic bile ducts with involvement of the pancreatic duct. Hepatogastroenterol, 1991; 38:413–418

149. Albores-Saavedra J, Alcantara-Vasquez A, Cruz-Ortiz H, Herrera-Goepfert R. The precursor lesions of invasive gallbladder carcinoma. Hyperplasia, atypical hyperplasia and carcinoma-in-situ. Cancer, 1980; 45:919–927

150. Albores-Saavedra J, Angeles-Angeles A, de Jesus Manrique J, Henson DE. Carcinoma-in-situ of the gallbldder. A clinicopathologic study of 18 cases. Am J Surg Pathol, 1984; 8:323–333

151. Albores-Saavedra J, Nadji M, Henson DE. Intestinal type adenocarcinoma of the gallbladder. A clinicopathologic and immunohistochemical study of seven cases. Am J Surg Pathol, 1986; 10:19–25

152. Albores-Saavedra J, Molberg K, Henson DE. Unusual malignant epithelial tumors of the gallbladder. Semin Diagn Pathol, 1996; 13:326–338

153. Albores-Saavedra J, Soriano J, Larraza-Hernandez O et al. Oat cell carcinoma of the gallbladder. Hum Pathol, 1984; 15:639–646

154. Wistuba I, Gazdar AF, Roa I et al. P53 protein over-expression in gallbladder carcinoma and its precursor lesions. An immunohistochemical study. Hum Pathol, 1996; 27:360–365

155. deGroen PC, Gores, GJ, LaRusso NF et al. Biliary tract cancers. N Engl J Med, 1999; 341:1368–1378

156. Miyazaki K, Date K, Imamura S et al. Familial occurrence of anomalous pancreaticobiliary duct union associated with gallbladder neoplasms. Am J Gastroenterol, 1989; 84:176–181

157. Kimura K, Ohto M, Saisho H et al. Association of gallbladder carcinoma and anomalous pancreaticobiliary ductal union. Gastroenterology, 1985; 89:1258–1265

158. Parker GW, Joffe N. Calcifying primary mucus-producing adenocarcinoma of the gallbladder. Br J Radiol, 1972; 45:468–469

159. Rogers LF, Lastra MP, Lin K-T et al. Calcifying mucinous adenocarcinoma of the gallbladder. Am J Gastroenterol, 1973; 59:441–445

160. Albores-Saavedra J, Nadji M, Henson DE et al. Enteroendocrine differentiation in carcinomas of the gallbladder and mucinous cystadenocarcinomas of the pancreas. Pathol Res Pract, 1988; 183:169–174

161. Yamaguchi K, Enjoji M. Carcinoma of the gallbladder. A clinicopathology of 103 patients and a newly proposed staging. Cancer, 1988; 62:1425–1432

162. Bittinger A, Altekrüger I, Barth P. Clear cell carcinoma of the gallbladder. A histological and immunohistochemical study. Path Res Pract, 1995; 191:1259–1265

163. Sugaya Y, Sugaya H, Kuronuma Y et al. A case of gallbladder carcinoma producing both alpha-fetoprotein (AFP) and carcinoembryonic antigen (CEA). Gastroenterol Jpn, 1989; 24:325–331

164. Vardaman C, Albores-Saavedra J. Clear cell carcinoma of the gallbladder and extrahepatic bile ducts. Am J Surg Pathol, 1995; 19:91–99

165. Nishihara K, Nagai E, Izumi Y et al. Adenosquamous carcinoma of the gallbladder. A clinicopathological immunohistochemical and flow cytometric study of twenty cases. Jpn J Cancer Res, 1994; 85:389–399

166. Suster S, Huszar M, Herezeg E et al. Adenosquamous carcinoma of the gallbladder with spindle cell features. A light microscopic and immunohistochemical study of a case. Histopathology, 1987; 11:209–214

167. Nishihara K, Takashima M, Haraguchi M et al. Adenosquamous carcinoma of the gallbladder with gastric foveolar-type epithelium. Pathol Internat, 1995; 45:250–256

168. Albores-Saavedra J, Cruz-Ortiz H, Alcantara-Vazques A et al. Unusual types of gallbladder carcinoma. Arch Pathol Lab Med, 1981; 105:287–293

169. Nishihara K, Tsuneyoshi M. Small cell carcinoma of the gallbladder. A clinicopathological, immunohistochemical and flow cytometrical study of 15 cases. Int J Oncol, 1993; 3:901–908

170. Iida Y, Tsutsumi Y. Small cell (endocrine cell) carcinoma of the gallbladder with squamous and adenocarcinomatous components. Acta Pathol Jpn, 1992; 22:119–125

171. Diebold-Berger S, Vaiton J-C, Pache, J-C et al. Undifferentiated carcinoma of the gallbladder. A report of a case with immunohistochemical findings. Arch Pathol Lab Med, 1995; 119:279–282

172. Guo K-J, Yamaguchi K, Enjoji M. Undifferentiated carcinoma of the gallbladder. A clinicopathologic, histochemical, and immunohistochemical study of 21 patients with a poor prognosis. Cancer, 1988; 61:1872–1879

173. Nishihara K, Tsuneyoshi M. Undifferentiated spindle cell carcinoma of the gallbladder. A clinicopathologic immunohistochemical and flow cytometric study of 11 cases. Hum Pathol, 1993; 24:1298–1305

174. Teh M, Wee A, Raju GC. An immunohistochemical study of p53 protein in gallbladder and extrahepatic bile duct/ampullary carcinomas. Cancer, 1994; 74:1542–1545

175. Wistuba II, Albores-Saavedra J. Genetic abnormalities involved in the pathogenesis of gallbladder carcinoma. J Hepatobiliary Pancreat Surg, 1999; 6:237–244

176. Wistuba I, Sugio K, Hung J et al. Allele-specific mutations involved in the pathogenesis of endemic gallbladder carcinoma in Chile. Cancer Res, 1995; 55:2511–2515

177. Yoshida S, Todoroki T, Ichikawa Y et al. Mutations of p16Ink 4/CDKN2 and p15Ink4B/MTS2 genes in biliary tract cancers. Cancer Res, 1995; 55:2756–2760

178. Lee CS, Pirdas A. Epidermal growth factor receptor immunoreactivity in gallbladder and extrahepatic biliary tract tumors. Path Res Pract, 1995; 191:1087–1091

179. Watanabe M, Asaka M, Tanaka J et al. Point mutation of K-ras gene codon 12 in biliary tract tumors. Gastroenterology, 1994; 107:1147–1153

180. Hanada K, Itoh M, Fujii K et al. K-ras and p53 mutations in stage I gallbladder carcinoma with an anomalous junction of the pancreaticobiliary duct. Cancer, 1996; 77:452–458

181. Rijken AM, Van Gulik TM, Polak MM et al. Diagnostic and prognostic value of incidence of K-ras codon 12 mutations in resected distal bile duct carcinoma. J Surg Oncol, 1998; 68:187–192

182. Barone GW, Schaefer RF, Counce JS et al. Gallbladder and gastric argyrophil carcinoid associated with a case of Zollinger–Ellison syndrome. Am J Gastroenterol, 1992; 87:392–394

183. Modlin IM, Sandor A. An analysis of 8305 cases of carcinoid tumors. Cancer, 1997; 79:813–829

184. Yamaguchi K, Kuroki S, Daimaru Y et al. Granular cell tumor of the gallbladder. Acta Pathol Jpn, 1985; 35:687–691

185. Yamashina M, Stemmerman GN. Granular cell tumor: Unusual cause for mucocele of gallbladder. Am J Gastroenterol, 1984; 79:701–703

186. Mihara S, Matsumoto H, Tokunaga F et al. Botryoid rhabdomyosarcoma of the gallbladder in a child. Cancer, 1982; 49:812–818

187. Dong X, DeMatos P, Prieto V et al. Melanoma of the gallbladder. A review of cases at Duke Medical Center. Cancer, 1999; 85: 32–37

188. Satoh H, Iyama A, Hidaka K et al. Metastatic carcinoma of the gallbladder from renal cancer presenting as intraluminal polypoid mass. Dig Dis Sci, 1991; 36:520–523

189. Weiss L, Harlos JP, Torhorst J et al. Metastatic patterns of renal carcinoma: an analysis of 687 necropsies. J Cancer Res Clin Oncol, 1988; 114:605–612

190. Henson DE, Albores-Saavedra J, Corle D. Carcinoma of the gallbladder. Histologic types, stage of disease, grade, and survival rates. Cancer, 1992; 70:1493–1497

191. American Joint Committee on Cancer Staging Manual, 6th edn, (eds, Greene F, Page D, Fleming I, et al.) NY: Springer, 2002

Vascular disorders

13

Ian R. Wanless

Vascular lesions are important in the pathogenesis of many acute and all chronic liver diseases. For example, widespread obstruction of small portal and hepatic veins leads to cirrhosis and arterial obstruction may cause ischaemic stricture in bile ducts. Although lesions of portal veins, hepatic veins, sinusoids, and arteries are usually discussed separately, they are not independent. Obstruction to the flow of blood at one level often leads to secondary lesions upstream and downstream from the initial lesion. In addition, obstruction of veins is followed by arterial dilatation and growth (angiogenesis). This chapter reviews anatomical lesions and pathophysiology of the hepatic circulation. Other sources review normal anatomy, physiology, pharmacology, and embryology.[1-6] There are several useful historical sources.[7-10]

Portal veins

Normal variations and congenital anomalies

The portal vein diameter is 0.6 to 1.2 cm in normal adults[11] and up to 1.9 cm in patients with portal hypertension.[12] The branches of the portal vein define the eight segments of the liver parenchyma.[13,14] Variants of the portal vein are uncommon. A branch of the left portal vein may supply a portion of the right lobe. An irregular system of veins, the parabiliary system, drains from the pancreatic or pyloric regions to supplement the parenchymal portal supply near the hilum.[15,16]

Rare anomalies of the portal vein can often be explained by persistence of portions of the vitelline veins.[17-20] The most common of these anomalies, *preduodenal portal vein*, is often accompanied by biliary atresia or anomalous origin of the hepatic artery.[21,22] *Hypoplasia* or *atresia* of the portal vein may be developmental or secondary to neonatal disease.[23] Portal vein atresia has been found in two cases with the multiple focal nodular hyperplasia syndrome.[24,25] Odievre et al.[26] found that non-hepatic malformations, often of a vascular nature, occurred in many children with non-cirrhotic portal hypertension. A mass of ectopic liver tissue may obstruct the portal vein.[27] Portal vein *aneurysm* is a rare congenital anomaly or response to portal hypertension, usually occurring in the extrahepatic vein.[28] *Anomalous pulmonary venous drainage* into a portal or hepatic vein has been reported,[29,30] usually in association with cardiac and other anomalies.

Extrahepatic portosystemic shunts (the Abernethy malformation) have been subtyped.[18,31,32] Type I has complete portal diversion to a systemic vein, usually the vena cava. Type Ia has absent portal vein, with splenic and superior mesenteric vein entering systemic veins separately. These patients are usually girls with cardiac or other congenital anomalies, including biliary atresia, oculoauriculovertebral dysplasia (Goldenhar syndrome), situs inversus, and polysplenia. Hepatic masses are frequent, usually described as focal nodular hyperplasia, but also hepatoblastoma, hepatocellular carcinoma, and adenoma.[32-36] In Type Ib the splenic and superior mesenteric veins join to form a portal vein prior to drainage into a systemic vein. This form usually occurs in boys without other associated anomalies or hepatic masses. Type II has partial diversion with a side-to-side portosystemic shunt. Type IIa is congenital, usually as an isolated malformation occurring in boys. Type IIb is acquired, usually induced by portal hypertension or trauma. Some type IIa cases may be the equivalent of persistent *ductus venosus* (Fig. 13.1).

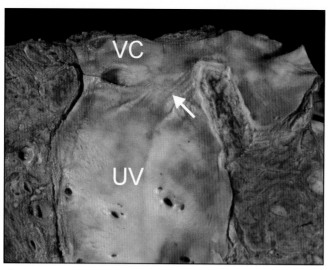

Fig. 13.1 • Patent ductus venosus (arrow) connecting the umbilical portion of the left portal vein (UV) with the inferior vena cava (VC). From Wanless et al.[475]

Intrahepatic portosystemic venous fistula may occur as a congenital anomaly[37] or secondary to portal hypertension, trauma, or rupture of a portal vein aneurysm.[38-40] Many reported cases had a single large channel between the right portal vein and vena cava.[41,42] Others had multiple peripheral intrahepatic shunts.[43] Large intrahepatic shunts may be accompanied by atrial septal defect, hypoplasia of intrahepatic portal vein branches, nodular hyperplasia, hepatocellular carcinoma, or steatosis.[19,44-48] Clinically, there is often portosystemic encephalopathy, hyperammonaemia, hypergalactosaemia, and elevated serum bile acids.

Patent umbilical vein is a special variant of portosystemic fistula. When associated with dilated periumbilical veins, abdominal bruit, hypoplasia of intrahepatic portal veins, and atrophy of the liver with little or no hepatic fibrosis, this condition has been called Cruveilhier–Baumgarten disease.[49] When the dilated veins are secondary to portal hypertension, the condition has been defined as Cruveilhier–Baumgarten syndrome.[49] In retrospect, it is likely that the reported patients with Cruveilhier–Baumgarten disease also had portal hypertension either from portal vein thrombosis or congenital hypoplasia of the intrahepatic portal veins[50] so that the distinction between the disease and the syndrome is of little value. The prominent periumbilical circulation in Cruveilhier–Baumgarten syndrome is usually fed by dilated paraumbilical veins.[49,51]

Intrahepatic arterioportal fistula is a rare condition that may present with portal hypertension, failure to thrive, or diarrhoea.[52-55] The fistula may be congenital, often in association with hepatic artery aneurysm,[56] or other vascular anomaly;[54] it may also be acquired from trauma[57] or needle biopsy,[58,59] or be associated with hepatocellular carcinoma invading the portal vein.[60,61] The lesions may cause aneurysmal dilatation of the portal vein and pulsatile retrograde portal vein flow. Secondary portal vein thrombosis and mesenteric ischaemia have been reported.[54] Arteriovenous shunts in extrahepatic splanchnic locations may also produce portal hypertension.[62,63] Arteriovenous malforma-tions, consisting of multiple vascular channels, are distinguished by greater difficulty in achieving therapeutic ablation.

Arteriovenous fistulas connecting to hepatic veins often present with congestive heart failure. They are usually caused by trauma but may be congenital or associated with hereditary haemorrhagic telangiectasis and pregnancy.[64-66] Small shunts may be detected by Doppler examination in patients with cirrhotic livers.[67]

Nomenclature and pathophysiology of portal hypertension

Portal hypertension arises because of obstruction to hepatic blood flow. Patients with portal hypertension are broadly divided into those with either presinusoidal or postsinusoidal obstruction on the basis of pressure measurements or clinical findings. The validity of the assumptions underlying this nomenclature has been questioned.[68] However, it is usually true that, in the absence of cirrhosis, varices, and splenomegaly are features of portal vein disease while ascites and hepatomegaly are features of hepatic vein disease.

Patients with *presinusoidal noncirrhotic portal hypertension* have usually been classified according to clinical or radiological features rather than by anatomical lesions or pathogenetic mechanisms. The classification used is largely dependent on the method of investigation. Splanchnic arteriograms viewed in the venous phase allow rather crude identification of the portal vein up to the second or third order branches. This technique allows division of cases into extrahepatic block and intrahepatic block. The term *cavernous transformation*, often considered as synonymous with extrahepatic block, refers to the presence of abundant collateral veins in the region of the original portal vein.[69]

Idiopathic portal hypertension is defined as non-cirrhotic portal hypertension in the absence of known cause of liver disease and with a patent extrahepatic portal vein.[70,71] This may be synonymous with intrahepatic portal vein block, although the lesions have not always been well documented. 'Hepatoportal sclerosis' is a term suggested by Mikkelsen et al. to describe fibrous intimal thickening of the portal vein or its branches in patients with non-cirrhotic portal hypertension.[72] 'Non-cirrhotic portal fibrosis' is the term chosen by a panel of Indian experts for the lesions in such patients.[73] Although these three terms are nearly synonymous, there have been differences in their application. Some cases with non-cirrhotic portal hypertension have been defined by the presence of hepatocellular nodules and called 'nodular regenerative hyperplasia' or 'partial nodular transformation'.

The early events in non-cirrhotic portal hypertension have not been fully documented because clinical manifestations occur long after vascular lesions have healed. Small biopsies often fail to demonstrate the vascular lesions. Large vessel lesions are well-documented only at autopsy or explantation.

The difficulty in appreciating portal vein lesions has caused some to wonder if sinusoidal lesions may be sufficient to cause portal hypertension.[74,75] This idea is supported by the occasional finding of portal hypertension in patients with sinusoidal compression or cellular infiltration as in steatosis,[76] acute hepatitis,[77] leukaemia,[78] mastocytosis,[79-81] Gaucher disease,[78] and agnogenic myeloid metaplasia.[82] However, portal hypertension in agnogenic myeloid metaplasia and in polycythaemia vera correlates with portal vein lesions and not with sinusoidal infiltration.[83] Furthermore, the rarity of portal hypertension in amyloidosis despite massive sinusoidal deposition[84] makes it unlikely that mild or moderate disease confined to the sinusoids produces clinical portal hypertension. It is likely that undocumented venous lesions are responsible for the portal hypertension occasionally found in these various conditions. In mastocytosis, occlusive lesions of portal and hepatic venules have been documented.[81]

Arterioportal fistulas may produce sufficiently high portal flow for clinically significant portal hypertension to develop in the absence of hepatic vascular obstruction.[52-54,62,85,86] It has been suggested that large spleens, in various diseases, may increase portal flow sufficiently to produce portal hypertension.[87] However, the response to splenectomy or splenic vein clamping has been variable, suggesting that a fixed intrahepatic vascular obstruction is often present in many of these patients.[83,88,89] This subject has been reviewed in detail.[52,90]

Acquired disease of large portal veins (portal vein thrombosis)

Portal vein disease is conveniently divided into hypoplasia, thrombosis, and local portal tract disease. A pathogenetic classification of portal vein disease is presented in Table 13.1. Large vessel disease is most commonly a result of thrombosis while small vessel disease may be caused either by propagation of thrombus or local portal tract inflammation.

Thrombosis of the portal vein is usually associated with the presence of a hypercoagulable state, vascular injury, or stasis (Table 13.2). Associated hypercoagulable states have included pregnancy, use of oral contraceptives, various myeloproliferative disorders,[91,92] prothrombin mutation G20210A,[92,93] protein C deficiency,[94] protein S deficiency,[95] lupus anticoagulant or cardiolipin antibodies, antithrombin III deficiency, heparin cofactor II deficiency, dysfibrinogenaemia, homocystinaemia,[96] homozygous methylenetetrahydrofolate reductase C677T genotype,[97] and elevated factor VIII.[98] The Leiden factor V mutation was associated with portal or mesenteric vein thrombosis in some studies[91,99] and not in others.[92,93,100,101] Some myeloproliferative disorders can only be diagnosed by demonstration of spontaneous erythroid colony formation in vitro.[102,103]

Inflammation of the portal vein (pylephlebitis) can be induced by: (i) infection, especially appendicitis, diverticulitis, or omphalitis; (ii) chemical injury initiated by pancreatitis, bile leak from primary sclerosing cholangitis, bile leak from transhepatic biliary drainage, oesophageal sclerotherapy, or infusion of hyperosmolar glucose into the umbilical vein; and (iii) accidental or surgical trauma. Portal vein thrombosis occurred in 8% of left lobe grafts in children.[104] Asymptomatic segmental portal vein thrombosis is frequent during acute cholecystitis.[105]

Stasis is a cause of portal vein thrombosis in cirrhosis, primary or secondary neoplasms, and retroperitoneal fibrosis. There is evidence of portal vein thrombosis in 0.6% of all patients with cirrhosis and 2–40% among those coming to transplantation.[106-112] Portal vein obstruction with tumour and/or thrombus also occurs in 23–70% of patients with hepatocellular carcinoma[107,110,113-115] and in 5–8% of patients with metastatic tumour in the liver.[107,116] Islet cell infusion is an emerging cause of portal vein thrombosis.[117,118]

The relative importance of these causal factors varies geographically. In Western countries and Japan, cirrhosis is the

Table 13.1	Pathogenetic classification of portal vein disease	
Pathogenesis	**Comments and examples**
1. *Primary agenesis or hypoplasia*	This is seen in childhood 'cavernous transformation' and with various congenital shunts. Hypoplasia of small portal veins may be present in congenital hepatic fibrosis.
2. *Thrombosis* a. Thrombosis of large portal veins	This includes most cases of 'cavernous transformation' and extrahepatic portal vein block. This may be secondary to inflammation, hypercoagulable states, or stasis.
b. Thrombosis of small portal veins (i) propagation from large portal vein thrombosis	This explains residual small portal vein obliteration after large portal vein thrombosis followed by recanalization. This includes many cases of idiopathic portal hypertension, non-cirrhotic portal fibrosis, hepatoportal sclerosis, and congenital hepatic fibrosis.
(ii) emboli or local thrombi	Local portal thrombosis is frequent secondary to hepatic vein thrombosis. Emboli may arise from pancreatic carcinoma or injected vinyl beads.
3. *Local portal tract disease* a. Primary portal phlebitis b. Primary arteritis c. Primary duct disease d. Primary portal tract disease, site uncertain	This includes some cases of idiopathic portal hypertension. Schistosomiasis, sarcoidosis, other granulomatous vasculitis, vinyl chloride, and other toxins. Polyarteritis nodosa, rheumatoid arteritis, systemic lupus erythematosus, systemic sclerosis. Primary biliary cirrhosis, primary sclerosing cholangitis, bacterial cholangitis. Chronic hepatitis, lymphoma.

Table 13.2 Causes of portal vein thrombosis

Hypercoagulable states
 Polycythaemia vera[83,92,102,484]
 Agnogenic myeloid metaplasia[83,92,102]
 Idiopathic thrombocytosis[70,82,92,102]
 Paroxysmal nocturnal haemoglobinuria[102,485]
 Chronic myeloid leukaemia[486]
 Subclinical myeloproliferative disease[91,102,103]
 Oral contraceptive therapy[98,487]
 Pregnancy[23]
 Lupus anticoagulant or antiphospholipid antibodies[383]
 Protein C deficiency[92,94,488,489]
 Protein S deficiency[92,94,95,490,491]
 Antithrombin III deficiency[492]
 Factor II G20210A[92,93,97]
 Factor V Leiden[91,99]
 Heparin cofactor II deficiency[493]
 Methylenetetrahydrofolate reductase (MTHFR) C677T genotype[97]
 Homocystinaemia[92,96]
 Elevated factor VIII[98]

Stasis or mass lesion
 Cirrhosis[107,111,128,494]
 Hepatocellular carcinoma[107,485]
 Carcinoma of pancreas[495,496]
 Splenectomy[497,498]
 Retroperitoneal fibrosis[499]
 Embolized beads

Vascular injury
 Umbilical sepsis[486]
 Pylephlebitis[68,484,500–502]
 Cholecystitis[105]
 Congenital hepatic fibrosis[124–126]
 Beçhet disease[126]
 Cytomegalovirus infection[503]
 Trauma[504,505]
 Catheterization[506]
 Oesophageal sclerotherapy[507,508]
 Schistosomiasis[154]
 Sarcoidosis[145,509]
 Inflammatory bowel disease[510–512]
 Islet cell infusion[117,118]

cause of portal vein thrombosis in 20–60% of cases[109,119] and myeloproliferative disorders account for 28–48% of cases.[91,102,103] Multiple risk factors, including local and systemic factors, are often present.[91,120] The high prevalence of non-cirrhotic portal hypertension and extrahepatic portal vein block in India may be related to the high incidence of omphalitis and of dehydration in that country.[121]

Recanalization after thrombosis of large portal veins has been documented by ultrasound and by histological examination.[109,111,122,123] Thrombus in large portal veins usually propagates to small veins which are less likely to recanalize. The transient nature of thrombotic occlusion in large vessels may explain why it has been so difficult to establish the importance of portal vein thrombosis in the genesis of non-cirrhotic portal hypertension. In the neonate, umbilical vein infection may induce fibrosis so that the portal vein

fails to enlarge as the body grows. This may explain why extrahepatic portal vein block is more common in children than in adults.

Congenital hepatic fibrosis is usually associated with portal hypertension. The small portal veins are decreased in number, a finding often attributed to hypoplasia. However, a large number of reported cases have evidence of portal vein thrombosis.[124–126] Polycystic liver disease is rarely associated with portal hypertension of uncertain pathogenesis.[127]

Portal vein thrombosis is often clinically silent. In the presence of cirrhosis or hepatic neoplasm, thrombosis may precipitate hepatic decompensation, variceal bleeding, or ascites.[128] Portal biliopathy is a syndrome of partial bile duct obstruction occurring in patients with portal hypertension, especially those with extrahepatic portal vein obstruction.[129,130] It is thought to be caused by: (i) compression of the extrahepatic bile duct by adjacent varices; or (ii) ischaemic duct injury. Some patients have choledocholithiasis as a cofactor or complication.[131] Portal vein flow decreases during carbon dioxide pneumoperitoneum induced during laparoscopic procedures. This may cause hepatic ischaemia in susceptible individuals.[132]

Acquired disease of small portal veins

Patients with portal hypertension because of obliteration of small portal veins may also have evidence of systemic microvascular disease as seen in rheumatoid arteritis,[133,134] myeloproliferative diseases,[83] systemic lupus erythematosus,[135] polyarteritis nodosa,[136] systemic sclerosis,[137] and monoclonal gammopathies,[138] or exposure to vasculotoxic chemicals, such as azathioprine, vinyl chloride, 'toxic oil', or arsenic (Table 13.3).*[139]

Obliteration of small portal veins may also occur early in the course of primary biliary cirrhosis,[140] primary sclerosing cholangitis, and sarcoidosis,[141,142] causing portal hypertension before the development of cirrhosis.

The genesis of portal hypertension in these various conditions can be explained by the concept of 'ménage à foie'.[143] This is the development of injury to one portal structure because of inflammation primarily directed at a neighbouring portal tract structure. Thus, local portal venous obliteration may be secondary to arteritis (Fig. 13.2) or to ductal inflammation, as in primary sclerosing cholangitis and primary biliary cirrhosis. The obliteration is usually confined to small portal veins. However, even large first and second-order portal vein branches may be obliterated by portal inflammation.[144]

Portal vein obliteration may be caused by sarcoid granulomas,[145] mineral oil granulomas,[146] and exposure to thorotrast[147] and other toxins (Table 13.3). Emboli or local thromboses are important in schistosomiasis, normal aging, and in congestive heart failure.[148] Idiopathic granulomatous vasculitis involving portal or hepatic venules is rare.[140]

---

* It is curious that Banti believed that arsenic was the only effective treatment for patients affected by his disease.

Table 13.3 Microvascular disease related to drugs and toxins

Histology	Obliterative portal venopathy	Sinusoidal fibrosis	Veno-occlusive disease*	Peliosis hepatis	Angiosarcoma	References
6-Thioguanine			++	+		341
Azathioprine	+	+	+	+		74, 256, 261, 266, 342
6-Mercaptopurine	+	+	+	+		74
BCNU			+			513
Hepatic radiation	+		++			255, 514
Dacarbazine			++			257
Oxaliplatin			+			265
Flurodeoxyuridine (intra-arterial)	+		+			264
Methotrexate		+		+		515
Senecia alkaloids		+	++			244
Cysteamine			+			259
Thorotrast	++	++	++	++	+	516, 517
Arsenic	++	+	+	+	+	172, 173, 516
Copper	+	+				518
Vinyl chloride	++	++			+	516
Vitamin A	+	++		+		310
'Toxic oil'	+	+				519
Anabolic and oestrogenic steroids, medroxyprogesterone				++	+	520
Corticosteroids				+		521
Tamoxifen				+		522

* Other drugs associated with VOD include busulfan, dimethylbusulfan, cytosine arabinoside, cyclophosphamide, indicine-N-oxide, mustine-HCl, adriamycin, urethane, vincristine, mitomycin-C, and etoposide.[253,523]

Ducts may also be injured by inflammation primarily involving the arteries and other portal tract structures. This could explain the elevated alkaline phosphatase commonly present in patients with temporal arteritis,[149] rheumatoid arteritis,[133] nodular regenerative hyperplasia,[150] idiopathic portal hypertension,[151] and sarcoidosis.[152]

Schistosomiasis

Schistosomiasis deserves special mention as the most common cause of portal hypertension in the world (see Chapter 9). In some endemic regions there is evidence of hepatic schistosomiasis in up to 18% of the population.[153] Eggs deposited in rectal veins float into the small portal veins <100 µm diameter, where a transient eosinophilic infiltrate is followed by a granulomatous reaction and fibrous obliteration of the veins. A PAS-positive remnant of egg cuticle is seen in one third of surgical wedge biopsies.[154] Clusters of small eggs are seen with *Schistosoma japonicum* and *Schistosoma mekongi*,[155] and larger single eggs with a lateral spine are seen with *Schistosoma mansoni* (Fig. 13.3). Although the primary lesion is in small portal veins, dense fibrosis of the medium and large portal tracts gives the typical gross appearance of Symmer's pipe-stem fibrosis.[154,156,157] This lesion is easily seen by ultrasonography allowing detailed demographic studies.[158,159] After treatment, ultrasound evidence of 'portal vein wall thickening' and splenomegaly abates in the majority of patients with moderate disease; improvement in patients with severe disease is less often observed.[160]

Idiopathic portal hypertension

In idiopathic portal hypertension small vessel lesions are dominant but large vein lesions are usually found when sought.[72,73,110] Most cases of idiopathic portal hypertension are probably a result of large portal vein thrombosis.[161] This possibility has been difficult to prove because large

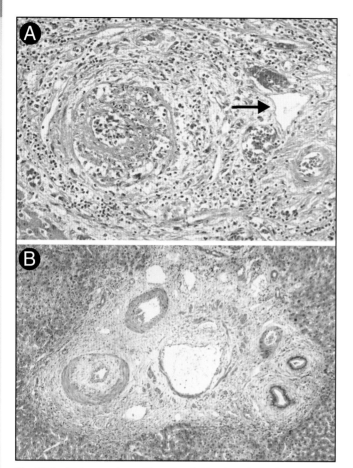

Fig. 13.2 • (A) Acute polyarteritis nodosa (left) with marked inflammation of the adjacent portal vein wall (arrow). H&E. **(B)** Healed arteritis and adjacent organized portal vein thrombosis. Haematoxylin–Phloxine–Saffron.

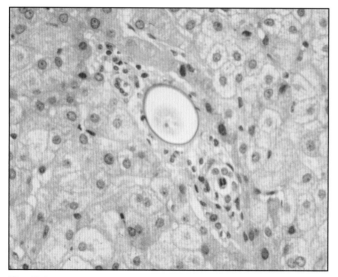

Fig. 13.3 • Egg of *Schistosoma japonicum* obstructing a small portal vein. H&E.

thrombi usually recanalize (see below), leaving a patent portal vein trunk and permanent narrowing or obliteration of the distal branches. The cause of the thrombosis varies, but many livers have evidence of regressed cirrhosis, suggesting that the thrombus occurred in the presence of cirrhosis.[161]

Pathology of portal vein disease

After thrombosis followed by organization, large veins may have subtle white intimal plaques or mural calcification. When recanalization is less complete the lumen may be obliterated or contain complex webs (Fig. 13.4). Portal veins larger than 200 µm in diameter have eccentric intimal fibrous thickening which may be layered, suggesting recurrent thrombosis. Small veins are commonly involved by extension of thrombus from larger vessels. After organization, veins less than 200 µm in diameter disappear as the wall becomes incorporated into fibrous scar, while large veins may have residual wall, best seen with the elastic-trichrome or Movat stains (Fig. 13.4).

Some small portal veins remain patent and become dilated if the supplying portal veins are patent, because the elevated portal pressure is transmitted to the small veins.[162,163] These dilated veins often expand outside the portal tract stroma into the adjacent parenchyma giving an 'ectopic' appearance (Fig. 13.5). It is a common error for the eye to recognize these 'supernormal' veins and to ignore the more subtle absence of veins. When evaluating the extent of obliteration of small portal veins, a quantitative approach is necessary because histologically identical lesions, but fewer in number, occur in elderly subjects without clinical portal hypertension.[164]

Multiple dilated collateral veins appear within the large and medium-sized portal tracts. Dilated vessels arise in part by enlargement of normal collateral portal venous channels and in part by dilatation of the artery-fed peribiliary plexus (see Chapter 1).[165,166] The number of small portal tract vessels is increased in extrahepatic portal vein obstruction and in cirrhosis but is decreased in idiopathic portal hypertension,[167] suggesting more severe injury to the small portal veins has occurred in the latter disease.

Specific causes of portal vein obstruction are suggested by finding chronic cholangitis, paucity of bile ducts, mineral oil or Thorotrast deposits, sarcoid granulomas, schistosome eggs (Fig. 13.3), healed arteritis (Fig. 13.2), or embolized beads (Fig. 13.4D).

Vascular occlusion causes remodelling of the parenchyma. Acute thrombosis of a small portal vein results in a pseudoinfarct (of Zahn) (Fig. 13.6).[168] Hepatocellular apoptosis may be seen after recent portal obstruction.[169] Obstruction of the portal vein trunk may lead to diffuse atrophy of the liver.[170] Partial recanalization or compensatory arterial dilatation allows regeneration of parts of the liver, especially near the hilum. The result may be a localized depression on the capsular surface, atrophy of a lobe,[171] partial nodular transformation, or nodular regenerative hyperplasia (see below). The Zahn infarct is a region of hepatocellular atrophy which has a congested appearance because of the enlarged sinusoidal volume. Many agents causing lesions in small portal veins, such as arsenic, vinyl chloride, and Thorotrast, also cause mild hepatocellular necrosis leading to incomplete septal cirrhosis,[172] possibly because they are capable of causing veno-occlusive disease[173] with secondary congestive parenchymal damage.

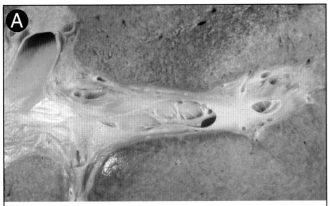

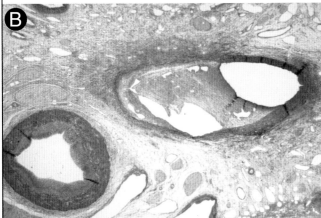

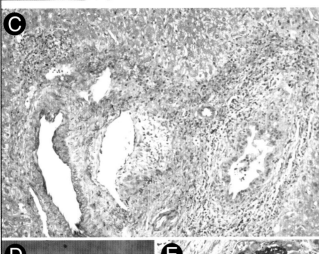

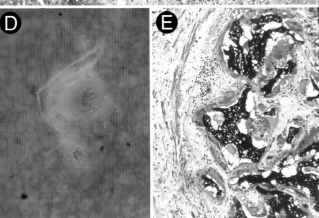

Table 13.4	Pathogenetic classification of hepatic vein disease
Pathogenesis	**Comments and examples**
1. *Thrombosis*	
a. Thrombosis of large hepatic veins	This includes Budd–Chiari syndrome. This may be secondary to inflammation, hypercoagulable states, or stasis (congestive heart failure).
b. Thrombosis of small hepatic veins	This includes residual small hepatic vein obliteration after recanalization of large hepatic vein thrombosis. It includes cases of Budd–Chiari syndrome in whom large vein obstruction cannot be documented using current imaging techniques.
2. *Non-thrombotic hepatic vein disease*	
a. Primary hepatic phlebitis	Granulomatous vasculitis (e.g. sarcoidosis) and toxins (e.g. pyrollizadine alkaloids, chemotherapy)
b. Secondary hepatic phlebitis	Chronic hepatitis and steatohepatitis
c. Congestive hepatic venopathy	Found in diseases where afferent flow exceeds outflow capacity, including schistosomiasis, EHPVO, NCPF, severe cirrhosis, and adjacent to neoplasms.

Hepatic veins

Normal variations and congenital anomalies

There is considerable variation in the anatomy of large hepatic veins, with accessory or absent veins seen in 10–14% of individuals.[22,174–176] Collateral drainage between anatomical segments is often sufficient to ameliorate hepatic necrosis after hepatic vein obstruction and to lessen peripheral oedema after thrombosis of the inferior vena cava.[177,178] The inferior right hepatic vein is often available to form collaterals because it enters the vena cava separately and escapes thrombosis of the main hepatic veins.

Nomenclature of hepatic vein obstruction

Hepatic vein obstruction can be classified according to the mechanism of obstruction or the size of vein involved (Table 13.4).[179] Thrombosis may involve large and/or small veins. Non-thrombotic injury affects only small veins in response to toxic injury,[180] local inflammation,[181] or

Fig. 13.4 • Post-thrombotic intimal fibrosis in portal veins of various sizes. **(A)** Portal vein webs several months after splenectomy in a patient with otherwise normal liver. **(B)** Web in large portal vein with partial fibrous occlusion. Elastic trichrome. From Tanaka et al.[227] **(C)** Medium-sized portal vein several weeks after thrombosis. Later lesions are so thoroughly organized that the original vein wall may not be recognizable. Elastic trichrome. **(D)** Liver with portal vein embolized by polyvinyl alcohol beads. Note that nodular regenerative hyperplasia has developed (left). The beads are largely phagocytosed by foreign body giant cells (right). The beads are black in this elastic–trichrome stain.

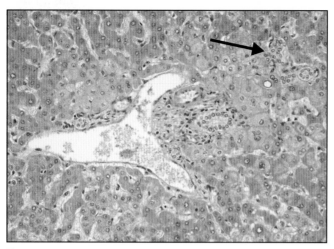

Fig. 13.5 • Ectopic portal vein in a patient with non-cirrhotic portal hypertension. An adjacent small portal tract has no vein (arrow). Haematoxylin–Phloxine–Saffron.

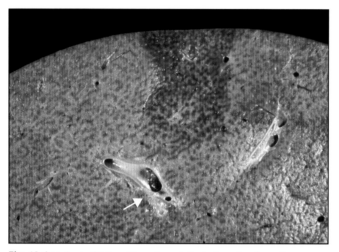

Fig. 13.6 • Infarct of Zahn with acute portal vein thrombus (arrow).

congestion (congestive hepatic venopathy).[182] Obliterative hepatic venopathy is a morphologic term for small hepatic vein obstruction independent of the mechanism of injury.

Hepatic vein thrombosis (Budd–Chiari syndrome)

Clinical findings

There is a broad clinical spectrum associated with hepatic vein thrombosis, usually referred to as the *Budd–Chiari syndrome*. The classic findings are hepatomegaly, ascites, abdominal pain, and varying degrees of hepatic dysfunction.[183] Severity of disease at presentation has declined in the last 20 years as milder cases are discovered with sensitive imaging techniques.[184,185] Formerly, the majority of patients presented with hepatic failure and median survival was less than 2 years in the absence of surgical therapy.[183,186–189] Fulminant hepatic failure may be the initial presentation when there is obstruction of all major hepatic veins.[190] Patients with involvement of only one or two of the hepatic veins may have only hepatomegaly and mild or

transient liver test abnormalities.[191] Bleeding varices are usually accompanied by cirrhosis or secondary portal vein thrombosis.[192] Extension of thrombus to small mesenteric veins may cause bowel infarction.[95,193]

The differential diagnosis includes constrictive pericarditis, which should be distinguished on clinical grounds as biopsy findings may be similar to those of hepatic vein obstruction.[194] Aggressive attempts to establish the diagnosis should be made, as anticoagulation therapy and/or surgical intervention often lead to prolonged survival.[186,195,196]

Aetiology and pathogenesis

Three-quarters of patients in American, British, and French series with Budd–Chiari syndrome have a recognized predisposing factor belonging to Virchow's triad (Table 13.5).[197,198] Such factors are less common in children and in Japanese adults.[186,199] The most common factor is a hypercoagulable state, especially a myeloproliferative disease such as polycythaemia vera or the Leiden mutation of factor V.[101,200] Other hypercoagulable states include paroxysmal nocturnal haemoglobinuria, oral contraceptive use, pregnancy, anticardiolipin antibodies,[189,201,202] antithrombin III deficiency, protein C deficiency, protein S deficiency, prothrombin mutant G20210A,[203] homozygous MTHFR C677T mutation,[204] and the 5q deletion myelodysplastic syndrome.[205] A large proportion of those with no obvious risk factor appear to have a subclinical myeloproliferative disorder characterized by spontaneous erythroid colony formation in vitro.[91,103,206] Pregnancy, oral contraceptive therapy, and trauma may unmask latent hypercoagulable states.[206] More than one risk factor may be detected in a patient.[91] Hypercoagulable states are often associated with thrombosis in arteries and veins of other organs, or in the allograft after liver transplantation.[91,207–210]

Vascular injury and stasis are other causes. The high prevalence in some developing countries suggests that infection, toxins,[186] or dehydration may have a role, especially in children[211] and postpartum women. In North America the common causes are polycythaemia (10%), paroxysmal nocturnal haemoglobinuria (7%), oral contraceptives (9%), pregnancy (10%), tumours (9%), and infections (9%).[189] Using the more sensitive colony formation assay, myeloproliferative disease was present in 45–80% of patients.[91,103,206] In India, the most commonly associated conditions are amoebic abscess (18%), pregnancy (15%), and hepatic neoplasm (13%).[212,213] In some patients, obstruction of the inferior vena cava occurs and may dominate the clinical picture.[214]

Tumours involving the vena cava or hepatic veins may present with hepatic outflow obstruction (Table 13.5). Hepatocellular carcinoma involves the major hepatic veins in 6–23% of cases.[114] Most patients with hepatic vein involvement by this tumour also have portal vein involvement.[114]

Budd–Chiari syndrome may be associated with a radiological appearance suggesting membranous obstruction or stricture of the inferior vena cava.[215–217] While some early investigators believed these lesions to be developmental anomalies causing hepatic vein thrombosis,[211,218]

Table 13.5	Causes of hepatic vein thrombosis

Hypercoagulable states
  Polycythaemia vera[197]
  Agnogenic myeloid metaplasia[83]
  Paroxysmal nocturnal haemoglobinuria[179,233,524,525]
  Promyelocytic leukaemia[526,527]
  Chronic myeloid leukaemia[528]
  Subclinical myeloproliferative disease[91,103,206]
  Undefined (e.g. history of thrombotic disease)[188]
  Oral contraceptive therapy[197,529–531]
  Pregnancy[212]
  Factor V Leiden[91,101,200]
  Lupus anticoagulant or anticardiolipin antibodies[91,201,202,219,532–536]
  Idiopathic thrombocytopenic purpura[197]
  Protein C deficiency[91,200,537]
  Protein S deficiency[91,200]
  Prothrombin 20210A[203,538]
  Methylenetetrahydrofolate reductase (MTHFR) C677T genotype[204]
  Antithrombin III deficiency[539,540]
  Plasminogen deficiency[221]
  Dysfibrinogenaemia[541]
  Systemic malignancy[542]

Stasis or mass lesion
  Membranous obstruction of inferior vena cava (see text)[211,218]
  Other congenital anomalies[186,543]
  Cirrhosis[188]
  Congestive heart failure[188]
  Constrictive pericarditis[544,545]
  Superior vena cava obstruction[546]
  Atrial myxoma[547]
  Sickle cell disease[548]
  Hepatocellular carcinoma[549,550]

  Renal cell carcinoma[551]
  Adrenal carcinoma[552]
  Hodgkin disease[349]
  Epithelioid haemangioendothelioma[553]
  Wilms tumour[554,555]
  Leiomyosarcoma or leiomyoma[550,556–558]
  Metastatic neoplasm[550]
  Hydatid cyst[559]
  Hepatic abscess, pyogenic or amoebic[183,560]
  Haematoma[561]

Vascular injury
  Trauma[192,207,562–564]
  Ventriculoatrial shunt[565]
  Catheterization[566]
  Sclerotherapy[507]
  Amyloidosis[567]
  Vasculitis or tissue inflammation[186]
  Tuberculosis[568]
  Fungal vasculitis[569,570]
  Behçet disease[126,571,572]
  Sarcoidosis[282,573]
  Idiopathic granulomatous venulitis[283]
  Filariasis[574]

Associations of uncertain mechanism
  Inflammatory bowel disease[188,575,576]
  Mixed connective tissue disease[577]
  Protein-losing enteropathy[578,579]
  Coeliac disease[580]
  Multiple myeloma[581]
  5q deletion syndrome and hypereosinophilia[205]

more recent histological,[199,213] and sequential radiological studies[219] suggest that these caval lesions are secondary to extension of hepatic vein thrombosis. Compression of the vena cava by an enlarged caudate lobe may precipitate this extension.[211,220] Acquired caval membranes have been documented after trauma.[221] Hepatocellular carcinoma occurs in 36–46% of patients with membranous obstruction of the vena cava and less often in hepatic vein obstruction with patent vena cava.[215,222,223]

The initial site of thrombosis cannot be determined from examination of established Budd–Chiari syndrome. However, my experience with subclinical hepatic vein thrombosis found incidentally at autopsy suggests that thrombi begin in sinusoids or terminal hepatic venules and propagate towards the large hepatic veins. The frequency of primary thrombosis in small hepatic vein branches is probably underestimated because this lesion is clinically silent until propagation to several large hepatic veins has occurred.[191,224]

Pathology

The acute lesions after hepatic vein thrombosis are dilatation of veins and sinusoids, and variable degrees of necrosis (Fig. 13.7). The sinusoids are congested and red blood cells infiltrate the space of Disse.[225] Acute or organizing thrombus is occasionally seen within small hepatic[189] or portal veins.[199] As disease advances, the sinusoids become collagenized and dilated and hepatocytes become atrophic and are lost. The small hepatic veins disappear as they are incorporated into septa which eventually link hepatic veins to form cirrhosis with relative sparing of the portal triads, so-called reversed lobulation cirrhosis or venocentric cirrhosis (Fig. 13.7C). It has been demonstrated that venocentric cirrhosis occurs when vascular obstruction is largely confined to hepatic veins. Secondary portal vein thrombosis is frequent in Budd–Chiari syndrome,[183,226] an event that leads to a venoportal type of cirrhosis, with parenchymal extinction and septa that involve perivenous and periportal regions.[227]

The liver remodels in a fashion dependent on the pattern of venous involvement. The left lobe is hypertrophied when the left vein is relatively spared. The caudate lobe becomes hypertrophied when the caudate lobe veins, which enter the vena cava directly, remain patent. Small regions of regeneration and hypertrophy commonly occur to form nodules or a ribbon of healthy hepatocytes surrounding the larger portal systems.[227–229] Lesions grossly similar to Zahn infarcts may be seen with localized hepatic vein thrombosis.[230]

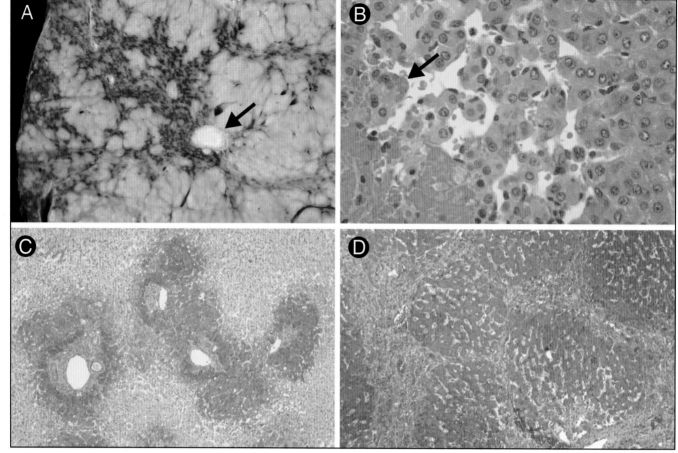

Fig. 13.7 • Hepatic vein thrombosis (Budd–Chiari syndrome). **(A)** Gross appearance shows a large hepatic vein obstructed by organized thrombus (arrow). There are large regions of parenchymal congestion and extinction. Residual parenchyma has regenerated to form nodules of various sizes. **(B)** There is marked congestion with dilated sinusoids and extravasation of red cells into the hepatocyte plates (arrow). H&E. **(C)** Venocentric type of cirrhosis. This type occurs when vascular obstruction is largely confined to hepatic veins. The regenerative nodules contain portal tracts having patent and dilated portal veins. Elastic trichrome. **(D)** Venoportal type of cirrhosis. This type occurs when there is obstruction of portal veins as well as hepatic veins. The result is extinction that involves periportal tissue so that portal tracts are incorporated into the fibrous septa. Note that most portal veins are obliterated. Elastic trichrome. From Wanless.[582]

Fibrous thickening and stenosis of the hepatic portion of the inferior vena cava is found in approximately 50% of cases of Budd–Chiari syndrome. The thickened region may form a thin valve-like membrane or may be several centimetres in length. Histologically, these lesions show thrombus in various stages of organization, often with calcification, and with no evidence of a pre-existing congenital membrane.[199]

Clinicopathological correlation

A normal biopsy, especially early in the course, does not exclude the diagnosis. However, most patients have evidence of histological chronicity soon after the onset of clinical symptoms, suggesting that recurrence and extension of thrombosis is the rule. Hepatic vein thrombosis presenting in the post-partum period does not usually have histological evidence of chronicity.[213,231]

Histological diagnosis can be difficult in chronic disease because congestion and reversed lobulation are focal and may not be seen in a small biopsy. Hepatic vein thrombosis should be considered in any cirrhotic liver with sinusoidal dilatation or prominent dilated vascular channels. Organized thrombi or fibrous obliteration of small hepatic veins may be histologically identical to the lesions of chronic veno-occlusive disease.[224,232] Haemosiderosis may occur, especially when there is coexistent paroxysmal nocturnal haemoglobinuria.[233]

Many surgeons use the liver biopsy to guide therapy, with the presence of necrosis suggesting the need for a shunt procedure and extensive fibrosis favouring the need for transplantation.[192,198] Although the risk of bleeding from the biopsy site is significant, the benefit in therapeutic guidance may justify the procedure even in the presence of coagulopathy and ascites. Accurate assessment requires at least two biopsies from different lobes because of the marked regional variation in severity found in this condition.[190] Histological and clinical improvement is often seen after a decompression procedure such as mesocaval shunt.[234] Repeat biopsies after therapy are recommended; CT guidance is useful to ensure that the specimens are obtained from the same sites on the repeat occasion. The appearance of regenerative nodules on imaging studies must be distinguished from malignancy.[227,235]

Congestive heart failure

Congestive heart failure is associated with dilatation of sinusoids and atrophy of zone 3 hepatocytes. Fibrosis is usually minimal with focal pericellular collagen. Fibrosis is probably secondary to obliteration of hepatic veins, judging from the close topographic correlation between these two lesions (Fig. 13.8 and 13.9).[148] Examples with severe fibrosis are histologically indistinguishable from Budd–Chiari syndrome. Nodular regenerative hyperplasia occasionally occurs in chronic passive congestion,[236] probably because of coexistent obliteration of small portal and hepatic veins (Fig. 13.8B).[148]

Veno-occlusive disease

Veno-occlusive disease (VOD) is a condition characterized by fibrous occlusion of small hepatic veins less than 1 mm in diameter without evident thrombosis or large hepatic vein obstruction.[230,237] Veno-occlusive disease is understood to be a response to various toxins. In the acute phase sinusoidal endothelial cell necrosis dominates and produces clinical dysfunction before fibrous venous lesions have developed. Thus the term 'sinusoidal obstruction syndrome' was suggested.[238] 'Veno-occlusive lesion' or 'VOD-like lesion'

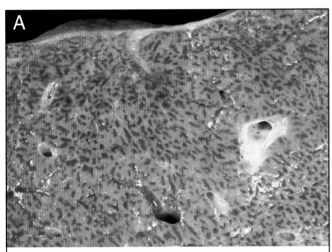

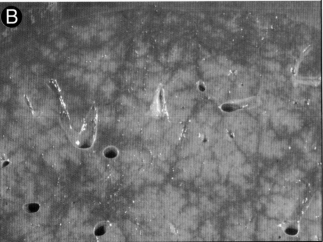

Fig. 13.8 • Chronic passive congestion with **(A)** diffuse 'nutmeg' pattern, and **(B)** nodular regenerative hyperplasia pattern.

are names often applied to histologically similar venous lesions found in any chronic liver disease. To avoid confusion with VOD, the descriptive term of 'obliterative hepatic venopathy' is recommended.

Aetiology and clinical findings

Hepatic injury presenting as abdominal pain and ascites after ingestion of plants or extracts of *Senecio* species was described in humans long before the actual vascular lesions were recognized (Chapter 14).[239–241] This disease, known variously as Senecio disease, serous hepatosis, heliotrope toxicosis, and Pictou cattle disease[242,243], has been reported in humans and livestock from many parts of the world. The apparent cause of this condition is ingestion of pyrrolizidine alkaloids derived mostly from *Senecio* species, *Crotalaria* species, *Heliotropium lasiocarpum*[244], or *Symphytum* species (comfrey).[245] Hepatotoxic pyrrolizidine alkaloids have been documented in more than 150 species of plants but there are several thousand potentially toxic species.[246] Alkaloid preparations of this type have been shown to produce marked hepatic congestion and venular endothelial necrosis in many rodents and ruminants. The pattern of toxicity in rats depends on the dose, with diffuse hepatocellular necrosis and pulmonary vascular injury occurring at doses higher than those producing VOD.[247] Hepatic tumours have been produced in rats.[248]

Reports of human toxicity have followed ingestion of the alkaloids in herbal teas or in epidemics caused by contaminated grain. The disease usually affects young children but adults are also susceptible. The onset may be acute or insidious. Acute disease is characterized by rapid onset of abdominal pain, hepatomegaly, and ascites, usually without jaundice, splenomegaly, or fever. Chronic disease may be indistinguishable from cirrhosis of other causes, with features of portal hypertension or hepatic failure.

An epidemic of VOD occurred in India after consumption of cereal contaminated with a *Crotalaria* species.[249] Of 188 cases found among 486 villagers, 49% died within 5 years, mostly in the first 6 months.[250] A similar outbreak occurred in Afghanistan affecting 23% of the local population after consumption of bread contaminated with *Heliotropium* plants.[251] Herbal tea made from *Heliotropium* is used in India for the treatment of psoriasis and other skin conditions.[213,244]

After bone marrow transplantation, symptomatic VOD occurs in up to 54% of patients.[252,253] The lesions are thought to be caused by the hepatic radiation and intense chemotherapy preceding the transplantation. Patients usually present in the 3 weeks after therapy with weight gain, thrombocytopenia, jaundice, hepatic failure, and increased aminotransferases and alkaline phosphatase. Ascites is present in 23% and peripheral oedema in 63% of patients.[253] Liver disease contributed to death in 25% of patients with symptomatic VOD.[253]

Hepatic radiation[254,255] and chemotherapeutic drugs given without bone marrow transplantation have been implicated (Table 13.3).[255–265] Azathioprine therapy has been associated with VOD, presenting insidiously with

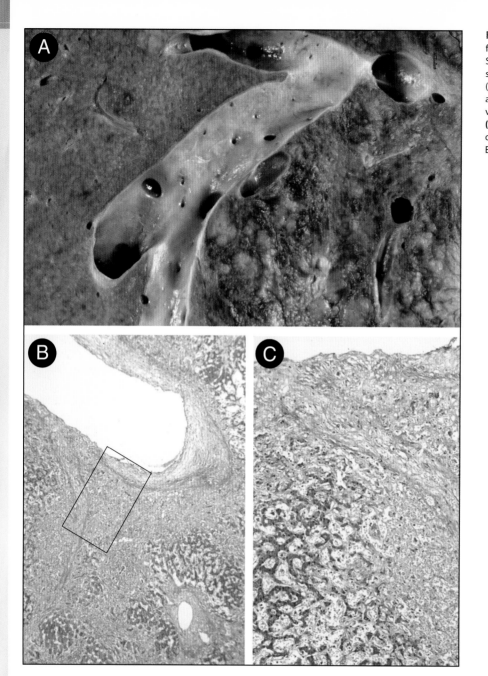

Fig. 13.9 • Hepatic fibrosis in chronic congestive failure. **(A)** The congestion and fibrosis is focal. Sections from the less affected region on the left showed normal hepatic veins and no fibrosis (not shown). **(B and C)** Section from the severely affected region shows obliteration of hepatic veins accompanied by sinusoidal fibrosis. **(C)** Higher magnification of box in **(B)** showing obstructed hepatic vein and sinusoidal fibrosis. Elastic trichrome. Panel **(A)** from Wanless et al.[148]

cholestasis or ascites after renal transplantation and, rarely, after azathioprine treatment of other conditions.[263] There is a striking male predominance among patients with VOD after azathioprine therapy.[266] Other associations include immunodeficiency states,[267] tyrosinaemia,[268] and cystinosis with cysteamine therapy.[259]

The pathogenesis of the lesions is believed to be a primary injury to the endothelial cells of sinusoids and small venules.[180,253,266] The mechanism of endothelial injury after cytotoxic drugs may involve depletion of cellular glutathione.[269,270] Patients with VOD related to a variety of insults may improve after cessation of the offending agent[260,262,266,271] or after portacaval shunt.[272,273]

Pathology

The early lesion is subintimal oedema and haemorrhage involving the sinusoids and small hepatic veins (Fig. 13.10).

Most affected veins are less than 300 μm in diameter. Thrombosis is usually not recognized, but fibrin deposits are often present on ultrastructural and immunochemical examination of acute lesions.[255,274] Sinusoidal congestion and hepatocellular necrosis may be severe with sparing of only a few periportal hepatocytes. In mild cases there may be patchy congestion in zone 3. Cholestasis is often prominent in chemotherapy-induced lesions.[263] The venous lesion heals with concentric or eccentric intimal fibrosis, fibrous obliteration, and occasionally multiple lumina. Angiomatoid endothelial proliferation has been described.[275] Zone 3 hepatocytes atrophy and sinusoidal fibrosis develops. Patients surviving for years may develop 'congestive cirrhosis' with relative sparing of the portal tracts,[230,237] but cirrhosis indistinguishable from other common forms can be expected on needle biopsy.[250] Regenerative nodules similar to those of nodular regenerative hyperplasia may be seen.[256,262,263,267,276] Obliteration of small portal veins has

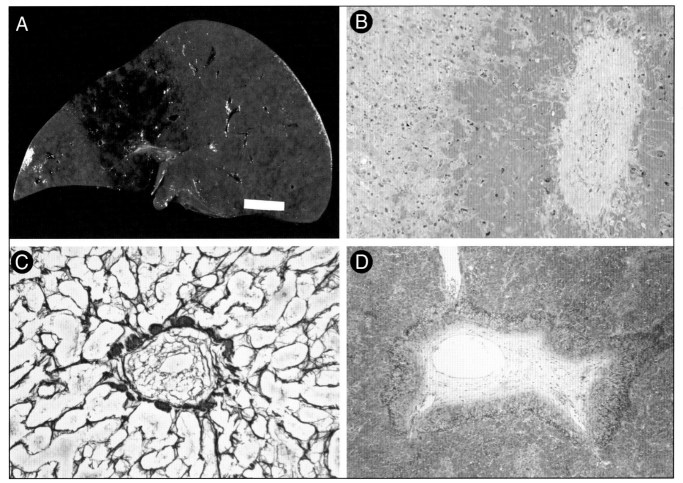

Fig. 13.10 • Veno-occlusive disease. **(A)** Patient with Hodgkin disease who developed peripheral oedema and ascites 3 weeks after bone marrow transplantation. Congestion and necrosis involves the mid-portion of the liver. Microscopic lesions were confined to veins less than 0.5 mm in diameter. **(B)** Zone 3 hepatocytes have been largely replaced by blood cells. A small hepatic vein contains macrophages and fibrous tissue. Haematoxylin–Phloxine–Saffron. **(C)** A child who received chemotherapy for Wilms tumour. The reticulin stain often highlights venous lesions that are otherwise invisible within zones of severe necrosis and haemorrhage. Reticulin stain. Courtesy of Professor Ken Fleming. **(D)** A patient who received mediastinal radiation for oesophageal carcinoma. At laparotomy, marked hepatic induration was confined to the left lobe. This lesion involves an hepatic vein 0.6 mm in diameter. Elastic trichrome. Courtesy of Dr Michele Weir.

been seen in some patients with VOD after irradiation[255] and peliosis hepatis has been reported in renal transplant recipients with VOD.[256]

After high-dose drug therapy, the lesions may develop within days of intensive therapy so that the veins are not fibrotic and the importance of the venous injury may not be recognized amid the intense haemorrhage.[257] Dacarbazine has been associated with acute thrombosis of small and medium-sized hepatic veins. Reaction to this drug may have an allergic component, as it typically occurs shortly after beginning the second course of therapy and is associated with eosinophils in portal tracts and hepatic vein walls and peripheral blood eosinophilia.[257]

Differential diagnosis

If the vascular lesions are missed on needle biopsy, marked congestion of sinusoids suggests VOD if the history is appropriate, with a differential diagnosis of constrictive pericarditis,[194] congestive heart failure, hepatic vein thrombosis, shock necrosis, and acetaminophen toxicity. In VOD,

secondary thrombosis may propagate to involve the large hepatic veins.[240] Conversely, thrombosis of large hepatic veins is often accompanied by fibrous obliteration of small hepatic veins with an appearance identical to VOD.[224,232] Thus, occasional patients are difficult to classify histologically.

Fibrous obliteration of small hepatic veins is frequently found in alcoholic and non-alcoholic cirrhosis.[277–279] In cirrhosis, the obliterated veins are usually incorporated into fibrous septa so that VOD-like lesions may not be recognized.

Hepatic vein phlebitis

Phlebitis is most often seen in acute[280] and chronic hepatitis, especially viral and autoimmune types,[181] steatohepatitis,[281] sarcoidosis (Fig. 13.11),[227,282] idiopathic granulomatous vasculitis (Fig. 13.12),[140,283] and virus-associated haemophagocytic syndrome.[284] Phlebitis and venous obstruction within regions of bacterial infection causes the ischaemic necrosis at the core of abscesses (Fig. 13.13).

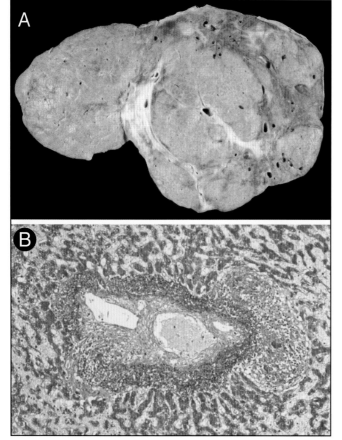

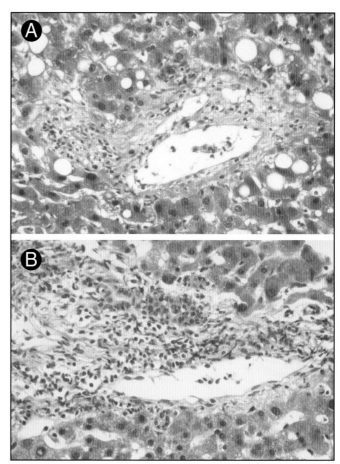

Fig. 13.11 • Sarcoidosis. **(A)** Vascular involvement is patchy causing an irregular distribution of parenchymal extinction. In this example most lesions are in the right lobe. Regeneration has caused a large perihilar nodule. **(B)** An hepatic vein with granulomas involving intima, media, and adventitia. Elastic trichrome. From Moreno-Merlo et al.[145]

Fig. 13.13 • Phlebitis adjacent to an abscess 3 cm in diameter. **(A)** Hepatic vein. **(B)** Portal vein. Masson's trichrome.

Congestive hepatic venopathy

This newly described lesion embodies a novel mechanism whereby subendothelial haemorrhage leads to obliterative hepatic venopathy. This mechanism explains the parenchymal extinction and fibrous septation that occurs in schistosomiasis, idiopathic portal hypertension, and adjacent to tumours (Fig. 13.14).[182] It also provides an alterative mechanism, in addition to thrombosis, for the development of regional parenchymal extinction in congestive heart failure[148] and severe cirrhosis.[111]

Sinusoids

Normal sinusoidal structure

Sinusoids are lined by modified endothelial cells containing fenestrations, 50–300 nm in diameter, which allow passage of lipoproteins and other large molecules but provide a barrier to blood cells (Chapter 1). The fenestrations are dynamic, responding to pharmacologic agents, pressure, and the quality of matrix in the space of Disse.[288,289] Sinusoidal endothelial cells have numerous bristle-coated pits, pinocytotic vacuoles, and absent Weibel–Palade bodies.[290] Kupffer cells reside in the lumen and are anchored to the underlying sinusoidal wall. Natural killer cells

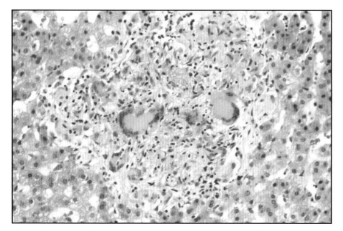

Fig. 13.12 • Granulomatous phlebitis with obliteration of an hepatic venule. Portal veins were also involved. The patient was a young man with vasculitic rash and hepatomegaly. H&E.

Prolapse of hepatocytes into hepatic venules was first described as an apparent response to testosterone therapy[285] but was subsequently described in idiopathic portal hypertension, incomplete cirrhosis, and regressing cirrhosis.[286,287] This prolapse is the healed state of obliterative venopathy involving terminal hepatic venules.[287]

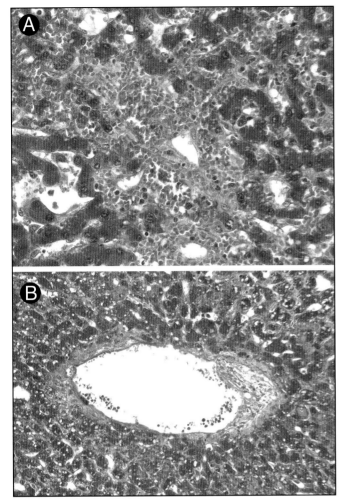

Fig. 13.14 • Congestive hepatic venopathy is a response to haemodynamic stress such as outflow block or hyperperfusion. These examples are in congested parenchyma adjacent to a tumour. There is marked intimal haemorrhage **(A)** and intimal fibrosis **(B)** as well as congestive sinusoidal injury with hepatocellular atrophy and dropout.

(pit cells) and mast cells may also be found in small numbers within the space of Disse.

Sinusoidal endothelial cells differ from venous and arterial endothelial cells in expressing a variety of markers, including CD32 and CD16 (receptors for the Fc fragment of IgG), aminopeptidase N, CD14, CD32, CD4, and CD54 (intercellular adhesion molecule-1, ICAM-1).[291] Other markers are absent, including laminin, factor VIII-related antigen, *Ulex europaeus agglutinin* I lectin, CD31 (platelet endothelial cell adhesion molecule-1; PECAM-1), CD34, CD62P (P-selectin), CD55 (decay-accelerating factor), and 1F10.[5,290] Normally there is almost no basement membrane, laminin, or collagen in the space of Disse.[292,293] Tenascin and fibronectin are normally present. In cirrhosis and other fibrotic states, collagen type IV and laminin are deposited in the spaces of Disse.[290,294,295] Sinusoidal endothelial expression of CD34 and CD31 is an indicator of angiogenesis seen focally in cirrhosis,[287,294,296] focal nodular hyperplasia,[297] and dysplastic nodules,[298] and more diffusely in hepatocellular carcinoma.[298] The expression of chemotactic cytokines on venous and sinusoidal endothelial cells may determine the pattern of inflammatory cell infiltration in various liver diseases.[299]

Stellate cells are found in the space of Disse. At rest, these cells contain 95% of the hepatic vitamin A.[300] Stellate cells are specialized fibroblasts which produce collagen in response to liver injury (Chapter 2). They have cytoplasmic processes that embrace the sinusoids and, when activated by endothelin-1 or other agonists, can contract to alter sinusoidal blood flow.[301,302]

Pericellular fibrosis

In alcoholic cirrhosis and in alcoholic liver disease with mild pericellular fibrosis there is a decrease in sinusoidal fenestrations, deposition of subendothelial basement membrane and collagen, loss of hepatocellular microvilli, increased expression of endothelial factor VIII, and binding of *Ulex europaeus agglutinin* I (UEA I) lectin to endothelial cells.[102,219,296,303] These findings are typical of arteries, veins, and non-hepatic capillaries and have been called *capillarization*.[294,304] Permeability of the sinusoidal wall may be significantly impaired by these changes.[305] Linear sinusoidal deposition of IgA is found in most biopsies from alcoholics and diabetics, and to a lesser degree in other diseases and in normal controls.[306] Sinusoidal binding of UEAI lectin or increased expression of factor VIII, CD31, and CD34 may be useful findings when small biopsies are otherwise not diagnostic of cirrhosis.[294,296] Pericellular fibrosis is delicate and often transient, being resorbed after cessation of the injury or compacted into septa if intervening hepatocytes are lost.[287]

Pericellular fibrosis is commonly seen in alcoholic liver disease, steatohepatitis of obesity and diabetes type II (non-alcoholic steatohepatitis; NASH),[307–309] chronic passive congestion, Budd–Chiari syndrome, diabetes mellitus type I,[293] Gaucher disease, congenital syphilis, vitamin A toxicity,[310,311] and mastocytosis.[81] Patients with idiopathic thrombocytopenic purpura or agnogenic myeloid metaplasia may have diffuse sinusoidal fibrosis, possibly caused by sinusoidal release of platelet-derived growth factor (Fig. 13.15).[312,313] Pericellular fibrosis can be seen in any cirrhotic liver, especially adjacent to portal tracts and septa, as part of the hepatic repair complex.[287] This represents residual collagen after resorption and remodelling of septa.

Congestive sinusoidal injury

Injury to the sinusoidal endothelium occurs in cirrhosis, hepatic vein outflow block, adjacent to neoplasms, and in small-for-size grafts (Fig. 13.14).[182] These are situations where there is imbalance of inflow and outflow in the sinusoidal microcirculation.

After transplantation, small grafts less than 30% of ideal liver weight often develop the small-for-size syndrome characterized by delayed function, cholestasis, and ascites.[314] These grafts have parenchymal haemorrhage and hepatocellular vacuolization. By electron microscopy there may be mitochondrial swelling and gaps between sinusoidal endothelial cells.[315] The lesion is a sinusoidal endothelial injury related to excessive portal vein flow with accompanying portal hypertension and shear stress. Lesions are

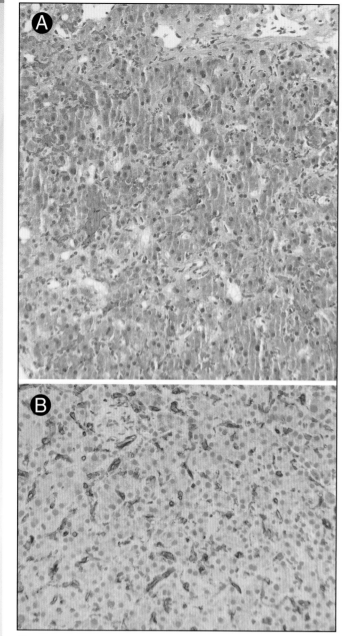

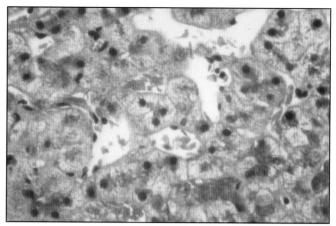

Fig. 13.16 • Sickle cell disease. Sinusoids are dilated and contain sickled red cells. There is slight sinusoidal fibrosis. Masson's trichrome.

Fig. 13.15 • Diffuse sinusoidal fibrosis. (A) This patient with idiopathic thrombocytopenic purpura developed ascites without cirrhosis (confirmed by subsequent autopsy). Masson's trichrome. (B) The fibrosis is accompanied by marked CD34 positivity of the sinusoidal endothelium.

ameliorated by shunt procedures designed to decrease portal vein pressure.[314,316,317]

Sinusoidal dilatation

Sinusoidal dilatation occurs when there is increased pressure in the hepatic veins or atrophy of hepatocytes, or disruption of the sinusoidal reticulin fibres. Frequent causes of sinusoidal dilatation are those diseases with outflow obstruction, including cardiac failure, constrictive pericarditis, hepatic vein thrombosis, and in severe cirrhosis. Erythrocytes may extravasate into the space of Disse and between hepatocytes.[225,318] Hyaline globules may be seen in zone 3 hepatocytes, typically in the presence of ischaemia

and cardiac failure.[319,320] Portal vein obstruction is another cause, as seen adjacent to neoplasms, in Zahn infarcts, and in nodular regenerative hyperplasia.

Sinusoidal dilatation after oral contraceptive therapy or in pregnancy usually occurs in zones 1 and 2.[321,322] It may be caused by angiogenesis with increased numbers of small arteries in portal tracts. Mild sinusoidal fibrosis, usually only seen by electron microscopy, has been reported in these conditions.[322,323]

In sickle cell disease there is often a mild elevation of aminotransferases, chronic cholestasis or, rarely, progressive hepatic failure.[324] Hepatic dysfunction does not appear to correlate temporally with crisis involving other organs.[325,326] Biopsies demonstrate sinusoids packed with sickled red cells and erythrophagocytosis (Fig. 13.16). Pericellular fibrosis is occasionally prominent.

Sinusoidal dilatation may also be seen as a result of nonspecific malnutrition in wasting illnesses such as malignancy, tuberculosis, and AIDS[327,328] and as a paraneoplastic lesion associated with renal cell carcinoma[329,330] and Hodgkin disease.[331] Sinusoidal dilatation induced by steroids and wasting illnesses may be a precursor to peliosis hepatis.

Peliosis hepatis

Peliosis is defined as cystic blood-filled spaces in the liver, spleen, lymph nodes, and other organs (Fig. 13.17).[332] Although the term was originally applied to macroscopic lesions (peliosis = dusky or purple), microscopic lesions are now often called peliosis. Microscopic peliosis hepatis is often confused with extreme sinusoidal dilatation or with 'evacuation of the liver cell plates', a lesion seen after zonal hepatocellular dropout but without loss of the normal reticulin fibres. To be called peliosis hepatis, lesions should have evidence of rupture of these fibres (Fig. 13.17E). Rupture may follow intrinsic weakness of the fibres of the wall (phlebectatic type) or may accompany focal hepatocyte necrosis (parenchymal type).[333,334] Initially, the spaces may have no endothelial lining, but re-endothelialization probably occurs rapidly. Thus, classification of lesions on the

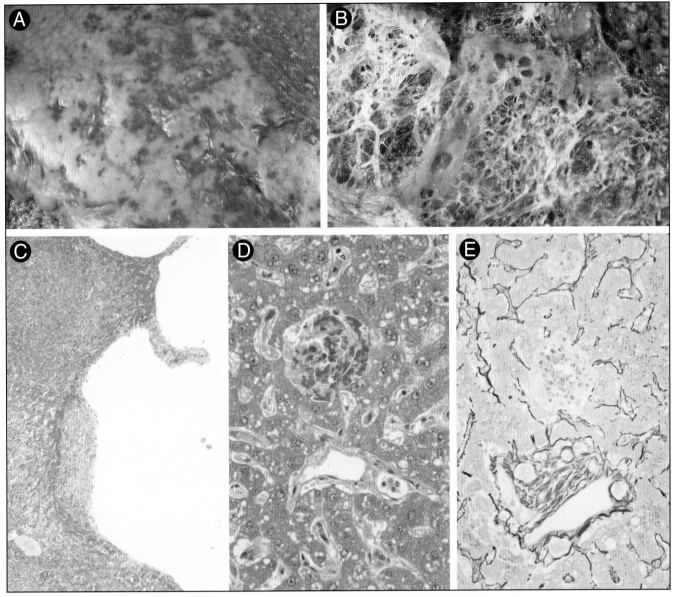

Fig. 13.17 • Peliosis hepatis, major and minor types. **(A–C)** This patient was a 30-year-old woman who had progressive enlargement on ultrasonography of mass lesions over 2 years. **(A)** The capsular surface shows multiple dark cavities. **(B)** On cut section the cavities are seen to range from minute to many centimetres in diameter. **(C)** The portal tracts protrude into the cavities, having been denuded of sinusoidal parenchyma. The interface of cavity and parenchyma shows absence of a fibrous wall. Masson's trichrome. (Details of this case have been published.)[583] **(D and E)** Minor peliosis in a patient who received chemotherapy for a malignant thymoma. This lesion, an incidental finding at autopsy, was not visible grossly. Reticulin stain shows lysis of reticulin fibres. Parallel sections, Masson's trichrome and reticulin.

basis of the presence or absence of endothelium is not warranted.[335] The lesions are randomly distributed without zonal preference.

It is appropriate to classify the lesions according to the apparent aetiology as this correlates with distinctive histological and clinical features. Macroscopic lesions are usually induced by anabolic, oestrogenic, or adrenocortical steroids and are often associated with splenic peliosis. Macroscopic peliosis hepatis has also been reported with a variety of chronic diseases such as malnutrition,[336] leukaemia,[337] tuberculosis,[332] leprosy,[338] vasculitis,[339] and AIDS.[340] Microscopic lesions occur in patients receiving thiopurines for renal transplantation, liver transplantation, or various malignancies.[341-343] Other associated drugs are listed in Table 13.3. and are considered in Chapter 14.

Peliotic lesions found in AIDS and other immunosuppressed patients are caused by rickettsial organisms (*Bartonella* species).[344-347] These lesions have a myxoid stroma which has a bluish haze on haematoxylin and eosin staining and contains clumps of organisms which stain with the Warthin–Starry technique. Patients often have peliosis of the spleen and lymph nodes and cutaneous angiomatous lesions. Hepatosplenomegaly and increased alkaline phosphatase are usually present and respond to antibiotics. This lesion should be distinguished from sinusoidal dilatation and Kaposi sarcoma, which also occur in AIDS.[328]

In hairy cell leukaemia, peliosis of liver and spleen may be the result of sinusoidal wall injury induced by tumour cells.[337] The unusual sinusoidal distribution of these cells is determined by the presence of vascular cell adhesion molecule-1 (VCAM-1) receptors on hepatic and splenic endothelium.[348] Peliosis hepatis also occurs within neoplasms such as adenoma and hepatocellular carcinoma. Peliosis hepatis of minor degree has rarely been associated with Hodgkin disease,[349] angioimmunoblastic lymphadenopathy,[350] myeloproliferative disorders,[351] and Waldenstrom's macroglobulinaemia with light chain deposition.[352]

Peliotic cysts lined by dysplastic or frankly malignant endothelial cells are seen in association with angiosarcoma. Livers with angiosarcoma also may have portal fibrosis and poorly-formed nodules of hepatocytes.[147] These nodules have been considered to be the result of hepatocellular dysplasia but may be nodular hyperplasia secondary to portal vascular obliteration.

Although peliosis hepatis is usually of no clinical significance, macroscopic peliosis of liver or spleen may rupture spontaneously or after trauma.[353,354] The lesions may be also be associated with cholestasis,[336,341] hepatic failure,[336,344] and, rarely, portal hypertension.[355]

Toxic microvascular injury

Drugs, alkalating agents and radiation may cause a variety of histological lesions involving the microvasculature (Table 13.3; and Chapter 14). These lesions include veno-occlusive disease, sinusoidal fibrosis, peliosis hepatis, obliterative portal venopathy, and nodular regenerative hyperplasia. Some patients have presented with portal hypertension.[356,357] Although patients are categorized according to the dominant clinical or histological finding, several lesions often occur together.[341,358] The dominant lesion appears to depend on host factors and drug dosage as well as the particular agent. The lesions are more common when the drugs are used in antineoplastic regimens than with lower immunosuppressive doses. High dose therapy tends to give acute or subacute VOD while low-dose therapy gives chronic lesions of VOD, non-cirrhotic portal hypertension, nodular regenerative hyperplasia, or sinusoidal fibrosis. Patients with cirrhosis and hepatocellular carcinoma who are radiated with ^{90}Yttrium beads often develop liver failure[266] and exhibit congestive changes on biopsy.[359]

Other sinusoidal lesions

Hepatic amyloidosis (see Chapter 17) is characterized by deposits within vessel walls, portal stroma, and spaces of Disse.[360] Diffuse sinusoidal wall thickening may be so marked as to cause atrophy and disappearance of hepatocytes. Rarely, one may see only small sinusoidal nodules of amyloid.[361] In AA disease, amyloid is found in portal vessels in 90% and sinusoids in 37%. In AL disease, deposits are found in portal vessels in 87% and in sinusoids in 75%.[360,362] Diffuse deposition causes hepatomegaly, cholestasis,[363] and, rarely, portal hypertension.[84]

Light chain disease may be associated with cholestasis and deposition of light chains in sinusoids and portal tracts. The deposits are PAS positive and may also be congophilic.[364]

Infiltration of sinusoids by cells may be of diagnostic value, but rarely causes clinical effects unless it is massive.[365]

Lymphoid infiltration is seen in viral and autoimmune hepatitis, phenytoin (and other) hepatotoxicity (see Chapter 14), allograft rejection, leukaemia, and lymphoma. Hairy cells may be demonstrated with B-cell markers, vimentin, and tartrate-resistant acid phosphatase.[366] Extramedullary haematopoiesis is seen in myeloproliferative disorders.[367] Characteristic cells are seen in *mastocytosis, Gaucher disease,* and metastatic infiltration by tumours. Mast cells may be demonstrated with tryptase and CD68.[368] Primary angioformative tumours (haemangiosarcoma and epithelioid haemangioendothelioma) characteristically grow along the sinusoidal wall replacing the original endothelium and causing hepatocellular atrophy and peliosis hepatis.

In disseminated intravascular coagulation and eclampsia, fibrin deposits may be seen in small portal veins, the media or lumen of arterioles, and sinusoids. Sinusoidal fibrin and secondary necrosis are most prominent in zone 1. When this lesion is severe, widespread infarction and rupture of the liver may occur. Sinusoidal microthrombi have been noted in the antiphospholipid syndrome.[369]

Ischaemic injury of the sinusoidal endothelial cells of the allograft is commonly seen immediately after liver transplantation and may be important in some cases of early graft dysfunction.[370,371] The endothelial cells are rounded up and may either recover or detach.

Arteries

Normal variations and congenital anomalies

Unlike the portal and hepatic veins, the hepatic artery exhibits considerable anatomical variation (Fig. 13.18) (Chapter 4) which may lead to inadvertent ligation with secondary duct strictures or allograft failure.[20,372–375] A variety of vascular anomalies may be found in the liver with diverse clinical presentations. Abnormal origin of the hepatic artery is frequent with biliary atresia.[22] Arteriovenous malformations of the spleen or liver may cause high portal blood flow and portal hypertension[53,85,376] and are discussed with portal vein disease. Intrahepatic arteriovenous fistulae in Osler–Weber–Rendu disease may be associated with high output cardiac failure, portal or pulmonary hypertension, and ascites.[377,378]

Diseases of hepatic arteries

The hepatic artery is susceptible to diseases found in other arteries. Atherosclerosis, hyaline arteriosclerosis, thrombotic and atheromatous embolism, transplant arteriopathy,[379] cryoglobulinaemia, monoclonal gammopathies, and amyloidosis may involve hepatic arteries but are rarely of clinical significance. Arterial injury may occur with polyarteritis nodosa, Takayasu arteritis, rheumatoid arteritis,[380] septic embolus, tuberculosis, syphilis, local infection, pancreatitis, or trauma. The histological appearance of these lesions is the same as in other organs. For example, temporal arteritis may be associated with giant cell arteritis in the liver.[149] Complications of arteritis or traumatic arterial

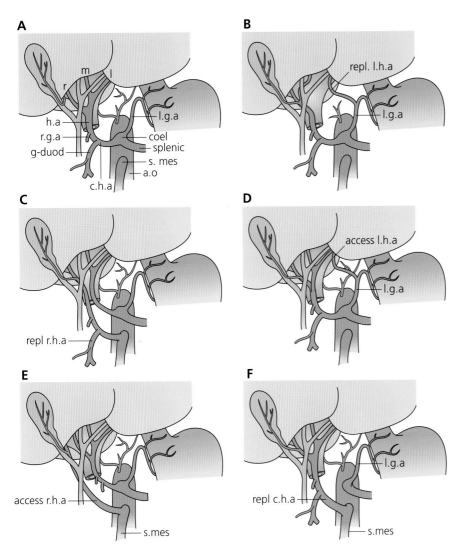

Fig. 13.18 • Variations in hepatic arterial blood supply and collaterals, after Michels[372] and Netter.[584] Abbreviations as follows: ha = hepatic artery; cha, rha, mha, lha = common, right, middle and left hepatic artery; rga, lga = right and left gastric artery; g-duod = gastroduodenal artery; ao = aorta; s.mes = superior mesenteric artery; coel = coeliac axis. (A) Most common patterns of arterial supply; 55% of dissections. (B) Replaced (repl) left hepatic artery; 10%. (C) Replaced right hepatic artery; 11%. (D) Accessory (access) left hepatic artery originating from left gastric artery; 8%. (E) Accessory right hepatic artery originating from superior mesenteric artery; 7%. (F) Replaced common hepatic artery; 2.5%.

lesions include aneurysmal dilatation, arterial rupture, arteriovenous fistula,[58,381] infarction, and various biliary lesions. Aneurysms most commonly involve the extrahepatic arteries.[382] Antiphospholipid syndrome may include hepatic artery thrombosis.[383] Arteritis involving small arteries and arterioles is easily missed and may heal without a trace of the original vessel.[133] Such lesions may cause fibrosis in small portal tracts with obliteration of adjacent portal veins and ducts.

Large and small bile ducts depend on arterial supply.[4,384] Small duct ischaemic disease has been reported after leukocytoclastic vasculitis,[385] Henoch–Schönlein purpura,[386] and Kawasaki disease.[387] Large duct ischaemic injury has been reported with polyarteritis, intra-arterial injection of alcohol or chemotherapeutic agents,[388,389] abdominal radiation,[390] laparoscopic cholecystectomy, and after liver transplantation.[391] Biliary injury of probable ischaemic origin has been associated with lupus anticoagulant and paroxysmal nocturnal haemoglobinuria.[392–394] The cholangiopathy of cytomegalovirus infection may have an ischaemic component.[395,396]

The biliary lesions may include stricture, cysts, rupture of bile duct or gallbladder, hydrops of the gallbladder, and hepatic artery–biliary fistula leading to haemobilia.[397–400]

After transplantation, hepatic artery thrombosis (HAT) may lead to necrosis of the biliary tree and present with progressive cholestasis, bile leak, hepatic abscesses, and loss of the graft. Some cases have mild cholestasis and hydropic ischaemic changes without progressive graft dysfunction.[401] Although usually evident within a few weeks of implantation, HAT may occur months or years later.[402,403] Risk factors for HAT include arterial anomalies requiring repair or conduits, advanced donor age, and, recipient history of smoking or postoperative CMV infection.[404]

Since the advent of percutaneous biliary drainage procedures several complications have become frequent clinical events. These include arteriovenous fistula, pseudoaneurysm, and portobiliary fistula with secondary peritoneal haemorrhage or haemobilia.[381,405] Percutaneous drainage tracts are lined by granulation tissue, usually with cytolysis secondary to direct bile exposure and organized thrombi in adjacent portal veins. Veins draining arteriovenous fistula are susceptible to secondary thrombosis.[58]

Acute hepatic ischaemia

Ischaemic necrosis may have a generalized zone 3 distribution or the circumscribed geographic pattern of an infarct, in which there is involvement of at least two contiguous acini.[406] The parenchyma is protected against ischaemia by its double blood supply. Most individuals can tolerate hepatic artery ligation without infarction.[407] Large infarcts are usually accompanied by obstruction of both artery and portal vein, but in 20% of cases there is portal vein thrombosis alone, and in 40% there is no identifiable vascular lesion (Fig. 13.19).[398,406,408] Infarcts also occur with combined portal and hepatic vein thrombosis[227] and combined hepatic artery and portal vein thrombosis.[383]

Zone 3 necrosis is much more common than infarction. The former occurs after shock[409] when arterial flow and portal vein oxygen saturation are decreased simultaneously. Although hepatic necrosis in shock is usually a zone 3 lesion, zone 2 may rarely be the site of maximum necrosis.[410] A polymorphonuclear infiltrate may be prominent in the healing phase, followed by perivenular fibrosis. Calcification of hepatocytes may occur early or late.[411] Coexistent atrophy of zone 3 hepatocytes suggests chronic right heart failure.[409] Zone 3 ischaemic necrosis may be very difficult to distinguish from toxic injury caused by acetaminophen or cocaine.[412]

The cirrhotic liver is susceptible to ischaemia because portal flow is impeded and the parenchyma is largely dependent on arterial flow. Marked transaminase elevation commonly occurs after variceal haemorrhage or other cause of hypotension.

Infarction in pregnancy may arise because of one or more events related to eclampsia, disseminated intravascular coagulation, hypovolaemic shock, or thrombosis of the hepatic artery, portal vein, or hepatic veins.[413] Antiphopholipid antibodies and HELLP syndrome are both associated with infarction in pregnancy.[414] In pre-eclampsia and eclampsia there may be fibrinoid necrosis of arteries in many organs (see Chapter 17).

Ischaemia occurring in the hepatic allograft is discussed in Chapter 16.

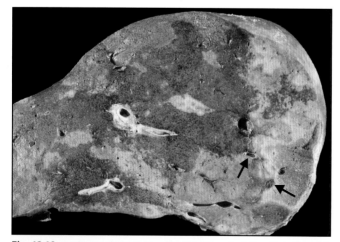

Fig. 13.19 • Multiple infarcts 8 days after liver transplantation. Note thrombi in a portal vein (left arrow) and hepatic vein (right arrow).

Parenchymal response to vascular obstruction—the two hit model

Vascular obstruction causes ischaemic changes characterized by either atrophy or parenchymal extinction.[415] Atrophy is recognized by a region with decreased hepatocyte size with little or no parenchymal fibrosis. Extinction is the loss of contiguous hepatocytes, usually with fibrosis of the parenchymal stroma.[111,181] These two responses are possible because the dual blood supply allows for two levels of ischaemia. Simple portal vein block leads to atrophy. If both the portal vein and the artery, or, more commonly, both the portal vein and the hepatic vein are obstructed, these two 'hits' cause contiguous hepatocytes in a region to die, leading to extinction. If hepatic veins alone are obstructed, as in Budd–Chiari syndrome and veno-occlusive disease, some zone 3 extinction occurs but zone 1 parenchyma often survives because drainage may be secured by local retrograde flow of arterial blood into patent portal veins (Fig. 13.7C).[227]

After atrophy or extinction, secondary hepatocellular hyperplasia occurs, often with the formation of well-defined regions of parenchyma called regenerative nodules.[416] If regenerative nodules are delimited by adjacent fibrous septa, they are called cirrhotic nodules. If nodules are delimited by atrophy, the lesion is called nodular hyperplasia (see below).[416] Hyperplasia and regenerative nodules occur in regions of parenchyma that have adequate arterial or portal venous supply, venous drainage, and bile drainage. The blood supply may be derived from residual patent portal veins or from dilatation and growth of arteries. When atrophy or extinction are multifocal and widespread, prototypic lesions are seen: the combination of atrophy and hyperplasia is called nodular regenerative hyperplasia; the combination of extinction and hyperplasia is called cirrhosis. All anatomical forms of chronic liver disease can be produced by vascular obstructive lesions in various combinations and distributions.[415]

Vascular lesions in cirrhosis

Hepatocellular necrosis precedes the development of cirrhosis. However, necrosis per se is not sufficient, as rapid regeneration allows restitution of normal liver architecture.[417] A single attack of acute hepatitis may lead to extinction and cirrhosis if there is sufficient obliteration of the vasculature.[418] Chronic hepatitis is the most frequent histological lesion leading to cirrhosis. A major paradox is that hepatocellular injury in chronic hepatitis is fairly uniform but the fibrotic lesions are focal, being confined to septa. This transition from diffuse activity to focal fibrosis is achieved by the chance obliteration of veins and/or sinusoids (Fig. 13.20).[415]

The development of extinction in chronic hepatitis may be recognized as bridging necrosis in very active cases, and as clusters of apoptotic and atrophic hepatocytes in less active cases.[169] After extinction lesions are organized, they may be recognized as septa or as short broad fibrous adhesions between hepatic veins and portal tracts (Fig. 13.20).[287]

The mechanism of vascular obstruction depends on the nature of the primary disease. In most forms of hepatitis, portal and hepatic vein phlebitis occurs as a bystander effect of inflammation in tissue adjacent to the veins. In Budd–Chiari syndrome and chronic congestive failure, thrombosis is the cause of the vascular obliteration.[148,227] Granulomatous phlebitis is important in sarcoidosis.[145] In chronic biliary disease, bile salt injury is the apparent cause of hepatic vein obliteration.[419]

Secondary venous obstruction in cirrhosis

In established cirrhosis, stasis commonly leads to secondary obstruction of portal and hepatic veins by congestive venopathy and/or thrombosis (Figure 13.21).[111,420] This obstruction causes a focal worsening of fibrosis and hepatocyte loss, known as focal (or regional) parenchymal extinction[111] or confluent hepatic fibrosis.[421] Portal vein thrombosis is an important complication leading to worsening of portal hypertension or hepatic failure.

Vascular shunts in cirrhosis

As cirrhosis develops, necrotic parenchyma is replaced with scar tissue containing vascular channels that shunt blood from the portal venous circulation to the systemic venous circulation (Fig. 13.20B6).[422,423] Other shunts develop between arteries and portal veins and between arteries and hepatic veins.[424] Although most intrahepatic portosystemic shunts are microscopic, approximately a quarter of cirrhotic patients have 1–2 mm diameter shunts visible on transhepatic portography.[425] Shunts have been demonstrated by Doppler ultrasonography examination.[67] Large shunts between portal veins and hepatic veins or inferior vena cava may rarely develop spontaneously. The associated encephalopathy may respond to embolization therapy.[43,426] Spontaneous splenorenal shunts also occur in patients with cirrhosis or portal vein block.[427,428] Intrahepatic venous shunts are often prominent in Budd–Chiari syndrome.[420,429] Dilated paraumbilical veins form significant collaterals in 11–25% of patients with portal hypertension,[430–432] explaining periumbilical bruits and the rare caput medusa. Retrograde portal vein flow may be a result of arterioportal shunts.[433–436]

Intrapulmonary shunts occur in approximately 20% of patients with cirrhosis or non-cirrhotic portal hypertension,[437–439] often in association with finger clubbing and hypoxia. Severe hypoxia is becoming a frequent indication for liver transplantation. The mechanism of the shunts is not certain but they are probably a pulmonary manifestation of the generalized vasodilation found in patients with portal hypertension (see Chapter 2). Pulmonary hypertension occurs in 2% of patients with portal hypertension, with or without cirrhosis.[440,441] The pulmonary lesion is plexogenic arteriopathy, thought to be the result of spasm-induced arterial necrosis which occurs in certain

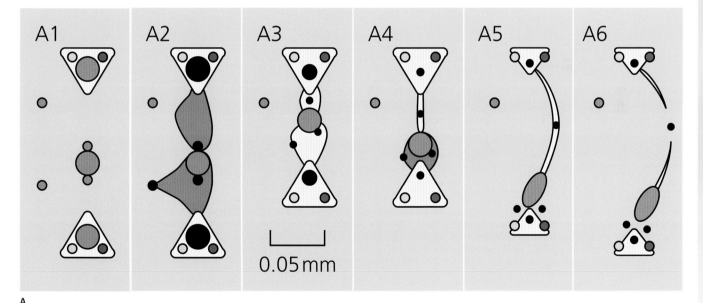

A

Fig. 13.20 • Tissue remodelling in cirrhosis. Events occurring during the development and regression of cirrhosis are depicted in the diagram (A) and are illustrated with photomicrographs in (B). (A1) Two normal acini. (A2) Obliteration of small portal and hepatic veins occurs early in the development of cirrhosis in response to local inflammatory damage. The supplied parenchyma becomes ischaemic. The size of the ischaemic region may be smaller than an acinus when obstruction is mostly at the sinusoidal level. (A3) Ischaemic parenchyma disappears with fibrosis and approximation of adjacent vascular structures. This approximation can be seen as venoportal adhesions (B1) and ectopic hepatic veins (B2). (A4) Fibrous septa develop in regions of extinction and in regions of sinusoidal fibrosis that undergo subsequent collapse. Sinusoidal fibrosis is thought to occur in advance of parenchymal collapse in certain diseases, especially in alcoholic disease (not shown but discussed elsewhere[415]). (A5) Septa are deformed and stretched by expansion of regenerating hepatocytes (B3). (A6) As septa are resorbed one sees perforation, thinning, and disappearance (B3). Trapped structures are released and are recognizable as remnants (B4 and B5). From Wanless et al.[287]

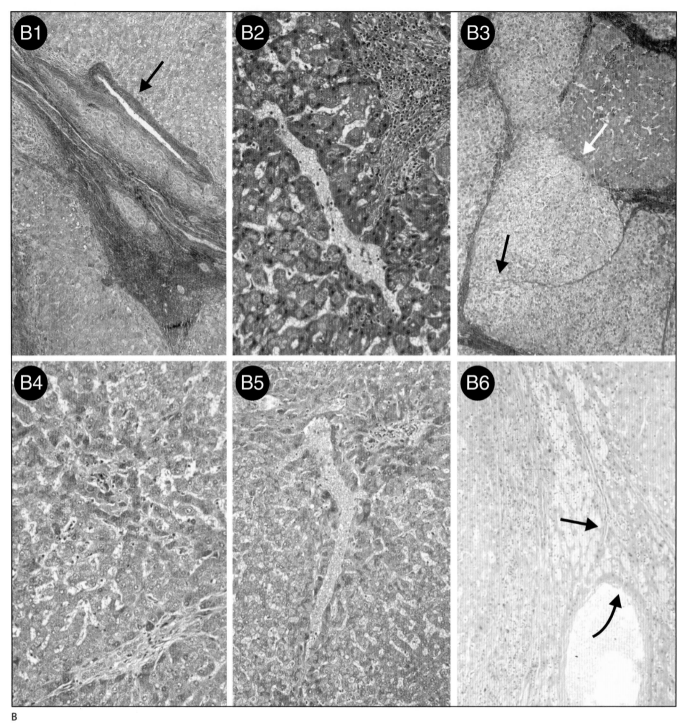

B

Fig. 13.20 • cont'd (B) Inactive cirrhosis, various livers. (B1) Venoportal adhesion. A medium hepatic vein (arrow) is tightly adherent to the adjacent portal tract. (B2) An 'ectopic' small hepatic vein approximated to a portal tract with a delicate septum. (B3) Several delicate septa with perforation (black arrow) and nearly total resorption (white arrow). (B4) Remnants of a portal tract and hepatic vein. Portal tract remnants usually lack portal veins (bottom) and hepatic vein remnants form rings of collagen (top), usually with migration of hepatocytes into the former lumina. (B5) Hepatic vein containing 'prolapsed' hepatocytes. (B6) A–V shunt in a region of telangiectasis. The artery (straight arrow) drains into dilated sinusoids and blood apparently then drains into the hepatic vein (curved arrow). B1–B5 Elastic trichrome, B6 H&E.

individuals in response to increased pulmonary blood flow (and pressure).[442] The mechanism of the pulmonary arterial constriction is uncertain but may be related to high levels of endothelin-1, impaired nitric oxide production, or decreased response to nitric oxide. Patients with hepatic schistosomiasis may develop pulmonary hypertension because of embolism of schistosoma ova through hepatic shunts to the lungs.[443]

Transjugular intrahepatic portosystemic shunts (TIPS)

Insertion of a metallic shunt between a large hepatic vein and a large portal vein is frequently performed to

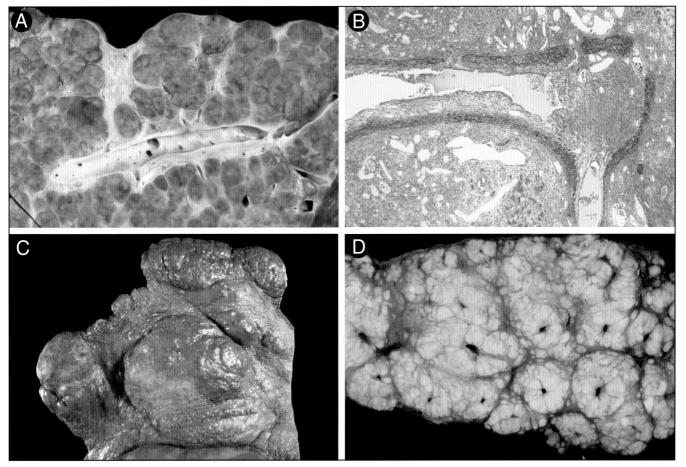

Fig. 13.21 • Regional parenchymal extinction in cirrhosis. **(A)** Small region of extinction is associated with obliteration of a medium hepatic vein. **(B)** Intimal fibrosis in a medium hepatic vein within a region of extinction. The irregular appearance in this example suggests post-thrombotic scar. Elastic trichrome. **(C)** Multiple large regions of extinction cause marked distortion of a lobe. **(D)** After widespread small and medium hepatic vein obliteration, regeneration is most dependent on the available hepatic vein drainage. The best drainage is close to the hepatic vein trunk, giving nodules or cylinders of regenerating tissue with the hepatic vein trunk at their cores. (a–c from Wanless et al.[111])

ameliorate portal hypertension. The wire mesh becomes covered with a pseudointima, usually beginning in the mid-portion and reaching completion within several weeks.[444–446] The endothelial cells have a phenotype similar to that of normal sinusoidal endothelial cells.[447] Complications include early thrombosis and late stenosis from fibromuscular hyperplasia. Thrombosis may predispose to fibromuscular hyperplasia.[445] Transection of a bile duct followed by bile-leak-induced thrombosis may initiate this sequence (Fig. 13.22).[448,449] Segmental ischaemic events, haematoma, and pseudoaneurysm may occur after the shunt procedure.[450–452]

Regression of cirrhosis

There is increasing evidence that cirrhosis is potentially reversible.[453–455] Within most cirrhotic livers, lesions indicative of regression can be found. These features are collectively called the *hepatic repair complex* (Fig. 13.20).[287] With time, septa become progressively more delicate and fragmented. Portal tracts and hepatic veins become separated from septa and appear as 'free' remnants in the parenchyma. Such portal tract remnants are recognized by the presence of arteries and ducts but there is usually no portal vein branch. Separated hepatic veins are often ectopic, being

located adjacent to portal tracts. Some hepatic vein remnants become filled with 'prolapsed' hepatocytes. Cirrhotic nodules enlarge by hepatocyte proliferation and by coalescence of adjacent nodules. The patterns seen, in sequence, are macronodular cirrhosis with delicate septa, incomplete septal cirrhosis, and nearly normal liver. If portal thrombosis had occurred in a cirrhotic liver that subsequently regressed, the end-stage of the liver would be non-cirrhotic portal hypertension, as seen with idiopathic portal hypertension.[161]

Nodular hyperplasia

Nodular hyperplasia refers to roughly spherical masses of hepatocytes demarcated by a transition to smaller hepatocytes rather than by fibrous septa. This lesion was formerly called nodular transformation. The nodules usually occur in one of two patterns, either small and widespread (diffuse) or large and few in number (focal).[150,228,416,456]

Diffuse nodular hyperplasia (nodular regenerative hyperplasia)

The term 'nodular regenerative hyperplasia' was originally applied to livers which had innumerable small nodules but

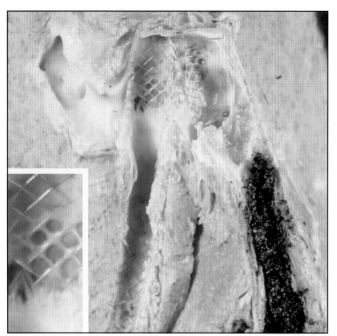

Fig. 13.22 • Cirrhotic liver with two transhepatic intrahepatic portosystemic shunts (TIPS). The first TIPS became obstructed (right) and a second was inserted (left). The first TIPS developed an intravenous bile leak that apparently caused a thrombotic obstruction. Biliary sludge has accumulated in the obstructed portion of the shunt. The inset shows a close-up of the left-hand shunt. Note regions of early and complete neointima formation.

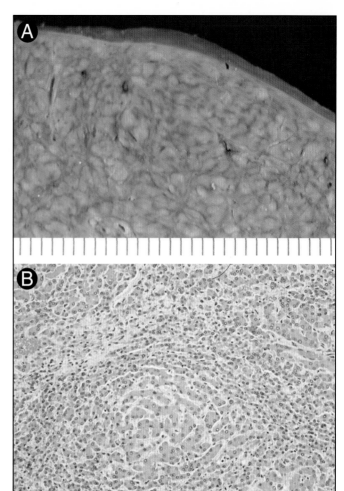

Fig. 13.23 • Nodular regenerative hyperplasia. The patient had acute polyarteritis nodosa in many organs (same patient as in Fig. 13.2a). **(A)** Most nodules are 1 mm in diameter, the size of a normal acinus. **(B)** Microscopic appearance with normal or atrophic cells in adjacent acini. H&E.

with minimal or no parenchymal fibrosis (Fig. 13.23).[150,236,456] The cells of the nodules are often arranged in double-cell plates surrounding a central portal supply. The nodules usually measure 1 mm in diameter but these may be accompanied by nodules up to several centimetres in diameter. The term 'diffuse nodular hyperplasia' is less specific and may be applied to livers with fibrous septa or cirrhosis. Nodular regenerative hyperplasia is invariably associated with obliteration of small portal veins[150] and occasionally small hepatic veins.[148,150,228] The pathogenesis is thought to be related to ischaemic atrophy with secondary nodular hyperplasia in regions with favourable blood flow.[150]

Nodular regenerative hyperplasia occurs in up to 5% of the elderly population, but with higher prevalence in patients with certain systemic disease that are associated with systemic vascular disease and local portal tract inflammation, such as polycythaemia, rheumatoid arthritis, and polyarteritis nodosa.[150,457] Symptomatic patients are usually discovered because of oesophageal varices, splenomegaly, or moderate elevation of alkaline phosphatase; ascites, when present, is usually mild.

Large regenerative nodules

In severely damaged livers regenerative nodules may develop in regions with favourable blood flow and adequate bile drainage.[458] The cause of the damage may be portal or hepatic vein thrombosis, massive necrosis, or cirrhosis. Large regions of hyperplasia with normal architecture represent segmental or lobar hyperplasia. Large regenerative nodules are distinctly larger than any nodules in surround-

ing tissues and generally measure at least 5 mm diameter. If most of the liver is composed of large cirrhotic nodules, the individual nodules would probably not receive scrutiny and macronodular cirrhosis would be an appropriate name.[416] Large regenerative nodules may account for many of the livers previously described under the term 'partial nodular transformation'.[150,459]

Large regenerative nodules are usually supplied by recognizable portal tracts. If there is prominent arterial branching, the lesions may resemble focal nodular hyperplasia or adenoma. Adenoma usually has no ductular elements, as shown by CK7 or CK19. However, there is a variant type of adenoma with ductular differentiation adjacent to the arterial supply.[460] Intense regenerative features, especially in Budd–Chiari syndrome, may lead to an erroneous diagnosis of hepatocellular carcinoma. Within cirrhotic livers, most nodules distinctly larger than background and measuring more than 8 mm are dysplastic nodules or carcinomas.

Lobar or segmental atrophy and hyperplasia

The term 'lobar atrophy' has been applied to the gross appearance of shrinkage of a lobe, usually without

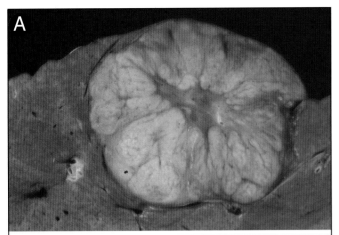

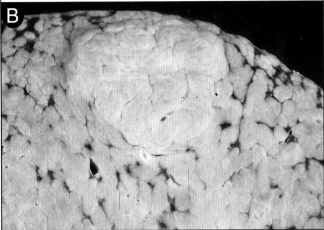

Fig. 13.24 • Focal nodular hyperplasia. **(A)** There is a characteristic central fibrous stalk region and radiating fibrous cords. The background liver appears to be normal. **(B)** Large regenerative nodules in Budd–Chiari syndrome are very similar to focal nodular hyperplasia.

consideration of the histological appearance. Severe tissue shrinkage occurs when there is hepatic vein obstruction with secondary parenchymal extinction and stromal fibrosis.[111] Portal vein obstruction causes much less tissue shrinkage with a decrease in size of hepatocytes and crowding of portal tracts (infarct of Zahn) but otherwise normal architecture.[169] Compensatory hyperplasia may expand whole lobes or segments, usually with a globular shape. Residual broad septation may produce deep capsular retraction that segments the liver, giving an appearance called *hepar lobatum*.[461] This is caused by metastatic breast carcinoma, Hodgkin disease, and syphilis. Shrinkage involving one or more lobes, usually the left, occurs in about 13% of cirrhotic livers, in 50% of livers with non-cirrhotic portal hypertension, and rarely in other conditions.[111,171,462]

Focal nodular hyperplasia

Focal nodular hyperplasia (FNH) is a localized region of hyperplasia within an otherwise normal, or nearly normal liver (Fig. 13.24).[297,463,464] The lesions typically have a central stellate fibrous region containing large arteries. Ducts are usually absent but a ductular reaction (ductular proliferation) may be prominent. The telangiectatic type of FNH has prominent dilatation of many intralesional sinusoids.[25] This

type has recently been shown to be monoclonal and therefore are better called 'variant adenomas'.[460,465] Variant forms without a central scar or ductules exist and are difficult to distinguish from adenomas and other types of large regenerative nodules.[464,466,467] FNH may be a hyperplastic response to an arteriovenous shunt or other local stimulus.[463,468–471]

Focal nodular hyperplasia occurs at all ages with a strong female predominance. Complications are uncommon. When lesions are multiple there is a high probability of associated lesions (multiple FNH syndrome), most commonly hepatic haemangiomas, meningiomas, astrocytoma, and arterial dysplasia in various organs.[25] FNH also occurs in hereditary haemorrhagic telangiectasia,[472] portal vein thrombosis,[473] congenital absence of the portal vein,[36,47,474] patent ductus venosus,[475,476] glycogen storage disease,[477,478] and rarely adjacent to various lesions including hydatid cyst,[479] haemangioma,[480] fibrolamellar carcinoma,[470,481,482] and epithelioid haemangioendothelioma.[483]

References

1. Ballet F. Hepatic circulation: potential for therapeutic intervention. Pharma Therapeutics, 1990; 47:281–328
2. Bomzon A, Blendis LM, eds. Cardiovascular complications of liver disease. Boca Raton: CRC Press, 1990
3. Okuda K, Benhamou JP, eds. Portal hypertension. Clinical and physiological aspects. Tokyo: Springer-Verlag, 1991
4. McCuskey RS. The hepatic microvascular system. In: Arias IM, Boyer JL, eds. The Liver: Biology and Pathobiology, 3rd edn. New York: Raven Press, 1994; pp. 1089–1106
5. Couvelard A, Scoazec JY, Dauge MC, Bringuier AF, Potet F, Feldmann G. Structural and functional differentiation of sinusoidal endothelial cells during liver organogenesis in humans. Blood, 1996; 87:4568–4580
6. Wanless IR. Physioanatomic considerations. In: Schiff L, Schiff ER, eds. Schiff's Diseases of the Liver, 10th edn. Philadelphia: JB Lippincott, 2006; (in press)
7. Child CG, III. The hepatic circulation and portal hypertension. Philadelphia: W.B. Saunders, 1954
8. Hunt AH. A contribution to the study of portal hypertension. Edinburgh: Livingstone, 1958
9. Marks C. The portal venous system. Springfield: C. C. Thomas, 1973
10. Rappaport AM, Wanless IR. Physioanatomic considerations. In: Schiff L, Schiff ER, eds. Diseases of the Liver, 7th edn. Philadelphia: JB Lippincott, 1993; pp. 1–41
11. Douglass BE, Baggenstoss AA, Hollinshead WH. The anatomy of the portal vein and its tributaries. Surg Gyn Obst, 1950; 91:562–576
12. Doust B, Pearce J. Gray-scale ultrasonic properties of the normal and inflamed pancreas. Radiology, 1976; 120:653–657
13. Elias H, Petty D. Gross anatomy of the blood vessels and ducts within the human liver. Am J Anat, 1952; 90:59–111
14. Strasberg SM. Terminology of liver anatomy and liver resections: coming to grips with hepatic Babel. J Am Coll Surg, 1997; 184:413–434
15. Couinaud C. The parabiliary venous system. Surg Radiol Anat, 1988; 10:311–316
16. Deneve E, Caty L, Fontaine C, Guillem P. Simultaneous aberrant left and right gastric veins draining directly into the liver. Ann Anat, 2003; 185:263–266
17. Shawker TH, Miller D. The persistent vitelline vein segment. Embryologic and ultrasound features. J Ultrasound Med, 1988; 7:681–685
18. Howard ER, Davenport M. Congenital extrahepatic portocaval shunts—the Abernethy malformation. J Pediatr Surg, 1997; 32:494–497
19. Yoshidome H, Edwards MJ. An embryological perspective on congenital portacaval shunt: a rare anomaly in a patient with hepatocellular carcinoma. Am J Gastroenterol, 1999; 94:2537–2539
20. Erbay N, Raptopoulos V, Pomfret EA, Kamel IR, Kruskal JB. Living donor liver transplantation in adults: vascular variants important

in surgical planning for donors and recipients. Am J Roentgenol, 2003; 181:109–114

21. Yamagiwa I, Ohta M, Obata K, Washio M. Case report of biliary atresia associated with preduodenal portal vein, ventricular septal defect and bilobed spleen. Zeitschrift Fur Kinderchirurgie, 1988; 43:108–109

22. Carmi R, Magee CA, Neill CA, Karrer FM. Extrahepatic biliary atresia and associated anomalies—etiologic heterogeneity suggested by distinctive patterns of associations. Am J Med Gen, 1993; 45:683–693

23. Webb LJ, Sherlock S. The aetiology, presentation and natural history of extra-hepatic portal venous obstruction. Q J Med, 1979; 48:627–639

24. Everson RB, Museles M, Henson DE, Grundy GW. Focal nodular hyperplasia of the liver in a child with hemihypertrophy. J Pediatrics, 1976; 88:985–987

25. Wanless IR, Albrecht S, Bilbao J, Frei JV, Heathcote EJ, Roberts EA, et al. Multiple focal nodular hyperplasia of the liver associated with vascular malformations of various organs and neoplasia of the brain: a new syndrome. Modern Pathol, 1989; 2:456–462

26. Odievre M, Pige G, Alagille D. Congenital abnormalities associated with extrahepatic portal hypertension. Arch Dis Child, 1977; 52:383–385

27. Matley PJ, Rode H, Cywes S. Portal vein obstruction by ectopic liver tissue. J Ped Surg, 1989; 24:1163–1164

28. Ohnishi K, Nakagawa T, Saito M, Nomura F, Koen H, Tamaru J, et al. Aneurysm of the intrahepatic branch of the portal vein. Report of two cases. Gastroenterology, 1984; 86:169–173

29. Bullaboy CA, Johnson DH, Azar H, Jennings RB, Jr. Total anomalous pulmonary venous connection to portal system: a new therapeutic role for prostaglandin E1? Pediatr Cardiol, 1984; 5:115–116

30. Duff DF, Nihill MR, McNamara DG. Infradiaphragmatic total anomalous pulmonary venous return. Review of clinical and pathological findings and results of operation in 28 cases. Br Heart J, 1977; 39:619–626

31. Morgan G, Superina R. Congenital absence of the portal vein: two cases and a proposed classification system for portasystemic vascular anomalies. J Pediatr Surg, 1994; 29:1239–1241

32. Kohda E, Saeki M, Nakano M, Masaki H, Ogawa K, Nirasawa M, et al. Congenital absence of the portal vein in a boy. Pediatr Radiol, 1999; 29:235–237

33. Marois D, van Heerden JA, Carpenter HA, Sheedy PFD. Congenital absence of the portal vein. Mayo Clin Proc, 1979; 54:55–59

34. Liver transplantation for hepatoblastoma in a child with congenital absence of the portal vein. Pediatr Radiol, 1989; 20:113–114

35. Motoori S, Shinozaki M, Goto N, Kondo F. Case report: congenital absence of the portal vein associated with nodular hyperplasia in the liver. J Gastroenterol Hepatol, 1997; 12:639–643

36. Guariso G, Fiorio S, Altavilla G, Gamba PG, Toffolutti T, Chiesura-Corona M, et al. Congenital absence of the portal vein associated with focal nodular hyperplasia of the liver and cystic dysplasia of the kidney. Eur J Pediatr, 1998; 157:287–290

37. Chagnon SF, Vallee CA, Barge J, Chevalier LJ, Le Gal J, Blery MV. Aneurysmal portahepatic venous fistula: report of two cases. Radiology, 1986; 159:693–695

38. Takayasu K, Moriyama N, Shima Y. Spontaneous portal-hepatic venous shunt via an intrahepatic portal vein aneurysm. Gastroenterology, 1984; 86:945–948

39. Tsukuda M, Yokomizo Y, Shima Y. Intrahepatic portal vein aneurysm with portal-hepatic venous shunt: case report. Acta Radiol Jpn, 1988; 48:304–307

40. Araki T, Ohtomo K, Kachi K, Monzawa S, Hihara T, Ohba H, et al. Magnetic resonance imaging of macroscopic intrahepatic portal-hepatic venous shunts. Gastrointest Radiol, 1991; 16:221–224

41. Park JH, Cha SH, Han JK, Han MC. Intrahepatic portosystemic venous shunt. Am J Roentgenol, 1990; 155:527–528

42. Papagiannis J, Kanter RJ, Effman EL, Pratt PC, Marcille R, Browning IB, et al. Polysplenia with pulmonary arteriovenous malformations. Pediatr Cardiol, 1993; 14:127–129

43. Mori H, Hayashi K, Fukuda T, Matsunaga N, Futagawa S, Nagasaki M, et al. Intrahepatic portosystemic venous shunt: occurrence in patients with and without liver cirrhosis. Am J Roentgenol, 1987; 149:711–714

44. Ohnishi K, Hatano H, Nakayama T, Kohno K, Okuda K. An unusual portal-systemic shunt, most likely through a patent ductus venosus. A case report. Gastroenterology, 1983; 85:962–965

45. Wanless IR, Lentz JS, Roberts EA. Partial nodular transformation of liver in an adult with persistent ductus venosus. Review with hypothesis on pathogenesis. Arch Pathol Lab Med, 1985; 109:427–432

46. Lalonde L, Van Beers B, Trigaux JP, Delos M, Melange M, Pringot J. Focal nodular hyperplasia in association with spontaneous

intrahepatic portosystemic venous shunt. Gastrointest Radiol, 1992; 17:154–156

47. Matsuoka Y, Ohtomo K, Okubo T, Nishikawa J, Mine T, Ohno S. Congenital absence of the portal vein. Gastrointest Radiol, 1992; 17:31–33

48. Uchino T, Matsuda I, Endo F. The long-term prognosis of congenital portosystemic venous shunt. J Pediatr, 1999; 135:254–256

49. Armstrong EL, Adams WL, Tragerman LJ, Townsend EW. The Cruveilhier-Baumgarten syndrome: review of the literature and report of two additional cases. Ann Intern Med, 1942; 16:113–149

50. Leger L, Lemaigre G, Richarme J, Chapuis Y. La maladio de Cruveilhier-Baumgarten: cas particulier d'hypertension portale essentielle. Presse Medicale, 1966; 74:1031–1036

51. Lafortune M, Constantin A, Breton G, Legare AG, Lavoie P. The recanalized umbilical vein in portal hypertension. A myth. Am J of Roentgenol, 1985; 144:549–553

52. Vauthey JN, Tomczak RJ, Helmberger T, Gertsch P, Forsmark C, Caridi J, et al. The arterioportal fistula syndrome: clinicopathologic features, diagnosis, and therapy. Gastroenterology, 1997; 113:1390–1401

53. Lamireau T, Chateil JF, Petit P, Portier F, Panuel M, Grenier N. Successful embolization of congenital intrahepatic arterioportal fistula in two infants. J Pediatr Gastroenterol Nutr, 1999; 29:211–214

54. Marchand V, Uflacker R, Baker SS, Baker RD. Congenital hepatic arterioportal fistula in a 3-year-old child. J Pediatr Gastroenterol Nutr, 1999; 28:435–441

55. Aithal GP, Alabdi BJ, Rose JD, James OF, Hudson M. Portal hypertension secondary to arterio-portal fistulae: two unusual cases. Liver, 1999; 19:343–347

56. Gryboski JD, Clemett A. Congenital hepatic artery aneurysm with superior mesenteric artery insufficiency: a steal syndrome. Pediatrics, 1967; 39:344–347

57. Wolf S, Berger H, Jauch KW. Arterioportal fistula with portal hypertension after liver trauma and resection: a case report and review of the literature. Hepatogastroenterology, 1998; 45:821–826

58. Hashimoto E, Ludwig J, MacCarty RL, Dickson ER, Krom RA. Hepatoportal arteriovenous fistula: morphologic features studied after orthotopic liver transplantation. Hum Pathol, 1989; 20:707–709

59. Jabbour N, Reyes J, Zajko A, Nour B, Tzakis AG, Starzl TE, et al. Arterioportal fistula following liver biopsy. Three cases occurring in liver transplant recipients. Dig Dis Sci, 1995; 40:1041–1044

60. Sachdeva R, Yapor M, Schwersenz A, Mitty H, Norton K, Rosh J, et al. Massive variceal bleeding caused by a hepatic artery-portal vein fistula: a manifestation of hepatocellular carcinoma in a 12-year-old. J Pediatr Gastroenterol Nutr, 1993; 16:468–471

61. Ngan H, Peh WC. Arteriovenous shunting in hepatocellular carcinoma: its prevalence and clinical significance. Clin Radiol, 1997; 52:36–40

62. McClary RD, Finelli DS, Croker B, Davis GL. Portal hypertension secondary to a spontaneous splenic arteriovenous fistula: case report and review of the literature. Am J Gastroenterol, 1986; 81:572–575

63. Baranda J, Pontes JM, Portela F, Silveira L, Amaro P, Ministro P, et al. Mesenteric arteriovenous fistula causing portal hypertension and bleeding duodenal varices. Eur J Gastroenterol Hepatol, 1996; 8:1223–1225

64. Nikolopoulos N, Xynos E, Vassilakis JS. Familial occurrence of hyperdynamic circulation status due to intrahepatic fistulae in hereditary hemorrhagic telangiectasia. Hepatogastroenterology, 1988; 35:167–168

65. Tomczak R, Helmberger T, Gorich J, Schutz A, Merkle E, Brambs HJ, et al. Abdominal arteriovenous and arterio-portal fistulas: etiology, diagnosis, therapeutic possibilities. Z Gastroenterol, 1997; 35:555–562

66. Stockx L, Raat H, Caerts B, Van Cutsem E, Wilms G, Marchal G. Transcatheter embolization of hepatic arteriovenous fistulas in Rendu-Osler-Weber disease: a case report and review of the literature. Eur Radiol, 1999; 9:1434–1437

67. Taylor CR, Garcia-Tsao G, Henson B, Case CQ, Taylor KJ. Doppler ultrasound in the evaluation of cirrhotic patients: the prevalence of intrahepatic arteriovenous shunting, and implications for diagnosis of hepatocellular carcinoma. Ultrasound Med Biol, 1997; 23:1155–1163

68. Wanless IR. The pathophysiology of non-cirrhotic portal hypertension: a pathologist's perspective. In: Boyer JL, Bianchi L, eds. Falk Symposium 44: Liver Cirrhosis. Proceedings of the VIIth international congress of liver diseases. Lancaster: MTP Press, 1987; pp. 293–311

69. Williams AO, Johnston GW. Cavernous transformation of the portal vein in rhesus monkeys. J Pathol Bacteriol, 1965; 90:613–618

70. Klemperer P. Cavernous transformation of the portal vein Its relation to Banti's disease. Arch Pathol Lab Med, 1928; 6:353–377

71. Okuda K, Kono K, Ohnishi K, Kimura K, Omata M, Koen H, et al. Clinical study of eighty-six cases of idiopathic portal hypertension and comparison with cirrhosis with splenomegaly. Gastroenterology, 1984; 86:600–610

72. Mikkelsen WP, Edmondson HA, Peters RL, Redeker AG, Reynolds TB. Extra- and intrahepatic portal hypertension without cirrhosis (hepatoportal sclerosis). Ann Surg, 1965; 162:602–618

73. Nayak NC. Pathology of noncirrhotic portal fibrosis of India. In: Okuda K, Omata M, eds. Idiopathic portal hypertension. Tokyo: University of Tokyo Press, 1983; pp. 37–47

74. Nataf C, Feldmann G, Lebrec D, C D, Descamps J-M, Rueff B, et al. Idiopathic portal hypertension (perisinusoidal fibrosis) after renal transplantation. Gut, 1979; 20:531–537

75. Tandon BN, Lakshminarayanan R, Bhargava S, Nayak NC, Sama SK. Ultrastructure of the liver in non-cirrhotic portal fibrosis with portal hypertension. Gut, 1970; 11:905–910

76. Vidins EI, Britton RS, Medline A, Blendis LM, Israel Y, H O. Sinusoidal calibre in alcoholic and nonalcoholic liver disease: Diagnostic and pathogenic implications. Hepatology, 1985; 5:408–414

77. Valla D, Flejou JF, Lebrec D, Bernuau J, Rueff B, Salzmann JL, et al. Portal hypertension and ascites in acute hepatitis: clinical, hemodynamic and histological correlations. Hepatology, 1989; 10:482–487

78. Blendis LM, Banks DC, Ramboer C, Williams R. Spleen blood flow and splanchnic haemodynamics in blood dyscrasia and other splenomegalies. Clin Sci, 1970; 38:73–84

79. Grundfest S, Cooperman AM, Ferguson R, Benjamin S. Portal hypertension associated with systemic mastocytosis and splenomegaly. Gastroenterology, 1980; 78:370–373

80. Horny HP, Kaiserling E, Campbell M, Parwaresch MR, Lennert K. Liver findings in generalized mastocytosis. A clinicopathologic study. Cancer, 1989; 63:532–538

81. Mican JM, Di Bisceglie AM, Fong TL, Travis WD, Kleiner DE, Baker B, et al. Hepatic involvement in mastocytosis: clinicopathologic correlations in 41 cases. Hepatology, 1995; 22:1163–1170

82. Shaldon S, Sherlock S. Portal hypertension in the myeloproliferative syndrome and the reticuloses. Am J Med, 1962; 32:758–764

83. Wanless IR, Peterson P, Das A, Boitnott JK, Moore GW, Bernier V. Hepatic vascular disease and portal hypertension in polycythemia vera and agnogenic myeloid metaplasia: a clinicopathological study of 145 patients examined at autopsy. Hepatology, 1990; 12:1166–1174

84. Melkebeke P, Vandepitte J, Hannon R, Fevery J. Huge hepatomegaly, jaundice, and portal hypertension due to amyloidosis of the liver. Digestion, 1980; 20:351–357

85. Donovan AJ, Reynolds TB, Mikkelsen WP, Peters RL. Systemic-portal arteriovenous fistulas: pathologic and hemodynamic observations in two patients. Surgery, 1969; 66:474–482

86. Alkim C, Sahin T, Oguz P, Temucin G, Cumhur T, Kirimlioglu V, et al. A case report of congenital intrahepatic arterioportal fistula. Am J Gastroenterol, 1999; 94:523–525

87. Williams R, Parsonson A, Somers K, Hamilton PJS. Portal hypertension in idiopathic tropical splenomegaly. Lancet, 1966; 1:329–333

88. Ohnishi K, Saito M, Sato S, Terabayashi H, Iida S, Nomura F, et al. Portal hemodynamics in idiopathic portal hypertension (Banti's syndrome). Gastroenterology, 1987; 92:751–758

89. Gusberg RJ, Peterec SM, Sumpio BE, Meier GH. Splenomegaly and variceal bleeding—hemodynamic basis and treatment implications. Hepatogastroenterology, 1994; 41:573–577

90. Morali GA, Blendis LM. Splenomegaly in portal hypertension: causes and effects. In: Okuda K, Benhamou JP, eds. Portal hypertension. Clinical and physiological aspects. Tokyo: Springer-Verlag, 1991; pp. 85–99

91. Denninger MH, Helley D, Valla D, Guillin MC. Prospective evaluation of the prevalence of factor V Leiden mutation in portal or hepatic vein thrombosis. Thromb Haemost, 1997; 78:1297–1298

92. Primignani M, Martinelli I, Bucciarelli P, Battaglioli T, Reati R, Fabris F, et al. Risk factors for thrombophilia in extrahepatic portal vein obstruction. Hepatology, 2005; 41:603–608

93. Chamouard P, Pencreach E, Maloisel F, Grunebaum L, Ardizzone JF, Meyer A, et al. Frequent factor II G20210A mutation in idiopathic portal vein thrombosis. Gastroenterology, 1999; 116:144–148

94. Harward TR, Green D, Bergan JJ, Rizzo RJ, Yao JS. Mesenteric venous thrombosis. J Vasc Surg, 1989; 9:328–333

95. Zigrossi P, Campanini M, Bordin G, Arceci F, Gamba G, Gnemmi PM, et al. Portal and mesenteric thrombosis in protein S (pS) deficiency. Am J Gastroenterol, 1996; 91:163–165

96. Buchel O, Roskams T, Van Damme B, Nevens F, Pirenne J, Fevery J. Nodular regenerative hyperplasia, portal vein thrombosis, and avascular hip necrosis due to hyperhomocysteinaemia. Gut, 2005; 54:1021–1023

97. Pinto RB, Silveira TR, Bandinelli E, Rohsig L. Portal vein thrombosis in children and adolescents: the low prevalence of hereditary thrombophilic disorders. J Pediatr Surg, 2004; 39:1356–1361

98. Julapalli VR, Bray PF, Duchini A. Elevated factor VIII and portal vein thrombosis. Dig Dis Sci, 2003; 48:2369–2371

99. Heresbach D, Pagenault M, Gueret P, Crenn P, Heresbach-Le Berre N, Malledant Y, et al. Leiden factor V mutation in four patients with small bowel infarctions. Gastroenterology, 1997; 113:322–325

100. Seixas CA, Hessel G, Ribeiro CC, Arruda VR, Annichino-Bizzacchi JM. Factor V Leiden is not common in children with portal vein thrombosis. Thromb Haemost, 1997; 77:258–261

101. Mahmoud AE, Elias E, Beauchamp N, Wilde JT. Prevalence of the factor V Leiden mutation in hepatic and portal vein thrombosis. Gut, 1997; 40:798–800

102. Valla D, Casadevall N, Huisse MG, Tuillez M, Grange JD, Muller O, et al. Etiology of portal vein thrombosis in adults: a prospective evaluation of primary myeloproliferative disorders. Gastroenterology, 1988; 94:1063–1069

103. Pagliuca A, Mufti GJ, Janossa-Tahernia M, Eridani S, Westwood NB, Thumpston J, et al. In vitro colony culture and chromosomal studies in hepatic and portal vein thrombosis—possible evidence of an occult myeloproliferative state. Quart J Med, 1990; 76:981–989

104. Corno V, Torri E, Bertani A, Guizzetti M, Lucianetti A, Maldini G, et al. Early portal vein thrombosis after pediatric split liver transplantation with left lateral segment graft. Transplant Proc, 2005; 37:1141–1142

105. Choi SH, Lee JM, Lee KH, Kim SH, Kim YJ, An SK, et al. Relationship between various patterns of transient increased hepatic attenuation on CT and portal vein thrombosis related to acute cholecystitis. Am J Roentgenol, 2004; 183:437–442

106. Stieber AC, Zetti G, Todo S, Tzakis AG, Fung JJ, Marino I, et al. The spectrum of portal vein thrombosis in liver transplantation. Ann Surg, 1991; 213:199–206

107. Albacete RA, Matthews MJ, Saini N. Portal vein thromboses in malignant hepatoma. Ann Int Med, 1967; 67:337–348

108. Monarca A, Natangelo R, Tavani E, Azzolini V. Cirrhosis and portal vein thrombosis [letter]. Gastroenterology, 1986; 90:509

109. Belli L, Sansalone CV, Aseni P, Romani F, Rondinara G. Portal thrombosis in cirrhosis. A retrospective analysis. Ann Surg, 1986; 302:286–291

110. Kage M, Arakawa M, Fukuda K, Kojiro M. Pathomorphologic study on the extrahepatic portal vein in idiopathic portal hypertension. Liver, 1990; 10:209–216

111. Wanless IR, Wong F, Blendis LM, Greig P, Heathcote EJ, Levy G. Hepatic and portal vein thrombosis in cirrhosis: possible role in development of parenchymal extinction and portal hypertension. Hepatology, 1995; 21:1238–1247

112. Nonami T, Yokoyama I, Iwatsuki S, Starzl TE. The incidence of portal vein thrombosis at liver transplantation. Hepatology, 1992; 16:1195–1198

113. Okuda K, Musha H, Yoshida T, Kanda Y, Yamazaki T, Jinnouchi S, et al. Demonstration of growing casts of hepatocellular carcinoma in the portal vein by celiac angiography: The thread and streaks sign. Radiology, 1975; 117:303–309

114. Nakashima T, Okuda K, Kojiro M, Atsuro J, Yamaguchi R, Sakamoto K, et al. Pathology of hepatocellular carcinoma in Japan. 232 consecutive cases autopsied in ten years. Cancer, 1983; 51:863–877

115. Pirisi M, Avellini C, Fabris C, Scott C, Bardus P, Soardo G, et al. Portal vein thrombosis in hepatocellular carcinoma: age and sex distribution in an autopsy study. J Cancer Res Clin Oncol, 1998; 124:397–400

116. Atri M, de Stempel J, Bret PM, Illescas FF. Incidence of portal vein thrombosis complicating liver metastasis as detected by duplex ultrasound. J Ultrasound Med, 1990; 9:285–289

117. Casey JJ, Lakey JR, Ryan EA, Paty BW, Owen R, O'Kelly K, et al. Portal venous pressure changes after sequential clinical islet transplantation. Transplantation, 2002; 74:913–915

118. Bucher P, Mathe Z, Bosco D, Becker C, Kessler L, Greget M, et al. Morbidity associated with intraportal islet transplantation. Transplant Proc, 2004; 36:1119–1120

119. Okuda K, Ohnishi K, Kimura K, Matsutani S, Sumida M, Goto N, et al. Incidence of portal. Gastroenterology, 1985; 89:279–286

120. Valla D, Denninger MH, Casadevall N, Chait Y, Hillaire S, Guillin MC, et al. Thrombose de la veine porte et des veines hepatiques: combinaisons d'affections thrombogenes multiples et de facteurs locaux (abstr). Gastroenterol Clin Biol, 1997; 21:731

121. Sarin SK. Non-cirrhotic portal fibrosis. Gut, 1989; 30:406–415

122. Benhamou JP. Transient portal hypertension. In: Okuda K, Benhamou JP, eds. Portal Hypertension. Clinical and Physiological Aspects. Tokyo: Springer-Verlag, 1991; pp. 363–364

123. Knockaert DC, Robaeys GK, Cox EJ, Marchal GJ. Suppurative pylethrombosis: a changing clinical picture. Gastroenterology, 1989; 97:1028–1030

124. Delamarre J, Fabre V, Remond A, Sevenet F, Tossou H, Capron JP. [Portal venous system calcifications. Study of 3 cases and review of the literature]. Gastroenterol Clin Biol, 1991; 15:254–260

125. Besnard M, Pariente D, Hadchouel M, Bernard O, Chaumont P. Portal cavernoma in congenital hepatic fibrosis. Angiographic reports of 10 pediatric cases. Pediatr Radiol, 1994; 24:61–65

126. Bayraktar Y, Balkanci F, Kayhan B, Uzunalimoglu B, Ozenc A, Ozdemir A, et al. Congenital hepatic fibrosis associated with cavernous transformation of the portal vein. Hepatogastroenterology, 1997; 44:1588–1594

127. Misra A, Loyalka P, Alva F. Portal hypertension due to extensive hepatic cysts in autosomal dominant polycystic kidney disease. South Med J, 1999; 92:626–627

128. Hunt AH, Whittard BR. Thrombosis of the portal vein in cirrhosis hepatis. Lancet, 1954; 1:281–284

129. Chandra R, Kapoor D, Tharakan A, Chaudhary A, Sarin SK. Portal biliopathy. J Gastroenterol Hepatol, 2001; 16:1086–1092

130. Perego P, Cozzi G, Bertolini A. Portal biliopathy. Surg Endosc, 2003; 17:351–352

131. Chiu B, Superina R. Extrahepatic portal vein thrombosis is associated with an increased incidence of cholelithiasis. J Pediatr Surg, 2004; 39:1059–1061

132. Eleftheriadis E, Kotzampassi K, Botsios D, Tzartinoglou E, Farmakis H, Dadoukis J. Splanchnic ischemia during laparoscopic cholecystectomy. Surg Endosc, 1996; 10:324–326

133. Reynolds WJ, Wanless IR. Nodular regenerative hyperplasia of the liver in a patient with rheumatoid vasculitis: a morphometric study suggesting a role for hepatic arteritis in the pathogenesis. J Rheumatol, 1984; 11:838–842

134. Thorne C, Urowitz M, Wanless IR, Roberts E, Blendis LM. Liver disease in Felty's syndrome. Am J Med, 1982; 73:35–40.

135. Kuramochi S, Tashiro Y, Torikata C, Watanabe Y. Systemic lupus erythematosus associated with multiple nodular hyperplasia of the liver. Acta Pathol Jpn, 1982; 32:547–560

136. Nakanuma Y, Ohta G, Sasaki K. Nodular regenerative hyperplasia of the liver associated with polyarteritis nodosa. Arch Pathol and Lab Med, 1984; 108:133–135

137. Russell ML, Kahn HJ. Nodular regenerative hyperplasia of the liver associated with progressive systemic sclerosis: a case report with ultrastructural observation. J Rheumatol, 1983; 10:748–752

138. Wanless IR, Solt L, Kortan P, Deck JHN, Gardiner GW, Prokipchuk EJ. Nodular regenerative hyperplasia of the liver associated with macroglobulinemia: A clue to the pathogenesis. Am J Med, 1981; 70:1203–1209

139. Banti G. Splenomegalie mit Lebercirrhose. Beitr z Path Anat u z Allg Path, 1898; 24:21–33

140. Nakanuma Y, Ohta G, Doishita K, Maki H. Granulomatous liver disease in the small hepatic and portal veins. Arch Pathol Lab Med, 1980; 104:456–458

141. Berger I, Katz M. Portal hypertension due to hepatic sarcoidosis. Am J Gastroenterol, 1973; 59:147–151

142. Deveney K, Goodman ZD, Epstein MS, Zimmerman HJ, Ishak KG. The histologic spectrum of hepatic sarcoidosis. A study of 100 cases. Mod Pathol, 1991; 4:91A

143. Wanless IR. Understanding non-cirrhotic portal hypertension: menage a foie (editorial). Hepatology, 1988; 8:192–193

144. Shimada H, Nihmoto S, Matsuba A, Nakagawara G. Acute cholangitis: a histopathologic study. J Clin Gastroenterol, 1988; 10:197–200

145. Moreno-Merlo F, Wanless IR, Shimamatsu K, Sherman M, Greig P, Chiasson D. The role of granulomatous phlebitis and thrombosis in the pathogenesis of cirrhosis and portal hypertension in sarcoidosis. Hepatology, 1997; 26:554–560

146. Wanless IR, Geddie WR. Lipogranulomata in liver and spleen: An autopsy series. Arch Pathol Lab Med, 1985; 109:283–286

147. Thomas LB, Popper H, Berk PD, Selikoff I, Falk H. Vinyl-chloride-induced liver disease. From idiopathic portal hypertension (Banti's syndrome) to angiosarcoma. N Engl J Med, 1975; 292:17–22

148. Wanless IR, Liu JJ, Butany J. Role of thrombosis in the pathogenesis of congestive hepatic fibrosis (cardiac cirrhosis). Hepatology, 1995; 21:1232–1237

149. Rousselet MC, Kettani S, Rohmer V, Saint-Andre JP. A case of temporal arteritis with intrahepatic arterial involvement. Pathol Res Pract, 1989; 185:329–331

150. Wanless IR. Micronodular transformation (nodular regenerative hyperplasia) of the liver: a report of 64 cases among 2500 autopsies and a new classification of benign hepatocellular nodules. Hepatology, 1990; 11:787–797

151. Nakanuma Y, Nonomura A, Hayashi M, Doishita K, Takayanagi N, Uchida T, et al. Pathology of the liver in 'idiopathic portal hypertension' associated with autoimmune disease. The Ministry of Health and Welfare Disorders of Portal Circulation Research Committee. Acta Pathologica Japonica, 1989; 39:586–592

152. Murphy JR, Sjogren MH, Kikendall JW, Peura DA, Goodman Z. Small bile duct abnormalities in sarcoidosis. J Clin Gastroenterol, 1990; 12:555–561

153. Homeida M, Ahmed S, Dafalla A, Suliman S, Eltom I, Nash T, et al. Morbidity associated with Schistosoma mansoni infection as determined by ultrasound: a study in Gezira, Sudan. Am J Trop Med Hyg, 1988; 39:196–201

154. Andrade ZA, Peixoto E, Guerret S, Grimaud JA. Hepatic connective tissue changes in hepatosplenic schistosomiasis. Hum Pathol, 1992; 23:566–573

155. Ohmae H, Sinuon M, Kirinoki M, Matsumoto J, Chigusa Y, Socheat D, et al. Schistosomiasis mekongi: from discovery to control. Parasitol Int, 2004; 53:135–142

156. Cheever AW, Andrade ZA. Pathological lesions associated with Schistosoma mansoni infection in man. Trans R Soc Trop Med Hyg, 1967; 61:626–639

157. Nash TE, Cheever AW, Ottesen EA, Cook JA. Schistosome infections in humans: perspectives and recent findings. Ann Int Med, 1982; 97:740–754

158. Homeida MA, el Tom I, Nash T, Bennett JL. Association of the therapeutic activity of praziquantel with the reversal of Symmers' fibrosis induced by Schistosoma mansoni. Am J Trop Med Hyg, 1991; 45:360–365

159. Doehring-Schwerdtfeger E, Mohamed-Ali G, Abdel-Rahim IM, Kardorff R, Franke D, Kaiser C, et al. Sonomorphological abnormalities in Sudanese children with Schistosoma mansoni infection: a proposed staging-system for field diagnosis of periportal fibrosis. Am J Trop Med Hyg, 1989; 41:63–69

160. Ohmae H, Tanaka M, Hayashi M, Matsuzaki Y, Kurosaki Y, Blas BL, et al. Improvement of ultrasonographic and serologic changes in Schistosoma japonicum-infected patients after treatment with praziquantel. Am J Trop Med Hyg, 1992; 46:99–104

161. Nakashima E, Kage M, Wanless IR. Idiopathic portal hypertension: Histologic evidence that some cases may be regressed cirrhosis with portal vein thrombosis. Hepatology, 1999; 30:218A

162. Fukuda K, Kage M, Arakawa M, Nakashima T. Portal vein or hepatic vein? A curious aberrant vasculature in the liver with idiopathic portal hypertension. Acta Pathologica Japonica, 1985; 35:885–897

163. Eckhauser FE, Appelman HD, Knol JA, Strodel WE, Coran AG, Turcotte JG. Noncirrhotic portal hypertension: Differing patterns of disease in children and adults. Surgery, 1983; 94:721–728

164. Wanless IR, Bernier V, Seger M. Intrahepatic portal sclerosis in patients without history of liver disease: an autopsy study. Am J Pathol, 1982; 106:63–70

165. Terada T, Hoso M, Nakanuma Y. Development of cavernous vasculatures in livers with hepatocellular carcinoma. An autopsy study. Liver, 1989; 9:172–178

166. Terada T, Ishida F, Nakanuma Y. Vascular plexus around intrahepatic bile ducts in normal livers and portal hypertension. J Hepatol, 1989; 8:139–149

167. Terada T, Hoso M, Nakanuma Y. Microvasculature in the small portal tracts in idiopathic portal hypertension. A morphological comparison with other hepatic diseases. Virchows Archiv-A Pathol Anat Histopathol, 1989; 415:61–67

168. Horrocks P, Tapp E. Zahn's 'infarcts' of the liver. J Clin Pathol, 1966; 19:475–478

169. Shimamatsu K, Wanless IR. Role of ischemia in causing apoptosis, atrophy, and nodular hyperplasia in human liver. Hepatology, 1997; 26:343–350

170. Putnam CW, Porter KA, Starzl TE. Hepatic encephalopathy and light and electron micrographic changes of the baboon liver after portal diversion. Ann Surg, 1976; 184:155–161

171. Watanabe M, Umekawa Y, Ueki K, Hirakawa H, Fukumoto S, Shimada Y. Laparoscopic observation of hepatic lobe atrophy. Endoscopy, 1989; 21:234–236

172. Nevens F, Fevery J, Van Steenbergen W, Sciot R, Desmet V, De Groote J. Arsenic and non-cirrhotic portal hypertension. A report of eight cases. J Hepatol, 1990; 11:80–85

173. Labadie H, Stoessel P, Callard P, Beaugrand M. Hepatic venoocclusive disease and perisinusoidal fibrosis secondary to arsenic poisoning. Gastroenterology, 1990; 99:1140–1143

174. Makuuchi M, Hasegawa H, Yamazaki S, Bandai Y, Watanabe G, Ito T. The inferior right hepatic vein: ultrasonic demonstration. Radiology, 1983; 148:213–217

175. Cosgrove DO, Arger PH, Coleman BG. Ultrasonic anatomy of hepatic veins. J Clin Ultrasound, 1987; 15:231–235

176. Mukai JK, Stack CM, Turner DA, Gould RJ, Petasnick JP, Matalon TA, et al. Imaging of surgically relevant hepatic vascular and segmental anatomy. Part 1. Normal anatomy. Am J Roentgenol, 1987; 149:287–292

177. Takayasu K, Moriyama N, Muramatsu Y, Goto H, Shima Y, Yamada T, et al. Intrahepatic venous collaterals forming via the inferior right hepatic vein in 3 patients with obstruction of the inferior vena cava. Radiology, 1985; 154:323–328

178. Ou QJ, Hermann RE. Hepatic vein ligation and preservation of liver segments in major resections. Arch Surg, 1987; 122:1198–1200

179. Ludwig J, Hashimoto E, McGill DB, van Heerden JA. Classification of hepatic venous outflow obstruction: ambiguous terminology of the Budd–Chiari syndrome. Mayo Clin Proc, 1990; 65:51–55

180. DeLeve LD, McCuskey RS, Wang X, Hu L, McCuskey MK, Epstein RB, et al. Characterization of a reproducible rat model of hepatic veno-occlusive disease. Hepatology, 1999; 29:1779–1791

181. Wanless IR. Thrombosis and phlebitis in the pathogenesis of portal hypertension and cirrhosis: the 2-hit hypothesis for the pathogenesis of chronic liver disease. In: Arroyo V, Bosch J, Bruguera M, Rodes J, eds. Therapy in Liver Diseases, 3rd edn. Barcelona: Masson, 1997; pp. 47–50

182. O'Shea A-M, Wanless IR. Tumor capsule formation in the liver: Importance of tumor ischemia and parenchymal ischemia. Mod Pathol, 2006; in press

183. Parker RGF. Occlusion of the hepatic veins in man. Medicine, 1959; 38:369–402

184. Langlet P, Escolano S, Valla D, Coste-Zeitoun D, Denie C, Mallet A, et al. Clinicopathological forms and prognostic index in Budd–Chiari syndrome. J Hepatol, 2003; 39:496–501

185. Wang ZG, Zhang FJ, Yi MQ, Qiang LX. Evolution of management for Budd–Chiari syndrome: a team's view from 2564 patients. ANZ J Surg, 2005; 75:55–63

186. Gentil-Kocher S, Bernard O, Brunelle F, Hadchouel M, Maillard JN, Valayer J, et al. Budd–Chiari syndrome in children: report of 22 cases. J Pediatr, 1988; 113:30–38

187. Tavill AS, Wood EJ, Creel L, Jones EA, Gregory M, Sherlock S. The Budd–Chiari syndrome. Correlation between hepatic scintigraphy and the clinical, radiological and pathological findings in, 19 cases of hepatic venous outflow obstruction. Gastroenterology, 1975; 68:509–518

188. Averbuch M, Aderka D, Winer Z, Levo Y. Budd–Chiari syndrome in Israel: predisposing factors, prognosis, and early identification of high-risk patients. J Clin Gastroenterol, 1991; 13:321–324

189. Mitchell MC, Boitnott JK, S K, Cameron JL, Maddrey WC. Budd–Chiari syndrome: Etiology, diagnosis and management. Medicine, 1982; 61:199–218

190. Bismuth H, Sherlock DJ. Portasystemic shunting versus liver transplantation for the Budd–Chiari syndrome. Ann Surg, 1991; 214:581–589

191. Valla D, Hadengue A, el Younsi M, Azar N, Zeitoun G, Boudet MJ, et al. Hepatic venous outflow block caused by short-length hepatic vein stenoses. Hepatology, 1997; 25:814–819

192. Millikan WJ, Jr, Henderson JM, Sewell CW, Guyton RA, Potts JR, 3d, Cranford CA, Jr, et al. Approach to the spectrum of Budd–Chiari syndrome: which patients require portal decompression? Am J Surg, 1985; 149:167–176

193. Hansen HJ, Christoffersen JK. Occlusive mesenteric infarction. A retrospective study of 83 cases. Acta Chir Scand Suppl, 1976; 472:103–108

194. Arora A, Tandon N, Sharma MP, Acharya SK. Constrictive pericarditis masquerading as Budd–Chiari syndrome. J Clin Gastroenterol, 1991; 13:178–181

195. Martin LG, Henderson JM, Millikan WJ, Jr, Casarella WJ, Kaufman SL. Angioplasty for long-term treatment of patients with Budd–Chiari syndrome. Am J Roentgenol, 1990; 154:1007–1010

196. Orloff MJ, Girard B. Long term results of treatment of Budd–Chiari syndrome by side to side portacaval shunt. Surg Gyn Obstet, 1989; 168:33–41

197. Klein AS, Sitzmann JV, Coleman J, Herlong FH, Cameron JL. Current management of the Budd–Chiari syndrome. Ann Surg, 1990; 212:144–149

198. Henderson JM, Warren WD, Millikan WJ, Jr, Galloway JR, Kawasaki S, Stahl RL, et al. Surgical options, hematologic

199. Kage M, Arakawa M, Kojiro M, Okuda K. Histopathology of membranous obstruction of the inferior vena cava in the Budd–Chiari syndrome. Gastroenterology, 1992; 102:2081–2090

200. Bhattacharyya M, Makharia G, Kannan M, Ahmed RP, Gupta PK, Saxena R. Inherited prothrombotic defects in Budd–Chiari syndrome and portal vein thrombosis: a study from North India. Am J Clin Pathol, 2004; 121:844–847

201. Asherson RA, Khamashta MA, Hughes GR. The hepatic complications of the antiphospholipid antibodies (editorial). Clin Exp Rheumatol, 1991; 9:341–344

202. Pelletier S, Landi B, Piette JC, Ekert P, Coutellier A, Desmoulins C, et al. Antiphospholipid syndrome as the second cause of non-tumorous Budd–Chiari syndrome. J Hepatol, 1994; 21:76–80

203. Bucciarelli P, Franchi F, Alatri A, Bettini P, Moia M. Budd–Chiari syndrome in a patient heterozygous for the G20210A mutation of the prothrombin gene [letter]. Thromb Haemost, 1998; 79:445–446

204. Li XM, Wei YF, Hao HL, Hao YB, He LS, Li JD, et al. Hyperhomocysteinemia and the MTHFR C677T mutation in Budd–Chiari syndrome. Am J Hematol, 2002; 71:11–14

205. Zylberberg H, Valla D, Viguie F, Casadevall N. Budd–Chiari syndrome associated with 5q deletion and hypereosinophilia. J Clin Gastroenterol, 1996; 23:66–68

206. Valla D, Casadevall N, Lacombe N, Varet B, Goldwasser E, Franco D, et al. Primary myeloproliferative disorders and hepatic vein thrombosis: a prospective study of erythroid colony formation in vitro in 20 patients with Budd–Chiari syndrome. Ann Intrn Med, 1985; 103:329–334

207. Campbell DA, Rolles K, Jameson N, O'Grady J, Wight D, Williams R, et al. Hepatic transplantation with perioperative and long term anticoagulation as treatment for Budd Chiari syndrome. Surg Gynecol Obstet, 1988; 166:511–518

208. Hirshfield G, Collier JD, Brown K, Taylor C, Frick T, Baglin TP, et al. Donor factor V Leiden mutation and vascular thrombosis following liver transplantation. Liver Transpl Surg, 1998; 4:58–61

209. Ruckert JC, Ruckert RI, Rudolph B, Muller JM. Recurrence of the Budd–Chiari syndrome after orthotopic liver transplantation. Hepatogastroenterology, 1999; 46:867–871

210. Cruz E, Ascher NL, Roberts JP, Bass NM, Yao FY. High incidence of recurrence and hematologic events following liver transplantation for Budd–Chiari syndrome. Clin Transplant, 2005; 19:501–506

211. Okuda K, Ostrow JD. Clinical conference: Membranous type of Budd–Chiari syndrome. J Clin Gastroenterol, 1984; 6:81–88

212. Khuroo M, Datta DV. Budd–Chiari syndrome following pregnancy. Report of 16 cases, with roentgenologic, hemodynamic and histologic studies of the hepatic outflow tract. Am J Med, 1980; 68:113–121

213. Bhusnurmath SR. Budd Chiari syndrome. In: Okuda K, ed. 2nd International Symposium on Budd–Chiari Syndrome, 1991; Kyoto, Japan: Annual Report of the Ministry of Health of Japan, 1991; pp. 280–293

214. Okuda K, Kage M, Shrestha SM. Proposal of a new nomenclature for Budd–Chiari syndrome: hepatic vein thrombosis versus thrombosis of the inferior vena cava at its hepatic portion. Hepatology, 1998; 28:1191–1198

215. Simson I. Membranous obstruction of the inferior vena cava and hepatocellular carcinoma in South Africa. Gastroenterology, 1982; 82:171–178

216. Wang ZG. Recognition and management of Budd–Chiari syndrome. Experience with 143 patients. Chin Med J-Peking, 1989; 102:338–346

217. Chang CH, Lee MC, Shieh MJ, Chang JP, Lin PJ. Transatrial membranotomy for Budd–Chiari syndrome. Ann Thoracic Surg, 1989; 48:409–412

218. Hirooka M, Kimura C. Membranous obstruction of the hepatic portion of the inferior vena cava. surgical correction and etiological study. Arch Surg, 1970; 100:656–663

219. Terabayashi H, Okuda K, Nomura F, Ohnishi K, Wong P. Transformation of inferior vena caval thrombosis to membranous obstruction in a patient with the lupus anticoagulant. Gastroenterology, 1986; 91:219–224

220. Mori H, Hayashi K, Amamoto Y. Membranous obstruction of the inferior vena cava associated with intrahepatic portosystemic shunt. Cardio Interven Radiol, 1986; 9:209–213

221. Balian A, Valla D, Naveau S, Musset D, Coue O, Lemaigre G, et al. Post-traumatic membranous obstruction of the inferior vena cava associated with a hypercoagulable state. J Hepatol, 1998; 28:723–726

222. Okuda K. Membranous obstruction of the inferior vena cava: etiology and relation to hepatocellular carcinoma. Gastroenterology, 1982; 82:376–379

evaluation, and pathologic changes in Budd–Chiari syndrome. Am J Surg, 1990; 159:41–50

223. Kew MC, McKnight A, Hodkinson J, Bukofzer S, Esser JD. The role of membranous obstruction of the inferior vena cava in the etiology of hepatocellular carcinoma in Southern African blacks. Hepatology, 1989; 9:121–125

224. Girardin MS, Zafrani ES, Prigent A, Larde D, Chauffour J, Dhumeaux D. Unilobar small hepatic vein obstruction: possible role of progestogen given as oral contraceptive. Gastroenterology, 1983; 84:630–635

225. Leopold JG, Parry TE, Storring FK. A change in the sinusoid-trabecular structure of the liver with hepatic venous outflow block. J Pathol, 1970; 100:87–98

226. Cho KJ, Geisinger KR, Shields JJ, Forrest ME. Collateral channels and histopathology in hepatic vein occlusion. Am J Roentgenol, 1982; 139:703–709

227. Tanaka M, Wanless IR. Pathology of the liver in Budd–Chiari syndrome: portal vein thrombosis and the histogenesis of veno-centric cirrhosis, veno-portal cirrhosis, and large regenerative nodules. Hepatology, 1998; 27:488–496

228. de Sousa JM, Portmann B, Williams R. Nodular regenerative hyperplasia of the liver and the Budd–Chiari syndrome. Case report, review of the literature and reappraisal of pathogenesis. J Hepatol, 1991; 12:28–35

229. Castellano G, Canga F, Solis-Herruzo JA, Colina F, Martinez-Montiel MP, Morillas JD. Budd–Chiari syndrome associated with nodular regenerative hyperplasia of the liver. J Clin Gastroenterol, 1989; 11:698–702

230. Bras G, Brandt KH. Vascular disorders. In: MacSween RNM, Anthony PP, Scheuer PJ, editors. Pathology of the liver, 2nd edn. Edinburgh: Churchill Livingstone, 1987; pp. 478–502

231. Cazals-Hatem D, Vilgrain V, Genin P, Denninger MH, Durand F, Belghiti J, et al. Arterial and portal circulation and parenchymal changes in Budd–Chiari syndrome: a study in 17 explanted livers. Hepatology, 2003; 37:510–519

232. Alpert LI. Veno-occlusive disease of the liver associated with oral contraceptives: case report and review of literature. Hum Pathol, 1976; 7:709–718

233. Valla D, Dhumeaux D, Babany G, Hillon P, Rueff B, Rochant H, et al. Hepatic vein thrombosis in paroxysmal nocturnal hemoglobinuria: a spectrum from asymptomatic occlusion of hepatic venules to fatal Budd–Chiari syndrome. Gastroenterology, 1987; 93:569–575

234. Cameron JL, Herlong HF, Sanfey H, Boitnott J, Kaufman SL, Gott VL, et al. The Budd–Chiari syndrome. Treatment by mesenteric–systemic venous shunts. Ann Surg, 1983; 198:335–346

235. Vilgrain V, Lewin M, Vons C, Denys A, Valla D, Flejou JF, et al. Hepatic nodules in Budd–Chiari syndrome: imaging features. Radiology, 1999; 210:443–450

236. Steiner PE. Nodular regenerative hyperplasia of the liver. Am J Pathol, 1959; 35:943–953

237. Bras G, Hill KR. Veno-occlusive disease of the liver. Essential pathology. Lancet, 1956; 2:161–163

238. DeLeve LD, Ito Y, Bethea NW, McCuskey MK, Wang X, McCuskey RS. Embolization by sinusoidal lining cells obstructs the microcirculation in rat sinusoidal obstruction syndrome. Am J Physiol Gastrointest Liver Physiol, 2003; 284:G1045–1052

239. Willmot FC, Robertson GW. Senecio disease, or cirrhosis of the liver due to senecio poisoning. Lancet, 1920; 2:848–849

240. Selzer G, Parker RGF. Senecio poisoning exhibiting as Chiari's syndrome. A report of 12 cases. Am J Pathol, 1951; 27:885–907

241. Bras G, Jelliffe DB, Stuart KL. Veno-occlusive disease of the liver with non-portal type of cirrhosis, occurring in Jamaica. Arch Pathol, 1954; 57:285–300

242. Adami JG. Pictou cattle disease. Montreal Med J, 1902; 31:105–117

243. Cushny AR. On the action of senecio alkaloids and the causation of the hepatic cirrhosis of cattle (Pictou, Molteno, or Winton disease). J Pharmacol Exptl Ther, 1910–1911; 2:531–548

244. Culvenor CC, Edgar JA, Smith LW, Kumana CR, Lin HJ. Heliotropium lasiocarpum Fisch and Mey identified as cause of veno-occlusive disease due to a herbal tea (letter). Lancet, 1986; 1:978

245. Bach N, Thung SN, Schaffner F. Comfrey herb tea-induced hepatic veno-occlusive disease. Am J Med, 1989; 87:97–99

246. Smith LW, Culvenor CCJ. Plant sources of hepatotoxic pyrrolizidine alkaloids. J Nat Prod, 1981; 44:129–144

247. Shubat PJ, Banner W, Huxtable RJ. Pulmonary vascular responses induced by the pyrrolizidine alkaloid monocrotaline in rats. Toxicon, 1987; 25:995–1002

248. Hirono I, Mori H, Haga M. Carcinogenic activity of symphytum officinale. J Nat Cancer Inst, 1978; 61:865–869

249. Tandon BN, Tandon HD, Tandon RK, Narndranathan M, Joshi YK. An epidemic of veno-occlusive disease of liver in central India. Lancet, 1976; 2:271–272

250. Tandon BN, Joshi YK, Sud R, Koshy A, Jain SK, Tandon HD. Follow-up of survivors of epidemic veno-occlusive disease in India (letter). Lancet, 1984; 1:730

251. Mohabbat O, Younos MS, Merzad AA, Srivastava RN, Sediq GG, Aram GN. An outbreak of hepatic veno-occlusive disease in north-western Afghanistan. Lancet, 1976; 2:269–271

252. McDonald GB, Sharma P, Matthews DE, Shulman HM, Thomas ED. The clinical course of 53 patients with venocclusive disease of the liver after marrow transplantation. Transplantation, 1985; 39:603–608

253. McDonald G, Hinds MS, Fisher LD, Schoch HG, Wolford JL, Banaji M, et al. Veno-occlusive disease of the liver and multiorgan failure after bone marrow transplantation: a cohort study of 355 patients. Ann Intern Med, 1993; 118:255–267

254. Reed GB, Cox AJ, Jr. The human liver after radiation injury. A form of veno-occlusive disease. Am J Pathol, 1966; 48:597–611

255. Fajardo LF, Colby TV. Pathogenesis of veno-occlusive liver disease after radiation. Arch Pathol Lab Med, 1980; 104:584–588

256. Liano F, Moreno A, Matesanz R, Teruel JL, Redondo C, Garcia-Martin F, et al. Veno-occlusive hepatic disease of the liver in renal transplantation: Is azathioprine the cause? Nephron, 1989; 51:509–516

257. Ceci G, Bella M, Melissari M, Gabrielli M, Bocchi P, Cocconi G. Fatal hepatic vascular toxicity of DTIC. Is it really a rare event? Cancer, 1988; 61:1988–1991

258. Shulman HM, McDonald GB, Matthews D, Doney KC, Kopecky KJ, Gauvreau JM, et al. An analysis of hepatic venocclusive disease and centrilobular hepatic degeneration following bone marrow transplantation. Gastroenterology, 1980; 79:1178–1191

259. Avner ED, Ellis D, Jaffe R. Veno-occlusive disease of the liver associated with cysteamine treatment of nephropathic cystinosis. J Pediatr, 1983; 102:793–796

260. D'Cruz CA, Wimmer RS, Harcke HT, Huff DS, Naiman JL. Veno-occlusive disease of the liver in children following chemotherapy for acute myelocytic leukemia. Cancer, 1983; 52:1803–1807

261. Katzka DA, Saul SH, Jorkasky D, Sigal H, Reynolds JC, Soloway RD. Azathioprine and hepatic venocclusive disease in renal transplant patients. Gastroenterology, 1986; 90:446–454

262. Read AE, Wiesner RH, LaBrecque DR, Tifft JG, Mullen KD, Sheer RL, et al. Hepatic veno-occlusive disease associated with renal transplantation and azathioprine therapy. Ann Intern Med, 1986; 104:651–655

263. Weitz H, Gokel JM, Loeschke K, Possinger K, Eder M. Veno-occlusive disease of the liver in patients receiving immunosuppressive therapy. Virchows Arch (Pathol Anat), 1982; 395:245–256

264. Nakhleh RE, Wesen C, Snover DC, Grage T. Venoocclusive lesions of the central veins and portal vein radicles secondary to intraarterial 5-fluoro-2'-deoxyuridine infusion. Hum Pathol, 1989; 20:1218–1220

265. Rubbia-Brandt L, Audard V, Sartoretti P, Roth AD, Brezault C, Le Charpentier M, et al. Severe hepatic sinusoidal obstruction associated with oxaliplatin-based chemotherapy in patients with metastatic colorectal cancer. Ann Oncol, 2004; 15:460–466

266. Haboubi NY, Ali HH, Whitwell HL, Ackrill P. Role of endothelial cell injury in the spectrum of azathioprine-induced liver disease after renal transplant: light microscopy and ultrastructural observations. Am J Gastroenterol, 1988; 83:256–261

267. Mellis C, Bale PM. Familial hepatic venoocclusive disease with probable immune deficiency. J Pediatr, 1976; 88:236–242

268. Jevtic MM, Thorp FK, Hruban Z. Hereditary tyrosinemia with hyperplasia and hypertrophy of juxtaglomerular apparatus. Am J Clin Pathol, 1974; 61:423–437

269. Shulman HM, Luk K, Deeg HJ, Shuman WB, Storb R. Induction of hepatic veno-occlusive disease in dogs. Am J Pathol, 1987; 126:114–125

270. DeLeve LD. Glutathione defense in non-parenchymal cells. Semin Liver Dis, 1998; 18:403–413

271. Kumana CR, Ng M, Lin HJ, Ko W, Wu PC, Todd D. Hepatic veno-occlusive disease due to toxic alkaloid herbal tea (letter). Lancet, 1983; 2:1360–1361

272. Eisenhauer T, Hartmann H, Rumpf KW, Helmchen U, Scheler F, Creutzfeldt W. Favourable outcome of hepatic veno-occlusive disease in a renal transplant patient receiving azathioprine, treated by portacaval shunt. Report of a case and review of the literature. Digestion, 1984; 30:185–190

273. Murray JA, LaBrecque DR, Gingrich RD, Pringle KC, Mitros FA. Successful treatment of hepatic venocclusive disease in a bone marrow transplant patient with side-to-side portacaval shunt. Gastroenterology, 1987; 92:1073–1077

274. Shulman HM, Gown AM, Nugent DJ. Hepatic veno-occlusive disease after bone marrow transplantation: Immunohistochemical

identification of the material within occluded central venules. Am J Pathol, 1987; 127:549–558

275. Burkhardt A, Klöppel G. Unusual obliterative disease of the hepatic veins in an infant. Virchows Arch (Pathol Anat), 1977; 375:225–232

276. Snover DC, Weisdorf S, Bloomer J, McGlave P, Weisdorf D. Nodular regenerative hyperplasia of the liver following bone marrow transplantation. Hepatology, 1989; 9:443–448

277. Goodman ZD, Ishak KG. Occlusive venous lesions in alcoholic liver disease: A study of, 200 cases. Gastroenterology, 1982; 83:786–796

278. Burt AD, MacSween RNM. Hepatic vein lesions in alcoholic liver disease: retrospective biopsy and necropsy study. J Clin Pathol, 1986; 39:63–67

279. Nakanuma Y, Ohta G, Doishita K. Quantitation and serial section observations of focal veno-occlusive lesions of hepatic veins in liver cirrhosis. Virchows Arch (Pathol Anat), 1985; 405:429–438

280. Lucke B. The pathology of acute hepatitis. Am J Pathol, 1944; 20:471

281. Wanless IR, Shiota K. The pathogenesis of nonalcoholic steatohepatitis and other fatty liver diseases: a four-step model including the role of lipid release and hepatic venular obstruction in the progression to cirrhosis. Semin Liver Dis, 2004; 24:99–106

282. Russi EW, Bansky G, Pfaltz M, Spinas G, Hammer B, Senning A. Budd–Chiari syndrome in sarcoidosis. Am J Gastroenterol, 1986; 81:71–75

283. Young ID, Clark RN, Manley PN, Groll A, Simon JB. Response to steroids in Budd–Chiari syndrome caused by idiopathic granulomatous venulitis. Gastroenterology, 1988; 94:503–507

284. Hoagland MH, Zinkham WH, Hutchins GM. Generalized venocentric lesions in the virus-associated hemophagocytic syndrome. Hum Pathol, 1986; 17:195–198

285. Paradinas FJ, Bull TB, Westaby D, Murray-Lyon IM. Hyperplasia and prolapse of hepatocytes into hepatic veins during longterm methyltestosterone therapy: possible relationships of these changes to the developement of peliosis hepatis and liver tumours. Histopathology, 1977; 1:225–246

286. Sasaki M, Nakanuma Y, Watanabe K. Hepatocellular prolapse of hepatic portal tracts and subendothelial space of central veins in idiopathic portal hypertension. Histopathology, 1995; 27:67–70

287. Wanless ir, Nakashima E, Sherman M. Regression of human cirrhosis: morphologic features and the genesis of incomplete septal cirrhosis. Arch Pathol Lab Med, 2000; 124:1599–1607

288. Nopanitaya W, Lamb JC, Grisham JW, Carson JL. Effect of Hepatic Venous Outflow Obstruction on Pores and Fenestration in Sinusoidal Endothelium. Br J Exp Pathol, 1976; 57:604–609

289. McGuire RF, Bissell DM, Boyles J, Roll FJ. Role of extracellular matrix in regulating fenestrations of sinusoidal endothelial cells isolated from normal rat liver. Hepatology, 1992; 15:989–997

290. Burt AD, Le Bail B, Balabaud C, Bioulac-Sage P. Morphologic investigation of sinusoidal cells. Semin Liver Dis, 1993; 13:21–38

291. Scoazec JY, Feldmann G. In situ immunophenotyping study of endothelial cells of the human hepatic sinusoid: results and functional implications. Hepatology, 1991; 14:789–797

292. De Leeuw AM, Brouwer A, Knook DL. Sinusoidal endothelial cells of the liver: fine structure and function in relation to age. J Electr Micro Tech, 1990; 14:218–236

293. Bernuau D, Guillot R, Durand AM, Raoux N, Gabreau T, Passa P et al. Ultrastructural aspects of the liver perisinusoidal space in diabetic patients with and without microangiopathy. Diabetes, 1982; 31:1061–1067

294. Babbs C, Haboubi NY, Mellor JM, Smith A, Rowan BP, Warnes TW. Endothelial cell transformation in primary biliary cirrhosis: a morphological and biochemical study. Hepatology, 1990; 11:723–729

295. Griffiths MR, Keir S, Burt AD. Basement membrane proteins in the space of Disse: a reappraisal. J Clin Pathol, 1991; 44:646–648

296. Tsui MS, Burroughs A, McCormick PA, Scheuer PJ. Portal hypertension and hepatic sinusoidal Ulex lectin binding. J Hepatol, 1990; 10:244–250

297. Fukukura Y, Nakashima O, Kusaba A, Kage M, Kojiro M. Angioarchitecture and blood circulation in focal nodular hyperplasia of the liver. J Hepatol, 1998; 29:470–475

298. Roncalli M, Roz E, Coggi G, Di Rocco MG, Bossi P, Minola E et al. The vascular profile of regenerative and dysplastic nodules of the cirrhotic liver: implications for diagnosis and classification. Hepatology, 1999; 30:1174–1178

299. Shields PL, Morland CM, Salmon M, Qin S, Hubscher SG, Adams DH. Chemokine and chemokine receptor interactions provide a mechanism for selective T cell recruitment to specific liver compartments within hepatitis C-infected liver. J Immunol, 1999; 163:6236–6243

300. Wanless IR. The cellular distribution of vitamin A in the liver. Liver, 1983; 3:403–409

301. Rockey D. The cellular pathogenesis of portal hypertension: stellate cell contractility, endothelin, and nitric oxide. Hepatology, 1997; 25:2–5

302. Rockey DC, Fouassier L, Chung JJ, Carayon A, Vallee P, Rey C et al. Cellular localization of endothelin-1 and increased production in liver injury in the rat: potential for autocrine and paracrine effects on stellate cells. Hepatology, 1998; 27:472–480

303. Taguchi K, Asano G. Neovascularization of pericellular fibrosis in alcoholic liver disease. Acta Pathologica Japonica, 1988; 38:615–626

304. Schaffner F, Popper H. Capillarization of hepatic sinusoids in man. Gastroenterology, 1963; 44:239–242

305. Mastai R, Laganiere S, Wanless IR, Giroux L, Rocheleau B, Huet PM. Hepatic sinusoidal fibrosis induced by cholesterol and stilbestrol in the rabbit: 2. Hemodynamic and drug disposition studies. Hepatology, 1996; 24:865–870

306. Nagore N, Scheuer PJ. Does a linear pattern of sinusoidal IgA deposition distinguish between alcoholic and diabetic liver disease? Liver, 1988; 8:281–286

307. Falchuk KR, Fiske SC, Haggitt RC, Federman M, Trey C. Pericentral hepatic fibrosis and intracellular hyalin in diabetes mellitus. Gastroenterology, 1980; 78:535–541

308. Le Bail B, Bioulac-Sage P, Senuita R, Quinton A, Saric J, Balabaud C. Fine structure of hepatic sinusoids and sinusoidal cells in disease. J Electr Micro Tech, 1990; 14:257–282

309. Latry P, Bioulac-Sage P, Echinard E, Gin H, Boussarie L, Grimaud JA et al. Perisinusoidal fibrosis and basement membrane-like material in the livers of diabetic patients. Human Pathology, 1987; 18:775–780

310. Zafrani ES, Bernuau D, Feldmann G. Peliosis-like ultrastructural changes of the hepatic sinusoids in human chronic hypervitaminosis A: report of 3 cases. Hum Pathol, 1984; 15:1166–1170

311. Russell RM, Boyer JL, Bagheri SA, Hruban Z. Hepatic injury from chronic hypervitaminosis A resulting in portal hypertension and ascites. N Engl J Med, 1974; 291:435–440

312. Lafon ME, Bioulac-Sage P, Balabaud C. Hepatic fibrosis in patients with idiopathic thrombocytopenic purpura. Liver, 1988; 8:24–27

313. Roux D, Merlio JP, Quinton A, Lamouliatte H, Balabaud C, Bioulac-Sage P. Agnogenic myeloid metaplasia, portal hypertension, and sinusoidal abnormalities. Gastroenterology, 1987; 92:1067–1072

314. Tucker ON, Heaton N. The 'small for size' liver syndrome. Curr Opin Crit Care, 2005; 11:150–155

315. Man K, Fan ST, Lo CM, Liu CL, Fung PC, Liang TB et al. Graft injury in relation to graft size in right lobe live donor liver transplantation: a study of hepatic sinusoidal injury in correlation with portal hemodynamics and intragraft gene expression. Ann Surg, 2003; 237:256–264

316. Troisi R, Ricciardi S, Smeets P, Petrovic M, Van Maele G, Colle I et al. Effects of hemi-portocaval shunts for inflow modulation on the outcome of small-for-size grafts in living donor liver transplantation. Am J Transplant, 2005; 5:1397–1404

317. Wang HS, Enomoto Y, Usuda M, Miyagi S, Asakura T, Masuoka H et al. Excessive portal flow causes graft nonfunction in small size liver transplantation: an experimental study in pigs. Transplant Proc, 2005; 37:407–408

318. Kanel GC, Ucci AA, Kaplan MM, Wolfe HJ. A distinctive perivenular hepatic lesion associated with heart failure. Am J Clin Patholo, 1980; 73:235–239

319. Klatt EC, Koss MN, Young TS, Macauley L, Martin SE. Hepatic hyaline globules associated with passive congestion. Arch Pathol Labo Med, 1988; 112:510–513

320. Holdstock G, Millward-Sadler GH. Hepatic changes in systemic disease. In: Wright R, Alberti KGMM, Karran S, Millward-Sadler GH, eds. Liver and biliary disease. London: WB Saunders, 1979; pp. 862

321. Winckler K, Poulsen H. Liver disease with periportal sinusoidal dilatation. A possible complication to contraceptive steroids. Scand J Gastroenterol, 1975; 10:699–704

322. Spellberg MA, Mirro J, Chowdhury L. Hepatic sinusoidal dilatation related to oral contraceptives. Am J Gastroenterol, 1979; 72:248–252

323. Balazs M. Sinusoidal dilatation of the liver in patients on oral contraceptives. Electron microscopical study of 14 cases. Exp Pathol, 1988; 35:231–237

324. Bauer TW, Moore GW, Hutchins GM. The liver in sickle cell disease: a clinicopathologic study of 70 patients. Am J Med, 1980; 69:833–837

325. Omata M, Johnson CS, Tong M, Tatter D. Pathological spectrum of liver diseases in sickle cell disease. Dig Dis Sci, 1986; 31:247–256

326. Mills LR, Mwakyusa D, Milner PF. Histopathologic features of liver biopsy specimens in sickle cell disease. Arch Pathol Lab Med, 1988; 112:290–294

327. Bruguera M, Aranguibel F, Ros E, Jr. Incidence and clinical significance of sinusoidal dilatation in liver biopsies. Gastroenterology, 1978; 75:474–478

328. Welch K, Finkbeiner W, Alpers CE, Blumenfeld W, Davis RL, Smuckler EA et al. Autopsy findings in the acquired immune deficiency syndrome. JAMA, 1984; 252:1152–1159

329. Delpre G, Ilie B, Papo J, Streifler C, Gefel A. Hypernephroma with nonmetastatic liver dysfunction (Stauffer syndrome) and hypercalcemia. Am J Gastroenterol, 1979; 72:239–247

330. Aoyagi T, Mori I, Ueyama Y, Tamaoki N. Sinusoidal dilatation of the liver as a paraneoplastic manifestation of renal cell carcinoma. Hum Pathol, 1989; 20:1193–1197

331. Bain BJ, Coghlan SJ, Chong KC, Roberts SJ. Hepatic sinusoidal ectasia in association with Hodgkin's disease. Postgrad Medi J, 1982; 58:182–184

332. Zak FG. Peliosis hepatis. Am J Pathol, 1950; 26:1–15

333. Zafrani ES. An additional argument for a toxic mechanism of peliosis hepatis in man. Hepatology, 1990; 11:322–323

334. Yanoff M, Rawson AJ. Peliosis hepatis. An anatomic study with demonstration of two varieties. Arch Pathol, 1964; 77:159–165

335. Wold LE, Ludwig J. Peliosis hepatis: two morphologic variants? Hum Pathol, 1981; 12:388–389

336. Simon DM, Krause R, Galambos JT. Peliosis hepatis in a patient with marasmus. Gastroenterology, 1988; 95:805–809

337. Zafrani ES, Degos F, Guigui B, Durand-Schneider AM, Martin N, Flandrin G et al. The hepatic sinusoid in hairy cell leukemia. An ultrastructural study of 12 cases. Hum Pathol, 1987; 18:801–807

338. Furata M, Asmaoto H, Kitachi M. A case of peliosis hepatis appearing in a patient with lepromatous leprosy. Nippon Rai Gakkai Zasshi, 1982; 51:22–27

339. Delas N, Faurel JP, Wechsler B, Adotti F, Leroy DO, Lemerez M. Association of peliosis and necrotizing vasculitis (letter). Nouv Presse Med, 1982; 11:2787

340. Scoazec JY, Marche C, Girard PM, Houtmann J, Durand-Schneider AM, Saimot AG et al. Peliosis hepatis and sinusoidal dilation during infection by the human immunodeficiency virus (HIV). An ultrastructural study. Am J Pathol, 1988; 131:38–47

341. Larrey D, Freneaux E, Berson A, Babany G, Degott C, Valla D et al. Peliosis hepatis induced by 6-thioguanine administration. Gut, 1988; 29:1265–1269

342. Degott C, Rueff B, Kreis H, DuBoust A, Potet F, Benhamou JP. Peliosis hepatis in recipients of renal transplants. Gut, 1978; 19:748–753

343. Scheuer PJ, Schachter LA, Mathur S, Burroughs AK, Rolles K. Peliosis hepatis after liver transplantation. J Clin Pathol, 1990; 43:1036–1037

344. Czapar CA, Weldon-Linne CM, Moore DM, Rhone DP. Peliosis hepatis in the acquired immunodeficiency syndrome. Arch Pathol Lab Med, 1986; 110:611–613

345. Perkocha LA, Geaghan SM, Yen TSB, Nishimura SL, Chan SP, Garcia-Kennedy R et al. Clinical and pathological features of bacillary peliosis hepatis in association with human immunodeficiency virus infection. N Eng J Med, 1990; 323:1581–1586

346. Ahsan N, Holman MJ, Riley TR, Abendroth CS, Langhoff EG, Yang HC. Peloisis hepatis due to Bartonella henselae in transplantation: a hemato-hepato-renal syndrome. Transplantation, 1998; 65:1000–1003

347. Dauga C, Miras I, Grimont PA. Identification of Bartonella henselae and B. quintana 16s rDNA sequences by branch-, genus- and species-specific amplification. J Med Microbiol, 1996; 45:192–199

348. Vincent AM, Burthem J, Brew R, Cawley JC. Endothelial interactions of hairy cells: the importance of alpha 4 beta 1 in the unusual tissue distribution of the disorder. Blood, 1996; 88:3945–3952

349. Bhaskar KVS, Joshi K, Banerjee CK, Rao RKS, Verma SC. Peliosis hepatis in Hodgkin's disease: an infrequent association (letter). Am J Gastroenterol, 1990; 85:628–629

350. Cadranel JF, Cadranel J, Buffet C, Fabre M, Pelletier G, d'Agay MF et al. Nodular regenerative hyperplasia of the liver, peliosis hepatis, and perisinusoidal fibrosis. Association with angioimmunoblastic lymphadenopathy and severe hypoxemia. Gastroenterology, 1990; 99:268–273

351. Lioté F, Yeni P, Teillet-Thiebaud F, Barge J, Devars Du Mayne JF, Flamant Y et al. Ascites revealing peritoneal and hepatic extramedullary hematopoiesis with peliosis in agnogenic myeloid metaplasia: case report and review of the literature. Am J Med, 1991; 90:111–117

352. Voinchet O, Degott C, Scoazec JY, Feldmann G, Benhamou JP. Peliosis hepatis, nodular regenerative hyperplasia of the liver, and light-chain deposition in a patient with Waldenstrom's macroglobulinemia. Gastroenterology, 1988; 95:482–486

353. Hayward SR, Lucas CE, Ledgerwood AM. Recurrent spontaneous intrahepatic hemorrhage from peliosis hepatis. Arch Surg, 1991; 126:782–783

354. Kubosawa H, Konno A, Komatsu T, Ishige H, Kondo Y. Peliosis hepatis. An unusual case involving the spleen and lymph nodes. Acta Pathologica Japonica, 1989; 39:212–215

355. Chawla SK, Patel HD, Mahadevia SD, LoPresti PA. Portal hypertension in peliosis hepatis: report of the first case. Am J Proctol Gastroenterol Col Rect Surg, 1980; 31:11–17

356. Yanagisawa N, Sugaya H, Yunomura K, Harada T, Hisauchi T. A case of idiopathic portal hypertension after renal transplantation. Gastroenterologia Japonica, 1990; 25:643–648

357. Fonseca V, Havard CW. Portal hypertension secondary to azathioprine in myasthenia gravis. Postgrad Med J, 1988; 64:950–952

358. Olsen TS, Fjeldborg O, Hansen HE. Portal hypertension without liver cirrhosis in renal transplant recipients. APMIS (Suppl.), 1991; 23:13–20

359. Geschwind JF, Salem R, Carr BI, Soulen MC, Thurston KG, Goin KA et al. Yttrium-90 microspheres for the treatment of hepatocellular carcinoma. Gastroenterology, 2004; 127:S194–205

360. Buck FS, Koss MN. Hepatic amyloidosis: morphologic differences between systemic AL and AA types. Hum Pathol, 1991; 22:904–907

361. French SW, Schloss GT, Stillwan AE. Unusual amyloid bodies in human liver. Am J Clin Pathol, 1981; 75:400–402

362. Looi LM, Sumithran E. Morphologic differences in the pattern of liver infiltration between systemic AL and AA amyloidosis. Hum Pathol, 1988; 19:732–735

363. Rubinow A, Koff RS, Cohen AS. Severe intrahepatic cholestasis in primary amyloidosis: a report of four cases and a review of the literature. Am J Med, 1978; 64:937–946

364. Faa G, Van Eyken P, De Vos R, Fevery J, Van Damme B, De Groote J et al. Light chain deposition disease of the liver associated with AL-type amyloidosis and severe cholestasis. J Hepatol, 1991; 12:75–82

365. Evans MA, Gastineau DA, Ludwig J. Relapsing hairy cell leukemia presenting as fulminant hepatitis. Am J Med, 1992; 92:209–212

366. Hoyer JD, Li CY, Yam LT, Hanson CA, Kurtin PJ. Immunohistochemical demonstration of acid phosphatase isoenzyme 5 (tartrate-resistant) in paraffin sections of hairy cell leukemia and other hematologic disorders. Am J Clin Pathol, 1997; 108:308–315

367. Pereira A, Bruguera M, Cervantes F, Rozman C. Liver involvement at diagnosis of primary myelofibrosis: a clinicopathological study of twenty-two cases. Eur J Haematol, 1988; 40:355–361

368. Li WV, Kapadia SB, Sonmez-Alpan E, Swerdlow SH. Immunohistochemical characterization of mast cell disease in paraffin sections using tryptase, CD68, myeloperoxidase, lysozyme, and CD20 antibodies. Mod Pathol, 1996; 9:982–988

369. Inam S, Sidki K, al-Marshedy AR, Judzewitsch R. Addison's disease, hypertension, renal and hepatic microthrombosis in 'primary' antiphospholipid syndrome. Postgrad Med J, 1991; 67:385–388

370. Kakizoe S, Yanaga K, Starzl TE, Demetris AJ. Evaluation of protocol before transplantation and after reperfusion biopsies from human orthotopic liver allografts: considerations of preservation and early immunological injury. Hepatology, 1990; 11:932–941

371. McKeown CM, Edwards V, Phillips MJ, Harvey PR, Petrunka CN, Strasberg SM. Sinusoidal lining cell damage: the critical injury in cold preservation of liver allografts in the rat. Transplantation, 1988; 46:178–191

372. Michels NA. Newer anatomy of liver- variant blood supply and collateral circulation. JAMA, 1960; 172:125–132

373. Halasz NA. Cholecystectomy and hepatic artery injuries. Arch Surg, 1991; 126:137–138

374. Balakhnin PV, Tarazov PG, Polikarpov AA, Suvorova Iu V, Kozlov AV. [Long-term regional chemotherapy for colorectal liver metastasis: significance of hepatic arterial anatomy in the surgical placement of the implantable infusion device]. Vopr Onkol, 2003; 49:588–594

375. Hwang S, Lee SG, Lee YJ, Park KM, Kim KH, Ahn CS et al. Donor selection for procurement of right posterior segment graft in living donor liver transplantation. Liver Transpl, 2004; 10:1150–1155

376. Van Way CW, Crane JM, Riddell DH, Foster JH. Arteriovenous fistula in the portal circulation. Surgery, 1971; 70:876–890

377. Brohée D, Franken P, Fievez M, Baudoux M, Henuzet C, Brasseur P et al. High-output right ventricular failure secondary to hepatic arteriovenous microfistulae. Selective arterial embolization treatment. Arch Int Med, 1984; 144:1282–1284

378. Danchin N, Thisse JY, Neimann JL, Faivre G. Osler-Weber-Rendu disease with multiple intrahepatic arteriovenous fistulas. Am Heart J, 1983; 105:856–859

379. Liu G, Butany J, Wanless IR, Cameron R, Greig P, Levy G. The vascular pathology of human hepatic allografts. Hum Pathol, 1993; 24:182–188

380. Hocking WG, Lasser K, Ungerer R, Bersohn M, Palos M, Spiegel T. Spontaneous hepatic rupture in rheumatoid arthritis. Arch Int Med, 1981; 141:792–794

381. Okuda K, Musha H, Nakajima Y, Takayasu K, Suzuki Y, Morita M et al. Frequency of intrahepatic arteriovenous fistula as a sequela to percutaneous needle puncture of the liver. Gastroenterology, 1978; 74:1204–1207

382. Song HY, Choi KC, Park JH, Choi BI, Chung YS. Radiological evaluation of hepatic artery aneurysms. Gastrointest Radiol, 1989; 14:329–333

383. Collier JD, Sale J, Friend PJ, Jamieson NV, Calne RY, Alexander GJ. Graft loss and the antiphospholipid syndrome following liver transplantation. J Hepatol, 1998; 29:999–1003

384. Douglas TC, Cutter WW. Arterial supply of the common bile duct. Arch Surg, 1948; 57:599–612

385. Kasper HU, Dries V, Drebber U, Stippel D, Reinhold K, Dienes HP. Florid ischemic cholangitis due to leucocytoclastic vasculitis. J Gastroenterol, 2004; 39:188–191

386. Viola S, Meyer M, Fabre M, Tounian P, Goddon R, Dechelotte P et al. Ischemic necrosis of bile ducts complicating Schonlein-Henoch purpura. Gastroenterology, 1999; 117:211–214

387. Bader-Meunier B, Hadchouel M, Fabre M, Arnoud MD, Dommergues JP. Intrahepatic bile duct damage in children with Kawasaki disease. J Pediatr, 1992; 120:750–752

388. Ludwig J, Kim CH, Wiesner RH, Krom RA. Floxuridine-induced sclerosing cholangitis: an ischemic cholangiopathy? Hepatology, 1989; 9:215–218

389. Batts KP. Ischemic cholangitis. Mayo Clin Proc, 1998; 73:380–385

390. Cherqui D, Palazzo L, Piedbois P, Charlotte F, Duvoux C, Duron JJ et al. Common bile duct stricture as a late complication of upper abdominal radiotherapy. J Hepatol, 1994; 20:693–697

391. Sanchez-Urdazpal L, Gores GJ, Ward EM, Maus TP, Buckel EG, Steers JL et al. Diagnostic features and clinical outcome of ischemic-type biliary complications after liver transplantation. Hepatology, 1993; 17:605–609

392. Kirby DF, Blei AT, Rosen ST, Vogelzang RL, Neiman HL. Primary sclerosing cholangitis in the presence of a lupus anticoagulant. Am J Med, 1986; 81:1077–1080

393. Le Thi Huong D, Valla D, Franco D, Wechsler B, De Gramont A, Auperin A et al. Cholangitis associated with paroxysmal nocturnal hemoglobinuria: another instance of ischemic cholangiopathy? Gastroenterology, 1995; 109:1338–1343

394. Dessailloud R, Papo T, Vaneecloo S, Gamblin C, Vanhille P, Piette JC. Acalculous ischemic gallbladder necrosis in the catastrophic antiphospholipid syndrome. Arthritis Rheum, 1998; 41:1318–1320

395. Burt AD, Scott G, Shiach CR, Isles CG. Acquired immunodeficiency syndrome in a patient with no known risk factors: a pathological study. J Clin Pathol, 1984; 37:471–474

396. Jacobson MA, Cello JP, Sande MA. Cholestasis and disseminated cytomegalovirus disease in patients with the acquired immunodeficiency syndrome. Am J Med, 1988; 84:218–224

397. Parangi S, Oz MC, Blume RS, Bixon R, Laffey KJ, Perzin KH et al. Hepatobiliary complications of polyarteritis nodosa. Arch Surg, 1991; 126:909–912

398. Haratake J, Horie A, Furuta A, Yamato H. Massive hepatic infarction associated with polyarteritis nodosa. Acta Pathologica Japonica, 1988; 38:89–93

399. Doppman JL, Dunnick NR, Girton M, Fauci AS, Popovsky MA. Bile duct cysts secondary to liver infarcts: report of a case and experimental production by small vessel hepatic artery occlusion. Radiology, 1979; 130:1–5

400. Noda M, Kusunoki M, Yanagai H, Yamamura T, Utsunomiya J. Hepatic artery-biliary fistula during infusion chemotherapy. Hepatogastroenterology, 1996; 43:1387–1389

401. Chen JW, Chen DZ, Lu GZ. Asymptomatic process of hepatic artery thrombosis in a patient after orthotopic liver transplantation. Hepatobiliary Pancreat Dis Int, 2004; 3:149–151

402. Gunsar F, Rolando N, Pastacaldi S, Patch D, Raimondo ML, Davidson B et al. Late hepatic artery thrombosis after orthotopic liver transplantation. Liver Transpl, 2003; 9:605–611

403. Leonardi MI, Boin I, Leonardi LS. Late hepatic artery thrombosis after liver transplantation: clinical setting and risk factors. Transplant Proc, 2004; 36:967–969

404. Vivarelli M, Cucchetti A, La Barba G, Bellusci R, De Vivo A, Nardo B et al. Ischemic arterial complications after liver transplantation in the adult: multivariate analysis of risk factors. Arch Surg, 2004; 139:1069–1074

405. Rankin RN, Vellet DA. Portobiliary fistula: occurrence and treatment. Can Ass Radiol J, 1991; 42:55–59

406. Wooling KR, Baggenstoss AH, Weir JF. Infarction of the liver. Gastroenterology, 1951; 17:479–493

407. Brittain RS, Marchioro TL, Hermann G, Waddell W, Starzl TE. Accidental hepatic artery ligation in humans. Am J Surg, 1964; 107:822–832

408. Chen V, Hamilton J, Qizilbash A. Hepatic infarction. Arch Pathol Lab Med, 1976; 100:32–36

409. Arcidi JM, Jr, Moore GW, Hutchins GM. Hepatic morphology in cardiac dysfunction. A clinicopathologic study of 1000 subjects at autopsy. Am J Pathol, 1981; 104:159–166

410. Bynum TE, Boitnott JK, Maddrey WC. Ischemic hepatitis. Dig Dis Sci, 1979; 24:129–135

411. Shibuya A, Unuma T, Sugimoto T, Yamakado M, Tagawa H, Tagawa K et al. Diffuse hepatic calcification as a sequela to shock liver. Gastroenterology, 1985; 89:196–201

412. Wanless IR, Dore S, Gopinath N, Tan J, Cameron R, Heathcote EJ et al. Histopathology of cocaine hepatotoxicity: report of four patients. Gastroenterology, 1990; 98:497–501

413. Dammann HG, Hagemann J, Runge M, Kloppel G. In vivo diagnosis of massive hepatic infarction by computed tomography. Dig Dis Sci, 1982; 27:73–79

414. Pauzner R, Dulitzky M, Carp H, Mayan H, Kenett R, Farfel Z et al. Hepatic infarctions during pregnancy are associated with the antiphospholipid syndrome and in addition with complete or incomplete HELLP syndrome. J Thromb Haemost, 2003; 1:1758–1763

415. Wanless IR. Physioanatomic considerations. In: Schiff L, Schiff ER, eds. Schiff's Diseases of the Liver, 8th edn. Philadelphia: JB Lippincott, 1999; pp. 3–37

416. International Working Party. Terminology of nodular hepatocellular lesions. Hepatology, 1995; 22:983–993

417. Karvountzis GG, Redeker AG, Peters RL. Long term follow-up studies of patients surviving fulminant viral hepatitis. Gastroenterology, 1974; 67:870–877

418. Wanless IR, Tanaka M. Determinants of hepatic regeneration after fulminant hepatic failure. Mod Pathol, 1999; 12:168A

419. Wanless IR, Shimamatsu K. The histogenesis of biliary cirrhosis. Mod Pathol, 1999; 12:169A

420. Millener P, Grant EG, Rose S, Duerinckx A, Schiller VL, Tessler FN et al. Color Doppler imaging findings in patients with Budd–Chiari syndrome: correlation with venographic findings. Am J Roentgenol, 1993; 161:307–312

421. Ohtomo K, Baron RL, Dodd GD, Federle MP, Miller WJ, Campbell WL et al. Confluent hepatic fibrosis in advanced cirrhosis—appearance at CT. Radiology, 1993; 188:31–35

422. Popper H. Pathologic aspects of cirrhosis. Am J Pathol, 1977; 87:228–264

423. Huet PM, Goresky CA, Villeneuve JP, Marleau D, Lough JO. Assessment of liver microcirculation in human cirrhosis. J Clin Invest, 1982; 70:1234–1244

424. Ohnishi K, Chin N, Sugita S, Saito M, Tanaka H, Terabayashi H et al. Quantitative aspects of portal-systemic and arteriovenous shunts within the liver in cirrhosis. Gastroenterology, 1987; 93:129–134

425. Ohnishi K, Chin N, Saito M, Tanaka H, Terabayashi H, Nakayama T et al. Portographic opacification of hepatic veins and (anomalous) anastomoses between the portal and hepatic veins in cirrhosis—indication of extensive intrahepatic shunts. Am J Gastroenterol, 1986; 81:975–978

426. Horiguchi Y, Kitano T, Imai H, Ohsuki M, Yamauchi M, Itoh M. Intrahepatic portal-systemic shunt: its etiology and diagnosis. Gastroenterologia Japonica, 1987; 22:496–502

427. Dilawari JB, Chawla YK. Spontaneous (natural) splenoadrenorenal shunts in extrahepatic portal venous obstruction: a series of 20 cases. Gut, 1987; 28:1198–1200

428. Dilawari JB, Raju GS, Chawla YK. Development of large splenoadrenorenal shunt after endoscopic sclerotherapy. Gastroenterology, 1989; 97:421–426

429. Menu Y, Alison D, Lorphelin JM, Valla D, Belghiti J, Nahum H. Budd–Chiari syndrome: US evaluation. Radiology, 1985; 157:761–764

430. Burcharth F. Percutaneous transhepatic portography. I. Technique and application. Am J Roentgenol, 1979; 132:177–182

431. Schabel SI, Rittenberg GM, Javid LH, Cunningham J, Ross P. The "bull's-eye" falciform ligament: a sonographic finding of portal hypertension. Radiology, 1980; 136:157–159

432. Okuda K, Matsutani S. Portal-systemic collaterals: anatomy and clinical implications. In: Okuda K, Benhamou JP, eds. Portal hypertension. Clinical and physiological aspects. Tokyo: Springer-Verlag, 1991; pp. 51–62

433. Viamonte MJ. Liver shunts. Am J Roentgenol, 1968; 102:773–775

434. Farrell R, Steinman A, Green WH. Arteriovenous shunting in a regenerating liver simulating hepatoma. Report of a case. Radiology, 1972; 102:279–280

435. Deutsch V, Adar R, Bogokowsky H, Itzchak Y, Mozes M. Diversion of the hepatic arterial flow into the portal vein in the Budd–Chiari syndrome. Blood Vessels, 1974; 11:96–100

436. Gorka W, Gorka TS, Lewall DB. Doppler ultrasound evaluation of advanced portal vein pulsatility in patients with normal echocardiograms. Eur J Ultrasound, 1998; 8:119–123

437. Krowka JK. Hepatopulmonary syndrome: an evolving perspective in the era of liver transplantation. Hepatology, 1990; 11:138–142

438. al-Moamary M, Altraif I. Hepatopulmonary syndrome associated with schistosomal liver disease. Can J Gastroenterol, 1997; 11:449–450

439. Herve P, Lebrec D, Brenot F, Simonneau G, Humbert M, Sitbon O et al. Pulmonary vascular disorders in portal hypertension. Eur Respir J, 1998; 11:1153–1166

440. Krowka MJ. Hepatopulmonary syndrome versus portopulmonary hypertension: distinctions and dilemmas. Hepatology, 1997; 25:1282–1284

441. Ramsay MA, Simpson BR, Nguyen AT, Ramsay KJ, East C, Klintmalm GB. Severe pulmonary hypertension in liver transplant candidates. Liver Transpl Surg, 1997; 3:494–500

442. Wanless IR. Coexistent pulmonary and portal hypertension: Yin and Yang. Hepatology, 1989; 10:255–257

443. Morris W, Knauer CM. Cardiopulmonary manifestations of schistosomiasis. Semin Respir Infect, 1997; 12:159–170

444. LaBerge JM, Ferrell LD, Ring EJ, Gordon RL, Lake JR, Roberts JP et al. Histopathologic study of transjugular intrahepatic portosystemic shunts. J Vasc Interv Radiol, 1991; 2:549–556

445. Ducoin H, El-Khoury J, Rousseau H, Barange K, Peron JM, Pierragi MT et al. Histopathologic analysis of transjugular intrahepatic portosystemic shunts. Hepatology, 1997; 25:1064–1069

446. Terayama N, Matsui O, Kadoya M, Yoshikawa J, Gabata T, Miyayama S et al. Transjugular intrahepatic portosystemic shunt: histologic and immunohistochemical study of autopsy cases. Cardiovasc Intervent Radiol, 1997; 20:457–461

447. Sanyal AJ, Mirshahi F. Endothelial cells lining transjugular intrahepatic portasystemic shunts originate in hepatic sinusoids: implications for pseudointimal hyperplasia. Hepatology, 1999; 29:710–718

448. LaBerge JM, Ferrell LD, Ring EJ, Gordon RL. Histopathologic study of stenotic and occluded transjugular intrahepatic portosystemic shunts. J Vasc Interv Radiol, 1993; 4:779–786

449. Jalan R, Harrison DJ, Redhead DN, Hayes PC. Transjugular intrahepatic portosystemic stent-shunt (TIPSS) occlusion and the role of biliary venous fistulae. J Hepatol, 1996; 24:169–176

450. Schweiger GD, Redick ML, Siegel EL, Harrison LA, Rosenthal SJ. Hepatic arterial pseudoaneurysm after placement of transjugular intrahepatic portosystemic shunt. J Ultrasound Med, 1997; 16:437–439

451. Ferguson JW, Tripathi D, Redhead DN, Ireland H, Hayes PC. Transient segmental liver ischaemia after polytetrafluoroethylene transjugular intrahepatic portosystemic stent-shunt procedure. J Hepatol, 2005; 42:145

452. Ochs A. Transjugular intrahepatic portosystemic shunt. Dig Dis, 2005; 23:56–64

453. Lewis DR, Burbige EJ, French SW. Reversal of cirrhosis in hemochromatosis following long-term phlebotomy. Gastroenterology, 1983; 84:1382

454. Dufour JF, DeLellis R, Kaplan MM. Regression of hepatic fibrosis in hepatitis C with long-term interferon treatment. Dig Dis Sci, 1998; 43:2573–2576

455. Iredale JP, Benyon RC, Pickering J, McCullen M, Northrop M, Pawley S et al. Mechanisms of spontaneous resolution of rat liver fibrosis. Hepatic stellate cell apoptosis and reduced hepatic expression of metalloproteinase inhibitors. J Clin Invest, 1998; 102:538–549

456. Stromeyer FW, Ishak KG. Nodular transformation (nodular "regenerative" hyperplasia) of the liver. Hum Pathol, 1981; 12:60–71

457. Nakanuma Y. Nodular regenerative hyperplasia of the liver: retrospective survey in autopsy series. J Clin Gastroenterol, 1990; 12:460–465

458. Wanless IR. Benign liver tumors. Clin Liver Dis, 2002; 6:513–526, ix

459. Sherlock S, Feldman CA, Moran B, Scheuer PJ. Partial nodular transformation of the liver with portal hypertension. Am J Med, 1966; 40:195–203

460. Paradis V, Benzekri A, Dargere D, Bieche I, Laurendeau I, Vilgrain V et al. Telangiectatic focal nodular hyperplasia: a variant of hepatocellular adenoma. Gastroenterology, 2004; 126:1323–1329

461. Qizilbash A, Kontozoglou T, Sianos J, Scully K. Hepar lobatum associated with chemotherapy and metastatic breast cancer. Arch Pathol Lab Med, 1987; 111:58–61

462. Benz EJ, Baggenstoss AH, Wollaeger EE. Atrophy of the left lobe of the liver. Arch Pathol, 1952; 53:315–330

463. Wanless IR, Mawdsley C, Adams R. On the pathogenesis of focal nodular hyperplasia of the liver. Hepatology, 1985; 5:1194–1200

464. Nguyen BN, Flejou JF, Terris B, Belghiti J, Degott C. Focal nodular hyperplasia of the liver: a comprehensive pathologic study of 305 lesions and recognition of new histologic forms. Am J Surg Pathol, 1999; 23:1441–1454

465. Bioulac-Sage P, Rebouissou S, Sa Cunha A, Jeannot E, Lepreux S, Blanc JF et al. Clinical, morphologic, and molecular features defining so-called telangiectatic focal nodular hyperplasias of the liver. Gastroenterology, 2005; 128:1211–1218

466. Terada T, Kitani S, Ueda K, Nakanuma Y, Kitagawa K, Masuda S. Adenomatous hyperplasia of the liver resembling focal nodular hyperplasia in patients with chronic liver disease. Virchows Arch A Pathol Anat Histopathol, 1993; 422:247–252

467. Matsushita M, Hajiro K, Suzaki T, Takakuwa H, Sawami H, Kusumi F et al. Focal nodular hyperplasia of the liver without central scar. Dig Dis Sci, 1995; 40:2407–2410

468. Kaji K, Kaneko S, Matsushita E, Kobayashi K, Matsui O, Nakanuma Y. A case of progressive multiple focal nodular hyperplasia with alteration of imaging studies. Am J Gastroenterol, 1998; 93:2568–2572

469. Lough J, Spicer P, Kinch R. Focal nodular hyperplasia of the liver. An electron microscopic study of the vascular lesions. Hum Pathol, 1980; 11:181–186

470. Wanless IR. Focal nodular hyperplasia of the liver: comments on the pathogenesis. Arch Pathol Lab Med, 2000; 124:1105–1107

471. Takayama A, Olshansky D, Wanless IR. Three-dimensional angioarchitecture of focal nodular hyperplasia and hypothesis on the pathogenesis. Mod Pathol, 2004; 17:313A

472. Wanless IR, Gryfe A. Nodular transformation of the liver in hereditary hemorrhagic telangiectasia. Arch Pathol Lab Med, 1986; 110:331–335

473. Bureau C, Peron JM, Sirach E, Selves J, Otal P, Vinel JP. Liver nodules ressembling focal nodular hyperplasia after portal vein thrombosis. J Hepatol, 2004; 41:499–500

474. De Gaetano AM, Gui B, Macis G, Manfredi R, Di Stasi C. Congenital absence of the portal vein associated with focal nodular hyperplasia in the liver in an adult woman: imaging and review of the literature. Abdom Imaging, 2004; 29:455–459

475. Wanless IR, Lentz JS, Roberts EA. Partial nodular transformation of liver in an adult with persistent ductus venosus. Arch Pathol Lab Med, 1985; 109:427–432

476. Jacob S, Farr G, De Vun D, Takiff H, Mason A. Hepatic manifestations of familial patent ductus venosus in adults. Gut, 1999; 45:442–445

477. Sakatoku H, Hirokawa Y, Inoue M, Kojima M, Yabana T, Sakurai M. Focal nodular hyperplasia in an adolescent with glycogen storage disease type I with mesocaval shunt operation in childhood: a case report and review of the literature. Acta Paediatr Jpn, 1996; 38:172–175

478. Pizzo CJ. Type I glycogen storage disease with focal nodular hyperplasia of the liver and vasoconstrictive pulmonary hypertension. Pediatrics, 1980; 65:341–343

479. Komisarof JA, Olthoff K, Siegelman ES, Lawton TJ, Furth EE. Focal nodular hyperplasia contiguous with an echinococcal cyst. Am J Gastroenterol, 1999; 95:1078–1081

480. Ndimbie OK, Goodman ZD, Chase RL, Ma CK, Lee MW. Hemangiomas with localized nodular proliferation of the liver. A suggestion on the pathogenesis of focal nodular hyperplasia. Am J Surg Pathol, 1990; 14:142–150

481. Saul SH, Titelbaum DS, Gansler TS, Varello M, Burke DR, Atkinson BF et al. The fibrolamellar variant of hepatocellular carcinoma. Its association with focal nodular hyperplasia. Cancer, 1987; 60:3049–3055

482. Saxena R, Humphreys S, Williams R, Portmann B. Nodular hyperplasia surrounding fibrolamellar carcinoma: a zone of arterialized liver parenchyma. Histopathology, 1994; 25:275–278

483. Bralet MP, Terris B, Vilgrain V, Bregeaud L, Molas G, Corbic M et al. Epithelioid hemangioendothelioma, multiple focal nodular hyperplasias and cavernous hemangiomas of the liver: an unusual association. Arch Pathol Lab Med, 1999; 123:846–849

484. Simonds JP. Chronic occlusion of the portal vein. Archives of Surgery, 1936; 33:397–424

485. McDermott WV, Bothe A, Clouse ME, Bern MM. Noncirrhotic portal hypertension in adults. Am J Surg, 1981; 141:514–518

486. Thompson EN, Sherlock S. The aetiology of portal vein thrombosis with particular reference to the role of infection and exchange transfusion. Quart J Med, 1964; 33:465–480

487. Capron JP, Lemay JL, Muir JF, Dupas JL, Lebrec D, Gineston JL. Portal vein thrombosis and fatal pulmonary thromboembolism associated with oral contraceptive treatment. J Clin Gastroenterol, 1981; 3:295–298

488. Orozco H, Guraieb E, Takahashi T, Garcia-Tsao G, Hurtado R, Anaya R et al. Deficiency of protein C in patients with portal vein thrombosis. Hepatology, 1988; 8:1110–1111

489. Valla D, Denninger MH, Delvigne JM, Rueff B, Benhamou JP. Portal vein thrombosis with ruptured oesophageal varices as presenting manifestation of hereditary protein C deficiency. Gut, 1988; 29:856–859

490. Klar E, Buhr H, Zimmermann R. Protein C deficiency with recurrent infarct of the small intestine. Chirurg, 1990; 61:59–62

491. Seifert M, Fleck U, Vogel G, Batz C, Basche S. Partial portal vein and mesenteric vein thrombosis in familial protein S deficiency. Chirurg, 1994; 65:1143–1147

492. Odegard QR, Abildgaard U. Antifactor Xa activity in thrombophilia. Studies in a family with AT-III deficiency. Scand J Hematol, 1977; 18:86–90

493. Schved JF, Gris JC, Aguilar-Martinez P, Birbes P, Carabalona P. Recurrent venous thromboembolism caused by heparin cofactor II deficiency. A case. Presse Med, 1991; 20:1211–1214

494. Chang HP, McFadzean AJS. Thrombosis and intimal thickening in the portal system of the liver in cirrhosis of the liver. J Pathol Bacteriol, 1965; 89:473–480

495. Die Goyanes A, Pack GT, Bowden L. Cancer of the body and tail of the pancreas. Rev Surg, 1971; 28:153–175

496. McDermott WV, Jr. Portal hypertension secondary to pancreatic disease. Ann Surg, 1960; 152:147–150

497. Bilbao JI, Rodriguez-Cabello J, Longo J, Zornoza G, P:aramo J, Lecumberri FJ. Portal thrombosis: percutaneous transhepatic treatment with urokinase—a case report. Gastrointest Radiol, 1989; 14:326–328

498. Perel Y, Dhermy D, Carrere A, Chateil JF, Bondonny JM, Micheau M et al. Portal vein thrombosis after splenectomy for hereditary stomatocytosis in childhood. Eur J Pediatr, 1999; 158:628–630

499. Mosimann F, Mange B. Portal hypertension as a complication of idiopathic retroperitoneal fibrosis. Br J Surg, 1980; 67:804

500. Lin CS. Suppurative pylephlebitis and liver abscess complicating colonic diverticulitis: report of two cases and review of literature. Mt Sinai J Med, 1973; 40:48–55

501. Slovis TL, Haller JO, Cohen HL, Berdon WE, Watts FB, Jr. Complicated appendiceal inflammatory disease in children: pylephlebitis and liver abscess. Radiology, 1989; 171:823–825

502. Nishimori H, Ezoe E, Ura H, Imaizumi H, Meguro M, Furuhata T et al. Septic thrombophlebitis of the portal and superior mesenteric veins as a complication of appendicitis: report of a case. Surg Today, 2004; 34:173–176

503. Inacio C, Hillaire S, Valla D, Denninger MH, Casadevall N, Erlinger S. Case report: cytomegalovirus infection as a cause of acute portal vein thrombosis. J Gastroenterol Hepatol, 1997; 12:287–288

504. Whipple AO. The problem of portal hypertension in relation to the hepatosplenopathies. Ann Surg, 1945; 122:449–475

505. Maddrey WC, Sen Gupta KP, Basu Mallik KC, Iber FL, Basu AK. Extrahepatic obstruction of the portal venous system. Surg Gynecol Obstet, 1968; 127:989–998

506. Lauridsen UB, Enk B, Gammeltoft A. Oesophageal varices as a late complication to neonatal umbilical vein catheterization. Acta Ped Scand, 1978; 67:633–636

507. Hunter GC, Steinkirchner T, Burbige EJ, Guernsey JM, Putnam CW. Venous complications of sclerotherapy for esophageal varices. Am J Surg, 1988; 156:497–501

508. Thatcher BS, Sivak MV, Ferguson DR, Petras RE. Mesenteric venous thrombosis as a possible complication of endoscopic sclerotherapy. Am J Gastroenterol, 1986; 81:126–129

509. Valla D, Pessegueiro-Miranda H, Degott C, Lebrec D, Rueff B, Benhamou JP. Hepatic sarcoidosis with portal hypertension. A report of seven cases with a review of the literature. Quart J Med, 1987; 63:531–544

510. Talbot RW, Heppell J, Dozois RR, Baert RW, Jr. Vascular complications of inflammatory bowel disease. Mayo Clin Proc, 1986; 61:140–145

511. Capron JP, Remond A, Lebrec D, Delamarre J, Dupas JL, Lorriaux A. Gastrointestinal bleeding due to chronic portal vein thrombosis in ulcerative colitis. Dig Dis Sc, 1979; 24:232–235

512. Aronson AR, Steinheber FU. Portal vein thrombosis in ulcerative colitis. NY State J Med, 1971; 71:2310–2311

513. McIntyre RE, Magidson JG, Austin GE, Gale RP. Fatal veno-occlusive disease of the liver following high-dose 1,3-Bis(2-chloroethyl)-1-nitrosourea (BCNU) and autologous bone marrow transplantation. Am J Clin Pathol, 1981; 75:614–617

514. Benesch M, McDonald GB, Schubert M, Appelbaum FR, Deeg HJ. Lack of cytoprotective effect of amifostine following HLA-identical sibling transplantation for advanced myelodysplastic syndrome (MDS): a pilot study. Bone Marrow Transplant, 2003; 32:1071–1075

515. Brick JE, Moreland LW, Al-Kawas F, Chang WWL, Layne RD, DiBartolomeo AG. Prospective analysis of liver biopsies before and after methotrexate therapy in rheumatoid patients. Semin Arthritis Rheum, 1989; 19:31–44

516. Popper H, Thomas LB, Telles NC, Faek H, Selikoff IJ. Angiosarcoma in man induced by vinyl chloride, thorotrast, and arsenic: comparison of cases with unknown etiology. Am J Pathol, 1978; 92:349–376

517. Okuda K, Omata M, Itoh Y, Ikezaki H, Nakashima T. Peliosis hepatis as a late and final complication of thorotrast liver disease. Report of five cases. Liver, 1981; 1:110–122

518. Pimental JC, Menezes AP. Liver disease in vineyard sprayers. Gastroenterology, 1977; 72:275–283

519. Solis-Herruzo JA, Vidal JV, Colina F, Santalla F, Castellano G. Nodular regenerative hyperplasia of the liver associated with the toxic oil syndrome: report of five cases. Hepatology, 1986; 6:687–693

520. Nadell J, Kosek J. Peliosis hepatis. Twelve cases associated with oral androgen therapy. Arch Pathol Lab Med, 1977; 101:405–410

521. Taxy JB. Peliosis: a morphological curiosity becomes an iatrogenic problem. Hum Pathol, 1978; 9:331–340

522. Loomus GN, Aneja P, Bota RA. A case of peliosis hepatis in association with tamoxifen therapy. Am J Clin Pathol, 1983; 80:881–883

523. McDonald GB, Sharma P, Matthews DE, Shulman HM, Thomas ED. Venocclusive disease of the liver after bone marrow transplantation: diagnosis, incidence and predisposing factors. Hepatology, 1984; 4:116–122

524. Leibowitz AI, Hartmann RC. The Budd–Chiari syndrome and paroxysmal nocturnal hemoglobinuria. Br J Haematol, 1981; 48:1–6

525. Bahr MJ, Schubert J, Bleck JS, Tietge UJ, Boozari B, Schmidt RE et al. Recurrence of Budd–Chiari syndrome after liver transplantation in paroxysmal nocturnal hemoglobinuria. Transpl Int, 2003; 16:890–894

526. Riccio JA, Colley AT, Cera PJ. Hepatic vein thrombosis (Budd–Chiari syndrome) in the microgranular variant of acute promyelocytic leukemia. Am J Clin Pathol, 1989; 92:366–371

527. Chillar RK, Paladugu RR. Hepatic vein thrombosis (acute Budd–Chiari syndrome) in acute leukemia. Am J Med Sci, 1981; 282:153–156

528. Wang Z, Zhu Y, Wang S, Pu L, Du Y, Zhang H et al. Recognition and management of Budd Chiari syndrome. A report of 100 cases. J Vasc Surg, 1989; 10:149–156

529. Lewis JH, Tice HL, Zimmerman HJ. Budd–Chiari syndrome associated with oral contraceptive steroids. Review of treatment of 47 cases. Dig Dis Sci, 1983; 28:673–683

530. Maddrey WC. Hepatic vein thrombosis (Budd–Chiari syndrome): possible association with the use of oral contraceptives. Semin Liver Dis, 1987; 7:32–39

531. Valla D, Le GM, Poynard T, Zucman N, Rueff B, Benhamou JP. Risk of hepatic vein thrombosis in relation to recent use of oral contraceptive: a case–control study. Gastroenterology, 1986; 90:807–811

532. Pomeroy C, Knodell RG, Swaim WR, Arneson P, Mahowald ML. Budd–Chiari syndrome in a patient with the lupus anticoagulant. Gastroenterology, 1984; 86:158–161

533. Farrant JM, Judge M, Thompson RP. Thrombotic cutaneous nodules and hepatic vein thrombosis in the anticardiolipin syndrome. Clin Exp Dermatol, 1989; 14:306–308

534. Van Steenbergen W, Beyls J, Vermylen J, Fevery J, Marchal G, Desmet V et al. Lupus anticoagulant and thrombosis of the hepatic veins (Budd–Chiari syndrome). Report of three patients and review of the literature. J Hepatol, 1986; 3:87–94

535. Asherson RA, Thompson RP, MacLachlan N, Baguley E, Hicks P, Hughes GR. Budd Chiari syndrome, visceral arterial occlusions, recurrent fetal loss and the "lupus anticoagulant" in systemic lupus erythematosus. J Rheumatol, 1989; 16:219–224

536. Nakamura H, Uehara H, Okada T, Kambe H, Kimura Y, Ito H et al. Occlusion of small hepatic veins associated with systemic lupus erythematosus with the lupus anticoagulant and anti-cardiolipin antibody. Hepatogastroenterology, 1989; 36:393–397

537. Couffinhal T, Bonnet J, Benchimol D, Dos Santos P, Besse P, Bricaud H. A case of the Budd Chiari syndrome attributed to a deficit in protein C. Eur Heart J, 1991; 12:266–269

538. De Stefano V, Chiusolo P, Paciaroni K, Teofili L, La Barbera EO, Casorelli I et al. Hepatic vein thrombosis in a patient with mutant prothrombin 20210A allele. Thromb Haemost, 1998; 80:519

539. Das M, Carroll S. Antithrombin III deficiency: an etiology of Budd–Chiari syndrome. Surgery, 1985; 97:242–245

540. McClure S, Dincsoy HP, Glueck H. Budd–Chiari syndrome and antithrombin III deficiency. American J Clin Pathol, 1982; 78:236–241

541. Min AD, Atillasoy EO, Schwartz ME, Thiim M, Miller CM, Bodenheimer HC, Jr. Reassessing the role of medical therapy in the management of hepatic vein thrombosis. Liver Transpl Surg, 1997; 3:423–429

542. Bandyopadhyay SK, Sarkar N, Ghosh S, Dasgupta S. Cholangiocarcinoma presenting with recurrent venous thrombosis. J Assoc Physicians India, 2003; 51:824–825

543. Correa de Araujo R, Bestetti RB, Oliveira JSM. An unusual case of Budd–Chiari syndrome—a case report. Angiology, 1988; 39:193–198

544. Lorenzo MJ, Gual Corts M, Morato Griera J. The syndrome of Budd–Chiari associated with constrictive pericarditis and complete thrombosis of the inferior vena cava. Rev Clin Esp, 1979; 152:407–410

545. Paul O, Castleman B, White PD. Chronic constrictive pericarditis: a study of 53 cases. Am J Med Sci, 1948; 216:361–377

546. Fonkalsurd EW, Linde LM, Longmire WPJ. Portal hypertension from idiopathic superior vena caval obstruction. JAMA, 1966; 196:115–118

547. Feingold ML, Litwak RL, Geller SS, Baron MM. Budd–Chiari syndrome caused by a right atrial tumor. Arch Inter Med, 1971; 127:292–295

548. Sty JR. Ultrasonography: hepatic vein thrombosis in sickle cell anemia. Am J Pediatr Hematol-Oncol, 1982; 4:213–215

549. Reynolds TB. Budd–Chiari syndrome. In: Schiff L, Schiff ER, eds. Diseases of the liver, 6th edn. Philadelphia: J.B. Lippincott, 1987; pp. 1466–1473

550. Fortner JG, Kallum BO, Kim DK. Surgical management of hepatic vein occlusion by tumor. Arch Surg, 1977; 112:727–728

551. Spapen HD, Volckaert A, Bourgain C, Braeckman J, Van Belle SJ. Acute Budd–Chiari syndrome with portosystemic encephalopathy as first sign of renal carcinoma. Br J Urol, 1988; 62:274–275

552. Carbonnel F, Valla D, Menu Y, Lecompte Y, Belghiti J, Rueff B et al. Acute Budd–Chiari syndrome as first manifestation of adrenocortical carcinoma. J Clin Gastroenterol, 1988; 10:441–444

553. Walsh MM, Hytiroglou P, Thung SN, Fiel MI, Siegel D, Emre S et al. Epithelioid hemangioendothelioma of the liver mimicking Budd–Chiari syndrome. Arch Pathol Lab Med, 1998; 122:846–848

554. Jose B, Narayan PI, Pietsch JB, Nagaraj HS, Patel CC, Bertolone SJ et al. Budd–Chiari syndrome secondary to hepatic vein thrombus from Wilm's tumor. Case report and literature review. J Kentucky Med Ass, 1989; 87:174–176

555. Kinmond S, Carter R, Skeoch CH, Morton NS. Nephroblastoma presenting with acute hepatic encephalopathy. Arch Dis Child, 1990; 65:542–543

556. Imakita M, Yutani C, Ishibashi-Ueda H, Hiraoka H, Naito H. Primary leiomyosarcoma of the inferior vena cava with Budd–Chiari syndrome. Acta Pathologica Japonica, 1989; 39:73–77

557. Lee PK, Teixeira OH, Simons JA, Goodman RL, Brais MP, Barber GG et al. Atypical hepatic vein leiomyoma extending into the right atrium: an unusual cause of the Budd–Chiari syndrome. Can J Cardiol, 1990; 6:107–110

558. Pollanen M, Butany J, Chiasson D. Leiomyosarcoma of the inferior vena cava. Arch Pathol Lab Med, 1987; 111:1085–1087

559. Koshy A, Bhusnurmath SR, Mitra SK, Mahajan KK, Datta DV, Aikat BK et al. Hydatid disease associated with hepatic outflow tract obstruction. Am J Gastroenterol, 1980; 74:274–278

560. Aikat BK, Bhusnurmath SR, Chhuttani PN, Datta DV. Hepatic vein obstruction—A retrospective analysis of 72 autopsies and biopsies. Ind J Med Res, 1978; 67:128–144

561. Nicoloff DM, Fortuny IE, Pewall RA. Acute Budd–Chiari syndrome secondary to intrahepatic hematoma following blunt abdominal trauma: Treatment by open intracardiac surgery. J Thorac Cardiovasc Surg, 1964; 47:225–229

562. Klein MD, Philippart AI. Posttraumatic Budd–Chiari syndrome with late reversibility of hepatic venous obstruction. J Pediatr Surg, 1979; 14:661–663

563. Hales MR, Scatliff JH. Thrombosis of the inferior vena cava and hepatic veins (Budd–Chiari syndrome). Ann Intern Med, 1966; 65:768–781

564. Chamberlain DW, Walter JB. The relationship of Budd–Chiari syndrome to oral contraceptives and trauma. Can Med Assoc J, 1969; 101:618

565. O'Shea PA. Inferior vena cava and hepatic vein thrombosis as a rare complication of ventriculoatrial shunt. J Neurosurg, 1978; 48:143–145

566. Estrada V, Gutierrez FM, Cortes M, Garcia-Gonzalez C, Estrada RV. Budd–Chiari syndrome as a complication of the catheterization of the subclavian vein (letter). Am J Gastroenterol, 1991; 86:250–251

567. Paliard P, Bretagnolle M, Collet P, Vannieuwenhyse A, Berger F. Inferior vena cava thrombosis with Budd–Chiari syndrome during the course of hepatic and digestive amyloidosis. Gastroenterol Clin Biol, 1983; 7:919–922

568. Victor S, Jayanthi V, Madanagopalan N. Budd Chiari syndrome in a child with hepatic tuberculosis. Indian Heart J, 1989; 41:279

569. Vallaeys JH, Praet MM, Roels HJ, Van Marck E, Kaufman L. The Budd–Chiari syndrome caused by a zygomycete. A new pathogenesis of hepatic vein thrombosis. Arch Pathol Laboratory Med, 1989; 113:1171–1174

570. Young RC. The Budd–Chiari syndrome caused by Aspergillus. Two patients with vascular invasion of the hepatic veins. Arch Intern Med, 1969; 124:754–757

571. al-Dalaan A, al-Balaa S, Ali MA, Huraib S, Amin T, al-Maziad A et al. Budd–Chiari syndrome in association with Behçet's disease. J Rheumatol, 1991; 18:622–626

572. Bismuth E, Hadengue A, Hammel P, Benhamou JP. Hepatic vein thrombosis in Behçet's disease. Hepatology, 1990; 11:969–974

573. Natalino MR, Goyette RE, Owensby LC, Rubin RN. The Budd–Chiari syndrome in sarcoidosis. JAMA, 1978; 239:2657–2658

574. Victor S. In: Okuda K, ed. 2nd International Symposium on Budd–Chiari Syndrome, 1991. Kyoto: Japan, 1991

575. Maccini DM, Berg JC, Bell GA. Budd–Chiari syndrome and Crohn's disease. An unreported association. Dig Dis Sci, 1989; 34:1933–1936

576. Brinson RR, Curtis WD, Schuman BM, Mills LR. Recovery from hepatic vein thrombosis (Budd–Chiari syndrome) complicating ulcerative colitis. Dig Dis Sci, 1988; 33:1615–1620

577. Cosnes J, Robert A, Levy VG, Darnis F. Budd–Chiari syndrome in a patient with mixed connective-tissue disease. Dig Dis Sci, 1980; 25:467–469

578. Shani M, Theodor E, Frand M, Goldman B. A family with protein-losing enteropathy. Gastroenterology, 1974; 66:433–445

579. Tsuchiya M, Oshio C, Asakura H, Ishii H, Aoki I, Miyairi M. Budd–Chiari syndrome associated with protein-losing enteropathy. Gastroenterology, 1978; 75:114–117

580. Marteau P, Cadranel JF, Messing B, Gargot D, Valla D, Rambaud JC. Association of hepatic vein obstruction and coeliac disease in North African subjects. J Hepatol, 1994; 20:650–653

581. Tsuji H, Murai K, Kobayashi K, Nishimura J, Sumiyoshi K, Akagi K et al. Multiple myeloma associated with Budd–Chiari syndrome. Hepatogastroenterology, 1990; 37 Suppl. 2:97–99

582. Wanless IR. Hepatic vascular disorders—pathology. In: Bloomer JR, Goodman ZD, Ishak KG, eds. Clinical and pathological correlations in liver disease. Washington: AFIP, ARP and AASLD, 1998; pp. 37–49

583. Muradali D, Wilson SR, Wanless IR, Greig PD, Cattral M, Cameron RG et al. Peliosis hepatis with intrahepatic calcifications. J Ultrasound Med, 1996; 15:257–260

584. Netter FH. Digestive system, part III: Liver, biliary tract and pancreas. New York: Colorpress, 1964

Hepatic injury due to drugs, chemicals and toxins

14

James H. Lewis   David E. Kleiner

Drug-induced liver injury: a penalty for progress

Hans Popper, MD

Importance of drug- and chemical-induced hepatic injury

Drug-induced liver disease (DILD) can produce all forms of acute, chronic, vascular and neoplastic hepatic diseases caused by other aetiologies.[1,2] In doing so, it represents both a great imitator and a diagnostic challenge, often requiring a high degree of clinical suspicion on the part of physicians and patients alike. The relative importance of hepatic injury due to various types of exposure to toxins and drugs has changed considerably over the years. Acute toxic injury, formerly an occupational and domestic hazard, is now mainly a domestic one.[1] At present, chlorinated hydrocarbons are an uncommon cause of injury in the home and poisoning by phosphorus has almost disappeared from the USA, but remains a problem in parts of the world where suicidal or accidental ingestion of rodenticides or fire crackers containing it still occurs. Mushroom poisoning accounts for several hundred cases of hepatic injury per year, mainly in California and Europe.[3] A cause of hepatotoxicity outstripping all others in the USA and UK, and of growing importance elsewhere, is the deliberate, as well as the unintended, overdose of acetaminophen (paracetamol).[4,5,6,7]

To most modern-day clinicians and pathologists, hepatic injury caused by adverse reactions to medicinal agents is more important than that caused by other substances. Regarded as a 'penalty for progress' by Popper nearly 4 decades ago,[8] adverse reactions to drugs have been increas-ing. Indeed, more than 600 medicinal, chemical and herbal agents by last count are recognized as producing hepatic injury.[1,9,10] Additionally, in the drug discovery industry, DILD is the most frequent cause of drug withdrawal, restrictions on use and failure to move forward in the development process.[11] The incidence of DILD has been estimated by various epidemiologic and population-based studies[4,12-23] (Table 14.1), and appears to be increasing. For example, in Japan, the number of cases of DILD reported during the period 1964–1973 increased more than 10-fold over the number seen in the previous decade.[13] In France, 10% of cases of apparent 'hepatitis' were due to drug-induced injury at a large centre, with the figure rising to over 40% in patients above the age of 50.[15] A recent study that attempted to better define the incidence of DILD over a three year period in the Dijon region of France, found an annual incidence of nearly 14 cases per 100 000 inhabitants; a rate that was 16 times higher than that based on spontaneous reports.[17] The drugs implicated by these clinicians trained in causality assessment in France included several well-described anti-infectious, psychotropic, hypolipidemic and antiflammatory agents (Table 14.2).

Drug-induced injury also assumes an important role in cases of acute liver failure (ALF). Notable recent examples of severe hepatocellular hepatotoxins include troglitazone,[24] fialuridine,[25] trovafloxacin[26] and bromfenac,[27] all of which resulted in regulatory action by the Foods and Drug Administration (FDA).[28] More than 50% of the estimated 2000 cases of fulminant hepatic failure estimated to occur each year in the USA are the result of adverse reactions to medicinal agents, with most instances being due to acetaminophen.[4,21] This figure correlates with recent data iden-

Table 14.1 Incidence of drug-induced liver disease

Author	Year	Setting	Incidence of DILD
Koff[12]	1970	Boston hospitals	2% of all jaundiced patients
Sameshine[13]	1974	Japan	10-fold increase between 1963 and 1974
Eastwood[14]	1971	USA	20% of all cases of jaundice in elderly patients
Benhamou[15]	1986	France	10% of all acute 'hepatitis' 43% of all hepatic injury in patients >50 yr
Friis[16]	1992	Denmark	47% of all drug-related adverse reactions (world-wide frequency of DILD 3–9%)
Sgro[17]	2003	France	13.9 cases per 100 000 inhabitants (by causality assessment) (16 fold greater than the spontaneously reported rate)
Byron[18]	1996	Canadian hospital-based practice	6% of >1200 consults
Garcia Rodriguez[19]	1997	UK general practice data	>100 per 100 000 (isoniazid, chlorpromazine) >10 <100 per 100 000 (Augmentin) <10 per 100 000 (most others)
Jmelnitzky[20]	2000	Latin American Hospital GI Service	5.6% of >10 000 consults
Ostapowicz[21]	2002	US Acute LFSG	39% due to acetaminophen (of 2000 cases/yr) 12% all other drugs
Russo[22]	2004	UNOS database of OLT	15% due to drugs and toxins (50% from acetaminophen)
Lee[4]	2004	Updated US ALFSG	50% due to acetaminophen
Galan[23]	2005	US tertiary referral centre	33% of patients presenting with acute hepatitis (0.8% of all consults)

Table 14.2 Most commonly reported causes of drug-induced liver disease

Series	Year	Drugs implicated most commonly in hepatic injury
Garcia-Rodriguez[19]	1997	Chlorpromazine, isoniazid > Augmentin
Jmelnitsky[20]	2000	Oral contraceptives, isonazid +/− rifampicin, sulfonamides, chlorpropamide, carbamazepine, amiodarone
Ostapowicz[21]	2002	Drugs causing acute liver failure: acetaminophen 39% of all cases; 13% all other drugs (e.g. isoniazid, troglitazone, bromfenac)
Clarkson[29]	2002	Anticonvulsants (VPA), anaesthetics, among causes of hepatic failure in children under age 17
Russo[22]	2004	Drugs implicated in OLT between 1990–2002: APAP 50% (of the 15% of all causes); others: isoniazid, PTU, phenytoin, VPA, herbals, nitrofurantoin, ketoconazole, disulfiram, troglitazone
Galan[23]	2005	Antimicrobials (44% by class) (e.g. augmentin, minocycline, nitrofurantoin, TMP-SMX, trovan); amiodarone (22% of all single drug causes)
Andrade[29a]	2005	Antimicrobials (32% overall; amoxicillin-clavulanate 12.8%), CNS agents (17%), musculoskeletal and NSAIDs (17%)
Bjornsson & Olsson[29b]	2005	Antibiotics (flucloxacillin, erythromycin), NSAIDs (diclofenac), anticonvulsants, anti-tuberculosis drugs, disulfiram

tifying acetaminophen as the leading cause of ALF leading to liver transplant in the USA[22] and the UK.[7] All other drugs accounted for only 12% of acute liver failure cases in the USA,[21] but represented about half of all liver transplants performed for acute drug or toxin-induced liver failure.[22] Children are also vulnerable to hepatic failure due to drugs. In a UK study of fatal reactions among patients age 16 years or less, hepatic failure was the most common cause of death among 331 cases reported to the Committee on Safety of Medicines Yellow Card programme.[29] Anticonvulsants (most often valproate), anesthetics and antibiotics were the most frequently cited classes of drug-induced liver failure. Two large registries from Spain[29a] and Sweden[29b], respectively, have confirmed the >10% risk of death or need for liver transplant from severe drug-induced hepatocellular injury (Table 14.2).

Drug-induced cholestatic injury appears to outrank causes of acute cholestasis due to gallstones and other aetiological factors, certainly among hospitalized individuals.[30,31] Drugs also are an important cause of chronic hepatic disease. They have been held responsible for instances of chronic autoimmune hepatitis, fatty liver disease, cirrhosis, chronic cholestasis, granulomatous disease and several vascular and neoplastic lesions of the liver.[2,30-34] Of increasing concern is the risk of acquiring chronic disease, particularly hepatic neoplasms, as a result of prolonged occupational exposure to toxic chemicals and of the ingestion of mycotoxins and other natural hepatotoxins [10,33-36] although in some cases, underlying chronic viral hepatitis B or C may be contributory.[37,38,39,40] Some drugs, notably anabolic and contraceptive steroids, have been incriminated in the causation of hepatic tumours.[41,42]

Building on the information described by our predecessors in the last edition of this textbook, we have attempted to update the clinical and pathologic aspects of new and old hepatotoxins alike. The summary information contained in this review is clearly dependent on the quality of the information contained in case reports and case-series. In some instances, ample data are available on which to draw conclusions. For many agents, however, the available information about hepatotoxicity remains sparse, and awaits further corroborating reports to confirm the association with, and the spectrum of, the liver injury. Where appropriate, the causal relationship of such reports is noted. In addition, for many of the well-described hepatotoxins, we have chosen to include only selected references; the interested reader is referred to the many excellent textbooks and recent monographs on the subject of DILD for additional citations.[1,43-47] PubMed and other Internet sources can provide the most current information on specific agents as well as FDA regulatory actions as they pertain to the hepatic safety of drugs and chemicals.

Classification of hepatotoxic agents

Zimmerman defined two main categories of agents that can produce hepatic injury: *intrinsic* (predictable or true) hepatotoxins; and *idiosyncratic* (unpredictable) hepatotoxins that only produce liver injury in a small proportion of exposed individuals who are unusually susceptible[1] (Table 14.3, Table 14.4). The pathophysiological mechanisms by which drugs injure the liver generally involves their interacting with or disrupting one or more of six main targets as reviewed by Lee[48] as discussed below (Table 14.5, Table 14.6).

Intrinsic hepatotoxins

Intrinsic hepatotoxins are recognized by the high incidence of hepatic injury in individuals exposed to them, the pro-

Table 14.3	Classification of hepatotoxic agents and major characteristics of each group					
Category	Incidence	Experimental Reproducibility	Dose dependent	Mechanism	Histological lesion	Examples
Intrinsic toxicity						
Direct				Direct physico-chemical destruction by peroxidation of		
Cytotoxic	High	Yes	Yes	hepatocytes	Necrosis and/or steatosis	Carbon tetrachloride, phosphorus
Cholestatic	High	Yes	Yes	ductal cells	Cholestasis Duct destruction	Paraquat
Indirect						
Cytotoxic	High	Yes	Yes	Interference with specific pathways or production of selective lesions in: hepatocytes	Necrosis and/or steatosis	See Table 14.5
Cholestatic	High	Yes	Yes	ductal cells	Cholestasis Duct destruction	Methylene dianiline
Host idiosyncrasy						
Immunological (Hypersensitivity)	Low	No	No	Drug allergy	Necrosis or cholestasis	Phenytoin, sulfonamides, paraminosalicylic acid, halothane,* chlorpromazine, augmentin
Metabolic	Low	No	No	Production of hepatotoxic metabolites	Necrosis or cholestasis	Isoniazid, valproic acid, diclofenac, troglitazone

* Features suggestive of both hypersensitivity and metabolic idiosyncrasy

Table 14.4 Features that distinguish intrinsic (predictable) hepatotoxins from those that produce hepatic injury as idiosyncratic (unpredictable) reactions

Feature	Intrinsic toxicity	Idiosyncratic toxicity	
Mechanism	Direct/Indirect physiochemical destruction	Aberrant metabolism (toxic reactive metabolite)	Hypersensitivity (drug allergy) (immune-mediated)
Risk of injury	very high (predictable)	low (unpredictable)	low (unpredictable)
Latency	hours (acute)	weeks-months (variable)	1–5 weeks (fixed)
Animal model	yes	no	no
Dose-dependency	yes	no	no
Positive response to rechallenge	NA	possibly (delayed)	expected (prompt)
Injury pattern	usually necrosis	broad spectrum	broad spectrum, granulomas
Clinical features	Acute liver failure	elevated LAEs, acute hepatitis, ALF	fever, rash,eosinophilia, arthralgias
Mortality rate	high*	variable*	variable*
Examples	APAP	INH, diclofenac, Troglitazone Ketoconazole	sulfonamides, ticyrnafen, sulindac vaproate, phenytoin, halothane

* hepatocellular jaundice is associated with a case-fatality rate or need for liver transplant of 10% or higher

Table 14.5 Putative biochemical and histological lesions produced by hepatotoxins

Biochemical lesion	Histological lesion	Agents*
A. Attachment to membrane receptors	Necrosis Peliosis hepatis	Phalloidin
B. Covalent binding of active metabolite to:		
1. Cytosol molecules		
a. Alkylation	Necrosis +/− steatosis	Dimethylnitrosamine, other nitrosamines, thioacetamide
b. Arylation	Necrosis +/− steatosis	Acetaminophen, bromobenzene, aflatoxin, amanitine, pyrrolizidine alkaloids
2. Nuclear molecules (DNA)		
a. Alkylation	Carcinoma; angiosarcoma	Ethionine, dimethylnitrosamine and other nitrosamines, thioacetamide, vinyl chloride
b. Arylation	Veno-occlusive disease	Aflatoxin, pyrrolizidine alkaloids
C. Binding or blockade of tRNA	Steatosis	Tetracycline, puromycin
D. Cofactor depletion:		
1. ATP	Steatosis; cirrhosis; carcinoma	Ethionine
2. UTP	Necrosis; steatosis	Galactosamine
E. Thiol group binding	Necrosis; steatosis; hepatoportal sclerosis angiosarcoma; carcinoma	Arsenicals, inorganic

* Individual agents may lead to other biochemical lesions as well

duction of a similar lesion in experimental animals, and the dose-dependence of the phenomena. The two types of intrinsic hepatotoxins are categorized as direct and indirect. Direct hepatotoxicity is epitomized as destruction of the structural basis of hepatocyte metabolism, whereas indirect hepatotoxicity is the secondary effect of changes in the structure of key metabolites, or in the structure, metabolism or function of hepatocytes.

Direct hepatotoxins

These agents, or their metabolic products, injure the hepatocyte and its organelles by a direct physiochemical effects; i.e., peroxidation of the membrane lipids or other chemical changes that lead to distortion or destruction of the membranes. Examples include carbon tetrachloride ($CC1_4$) and some other chlorinated aliphatic hydrocarbons, the white

Table 14.6 Targets of drug-induced liver injury

Target	Hepatocyte injury	Mechanism
Hepatocyte membrane	blebbing, rupture, cell lysis	disassembly of actin fibrils
Canaliculus	loss of villous processes	Interruption of transport pumps
Endoplasmic reticulum	cytochrome P-450 system	creation of nonfunctioning adducts
Vesicles	attack by T cells	immune response by cytolytic T cells and cytokines
Nuclear chromatin	apoptosis	activation of TNF or FAS triggers a cascade of intercellular caspases
Mitochondria	impaired oxidation and respiratory chain enzymes	lactic acidosis, reactive oxygen species

after Lee[48]

allomorph of phosphorus, ferrous salts and copper salts.[1] No currently available medicinal agents are found in this category, although at one time $CC1_4$ and chloroform ($CHC1_3$) were employed in clinical medicine. Direct hepatotoxins characteristically produce cytotoxic injury by damageing or destroying hepatocytes, although they may also injure Kupffer and hepatic stellate cells. At least one direct toxin, paraquat, produces cholestasis by leading to bile-duct destruction, probably by peroxidative injury.[49]

Indirect hepatotoxins

Agents in this category produce hepatic injury by interference with a specific metabolic pathway or process or by selectively damaging cell components. The hepatic damage produced may be mainly cytotoxic and expressed as steatosis or necrosis, or mainly cholestatic and expressed as impaired bile flow.

Cytotoxic indirect hepatotoxins

These cause injury by interfering with metabolic pathways or molecules essential for parenchymal cell integrity.

In this group are drugs, botanical hepatotoxins and compounds that are mainly of experimental interest. The lesions induced by these agents lead to steatosis, necrosis or both.

Hepatic steatosis is usually the result of defective disposal of lipid by the liver, either impaired egress of triglycerides or impaired oxidation of fatty acids by the hepatocyte in what has been termed the 'two-hit' hypothesis.[50]

Among agents causing steatosis, *ethionine* competes with methionine for available adenosine triphosphate (ATP), interferes with the utilization of methionine, and ethylates compounds that should be methylated. The resultant deficient synthesis of the apoprotein moiety and defective assembly of the VLDL needed to remove lipid from the liver leads to steatosis.[1] Puromycin also causes steatosis by interfering with protein synthesis. It blocks synthesis by attachment to the ribosome in place of the normally attached activated tRNA. This leads to the formation of incomplete proteins truncated by a terminal puromycin molecule. Tetracycline in high doses also leads to rapid inhibition of movement of lipid from the liver and to steatosis, in part by

impaired mitochondrial oxidation of fatty acids.[51] It also may impair movement of lipid from the liver related to the known ability of tetracycline to interfere with protein synthesis, through binding of tRNA or interference with some other element of the complex system of synthesis of the VLDL. It is apparent that drugs that cause microvesicular steatosis lead to impaired mitochondrial oxidation of fatty acids as an important pathogenic factor.[52]

Alcohol also warrants classification as an indirect hepatotoxin (Chapter 6). It causes steatosis by a number of adverse effects on hepatocyte metabolism. It also can lead to necrosis, perhaps by the necrogenic effect of acetaldehyde and by increasing oxygen requirements of hepatocytes.[53,54]

Cholestatic indirect hepatotoxins

These produce jaundice or impair liver function by selective interference with hepatic mechanisms for excretion of substances into the canaliculus or uptake from the blood. In this category are icterogenin (an alkaloid of the plant *Lippia rhemani*), the C-17 alkylated anabolic and contraceptive steroids and lithocholic acid. Also included in this category are agents that can produce hyperbilirubinaemia by selective interference with the sinusoid/hepatocyte uptake of, or with the conjugation of, bilirubin; examples are flavaspidic acid, cholecystographic dyes, rifampicin and novobiocin.[1,30,31] The cholestatic effects of ethinyloestradiol apparently include inhibition of uptake of bile acids at the sinusoidal membrane, and probably, impaired canalicular excretion and even regurgitation through the 'tight junction'.[55]

Idiosyncratic hepatic injury

Agents that injure the liver unpredictably in only specially susceptible individuals also appear to fall into two categories. As characterized by Zimmerman,[1] the mechanism for the injurious action of one group appears to be hypersensitivity or allergy (immunological idiosyncrasy); while the mechanism for the other appears to be a metabolic aberration of the host that permits production or accumulation of damaging amounts of hepatotoxic metabolites (metabolic idiosyncrasy) (Tables 14.3, 14.4). Some drugs seem able to produce hepatic injury by either mechanism. For example, in the majority of cases of liver damage induced by isoniazid appear to result from toxic metabolites, but in a minority of cases the liver damage is accompanied by fever and eosinophilia and may be presumed to result from hypersensitivity.[56]

Hypersensitivity-related injury

Immunological idiosyncrasy (so-called drug allergy), is the presumptive mechanism for the hepatic injury which develops after a relatively short, fixed sensitization period of 1–5 weeks, recurs promptly on re-administration of the agent, and tends to be accompanied by the clinical hallmarks of hypersensitivity. These may include fever, rash and eosinophilia, lymphocytosis, 'atypical lymphocytes' and an eosinophil-rich or granulomatous inflammatory infiltrate in the liver. These features, however, provide only circumstantial evidence for hypersensitivity.

Recent studies have offered more convincing evidence for the role of immunological factors in some forms of drug-induced injury. Halothane-induced hepatic injury has been found to be accompanied by the development of antibodies and sensitized T-cells that react with rabbit hepatocytes that have been modified by an oxidative metabolite of halothane.[57] Furthermore, patients with hepatic injury induced by ticrynafen (tienilic acid) have been found to have antibodies that react with ticrynafen-altered hepatocyte proteins.[58] One such antibody reacts with microsomes. This anti-liver kidney microsomal antibody type 2 (anti-LKM2), appears to be an antibody to the cytochrome P450 isoform involved in metabolism of ticrynafen (see section on *chronic hepatitis*). These studies provide suggestive evidence that the pathogenesis of the injury in halothane and ticrynafen injury is the consequence of conversion of hepatocyte protein to neoantigen by reaction with a metabolite of the drug and that the ensuing immunological reaction, humoral or cell-mediated, leads to hepatic injury.[59] However, even among individuals possessing these autoantibodies, liver injury appears to be rare. For example, despite the presence of serum antibodies to halothane and other anesthetics in 158 paediatric anesthesiologists, only a single individual developed liver injury.[60]

The concept that drug hypersensitivity per se will lead to hepatic injury appears to be an oversimplification. Generalized hypersensitivity caused by some drugs (e.g. penicillin) almost never includes liver injury, while that caused by others (e.g. phenytoin) includes liver disease with appreciable frequency.[1] Other drugs (e.g. chlorpromazine) may cause liver damage with or without associated features suggestive of drug allergy. Furthermore, while chlorpromazine (CPZ) causes overt liver disease in less than 1% of recipients, it can induce a much higher incidence (35–50%) of subclinical hepatic dysfunction.[61] As opined by Zimmerman, these figures are too high to permit the assumption that hypersensitivity alone is the mechanism for the hepatic abnormality. With other observations, they have led to the hypothesis that a mildly adverse effect of an agent on the liver, when accompanied by generalized hypersensitivity, may lead to overt hepatic injury. The demonstration that CPZ can produce injury in in vitro models and cholestatic injury in experimental animals are consistent with this hypothesis.[1]

Hypersensitivity-mediated reactions may result from a metabolic defect as postulated by the observations of Spielberg and co-workers.[62,63] They found that patients who had sustained hepatic injury in a hypersensitivity type reaction to phenytoin had an apparent defect in converting the active metabolite (arene oxide) to the inactive dihydriol. The active metabolite presumably could serve as a hapten or could be cytotoxic. Other potential genetic predispositions to developing DILD are given in Table 14.7; although they remain largely unproven possibilities.[64,65] With the burgeoning field of pharmacogenomics, it is expected that our ability to identify susceptible individuals will

Table 14.7	Proposed genetic predisposition to DILD
Hepatotoxic agent	**Possible predisposing metabolic factor**
Perhexiline	Poor metabolizer of debrisoquine and/or dextromethorphan (seen In 5–10% of Europeans) from CYP2D6 deficiency
Sulfonamides, dihydralazine	Slow acetylation due to deficiency of N-acetyltransferase 2 activity
Atrium (meprobamate)	Poor metabolizer of S-mephenytoin from CYP2C19 deficiency
Chlorpromazine	Sulfoxidation deficiency; poor metabolizer of S-carboxy-L-methyl- cysteine and/or extensive metabolizer of sparteine
Halothane	Postulated familial susceptibility of epoxide hydrolase deficiency
Amineptine	Postulated familial susceptibility; extensive detromethorphan oxidation capacity; genetic deficiency of a yet to be identified cell defence mechanism
Acetaminophen	Deficiency of glutathione synthetase
Isoniazid	Deficiency of glutathione -S-transferase due to mutations at GST M1 and GST T1 loci; and N-acetyltransferase 2 (NAT2) polymorphisms

after references 62, 64

permit a greater understanding of the mechanisms involved as well as a means to avoid serious toxicity in such patients.[66,67]

Toxic metabolite-dependent

Idiosyncratic hepatic injury that is not accompanied by clinical hallmarks of hypersensitivity, is not promptly reproduced by readministration of the drug and which may appear after widely varying periods of exposure to the drug (often several months), is generally assumed to result from metabolic rather than immunological mechanisms. Convincing evidence for some agents with demonstrated metabolic idiosyncrasy includes perhexiline maleate, valproic acid, isoniazid, and iproniazid.[1] For the

majority of other agents, however, the cause remains undefined.

The morphological patterns of toxic hepatic injury

The diagnosis of drug and toxic hepatic injury begins with careful morphologic evaluation of the liver for the types cellular injury as well as the overall pattern (Table 14.8). While it is true that hepatoxicity can replicate essentially every other type of liver disease, individual hepatotoxins display a more limited range of injury. Thus, identification of the pattern of injury can be very helpful in both including and excluding hepatotoxicity as the cause of liver dys-

Table 14.8	Morphological patterns of toxic hepatic injury

Type of injury	Examples of agents
Necroinflammatory	
Acute coagulative (zonal) necrosis	
Perivenular (Zone 3)	CCl_4, acetaminophen, halothane
Mid (Zone 2)	Ngaione, frusemide
Periportal (Zone 1)	Allylformate, albitocin
Acute hepatitis-like	Isoniazid, sulphonamides, halothane, diclofenac
Mononucleosis-like	Phenytoin, para-aminosalicylate, dapsone
Chronic hepatitis-like	Oxyphenisatin, methyldopa, nitrofurantoin, dantrolene, clometacine, papaverine, sulphonamides
Granulomatous	
Cholestatic	
Acute intrahepatic cholestasis ('bland cholestasis')	C-17 alkylated anabolic and contraceptive steroids
Hepatocanalicular ('pericholangitic')	CPZ, TPN, erythromycin estolate, organic arsenicals
Chronic intrahepatic cholestasis (ductopenic, PBC-like)	CPZ, haloperidol, imipramine, organic arsenicals, thiabendazole, tolbutamide
Biliary sclerosis (PSC-like)	Floxuridine by hepatic artery perfusion
Mixed hepatocellular-cholestatic injury	
Steatosis	
Microvesicular	Ethionine, tetracycline, phosphorus, ethanol
Macrovesicular	Ethanol, MTX
Steatohepatitis-like	Perhexiline maleate, amiodarone
Phospholipidosis	Amiodarone
Vascular	
Sinusoidal dilitation	Oral contraceptives
Peliosis hepatis	Anabolic steroids, vinyl chloride, arsenicals
Sinusoidal obstuction syndrome/Veno-occlusive disease	pyrrolizidine alkaloids, antineoplastic agents
Hepatic vein thrombosis (Budd-Chiari syndrome)	Contraceptive steroids
Hepato-portal sclerosis	Arsenicals, copper sulphate, antineoplastic agents
Nodular regenerative hyperplasia	6-Thioguanine, azathioprine
Fibrosis/cirrhosis	Methotrexate, drugs which cause chronic injury
Neoplasms	
Hepatocellular adenoma	OCs, anabolic steroids
Hepatocellular carcinoma	Anabolic steroids, TPN, OCs, Th-O, vinyl chloride
Cholangiocarcinoma	
Angiosarcoma	Th-O, vinyl chloride, As, $CuSO_4$, anabolic steroids

(a) Massive and sub-massive necrosis may result in severe forms of zonal or non-zonal necrosis

CCl_4 = carbon tetrachloride; CPZ = chlorpromazine; MTX = methotrexate; As = arsenic; Th-O = Thorotrast; OCs = oral contraceptives; DES = diethylstilboestrol; TPN = total parenteral nutrition; PBC = primary biliary cirrhosis; PSC = primary sclerosing cholangitis

function. Hepatotoxins may injure any or all of the cell types found in the liver, but particular attention should be paid to hepatocytes, bile duct cells and endothelial cells. Ultimately the type of cellular injury will depend on the particular agent involved. Table 14.6 summarizes major types of cellular injury.[48] Cell injury may result in necrosis, apoptosis, cholestasis, steatosis, cytoplasmic inclusions, or pigment accumulation depending on the degree of injury and the cellular elements involved. Cellular injury may vary across the hepatic lobule and may affect the different cell types in different ways. The overall outcome is a pattern of injury that is characteristic of the agent involved, and this pattern may modified by the genetic and biochemical background of the host as well as the response of the host's immune system to the injury. As complex as this seems, there are a limited number of major morphological patterns of drug and toxin injury and these are listed in Table 14.8. Definition of the forms of injury produced by the intrinsic hepatotoxins has been relatively simple, since the hepatic damage can be reproduced in experimental animals. Characterization of the forms of idiosyncratic injury, however, has been more difficult, and has depended on collation of material from reports of individuals and groups of cases.[1,68,69]

Necroinflammatory injury

Toxic injury which comes to clinical attention frequently takes the form of either necroinflammatory injury or cholestatic injury. In toxicity, which is mainly necroinflammatory, the relative degree of cell death and inflammation may vary from lesions that are almost entirely necrotic with little inflammation to those, which may mimic chronic viral or autoimmune hepatitis. Most intrinsic toxins produce predominantly cytotoxic rather than cholestatic injury. Idiosyncratic injury caused by some drugs is cholestatic and by others is cytotoxic. Some drugs characteristically produce a mixed pattern of injury, with both hepatocellular and cholestatic injury. The necrosis observed in necroinflammatory injury may be non-zonal, zonal or massive. As a general rule, the necrosis produced by intrinsic hepatotoxins is zonal (Figs 14.1–14.3, 14.5), while that produced by idiosyncratic injury is usually non-zonal (Figs 14.4, 14.6–14.8). Extreme degrees of both zonal and non-zonal necrosis can result in massive necrosis (Fig. 14.6).

Cytotoxic injury: necrosis and cell death (apoptosis)

Individual cells involved in necroinflammatory injury can undergo a variety of changes. Cell death can occur by two processes: *necrosis* and *apoptosis* (Chapter 2).[48,70,71] Necrosis refers to destructive disintegration of the cell, apparently initiated by plasma membrane injury and yielding only debris. Apoptosis (programmed cell death) is an evolving disintegration including cell shrinkage, nuclear fragmentation, condensation of chromatin and the production of cytoplasmic blebs yielding distinct fragments of the cells or entire condensed shrunken cells. The condensed cells are

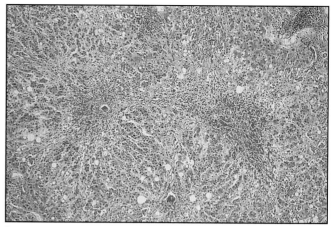

A

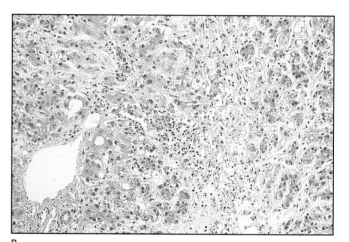

B

Fig. 14.1 • Carbon tetrachloride toxicity. Both figures from same case. **(A)** Bridging perivenular necrosis. Note focal steatosis in preserved parenchyma. H&E. **(B)** There is drop-out of liver cells in the perivenular zone and neutrophilic infiltration of the residual stroma. H&E.

referred to as *apoptotic* or *free acidophilic bodies*. Apoptosis has been whimsically described as 'cell suicide' and necrosis as 'cell murder'. The mechanisms for the two are different. Activation of apoptotic pathways involves tumour necrosis factor alpha receptor or Fas-mediated release of intercellular caspases that eventuate in cell death.[72]

Necrosis results when there is massive injury to the cells. Frequently this is due to massive injury to the cell membrane and organelles. Apoptosis may occur when the cell suffers similar direct injury, but in lesser degrees. Thus, apoptotic hepatocytes are sometimes seen adjacent to zones of confluent necrosis. Apoptosis may also result from immune-mediated injury, in which cytotoxic T-cells, antibodies or cytokines initiate the apoptotic pathway. Ballooning hepatocellular changes, steatosis, Mallory body formation may also be seen as components of necroinflammatory injury, depending on the injurious agent. The presence of cholestasis (either canalicular or hepatocellular) should lead the pathologist to consider agents that cause mixed injury (discussed below).

Acute coagulative (zonal) necrosis

Zonal necrosis may involve the perivenular (zone 3), peri-portal (zone 1) or mid-zone (zone 2) depending on the

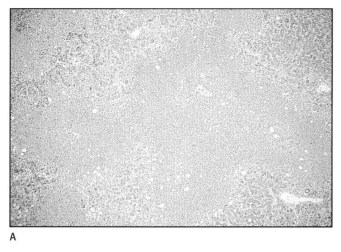

A

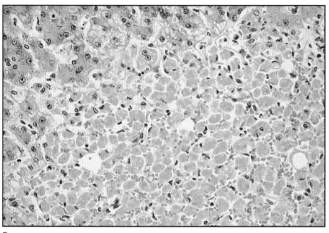

B

Fig. 14.2 • Paracetamol (acetaminophen) toxicity. **(A)** Confluent coagulative necrosis involving the perivenular and mid-zones. H&E. **(B)** Coagulated hepatocytes are shrunken, eosinophilic, more or less rounded and have lost their nuclei. H&E.

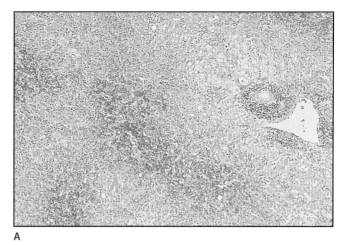

A

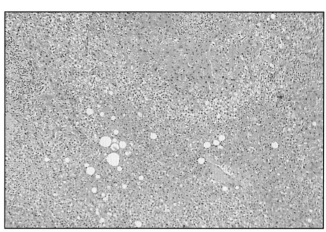

B

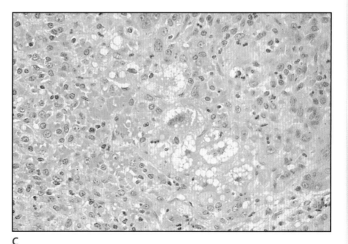

C

Fig. 14.3 • Mushroom toxicity. All figures from same case. **(A)** Bridging perivenular necrosis with marked sinusoidal congestion. Masson's trichrome. **(B)** Haematoxylin and eosin-stained section. **(C)** Higher magnification showing drop-out of liver cells and stromal inflammation. Note macrovesicular steatosis of residual hepatocytes. H&E.

agent and is usually the result of intrinsic toxins (Table 14.9). However, there are exceptions. The experimental necrosis produced by the intrinsic toxin galactosamine is non-zonal rather than zonal.[73] Conversely, in the idiosyncratic injury caused by halothane and other halogenated anaesthetics (Fig. 14.4), the necrosis is often perivenular and is strikingly similar to that of carbon tetrachloride, an intrinsic toxin. Histologically, there is confluent coagulative necrosis that involves the liver evenly, striking the same distribution in each acinus. Usually there is little inflammatory infiltrate except as a secondary response to the necrosis. As the injury becomes more severe it will extend to involve other zones with bridging necrosis. Massive necrosis of the zonal type tends to retain its zonal character. For example a rim of hepatocytes might remain adjacent to the portal areas in severe toxicity from an agent that affects zone 3 first.

Perivenular (zone 3) necrosis is the most common type of zonal necrosis and is the characteristic lesion produced by a number of intrinsic toxins (Figs 14.1–14.3). The toxins in this category that are relevant to human disease include CCl₄ (Fig. 14.1), CHCl₃, copper salts, pyrrolizidine alkaloids, tannic acid, the toxins of *Amanita phalloides* (Fig. 14.3) among others.[1] Paracetamol in high doses may become an intrinsic hepatotoxin that can cause perivenular necrosis (Fig. 14.2). Perivenular necrosis induced by some agents (pyrrolizidine alkaloids, aflatoxin B in some species) is accompanied by injury to the hepatic veins or venules, adding a haemorrhagic component to the necrosis.[1,74,75]

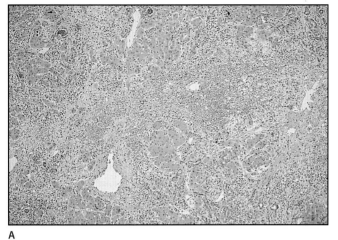

A

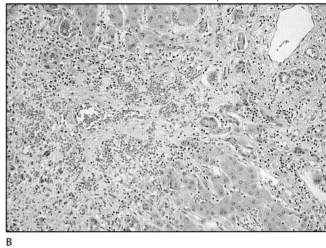

B

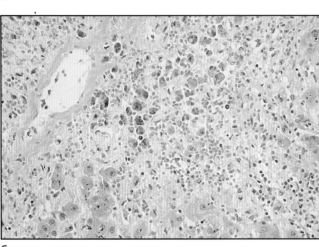

C

Fig. 14.4 • Halothane injury. All figures from same case. **(A)** Bridging perivenular necrosis. H&E. **(B)** A bridge of necrosis ('central to portal'). Note periportal cholangiolar reaction and the moderate inflammatory response. H&E. **(C)** There is drop-out of liver cells in the perivenular zone, ceroid pigment accumulation in hypertrophied Kupffer cells, and mononuclear cell infiltration. H&E.

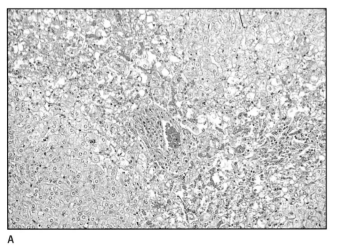

A

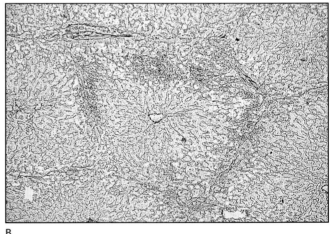

B

Fig. 14.5 • Phosphorus toxicity. All figures from same case. **(A)** Periportal hepatocytes have dropped out and there is sinusoidal dilatation and congestion. H&E. **(B)** Bridging periportal necrosis. Manuel reticulin.

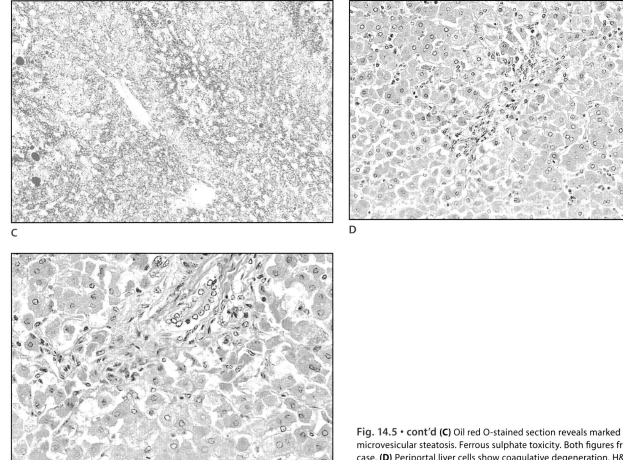

C

D

E

Fig. 14.5 • cont'd (C) Oil red O-stained section reveals marked microvesicular steatosis. Ferrous sulphate toxicity. Both figures from same case. **(D)** Periportal liver cells show coagulative degeneration. H&E. **(E)** Liver cells in the periportal zone are shrunken, angulated and more eosinophilic than normal. H&E.

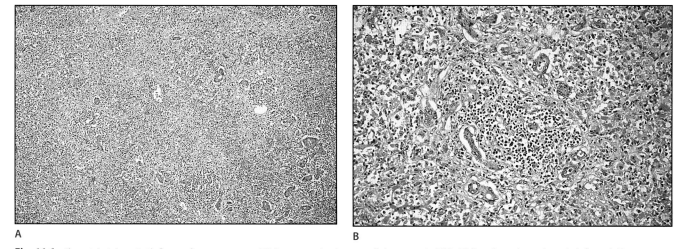

A

B

Fig. 14.6 • Phenytoin injury. Both figures from same case. **(A)** Acute massive hepatocellular necrosis. H&E. **(B)** Portal area is moderately inflamed. Note periportal ductutar reaction with inflammatory cell infiltration. All liver cells have dropped out. H&E.

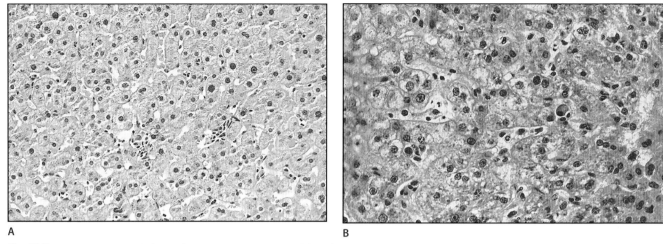

A

B

Fig. 14.7 • Phenytoin injury. Both figures from same case. **(A)** Two small foci of necrosis. H&E. **(B)** Sinusoidal acidophilic body and mild ballooning of hepatocytes. H&E.

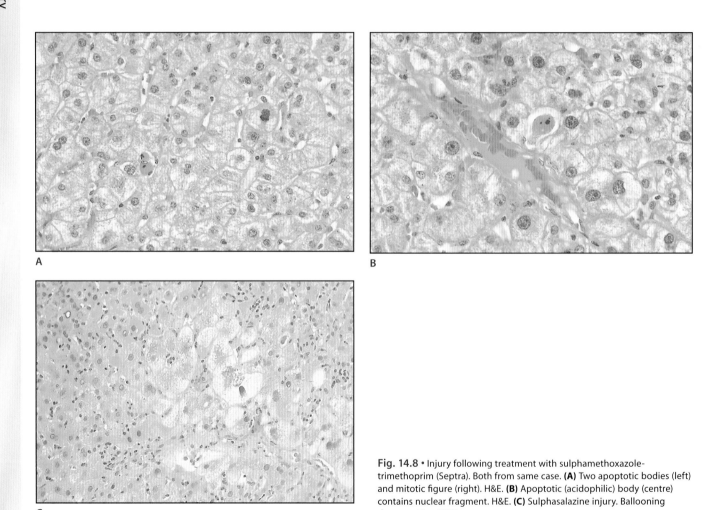

A

B

C

Fig. 14.8 • Injury following treatment with sulphamethoxazole-trimethoprim (Septra). Both from same case. **(A)** Two apoptotic bodies (left) and mitotic figure (right). H&E. **(B)** Apoptotic (acidophilic) body (centre) contains nuclear fragment. H&E. **(C)** Sulphasalazine injury. Ballooning degeneration. H&E.

Table 14.9	Agents associated with zonal and diffuse necrosis*

2-Chloropropane (Z3)	Isoniazid (ZN)
2-Nitropropane (D)	Ketoconazole (Z3)
Aflatoxins (Z1, Z3)	Lovastatin (Z3)
Albitocin (Z1)	Luteoskyrin (Z3)
Alloxan (Z1)	Manganese compounds (Z1)
Allyl compounds (Z1)	Methoxyflurane (ZN)
Amanitin (Z3)	Methyldopa (Z3)
Aniline (D)	Metoprolol (Z3)
Arsenic compounds (Z3, D)	Mithramycin (Z3)
B. cereus toxin (Z2)	Mushrooms (Z3, D)
Beryllium (Z2)	Naphthalene (Z3)
Bromobenzene (Z3)	Ngaione (Z2)
Carbon tetrachloride (Z3)	P. vulgaris endotoxin (Z1)
Chlorinated Benzenes (Z3, D)	Para-aminosalicylic acid (Z1)
Chlorinated diphenyls (D)	Paracetamol (Z3)
Chlorinated naphthalene (D)	Paraquat (Z3)
Chloroform (Z3)	Phalloidin (Z3)
Chloroprene (Z3)	Phenelzine (D)
Cocaine (Z1, Z3)	Phosphorus (Z1)
Copper sulphate (Z3)	Piroxicam (D)
DDT (Z3)	Propylthiouracil (Z3)
Desipramine (ZN)	Pyrrolizidine alkaloids (Z3)
Dichloropropane (Z3)	Quinidine (ZN)
Dimethylnitrosamine (Z3)	Rifampin (ZN)
Dinitrobenzone (Z3, D)	Rubratoxin (Z3)
Dinitrotoluene (Z3, D)	Selenium (D)
Dioxane (Z2, D)	Sporidesmin (Z1)
Diptheria toxin (Z3)	Sulindac (ZN)
Ethionamide (Z3)	Sulphasalazine (ZN)
Ethylene dibromide (Z3)	Synthaline (Z1)
Ethylene dichloride (Z3)	Tannic acid (Z3)
Ferrous sulphate (Z1)	Tetrachloroethane (Z3, D)
Galactosamine (D)	Tetrachloroethylene (Z3)
Halogenated Hydrocarbons (Z3, D)	Thioacetamide (Z3)
Halothane (Z3)	Tolazamide (ZN)
Imipramine (ZN)	Trichloroethylene (Z3)
Indomethacin (ZN)	Tricrynafen (Z3)
Iodoform (Z3)	Trinitrotoluene (Z3, D)
Islandicum (Z3)	Urethane (Z3)
	Valproic acid (Z3)

* D, diffuse (pan-acinar) necrosis; Z1, zone 1 necrosis; Z2, zone 2 necrosis; Z3, zone 3 necrosis; ZN, zonal necrosis

A few agents characteristically produce periportal (zone 1) necrosis (Fig. 14.5); in this category are known toxins such as phosphorus,[76,77] poisonous doses of ferrous sulphate,[78] ingestion of concentrated (90%) acetic acid,[79] allyl alcohol and its esters,[80] the endotoxin of *Proteus vulgaris*,[1] as well as adverse reactions to some drugs (e.g. halothane).[56]

A few agents produce mid-zonal necrosis in experimental animals. These include ngaione, beryllium, frusemide and, in hyperthyroid animals, CCl_4 and $CHCl_3$.[1] Mid-zonal necrosis in isolation is a rare lesion in humans.

The zonality of necrosis may be related to the mechanism of injury. The perivenular location of the lesion induced by CCl_4, by bromobenzene, and by paracetamol appears to reflect the concentration in that zone of the enzyme systems

responsible for the conversion of these agents to hepatotoxic metabolites.[81] The periportal necrosis of ferrous sulphate toxicity in children is presumed to be a direct cytopathic effect of the high concentration of iron reaching the liver via the portal vein.[78]

Acute hepatitis-like injury

Another common pattern of acute hepatoxicity is that of multiple small areas of degeneration or 'spotty' necrosis, similar to acute hepatitis (Table 14.10). It is most often the result of an idiosyncratic drug injury. There is a predominantly lobular, lymphocytic infiltrate with scattered apoptotic hepatocytes. Increased numbers of eosinophils can be seen, which may help suggest the diagnosis of toxic liver injury. There may be other evidence of hepatocellular injury, such as ballooning degeneration and steatosis and regenerative changes such as mitoses, hepatocyte rosette formation and the proliferation of ductular hepatocytes. When severe, there may be areas of confluent necrosis from extensive apoptotic cell death. The massive necrosis that results from drugs in this category of injury may mimic zonal necrosis, particularly zone 3 necrosis, since the injury is sometimes more severe in the peri-venular zone (Figs 14.4 and 14.6). Reticulin stains will show the zones of collapse but usually true fibrosis is not yet present at the time of biopsy (or death).

There is a second acute hepatitis pattern that most resembles the hepatitis of Epstein–Barr virus infection. In this pattern there is sinusoidal beading of lymphocytes similar to the mononucleosis hepatitis of EBV; granulomas and eosinophils can be seen. The archetypical drug that causes this pattern of injury is phenytoin (Figs 14.7 and 14.9), although it can also cause cholestatic and mixed injury patterns.[82,83] Other drugs reported to give this pattern include para-amino salicylate, dapsone and the sulphonamides.[69]

Subacute hepatic necrosis is a form of chronic necroinflammatory disease, which is an insidious and subclinical form of liver injury. Subacute hepatic necrosis was a dreaded occupational disease of the defence industries during both World Wars, a consequence of prolonged exposure to tetrachloroethane, trinitrotoluene, chlorinated biphenyl-chloronaphthalene mixtures or dinitrobenzene.[1,9,84] These occupationally-associated injuries are now virtually obsolete. Subacute hepatic necrosis, however, also can result from long-term administration of isoniazid[85,86] or methyldopa,[87,88] and was seen in recipients of cinchophen.[89] The histological features include varying degrees of necrosis, fibrosis and regeneration (Fig. 14.10).

Chronic hepatitis-like injury

Many of the drugs that are known to cause an acute hepatitis-like pattern are also responsible for a pattern of injury that resembles chronic hepatitis (Table 14.10). This is characterized by a necroinflammatory infiltrate that is mainly portal and periportal in distribution. The portal inflammation is mixed, but composed predominantly of lymphocytes and macrophages. There is interface hepatitis associated with variable periportal fibrosis. There is also lobular inflammation in the form of spotty necrosis and scattered

Table 14.10 Agents that cause acute and chronic hepatitis-like patterns

Acute (lobular-predominant) hepatitis		Chronic hepatitis
Acetylsalicylic acid	Lergotrile	Acetylsalicylic acid*
Amiodarone	Lisinopril	Chlorpromazine
Amitryptyline	Mercaptopurine	Clometacin
Aprindine	Methimazole	Dantrolene
Asparaginase	Methotrexate	Diphenylhydantoin
Aureomycin	Methoxyflurane	Doxidan
Benzarone	Methyldopa	Erythromycin
Bupropion	Minocycline	Etretinate
Captopril	Mitomycin C	Haloperidol
Carbamazepine	Naproxen	Halothane
Carbenicillin	Niacin	Isoniazid
Cephalosporin	Nicotinic acid	Methyldopa
Chemotherapeutic agents	Nitrofurantoin	Nicotinic acid
Chenodeoxycholic acid	Oxacillin	Nitrofurantoin
Chlorpromazine	Oxaprozin	Oxacillin
Cimetidine	Oxyphenacetin	Oxyphenacetin
Cis platinum	Oxyphenisatin	Paracetamol*
Clarithromycin	Papaverine	Pentamidine
Clometacin	Para-aminosalicylic acid	Perhexiline maleate
Cocaine	Pemoline	Procainamide
Cromolyn	Perhexiline maleate	Propylthiouracil
Danazol	Phenazopyridine	Sulphonamides
Dantrolene	Phenobarbitol	Tolazamide
Dapsone	Phenothiazines	
Desipramine	Phenylbutazone	
Diazepam	Phenytoin	
Diclofenac	Pirprofen	
Dihydralazine	Probenecid	
Diphenylhydantoin	Procainamide	
Disopyramide	Propylthiouracil	
Disulfiram	Rifampin	
Enflurane	Spironolactone	
Ethanol	Streptokinase	
Etretinate	Sulindac	
Fenofibrate	Suloctidil	
Fluorodeoxyuridine	Sulphadiazine	
Germander	Sulphadoxine-	
Glyburide	pyrimethamine	
Gold	Sulphamethoxazole	
Halogenated	Sulphasalazine	
Hydrocarbons	Sulphonamides	
Haloperidol	Tolazamide	
Halothane	Toxic oil (Rapeseed)	
Hydralazine	Trazodone	
Hydrochlorothiazide	Tricrynafen	
Ibuprofen	Troglitazone	
Indomethacin	Verapamil	
Isoniazid	VP-16	
Ketoconazole		

* evidence for chronic injury remains scant and controversial

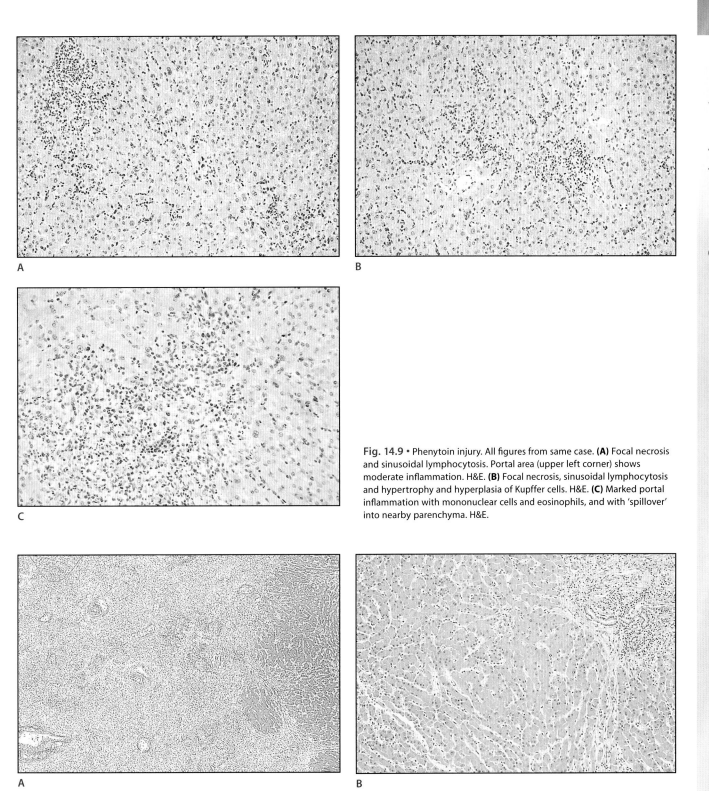

Fig. 14.9 • Phenytoin injury. All figures from same case. **(A)** Focal necrosis and sinusoidal lymphocytosis. Portal area (upper left corner) shows moderate inflammation. H&E. **(B)** Focal necrosis, sinusoidal lymphocytosis and hypertrophy and hyperplasia of Kupffer cells. H&E. **(C)** Marked portal inflammation with mononuclear cells and eosinophils, and with 'spillover' into nearby parenchyma. H&E.

Fig. 14.10 • Isoniazid injury. Both figures from same case. **(A)** Area of multiacinar necrosis (left) and residual parenchyma (right). Masson trichrome. **(B)** Residual parenchyma shows thick liver plates indicative of regeneration. H&E.

apoptotic hepatocytes may be seen. The fibrosis is progressive, at least as long as the injury persists, and can result in cirrhosis. Hepatocytes may show degenerative changes or steatosis as in acute hepatitis. Cholestasis is not a feature of chronic viral hepatitis until late in the disease, and its presence should alert the pathologist to the possibility of drug injury (or a second process).

Drug-induced chronic hepatitis may be subdivided into several categories (Table 14.11). One category consists of drugs that have been associated with a syndrome similar to autoimmune hepatitis type 1 (AIH-1) with the presence of serum anti-nuclear or anti-smooth muscle (actin) antibodies along with hyperglobulinaemia. Recognition that drug-induced injury can mimic AIH came some thirty years ago

Table 14.11 Categories of drug-induced chronic autoimmune hepatitis[a]

	Serology[b]
Type I. *Syndrome resembling autoimmune hepatitis type 1 (AIH-1)*	
Multiple cases:	
Clometacine	ASMA, Anti-DNA
Methyldopa	ANA (16%), ASMA 35%
Minocycline	ANA, Anti-DNA
Nitrofurantoin	ANA (80%), ASMA (72%)
Oxyphenisatin	ANA (67%), ASMA (67%)
Few cases (<5):	
Benzarone	ASMA
Diclofenac	ANA
Ecstasy (3,4-methylenedioxymethamphetamine)	ANA
Fenofibrate	ANA
Germander	ANA, ASMA
Papaverine	ANA, ASMA
Pemoline	ANA, antimicrosomal
Propylthiouracil	ANA
Type II. *Syndrome resembling autoimmune hepatitis type 2 (AIH-2) or acute hepatitis*	
Dihydralazine	Anti-CYP1A2
Tienilic acid (ticrynafen)	Anti-CYP2C9 (LKM2)
Halothane	Anti-carboxylesterase, anti-protein disulfide isomerase
Iproniazid	Anti-microsomal Ab 6
Type III. *Syndrome with histology of chronic hepatitis but no autoantibodies*	
Etretinate	
Lisinopril	
Sulphonamides	
Trazadone	
Uracil (in combination with tegafur and tamoxifen)	

(a) Modified from Lewis & Zimmerman (In Krawitt et al. eds. Autoimmune liver diseases 2nd ed. 1998 Elsevier, pp. 629–49)

(b) ASMA = antismooth muscle antibodies; ANA = antinuclear antibodies

with reports of the lesion in patients taking *oxyphenisatin*, an ingredient of laxative preparations no longer in use in the USA.[90] Thereafter, the syndrome was reported in those treated with nitrofurantoin,[91] methyldopa,[92,93] clometacine,[94] fenofibrate,[95] diclofenac,[96] papaverine,[97] pemoline,[98] and minocycline.[99] Several of these drugs have led to multiple cases with biochemical, serological and histological features very similar to AIH, providing convincing evidence for the reality of the phenomenon referred to as *drug-induced autoimmune hepatitis type 1 (DrAIH-1)*. For the others, only occasional instances of the syndrome have been attributed to each of the respective agents.[100] Not all recipients of the drugs implicated in causing an autoimmune type of hepatitis show the expected autoantibodies. Almost 20% of patients with nitrofurantoin-associated chronic hepatitis, and at least 40% of patients with methyldopa-induced chronic hepatitis are seronegative. This may reflect the diligence with which autoantibodies are sought, the methodology used to detect them or a different mechanism of injury in the seronegative cases.

A second group of agents includes dihydralazine and tienilic acid that lead to acute or chronic hepatitis accompanied by a different form of autoimmune response to drug-induced AIH-1. The antibodies here are directed against microsomal components similar to that of AIH-2. These are CYP2C9 (also called LKM2) in tienilic acid-induced disease[58] and the isoform CYP1A2 (a liver microsomal protein (LM)) in hydralazine-induced hepatitis. The isoforms are involved in the metabolism of the respective drug and it may be presumed that, in the process of biotransformation of the drug, an effect of the drug metabolite on the enzyme protein renders it a neoantigen. Hyperglobulinaemia is less characteristic of this entity. We have called this *drug-induced autoimmune hepatitis type 2 (DrAIH-2)*.

Autoimmune markers may be associated with drug reactions other than chronic hepatitis. Tienilic acid-induced injury and dihydralazine-induced injury, whether acute or chronic, may be accompanied by the antimicrosomal antibodies listed in Table 14.11. Antinuclear antibodies may accompany chronic cholestatic injury induced by flucloxacillin and the reaction to aniline-contaminated rapeseed oil in the 'toxic oil syndrome' reported from Spain. They also may mark drug reactions without hepatic disease, as in the drug-induced systemic lupus erythematosus syndrome induced by hydralazine.[101]

Drugs in a third group (*Dr(A)IH-3*) have been associated with a more non-descript or insufficiently characterized form of chronic hepatitis, apparently not accompanied by autoimmune serological markers. Clinical presentation has been oligosymptomatic with elevated aminotransferase levels leading to biopsy and a diagnosis of clinically presenting acute hepatitis but with histological features of chronic hepatitis.

Drug-induced AIH-1 is characterized histologically by intense portal and periportal inflammation with infiltration by lymphocytes, plasma cells and eosinophils in varying combinations. Interface hepatitis is usually marked (Fig. 14.23(A),(B)). The inflammation may be accompanied by fibrosis extending into the parenchyma or encircling islands of cells, and there may be degeneration and necrosis in other parts of the parenchyma; in some patients there may be bridging fibrosis or cirrhosis, a picture indistinguishable from idiopathic autoimmune hepatitis. Drug-induced AIH-2 also shows interface hepatitis and portal inflammation, but the intensity of the necroinflammation is less severe. Furthermore, the inflammation is not marked by a profusion of plasma cells.

Granulomatous injury

Granulomatous inflammation is observed in a large number of drug-associated injuries[102] (Table 14.12). Granulomas may be seen alone or associated with other types of hepatic injury (Fig. 14.11), including acute and chronic hepatitis, cholestasis and steatosis. In one study approximately 30% of instances of hepatic granulomas were attributed to medicinal agents.[103] Drug-induced hepatic granulomas have no specific features that distinguish them from those of sarcoidosis or other causes of non-caseating epithelioid granulomas, although the presence of eosinophils should suggest the possibility of a drug injury. Fibrin ring granulomas have been attributed to allopurinol.[104] Granulomas due to BCG, whether resulting from vaccination or from instillation into the urinary bladder for treatment of carcinoma, may contain acid-fast bacilli.[105] Systemic granulomatous disease does not preclude the possibility of drug-induced granulomas, since sarcoid-like granulomas have been reported in the liver, lungs and other organs as a result of chronic exposure to metals such as beryllium,[106] copper,[107] and aluminium.[108] Drug-induced granulomatous hepatitis may be related to hypersensitivity, particularly when associated with tissue eosinophilia[2] Prominence of eosinophils in the sinusoids, however, is usually a reflection of peripheral eosinophilia.[61,109]

Cholestatic injury

Acute intrahepatic cholestasis

Some agents lead to injury that mainly spares the parenchyma and instead causes arrested bile flow[30,31,33] (Tables 14.13, 14.14). This mild form of cholestatic injury consists mainly of bile accumulation in the cytoplasm of liver cells (hepatocellular cholestasis) and in canaliculi (canalicular cholestasis). Hepatocellular cholestasis is frequently marked by cell swelling, and the bile itself may be difficult to identify without the use of special stains. Iron and copper stains may both be more useful in this regard than a hematoxylin

Table 14.12	Drugs that can lead to hepatic granulomas
Acetylsalicylic acid	Mineral oil
Actiretin	Nitrofurantoin
Allopurinol	Nomifensine
Amoxicillin-Clavulinate	Norethindrone
Aprindine	Norethynodrel
Azapropazone	Norgestrel
Barium salts	Oral contraceptives
BCG	Oxacillin
Beryllium	Oxyphenbutazone
Carbamazepine	Oxyphenisatin
Carbutamide	Papaverine
Cephalexin	Paracetamol
Cephalosporin	Penicillin
Chinidin	Phenazone
Chlorpromazine	Phenothiazines
Chlorpropamide	Phenprocoumon
Clavulanic acid	Phenylbutazone
Clometacin	Phenytoin
Contraceptive steroids	Polyvinyl pyrrolidone
Copper sulphate	Prajmalium
Dapsone	Probenecid
Detajmium tartrate	Procainamide
Diazepam	Procarbazine
Didanosine	Pronestyl
Diltiazem	Quinidine
Dimethicone	Quinine
Diphenylhydantoin	Ranitidine
Disopyramide	Salicylazosulfapyridine
Feprazone	Silica
Glibenclamide	Succinylsulphathiazole
Glyburide	Sulphadiazine
Gold	Sulphadimethoxine
Green-lipped mussel	Sulphadoxine-
(Seatone)	pyrimethamine
Halogenated	Sulphanilamide
Hydrocarbons	Sulphasalazine
Halothane	Sulphathiazole
Hydralazine	Sulphonamides
Imipramine	Sulphonylurea
Interferon	Tacrine
Isoniazid	Thorotrast
Mestranol	Tocainide
Metahydrin	Tolbutamide
Methimazole	Trichlormethiazide
Methotrexate	Trimethoprim-
Methyldopa	Sulphamethoxazole
Metolaxone	Verapamil
Metolazone	

and eosin stained section because of their light counterstains that allow the bile pigment to be more easily seen. An iron stain is doubly useful in that it can be used to distinguish iron (blue) from lipofuschin (granular and dirty brown) from bile (pale green to greenish brown). The cholestasis is usually most prominent in zone 3, and one should be careful to exclude other processes that may result in zone 3 cholestasis. There is sometimes a mild degree of parenchymal injury and inflammation (particularly portal inflammation) associated with acute cholestasis. This occurs

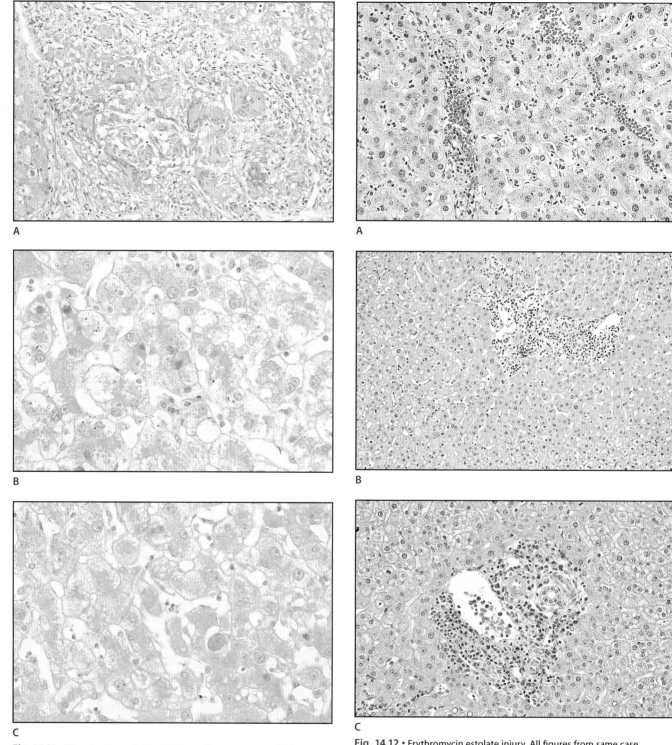

Fig. 14.11 • Phenylbutazone injury. All figures from same case. **(A)** Large, non-caseating granuloma in portal area. H&E. **(B)** Ballooning degeneration of liver cells and marked cholestasis. H&E. **(C)** Cytoplasmic cholestasis, ballooning and sinusoidal acidophilic body. H&E.

Fig. 14.12 • Erythromycin estolate injury. All figures from same case. **(A)** Marked cholestasis in perivenular zone. Note acidophilic body, mild to moderate ballooning and anisonucleosis. H&E. **(B)** Portal area is infiltrated with a moderate number of inflammatory cells. There is one acidophilic body (lower left). H&E. **(C)** Moderate portal inflammation with many eosinophils. Note mitoses to left. H&E.

with, for example, the cholestatic injury associated with chlorpromazine and erythromycin estolate (Fig. 14.12) but rarely in the cholestasis associated with steroids (Fig. 14.13). Intrahepatic cholestasis accompanied by portal inflammation has been called the 'cholangiolitic' or 'hypersensitivity' type of cholestasis,[30,31] while the cholestasis occurring with little or no portal tract inflammation has been termed 'bland' or 'steroid' type cholestasis[41] (Fig. 14.13). Different drugs may also lead to different distributions of bile accumulation. Chlorpromazine is associated with both hepatocellular and canalicular cholestasis while steroids are typically associated with pure canalicular cholestasis.

Table 14.13 Types of cholestatic injury caused by drugs				
Features	Canalicular (e.g. C-17 alkylated steroids—anabolic, contraceptive)	Hepatocanalicular (e.g. Chlorpromazine Erythromycin, Augmentin)	Ductal (e.g. Benoxaprofen)	Cholangiodestructive (e.g. Paraquat, FUDR Infusion)
Clinical evidence of hypersensitivity	No	Frequent	No	No
Biochemical				
AST-ALT (fold increased)	1–8	2–10	2–10	2–10
Alkaline phosphatase	1–3	3–10	>3	>3
Histological				
Bile casts	+	+	++ (canalicular, ductal)[c]	+
Portal inflammation	0	++ (especially early)	+/–	+
Duct destruction	0	+	+/–	++
Association[a]				
Adenoma	+	–	0	0
Carcinoma	+	–	0	0
Chronic cholestasis	±	+	±	0 or +[d]
Peliosis hepatis	+	+	–	±
Other terms	Bland cholestasis Steroid jaundice	Cholangiolitic Hypersensitivity cholestasis	Cholangiolar/vanishing bile duct syndrome	Biliary sclerosis[b]

(a) As a possible consequence
(b) A lesion caused by floxuridine resembles sclerosing cholangitis; referred to as biliary sclerosis
(c) In canaliculi, ductules and interlobular ducts
(d) No chronic cholestasis in paraquat poisoning, that is usually fatal, but chronic cholestasis is typical of floxuridine injury
+ = occurs; 0 = does not occur; ± = uncertain

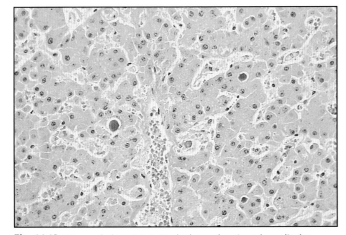

Fig. 14.13 • Oxymetholone injury. Marked cytoplasmic and canalicular perivenular cholestasis. H&E.

Cholangiolar cholestasis similar to that seen with sepsis may be caused by benoxaprofen. Sometimes, the acute intrahepatic cholestasis is accompanied by acute cholangitis,[69] which in turn may lead to chronic duct injury and loss.

Acute hepatocellular and cholestatic injury

When acute intrahepatic cholestasis is associated with an acute hepatitic injury, the result is a mixed form of hepatic injury. This is a common manifestation of drug-induced liver injury and should strongly suggest a drug aetiology when present (Table 14.14). Zimmerman has divided this injury into three types: mixed-hepatocellular, mixed-cholestatic and mixed-hepatocanalicular, depending on which part of the injury seems to predominate.[30]

Chronic cholestatic injury

Drug-induced chronic cholestatic injury may take a variety of forms, but the central feature is chronic injury to the intrahepatic ducts. The injury may mimic primary biliary cirrhosis or primary sclerosing cholangitis or the ducts may be destroyed by direct injury as exemplified by the changes (Fig. 14.15) of paraquat poisoning.[49,110] Chronic cholestasis with duct damage may occur with a number of therapeutic drugs, e.g. chlorpromazine, chlorpropamide, sulpha-methoxazole-trimethoprim, amoxicillin-clavulanate and others (Table 14.14). Indeed, ductal injury may accompany hepatocanalicular cholestasis and can lead to drug-induced vanishing bile-duct syndrome.[111,112,113] A syndrome that resembles primary biliary cirrhosis has followed acute cholestasis due to chlorpromazine, prochlorperazine, amitryptiline, imipramine, organic arsenicals, tolbutamide, ajmaline amongst others[30,31] (Table 14.14). The degree of duct destruction ('vanishing bile-duct syndrome') and portal inflammation tend to be less prominent in the drug-induced syndrome than in primary biliary cirrhosis (Fig. 14.16, Table 14.15).

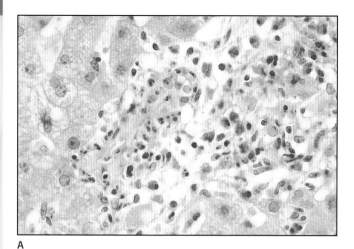

A

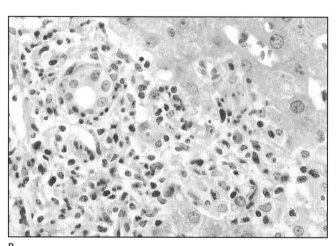

B

Fig. 14.14 • Phenytoin injury. Both figures from same case. **(A)** Acute cholangiolitis and portal inflammation with many neutrophils. H&E. ×450. **(B)** Acute cholangitis (left upper corner). H&E. ×450.

Biliary sclerosis

Biliary sclerosis is the term that has been applied to the biliary tree injury produced by hepatic arterial infusion therapy with floxuridine (FUDR) for metastatic carcinoma[114,115] and from the use of scolicides for treatment of echinococcal cysts.[116] The incidence with FUDR appears to be high, and the lesion consists of blebs and oedema in the duct epithelial surface and compression and distortion of the duct lumen (Fig. 14.17). Ludwig et al.[117] have attributed the ductal injury to occlusive arterial injury and have labelled it an 'ischaemic cholangiopathy' (Chapter 11). On cholangiography, the lesion resembles primary sclerosing cholangitis.

Steatosis and steatohepatitis

Non-alcoholic fatty liver disease (NAFLD) is a rubric currently used to encompass all forms of liver disease that have some degree of steatosis and in which alcohol and other known liver diseases do not play a role.[118] NAFLD is most often associated with glucose-intolerance or insulin-resistance; the estimated prevalence of NAFLD is very high, and up to 5% of the general population may have some

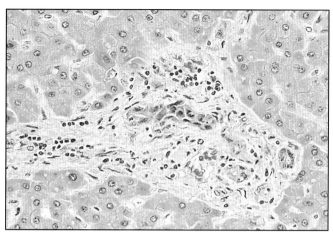

Fig. 14.15 • Paraquat toxicity. Bile-duct degeneration. H&E.

form of NAFLD.[119] Consequently, the presence of steatosis in the liver biopsy is not a very specific finding, particularly when present in only a mild to moderate degree. Nevertheless, steatosis has been associated with a large number of agents (Table 14.16) and may be seen combined with other forms of liver injury, such as zonal necrosis.[1]

Two main types of steatosis occur-macrovesicular and microvesicular, and both may be present simultaneously in various combinations. *Microvesicular steatosis* is generally associated with acute presentations and is characterized by a foamy change in the hepatocyte cytoplasm composed of tiny fat droplets that do not displace the nucleus (Fig. 14.18). Drug-induced microvesicular steatosis has been observed with tetracycline,[120,121] valproic acid,[122,123] some nucleoside analogues,[25,124,125] and salicylates (Reye syndrome).[126] Non-therapeutic toxins associated with microvesicular steatosis include ackee poisoning in children from hypoglycin A (Jamaican vomiting sickness),[127] occupational toxicity from dimethylformamide,[128] and cocaine abuse.[129] In at least some of these toxicities, mitochondrial injury is a common theme and some are associated with lactic acidosis and uncoupling of oxidative phosphorylation.

In *macrovesicular steatosis*, the hepatocytes contain a medium or large-size cytoplasmic fat droplet that displaces the nucleus to the periphery. Frequently multiple vacuoles of varying sizes are observed in a single cell. This mixed form of steatosis is probably more related to macrovesicular steatosis than microvesicular steatosis. Macrovesicular steatosis is characteristic of alcohol abuse, methotrexate injury and a number of other agents (Fig. 14.18). The steatosis may be the sole finding or may be associated with varying degrees of inflammation and necrosis. The combination of zonal necrosis and steatosis is observed with a number of toxic agents, including halogenated hydrocarbons, tannic acid and arsenicals.[1,34] Glucocorticoid steatosis is frequently bland, while methotrexate-related steatosis can lead to fibrosis and cirrhosis.[130] There are differences in the zonal distribution of fat of different toxic aetiologies. Phosphorus leads mainly or initially to accumulation of fat in the periportal zone, while tetracycline and alcohol lead predominantly or initially to perivenular steatosis.[1]

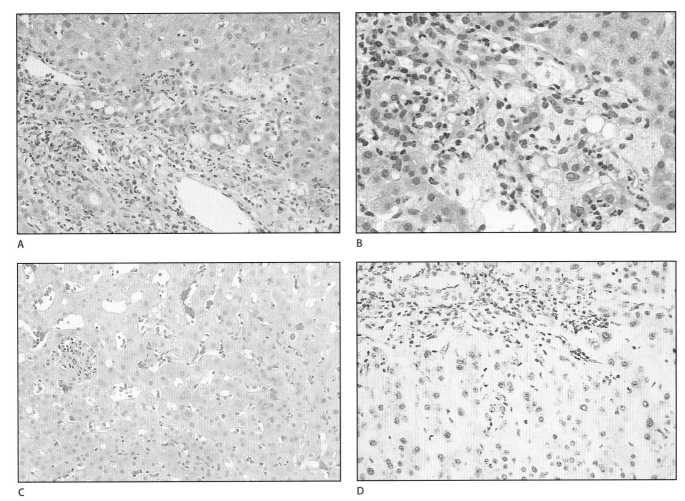

A

B

C

D

Fig. 14.16 • Chlorpromazine-induced chronic cholestasis. All figures from same case. **(A)** Marked portal inflammation (neutrophils, eosinophils) and acute cholangiolitis. H&E. **(B)** Periportal focus of pseudoxanthomatous transformation. H&E. **(C)** Moderate cholestasis and focal necrosis (left).H&E. **(D)** Moderate copper accumulation (red granules) in periportal liver cells. Rhodanine.

Table 14.14	Acute and chronic cholestasis and vanishing bile duct syndrome (VBDS) caused by medicinal agents		

Acute intrahepatic cholestasis	Chronic cholestasis	Combined hepatocellular-cholestatic injury	
Allopurinol	Aceprometazine	Acetohexamide	Ketoconazole
Androgens	Ajmaline (and related drugs)	Allopurinol	Lovastatin
Aprindine	Amineptine	Aminoglutethimide	Meglumine
Aureomycin	Amitryptyline	Aminosalicylic acid	Meprobamate
Captopril	Amoxicillin-Clavulinate	Amitryptyline	Mercaptopurine
Carbamazepine	Ampicillin	Amoxicillin-Clavulinate	Methyldopa
Chloramphenicol	Arsenic compounds	Aprindine	Naproxen
Chlordiazepoxide	Azathioprine	Atenolol	Niacin
Chlorozotocin	Barbiturates	Aureomycin	Nicotinic acid
Chlorpromazine	Carbamazepine	Azathioprine	Nifedipine
Chlorpropamide	Carbutamide	Benoxaprophen	Nitrofurantoin
Cimetidine	Chlorpromazine	Captopril	Nomifensine
Contraceptive steroids	Chlorpropamide	Carbamazepine	Oxacillin
Cyclosporin	Chlorthiazide	Carbarsone	Oxaprozin
Danazol	Cimetidine	Carbimazole	Oxyphenacetin
Diazepam	Cromolyn	Carisoprodol	Papaverine
Diphenylhydantoin	Cyamemazine	Cefadroxil monohydrate	Para-aminosalicylic acid
Disopyramide	Cyproheptadine	Cefazolin sodium	Paracetamol
Erythromycin	Diazepam	Cephalosporin	Penicillamine
Ethchlorvynol	Dicloxacillin	Chemotherapeutic agents	Penicillin
Fluoxymesterone	Erythromycin	Chlorambucil	Perphenazine
Gold	Flucloxacillin	Chloramphenicol	Phenobarbitol

Table 14.14 Acute and chronic cholestasis and vanishing bile duct syndrome (VBDS) caused by medicinal agents—cont'd

Acute intrahepatic cholestasis	Chronic cholestasis	Combined hepatocellular-cholestatic injury	
Haloperidol	Glycyrrhizin	Chlordiazepoxide	Phenothiazines
Iprindole	Haloperidol	Chlorpromazine	Phenylbutazone
Mercaptopurine	Ibuprofen	Chlorpropamide	Phenytoin
Mestranol	Imipramine	Chlortetracycline	Piperazine
Methandrostenolone	Itraconazole	Chlorthalidone	Piroxicam
Methimazole	Methylenediamine	Chlorthiazide	Pizotyline
Methyldopa	Methyltestosterone	Cimetidine	Polythiazide
Methyltestosterone	Norandrostenolone	Cis platinum	Prajmalium
Nitrofurantoin	Oral contraceptives	Clarithromycin	Procainamide
Norethindrone	Paracetamol	Clavulanic acid	Prochloperazine
Norethynodrel	Phenylbutazone	Clometacin	Propoxyphene
Norgestrel	Phenytoin	Clorazepate	Quinethazone
Oestrogens, synthetic	Piroxicam	Cyclosporin	Quinidine
Oral contraceptives	Prochloperazine	Dacarbazine	Ranitidine
Oxymethalone	Sporidesmin	Dantrolene	Rifampin
Para-aminosalicylic acid	Sulphonylurea	Dapsone	Sulfones
Perphenazine	Sulpiride	Diazepam	Sulindac
Phenobarbitol	Tetracycline	Diclofenac	Sulphadiazine
Phenothiazines	Thiabendazole	Diphenylhydantoin	Sulphamethoxazole
Phenylbutazone	Tiopronin	Disopyramide	Sulphasalazine
Piroxicam	Tolazamide	Doxidan	Sulphonamides
Prochloperazine	Tolbutamide	Enalapril	Tamoxifen
Sulfamethoxazole	Toxic oil (Rapeseed)	Erythromycin	Thiabendazole
Sulphadiazine	TPN	Ethchlorvynol	Thiopental sodium
Sulphonamides	Trifluoperazine	Ethionamide	Thiopentone
Tamoxifen	Troleandomycin	Flucloxacillin	Thioridazine
Thioridazine	Xenelamine	Fluorodeoxyuridine	Ticlopidine
Tolbutamide		Fluoxymesterone	Tocainide
Warfarin sodium		Fluphenazine	Tolazamide
		Flurazepam	Tolbutamide
	PBC-like	Flutamide	Toxic Oil (Rapeseed)
	Chlorpromazine	Glibenclamide	TPN
	Cromolyn	Gold	Tranylcypromine
	Practolol	Griseofulvin	Triazolam
	Thiabendazole	Halogenated	Trifluoperazine
	Tolbutamide	Hydrocarbons	Trimethobenzamide
		Haloperidol	Trimethoprim
		Halothane	Trimethoprim-Sulphamethoxazole
	PSC-like	Hycanthone	Tripelennamine
	Floxuridine	Hydralazine	Troleandomycin
	Scolicides	Hydrochlorothiazide	Valproic acid
		Ibuprofen	Verapamil
		Imipramine	Zimelidine
		Indomethacin	
		Iodipamide meglumine	
		Iproclozide	
		Isocarboxazid	
		Isoniazid	

Characteristics	Primary biliary cirrhosis	Drug-induced chronic cholestasis
Associated diseases	Sicca syndrome, other 'collagen' diseases	Irrelevant
Drug intake	Irrelevant	Phenothiazine Organic arsenicals Tolbutamide Other cholestasis-producing drugs (Table 14.14)
Age	Middle-aged	All ages
Gender	Women 9 : 1	Both
Onset	Insidious	Acute
Anitimitochondrial antibody	Positive (95%)	Negative
Symptoms		
Pruritus	+	+
Jaundice	Late feature	Early feature
Signs		
Melanoderma	+	
Jaundice[a]	− or +	+
Xanthomas	+ or −	+ or − (transient)
Hepatomegaly	+ or −	+ or −
Splenomegaly	+ or −	+ or −
Biochemical		
Total serum bilirubin	1–5 mg/dl	1–20 mg/dl
AST/ALT (fold increased)	1–5	1–5
Alkaline phosphatase	3–10	3–10
Cholesterol	Increased	Increased
β-globulin	Increased	Increased
IgM globulin	Increased	?
Histological		
Non-suppurative cholangitis	+	−
Ductopenia (VBDS)	+	+
Hepatic granulomas	+	−
Copper in hepatocytes	+	+
Cirrhosis	+/−	+/−
Prognosis	Variable[b]	Good

(a) Jaundice is usually slight and tends to occur relatively late in the course of primary biliary cirrhosis, while it is early in the course of drug-induced chronic cholestasis

(b) In most instances, outcome is eventually poor + = usually present; − = usually absent; +/− = present but of slight degree

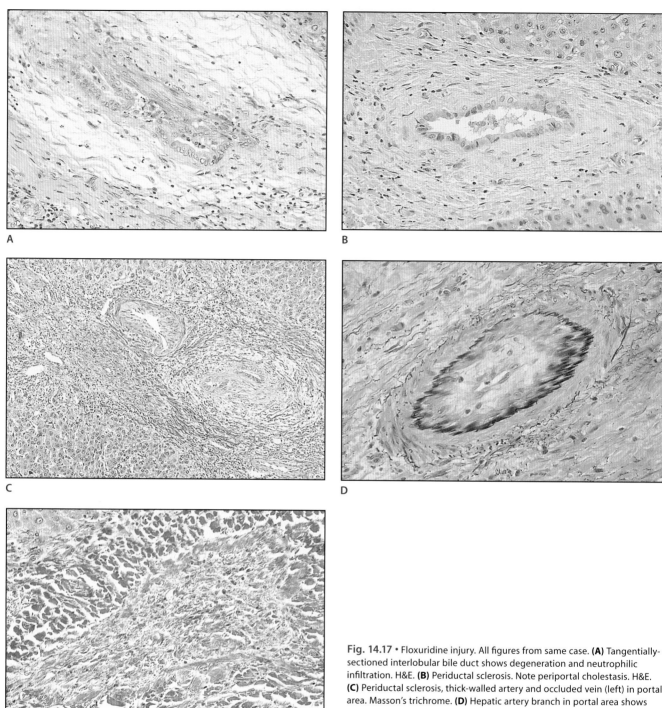

Fig. 14.17 • Floxuridine injury. All figures from same case. **(A)** Tangentially-sectioned interlobular bile duct shows degeneration and neutrophilic infiltration. H&E. **(B)** Periductal sclerosis. Note periportal cholestasis. H&E. **(C)** Periductal sclerosis, thick-walled artery and occluded vein (left) in portal area. Masson's trichrome. **(D)** Hepatic artery branch in portal area shows marked intimal thickening with almost complete occlusion of the lumen, medial hypertrophy and a thickened elastica. Musto. **(E)** Portal vein branch shows old fibrotic occlusion. Masson's trichrome.

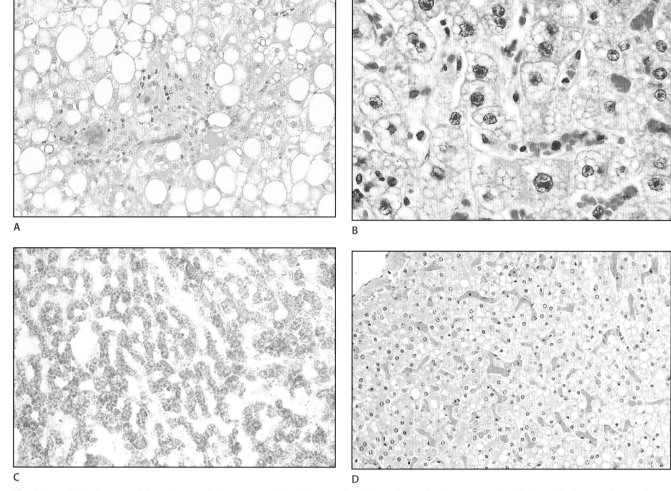

Fig. 14.18 • **(A)** Methotrexate injury. Macrovesicular steatosis. H&E. **(B)** Tetracycline injury. Microvesicular steatosis. H&E. **(C)** Liver cells show marked small droplet steatosis. Oil red O stain. **(D)** Asparaginase injury. Lipid vacuoles in liver cells are of medium size. H&E.

Table 14.16 Agents that produce steatosis and/or phospholipidosis

Steatosis (type)*		Steatohepatitis	Phospholipidosis
2-Chloropropane	Carbon tetrachloride (macro)	Amiodarone	Amiodarone
Acetylsalicylic acid (both)	Chlorinated diphenyls	Corticosteroids	Amitryptyline
Aflatoxins (micro)	Chlorinated naphthalene	Ethanol	Chloramphenicol
Amanitin (macro)	Chloroform (macro)	Methotrexate	Chloroquine
Amineptine (micro)	Chloroprene	Naproxen	Chlorphenteramine
Amiodarone (micro)	Chlortetracycline (micro)	Oestrogens, synthetic	Chlorpromazine
Antiemetics (micro)	Chromates (macro)	Perhexiline maleate	Coralgil
Antimony	Cis platinum (macro)	Spironolactone	Gentamycin
Arsenic compounds	Clometacin (macro)	Sulphasalazine	Ketoconazole
Asparaginase (macro)	Cocaine (both)		Oestrogens, synthetic
Azacytidine	Contraceptive steroids		Perhexiline maleate
Azaserine	Corticosteroids (macro)		Promethazine
Azauridine	Cortisone (macro)		Thioridazine
B. cereus toxin	Cyanamide (macro)		TPN
Barium salts	Dantrolene (macro)		Trimethoprim-Sulphamethoxazole
Bleomycin (macro)	DDT		
Blood alchohol level	Demeclocycline (micro)		
Borates (both)	Desferrioxamine (micro)		
Bromobenzene	Dichloroethylene (macro)		
Cadmium (macro)	Dichloropropane		
Calcium hopantenate	Didanosine (micro)		
Camphor (micro)	Dimethylformamide (both)		
Carbon disulphide	Dimethylhydrazine		

Table 14.16	Agents that produce steatosis and/or phospholipidosis—cont'd

Steatosis (type)*

Dimethylnitrosamine	Naphthalene
Dinitrobenzone	Naproxen
Dinitrotoluene	Nifedipine
Ethanol (both)	Nitrofurantoin (macro)
Ethionine (both)	Oestrogens, synthetic
Ethyl bromide (macro)	Organic solvents (macro)
Ethyl chloride (macro)	Orotic acid (macro)
Ethylene dibromide	Oxytetracycline (micro)
Ethylene dichloride	Paracetamol (macro)
Etretinate (macro)	Pennyroyal oil (micro)
Fialuridine (both)	Pentanoic acid (micro)
Flectol H	Perhexiline maleate (macro)
Flurazepam (macro)	Phalloidin (micro)
Galactosamine	Phosphorus (both)
Gold (macro)	Piroxicam (micro)
Halogenated Hydrocarbons (macro)	Pirprofen (micro)
Hydralazine (macro)	Puromycin
Hydrazine	Pyrrolizidine alkaloids (micro)
Hypoglycin A (micro)	Rare Earths (Low atomic #)
Ibuprofen (both)	Rifampin (macro)
Indinivir	Rolitetracycline (micro)
Indomethacin (macro)	Safrole
Iodoform	Salicylate intoxication (micro)
Islandicum	Spironolactone
Isoniazid (macro)	Sulindac (macro)
Ketoprofen (micro)	Sulphasalazine (macro)
Luteoskyrin	Synthaline
Margosa oil (micro)	Tamoxifen (macro)
Mefloquine	Tannic acid (macro)
Mercury	Terramycin
Methimazole (macro)	Tetrachloroethane (macro)
Methotrexate (macro)	Tetrachloroethylene (macro)
Methyl bromide (macro)	Tetracycline (micro)
Methyl chloride (macro)	Thallium compounds (micro)
Methyl chlorobromide	Tolmetin (micro)
Methyl dichloride (macro)	TPN (macro)
Methyl salicylate (micro)	Trichloroethylene (macro)
Methylchloroform	Trinitrotoluene
Methyldopa (macro)	Uranium compounds (macro)
Microcycline (macro)	Valproic acid (both)
Minocycline (macro)	Vitamin A (micro)
Mitomycin C (macro)	Warfarin sodium (both)
Mushrooms (both)	Zidovudine (macro)

* Micro = microvesicular steatosis; macro = macrovesicular; when specifically defined in pathological studies

Non-alcoholic steatohepatitis (NASH)

Steatohepatitis caused by drugs and toxins has essentially the same histologic features as other forms of steatohepatitis.[131] The basic pattern of injury is a zone 3 hepatocellular injury characterized by hepatocellular ballooning, and Mallory body formation with variable lobular inflammation (Fig. 14.19). Portal inflammation may also be present. The associated fibrosis is typically perisinusoidal and perivenular at first, but can progress to bridging fibrosis and cirrhosis. Many of the drugs that have been associated with steatohepatitis and Mallory body formation are also associated with phospholipidosis. The drugs in current use chiefly responsible for the entity are perhexiline maleate[132] and amiodarone.[133] Steatohepatitis or Mallory bodies (without phospholipidoses) have also been produced by diethylstilboesterol,[134] prednisolone,[135] nifedipine,[136] tamoxifen,[137] didanosine[138] (and, of course, by alcohol[53,54]) (Table 14.16). Some of these drugs, notably tamoxifen, methotrexate, corticosteroids, diethylstilbestrol and oestrogens, seem to have

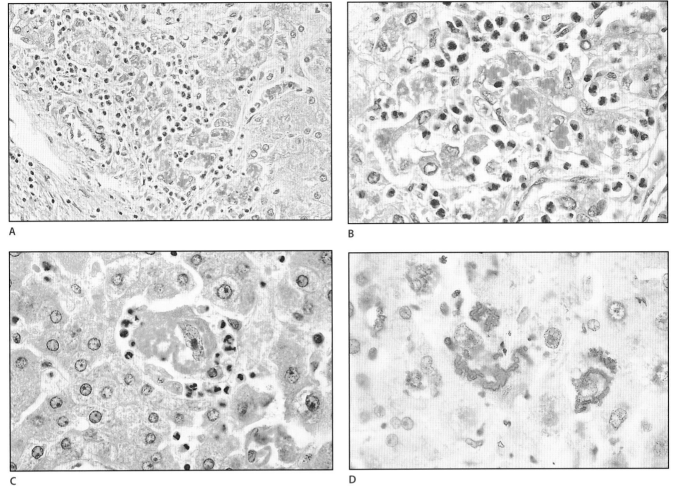

Fig. 14.19 • Amiodarone injury. All figures from same case. **(A)** Periportal liver cells contain Mallory bodies and are surrounded by neutrophils. Same case illustrated in Fig. 14.20(b). H&E. **(B)** High power view of Mallory bodies. **(C)** Neutrophil 'satellitosis', the body is rope-like and includes the nucleus of a lysed liver cell. H&E. **(D)** Mallory bodies (light brown) are demonstrated by immunostaining for ubiquitin.

their effect by exacerbating underlying steatohepatitis. Some of the antiretroviral drugs have been associated with a syndrome of dyslipidemia, fat maldistribution and insulin resistance that has been termed HIV-associated lipodystrophy syndrome or HIV-associated metabolic and morphological abnormality syndrome (HAMMAS).[139] The steatosis and steatohepatitis that have been observed in patients with HIV infection may be more related to the induction of HAMMAS than to a direct toxic effect on the liver. The drugs implicated in HAMMAS are ritonavir, amprenavir, nelfinavir, indinavir, saquinavir, atazanavir and the combination drug lopinavir/ritonavir.

Phospholipidosis

Phospholipidosis is an additional form of lipid accumulation that may be drug-induced. The lesion was first recognized in Japan in 1969 as a complication of the early coronary vasodilator diethylaminoethoxyhexoestrol;[140] Phospholipidosis is characterized by enlarged, foamy or granular hepatocytes by light microscopy (Fig. 14.20(A), (B)); lamellated or crystalloid inclusions can be seen by electron microscopy (Fig. 14.20(C)).[141] There are similar changes in Kupffer cells and in cells at extrahepatic sites.[142]

The lesion resembles the changes seen in inborn disorders of phospholipid metabolism and can lead to cirrhosis. It has since been seen in patients taking Coralgil, perhexiline maleate[143,144] or amiodarone,[145,146] and has been reproduced in experimental animals by amphiphilic compounds.[147,148] Indeed, the amphiphilic character of the drugs appears to account for the accumulation of phospholipids in lysosomes of hepatocytes and other cells. The drugs bind to phospholipids and inhibit their hydrolysis by lysosomal phospholipase A. The full-blown lesion requires several months to develop, but early changes occur after only several doses. It is not clear whether the cirrhosis is a consequence of the accumulation of phospholipids or the result of other cytological injury. Many of these drugs are also associated with steatohepatitis and may develop fibrosis by a mechanism similar to those with others forms of NASH. There are some drugs, however, that cause phospholipidosis but not steatohepatitis (Table 14.16).

Fibrosis and cirrhosis

Fibrosis and cirrhosis may result from a variety of drug and toxin-induced injuries. Agents which cause chronic hepatitis, chronic cholestasis and steatohepatitis may all have

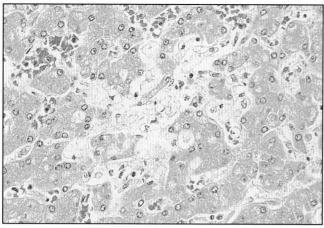

A

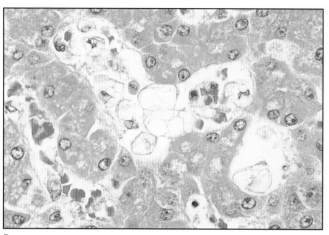

B

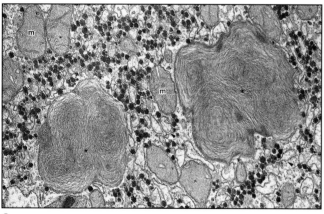

C

Fig. 14.20 • Amiodarone-induced phospholipidosis. **(A)** Cluster of foam cells. H&E. **(B)** Same case illustrated in Fig. 14.19(A). Foam cells in hepatic sinusoid. H&E. **(C)** Electron micrograph of hepatocytes in aminodarone-associated phospholipidosis showing two membrane-bound lysosomal structures (asterisks) in a hepatocyte. These structures are composed of densely-packed concentric membranous arrays with a fingerprint pattern and are identical to those described in phospholipidosis. Note also altered mitochondria (m) with reduced cristae and increased matrix density and vesiculated smooth endoplasmic reticulum (arrowheads). Lead citrate, ×36 900. Courtesy of Dr M J Phillips.

cirrhosis as an end point.[1] We are unaware, however, of any examples of acute hepatic injury in humans that has led to cirrhosis after biochemical and clinical resolution of the acute injury following drug discontinuation. This is similar, for example, to the expected course seen after acute viral hepatitis A.[149]

Periportal fibrosis occurs in drug-induced chronic hepatitis and chronic cholestasis induced by a number of other drugs (Tables 14.10 and 14.14). Methotrexate can lead to periportal fibrosis when used in the treatment of leukaemia,[150] and to both periportal and intralobular fibrosis (and even cirrhosis) when used in the long-term therapy of psoriasis and, rarely of rheumatoid arthritis[130,151,152] (Fig. 14.21). Hypervitaminosis A[153] discussed below, can lead to perivenular fibrosis. This is accompanied by marked hypertrophy of the hepatic stellate cells, atrophy of hepatocytes, veno-occlusive lesions and sinusoidal dilatation (Fig. 14.22).

Macronodular and micronodular cirrhosis,[2,34] congestive hepatopathy resembling cardiac cirrhosis,[154] and a biliary cirrhosis-like lesion[155,156,157] can all result from toxin- or drug-induced liver damage. Macronodular or micronodular cirrhosis may be a sequel to continued or repetitive injury or the result of subacute necrosis, or chronic necroinflammatory disease[1] (Fig. 14.23). A single episode of necrosis may leave architectural distortion, but cirrhosis does not occur. A single episode of zonal necrosis in experimental animals (e.g. CC1₄ poisoning), even when extensive, is followed by complete histological restitution in surviving animals.[158]

The most important path to drug-induced cirrhosis occurs via the lesions of chronic hepatitis (Fig. 14.23), subacute necrosis (Fig. 14.10) and phospholipidosis-steatohepatitic injury (Figs 14.19 and 14.20). Biliary cirrhosis may occur as a sequel to acute intrahepatic cholestasis with bile-duct loss (Fig. 14.16, Table 14.15), and as noted above an obstructive biliary cirrhosis type of injury can be a consequence of the biliary sclerosis produced by hepatic artery infusion of floxuridine (Fig. 14.17).

Vascular lesions

A number of important vascular lesions can be produced by drugs (Table 14.17).[75,159] Two involve blockade of efferent blood flow with and congestive hepatopathy, leading to perivenular necrosis; when severe, mid-zone necrosis also occurs. Prolonged occlusion leads to fibrotic bridging between adjacent hepatic vein branches and a picture resembling cardiac cirrhosis. The two occlusive lesions are thrombosis of the hepatic veins (Fig. 14.24) and fibrotic occlusion of the hepatic venules and sinuosoids (Fig. 14.25). Additional lesions include peliosis hepatis (Fig. 14.26) sinusoidal dilatation (Fig. 14.27), perisinusoidal fibrosis (Fig. 14.22) and hepatoportal sclerosis (Fig. 14.28). Abnormal blood flow that results from a number of these lesions may cause irregular regeneration, resulting in nodular regenerative hyperplasia (Fig.14.29). It has been suggested that these lesions are linked by a common pathway of endothelial cell injury.[160]

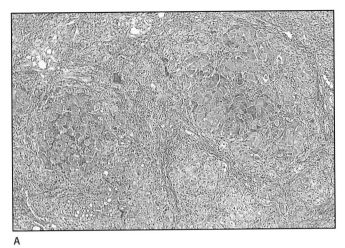

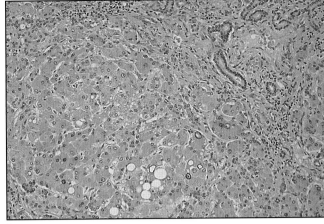

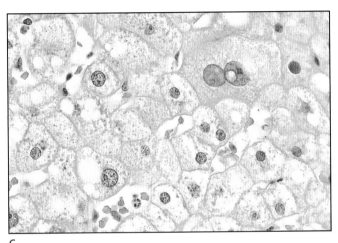

Fig. 14.21 • Methotrexate-induced micronodular cirrhosis. **(A)** Masson trichrome. **(B)** Same case illustrated in (A). Segment of micronodule reveals mild portal inflammation, patchy steatosis, glycogenated nuclei and moderate anisonucleosis. H&E. **(C)** Methotrexate-induced anisonucleosis. H&E.

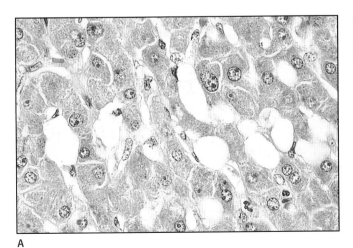

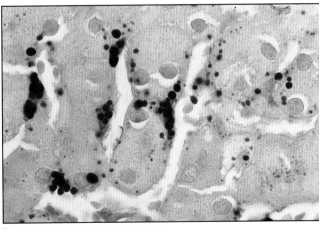

Fig. 14.22 • Hypervitaminosis A. All figures from same case. **(A)** Markedly hypertrophied hepatic stellate cells consist of clusters of faintly outlined fat vacuoles and distorted eccentrically-located nuclei. H&E. **(B)** Perisinusoidal location of stellate cells is demonstrated by use of lipid stain. Osmium tetroxide post-fixation.

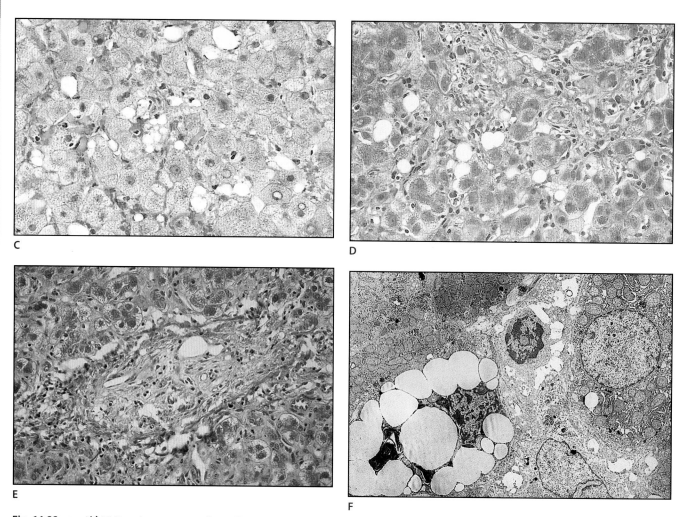

Fig. 14.22 • cont'd (C) Vacuoles represent stellate cells jammed in space of Disse. Masson trichrome. **(D)** More extensive fibrosis in perivenular zone. Masson. **(E)** Occluded terminal hepatic terminal hepatic venule. Masson trichrome. **(F)** Markedly hypertrophied stellate cell (lower left) contains numerous lipid vacuoles and an eccentrically-located nucleus with scalloped margins. Electron micrograph, ×14 000.

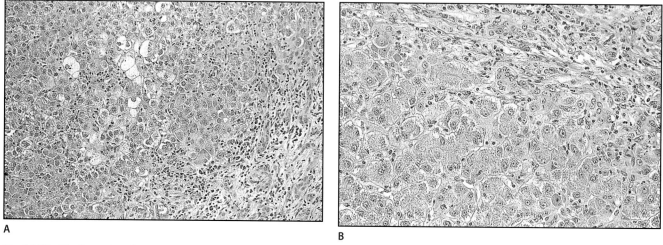

Fig. 14.23 • Nitrofurantoin-induced chronic hepatitis. Both (A) and (B) from same case. **(A)** Periportal ductular proliferation and interface hepatitis (bottom and right). Hepatocytes show patchy ballooning degeneration. H&E. **(B)** Scattered acidophilic bodies and mild to moderate ballooning in periportal area. H&E. Pemoline-induced chronic hepatitis. Figures (C)–(E) from same case.

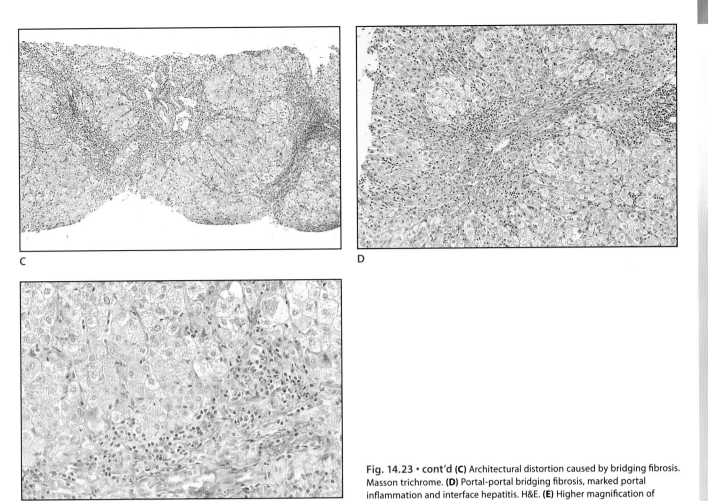

Fig. 14.23 • cont'd **(C)** Architectural distortion caused by bridging fibrosis. Masson trichrome. **(D)** Portal-portal bridging fibrosis, marked portal inflammation and interface hepatitis. H&E. **(E)** Higher magnification of periportal interface hepatitits. H&E.

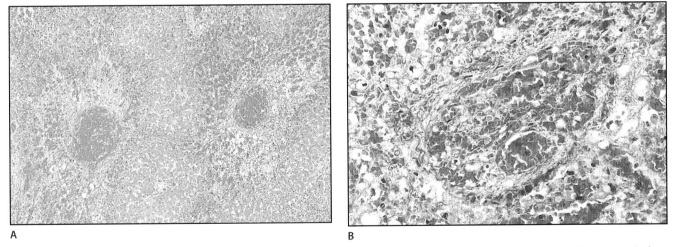

Fig. 14.24 • Hepatic vein thrombosis associated with long-term use of oral contraceptive. Both figures from same case. **(A)** Recent thrombi in two terminal hepatic venules with perivenular zone necrosis and marked sinusoidal dilatation and congestion. H&E. **(B)** Thrombosed and recanalized terminal hepatic venule. Masson trichrome.

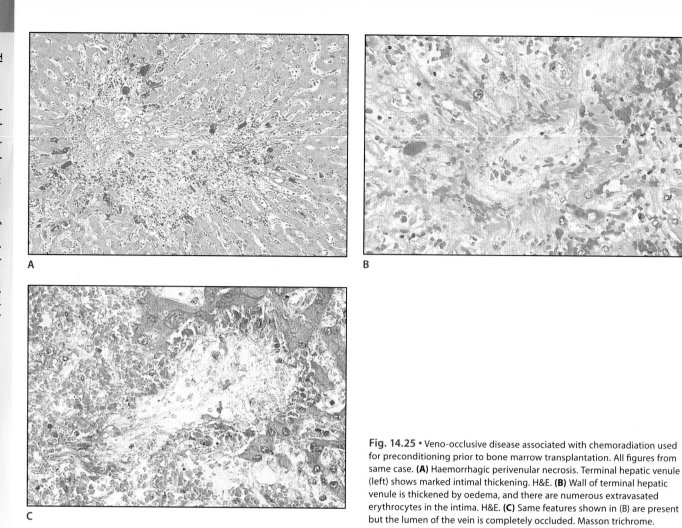

A

B

C

Fig. 14.25 • Veno-occlusive disease associated with chemoradiation used for preconditioning prior to bone marrow transplantation. All figures from same case. **(A)** Haemorrhagic perivenular necrosis. Terminal hepatic venule (left) shows marked intimal thickening. H&E. **(B)** Wall of terminal hepatic venule is thickened by oedema, and there are numerous extravasated erythrocytes in the intima. H&E. **(C)** Same features shown in (B) are present but the lumen of the vein is completely occluded. Masson trichrome.

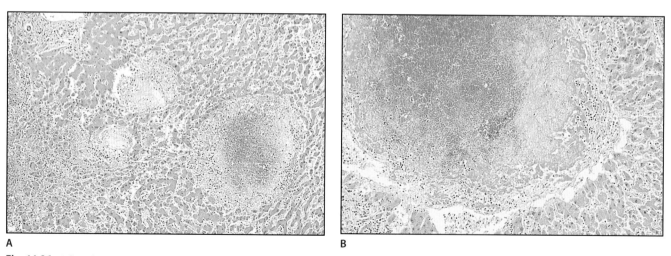

A

B

Fig. 14.26 • Peliosis hepatis associated with oxymetholone therapy given to patient with aplastic anaemia. Both figures from same case. **(A)** Peliotic cavities are of variable size. H&E. **(B)** Blood in cavity is clotted, with fibrin accumulation at the periphery of the cavity. The cavity has no endothelial lining. H&E.

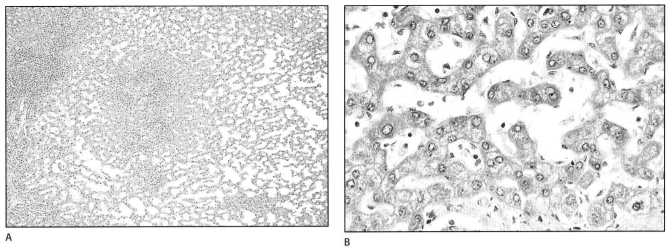

Fig. 14.27 • Sinusoidal dilatation associated with long-term use of oral contraceptive. Both figures from same case. **(A)** Note portal area in centre of field. H&E. **(B)** Atrophy of liver plates and striking sinusoidal dilatation. H&E.

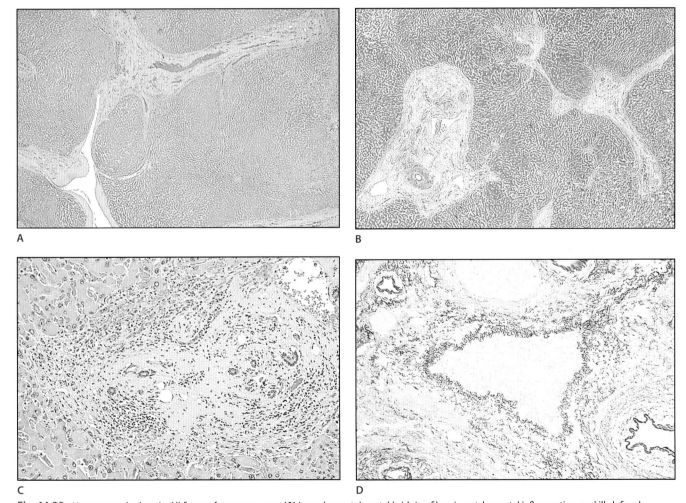

Fig. 14.28 • Hepatoportal sclerosis. All figures from same case. **(A)** Irregular portal-portal bridging fibrosis, patchy portal inflammation, and ill-defined nodularity of the parenchyma. H&E. There was no known cause for this lesion, as is often true of hepatoportal sclerosis. The lesion is typical of that seen after long-term exposure to inorganic trivalent arsenic. **(B)** Markedly expanded acellular portal area (left) and portal-portal fibrous bridge (right). Masson trichrome. **(C)** Expanded portal area lacks portal vein branches with a diameter corresponding to its size. There is patchy infiltration with lymphocytes and plasma cells. H&E. **(D)** Occluded portal vein branch is readily identified by an elastic stain. Orcein.

Table 14.17 Vascular lesions of the liver caused by drugs

VOD/SOS*	Peliosis	Sinusoidal dilatation	Hepatic vein thrombosis
Actinomycin D	Androgens	Androgens	Contraceptive steroids
Adriamycin	Arsenic compounds	Azathioprine	Cyclophosphamide
Aflatoxins	Azathioprine	Carmustine	Dacarbazine
Arsenic compounds	Busulfan	Contraceptive steroids	Vincristine
Azathioprine	Chemotherapeutic agents	Dacarbazine	
BCNU	Contraceptive steroids	Daunorubicin	
Busulfan	Corticosteroids	Metoclopramide	
Carboplatin	Danazol	Mitomycin C	
Chemotherapeutic agents	Diethylstilbestrol	Thioguanine	
Cis platinum	Estrone sulfate	Valproic acid	
Contraceptive steroids	Fluoxymesterone	Vinblastine	
Cyclophosphamide	Glucocorticoids	Vitamin A	
Cysteamine	Hydroxyprogesterone		
Cytarabine	Hydroxyurea		
Cytosine arabinoside	Medroxyprogesterone		
Dacarbazine	Mercaptopurine		
Dacarbazine	Methandrostenolone		
Danazol	Methotrexate		
Daunorubicin	Methyltestosterone		
Dimethylbusulfan	Oestrogens, synthetic		
Dimethylnitrosamine	Phalloidin		
Estramustine	Tamoxifen		
Floxuridine	Testosterone		
Fluorodeoxyuridine	Thioguanine		
Indicine	Thorotrast		
Mate tea	Vinyl Chloride		
Mechlorethamine	Vitamin A		
Mercaptopurine			
Mitomycin C	**NRH***	**Hepato-portal sclerosis**	**Vasculitis**
Pyrrolizidine alkaloids			
Tamoxifen	Androgens	Arsenic compounds	Allopurinol
Thioguanine	Chemotherapeutic agents	Contraceptive steroids	Chlorpropamide
Urethane	Contraceptive steroids	Ethanol	Chlorthiazide
Vinblastine	Copper sulphate	Vinyl Chloride	Penicillin
Vincristine	Corticosteroids		Phenylbutazone
	Ethanol		Phenytoin
	Thorotrast		Sulphonamides
	Toxic Oil (Rapeseed)		
	Vinyl Chloride		

* VOD/SOS: Veno-occlusive disease/Sinusoidal obstruction syndrome; NRH: Nodular regenerative hyperplasia

Hepatoportal sclerosis and nodular regenerative hyperplasia (NRH)

Strategic deposition of collagen in the periportal area and space of Disse, accompanied by reduction of portal vein calibre or obliteration of the portal vein can lead to portal hypertension (Fig. 14.28). This 'non-cirrhotic portal hypertension' has been termed *hepatoportal sclerosis*.[161] Instances of non-cirrhotic portal hypertension have been attributed to chronic exposure to inorganic arsenicals,[162] vinyl chloride,[163] and copper sulphate[164] as well as to alcoholic liver disease[165] (Chapter 6). Non-cirrhotic portal hypertension can result from vitamin A intoxication (Fig. 14.22). Several protocols employed to prepare patients for bone marrow transplantations or to treat neoplastic disease have led to non-cirrhotic portal hypertension by producing hepatoportal sclerosis[166] or nodular regenerative hyperplasia (NRH).[167–169] NRH has also been associated with the use of azathioprine in transplantation,[170,171] and mercaptopurine and 6-thioguanine for Crohn disease[172] (Fig. 14.29). This lesion can be difficult to recognize in routinely stained sections. However, careful examination of reticulin preparations will demonstrate nodules of enlarged hepatocytes arranged in cords that are more than 2 cells thick and which are not organized into parallel plates. Between regenerating nodules, the hepatocytes are atrophic and compressed; there may be no fibrosis or only a small amount of sinusoidal fibrosis in the areas of hepatocyte atrophy.

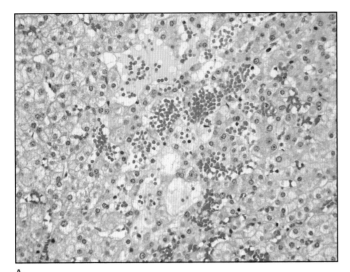

A

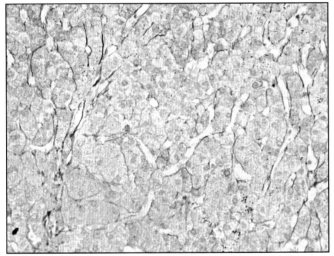

B

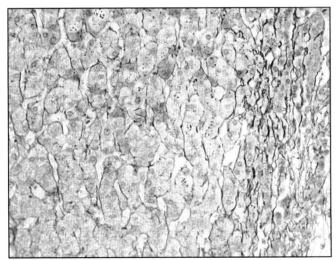

C

Fig. 14.29 • 6-Thioguanine injury causing nodular regenerative hyperplasia in a patient with ulcerative colitis. All figures from the same case. **(A)** Sinusoidal dilatation with compressed hepatocytes in between widened vascular spaces. H&E. **(B)** Focus of regeneration. Note the widened, anastomosing liver cell plates. Reticulum. **(C)** Zone of regeneration adjacent to a zone of compression. The reticulum fibres are pressed together and the hepatocytes are also flattened. Reticulin.

Hepatic vein thrombosis

Certain chemotherapuetic agents and oral contraceptives have been implicated in causing hepatic vein thrombosis (Fig. 14.24). At least 100 cases have been reported in patients taking oral contraceptives and have been attributed to the thrombogenic effects of contraceptive steroids.[75,173-176] Many of the patients appear to have had overt or latent myeloproliferative disease, but a third of cases have not. According to Valla et al.,[174] the risk of developing hepatic vein thrombosis seems to be increased two-fold in women taking oral contraceptives. Incrimination of oral contraceptives as a cause of Budd–Chiari syndrome, however, is controversial.

Sinusoidal obstruction syndrome (SOS)/ veno-occlusive disease (VOD)

Veno-occlusive disease is a pattern of liver injury in which there is obliteration of small hepatic veins by loose, oedematous connective tissue that appears between the endothelium and the underlying normal collagen matrix, narrowing the lumen. This is associated with endothelial injury in the sinusoids, particularly in zone 3 with the accumulation of cell debris, trapped red cells and extracellular matrix in the sinusoids; there is frequently necrosis of the perivenular hepatocytes. Because of the key role played by sinusoidal obstruction in the pathophysiology, the term *sinusoidal obstruction syndrome* has been suggested as an alternative name for this process. Injury and occlusion of the efferent hepatic venules has long been known to be produced by pyrrolizidine alkaloids.[74,177] The initial lesion is perivenular necrosis accompanied and followed by progressive fibrotic decrease in venule calibre (Fig. 14.25). It causes hepatic congestion and can lead to a fatal congestive cirrhosis, to an arrested lesion, or even to reversal.[178,179]

The clinical features resemble those of the Budd–Chiari syndrome produced by hepatic vein thrombosis. In addition to the alkaloids, causal agents include urethane, thioguanine, azathioprine and a number of other oncotherapeutic agents, as well as irradiation.[180-183] The use of multiple chemotherapuetic agent or combination chemotherapy and radiotherapy seem to be more toxic than the use of any single agent. The most important cause today is myeloablative conditioning treatment associated with bone marrow transplantation,[184,185] but the incidence of SOS/VOD has fallen due to changes in bone marrow transplant protocols and the advent of non-myeloblative regimens.

Peliosis hepatis and sinusoidal dilatation

Peliosis hepatitis consists of large blood-filled cavities not lined by endothelium (Fig. 14.26). It has been of recognized clinical significance only since the middle of the 20th century.[75] The lesion has been produced in experimental animals by administration of phalloidin.[186] Phalloidin has a special proclivity for injury to membranes; this is consistent with the theory that the lesion reflects damage to sinusoidal supporting membranes.

Incriminated causes of the lesion in humans include anabolic steroids,[187,188] diethylstilboestrol[189] contraceptive steroids,[190,191] tamoxifen[192] and azathioprine,[193,194] vitamin A[195] and thorotrast[196] (Table 14.17). Of practical importance is the observation of marked *sinusoidal dilatation* in livers that show peliosis hepatis, even in sites remote from the cavitary lesions. Furthermore, anabolic and contraceptive steroids can lead to sinusoidal dilatation, even when no peliosis has developed.[197] Indeed, a characteristic lesion of prominent dilatation of periportal sinusoids (Fig. 14.27) has been described in patients taking contraceptive steroids.[198] Ultrastructurally, the lesion is characterized by striking perisinusoidal fibrosis and proliferation and 'enhanced activity' of sinusoidal endothelial cells and perisinusoidal stellate cells.[199]

Hepatic neoplasia

The histopathology of drug-induced hepatic neoplasia is indistinguishable from the non-drug-induced tumours. Both benign and malignant tumours of the liver have been associated with drugs and toxins[200,201] (see Chapter 15 and Table 14.18).

Benign tumours

Hepatocellular adenoma, a lesion almost entirely restricted to females in the child-bearing years, was an extremely uncommon tumour prior to the era of oral contraceptives.[202,203,204] Convincing evidence for a causal effect is the reported regression of this tumour following withdrawal of oral contraceptives, and the large case-control epidemiological study of Rooks et al.[205] There is no relationship between focal nodular hyperplasia and contraceptive steroids.[206]

Malignant tumours

Thorotrast has produced hepatocellular and cholangiocellular carcinomas, both as well as angiosarcoma, lesions that may be due to the radioactivity rather than the chemical toxicity of the agent.[207] Epidemiological studies suggest that mycotoxins as well as synthetic chemicals encountered occupationally may also be carcinogenic in man.[35,36,208]

Several medicinal agents have come under suspicion as possible hepatocarcinogens. Development of hepatocellular carcinoma in at least 40 long-term recipients of anabolic steroids have made these agents suspect.[41] Contraceptive steroids have also been incriminated in the development of hepatocellular carcinoma.[42,209–211] Tamoxifen and danazol have been implicated in hepatic carcinogenesis, as discussed later.

Angiosarcoma has been reported in individuals with occupational exposure to vinyl chloride.[212–214] This rare tumour also developed in vintners with long exposure to inorganic arsenic, in patients with psoriasis treated with arsenicals or in individuals who had ingested arsenic-contaminated water or had had other environmental exposures,[215–217] and in patients who had been injected with thorotrast.[218–220] Other drugs incriminated rarely as causes of this tumour include androgenic-anabolic steroids,[221,222] diethylstilboestrol[223] and phenelzine.[224]

Other drug-associated morphological changes

Subcapsular haematoma

This lesion, which may rupture, has been reported in a number of patients taking oral anticoagulants (warfarin, streptokinase),[225,226] and in one patient who abused anabolic steroids.[227]

Hepar lobatum

Reported as a complication of chemotherapy for metastatic carcinoma, this lesion has been attributed to regression of the tumour nodules with subsequent tissue collapse, fibrosis and scar contraction.[228] Possibly related to this lesion are reports of abnormal imaging findings resembling cirrhosis in patients with metastatic breast or gastric carcinoma treated with systemic chemotherapy.[229–231]

Adaptive changes

Ground-glass hepatocytes may develop in patients on long-term therapy with some drugs (Fig. 14.30). This change was first reported by Klinge and Bannasch[232] in patients on long-term therapy with chlorpromazine and barbiturates. Other drugs that have been implicated include azathioprine, steroids, phenytoin,[82] resorcin and some analgesics.[233] The change was attributed to a marked, diffuse hypertrophy of

Table 14.18	Hepatic neoplasia caused by drugs and chemicals

Hepatocellular adenoma	Hepatocellular carcinoma	Cholangiocarcinoma	Angiosarcoma
Androgens	Aflatoxins	Androgens	Androgens
Contraceptive steroids	Androgens	Contraceptive steroids	Arsenic compounds
Danazol	Arsenic compounds	Isoniazid	Contraceptive steroids
Methyltestosterone	Contraceptive steroids	Methyldopa	Copper sulphate
Oestrogens, synthetic	Ethanol	Oestrogens, synthetic	Diethylstilbestrol
Oxymethalone	Methotrexate	Thorotrast	Phenelzine
Toxic oil (Rapeseed)	Methyltestosterone		Thorotrast
	Oestrogens, synthetic		Vinyl chloride
	Thorotrast		

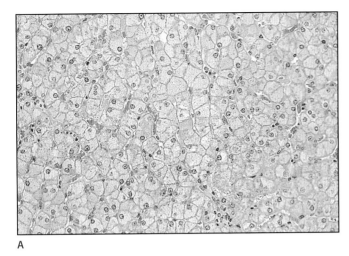

A

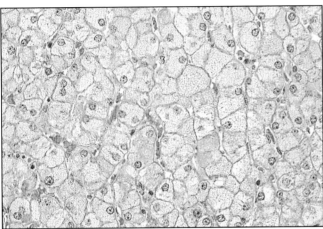

B

Fig. 14.30 • Enzymic induction associated with long-term therapy with phenytoin. Both figures from same case. **(A)** Liver cells are markedly enlarged and have a lightly stained, very finely vesiculated cytoplasm. H&E. **(B)** Higher magnification of induced hepatocytes. Nuclei are located either centrally or eccentrically. H&E.

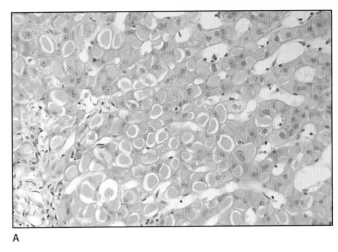

A

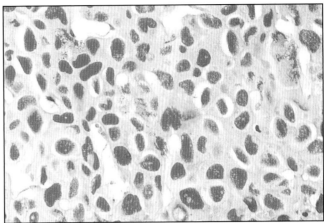

B

Fig. 14.31 • Cyanamide-induced injury. Both figures from same case. **(A)** Periportal liver cells contain large, eosinophilic (ground-glass) inclusions surrounded by an artifactual space. H&E. **(B)** Inclusions are still strongly PAS-positive after diastase digestion.

the smooth endoplasmic reticulum (SER) by Klinge and Bannasch, and this has been confirmed by ultrastructural studies.[234] It is associated with increased activity of microsomal NADPH cytochrome c reductase.[235] Drug-associated ground glass cell change may be differentiated from the ground glass cells of chronic hepatitis B both by special stains (aldehyde fuchsin, Victoria blue and orcein), and by immunohistochemistry.

The prognostic significance of drug-induced ground-glass transformation is not known. It is accompanied by elevated levels of gamma-glutamyltransferase and is believed to account for the hepatomegaly commonly observed in patients on anticonvulsant and other drugs. It is not associated with acute or chronic injury that may be caused by the same drug, and there are no long-term studies of patients with this drug-induced hepatic change. A dramatic form of ground-glass change (Fig. 14.31) has been noted in patients undergoing alcohol aversion therapy.[236] At first attributed to disulfiram, it now appears more clearly associated with cyanamide treatment. The change differs from that described in the foregoing paragraphs, in that the cyanamide-associated altered cells contain ground-glass 'inclusion bodies' that are periodic acid-Schiff (PAS)-positive and

resist diastase digestion (Fig. 14.31(B)), unlike the ground-glass cells of HBsAg carriers which are PAS-negative.[237] Ultrastructurally, the inclusions are composed of glycogen beta granules, secondary lysosomes, lipid vesicles and residues of degenerating organelles; this lesion can apparently lead to cirrhosis.[238]

Pigment deposits

Several types of pigmentary deposits may follow exposure to exogenous chemicals. These include lipofuscin, haemosiderin, Thorotrast, gold, titanium, mercury, silver, polyvinylpyrrolidone and bilirubin.[2,68,69]

Lipofuscin, the least significant of these, occurs normally in the lysosomes of the perivenular hepatocytes; it is more prominent in elderly people (Fig. 14.32). It also is increased in patients on various long-term medications, such as phenacetin, *Cascara sagrada* and chlorpromazine,[2,68] as well as anticonvulsant therapy.[82] Lipofuscin accumulation is prominent in Kupffer cells following recent hepatocellular injury, and increased deposits may follow intravenous infusion of fat emulsions.[239,240]

Black pigment granules in the liver (Fig. 14.33) may reflect the presence of gold as a residue of use of *gold compounds* for

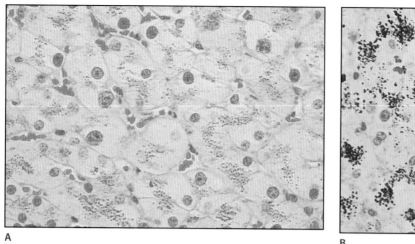

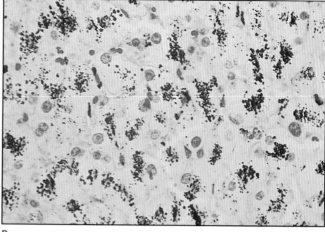

Fig. 14.32 • Excess lipofuscin accumulation in liver cells in patient on long-term chlorpromazine therapy. Both figures from same case. **(A)** H&E. **(B)** Pigment accumulation is well demostrated by the Fontana stain.

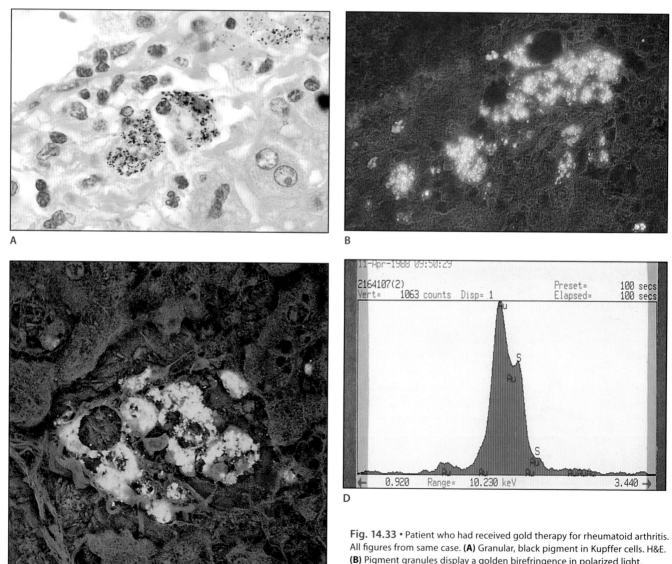

Fig. 14.33 • Patient who had received gold therapy for rheumatoid arthritis. All figures from same case. **(A)** Granular, black pigment in Kupffer cells. H&E. **(B)** Pigment granules display a golden birefringence in polarized light. **(C)** The pigment granules are readily identified by scanning electron microscopy using the back scatter technique. ×1500. **(D)** X-ray microanalysis reveals the presence of the elements gold and sulphur in the pigment granules.

treatment of rheumatoid arthritis,[241,242] *titanium* which may be found in parenteral drug abusers,[243] or *mercuric sulphide* in chronic mercury poisoning following ingestion of a laxative preparation containing mercurous chloride.[244] Dark brown pigment granules containing *silver* were reported in a patient with argyria.[245]

Haemosiderin deposits are seen in several forms of chemical and other causes of hepatic injury.[246] In dietary iron overload ('Bantu' siderosis), haemosiderin accumulates in hepatocytes, Kupffer cells and macrophages (Chapter 5). Similar deposits are seen in the hepatocytes of patients with porphyria cutanea tarda resulting from drugs or toxins, e.g. hexachlorobenzene.[247] Hepatic haemosiderosis has been reported in patients on long-term haemodialysis who had received parenteral iron[248] (Fig. 14.34). Transfusional haemosiderosis is discussed in Chapter 5. Rare cases of iron overload have been attributed to excess ingestion of iron preparations.[249] Parenteral iron overload in animal models is thought to lead to oxidative stress.[250]

Thorotrast, a formerly used radioactive contrast medium, remains in the livers of patients many years after its administration. It appears as glistening, greyish-brown granules engorging macrophages or lying free in dense fibrous tissue[251] (Fig. 14.35).

Polyvinylpyrrolidone (PVP) is a water-soluble, hydrophilic, high-molecular-weight product of the polymerization of vinylpyrrolidone. During World War II it was used as a plasma expander and continues to be used as a retarding agent for drugs injected subcutaneously.[252] A substantial amount of the compound is stored in cells of the reticuloendothelial system for many years, but long-term sequelae have not been reported. In the liver, PVP accumulates in markedly hypertrophied Kupffer cells and portal macrophages; the former may be converted into multinucleated giant cells, but granuloma formation does not occur. The affected cells have a granular, basophilic cytoplasm. The PVP stains positively with Lugol's iodine solution (mahogany brown), Congo red and Sirius red. Unlike amyloid deposits, Congo red stained-PVP does not display apple-green birefringence. Ultrastructurally, Kupffer cells contain

vacuoles surrounded by a membrane; granular or thread-like material may be present in the vacuoles.

Bilirubin is, of course, the pigment most likely to be seen in patients with drug-induced hepatic injury. In intrahepatic cholestasis it is particularly prominent in canaliculi of the perivenular zone, and may also be present in hepatocytes and in Kupffer cells (Fig. 14.13).

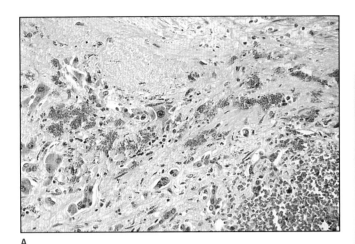

A

B

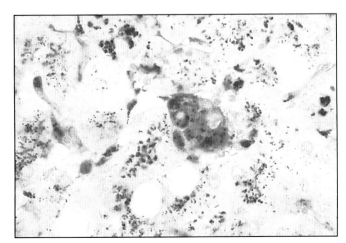

Fig. 14.34 • Marked haemosiderosis (reticuloendothelial and hepatocellular) in patient on renal haemodialysis who had received intramuscular iron therapy. Mallory stain for iron.

C

Fig. 14.35 • Thorotrast. All figures from same case. **(A)** Coarsely granular deposits of Thorotrast are pink-brown in colour, and are surrounded by dense fibrous tissue. H&E. **(B)** Thorotrast particles are readily identified by scanning electron microscopy. ×3000. **(C)** Element thorium is identified in Thorotrast deposits by X-ray microanalysis.

Mild non-specific changes

Finally, drugs may cause serum biochemical changes sufficient to generate a liver biopsy, yet not cause much in the way of diagnosable changes. There may be minimal or mild steatosis, rare apoptotic bodies, scattered pigmented macrophages or spotty necrosis. Like the adaptation changes noted above, it is unclear whether there is potential for more serious injury if the drug is continued. At least in the case of methotrexate, a biopsy showing such mild changes would be reassurance that the drug could be continued, but it is difficult to extend that generalization to therapeutics that are less well understood.

Biochemical, functional and clinical manifestations of hepatotoxicity

The biochemical manifestations of hepatotoxicity reflect the histological patterns of injury (Table 14.19). Toxic necrosis leads to biochemical changes and to clinical features similar to those of acute viral hepatitis.[253] Toxic steatosis leads to qualitatively similar, but quantitatively more modest abnormalities. The histological pattern and biochemical signature of cholestasis mimic those of biliary tract obstruction.[254]

Hepatocellular necrosis leads to the release into the blood of high levels of enzymes. Most extensively studied, in this regard, are the levels of the aminotransferases (ALT, AST) which may be increased to values that are 10 to 1000 times normal values;[255] but a number of other enzymes also reflect the change sensitively [1] In contrast to the logarithmic increase in levels of aminotransferases, the values for serum alkaline phosphatase, 5'-nucleotidase and leucine aminopeptidase increase no more than one- to three-fold in response to necrosis.

Depressed levels of plasma coagulation factors (INR, factor VIII levels, etc) are characteristic of severe hepatic necrosis, with the most useful clinical clues to the severity of necrosis being the prothrombin time (INR) and bilirubin levels.[256] Albumin levels do not change appreciably in the early phase of acute necrosis. Hypo-albuminaemia ensues only late in the clinical course, or in association with subacute or chronic disease. Globulin levels also may stay unchanged, although in subacute and chronic disease the gamma globulin fraction may increase somewhat. Indeed in the drug-induced chronic hepatitis that mimics autoimmune hepatitis, gamma globulin levels may be strikingly increased.[257] Plasma cholesterol levels tend to be low or normal in acute hepatic necrosis.

Microvesicular steatosis leads to less dramatic biochemical evidence of hepatic injury than acute necrosis. In tetracycline toxicity, values for the serum aminotransferases increase to 5-to 20-fold the upper limit of normal. Bilirubin levels are only modestly increased as are values for alkaline phosphatase. Prolonged prothrombin times are characteristic. Hypoglycaemia may be prominent. Macrovesicular steatosis leads to even lesser abnormalities.[258]

Cholestatic injury is manifest clinically by jaundice and itching.[259] The aminotransferase levels in the two types of cholestasis do not differ appreciably, but the alkaline phosphatase levels do. In hepatocanalicular cholestasis, alkaline phosphatase may be increased 3- to 10-fold the normal level and the cholesterol values also are increased, whereas in the canalicular type the alkaline phosphatase increases are less

Table 14.19	Histological types of acute toxic hepatic injury and associated biochemical and clinical aspects*				
Histological lesion	**Biochemical abnormalities in serum**				
	AST and ALT	**Alk phosphatase**	**Cholesterol**	**Clinical aspects**	**Examples**
I. Cytotoxic					
Zonal necrosis	10–500*	1–2*	Normal or low	Hepatic and renal failure	Carbon tetrachloride, poisonous mushrooms, paracetamol, halothane
Diffuse necrosis	10–200*	1–2*	Normal or low	Severe hepatitis-like illness	Isoniazid, methyldopa, halothane
Steatosis	5–20*	1–2*	Normal or low	Resembles fatty liver of pregnancy and Reye syndrome	Tetracycline
II. Cholestatic					
With portal tract inflammation (hepatocanalicular)	1–10*	1–10*	High	Resembles obstructive jaundice	Chlorpromazine, erythromycin estolate
Without portal tract inflammation (canalicular)	1–5*	1–3*	Normal or high	Resembles obstructive jaundice	Anabolic and contraceptive steroids
III. Mixed (mixtures of cytotoxic and cholestatic injury)	10–100*	1–10*	Normal or high	May resemble hepatitis or obstructive jaundice	Phenylbutazone, para-aminosalicylic, sulphonamides, acids

* Degree of abnormality indicated as fold increases

than three-fold and the cholesterol level is usually normal.[29,30]

Toxic porphyria may accompany several forms of hepatic injury. The hepatic steatosis, necrosis and cirrhosis produced in humans and experimental animals by hexachlorobenzene[34] is accompanied by a form of porphyria resembling porphyria cutanea tarda.

Tolerance

Many drugs capable of causing acute hepatocellular injury lead to an appreciable rise in ALT and AST values that either do not progress or normalize despite continuation of the agent. This phenomenon has been called hepatocyte 'tolerance', implying a form of adaptation that takes place to prevent more severe injury.[1,33] Although the actual mechanism of such tolerance is unknown, it is thought to represent an upregulation of cytoprotective cytokines or suppression of necrogenic factors.[260–262] Usually no histologic correlation of these mild enzymes elevations is available; liver biopsy is rarely done if the elevated ALT values are clinically silent and reversible. Table 14.20 lists drugs associated with ALT elevations that conform to the concept of 'tolerance'. As can be seen, ALT elevations may be very frequently observed, yet the risk of progression to severe hepatic injury from agents acting through metabolic idiosyncrasy remains low.[33]

Some of the clinical manifestations of drug-induced hepatic injury are systemic and extrahepatic. Fever, rash and eosinophilia may precede or accompany the hepatic injury, presumably reflecting the immunological idiosyncrasy responsible for the injury. Indeed, the hypersensitivity syndrome (formerly referred to as the *pseudomononucleosis* syndrome of fever, rash, lymphadenopathy and lymphocytosis with 'atypical' lymphocytes, accompanied by haematological changes resembling those of infectious mononucleosis in the blood), is a classical reaction to injury by phenytoin,

sulphonamides, dapsone, para-aminosalicylic acid and a number of other drugs.[1,62,63,263] Renal injury may occur as a result of nephrotoxic metabolites, e.g. methoxyflurane,[101] or as a manifestation of generalized hypersensitivity.[265]

The syndrome patterns characteristic of acute poisoning due to $CC1_4$, phosphorus, iron, hepatotoxic mushrooms and acetaminophen (paracetamol), tend to consist of three distinct phases: (i) immediate with severe neurological or gastrointestinal manifestations; (ii) a period of relative well-being; (iii) a phase of overt hepatic injury often accompanied by renal failure[1] This sequence is listed in Table 14.21. These acute hepatotoxins produce initial symptoms within a few hours of exposure, although those associated by ingestion of toxic mushrooms may be delayed for several hours.[3]

Analysis of hepatotoxic reactions according to the circumstances of exposure

Occupational and domestic hepatotoxins

Occupational and environmental hepatotoxicity has been recognized for more than a century, with workers exposed to a wide variety of solvents and chemicals used in the production of munitions and other materials during the First and Second World Wars emphasizing the risks involved.[1,9,33,34,266] While industrial exposure to hepatotoxic chemicals is less of an occupational hazard today, many of these agents remain important experimental tools in the study of mechanisms and the prevention of hepatotoxicity, and reports of toxicity from chemical agents have not disappeared. For example, recent reports of non-alcoholic steatohepatitis in workers chronically exposed to several volatile *petrochemical products* (including $CC1_4$, chloroform, dimethylformamide, methanol, toluene, trinitrotoluene and tetrachlorethane, to name but a few), attest to the ongoing presence of chemical injury in the workplace.[267–273]

Among thousands of chemical compounds in commercial and industrial use, several hundred are listed as causing liver injury by the National Institute for Occupational Safety and Health (NIOSH).[10] The National Library of Medicine also maintains a database on chemical toxins in its Toxicology and Environmental Health Information Program (TEHIP) that serves as another important resource of information.[37] Toxic exposure to chemical agents occurs most often from inhalation or absorption from the skin, and less often after oral ingestion via the gastrointestinal tract or via parenteral means. As a majority of chemical toxins are lipid soluble, once absorbed they can easily cross biological membranes to reach their target organ(s), including the liver.[9,34] The clinical syndrome associated with hepatotoxic chemical exposure is usually acute cytotoxic injury (as seen with $CC1_4$ and phosphorus) that typically consists of three distinct phases similar to that observed after an acetaminophen overdose or ingestion of toxic mushrooms,[1,34] (Table 14.20), or less commonly as acute cholestatic injury (as seen

Table 14.20	Tolerance: prevalence of subclinical liver-associated enzyme elevations ('tolerance') for various drugs
Prevalence	**Examples**
25–50%	Tacrine
20–25%	Chlorpromazine, triacetyloleandomycin, phenytoin, amiodarone, perhexiline, papaverin, cisplatin, nicotinic acid, valproic acid, 6-MP
10–20%	Isoniazid, ketoconazole, androgens, erythromycin estolate, etretinate, ximelagatran
5–10%	Penicillamine, chenodeoxycholate, flucytosine, disulfiram, most NSAIDs
<5%	HMG-CoA reductase inhibitors (statins), salicylates, gold salts, sulfonamides, dantrolene, sulfonylureas, quinidine, thiabendazole, ticarcillin, ethionamide, tricyclic antidepressants

after Lewis[33]

6-MP = 6-mercaptopurine; NSAIDs = non-steroidal anti-inflammatory drugs

Table 14.21 Phases of acute hepatic injury from chemical hepatotoxins

Phase of injury	APAP	Phosphorus	Amanita phalloides	CCl₄
I. 1–24 hr				
Onset	Immediate	Immediate	Delayed 6–20 hr	Immediate
A, N, V, D	+	4+	4+	+
Shock	–	+	+/–	–
Neuro symptoms	–	+	+/–	–
II. 24–72 hr				
Latent period	+	+/–	+	+
III. >72 hr				
Jaundice	+	+	+	+
Hepatic failure	+	+	+	+
Renal failure	+	+	+	+
Maximum AST/ALT	1000X	100X*	500X	500X
Zonal necrosis	3	1	3	3
Steatosis	no	4+	+	+
Case-fatality rate	5–15%	25–50%	20–25%	20–25%

* often < 10X

APAP = paracetamol, acetaminophen; CCl₄ = carbon tetrachloride
A = anorexia; N = nausea; V = vomiting; D = diarrhoea

with methylenedianaline, the agent responsible for Epping jaundice).[274,275] Many chemicals (e.g. vinyl chloride) are also carcinogenic, and the development of hepatic malignancies has been part of the clinicopathologic spectrum of chemical injury.[2,34]

Hepatotoxins still encountered in the home include some of the well-known industrial toxins, e.g. CCl₄, and other chemicals such as phosphorus, copper salts, and camphor. *Camphor* is a home remedy that is highly toxic to the gastrointestinal and nervous systems and its use has been reported to lead to abnormal liver function tests and hepatic steatosis.[276] Chronic ingestion by a 6-month-old child has led to Reye-like syndrome.[277]

Large overdoses of ordinarily safe drugs, e.g. acetaminophen (paracetamol) and ferrous salts, are discussed later. Mycotoxins and other botanical agents such as poisonous mushrooms are still an important cause of acute hepatic injury in some parts of the world.[3,278–280] Food contaminated with aflatoxins has been implicated in acute hepatic disease and, on epidemiological grounds, in the aetiology of hepatocellular carcinoma.[35,281,282] Consumption of plants containing pyrrolizidine alkaloids has long been known to cause acute and chronic hepatic disease, and continues to be responsible for epidemics of veno-occlusive injury.[74,283,284] Herbal remedies and agents used in illicit substance abuse are discussed below, as are foods contaminated with toxic chemicals, and various pesticides and herbicides.

Chemicals and environmental agents causing hepatic injury

The clinicopathological spectrum of several chemical hepatotoxins is given in Table 14.22, and additional details of

their hepatotoxicity can be found in a number of recent reviews.[1,9,34,43] The following sections describes the best-described chemical hepatotoxins in more detail.

Carbon tetrachloride and other chlorinated aliphatic hydrocarbons

Carbon tetrachloride is a classic example of a zone 3 hepatotoxin (Fig. 14.1) causing necrosis leading to hepatic failure. Injury is mediated by its metabolism to a toxic trichloromethyl radical catalyzed by CYP 2E1.[285] Alcohol potentiates the injury via induction of this cytochrome.[286] Although it was used as a vermifuge in the first part of the 20th century, most cases have been the result of industrial or domestic accidents, such as inhalation of CCl₄-containing dry cleaning fluids, use as a household reagent, or after ingestion by alcoholics who have been known to mistake it for a potable beverage.[1] At the cellular level, direct damage to cellular membranes results in leakage of intracellular enzymes and electrolytes leading to calcium shifts and lipid peroxidation.[285] Hepatic steatosis develops as a result of triglyceride accumulation from haloalkylation-dependent inhibition of lipoprotein micelle transport out of the hepatocyte and increases with the continuous supply of free fatty acids from the blood.[287] The relative toxicity of CCl₄ compared to other haloalkanes and haloalkenes correlates inversely with the level of bond dissociation energy, the number of halogen atoms, and the chain length[1,287] (Table 14.23). Although complete clinical and histological recovery from CCl₄-induced liver damage was the rule with more modest exposures, supervening renal failure from acute tubular necrosis and gastrointestinal haemorrhage were associated with a case-fatality rate of 10–25%.[1,288]

Table 14.22	Clinico-pathologic spectrum of chemical hepatotoxins

I.	**Acute injury**	
	A. Necrosis:	CCl$_4$ and other haloalkanes
		Haloaromatics, nitroaromatics, nitroaliphatics,
		Hydrochlorofluorocarbons
		Phosporus, iron, copper salts, inorganic arsenic
		Cocaine, ecstasy, phencyclidine
	B. Microvesicular steatosis	Dimethylformamide
		Hypoglycin
		Hydrazine
		Toluene, xylene
		Chlordecone
		Cocaine, boric acid, thallium
	C. Cholestasis	Methylene dianiline
		Paraquat
		Aniline-rapeseed oil
		Dinitrophenol
		Alpha-naphthylisocyanate (ANIT)
II.	**Subacute injury**	
	A. Necrosis	Trinitrotoluene (TNT)
	B. VOD	Pyrrolizidine alkaloids, arsenic, thorium dioxide
	C. Toxic cirrhosis	Tetrachlorethane
		Hexachlorobenzene, PCBs
	D. Peliosis	Dioxin
III.	**Chronic injury**	
	A. Cirrhosis	Chloroaliphatics, TNT, arsenic, pyrrolizidine alkaloids
	B. Hepatoportal sclerosis	Arsenic, vinyl chloride
IV.	**Neoplastic**	
	A. Hepatocellular carcinoma	Arsenic, aflatoxins, thorium dioxide
	B. Angiosarcoma	Vinyl chloride, thorium dioxide, arsenic
	C. Haemangioendothelioma	Arsenic

Table 14.23	Relative hepatotoxicity of haloalkane compounds

Compound	Relative toxicity
CCl$_4$	4+
Tetrachlorethane	4+
Chloroform	2+
Trichloroethylene	1–2+
1,1,2-trichloroethane	1–2+
Tetrachloroethylene	+
1,1,1-trichloroethane	+
Dichloromethane	+/–
Dibromomethane	+/–
Methylchloride	–

4+ maximal injury; – denotes trivial or no injury

Chloroform remains an important experimental hepatotoxin; its use as an anesthetic has long been abandoned[26] (see below). **1,1,2-trichloroethane** (methylchloroform) and **tetrachloroethane** are less potent haloalkane hepatotoxins that found use as solvents for components of varnish used to cover fabrics of airplane covers during the First and Second World Wars.[289] Inhalational or percutaneous exposure led to subacute hepatic necrosis, with susceptibility increased in females and alcoholics.[1] There are a number of reports of injury with **1,1,1-trichloroethane**, including chronic hepatitis.[290] Only trivial hepatotoxicity has been reported for **dichloromethane** and **dibromoethane**, and **methyl chloride** appears to be free of liver injury.[1]

Hydrochlorofluorocarbons (HCFCs) caused liver injury in industrial workers exposed to dichlorotrifluoroethane (HCFC 123) and 1-chloro-tetrafluoroethane (HCFC 124), both of which are metabolized to reactive trifluoroacetyl halide intermediates similar to those implicated in halothane hepatoxicity. Zone 3 necrosis was present on biopsy, and autoantibodies against cytochrome P450 2E1 or P58 were detected in the serum. As with halothane, potentiation of HCFC liver toxicity is seen with ethanol-induced CYP 2E1 activity in animal models.[291,292]

Vinyl chloride and other chlorinated ethylenes

Vinyl chloride monomer (VCM, monochloroethylene) exposure previously occurred in polymerization plants where vinyl chloride was heated to form polylvinyl chloride (PVC) in the manufacturing of plastics, leading to inhalation of the toxic gas in the process.[1] VCM is ubiquitous in the environment and has been estimated by the EPA to exist in at least 10% of toxic waste sites.[9] Although PVCs appear to be non-toxic per se, liver damage from VCM has been described in the form of several types of chronic liver injury from long-term exposure, including nodular subcapsular fibrosis, sinusoidal dilatation, peliosis hepatics, and periportal fibrosis associated with portal hypertension.[34,43] Milder forms of injury have also been described, which were reversible within 6–24 months of avoiding exposure with instances of relapse after re-exposure.[293] In workers with hepatitis B or C infection, a higher prevalence of elevated ALT values was seen in those with a high exposure to VCM compared to those with a lower exposure, a finding not observed among those without a viral hepatitis infection.[294]

VCM is carcinogenic in animals and humans, with the first reports of angiosarcoma among workers in rubber plants appearing in 1974.[295] Tumours developed after a mean latency of 25 years of exposure[296] with the risk related to the time and extent of contact.[297] Alcohol enhances the hepatocarcinogenicity of VCM in rodents, and possibly in humans, by the induction of CYP 2E1 responsible for its conversion to a toxic or carcinogenic metabolite (e.g. 2-chloroethylene oxide).[286] A history of vinyl chloride exposure was found to be present in 15 to 25% of all cases of hepatic angiosarcoma reported in the late 1970s.[298] Efforts to reduce occupational exposure to VCM have resulted in a marked decrease in the incidence of angiosarcoma. In recent studies, no excess number of cases of angiosarcoma were observed among 757 workers, although those with the highest exposure had a four-fold increased risk of periportal fibrosis, which may be a precursor lesion to angiosarcoma.[299] Reports of hepatocellular carcinoma linked to chronic VCM exposure have been confounded by the presence of chronic hepatitis B infection, especially in China and south-east Asia, although a possible interaction between the two cannot be excluded.[300] In those working in PVC plants, regular biochemical monitoring of liver tests is conducted; individuals with persistent abnormalities are removed from workplace exposure.[294,299]

Trichloroethylene (TCE) leads to a similar but often less severe clinical syndrome as seen with CCl_4, with exposure the result of accidental industrial exposure or from sniffing the chemical.[301,302] Once used as an anaesthetic, it now has a role as a solvent , spot remover and degreaser. **Vinylidene chloride (VDC)** is another intermediate used in the production of plastics that targets the liver.[9]

Non-halogenated organic compounds

In general, these agents, including aliphatic hydrocarbons, cycloparaffins, esters, ethers and ketones, produce trivial or no hepatic injury in animals and humans.[1] Most aromatic hydrocarbons also appear devoid of significant hepatotoxic potential. **Benzene** has been associated with minor hepatic injury in animals. **Toluene** led to steatosis and necrosis in a 'glue sniffer'.[303] It caused elevations in gamma glutamy-transpeptidase after industrial exposure. **Xylene** can cause mild steatosis and **styrene** (vinyl benzene) has led to elevated aminotransferases after prolonged exposure. **Tetralan** and **decalin** have produced steatosis and necrosis in animals, but not in humans.[1,34]

Trinitrotoluene (TNT) and other nitroaromatic compounds

TNT (nitroglycerin) has been known to be hepatotoxic since World War I when munitions workers developed severe acute and subacute necrosis, with a case-fatality rate of more than 25%.[304] The incidence of hepatotoxicity during World War II was lower, with approximately 1 in 500 workers affected, while the estimated incidence of associated toxicities, methemoglobinemia and aplastic anaemia, being as much as fifty times higher than liver injury.[305] The syndrome of subacute hepatic necrosis was preceded by a latent period of 2–4 months of regular exposure to TNT. Percutaneous absorption through the skin was the major source of exposure, with lesser contributions from inhaling toxic fumes and ingesting contaminated food. In some patients, rapidly progressive liver failure and death within days to months was observed, with massive hepatic necrosis at autopsy.[306] In others, the subacute injury progressed to the development of micronodular cirrhosis after several months.[1]

Nitrobenzene and **dinitrobenzene** are also potent hepatotoxins described during World War I. Ingestion of **dinitrophenol** has been associated with necrosis and intrahepatic

cholestasis, possibly owing to its uncoupling of oxidative phosphorylation.[34,307]

Nitroaliphatic compounds

These agents, including **nitromethane, nitroethane,** and **nitropropane,** cause variable degrees of hepatic injury. 2-nitropropane (2-NP) caused fatal massive hepatic necrosis after occupational exposure as a solvent, fuel additive, varnish remover and rocket propellant.[308] Toxic hepatitis associated with the chronic inhalation of propane and butane has been reported.[309] In animals, intraperitoneal injection of 2-NP induced perivenular necrosis, steatosis and mitochondrial abnormalities after 24 hours.[310] Minor degrees of zone 3 necrosis and steatosis have been observed in animals exposed to nitromethane and nitroethane. Both 1-NP and 2-NP are mutagenic potential human carcinogens.[311]

Polychlorinated biphenyls and other halogenated aromatic compounds

Polychlorinated biphenyls (PCBs) are mixtures of tri-chloro-, tetrachloro-, pentachloro- and hexachloro- derivatives of biphenyls, naphthalenes and triphenyls used in the manufacture of electrical transformers, condensers, and industrial fluids. Acute and chronic hepatotoxicity was seen during World War II and resembled that due to TNT.[9,34] Inhalation of toxic fumes released by the melting of PCBs and **chloronaphthalene** mixtures during soldering of electrical materials was the most common means of exposure.[1] Liver injury appeared to correlate with the number of chlorine molecules.[312] Liver damage appeared as early as seven weeks after initial exposure. Skin lesions, known as chloracne, usually preceded the hepatic injury. Death occurred within two weeks in fulminant cases with massive necrosis, or after 1–3 months in subacute injury; cirrhosis developed in some who survived the acute injury 1. **Polybrominated biphenyls (PBBs)** appear to more toxic and more potent enzyme inducers compared to PCBs. Consumption of milk and meat from livestock given feed mistakenly contaminated by a PBB led to hepatomegaly and minor abnormalities of liver function tests in exposed persons.[313]

Miscellaneous chemical compounds

Dimethylformamide is a widely used solvent used in the synthetic resin and leather industries that causes dose-related massive necrosis in animals[314] and is capable of producing focal hepatic necrosis and microvesicular steatosis in humans, the severity of which correlates with the duration of occupational exposure.[315] Most individuals with prolonged exposure (greater than 1 year) had symptomatic disease that slowly resolved when they were removed from the workplace. Re-exposure in one individual produced recurrent injury.[268] In a series of workers from Italy, 23% had liver function test abnormalities and 50% reported disulfiram-like symptoms.[270] DMF is metabolized by the P-450 system into N-methylformamide,[316] and alcohol appears to have a synergistic effect,[269] as do both the hepatitis B surface antigen carrier state and a high BMI.[317]

Hydrazine and its derivatives are experimental hepatotoxins and carcinogens. In humans, steatosis and focal necrosis have been reported.[1] **Bromoalkanes** and **iodoalkanes** have been used in insecticides and aircraft fuels, with rare reports of hepatic injury.[318] **Ethylene dibromide** (dibromoethane) produces zone 3 necrosis in experimental animals with at least one instance of necrosis after an attempted suicidal ingestion . Occupational exposure has been linked to fatal toxicity,[319] which may be potentiated by the concomitant use of disulfiram.[1]

Hepatotoxic metals

Iron

Accidental iron poisoning has been described for more than half a century, with upwards of 5000 cases reported to occur in the USA annually.[1] Most cases occur in young children who mistake iron supplements for sweets,[320] and the severity of injury depends on the dose ingested. Ingestion of <20 mg/kg of elemental iron is unlikely to produce serious toxicity, whereas doses >200 mg/kg can be fatal.[1] Iron, per se, is not hepatotoxic, but ferric and ferrous ions acting through free radicals and lipid peroxidation can cause membrane disruption and necrosis.[321] Clinically evident liver injury is uncommon in most instances. Periportal necrosis may be seen in the most severe cases (Fig. 14.5(D),(E)).[1]

Phosphorus

Poisoning by white phosphorus is rare since its use in fireworks and matches was outlawed more than 60 years ago.[77,322,323] Cases reported since then have usually been the result of ingestion of rat or cockroach poison.[1] Symptoms of severe gastrointestinal and neurotoxicity develop shortly after ingestion with death occurring within 24 hours. Phosphorescence of the vomitus and stools and a typical garlic-like odour on the breath are characteristic when present. Histologically, the liver may show only steatosis, initially in the periportal and then diffuse (Fig. 14.5(A)–(C)). Necrosis may, however, be present and is also predominantly periportal in distribution.[77]

Copper salts

Acute poisoning by copper leads to a syndrome resembling iron toxicity. Ingestion of toxic amounts (1–10 mg) is usually seen with suicidal intent, especially on the Indian subcontinent.[324] Acute copper toxicity may result from ingestion (either suicidal or accidental) of copper sulphate, from its use (in the past) as an emetic or for the treatment of burns, and from the release of copper ions (from equipment such as tubing made of copper) in an acid pH, for example, malfunctioning haemodialysis equipment, or from high levels of copper in drinking water.[325] Histologically there is perivenular necrosis and cholestasis in the deeply jaundiced patients, but only focal necrosis or no changes in mildly jaundiced patients; non-cirrhotic portal hypertension has been described.[164] Serum copper levels are markedly elevated in acute copper intoxication, as is serum caeruloplasmin; the concentrations of copper in the liver can be very high.[324]

Gastrointestinal erosions, renal tubular necrosis, and rhabdomyolysis often accompany hepatic (zone 3) necrosis, occurring by the 2nd or 3rd day. Jaundice results from both hepatic injury and acute haemolysis produced by high blood copper levels.[326] Mortality rates are around 15%.[1]

Chronic copper toxicity can be hereditary (Wilson disease) or acquired (Chapter 5). In humans, acquired toxicity can result from occupational or domestic exposure. An example of the former is the chronic exposure of vineyard workers to fungicide sprays containing copper sulphate.[164] The resultant hepatic injury includes non-caseating granulomas, parenchymal and periportal fibrosis, cirrhosis and rarely, angiosarcoma. Copper poisoning remains a hazard in rural parts of the world.[327] Of interest are reports of several children who developed an illness, clinically and histopathologically resembling Indian childhood cirrhosis (p. 254), from the chronic ingestion of well water contaminated with high levels of copper. The copper was leached from copper pipes into drinking water delivered to the children's homes. Early exposure to copper appears to be crucial, since siblings exposed after 9 months of age, and the parents who drank the same water, did not develop the disease.[328]

Other support for excess dietary copper as a cause of non-Indian childhood cirrhosis after years of exposure is found in observations of *endemic Tyrolean infantile cirrhosis* that is transmitted by autosomal recessive inheritance but which requires the additional risk factor of excess dietary copper (from cow's milk contaminated with copper leached from untinned copper or brass vessels) for its expression. The disease was eradicated when the untinned copper containers were replaced by modern industrial vessels.[329]

Thorium dioxide (Thorotrast)

The colloidal preparation of thorium dioxide was used as an intravenous contrast medium for radiographic procedures in the first half of the 20th century, with estimates of >50 000 patients being exposed before it was abandoned in 1955.[1] A large number of reports have appeared describing tumours of the liver and, less frequently, of other organs, as well as lympho- and myeloproliferative syndromes and non-neoplastic lesions of the liver.[218,330–333] The lesion that has drawn most attention is angiosarcoma, after latency periods of 20–40 years[219,220,330–332] but cholangiocarcinoma and hepatocellular carcinomas have been attributed to Thorotrast with almost equal frequency.[332–335] Hepatic leiomyosarcoma has also been reported.[336] Non-malignant hepatic lesions attributed to Thorotrast include periportal fibrosis, veno-occlusive lesions and cirrhosis. The fibrosis is particularly marked in the subcapsular region. An additional lesion of note is peliosis hepatis, which may be fatal.[337] Given the extraordinarily long half-life of the compound (hundreds of years), which is a radioactive alpha emitter, exposed individuals remain at risk for the development of leuaemia in addition to liver cell tumours.[208,332] Histologically, thorium dioxide is found in Kupffer cells and macrophages as dark brown refractile granules approximately 10 μm in diameter (Fig. 14.35), often in clusters, which can be confirmed by spectrographic analysis. They are illuminated by phase contrast clearly defined by scanning electron microscopy; the thorium dioxide in the particles can be definitively identified by energy dispersive X-ray analysis.[331,338] (Fig. 14.35(C)).

Other metals

Cadmium is an experimental hepatotoxin that produces hepatic necrosis and cirrhosis and that can enhance the hepatotoxicity of endotoxin in laboratory animals.[1,339] There is no evidence that exposure to cadmium causes significant human injury.[1]

Beryllium has led to midzonal (zone 2) necrosis, the result of phagocytosis of insoluble beryllium phosphate (formed by the reaction of beryllium with phosphate in the blood) by Kupffer cells. The Kupffer cells undergo necrosis, releasing beryllium, and possibly cytokines.[1] Chronic industrial exposure, usually by inhalation of high concentrations of oxide or phosphorus mixtures, is associated with the formation of hepatic (and pulmonary) granulomas.[340]

Experimental hepatotoxins

Hepatocellular toxins

Carbon tetrachloride (CCl4) continues to be used in experimental models of hepatotoxicity to help identify the mechanisms associated with acute injury.[341] A trichloromethyl radical (CCl_3) that binds to cellular proteins, lipids and nucleic acids is formed after metabolism by CYP2E1, 2B1, 2B2 and possibly 3A. Chemicals that induce these cytochromes can potentiate the toxicity of CCl_4. When CCl_3 reacts with oxygen, a reactive trichloromethyoxyperoxy radical is formed that destroys polyunsaturated fatty acids in the process of lipid peroxidation, leading to the characteristic fatty degeneration that accompanies hepatic necrosis.[285] CCl_4 activates tumour necrosis factor, nitric oxide and transforming growth factors that contribute to cell destruction and fibrosis. In addition, adducts that are formed between CCl_3 and DNA are thought to be possible initiators in the development of hepatocellular carcinoma.[342]

Cholestatic hepatotoxins

Several naturally occurring and synthetic agents are associated with acute cholestatic injury and are used in the study of experimental hepatotoxicity.[30,31] Historically, many of these compounds produced a form of facial eczema in ruminants that was later attributed to the effects of **phylloerythrin,** a product of chlorophyll degraded in the rumen of these animals leading to photosensitization as a result of its accumulation from cholestatic injury.[343] **Icterogen** is a triterpene-pentacyclic alkaloid that is a chemical analogue of C-17 alkylated steroids that structurally resembles anabolic and contraceptive steroids. Inhibition of canalicular Na+,

K+-ATPase produces cholestatic injury within 24–48 hr of administration.[29] **Sporidesmin,** derived from the fungus *Phithomyces chartarum,* disrupts canalicular membranes and microvilli. **Cytochalasin B** is another fungal alkaloid that also impairs canalicular function. **Phalloidin** is a potent hepatotoxin found in certain mushrooms that causes necrosis and steatosis in high doses, and impairs bile flow when given in low doses for several days[344] (see Hepatotoxic mushrooms, p. 695). **Endotoxin** has a cholestatic effect in isolated perfused liver and other models,[345] inhibiting both bile acid-independent and dependent flow, possibly mediated by tumour necrosis factor.[346] Severe sepsis attributed to bacterial endotoxin is characterized histologically by inspissated bile casts in cholangioles. Endotoxin has been shown to potentiate the hepatotoxicity of cocaine in mice, via the formation of increased levels of nitric oxide promoting oxidative stress.[347]

Lithocholic acid (LCA) has been utilized as a model for cholestasis for more than 60 years. Derived from the conversion of chenodeoxycholic acid by intestinal bacteria, LCA produces cholestasis within 2–4 hours as a single bolus, with jaundice apparent by 4 hours , and hepatocyte damage within 12 hours. Ultrastructural changes include damage to bile canaliculi and loss of microvilli, with focal areas of necrosis that become filled with blood and resemble peliosis. Chronic administration leads to ductular proliferation and cirrhosis in some species.[1,348]

Alpha-naphthylisothiocyanate (ANIT) produces necrosis of interlobular bile ducts and ductules along with portal inflammation in rats given high doses.[26] Long-term administration leads to bile duct proliferation, periductal inflammation and biliary cirrhosis,[349] with variable species-specific susceptibility. ANIT undergoes metabolism via the P450 system.[350] Agents such as phenobarbital enhance the metabolism of ANIT and increase its cholestatic effect. In contrast, agents that inhibit protein synthesis reduce the cholestatic injury.[1]

Heptatotoxic agents in the environment and food supply

Hepatotoxic pesticides

While exposure to insecticides, herbicides and other pesticides in the environment is common, acute liver injury from these compounds, many of which are chlorinated hydrocarbons, is rare.[351] Ingestion of large amounts of DDT or chlordane have occasionally been reported to cause a clinical syndrome of hepatic necrosis similar to that seen with CCl_4. With other pesticides, neurologic and systemic toxicity, rather than acute hepatotoxicity dominate the clinical picture.[1] The P-450 cytochrome enzyme inducing effects of some of these agents can enhance the toxicity of other agents.[352]

Dichlorodiphenyltrichloroethane (DDT) and other organochlorines (aldrin, amitrole, chlordane, dieldrin, lindane, mirex) accumulate in fat deposits, and to a lesser extent, in the liver after prolonged exposure. Despite the concern that DDT might lead to occupational hepatotoxicity, there is almost no evidence of liver damage from chronic contact.[1] Similarly, there is scant direct evidence that DDT is carcinogenic in humans. Most attention has focused on **Agent Orange** (2,4-dichlorophenoxyacetic acid), the defoliant widely used in Vietnam. Acute hepatitis has been reported after chronic exposure from licking a contaminated golf ball.[353] In animals, **dioxin** (tetrachlorodibenzo-p-dioxin) has produced progressive sinusoidal dilatation and peliosis hepatis.[354] Some suspect that contaminating doxins may be have been responsible for the toxic effects in humans alleged to be from Agent Orange.[355] Indeed, more recent studies have concluded that any chronic liver injury among Vietnam veterans was more likely to be related to viral infections or alcohol rather than Agent Orange.[39]

Dichloridedimethyldipyridlium (paraquat) has been implicated in several instances of poisoning, many as the result of attempted suicides, and occasionally due to homicides.[356,357] Ingestion of 2–25 grams of the liquid concentrate has produced severe toxicity, and dermal exposure has also been sufficient to cause liver injury.[358,359] Many patients have severe vomiting, and profuse diarrhoea leading to hypokalemia, and often show evidence of oral, pharyngeal and esophageal caustic lesions (stomatitis) after ingestion. Death results from a combination of renal, respiratory, cardiac and hepatic failure with mortality rates as high as 70%, often within the first 48 hours.[356] Histopathological changes include zone 3 necrosis and rather unique injury to small and medium-sized interlobular bile ducts that occurs in a biphasic pattern (Fig. 14.15). It is thought that hepatocellular injury becomes cholangiocellular in nature with jaundice after the initial 48 hours, with bile duct injury being a direct corrosive effect of paraquat.[49]

Chlordecone (kepone) has been shown to impair biliary excretion , and lipid transport and storage,[360] but neurological toxicity appears to dominate the clinical picture. Occupational exposure has led to hepatic steatosis and abnormal liver function tests, and chronic exposure is hepatocarcinogenic in rodents.[361] Steatosis is seen in rodents exposed to **chlordane**.[362] **Hexochlorobenzene** was associated with an epidemic of porphyria cutanea tarda and liver injury from contaminated grain[363] (see under contaminated foods, p. 696).

Inorganic arsenic has long been used as a homicidal or suicidal agent,[364] and toxic exposure also followed ingestion of Fowler's solution (arsenic trioxide) used in the past as a treatment for psoriasis and asthma. Other sources of exposure come from contaminated ground and well water and homemade alcohol. Doses >3 grams can cause death in 1–3 days, with hepatic injury generally overshadowed by more prominent gastrointestinal, neurological and vascular effects.[1,34] Necrosis of capillary walls causes congestion and haemorrhagic necrosis of the gastrointestinal tract leading to severe nausea, vomiting and diarrhoea, and is also thought to produce a lesion in the liver resembling veno-occlusive disease.[365] Severe steatosis and varying degrees of necrosis have been observed.[1] More than 90% of a group of 248 patients who consumed contaminated drinking water for up to 15 years were shown to develop non-cirrhotic portal hypertension.[366]

Occupational exposure to arsenic is still observed among vineyard workers, farmers and gold miners,[367] although its use as an insecticide has been curtailed since the 1940s. Lumber treated with chromated copper arsenate as a preservative may be an additional source of exposure.[368] The clinical syndrome associated with arsenicosis includes skin lesions (blackfoot disease), anaemia, diabetes mellitus, hearing loss, neurobehavioural disorders, and cardiovascular diseases in addition to benign and malignant liver disease.[369] Chronic hepatic injury, including cirrhosis and non-cirrhotic portal hypertension, may be precursor lesions to hepatic malignancies, including angiosarcoma, hemangioendothelioma and hepatocellular carcinoma.[370,371] The lifetime mortality risk from hepatocellular carcinoma and other malignancies (bladder and lung) in persons chronically exposed to arsenic in drinking water from countries such as Bangladesh, Egypt and Taiwan is more than doubled.[217,372] In animals, initial alterations in liver function are associated with decreased glutathione and antioxidant store; continued exposure leads to fatty liver and hepatic fibrosis by 15 months.[373,374]

Hepatotoxicity of herbal products and botanical and environmental hepatotoxins

The use of vitamins, dietary supplements, food additives, and herbal and non-proprietary remedies collectively referred to as **complementary and alternative medicines (CAM)** continue to increase around the world.[375,376,377] In the USA, the use of alternative medicines rose from 34% of the population in 1990 to 42% in 1997, with nearly 20% taking complementary medicines at the same time as conventional prescriptions.[378] The use of herbal products is even more popular among patients with chronic liver disease,[379,380] including patients who have undergone liver transplantation,[381] despite the absence of controlled clinical trials from which we might assess safety and efficacy in these settings.[382]

Many botanical substances contained in so-called 'health foods'; dietary and weight loss supplements and herbal products are, in some instances, potent hepatotoxins, which may lead to acute liver failure.[375–377,383] Examples of hepatotoxic mushrooms, fruits and other foodstuffs, including grains and nuts contaminated by fungal mycotoxins or other potentially injurious compounds, are discussed below (see Botanical and environmental hepatotoxins, p. 697). Potentially hepatotoxic herbal products, including the pyrrolizidine alkaloids (an important cause of veno-occlusive disease), germander, pennyroyal, mistletoe, and some of the constituents of Chinese traditional remedies, and food supplements, including potentially hepatotoxic vitamins, will be discussed under the heading of Hepatotoxic herbal and related products (see p. 697).

Hepatotoxic mushrooms

There are about 100 poisonous varieties of mushrooms among the more than 5000 species.[384] In the USA more than

8000 mushroom poisonings were reported in 2001,[385] with greater than 90% of cases of fatal poisonings due to Amanita phylloides (death cap) or A. verna (destroying angel), found in the pacific northwest and the eastern USA.[3,386] A fatal dose can involve the ingestion of a single 50 g mushroom,[387] the consequence of one of the most potent and lethal biological toxins in nature.[388] Alpha amatoxin is thermostable and can resist drying for years, and is not inactivated by cooking. Rapidly absorbed via the GI tract, the amatoxin travels within the enterohepatic circulation to reach the hepatocytes where it inhibits production of mRNA and protein synthesis, leading to necrosis.[389] A second toxin, phalloidin, is responsible for the GI distress that precedes the hepatic and CNS injury.[278,390] Phalloidin disrupts cell membranes by interfering with actin polymerization, and leads to severe gastroenteritis. In contrast to the injury seen with CCl$_4$ and phosphorus, the latent period is often longer (6–20 hours). Intense abdominal pain, vomiting and diarrhoea develop, with hepatocellular jaundice and renal failure occurring over the next 24–48 hours, followed by convulsions and coma by 72 hours.[1,3,278,386,387,390] The characteristic hepatic lesion is prominent steatosis and zone 3 necrosis with nucleolar inclusions seen on electron microscopy[391] (Fig. 14.3).

In a case-series of 8 patients reported by Rengstoroff et al.,[278] mean AST was 5488 IU/L(range 1486–12 340), mean ALT was 7618 (range 3065–15 210), and bilirubin was 10.5 mg% (range 1.8–52), peaking at day 4–5. Although mortality traditionally has been high, especially when the ALT has exceeded 1000 IU/L, and emergency liver transplantation is often required,[279,391,392] all of their patients survived with conservative management, which included nasogastric lavage with activated charcoal, penicillin G, acetylcysteine [NAC] and the use of milk thistle (silybum marianum). However, in a review of 2108 amatoxin poisonings over a 20 year period in the USA and Europe, penicillin G, either alone or in combination with other agents produced limited benefit, despite being hepatoprotective in animals.[280] Other treatments include plasmapheresis.[393] Current estimates on mortality rates in the past 20 years are significantly lower than the 30–50% in the pre-liver transplant era.[64,394]

Other hepatotoxic foodstuffs

The unripe fruit of the **ackee tree** (Blighia surpida), native to Jamaica, contains a cholestatic hepatotoxin, hypoglycin A, that produces a clinical syndrome of GI distress and microvesicular steatosis known as Jamaican vomiting sickness that resembles Reye syndrome.[80,395,396] Cholestatic jaundice has been described after chronic ingestion.[397]

Cycasin is a potent hepatotoxin and carcinogen found in the fruit of the cycad tree (Cycas circinalis, C. revoluta). A small epidemic of acute hepatic injury attributable to the ingestion of cycad nuts was reported from Japan.[398] The purported toxin is methylazoxymethanol, which is normally eliminated or rendered inactive in preparing the nuts prior to eating.[398]

Aflatoxins are a family of mycotoxins found in Aspergillus flavus and related fungi that are ubiquitous in the tropics and subtropical regions. They contaminate peanuts, cashews, soybeans and grains stored under warm, moist conditions, and are well-known hepatotoxins and hepatocarcinogens.[34] Aflatoxin B1, a potent inhibitor of RNA synthesis, is the most hepatotoxic.[399] Reactive metabolites are formed by P450 metabolism; malnutrition is a possible potentiating factor (perhaps due to glutathione depletion). When consumed in large quantities, it is responsible for a clinical syndrome characterized by a prodrome of fever, malaise, anorexia and vomiting followed by jaundice. Portal hypertension with splenomegaly and ascites may develop over the next few weeks. In large epidemics, mortality rates have approached 25% and are dose-related.[400] Zone 3 necrosis without significant inflammation is the characteristic lesion. Other histological findings include cholestasis, microvesicular steatosis, and bile duct proliferation.[30]

The risk of hepatocellular carcinoma has been well-confirmed and is directly related to the amount of aflatoxin consumed, especially in sub-Saharan Africa and eastern China where wheat often exceeds rice as a staple in the diet.[401] Alcohol and possibly exposure to DDT appear to play an enhancing role in the hepatocarcinogenesis of rats exposed to aflatoxin B1.[402] Perhaps an even more important cofactor is the interaction between aflatoxin and the hepatitis B virus.[403] The frequency of a mutation in the p53 tumour suppressor gene has been directly correlated to the development of hepatocellular carcinoma in these regions as compared to the rarity of this mutation in HCC from Western countries.[404]

Kodo millet (Paspalum scrobiculatum) is a staple food found in northern India that is frequently contaminated by Aspergillus tamarii, which produces acute hepatic injury and preneoplastic changes due to another mycotoxin, cyclopiazonic acid.[405]

Epidemics of hepatic injury from adulterated cooking oils and contaminated foods

A number of contaminated foodstuffs and cooking oils have been associated with epidemics of hepatotoxicity. While they are now largely of historical interest they are included as examples of the types of contaminations that can occur.

Spanish toxic oil syndrome occurred in 1981 after exposure of up to 100 000 Spaniards to rapeseed cooking oil that was contaminated by anilines and acetanilides.[406] Nearly 20 000 individuals became ill, many of whom had hepatic injury.[406] Overall, approximately 2500 people died.[407] The disease was characterized by pulmonary oedema, pulmonary hypertension, rash, myalgias, eosinophilia, joint contractures, scleroderma, sicca syndrome, polyneuropathy and Raynaud disease, with an immunological pathogenesis suspected.[408] Among a cohort of 332 patients followed for up to 8 years, hepatic injury developed in 43%.[409] A mixed cholestatic-hepatocellular injury pattern was seen biochemically. The histopathological changes were those of a cholestatic hepatitis that resembled chlorpromazine-induced liver injury.[410] Of 24 patients studied by Solis-Herruzo et al.,[411] 11 had necroinflammatory bile-duct lesions; nodular regenerative hyperplasia was also noted.

Epping jaundice refers to an epidemic of toxic liver injury that has occurred in Epping, England in 1965.[274,412] It involved 84 persons who had eaten bread contaminated with methylenedianiline (MDA) that had spilled onto the floor of a van carrying flour. Occupational exposure has been described from the use of MDA as a hardener for epoxy resins,[413] and accidental ingestion occurred when methylenedianiline was mistaken for Ecstasy (methylenedioxymethamphetamine, (also referred to as MDMA or MDA on the street).[414] The clinical syndrome consists of cholestatic jaundice preceded by abdominal pain and fever, resembling biliary colic, beginning a few hours of ingestion. Liver biopsies performed in some patients revealed Kupffer cell hyperplasia with portal inflammation but little or no necrosis.[274] Most individuals recovered within 4–6 weeks, with jaundice lasting up to 4 months in a few. The mechanism of injury was thought to be a chemically induced cholangitis, possibly as a result of a hypersensitivity reaction. Most individuals had no long-term health consequences, although one person developed cholangiocarcinoma.[415,416]

Yusho oil disease in western Japan, and a related epidemic referred to as **Yu-Cheng** in Taiwan, involved nearly 2000 individuals who had eaten rice prepared in oil contaminated by PCBs, dioxins and polychlorinated dibenzofurans (PCDFs) in 1968 . It was characterized by chloracne, skin hyperpigmentation and neuropathy with jaundice reported in approximately 10%.[417] Exposed individuals still harbour high levels of these agents more than 26 years after the outbreak.[418]

Hexochlorobenzene contamination of wheat in the 1950s led to an epidemic of toxic porphyria cutanea tarda and severe liver disease involving more than 3000 Turkish Kurds, with a mortality rate that exceeded 10%. This fungicide had been added to seed grain that was diverted to use for food during a famine.[419,420]

Hepatotoxic drug abuse

By far the most commonly abused drug is **alcohol**. Its toxic affects on the adult liver are discussed in Chapter 6.

Cocaine is a dose- and time-dependent hepatotoxin in mice manifested by elevated aminotransferase levels and by necrosis and steatosis.[421,422] Numerous reports attest to its hepatotoxic potential in humans.[423,424] Acute cocaine intoxication involved the liver in 60% of patients reported by Silva et al.,[425] many of whom had elevated ALT values >1000 IU/L. Associated features include rhabdomyolysis, hypotension, hyperpyrexia, disseminated intravascular coagulation and renal failure.[423–425] Hepatic and other organ injury is likely the result of toxic metabolites (e.g. norcocaine nitroxide) formed via CYP2E1 and CYP2A,[426] which helps explain the enhanced hepatotoxicity seen in those who also abuse alcohol.[286]

Necrosis has been described as zonal, but the zone involved has varied, apparently according to strain of mouse and status of the P450 system.[421,427,428] In man, minor elevations of the aminotransferases are common in non-

parenteral cocaine users.[429] More severe injury is characterized by coagulative necrosis involving the perivenular and mid-zones or all three zones, and microvesicular steatosis.[421,423,424]

Amphetamines have long been suspected to cause hepatic injury when taken as a form of drug abuse, but evidence for this is scant.[430] However, **ecstasy** (3,4 methylenedioxymethamphetamine) is a euphorigenic and psychedelic amphetamine derivative that can lead to hepatic necrosis as part of a heat-stroke-like syndrome that occurs as a result of exhaustive dancing in hot nightclubs.[431,432,433] The injury can be fatal, and has necessitated liver transplantation in some instances.[434,435] Hepatic injury may be related to apoptosis,[436] or disruption of thiol homeostasis resulting in loss of protein function.[437] The role of P450 enzymes in the toxicity of this and other so-called 'designer drugs' maybe related to specific genetic polymorphisms of CYP2D6 or other cytochromes.[438] Both cholestatic and hepatocellular injuries have been described. Chronic hepatitis with and without autoimmune features has also been attributed to this agent.[439,440]

Phencyclidine ('angel dust') is another stimulant that has led to hepatic injury as part of a malignant hyperthermia syndrome producing zone 3 necrosis with congestion reminiscent of shock liver.[441] Phencyclidine potentiates cocaine hepatotoxicity in animals, in part by depleting glutathione.[442]

Veno-occlusive disease-like lesions have been described in intravenous abusers of **heroin**.[443] The changes included inflammation of the wall of terminal hepatic venules with fibrosis and sinusoidal dilatation. Patients who stopped abusing heroin had fibrous thickening of the veins and perisinusoidal fibrosis. It is considered to be a direct cytopathic effect of heroin.

Although there are few reports of serious toxic effects from smoking or ingesting **marijuana,**[444] intravenous usage is hazardous. Four cases of dose-related, multisystem injury were reported by Payne and Brand.[445] The findings included fulminant gastroenteritis, hypoalbuminaemia, acute renal failure, pancytopenia and a toxic hepatitis-like injury confirmed by serial biopsy.

Inhalation of **chloroform, trichloroethylene** and related compounds can lead to perivenular zone necrosis and or steatosis.[1] '**Glue sniffing**' and inhalation of other euphorogenic intoxicating agents also may lead to hepatic disease. These agents may, however, contain non-hepatotoxic (e.g. acetone) or only mildly hepatotoxic (e.g. toluene) agents.

No important direct hepatotoxic effects can be ascribed to the **opiates**.[1]

Hepatotoxic herbal remedies and related products

Paralleling the rise in herbal therapy usage have been reports of hepatotoxicity with many components of these agents as reviewed by several recent authors.[64,375–377,446,447] They are reported to lead to both acute and chronic hepatic injury, that may be hepatocellular (necrosis, steatosis, chronic hepatitis, cirrhosis), cholestatic or vascular (veno-occlusive disease) in nature. While the safety record of many herbal products is generally favourable, serious toxicity may result from others, including Chinese proprietary medicines, whose constituents often contain small amounts of Western medicines, arsenic, or cadmium.[377] Herbal products are available through mail order or the Internet and in some countries do not conform to the high standards of manufacturing required for pharmaceutical products, nor do they all undergo tests of purity.[377] As a result, warnings have been issued for a number of agents, and in a few instances, the FDA and other health authorities have requested their removal from the marketplace. It is therefore important to consider self-prescribing with herbal agents whenever investigating cases of liver injury, and for clinicians to inquire about the ingestion of herbal remedies as a routine part of a patient's drug history. Underscoring the importance of herbal hepatotoxicity, Estes et al.[383] and Neff et al.[448] have reported an association with several commonly promoted weight loss and other herbal products in their series of patients with acute liver failure who were evaluated for, and in some cases received a liver transplant. The use of herbal agents (including Lipokinetix, skullcap, Ma huang, chaparral, and kava kava) was noted in 50% of the acute liver failure cases collected by Estes et al.[383] over a two-year period. Six of 10 individuals underwent transplantation; three died prior to transplant and only one patient recovered spontaneously.

Table 14.24 lists various herbal remedies that have been implicated as causing hepatic injury, according to their purported hepatotoxic constituent and the nature of the liver disease they cause. As with other classes of drugs and chemicals, isolated case reports in which an association with liver injury has been made may not always be causally related, as some authors have acknowledged.[449,450,451]

Pyrrolizidine alkaloids (PA)

These are extremely common, being found in about 3% of all flowering plant species throughout the world, and their ingestion, often as medicinal teas, can produce acute and chronic forms of liver disease, including veno-occlusive disease (VOD), now referred to as sinusoidal obstructive syndrome (SOS) in humans as well as livestock.[74,160] VOD was first reported in the 1950s as a disease of Jamaican children who developed acute abdominal distention with marked hepatomegaly and ascites that resembled Budd–Chiari syndrome.[452] The aetiopathological event was perivenular congestion with occlusion of the hepatic venules leading to a form of congestive cirrhosis that Bras and colleagues linked to the drinking of 'bush teas', largely made from plants of the *Senecio, Heliotopium* and *Crotalaria* species, taken as a folk remedy for acute childhood illnesses. **Comfrey** (*Symphytum officinale*) remains commercially available despite being a dose-dependent hepatotoxin.[453] Hepatotoxic PAs are cyclic diesters and some forms (e.g. fulvine and monocrotaline) cause both liver and lung injury.[74] The mechanism of injury is postulated to be impairment of nucleic acid synthesis by reactive metabolites of PAs generated by hepatic microsomes, leading to progressive

loss of sinusoidal cells with haemorrhage, as well as injury to the terminal hepatic venule endothelium with fibrin deposition.[446,454,455] In certain parts of the world, ingestion of PA-contaminated grains and bread have led to large epidemics of VOD, most notably in Afghanistan where nearly 8000 persons and innumerable sheep were affected.[283]

VOD (SOS) may take the form of acute, subacute or chronic injury. In the acute form, there is zone 3 necrosis and sinusoidal dilatation leading to a Budd–Chiari-like syndrome with abdominal pain and the rapid onset of ascites within 3–6 weeks of ingestion. In Jamaica, a rapidly fatal course due to liver failure was observed in 15–20% of individuals, with the prognosis worst in adults.[452] About half of acute cases recovered spontaneously and the remainder underwent a transition to more chronic injury. In the subacute and chronic forms, perivenular fibrosis and bridging between terminal hepatic veins led to a form of cirrhosis similar to that seen with chronic passive hepatic congestion (so-called cardiac cirrhosis). At one time, this form of injury accounted for one-third of the cases of cirrhosis seen in Jamaica, with death due to complications of portal hypertension.[34] Certain PAs, such as comfrey extracts, are also hepatocarcinogenic, inducing mutations of the *p53* gene, akin to aflatoxins.[74]

Germander

The blossoms of plants from the *Labiatae* family (*Teucrium chamaedrys*) were used for years in herbal teas for various purposes and in the mid-1980s as capsules for weight reduction in France and other European nations.[456] Several dozen cases of liver injury, including fatal hepatic failure, forced its withdrawal from the French marketplace in 1992.[457] Most patients were middle-aged women who had ingested germander for three to 18 weeks, and developed acute hepatocellular injury. The injury usually resolved within 1.5 to 6 months after the germander was discontinued, with prompt recurrence after rechallenge documented in many individuals.[312] At least one fatal case has been described.[458] In a few instances, chronic hepatitis developed after prolonged exposure, often associated with autoantibodies[459] and a case of severe cholangiolitic hepatitis was reported.[446]

Germander hepatotoxicity is an interplay of toxic metabolites and immunoallergic mechanisms. Germander is composed of several compounds, including glycosides, flavonoids, and furan-containing diterpenoids, all of which are converted by the P450 system (especially CYP3A) into reactive metabolites.[460] Covalent binding to cellular proteins, depletion of hepatic glutathione, apoptosis and cytoskeleton membrane injury (blebs) cause cell disruption in animal models.[461,462] Epoxide hydrolase on plasma membranes is a target of antibodies found in the sera of patients who drank germander teas for long periods of time.[463]

Reports of liver injury have appeared with other species of *Teucrium*. *T. capitatum* was reported to cause acute cholestatic hepatitis in a 62 year old man four months after taking the herbal therapy for hypercholesterolemia and hyperglycemia.[464] *T. polium* caused acute cholestatic hepati-

Table 14.24	Hepatotoxic herbal remedies			
Remedy	**Use**	**Source**	**Hepatotoxic component**	**Type of liver injury**
Barakol	anxiolytic	*Cassia siamea*	?	reversible hepatitis/cholestasis
Black cohosh	menopausal syndrome	*Cimicifuga racemosa*	?	fulminant hepatitis
'Bush tea', herbal teas, fever		*Senecio, heliotropium, crotalaria sp.*	Pyrrolizidine alkaloids	VOD
Cascara sagrada	laxative	—	Anthracene glycoside	cholestatic hepatitis
Chaso/onshido	weight loss	—	N-nitro-fenfluramine	acute hepatitis, ALF
Chaparral leaf	'liver tonic' burn salve, weight loss	*Larrea tridenta* (greasewood, creosote bush)	Nordihydroguaiarectic acid	acute/chr hepatitis, ALF
Chinese medicines Ma-huang Jin bu huan	weight loss sleep aid, analgesic	*Ephedra sp.* *Lycopodium serratum*	Ephedrine levo-tetrahydropalmitine?	acute hepatitis, AIH, ALF acute or chronic hepatitis/cholestasis; steatosis H-cell necrosis, chols.,steatosis, granulomas
Syo-saiko-to Shou-wu-pian		*Scutellaria* root *Polygonum multiflorum*		acute hep or cholestasis
Comfrey	herbal tea	*Symphytum sp.*	Pyrrolizidine alkaloid	acute VOD; cirrhosis
Germander	weight loss; fever	*Teucrium chamaedrys* *T. capitatum* *T. polium*	diterpenoids, epoxides	acute/chr. hepatitis autoimmune injury? ALF
Greater celandine	gallstones, IBS	*Chelidonium majus*		chol hep, fibrosis
Impila	multiple uses	*Callilepsis laureola*	potassium atractylate	necrosis
Kava kava	anxiolytic	*Piper methysticum*	kava lactone, pyrone	acute hep/chol; ALF
Lipokinetix	weight loss	lichen alkaloid	usnic acid	acute hep, J; ALF
Mistletoe	asthma, infertility	*Viscus album*		hepatitis (combined with skullcap)
Oil of cloves	dental pain	various foods, oils	Eugenol	zonal necrosis
Pennyroyal (squawmint oil)	abortifacient	*Hedeoma pulegoides* *Mentha pulegium*	pulegone, monoterpenes	severe necrosis
Prostata	prostatism	multiple sources	?	chronic cholestasis
Senna	laxative	*Cassia angustifolia*	sennoside alkaloids; anthrone	acute hepatitis
Sassafras	herbal tea	*Sassafras albidum*	safrole	HCC (in animals)
Skullcap	anxiolytic	*Scutellaria*	diterpenoids	hepatitis
Kombucha	weight loss	lichen alkaloid	usnic acid	acute hepatitis
Valerian	sedative	*Valeriana officinalis*	?	elevated LFTs

? = unknown or unidentified   ALF = acute liver failure   J = jaundice   AIH = autoimmune hepatitis   H-cell = hepatocellular   hep = hepatitis   chol = cholestasis   VOD = venoocclusive disease   IBS = irritable bowel syndrome   chr. = chronic   HCC = hepatocellular carcinoma   LFTs = liver function tests

tis associated with antimitochondrial antibodies that later disappeared.[465]

Chaparral

The leaf of this desert shrub known as greasewood or creosote bush (*Larrea tridentata*) is ground into a tea or used in capsules or tablets for various ailments. Multiple reports of hepatitis have appeared, most occurring within 1–12 months of use, and resolving within a few weeks to months of discontinuation.[466] Among 13 cases reported to the FDA, acute hepatocellular or cholestatic injury was observed, with two cases of fulminant hepatitis requiring transplantation, and progression to cirrhosis in 4 individuals.[467] Estes et al.[383] also reported irreversible acute liver failure. It is postulated that its active ingredient, nordihydroguaiaretic acid, an inhibitor of cycloxygenase and lipoxygenase pathways, is the likely cause of hepatic injury,[446] although the mechanism might also involve phytoestrogen-induced effects on the liver.[383] At least one case with a documented rechallenge has appeared, suggesting a possible role for immunoallergy.[468]

Pennyroyal

The leaves of *Hedeoma pulgoides* or *Mentha pulegium* (squawmint oil) contain pulegone and smaller amounts of other monoterpene ketones that are formed into oils, tablets and home-brewed mint teas. Oxidative metabolites of pulegone (e.g. menthofuran) bind to cellular proteins and deplete hepatic glutathione, leading to liver injury.[469] Cases of hepatocellular injury, including fatal necrosis, are described, several of whom had associated gastrointestinal and CNS toxicity within just a few hours of ingestion.[469,470] In animals, inhibiting pulegone metabolism via the P450 system (utilizing disulfiram and cimetidine) limits pennyroyal hepatotoxicity.[471]

Chinese herbal medications

Chinese herbal medicines have been used for centuries, and continue to be widely employed, finding increased usage in the West. While many therapies appear safe, a few have been associated with liver injury and are described below.

Jin Bu Huan (*Lycopodium serratum*) is a traditional herbal remedy that has been used as a sedative and an analgesic. Woolf et al.[472] described acute hepatitis in 7 adults in the Los Angeles area after a mean latency of 20 weeks after starting the agent. Liver biopsies from a small number of patients showed a range of changes including lobular hepatitis with prominent eosinophils in one patient and mild hepatitis with microvesicular steatosis and fibrotic expansion of the portal tracts in a patient who had taken the herbal remedy for 12 months. The injury resolved within a mean of 8 weeks in this series. In two patients, rechallenge was associated with an abrupt recurrence of liver injury. All patients were taking doses within the recommended range. Other than female predominance, no predisposing factors were evident. Liver enzymes showed 20- to 50-fold increases in serum ALT levels with minor increases in the alkaline phosphatase, except for one patient with cholestasis. The mechanism of injury is unclear. The presence of levo-tetrahydropalmatine, a compound with structural similarity to pyrrolizidine alkaloids, is a potent neuroactive substance[473] but is of unproven hepatotoxic potential.[377] Both adults and children have been affected[473] and a case of possible chronic hepatitis has been described.[474] The FDA has banned the importation of Jin Bu Huan Anodyne tablets into the USA.[377]

Syo-saiko-to (Xiao-chai-hu-tang, Dai-saiko-to) contains several ingredients, including scutellaria root (skullcap), which is a postulated hepatotoxin. Several reports of liver injury have appeared, including hepatocellular necrosis, microvesicular steatosis, cholestasis and granuloma formation, and it may have triggered a flare of autoimmune hepatitis in one patient.[475,476] Reversible acute hepatitis or

cholestasis has followed the consumption of **Shou-wu-pian,** a product derived from *Polygonum multiflorum*.[477,478]

Ma-huang, derived from plants of the Ephedra species, has been reported to cause (or be a cofactor for) acute, sometimes severe, hepatitis, leading to acute liver failure requiring liver transplantation.[383,448,450,451]

In the series of 12 patients presenting to transplant centres with liver failure from the use of weight loss agents (see above), 10 were taking a formulation containing Ma-huang.[448] In the report by Borum,[451] the agent may have induced autoimmune hepatitis. The active constituent, ephedrine, has been linked predominantly to severe adverse cardiovascular and central nervous system effects, including some fatalities when used as a stimulant and weight loss aid.[479,480] As a result, the FDA followed Canadian authorities by issuing a ruling that ephedra-containing products present an unreasonable risk and should be avoided.[481] The mechanism for the hepatic injury is unknown.[482]

Chaso and Onshido are Chinese herbal dietary weight loss supplements that were the subject of a report of severe liver injury.[483] Twelve patients were described, with a mean ALT level of 1978 IU/L. Two individuals developed fulminant hepatic failure, one of whom died and the other who survived after receiving a liver transplant. These products contain N-nitroso-fenfluramine, a derivative of the appetite suppressant, fenfluramine, that was withdrawn from the market a few years ago. It was suspected that this ingredient was the hepatotoxic component, as it has been associated with other instances of hepatic injury.[484]

A related dietary supplement used for weight loss, **Lipokinetix,** is composed of norephedrine, sodium usniate (usnic acid), diiodothyronine, yohimbine and caffeine. It has been associated with acute hepatitis leading to including fulminant hepatic failure requiring liver transplantation.[383] Favreau et al.[485] described a case-series of 7 previously healthy patients who developed acute hepatitis after a latent period of less than 4 weeks in 5 patients and 8–12 weeks in the other two. Mean ALT elevations were 4501 IU/L, and urea bilirubin was 6.5 mg/dl. No evidence of immunoallergy (e.g. rash, fever, eosinophilia) was evident. All recovered spontaneously. Although the authors could not identify any single component of Lipokinetix as being responsible for the injury, the FDA has issued a warning that individuals not use Lipokinetix due to its inherent danger of liver toxicity.[486]

A report of fulminant liver failure necessitating emergency liver transplantation in a previously healthy 28 year old non-obese woman who had taken an over the counter preparation of **usnic acid** for weight loss[487] suggests that this agent may be the hepatotoxic component. Usnic acid is a lichen alkaloid that has been shown to be toxic to a number of biological systems leading to hepatic injury in animals by uncoupling oxidative phosphorylation in mitochondria and triggering oxidative stress.[488] Usnic acid is also a component of **Kombucha** tea, and reports of hepatic injury have been reported with its use.[489]

Given the proliferation of dietary supplements that have been introduced into the marketplace, and the apparent risk of hepatotoxicity seen with some of them, the Center for Natural Product Research of the Food and Drug Administration hosted a workshop to review the possible mechanisms of injury and to predict the frequency of liver injury from these various botanical products.[490] It is hoped that such efforts will lead to a better understanding of the risks and improved tools for predicting such injury in the future.

Kava kava

This natural sedative and anxiolytic agent, derived from the root of the pepper plant (*Piper methysticum*), was the subject of a recent FDA consumer alert[377] after being banned in the European Union and Canada[491] due to severe hepatotoxicity, including fatal liver failure.[383,492–495] Clouatre et al.[451] reviewed 78 cases of hepatic injury reported to the FDA, which included 11 patients who developed liver failure requiring transplantation, and 4 deaths, and questioned the causality in some cases. Kavalactone has been shown to inhibit P450 cytochromes, deplete hepatic glutathione content, and possibly inhibit cyclooxygenase,[496] although the hepatotoxic component may be the major kava alkaloid, pipermethystine.

Barakol

This extract of *Cassia siamea*, is a natural anxiolytic frequently used in Thailand. It was incriminated as a cause of liver injury in 12 patients, nine of whom developed cholestasis, and three with asymptomatic elevations of transaminases.[497] Two individuals had recurrence of abnormal LFTs after rechallenge, but all 12 had complete resolution of the injury within 20 weeks of stopping Barakol. Liver biopsy in three individuals showed interface hepatitis.

Greater celandine

This preparation of *Chelidonium majus* is used in the management of dyspepsia, gallstones and the irritable bowel syndrome. Several reports describe acute cholestatic hepatitis with ALT up to 1000 IU/L and alkaline phosphatase three-fold elevated.[498] Recovery was complete within 2–6 months of discontinuation; unintentional rechallenge produced a flare of hepatitis in one patient. The toxic component of greater celandine has not been identified.[377]

Black cohosh

This agent, derived from *Cimicifuga racemosa*, is used to allieve menopause symptoms. It has been the subject of several reports of fulminant hepatic failure requiring liver transplantation.[499,500]

Breynia officinalis

This poisonous species of *Euphorbiaceae* caused symptomatic hepatitis in 19 patients after it was mistakenly substi-

tuted for a similar plant (*Securinega suffruticosa*) used as an ingredient for a medicinal soup to treat musculoskeletal symptoms.[501] Diarrhoea, nausea, vomiting, abdominal pain, and chills were reported along with hepatocellular liver injury that developed over 2–12 days. The median ALT level was 647 IU/L. Jaundice was not a prominent feature. With supportive measures, the hepatic manifestations resolved over a six month period.

Herbal laxatives

Cholestatic hepatitis complicated by portal hypertension was reported after ingestion of *Cascara sagrada*. Anthracene glycoside or possibly another component of this laxative agent was thought to be responsible.[502]

Senna (*Cassia angustifolias*)

Senna has been associated with hepatocellular injury after long-term use.[503] It is metabolized to antron, which is structurally similar to danthrone, an agent that in combination with dioctyl calcium sulphosuccinate led to chronic hepatitis.[504]

Mistletoe

This plant (*Viscus album*) is used to treat asthma and epilepsy. In combination with skullcap it has been reported to cause reversible hepatitis.[505] In animals, skullcap causes hepatic injury attributed to diterpenoids that act similarly to those implicated in germander hepatotoxicity.[506]

Valerian

This anxiolytic agent derived from *Valeriana officinalis* has caused abnormal liver function tests, although its hepatotoxic potential remains controversial.[377]

Prostata

A report of chronic cholestatic hepatitis has appeared with this agent used to treat prostate problems.[507] It is composed of several agents, including zinc picolinate, ginseng, bee pollen, and *Pygeum africanum*. The specific hepatotoxic component, however, has not yet been identified.[377]

Impila

This traditional medicine, known in South Africa as 'Zulu remedy', contains *Callilepsis laureola*. It has been associated with fatal acute liver and kidney failure heralded by the acute onset of abdominal pain and diarrhoea. A case-fatality rate as high as 90% within 5 days is reported, with the toxic component possibly being related to potassium atractylate.[508,509] Histologically there is zonal (zones 3 and 2) coagulative necrosis.

Oil of cloves

Used for the relief of dental pain, clove oil contains eugenol and methyleugenol, phenylpropenes found in various food products, essential oils, spices and clove cigarettes.[510] A few reports of severe, sometimes fatal, acute hepatic necrosis in association with coagulopathy (including disseminated intravascular coagulation) have appeared, most often after toxic exposure in children.[511,512] The clinical syndrome has resembled acute acetaminophen toxicity, and N-acetylcysteine has been used successfully in association with other supportive measures.[511]

Hepatotoxic vitamins

Hypervitaminosis A

Vitamin A is a dose- and duration-dependent hepatotoxin capable of causing injury ranging from asymptomatic elevations in hepatic enzymes with minor histologic changes, to perisinusoidal fibrosis leading to non-cirrhotic portal hypertension, and in some cases, cirrhosis.[513,514] It is estimated that about one-third of the US population takes vitamin supplements containing vitamin A, with as many as 3% of products providing a daily dose of 25 000 IU or more.[515,516] Most cases of hypervitaminosis A occur as a result of self-ingestion rather than intentional overdoses, with all age groups represented.[153] While the average daily dose of vitamin A in reported cases of liver disease has been nearly 100 000 IU, over an average duration of 7.2 years, for a mean cumulative dose of 229 million units,[513,517] liver injury has been described with lower daily doses of 10 000 to 45 000 IU,[518,519] and cirrhosis has occurred after a daily intake of only 25 000 IU for 6 years or longer.[517,519] Long-term use of low dose vitamin A supplements (250–5000 retinol equivalents/day) does not appear to present a risk for toxicity.[520]

The severity of liver disease depends on the duration as well as the dose, and the fibrotic process may continue from the slow release of hepatic stores despite discontinuation of vitamin A due to its long half-life in the liver (50 days to 1 year).[153,521] Genetic factors may play a role as illustrated by apparent familial hypervitaminosis A developing in 4 siblings all ingesting large doses for congenital ichthyosis.[522] Toxicity in persons who consume large amounts of fresh liver (such as native Alaskans who eat large amounts of polar bear liver) have been reported for decades.[523,524] Water-soluble, emulsified and solid formulations of vitamin A have been found to be as much as 10 times more toxic than oil-based preparations.[525]

Stellate cells are the body's main site of storage of vitamin A (retinol), and hepatotoxicity from vitamin A has been attributed to activation of these cells resulting in hyperplasia and hypertrophy that in turn produces sinusoidal obstruction, along with increased collagen synthesis leading to portal hypertension.[526,527] Beta carotene, a precursor of vitamin A, can interact with ethanol which impairs its conversion to retinol and can result in hepatotoxicity. Retinol itself is metabolized to several metabolites, some of which

are locally toxic from intrinsic or environmentally-mediated mechanisms.[528]

The histopathological spectrum of hypervitaminosis A-related liver disease includes stellate cell hyperplasia and hypertrophy after acute and subacute intoxication following high-dose ingestion, and non-cirrhotic portal hypertension with perisinusoidal fibrosis, or cirrhosis following chronic consumption of 'therapeutic' doses[514,517] (Fig. 14.22). Rare cases of peliosis hepatitis have been attributed to hypervitaminosis A.[529]

Liver biopsy specimens show increased storage of vitamin A as characteristic greenish autofluorescence after irradiation with ultraviolet light.[2,517] The excess vitamin A is stored initially in stellate cells that lie in the space of Disse; and become hyperplastic and hypertrophic. Under light microscopy, the enlarged clear stellate cells compress the hepatic sinusoids and give rise to a 'Swiss cheese', or honeycombed, appearance.[517] Hepatocellular injury is usually minor, with microvesicular steatosis and focal degeneration, without significant necrosis or inflammation. Hepatic fibrosis is the other striking histologic feature. It begins in a perisinusoidal distribution and most likely arises from activated stellate cells that transform into myofibroblasts.[518,526] In the series reported by Geubel et al.,[517] cirrhosis was present in 59%, chronic hepatitis in 34%, microvesicular steatosis in 21%, perisinusoidal fibrosis in 14% and peliosis in 3%.

The clinical features of hypervitaminosis A are varied and can involve several different organ systems (Table 14.25).

Table 14.25	Clinical manifestations of hypervitaminosis A
Gastrointestinal	Anorexia, weight loss, nausea, vomiting, abdominal pain
	Hepatosplenomegaly (35–50%)
	Glossitis, cheilosis
	Jaundice, ascites (12%)
Skin	Dry, cracked, desquamation
	Hair loss, brittle cracked nails
	Pruritus
Neuro-ophthalmic	Headache
	Diplopia, strabismus, nystagmus
	Papilloedema
	Pseudotumour cerebri
Musculoskeletal	Myopathy, bone pain
	Arthropathy, joint stiffness
	Hypercalcemia (from bone resorption)
	Growth retardation (premature closure of growth plates)
	Calcification of joints, tendons
Renal	Polydipsia, polyuria
Haematological	Anaemia
	Hypersplenism (neutropenia, thrombocytopenia)
	Lymphadenopathy
General	Fatigue (35%), insomnia, irritability

After references 1, 282, 283, 293

Hepatomegaly is common, and in severe cases, spleno-megaly and ascites may be evident. Cases with portal hypertension can present with bleeding oesophageal varices.[514,529] Liver tests are abnormal in two thirds of cases, but the changes are non-specific, with only modest elevations in aminotransferases and alkaline phosphatase. In advanced cases, low serum albumin, hyperglobulinemia (especially IgM), hyperbilirubinemia, and prolongation of prothrombin time may be present[516–518]

The diagnosis of hypervitaminosis A rests on obtaining the relevant dietary and medication history and on clinical suspicion given the diverse manifestations of the syndrome. Plasma vitamin A levels may be normal, and it is more reliable to demonstrate increased hepatic storage of vitamin A and characteristic histology. Serum levels of retinol do not correlate with vitamin A stores in the liver in patients with fibrosis and even cirrhosis.[530,531] The average duration of vitamin A intake before diagnosis is 18 months, but in some cases diagnosis is delayed for several years because of failure to suspect the cause of liver injury.[517,532,533]

Gradual resolution of symptoms and normalization of liver enzymes occur after discontinuation of vitamin A ingestion in less severe cases, but deterioration may continue in cases of severe intoxication, particularly when cirrhosis is already present.[153] Features of liver failure and established cirrhosis at the time of diagnosis indicate a poor prognosis, and liver transplantation may be required.[153,513] Alcohol should be avoided because of possible potentiation of hepatotoxicity,[528,534] and vitamin A supplements generally should be avoided in other types of liver disease because of possible accentuation of hepatic injury and fibrosis.[515] The use of red palm fruit oil has been advocated as a safer source of vitamin A owing to a lack of toxicity.[535]

Other vitamins

Vitamin E (tocopherol) taken in daily doses of >1 gram has been associated with elevated aminotransferase levels in patients who underwent liver transplantation for PBC . The enzyme elevations were reversible within 4–8 weeks after the vitamin E was discontinued.[381] Of interest is the fact that troglitazone, a tocopherol derivative[536] has been associated with severe hepatic injury (p. 649).

Niacin (nicotinic acid) is discussed under cholesterol-lowering agents. The extended release formulations are more likely to cause liver injury than crystalline forms.[537]

Liver disease due to medicinal agents

There is an interesting relationship between the pharmacological category of a drug and the type of hepatic injury that it can produce. General anaesthetics, many of the drugs used to treat rheumatic and musculoskeletal disease, the hydrazine antidepressants and most anticonvulsants produce cytotoxic injury. Most neuroleptic drugs, and some antithyroid and antidiabetic agents, produce cholestatic injury. Other antithyroid and antidiabetic agents lead to cytotoxic injury. Anabolic and contraceptive steroids also produce cholestasis, albeit of a somewhat different category than do the neuroleptics. The diversity of drugs employed in cardiovascular and microbial disease precludes such generalizations.[1]

Liver disease caused by anaesthetic agents

The volatile inhalational anaesthetics in current use are derivatives of some of the most potent (now regarded as classical) chemical hepatotoxins developed for medicinal purposes (Table 14.26). All produce a cytotoxic type of injury with none leading to cholestasis. Chloroform, the original haloakane anaesthetic, has long since been abandoned, but remains an important experimental hepatotoxin, as does carbon tetrachloride, trichlorethylene, vinyl ether and tribromoethanol.[1,285] Halothane, introduced in the 1950s as a safer, non-explosive alternative to ether and other agents in use at the time, is a haloakane compound that produced a well-described but rare syndrome of acute hepatotoxicity, usually following a known or inadvertent repeat exposure.[538,539] The anaesthetics that followed (methoxyflurane, enflurane, isoflurane) have all been implicated as a cause of similar injury, albeit much less commonly than halothane, with only a few instances reported for the newest agents, sevoflurane and desflurane.[540,541] The lower incidence of hepatic injury seen with each of these newer anesthetics relates to their proportionally lower degree of metabolism.[542,543] In the USA, halothane is rarely used today, but continues to be employed in other countries.[544,545] It remains an important agent elucidating immunologic-mediated liver injury, with much seminal work having been focused on the production of trifluoroacetyl components that act as in the history of haptens.[57]

Halothane-induced liver injury

Although the retrospective National Halothane Study, which was published in 1966, is often cited as the basis for exonerating halothane as a cause of hepatotoxicity,[546] even when used for patients with underlying hepatobiliary disease, its design (and therefore its conclusions) has been criticized as being seriously flawed.[1] Nearly 1000 cases were reported from around the world during the 1960s and 1970s[538,547–553] and what emerges is a fairly uniform clinical syndrome of postoperative fever, eosinophilia, jaundice and hepatic necrosis with a high case-fatality rate occurring a few days or weeks after anaesthesia, usually after repeat exposure to halothane.[1] Despite such convincing evidence, acceptance of halothane as the cause of hepatic injury came slowly, especially among anaesthesiologists, and even today, some continue to regard 'halothane hepatitis' as a controversial entity.[554] However, given the sizeable database describing a reproducible clinical syndrome, the presence of antibodies suspected in the pathogenesis of the injury, and observations from deliberate or inadvertent rechallenge, it is difficult, if not impossible, to ignore a causal relationship.[1,43] Rare cases of halothane-induced liver injury have occurred after workplace exposure among anaesthesiologists, surgeons, nurses, and laboratory staff, and after halothane

Table 14.26 Hepatotoxic potential of general anaesthetics

Hepatotoxicity	Agents	Lesion	
		Steatosis	Necrosis
I. Intrinsic hepatotoxins	Chloroform	+	PV
	Trichlorethylene	+	PV
	Vinyl ether	−	PV
	Tribromoethyl alcohol	−	PV
II. Agents hepatotoxic only as idiosyncratic reactions	Halothane	−	PV, M
	Methoxyflurane	−	PV, M, D
	Fluroxene	−	PV, M, D
	Enflurane	−	PV, M, D
	Isoflurane	+	PV
	Desflurane	−	D
	Sevoflurane	−	D
II. Agents that seem virtually free of potential for significant hepatic injury in man	Cyclopropane	−	−
	Ether	−	−
	Nitrous oxide	−	−

PV = perivenular (acinar zone 3); M = massive; D = diffuse and hepatitis-like; + = variable and usually slight; − = no injury

sniffing for 'recreational' use. In this situation antibodies can be demonstrated, indicating prior exposure.[60,555,556]

Two types of postoperative liver injury have been associated with halothane. A *minor form* of injury is seen in 10–30% of patients who develop mild asymptomatic elevations in the serum ALT values between the first and tenth postoperative day, the risk being higher after a second (or more) exposure to halothane than with subsequent use of agents like enflurane, isoflurane, and desflurane.[557,558] There is no evidence of immune activation in these patients[559] or in animal models.[560] The *major form* of halothane-induced hepatotoxicity is a rare, dose-independent severe hepatic drug reaction with elements of immunoallergy and metabolic idiosyncrasy. After an initial exposure to halothane, the frequency is low, estimated to be about one per 10 000 exposed persons,[561] but increases to about one per 1000 after two or more exposures, especially when the repeat anesthesia occurred within a few weeks.[562,563] Typically, zone 3 necrosis is seen histologically,[564] and the case-fatality rate ranged between 14% and 71% in the pre-liver transplant era.[1]

Clinical and laboratory features

Classical halothane hepatitis presents as a hypersensitivity reaction with delayed postoperative fever (5 to 14 days after anesthesia), accompanied by rash, eosinophilia and jaundice, which is usually preceded or accompanied by symptoms of hepatitis.[1] The time interval is significantly shortened with repeat exposures. Severe hepatocellular necrosis is accompanied by serum ALT levels typically exceeding 1000 U/L and sometimes much higher. The serum bilirubin level is increased according to severity, and the prothrombin time/INR is prolonged in severe cases. In liver failure, hypoglycemia and metabolic acidosis occur, and in the terminal phase, the serum ALT level decreases as

a result of impaired hepatic protein synthesis and loss of hepatic parenchyma. Renal failure may develop as part of the hepatorenal syndrome, but acute tubular necrosis may result from a nephrotoxic effect of halothane, as has been even better documented for methoxyflurane (see below).

Risk factors associated with halothane hepatitis

Susceptibility to halothane hepatitis has been associated with a number of host-related factors.[1] The reaction is rare but well-described in childhood[565] with estimates of patients under the age of 10 representing only 3% of the total, and cases occurring under the age of 30 being recorded in only 7% of a Swedish series.[549] It tends to be more severe in individuals over the age of 40 years. Two thirds of cases have been in women, and repeated exposure to halothane (especially within just a few weeks or months) is a feature documented in as many as 90% of cases.[1] The time between exposures has been reported to be as long as 28 years.[566] After repeat exposure, the onset of hepatitis is earlier, and more severe. Obesity is another risk factor, possibly related to increased storage of halothane in body fat.[560] The induction of P450 enzymes (especially CYP 2E1) has been produced experimentally with Phenobarbital,[567] alcohol,[568] and isoniazid.[569] In contrast to Phenobarbital, other anticonvulsants have differing effects on halothane, with valproate inhibiting and phenytoin having no specific effect on halothane hepatotoxicity.[570] Inhibition of CYP 2E1 by single-dose disulfiram has been suggested as a possible means of preventing halothane hepatitis by preventing the production of the metabolite responsible for its neoantigen formation.[571,572]

A genetic predisposition to halothane-induced liver injury is evident in guinea pigs,[560] and there are data in humans suggesting a familial predisposition, based on several closely related family members, all of whom experienced halothane hepatitis.[573] Njoku et al.[60] investigated the presence of serum antibodies to volatile anesthetics in paediatric anaesthestiologists. Much like halothane-induced hepatitis patients, they were found to have higher levels of serum autoantibodies to CYP2E1 and to endoplasmic reticulum protein (ERp58) compared to general anaesthesiologists and to controls who had never been exposed to inhalational anaesthetics. Female anaesthesiologists had higher levels than their male counterparts, although only one female paediatric anaesthesiologist developed liver injury out of a total of 158 anaesthesiologists in the study. The authors concluded that the autoantibodies in serum appear to only rarely have a pathologic role. Although much interest has surrounded use of an antibody test[574] there is no readily available diagnostic test for halothane hepatitis.[1,541]

Liver histology

The hepatic injury is cytotoxic, comprising necrosis and steatosis. There are some differences in the literature regarding the type of necrosis. Massive necrosis, zonal necrosis, or diffuse hepatitis-like degeneration and necrosis have each been reported. It is our view that perivenular zone necrosis, resembling that of CCl_4 as described by Morgenstern et al.[575] and Peters et al.[576] is the most characteristic lesion, particularly in patients whose prior exposure was recent (Fig. 14.4). Even in cases which are described as massive necrosis, there is often a remnant of residual tissue in the periportal zone suggesting that the lesion is severe zonal rather than massive necrosis. In a study of 77 cases of halothane hepatitis reviewed by the Armed Forces Institute of Pathology,[564] massive or submassive necrosis involving zone 3 was present in all autopsy specimens, while biopsy material revealed a broader range of injury from spotty necrosis in about one-third of cases and zone 3 necrosis in two-thirds. Uncommonly, instances of periportal necrosis have been seen. Sections obtained by biopsy in mild or moderately severe illness, however, may reveal diffuse spotty necrosis, apoptotic bodies and mononuclear infiltration, changes that may be indistinguishable from those of viral hepatitis. Even in moderately severe injury, however, biopsy sections usually show zonal injury (Fig. 14.4). Furthermore, the sharp demarcation of the areas of necrosis in halothane injury is an infrequent feature of fatal cases of viral hepatitis. In general, inflammatory infiltration is less prominent in halothane-induced injury than in viral hepatitis, although the liver from some patients may show a prominent, eosinophilic inflammatory response. Granulomatous inflammation is also described.[577,578]

Pathogenesis

Halothane injury appears to occur by one or more of three potential mechanisms; immunologically-mediated, production of hepatotoxic metabolites, and halothane-associated hypoxia, in decreasing order of importance.[1] Evidence for the role of hypersensitivity is found in the increased susceptibility and shortened latency after repeat exposure, the hallmark symptoms and signs of drug allergy (fever, rash, eosinophilia and granuloma formation), and the demon-

stration of neoantigens and antibodies. Halothane oxidation yields trifluoroacetylchloride that acts on hepatocyte proteins to produce neoantigen formation responsible for the major form of injury. In contrast, reductive pathways produce free radicals that can act as reactive metabolites that may have a role in causing minor injury. A unifying hypothesis set forth by Zimmerman[1] suggests that halothane injury is most likely the result of immunological enhancement of perivenular necrosis produced by the reductive metabolite(s). Accordingly, the hepatotoxic potential of halothane depends on the susceptibility of the patient and factors that promote production of hepatotoxic or immunogenic metabolites.[1]

Course and outcome

Mortality rates were high in early series, although with the advent of liver transplantation, many patients have been treated successfully.[544] When spontaneous recovery occurs, symptoms usually resolve within 5 to 14 days, and recovery is usually complete within several weeks.[1,579] While an immunological mechanism has been invoked in the pathogenesis of halothane hepatitis,[580,581] immunosuppressive agents have only rarely been reported to successfully alter the outcome.[582] A few reports have implicated halothane as the cause of chronic hepatitis,[583,584,585] but it is unclear whether these are cases of repeated halothane exposure with continuing or intermittent liver injury, or cases of chronic hepatitis attributable to other aetiologies and exacerbated by surgery and anaesthesia. For example, autoimmune hepatitis seems more likely to have been the cause in the case reported by Kronberg et al.[584]

Adverse prognostic factors include older age (>40 years), obesity, severe coagulopathy, bilirubin >20 mg/dL, and a shorter interval to the onset of jaundice.[1,548] As many as two thirds of cases occurred in persons with a history of previous reactions to halothane, and the majority of cases were associated with repeated use of halothane within 28 days, especially in obese, middle-aged women.[548] Halothane-induced liver disease might have been prevented in many reported cases had greater attention been paid to the previous anesthetic history and adherence to safety guidelines.[586] Because halothane may leach out of the tubing of anaesthetic devices, prevention of recurrence in sensitized patients requires that the equipment used for anaesthesia should never have been exposed to halothane. Cross-sensitivity between halothane and other haloalkane anesthetics is best documented for methoxyflurane, an agent that is no longer in use. Cross-reactivity also was reported with enflurane and possibly for isoflurane, as described later, but has not been reported for desflurane and sevoflurane (see below).

Other anaesthetic agents associated with hepatic injury

The likelihood that individual haloalkane anesthetics will cause liver injury appears to be related to the extent to which they are metabolized by hepatic CYP enzymes: 20–30% for halothane, >30% for methoxyflurane, 2% for enflurane, 1% for sevoflurane, and 0.2% or less for isoflurane and desflurane.[541,543] Likewise, the extent of acylation of hepatic proteins in rats exposed to anaesthetic concentrations of these agents for 8 hours was greatest for halothane, followed by enflurane, isoflurane, and desflurane.[541] Accordingly, the estimated frequency of hepatitis from these newer agents is much less than that for halothane (Table 14.27).

Methoxyflurane caused hepatotoxicity similar to halothane hepatitis, with cross-sensitivity to halothane and enflurane and a high frequency of nephrotoxicity that led to its withdrawal.[264] The necrosis of methoxyflurane jaundice is also usually in perivenular, although it may be massive. The renal lesion apparently results from the toxic effects on the renal tubule of fluoride liberated from the methoxyflurane.[587]

Enflurane caused a clinical syndrome similar to that for halothane, with the onset of fever within 3 days and jaundice in 3 to 19 days after anesthesia,[588] although the estimated incidence of enflurane-induced liver injury is much lower, in the order of 1 in 800 000 exposed patients.[589] The usual lesion is also perivenular necrosis, and the clinical and biochemical features resemble those of halothane injury. While the causality of many of the cases of enflurane hepatotoxicity was challenged,[590] previous exposure to either enflurane or halothane in two-thirds of patients, and cases with a documented positive rechallenge confirmed the likelihood that enflurane was indeed the cause.[1,540,588]

Despite its very low rate of metabolism,[542] numerous instances of **isoflurane**-associated liver injury have been reported[591–602] since it was introduced in the 1980s. While an FDA Advisory Committee concluded that no association between isoflurane and severe hepatotoxicity could be proven at a 1986 meeting,[592] subsequent reports in which serious and fatal hepatotoxicity were described after repeated exposure to isoflurane in the absence of other potential causes of liver injury,[593,594,597–599] or where isoflurane had been administered after possible previous sensitization by halothane[593,597–599] or enflurane[595] demonstrated that isoflurane was the likely cause. In one instance, cross sensitivity was suspected 22 years after an initial exposure to enflurane.[599] Trifluoroacetylated liver proteins have been detected in patients with suspected isoflurane liver toxicity,[594,600] although their presence does not confirm isoflurane as the cause.[603] As no antibodies had been demonstrated in rats, consistent with the very small degree to which the drug is metabolized (<0.2%),[542] isoflurane should be regarded as a possible, but rare, idiopathic hepatotoxin, whose pathogenic mechanism remains largely undefined.

The newest haloalkane anesthetics, **desflurane** and **sevoflurane,** appear to be essentially free of adverse hepatic effects. Desflurane undergoes minimal biotransformation compared to isoflurane[604] and was not associated with the development of TFA antibodies in exposed rats.[542] Only isolated reports have noted an association between liver injury and desflurane anesthesia;[605–607] one of which reportedly developed after a third anaesthetic exposure with desflurane following prior isoflurane and sevoflurane within a one year time frame.[607] In contrast to the rarity of liver injury, desflurane has been associated with cardiovascular toxicity and delayed malignant hyperthermia.[608,609] The biotransformation of sevoflurane is also minimal in in vivo models,[610] and only rare reports have implicated this agent in postoperative hepatic dysfunction, despite its extensive use in Japan, although they have not been well documented.[611,612]

Anaesthetics that are apparently devoid of any significant hepatotoxic potential include ether, nitrous oxide, and cyclopropane, owing to their lack of halogen moieties.[1]

Psychotropic and anticonvulsant drugs

There is an apparent correlation between the form of injury and the therapeutic category of the drugs in this group (Table 14.28). For example, chlorpromazine and other neuroleptics produce mainly cholestatic injury. Monoamine oxidase inhibitor hydrazine antidepressants and most anticonvulsants cause cytotoxic injury, although phenobarbital and carbamazepine cause either cholestatic or cytotoxic injury. The tricyclic antidepressants cause injury that appears to be more variable in character, both hepatocellular and cholestatic injury having been reported.[1] The mechanism for hepatic injury often relates to the fact that these agents are highly fat-soluble and undergo transformation and metabolism in the liver that may lead to hepatic dysfunction or toxic metabolites.[613] Representative examples from each drug class are described in more detail below.

Table 14.27	Metabolism and incidence of hepatotoxicity with anaesthetics			
Agent	**% metabolized**	**Incidence**	**Cross-sensitivity**	**Other features**
Halothane	20–30%	1–1.5 per 1000*	yes	
Methoxyflurane	>30%	low	yes	nephrotoxicity
Enflurane	2%	1 in 800 000	yes	similar to halothane
Isoflurane	0.2%	very rare	yes	similar to halothane
Desflurane	<0.2%	isolated reports	yes?	cardiac toxicity, malignant hyperthermia
Sevoflurane	minimal	rare reports	?	—

* risk after multiple exposures; risk after first exposure = 0.3–1.5 per 10 000; ? = uncertain

Antipsychotic drugs

Chlorpromazine (Thorazine)

Jaundice occurs in approximately 1% of all patients who receive this drug, usually after just a few weeks of exposure.[1] A period of 1–5 weeks of drug administration precedes the development of jaundice in 90% of cases[614] and re-administration of small doses leads to prompt recurrence of hepatic dysfunction or jaundice in approximately half of the patients.[614] The hepatic injury is primarily cholestatic, of the hepatocanalicular type. Severe pruritis is common with eosinophilia in up to 40% and rarely agranulocytosis and thrombocytopenia. Bilirubin levels are increased as much as 15 mg/dL with alkaline phosphatase 10–12× elevated, aminotransferases as high as 8-fold and cholesterol between 300–800 mg/dL. Asymptomatic elevations of liver enzymes that do not progress to serious injury occur in as many as 50% of patients.[30]

From a review of cases examined at the AFIP, the histopathological spectrum of injury includes prominent zone 3 bilirubinostasis in most patients with only mild hepatocyte degeneration and necrosis and occasional apoptotic bodies.[61] The inflammatory response, mainly in portal areas, is usually rich in eosinophils, and is prominent only early in the course of the illness[61] (Fig. 14.16). A small proportion of patients develop hepatic necrosis and high aminotransferase levels, as well as prominent cholestasis and high alkaline phosphatase levels (mixed-jaundice).[1]

The prognosis of chlorpromazine jaundice is generally good. Two-thirds of the patients recover within 8 weeks.[61] Most of the remainder require 2–12 months to return to normal, although there have been a number of reported instances of a prolonged cholestatic syndrome, and with some patients, histological features that have resembled those of primary biliary cirrhosis (vanishing bile duct syndrome).[30,61,615–617] Chronic cholestasis also has been attributed to **prochlorperazine**[61,156,618] and **haloperidol**.[61,109,619]

The clinical features of chlorpromazine-induced jaundice and the prompt recurrence of hepatic abnormality in many of those given a challenge dose suggest that hypersensitivity is responsible for the hepatic injury,[614] with an immunological reaction aimed at one or more of the multiple (>170) chlorpromazine metabolites. Intrinsic toxicity may also occur. The mechanism of cholestasis relates to the drug's ability to impair or disrupt several membrane and bile flow systems.[620,621] Impaired sulphoxidation, HLA DR6 pheno-

Table 14.28	Hepatic injury produced by psychotropic drugs			
Drug	**Type of injury(a)**		**Drug**	**Type of injury(b)**
I. Neuroleptics			II. Antidepressants	
A. Phenothiazines			A. Monoamine oxidase inhibitors(e)	
Chlorpromazine			1. Hydrazine derivatives	
Carphenazine			Iproniazid	
Cyamamazine	Cholestatic or mixed		Isocarboxazide	
Fluphenazine			Nialamide	
Laevopromazine			Phenelzine	Hepatocellular
Mepazine			Pheniprazine	
Perphenazine			Phenoxypropazine	
Prochlorperazine			Privaloylbenzylhydrazine	
Promazine©			Mebanazine	
Thioridazine			2. Non-hydrazine derivatives	
Trifluperazine			Tranylcypromine(d)	Hepatocellular
B. Thioxanthenes(d)			Toloxatone	Hepatocellular
Chlorprothixene				
Chlorpenthixol	Cholestatic or		B. Tricyclic antidepressants	
Thiothixene	hepatocellular		Amoxapine	
C. Butyrophenones			Amineptine	
Haloperidol	Cholestatic or		Amitryptiline	
	hepatocellular		Nortryptiline	
			Protryptiline	
			Clomipramine	Cholestatic or hepatocellular
			Doxepine	
			Imipraminer	
			Iprindole	
			Nitroxazepine	
			Trimipramine	
			Tianeptine	
			C. Tetracyclic antidepressants	
			Mainserine	Cholestatic
			Maprotiline	Cholestatic

Table 14.28 Hepatic injury produced by psychotropic drugs—cont'd

Drug	Type of injury[a]	Drug	Type of injury[b]
D. Anxiolytics		**D. Other antidepressants**	
Benzodiazepines[d]		Nomifensine	Hepatocellular
Alprazolam		Trazodone	Hepatocellular or cholestatic
Chlordiazepoxide[f]	Cholestatic or	Femoxitene	Hepatocellular
Diazepam	hepatocellular	Viloxazine	Hepatocellular
Flurazepam		Bupropion	Hepatocellular (rare)
Triazolam		Fluoxetine	Hepatocellular
		Paroxetine	Hepatocellular
		Sertraline	Hepatocellular
		Sulpiride	Cholestatic
E. Other antipsychotics			
Risperidone	Hepatocellular		
Clozapine	H-epatocellular or cholestatic		
Loxapine	Hepatocellular		
F. Anticonvulsants			
Carbamazepine	Hepatocellular, cholestatic, or mixed		
Mephenytoin	Hepatocellular, mixed		
Paramethadione	Hepatocellular, mixed		
Phenacemide	Hepatocellular, mixed		
Phenytoin	Hepatocellular, mixed		
Phenobarbital	Hepatocellular, mixed or cholestatic		
Phethenylate sodium	Hepatocellular		
Progabide	Hepatocellular		
Trimethadione	Hepatocellular, mixed		
Valproic acid	Hepatocellular		
Lamotrigine	Hepatocellular		

(a,b) Cholestatic injury-consists mainly of bilirubin casts in canaliculi, usually with portal inflammatory infiltrate and with or without mild parenchyma injury; hepatocellular injury—consists mainly of necrosis with or without inflammation; mixed injury—consists of both hepatocellular and cholestatic injury. See Table 14.19 for biochemical features
(c) Very few reports of injury to our knowledge
(d) Too few cases for clear picture
(e) Use of all in this group, except isocarboxazide and phenelzine, has been abandoned
(f) Rare instances of hepatocellular injury in recipients of chlordiazepoxide plus other drugs

type and chronic alcoholism are among the factors that may enhance susceptibility for hepatotoxicity.[622,623,624]

Risperidone

This benzisoxazole derivative has been occasionally associated with abnormal liver function tests, steatosis and steatohepatitis.[625-628] **Clozapine** causes elevated transaminases in up to 31% of recipients that usually resolve within 3–5 months.[629] Histologically, hepatocellular injury, cholestasis and fulminant hepatic failure have been reported.[630]

Antidepressants

Monoamine oxidase inhibitors

Iproniazid (Marsilid) and other hydrazine derivatives can produce severe hepatic injury in susceptible individuals, and their use has been largely abandoned.[1] Iproniazid was the earliest of these drugs and it was estimated by Rosenblum et al.[631] to produce jaundice in approximately 1% of recipients. The clinical, biochemical and histological features indicated hepatocellular injury with a case fatality rate of

about 15%. The liver showed extensive, diffuse parenchymal degeneration and necrosis; in some cases, bilirubin casts were prominent.[631] In some instances there was a predominant perivenular necrosis. Where massive necrosis developed, the lesion resembled that of fatal viral hepatitis. The inflammatory response was usually sparse. The suggestion of Rosenblum et al.[631] that the mechanism for the hepatic injury is the production of hepatotoxic metabolites of iproniazid found support in the experimental studies of Mitchell and Jollow.[632] Presumably, the responsible metabolites are formed or accumulate in greater amounts in susceptible persons. The hepatic injury produced by other antidepressant hydrazides (e.g. **phenelzine, isocarboxazid**) are less hepatotoxic than was iproniazid. Of the nonhydrazine antidepressants, **tranylcypromine** (Parnate)[633] has a low incidence of hepatocellular injury.

Tricyclic antidepressants

The injury induced by the tricyclic group may be cholestatic or cytotoxic.[1,634] **Amitiptyline** and **Imipramine** may cause severe cholestatic hepatitis with ductopenia.[634] **Sulpride,** a dibenzodiazepine antidepressant is also reported to trigger a symptomatic primary biliary cirrhosis-like syndrome.[635]

SSRIs

Among the serotonin reuptake inhibitors, **fluoxetine** has led to asymptomatic increases in liver enzymes in 0.5% of recipients, as well as to several instances of acute hepatitis.[636-639] **Paroxetine** also has been associated with reversible hepatitis.[640] Reports of reversible hepatic injury with **sertaline** and **venlafaxine** also have appeared.[641-644] To date, **duloxetine** and **escitalapram** appear to be free of hepatic injury, although a case of acute hepatitis has been reported with **citalopram**.[645]

Other antidepressants

Nefazodone (Serzone) is a phenylpiperazine derivative that inhibits the presynaptic uptake of serotonin. While structurally similar to **trazodone**, which is associated with mild reversible hepatotoxicity,[646] nefazodone injury is more severe, with several instances of fulminant hepatic failure having been reported,[647] and it was subsequently withdrawn from use in Europe[648] and its use has been severely restricted elsewhere.[647-651] The mechanism appears to be metabolic idiosyncrasy, possibly due to reactive quinone-imine metabolites,[652] with injury occurring 6–28 weeks after the start of therapy.[649-651]

Reports of hepatic injury from **buproprion** are scant.[653] Alvaro et al.[654] reported acute reversible cholestatic hepatitis with positive antinuclear antibodies and bile duct injury on biopsy. One case reporting extremely high aminotransferases suggested ischaemic hepatitis.[655] Reversible cholestatic Injury has been reported with **mirtazapine**.[656]

Anticonvulsants (Table 14.28)

Several anticonvulsant agents have led to toxic hepatitis.[1,657] Mephenytoin and phenacemide are two agents that were abandoned due to a high incidence of liver failure.[1] The drugs in current use all have been associated with instances of severe injury, although the frequent use of multiple drugs in patients whose convulsions are difficult to control, complicates incrimination of individual drugs. Nevertheless, the role of a number of them in producing hepatic injury and the character of the injury has become quite clear.[658]

Phenobarbital

This has been employed as an anticonvulsant since 1918, as well as an anxiolytic agent, and has been incriminated in relatively few cases of hepatic injury despite its widespread use.[1] More frequently, as an enzyme inducer, it leads to increases to asymptomatic elevations in gamma-GT.[659] Both hepatocellular and cholestatic injury has been described, usually accompanied by features of hypersensitivity.[660] Massive hepatic necrosis was reported in a 2-year-old child after administration of phenobarbital.[661]

Phenytoin

While hundreds of cases of hepatic injury have been reported, the incidence of jaundice in recipients of phenytoin (diphenylhydantoin) appears to be low.[1,657] However, the mortality rate of the full-blown syndrome of generalized hypersensitivity and jaundice appears to be approximately 30%.[1,662-666] The hepatic damage is predominantly cytotoxic, although cholestasis may be prominent and warrants designation of the injury as mixed-hepatocellular.[1] It is generally seen after a few days to 2 months with ALT levels up to 100× normal, and lesser elevations of alkaline phosphatase. Less dramatic hepatic injury also may be caused by phenytoin as reflected by abnormal levels of transaminases recorded in about 20% of patients taking the drug.[1] Granulomatous inflammation has been described.[82,101,664] Alkaline phosphatase levels are elevated in almost all patients taking the drug, even in the absence of other evidence of hepatic injury. These elevations reflect the relative deficiency of vitamin D secondary to its enhanced turnover due to induction of P-450 by phenytoin. The regular elevation of aGT levels also reflect the induction.[1]

The liver shows diffuse degeneration, multifocal or even massive necrosis and multiple apoptotic bodies accompanied by a rich inflammatory response.[82] The latter often includes clusters of eosinophils or lymphocytes, and at times focal aggregates of hyperplastic Kupffer cells having a granulomatoid appearance.[82] The hepatic lesion, with lymphocyte 'beading' in sinusoids, granulomatoid changes and frequent hepatocyte mitoses, may resemble that of infectious mononucleosis (Figs 14.6, 7, 9).[82,263] Indeed, in some instances, severe generalized hypersensitivity, rather than hepatic failure per se, appears responsible for the devastating clinical syndrome. A systemic granulomatous vasculitis involving the liver, spleen and kidneys,[666] as well as 'periarteritis nodosa' associated with exfoliative dermatitis,[667] have been reported. In addition, lymphadenopathy with a spectrum of changes from benign to malignant lymphomas,[668] and bone marrow injury[669] may accompany the liver damage.

The symptoms, signs and laboratory features offer strong clinical support for the view that the hepatic injury is a manifestation of drug hypersensitivity.[662,663] Indeed, the 'pseudomononucleosis' syndrome of lymphadenopathy, lymphocytosis and circulating atypical lymphocytes, resembling serum sickness[1,82,665] has been termed the anticonvulsant (antiepileptic) hypersensitivity syndrome (AHS) by Shear and colleagues[62,63,670,671] and others.[672,673] Almost all patients develop a generalized rash that may become exfoliative. The immunological reaction is possibly triggered by an active metabolite of phenytoin which susceptible persons are unable to metabolize normally.[62,673] The susceptibility is apparently genetic; possibly a deficiency of arene oxide.[62,671]

Carbamazepine

This has led to several forms of hepatic injury, often as part of a hypersensitivity syndrome within 4 weeks of exposure. Among the estimated 250 cases of overt hepatic injury attributed to this drug, cholestatic and hepatocellular injury as well as hepatic granulomas have all been reported.[674-678] Fatal reactions are reported in 10–15% of cases. Cholestatic injury may fail to subside for many months or even lead to chronic cholestasis with disappearance of intrahepatic bile ducts (VBDS).[678,679] Multiple hepatocellular adenomas occurred in a patient who had been treated with carbamazepine for 14 years.[680]

Neonatal cholestasis from fetal exposure during pregnancy and breast-feeding has been reported.[681]

The morphological changes have been hepatocellular in about 25% of cases, cholestatic in about 30%, and mixed in the rest. Granulomatous hepatitis is present in up to 75% of biopsy specimens.[682] A few of the hepatocellular cases have had massive necrosis while others have shown lesser degrees of necrosis. Some of the cholestatic cases have shown prominent cholangitis[677] and, as noted earlier, chronic cholestasis with disappearance of bile ducts has been recorded.[678,679] Cross-reactions between phenytoin and carbamazepine are to be expected, since the metabolic defect responsible for susceptibility to the former drug, also enhances susceptibility to the latter.[683] Hypersensitivity is the likely mechanism, with susceptibility related to one or more genetic polymorphisms.[670,671]

Valproic acid

This has led to severe hepatic injury; at least 100 fatal cases and 25 recovered ones have been reported.[122,123,684,685] The liver has shown microvesicular steatosis, necrosis or both, as well as cirrhosis in some instances (Fig. 14.36).[122] The microvesicular steatosis seems clearly ascribable to the valproic acid, since a similar lesion can be produced in experimental animals by the agent,[686,687] but the role of valproic acid and other drugs taken concurrently, in the production of the necrosis, is not clear.[122] The syndrome develops after 3 to 6 months of therapy; it is characterized by somnolence, hyperammonaemia, coma and coagulopathy. The injury appears to be due to a metabolite of the drug. Children, and particularly infants below the age of 2, are more susceptible than adults.[122,685,688] Hepatic injury is often associated with nausea, vomiting, abdominal pain and increased seizure activity, including status epilepticus in 40–60%.[658,685] The development of carnitine deficiency after long-term use has been suggested as a possible contributing mechanism.[689] A novel metabolite, valproyldephosphoCoA, has been proposed as a possible cause of its inibition of fatty acid beta oxidation.[690]

Felbamate

This has been incriminated in a number of instances of hepatic injury. The injury has been hepatocellular with some cases of fulminant hepatic failure.[691–693] In animals, a reactive metabolite, 2-phenylpropenal, is a potent immunogen.[694] A high incidence of aplastic anaemia has severely limited its use.[695]

Lamotrigene

This is a phenyltriazine agent that causes skin rashes in 3–10%, often in association with fever and eosinophilia as part of the anticonvulsant hypersensitivity syndrome,[696] but infrequently leads to instances of hepatic injury.[697,698] A few reports of fulminant hepatic failure, some fatal, have been

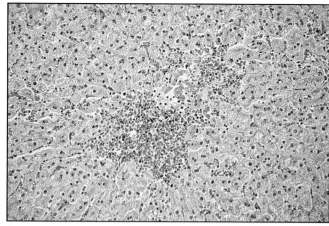

A

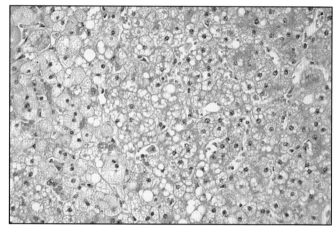

B

Fig. 14.36 • Valproate-associated injury. **(A)** Perivenular zone necrosis. Preserved liver cells show microvesicular steatosis. H&E. **(B)** Higher magnification of steatosis in case illustrated in (A).

reported.[699,700] In one fatal case, a subacute course of progressive liver damage was documented in serial liver biopsies, with an initial biopsy showing approximately 50% hepatocyte necrosis. At autopsy massive hepatic necrosis with extensive bile duct proliferation was seen.[700] A possible delayed hypersensitivity mechanism was postulated.

Drugs used in other neurological disorders

Pemoline, an adrenergic agent, was used to treat attention deficit disorder and narcolepsy, but was withdrawn after being implicated in dozens of cases of acute, sometimes fatal, hepatic injury possibly mediated by toxic metabolites.[701,702] Chronic autoimmune injury was also reported suggesting immunologic mechanisms.[703]

Tacrine, an acetylcholinesterase inhibitor used for the treatment of Alzheimer's disease, has significant hepatotoxic potential. In the doses employed, it has been found to lead to a 40–50% incidence of elevated aminotransferase levels, about half of which have been more than three-fold the normal.[704] About 2% of patients have ALT elevations of 20-fold or higher, but the drug was rarely associated with liver failure.[704,705] Mechanisms underlying tacrine-induced hepatotoxicity initially focused on possible P450-mediated reactive metabolites;[706,707] but more recently have evaluated alterations in hypoxia-reoxygenation mediated by the sympathetic nervous system;[708] alterations in hepatocytes membrane fluidity;[709] and possible (genetic?) deficiencies in glutathione-S-transferase.[710] **Levodopa** has led to elevated liver enzymes, but cases of overt hepatic injury are extremely rare.[1] **Riluzole,** an antiglutamate agent used in the treatment of amyotrophic lateral sclerosis, has been implicated in three instances of acute hepatitis that all resolved after withdrawal of the drug.[711,712] **Lergotrile mesylate,** a dopaminergic ergot derivative with apparent therapeutic promise in Parkinson's disease was abandoned because of a 50% incidence of abnormal alanine aminotransferase levels.[1] The drug led to spotty necrosis and to distinctive mitochondrial changes ultrastructurally.[713] **Tolcapone,** a catechol-O-methyl transferase (COMT) inhibitor used to enhance the effect of levodopa for the treatment of Parkinson's disease, has led to several instances of severe hepatocellular injury, including fulminant liver failure.[714–717] As a result, it was withdrawn from use in Europe,[718] its use is severely restricted elsewhere.[718,719] and it has been largely replaced by newer COMT inhibitors such as **entacapone** that does not require LFT monitoring.[720] Tolcapone is lipophilic and can cause mitochondrial injury. Swelling, reduced matrix density and loss of cristae has been described,[721] similar to changes seen with valproate.[722]

Anti-inflammatory agents and other drugs used in musculoskeletal disease

As a class, the non-steroidal anti-inflammatory drugs (NSAIDs) are a leading cause of DILD[723,724] (Table 14.29). In Denmark, NSAID-related liver injury accounted for 9% of all drug-induced injury reports between 1978 and 1987.[6] Indeed, the past few decades have seen a sharp focus on the hepatic injury induced by the NSAIDS, generated most recently by the fatal hepatic injury noted in patients taking bromfenac.[27]

Numerous other NSAIDs have been developed or introduced into clinical practice only to be abandoned during premarket evaluation or after approval due to serious liver injury.[1,89,723] For example, **Cinchophen,** once used to treat rheumatic disease and gout, fell into disuse a half-century ago[89,725] but remains of interest as the first agent reported to produce idiosyncratic hepatic injury and as the prototype of drug-induced hepatocellular jaundice.[1] Indeed, reports of cinchophen-associated hepatic injury continued to appear.[726] The reported mortality was high, approaching 50%.[89,725] Fatal cases showed acute or subacute hepatic necrosis.[89] In those with a prolonged course the liver was described as showing a 'toxic cirrhosis'.[727] However, it was not until the withdrawal of benoxaprofen in 1982 because of reports of fatal jaundice in the UK that attention was intensively focused on NSAIDs as a group, culminating in the FDA Arthritis Drug Advisory Committeee concluding that hepatic injury should be considered a class effect , with a designation that elevations in AST and ALT occur in 5–15%.[728] This uniform designation of hepatic injury obscures the many individual differences found within and among

the various NSAID classes with regard to the character and mechanism of injury.[1,723,724] Some of the drugs produce cytotoxic injury, while others lead to cholestasis (Table 14.27). The biochemical changes seen with NSAID-associated liver injury reflect the histological pattern of damage.

It should be remembered that the underlying rheumatic disease being treated also may adversely affect the liver, leading at times to diagnostic confusion.[724] Hepatic involvement in systemic lupus erythematosis is present in up to 20% with twofold elevations in liver-associated enzymes. Biochemical abnormalities are also seen in Felty syndrome, Sjögrens syndrome, progressive systemic sclerosis, polyarteritis nodosa, essential mixed cryoglobulinemia (which may be associated with chronic hepatitis C), polymyalgia rheumatica, Reiters syndrome and occasionally even osteoarthritis.[729,730]

Salicylates

Aspirin (acetylsalicylic acid)

This has been associated with several hundred cases of hepatic injury since the 1970s, although this represented a delay of more than 75 years before its hepatotoxic potential was truly appreciated.[1] Liver damage is primarily hepatocellular with AST/ALT levels elevated 5 to 40 times normal. In general, it is clinically mild and reversible. Bilirubin levels usually remain normal or are only minimally elevated with overt jaundice in fewer than 5% of cases. Liver biopsy characteristically shows areas of focal necrosis with a mild inflammatory response in portal areas. Ultrastructural changes include increased numbers of lysosomes, peroxisomes and mitochondria with dilatation of the smooth and rough endoplasmic reticulum.[731]

Aspirin injury is both dose- and blood concentration-dependent, consistent with intrinsic toxicity. Levels above 15 mg/dl can lead to high aminotransferase levels, hyperbilirubinaemia and biopsy evidence of parenchymal injury in up to 50% of patients.[732] These aspirin levels in the serum are achieved with the full dosage employed to treat rheumatic fever, acute rheumatoid arthritis and systemic lupus erythematosus. The phenomenon appears to depend on the salicylate moiety since it has been observed with aspirin, choline salicylate and sodium salicylate.[723,731] Patients with active juvenile rheumatoid arthritis and active systemic lupus erythematosus seem particularly vulnerable to aspirin-induced injury, but patients with inactive disease and normal subjects may also be affected.[733,734,735] No gender differences have been found, but hypoalbuminaemia appears to enhance susceptibility,[736] as does pre-existing chronic liver disease where more salicylate is free to distribute to the liver.[737,738] The major metabolites of aspirin are salicyluric and sulicylphenolic glucuronide. It has been suggested that these pathways are readily saturated in children, as well as adults, leading to the accumulation of an otherwise minor non-toxic metabolite that may become responsible for hepatic injury. The exact mechanism may involve lipid peroxidation, mitochondrial damage, hydroxyl radical scavenging, or injury to hepatocyte membranes.[723,731]

Table 14.29 Hepatic injury produced by non-steroidal anti-inflammatory drugs (NSAIDs) and other agents used to treat rheumatic and myotonic disease

Agents	Type of injury[a]	Mechanism
Allopurinol	H-Cell or cholestasis, granulomas	hypersensitivity
Benorilate	Zone 3 necrosis	Intrinsic toxicity
Benoxaprofen[c]*	cholestatic jaundice	metabolic idiosyncrasy
Bromfenac*	H-Cell, massive necrosis	metabolic idiosyncrasy
Celecoxib	H-cell (rare)	unknown
Chlorzoxazone	H-Cell	
Cinchophen[c]*	H-Cell necrosis	metabolic idiosyncrasy
Clometacine[c]	autoimmune CH, granulomas, cholestasis	hypersensitivity
Colchicine[d]	steatosis (rare)	high doses
Dantrolene	H-Cell[c] necrosis (severe)	metabolic idiosyncrasy
Diclofenac	acute H-Cell, chronic autoimmune	metabolic idiosyncrasy
Diflunisal	cholestasis, mixed	hypersensitivity?
Droxicam	Cholestasis	hypersensitivity?
Etodolac	H-Cell necrosis	metabolic idiosyncrasy?
Fenbufen*	H-Cell	
Fenclozic acid[b]*	H-Cell	
Fenoprofen[b]	cholestatic jaundice (rare)	hypersensitivity?
Flurbiprofen	H-Cell jaundice (rare)	hypersensitivity?
Gold Preparations	cholestasis or H-Cell	hypersensitivity
Ibufenac[c]*	H-Cell	metabolic Idiosyncrasy
Ibuprofen	H-Cell or mixed (rare), steatosis	hypersensitivity?
Indomethacin	H-Cell necrosis, microvesicular steatosis, cholestasis	metabolic idiosyncrasy
Ketoprofen	H-Cell jaundice (rare)	metabolic idiosyncrasy?
Ketorolac	none reported	
Meclofenamic acid	H-cell (minor)	unknown
Mefenamic acid	H-Cell necrosis (rare)	unknown
Methotrexate	steatosis, fibrosis	dose-, frequency-related
	acute hepatitis	large oncotherapeutic doses
Naproxen	cholestasis or H-Cell	hypersensitivity?
Nimesulide*	H-cell necrosis (severe)	hypersensitivity?
Oxaprozin	H-cell	metabolic idiosyncrasy?
Oxyphenbutazone[e]	H-Cell necrosis, granulomas	hypersensitivity
Paracetamol	H-Cell necrosis	Intrinsic toxicity
Penicillamine	Cholestasis	hypersensitivity
Phenylbutazone[e]*	H-Cell necrosis, steatosis, or cholestasis, granulomas	hypersensitivity or metabolic idiosyncrasy in high doses
Piroxicam[b]	H-Cell necrosis or cholestasis	hypersensitivity
Pirprofen	H-Cell	hypersensitivity?
Probenecid	dose-related jaundice,	Intrinsic toxicity
	rare H-Cell necrosis	metabolic Idiosyncrasy?
Rofecoxib	H-Cell (rare)	unknown
Salicylates	acute H-Cell, Reye syndrome	Intrinsic toxicity
Salsalate	minor H-cell	unkown
Sodium,choline salicylates	minor	hypersensitivity
Sulindac	cholestasis or mixed; H-Cell (25%)	hypersensitivity
Tolmetin[b]	H-Cell jaundice, steatosis	metabolic idiosyncrasy?
Zoxazolamine	H-Cell necrosis (massive)	metabolic idiosyncrasy

after Lewis[723,724]

(a) H-Cell = hepatocellular; choles = cholestatic; CH = chronic hepatitis

(b) Too few cases reported for clear picture

(c) Largely or completely withdrawn from clinical use

(d) Hepatic injury observed mainly in experimental animals

(e) Can cause granulomas

* agent withdrawn due to hepatotoxicity

Epidemiological studies have demonstrated a strong association between aspirin use and Reye syndrome in children with influenza or varicella, although adults can also be affected.[739,740] A striking decline in the incidence of Reye syndrome in the USA paralleled the decrease in aspirin use.[741] The mechanism by which aspirin interacted with the viral illness to produce the microvesicular steatosis associated with Reye syndrome is unclear, although the association might be the result of one of several defects in ammonia metabolism.[742]

Other salicylates

Diflunisal, a diflurophenyl derivative of salicylate, has been associated with hepatic injury. At least one instance of cholestatic[743] and three of mixed-hepatocellular[744] injury have been reported. **Benorylate**, an acetamoniphen ester of acetylsalicylic acid has caused perivenular necrosis.[745] **Salsalate** has caused aminotransferase elevations, but serious liver injury appears unlikely.[746]

Acetic acid derivatives

Ibufenac, which was withdrawn from use, produced abnormal liver function tests in about 30% and jaundice in about 5% of patients.[747] The jaundice was hepatocellular with high transaminase levels. The liver showed necrosis and there were instances of fatal liver disease.[748] A closely related drug, **ibuprofen** (see below), appears to have a much lower incidence of hepatic injury, but cases of severe hepatocellular damage have been reported.[723,749,750,751]

Diclofenac, a widely used NSAID, has been incriminated in more than 250 instances of hepatic injury, occurring with a frequency that appears to exceed that of all other NSAIDs except sulindac.[723,752,753] A study of 180 cases reported to the US Food and Drug Administration[753] found that most have been hepatocellular (zone 3 necrosis) or mixed injury, but cases of intrahepatic cholestasis represent about 8% of the total.[753,754] Granulomas were rarely found , but a few individuals had changes consistent with chronic hepatitis in the available histologic material.[753] A majority of patients present with fatigue anorexia and nausea, half of whom are also jaundiced. A delayed onset of injury (up to 3 months), and a late response to rechallenge suggest metabolic idiosyncrasy, and a reactive metabolite has been postulated.[755–757] Recovery is usually prompt after the drug is withdrawn, but fulminant hepatic failure with a case fatality rate of 8% among icteric cases attests to the severity of the injury.[753] The average age of affected patients is 60 years and women with osteoarthritis appear to be most susceptible. Instances resembling autoimmune hepatitis with positive antinuclear antibodies also have been recorded.[753]

Indomethacin has led to a few instances of jaundice; the injury is usually hepatocellular. Necrosis may be zonal or massive and may be accompanied by microvesicular steatosis.[758–760]

Clometacine, an isomer of indomethacin which has been used mainly in France, has led to a number of instances of acute or chronic hepatocellular injury.[94,761] The cases of chronic injury have resembled autoimmune hepatitis[762] and

have led to cirrhosis in some cases.[763] Immunological idiosyncrasy is the presumed mechanism in most cases.[764]

Sulindac, structurally similar to indomethacin, has been incriminated in more than 100 instances of hepatic injury, mostly cholestatic but some hepatocellular.[765] Circumstances and associated clinical features suggest the mechanism is hypersensitivity, with injury occurring within 4 to 8 weeks of starting the drug. Recovery occurs within 1–2 months, but may be delayed up to 7 months.[766] Case fatality rates of about 5% related to generalized hypersensitivity which can include Stevens–Johnson syndrome.[765] Cholelithiasis with sulindac metabolites identified in one of the intrahepatic stones has been reported,[767] as has pancreatitis,[768] which may contribute to the jaundice that is seen with the drug. While it is reported to have renal-sparing effects compared to other NSAIDs,[769] its use in cirrhosis is not recommended.[724]

Bromfenac, intended for the short-term management of acute pain, led to fatal hepatic necrosis and/or the need for liver transplantation when used for prolonged periods (average of 3 months).[27,770–772] As a result it was withdrawn by its manufacturer in 1998.[724,773] Massive and submassive necrosis was seen histologically.[27] The mechanism was probably metabolic idiosyncrasy, as no hallmarks of hypersensitivity were reported.[724]

Propionic acid derivatives

Benoxaprofen was withdrawn from clinical use in the USA and UK after it was found to lead to a number of instances of a fatal syndrome characterized by cholestatic jaundice and renal failure (Fig. 14.37).[723,774,775] The fatal outcome was curious since cholestatic jaundice rarely leads to death. Accordingly, Prescott et al.[776] suggested that impaired hepatic and renal excretion might have combined to produce lethal blood levels. The half-life of the drug was prolonged in patients over 40 years,[777] possibly contributing to the injury seen almost exclusively in the elderly. Histologically, it produced perivenular cholestasis with characteristic inspissated bile casts.[34] **Naproxen** has lead to instances of hepatocellular injury including cases of massive necrosis.[778,779] It also has led to cases of cholestatic and mixed-jaundice.[724]

A derivative of ibufenac, **ibuprofen** rarely causes hepatic injury.[724] Of interest is a report of reversible ibuprofen-induced hepatotoxicity (manifested by raised aminotransferases) in three patients with chronic hepatitis C,[780] although no corroborating cases have appeared. Instances of cholestatic injury with vanishing bile ducts and chronic cholestasis have been described.[781,782] Laurent et al.[750] reported a case of sub-fulminant hepatitis after ibuprofen overdose that required liver transplantation. An instance of fatal injury with microvesicular steatosis has been attributed to the drug.[751] **Fenbufen**,[783,784] **oxaprozin**,[785] **etodolac**[786] and **ketoprofen**[724] have each been incriminated in instances of hepatic injury, mainly hepatocellular. **Pirprofen** has been involved in at least 14 published cases of hepatocellular injury, four fatal.[787,788] Most of the patients were female and over 60 years of age. The lesion is usually non-zonal necro-

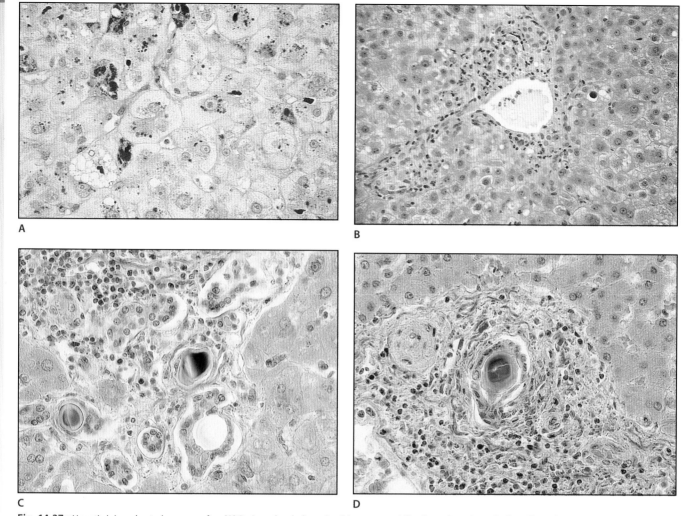

Fig. 14.37 • Hepatic injury due to benoxaprofen. **(A)** Perivenular cholestasis with numerous bile plugs: there is marked swelling of hepatocytes with some cytoplasmic vacuolation; there are mild reactive inflammatory changes with some ceroid-laden macrophages. PAS-diastase. **(B)** Same case as (A); cholestasis was panacinar; note bile plugs in cholangioles and a mild cholangiolitis. H&E. **(C)** and **(D)** Autopsy liver in a further case showing inspissated bile plugs in cholangioles and bile ducts. van Gieson.

sis, accompanied in some cases by microvesicular steatosis. This agent is not available in the USA.

Oxicams

Piroxicam has led to instances of hepatocellular injury, some fatal,[789–791] as well as to cases of cholestasis.[792] It also has been implicated in cases of pancreatitis.[515] Eosinophilia suggests an immunoallergic mechanism.[724] Reports of toxic epidermal necrolysis in association with **Isoxicam** forced its withdrawal from clinical use.[724]

Pyrazolone derivatives

Phenylbutazone was associated with more than 100 cases of hepatic injury, with an incidence of overt hepatotoxicity of 1–5%, and jaundice occurred in 0.25% of recipients prior to the drug being withdrawn from human use.[793] It is still available in veterinary medicine.[794] The mechanism appears to be hypersensitivity.[793] The injury was hepatocellular in at least two-thirds of the patients, with a case-fatality rate of 25% for those with severe necrosis. However, instances of cholestatic jaundice also occurred;[793] some of these have shown granulomas, especially in the portal areas[795] (Fig. 14.11). **Oxyphenbutazone** apparently produces a similar injury, and is also not currently marketed.[724]

Other agents

Shortly after the introduction of **methotrexate** 40 years ago for the treatment of leukaemia, hints that it might be hepatotoxic appeared.[796,797] Subsequently, even more convincing evidence of the hepatotoxicity of this agent came from its use for the treatment of psoriasis where there have been many reports of psoriatic patients who developed cirrhosis, fibrosis or fatty liver.[130,798–800] The likelihood of liver damage seems directly related to duration of therapy and inversely related to the length of the interval between doses.[801,802] Daily small doses at weekly intervals are more likely to lead to liver damage than are larger less frequent doses.[130] The role of cofactors such as age, obesity and alcoholism was stressed in the study of Nyfors and Poulsen.[799] Indeed, it has become increasingly clear that significant hepatic injury is uncommon in the non-drinking, non-obese, non-diabetic patient. The biochemical changes produced by small weekly doses of methotrexate taken for psoriatic and rheumatoid arthritis are usually mild and may be misleading in relation to the hepatic damage.[130,803] Liver enzymes do not appear to correlate with methotrexate blood levels or with clinical efficacy.[804]

Histological changes include steatosis, ballooning degeneration and necrosis of hepatocytes, fibrosis and ultimately cirrhosis[798-800] (Fig. 14.18A, 14.21). Portal inflammation is usually moderate and consists of lymphocytes, macrophages and neutrophils. Hepatocyte nuclei are usually hyperchromatic, pleomorphic and vacuolated (Fig. 14.21(C)). Thus far, relatively little hepatic injury has been noted in rheumatoid arthritis patients, apparently less than that recorded in treated psoriatic patients.[130] Series of arthritic patients monitored for injury have revealed only steatosis and some fibrosis,[805,806] although instances of severe hepatic disease have been recorded,[807,808,809] including cases of cirrhosis.[810]

Prevention of injury in patients with psoriasis or arthritis treated with methotrexate requires adherence to a few principles. In patients who take alcohol regularly or who are obese diabetics, use of small doses of the drug and administration of the drug no more frequently than weekly, minimizes the likelihood of hepatic injury.[130,811] Monitoring for injury in the treatment of psoriasis still often requires performing baseline and serial liver biopsies, since biochemical or other non-invasive methods are insufficiently sensitive. The frequency of monitoring has been based on cumulative dose, with varying figures of 1.5–2.0 g, 2–4 g, and 4 g recommended for the interval between biopsies.[812] In contrast, current guidelines for using MTX in RA recommend liver biopsy only if significant hepatic disease is thought to be present.[813] Indeed, a survey of rheumatologists found that serious hepatotoxicity in RA patients was very low.[814]

Leflunamide has been reviewed for hepatotoxicity by the FDA[815] but published reports are rare. No significant abnormalities in liver functions tests were reported in clinical trials with leflunamide alone,[816] or in combination with methotrexate.[817]

Gold compounds have led to a number of instances of hepatic injury.[818-821] Cholestatic and, less frequently, hepatocellular injury have been reported. Fatalities have occurred among the cases of hepatocellular injury, but the prognosis among the cholestatic cases has been good, although at least one case has evolved into vanishing bile duct syndrome.[822] Some of the reported cases have appeared to reflect immunological idiosyncrasy; others, especially those with hepatocellular injury, may reflect metabolic idiosyncrasy.[1] In rare instances, prolonged treatment with a gold preparation may lead to accumulation of the metal within lysosomes and ultimate rupture of the lysosomes with resulting hepatic necrosis.[823] Gold accumulates in reticuloendothelial cells in the form of a black pigment[241,242] (Fig. 14.33).

Penicillamine has been used for treatment of rheumatoid arthritis, in addition to its more common use in Wilson disease. It has been incriminated in at least 20 cases of intrahepatic cholestasis, the mechanism being hypersensitivity.[824-826] A case with hepatotoxicity and associated fatal myelotoxicity has appeared.[827]

Nimesulide, a COX-2 preferential inhibitor, has been implicated in numerous reports of liver injury, including acute hepatitis,[828] cholestatic hepatitis,[829] and several instances of fulminant hepatic failure.[830-835] Although it is a sulphonamide derivative, eosinophilia has been described in a minority of patients,[832] suggesting metabolic idiosyncrasy rather than hypersensitivity is the mechanism. Most patients have been women. The other members of the COX-2 inhibitor family have rarely been shown to produce hepatic injury, although case reports have appeared with **celecoxib.**[836,837]

Allopurinol has been incriminated in many instances of hepatic injury. These include minor hepatic dysfunction,[1] hepatic granulomas (with or without a fibrin ring),[104,838-840] cholestasis and some cases of hepatic necrosis.[841-843] The cases of necrosis have been accompanied by manifestations of systemic hypersensitivity.[844]

Colchicine, despite its long use in the treatment of gout, has shown little evidence of hepatic injury in humans.[1] Very high blood levels can lead to a generalized reaction that includes injury to bone marrow, gastrointestinal tract, liver and other organs.[845] Large doses can lead to microvesicular steatosis in experimental animals[846] and in man.[847] The ability of colchicine to arrest mitosis may yield multiple mitotic figures in the liver.[2]

Zoxazolamine, briefly in use as a muscle relaxant several decades ago, produced severe hepatic necrosis in recipients, leading to its abandonment.[848]

Dantrolene, which was introduced for the treatment of severe muscle spasm associated with grave neurological disease, can also produce cytotoxic hepatic injury. Both acute and subacute hepatic necrosis have been reported.[849,850] The subacute lesion has resembled chronic hepatitis, while the acute lesion has resembled that produced by cinchophen, iproniazid and zoxazolamine. Overt hepatic injury which occurs in about 0.5% of recipients, tends to spare children below the age of 10 and adults taking daily doses below 200 mg. It usually does not appear until at least 6 weeks after starting the drug.[1]

Chlorzoxazone, a muscle-relaxant structurally similar to dantrolene, has produced cases of severe hepatic necrosis.[851]

Agents employed in the treatment of endocrine disease

A number of hormonal agents and their derivatives and drugs used in the treatment of diabetes and other endocrine diseases can produce hepatic dysfunction and jaundice (Table 14.30). These include the oral hypoglycemics in the thiazolidinedione class, thiourea derivatives used to treat thyroid disease, the C-17 alkylated anabolic steroids and oral contraceptive agents, as well as several other agents that can play endocrine or quasi-endocrine roles.[1]

Table 14.30 Hepatic injury produced by hormonal derivatives and other agents used in endocrine disease

Agent	Type of injury*	Other lesions
Steroids and associated agents		
Anabolic-Androgen (C-17)	Ch-Can	See Table 14.14
Oral contraceptives	Ch-Can	
Tamoxifen	Ch-Can	Peliosis hepatis
Danazol	Ch-Can	Carcinoma
Glucocorticoids	—	Steatosis
Oral hypoglycaemics		
Sulfonylureas		
Acetohexamide	H-Cell-M	
Azepinamide	H-Cell-M	
Carbutamide	H-Cell-M (ALF)	
Chlorpropamide	Ch-H-Can	
Glibenclamide	Ch-H-Can	
Metahexamide	H-Cell-M (ALF)	Chronic cholestasis
Tolazemide	Ch-H-Can	Chronic cholestasis
Tolbutamide	Ch-H-Can	Chronic cholestasis, VBDS
Thiazolidinediones		
Troglitazone	H-Cell (ALF)	
Rosiglitazone	H-Cell	
Pioglitazone	Ch-Can	
Others		
Acarbose (glucosidase)	H-cell (rare)	
Metformin (Biguanide)	Ch-H-can (rare)	Lactic acidosis
Antithyroid drugs		
Carbimazole	Ch-H-Can	
Methimazole	Ch-H-Can	
Thiouracil	Ch-H-Can	
Propylthiouracil	H-Cell (ALF)	Chronic hepatitis

* Ch-Can = Cholestasis, canalicular type; Ch-H-Can = Cholestasis, hepatocanalicular type; H-Cell-M = Hepatocellular injury, mixed, i.e. with prominent cholestasis; VBDS = vanishing bile duct syndrome; ALF = acute liver failure

Oral hypoglycaemic drugs

Sulphonylureas

Among the older agents, hepatic injury occurred in 0.5–1% of recipients of **carbutamide or metahexamide.**[1] The incidence of jaundice among patients taking **acetohexamide** appears to have been lower.[852] **Tolbutamide,** despite its extremely wide use, has been incriminated in only a few instances of jaundice.[853] The jaundice of **chlorpropamide** has been cholestatic (hepatocanalicular); that of metahexamide, acetohexamide and carbutamide appears to have been mixed-hepatocellular.[1] The few reported examples of tolbutamide jaundice have been cholestatic. Gregory et al.[853] described a case of prolonged jaundice with features resembling those of primary biliary cirrhosis and a fatal outcome. **Tolazamide** has also been incriminated in chronic cholestasis.[1] Sulphonylurea derivatives also can produce granulomas in the absence of other evidence of hepatic injury.[854]

Gliburide has rarely been associated with liver toxicity.[1] **Gliclazide** caused injury associated with cholestasis and lobular portal inflammation and prominent eosinophils in a patient with underlying cirrhosis presenting with a rash and peripheral eosinophilia.[855] Lesions associated with other sulphonylurea derivatives are listed in Table 14.30. An epidemiological study by Chan et al.[856] suggests that all hypoglycemic agents are capable of causing severe liver injury.

Thiazolidinediones

Troglitazone is an oral hypoglycaemic agent in the new class of thiazolidinediones that was incriminated in a number of cases of severe or fatal hepatocellular injury soon after marketing in the USA.[24,857–863] Acute injury generally developed within the first 6 months of use, and was not associated with hypersensitivity features. Although the exact mechanism of injury has not been determined, several theories have been proposed.[864] According to Chojkier,[865] however, there is no evidence that troglitazone accumulates in the liver, stimulates oxidative stress, causes pathological apoptosis or mitochondrial injury, provokes steatohepatitis, or causes 'silent' injury. The mechanism appears to be metabolic idiosyncrasy, possibly related to P450 or other genetic susceptibilities.[865] For example, metabolic activation may involve the formation of a reactive sulphonium ion from a sulphoxide reaction mediated by the cytochrome P450 system.[866] A hint of its hepatotoxic potential was suggested in retrospect, by the incidence of ALT levels exceeding 3 times the upper limit of normal in nearly 2% of clinical trial recipients,[867,868] some of whom had associated jaundice.[869]

Despite numerous attempts to ensure liver function test monitoring by physicians, the rate of testing proved to be unacceptably low given the incidence of fulminant liver failure in approximately one in 10 000 recipients,[870,871] and the drug was withdrawn by the manufacturer about 3 years following approval, with the knowledge that the two second generation thiazolidinediones, **rosiglitazone** and **pioglitazone,** had been marketed for a year without an apparent increased risk of liver failure.[868,872,873] Histological descriptions of massive and submassive necrosis from troglitazone are taken mostly from reports filed with the FDA,[869,874] as summarized by Faich & Moseley,[863] and from several published cases.[24,857–862]

Troglitazone injury was predominantly hepatocellular (Fig. 14.38); cholestatic injury being much less frequent.[865,875] Biopsy material is generally lacking from less serious instances of acute hepatitis not culminating in death or transplantation. No substantiated reports of chronic hepatitis are known,[865] although NASH secondary to diabetes can lead to 'cryptogenic' cirrhosis,[876] which in some patients may confound the issue. There is no evidence that patients who were exposed to troglitazone are at any risk for developing cirrhosis or liver cancer.[865]

While a few cases of hepatocellular injury[877,878] and possible cholestatic injury[879,880] have been reported with **rosiglitazone,** no substantiated deaths have been reported and other causes may have been responsible.[881–884] Likewise,

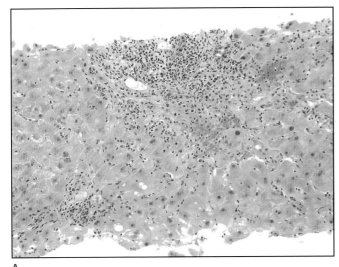

A

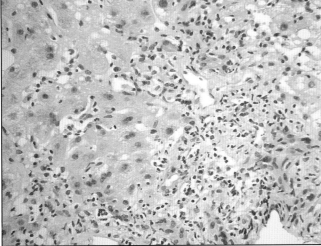

B

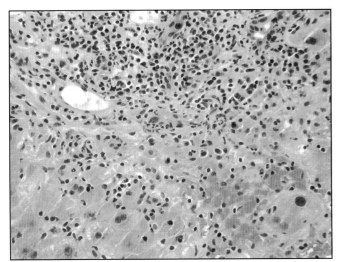

C

Fig. 14.38 • Troglitazone-associated injury. **(A)** Medium magnification view of portal area with an acute and chronic infiltrate, ductular reaction and drop-out of hepatocytes. Apoptotic hepatocytes and spotty inflammation are seen in the adjacent lobule. There is only minimal steatosis. H&E. **(B)** Portal area with interface hepatitis and ductular reaction. H&E. **(C)** Periportal haemorrhage with hepatocyte dropout and ductular reaction. H&E. Photomicrographs courtesy of Dr Joel Greenson.

pioglitazone appears relatively devoid of hepatocellular damage, although a few instances of reversible cholestatic, hepatocellular or mixed injury have been published.[885–887] Both agents may cause fluid overload and exacerbate oedema, and some of the enzyme elevations may reflect drug-induced congestive heart failure.[888] Both drugs have been used safely in patients with a history of previous troglitazone-related hepatic injury.[889,890]

Other agents

Acarbose is a recently introduced agent which inhibits intestinal glucosidases, thereby blunting post absorptive hyperglycaemia. It has been incriminated in cases of hepatocellular injury.[891,892] High doses of acarbose, alone or in combination with ethanol, can potentiate CCl_4 and acetaminophen (paracetamol) hepatotoxicity in rats by inducing hepatic CYP2E1.[893]

Only isolated instances of hepatic injury, including cholestasis associated with jaundice and pruritus, have been ascribed to **biguanides,** such as **metformin.**[894–896] The risk of lactic acidosis with metformin remains unsubstantiated,[897] in contrast to **Phenformin,** whose use was associated with fatal lactic acidosis.[898] To our knowledge, phenformin has led to only one case of hepatic damage,[1] which is somewhat a surprise, since it is structurally related to the hepatotoxic agent **synthalin.**[1]

Repaglinide has been associated with mild hepatitis.[899]

Thiourea derivatives for thyroid disease

There appear to be differences between the type of injury produced by different derivatives of thiourea.[1] The instances of jaundice induced by **methimazole, carbimazole and methylthiouracil** appear to have been cholestatic (hepatocanalicular or mixed hepatocanalicular).[900,901] Of interest is the precipitation of acute liver failure in a chronic hepatitis B carrier treated with methimazole.[902]

Cases of hepatotoxicity reported in recipients of **propylthiouracil** have been hepatocellular; with several instances of fulminant hepatic failure In children and adults,[903–910] placing this agent in the top tier of drugs leading to emergency liver transplant.[22] Several other patients have had features of chronic hepatitis.[1,911,913] The association of rash, fever, eosinophilia and neutropenia with hepatic injury suggests that the mechanism for the hepatotoxicity of the thiourea derivatives is hypersensitivity.[1,904,909]

Anabolic and contraceptive steroids

The hepatic effects of the C-17 alkylated anabolic steroids and of the oral contraceptive steroids have much in common. Both groups of drugs are intrinsic hepatotoxins capable of producing acute cholestatic jaundice. Both have led to instances of **peliosis hepatis**[187,189–191,913] (Fig. 14.26), and sinusoidal dilatation,[197,198] and have been implicated in the development of hepatocellular adenoma[202–205] and carcinoma[42,209–212] (Table 14.31). The Budd–Chiari syndrome is apparently related to the thrombogenic effect of the oestrogenic component of the contraceptive preparations.[173,174]

Table 14.31	Adverse effects associated with alkylated steroids	
	Anabolic	**Contraceptive**
Acute cholestasis	+	+
Chronic cholestasis	?	?
Budd-Chiari syndrome	−	+
Hepatocellular carcinoma	+	±
Cholangiocellular carcinoma	±	−
Adenoma	±	+
Nodular regenerative hyperplasia	±	±
Focal nodular hyperplasia	−	−
Peliosis hepatis	+	±
Sinusoidal dilatation(a)	±	+
Lithogenesis	−	±

+ = Association definite; ± = association possible; − = no association
(a) Dilatation associated with contraceptive steroids in periportal zone; dilatation possibly associated with anabolic steroids in perivenular zone

The structure of these agents is important to their toxicity. The presence of an alkyl or ethinyl group in the C-17 position appears to be essential for the production of cholestatic jaundice.[1,30] Testosterone does not lead to jaundice or impaired hepatic function.[30] Unsaturation of ring A, a characteristic of native oestrogens, appears to enhance the adverse effect of steroids on hepatic function, as may be deduced from the greater potency of the oestrogenic than of the progestogenic component of contraceptive preparations.[914]

The incidence of jaundice in patients who receive anabolic steroids appears to be very low, although hepatic dysfunction occurs in almost all patients who take them in sufficiently large doses. However, in patients treated for aplastic anaemia the incidence exceeds 15%. In most of the patients in whom jaundice developed the drug had been taken for 1–6 months.[41]

The impression gained from the anabolic steroid phenomenon, that individual susceptibility permits a mildly adverse effect to be translated into the development of jaundice, is even more apparent with respect to the contraceptive steroids. The latter are far more likely to lead to jaundice in women who have a personal or familial history of jaundice of pregnancy.[915,916] This, and the clustering of cases of 'pill jaundice' in Chile[917] and Scandinavia,[918] suggest a genetic susceptibility to this type of hepatic injury.[30] The jaundice appears to result from selective interference with transport of bile acids across the sinusoidal membrane of the hepatocyte and perhaps of constituents of bile across the canalicular membrane.[30,55,919] There is evidence that they interfere with both bile-salt-dependent and bile-salt-independent flow.[55,919] The histological features are those of the cholestasis with no portal area inflammation, and little or no parenchymal injury. Death has been reported only in patients

who were debilitated or had other disease.[1,30] In most patients jaundice has subsided promptly, although a case of a destructive cholangitis[920] and another of 'biliary cirrhosis'[921] have been attributed to methyltestosterone.

Both **stilboestrol** and **diethylstilboestrol** appear to have the potential for producing parenchymal injury. Lesions produced by large doses include necrosis and steatosis,[1] and one instance of non-alcoholic steatohepatitis.[134]

Hepatoneoplastic potential of steroids

Hepatocellular carcinoma has been reported in several dozen recipients of the alkylated anabolic steroids[41] and in at least as many patients who had been taking contraceptive steroids.[30,41,42,204,209,922] In view of the large number of women who have taken contraceptives, and the relatively limited number of patients who have used alkylated anabolic steroids, hepatocarcinogenesis would appear to be more readily attributable to anabolic than to contraceptive steroids.[41]

Hepatocellular adenoma seems clearly relatable to use of contraceptive steroids. Hundreds of cases have now been recorded.[30,41,202–205] Almost all of those in the files of the Armed Forces Institute of Pathology (AFIP) have presented since the introduction of 'the pill' and almost all patients with this tumour have been users of it—a far more convincing relationship to the steroid than that of focal nodular hyperplasia.[204,209] Instances of hepatocellular adenoma also have been attributed to anabolic steroids.[41] A few cases of nodular regenerative hyperplasia have been attributed to the use of contraceptive or androgenic-anabolic steroids.[204,923] The histological features of these tumours are considered in Chapter 15.

Reports of hepatic angiosarcoma in recipients of oestrogenic and androgenic compounds have also appeared.[30,204,212,924] Several instances of intrahepatic *cholangiocarcinoma* have been reported in patients taking androgenic-anabolic steroids.[204,923]

Oestrogen receptor modulators

Raloxifene, a selective oestrogen receptor modulator, has been implicated in an instance of a hepatitis-like injury associated with a rash and eosinophilia.[925]

Anti-oestrogens

Tamoxifen, an anti-oestrogen chemically related to stilboestrol, has been reported to lead to cholestatic and mixed jaundice[926] and to peliosis hepatis,[192] but appears most commonly to cause or contribute to hepatic steatosis and non-alcoholic steatohepatitis,[927,928–932] Asymptomatic abnormal liver function tests are commonly seen,[930] but generally resolve after the drug is discontinued. Progression to cirrhosis has been described, but is rare.[928] In animals, nodular regenerative hyperplasia has been reported.[933]

Clomiphene, an ovulation-inducing agent employed to treat fertility, has been implicated in two instances of tumourigenesis. One involved the occurrence of a hepatoblastoma in an infant whose mother had received the agent.[934] The other involved development of an hepatocellular adenoma in a woman who had been taking the drug for 2 years.[935]

Cyclofenil has been implicated in the development of biochemical evidence of hepatic injury in at least 35% of recipients[936,937] and of overt hepatitis in 1% of treated patients.[936]

Anti-androgens

Flutamide, a synthetic anti-androgen used in the treatment of prostate cancer, has led to asymptomatic elevations of serum transaminases, mixed cholestatic and hepatocellular injury, and several examples of severe hepatic necrosis with fulminant liver failure.[938–944] There appears be to an increased risk of flutamide liver injury in patients with underlying chronic hepatitis B.[945]

Cyproterone, another anti-androgen used for prostate cancer, has been implicated in a number of instances of severe, sometimes fatal, hepatocellular damage,[946,947,948] and to biochemical evidence of injury in up to 25% of recipients.[943,944]

Anti-hypophyseal drugs

Danazol, a compound structurally related to the C-17 anabolic steroids, also can lead to cholestatic jaundice.[949,950] It has been implicated in a fatal case of peliosis hepatitis,[951] and in several cases of hepatocellular adenoma,[952,953,954] and hepatocellular carcinoma.[955,956]

Octreotide, an analogue of somatostatin, has been implicated in an instance of hepatocellular injury.[957] However, as it is usually given to patients with underlying portal hypertension, differentiating acute drug-induced injury from the underlying liver disease being treated may be difficult.

Antimicrobial agents

A number of agents in this category can produce hepatic dysfunction or jaundice.[958,959] The form of injury and the presumed mechanism are shown in Table 14.32.

Tetracyclines

Tetracyclines produce a characteristic microvesicular steatosis, resembling the fatty liver of pregnancy or of Reye syndrome[1,960] (Fig. 14.18(B),(C)). Hepatocytes contain many small sudanophilic fat droplets. There is little or no necrosis and little cholestasis. The microvesicular steatosis of tetracycline has been reproduced in experimental animals.[961]

The clinically significant syndrome of severe steatosis with hepatic failure occurs in patients who have received the drug intravenously in a dose of 1.5 g/day or more, particularly if the recipient is in the last trimester of pregnancy or has renal disease.[962] While pregnancy appears to enhance susceptibility to tetracycline-induced hepatic injury, nonpregnant females and males are also susceptible.[119] The clinical manifestations include nausea, vomiting and abdominal pain, possibly related to the frequently associated pancreatitis. Jaundice is rarely intense. Most of the reported patients have died.[1,119,962] Less severe cases probably were unrecognized or unrecorded.

The mechanism for the liver damage is clearly that of intrinsic hepatotoxicity. The lesion appears to be mainly the result of inhibition of transport of lipid from the liver and impaired mitochondrial oxidation of fatty acids.[120,961,963]

Tetracycline-induced microvesicular steatosis has lost its practical importance, since intravenous administration of the drug is today rarely used. However, tetracycline has been implicated in chronic cholestasis accompanied by depletion of interlobular bile ducts (vanishing bile-duct syndrome).[964]

Minocycline, a derivative of tetracycline, can also produce steatosis, although in at least one reported case it was macrovesicular.[965] In addition, an entirely different form of hepatic injury has been induced by oral minocycline. Given for treatment of adolescent acne, oral minocycline has been implicated in several dozen cases of hepatocellular injury, some acute and some with features of chronic hepatitis, many with accompanying features of autoimmune injury including auto-antibodies.[99,966–971] Three separate clinical presentations have been observed: a rapid onset serum sickness-like illness associated with fever, myalgias, arthralgias and rash occurring a mean of 15 days after administration; a hypersensitivity syndrome with exfoliative dermatitis and eosinophilia that occurs within 3–4 weeks of exposure; and a chronic drug-induced lupus-like syndrome that presents after a year or more of administration with jaundice, malaise, polyarthralgias, fever and the presence of autoantibodies (usually antinuclear), with typical autoimmune hepatitis features on liver biopsy.[968–971] Women under age 40 years are most susceptible with a latency period about half as long as that seen in males.[971] While most cases resolve after the drug is discontinued, immunosuppressive therapy has been required in some patients.[968]

Macrolides/ketolides

Erythromycin estolate was for many years considered to be the only erythromycin derivative which produced jaundice.[1,30,972] It is now clear that erythromycin ethylsuccinate,[973] erythromycin propionate,[972] perhaps erythromycin stearate[974] or even erythromycin base,[972,975] can produce the same syndrome and lesion. Jaundice occurs in about 1–2% of adults taking erythromycin estolate but very rarely in children taking the drug.[30] The jaundice is hepatocanalicular with high values for alkaline phosphatase and modestly elevated aminotransferase values. Liver biopsy usually shows only bile casts and prominent portal inflammatory infiltration, often rich in eosinophils.[972] Erythromycin lactobionate, administered intravenously, has been incriminated in a case of severe hepatic necrosis.[976] Ultrastructural changes include dilatation and effacement of canaliculi and microvilli. Hyperplasia of the Golgi apparatus and smooth endoplasmic reticulum has also been demonstrated, as has mitochondrial injury.[972]

The fever, rash and blood and tissue eosinophilia in up to 60% of cases have led to the inference that it is a manifestation of hypersensitivity.[1,30] However, the high incidence of hepatic dysfunction in patients taking erythromycin estolate, and the demonstration that it is damaging to suspensions of hepatocytes in vitro[977] and the ex vivo perfused liver,[978] suggest that intrinsic hepatotoxicity of the agent may contribute to the injury. The onset of symptoms generally occurs between 5 and 20 days after the start of therapy, with individuals who have been previously treated having a shortened latent period. About half of cases are icteric, with bilirubin values as high as 50 mg/dL. Abdominal pain is common and may mimic acute cholecystitis.[31,979] Jaundice usually subsides within 2–5 weeks after the drug is stopped, but prolonged cholestasis and the vanishing bile duct syndrome are described.[31,111]

Telithromycin, a newly approved agent for the treatment of upper respiratory infections, was associated with a few instances of mild reversible cholestatic hepatitis in clinical trials.[980]

Azithromycin has been associated with intrahepatic cholestasis biochemically and on histology.[981–983]

Clarithromycin and **roxithromycin** have also been reported to cause cholestatic hepatitis.[984,985]

Triacetyloleandomycin (troleandomycin) produced jaundice in 4% and biochemically detected hepatic dysfunction in over 50% of a group of patients who had taken 2 g daily for 2 or more weeks.[986] Characteristically, the injury due to this drug is mixed, with both cytotoxic and cholestatic features, the latter predominating. Triacetyloleandomycin or a metabolite appears to be a mild intrinsic hepatotoxin. Metabolic differences between different individuals presumably determine the extent of hepatic injury. Patients taking both this drug and oral contraceptives appear to be more likely to develop jaundice than those taking either preparation alone.[987]

Chloramphenicol jaundice has been reported in a number of patients. The scant data available suggest that both hepatic parenchymal necrosis and cholestasis can occur. The mechanism for the apparent hepatotoxicity is unclear.[1]

Novobiocin, now little used, can produce unconjugated hyperbilirubinaemia, apparently by blockade of conjugation.[1] Accordingly, it should be categorized as a mild intrinsic hepatotoxin. Rare instances of hepatic necrosis due to idiosyncrasy have been described.[988]

Penicillins

Penicillin commonly leads to generalized hypersensitivity, but rarely to hepatic injury.[1] Among the countless number of patients who have been given penicillin, very few instances of liver damage have been reported.[989–991] Several semisynthetic derivatives (Table 14.32), such as **oxacillin, carbenicillin, and ampicillin,** seem to produce jaundice or biochemical evidence of hepatic injury more commonly.[992–994] **Cloxacillin, dicloxacillin** and **floxacillin** have led to multiple instances of cholestatic hepatitis.[995–997] Flucloxacillin seems to produce hepatic injury with a higher frequency.[998] A number of cases of flucloxacillin-induced

cholestasis have remained chronic for up to 6 months, and the drug is now recognized as a cause of the vanishing bile-duct syndrome.[999,1000]

The combination drug, **amoxicillin-clavulanate** (*Augmentin*) has led to many instances of cholestatic injury.[1001–1004] Indeed, it appears to be the most commonly encountered cause of cholestasis among antibiotics,[30] and has produced at least one case of chronic cholestasis.[1005] The incidence has been estimated to be one case of jaundice in 78 000 prescriptions, according to a Scottish study.[1006] In contrast to many other drug classes, older males appear to be predisposed to injury, with an incidence that is several fold higher when two or more courses of therapy have been prescribed.[1002] The mean onset of jaundice among 22 cases from Scotland was 17 days after the start of therapy,[1006] but a delay of up to 6–7 weeks has been reported,[1007] with hypersensitivity features present in up to two-thirds of cases. Interstitial nephritis and sialadenitis have accompanied some instances of amoxicillin-clavulanate injury.[1008] Clavulanate is considered the hepatotoxic component, as the combination is more hepatotoxic than amoxicillin aline.[1009] Hepatic injury has also been reported with the combination of **ticarcillin** and clavulanate.[1010] An immuno-allergic mechanism seems likely, and a higher frequency of certain HLA haplotypes has been found as one possible predisposing factor (DRB1*1501-DRB5*0101-DQB1*0602).[1006,1011] Histologically, centrilobular cholestasis with a mixed portal inflammatory infiltrate, variable portal oedema and interlobular bile duct injury with bile duct proliferation is described.[1008] A case of granulomatous hepatitis also has been attributed to this combination drug.[1012] Recovery is the general rule within 1–4 months, although fatal outcomes have been reported.[1008]

Cephalosporins

These agents are associated with formation of biliary sludge that can cause symptoms of cholecystitis.[1013] Less commonly cholestatic hepatitis reported.[1014] Progressive cholestasis has been reported with **clarithromycin.**[1015]

Fluoroquinolones

Injury by these agents may be either cholestatic or hepatocellular, and the mechanism is likely hypersensitivity. Implicated drugs have included **norfloxacin, ciprofloxacin, levofloxacin, ofloxacin, trovafloxacin** and **nalidixic acid.**[1,1016–1020] Granulomatous hepatitis was described with norfloxacin[1021] and prolonged cholestasis with ciprofloxacin.[1022] **Gatifloxacin** has been reported to cause severe hepatocellular injury,[1023] possibly associated with pancreatitis.[1024]

In the case of trovofloxacin, severe hepatic injury has restricted its use to inpatients under the direction of infectious disease experts.[1025,1026] Reversible trovofloxacin-associated acute hepatocellular injury with peripheral and histologic eosiniphilia has been described.[1027] Liver biopsy in these patients revealed perivenular and focal periportal necrosis with eosinophilic infiltration (Fig. 14.41).[1027] Trovofloxacin has a difluorophenyl substitution of position N-1 of the naphthyridone ring that is implicated in the development of hypersensitivity reactions.[1028] A similar structure is seen with **temafloxacin,** which may account for its immunoallergic manifestations.[1029] In contrast, the other quinolones have a different chemical structure, and/or differences in P450 metabolism,[1030] although eosinophilia has been described with their injury.[1020]

Sulphonamides

These agents have been incriminated in hundreds of instances of hepatic injury.[1] Many have shown hepatic necrosis and hepatocellular jaundice, although reports of cholestatic jaundice and granulomas have been described. The hepatic damage caused by these agents appears to be mixed-hepatocellular and the mechanism involves hypersensitivity, including instances of Steven–Johnson syndrome.[1031–1033] Affected individuals may be predisposed by aberrant production and detoxification of hydroxylamine derivatives.[1034,1035,1036] Prompt recurrence of injury is seen on rechallenge, and some patients have developed fulminant hepatitis.[1037,1038]

The **sulphamethoxazole-trimethoprim** combination (Bactrim, Septra) has led to a number of instances of acute cholestatic and hepatocellular injury (Fig. 14.8(A),(B)) (in some cases accompanied by pancreatitis[1039,1040]) although the injury appears to be more commonly cholestatic.[30,31] Indeed, chronic cholestasis with the vanishing bile duct syndrome has been reported,[1041,1042] as has phospholipidosis in one patient.[1043] Fulminant hepatic failure requiring liver transplantation has been reported;[1038] although the height of the enzymes (AST > 23 000 and ALT > 11 000) suggest possible shock liver. While the clinical inference has led to implicating the sulphonamide component in the injury,[1032] there is evidence that the trimethoprim can contribute.[1044] A significantly higher incidence of hypersensitivity reactions is found in HIV-positive patients receiving SMX-TMP compared to the general population (up to 70% vs 3%).[260,1045–1047]

The hepatic injury attributed to **sulphasalazine,** including massive necrosis,[1037] is thought to be related to its content of sulphapyridine[1048] (Fig. 14.8(C)). Cholestatic injury attributed to **mesalazine** therapy for Crohn disease was reported by Stoschus et al.[1049] Injury due to other sulphonamide-containing preparations is shown in Table 14.32.

Sulphones, long used in the treatment of leprosy, appear to produce hepatic injury more often than do the sulphonamides. The incidence has been reported to be about 5% in recipients of the prototypic compound, 4,4′-diamino-diphenylsulphone (**dapsone**).[1050] Jaundice appears to be mixed-hepatocellular. The mechanism for the hepatic injury is not clear, presumably hypersensitivity, as injury is seen within the first two weeks of beginning treatment, and has led to fatal hepatitis. The histological changes include inflammation with sinusoidal beading and non-zonal necrosis.

Nitrofurantoin causes mainly acute hepatocellular injury, but it may be cholestatic or mixed.[1051] The drug appears to have led to a number of instances of chronic hepatitis resembling autoimmune hepatitis,[91] and less often to a cholestatic injury or a granulomatous hepatitis[1051,1052] (Fig. 14.23(A),(B)). Hypersensitivity features are often present.

Antituberculous drugs

Clarification of the aetiological role of a particular agent in this group as the cause of hepatic injury has been complicated by the frequent use of several drugs in combination. Nevertheless, observations recorded from the period when para-aminosalicylic acid (PAS) was employed alone or with streptomycin, and the more recent practice of treating 'tuberculin converters' with isoniazid (INH) alone, has permitted some deductions regarding the ability of each of these agents to produce hepatic injury.[1] Streptomycin and dihydrostreptomycin appear to be free of hepatotoxic potential, but PAS can cause liver damage.[1053] Ethambutal leads to very rare instances of cholestatic jaundice.[1054] Rifampin also has been implicated in cases of hepatic injury.[1055] It appears to potentiate the ability of INH to produce hepatic injury and vice versa.[1056] By far the most important members of this group with regard to hepatotoxicity is INH.[56,85,86,1057] Similar injury is caused by its congeners, pyrazinamide[1058] and ethionamide.[1059]

Para-aminosalicylic acid (PAS)

Hepatic injury is part of a generalized hypersensitivity which occurs in 0.3–5% of patients taking the drug. While the decreased use of PAS has diminished the immediate relevance of its hepatotoxic effects, the syndrome of hepatic injury is an important and classical one and warrants description. PAS-associated injury appears after 1–5 weeks of therapy; it includes fever, rash, eosinophilia, lymphadenopathy and often, atypical circulating lymphocytes ('pseudomononucleosis').[1053] Approximately 25% of patients with this generalized hypersensitivity developed jaundice and biochemical evidence of mixed hepatocellular hepatic injury. The histological changes included prominent inflammation, with sinusoidal beading accompanying the diffuse degeneration, necrosis and cholestasis. Necrosis was massive in fatal cases. In some non-fatal cases there was striking periportal necrosis.[1]

Isoniazid (INH)

This apparently showed only a slight potential for producing hepatic injury during almost 2 decades of its clinical use.[85,86,1057] Despite the huge number of recipients of INH, only a few instances of jaundice had been attributed to it prior to 1972, and these were usually in patients who also had been taking other drugs. In that year, however, Garibaldi et al.[1060] reported 19 instances of hepatocellular injury, most of them accompanied by jaundice, out of 2321 patients taking INH for chemoprophylaxis. These authors also cited a number of other previously unreported instances of INH hepatotoxicity described to them by other physicians. Since then, numerous other reports have appeared,[85,86] although the rate of hepatotoxicity from isoniazid preventive therapy remains low—0.10% for patients starting treatment and 0.15% for those completing treatment.[1061] Injury appears to be related to the age of the recipient; the incidence is very low under the age of 20, but rises to greater than 2% in patients above 50.[86,1062] Hepatitis B may increase the risk of injury.[1063] The clinical features and experimental data support the view that metabolic idiosyncrasy leading to toxic hydrazine metabolites is responsible for the injury.[1057] INH is metabolized to hepatotoxic intermediates by N-acetyltransferase. Huang et al.[1064] demonstrated that in addition to older age, a slow acetylator phenotype of the NAT gene places individuals at increased risk of liver injury. Among 224 patients, 15% overall developed hepatotoxicity in their series; more than twice as many having a slow acetylator phenotype (26% vs 11%). Higher transaminase levels were also seen in the slow acetylators.[1064]

Examination of liver biopsies has revealed diffuse degeneration and necrosis, and fatal cases have shown massive necrosis[86] (Fig. 14.10). In a few patients biopsy has shown changes consistent with chronic hepatitis, although there are too few cases to draw any firm conclusions about chronic injury.[86] The fatality rate is in excess of 10% of icteric cases with fulminant hepatitis, and INH has been responsible for more liver transplants due to drug injury than all other medications except acetaminophen.[21,22,85,86]

Minor elevations (less than three-fold) of serum aminotransferase levels occur in 10–20% of patients during the first 2 months of INH therapy; and yet, in most of these, the abnormality does not progress or may even subside despite continued administration of the drug.[1057,1065] Such patients show minor histological abnormalities on biopsy.[1065]

Rifampin

A number of patients have developed jaundice while taking rifampin and INH, whereas jaundice due to rifampin alone is rare.[1055] Earlier reports suggested that rifampin and INH together may be more hepatotoxic than either alone, supported by the study of Hugues and his colleagues[1066] who found that rats developed hepatic necrosis when given rifampin and INH together, but not when given either drug alone. Current views consider that most rifampin toxicity consists of enhancement of INH toxicity due to rifampin induction of P-450.[1067]

Hepatic injury in recipients of rifampin and INH appears during the first month of therapy.[1055] Patients with active tuberculosis or who have AIDS are more susceptible to hepatotoxicity from rifampin and INH than are other patients.[1056] The injury of rifampin and INH is mainly hepatocellular, although cholestasis may be present.[1055] Hepatocellular degeneration and necrosis are characteristic and tend to be most marked in the perivenular zone. The inflammatory response to the combination appears to be more prominent than that in INH injury.[1055] Some reports suggest that the prognosis is guarded, with a high case fatality rate, while others suggest that the disease is relatively mild.[1055]

Presumably unrelated to this hepatic injury is the ability of rifampin to produce unconjugated hyperbilirubinaemia and impaired BSP excretion in experimental animals and humans. Apparently the drug competes with other substances cleared by the liver for excretion into bile or uptake from sinusoidal blood by the hepatocyte.[1068]

Pyrazinamide

This has a risk of hepatotoxicity equal to or greater than that for INH. Because of several reports of severe liver injury (including hospitalization, the need for liver transplant and case-fatalities) seen with the combination of PZA and rifampicin, the CDC has cautioned against the use of this regimen for the treatment of latent TB.[1058,1069–1071] Indeed, the American Thoracic Society and the Infectious Diseases Society of America joined the CDC in recommending that this combination not be used except as part of a multidrug combination for active tuberculosis.[1069] The risk of hepatitis from PZA+RFP has been found to be three-fold higher compared to INH.[1058] We have reported a patient who developed acute reversible autoimmune hepatitis and thyroiditis after the start of prophylactic therapy with PZA+RFP for a documented PPD conversion.[1072]

Antifungal agents

Griseofulvin produces hepatic necrosis, hepatocellular carcinoma and toxic porphyria in mice.[1073] Denk et al.[1074] have described formation of Mallory bodies in mice given griseofulvin. Humans have developed porphyrinuria and those with acute intermittent porphyria in remission may experience a relapse while taking the drug.[1075] We are aware of only isolated reports of cholestatic jaundice due to the drug.[1076]

Ketoconazole, an azole derivative, has been reported to lead to more than 100 instances of hepatocellular injury and a much smaller number of cases of apparent cholestatic injury.[1077–1079] The incidence of jaundice appears to be low; based on apparent usage, it has been estimated to range from 0.01 to 0.1%.[1079] Minor abnormalities of liver function tests occur in about 10% of recipients.[1079] **Fluconazole** can lead to a 15–20% incidence of elevated transaminase and to rare cases of jaundice and severe hepatitis.[1080,1081] **Itraconazole** has led to hepatocellular and cholestatic injury,[1082,1083] and is a more potent hepatotoxin than fluconazole in animals.[1084]

Fluocytosine is converted to 5-fluorouracil, a transformation on which its antifungal activity depends. Data on the hepatic effects of this drug are scant; it appears to lead to transient elevations of serum aminotransferase levels in 10% of recipients and has been incriminated in hepatic necrosis.[1,1085]

Terbinafine, a synthetic antimycotic agent of the alylamine class, has been reported to lead to cholestatic injury, including the VBDS, to a mixed hepatocellular-cholestatic injury, and to submassive hepatocellular necrosis with liver failure.[1086–1090] Injury has been linked to the allylic aldehyde metabolite of the compound (7,7-dimethylhept-2-ene-4-ynal).[1091]

Amphotericin B has rarely caused hepatic injury; one case convincingly proved by withdrawal and readministration.[1092,1093]

Antiviral agents

Highly active anti-retroviral therapy (HAART) drugs

Drugs for the treatment of HIV/AIDS have produced a wide spectrum of liver injury, from mild hepatocellular damage to fatal steatosis associated with lactic acidosis depending on the drug class (Table 14.33).[1094-1098] The mechanism of injury also varies, with mitochondrial damage suspected for several nucleoside reverse transcription inhibitors (NRTIs)[1099-1101] and hypersensitivity most commonly observed with the non-NRTIs, e.g. nevirapine.[1094,1099] Coexisting chronic viral hepatitis B and C is associated with an increased risk of hepatotoxicity with HAART agents.[1094,1097,1102,1103]

Zidovudine (azidothymidine, AZT) has led to abnormal liver function tests, to cholestatic jaundice, to hepatocellular injury and to massive hepatic steatosis and lactic acidosis in several patients.[1094,1096,1104] Chariot et al.[1105] and others have shown that the latter injury is related to mitochondrial DNA depletion.[1094]

Didanosine leads to a high incidence of elevated aminotransferase levels, and has been incriminated to instances of hepatic failure accompanied by microvesicular steatosis.[1106] Combination therapy for HIV infection with didanosine and stavudine has also led to a Reye-syndrome-like

Table 14.32	Hepatic injury produced by antimicrobial agents			
Agent	**Type of injury (a)**		**Agent**	**Type of injury**
Antibiotics			*Antimetazoal and antiprotozoal agents*	
Chloramphenicol	H-Cell, M		Antimonials	Steatosis
Cephalosporins	Ch		Amodiaquine	H-Cell
Clindamycin	H-Cell		Hycanthone	H-Cell
Erythromycins[(b)]	Ch		Mepacrine[(f)]	Ch
Penicillins[(c)]			Niclofan	Ch
G	?		Thiabendazole	Ch[(d)]
Amoxicillin	AT			
Amoxicillin-clavulanic acid	Ch		*Antituberculous*	
Ampicillin	H-Cell		Cycloserine	AT
Carbenicillin	AT		Ethionamide	H-Cell
Oxacillin	Ch		Isoniazid	H-Cell
Cloxacillin, dicloxacillin	Ch		p-Aminosalicylate	H-Cell
Tetracyclines	Steatosis, CH		Pyrazinamide	H-Cell
			Rifampicin	H-Cell[(h)]
Synthetic drugs			Thiosemicarbazone	H-Cell
Fluoroquinolones	H-Cell, Ch			
Arsenicals, organic	Ch[(d)]			
Nitrofurantoin	H-Cell, Ch, CH			
Sulphonamides	H-Cell, M, CH			
Sulphones	H-Cell			
Sulphomethoxazole-trimethoprim	Ch, H-Cell			
Antifungal agents				
Amphotericin[(e,f)]	H-Cell			
5-Fluorocytosine[(f)]	Ch			
Griseofulvin[(g)]	Ch			
Hydroystilbamidine	H-Cell			
Ketoconazole	H-Cell			
Fluconazole	J			
Intraconazole	Ch, H-Cell			
Pentamidine[(f)]	H-Cell			
Terbinafine				

(a) Ch = cholestatic injury; bilirubin casts in canaliculi with or without portal inflammation and with or without mild parenchymal injury; H = cell, hepatocellular injury, mainly degeneration and necrosis with or without inflammation; M = mixed type; J = jaundice, details not clear; PBC = primary biliary cirrhosis; CH = chronic hepatitis

(b) All erythromycins except base

(c) Natural penicillin rarely leads to hepatic injury. Semi-synthetic ones are more likely to do so

(d) Can lead to chronic cholestasis (PBC-like)

(e) Hardly any convincing cases

(f) Too few cases for clear picture

(g) Cause necrosis, fat, carcinoma, and Mallory bodies in mice

(h) Dose related dysfunction leading to hyperbilirubinaemia

Table 14.33 Anti-retroviral agents

Class	Injury pattern	Risk with hepatitis B or C	Comment
A. Nucleoside reverse transcriptase Inhibitors (NRTIs)			
Lamivudine (Epivir)	↑ AT	yes (Hep B)	flare in AT after discontinuation
Stavudine (d4T) (Zerit)	H-cell, jaundice rare	no reports	mean latency 8 months
Zidovudine (AZT) (Retrovir)	H-cell, steatosis	no reports	lactic acidosis, pancreatitis after mean latency of 8 months; Inc risk in women and obesity
Didanosine (Videx)	steatosis, ↑ AT	no reports	fatal lactic acidosis with steatosis (rare)
Abacavir (Ziagen)	steatosis, ↑ GGT	no reports	lactic acidosis with steatosis (class labelling)
Zalcitabine (ddC, hivid)	no reports	no reports	—
B. Nonnucleoside reverse transcriptase Inhibitors (NNRTIs)			
Nevirapine (Viramune)	H-cell, ALF	yes	hypersensitivity reaction with Rash, eosinophilia w/i 3 weeks
Delavirdine (Rescriptor)	no reports	yes	↑ concentration of protease inhibitors
Efavirenz (Sustiva)	H-cell	yes	AT monitoring recommended*
C. Protease Inhibitors (PI)			
Indinavir (Crixivan)	H-cell, steatosis	yes	unconjugated hyperbilirubinemia
Ritonavir (Norvir)	H-cell	yes	acute hepatitis + jaundice in 5–10%
Lopinovir (Kaletra)	H-cell	yes	AT monitoring recommended*
Saquinavir (Fortovase, Invirase)	↑ AT	yes	—
Nelfinavir (Viracept)	no reports	yes	—
Amprenavir (Agenerase)	no reports	?	↑ AUC In cirrhosis
Atazanavir (Reyataz)	H-cell	yes	AT monitoring recommended*

* enzyme monitoring recommended, especially in co-infected hepatitis B or C patients
↑ AT = elevated AST/ALT; ALF = acute liver failure; AUC = area under the curve

---

illness with microvesicular steatosis and may be associated with the formation of Mallory bodies.[1107] Severe hepatitis has been described in patients with AIDS who were treated with **indinavir;** liver biopsy from one of them revealed microvesicular steatosis, fibrosis and inflammatory eosinophilic infiltrates.[1108]

Nevirapine has been associated with the highest rate of severe hepatotoxicity among the HAART agents,[1094,1096,1099,1110] although a review of several large clinical trials disputes this assertion.[1110] Overall, a 1% incidence of hepatotoxicity, including fulminant hepatic failure and Stevens–Johnson syndrome has been reported,[1111] secondary to hypersensitivity mechanisms within 3 weeks of starting therapy. High serum nevirapine levels and coinfection

with viral hepatitis were important risk factors for acute hepatic injury in a study by Gonzalez et al.[1112] Its use in post-exposure prophylaxis in healthy individuals is not recommended.[1111,1113]

Ritonavir has been reported to lead to severe hepatotoxicity in patients with HIV infection who were also infected with hepatitis C or B viruses.[1103,1114] The other PIs are less likely to cause hepatotoxicity[1103,1115] (Table 14.33).

Drugs for the treatment of chronic hepatitis B and C

A trial of **fialuridine** (fluoroiodoarabinofuranosyluracil), a nucleoside analogue for treatment of chronic hepatitis B, was halted because of the sudden development of hepatic failure, lactic acidosis and death in five patients.[25]

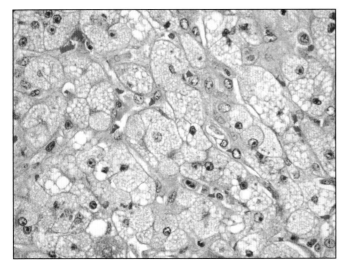

Fig. 14.39 • Fialuridine-associated injury. There is diffuse, microvesicular steatosis. Note the variation in droplet size from cell to cell. There is little inflammation and only rare apoptotic hepatocytes (not shown). H&E.

Histopathological changes included diffuse microvesicular steatosis, glycogen depletion, cholestasis and ductular proliferation (Fig. 14.39). Marked mitochondrial injury was noted ultrastructurally.[25]

Two patients with chronic hepatitis C developed acute hepatitis with marked transaminase elevations and jaundice 3–5 months after initiation of **α-interferon** therapy.[1116] Another patient with chronic hepatitis C developed hepatic failure for which he was successfully transplanted, and was alive and well 16 months later.[1117] Fatal hepatic decompensation also has been reported in several patients with chronic hepatitis B following treatment with α-interferon.[1118] Transient autoimmune hepatitis developed in one patient with chronic hepatitis B treated with α-interferon.[1119] Three other patients with type-1 autoimmune hepatitis, erroneously diagnosed as chronic hepatitis C, had an exacerbation of their liver disease when treated with α-interferon.[1120] α-2β interferon led to the acute vanishing bile-duct syndrome in two patients treated for recurrent HCV infection after liver transplantation.[1121] Epithelioid granulomas have been reported in patients with chronic hepatitis C treated with α-interferon,[1122] but they have been found in a small percentage of patients regardless of therapy.[1123] It is of interest to note that α-interferon therapy has been incriminated in the development of pulmonary sarcoidosis in three patients with chronic hepatitis C.[1124]

Miscellaneous antiviral agents

Idoxuridine has been reported to produce cholestatic jaundice,[1125] as well as instances of serum ALT elevations to a degree that suggests hepatocellular injury.[1126] **Xenalamine** has led to instances of cholestatic jaundice,[1127] and **cytosine arabinoside** has led to jaundice of uncertain type.[1128] Drugs used to treat herpesvirus infections (e.g. **acyclovir, famciclivir**) and those used in the management of influenza (e.g. **zanamivir, amantadine**) have not been reported to cause significant, if any, hepatotoxicity.[1098]

Antiprotozoal and antihelminthic agents

Most of the agents employed to treat malaria, amoebiasis and other protozoal diseases have had little overt hepatotoxic effect.[1] **Amodiaquine,** an antimalarial, has led to a number of instances of severe hepatitis, several fatal.[1129] **Pentamidine,** used for the treatment of *Pneumocystis carinii* pneumonia in patients with AIDS, has led to a 30% incidence of elevated transaminase levels.[1130] **Metronidazole** has been implicated in instances of cholestatic hepatitis confirmed by rechallenge.[1131] Other antiprotozoal agents reported to produce hepatic injury are listed in Table 14.32.

Chlorinated hydrocarbons and organic antimonials, long used as antihelminthics, are known to cause hepatic injury. **Hycanthone,** employed for the treatment of schistosomiasis, has also been found to produce hepatocellular injury and, in some cases, fatal necrosis.[1132] **Thiabendazole** has produced intrahepatic cholestasis, in some instances progressing to the vanishing bile-duct syndrome[1133] and even cirrhosis.[1134] **Niclofolan** has been incriminated in the causation of cholestatic jaundice.[1135] **Piperazine** has been reported to cause acute hepatocellular injury.[1136] **Albendazole**[1137] and **mebendazole**[1138] also have been reported to produce hepatic injury.

Drugs used in cardiovascular diseases

A number of the drugs which are employed in the treatment of cardiac disease, hypertension and atherosclerosis and anticoagulants can produce hepatic injury (Table 14.34). A few warrant special comment.

Anticoagulants

Phenindione has led to well over 100 instances of generalized hypersensitivity. About 10% of these were accompanied by jaundice, which had both cholestatic and hepatocellular features.[1139] The approximately 10% case-fatality-rate was mainly due to generalized hypersensitivity rather than to liver failure. **Acenocoumarol**[1140] and **warfarin**[1141,1142] also have been incriminated in instances of cholestatic injury. **Dicoumarol** has led to fulminant hepatitis.[1143] Cases of acute (sometimes fatal) as well as chronic hepatitis have been attributed to **phenprocoumon.**[1144,1145]

Unfractionated and low molecular weight **heparins** are associated with a high frequency (up to 80%) of low level aminotransferase elevations that are seen early in the course of therapy.[1146,1147] Occasionally, elevated alkaline phosphatase without jaundice reflecting cholestatic injury is seen.[1148,1149] **Ticlopidine,** an antiplatelet agent, has been incriminated in several instances of a cholestatic hepatitis, including prolonged cholestasis for over a year.[1150,1151,1152] A positive T-cell stimulation test suggests an immune mechanism.[1152]

Ximelagatran, the first oral thrombin inhibitor, is approved in Europe for the prevention of venous thromboembolism (VTE) after knee and hip replacement surgery, and is being considered for several other indications, includ-

Table 14.34 Types of hepatic injury produced by various agents used to treat cardiovascular disease

Agents	Types of injury[a]	Agents	Types of injury[a]
Anti-anginal		*Beta blockers*	
Benziodarone	H-Cell	Acebutalol	H-Cell
Coralgil[i]	H-Cell[b]	Atenolol	Ch
Perhexiline	H-Cell[b]	Labetalol	H-Cell
Nitroglycerine	AT	Metoprolol	H-Cell
		Propanolol	H-Cell
Anti-arrythmics			
Ajmaline[e]	Ch, Chronic Ch	*Calcium blockers*	
Aprindine	H-Cell, M	Bepridil	H-Cell
Disopyramide	Ch, M	Diltiazem	H-Cell
Encainide	H-Cell	Nifedipine	H-Cell,Ch,M[b,c,d]
Flecainide	AT, H-Cell	Nicardipine	H-Cell
Mexiletine	H-Cell	Verapamil	H-Cell
Procainamide	H-Cell, M[c]		
Popafenone	Ch	*Diuretics*	Ch
Quinidine	H-Cell[c]	Chlorthalidone	Ch
Tocainide	H-Cell	Furosemide	H-Cell[c]
Amiodarone	H-cell[b]	Quinethazone	Ch
		Thiazides	Ch
		Ticrynafen	H-Cell[d]
Antithrombotics			
Acenocoumarol	H-Cell, M	*Lipid lowering*	
Dipyramidole	H-Cell	Cholestryramine	AT
Heparin	AT	Clofibrate	Ch
Phenindione	Ch	Fenofibrate	Ch, M
Phenoprocoumon	H-Cell, M	Gemfibrozil	AT
Sulphinpyrazole	O	Lovastatin	H-Cell
Streptokinase	AT[g]	Simvastatin	H-Cell
Ticlopidene	H-Cell, Ch, M	Pravastatin, atorvastatin	Ch, AT
Warfarin sodium	Ch[f,g]	Nicotinic acid	H-Cell
Dicoumarol	H-Cell		
Ximelagatran	H-cell, AT		
		Miscellaneous	
Antihypertensives		Nafronyl	H-Cell
Captopril	Ch, M, H-Cell	Papaverine	H-Cell[d]
Dihydralazine	H-Cell[c]	Pentoxifylline	H-Cell[h]
Enalapril	M		
Hydralazine	H-Cell[c]		
Methyldopa	H-Cell[c,d]		

(a) Ch, cholestatic injury; consists mainly of bilirubin casts in canaliculi, usually with portal inflammatory infiltrate and with or without mild, parenchymal injury; H-cell = hepatocellular lesion that consists mainly of necrosis with or without inflammation; M = mixed; AT = abnormal transaminase levels

(b) Lesions may include Mallory bodies, phospholipidosis or both and may lead to cirrhosis

(c) Also lead to hepatic granulomas

(d) Can lead to chronic hepatitis

(e) Includes congeners; prajmaline, detajmium. All three can lead to a chronic cholestatic syndrome resembling primary biliary cirrhosis

(f) Also lead to microvesicular steatosis in large doses

(g) Also had led to haematomas and rupture of the liver

(h) None published

(i) Trade name for 4,'4 diethylaminoethoxyhexestrol, a Japanese drug no longer in use

ing chronic atrial fibrillation and the long-term prevention of stroke and thromboembolism. Clinical trials involving greater than 15 000 on the drug (more than 3500 for >12 months) revealed an incidence of elevated ALT > 3X normal in 7.9% of patients, a few of whom had associated jaundice (0.5%). Nearly all instances of ALT elevations were asymptomatic and resolved whether or not the drug was stopped. More than 90% occurred within 6 months of starting the medication. Three individuals died from liver injury, one of whom had histological evidence of submassive hepatic necrosis.[1153–1156] The deaths, however, were due to massive gastrointestinal haemorrhage in two (due in one patient to a duodenal ulcer that bled well after ximelagatran was stopped), and from acute reactivation of chronic hepatitis B in the third.[1157] In part because of the potential risk of hepatic failure, an FDA advisory committee did not recommend approval in the USA in a September 2004 meeting.[1158]

Antiarrythmics

Despite 60 years of clinical use, **quinidine** was not recognized to cause hepatic injury until 1969.[1] Since then a number of cases have been reported.[1159–1161] Patients have had a syndrome ushered in with fever within 6–12 days of initiation of treatment. In most cases, readministration of a single dose of quinidine led to prompt recurrence of fever and to elevated transaminase levels. The injury is hepatocellular with degeneration and focal necrosis. Liver biopsy has shown granulomas in several patients.[1162]

Procainamide may rarely cause hepatic injury.[1163] In these patients the injury appeared to be mixed-hepatocellular. **Aprindine,** an antiarrhythmic agent with local anaesthetic properties similar to those of procainamide, has been reported to cause hepatic injury with both hepatocellular and cholestatic features.[1164] **Disopyramide** can lead to a cholestatic or mixed injury.[1165]

Amiodarone is a potent anti-arrhythmic with the potential for serious side-effects. The phospholipidosis that this drug can produce is described in an earlier section of this chapter, as are the changes simulating alcoholic liver disease.[133,145,1166] The phospholipidosis depends on the dose and duration of intake as well as, presumably, susceptibility. In a small proportion of recipients of the drug, Mallory bodies with satellitosis with or without steatosis develop[133,1167] (Figs 14.19, 14.20). Whereas the pseudoalcoholic changes usually occur in patients with phospholipidosis, they may precede the latter. Indeed, the two lesions may be presumed to be of different pathogenesis, since each may occur independently of the other[1168] (Table 14.16). In addition, there have been several cases of acute hepatocellular injury after parenteral administration,[1169–1172] although the vehicle (polysorbate 80) has been suggested as the causative component by some authors.[1173,1174] Cholestatic jaundice has been reported,[1175] presumed to be due to immunological idiosyncrasy, as well as a case of microvesicular steatosis.[1176] Minor injury, expressed as abnormal liver function tests (transaminase), occurs in about 25% of recipients.[145] Since amiodarone can remain in the body for months, abnormalities may be slow in subsiding. Dogs develop a similar hepatopathy.[1177] Histologically, aggregates of swollen granular cells (macrophages) containing phospholipid membranous inclusions are seen.[1167,1178,1179] They are also known as 'foam cells'.[133]

Ajmaline, an alkaloid derived from the root of *Rauwolfia serpentina*, is closely related to quinidine in structure and has found similar clinical applications. This drug and several derivatives have been incriminated in a number of instances of jaundice.[1180] In most patients the jaundice has been cho-

lestatic with high levels of alkaline phosphatase, modestly elevated transaminase values, and evidence of cholestasis on biopsy. A number of cases became chronic and developed bile-duct injury with a syndrome resembling primary biliary cirrhosis.[1180]

Propafenone has been associated with acute cholestatic hepatitis.[1181,1182]

Antihypertensives

Methyldopa has led to hepatic injury in at least 80 reported cases during almost two decades of widespread clinical use.[1183] Presumably, there were many unreported cases. The available data suggest that the incidence of overt hepatic disease is well under 1% but that trivial injury reflected by biochemical abnormalities and apparent hepatic dysfunction is more frequent. The hepatic disease has been acute in 85% of recorded cases. The predominant injury has been hepatocellular, resembling that of acute viral hepatitis.[1183] There has usually been a prodromal period of anorexia, malaise and fever, followed in a few days by frank jaundice. Values for AST in most patients have ranged up to 3000 IU/l. Levels of serum alkaline phosphatase have been elevated in almost all patients, but have normally been less than three-times normal.

Coombs-positive haemolytic anaemia occurs in 3% of patients with hepatic injury, a figure similar to the overall incidence in recipients of methyldopa. Lupus erythematosus cells may be demonstrable, and serum antinuclear and anti-smooth muscle antibodies may be transiently present.[1184] The majority of recipients of the drug who develop acute hepatocellular injury, however, have not shown these auto-immune serological markers. Blood eosinophilia also has been rare.

The histological changes resemble those of acute viral hepatitis. Ballooning degeneration, 'free' acidophilic bodies and areas of necrosis are characteristic. The inflammatory response tends to be concentrated in the portal and periportal zones. It consists mainly of lymphocytes and other mononuclear cells with some neutrophils. Tissue eosinophilia is uncommon. Prominence of plasma cells is also not characteristic of the acute form of injury, but is seen in the patients who develop chronic hepatitis. Bridging necrosis extending between portal areas and from portal to central areas was prominent among the patients of Maddrey and Boitnott;[87] and several reported patients have had severe subacute hepatic necrosis.[87,88]

The prognosis of the acute form of hepatocellular injury due to methyldopa approximates that of other forms of drug-induced hepatocellular damage. Approximately 10% of the reported patients with acute hepatic injury have died.[1] In non-fatal cases, recovery is usually prompt after discontinuation of the drug and jaundice disappears in 3–8 weeks. A chronic syndrome which in all regards resembles that of the autoimmune type of chronic hepatitis has been attributed to methyldopa.[92,93,1183] Biopsy has revealed confluent areas of parenchymal necrosis and collapse, condensation of reticulin and an intense inflammatory response in the portal and periportal areas. The inflammatory cells have consisted of lymphocytes, plasma cells, and varying numbers of eosinophils. Biopsy specimens from some patients have shown fibrous septum formation, and several have had pattern of frank macronodular cirrhosis in a setting of chronic necroinflammatory disease.[88] The clinical features, like those of other forms of autoimmune hepatitis, have been a mixture of acute and chronic hepatic disease. Some patients had already developed clinical evidence of cirrhosis when first diagnosed with liver disease. Others presented with apparently acute hepatocellular injury, only to have the biopsy reveal chronic hepatitis.[1183]

The calcium channel blockers **nifedipine, diltiazem, verapamil,** and **amlodipine** have been incriminated in instances of hepatic injury (Table 14.34), both hepatocellular and cholestatic.[1185,1186,1187] Each has led to hepatocellular injury. Nifedipine and diltiazem have been reported to induce the formation of Mallory bodies.[1188] Diltiazem has led to hepatic granulomas.[1189]

Among the angiotensin-converting enzyme inhibitors, **captopril** and **enalapril** have led to both cholestatic and hepatocellular jaundice, more commonly cholestatic.[1190–1192] Acute liver failure has been reported with enalapril.[1193] The congener, **lisinopril**, has led to hepatocellular jaundice with fulminant hepatic failure,[1194] and to chronic hepatitis.[1195] **Ramipril** has led to cholestatic injury with jaundice, with a protracted course with recovery after one year in at least one instance.[1196]

Several **beta blockers** have been incriminated in hepatic injury. These include **labetalol**, which has led to cases of hepatocellular jaundice, a number of which have been fatal,[1197] **acebutolol** which also led to hepatocellular jaundice[1198] and **atenolol**, which has been reported to lead to cholestasis.[1199]

Losartan, a non-peptide angiotensin II type 1 receptor used for treatment of hypertension, has led to one instance of a severe hepatocellular injury.[1200] **Candesartan** caused reversible bile stasis, portal cholangitis and ductopenia in a patient presenting with abdominal pain and jaundice.[1201] Chronic cholestasis was also reported with **irbesartan**.[1202]

Hydralazine and its congener **dihydralazine** has been reported to lead to perivenular zone necrosis,[1203] and to cholangitis and a granulomatous reaction.[1204]

Drugs for the treatment of hyperlididemia

Clofibrate appears to have few important adverse effects on the liver. It leads to mild and transient increases in transaminase and to impaired hepatic excretory function,[1] possibly through effects on mitochondria.[1205] It has been reported to lead to cholestatic injury[1206] and to hepatic granulomas.[1207] Clofibrate may have hepatoprotective properties.[1208] **Fenofibrate** has been reported to lead to instances of cholestasis and of chronic hepatitis.[1209] While clofibrate and its congeners have induced peroxisomal proliferation and carcinoma in experimental animals, there is no evidence that either of these occur in humans.[1]

Nicotinic acid and its derivatives have caused biochemical evidence of hepatic dysfunction in about one-third and jaundice in 3–5% of long-term recipients.[1210–1212] The long-

acting preparation appears to be particularly prone to cause the injury, which usually resolves within one month of discontinuation, although severe necrosis and fulminant hepatic failure has occurred.[1210,1212] The demonstration of parenchymal degeneration and necrosis on biopsy, and the high serum levels of ALT in these cases indicate hepatocellular injury.[1211]

Several **hydroxymethylglutaryl CoA (HMGCoA) reductase inhibitors (statins), lovastatin,[1213] simvastatin,[1214] pravastatin,[1215] fluvastatin** and **atorvastatin**[1216,1217] have been implicated in cases of mild hepatocellular or cholestatic injury. Elevations in ALT rarely exceeding 3-fold are seen in about 5% of patients, often resolving (or at least not progressing) despite continued treatment.[1218,1219] Studies in animals suggest that the ALT elevations are due to the inhibition of mevalonic acid in the cholesterol synthesis cascade.[1220] The newest statin, **rosuvastatin**, had an incidence of ALT elevations identical to placebo in clinical trials.[1221] Similarly, no difference in the incidence of ALT > 3X was found In a large prospective analysis of nearly 20 000 patients.[1222] **Cervistatin** (Baycol) was withdrawn after an increased risk of renal failure and muscle injury (rhabdomyolysis) was observed compared with other agents in this class, especially when taken with a fibrate.[1223] While ALT monitoring has been proposed for the class, its cost-effectiveness has been called into question given the rarity of serious liver injury seen with these drugs.[1219,1224,1225] The use of statins has been demonstrated to be safe in patients with underlying NASH and other chronic liver diseases.[1226,1227]

Diuretics

Rare instances of jaundice, apparently hepatocanalicular, have been observed in patients taking **thiazide** diuretics.[1] **Quinethazone, ethacrynic acid, chlorthalidone** and **frusemide** have been reported rarely to lead to jaundice, perhaps due to hypersensitivity.[1] Mitchell and Jollow[632] showed that large doses of furosemide led to mid-zonal necrosis in rats. Their studies demonstrated clearly that the injury was caused by a metabolite of the drug. An experimental, light microscopic and ultrastructural study of furosemide injury in mice revealed perivenular zone necrosis, and suggested an important role for the plasma membrane in the development of hepatic damage.[1228]

Ticrynafen (tienilic acid) is a uricosuric diuretic that caused severe acute hepatocellular injury with fatal necrosis, and instances of chronic hepatitis and cirrhosis that forced its withdrawal from clinical use soon after its introduction in the USA.[1229,1230] It remains a prototypical example of hepatic injury caused by immunoallergic mechanisms.[1231]

Antineoplastic and immunosuppressive agents

Several forms of hepatic injury are particularly characteristic of some oncotherapeutic and immunosuppressive agents (Table 14.35) including steatosis and steatohepatitis seen

Table 14.35 Some hepatic lesions produced by oncotherapeutic agents

	Biochemical(a)	Fat	Necrosis	Cholestasis	VOD	Peliosis
Aclarubicin	AT	–	–	–	–	–
Actinomycin D(b)	H-Cell	+	+	–	+	–
Aminoglutethamide	Chol	–	–	+	–	–
Amsacrine(c)	H-Cell/Chol	+	+	+	–	–
Anabolic Steroids	Chol	–	–	+	–	+
Asparaginase	H-Cell	+	(+)(d)	–	–	–
Azathioprine(e,f)	H-Cell/Chol	–	+	+	+	+
Bleomycin	H-Cell(d)	+	–	–	–	–
Busulfan	Chol	–	–	+	+(b)	+
Carmustine	H-Cell	+	+	–	–	–
Chlorambucil	H-Cell	–	+	–	–	–
Chloropurine	H-Cell	–	+	–	–	–
Cisplatin	H-Cell	+	+	–	–	–
Cyclophosphamide	Chol	–	–	+	+	+
Cyclosporin	Chol	–	–	+	–	–
Cytoxan	H-Cell	–	+	–	–	–
Cytarabine	H-Cell	–	+	–	+(b)	–
Dacarbazine	H-Cell	–	+	–	+	–
Daunorubicin	H-Cell(b)	–	+	–	+(b)	–
Dichloromethotrexate	H-Cell	+	+	–	–	–
Diethylstiboestrol(d)	H-Cell	+	–	–	–	–
Doxorubicin	H-Cell	–	+	–	+(b)	–
Oestrogens (Steroid)	Chol	–	–	–	+/–	+
Etoposide	H-Cell	–	+	–	–	–
Floxuridine(j)	Chol/H-Cell	–	–	+	+	–
Gemcitabine	H-cell, AT		+			
Gemtuzumab	H-cell		+		+	
Homoharringtonine	AT					
Hydrazines	H-Cell	+	+	–	–	–
Hydroxyprogesterone	Chol	–	–	+	–	–
Hydroxyurea	H-Cell	–	–	–	–	+
Indicine-N oxide	H-Cell	–	+	–	+	–
Interferons	AT	–	–	–	–	–
Interleukin-2(i)	Chol	+	+	+	–	–
Medroxyprogesterone	Chol	–	–	+	–	–
Melphalan	AT	–	–	–	–	–
Mercaptopurine	H-Cell/Chol	–	+	+	–	–
Methotrexate	H-Cell	+	+(g)	–	–	–
Mithramycin	H-Cell	–	+	–	–	–
Mitomycin	H-Cell	+	–	–	+	–
Mitoxantrone	AT	–	–	–	–	–
Monomethylformamide	H-Cell	+	+	–	–	–
Procarbazine	H-Cell(b)	–	–	–	–	–
Semustine	AT	–	–	–	–	–
Streptozotocin	H-Cell	+	+	–	–	–
Tamoxifen	H-cell, chol	+	–	+	–	+
Teniposide	H-Cell	–	+	–	–	–
Thioguanine	H-Cell	–	+	+	+	–
Thiotepa(h)	H-Cell	+	+	–	–	–
Urethane	H-Cell	–	+	–	+	–
Vinca alkaloids	H-Cell(b)	–	+(b)	–	+(b)	–

(a) Pattern of injury: H-Cell = hepatocellular; Chol = cholestatic; H-Cell/Chol = either; AT = elevated aminotransferase levels; PL = phospholipidosis; VOD = veno-occlusive disease

(b) Only when given with other agents or radiotherapy

(c) Cholestasis is the more characteristic lesion

(d) Minor component of lesion

(e) Can cause chronic cholestatisis

(f) Can cause chronic hepatitis

(g) In large parenteral doses

(h) Periportal injury resembling that of phosphorus poisoning

(i) Pattern of injury is consistently cholestatic. Histological changes show more variation

(j) Characteristic injury is sclerosing cholangitis when drug is administered by pump infusion into hepatic artery with antimetabolites and antioestrogens, and veno-occlusive disease, similar to that seen with the pyrrolizidine alkaloids (Fig. 14.25).[1232–1234] Some antineoplastic drugs appear to spare the liver altogether, or produce hepatic injury only rarely as a result of host idiosyncrasy.[1,1235]

Antimetabolites and related agents

Some antimetabolites and antibiotics are intrinsic hepatotoxins with a dose-related ability to produce liver damage. In this category are methotrexate, some antipyrimidine and antipurine compounds, asparaginase and a number of antineoplastic antibiotics.

Treatment of neoplastic disease with large doses of **methotrexate** can lead to acute injury, even necrosis, but the incidence is low.[797,1236] Cirrhosis is even less likely to be a problem, since prolonged therapy is not usual. Light microscopic and ultrastructural changes in patients on methotrexate therapy are described by many investigators.[1234] The use of methotrexate in non-malignant disease is discussed under NSAIDs (p. 711).

Azauridine and azacytidine are pyrimidine antagonists that have been shown to produce steatosis and necrosis in experimental animals.[1237] **Cytosine arabinoside** (cytarabine) has been reported to produce cholestatic jaundice in a few case reports; apparently mild.[1238] **5-fluorouracil** can produce hepatic injury when given intravenously but not orally.[1239]

Floxuridine (FUDR) given by pump-infusion via the hepatic artery for treatment of colonic carcinoma metastatic to the liver has led to a high incidence of sclerosing cholangitis[114,115,117] (Fig. 14.17). The blebbing, necrosis, inflammation and distortion of the biliary tree has been called an 'ischaemic cholangiopathy' since it appears to result from injury to branches of the hepatic artery[117] (Fig. 14.17(D)).

Azaserine is a glutamine antagonist which inhibits purine synthesis. It produces steatosis as well as some liver cell necrosis.[1240] **6-mercaptopurine**, an agent which may also be used as an immunosuppressant, may produce hepatocellular or cholestatic injury, with jaundice in 6–40% of recipients.[1241–1243] While cholestasis is prominent in some patients, the predominant injury is hepatocellular, and fatal hepatic necrosis has occurred. Possible potentiation of the hepatotoxicity of mercaptopurine by doxorubicin has been suggested because of the frequency and severity of hepatic injury when these two drugs are used in combination for the treatment of refractory leukaemia.[1244,1245] **6-chloropurine** has led to similar hepatic injury.[1] **Thioguanine** has been reported to cause jaundice, veno-occlusive disease and NRH[1,1233] (Fig. 14.29).

Azathioprine, a derivative of mercaptopurine used mainly as an immunosuppressant, has led to a few reported instances of cholestatic injury, and also has been incriminated in a number of instances of hepatocellular or mixed injury.[1246] This drug also can lead to striking sinusoidal dilatation,[1247] peliosis hepatis[193] and veno-occlusive disease.[1248] Nodular regenerative hyperplasia is also reported, with a possible mechanism common to all forms of the injury being endothelial cell damage with leakage of red blood cells into the space of Disse, resulting in progressive fibrosis.[1249] Clinically, VOD (sinusoidal obstruction syndrome) presents as the rapid onset of ascites with other features of portal hypertension. Markedly elevated ALT , bilirubin and alkaline phosphatase levels can be seen. Those with severe VOD have a poor outcome marked by a high case-fatality.[59,160] A possible role for azathioprine in the development of hepatocellular carcinoma in two renal transplant recipients has been raised by Sacian et al.[1250]

L-asparaginase, although an enzyme, behaves like an antimetabolite. It catalyses the deamination of asparagine, thus depriving the neoplastic cell of this amino acid and blocking protein synthesis. Presumably, the steatosis which asparaginase produces in 60 to 90% of recipients (Fig. 14.18(D)) depends on the same mechanism, although some authors have attributed the hepatic injury to a contaminant of the enzyme.[1251]

Some **antineoplastic antibiotics** produce necrosis, while others cause steatosis, presumably by mechanisms related to their antineoplastic effects.[1233,1234] Nevertheless, some potent cytostatic agents (**actinomycin D, cycloheximide, daunorubicin**) cause necrosis of bone marrow and intestinal mucosa, but not hepatic lesions. The potentiation of hepatic injury of 6-mercaptopurine by **adriamycin (doxorubicin)**, however, has been noted previously.[1252] Similarly, severe liver toxicity may follow the administration of **actinomycin D** after nephrectomy and irradiation for Wilms tumour.[1253] Doxorubicin itself has led to hepatic necrosis.[1252] Adverse effects of other oncotherapeutic antibiotics are shown in Table 14.35.

Alkaloids

The vinca alkaloids, **vincristine** and **vinblastine,** differ from each other somewhat in their toxic side effects, but both lead to little hepatic injury in man or experimental animals.[1] One early report drew attention to the small areas of hepatic necrosis observed at autopsy in patients who had been treated with vincristine.[1254] El Saghir and Hawkins[1255] observed transient serum enzyme elevations in a patient on vincristine therapy. Coupled with radiation, these agents can apparently lead to necrosis.[1256]

Interleukin-2, IL-2 used for the treatment of renal cell carcinoma, melanoma and other malignancies, has led to severe intrahepatic cholestasis,[1257] and to abnormal liver function tests associated with portal and sinusoidal lymphocytic infiltrates, focal necrosis and cholestasis in a series of cases.[1258,1259] **IL-6** an agent used for colon cancer, has demonstrated zone 3 ballooning and cholestasis in animals[1260], and in humans (Fig. 14.40).

Alkylating agents

Five groups of alkylating agents have been utilized in the treatment of neoplastic diseases—the nitrogen mustards, ethyleneamines, alkyl sulphonates (busulphan, dimethylbusulphan), the nitrosoureas, and the triazines (dacarbazine, procarbazine).[796] As nearly as can be ascertained from

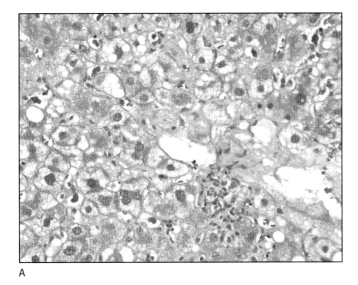

A

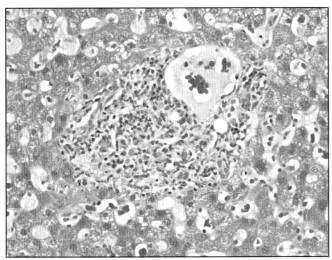

B

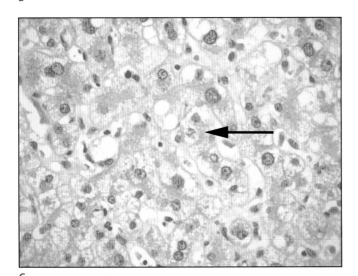

C

Fig. 14.40 • Interleukin-6-associated injury. All figures from the same case. **(A)** Zone 3 injury with mixed micro and macrovesicular steatosis and cell swelling with focal spotty inflammation. H&E. **(B)** Rare portal areas showed significant lymphohistiocytic infiltration with focal interface hepatitis. H&E. **(C)** Hepatocellular bile stasis (arrow)was seen best in the iron stain. Iron.

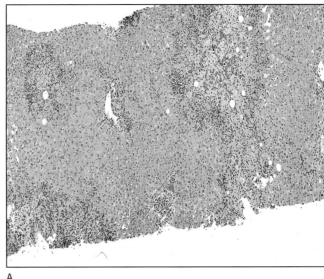

A

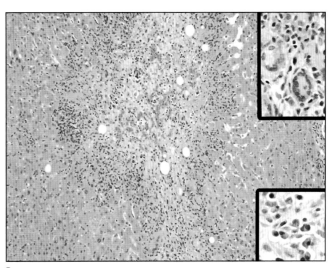

B

Fig. 14.41 • Trovofloxacin-associated injury. All figures from the same case. **(A)** At low magnification there is prominent zone 3 necrosis with a marked inflammatory infiltrate. The portal areas show mild infiltration with little periportal injury. H&E. **(B)** Higher magnification of the zone 3 injury. The inflammation has a granulomatous character, with giant cells and eosinophils (inset, upper right) and plasma cells (inset, lower right). H&E. Photomicrographs courtesy of Dr Zachary Goodman.

the available literature, the ethyleneamine derivatives have not been incriminated in the production of liver damage.[796]

Among the nitrogen mustards, the prototypic **mechlorethamine and melphalan** also seem free of responsibility for hepatic injury, although several other members of the group have led to liver damage.[796,1233] Hepatocellular injury, associated in one case with massive necrosis, has been reported after the use of **cyclophosphamide** when given postoperatively for breast cancer,[1261] or for treatment of lupus erythematosus[1262] or Wegeners granulomatosis.[1263] Cumulative hepatotoxicity (acute hepatitis) was reported after continuous low-dose therapy for Sjögren syndrome for 24 months.[1264] Hepatocellular necrosis was also reported in patients with vasculitis who were treated with cyclophosphamide preceded by azathioprine.[1265] A case of veno-occlusive disease involving both terminal hepatic venules and portal vein branches was reported by Modzelewski et al.[1266] (Fig. 14.25). **Chlorambucil** has been incriminated in several instances of hepatocellular jaundice.[1260] Cholestatic jaundice, hepatitis, and nodular regenerative hyperplasia have been attributed to an alkyl sulphonate (**busulphan**).[1267] High doses have led to veno-occlusive disease.[1233] In reference to the *nitrosoureas*, the parent compound **carmustine (BCNU)** has led to hepatic dysfunction in up to 25% of recipients. **Lomustine (CCNU)** and **semustine** have also led to elevated serum transaminase.[1234]

Other anti-tumour agents

Cisplatin is associated with a relatively low incidence of steatosis, cholestasis and less frequently, hepatocellular injury.[1234] **Gemcitabine** leads to transaminase elevations in over half of patients, in some >10-fold normal.[1234] It was recently reported to cause severe cholestatic hepatitis in a patient with metastatic breast cancer.[1268] **Gemtuzumab ozogamicin** (Mylotarg) is a monoclonal antibody conjugate directed against blast cells in used in the treatment of acute myeloid leukaemia. It has been associated with veno-occlusive disease (sinusoidal obstruction syndrome (SOS)) that can be fatal without stem cell transplantation.[1269,1270] Even among those undergoing pre-treatment stem cell transplantation, mortality rates from SOS have been >10%.[1271] Other monoclonal antibody therapies used in the treatment of malignancy are reviewed by Cersosimo.[1272]

Imatinib mesylate (Gleevec) was recently approved for the treatment of CML and gastrointestinal stromal tumours (GIST). A few reports of liver injury have started to appear.[1273]

Urethane, formerly used to treat leukaemia and multiple myeloma, is a known experimental hepatotoxin and hepatocarcinogen.[1274] It has produced perivenular necrosis and fibrosis in association with injury to the efferent hepatic veins and venules.[1274] The histological changes and syndrome resemble the veno-occlusive disease of pyrrolizidine toxicity.

Anti-androgens and anti-oestrogens used in the management of prostate, breast and gynecological malignancies are discussed under Hormonal agents (see p. 715). Before leaving this section note should be made of the reactivation or development of hepatic decompensation of chronic hepatitis B by withdrawal of cytotoxic chemotherapy or immunosuppressive therapy.[1275,1276] A similar phenomenon has been reported in chronic hepatitis C.[1277]

Drugs used in gastrointestinal disease

H₁-receptor antagonists

A number of antihistamines have been incriminated in liver injury. Isolated instances of cholestatic or mixed-jaundice have been attributed to **chlorpheniramine**,[1278] **cyclizine**,[1279] **trimethobenzamide**,[1280] **cyproheptadine**,[1281] **terfenadine**,[1282] and **tripelennamine**.[1] **Loratidine** has been incriminated in an instance of subfulminant liver failure.[1283] **Cetirizine** has been implicated in hepatocellular

injury.[1284,1285] Liver biopsy findings of diffuse portal tract and lobular inflammation with a prominent eosinophilic infiltrate were described in a patient with two prior episodes associated with cetirizine use, and a positive lymphocyte stimulation test suggesting hypersensitivity as the mechanism.[1285]

Acid suppressive agents

Histamine (H₂) receptor antagonists

These widely used agents, including **cimetidine, ranitidine, famotidine** and **nizatidine,** appear to have a very low incidence of hepatic injury.[1286,1287] Cimetidine and ranitidine have been incriminated in clinically evident hepatocellular, cholestatic and mixed injury.[1286,1288,1289] A case of fatal hepatitis associated with ranitidine has been reported,[1290] although several other drugs were also being taken, making causality difficult. Luyendyk et al.[1291] described fibrin deposition in the livers of animals with ranitidine hepatotoxicity. The injury was abolished by rats pre-treated with LPS heparin. Prolonged cholestasis[1292] and chronic hepatitis[1293] have each been reported with cimetidine therapy. Other H₂ receptor antagonists not in clinical use, that appear to have led to significant hepatic injury, include **ebrotidine,** which was implicated in several cases of perivenular zone necrosis, massive necrosis, persistently abnormal liver tests after acute hepatitis, and cirrhosis,[1294,1295] as well as **oxmetidine**[1296] and **zaltidine**.[1297]

Proton pump inhibitors (PPIs)

At least two well-documented cases of hepatotoxicity related to **omeprazole** have been reported.[1298,1299] A patient with fulminant hepatitis on omeprazole was also taking aspirin, diltiazem and atenelol.[1300] Another case where causality was unclear involved a patient with congestive cardiac failure who had been taking omeprazole for years.[1301] Similar difficulties in establishing a causal relationship to **rabeprazole** was cited by Andrade & Lucena.[1302] Liver injury from the other PPIs is infrequent.[1287]

Laxatives

The agent **oxyphenisatin** had been in use as a component of laxative preparations for many years, when it was first recognized as a cause of hepatic disease. Within 3–4 years more than 100 cases had been identified.[1303–1305] About two-thirds of these presented with chronic hepatitis, while the remainder apparently had acute disease.[1306] The injury is the prototype of drug-induced autoimmune chronic hepatitis.

The majority of patients were women. Those with acute liver damage presented with anorexia, fatigue and jaundice, often accompanied by slight upper abdominal distress.[1305,1306] A similar presentation also was found in some patients with chronic liver damage, although most had an insidious onset. Chronic liver injury seemed particularly to develop in patients who continued taking oxyphenisatin after jaundice had appeared and been ignored, or where the relationship to the drug had been overlooked.[1307] Serological features, typical for autoimmune hepatitis, including lupus erythmatosus cells, anti-nuclear and anti-smooth muscle antibodies, were observed in patients with the chronic syndrome.

The histological changes in oxyphenisatin-induced disease ranged from those typical for acute hepatitis, through changes classical for chronic hepatitis, to frank cirrhosis.[1303–1307] Patients with the acute syndrome showed diffuse hepatocellular necrosis, apoptotic bodies, lobular disarray, Kupffer-cell prominence and inflammation, mainly portal. The pattern resembled that of acute viral hepatitis, although cholestasis and steatosis appeared to be more prominent in oxyphenisatin jaundice. Patients with the syndrome of chronic hepatitis may show subacute hepatic necrosis.[1307] More often the changes were those classical for chronic hepatitis with interface hepatitis, portal and periportal inflammation (with plasma cells and lymphocytes), 'rosette' formation and periportal architectural distortion. A number of patients had frank cirrhosis.

The prognosis in most patients with acute injury was good. Withdrawal of the drug usually led to prompt improvement, although instances of progression of disease even after stopping the drug have been described. Even patients with chronic disease usually improved after the drug was stopped, but some continued to show active disease.[1303–1307] Use of oxyphenisatin has been largely abandoned.

Senna and cascara sagrada are reviewed under *Herbal therapies*.

Drugs used to treat inflammatory bowel disease

Sulphasalazine—a combination of sulphapyridine and 5-aminosalicylate—has been implicated in over 70 instances of hepatic injury.[1308–1312] Injury has been more frequently hepatocellular than cholestatic, although either may occur. In about 10% of cases, the hepatic injury is severe enough to lead to massive necrosis and death. The necrosis is non-zonal, being similar to that of other forms of sulphonamide-associated injury. One of the patients with sulphasalazine liver injury had a mononucleosis-like syndrome,[1313] and granulomatous hepatitis has been reported.[1314]

Reactions to sulphasalazine had been assumed to be due to the sulphonamide component. However, there are reports of similar injury due to **5-aminosalicylate (mesalamine)** formulations alone.[1315–1317]

6-Mercaptopurine, and **azathiprine** used for the treatment of Crohn disease, has led to several instances of hepatic injury.[1318]

The anti-tumour necrosis factor agents, **inflixamab and etanercept,** do not appear to be inherently hepatotoxic, but case reports have appeared associated with a positive antinuclear antibody.[1319] Infliximab, a chimeric monoclonal antibody to tumour necrosis factor used in the management of Crohn disease and rheumatoid arthritis, has been associated with a few reports of cholestasis and acute hepatitis with prominent bile duct injury.[1320,1321] In addition, enzyme flares have been seen in patients with underlying hepatitis B.[1322] In contrast, these agents were being investigated for the treatment of alcoholic hepatitis, although an increased rate of infectious complications was seen with the use of Inflixamab in clinical trials.[1323]

Analgesic drugs

Acetaminophen (paracetamol, N-acetyl-p-aminophenol [APAP])

This widely used mild analgesic has virtually no side-effects when taken in the usual therapeutic doses. However, it produces severe hepatic necrosis when large doses are ingested, usually in an attempted suicide,[4,255,1324–1327] but increasingly as inadvertent overdoses in adults and children.[1324,1328,1329] APAP is the most common cause of acute liver failure in the USA and other nations, and leads to liver transplantation more often than any other drug-related cause of liver failure.[4,22] Doses taken in suicidal attempts have ranged from a minimum of 7.5–10 g to more than 70 g.[1324,1327] Histological changes in the liver in the majority of cases consist of perivenular zone 3 necrosis and sinusoidal congestion, at times accompanied by steatosis (Fig. 14.2). This zonality reflects the role of CYP2E1 in the formation of the toxic metabolite formed, and the lower levels of GSH located in this part of the liver acinus. Submassive and massive (panacinar) necrosis may be present in severe cases.[1330] One example each of a cholestatic injury and a granulomatous hepatitis have been attributed to the drug.[1331] In patients who recover without the need for liver transplantation, complete resolution of the injury (without fibrosis) is to be expected.[1332]

Biochemical features of importance include striking elevations of transaminase levels, hypoprothrombinaemia and, in severe injury, lactic acidosis. Aminotransferase levels range from 50- to 1000-fold increases and the injury progresses through three well-defined stages. The seminal studies of Mitchell and others[81] demonstrated that a metabolite of the drug (N-acetyl-p-benzoquinone imine (NAPQI)), leads to the necrosis, apparently as a consequence of its covalent binding to tissue macromolecules. Necrosis occurs only when the quantity of drug taken yields amounts of metabolite that exceed the binding capacity of tissue glutathione. Subclinical elevations of ALT are not well-described, and chronic hepatitis from APAP remains unsubstantiated.[1332]

A number of potential factors appear to influence the susceptibility of acute APAP injury, including regular alcohol ingestion, fasting and malnutrition (that reduce hepatic glutathione concentrations), and drug-drug interactions (INH, rifampin and anticonvulsants),[1324] although Rumack has called many of these relationships into question.[1333] For example, the amount of alcohol ingestion that may predispose to injury from therapeutic doses is not known. While the majority of cases of APAP-induced hepatic necrosis appear to have resulted from large suicidal overdose of the drug, a number of cases have been the result of 'misadventures' involving doses in the therapeutic range.[1324,1328,1329] For the most part, these have involved alcoholic patients in whom the inducing effect of alcohol on CYP2E1 was held responsible for increased production of the hepatotoxic metabolite. Depletion of glutathione secondary to alcoholism is also considered to play a role.[1328] In contrast, acute alcohol intoxication does not appear to predispose to APAP injury.[1334] A number of authorities still regard the concept of 'therapeutic misadventure' (as coined by Zimmerman) as being controversial (if not unlikely) when it comes to truly therapeutic doses of APAP leading to fulminant hepatic failure.[1333] Perhaps it should be renamed 'unintentional overdose' to distinguish an accidental ingestion taken with therapeutic intent (which in fact may exceed 4 g/day) from a deliberate overdose taken with suicidal intent. Daily doses of 2 g or less appear safe for use, even in patients with chronic liver disease. Children are at risk from the use of adult formulations given in an unintentional overdose.[1329]

The prognosis of a suicidal overdose is similar to that of acute hepatic necrosis induced by other drugs. Approximately 10% of all patients who have taken an overdose and up to 25% of those who develop hepatic injury develop hepatic failure. In contrast, those in whom an accidental or inadvertent overdose has occurred typically present much later in the course of the injury, and mortality rates have been higher.[255] For acute ingestions recognized (or brought to medical attention) early in phase I, the prognosis seems to correlate with peak levels of unmetabolized drug measured between 4 and 15 hours after ingestion based on nonograms developed by Rumack and colleagues.[1332,1335] Treatment with N-acetyl cystene administered early in the course has reduced mortality rates down to <10%, with near complete protection against severe hepatic injury developing when the antidote is given within 12 hours of ingestion.[255,1332]

APAP may also play a role in cases of 'idiopathic' acute liver failure seen in the USA and abroad, based on the finding by Lee and colleagues of APAP protein adducts in the serum of about 20% of these cases. Moreover, APAP ingestion may contribute to the hepatic injury of viral hepatitis.[4]

Aspirin

The effects of this agent are discussed in the section on NSAIDs.

Propoxyphene

This widely used analgesic has been incriminated in rare instances of hepatic injury. Several cases of cholestatic injury have now been recorded.[1336]

Miscellaneous drugs

Etretinate

A number of patients receiving the aromatic retinoid derivative of vitamin A for the treatment of psoriasis have developed liver abnormalities including elevations of liver function tests, cholestasis, periportal fibrosis, chronic hepatitis and even cirrhosis.[1337–1339] The latent period has ranged from 1 to 6 months. That hypersensitivity may be the mechanism for the injury in some cases is suggested by the associ-

ated eosinophilia and fever in some cases. Reappearance of etretinate-induced liver injury upon challenge also has been demonstrated.[1338] **Acitretin,** a metabolite of etretinate, also has been reported to cause severe hepatic injury that progressed to cirrhosis.[1340]

Total parenteral nutrition (TPN)

Most instances of TPN-related liver injury have occurred in infants,[1341,1342] but adults also may be affected.[1343–1345] Risk factors in infants include prematurity, low birth weight and sepsis. However, prolonged duration of treatment may be the most important factor.[1346] One or more components of the TPN solution may be directly toxic to the liver, in particular the amino acids or micronutrients in the solution. Recent experimental evidence suggests that methionine, manganese and phytosterols may be responsible;[1345,1346] deficiencies of taurine, choline or carnitine may also play a role.[1345,1346]

The histological changes of TPN injury include intrahepatic cholestasis, ballooning and scattered apoptotic bodies, presence of lipofuscin pigment in hypertrophied Kupffer cells, variable periportal ductular proliferation and fibrosis and, in some cases, a biliary-type micronodular cirrhosis. Steatosis is less common in infants than in adults.[1342,1345,1346] Other hepatobiliary complications have included phospholipidosis in a number of adult patients,[1347] an instance of the Budd–Chiari syndrome in a premature infant,[1348] cases of hepatocellular carcinoma in children, one with cirrhosis[1349] and one without,[1350] and cholelithiasis in both children and adults.[1345,1346,1351]

Drugs used in hepatic, renal, cardiac and bone marrow transplantation

Recognizing and confirming drug-induced injury in the transplant setting may be quite challenging given the number of confounding factors. Changes in liver enzymes and histological abnormalities may have more than one aetiology (e.g. acute or chronic rejection; graft versus host disease, recurrent viral or autoimmune hepatitis, etc.) that must be differentiated from possible drug injury. Moreover, cyclosporin, tacrolimus and sirolimus are metabolized by CYP3A, and are substrates for p-glycoprotein in the liver and intestine; they are subject to drug-drug interactions that may lead to various forms of toxicity.[1352] Nevertheless, a few general comments can be made regarding the most commonly used agents.

Cyclosporin hepatotoxicity has been reported in renal allograft recipients,[1353] heart transplant recipients,[1354] and liver allograft recipients.[1355] Liver injury has also been reported when cyclosporin was used for treatment of endogenous uveitis, with the latent period averaging 5.5 months, and mild-moderate elevations in alkaline phosphatase being the predominant biochemical abnormality.[1356] In general, the hepatotoxicity has been predominantly cholestatic and mild. Cyclosporin tissue levels in recipients of liver allografts were high in one study[1355] and correlated with increased gamma glutamyl transpeptidase levels, implying dose-related toxicity.[1356] Liver biopsy specimens from the patients showed hypertrophy of bile ductal epithelial cells with cytoplasmic vacuoles, and the presence of 'foamy' material in sinusoids.[1356] Granulomatous hepatitis is also reported. Cyclosporin induces cholestasis in the rat liver by decreasing both bile flow and bile salt secretion, and by altering membrane permeability to calcium.[1357] In humans, biliary sludge or gallstone formation is reported in up to 30% of transplant patients,[1352] depletion of antioxidant activity has been suggested as a possible mechanism of injury.[1358]

Tacrolimus (FK 506, Prograf) led to hepatic dysfunction in about 10% of kidney transplant recipients.[1352] In liver transplant patients, elevations in ALT and alkaline phosphatase (up to 10 fold) have been reported to occur after a latency of 6–24 weeks.[1359] Liver biopsies have shown perivenular hepatocellular necrosis and drop-out.[1360]

Sirolimus has been associated with elevations in alkaline phosphatase and aminotransferases that were not significantly different from placebo or azathioprine in clinical trials.[1352] At least one case of acute hepatic injury has appeared.[1361]

Corticosteroids are associated with macrovesicular steatosis, thought to be related to increased levels of free fatty acids associated with their use. Overt hepatic injury appears to be rare, if it occurs at all.[1]

Disulfiram, used in aversion therapy for alcoholism, has been incriminated in several dozen reported instances of hepatic injury.[1362–1364] The injury has been mainly hepatocellular; in many instances leading to fulminant hepatic failure with a high fatality rate.[1,1364,1365] About 25% of recipients have developed abnormal LFTs,[1366] suggesting some degree of intrinsic hepatotoxic potential, although positive rechallenge cases imply immunological idiosyncrasy.[1] Injury generally occurs within the first 8 weeks with transaminase elevations up to 100-fold, and jaundice in many cases. Recovery is usually seen within 1–2 months after the drug is withdrawn.

Cyanamide, as noted earlier, can lead to a dramatic form of ground glass change resembling Lafora bodies (Fig. 14.31), and the lesion can lead to cirrhosis.[236]

Ritodrine, a tocolytic β2-adrenergic agonist agent used to delay or abolish preterm labour, has been implicated in liver function test abnormalities and in two instances of liver injury.[1367]

Microcystins, produced by cyanobacteria (blue-green algae) growing in water used for haemodialysis in a haemodialysis centre in Brazil, led to liver failure and death of 26 patients.[1368] Liver tissue from 16 of the patients revealed disruption of liver plates, extensive necrosis, apoptosis, severe cholestasis, cytoplasmic vacuolization and a mixed leucocyte infiltrate.[1368]

Zafirlukast, a leukotriene receptor antagonist used in the treatment of asthma, has been reported to cause a number of instances of fulminant liver failure.[1369–1373] Submassive necrosis with eosinophilia has been described.[1370]

Propafenone has been associated with acute reversible cholestatic hepatitis along with the development of positive anti-nuclear antibodies in a few patients.[1374,1375]

Thalidomide has caused reversible hepatocellular jaundice in a patient with stable hepatitis C being treated for hairy cell leukaemia. The reaction resolved after thalidomide was withdrawn.[1376]

Diagnostic considerations in causality assessment in DILD

A detailed history is essential for adequate evaluation of drug-induced or toxic liver injury. This must include the use of herbal preparations and substance abuse, past or present as well as over-the-counter products. If a therapeutic drug is suspected, the history should document the dosage, route of administration, and duration of therapy of the suspect drug and any other concomitantly administered drugs. When a toxin is being considered the amount, duration, and type of exposure (ingestion, inhalation, absorption from the skin or mucous membranes) are all extremely important in the evaluation of a given case.

The interval of time from the beginning of drug therapy or exposure to a toxin to the development of symptoms or signs heralding the onset of the injury ('latent period') must be estimated. In some instances, it is possible to pinpoint the onset by the occurrence of a symptom complex, such as a 'flu-like' syndrome, various gastrointestinal complaints, or fever followed by a rash while the patient is taking a drug. On the other hand, such symptoms and signs may be difficult to unravel from those of the underlying disease, in which case reliance must be placed on the subsequent appearance of jaundice or abnormal results of liver function tests. When determined, the latent period should fall within the previously accepted range of time for injury for a particular drug (or class of drugs); for example, a few days after a second or multiple exposure to halothane; 1–4 weeks for injury associated with chlorpromazine, erythromycin or phenytoin; and anywhere from 5 weeks to a year for a drug such as isoniazid. In patients with chronic liver disease (chronic hepatitis, cirrhosis) on long-term drug therapy the onset of the illness may be difficult if not impossible to determine.

Without question, the most important aspect of the investigation of a possible drug-induced or toxic injury is to rule out other causes of liver disease by careful assessment of all the clinical, morphological, radiological, biochemical and serological findings. The possibility of a drug or toxic insult superimposed on another, pre-existing liver disease, also should be considered. It is worth noting that drugs also can exacerbate or reactivate a pre-existing liver disease, for example the reactivation of chronic hepatitis B or hepatitis C infection by withdrawal (or initiation) of cancer chemotherapy, α-interferon or corticosteroid therapy. Additionally, the presence of chronic viral hepatitis may predispose to injury from antiretroviral agents and drugs used to treat tuberculosis. Pretreatment with anticonvulsants, particularly Phenobarbital, is associated with a greater risk of development of halothane-induced liver damage. Both starvation and chronic alcoholism appear to predispose to APAP-induced liver injury. In general, however, the presence of underlying liver disease does not seem to increase the risk of drug-induced hepatotoxicity.[1377]

Although most drugs or toxins generally lead to one type of injury, the simultaneous occurrence of two or more injuries should be borne in mind. The anabolic steroids, for example, can cause peliosis hepatis and intrahepatic cholestasis, and some affected livers may also exhibit haemosiderosis from multiple blood transfusions used in the treatment of an underlying anaemia. Another example of simultaneous multiple injuries has been observed with phenylbutazone which can induce hepatic granulomas that, in some patients, may be associated with a hepatocellular/cholestatic injury. Perhexilene maleate and amiodarone can induce steatohepatitis with Mallory bodies, as well as a phospholipidosis. It must be kept in mind that some drugs may injure the liver as well as other organs simultaneously, e.g. kidney, bone marrow, lung. Some drug-induced injuries, such as pancreatitis, biliary sludge or cholelithiasis, can have secondary effects on the liver that are independent of direct hepatotoxicity, e.g. obstructive jaundice.

Use of the offending drug should be immediately discontinued if severe hepatic injury is suspected or if clinico-pathological correlation establishes with reasonable certainty that a drug is a possible or probable cause of hepatic injury. More often than not, this is followed by prompt clinical and biochemical improvement, providing further presumptive evidence of a drug-induced aetiology. Ultimate proof of a cause-and-effect relationship requires rechallenge with the suspected drug; today, rechallenge is conducted only when the need for the drug clearly exceeds the risk.[33] Other, less risky and more sensitive methods of diagnosis are likely to be increasingly utilized in the future. Lymphocyte transformation studies, macrophage inhibition factor tests, anticytoplasmic organelle autoantibodies[1378] and specific T-cell reactivity associated with drug-induced liver injury[1379] remain of limited utility except in highly specialized centres.

The astute clinician and pathologist will recognize that the broad spectrum of hepatic lesions associated with medicinal agents and chemicals demands an ever-present vigilance be maintained whenever confronted with possible drug-induced liver disease. Given the wide range of clinical circumstances that may be encountered when attempting to determine an individual drug's role in the development of liver injury, performing a thorough causality assessment assumes an even greater importance, especially given the need to accurately define the ever-expanding hepatotoxicity database.[1380,1381] A number of causality assessment methodologies have been validated, and can prove beneficial when attempting to determine a causal relationship between a drug and hepatotoxicity.[1380–1386]

Acknowledgements

We are indebted to the originators of this chapter, Hyman J. Zimmerman and Kamal G. Ishak, for developing and advancing the format of a clinical-pathological correlation to best describe the various forms of drug-induced liver injury. They were our friends and mentors for more than 20 years, and we are honoured to have been named as their successors, and have strived to update the information contained in the last edition of this textbook in a manner in which we hope they would have approved. No doubt their influence will continue to guide our approach to drug-induced liver disease for years to come.

References

1. Zimmerman HJ. Hepatotoxicity: the adverse effects of drugs and other chemicals on the liver, 2nd edn. Philadelphia: Lippincott, Williams & Wilkins, 1999
2. Ishak KG, Zimmerman HJ. Morphologic spectrum of drug-induced hepatic disease. Gastroenterol Clin North Am, 1995; 24:759–786
3. Bartoloni ST, Omer F, Giannini A et al. Amanita poisoning: a clinical-histopathological study of 64 cases of intoxication. Hepatogastroenterology, 1985; 32:229–231
4. Lee WM. Acetaminophen and the U.S. Acute Liver Failure Study Group: lowering the risks of hepatic failure. Hepatology, 2004; 40:6–9
5. Rumack BH. Acetaminophen hepatotoxicity: the first 35 years. J Toxicol Clin Toxicol, 2002; 40:3–20
6. Bromer MQ, Black M. Acetaminophen hepatotoxicity. Clin Liver Dis, 2003; 7:351–368
7. Bernal W. Changing patterns of causation and the use of transplantation in the United Kingdom. Semin Liver Dis, 2003; 23:227–237
8. Popper H, Rubin E, Gardiol D et al. Drug-induced liver disease: a penalty for progress. Arch Intern Med, 1965; 115:128–136
9. Tolman KG, Sirrine RW. Occupational hepatotoxicity. Clin Liver Dis, 1998; 2:563–589
10. National Institute for Occupational Safety and Health (NIOSH). Pocket guide to chemical hazards, January 2003. Publication No. 97–140. Government Printing Office, Pittsburgh, PA
11. Clinical White Paper: Drug-induced liver toxicity. CDER-PhRMA-AASLD November 2000; accessed via www.fda.gov/cder/livertox/postmarket.pdf
12. Koff RS, Gardner P, Harinasuta U, Pihl CO. Profile of hyperbilirubinemia in three hospital populations. Clin Res, 1970; 18:680–681
13. Sameshine Y, Shiozaki Y, Mizuno T et al. Clinical statistics on drug-induced liver injuries: drug-induced liver injuries in Japan in the last 30 years. Jpn J Gastroenterol, 1974; 71:799
14. Eastwood HOH. Causes of jaundice in the elderly: a survey of diagnosis and investigation. Gerontol Clin, 1971; 13:69–81
15. Benhamou JP. Drug-induced hepatitis: clinical aspects. In: Fillastre JP, ed. Hepatotoxicity of drugs. Rouen: University de Rouen, 1985: pp 22–30
16. Friis H, Andreasen PB. Drug-induced hepatic injury: an analysis of 1100 cases reported to the Danish Committee on Adverse Drug Reactions between 1978 and 1987. J Intern Med, 1992; 232:133–138
17. Sgro C, Clinard F, Ouazir K et al. Incidence of drug-induced hepatic injuries: a French population based study. Hepatology, 2002; 36:451–455
18. Byron D, Minuk GY. Clinical hepatology: profile of an urban hospital-based practice. Hepatology, 1996; 24:813–815
19. Garcia Rodriguez LA, Ruigomez A, Jick H. A review of epidemiologic research on drug-induced acute liver injury using the general practice research data base in the United Kingdom. Pharmacotherapy, 1997; 17:721–728
20. Jemlnitzky AC, Guidi M, Bologna A et al. Clinical-epidemiological significance of drug hepatotoxicity in liver disease consultation. Acta Gastroenterol Latinoam, 2000; 30:77–84
21. Ostapowicz G, Fontana RJ, Schiodt FV et al. Results of a prospective study of acute liver failure at 17 tertiary care centers in the United States. Ann Intern Med, 2002; 137:947–954
22. Russo MW, Galanko JA, Shrestha R et al. Liver transplantation for acute liver failure from drug-induced injury in the United States. Liver Transplantation, 2004; 10:1018–1023
23. Galan MV, Potts JA, Silverman AL et al. Hepatitis in a United States tertiary referral center. J Clin Gastroenterol, 2005; 39:64–67
24. Kohlroser J, Mathai J, Reichheld J et al. Hepatotoxicity due to troglitazone: report of two cases and review of adverse events

reported to the United States Food and Drug Administration. Am J Gastroenterol, 2000; 95:272–276

25. Kleiner DE, Gaffey MJ, Sallie R et al. Histopathologic changes associated with fialuridine hepatotoxicity. Mod Pathol, 1997; 10:192–199

26. Chen HJL, Block KJ, Maclean JA. Acute eosinophilic hepatitis from trovafloxacin. N Engl J Med, 2000; 342:359–360

27. Fontana RJ, McCashland TM, Benner KG et al. Acute liver failure associated with prolonged use of bromfenac leading to liver transplantation. The Acute Liver Failure Study Group. Liver Transpl Surg, 1999; 5:480–484

28. Drug induced liver injury conference, Chantilly, Virginia, February 12–13, 2001 via website: fda.gov/cder/livertox/default.htm

29. Clarkson A, Choonara I. Surveillance for fatal suspected adverse drug reactions in the UK. Arch Dis Child, 2002; 87:462–466

29a. Andrade RJ, Lucena MI, Fernandez MC, et al. Drug-induced liver injury: An analysis of 461 incidences submitted to the Spanish registry over a 10-year period. Gastroenterology, 2005; 129:512–521.

29b. Björnsson E, Olsson R. Outcome and prognostic markers in severe drug-induced liver disease. Hepatology, 2005; 42:481–489.

30. Lewis JH, Zimmerman HJ. Drug- and chemical-induced cholestasis. Clin Liver Dis, 1999; 3:433–464

31. Mohi-ud-din R, Lewis JH. Drug- and chemical-induced cholestasis. Clin Liver Dis, 2004; 8:95–132

32. Strader DH, Seeff LB. Drug-induced chronic liver disease. In: Black M, ed. Clinics in liver disease. Philadelphia: Saunders, 1998: pp 501–522

33. Lewis JH. Drug-induced liver disease. Med Clin North Am, 2000; 84:1275–1311

34. Zimmerman HJ, Lewis JH. Chemical- and toxin-induced hepatotoxicity. Gastroenterol Clin North Am, 1995; 24:1027–1045

35. Lai DY, Wso Y-T. Naturally occurring carcinogens: an overview. Environ Carcinog Rev, 1987; 5:12–143

36. Wogan GN. Aflatoxins as risk factors for hepatocellular carcinoma in humans. Cancer Res, 1992; 32(Suppl):2114s–2116s

37. Wexler P. The U.S. National Library of Medicine's Toxicology and Environmental Health Information Program. Toxicology, 2004; 198:161–168

38. Wong RH, Chen PC, Wang JD et al. Interaction of vinyl chloride monomer exposure and hepatitis B viral infection on liver cancer. J Occup Environ Med, 2003; 45:379–383

39. Tamburro CH. Chronic liver injury in phenoxy herbicide-exposed Vietnam veterans. Environ Res, 1992; 59:175–188

40. Cordier S, Le TB, Verger P et al. Viral infections and chemical exposures as risk factors for hepatocellular carcinoma in Vietnam. Int J Cancer, 1993; 55:196–201

41. Ishak KG, Zimmerman HJ. Hepatotoxic effects of the anabolic androgenic steroids. Semin Liver Dis, 1987; 7:230–238

42. Neuberger J, Forman D, Doll R, Williams R. Oral contraceptives and hepatocellular carcinoma. BMJ, 1986; 292:355–357

43. Farrell GC. Drug-induced liver disease. Edinburgh: Churchill Livingstone, 1994

44. Phillips MJ, Poucell S, Patterson J, Valencia P. The liver. An atlas and text of ultrastructural pathology. New York: Raven Press, 1987

45. Kaplowitz N, DeLeve LD, eds. Drug-induced liver disease. New York: Marcel Dekker, 2003

46. Lefkowitch JH, ed. Liver histopathology. Clin Liver Dis, 2002; 6:xv–xix

47. Cameron RG, Feuer G, de la Iglesia FA, eds. Drug-induced hepatotoxicity. Berlin: Springer-Verlag, 1996

48. Lee WM. Drug-induced hepatotoxicity. N Engl J Med, 2003; 349:474–485

49. Mullick FG, Ishak KG, Mahabir R, Stromeyer FW. Hepatic injury associated with paraquat toxicity in humans. Liver, 1981; 1:209–221

50. Day CP, James OF. Steatohepatitis: a tale of two 'hits'? (editorial). Gastroenterology, 1998; 114:842–845

51. Freneaux E, Labbe G, Letteron P et al. Inhibition of the mitochondrial oxidation of fatty acids by tetracycline in mice and in man: possible role of microvesicular steatosis induced by this antibiotic. Hepatology, 1988; 8:1056–1062

52. Pessayre D, Mansouri A, Haouzi D et al. Hepatotoxicity due to mitochondrial dysfunction. Cell Biol Toxicol, 1999; 15:367–373

53. Lieber CS. New concepts of the pathogenesis of alcoholic liver disease lead to novel treatments. Curr Gastroenterol Rep, 2004; 6:60–65

54. Lieber CS. The discovery of the microsomal ethanol oxidizing system and its physiologic and pathologic role. Drug Metab Rev, 2004; 36:511–529

55. Bohan A, Boyer JL. Mechanisms of hepatotoxicity transport of drugs: implications for cholestatic drug reaction. Semin Liver Dis, 2002; 22:123–136

56. Mitchell JR, Zimmerman HJ, Ishak KG et al. Isoniazid liver injury. Clinical spectrum, pathology and probable pathogenesis. Ann Intern Med, 1976; 84:181–192

57. Vergani D, Mieli-Vergani G, Alberti A et al. Antibodies to the surface of halothane-altered rabbit hepatocytes in patients with severe halothane-associated hepatitis. N Engl J Med, 1980; 303:66–71

58. Neuberger J, Williams R. Immune mechanisms in tienilic associated hepatotoxicity. Gut, 1989; 30:515–519

59. Beaune P, Dansette PM, Nansuy D et al. Human antiendoplasmic reticulum autoantibodies in a drug-induced hepatitis are directed against a human cytochrome P450 that hydroxylates the drug. Proc Natl Acad Sci USA, 1987; 84:551–555

60. Njoku DB, Greenberg RS, Bourdi M et al. Autoantibodies associated with volatile anesthetic hepatitis found in the sera of a large cohort of pediatric anesthesiologists. Anesth Analg, 2002; 94:243–249

61. Ishak KG, Irey NS. Hepatic injury associated with the phenothiazines: clinicopathologic and follow-up study of 36 patients. Arch Pathol, 1972; 93:283–304

62. Shear NH, Spielberg S, Cannon M, Miller AR. Anti-convulsant hypersensitivity syndrome. J Clin Invest, 1988; 82:1826–1832

63. Schlienger RG, Shear NM. Antiepileptic drug hypersensitivity syndrome. Epilepsia, 1988; 39(suppl 7):s3–s7

64. Larrey D, Pageaux GP. Hepatotoxicity of herbal remedies and mushrooms. Semin Liver Dis, 1995; 15:183–188

65. Hippius M, Buchardt C, Farker K et al. Adverse drug reaction monitoring in Jena. Relevance of polymorphic drug metabolizing enzymes for inducing adverse drug reactions. Exp Toxicol Pathol, 2003; 54:417–421

66. Weinshilboum R. Inheritance and drug response. N Engl J Med, 2003; 348:529–537

67. Evans WE, McLeod HL. Pharmacogenomics—drug disposition, drug targets, and side effects. N Engl J Med, 2003; 348:538–549

68. Ishak KG. The liver. In: Riddell RH, ed. Pathology of drug-induced and toxic diseases. New York: Churchill Livingstone, 1982: pp 457–513

69. Goodman ZD. Drug hepatotoxicity. Clin Liver Dis, 2002; 6:381–397

70. Kaplowitz N. Mechanisms of cell death and relevance to drug hepatotoxicity. In: Kaplowitz N, DeLeve LD, eds. Drug-induced liver disease. New York: Marcel Dekker, 2003

71. Granville DJ, Carthy CM, Hunt DWC, McManus BM. Apoptosis: molecular aspects of cell death and disease. Lab Invest, 1998; 78:893–913

72. Reed JC. Apoptosis-regulating proteins as targets for drug discovery. Trends Mol Med, 2001; 7:314–319

73. Docker K, Keppler D. Galactosamine induced liver injury. Prog Liver Dis, 1972; 4:183–199

74. Chojkier M. Hepatic sinusoidal-obstruction syndrome: toxicity of pyrrolizidine alkaloids. J Hepatol, 2003; 39:437–446

75. Gitlin N. Drug-induced hepatic vascular abnormalities. Clin Liver Dis, 1998; 2:591–606

76. Rodriguez-Iturbe B. Acute yellow-phosphorus poisoning. N Engl J Med, 1971; 284:157

77. Salfelder K, Doehnert HR, Doehnert G, Sauerteg K, Deliscano TR, Fabrega SE. Fatal phosphorus poisoning. A study of forty-five autopsy cases. Beitr Pathol, 1972; 147:321–340

78. Pestaner JP, Ishak KG, Mullick FG, Centeno J. Ferrous sulfate toxicity. A review of autopsy findings. Biol Trace Elem Res, 1999; 70:1–8

79. Kamijo Y, Soma K, Iwabuchi K, Ohwada T. Massive noninflammatory periportal liver necrosis following concentrated acetic acid ingestion. Arch Pathol Lab Med, 2000; 124:127–129

80. Rees KR, Tarlow MJ. The hepatotoxic action of allyl formate. Biochem J, 1985; 104:757–761

81. Mitchell JR, Jollow DJ, Potter WZ. Acetaminophen induced hepatic necrosis. I. Role of drug metabolism. J Pharmacol Exp Ther, 1973; 187:185–194

82. Mullick FG, Ishak KG. Hepatic injury associated with diphenylhydantoin therapy: a clinicopathologic study of 20 cases. Am J Clin Pathol, 1980; 74:442–452

83. Prosser TR, Lander RD. Phenytoin-induced hypersensitivity reactions. Clin Pharm, 1987; 6:728–734

84. Bridge JC, Swanston C, Lane RE, Davie TB. Discussion on trinitrotoluene poisoning. Proc R Soc Med, 1943; 35:553–560

85. Maddrey WC, Boitnott JK. Isoniazid hepatitis. Ann Intern Med, 1973; 79:1–12

86. Black M, Mitchell JR, Zimmerman HJ, Ishak KG, Epler GR. Isoniazid-associated hepatitis in 114 patients. Gastroenterology, 1975; 69:289–302

87. Maddrey WC, Boitnott JK. Severe hepatitis from methyldopa. Gastroenterology, 1975; 68:351–360

88. Schweitzer IL, Peters RL. Acute submassive hepatic necrosis due to methyldopa: a case demonstrating possible initiation of chronic liver disease. Gastroenterology, 1974; 66:1203–1211

89. Palmer WL, Woodall PS, Wang KC. Cinchophen and toxic necrosis of the liver: a survey of the problem. Trans Am Assoc Physicians, 1936; 51:381–393

90. Reynolds TB. Laxative liver disease. In: Gerok W, Sickinger K, eds. Drugs and the liver. Stuttgart: FK Schattauer-Verlag, 1975: pp 319–325

91. Sharp JR, Ishak KG, Zimmerman HJ. Chronic active hepatitis and severe hepatic necrosis associated with nitrofurantoin. Ann Intern Med, 1980; 92:14–19

92. Goldstein GB, Lam KC, Mistilis SP. Drug-induced active chronic hepatitis. Am J Dig Dis, 1973; 18:177–184

93. Shalev O, Mosseri M, Ariel I, Stalikowicz R. Methyldopa-induced immune hemolytic anemia and chronic active hepatitis. Arch Intern Med, 1983; 143:592–593

94. Pariente EA, Hamoud A, Goldfain D et al. Clometacine hepatitis. Retrospective study of 30 cases. A model of drug-induced autoimmune hepatitis. Gastroenterol Clin Biol, 1989; 13:769–774

95. Bernard PH, Lamouliatte H, Bail B. Chronic active hepatitis induced by fenofibrate. Gastroenterol Clin Biol, 1994; 18:1048

96. Scully LJ, Clarke D, Barr RJ. Diclofenac-induced hepatitis in three cases with features of autoimmune chronic active hepatitis. Dig Dis Sci, 1993; 38:744–751

97. Poupon R, Longchal C, Darnis F. Hépatite chronique associée à la prise prolongée de papaverine. Gastroenterol Clin Biol, 1978; 2:305–308

98. Sterling MJ, Kane MJ, Grace ND. Pemoline-induced autoimmune hepatitis. Am J Gastroenterol, 1996; 91:2233–2234

99. Gough A, Chapman S, Wapoff K et al. Minocycline-induced autoimmune hepatitis and systemic lupus erythematosus syndrome. BMJ, 1996; 312:169–172

100. Liu Z-X, Kaplowitz N. Immune-mediated drug-induced liver disease. Clin Liver Dis, 2002; 6:755–774

101. Lewis JH, Zimmerman HJ. Drug-induced autoimmune liver disease. In: Krawitt EL, Wiesner RH, Nishioka M, eds. Autoimmune liver disease, 2nd edn. New York: Elsevier, 1998: pp 629–650

102. Ishak KG. Granulomas of the liver. Adv Pathol Lab Med, 1995; 8:247–361

103. McMaster KR, Hennigar GR. Drug-induced granulomatous hepatitis. Lab Invest, 1981; 44:61–73

104. Stricker BHC, Block AP, Babany G et al. Fibrin ring granulomas and allopurinol. Gastroenterology, 1989; 96:119–123

105. Proctor DD, Chopra S, Rubenstein SC, Jokela JA, Uhl L. Mycobacteremia and granulomatous hepatitis following initial intravesical bacillus Calmette-Guerin instillation for bladder carcinoma. Am J Gastroenterol, 1993; 88:1112–1115

106. Stoeckle JD, Hardy HL, Weber AL. Chronic beryllium disease. Long-term follow-up of sixty cases and selective review of the literature. Am J Med, 1986; 46:545–561

107. Pimentel JC, Menezes AP. Liver granulomas containing copper in vineyard sprayer's lung. A new etiology of hepatic granulomatosis. Am Rev Respir Dis, 1975; 111:189–195

108. Kurumaya H, Kono N, Nakanuma Y et al. Hepatic granulomata in long-term hemodialysis patients with hyperaluminuemia. Arch Pathol Lab Med, 1989; 113:1132–1134

109. Fuller CM, Yassinger S, Donlon P et al. Haloperidol-induced liver disease. West J Med, 1977; 127:515–518

110. Matsumoto T, Matsumori H, Kuwabara N, Fukuda Y, Ariwa R. A histopathological study of the liver in paraquat poisoning: an analysis of fourteen autopsy cases with emphasis on bile duct injury. Acta Pathol Jpn, 1980; 30:859–870

111. Degott C, Feldmann G, Larrey D et al. Drug-induced prolonged cholestasis in adults: a histological semiquantiative study demonstrating ductopenia. Hepatology, 1992; 15:244–251

112. Desmet VJ. Vanishing bile duct syndrome in drug-induced disease. J Hepatol, 1997; 26(Suppl 1):31–35

113. Geubel AP, Sempoux C, Rahie J. Bile duct disorders. Clin Liver Dis, 2003; 7:295–309

114. Hohn D, Rayner AA, Economou JS, Ignoffo RJ, Lewis DJ, Stagg RJ. Toxicities and complications of implanted pump hepatic arterial and intravenous floxuridine infusion. Cancer, 1986; 57:465–470

115. Doria MI, Shepard KV, Levin B, Riddell RH. Liver pathology following hepatic arterial infusion chemotherapy. Cancer, 1986; 58:855–861

116. Castellano G, Moreno-Sanchez D, Guitierrez J et al. Caustic sclerosing cholangitis. Report of four cases and a cumulative review of the literature. Hepatogastroenterology, 1994; 41:458–470

117. Ludwig J, Kim CH, Wiesner RH, Krom RA. Floxuridine-induced sclerosing cholangitis: An ischemic cholangiopathy? Hepatology, 1989; 9:215–218

118. Stravitz and Sanyal CLD, 2003; 7:435

119. McCullough AJ. Update on nonalcoholic fatty liver disease. J Clin Gastroentero, 2002; 34:255–262

120. Peters RL, Edmondson HA, Mikkelsen W, Tatter D. Tetracycline induced fatty liver in non-pregnant patients. Am J Surg, 1967; 113:622–632

121. Schenker S, Breen KJ, Heimberg M. Pathogenesis of tetracycline induced fatty liver. In: Gerok W, Sickinger K, eds. Stuttgart: FK Schattauer-Verlag, 1972: pp 269–280

122. Zimmerman HJ, Ishak KG. Valproate-induced hepatic injury. Analysis of 23 fatal cases. Hepatology, 1982; 2:591–597

123. Eadie MJ, Hooper WD, Dickinson RG. Valproate-associated hepatotoxicity and its biochemical mechanism. Med Toxicol, 1988; 3:85–106

124. Chariot P, Drogou I, de Lacroix-Szmania I et al. Zidovudine induced mitochondrial disorder with massive liver steatosis, myopathy, lactic acidosis, and mitochondrial DNA depletion. J Hepatol, 1999; 30:156–160

125. Ogedegbe AO, Sulkowski MS. Antiretroviral-associated liver injury. Clin Liver Dis, 2003; 7:475–499

126. Starko KM, Mullick FG. Hepatic and cerebral pathology findings in children with fatal salicylate intoxication: further evidence for a causal relation between salicylate and Reye's syndrome. Lancet, 1983; i:326–329

127. Tanaka K, Kean EK, Johnson B. Jamaican vomiting sickness. Biochemical investigation of two cases. N Engl J Med, 1976; 295:461–467

128. Redlich CA, West AB, Fleming L, True LD, Cullen MR, Riely CA. Clinical and pathological characteristics of hepatotoxicity associated with occupational exposure to dimethylformamide. Gastroenterology, 1990; 99:748–757

129. Wanless IR, Dore S, Gopinath N et al. Histopathology of cocaine hepatotoxicity. Report of four patients. Gastroenterology, 1990; 98:497–501

130. Lewis JH, Schiff ER. Methotrexate-induced chronic liver injuries: guidelines for detection and prevention. The AGC Committee on FDA-related matters. Am J Gastroenterol, 1988; 83:1337–1345

131. Zimmerman HJ, Ishak KG. Non-alcoholic steatohepatitis and other forms of pseudoalcoholic liver disease. In: Hall P, ed. Alcoholic liver disease, 2nd edn. London: Edward Arnold, 1994: pp 175–198

132. Poupon R, Rosenztajn L, Prudhomme de Saint-Maur P, Lageron A, Gombeau T, Darnis F. Perhexiline maleate-associated hepatic injury: prevalence and characteristics. Digestion, 1980; 20:145–150

133. Lewis JH, Mullick FG, Ishak KG et al. Histopathological analysis of suspected amiodarone hepatotoxicity. Hum Pathol, 1990; 221:59–67

134. Seki K, Minami Y, Nishikawa M et al. 'Nonalcoholic steatohepatitis' induced by massive doses of synthetic estrogen. Gastroenterol Jpn, 1983; 18:197–203

135. Koike R. Subacute severe steatohepatitis during prednisolone therapy for systemic lupus erythematosus [letter]. Am J Gastroenterol, 1999; 94:3379

136. Babany G, Uzzan F, Larrey D et al. Alcoholic-like liver lesions induced by nifedipine. J Hepatol, 1989; 9:252–255

137. Oien KA, Moffat D, Curry GW, Redeker AG, Reynolds TB. Cirrhosis with steatohepatitis after adjuvant tamoxifen. Lancet, 1999; 353:36–37

138. Hu B, French SW. 2', 3'-dideoxyinosine-induced Mallory bodies in patients with HIV. Am J Clin Pathol, 1997; 108:280–283

139. Bodasing N, Fox R. HIV-associated lipodystrophy syndrome: description and pathogenesis. J Infection, 2003; 46:149–154

140. Shikata T, Oda T, Naito C et al. Phospholipid fatty liver: a proposal of a new concept and its electron microscopical study. Acta Pathol Jpn, 1970; 20:467–486

141. Poucell S, Ireton J, Valencia-Mayoral P et al. Amiodarone-associated phospholipidosis and fibrosis of the liver: light, immunohistochemical and electron microscopic studies. Gastroenterology, 1984; 86:926–936

142. Lullmann H, Lullman-Rauch R, Wasserman O. Drug-induced phospholipidosis. CRC Crit Rev Toxicol, 1975; 4:185–218

143. Forbes GB, Rake MD. Liver damage due to perhexiline maleate. J Clin Pathol, 1984; 32:1282–1285

144. Pessayre D, Bichara M, Feldmann G, Degott C, Patet F, Benhamou JP. Perhexiline maleate-induced cirrhosis. Gastroenterology, 1979; 76:170–177

145. Lewis JH, Ranard RC, Caruso A et al. Amiodarone hepatotoxicity: prevalence and clinopathologic correlations among 104 patients. Hepatology, 1989; 9:679–685

146. Simon JB, Manley PN, Brien JF, Armstrong PN. Amiodarone hepatotoxicity simulating alcoholic liver disease. N Engl J Med, 1984; 311:167–172

147. Shajkl NA, Downer E, Butany J. Amiodarone: an inhibitor of phospholipase activity. A comparative study of the inhibiting activity of amiodarone, chloroquine and chlorpromazine. Mol Cell Biochem, 1987; 76:163–172

148. Hostetler NY, Giordano JR, Hoyumpa AM Jr, Jellison EJ. In vitro inhibition of lysosomal phospholipase A of rat lung by amiodarone and desethylamiodarone. Biochem Biophys Acta, 1988; 959:316–321

149. Chuttani HK, Sidhu AS, Wig KL, Gupta DN, Ranalingaswami V. Follow-up study of cases from the Delhi epidemic of infections hepatitis of 1955–6. Brit Med J, 1966; 2:676–679

150. Hutter RV, Shipkey FH, Tan CT, Murphy ML, Chowdhury M. Hepatic fibrosis in children with acute leukemia: a complication of therapy. Cancer, 1960; 13:288–307

151. Zachariae H, Kragballe K, Sogaard H. Methotrexate induced liver cirrhosis. Br J Dermatol, 1980; 102:407–412

152. Gilbert SC, Klintman G, Menter A, Silverman A. Methotrexate induced cirrhosis requiring liver transplantation in three patients with psoriasis. Arch Intern Med, 1990; 150:889–891

153. Leo MA, Lieber CS. Hypervitaminosis A: a liver lover's lament. Hepatology, 1988; 8:412–417

154. Brooks SEH, Miller CG, McKenzie K, Audretsch JJ, Bras G. Acute veno-occlusive disease of the liver. Arch Pathol, 1970; 89:507–520

155. Walker CO, Combes B. Biliary cirrhosis induced by chlorpromazine. Gastroenterology, 1966; 51:631–640

156. Lok AS, Ng IO. Prochlorperazine-induced chronic cholestasis. J Hepatol, 1988; 6:369–373

157. Hurt P, Wegmann T. Protracted largactil jaundice deepening into primary biliary cirrhosis. Acta Hepatol Splenol, 1961; 8:87–95

158. Cameron GR, Karunaratne WAE. Carbon tetrachloride cirrhosis in relation to liver regeneration. J Pathol Bacteriol, 1936; 42:1–13

159. Zafrani ES, Pinaudeau Y, Dhumeaux D. Drug-induced vascular lesions of the liver. Arch Intern Med, 1983; 143:495–502

160. DeLeve LD, Shulman HM, McDonald GB. Toxic injury to hepatic sinusoids: sinusoidal obstruction syndrome (veno-occlusive disease). Semin Liver Dis, 2002; 22:27–41

161. Mikkelsen WP, Edmondson HA, Peters RI et al. Extra and intrahepatic portal hypertension without cirrhosis (hepatoportal sclerosis). Ann Surg, 1965; 162:602–620

162. Nevens F, Fevery J, Van Steenbergen W, Sciot R, Desmet V, De Groote J. Arsenic and non-cirrhotic portal hypertension. J Hepatol, 1990; 11:80–85

163. Popper H, Thomas LB. Alterations of liver and spleen among workers exposed to vinyl chloride. Ann N Y Acad Sci, 1975; 246:172–194

164. Pimentel JC, Menezes AP. Liver disease in vineyard sprayers. Gastroenterology, 1977; 72:275–283

165. Goodman ZD, Ishak KG. Occlusive venous lesions in alcoholic liver disease. A study of 200 cases. Gastroenterology, 1982; 83:786–796

166. Shepherd P, Harrison DJ. Idiopathic portal hypertension associated with cytotoxic drugs. J Clin Oncol, 1990; 43:206–210

167. Snover DC, Weisdorf S, Bloomer J, McGlane P, Weisdorf D. Nodular regenerative hyperplasia of the liver following bone narrow transplantation. Hepatology, 1989; 9:443–448

168. Stromeyer FW, Ishak KG. Nodular transformation (nodular 'regenerative' hyperplasia) of the liver: a clinicopathologic study of 30 cases. Hum Pathol, 1981; 12:60–70

169. Rosen AA, Iseri O, Fishbein G, Knodell RG. Nodular regenerative hyperplasia: a cause of ascites and hepatomegaly after chemotherapy for leukemia. Am J Gastroenterol, 1991; 86:86–88

170. Buffet C, Cantarovitch M, Pelletier G et al. Three cases of nodular regenerative hyperplasia of the liver following renal transplantation. Nephrol Diag Transplant, 1988; 3:327–330

171. Jones MC, Best PV, Catto GRD. Is nodular regenerative hyperplasia of the liver associated with azathioprine therapy after renal transplantation? Nephrol Dial Transplant, 1988; 3:331–333

172. Geller SA, Dubinsky MC, Poordad FF et al. Early hepatic nodular hyperplasia and submicroscopic fibrosis associated with 6-thioguanine therapy in inflammatory bowel disease. Am J Surg Pathol, 2004; 28:1204–1211

173. Lewis JH, Tice H, Zimmerman HJ. Budd–Chiari syndrome associated with oral contraceptive steroids. Review of treatment of 47 cases. Dig Dis Sci, 1983; 38:673–683

174. Valla D, Le MG, Poynard T, Zucman N, Rueff B, Benhamou JP. Risk of hepatic vein thrombosis in relation to recent use of oral contraceptives. A case control study. Gastroenterology, 1986; 90:807–811

175. Maddrey WC. Hepatic vein thrombosis (Budd–Chiari syndrome): possible association with the use of oral contraceptives. Semin Liver Dis, 1987; 7:32–39

176. Valla D, Casadevall N, Lacombe C et al. Primary myeloproliferative disorder and hepatic vein thrombosis in 20 patients with Budd–Chiari syndrome. Ann Intern Med, 1985; 103:329–334

177. McLean EK. The toxic actions of pyrrolizidine (Senecio) alkaloids. Pharmacol Rev, 1970; 22:429–483

178. Shulman HM, Fisher LB, Schoch HG et al. Veno-occlusive disease of the liver after marrow transplantation: histological correlates of clinical signs and symptoms. Hepatology, 1994; 19:1171–1181

179. Wanless IR, Wong F, Blendis LM et al. Hepatic and portal vein thrombosis in cirrhosis: possible role in development of parenchymal extinction and portal hypertension. Hepatology, 1995; 21:1238–1247

180. Modzelewski JR Jr, Daeschner C, Joshi VV, Mullick FG, Ishak KG. Veno-occlusive disease of the liver induced by low-dose cyclophosphamide. Mod Pathol, 1994; 7:967–972

181. Kane S, Cohen SM, Hart J. Acute sinusoidal obstruction syndrome after 6-thioguanine therapy for Crohn's disease. Inflamm Bowel Dis, 2004; 10:652–654

182. Fajardo LF, Colby TV. Pathogenesis of veno-occlusive liver disease after radiation. Arch Pathol Lab Med, 1980; 104:584–588

183. Sempoux C, Horsmans Y, Geubel A et al. Severe radiation-induced liver disease following localized radiation therapy for biliopancreatic carcinoma: activation of hepatic stellate cells as an early event. Hepatology, 1997; 26:128–134

184. McDonald GB, Hinds MS, Fisher LD et al. Veno-occlusive disease of the liver and multiorgan failure after bone marrow transplantation: a cohort study of 355 patients. Ann Intern Med, 1993; 118:255–267

185. Lee JL, Gooley T, Bensinger W et al. Veno-occlusive disease of the liver after busulfan, melphalan, and thiotepa conditioning therapy: incidence, risk factors, and outcome. Biol Blood Marrow Transplant, 1999; 5:306–315

186. Tuchweber B, Kovacs K, Khandekar JD, Gorg BD. Peliosis-like changes induced by phalloidin in rat liver: a light and electron microscopic study. J Med (Basel), 1973; 4:327–345

187. Bagheri SA, Boyer JL. Peliosis hepatis associated with androgenic-anabolic steroid therapy: a severe form of hepatic injury. Ann Intern Med, 1974; 81:610–618

188. Nadell J, Kosek J. Peliosis hepatis. Twelve cases associated with oral androgen therapy. Arch Pathol Lab Med, 1977; 101:405–410

189. Puppala AR, Ro JA. Possible association between peliosis hepatis and diethylstilboesterol. Postgrad Med, 1979; 65:277–281

190. Schonberg LA. Peliosis hepatis and oral contraceptives. J Reprod Med, 1982; 27:753–756

191. Staub PG, Leibowitz CB. Peliosis hepatis associated with oral contraceptive use. Australas Radiol, 1996; 40:172–174

192. Loomus GN, Aneja P, Bota RA. A case of peliosis hepatis in association with tamoxifen therapy. Am J Clin Pathol, 1983; 80:881–883

193. Degott C, Rueff B, Kreis H et al. Peliosis hepatis in recipients of renal transplants. Gut, 1978; 19:748–753

194. Cavalcanti R, Pol S, Carnot F et al. Impact and evolution of peliosis hepatis in renal transplant recipients. Transplantation, 1994; 58:315–316

195. Zafrani ES, Bernuau D, Feldmann G. Peliosis-like ultrastructural changes of the hepatic sinusoids in human chronic hypervitaminosis A: report of three cases. Hum Pathol, 1984; 15:1166–1170

196. Okuda K, Omata M, Itoh Y et al. Peliosis hepatis as a late and fatal complication of thorotrast liver disease. Report of five cases. Liver, 1981; 1:110–122

197. Balazs M. Sinusoidal dilatation of the liver in patients on oral contraceptives. Electron microscopical study of 14 cases. Exp Pathol, 1988; 35:231–237

198. Winkler K, Christoffersen P. A reappaisal of Poulsen's disease (hepatic zone 1 sinusoidal dilatation). APMIS, 1991; 23(Suppl):86–90

199. Zafrani ES, Cazier A, Baudelot AM et al. Ultrastructural lesions of the liver in human peliosis. A report of 12 cases. Am J Pathol, 1984; 114:349–359

200. Wanless IR. Benign liver tumors. Clin Liver Dis, 2002; 6:513–526

201. Suriawinata AA, Thung SN. Malignant liver tumors. Clin Liver Dis, 2002; 6:527–554

202. Edmondson HA, Henderson B, Benton B. Liver cell adenomas associated with use of oral contraceptives. N Engl J Med, 1976; 294:470–472

203. Mays ET, Christofferson W. Hepatic tumors induced by sex steroids. Semin Liver Dis, 1984; 4:147–158

204. Ishak KG. Hepatic lesions caused by anabolic and contraceptive steroids. Semin Liver Dis, 1981; 1:116–128

205. Rooks JB, Ory HW, Ishak KG et al. Epidemiology of hepatocellular adenoma. The role of oral contraceptive use. JAMA, 1979; 242:644–648

206. Mathieu D, Kobeiter H, Cherqui D, Rahmouni A, Dhumeaux D. Oral contraceptive intake in women with focal nodular hyperplasia of the liver. Lancet, 1998; 352:1679–1680

207. dos Santos Silva I, Malveiro F, Jones ME et al. Mortality after radiological investigation with radioactive Thorotrast: a follow-up study of up to fifty years in Portugal. Radiat Res, 2003; 159:521–534

208. Lu SN, Chow NH, Wu WC et al. Characteristics of hepatocellular carcinoma in a high arsenicism area in Taiwan: a case-control study. J Occup Environ Med, 2004; 46:437–441

209. Ishak KG. Hepatic neoplasms associated with contraceptive and anabolic steroids. In: Lingeman CH, ed. Carcinogenic hormones. Berlin: Springer-Verlag, 1979: pp 73–128

210. Henderson BE, Preston-Marin S, Edmondson HA, Peters RL, Pike MC. Hepatocellular carcinoma and oral contraceptives. Br J Cancer, 1983; 48:437–440

211. Forman D, Vincent TJ, Doll R. Cancer of the liver and the use of oral contraceptives. BMJ, 1986; 292:1357–1361

212. Yamada S, Hosoda S, Tatero H, Kido C, Takahashi S. Survey of Thorotrast-associated liver cancers in Japan. J Nat Cancer Inst, 1983; 70:31–35

213. Heath CW Jr, Falk H, Creech JL Jr. Characteristics of cases of angiosarcoma of the liver among vinyl chloride workers in the United States. Ann N Y Acad Sci, 1975; 246:231–236

214. Mack L, Delmore F, Creech JL Jr et al. Clinical and morphologic features of hepatic angiosarcoma in vinyl chloride workers. Cancer, 1976; 37:149–163

215. Falk H, Caldwell GG, Ishak KG, Thomas LB, Popper H. Arsenic-related angiosarcoma. Am J Indust Med, 1981; 2:43–50

216. Kasper ML, Schoenfield L, Strom RL, Theologides A. Hepatic angiosarcoma and bronchoalveolar carcinoma-induced by Fowler's solution. JAMA, 1984; 252:3407–3408

217. Chen Y, Ahsan H. Cancer burden from arsenic in drinking water in Bangladesh. Am J Public Health, 2004; 94:741–744

218. Baxter PJ, Langlands AO, Anthony PP, MacSween RNM, Scheuer PJ. Angiosarcoma of the liver: a tumour for the late effects of Thorotrast in Great Britain. Br J Cancer, 1980; 41:446–452

219. Falk H, Herbert J, Crowley S et al. Epidemiology of hepatic angiosarcoma in the United States: 1964–1974. Environ Health Perspect, 1981; 41:107–113

220. Kojiro M, Nakashima T, Ito Y et al. Thorium dioxide related angiosarcoma of the liver. Pathomorphologic study of 29 autopsy cases. Arch Pathol Lab Med, 1985; 109:853–857

221. Ishak, KG, Anthony PP, Sobin LH. Histological typing of tumors of the liver, 2nd edn. Berlin: Springer, 1994

222. Falk H, Thomas LB, Popper H, Ishak KG. Hepatic angiosarcoma associated with androgenic-anabolic steroids. Lancet, 1979; ii:1120–1123

223. Hoch-Ligeti C. Angiosarcoma of the liver associated with diethylstilbesterol. JAMA, 1978; 240:1510–1511

224. Daneshmend TK, Scott GL, Bradfield JWB. Angiosarcoma of the liver associated with phenelzine. BMJ, 1979; 6:1679

225. Willis SM, Bailey SR. Streptokinase-induced subcapsular hematoma of the liver. Arch Intern Med, 1984; 144:2084–2085

226. Erichsen C, Sndenaa K, Streide JA, Andersen E, Tysvoer A. Spontaneous liver hematomas induced by anti-coagulation therapy. A case report and review of the literature. Hepato-gastroenterol, 1993; 40:402–406

227. Schumacher J, Müller G, Klotz K-K. Large hepatic hematoma and intra-abdominal hemorrhage associated with abuse of anabolic steroids [letter]. N Engl J Med, 1999; 340:1123–1124

228. Gravel DH, Begin LR, Brisson M-L, Lamoureux E. Metastatic carcinoma resulting in hepar lobatum. Am J Clin Pathol, 1996; 105:621–627

229. Shikhoda A, Baird S. Morphologic changes of the liver following chemotherapy for metastatic breast carcinoma: CT findings. Abdom Imaging, 1994; 19:39–42

230. Shreiner SA, Gorman B, Stephens DH. Chemotherapy-related hepatotoxicity causing imaging findings resembling cirrhosis. Mayo Clin Proc, 1998; 73:780–783

231. Chin NW, Chapman I, Jimenez FA. Complete chemotherapeutic regression of hepatic metastases with resultant hepar lobatum. Am J Gastroenterol, 1987; 82:149–151

232. Klinge O, Bannasch P. Zur Vermehrung des glatten endoplasmatischen Retikulum in Hepatocyten Menschlicher Leberpunktate. Verhandl Dtsch Gesell Pathol, 1968; 52:568–573

233. Winkler K, Junge U, Creutzfeldt W. Ground-glass hepatocytes in unselected liver biopsies. Ultrastructure and relationship to hepatitis B surface antigen. Scand J Gastroenterol, 1976; 11:167–170

234. Jezequel AM, Librari ML, Mosca P, Novelli G, Lorenzini I, Orlandi F. Changes induced in human liver by long-term anticonvulsant therapy. Functional and ultrastructural data. Liver, 1984; 4:307–317

235. Pamperl H, Grande W, Fridrich L et al. Influence of long-term anticonvulsant treatment on liver ultrastructure in man. Liver, 1984; 4:294–310

236. Vazquez JJ, Guillen FJ, Zozaya-Lahoz M. Cyanamide-induced liver injury. A predictable lesion. Liver, 1983; 3:225–231

237. Wang HC, Wu HC, Chen CF et al. Different types of ground glass hepatocytes in chronic hepatitis B virus infection contain specific pre-S mutants that may induce endoplasmic reticulum stress. Am J Pathol, 2003; 163:2441–2449

238. Vazquez JJ. Ground-glass hepatocytes: light and electron microscopy. Characterization of the different types. Histol Histopathol, 1990; 5:379–386

239. Koga Y, Swanson VL, Hays DM. Hepatic 'intravenous fat pigment' in infants and children receiving lipid emulsion. J Pediatr Surg, 1976; 10:641–648

240. Passwell JH, David R, Katznelson D, Cohen BE. Pigment deposition in the reticuloendothelial system after fat emulsion infusion. Arch Dis Child, 1976; 51:366–368

241. Landas SK, Mitros FA, Furst DE et al. Lipogranulomas and gold in the liver in rheumatoid arthritis. Am J Surg Pathol, 1992; 16:171–174

242. Al-Talib RK, Wright DH, Theaker JM. Orange-red birefringence of gold particles in paraffin wax embedded sections: an aid to the diagnosis of chrysiasis. Histopathology, 1994; 24:176–178

243. Coelho Filho JC, Moreira RA, Crocker PR, Levison DA. Identification of titanium pigment in drug addicts tissues. Histopathology, 1991; 19:190–192

244. Wands JR, Weiss SW, Yardley JH, Maddrey WC. Chronic inorganic mercury poisoning due to laxative abuse. A clinical and ultrastructural study. Am J Med, 1974; 57:92–101

245. Rauber G, Duprez A, Bibas H. Argyrisme avec localisation hépatique. Méd Chir Dig, 1981; 10:319–320

246. Ludwig J, Hashimoto E, Porayko MK et al. Hemosiderosis in cirrhosis: a study of 447 native livers. Gastroenterology, 1997; 112:882–888

247. Ockner RK, Schmid R. Acquired porphyria in man and rat due to hexachlorobenzene intoxication. Nature (London), 1961; 189:499–502

248. Ali M, Fayemi Riglusi R, Frasuno J, Marsden T, Malcolm D. Hemosiderosis in hemodialysis patients: an autopsy study of 50 cases. JAMA, 1980; 244:343–345

249. Hennigar GR, Greene WB, Walker EM et al. Hemochromatosis caused by excessive vitamin iron intake. Am J Pathol, 1979; 96:611–624

250. Brown KE, Dennery PA, Ridnour LA et al. Effect of iron overload and dietary fat on indices of oxidative stress and hepatic fibrogenesis in rats. Liver Int, 2003; 23:232–242

251. Yamasaki K, Yamasaki A, Tosaki M et al. Tissue distribution of Thorotrast and role of internal irradiation in carcinogenesis. Oncol Rep, 2004; 12:733–738

252. Reske-Nielsen E, Bojsen-Moller M, Vetner M et al. Polyvinylpyrrolidone storage disease: light microscopical, ultrastructural and chemical verification. Acta Pathol Microbiol Scand, 1976; 84:397–405

253. Reichling J, Kaplan M. Clinical use of serum enzymes in liver disease. Dig Dis Sci, 1988; 33:1601–1614

254. Sotil EU, Jensen DM. Serum enzymes associated with cholestasis. Clin Liver Dis, 2004; 8:41–54

255. Schiodt FV, Rochling FA, Casey DL, Lee WM. Acetaminophen toxicity in an urban county hospital. N Engl J Med, 1997; 337:1112–1117

256. Vale JA, Proudfoot AT. Paracetamol (acetaminophen) poisoning. Lancet, 1995; 346:547–552

257. McFarlane IG. Autoimmune hepatitis: diagnostic criteria, subclassifications, and clinical features. Clin Liver Dis, 2002; 6:605–621

258. Zimmerman HJ, Ishak KG. General aspects of drug-induced liver disease. Gastroenterol Clin North Am, 1995; 24:739–757

259. Bergasa NV, Jones EA. The pruritus of cholestasis. Semin Liver Dis, 1993; 13:319–327

260. Bissell DM, Gores GJ, Laskin DL, Hoofnagle JH. Drug-induced liver injury: mechanisms and test systems. Hepatology, 2001; 33:1009–1013

261. Bourdi M, Reilly TP, Elkahloun AG et al. Macrophage migration inhibitory factor in drug-induced liver injury: a role in susceptibility and stress responsiveness. Biochem Biophys Res Commun, 2002; 294:225–230

262. Reilly TP, Brady JN, Marchick MR et al. A protective role for cyclooxygenase-2 in drug-induced liver injury in mice. Chem Res Toxicol, 2001; 14:1620–1628

263. Harinasuta U, Zimmerman HJ. Diphenylhydantoin sodium hepatitis. JAMA, 1968; 203:1015–1018

264. Joshi PH, Conn HO. The syndrome of methoxyflurane-associated hepatitis. Ann Intern Med, 1974; 80:395–401

265. Neuberger J. Immune mechanisms in drug hepatotoxicity. Clin Liver Dis, 1998; 2:471–482

266. Jennings RB. Fatal fulminant acute carbon tetrachloride poisoning. AMA Arch Pathol, 1955; 59:269–284

267. Cotrim HP, Andrade ZA, Parana R, Portugal M, Lyra LG, Freitas LAR. Nonalcoholic steatohepatitis: a toxic liver disease in industrial workers. Liver, 1999; 19:299–304

268. Nomiyama T, Uehara M, Miyauchi H et al. Causal relationship between a case of severe hepatic dysfunction and low exposure concentrations of N,N-dimethylformamide in the synthetics industry. Ind Health, 2001; 39:33–36

269. Wrbitsky R. Liver function in workers exposed to N,N-dimethylformamide during the production of synthetic textiles. Int Arch Occup Environ Health, 1999; 72:19–25

270. Fiorito A, Larese F, Molinari S et al. Liver function alterations in synthetic leather workers exposed to dimethylformamide. Am J Ind Med, 1997; 32:255–260

271. Maroni M, Mocci F, Visentin S et al. Periportal fibrosis and the liver ultrasonography findings in vinyl chloride workers. Occup Environ Med, 2003; 60:60–65

272. Boucher R, Hanna C, Rusch GM et al. Hepatotoxicity associated with overexposure to 1,1-dichloro-2,2,2-trifluoroethane (HCFC-123). AIHA J, 2003; 64:68–79

273. Hoet P, Graf MLM, Bourdi M et al. Epidemic of liver disease caused by hydrochlorofluorocarbons used as ozone-sparing substitutes of chlorofluorocarbons. Lancet, 1997; 350:556–559

274. Kopelman H, Scheuer PJ, Williams R. The liver lesion in Epping jaundice. Quart J Med, 1966; 35:553–564

275. McGill DB, Motto JD. An industrial outbreak of toxic hepatitis due to methylenedianiline. N Engl J Med, 1974; 291:278–282

276. Siegel E, Wason S. Camphor toxicity. Pediatr Clin North Am, 1986; 33:375–379

277. Jimenez JF, Brown AL, Arnold WC, Byrne WJ. Chronic camphor ingestion mimicking Reye's syndrome. Gastroenterology, 1983; 84:394–398

278. Rengstorff DS, Osorio RW, Bonacini M. Recovery from severe hepatitis caused by mushroom poisoning without liver transplantation. Clin Gastroenterol Hepatol, 2003; 1:392–396

279. Broussard CN, Aggarwal A, Lacey SR et al. Mushroom poisoning—from diarrhea to liver transplantation. Am J Gastroenterol, 2001; 96:3195–3198

280. Enjalbert F, Rapior S, Nouguier-Soule J et al. Treatment of amatoxin poisoning: 20-year retrospective analysis. J Toxicol Clin Toxicol, 2002; 40:715–757

281. Krishnamachari KAVR, Bhat RV, Nagarajan V, Tilak TBG. Hepatitis due to aflatoxicosis. An outbreak in western India. Lancet, 1975; i:1061–1063

282. Wogan GN. Aflatoxin exposure as a risk factor in the etiology of hepatocellular carcinoma. In: Okuda K, Tabor E, eds. Liver cancer. New York: Churchill Livingstone, 1997: pp 51–58

283. Mohabbat O, Srivastava RN, Sediq GG, Merzad AA, Aram GM. An outbreak of hepatic veno-occlusive diseases in north-western Afghanistan. Lancet, 1976; ii:269–271

284. Tandon BN, Tandon RK, Tandon HD, Narndranathan M, Joshi YK. An epidemic of veno-occlusive disease of liver in central India. Lancet, 1976; ii:271–272

285. Weber LW, Boll M, Stampfl A. Hepatotoxicity and mechanism of action of haloalkanes: carbon tetrachloride as a toxilogical model. Crit Rev Toxicol, 2003; 33:105–136

286. Zimmerman HJ. Effect of alcohol on other hepatotoxins. Alcohol Clin Exp Res, 1986; 10:3–15

287. Recknagel RO, Glende EA Jr, Dolak JH et al. Mechanisms of carbon tetrachloride toxicity. Pharmacol Ther, 1989; 43:139–154

288. Williams AT, Burk RF. Carbon tetrachloride hepatotoxicity: an example of free radical-mediated injury. Semin Liver Dis, 1990; 10:279–284

289. Gurney R. Tetrachlorethane intoxication: early recognition of liver damage and means of prevention. Gastroenterology, 1943; 1:1112

290. Croquet V, Fort J, Oberti F et al. 1,1,1-Trichloroethane-induced chronic active hepatitis. Gastroenterol Clin Biol, 2003; 27:120–122

291. Lind RC, Gandolfi AJ, Hall PD. Biotransformation and hepatotoxicity of HCFC-123 in the guinea pig: potentiation of hepatic injury by prior glutathione depletion. Toxicol Appl Pharmacol, 1995; 134:175–181

292. Hoet P, Buchet JP, Sempoux C et al. Potentiation of 2,2-dichloro-1,1,1-trifluoroethane (HCFC-123)-induced liver toxicity by ethanol in guinea pigs. Arch Toxicol, 2002; 76:707–714

293. Ho SF, Phoon WH, Gan SL et al. Persistent liver dysfunction among workers at a vinyl chloride monomer polymerization plant. J Soc Occup Med, 1991; 41:10–16

294. Hsieh HI, Wang JD, Chen PC et al. Synergistic effect of hepatitis virus infection and occupational exposures to vinyl chloride monomer and ethylene dichloride on serum aminotransferase activity. Occup Environ Med, 2003; 60:774–778

295. Creech JL Jr, Johnson MN. Angiosarcoma of the liver in the manufacture of polyvinyl chloride. J Occup Med, 1974; 16:150–151

296. Jones RD, Smith DM, Thomas PG. A mortality study of vinyl chloride monomer workers employed in the United Kingdom in 1940–1974. Scand J Work Environ Health, 1988; 14:153–160

297. Du CL, Wang JD. Increased morbidity odds ratio of primary liver cancer and cirrhosis of the liver among vinyl chloride monomer workers. Occup Environ Med, 1998; 55:528–532

298. Brady J, Liberatore F, Harper P et al. Angiosarcoma of the liver: an epidemiologic survey. J Natl Cancer Inst, 1977; 59:1383–1385

299. Berk PD, Martin JF, Young RS et al. Vinyl chloride-associated liver disease. Ann Intern Med, 1976; 84:717–731

300. Wong RH, Chen PC, Wang JD et al. Interaction of vinyl chloride monomer exposure and hepatitis B viral infection on liver cancer. J Occup Environ Med, 2003; 45:379–383

301. DeFalque RJ. Pharmacology and toxicology of trichloroethylene: a critical review of the world literature. Clin Pharmacol Ther, 1965; 2:665–668

302. Clearfield HR. Hepatorenal toxicity from sniffing spot-remover (trichloroethylene). Am J Dig Dis, 1970; 15:851–861

303. Meadows R, Verghese A. Medical complications of glue sniffing. South Med J, 1996; 89:455–462

304. Martland HS. Trinitrotoluene poisoning. JAMA, 1917; 2:835–837

305. McConnell WJ, Flinn RH. Summary of 22 trinitrotoluene fatalities in World War II. J Indust Hyg Toxicol, 1946; 28:76–86

306. Davie TB. The pathology of T.N.T. poisoning. Proc R Soc Med (Lond), 1942; 35:553–560

307. Moridani MY, Siraki A, O'Brien PJ. Quantitative structure toxicity relationships for phenols in isolated rat hepatocytes. Chem Biol Interact, 2003; 145:213–223

308. Harrison R, Letz G, Pasternack G et al. Fulminant hepatitis after occupational exposure to 2-nitropropane. Ann Intern Med, 1987; 107:466–468

309. Aydin Y, Ozcakar L. Occupational hepatitis due to chronic inhalation of propane and butane gases. Int J Clin Pract, 2003; 57:546

310. Zitting A, Savolainen H, Nickels J. Acute effects of 2-nitropropane on rat liver and brain. Toxicol Lett, 1981; 9:237–246

311. Cunningham ML, Matthews HB. Relationship of hepatocarcinogenicity and hepatocullar proliferation induced by mutagenic noncarcinogens vs carcinogens. II. 1- vs 2-nitropropane. Toxicol Appl Pharmacol, 1991; 110:505–513

312. Kimbrough RD. Human health effects of polychlorinated biphenyls (PCBs) and polybrominated biphenyls (PBBs). Annu Rev Pharmacol, 1987; 27:87–111

313. Fries GF. The PBB episode in Michigan. An overall appraisal. CRC Crit Rev Toxicol, 1985; 16:105–156

314. Senoh H, Katagiri T, Arito H et al. Toxicity due to 2- and 13-wk inhalation exposures of rats and mice to N,N-dimethylformamide. J Occup Health, 2003; 45:365–375

315. Wang JD, Lai MY, Chen JS et al. Dimethylformamide-induced liver damage among synthetic leather workers. Arch Environ Health, 1991; 46:161–166

316. Koh SB, Cha BS, Park JK et al. The metabolism and liver toxicity of N,N-dimethylformamide in the isolated perfused rat liver. Yonsei Med J, 2002; 43:491–499

317. Luo JC, Kuo HW, Cheng TJ et al. Abnormal liver function associated with occupational exposure to dimethylformamide and hepatitis B virus. J Occup Environ Med, 2001; 43:474–482

318. Van Haaften AB. Acute tetrabromoethane (acetylene tetrabromide) intoxication in man. Am Indust Hyg Assoc J, 1969; 30:251

319. Letz GA, Pond SM, Osterloh JD. Two fatalities after occupational exposure to ethylene dibromide. JAMA, 1984; 252:2428–2431

320. Gleason W, DeMello DE, DeCastro FJ et al. Acute hepatic failure in severe iron poisoning. J Pediatr, 1979; 95:138–140

321. Britton RS. Metal-induced hepatotoxicity. Semin Liver Dis, 1996; 16:3–12

322. Diaz-Rivera RS, Collazo PJ, Pons ER et al. Acute phosphorus poisoning in man. A study of 56 cases. Medicine, 1950; 29:269–298

323. Pande TK, Pandey S. White phosphorus poisoning—explosive encounter. J Assoc Physicians India, 2004; 52:249–250

324. Chutani HR, Gupta PS, Gulati S et al. Acute copper sulfate poisoning. Am J Med, 1965; 29:849–854

325. Zimmerman HJ, Ishak KG. Non-alcoholic steatohepatitis and other forms of pseudoalcoholic liver disease. In: Hall P, ed. Alcoholic liver disease. Pathology and pathogenesis, 2nd edn. London: Edward Arnold, 1995: pp 175–198

326. Jantsch W, Kulig K, Rumack BH. Massive copper sulfate ingestion resulting in hepatotoxicity. J Toxicol Clin Toxicol, 1984; 22:585–588

327. Singh D, Dewan I, Pandey AN et al. Spectrum of unnatural fatalities in the Chandigarh zone of north-west India—a 25 year autopsy study from a tertiary care hospital. J Clin Forensic Med, 2003; 10:145–152

328. Müller-Höcker J, Summer KH, Schramel P, Rodeck B. Different pathomorphologic patterns in exogenous infantile copper intoxication of the liver. Pathol Res Proct, 1998; 194:377–384

329. Müller T, Feichtinger H, Berger H, Müller W. Endemic Tyrolean infantile cirrhosis: an ecogenetic disorder. Lancet, 1996; 347:877–880

330. Da Motta CL, Da Silva Horta J, Tavares MH. Prospective epidemiological study of Thorotrast exposed patients in Portugal. Environ Res, 1979; 18:152–153

331. Ishak KG. Malignant mesenchymal tumors and pseudotumors and some other nonhepatocellular tumors of the liver. In: Okuda K, Tabor E, eds. Liver cancer. New York: Churchill Livingstone, 1997: pp 291–314

332. Ito Y, Kojiro N, Nakashima T et al. Pathomorphologic characteristics of 102 cases of Thorotrast-related hepatocellular carcinoma, cholangiocarcinoma and hepatic angiosarcoma. Cancer, 1988; 62:1153–1162

333. Shaib Y, El-Serag HB. The epidemiology of cholangiocarcinoma. Semin Liver Dis, 2004; 24:115–125

334. Rubel LR, Ishak KG. Thorotrast associated cholangiocarcinoma. Cancer, 1982; 50:1408–1415

335. Andersson M, Storm HH. Cancer incidence among Danish Thorotrast-exposed patients. J Natl Cancer Inst, 1992; 84:1318–1325

336. Shurbaji MS, Olson LJ, Kahajda P. Thorotrast-associated hepatic leiomyosarcoma and cholangiocarcinoma. Hum Pathol, 1987; 18:254

337. Okuda K, Omata M, Itoh Y, Ikezaki H, Nakashima T. Peliosis hepatis as a late and fatal complication of Thorotrast liver disease: Report of five cases. Liver, 1981; 1:110–122

338. Ishak KG. Applications of scanning electron microscopy in the study of liver disease. Prog Liver Dis, 1986; 8:1–32

339. Brzoska MM, Moniuszko-Jakoniuk J, Pilat-Marcinkiewicz B et al. Liver and kidney function and histology in rats exposed to cadmium and ethanol. Alcohol Alcoholism, 2003; 38:2–10

340. Stoeckle JD, Hardy HL, Weber AL. Chronic beryllium disease: long-term follow-up of sixty cases and selective review of the literature. Am J Med, 1969; 46:545–561

341. Plaa GL. Chlorinated methanes and liver injury: highlights of the past 50 years. Annu Rev Pharmacol Toxicol, 2000; 40:42–65

342. Beddowes EJ, Faux SP, Chipman JK. Chloroform, carbon tetrachloride and glutathione depletion induce secondary genotoxicity in liver cells via oxidative stress. Toxicology, 2003; 187:101–115

343. Clare NT. Photosensitivity diseases in New Zealand. N Z J Agricult Res, 1959; 2:1249

344. Ishizaki K, Kinbara S, Miyazawa N et al. The biochemical studies on phalloidin-induced cholestasis in rats. Toxicol Lett, 1997; 90:29–34

345. Utili R, Abernathy CO, Zimmerman HJ et al. Cholestatic effects of Escherichia coli endotoxin on the isolated perfused rat liver. Gastroenterology, 1976; 70:248–253

346. Whiting JF, Green RM, Rosenbluth AB et al. Tumor necrosis factor-alpha decreases hepatocyte bile salt uptake and mediates endotoxin-induced cholestasis. Hepatology, 1995; 22(4 Pt 1):1273–1278

347. Labib R, Turkall R, Abdel-Rahman MS. Endotoxin potentiates cocaine-mediated hepatotoxicity by nitric oxide and reactive oxygen species. Int J Toxicol, 2003; 22:305–316

348. Hofmann AF. Detoxification of lithocholic acid, a toxic bile acid: relevance to drug hepatotoxicity. Drug Metab Rev, 2004; 36:703–722

349. Goldfarb S, Singer K, Popper H. Experimental cholangitis due to alpha-naphthylisothiocyanate (ANIT). Am J Pathol, 1962; 40:685–695

350. Lee MS. Oxidative conversion of isothiocyanates to isocyanates by rat liver. Environ Health Perspect, 1994; 102(Suppl 6):115–118

351. Guzelian P. Hepatic injury due to environmental agents. Clin Lab Med, 1984; 4:483–488

352. Wyde ME, Bartolucci E, Ueda A et al. The environmental pollutant 1,1-dichloro-2,2-bis (p-chlorophenyl)ethylene induces rat hepatic cytochrome P450 2B and 3A expression through the constitutive androstane receptor and pregnane X receptor. Mol Pharmacol, 2003; 64:474–481

353. Leonard C, Burke CM, O'Keane C et al. 'Golf ball liver': agent orange hepatitis. Gut, 1997; 40:687–688

354. Niittynen M, Tuomisto JT, Auriola S et al. 2,3,7,8-Tetrachlorodibenzo-p-dioxin (TCDD)-induced accumulation of biliverdin and hepatic peliosis in rats. Toxicol Sci, 2003; 71:112–123

355. Michalek JE, Ketchum NS, Longnecker MP. Serum dixide and hepatic abnormalities in veterans of Operation Ranch Hand. Ann Epidemiol, 2001; 11:304–311

356. Botella de Maglia J, Belenguer Tarin JE. Paraquat poisoning. A study of 29 cases and evaluation of the effectiveness of the 'Caribbean scheme.' Med Clin (Barc), 2000; 115:530–533

357. Stephens BG, Moormeister SK. Homicidal poisoning by paraquat. Am J Forensic Med Pathol, 1997; 18:33–39

358. Tungsanga K, Chusilp S, Israsena S et al. Paraquat poisoning: evidence of systemic toxicity after dermal exposure. Postgrad Med J, 1983; 59:338–339

359. Bateller R, Bragulat E, Nogue S et al. Prolonged cholestasis after acute paraquat poisoning through skin absorption. Am J Gastroenterol, 2000; 95:1340–1343

360. Carpenter HM, Hedstrom OR, Siddens LK et al. Ultrastructural, protein, and lipid changes in liver associated with chlordecone treatment of mice. Fundam Appl Toxicol, 1996; 34:157–164

361. Guzelian P. Comparative toxicology of chlordecone (Kepone) in humans and experimental animals. Annu Rev Pharmacol, 1982; 22:89–113

362. Ogata M, Izushi F. Effects of chlordane on parameters of liver and muscle toxicity in man and experimental animals. Toxicol Lett, 1991; 56:327–337

363. Taylor JR, Selhorst IB, Houff SA et al. Chlordecone intoxication in man: I. Clinical observations. Neurology, 1978; 28:626–630

364. Poklis A, Saady JJ. Arsenic poisoning: acute or chronic? Suicide or murder? Am J Forensic Med Pathol, 1990; 11:226–232

365. Labadie H, Stoessel P, Callard P et al. Hepatic veno-occlusive disease and perisinusoidal fibrosis secondary to arsenic poisoning. Gastroenterology, 1990; 99:1140–1143

366. Santra A, Das Gupta J, De BK et al. Hepatic manifestations in chronic arsenic toxicity. Indian J Gastroenterol, 1999; 18:152–155

367. Eisler R. Arsenic hazards to humans, plants, and animals from gold mining. Rev Environ Contam Toxicol, 2004; 180:133–165

368. Rice KC, Conko KM, Hornberger GM. Anthropogenic sources of arsenic and copper to sediments in a suburban lake, Northern Virginia. Environ Sci Technol, 2002; 36:4962–4967

369. Guha Mazumder. Chronic arsenic toxicity: clinical features, epidemiology, and treatment: experience in West Bengal. J Environ Sci Health Part A Tox Hazard Subst Environ Eng, 2003; 38:141–163

370. Tchounwou PB, Centeno JA, Patlolla AK. Arsenic toxicity, mutagenesis, and carcinogenesis—a health risk assessment and management approach. Mol Cell Biochem, 2004; 255:47–55

371. Cui X, Li S, Shraim A et al. Subchronic exposure to arsenic through drinking water alters expression of cancer-related genes in rat liver. Toxicol Pathol, 2004; 32:64–72

372. el Zayadi A, Khalil A, Samny N. Hepatic angiosarcoma among Egyptian farmers exposed to pesticides. Hepatogastroenterology, 1986; 33:148–150

373. Kannan GM, Flora SJ. Chronic arsenic poisoning in the rat: treatment with combined administration of succimers and an antioxidant. Ecotoxicol Environ Saf, 2004; 58:37–43

374. Guha Mazumder. Arsenic and liver disease. J Indian Med Assoc, 2001; 99:311–320

375. Stickel F, Egerer G, Seitz HK. Hepatotoxicity of botanicals. Public Health Nutr, 2000; 3:113–124

376. Stedman C. Herbal hepatotoxicity. Semin Liver Dis, 2002; 22:195–206

377. Schiano TD. Hepatotoxicity and complementary and alternative medicines. Clin Liver Dis, 2003; 7:453–473

378. Kessler RC, Davis RB, Foster DF et al. Long-term trends in the use of complementary and alternative medical therapies in the United States. Ann Intern Med, 2001; 135:262–268

379. Seeff LB, Lindsay KL, Bacon BR et al. Complementary and alternative medicine in chronic liver disease. Hepatology, 2001; 34:595–603

380. Fogden E, Neuberger J. Alternative medicines and the liver. Liver Int, 2003; 23:213–220

381. Neff GW, O'Brien C, Montalbano M et al. Consumption of dietary supplements in a liver transplant population. Liver Transplant, 2004; 10:881–885

382. Levy C, Seeff L, Lindor K. Use of herbal supplements for chronic liver disease. Clin Gastroenterol Hepatol, 2004; 2:947–956

383. Estes JD, Stolpman D, Olyaei A et al. High prevalence of potentially hepatotoxic herbal supplement use in patients with fulminant hepatic failure. Arch Surg, 2003; 138:852–858

384. Ellenhorn MJ, Barceloux DG. Medical toxicology: diagnosis and treatment of human poisoning. New York: Elsevier, 1988: pp 1324–1327

385. Litovitz L, Klein-Schwartz W, Rodgers GC et al. 2001 annual report of the American Association of Poison Control Centers Toxic Exposure Surveillance System. Am J Emerg Med, 2002; 20:391–452

386. Nordt SP, Manoguerra A, Clark RF. 5-Year analysis of mushroom exposures in California. West J Med, 2000; 173:314–317

387. Centers for Disease Control and Prevention. *Amanita phalloides* mushroom poisoning—Northern California, January 1997. JAMA, 1997; 278:16–17

388. Vetter J. Toxins of Amanita phalloides. Toxicon, 1998; 36:13–24

389. Kroncke KD, Fricker G, Meier PJ et al. Alpha-amanitin uptake into hepatocytes. J Biol Chem, 1986; 261:12562–12567

390. Berger KJ, Guss DA. Mycotoxins revisited: Part I. J Emerg Med, 2005; 28:53–62

391. Klein AS, Hart J, Brems JJ et al. *Amanita* poisoning: treatment and the role of liver transplantation. Am J Med, 1989; 86:187–193

392. Montanini S, Sinardi, D, Pratico C et al. Use of acetylcysteine as the life-saving antidote in Amanita phalloides (death cap) poisoning. Case report on 11 patients. Arzneimittelforschung, 1999; 49:1044–1047

393. Jander S, Bischoff J, Woodcock BG. Plasmapheresis in the treatment of Amanita phalloides poisoning II. A review and recommendations. Ther Apher, 2000; 4:308–312

394. Faybik P, Hetz H, Baker A et al. Extracorporeal albumin dialysis in patients with Amanita phalloides poisoning. Liver Int, 2003; 23(Suppl 3):28–33

395. Ware GM. Method validation study of hypoglycin A determination in ackee fruit. J AOAC Int, 2002; 85:933–937

396. Toxic hypoglycemic syndrome—Jamaica, 1989–1991. MMWR Morb Mortal Wkly Rep, 1992; 41:53–55

397. Larson J, Vender R, Camuto P. Cholestatic jaundice due to ackee fruit poisoning. Am J Gastroenterol, 1994; 89:1577–1578

398. Fukunishi R. Acute hepatic lesions induced by cycasin. Acta Pathol Jpn, 1973; 23:639–646

399. Butler WH. Liver injury induced by aflatoxin. Prog Dis, 1970; 3:408–418

400. Tandon HD, Tandon BN, Ramalingaswami V. Epidemic of toxic hepatitis in India of possible mycotoxin origin. Arch Pathol Lab Med, 1978; 102:372–376

401. Tanaka T, Nishikawa A, Iwata H et al. Enhancing effect of ethanol on aflatoxin B1-induced hepatocarcinogenesis in male ACI/N rats. Jpn J Cancer Res, 1989; 80:526–530

402. Angsubhakorn S, Pradermwong A, Phanwichien K et al. Promation of aflatoxin B1-induced hepatocarcinogenesis by dichlorodiphenyl trichloroethane (DDT). Southeast Asian J Trop Med Public Health, 2002; 33:613–623

403. Kew MC. Synergistic interaction between aflatoxin B1 and hepatitis B virus in hepatocarcinogenesis. Liver Int, 2003; 23:405–409

404. Aguilar F, Harris CC, Sun T et al. Geographic variation of p53 mutational profile in nonmalignant human liver. Science, 1994; 264:1317–1319

405. Antony M, Shukla Y, Janardhanan KK. Potential risk of acute hepatotoxicity of kodo poisoning due to exposure to cyclopiazonic acid. J Ethnopharmacol, 2003; 87:211–214

406. Solis-Herruzo JA, Castellano C, Colina F et al. Hepatic injury in the toxic oil syndrome caused by ingestion of adulterated cooking oil (Spain 1981). Hepatology, 1984; 4:131–139

407. Sanchez-Porro Valades P, Posada de la Paz M, de Andres Copa P et al. Toxic oil syndrome: survival in the whole cohort between 1981 and 1995. J Clin Epidemiol, 2003; 56:701–708

408. Diggle GE. The toxic oil syndrome: 20 years on. Int J Clin Pract, 2001; 55:371–375

409. Alonso-Ruiz A, Calabozo M, Perez-Ruiz F et al. Toxic oil syndrome. A long-term followup of a cohort of 332 patients. Medicine, 1993; 72:285–295

410. Diaz de Rojas F, Castro GM, Abaitua BI et al. Hepatic injury in the toxic oil syndrome. Hepatology, 1985; 5:166–174

411. Solis-Herruzo JA, Vidal JV, Colina F et al. Nodular regenerative hyperplasia of the liver associated with the toxic oil syndrome. Hepatology, 1986; 6:687–693

412. McGill DB, Motto JD. An industrial outbreak of toxic hepatitis due to methylenedianiline. N Engl J Med, 1974; 291:278–282

413. Bastian PG. Occupational hepatitis caused by methylenedianiline. Med J Aust, 1984; 141:533–535

414. Tillmann HL, van Palt FN, Martz W et al. Accidental intoxication with methylene dianiline p,p'-diaminodiphenylmethane: acute liver damage after presumed ecstasy consumption. J Toxicol Clin Toxicol, 1997; 35:35–40

415. Nichols L. The Epping jaundice outbreak: mortality after 38 years of follow-up. Int Arch Occup Environ Health, 2004; 77:592–594

416. Hall AJ, Harrington JM, Waterhouse JA. The Epping jaundice outbreak: a 24 year follow up. J Epidemiol Community Health, 1992; 46:327–328

417. Yoshimura T. Yusho in Japan. Ind Health, 2003; 41:139–148

418. Tukunga S, Kataoka K. Association between blood concentration of polychlorinated biphenyls and manifestations of symptoms and signs in chronic 'Yusho' patients from 1986 to 1997. Fuuoka Igaku Zasshi, 2001; 92:122–133

419. Peters HA. Hexachlorobenzene poisoning in Turkey. Fed Proc, 1976; 35:2400–2403

420. Can C, Nigogosyan G. Acquired toxic porphyria cutanea tarda due to hexachlorobenzene: report of 348 cases caused by this fungicide. JAMA, 1963; 183:88–91

421. Kanel GC, Cassidy W, Shuster L et al. Cocaine-induced liver cell injury: comparison of morphological features in man and in experimental models. Hepatology, 1990; 11:646–651

422. Kloss MW, Rosen GM, Rauckman EJ. Cocaine-mediated hepatotoxicity. A critical review. Biochem Pharm, 1984; 33:169–173

423. Wanless IR, Dore S, Gopinath N et al. Histopathology of cocaine hepatotoxicity: report of four patients. Gastroenterology, 1990; 98:497–501

424. Perino LE, Warren GH, Levine JS. Cocaine-induced hepatotoxicity in humans. Gastroenterology, 1987; 93:176–180

425. Silva MO, Roth D, Reddy KR et al. Hepatic dysfunction accompanying acute cocaine intoxication. J Hepatol, 1991; 12:312–315

426. Aoki K, Takimoto M, Ota H et al. Participation of CYP2A in cocaine-induced hepatotoxicity in female mice. Pharmacol Toxicol, 2000; 87:26–32

427. Mallat A, Dhumeaux D. Cocaine and the liver. J Hepatol, 1991; 12:275–278

428. Powell CJ, Charles SJ, Mullervy J. Cocaine hepatotoxicity: a study on the pathogenesis of periportal necrosis. Int J Exp Pathol, 1994; 75:415–424

429. Kothur R, Marsh F, Posner G. Liver function in nonparenteral cocaine users. Arch Intern Med, 1991; 151:1126–1128

430. Jones AL, Jarvie DR, McDermid G et al. Hepatocellular damage following amphetamine intoxication. Clin Toxicol, 1994; 34:435

431. Henry JA, Jeffreys KJ, Dawling S. Toxicity and deaths from 3,4-methylenedioxymethamphetamine ('ecstasy'). Lancet, 1992; 340:384–387

432. Tillman HL, VanPelt FNAM, Martz W et al. Accidental intoxication with methylene dianiline p,p'-diaminodiphenylmethane: acute liver damage after presumed ecstasy consumption. Clin Toxicol, 1997; 35:35–40

433. Dykhuizen RS, Smith CC, Brunt PW et al. Ecstasy induced hepatitis mimicking viral hepatitis. Gut, 1995; 36:939–941

434. Garbino J, Henry JA, Mentha G et al. Ecstasy ingestion and fulminant hepatic failure: liver transplantation to be considered as a last therapeutic option. Vet Human Toxicol, 2001; 43:99–102

435. Kramer L, Bauer E, Schenk P et al. Successful treatment of refractory cerebral edema in ecstasy/cocaine-induced fulminant liver failure using a new high-efficacy liver detoxification device (FPSA-Prometheus). Wien Klin Wochenschr, 2003; 115:599–603

436. Montiel-Duarte C, Varela-Rey M, Oses-Prieto JA et al. 3,4-Methylenedioxymethamphetamine ('Ecstasy') induces apoptosis of cultured rat liver cells. Biochim Biophys Acta, 2002; 1588(1):26–32

437. Carvalho M, Milhazes N, Remiao F et al. Hepatotoxicity of 3,4-methylenedioxyamphetamine and alpha-methyldopamine in isolated rat hepatocytes: formation of glutathione conjugates. Arch Toxicol, 2004; 78:16–24

438. Maurer HH, Kraemer T, Springer D et al. Chemistry, pharmacology, toxicology, and hepatic metabolism of designer drugs of the amphetamine (ecstasy), piperazine, and pyrrolidinophenone types: a synopsis. Ther Drug Monit, 2004; 26:127–131

439. Khakoo SI, Coles CJ, Armstrong JS et al. Hepatotoxicity and accelerated fibrosis following 3,4-methylenedioxymetamphetamine ('Ecstasy') usage. J Clin Gastroenterol, 1995; 20:244–247

440. Fidler H, Dhillon A, Gertner D et al. Chronic ecstasy (3,4-methylenedioxymetamphetamine) abuse: a recurrent and unpredictable course of severe acute hepatitis. J Hepatol, 1996; 25:563–566

441. Armen R, Kanel G, Reynolds T. Phencyclidine-induced malignant hyperthermia causing submassive liver necrosis. Am J Med, 1984; 77:167–172

442. Reid MJ, Bornheim LM. The effects of phencyclidine pretreatment on cocaine-mediated hepatotoxicity in mice. Toxicol Appl Pharmacol, 2001; 172:194–202

443. Trigueiro de Araujo MS, Gerard F, Chossegros P, Porto LC, Berlet P, Grimaud J-A. Vascular hepatotoxicity related to heroin addiction. Virchows Arch A Pathol Anat, 1990; 417:497–503

444. Borini P, Guimaraes RC, Borini SB. Possible hepatotoxicity of chronic marijuana usage. Sao Paulo Med J, 2004; 122:110–116

445. Payne RJ, Brand SN. The toxicity of intravenously used marihuana. JAMA, 1975; 233:351–354

446. Larrey D. Hepatotoxicity of herbal remedies. J Hepatol, 1997; 26(Suppl 1):47–51

447. Dasgupta A. Review of abnormal laboratory test results and toxic effects due to use of herbal medicines. Am J Clin Pathol, 2003; 129:127–137

448. Neff GW, Reddy KR, Durazo FA et al. Severe hepatotoxicity associated with the use of weight loss diet supplements containing ma huang or usnic acid. J Hepatol, 2004; 41:1062–1064

449. Clouatre DL. Kava kava: examining new reports of toxicity. Toxicol Lett, 2004; 150(1):85–96

450. Nadir A, Agarwal S, King PD et al. Acute hepatitis associated with the use of a Chinese herbal product, ma-huang. Am J Gastroenterol, 1996; 91:1436–1438

451. Borum ML. Fulminant exacerbation of autoimmune hepatitis after the use of ma huang. Am J Gastroenterol, 2001; 96:1654–1655

452. Bras G, Jelliffe DB, Stuart KL. Veno-occlusive disease of the liver with non-portal type of cirrhosis occurring in Jamaica. Arch Pathol, 1954; 57:285–300

453. Yeong ML, Clark SP, Waring JM et al. The effects of comfrey derived pyrrolizidine alkaloids on rat liver. Pathology, 1991; 23:35–38

454. DeLeve LD, McCuskey RS, Wang X et al. Characterization of a reproducible rat model of hepatic veno-occlusive disease. Hepatology, 1999; 29:1779

455. Copple BL, Ganey PE, Roth RA. Liver inflammation during monocrotaline hepatotoxicity. Toxicology, 2003; 190:155–169

456. Perez Alvarez J, Saez-Royuela F, Gento Pena E et al. Acute hepatitis due to ingestion of Teucrium chamaedrys infusions. Gastroenterol Hepatol, 2001; 24:240–243

457. Larrey D, Vial T, Pauwels A et al. Hepatitis after germander (Teucrium chamaedrys) administration: another instance of herbal medicine hepatotoxicity. Ann Intern Med, 1992; 117:129–132

458. Mostefa-Kara N, Pauwels A, Pines E et al. Fatal hepatitis after herbal tea. Lancet, 1992; 340:674

459. Ben Yahia M, Mavier P, Metreau JM et al. Chronic active hepatitis and cirrhosis induced by wild germander. 3 cases. Gastroenterol Clin Biol, 1993; 17:959–962

460. Lekehal M, Pessayre D, Lereau JM et al. Hepatotoxicity of the herbal medicine germander: metabolic activation of its furano diterpenoids by cytochrome P450 3A depletes cytoskeleton-associated protein thiols and forms plasma membrane blebs in rat hepatocytes. Hepatology, 1996; 24:212–218

461. Loeper J, Descatoire V, Letteron P et al. Hepatotoxicity of germander in mice. Gastroenterology, 1994; 106:464–472

462. Fau D, Lekehal M, Farrell G et al. Diterpenoids from germander, an herbal medicine, induce apoptosis in isolated rat hepatocytes. Gastroenterology, 1997; 113:1334–1346

463. De Berardinis V, Moulis C, Maurice M et al. Human microsomal epoxide hydrolasew is the target of germander induced autoantibodies on the surface of human hepatocytes. Mol Pharmacol, 2000; 58:542–551

464. Dourakis S, Papanikolaou IS, Tzemanakis EN et al. Acute hepatiotis associated with herb (Teucrium capatatum L.) administration. Eur J Gastroenterol Hepatol, 2002; 14:693–695

465. Polymeros D, Kamberoglou D, Tzias V. Acute cholestatic hepatitis caused by Teucrium polium (golden germander) with transient appearance of antimitochondrial antibody. J Clin Gastroenterol, 2002; 34:100–101

466. Gordon DW, Rosenthal G, Hart J et al. Chaparral ingestion. The broadening spectrum of liver injury caused by herbal medications. JAMA, 1995; 273:489–490

467. Sheikh NM, Philen RM, Love LA. Chaparral-associated hepatotoxicity. Arch Intern Med, 1997; 157:913–919

468. Batchelor WB, Heathcoat J, Wanless IR. Chaparral-induced hepatic injury. Am J Gastroenterol, 1995; 90:831–833

469. Anderson IB, Mullen WH, Meeker JE et al. Pennyroyal toxicity: measurement of toxic metabolite levels in two cases and review of the literature. Ann Intern Med, 1996; 124:726–734

470. Bakerink JA, Gospe SM Jr, Dimand RJ et al. Multiple organ failure after ingestion of pennyroyal oil from herbal tea in two infants. Pediatrics, 1996; 98:944–947

471. Sztajnkrycer MD, Otten EJ, Bond GR et al. Mitigation of pennyroyal oil hepatotoxicity in the mouse. Acad Emerg Med, 2003; 10:1024–1028

472. Woolf GM, Petrovic LM, Rojter SE et al. Acute hepatitis associated with the Chinese herbal product Jin Bu Huan. Ann Intern Med, 1994; 121:729–735

473. Horowitz RS, Feldhaus K, Dart RC et al. The clinical spectrum of Jin Bu Huan toxicity. Arch Intern Med, 1996; 156:899–903

474. Picciotti A, Campo N, Brizzolara R et al. Chronic hepatitis induced by Jin Bu Huan. J Hepatol, 1998; 28:165–167

475. Itoh S, Marutani K, Nishijima T et al. Liver injuries induced by herbal medicine, syo-saiko-to (xiao-chai-hu-tang). Dig Dis Sci, 1995; 40:1845–1848

476. Kamiyama T, Nouchi T, Kojima S et al. Autoimmune hepatitis triggered by administration of an herbal medicine. Am J Gastroenterol, 1997; 92:703–704

477. Park GJ, Mann SP, Ngu MC. Acute hepatitis induced by Shou-Wu-Pian, a herbal product derived from Polygonum multiflorum. J Gastroenterol Hepatol, 2001; 16:115–117

478. Mazzanti G, Battinelli L, Daniele C et al. New case of acute hepatitis following the consumption of Shou Wu Pian, a Chinese herbal product derived from Polygonum multiflorum [letter]. Ann Intern Med, 2004; 140:W30

479. Shekelle PG, Hardy ML, Morton SC et al. Efficacy and safety of ephedra and ephedrine for weight loss and athletic performance: a meta-analysis. JAMA, 2003; 289:1537–1545

480. Miller SC. Safety concerns regarding ephedrine-type alkaloid-containing dietary supplements. Mil Med, 2004; 169:87–93

481. Rados C. Ephedra ban: no shortage of reasons. FDA Consumer, 2004; 38(2):6–7

482. Lee MK, Cheng BWH, Che CT, Hsieh DPH. Cytoxicity assessment in Ma-huang (Ephedra) under different conditions of preparation. Toxicol Sci, 2000, 56:424–430

483. Adachi M, Saito H, Kobayashi H et al. Hepatic injury in 12 patients taking the herbal weight loss aids Chaso or Onshido. Ann Intern Med, 2003; 139:488–492

484. Kawaguchi T, Harada M, Arimatsu H et al. Severe hepatotoxicity associated with a N-nitrosofenfluramine-containing weight-loss supplement: report of three cases. J Gastroenterol Hepatol, 2004; 19:349–350

485. Favreau JT, Ryu ML, Braunstein G et al. Severe hepatotoxicity associated with the dietary supplement LipoKinetix. Ann Intern Med, 2002; 136:590–595

486. Food and Drug Administration 2001 Safety Information Summaries. Online. Available: http://www.fda.gov/medwatch/safety/2001/safety01.htm#lipoki

487. Durazo FA, Lassman C, Han SHB et al. Fulminant liver failure due to usnic acid for weight loss. Am J Gastroenterol, 2004; 99:950–952

488. Han D, Matsumaru K, Rettori D et al. Usnic acid-induced necrosis of cultured mouse hepatocytes: inhibition of mitochondrial function and oxidative stress. Biochem Pharmacol, 2004; 67:439–451

489. Perron AD, Patterson JA, Yanofsky NN. Kombucha 'mushroom' hepatotoxicity. Ann Emerg Med, 1995; 26:660–661

490. Willett KL, Roth RA, Walker L. Workshop overview: hepatotoxicity assessment for botanical dietary supplements. Toxicol Sci, 2004; 79:4–9

491. Schulze J, Raasch W, Siegers CP. Toxicity of kava pyrones, drug safety and precautions—a case study. Phytomedicine, 2003; 10(Suppl 4):68–73

492. Hepatic toxicity possibly associated with kava-containing products—United States, Germany, and Switzerland, 1999–2002. MMWR Morb Mortal Wkly Rep, 2002; 51:1065

493. Humbertson CL, Akhtar J, Krenzelok EP. Acute hepatitis induced by kava kava. J Toxicol Clin Toxicol, 2003; 41:109–113

494. Russmann S, Barguil Y, Cabalion P et al. Hepatic injury due to traditional aqueous extracts of kava root in New Caledonia. Eur J Gastroenterol Hepatol, 2003; 15:1033–1036

495. Stickel F, Baumuller HM, Seitz K et al. Hepatitis induced by Kava (Piper methysticum rhizome). J Hepatol, 2003; 39:62–67

496. Nerurkar PV, Dragull K, Tang CS. In vitro toxicity of kava alkaloid, pipermethystine, in HepG2 cells compared to kavalactones. Toxicol Sci, 2004; 79:106–111

497. Hongsirinirachorn M, Threeprasertsuk S, Chutaputti A. Acute hepatitis associated with Barakol. J Med Assoc Thai, 2003; 86(Suppl 2):S484–489

498. Stickel F, Poschl G, Seitz HK, et al. Acute hepatitis induced by greater celandine (Chelidonium majus). Scand J Gastroenterol, 2003; 38:565–568

499. Whiting PW, Clouston A, Kerlin P. Black cohosh and other herbal remedies associated with acute hepatitis. Med J Aust, 2002; 177:440–443

500. Lontos S, Jones RM, Angus PW et al. Acute liver failure associated with the use of herbal preparations containing black cohosh [letter]. Med J Aust, 2003; 179:390–391

501. Lin TJ, Su CC, Lan CK et al. Acute poisonings with Breynia officinalis—an outbreak of hepatotoxicity. J Toxicol Clin Toxicol, 2003; 41:591–594

502. Nadir A, Reddy D, Van Thiel DH. Cascara sagrada-induced intrahepatic cholestasis causing portal hypertension: case report and review of herbal hepatotoxicity. Am J Gastroenterol, 2000; 95:3634–3637

503. Woolf GM. Senna-induced hepatotoxicity. Hepatology, 1999; 550A:1560

504. Tolman KG, Sannella JJ, Freston JW. Possible hepatotoxicity of Doxidan. Ann Intern Med, 1976; 84:290

505. Harvey J, Colin-Jones DG. Mistletoe hepatitis. BMJ (Clin Res Ed), 1981; 282(6259):186–187

506. Haouzi D, Lekehal M, Moreau A et al. Cytochrome P450-generated reactive metabolites cause mitochondrial permeability transition, caspase activation and apoptosis in rat hepatocytes. Hepatology, 2000; 32:303

507. Hamid V, Rojter S, Vierling J. Protracted cholestatic hepatitis after the use of Prostata [letter]. Ann Intern Med, 1997; 127:169

508. Stewart MJ, Steenkamp V, van der Merwe S et al. The cytotoxic effects of a traditional Zulu remedy, impila (Callilepsis laureola). Hum Exp Toxicol, 2002; 21:643–647

509. Hamouda C, Hedhili A, Ben Saleh N et al. A review of acute poisoning from Atractylis gummifera L. Vet Hum Toxicol, 2004; 46:144–146

510. Schecter A, Lucier GW, Cunningham ML et al. Human consumption of methyleugenol and its elimination from serum. Environ Health Perspect, 2004; 112:678–680

511. Eisen JS, Koren G, Juurlink DN et al. N-acetylcysteine for the treatment of clove oil-induced fulminant hepatic failure. J Toxicol Clin Toxicol, 2004; 42:89–92

512. Brown SA, Biggerstaff J, Savidge GF. Disseminated intravascular coagulation and hepatocellular necrosis due to clove oil. Blood Coagul Fibrinolysis, 1992; 3:665–668

513. Jacques EA, Buschmann RJ, Layden TJ. The histopathologic progression of vitamin A-induced hepatic injury. Gastroenterology, 1979; 76:599–602

514. Russell RM, Boyer JL, Bagheri SA et al. Hepatic injury from chronic hypervitaminosis A resulting in portal hypertension and ascites. N Engl J Med, 1974; 291:435

515. Bendich A, Langseth L. Safety of vitamin A. Am J Clin Nutr, 1989; 49:358–371

516. Hathcock JN, Hattan DG, Jenkin MY et al. Evaluation of vitamin A toxicity. Am J Clin Nutr, 1990; 52:183–202

517. Geubel AP, De Galocsy C, Alves N et al. Liver damage caused by therapeutic vitamin A administration: estimation of dose-related toxicity in 41 cases. Gastroenterology, 1991; 100:1701–1709

518. Farrell GC, Bhathal PS, Powell LW. Abnormal liver function in chronic hypervitaminosis A. Am J Dig Dis, 1977; 22:724–728

519. Kowalski TE, Falestiny M, Furth E et al. Vitamin A hepatotoxicity: a cautionary note regarding 25,000 IU supplements. Am J Med, 1994; 97:523–528

520. Johnson EJ, Krall EA, Dawson-Hughes B et al. Lack of an effect of multivitamins containing vitamin A on serum retinyl esters and liver function tests in healthy women. J Am Coll Nutr, 1992; 11:682–686

521. Jorens PG, Michielsen PP, Pelckmans PA et al. Vitamin A abuse: development of cirrhosis despite cessation of vitamin A. A six-year clinical and histopathologic follow-up. Liver, 1992; 12:381–386

522. Sarles J, Scheiner C, Sarran M et al. Hepatic hypervitaminosis A: a familial observation. J Pediatr Gastroenterol Nutr, 1990; 10:71–76

523. Rodahl K, Moore T. The vitamin A content and toxicity of bear and seal liver. Biochem J, 1943; 37:166–168

524. Inkeles SB, Conner WE, Illingworth DR. Hepatic and dermatologic manifestations of chronic hypervitaminosis A in adults. Report of two cases. Am J Med, 1986; 80:491

525. Myhre AM, Carlsen MH, Bohn SK et al. Water-miscible, emulsified, and solid forms of retinol supplements are more toxic than oil-based preparations. Am J Clin Nutr, 2003; 78:1152–1159

526. Hautekeete ML, Geerts A. The hepatic stellate (Ito) cell: its role in human liver disease. Virchows Arch, 1997; 430:195–207

527. Senoo H. Structure and function of hepatic stellate cells. Med Electron Microsc, 2003; 37:3–15

528. Leo MA, Lieber CS. Alcohol, vitamin A, and β-carotene: adverse interactions, including hepatotoxicity and carcinogenicity. Am J Clin Nutr, 1999; 69:1071–1085

529. Zafrani ES, Bernuau D, Feldmann G. Peliosis-like ultrastructural changes of the hepatic sinusoids in human chronic hypervitaminosis A: report of three cases. Hum Pathol, 1984; 15:1166

530. Croquet V, Pilette C, Lespine A et al. Hepatic hyper-vitaminosis A: importance of retinyl ester level determination. Eur J Gastroenterol Hepatol, 2000; 12:361–364

531. Ukleja A, Scolapio JS, McConnell JP et al. Nutritional assessment of serum and hepatic vitamin A levels in patients with cirrhosis. JPEN J Parenter Enteral Nutr, 2002; 26:184–188

532. Levine PH, Delgado Y, Theise ND et al. Stellate-cell lipidosis in liver biopsy specimens. Recognition and significance. Am J Clin Pathol, 2003; 119:254–258

533. Bioulac-Sage P, Quinton A, Saric J et al. Chance discovery of hepatic fibrosis in a patient with asymptomatic hypervitaminosis A. Arch Pathol Lab Med, 1988; 112:505–509

534. Friedman SL. Stellate cell activation in alcoholic fibrosis—an overview. Alcohol Clin Exp Res, 1999; 23:904–910

535. Benade AJ. A place for palm fruit oil to eliminate vitamin A deficiency. Asia Pac J Clin Nutr, 2003; 12:369–372

536. Kuzuya T. The development of thiazolidinedione drugs as anti-diabetic agents. Nippon Rinsho, 2000; 58:364–369

537. Guyton JR. Extended-release niacin for modifying the lipoprotein profile. Expert Opin Pharmacother, 2004; 5:1385–1398

538. Inman WH, Mushin WW. Jaundice after repeated exposure to halothane: a further analysis of reports to the Committee on Safety of Medicines. BMJ, 1978; 2:1455–1456

539. Ray DC, Drummond GB. Halothane hepatitis. Br J Anaesth, 1991; 67:84–99

540. Holt C, Csete M, Martin P. Hepatotoxicity of anesthetics and other central nervous system drugs. Gastroenterol Clin North Am, 1995; 24:853–874

541. Kenna JG. Mechanism, pathology, and clinical presentation of hepatotoxicity of anesthetic agents. In: Kaplowitz N, DeLeve L, eds. Drug-induced liver disease. New York: Marcel Dekker, 2003: pp 405–424

542. Njoku D, Laster MJ, Gong DH et al. Biotransformation of halothane, enflurane, isoflurane, and desflurane to trifluoroacetylated liver proteins: association between protein acylation and hepatic injury. Anesth Analg, 1997; 84:173–178

543. Reichle FM, Conzen PF. Halogenated inhalational anaesthetics. Best Pract Res Clin Anaesthesiol, 2003; 17:29–46

544. Lo SK, Wendon J, Mieli-Vergani G et al. Halothane-induced acute liver failure: continuing occurrence and use of liver transplantation. Eur J Gastroenterol Hepatol, 1998; 10:635–639

545. Voigt MD, Workman B, Lombard C et al. Halothane hepatitis in a South African population—frequency and influence of gender and ethnicity. S Afr Med J, 1997; 87:882–885

546. Summary of the National Halothane Study. Possible association between halothane anesthesia and postoperative hepatic necrosis. JAMA, 1966; 197:775–788

547. Walton B, Simpson BR, Strunin L et al. Unexplained hepatitis following halothane. BMJ, 1976; 1(6019):1171–1176

548. Moult PJ, Sherlock S. Halothane-related hepatitis. A clinical study of twenty-six cases. Q J Med, 1975; 44:99–114

549. Böttiger LE, Dalén E, Hallén B: Halothane-induced liver damage: an analysis of the material reported to the Swedish Adverse Drug Reaction Committee, 1966–1973. Acta Anaesthesiol Scand, 1976; 20:40–46

550. Oikkonen M, Rosenberg PH. Liver damage after halothane anaesthesia: analysis of cases in Finnish hospitals in 1972–1981. Ann Chir Gynaecol, 1984; 73:28–33

551. Trey C, Lipworth L, Chalmers T et al. Fulminant hepatic failure: presumable contribution to halothane. N Engl J Med, 1968; 279:798–801

552. Stock JG, Strunin L. Unexplained hepatitis following halothane. Anesthesiology, 1985; 63:424–439

553. Neuberger J. Halothane and hepatitis. Incidence, predisposing factors and exposure guidelines. Drug Saf, 1990; 5:28–38

554. Dykes MH. Postoperative hepatic dysfunction in perspective. 1970. Int Anesthesiol Clin, 1998; 36:155–162

555. Neuberger J, Vergani D, Mieli-Vergani G et al. Hepatic damage after exposure to halothane in medical personnel. Br J Anaesth, 1981; 53:1173–1177

556. Varma RR, Whitsell RC, Iskandarani MM. Halothane hepatitis without halothane: role of inapparent circuit contamination and its prevention. Hepatology, 1985; 5:1159–1162

557. Wright R, Eade OE, Chisholm M et al. Controlled prospective study of the effect on liver function of multiple exposures to halothane. Lancet, 1975; 1:817–820

558. Trowell J, Peto R, Smith AC. Controlled trial of repeated halothane anaesthetics in patients with carcinoma of the uterine cervix treated with radium. Lancet, 1975; 1:821–824

559. Sakaguchi Y, Inaba S, Irita K et al. Absence of antitrifluoroacetate antibody after halothane anaesthesia in patients exhibiting no or mild liver damage. Can J Anaesth, 1994; 41:398–403

560. Bourdi M, Amouzadeh HR, Rushmore TH et al. Halothane-induced liver injury in outbred guinea pigs: role of trifluoroacetylated protein adducts in animal susceptibility. Chem Res Toxicol, 2001; 14:362–370

561. Cousins MJ, Plummer JL, Hall PD. Risk factors for halothane hepatitis. Aust N Z J Surg, 1989; 59:5–14

562. Hughes M, Powell LW. Recurrent hepatitis in patients receiving multiple halothane anesthetics for radium treatment of carcinoma of the cervix uteri. Gastroenterology, 1970; 58:790–797

563. Davis P, Holdsworth CD. Jaundice after multiple halothane anesthetics administered during the treatment of carcinoma of the uterus. Gut, 1973; 14:566–568

564. Benjamin SB, Goodman ZD, Ishak KG et al. The morphologic spectrum of halothane-induced hepatic injury: analysis of 77 cases. Hepatology, 1985; 5:1163–1171

565. Kenna JG, Neuberger J, Mieli-Vergani G et al. Halothane hepatitis in children. BMJ (Clin Res Ed), 1987; 294:1209–1211

566. Martin JL, Dubbink DA, Plevak DJ et al. Halothane hepatitis 28 years after primary exposure. Anesth Analg, 1992; 74:605–608

567. Jee RC, Sipes IG, Gandolfi AJ et al. Factors influencing halothane hepatotoxicity in the rat hypoxic model. Toxicol Appl Pharmacol, 1980; 52:267–277

568. Takagi T, Ishii H, Takahashi H et al. Potentiation of halothane hepatotoxicity by chronic ethanol administration in rat: an animal model of halothane hepatitis. Pharmacol Biochem Behav, 1983; 18(Suppl 1):461–465

569. Lind RC, Gandolfi AJ, Hall PM. Isoniazid potentiation of a guinea pig model of halothane-associated hepatotoxicity. J Appl Toxicol, 1990; 10:161–165

570. Nomura F, Hatano H, Ohnishi K et al. Effects of anticonvulsant agents on halothane-induced liver injury in human subjects and experimental animals. Hepatology, 1986; 6:952

571. Kharasch ED, Hankins D, Mautz D et al. Identification of the enzyme responsible for oxidative halothane metabolism: implications for prevention of halothane hepatitis. Lancet, 1996; 347:1367–1371

572. Spracklin DK, Emery ME, Thummel KE et al. Concordance between trifluoroacetic acid and hepatic protein trifluoroacetylation after disulfiram inhibition of halothane metabolism in rats. Acta Anaesthesiol Scand, 2003; 47:765–770

573. Farrell GC, Prendergast D, Murray M. Halothane hepatitis. Detection of a constitutional susceptibility factor. N Engl J Med, 1985; 313:1310–1314

574. Smith GC, Kenna JG, Harrison et al. Autoantibodies to hepatic microsomal carboxylesterase in halothane hepatitis. Lancet, 1993; 342:963–964

575. Morgenstern L, Sacks HJ, Marmer MJ. Postoperative jaundice associated with halothane anesthesia. Surg Gynecol Obst, 1965; 121:728–732

576. Peters RL, Edmondson HA, Reynolds TB, Meister JC, Curphey TJ. Hepatic necrosis associated with halothane anesthesia. Am J Med, 1967; 47:748–764

577. Shah IA, Brandt H. Halothane-associated granulomatous hepatitis. Digestion, 1983; 28:245–249

578. Dordal E, Glagov S, Orlando RA et al. Fatal halothane hepatitis with transient granuloma. N Engl J Med, 1970; 283:357–359

579. Miller DJ, Dwyer J, Klatskin G. Halothane hepatitis: benign resolution of a severe lesion. Ann Intern Med, 1978; 89:212–215

580. Kenna JG, Neuberger J, Williams R. Specific antibodies to halothane-induced liver antigens in halothane-associated hepatitis. Br J Anaesth, 1987; 59:1286–1290

581. Martin JL, Kenna JG, Martin BM et al. Halothane hepatitis patients have serum antibodies that react with protein disulfide isomerase. Hepatology, 1993; 18:858–863

582. Moore DH, Benson GD. Prolonged halothane hepatitis. Prompt resolution of severe lesion with corticosteroid therapy. Dig Dis Sci, 1986; 31:1269–1272

583. Thomas FB. Chronic aggressive hepatitis induced by halothane. Ann Intern Med, 1974; 81:487–489

584. Kronberg IJ, Evans DTP, Mackay IR et al. Chronic hepatitis after successive halothane anesthetics. Digestion, 1983; 27:123–128

585. Klatskin G, Kimberg DV. Recurrent hepatitis attributable to halothane sensitization in an anesthetist. N Engl J Med, 1969; 280:515

586. Neuberger J. Halothane hepatitis. Eur J Gastroenterol Hepatol, 1998; 10:631–633

587. Mazze RI, Cousins MJ. Renal toxicity of anesthetics: with specific reference to the nephrotoxicity of methoxyflurane. Can Anaesth Soc J, 1973; 20:64–80

588. Lewis JH, Zimmerman HJ, Ishak KG et al. Enflurane hepatotoxicity. A clinicopathologic study of 24 cases. Ann Intern Med, 1983; 98:984–992

589. Brown BR, Gandolfi AJ. Adverse effects of volatile anaesthetics. Br J Anaesth, 1987; 59:14–23

590. Eger EI II, Smuckler EA, Ferrell LD et al. Is enflurane hepatotoxic? Anesth Analg, 1986; 65:21–30

591. Zimmerman HJ. Even isoflurane. Hepatology, 1991; 13:1251–1253

592. Stoelting RK, Blitt CD, Cohen PJ et al. Hepatic dysfunction after isoflurane anesthesia. Anesth Analg, 1987; 66:147–153

593. Scheider DM, Klygis LM, Tsang T-K et al. Hepatic dysfunction after repeated isoflurane administration. J Clin Gastroenterol, 1993; 17:168–170

594. Sinha A, Clatch RJ, Stuck G et al. Isoflurane hepatotoxicity: a case report and review of the literature. Am J Gastroenterol, 1996; 91:2406–2409

595. Weitz J, Kienle P, Bohrer H et al. Fatal hepatic necrosis after isoflurane anaesthesia. Anaesthesia, 1997; 52:892

596. Gelven PL, Cina SJ, Lee JD, Nichols CA. Massive hepatic necrosis and death following repeated isoflurane exposure: case report and review of the literature. Am J Forensic Med Pathol, 1996; 17:61

597. Hasan F. Isoflurane hepatotoxicity in a patient with a previous history of halothane-induced hepatitis. Hepatogastroenterology, 1998; 45:518–522

598. Turner GB, O'Rourke D, Scott GO et al. Fatal hepatotoxicity after re-exposure to isoflurane: a case report and review of the literature. Eur J Gastroenterol Hepatol, 2000; 12:955–959

599. Martin JL, Keegan MT, Vasdev GMS et al. Fatal hepatitis associated with isoflurane exposure and CYP2A6 autoantibodies. Anesthesiology, 2001; 95:551–553

600. Njoku DB, Shrestha S, Soloway R et al. Subcellular localization of trifluoroacetylated liver proteins in association with hepatitis following isoflurane. Anesthesiology, 2002; 96:757–761

601. Malnick SD, Mahlab K, Borchardt J et al. Acute cholestatic hepatitis after exposure to isoflurane. Ann Pharmacother, 2002; 36:261–263

602. Turner GB, O'Rourke D, Scott GO et al. Fatal hepatotoxicity after re-exposure to isoflurane: a case report and review of the literature. Eur J Gastroenterol Hepatol, 2003; 12:955–959

603. Wark HJ. Hepatic failure after cardiopulmonary bypass is unlikely to be isoflurane hepatitis [letter]. Anesthesiology, 2002; 97:1323–1324

604. Ghantous HN, Fernando J, Gandolfi AJ et al. Mininal biotransformation and toxicity of desflurane in guinea pig liver slices. Anesth Analg, 1991; 72:796–800

605. Martin JL, Plevak DJ, Flannery KD et al. Hepatotoxicity after desflurane anesthesia. Anesthesiology, 1995; 83:1125–1129

606. Berghaus TM, Baron A, Geier A et al. Hepatotoxicity following desflurane anesthesia. Hepatology, 1999; 29:613–614

607. Chung PC, Chiou SC, Lien JM et al. Reproducible hepatic dysfunction following separate anesthesias with sevoflurane and desflurane. Chang Gung Med J, 2003; 26:357–362

608. Scholz J, Tonner PH. Critical evaluation of of the new inhalational anesthetics desflurane and sevoflurane. Anaesthesiol Reanim, 1997; 22:15–20

609. Hoenemann CW, Halene-Holtgraeve TB, Booke M et al. Delayed onset of malignant hyperthermia in desflurane anesthesia. Anesth Analg, 2003; 96:165–167

610. Ghantous HN, Fernando J, Gandolfi AJ et al. Sevoflurane is biotransformed by guinea pig slices but causes minimal cytotoxicity. Anesth Analg, 1992; 75:436–440

611. Ogawa M, Doi K, Mitsufuji T et al. Drug induced hepatitis following sevoflurane anesthesia in a child. Jpn J Anesth, 1991; 40:1542–1545

612. Shichinohe Y, Masuda Y, Takahashi H et al. A case of postoperative hepatic injury after sevoflurane anesthesia. Jpn J Anesth, 1992; 41:1802–1805

613. Keeffe EB, Blankenship NM, Scharschmidt BF. Alteration of rat liver plasma membrane fluidity and ATPase activity by chlorpromazine hydrochloride and its metabolites. Gastroenterology, 1980; 79:222–231

614. Hollister LE. Allergy to chlorpromazine manifested by jaundice. Am J Med, 1957; 23:870–879

615. Read AE, Harrison CV, Sherlock S. Chronic chlorpromazine jaundice with particular reference to its relationship to primary biliary cirrhosis. Am J Med, 1961; 31:249

616. Levine RA, Briggs GW, Lowell DM. Chronic chlorpromazine cholangiolitic hepatitis. Report of a case with immunofluorescent studies. Gastroenterology, 1966; 50:665–670

617. Moradpuor D, Altorfer J, Flury R et al. Chlorpromazine-induced vanishing bile duct syndrome leading to biliary cirrhosis. Hepatology, 1994; 20:1437–1441

618. Mindikoglu AL, Anantharaju A, Hartman GG et al. Prochlorperazine-induced cholestasis in a patient with alpha-1-antitrypsin deficiency. Hepatogastroenterology, 2003; 50:1338–1340

619. Dincsoy HP, Saelinger DA. Haloperidol-induced chronic cholestatic liver disease. Gastroenterology, 1982; 83:694–700

620. Akerboom T, Schneider I, Vom Dahl S et al. Cholestasis and changes of portal pressure caused by chlorpromazine in the perfused rat liver. Hepatology, 1991; 13:216–221

621. Utili R, Tripodi MF, Abernathy CO et al. Effects of bile salt infusion of chlorpromazine-induced cholestasis in the isolated perfused rat liver. Proc Soc Exp Biol Med, 1992; 199:49–53

622. Watson RGP, Olomu A, Clements D et al. A proposed mechanism for chlorpromazine jaundice: defective hepatic sulphoxidation combined with rapid hydroxylation. J Hepatol, 1988; 7:72–78

623. Utili R, Abernathy CO, Zimmerman HJ et al. Endotoxin protects against chlorpromazine-induced cholestasis in the isolated perfused rat liver. Gastroenterology, 1981; 80:673–680

624. Teschke R, Stutz G, Moreno F. Cholestasis following chronic alcohol consumption: enhancement after an acute dose of chlorpromazine. Biochem Biophys Res Commun, 1980; 94:1013–1020

625. Benazzi F. Risperidone-induced hepatotoxicity. Pharmacopsychiatry, 1998; 31:241

626. Kumra S, Herion D, Jacobsen LK et al. Case study: risperidone-induced hepatotoxicity in pediatric patients. J Am Acad Child Adolesc Psychiatry, 1997; 36:701–705

627. Phillips EJ, Liu BA, Knowles SR. Rapid onset of risperidone-induced hepatotoxicity. Ann Pharmacother, 1998; 32:843

628. Szigethy E, Wiznitzer M, Branicky LA et al. Risperidone-induced hepatotoxicity in children and adolescents? A chart review study. J Child Adolesc Psychopharmacol, 1999; 9:93–98

629. Lieberman JA. Maximizing clozapine therapy: managing side effects. J Clin Psychiatry, 1998; 59(Suppl 3):38–43

630. Macfarlane B, Davies S, Mannan K et al. Fatal acute fulminant liver failure due to clozapine: a case report and review of clozapine-induced hepatotoxicity. Gastroenterology, 1997; 112:1707–1709

631. Rosenblum LE, Korn RJ, Zimmerman HJ. Hepatocellular jaundice as a complication of iproniazid therapy. Arch Intern Med, 1960; 105:583–593

632. Mitchell JR, Jollow DJ. Metabolic activation of drugs to toxic substances. Gastroenterology, 1975; 68:392–410

633. Brandt C, Hoffbauer FW. Liver injury associated with tranylcypromine therapy. JAMA, 1964; 188:752–753

634. Short MH, Burns JM, Harris ME. Cholestatic jaundice during imipramine therapy. JAMA, 1968; 206:1791–1792

635. Villari D, Rubino F, Corica F et al. Bile ductopenia following therapy with sulpiride. Virchows Arch, 1995; 427:223–226

636. Cai Q, Benson MA, Talbot TJ et al. Acute hepatitis due to fluoxetine therapy. Mayo Clin Proc, 1999; 74:692–694

637. Capella D, Bruguera M, Figueras A et al. Fluoxetine-induced hepatitis: why is postmarketing surveillance needed? Eur J Clin Pharmacol, 1999; 55:545–546

638. Bobichon R, Bernard G, Mion F. Acute hepatitis during treatment with fluoxetine. Gastroenterol Clin Biol, 1993; 17:406–407

639. Friedenberg FK, Rothstein KD. Hepatitis secondary to fluoxetine treatment. Am J Psychiatry, 1996; 153:580

640. Azaz-Livshits T, Hershko A, Ben-Chetrit E. Paroxetine associated hepatotoxicity: a report of 3 cases and a review of the literature. Pharmacopsychiatry, 2002; 35:112–115

641. Hautekeete ML, Colle I, van Vlierberghe H et al. Symptomatic liver injury probably related to sertraline. Gastroenterol Clin Biol, 1998; 22:364–365

642. Horsmans Y, De Clercq M, Sempoux C. Venlafaxine-associated hepatitis. Ann Intern Med, 1999; 130:944

643. Cardona X, Avila A, Castellanos P. Venlafaxine-associated hepatitis. Ann Intern Med, 2000; 132:417

644. Cardona X, Avila A, Castellanos P. Venlafaxine-associated hepatitis. Ann Intern Med, 2000; 132:417

645. Lopez-Torres E, Lucena MI, Seoane J et al. Hepatotoxicity related to citalopram. Am J Psychiatry, 2004; 161:923–924

646. Fernandes NF, Martin RR, Schenker S. Trazodone-induced hepatotoxicity: a case report with comments on drug-induced hepatotoxicity. Am J Gastroenterol, 2000; 95:532–535

647. Aronoff S, Rosenblatt S, Braithwaite S et al. Pioglitazone hydrochloride monotherapy improves glycemic control in the treatment of patients with type 2 diabetes: a 6-month randomized placebo-controlled dose-response study. The Pioglitazone 001 Study Group. Diabetes Care, 2000; 23:1605–1611

648. Edwards R. Withdrawing drugs: nefazodone, the start of the latest saga. Lancet, 2003; 361:1240

649. Aranda-Michel J, Koehler A, Bejarano PA et al. Nefazodone-induced liver failure: report of three cases. Ann Intern Med, 1999; 130:285–288

650. Eloubeidi MA, Gaede JT, Swaim MW. Reversible nefazodone-induced liver failure. Dig Dis Sci, 2000; 45:1036–1038

651. Schirren CA, Barretton G. Nefazodone-induced acute liver failure. Am J Gastroenterol, 2000; 95:1596–1597

652. Kalgutkar AS, Vaz AD, Lame ME et al. Bioactivation of the nontricyclic antidepressant nefazodone to a reactive quinone-imine species in human liver microsomes and recombinant cytochrome P450 3A4. Drug Metab Dispos, 2005; 33(2):243–253

653. Oslin DW, Duffy K. The rise of serum aminotransferases in a patient treated with bupropion. J Clin Psychopharmacol, 1993; 13:364–365

654. Alvaro D, Onetti-Muda A, Moscatelli R et al. Acute cholestatic hepatitis induced by bupropion prescribed as pharmacological support to stop smoking. A case report. Dig Liver Dis, 2001; 33:703–706

655. Hu Ke-Qin, Tiyyagura L, Kanel G et al. Acute hepatitis induced by bupropion. Dig Dis Sci, 2000; 45:1872–1873

656. Hui CK, Yuen MF, Wong WM et al. Mirtazapine-induced hepatotoxicity. J Clin Gastroenterol, 2002; 35:270–271

657. Saeian K, Reddy KR. Hepatotoxicity of psychotropic drugs and drugs of abuse. In: Kaplowitz N, DeLeve LD, eds. Drug-induced liver disease. New York: Marcel Dekker, 2003: pp 447–470

658. Leeder JS, Pirmohamed M. Anticonvulsant agents. In: Kaplowitz N, DeLeve LD, eds. Drug-induced liver disease. New York: Marcel Dekker, 2003: pp 425–446

659. Park BK, Wilson AC, Kaatz G et al. Enzyme induction by phenobarbitone and vitamin K1 disposition in man. Br J Clin Pharmacol, 1984; 18:94–97

660. Evans WE, Self TH, Weisburst MR. Phenobarital-induced hepatic dysfunction. Drug Intell Clin Pharm, 1976; 10:439–443

661. Mockli G, Crowley M, Stern R, Warnock ML. Massive hepatic necrosis after administration of phenobarbital. Am J Gastroenterol, 1989; 84:820–822

662. Haruda F. Phenytoin hypersensitivity: Thirty eight cases. Neurology, 1979; 29:1480–1485

663. Aaron JS, Bank S, Ackert G. Diphenylhydantoin-induced hepatotoxicity. Am J Gastroenterol, 1985; 80:200–202

664. Cook IF, Shilkin KB, Reed WD. Phenytoin induced granulomatous hepatitis. Aust N Z J Med, 1981; 11:539–541

665. Brown M, Schubert T. Phenytoin hypersensitivity, hepatitis and mononucleosis syndrome. J Clin Gastroenterol, 1986; 4:469–477

666. Gaffey CM, Chun B, Harvey JC, Manz HJ. Phenytoin-induced systemic vasculitis. Arch Pathol Lab Med, 1986; 110:131–135

667. Van Wyk JJ, Hoffmann CR. Periarteritis nodosa. A case of fatal exfoliative dermatitis resulting from 'dilantin sodium' sensitization. Arch Intern Med, 1948; 81:605–611

668. Abbondanzo SL, Irey NS, Frizzera G. Dilantin-associated lymphadenopathy. Spectrum of histopathologic patterns. Am J Surg Pathol, 1995; 19:675–686

669. Easton JD. Potential hazards of hydantoin use. Ann Intern Med, 1972; 77:998–999

670. Knowles SR, Shapiro LE, Shear NH. Anticonvulsant hypersensitivity syndrome: incidence, prevention and management. Drug Saf, 1999; 21:489–501

671. Spielberg SP, Gordan GD, Bake DA et al. Predisposition to phenytoin hepatotoxicity assessed in vitro. N Engl J Med, 1981; 305:722–727

672. Bessmertny O, Hatton RC, Gonzalez-Peralta RTP. Antiepileptic hypersensitivity syndrome in children. Ann Pharmacother, 2001; 35:533–538

673. Galindo PA, Borja J, Gomez E et al. Anticonvulsant drug hypersensitivity. J Investig Allergol Clin Immunol, 2002; 12:299–304

674. Hadzie N, Portmann B, Davies ET, Mieli-Vergani G. Acute liver failure induced by carbamazepine. Arch Dis Child, 1990; 65:315–317

675. Bertram PD, Taylor RJ. Carbamazepine hepatotoxicity: Clinical and histopathological features. Am J Gastroenterol, 1980; 74:78–83

676. Levy M, Goodman MW, Van Dyne BJ, Sumner HW. Granulomatous hepatitis secondary to carbamazepine. Ann Intern Med, 1981; 95:64–65

677. Larrey D, Hadengue A, Pessayre D. Carbamazepine-induced acute cholangitis. Dig Dis Sci, 1987; 32:554–557

678. Forbes GM, Jeffrey GP, Shilkin KB, Reed WD. Carbamazepine hepatotoxicity: another case of the vanishing bile duct syndrome. Gastroenterology, 1992; 102:1385–1388

679. Ramos AM, Gayotto LC, Clemente CM et al. Reversible vanishing bile duct syndrome induced by cabamazepine. Eur J Gastroenterol Hepatol, 2002; 14:1019–1022

680. Tazawa K, Yasuda M, Ohtani Y, Makuuchi H, Osamura RY. Multiple hepatocellular adenomas associated with long-term carbamazepine. Histopathology, 1999; 35:86–95

681. Frey B, Braegger CP, Ghelfi D. Neonatal cholestatic hepatitis from carbamazepine exposure during pregnancy and breast feeding. Ann Pharmacother, 2002; 36:644–647

682. Williams SJ, Ruppin DC, Grierson JM, Farrell GC. Carbamazepine hepatitis: the clinicopathological spectrum. J Gastroenterol Hepatol, 1986; 1:159–163

683. Kalapos MP. Carbamazepine-provoked hepatotoxicity and possible aetiopathologic role of glutathione in the events. Retrospective review of old data and call for new investigation. Adverse Drug React Toxicol Rev, 2002; 1:123–141

684. Powell-Jackson PR, Tredger JM, Williams R. Hepatotoxicity to sodium valproate. A review. Gut, 1984; 25:673–684

685. Scheffner D, Konig S, Rauterberg-Ruland I et al. Fatal liver failure in 16 children with valproate therapy. Epilepsia, 1988; 29:530–542

686. Lewis JH, Zimmerman HJ, Garrett CT, Rosenburg E. Valproate-induced hepatic steatogenesis in rats. Hepatology, 1982; 2:870–873

687. Kesterson JW, Granneman GR, Machinist JM. The hepatotoxicity of valproic acid and its metabolites in rats. I. Toxicology, biochemical and histopathologic studies. Hepatology, 1984; 4:1143–1152

688. Konig SA, Schenk M, Sick C et al. Fatal liver failure associated with valproate therapy in a patient with Friedreich's disease: review of valproate hepatotoxicity in adults. Epilepsia, 1999; 40:1036–1040

689. Romero-Falcon A, de la Santa-Belda E, Garcia-Contreras R et al. A case of valproate-associated hepatotoxicity treated with L-carnitine. Eur J Intern Med, 2003; 14:338–340

690. Silva MF, Ijlst L, Allers P et al. Valproyl-dephosphoCoA: a novel metabolite of valproate formed in vitro in rat liver mitochondria. Drug Metab Dispos, 2004; 32:1304–1310

691. Anon. Acute liver failure linked to felbamate (News). Am J Hosp Pharm, 1994; 51:2882

692. Pellock JM. Felbamate. Epilepsia, 1999; 40(Suppl 5):S57–62

693. O'Neil MG, Perdun CS, Wilson MB et al. Felbamate-associated fatal acute hepatic necrosis. Neurology, 1996; 46:1457–1459

694. Popovic M, Nierkens S, Pieters R et al. Investigating the role of 2-phenylpropenal in felbamate-induced idiosyncratic drug reactions. Chem Res Toxicol, 2004; 17:1568–1576

695. Pellock JM, Brodie MJ. Felbamate: 1997 update. Epilepsia, 1997; 38:1261–1264

696. Schlienger RG, Knowles SR, Shear NH. Lamotrigine-associated anticonvulsant hypersensitivity syndrome. Neurology, 1998; 51:1172–1175

697. Fayad M, Choueiri R, Mikati M. Potential hepatotoxicity of lamotrigine. Pediatr Neurol, 2000; 22:49–52

698. Sauve G, Bresson-Hadni S, Prost P et al. Acute hepatitis after lamotrigine administration. Dig Dis Sci, 2000; 45:1874–1877

699. Makin AJ, Fitt S, Williams R et al. Fulminant hepatic failure induced by lamotrigine. BMJ, 1995; 311(7000):292

700. Overstreet K, Costanza C, Behling C et al. Fatal progressive hepatic necoris associated with lamotrigine treatment: a case report and literature review. Dig Dis Sci, 2002; 47:1921–1925

701. Nehra A, Mullick F, Ishak KG et al. Pemoline associated hepatic injury. Gastroenterology, 1990; 99:1517–1519

702. Safer DJ, Zito JM, Gartdner JE. Pemoline hepatotoxicity and postmarketing surveillance. J Am Acad Child Adolesc Psychiatry, 2001; 40:622–629

703. Sterling MJ, Kane M, Grace ND. Pemoline induced autoimmune hepatitis. Am J Gastroenterol, 1996; 91:2233–2234

704. Watkins PB, Zimmerman HJ, Knapp MJ et al. Hepatotoxic effects of tacrine administration in patients with Alzheimer's disease. JAMA, 1994; 271:992–998

705. Gracon SI, Knapp MJ, Berghoff WG et al. Safety of tacrine: clinical trials, treatment IND, and postmarketing experience. Alzheimer Dis Assoc Disord, 1998; 12:93–101

706. Madden S, Woolf TF, Pool WF et al. An investigation into the formation of stable, protein-reactive and cytotoxic metabolites

707. from tacrine in vitro. Studies with human and rat liver microsomes. Biochem Pharmacol, 1993; 46:13–20

707. Fontana RJ, Turgeon DK, Woolf TF et al. The caffeine breath test does not identify patients susceptible to tacrine hepatotoxicity. Hepatology, 1996; 23:1429–1435

708. Stachlewitz RF, Arteel GE, Raleigh JA et al. Development and characterization of a new model of tacrine-induced hepatotoxicity: role of the sympathetic nervous system and hypoxia-reoxygenation. J Pharmacol Exp Ther, 1997; 282:1591–1599

709. Galisteo M, Rissel M, Sergent O et al. Hepatotoxicity of tacrine: occurrence of membrane fluidity alterations without involvement of lipid peroxidation. J Pharmacol Exp Ther, 2000; 294:160–167

710. Simon T, Becquemont L, Mary-Krause M et al. Combined glutathione-S-transferase M1 and T1 genetic polymorphism and tacrine hepatotoxicity. Clin Pharmacol Ther, 2000; 67:432–437

711. Castells LI, Gamez J, Guardia J. Icteric toxic hepatitis associated with riluzole. Lancet, 1998; 351:648

712. Remy A-J, Camu W, Ramos J, Blane P, Larrey D. Acute hepatitis after riluzole administration. J Hepatol, 1999; 30:527–530

713. Teychenne PF, Jones EA, Ishak KG et al. Hepatocellular injury with distinctive mitochondrial changes induced by lergotrile mesylate: a dopaminergic ergot derivative. Gastroenterology, 1979; 76:575

714. Assal F, Spahr L, Hadengue A, Rubbici-Brandt L, Burkhard PR. Tolcapone and fulminant hepatitis. Lancet, 1998; 352:958

715. Waters CH, Kurth M, Bailey P et al. Tolcapone in stable Parkinson's disease: efficacy and safety of long term treatment. Neurology, 1997; 49:665–671

716. Spahr L, Rubbia-Brandt L, Burkhard PR et al. Tolcapone-related fulminant hepatitis. Dig Dis Sci, 2000; 45:1881–1884

717. Watkins P. COMT inhibitors and liver toxicity. Neurology, 2000; 55(11 Suppl 4):S51–S52; discussion S53–S56

718. Borges N. Tolcapone-related liver dysfunction: implications for use in Parkinson's disease therapy. Drug Saf, 2003; 26:743–747

719. Olanow CW. Tolcapone and hepatotoxic effects. Tasmar Advisory Panel. Arch Neurol, 2000; 57:263–267

720. Benabou R, Waters C. Hepatotoxic profile of catechol-O-methyltransferase inhibitors in Parkinson's disease. Expert Opin Drug Saf, 2003; 2:263–267

721. Haasio K, Lounatmaa K, Sukura A. Entacapone does not induce conformational changes in liver mitochondria or skeletal muscle in vivo. Exp Toxicol Pathol, 2002; 54:9–14

722. Sobaniec-Lotowska ME. Effects of long term administration of the antiepileptic drug sodium valproate upon the ultrastructure of hepatocytes in rats. Exp Toxic Pathol, 1997; 49:225–232

723. Lewis JH. NSAID-induced hepatotoxicity. Clin Liver Dis, 1998; 2:543–561

724. Lewis JH. Nonsteroidal anti-inflammatory drugs: pathology and clinical presentation of hepatotoxicity. In: Kaplowitz N, DeLeve LD, eds. Drug-induced liver disease. New York: Marcel Dekker, 2003: pp 377–404

725. Hueper WE. Cinchophen (Atophan): a critical review. Medicine, 1948; 27:43–103

726. Cutrin Prieto C, Nieto Pol E, Batalla Eiras A et al. Toxic hepatitis from cinchophen. Report of 3 cases. Med Clin (Barc), 1991; 97:104–106

727. Weir JF, Comfort MW. Toxic cirrhosis caused by cinchophen. Arch Intern Med, 1933; 52:685–724

728. Paulus HE. Arthritis Advisory Committee meeting. Arthritis Rheum, 1981; 25:1124–1125

729. O'Brien WM. Long-term efficacy and safety of tolmetin sodium in treatment of geriatric patients with rheumatoid arthritis and osteoarthritis: a retrospective study. J Clin Pharmacol, 1983; 23:309

730. Weinblatt ME, Tesser JR, Gilliam JH et al. The liver in rheumatic disease. Semin Arthritis Rheum, 1982; 11:399

731. Zimmerman HJ. Effects of aspirin and acetaminophen on the liver. Arch Intern Med, 1981; 141:333–342

732. Russell AS, Sturge RA, Smith MA. Serum transaminases during salicylate therapy. BMJ, 1971; 2:428–429

733. Seaman WE, Ishak KG, Plotz PH. Aspirin-induced hepatotoxicity in patients with systemic lupus erythematosus. Ann Intern Med, 1974; 80:1–8

734. Seaman WE, Ploitz PH. Effect of aspirin of liver tests in patients with rheumatoid arthritis or systemic lupus erythematosus and in normal volunteers. Arthritis Rheum, 1974; 19:155–160

735. Schaller JG. Chronic salicylate administration in juvenile rheumatoid arthritis: asprin hepatotoxicity and its clinical significance. Pediatrics, 1978; 4:916–925

736. Gitlin N. Salicylate hepatotoxicity: the potential role of hypoalbuminemia. J Clin Gastroenterol, 1980; 2:381–385

737. Lewis JH. Hepatic toxicity of nonsteroidal anti-inflammatory drugs. Clin Pharm, 1984; 3:128

738. Okamura H, Ichikawa T, Obayashi K et al. Studies on aspirin-induced hepatic injury. Recent Adv Gastroenterol, 1967; 3:223

739. Meythaler JM, Varma RR. Reye's syndrome in adults: diagnostic considerations. Arch Intern Med, 1987; 147:61

740. Peters LJ, Wiener GJ, Gilliam J et al. Reye's syndrome in adults: a case report and review of the literature. Ann Intern Med, 1986; 146:2401

741. Remington PL, Rawley D, McGee H et al. Decreasing trend in Reye's syndrome and aspirin use in Michigan, 1979 to 1984. Pediatrics, 1986; 77:93

742. White JM. Reye's syndrome and salicylates [letter]. JAMA, 1987; 258:3117

743. Warren JS. Diflunisal-induced cholestatic jaundice. BMJ, 1978; 2:736–737

744. Cook DJ, Achong MR, Murphy FR. Three cases of diflunisal hypersensitivity. Can Med Assoc J, 1988; 138:1029–1030

745. Symon DN, Gray ES, Hanmer OJ et al. Fatal paracetamol poisoning from benorylate therapy in a child with cystic fibrosis. Lancet, 1982; 2:1153

746. Lewis HJ, Zimmerman HJ. NSAID hepatotoxicity. IM Intern Med, 1996; 17:45–67

747. Thompson M, Stephenson P, Percy JS. Ibufenac in the treatment of arthritis. Ann Rheum Dis, 1964; 23:397–404

748. Hart FD, Boardman PL. Ibufenac (4-isobutylphenyl acetic acid). Ann Rheum Dis, 1965; 24:61–65

749. Zimmerman HJ. Update of hepatotoxicity due to classes of drugs in common clinical use: nonsteroidal anti-inflammatory drugs, antibiotics, antihypertensives, and cardiac and psychotropic agents. Semin Liver Dis, 1990; 10:322

750. Laurent S, Rahier J, Geubel AP, Lerut J, Horsmans Y. Subfulminant hepatitis requiring liver transplantation following ibuprofen overdose. Liver, 2000; 20:93–94

751. Bravo JF, Jacobson MP, Mertens BF. Fatty liver and pleural effusion with ibuprofen therapy. Ann Intern Med, 1977; 87:200–201

752. Purcell P, Henry D, Melville G. Diclofenac hepatitis. Gut, 1991; 32:1381–1385

753. Banks T, Zimmerman HJ, Harter J, Ishak KG. Diclofenac-associated hepatic injury: analysis of 181 cases. Hepatology, 1995; 22:245–249

754. Hackstein H, Mohl W, Püschel W, Stallmach A, Seitz M. Acute cholestatic hepatitis associated with diclofenac. Z Gastroenterol, 1999; 36:385–389

755. Aithal GP, Ramsay L, Daly AK et al. Hepatic adducts, circulating antibodies, and cytokine polymorphisms in patients with diclofenac hepatotoxicity. Hepatology, 2004; 39:1430–1440

756. Tang W. The metabolism of diclofenac—enzymology and toxicology perspectives. Curr Drug Metab, 2003; 4:319–329

757. Grillo MP, Hua F, Knutson CG et al. Mechanistic studies on the bioactivation of diclofenac: identification of diclofenac-S-acyl-glutathione in vitro in incubations with rat and human hepatocytes. Chem Res Toxicol, 2003; 16:1410–1417

758. Balduck N, Otten J, Verbruggen L et al. Sudden death of a child with juvenile chronic arthritis, probably due to indomethacin. Eur J Pediatr, 1987; 146:620

759. Fenech FF, Bannister WH, Grech JL. Hepatitis with biliverdinaemia in association with indomethacin therapy. BMJ, 1967; 3:155–156

760. Kelsey WM, Scharyj M. Fatal hepatitis probably due to indomethacin. JAMA, 1967; 199:586–587

761. Metreau JM, Andre C, Zafrani ES et al. Hepatites chroniques actives associees a des anticorps anti-DNA natif: frequence de l'etiologie medicamenteuse. Gastroenterol Clin Biol, 1984; 8:833

762. Pessayre D, Degos F, Feldmann G et al. Chronic active hepatitis and giant multinucleated hepatocytes in adults treated with clometacin. Digestion, 1982; 22:66–72

763. Meyer C, Chassagnon C. Un noveau cas mortel de cirrhose due a la clometacine. J Med Lyon, 1984; 251:339

764. Islam S, Mekhloufi F, Paul JM et al. Characteristics of clometacin-induced hepatitis with special reference to the presence of anti-actin cable antibodies. Autoimmunity, 1989; 2:213–221

765. Tarazi EM, Harter JG, Zimmerman HJ et al. Sulindac-associated hepatic injury: analysis of 91 cases reported to the Food and Drug Administration. Gastroenterology, 1992; 104:569–574

766. Whittaker SJ, Amar JN, Wanless IR et al. Sulindac hepatotoxicity. Gut, 1982; 23:875–877

767. Tokumine F, Sunagawa T, Shiohira Y et al. Drug-associated cholelithiasis: a case of sulinadac stone formation and the incorporation of sulinadac metabolites into the gallstones. Am J Gastroenterol, 1999; 94:2285–2288

768. Leriche A, Vyberg M, Kirkegaard E. Acute cholangitis and pancreatitis associated with sulindac (Clinoril). Histopathology, 1987; 11:647–653

769. Laffi G, Daskalopoulos G, Kronborg I et al. Effects of sulindac and ibuprofen in patients with cirrhosis and ascities: an explanation for the renal-sparing effect of sulindac. Gastroenterology, 1986; 90:182–187

770. Hunter EB, Johnston PE, Tanner G, Pinson W, Award JA. Bromfenac (Duract)-associated hepatic failure requiring liver transplantation. Am J Gastroenterol, 1999; 94:1300–1301

771. Moses PL, Schoeder B, Alkhatib O, Ferrentino N, Suppan T, Lidofsky SD. Severe hepatotoxicity associated with bromfenac sodium. Am J Gastroenterol, 1999; 94:1393–1396

772. Rabkin JM, Smith MJ, Orloff SL et al. Fatal fulminant hepatitis associated with bromfenac use. Ann Pharmacother, 1999; 33:945–947

773. Skjodt NM, Davies NM. Clinical pharmacokinetics and pharmacodynamics of bromfenac. Clin Pharmacokinet, 1999; 36:399–408

774. Taggert HM, Allerdice JM. Fatal cholestatic jaundice in elderly patients taking benoxaprofen [letter]. BMJ, 1982; 284:1372

775. Goudie BM, Birnie GF, Watkinson G, MacSween RNM, Kissen LH, Cunningham NE. Jaundice associated with the use of benoxaprofen. Lancet, 1982; i:959

776. Prescott LP, Leslie PJ, Padfield P. Side effects of benoxaprofen. BMJ, 1982; 284:1783

777. Hamdy RC, Murnane B, Perera N et al. The pharmacokinetics of benoxaprofen in elderly subjects. Eur J Rheumatol Inflamm, 1982; 5:69–75

778. Law IP, Knight H. Jaundice associated with naproxen [letter]. N Engl J Med, 1976; 295:1201

779. Giarelli L, Falconieri G, Delendi M. Fulminant hepatitis following naproxen administration. Hum Pathol, 1986; 17:1079

780. Riley TR, Smith JP. Ibuprofen-induced hepatotoxicity in patients with chronic hepatitis C: a case series. Am J Gastroenterol, 1998; 93:1563–1565

781. Alam I, Ferrell LD, Bass NM. Vanishing bile duct syndrome temporally associated with ibuprofen use. Am J Gastroenterol, 1996; 91:1626–1630

782. Srivastava M, Perez-Atayde A, Jonas MM. Drug-associated acute-onset vanishing bile duct and Stevens-Johnson syndrome in a child. Gastroenterology, 1998; 115:743–746

783. Crossley RJ. Side effects and safety data for fenbufen. Am J Med, 1983; 75:84–90

784. Becker A, Hoffmeister RT. Fenbufen, a new non-steroidal anti-inflammatory agent in rheumatoid arthritis, its efficiency and toxicity. J Int Med Res, 1980; 8:333–338

785. Zimmerman HJ. Hepatic effects of oxaprozin. Semin Arthritis Rheum, 1986; 15:35–42

786. Mabee CL, Mabee SW, Baker PB et al. Fulminant hepatic failure associated with etodolac use. Am J Gastroenterol, 1995; 90:659–661

787. Danan G, Trunet P, Bernuau J et al. Pirprofen-induced fulminant hepatitis. Gastroenterology, 1985; 89:210–213

788. De Herder WW, Scherder P, Purnode A et al. Pirprofen-associated hepatic injury. J Hepatol, 1987; 4:127–132

789. Lee SM, O'Brien CJ, Williams R, Whitaker S, Gould SR. Subacute hepatic necrosis induced by piroxicam. BMJ, 1986; 293:540–541

790. Planas R, Leon RD, Quer JC, Barranco C, Bruguera M, Gassull MA. Fatal submassive necrosis of the liver associated with piroxicam. Am J Gastroenterol, 1990; 5:468–470

791. Paterson D, Kerlin P, Walker N et al. Piroxicam induced submassive necrosis of the liver. Gut, 1992; 33:1436–1438

792. Hepps KS, Maliha GM, Estrada R et al. Severe cholestatic jaundice associated with piroxicam. Gastroenterology, 1991; 101:1737–1740

793. Benjamin S, Ishak KG, Zimmerman HJ, Grushka A. Phenylbutazone liver injury: a clinical-pathologic survey of 23 cases and review of the literature. Hepatology, 1981; 1:255–263

794. Carpenter SL, McDonnell WM. Misuse of veterinary phenylbutazone. Arch Intern Med, 1995; 155:1229–1231

795. Ishak KG, Kirchner JP, Dhar JK. Granulomas and cholestatic-hepatocellular injury associated with phenylbutazone. Report of two cases. Am J Dig Dis, 1977; 22:611–617

796. Zimmerman HJ. Hepatotoxic effect of oncotherapeutic agents. Prog Liver Dis, 1986; 8:621–642

797. Locasciulli A, Mura R, Fraschini D et al. High dose methotrexate administration and acute liver damage in children treated for acute lymphoblastic leukemia. A propective study. Haematologica, 1992; 77:49–53

798. Dahl MGC, Gregory MM, Scheuer PJ. Liver damage due to methotrexate in patients with psoriasis. BMJ, 1971; 1:625–630

799. Nyfors A, Poulsen H. Liver biopsies from psoriasis related to methotrexate. Acta Pathol Microbiol Scand, 1976; 84:253–261

800. Roenigk HR Jr, Bergfeld WF, St Jacques R, Owens FJ, Hawk WA. Hepatotoxicity of methotrexate in the treatment of psoriasis. Arch Dermatol, 1971; 103:250–261

801. Weinstein C, Roenigk H, Maibach H et al. Psoriasis—liver methotrexate interactions. Arch Dermatol, 1980; 108:36–42

802. Dahl MGC, Gregory MM, Scheuer PJ. Methotrexate hepatotoxicity in psoriasis—comparison of different dose regimens. BMJ, 1972; 1:654–656

803. Lewis JH. Monitoring for methotrexate hepatotoxicity in patients with rheumatoid arthritis: another hepatologist's perspective. J Rheumatol, 1997; 24:1459–1460

804. Findings: Arthritis Drug Ban Urged. Washington Post, March 29, 2002: A8

805. Kremer JM, Lee RG, Tolman KG. Liver histology in patients with rheumatoid arthritis undergoing long term treatment with methotrexate. Arthritis Rheum, 1989; 132:121–127

806. Kremer JM, Kaye GI, Kaye NW, Ishak KG, Axiotis CA. Light and electron microscopic analysis of sequential liver biopsy samples from patients with rheumatoid arthritis receiving long term methotrexate therapy. Arthritis Rheum, 1995; 38:1194–1203

807. Rau R, Karger T, Herborn G, Frenzel H. Liver biopsy findings on patients with rheumatoid arthritis undergoing long term treatment with methotrexate. J Rheumatol, 1989; 4:489–493

808. Shergy WJ, Polisson RP, Caldwell DS, Rice JR. Methotrexate-associated hepatotoxicity: retrospective analysis of 210 patients with rheumatoid arthritis. Am J Med, 1988; 85:771–774

809. Kujala GA, Shamma'a JM, Chang WL, Brick JE. Hepatitis with bridging fibrosis and reversible hepatic insufficiency in a woman with rheumatoid arthritis taking methotrexate. Arthritis Rheum, 1990; 33:1037–1041

810. ter Borg EJ, Seldenrijk CA, Timmer R. Liver cirrhosis due to methotrexate in a patient with rheumatoid arthritis. Nether J Med, 1996; 49:244–246

811. Reuben A. Methotrexate controversies. In: Kaplowitz N, DeLeve LD, eds. Drug-induced liver disease. New York: Marcel Dekker, 2003: pp 653–676

812. Roenigk HH Jr, Auerbach R, Maibach HI et al. Methotrexate in psoriasis: revised guidelines. J Am Acad Dermatol, 1988; 19(1 Pt 1):145–156

813. Kremer JM, Alarcon GS, Lightfoot RW Jr et al. Methotrexate for rheumatoid arthritis. Suggested guidelines for monitoring liver toxicity. American College of Rheumatology. Arthritis Rheum, 1994; 37:316–328

814. Yazici Y, Erkan D, Paget SA. Monitoring by rheumatologists for methotrexate-, etanercept-, infliximab-, and anakinra-associated adverse events. Arthritis Rheum, 2003; 48:2769–2772

815. Fathi NH, Mitros F, Hoffman J et al. Longitudinal measurement of methotrexate liver concentrations does not correlate with liver damage, clinical efficacy, or toxicity during a 3.5 year double blind study in rheumatoid arthritis. J Rheumatol, 2002; 29:2092–2098

816. Kremer JM, Genovese MC, Cannon GW et al. Concomitant leflunomide therapy in patients with active rheumatoid arthritis despite stable doses of methotrexate. Ann Intern Med, 2002; 137:726–733

817. Sanders S, Harisdangkul V. Leflunomide for the treatment of rheumatoid arthritis and autoimmunity. Am J Med Sci, 2002; 323:190–193

818. Schenker S, Olson KN, Dunn D, Breen KJ, Combes B. Intrahepatic cholestasis due to therapy of rheumatoid arthritis. Gastroenterology, 1973; 64:622–629

819. Favreau M, Tannenbaum H, Lough J. Hepatic toxicity associated with gold therapy. Ann Intern Med, 1977; 87:717–719

820. Pessayre D, Feldman G, Degott C et al. Gold salt-induced cholestasis. Digestion, 1979; 19:56–64

821. Watkins PB, Schade R, Mills AS, Carithers RL Jr, Van Thiel DH. Fatal hepatic necrosis associated with parenteral gold therapy. Dig Dis Sci, 1988; 33:1025–1029

822. Basset C, Vadrot J, Denis J et al. Prolonged cholestasis and ductopenia following gold salt therapy. Liver Int, 2003; 23:89–93

823. Fleischner GM, Morecki I, Manaichi T, Hayaski H, Sternlieb I. Light and electron microscopical study of a case of gold salt induced hepatotoxicity. Hepatology, 1991; 14:422–423

824. McLeod BD, Kinsella TD. Cholestasis associated with D-penicillamine for rheumatoid arthritis. Can Med Assoc J, 1979; 120:965

825. Gefel D, Harats N, Lijovetsky G, Eliakim M. Cholestatic jaundice associated with D-penicillamine therapy. Scand J Rheumatol, 1985; 14:303–306

826. Deutscher J, Kiess W, Scheerschmidt G et al. Potential hepatotoxicity of penicillamine treatment in three patients with Wilson's disease. J Pediatr Gastroenterol Nutr, 1999; 29:628

827. Fishel B, Tishler M, Caspi D et al. Fatal aplastic anaemia and liver toxicity caused by D-penicillamine treatment of rheumatoid arthritis. Ann Rheum Dis, 1989; 48:609–610

828. Van Steenbergen W, De Bondt PP, Staessen D et al. Nimesulide-induced acute hepatitis: evidence from six cases. J Hepatol, 1998; 29:135–141

829. Romero-Gómez M, Nevado-Santos M, Otero-Fernandez MA, Fovello MK, Suárez-Garcia E, Castro-Fernández M. Acute cholestatic hepatitis induced by nimesulide. Liver, 1999; 19:164–165

830. McCormick PA, Kennedy P, Curry M, Traynor O. COX-2 inhibitor and fulminant hepatic failure. Lancet, 1999; 353:40–41

831. Andrade RJ, Lucena MI, Fernandez MC, Gonzalez M. Fatal hepatitis associated with nimesulide [letter]. J Hepatol, 2000; 32:174

832. Traversa G, Bianchi C, Da Cas R et al. Cohort study of hepatotoxicity associated with nimesulide and other non-steroidal anti-inflammatory drugs. BMJ, 2003; 327:18–22

833. Rodrigo L, de Francisco R, Perez-Pariente JM et al. Nimesulide-induced severe hemolytic anemia and acute liver failure leading to liver transplantation. Scand J Gastroenterol, 2002; 37:1341–1343

834. Weiss P, Mouallem M, Bruck R et al. Nimesulide-induced hepatitis and acute liver failure. Isr Med Assoc J, 1999; 1:89–91

835. Boelsterli UA. Mechanisms of NSAID-induced hepatotoxicity: focus on nimesulide. Drug Saf, 2002; 25:633–648

836. Grieco A, Miele L, Giorgi A. Acute cholestatic hepatitis associated with celecoxib. Ann Pharmacother, 2002; 36:1887–1889

837. Galan MV, Gordon SC, Silverman AL. Celecoxib-induced cholestatic hepatitis. Ann Intern Med, 2001; 134:254

838. Vanderstigel M, Zafrani ES, Legone JL et al. Allopurinol hypersensitivity syndrome as cause of hepatic doughnut-ring granulomas. Gastroenterology, 1986; 90:188–190

839. Tjwa M, De Hertogh G, Neuville B et al. Hepatic fibrin-ring granulomas in granulomatous hepatitis: report of four cases and review of the literature. Acta Clin Belg, 2001; 56:341–348

840. Esperitu CR, Alaln J, Glueckauf LG, Lubin J. Allopurinol-induced granulomatous hepatitis. Am J Dig Dis, 1976; 21:804–806

841. Boyer TD, Sun N, Reynolds TB. Allopurinol hypersensitivity and liver damage. West J Med, 1977; 126:143–147

842. Al-Kawas FH, Seeff LB, Berendson RA, Zimmerman HJ, Ishak KG. Allopurinol hepatotoxicity. Report of two cases and review of the literature. Ann Intern Med, 1981; 95:588–590

843. Hande KR, Noone KR, Stone WJ. Severe allopurinol toxicity: description and guidelines for prevention in patients with renal insufficiency. Am J Med, 1984; 76:47–56

844. Sommers LM, Schoene RB. Allopurinol hypersensitivity syndrome associated with pancreatic exocrine abnormalities and new-onset diabetes mellitus. Arch Intern Med, 2002; 162:1190–1192

845. Murray SS, Kramlinger KG, McMichan JC, Mohr DN. Acute toxicity after excessive ingestion of colchicine. Mayo Clin Proc, 1983; 58:528–532

846. Stein O, Stein Y. Colchicine-induced inhibition of very low density lipoprotein release by rat liver in vivo. Biochim Biophys Acta, 1973; 306:142

847. Hoang C, Lavergne A, Bismuth C, Fournier PE, Leclerc JP, Le Charpentier Y. Lésions viscérales histologiques de intoxications aiguës mortelles à la colchicine. A propos de 12 observations. Ann Pathol, 1982; 2:229–237

848. Carr HJ Jr, Knauer F. Death due to hepatic necrosis in a patient receiving zoxazolamine. N Engl J Med, 1961; 264:977–979

849. Utili R, Boitnott J, Zimmerman HJ. Dantrolene-associated hepatic injury. Incidence and character. Gastroenterology, 1977; 72:610–616

850. Chan CH. Dantrolene sodium and hepatic injury. Neurology, 1990; 40:427–432

851. Powers BJ, Cattau EL, Zimmerman HJ. Chlorzoxazone hepatotoxic reactions. Arch Intern Med, 1986; 146:1183–1186

852. Goldstein MJ, Rothenberg AJ. Jaundice in a patient receiving acetohexamide. N Engl J Med, 1966; 275:97–99

853. Gregory DH, Zaki GF, Sarosi GA, Carey JB. Chronic cholestasis following prolonged tolbutamide administration. Arch Pathol, 1967; 84:194–201

854. Bloodworth JMB Jr. Morphologic changes associated with sulfonylurea therapy. Metabolism, 1963; 12:287–301

855. Chitturi S, Le V, Kench J et al. Gliclazide-induced hepatitis with hypersensitivity features. Dig Dis Sci, 2002; 47:1107–1110

856. Chan KA, Truman A, Gurwitz JH et al. A cohort study of the incidence of serious acute liver injury in diabetic patients treated with hypoglycemic agents. Arch Intern Med, 2003; 163:728–734

857. Li H, Heller DS, Leevy CB et al. Troglitazone-induced fulminant hepatitis: report of a case with autopsy findings. J Diabetes Complications, 2000; 14:175–177

858. Shibuya A, Watanabe M, Fujita Y et al. An autopsy case of troglitazone-induced fulminant hepatitis. Diabetes Care, 1998; 21:2140–2143

859. Gitlin N, Julie NI, Spurr C, Lim KN, Juarbe HM. Two cases of severe clinical and histologic hepatotoxicity associated with troglitazone. Ann Intern Med, 1998; 129:36–38

860. Neuschwander-Tetri BA, Isley WL, Oki JC et al. Troglitazone-induced hepatic failure leading to liver transplantation. Ann Intern Med, 1998; 129:38–41

861. Fukano M, Amano S, Sato J et al. Subacute hepatic failure associated with a new antidiabetic agent, troglitazone: a case report with autopsy examination. Hum Pathol, 2000; 31:250–253

862. Murphy EJ, Davern TJ, Shakil AO et al. Troglitazone-induced fulminant hepatic failure. Acute Liver Failure Study Group. Dig Dis Sci, 2000; 45:549–553

863. Faich GA, Moseley RH. Troglitazone (Rezulin) and hepatic injury. Pharmacoepidemiol Drug Saf, 2001; 10:537–547

864. Smith MT. Mechanisms of troglitazone hepatotoxicity. Chem Res Toxicol, 2003; 16:679–687

865. Chojkier M. Troglitazone and liver injury: in search of answers. Hepatology, 2005; 41:237–246

866. He K, Talaat RE, Pool WF et al. Metabolic activation of troglitazone: identification of a reactive metabolite and mechanisms involved. Drug Metab Dispos, 2004; 32:639–646

867. Watkins PB, Whitcomb RW. Hepatic dysfunction associated with troglitazone. N Engl J Med, 1998; 338:916–917

868. Tolman KG, Chandramouli J. Hepatotoxicity of the thiazolidinediones. Clin Liver Dis, 2003; 7:369–379

869. Graham DJ, Drinkard CR, Shatin D. Incidence of idiopathic acute liver failure and hospitalized liver injury in patients treated with troglitazone. Am J Gastroenterol, 2003; 98:175–179

870. Graham DJ, Drinkard D, Shatin D et al. Liver enzyme monitoring in patients treated with troglitazone. JAMA, 2001; 296:831–833

871. Lindsey C, Graham M, McMurphy J. A retrospective review of thiazolidinediones with development of troglitazone conversion protocol. Sci World J, 2003; 3:477–483

872. Lebovitz HE, Kreider M, Freed MI. Evaluation of liver function in type 2 diabetic patients during clinical trials: evidence that rosiglitazone does not cause hepatic dysfunction. Diabetes Care, 2002; 25:815–821

873. Scheen AJ. Thiazolidinediones and liver toxicity. Diabetes Metab, 2001; 27:305–313

874. Graham DJ, Green L, Senior JR et al. Troglitazone-induced liver failure: a case study. Am J Med, 2003; 114:299–306

875. Menon KV, Angulo P, Lindor KD. Severe cholestatic hepatitis from troglitazone in a patient with nonalcoholic steatohepatitis and diabetes mellitus. Am J Gastroenterol, 2001; 96:1631–1634

876. Caldwell SH, Oelsner DH, Iezzoni JC et al. Cryptogenic cirrhosis: clinical characterization and risk factors for underlying disease. Hepatology, 1999; 29:664–669

877. Forman LM, Simmons DA, Diamond RH. Hepatic failure in a patient taking rosiglitazone. Ann Intern Med, 2000; 132:118–121

878. Al-Salman J, Arjomand H, Kemp DG et al. Hepatocellular injury in a patient receiving rosiglitazone: a case report. Ann Intern Med, 2000; 132:121–124

879. Hachey DM, O'Neil MP, Force RW. Isolated elevation of alkaline phosphatase level associated with rosiglitazone. Ann Intern Med, 2000; 133:752

880. Bonkovsky HL, Azar R, Bird S et al. Severe cholestatic hepatitis caused by thiazolidinediones. Dig Dis Sci, 2002; 47:1632–1637

881. Freid J, Everitt D, Boscia J. Rosiglitazone and hepatic failure [letter]. Ann Intern Med, 2000; 132:164

882. Novak D, Lewis JH. Drug-induced liver disease. Curr Opin Gastroenterol, 2003; 19:203–215

883. Kaplowitz N, Lewis JH, Watkins PB. Did this drug cause my patient's hepatitis? Ann Intern Med, 2003; 138:159–160

884. Isley WL, Oki JC. Rosiglitazone and liver failure. Ann Intern Med, 2000; 133:393–394

885. May LD, Lefkowitch JH, Kram MT. Mixed hepatocellular-cholestatic liver injury after pioglitazone therapy. Ann Intern Med, 2002; 136:449–452

886. Pinto AG, Cummings OW, Chalasani N. Severe but reversible cholestatic liver injury after pioglitazone therapy [letter]. Ann Intern Med, 2002; 137:857

887. Chase MP, Yarze JC. Pioglitazone-associated fulminant hepatic failure. Am J Gastroenterol, 2003; 97:502

888. Cheng AY, Fantus IG. Thiazolidinedione-induced congestive heart failure. Ann Pharmacother, 2004; 38:817–820

889. Lenhard MJ, Funk WB. Failure to develop hepatic injury from rosiglitazone in a patient with a history of troglitazone-induced hepatitis. Diabetes Care, 2001; 24:168–169

890. Kane MP, Busch RS, Bakst G et al. Substitution of pioglitazone for troglitazone in patients with type 2 diabetes. Endocr Pract, 2004; 10:18–23

891. Andrade RJ, Lucenga MI, Rodriguez-L, Mendizabel M. Hepatic injury caused by acarbose [letter]. Ann Intern Med, 1996; 124:931

892. Carrascosa M, Pascual F, Aresti S. Acarbose-induced acute severe hepatotoxicity [letter]. Lancet, 1997; 349:698–699

893. Wang P-Y, Kaneko T, Wang Y, Sato A. Acarbose alone or in combination with ethanol potentiates the hepatotoxicity of carbon tetrachloride and acetaminophen in rats. Hepatology, 1999; 29:161–165

894. Deutsch M, Kountouras D, Dourakis SP. Metformin hepatotoxicity. Ann Intern Med, 2004; 140:W25

895. Babich MM, Pike I, Shiffman ML. Metformin-induced acute hepatitis. Am J Med, 1998; 104:490–492

896. Nammour EE, Fayad NF, Peikin SR. Metformin-induced cholestatic hepatitis. Endocr Pract, 2003; 9:307–309

897. Salpeter SR, Greyber E, Pasternak GA et al. Risk of fatal and nonfatal lactic acidosis with metformin use in type 2 diabetes mellitus: systematic review and meta-analysis. Arch Intern Med, 2003; 163:2594–2602

898. Gan SC, Barr J, Arieff AI, Pearl RG. Biguanide-associated lactic acidosis. Case report and review of the literature. Arch Intern Med, 1992; 152:2333–2336

899. Nan DN, Hernandez LJ, Fernandez-Ayala M et al. Acute hepatotoxicity caused by repaglinide. Ann Intern Med, 2004; 141:823

900. Schmidt G, Boersch G, Mueller KM, Wegener M. Methimazole associated cholestatic liver injury: case report and brief literature review. Hepatogastroenterology, 1986; 33:244–246

901. Sadoul JL, Canivet B, Freychet P. Toxic hepatitis induced by antithyroid drugs: four cases including one with cross-reactivity between carbimazole and benzylthiouracil. Eur J Med, 1993; 2:473–477

902. Kang H, Choi JD, Jung G et al. A case of methimazole-induced acute hepatic failure in a patient with chronic hepatitis B carrier. Korean J Intern Med, 1990; 5:69–71

903. Bloch CA, Jenski LJ, Balistreri WF. Propylthiouracil-associated hepatitis. Arch Intern Med, 1985; 145:2129–2130

904. Mihas AA, Holley P, Koff RS, Hirschowitz BI. Fulminant hepatitis and lymphocyte sensitization due to propylthiouracil. Gastroenterology, 1976; 70:770–774

905. Limage A, Ruffolo PR. Propylthiouracil-induced fatal hepatic necrosis. Am J Gastroenterol, 1987; 82:152–154

906. Ruiz JK, Rossi GV, Vallejos HA et al. Fulminant hepatic failure associated with propylthiouracil. Ann Pharmacother, 2003; 37:224–228

907. Deidiker R, deMello DE. Propylthiouracil-induced fulminant hepatitis: case report and review of the literature. Pediatr Pathol Lab Med, 1996; 16:845–852

908. Ichiki Y, Akahoshi M, Yamashita N et al. Propylthiouracil-induced severe hepatitis: a case report and review of the literature. J Gastroenterol, 1998; 33:747–750

909. Kim HJ, Kim BH, Han YS et al. The incidence and clinical characteristics of symptomatic propylthiouracil-induced hepatic injury in patients with hyperthyroidism: a single-center retrospective study. Am J Gastroenterol, 2001; 96:165–169

910. Jonas MM, Eidson MS. Propylthiouracil hepatotoxicity: two pediatric cases and review of the literature. J Pediatr Gastroenterol Nutr, 1988; 7:776–779

911. Fedotin MS, Lefer LG. Liver disease caused by propylthiouracil. Arch Intern Med, 1975; 135:319–321

912. Williams KV, Nayak S, Becker D et al. Fifty years of experience with propylthiouracil-associated hepatotoxicity: what have we learned? J Clin Endocrinol Metab, 1997; 82:1727–1733

913. Taxy JB. Peliosis: a morphologic curiosity becomes an iatrogenic problem. Hum Pathol, 1978; 9:331–340

914. Urban E, Frank BW, Kern F Jr. Liver dysfunction with mestranol but not with norethynodrel in a patient with enovid-induced jaundice. Ann Intern Med, 1968; 68:598–602

915. Holzbach RT, Sanders JH. Recurrent intrahepatic cholestasis of pregnancy: observations on pathogenesis. JAMA, 1965; 193:542–544

916. Metreau JM, Dhumeaux D, Bethelot P. Oral contraceptives and the liver. Digestion, 1972; 7:318–335

917. Orellana-Alcalde JM, Dominguez JP. Jaundice and oral contraceptive drugs. Lancet, 1966; ii:1278–1280

918. Eisalo A, Jarvinen PA, Luukkainen T. Hepatic impairment during the intake of contraceptive pills. Clinical trial with post-menopausal women. BMJ, 1964; 2:426–427

919. Hutchins GF, Gollan JL. Recent developments in the pathophysiology of cholestasis. Clin Liver Dis, 2004; 8:1–26

920. Hartleb M, Nowak A. Severe jaundice with destructive cholangitis after administration of methyltestosterone. Am J Gastroenterol, 1990; 85:766–767

921. Glober GA, Wilkerson JA. Biliary cirrhosis following the administration of methyltestosterone. JAMA, 1968; 204:170–173

922. Anthony PP. Hepatoma associated with androgenic steroids. Lancet, 1975; i:685–686

923. Stromeyer FW, Smith DH, Ishak KG. Anabolic steroid therapy and intrahepatic cholangiocarcinoma. Cancer, 1979; 43:440–443

924. Ham JM, Pirola RC, Crouch RI. Hemangioendothelial sarcoma of the liver associated with long-term estrogen therapy in man. Dig Dis Sci, 1980; 25:879–883

925. Vilches AR, Perez V, Suchecki DE. Raloxifene-associated hepatitis. Lancet, 1998; 352:1524–1525

926. Blackburn AM, Amiel SA, Millis RR, Rubens RD. Tamoxifen and liver damage. BMJ, 1984; 289:288

927. Pinto HC, Baptista A, Camilo ME et al. Tamoxifen-associated steatohepatitis: report of three cases. J Hepatol, 1995; 23:95–97

928. Oien KA, Moffat D, Curry GW et al. Cirrhosis with steatohepatitis after adjuvant tamoxifen [letter]. Lancet, 1999; 356:36–37

929. Elefsiniotis IS, Pantazis KD, Ilias A et al. Tamoxifen induced hepatotoxicity in breast cancer patients with pre-existing liver steatosis: the role of glucose intolerance. Eur J Gastroenterol Hepatol, 2004; 16:593–598

930. Murata Y, Ogawa Y, Saibara T et al. Unrecognized hepatic steatosis and non-alcoholic steatohepatitis in adjuvant tamoxifen for breast cancer patients. Oncol Rep, 2000; 7:1299–1304

931. Cai Q, Bensen M, Greene R et al. Tamoxifen-induced transient multifocal hepatic fatty infiltration. Am J Gastroenterol, 2000; 95:277–279

932. Nemoto Y, Saibara T, Ogawa Y et al. Tamoxifen-induced nonalcoholic steatohepatitis in breast cancer patients treated with adjuvant tamoxifen. Intern Med, 2002; 41:345–350

933. Wilking N, Isaksson E, von Schoultz E. Tamoxifen and secondary tumours. An update. Drug Saf, 1997; 16:104–117

934. Melamed I, Bujanover Y, Hammer J, Spirer Z. Hepatoblastoma in an infant born to a mother after hormonal treatment for sterility. N Engl J Med, 1982; 307:820

935. Carrasco D, Barrachina M, Prieto M, Berenguer J. Clomiphene citrate and liver-cell adenoma. N Engl J Med, 1984; 310:1120–1121

936. Olsson R, Tyllstrom J, Zettergren L. Hepatic reactions to cyclofenil. Gut, 1983; 24:260

937. Bouvet B, Rosas P, Paliard P, Brette R, Trepo C. Hepatite ague du au cyclofenil (Ondoyne). A propos de deux cas. Gastroenterol Clin Biol, 1985; 9:941–943

938. Dourakis SP, Alexopoulou AA, Hadziyannis SJ. Fulminant hepatitis after flutamide treatment. J Hepatol, 1994; 20:350–353

939. Andrade RJ, Lucena MI, Fernandez MC et al. Fulminant liver failure associated with flutamide therapy for hirsutism [letter]. Lancet, 1999; 353:983

940. Thole Z, Manso G, Salgueiro E et al. Hepatotoxicity induced by antiandrogens: a review of the literature. Urol Int, 2004; 73:289–295

941. Lin AD, Chen KK, Lin AT et al. Antiandrogen-associated hepatotoxicity in the management of advanced prostate cancer. J Chin Med Assoc, 2003; 66:735–740

942. Famularo G, De Simone C, Minisola G et al. Flutamide-associated acute liver failure. Ann Ital Med Int, 2003; 18:250–253

943. Cetin M, Demirci D, Unal A et al. Frequency of flutamide induced hepatotoxicity in patients with prostate carcinoma. Hum Exp Toxicol, 1999; 18:137–140

944. Pontiroli L, Sartori M, Pittau S et al. Flutamide-induced acute hepatitis: investigation on the role of immunoallergic mechanisms. Ital J Gastroenterol Hepatol, 1998; 30:310–314

945. Pu YS, Liu CM, Kao JH et al. Antiandrogen hepatotoxicity in patients with chronic viral hepatitis. Eur Urol, 1999; 36:293–297

946. Blake JC, Sawyer AM, Dooley JS, Scheuer PJ, McIntyre N. Severe hepatitis caused by cyproterone acetate. Gut, 1990; 31:556–557

947. Giordano N, Nardi P, Santacroce C et al. Acute hepatitis induced by cyproterone acetate. Ann Pharmacother, 2001; 35:1053–1055

948. Friedman G, Lamoureux E, Sherker AH. Fatal fulminant hepatic failure due to cyproterone acetate. Dig Dis Sci, 1999; 44:1362–1363

949. Boue F, Caffin B, Delfrasissy JF. Danazol and cholestatic hepatitis. Ann Intern Med, 1986; 105:139–140

950. Silva MO, Reddy R, McDonald T, Jeffers LJ, Schiff ER. Danazol-induced cholestasis. Am J Gastroenterol, 1989; 84:426–428

951. Makdisi WJ, Cherian R, Vanvelhuizen PJ, Talley RL, Stark SP, Dixon AY. Fatal peliosis of the liver and spleen in a patient with agnogenic myeloid metaplasia treated with danazol. Am J Gastroenterol, 1995; 90:317–318

952. Fermand JP, Levy Y, Bouscary D. Danazol-induced hepatocellular adenoma. Am J Med, 1990; 88:529–530

953. Kahn H, Manzarbeitia C, Theise N, Schwartz M, Miller C, Tung ST. Danazol-induced hepatocellular adenomas. A case report and review of the literature. Arch Pathol Lab Med, 1991; 115:1054–1057

954. Bork K, Pitton M, Harten P, Koch P. Hepatocellular adenomas in patients taking danazol for hereditary angio-oedema. Lancet, 1999; 353:1066–1067

955. Buamah PK. An apparent danazol-induced primary hepatocellular carcinoma. J Surg Oncol, 1985; 28:114–116

956. Crampon D, Barnoud R, Durand M et al. Danazol therapy: an unusual aetiology of hepatocellular carcinoma. J Hepatol, 1998; 29:1035–1036

957. Arosio M, Bazzoni N, Ambrosi B, Faglia G. Acute hepatitis after treatment of acromegaly with octreotide [letter]. Lancet, 1988; i:1498

958. Cameron RG, Feuer G, de la Iglesia FA, eds. Drug-induced hepatotoxicity. Berlin: Springer-Verlag, 1996

959. Thiim M, Friedman LS. Hepatotoxicity of antibiotics and antifungals. Clin Liver Dis, 2003; 7:381–399

960. Combes B, Whalley PJ, Adams RH. Tetracycline and the liver. Prog Liver Dis, 1972; 4:589–596

961. Breen K, Schenker S, Heimberg M. The effect of tetracycline on the hepatic secretion of triglyceride. Biochim Acta, 1972; 270:429–434

962. Kunelis CT, Peters JL, Edmondson HA. Fatty liver of pregnancy and its relationship to tetracycline therapy. Am J Med, 1965; 38:359–377

963. Freneaux E, Labbe G, Letteron P et al. Inhibition of the mitochondrial oxidation of fatty acids by tetracycline in mice and in man: possible role in microvesicular steatosis induced by this antibiotic. Hepatology, 1988; 8:1056–1062

964. Hunt CM, Washington K. Tetracycline-induced bile duct paucity and prolonged cholestasis. Gastroenterology, 1994; 107:1844–1847

965. Burette A, Finet C, Prigogine T et al. Acute hepatic injury associated with minocycline. Ann Intern Med, 1984; 44:1491–1492

966. Malcolm A, Heap TP, Eckstein RP, Lunzer MR. Minocycline-induced liver injury. Am J Gastroenterol, 1996; 91:1641–1643

967. Golstein PE, Deviere J, Cremer M. Acute hepatitis and drug-related lupus induced by minocycline treatment. Am J Gastroenterol, 1997; 92:143–146

968. Teitelbaum JE, Perez-Atayde AR, Cohen M et al. Minocycline-related autoimmune hepatitis: case series and literature review. Arch Pediatr Adolesc Med, 1998; 152:1132–1136

969. Goldstein NS, Bayati N, Silverman AL, Gordon SC. Minocycline as a cause of drug-induced autoimmune hepatitis. Report of four cases and comparison with autoimmune hepatitis. Am J Clin Pathol, 2000; 114:591–598

970. Knowles SR, Shapiro L, Shear NH. Serious adverse reactions induced by minocycline. Report of 13 patients and review of the literature. Arch Dermatol, 1996; 132:934–939

971. Lawrenson RA, Seaman HE, Sundstrom A et al. Liver damage associated with minocycline use in acne: a systematic review of the published literature and pharmacovigilance data. Drug Saf, 2000; 23:333–349

972. Zafrani ES, Ishak KG, Rudzki C. Cholestatic and hepatocellular injury associated with erythromycin esters: report of nine cases. Am J Dig Dis, 1979; 24:385–396

973. Diehl AM, Latham P, Boitnott JK et al. Cholestatic hepatitis from erythromycin ethlysuccinate. Am J Med, 1984; 76:931–934

974. Hosker JP, Jewell DP. Transient, selective factor X deficiency and acute liver failure following chest infection treated with erythromycin. Postgrad Med J, 1983; 59:514–515

975. Inman WH, Rawson NS. Erythromycin estolate and jaundice. BMJ, 1983; 286:1954–1955

976. Ghoulson CF, Warren GH. Fulminant hepatic failure associated with intravenous erythromycin lactobionate. Arch Intern Med, 1990; 150:215–218

977. Zimmerman HJ, Kendler J, Libber S, Lukacs L. Hepatocyte suspensions as a model for demonstration of drug hepatotoxicity. Biochem Pharmacol, 1974; 23:2187–2189

978. Kendler J, Anuras S, Laborda O, Zimmerman HJ. Perfusion of the isolated rat liver with erythromycin estolate and other derivatives. Proc Soc Exp Biol Med, 1972; 139:1272–1275

979. Brown RA. Two cases of untoward reaction after 'Isolone'. BMJ, 1963; 2:913–914

980. Spiers KM, Zervos MJ. Telithromycin. Expert Rev Anti Infect Ther, 2004; 2:685–693

981. Suriawinata A, Min AD. A 33-year-old woman with jaundice after azithromycin use. Semin Liver Dis, 2002; 22:207–212

982. Chandrupatla S, Demetris AJ, Rabinowitz M. Azithromycin-induced intrahepatic cholestasis. Dig Dis Sci, 2002; 47:2186–2188

983. Longo G, Valenti C, Gandini G et al. Azithromycin-induced intrahepatic cholestasis. Am J Med, 1997; 102:217–218

984. Pedersen FM, Bathum L, Fenger C. Acute hepatitis and roxithromycin. Lancet, 1993; 341:251–252

985. Wallace RJ Jr, Brown BA, Griffith DE. Drug intolerance to high-dose clarithromycin among elderly patients. Diagn Microbiol Infect Dis, 1993; 16:215–221

986. Zimmerman HJ. Intrahepatic cholestatis. Arch Intern Med, 1979; 139:1038–1045

987. Haber I, Hebens H. Cholestatic jaundice after troleandomycin and oral contraceptives. The diagnostic value of gamma glutamyl transpeptidase. Acta Gastroenterol Belg, 1980; 43:425–477

988. Bridges RA, Berendes H, Good RA. Serious reactions to novobiocin. J Pediatr, 1957; 50:579–585

989. Goldstein LI, Ishak KG. Hepatic injury associated with penicillin therapy. Arch Pathol, 1974; 98:114–117

990. Williams CN, Malatjalian DA. Severe penicillin-induced cholestasis in a 91-year-old woman. Dig Dis Sci, 1981; 26:470–473

991. Onate J, Montejo M, Aguirrebengoa K et al. Hepatotoxicity associated with penicillin V therapy. Clin Infect Dis, 1995; 20:474–475

992. Dismukes WE. Oxacillin-induced hepatic dysfunction. JAMA, 1973; 226:861–863

993. Knirsch AK, Gralla EJ. Abnormal serum transaminase levels after parenteral ampicillin and carbenicillin administration. N Engl J Med, 1970; 282:1081–1084

994. Wilson FM, Belamaric J, Lauter CB, Lerner AM. Anicteric carbenicillin hepatitis: eight episodes in four patients. JAMA, 1975; 232:818–821

995. Kleinman MS, Presberg JE. Cholestatic hepatitis after dicloxacillin-sodium therapy. J Clin Gastroenterol, 1986; 8:77

996. Victorino RM, Maria VA, Correoa AP, de Moura C. Floxacillin-induced cholestatic hepatitis: evidence of lymphocyte sensitization. Arch Intern Med, 1987; 147:987–989

997. Bengtsson F, Floren CH, Hagerstrand I. Flucloxacillin-induced cholestatic liver damage. Scand J Infect Dis, 1985; 17:125–128

998. Derby LE, Jick H, Henry DA, Dean AD. Cholestatic hepatitis associated with flucloxacillin. Med J Aust, 1993; 158:596–600

999. Turner IB, Eckstein RP, Riley JW, Lunzer MR. Prolonged hepatic cholestasis after flucloxacillin therapy. Med J Aust, 1989; 151:701–705

1000. Miros M, Kerlin P, Walker N, Harris O. Flucloxacillin induced delayed cholestatic hepatitis. Aust N Z J Med, 1990; 20:251–253

1001. Reddy KR, Brillant P, Schiff ER. Amoxicillin-clavulanate potassium-associated cholestasis. Gastroenterology, 1989; 96:1135–1141

1002. Garcia-Rodriguez LA, Stricker BH, Zimmerman HJ. Risk of acute liver injury associated with the combination of amoxicillin and clavulanic acid. Arch Intern Med, 1996; 156:1327–1232

1003. Larrey D, Vial T, Micaleff A et al. Hepatitis associated with amoxycillin-clavulanic acid combination: report of 15 cases. Gut, 1992; 33:368–371

1004. Stricker BH, Van den Broek JW, Keuning J et al. Cholestatic hepatitis due to antibacterial combination of amoxicillin and clavulanic acid (augmentin). Dig Dis Sci, 1989; 34:1576–1580

1005. Ryley NG, Fleming KA, Chapman RWG. Focal destructive cholangiopathy associated with amoxycillin/clavulanic acid (Augmentin). J Hepatol, 1995; 23:278–282

1006. O'Donohue J, Oien KA, Donaldson P et al. Co-amixoclav jaundice: clinical and histological features and HLA class II association. Gut, 2000; 47:717–720

1007. Mari JY, Guy C, Beyens MN, Ollagnier M. [Delayed drug-induced hepatic injury. Evoking the role of amoxicillin-clavulinic acid combination.] Therapie, 2000; 55:699–704

1008. Hautekeete ML, Brenard R, Harsmans Y et al. Liver injury related to amoxicillin-clavulanic acid interlobular bile-duct lesions and extrahepatic manifestations. J Hepatol, 1995; 22:71–77

1009. Caballero Plasencia AM, Valenzuela Barranco M, Martin Ruiz JL et al. [Hepatotoxicity caused by amoxicillin, clavulanic acid or both?] Gastroenterol Hepatol, 1997; 20:45–46

1010. Sweet JM, Jones MP. Intrahepatic cholestasis due to ticarcillin-clavulanate. Am J Gastroenterol, 1995; 90:675–676

1011. Hautekeete ML, Horsmans Y, Van Waeyenberge C et al. HLA association of amoxicillin-clavulanate-induced hepatitis. Gastroenterology, 1999; 117:1181–1186

1012. Silvain C, Fort E, Levillain P, Labat-Labourdette J, Beauchant M. Granulomatous hepatitis due to a combination of amoxicillin and clavulanic acid. Dig Dis Sci, 1992; 37:150–152

1013. Bor O, Dinleyici EC, Kebapci M et al. Ceftriaxone-associated biliary sludge and pseudocholelithiasis during childhood: a prospective study. Pediatr Int, 2004; 46:322–324

1014. Eggleston SM, Belandres MM. Jaundice associated with cephalosporin therapy. Drug Intell Clin Pharm, 1985; 19:553–555

1015. Fox JC, Szyjkowkski RS, Sanderson SO. Progressive cholestatic liver diseasee associated with clarithromycin treatment. J Clin Pharmacol, 2002; 42:676–689

1016. Lucena MI, Andrade RA, Sanchez-Martinez H, Perez-Serrano JM, Gomez-Outes A. Norfloxacin-induced cholestatic jaundice [letter]. Am J Gastroenterol, 1998; 93:2309–2311

1017. Food and Drug Administration Public Health Advisor, 9 June 1999. Trovan (Trovafloxacin/alatrovafloxacin mesylate). http://www.fda.gov/cder/news/trovanadvisory/htm.

1018. Spahr L, Rubbia-Brandt L, Marinescu O et al. Acute fatal hepatitis related to levofloxacin. J Hepatol, 2001; 35:308–309

1019. Villeneuve JP, Davies C, Cote J. Suspected ciprofloxacin-induced hepatotoxicity. Ann Pharmacother, 1995; 29:257–259

1020. Gonzales Carro P, Legaz Huidrobro ML, Pinardo Zabala A et al. Fatal subfulminant hepatic failure with ofloxacin. Am J Gastroenterol, 2000; 95:1606

1021. Bjornsson E, Olsson R, Remotti H. Norfloxacin-induced eosinophilic necrotizing granulomatous hepatitis. Ann J Gastroenterol, 2000; 95:3660–3664

1022. Bataille L, Rahier J, Geubel A. Delayed and prolonged cholestatic hepatitis with ductopenia after long-term ciprofoxacin therapy for Crohn's disease. J Hepatol, 2002; 37:696–699

1023. Coleman CI, Spencer JV, Chung JO et al. Possible gatifloxacin-induced fulminant hepatic failure. Ann Pharmacother, 2002; 36:1162–1167

1024. Henann NE, Zambie MF. Gatifloxacin-associated acute hepatitis. Pharmacotherapy, 2001; 21:1579–1582

1025. Cheung O, Chopra K, Yu T et al. Gatifloxacin-induced hepatotoxicity and acute pancreatitis. Ann Intern Med, 2004; 140:73–74

1026. Lazarczyk DA, Goldstein NS, Gordon SC. Trovafloxacin hepatotoxicity. Dig Dis Sci, 2001; 46:925–926

1027. Lucena MI, Andrade RJ, Rodrigo L et al. Trovafloxacin-induced acute hepatitis. Clin Infect Dis, 2000; 30:401–402

1028. Garey KW, Amsden GW. Trovafloxacin: an overview. Pharmacotherapy, 1999; 19:21–34

1029. Blum MD, Graham DJ, Temafloxacin syndrome: review of 95 cases. Clin Infect Dis, 1994; 186:946–950

1030. Ball P, Mandel L, Niki Y et al. Comparative tolerability of the newer fluoroquinolone antibacterials. Drug Saf, 1999; 21:407–421

1031. Azinge NO, Garrick GA. Stevens-Johnson syndrome (erythema multiforme) following ingestion of trimethoprim-sulfamethoxazole on two separate occasions in the same person: a case report. J Allergy Clin Immunol, 1978; 62:125–126

1032. Dujvone CA, Chan CH, Zimmerman HJ. Sulfonamide hepatic injury. Review of the literature and report of a case due to sulfamethoxazone. N Engl J Med, 1967; 277:785–788

1033. Mainra RR, Card SE. Trimethoprim-sulfamethoxazole-associated hepatotoxicity—part of a hypersensitivity syndrome. Can J Clin Pharmacol, 2003; 10:175–178

1034. Naisbitt DJ, Hough SJ, Gill HJ et al. Cellular disposition of sulphamethoxazole and its metabolites: implications for hypersensitivity. Br J Pharmacol, 1999; 126:1393–1407

1035. Naisbitt DJ, Gordon SF, Pirmohamed M et al. Antigenicity and immunogenicity of sulphamethoxazole: demonstration of metabolism-dependent haptenation and T-cell proliferation in vivo. Br J Pharmacol, 2001; 133:295–305

1036. Farrell J, Naisbitt DJ, Drummond NS et al. Characterization of sulfamethoxazole and sulfamethoxazole metabolite-specific T-cell responses in animals and humans. J Pharmacol Exp Ther, 2003; 306:229–237

1037. Rubin R. Sulfasalazine-induced fulminant hepatic failure and necrotizing pancreatitis. Am J Gastroenterol, 1994; 89:789–791

1038. Zaman F, Ye G, Abreo KD et al. Successful orthotopic liver transplantation after trimethoprim-sulfamethoxazole associated fulminant liver failure. Clin Transplant, 2003; 17:461–464

1039. Alberti-Flor JJ, Hernandez ME, Ferrer JP, Howell S, Jeffers L. Fulminant liver failure and pancreatitis associated with the use of sulfamethoxazole-trimethoprim. Gastroenterology, 1989; 84:1577–1579

1040. Brett AS, Shaw SV. Simultaneous pancreatitis and hepatitis associated with trimethoprin-sulfamethoxazole. Am J Gastroenterol, 1999; 94:267–268

1041. Kowdley KV, Keeffe EB, Fawaz KA. Prolonged cholestasis due to trimethoprim-sulfamethoxazole. Gastroenterology, 1992; 102:2148–2150

1042. Yao F, Behling CA, Saab S, Li S et al. Trimethoprim-sulfamethoxazole-induced vanishing bile duct syndrome. Am J Gastroenterol, 1997; 92:167–169

1043. Munoz JJ, Martinez-Hernandez A, Maddrey WC. Intrahepatic cholestasis and phospholipidosis associated with the use of trimethoprim-sulfamethoxazole. Hepatology, 1980; 12:342–347

1044. Tanner AR. Hepatic cholestasis induced by trimethoprim. BMJ, 1986; 293:1072–1073

1045. Cribb AE. Adverse reaction to sulfonamide-trimethoprim. Adverse Drug React Toxicol Rev, 1996; 15:49–50

1046. van der Ven AJ, Vree TB, Koopmans PP et al. Adverse reactions to co-trimoxazole in HIV infection: a reappraisal of the glutathione-hydroxylamine hypothesis. J Antimicrob Chemother, 1996; 73:55–60

1047. Montanaro A. A sulfonamide allergy. Immunol Allergy Clin North Am, 1998; 18:843–849

1048. Fich A, Schwartz J, Braverman D, Zafrani A, Rochmilewitz D. Sulfasalazine hepatotoxicity. Am J Gastroenterol, 1984; 79:401–402

1049. Stoschus B, Meybehm M, Spengler U, Scheurlan C, Sauerbruch T. Cholestasis associated with mesalazine therapy in a patient with Crohn's disease. J Hepatol, 1997; 26:425–428

1050. Johnson DA, Cattau EL, Kuritsky JN, Zimmerman HJ. Liver involvement in the sulfone syndrome. Arch Intern Med, 1986; 146:875–877

1051. Goldstein LI, Ishak KG, Burns W. Hepatic injury associated with nitrofurantoin therapy. Am J Dig Dis, 1974; 19:987–998

1052. Sippel PJ, Agger WA. Nitrofurantoin-induced granulomatous hepatitis. Urology, 1981; 18:177–178

1053. Sochocky S. Acute hepatitis due to para-aminosalicylic acid. Br J Clin Pract, 1971; 25:179–182

1054. Gulliford M, Mackey AD, Prowse K. Cholestatic jaundice caused by ethambutol. BMJ, 1986; 292:866–867

1055. Scheuer PJ, Summerfield JA, Lal S, Sherlock S. Rifampicin hepatitis. A clinical and histological study. Lancet, 1974; i:421–425

1056. Ozick LA, Jacob L, Comer GM et al. Hepatotoxicity from isoniazid and rifampin in inner-city AIDS patients. Am J Gastroenterol, 1995; 90:1978–1980

1057. Fernandez-Villar A, Sopena B, Fernandez-Villar J et al. The influence of risk factors on the severity of anti-tuberculosis drug-induced hepatotoxicity. Int J Tuberc Lung Dis, 2004; 8:1499–1505

1058. McNeill L, Allen M, Estrada C et al. Pyrazinamide and rifampin vs isoniazid for the treatment of latent tuberculosis: improved completion rates but more hepatotoxicity. Chest, 2003; 123:102–106

1059. Conn HO, Binder HJ, Orr HD. Ethionamide-induced hepatitis. A review with a report of an additional case. Am Rev Respir Dis, 1964; 90:542–552

1060. Garibaldi RA, Drusin RE, Ferebee SH, Gregg MB. Isoniazid-associated hepatitis: report of an outbreak. Am Rev Respir Dis, 1972; 106:357–365

1061. Nolan CM, Goldberg SV, Buskin SE. Hepatotoxicity associated with isoniazid preventive therapy. A 7-year survey from a public health tuberculosis clinic. JAMA, 1999; 281:1014–1018

1062. Teleman MD, Chee CB, Earnest A et al. Hepatotoxicity of tuberculosis chemotherapy under general program conditions in Singapore. Int J Tuberc Lung Dis, 2002; 6:699–705

1063. Patel PA, Voigt MD. Prevalence and interaction of hepatitis B and latent tuberculosis in Vietnamese immigrants to the United States. Am J Gastroenterol, 2002; 97:1198–1203

1064. Huang YS, Chern HD, Su WJ et al. Polymorphism of the N-acetyltransferase 2 gene as a susceptibility risk factor for antituberculosis drug-induced hepatitis. Hepatology, 2002; 35:883–889

1065. Scharer L, Smith JP. Serum transaminase elevations and other hepatic abnormalities in patients receiving isoniazid. Ann Intern Med, 1969; 71:1113–1120

1066. Hugues FC, Marche C, Marche J. Effects hepatobiliares de l'association rifamipicine-isoniazide. Therapie, 1969; 24:899

1067. Pessayre D. Present views on isoniazid and isoniazid-rifampin hepatitis. Aggressologie, 1982; 23:13

1068. Capelle P, Dhumeaux D, Mora M et al. Effect of rifampicin on liver function in man. Gut, 1972; 13:366–371

1069. Centers for Disease Control and Prevention: American Thoracic Society. Update: adverse event data and revised American Thoracic Society/CDC recommendations against the use of rifampin and pyrazinamide for treatment of latent tuberculosis infection—United States, 2003. MMWR Morb Mortal Wkly Rep, 2003; 52:735–739

1070. Kunimoto D, Warman A, Beckon A et al. Severe hepatotoxicity associated with rifampin-pyrazinamide preventive therapy requiring transplantation in an individual at low risk for hepatotoxicity. Clin Infect Dis, 2003; 36:e158–e161

1071. Yee D, Valiquette C, Pelletier M. Incidence of serious side effects from first line antiTB drugs among patients treated for active TB. Am J Respir Crit Care Med, 2003; 167:1472–1477

1072. Khokhar O, Gange C, Clement S, Lewis J. Autoimmune hepatitis and thyroiditis associated with rifampin and pyrazinamide prophylaxis: an unusual reaction. Dig Dis Sci, 2005; 50:207–211

1073. Matillin A, Molland EA. A light and electron microscope study of the liver in case of erythrohepatic protopoporhyria and griseofulvin-induced porphyria in mice. J Clin Pathol, 1974; 27:698–709

1074. Denk H, Gschnait F, Wolff K. Hepatocellular hyaline (Mallory bodies) in long term griseofulvin-treated mice. A new experimental model for the study of hyaline formation. Lab Invest, 1975; 32:773–776

1075. Berman A, Franklin RL. Precipitation of acute intermittent porphyria by griseofulvin therapy. JAMA, 1968; 188:466

1076. Chiprut RO, Viteri A, Jamroz C, Dyck WP. Intrahepatic cholestasis after griseofulvin administration. Gastroenterology, 1976; 70:1141–1143

1077. Lewis JH, Zimmerman HJ, Benson GD, Ishak KG. Hepatic injury associated with ketoconazole therapy. Gastroenterology, 1984; 86:503–513

1078. Stricker BH, Blok AP, Bronkhorst FB, Van Parys GE. Ketoconazole-associated hepatic injury. A clinicopathological study of 55 cases. J Hepatol, 1986; 3:399–406

1079. Lake-Bakaar G, Scheuer PJ, Sherlock S. Hepatic reactions associated with ketoconazole in the United Kingdom. BMJ, 1987; 294:419–422

1080. Ikemoto H. Clinical study of fluconazole for treatment of mycoses. Diag Microbiol Infect Dis, 1989; 12(Suppl):239S–247S

1081. Bronstein JA, Gros P, Hernandez E et al. Fatal acute hepatic necrosis due to dose-dependent fluconazole hepatotoxicity. Clin Infect Dis, 1997; 25:1266–1267

1082. Talwalkar JA, Soetikno RE, Carr-locke DL, Berg CL. Severe cholestasis related to itraconazole for the treatment of onychomycosis. Am J Gastroenterol, 1999; 94:3632–3633

1083. Gupta AK, Chwetzoff E, Del Rosso J et al. Hepatic safety of itraconazole. J Cutan Med Surg, 2002; 6:210–213

1084. Somchit N, Norshahida AR, Hasiah AH et al. Hepatotoxicity induced by antifungal drugs itraconazole and fluconazole in rats: a comparative in vivo study. Hum Exp Toxicol, 2004; 23:519–525

1085. Vermes A, Guchelaar HJ, Dankert J. Flucytosine: a review of its pharmacology, clinical indications, pharmacokinetics, toxicity and drug interactions. J Antimicrob Chemother, 2000; 46:171–179

1086. Fernandes NF, Geller SA, Fong T-L. Terfinafine hepatotoxicity: Case report and review of the literature. Am J Gastroenterol, 1998; 93:549–460

1087. Lazarus GA, Papatheodoridis GV, Dellatetsima JA, Tassopoulus NC. Terbinafine-induced cholestatic liver disease. J Hepatol, 1996; 24:753–756

1088. Agarwal K, Manas DM, Hudson M. Terbinafine and fulminant hepatic failure [letter]. N Engl J Med, 1999; 340:1292–1293

1089. Anania FA, Rabin L. Terbinafine hepatotoxicity resulting in chronic biliary ductopenia and portal fibrosis. Am J Med, 2002; 112:741–742

1090. Lovell MO, Speeg KV, Havranek RD et al. Histologic changes resembling acute rejection in a liver transplant patient treated with terbinafine. Hum Pathol, 2003; 34:187–189

1091. Ajit C, Suvannasankha A, Zaeri N et al. Terbinafine-associated hepatotoxicity. Am J Med Sci, 2003; 325:292–295

1092. Carnecchia BM, Kurtzke JM. Fatal toxic reaction to amphotericin B in cryptococcal meningo-encephalitis. Ann Intern Med, 1960; 53:1027–1036

1093. Miller MA. Reversible hepatotoxicity related to amphotericin B. Can Med Ass J, 1984; 131:1245–1247

1094. Nunez M, Soriano V. Hepatotoxicity of antiretrovirals: incidence, mechanisms and management. Drug Saf, 2005; 28:53–66

1095. Powderly WG. Antiretroviral therapy in patients with hepatitis and HIV: weighing risks and benefits. Clin Infect Dis, 2004; 38(Suppl 2):S109–S113

1096. Ogedegbe AO, Sulkowski MS. Antiretroviral-associated liver injury. Clin Liver Dis, 2003; 7:475–499

1097. Kontorinis N, Dieterich D. Hepatotoxicity of antiretroviral therapy. AIDS Rev, 2003; 5:36–43

1098. Bonacini M. Hepatic injury from antiviral agents. In: Kaplowitz N, DeLeve LD, eds. Drug-induced liver disease. New York: Marcel Dekker, 2003: pp 519–548

1099. Kontorinis N, Dieterich DT. Toxicity of non-nucleoside analogue reverse transcriptase inhibitors. Semin Liver Dis, 2003; 23:173–182

1100. Pol S, Lebray P, Vallet-Pichard A. HIV infection and hepatic enzyme abnormalities: intricacies of the pathogenic mechanisms. Clin Infect Dis, 2004; 38(Suppl 2):S65–S72

1101. Kamal MA, French SW. Drug-induced increased mitochondrial biogenesis in a liver biopsy. Exp Mol Pathol, 2004; 77:201–204

1102. Benhamou Y. Antiretroviral therapy and HIV/hepatitis B virus coinfection. Clin Infect Dis, 2004; 38(Suppl 2):S98–S103

1103. Sulkowski MS. Drug-induced liver injury associated with antiretroviral therapy that includes HIV-1 protease inhibitors. Clin Infect Dis, 2004; 38(Suppl 2):S90–S97

1104. Dubin G, Braffman MN. Zidovudine-induced hepatotoxicity. Ann Intern Med, 1989; 110:85–86

1105. Chariot P, Drogou I, de Lacroix-Szmania I et al. Zidovudine induced mitochondrial disorder with massive liver steatosis, myopathy, lactic acidosis, and mitochondrial DNA depletion. J Hepatol, 1999; 30:156–160

1106. Lai KK, Gang DL, Zawacki JK, Cooley TP. Fulminant hepatic failure associated with 2',3'-dideoxyinosine (ddI). Ann Intern Med, 1991; 115:283–284

1107. Finkle HI. Hepatic mitochondrial toxicity from nucleoside analog therapy [letter]. Arch Pathol Lab Med, 1999; 123:189

1108. Bräu N, Leaf HL, Wieczorek RL, Margolis DM. Severe hepatitis in three AIDS patients treated with indinavir. Lancet, 1997; 349:924–925

1109. de Maat MM, ter Heine R, van Gorp EC et al. Case series of acute hepatitis in a non-selected group of HIV-infected patients on nevirapine-containing antiretroviral treatment. AIDS, 2003; 17:2209–2214

1110. Stern JO, Robinson PA, Love J et al. A comprehensive hepatic safety analysis of nevirapine in different populations of HIV infected patients. J Acquir Immune Defic Syndr, 2003; 34(Suppl 1):S21–S33

1111. Johnson S, Chan J, Bennett CL. Hepatoxicity after prophylaxis with a nevirapine-containing antiretroviral regimen. Ann Intern Med, 2002; 137:146–147

1112. Gonzales de Requena D, Nunez M, Jiminez-Nacher I et al. Liver toxicity caused by nevirapine. AIDS, 2002; 16:290–291

1113. Patel SM, Johnson S, Belknap SM et al. Serious adverse cutaneous and hepatic toxicities associated with nevirapine use by non-HIV-infected individuals. J Acquir Immune Defic Syndr, 2004; 35:120–125

1114. Sulkowski MS, Thomas DL, Chaisson RE, Moore RD. Hepatotoxicity associated with antiretroviral therapy in adults infected with human immunodeficiency virus and the role of hepatitis C or B virus infection. JAMA, 2000; 283:74–80

1115. Sulkowski MS, Mehta SH, Chaisson RE et al. Hepatotoxicity associated with protease inhibitor-based antiretroviral regimens with or without concurrent ritonavir. AIDS, 2004; 18:2277–2284

1116. Cervoni J-P, Degos F, Marcellin P, Erlinger S. Acute hepatitis induced by a-interferon associated with viral clearance, in chronic hepatitis C. J Hepatol, 1997; 27:1113–1116

1117. Lock G, Reng CM, Graeb C. Interferon-induced hepatic failure in a patient with hepatitis C. Am J Gastroenterol, 1999; 94:2570–2571

1118. Janssen HLA, Brouwer JT, Nevens F et al. Fatal hepatic decompensation with interferon alpha. BMJ, 1993; 306:107–108

1119. Cianciara J, Laskus T. Development of transient autoimmune hepatitis during interferon treatment of chronic hepatitis B. Dig Dis Sci, 1995; 40:1842–1844

1120. Papo T, Marcellin P, Bernuau J, Durand F, Poynard T, Benhamou J-P. Autoimmune chronic hepatitis exacerbated by alpha-interferon. Ann Intern Med, 1992; 116:51–53

1121. Dousset B, Conti F, Houssin D, Calmus Y. Acute vanishing bile duct syndrome after interferon therapy for recurrent HCV infection in liver-transplant recipients [letter]. N Engl J Med, 1994; 330:1160–1161

1122. Veerabagu MP, Finkelstein SD, Rabinowitz M. Granulomas in a patient with chronic hepatitis C treated with interferon-a. Dig Dis Sci, 1997; 42:1445–1448

1123. Goldin RD, Levine TS, Foster GR, Thomas HC. Granulomas and hepatitis C. Histopathology, 1996; 28:265–267

1124. Hoffmann RM, Jung M-C, Motz R et al. Sarcoidosis associated with interferon-a therapy for chronic hepatitis C. J Hepatol, 1998; 28:1058–1063

1125. Dayan AD, Lewis PD. Idoxuridine and jaundice. Lancet, 1969; ii:1073

1126. Breeden CJ, Hall TC, Tyler HR. Herpes simplex encephalitis treated with systemic 5-iodo-2'-deoxyuridine. Ann Intern Med, 1966; 65:1050–1056

1127. Herbeuval R, Rauber G, Dornier R. Hepatite cholostatique a la xenalamine. Therapie, 1966; 21:781–786

1128. Hryniuk W, Foerster J, Shojania M, Chow A. Cytarabine for herpes virus infections. JAMA, 1972; 219:715–718

1129. Bernuau J, Larrey D, Campillo B et al. Amodiaquine-induced fulminant hepatitis. J Hepatol, 1988; 6:109–112

1130. Wharton JM, Coleman DL, Wofsy CB et al. Trimethoprim-sulfamethoxazole or pentamidine for Pneumocystis carinii pneumonia in the acquired immunodeficiency syndrome. Ann Intern Med, 1986; 105:37–44

1131. Bjornsson E, Nordlinder H, Olsson R. Metronidazole as a probable cause of severe liver injury. Hepatogastroenterology, 2002; 49:252–254

1132. Farid Z, Smith JH, Bassily S, Sparks HA. Hepatotoxicity after treatment of schistosomiasis with hycanthone. BMJ, 1972; 2:88–89

1133. Manivel JC, Bloomer JR, Snover DC. Progressive bile duct injury after thiabendazole administration. Gastroenterology, 1987; 93:245–249

1134. Roy MA, Nugent FW, Aretz Ht. Micronodular cirrhosis after thiabendazole. Dig Dis Sci, 1989; 34:938–941

1135. Reshet R, Lok A, Sherlock S. Cholestatic jaundice in fascioliasis treated with niclofolan. BMJ, 1982; 285:1243–1244

1136. Hamlyn AN, Morris JS, Sarkany I, Sherlock S. Piperazine hepatitis. Gastroenterology, 1976; 70:1144–1147

1137. Jagota SL. Jaundice due to albendazole. Indian J Gastroenterol, 1989; 8:58–60

1138. Jung U, Mahr W. Mebendazole hepatitis. Z Gastroenterol, 1983; 21:736–741

1139. Perkins J. Phenindione jaundice. Lancet, 1962; i:125–127

1140. De Bryne ELE, Bac DJ, de Man RA, Dees A. Jaundice associated with acenocoumarol exposure. Nether J Med, 1998; 52:187–189

1141. Adler E, Benjamin SB, Zimmerman HJ. Cholestatic hepatic injury related to warfarin exposure. Arch Intern Med, 1986; 146:1837–1839

1142. Höhler T, Schmütgen M, Helmreich-Becker I, Mayer Zum Büschanfelde K-H. Drug-induced hepatitis: a rare complication of oral anticoagulants. J Hepatol, 1994; 21:447–449

1143. Castedal M, Aldenborg F, Olsson R. Fulminant hepatic failure associated with dicoumarol therapy. Liver, 1998; 18:67–69

1144. Seidl C, Thomsen R, Lohse A, Grouls V. Phenprocoumon-associated hepatitis. A rare complication of oral anticoagulation. Leber Magen Darm, 1998; 28:178–182

1145. Schimanski CC, Burg J, Mohler M et al. Phenprocoumon-induced liver disease ranges from mild acute hepatitis to (sub-) acute liver failure. J Hepatol, 2004; 41:67–74

1146. Dukes GE Jr, Sanders SW, Russo J Jr et al. Transaminase elevations in patients receiving bovine or porcine heparin. Ann Intern Med, 1984; 100:646–650

1147. Al-Mekhaizeem KA, Sherker AH. Heparin-induced hepatotoxicity. Can J Gastroenterol, 2001; 15:527–530

1148. Manfredini R, Boari B, Regoli F et al. Cholestatic liver reaction and heparin therapy. Arch Intern Med, 2000; 160(2):3166

1149. Olsson R, Leonhardt T. Cholestatic liver reaction during heparin therapy. J Intern Med, 1991; 229:471–473

1150. Iqbal M, Goenka P, Young MF, Thomas E, Borthwick TR. Ticlopidine-induced cholestatic hepatitis. Report of three cases and review of the literature. Dig Dis Sci, 1998; 43:2223–2226

1151. Amaro P, Nunes A, Macoas F et al. Ticlopidine-induced prolonged cholestasis: a case report. Eur J Gastroenterol Hepatol, 1999; 11:673–676

1152. Skurnik YD, Tcherniak A, Edlan K et al. Ticlopidine-induced cholestatic hepatitis. Ann Pharmacother, 2003; 37:371–375

1153. Eriksson H. Treatment of venous thromboembolism and long-term prevention of recurrence: present treatment options and ximelagatran. Drugs, 2004; 64(Suppl 1):37–46

1154. Rosencher N. Ximelagatran, a new oral direct thrombin inhibitor, for the prevention of venous thromboembolic events in major elective orthopaedic surgery. Efficacy, safety and anaesthetic considerations. Anaesthesia, 2004; 59:803–810

1155. Albers GW, Diener HC, Frison L et al.; SPORTIF Executive Steering Committee for the SPORTIF V Investigators. Ximelagatran vs warfarin for stroke prevention in patients with nonvalvular atrial fibrillation: a randomized trial. JAMA, 2005; 293:690–698

1156. Schulman S, Wahlander K, Lundstrom T et al. Secondary prevention of venous thromboembolism with the oral direct thrombin inhibitor ximelagatran. N Engl J Med, 2003; 349:1713–1721

1157. Lee WM, Larrey D, Olsson R, Lewis JH et al. Hepatic findings in long-term clinical trials of ximelagatran. Drug Saf (in press)

1158. Lazerow SK, Abdi MS, Lewis JH. Drug-induced liver disease. Curr Opin Gastroenterol, 2004; 21:283–292

1159. Geltner D, Chajek T, Rubinger D, Levij IS. Quinidine hypersensitivity and liver involvement. A survey of 32 patients. Gastroenterology, 1976; 70:650–652

1160. Koch MJ, Seeff LB, Crumley CE, Rabin L, Burns WA. Quinidine hepatotoxicity: a report of a case and review of the literature. Gastroenterology, 1976; 70:1136–1140

1161. Farver DK, Lavin MN. Quinine-induced hepatotoxicity. Ann Pharmacother, 1999; 33:32–34

1162. Chajek T, Lehrer B, Geltner D, Levij IS. Quinidine-induced granulomatous hepatitis. Ann Intern Med, 1974; 81:774–776

1163. Worman HJ, Ip JH, Winters SL et al. Hypersensitivity reaction associated with acute hepatic dysfunction following a single intravenous dose of procainamide. J Intern Med, 1992; 232:361

1164. Herlong HF, Reid PR, Boitnott JK, Maddrey WC. Aprindine hepatitis. Ann Intern Med, 1978; 89:359–361

1165. Meinertz T, Langer KH, Kasper W, Just H. Disopyramide-induced intrahepatic cholestasis. Lancet, 1977; ii:828–829

1166. Babany G, Mallat A, Zafrani ES et al. Chronic liver disease after low daily doses of amiodarone. Report of three cases. J Hepatol, 1986; 3:228–232

1167. Poucell S, Ireton J, Valencia-Mayoral P et al. Amiodarone-associated phospholipidosis and fibrosis of the liver. Light, immunohistochemical, and electron microscopic studies. Gastroenterology, 1984; 86(5 Pt 1):926–936

1168. Guigui B, Perrot S, Berry JP et al. Amiodarone-induced hepatic phospholipidosis: a morphological alteration independent of pseudoalcoholic liver disease. Hepatology, 1988; 8:1063–1068

1169. Pye M, Northcote RJ, Cobbe SM. Acute hepatitis after parenteral amiodarone administration. Br Heart J, 1988; 59:690–691

1170. Kalantzis N, Gabriel P, Mouzas J et al. Acute amiodarone-induced hepatitis. Hepatogastroenterology, 1991; 38:71–74

1171. Bravo AE, Drewe J, Schlienger RG et al. Hepatotoxicity during rapid intravenous loading with amiodarone: description of three cases and review of the literature. Crit Care Med, 2005; 33:128–134

1172. Gonzalez GA, Garcia Sanchez MV, La Mata Garcia MD et al. Early-onset acute toxic induced by intravenous amiodarone administration. Gastroenterol Hepatol, 2002; 25:392–394

1173. Rhodes A, Eastwood JB, Smith SA. Early acute hepatitis with parenteral amiodarone: a toxic effect of the vehicle? Gut, 1993; 34:565–566

1174. Giannasttasio F, Salvio A, Varriale M. Three cases of severe acute hepatitis after parenteral administration of amiodarone: the active ingredient is not the only agent responsible for hepatotoxicity. Ann Ital Med Int, 2002; 17:180–184

1175. Change C-C, Petrelli M, Tomashefski JF, McCullough AJ. Severe intrahepatic cholestasis caused by amiodarone toxicity after withdrawal of the drug. A case report and review of the literature. Arch Pathol Lab Med, 1999; 123:251–256

1176. Jones DB, Mullick FG, Hoofnagle JH, Baranski B. Reye's syndrome-like illness in a patient receiving amiodarone. Am J Gastroenterol, 1988; 83:967–969

1177. Jacobs G, Calvert C, Kraus M. Hepatopathy in 4 dogs treated with amiodarone. J Vet Intern Med, 2000; 14:96–99

1178. Shepherd NA, Dawson AM, Crocker PR, Levison DA. Granular cells as a marker of early amiodarone hepatotoxicity: a pathological and analytical study. J Clin Pathol, 1987; 40:418–423

1179. Jain D, Bowlus CL, Anderson JM, Robert ME. Granular cells as a marker of early amiodarone hepatotoxicity. J Clin Gastroenterol, 2000; 31:241–243

1180. Larrey D, Pessayre D, Duhamel G et al. Prolonged cholestasis after ajmaline-induced acute hepatitis. J Hepatol, 1986; 2:81–87

1181. Cocozzella D, Curciarello J, Corallini O et al. Propafenone hepatotoxicity: report of two new cases. Dig Dis Sci, 2003; 48:354–357

1182. Gandolfi A, Rota E, Zanghieri G et al. [Acute cholestatic hepatitis caused by propafenone. Report of a case and review of the literature.] Recenti Prog Med, 2001; 92:197–199

1183. Rodman JS, Deutsch DJ, Gutman SI. Methyldopa hepatitis. A report of six cases and review of the literature. Am J Med, 1976; 60:941–948

1184. Toghill PJ, Smith PG, Benton P, Brown RC, Matthews HL. Methyldopa liver damage. BMJ, 1974; 3:545–548

1185. Shaw DR, Misan GH, Johnson RD. Nifedipine hepatitis. Aust N Z J Med, 1987; 17:447–448

1186. Burgunder J-M, Abernethy DR, Lauterberg BH. Liver injury due to verapamil. Hepatogastroenterology, 1988; 35:169–170

1187. Lafuente NG, Egea AM. Calcium channel blockers and hepatotoxicity. Am J Gastroenterol, 2000; 95:2145

1188. Beaugrand M, Denis J, Callard P. Tous les inhibiteurs calciques peuvent-ils entraîner des lésions d'hépatite alcoolique (HA). Gastroenterol Clin Biol, 1987; 11:76

1189. Toft E, Vyberg M, Therkelsen K. Diltiazem-induced granulomatous hepatitis. Histopathology, 1991; 18:474–475

1190. Rahmat J, Gelfand RL, Gelfand MC, Winchester JF, Schreiner GE, Zimmerman HJ. Captopril-associated cholestatic jaundice. Ann Intern Med, 1985; 102:56–58

1191. Nissan A, Spira RM, Sror D, Ackerman Z. Captopril-associated 'pseudocholangitis'. A case report and review of the literature. Arch Surg, 1996; 131:670–671

1192. Rosellini SR, Costa PL, Gaudio M, Saragoni A, Miglio F. Hepatic injury related to enalapril [letter]. Gastroenterology, 1989; 97:810

1193. Jeserich M, Ihling C, Allgaier HP et al. Acute liver failure due to enalapril. Herz, 2000; 25:689–693

1194. Larrey O, Babany G, Bernuacc J et al. Fulminant hepatitis after lisinopril. Gastroenterology, 1990; 99:1832–1833

1195. Droste HT, de Vries RA. Chronic hepatitis caused by lisinopril. Nether J Med, 1995; 46:95–98

1196. Yeung E, Wong FS, Wanless IR et al. Ramipril-associated hepatotoxicity. Arch Pathol Lab Med, 2003; 127:1493–1497

1197. Clark JA, Tanner LA, Zimmerman HJ. Labetalol and hepatocellular reactions. Ann Intern Med, 1990; 113:210

1198. Tanner LA, Bosco LA, Zimmernan HJ. Hepatic toxity after acebutolol therapy. Ann Intern Med, 1989; 111:533–534

1199. Schwartz MS. Atenolol-associated cholestasis. Am J Gastroenterol, 1989; 184:1084–1088

1200. Bosch X. Losartan-induced hepatotoxicity [letter]. JAMA, 1997; 278:1572

1201. Basile G, Villari D, Gangemi S et al. Candesartan cilexetil-induced severe hepatotoxicity. J Clin Gastroenterol, 2003; 36:273–275

1202. Andrade RJ, Lucena MI, Fernandez MC et al. Cholestatic hepatitis related to use of irbesartan: a case report and a literature review of angiotensin II antagonist-associated hepatotoxicity. Eur J Gastroenterol Hepatol, 2002; 14:887–890

1203. Pariente EA, Pessayre D, Bernuau J, Degott C, Benhamou J-P. Dihydralazine hepatitis. Report of a case and review of the literature. Digestion, 1983; 27:47–52

1204. Myers JL, Augur NA. Hydralazine-induced cholangitis. Gastroenterology, 1984; 87:1185–1188

1205. Qu B, Li QT, Wong KP et al. Mechanism of clofibrate hepatotoxicity: mitochondrial damage and oxidative stress in hepatocytes. Free Radic Biol Med, 2001; 31:659–669

1206. Valdes M, Jacobs WH. Intrahepatic cholestasis following the use of Atromid-s. Am J Gastroenterol, 1976; 66:69

1207. Pierce EH, Chesler DL. Possible association of granulomatous hepatitis with clofibrate therapy. N Engl J Med, 1978; 299:314

1208. Chen C, Hennig GE, Whiteley HE et al. Protection against acetaminophen hepatotoxicity by clofibrate pretreatment: role of catalase induction. J Biochem Mol Toxicol, 2002; 16:227–234

1209. Pichon N, Vincensini JF, Roziere A et al. [Acute cytolytic and cholestatic hepatitis induced by fenofibrate.] Gastroenterol Clin Biol, 2003; 27:947–949

1210. Mullen KE, Greenson JK, Mitchell MC. Fulminant hepatic failure after ingestion of sustained release nicotinic acid. Ann Intern Med, 1989; 111:253–255

1211. Parra JL, Reddy KR. Hepatotoxicity of hypolipidemic drugs. Clin Liver Dis, 2003; 7:415–433

1212. Pieper JA. Overview of niacin formulations: differences in pharmacokinetics, efficacy, and safety. Am J Health Syst Pharm, 2003; 60(13 Suppl 2):S9–S14

1213. Raveh D, Arnon R, Israeli A, Eisenberg S. Lovastatin-induced hepatitis. Isr J Med Sci, 1992; 28:101–102

1214. Koornstra JT, Ottervanger JP, Fehmers MC et al. Clinically manifest liver lesions during use of simvastatin. Ned Tijdschr Geneeskd, 1996; 140:846–848

1215. Hartleb M, Rymarczyk G, Januszewski K. Acute cholestatic hepatitis associated with pravastatin. Am J Gastroenterol, 1999; 94:1388–1390

1216. Nakad A, Bataille L, Hamoir V, Sempoux C, Horsmans Y. Atorvastatin-induced acute hepatitis with absence of cross-toxicity with simvastatin. Lancet, 1999; 353:1763–1764

1217. Gershovich OE, Lyman AE Jr. Liver function abnormalities and pruritus in a patient treated with atorvastatin: case report and review of the literature. Pharmacotherapy, 2004; 24(1):150–154

1218. Bottorff M, Hansten P. Long-term safety of hepatic hydroxymethyl glutaryl coenzyme A reductase inhibitors. Arch Intern Med, 2000; 160:2273–2280

1219. Tolman KG. Defining patient risks from expanded preventive therapies. Am J Cardiol, 2000; 85:15E–19E

1220. Kornbrust DJ, MacDonald JS, Peter CP et al. Toxicity of the HMG-coenzyme A reductase inhibitor, lovastatin, to rabbits. J Pharmacol Exp Ther, 1989; 248:498–505

1221. Jones PH, Davidson MH, Stein EA et al. Comparison of the efficacy and safety of rosuvastatin versus atorvastatin, simvastatin, and pravastatin across doses (STELLAR trial). Am J Cardiol, 2003; 92:152–160

1222. Pfeffer MA, Keech A, Sacks FM et al. Safety and tolerability of pravastatin in long-term clinical trials. Circulation, 2002; 105:2341–2346

1223. Graham DJ, Staffa JA, Shatin D et al. Incidence of hospitalized rhabdomyolysis in patients treated with lipid-lowering drugs. JAMA, 2004; 292:2585–2590

1224. Smith CC, Bernstein LI, Davis RB et al. Screening for statin-related toxicity: the yield of transaminase and creatine kinase measurements in a primary care setting. Arch Intern Med, 2003; 163:688–692

1225. Sniderman AD. Is there value in liver function test and creatine phosphokinase monitoring with statin use? Am J Cardiol, 2004; 94(9A):30F–34F

1226. Chalasani N, Hall SD. Statin-induced hepatotoxicity [reply]. Gastroenterology, 2004; 127:1278–1279

1227. Kiortsis DN, Nikas S, Hatzidimou K et al. Lipid-lowering drugs and serum liver enzymes: the effects of body weight and baseline enzyme levers. Fundam Clin Pharmacol, 2003; 17:491–494

1228. Walker RM, McElligott TF. Furosemide induced hepatotoxicity. J Pathol, 1981; 135:301–314

1229. Manier JW, Chang WW, Kirchner JP, Beltaos E. Hepatotoxicity associated with ticrynafen—a uricosuric diuretic. Am J Gastroenterol, 1982; 77:401–404

1230. Zimmerman HJ, Lewis JH, Ishak KG, Maddrey WC. Ticrynafen-associated hepatic injury: analysis of 340 cases. Hepatology, 1984; 4:315–323

1231. Neuberger J, Williams R. Immune mechanisms in tienilic acid associated hepatotoxicity. Gut, 1989; 30:515–519

1232. Nakhleh RE, Ween C, Snover DC, Grage T. Venoocclusive lesions of the central veins and portal vein radicles secondary to 5-fluoro-2–deoxyuridine infusion. Hum Pathol, 1989; 20:1218–1220

1233. King PD, Perry MC. Hepatotoxicity of chemotherapeutic and oncologic agents. Gastroenterol Clin North Am, 1995; 24:969–990

1234. DeLeve LD. Cancer chemotherapy. In: Kaplowitz N, DeLeve LD, eds. Drug-induced liver disease. New York: Marcel Dekker, 2003: pp 593–632

1235. Schein PS, Winokur SH. Immunosuppressive and cytotoxic chemotherapy: long-term complications. Ann Intern Med, 1975; 82:84–95

1236. McIntosh S, Davidson DL, O'Brien RT, Pearson HA. Methotrexate hepatotoxicity in children with leukemia. J Pediatr, 1977; 90:1019–1021

1237. Bellet RE, Mastrangelo MJ, Engstrom PF, Custer RP. Hepatotoxicity of 5-azacytidine. A clinical and pathologic study. Neoplasma, 1973; 20:303–309

1238. Ganesan TS, Barnett MJ, Amos RJ et al. Cytosine arabinoside in the management of recurrent leukemia. Hematol Oncol, 1987; 5:65–69

1239. Bateman JR, Pugh RP, Cassidey FR, Marshal GJ, Irwin LE. 5-Fluorouracil given once weekly: comparison of intravenous and oral administration. Cancer, 1971; 78:907–913

1240. Hruban Z, Swift H, Slesers R. Effect of azaserine on the fine structure of the liver and pancreatic acinar cells. Cancer Res, 1965; 25:708–723

1241. Shorey J, Schenker S, Suki WN, Combes B. Hepatotoxicity of mercaptopurine. Arch Intern Med, 1968; 122:54–58

1242. Nygaard U, Toft N, Schmiegelow K. Methylated metabolites of 6-mercaptopurine are associated with hepatotoxicity. Clin Pharmacol Ther, 2004; 75:274–281

1243. Kontorinis N, Agarwal K, Gondolesi G et al. Diagnosis of 6-mercaptopurine hepatotoxicity post liver transplantation utilizing metabolite assays. Am J Transplant, 2004; 4:1539–1542

1244. Minow RA, Stern MH, Casey JH, Rodriguez V, Luna M. Clinicopathological correlation of liver damage in patients treated with 6-mercaptopurine and adriamycin. Cancer, 1976; 38:1524–1528

1245. Rodriguez V, Bodey GP, McCredie KB et al. Combination 6-mercaptopurine-adriamycin in refractory adult acute leukemia. Clin Pharm Ther, 1975; 18:462–466

1246. DePinto RO, Goldberg CS, Lefkowtich JH. Azathioprine and the liver. Evidence favoring idiosyncratic mixed cholestatic-hepatocellular injury in man. Gastroenterology, 1984; 86:162

1247. Adler M, Delhaye M, Deprez C et al. Hepatic vascular disease after kidney transplantation. Report of two cases review of the literature. Nephrol Dial Transplant, 1987; 2:183

1248. Marubbio AT, Danielson B. Hepatic veno-occlusive disease in a renal transplant patient receiving azathioprine. Gastroenterology, 1975; 69:739–743

1249. Haboubi NY, Ali HH, Whitwell HL et al. Role of endothelial cell injury in the spectrum of azathioprine-induced liver disease after renal transplant: light microscopy and ultrastructural observations. Am J Gastroenterol, 1988; 83:256–261

1250. Sacian K, Franco J, Komorowski RA, Adams MB. Hepatocellular carcinoma after renal transplantation in the absence of cirrhosis of viral hepatitis: a case series. Liver Transplant Surg, 1999; 5:46–49

1251. Haskell CM, Canellos GP, Leventhal BG et al. L-asparaginase. Therapeutic and toxic effects in patients with neoplastic disease. N Engl J Med, 1969; 281:1028–1034

1252. Aviles A, Herrera J, Ramos E, Ambriz R, Aguirre J, Pizzuto J. Hepatic injury during doxorubicin therapy. Arch Pathol Lab Med, 1984; 108:912–913

1253. McVeagh P, Ekert H. Hepatotoxicity of chemotherapy following nephrectomy and radiation therapy for right-sided Wilms' tumor. J Pediatr, 1975; 87:627–628

1254. Costa G, Hreshchyshyn MM, Holland JF. Initial clinical studies with vincristine. Cancer Chemother Rep, 1962; 24:39–44

1255. El Saghir NS, Hawkins KA. Hepatotoxicity following vincristine therapy. Cancer, 1984; 54:2006–2008

1256. Hansen MM, Ranek L, Walbon S, Nisson NI. Fatal hepatitis following irradiation and vincristine. Acta Med Scand, 1982; 212:171–174

1257. Fisher B, Keenan AM, Garra BS et al. Interleukin-2 induces profound reversible cholestasis: a detailed analysis in treated patients. J Clin Oncol, 1989; 7:1852–1862

1258. Kragel AH, Travis WD, Feinberg L et al. Pathologic findings associated with interleukin-2-based immunotherapy for cancer: a postmortem study of 19 patients. Hum Pathol, 1990; 21:493–502

1259. Hoffman M, Mittelman A, Dworkin B et al. Severe intrahepatic cholestasis in patients treated with recombinant interleukin-2 and lymphokine activated killer cells. J Cancer Res Clin Oncol, 1989; 115:175–178

1260. Kovalovich K, DeAngelis RA, Li W et al. Increased toxin-induced liver injury and fibrosis in interleukin-6-deficient mice. Hepatology, 2000; 31:149–159

1261. Aubrey DA. Massive hepatic necrosis after cyclophosphamide [letter]. BMJ, 1970; 3:588

1262. Bacon AM, Rosenberg SA. Cyclophosphamide hepatotoxicity in a patient with systemic lupus erythamatosus. Ann Intern Med, 1982; 97:62–63

1263. Snyder LS, Heigh RI, Anderson ML. Cyclophosphamide-induced hepatotoxicity in a patient with Wegener's granulomatosis. Mayo Clin Proc, 1993; 68:1203–1204

1264. Mok C-C, Wong W-M, Shek T W-H, Ho C T-K, Lau C-S, Lai C-L. Cumulative hepatotoxicity induced by continuous low-dose cyclophosphamide therapy. Am J Gastroenterol, 2000; 95:845–846

1265. Shaunak S, Munro JM, Weinbren K, Walport MJ, Cox TM. Cyclophosphamide-induced liver necrosis: a possible interaction with azathioprine. Q J Med (New Series), 1988; 67:309–317

1266. Modzelewski JR Jr, Doeschner C, Joshi VV, Mullick FG, Ishak KG. Veno-occlusive disease of the liver induced by low-dose cyclophosphamide. Mod Pathol, 1994; 7:967–972

1267. Morris LE, Guthrie TH. Busulfan-induced hepatitis. Am J Gastroenterol, 1988; 83:682–683

1268. Robinson K, Lambiase L, Li J et al. Fatal cholestatic liver failure associated with gemcitabine therapy. Dig Dis Sci, 2003; 48:1804–1808

1269. Giles FJ, Kantarjian HM, Kornblau SM et al. Mylotarg (gemtuzumab ozogamicin) therapy is associated with hepatic venoocclusive disease in patients who have not received stem cell transplantation. Cancer, 2001; 92:406–413

1270. Cohen AD, Luger SM, Sickles C et al. Gemtuzumab ozogamicin (Mylotarg) monotherapy for relapsed AML after hematopoietic stem cell transplant: efficacy and incidence of hepatic veno-occlusive disease. Bone Marrow Transplant, 2002; 30:23–28

1271. Rajvanshi P, Shulman HM, Sievers EL, McDonald GB. Hepatic sinusoidal obstruction after gemtuzumab ozogamicin (Mylotarg) therapy. Blood, 2002; 99:2310–2314

1272. Cersosimo RJ. Monoclonal antibodies in the treatment of cancer, Part 2. Am J Health Syst Pharm, 2003; 60:1631–1641

1273. Ayoub WS, Geller SA, Tran T et al. Imatinib (Gleevec)-induced hepatotoxicity. J Clin Gastroenterol, 2005; 39:75–77

1274. Choudari Kommineni VR, Greenblatt M, Vesselinovitch SD, Mihailovich N. Urethane carcinogenesis in rats. Importance of age and dose. J Natl Cancer Inst, 1970; 45:687–696

1275. Hoofnagle JH, Dusheiko GM, Schafer DF. Reactivation of chronic hepatitis B virus infection by cancer chemotherapy. Ann Intern Med, 1982; 94:447–449

1276. Pinto PC, Hu E, Bernstein-Singer M, Pinter-Brown L, Govindarajan S. Acute hepatic injury after the withdrawal of immunosuppressive chemotherapy in patients with hepatitis B. Cancer, 1990; 65:878–884

1277. Vento S, Cainelli F, Mirandola F et al. Fulminant hepatitis on withdrawal of chemotherapy in carriers of hepatitis C virus. Lancet, 1996; 347:92–93

1278. Pagani A, Rizzetto M. Clofeniramine hepatotoxicity. Ital J Gastroenterol, 1987; 19:179

1279. Kew MC, Segel J, Zoutendyk A. Hypersensitivity hepatitis associated with administration of cyclizine. BMJ, 1973; 2:307

1280. Borda I, Jick H. Hepatitis following the administration of trimethobenzamide hydrochloride. Arch Intern Med, 1967; 120:371–373

1281. Larrey D, Geneve J, Pessayre D, Machaykhi J-P, Degott C, Benhamou J-P. Prolonged cholestasis after cyproheptadine-induced acute hepatitis. J Clin Gastroenterol, 1987; 9:102–104

1282. Sahai A, Villeneuve JP. Terfenadine-induced hepatitis. Lancet, 1996; 348:552–553

1283. Schiano TD, Bellary SV, Cassidy MJ et al. Subfulminant liver failure and severe hepatotoxicity caused by loratadine use. Ann Intern Med, 1996; 9:738

1284. Watanabe M, Kohge N, Kaji T. Severe hepatitis in a patient taking cetirizine. Ann Intern Med, 2001; 1354:142–143

1285. Pompili M, Basso M, Grieco A et al. Recurrent acute hepatitis associated with use of cetirizine. Ann Pharmacother, 2004; 38:1844–1847

1286. Lewis JH. Hepatic effects of drugs used in the treatment of peptic ulcer disease. Am J Gastroenterol, 1987; 82:987–1003

1287. Bashir RM, Lewis JH. Hepatotoxicity of drugs used in the treatment of gastrointestinal disorders. Gastroenterol Clin North Am, 1995; 24:937–967

1288. Garcia Rodriguez LA, Wallander MA, Stricker BH. The risk of acute liver injury associated with cimetidine and other acid-suppressing anti-ulcer drugs. Br J Clin Pharmacol, 1997; 43:183–188

1289. Ramrakhiani S, Brunt EM, Bacon BR. Possible cholestatic injury from ranitidine with a review of the literature. Am J Gastroenterol, 1998; 93:822–826

1290. Ribeiro JM, Lucas M, Baptista A et al. Fatal hepatitis associated with ranitidine. Am J Gastroenterol, 2000; 95:559–560

1291. Luyendyk JP, Maddox JF, Green CD et al. Role of hepatic fibrin in idiosyncrasy-like liver injury from lipopolysaccharide-ranitidine coexposure in rats. Hepatology, 2004; 40:1342–1351

1292. Boyd PT, Lepre F, Dickey JD. Chronic active hepatitis associated with cimetidine. BMJ, 1989; 298:324–325

1293. Clarke B, Yoong A. Prolonged cholestasis and cimetidine [letter]. Dig Dis Sci, 1987; 32:333

1294. Andrade RJ, Lucena MI, Martin-Vivaldi R et al. Acute liver injury associated with use of ebrotidine, a new H2-receptor antagonist. J Hepatol, 1999; 31:641–646

1295. Pineda JA, Larrauri J, Macias J et al. Rapid progression to liver cirrhosis of toxic hepatitis due to ebrotidine [letter]. J Hepatol, 1999; 31:777–779

1296. Zimmerman HJ, Jacob L, Bassan H et al. Effects of H2-blocking agents on hepatocytes in vitro: correlation with potential for causing hepatic disease in patients. Proc Soc Exp Biol Med, 1986; 182:511–514

1297. Farup PG. Zaltidine: an effective but hepatotoxic H2-receptor antagonist. Scand J Gastroenterol, 1988; 23:655–658

1298. Navarro JF, Gallego E, Aviléz J. Recurrent severe acute hepatitis and omeprazole. Ann Intern Med, 1997; 127:1135–1136

1299. Romero-Gómez M, Otero MA, Suárez-Garcia E, Garcia-Diaz E, Fobelo MJ, Castro-Fernández M. Acute hepatitis related to omeprazole [letter]. Am J Gastroenterol, 1999; 94:1119–1120

1300. Jocken V, Kirkpatrick R, Sorenson J et al. Fulminant hepatic failure related to omeprazole. Am J Gastroenterol, 1993; 87:523–525

1301. Christe C, Stoller R, Vogt N. Omeprazole-induced hepatotoxicity? A case report. Pharmacoepidemiol Drug Saf, 1998; 7(Suppl 1): S41–S44

1302. Andrade RJ, Lucena MI. Acute fulminant hepatitis after treatment with rabeprazole and terbinafine: is rabeprazole the culprit? Arch Intern Med, 2002; 162:360–361

1303. Reynolds TB, Peters RL, Yamada S. Chronic active and lupoid hepatitis caused by a laxative oxyphenisation. N Engl J Med, 1971; 285:813

1304. Delchier JC, Metreau JM, Levy VG et al. [Oxyphenisatin, a laxative responsible for chronic hepatitis and cirrhosis, still marketed in France.] Nouv Presse Med, 1979; 8:2955–2958

1305. Merker HJ, Henning H, Vogel HM. [Electron microscopy picture of oxyphenisatin-induced liver damage.] Z Gastroenterol, 1976; 14:779–795

1306. Dietrichson O, Juhl E, Nielsen JO et al. The incidence of oxyphenisatin-induced liver damage in chronic non-alcoholic liver disease. A control investigation. Scand J Gastroenterol, 1974; 9:473

1307. Reynolds JD, Wilber RD. Chronic active hepatitis associated with oxyphenisatin. Am J Gastroenterol, 1972; 57:566–570

1308. Sotolongo RP, Neefe LI, Rudzki C et al. Hypersensitivity reaction to sulfasalazine with severe hepatotoxicity. Gastroenterology, 1978; 75:95–99

1309. Fich A, Schwartz J, Braverman D, Zifroni A, Rachmilewitz D. Sulfasalazine hepatotoxicity. Am J Gastroenterol, 1984; 79:401–402

1310. Ribe RJ, Benkov KJ, Thung SN, Shen SC, Le Leioko NS. Fatal massive hepatic necrosis: a probable hypersensitivity reaction to sulfasalazine. Am J Gastroenterol, 1986; 81:205–208

1311. Boyer DL, Ulysses B, Li K, Fyda JN, Friedman RA. Sulfasalazine-induced hepatotoxicity in children with inflammatory bowel disease. J Pediatr Gastroenterol Nutr, 1989; 8:528–532

1312. Rubin R. Sulfasalazine-induced hepatic failure and necrotizing pancreatitis. Am J Gastroenterol, 1994; 89:789–791

1313. Carr-Locke DL, Ali M. Glandular fever-like illness associated with sulphasalazine. Postgrad Med J, 1982; 58:665–666

1314. Nahmias A. Reversible sulfasalazine-induced granulomatous hepatitis. J Clin Gastroenterol, 1981; 3:193–198

1315. Deltenre P, Berson A, Marcellin P, Degott C, Biour M, Pessayre D. Mesalazine (5-aminosalicylic acid) induced chronic hepatitis. Gut, 1999; 44:886–888

1316. Hautekeete ML, Bourgeois N, Potvin P et al. Hypersensitivity with hepatotoxicity to mesalazine after hypersensitivity to sulfasalazine. Gastroenterology, 1992; 103:1925–1927

1317. Ransford RA, Langman MJ. Sulphasalazine and mesalazine: serious adverse reactions re-evaluated on the basis of suspected adverse reaction reports to the Committee on Safety of Medicines. Gut, 2002; 51:536–539

1318. Gross R, Scapa E. Hepatotoxicity of 6-mercaptopurine in Crohn's disease [letter]. Am J Gastroenterol, 1992; 87:1885–1886

1319. Menghini VM, Amindra SA. Infliximab-associated reversible cholestatic liver disease. Mayo Clin Proc, 2001; 76:84–86

1320. Menghini VF, Arora AS. Infliximab-associated reversible cholestatic liver disease. Mayo Clin Proc, 2001; 76:84–86

1321. Saleem G, Li SC, MacPherson BR. Hepatitis with interface inflammation and IgG, IgM, and IgA anti-double-stranded DNA antibodies following infliximab therapy. Arthritis Rheum, 2001; 44:1966–1968

1322. Michel M, Duvoux C, Hezode C et al. Fulminant hepatitis after infliximab in a patient with hepatitis B virus treated for adult onset Still's disease. J Rheumatol, 2003; 30:1624–1625

1323. Naveau S, Chollet-Martin S, Dharancy S et al. A double-blind randomized controlled trial of infliximab associated with prednisolone in acute alcoholic hepatitis. Hepatology, 2004; 39:1390–1397

1324. Zimmerman HJ. Acetaminophen hepatoxicity. Clin Liver Dis, 1998; 2:533–541

1325. Black M. Acetaminophen hepatotoxicity. Annu Rev Med, 1984; 35:577–593

1326. Bromer MQ, Black M. Acetaminophen hepatotoxicity. Clin Liver Dis, 2003; 7:351–367

1327. Rumack BH. Acetaminophen hepatotoxicity: the first 35 years. J Toxicol Clin Toxicol, 2002; 40:3–20

1328. Zimmerman HJ, Maddrey WC. Acetaminophen (paracetamol) hepatotoxicity with regular intake of alcohol: analysis of instances of therapeutic misadventure. Hepatology, 1995; 22:767–773

1329. Heubi JE, Barbacci MB, Zimmerman HJ. Therapeutic misadventures with acetaminophen: hepatoxicity after multiple doses in children. J Pediatr, 1998; 132:22–27

1330. Portmann B, Talbot IC, Day DW et al. Histopathological changes in the liver following a paracetamol overdose: correlation with clinical and biochemical parameters. J Pathol, 1975; 2:579–585

1331. Lindgren A, Aldenborg F, Norkrans G, Olaison L, Olsson R. Paracetamol-induced cholestatic injury and granulomatous liver injury. J Intern Med, 1997; 241:435–439

1332. Lee WM, Ostapowicz G. Acetaminophen: pathology and clinical presentation of hepatotoxicity. In: Kaplowitz N, DeLeve LD, eds. Drug-induced liver disease. New York: Marcel Dekker, 2003: pp 327–344

1333. Rumack BH. Acetaminophen misconceptions. Hepatology, 2004; 40:10–15

1334. Prescott LF. Paracetamol, alcohol and the liver. Br J Clin Pharmacol, 2000; 49:291–301

1335. Rumack BH, Peterson RG. Acetaminophen overdosage: incidence, diagnosis, and management in 416 patients. Pediatrics, 1978; 62:880–886

1336. Bergeron L, Guy C, Ratrema M et al. [Dextropropoxyphene hepatotoxicity: four cases and literature review.] Therapie, 2002; 57:464–472

1337. Khouri MR, Saul SH, Dlugosz AA, Soloway RD. Hepatocanalicular injury associated with vitamin A derivative etretinate, an idiosyncratic hypersensitivity reaction. Dig Dis Sci, 1987; 32:1207–1211

1338. Weiss V, Spinowitz A, Buys CM, Nemehausky BA, West DP, Emmons KM. Chronic active hepatitis associated with etretinate therapy. Br J Dermatol, 1985; 112:591–597

1339. Kamm MA, Davies DJ, Breen KJ. Acute hepatitis due to etretinate. J Gastroenterol Hepatol, 1988; 3:663–666

1340. van Ditzhuijsen TJM, van Haelst UJGM, van Dooren-Greebe RJ, van de Karkhof PCM, Yap SH. Severe hepatotoxic reaction with progression to cirrhosis after use of novel retinoid (acetretin). J Hepatol, 1990; 11:185–188

1341. Whitington PF. Cholestasis associated with parenteral nutrition in infants. Hepatology, 1985; 5:693

1342. Mullick FG, Moran CA, Ishak KG. Total parenteral nutrition: a histopathologic analysis of the liver changes in 20 children. Mod Pathol, 1994; 7:190–194

1343. Fleming CR. Hepatobiliary complications in adults receiving nutrition support. Dig Dis Sci, 1994; 12:191–198

1344. Briones ER, Iber FL. Liver and biliary tract changes and injury associated with total parenteral nutrition: pathogenesis and prevention. J Am Coll Nutr, 1995; 14:219–228

1345. Bashir RM, Lipman TO. Hepatobiliary toxicity of total parenteral nutrition in adults. Gastroenterol Clin North Am, 1995; 24:1003–1025

1346. Kwan V, George J. Liver disease due to parenteral and enteral nutrition. Clin Liver Dis, 2004; 8:893–913

1347. Degott C, Messing B, Moreau D et al. Liver phospholipidosis induced by parenteral nutrition: histologic, histochemical, and ultrastructural investigations. Gastroenterology, 1988; 95:183–191

1348. McLead RE, Birken G, Wheller JJ, Hansen NB, Bickers RG, Menke JA. Budd-Chiari syndrome in a premature infant receiving total parenteral nutrition. J Pediatr Gastroenterol Nutr, 1986; 5:655–658

1349. Vileisis RA, Sorensen K, Gonzalez-Crussi F, Hunt CE. Liver malignancy after parenteral nutrition. J Pediatr, 1982; 100:88–90

1350. Patterson K, Kapur SP, Chandra RS. Hepatocellular carcinoma in a noncirrhotic infant after prolonged parenteral nutrition. J Pediatr, 1985; 106:797–800

1351. Pitt HA, King III W, Mann LL et al. Increased risk of cholelithiasis with prolonged total parenteral nutrition. Am J Surg, 1983; 145:106–111

1352. Hebert MF, Taylor SL, Carithers RL. Immunomodulating agents and the transplant situation. In: Kaplowitz N, DeLeve LD, eds. Drug-induced liver disease. New York: Marcel Dekker, 2003: pp 633–651

1353. Klintmalm GBG, Iwatsuki S, Starzl TE. Cyclosporin A hepatotoxicity in 66 renal allograft recipients. Transplantation, 1981; 32:488–489

1354. Myara A, Cadranel JF, Dorent R et al. Cyclosporin A-mediated cholestasis in patients with chronic hepatitis after heart transplantation. Eur J Gastroenterol Hepatol, 1996; 8:267–271

1355. Wisecarver JL, Earl RA, Timmins PW et al. Histologic changes in liver allograft biopsies associated with elevated whole blood and tissue cyclosporine concentrations. Mod Pathol, 1992; 5:611–615

1356. Kassianides C, Nussenblatt R, Palestine AG, Mellow SD, Hoofnagle JH. Liver injury from cyclosporine A. Dig Dis Sci, 1990; 35:693–697

1357. Chan FKL, Shaffer EA. Cholestatic effects of cyclosporine in the rat. Transplantation, 1997; 63:1574–1578

1358. Durak I, Ozbek H, Elgun S. Cyclosporine reduces hepatic antioxidant capacity: protective roles of antioxidants. Int Immunopharmacol, 2004; 4:469–473

1359. Fisher A, Mor E, Hytiroglou P et al. FK506 hepatotoxicity in liver allograft recipients. Transplantation, 1995; 59:1631–1632

1360. Hytiroglou P, Lee R, Sharma K et al. FK 506 versus cyclosporine as primary immunosuppressive agent for orthotopic liver allograft recipients: histologic and immunopathologic observations. Transplantation, 1993; 56:1389–1394

1361. Neff GW, Ruiz P, Madariaga JR et al. Sirolimus-associated hepatotoxicity in liver transplantation. Ann Pharmacother, 2004; 38:1593–1596

1362. Eisen HJ, Ginsberg AL. Disulfiram-hepatotoxicity. Ann Intern Med, 1975; 83:673–674

1363. Nassberger L. Disulfiram-induced hepatitis—a report of a case and review of the literature. Postgrad Med J, 1984; 60:639–641

1364. Berlin RG. Disulfiram hepatotoxicity: a consideration of its mechanism and clinical spectrum. Alcohol Alcohol, 1989; 24:241–245

1365. Forns X, Caballeria J, Bruguera M et al. Disulfiram-induced hepatitis. Report of four cases and review of the literature. J Hepatol, 1994; 21:853–857

1366. Sellers EM, Naranjo CA, Peachey JE. Drug therapy: drugs to decrease alcohol consumption. N Engl J Med, 1981; 305:1255–1262

1367. Ceriani R, Borroni G, Bissoli F. Ritodrine-related hepatic injury. Case reports and review of the literature. Ital J Gastroenterol Hepatol, 1998; 30:315–317

1368. Jochimsen EM, Carmichael WW, Cardo DM et al. Liver failure and death after exposure to microcystins at a hemodialysis center in Brazil. N Engl J Med, 1998; 338:873–878

1369. Grieco AJ, Burnstein-Stein J. Oral montelukast versus inhaled salmeterol to prevent exercise-induced bronchoconstriction. Ann Intern Med, 2000; 133:392–393

1370. Reinus JF, Persky S, Burkiewicz JS et al. Severe liver injury after treatment with leukotriene receptor antagonist zafirlukast. Ann Intern Med, 2000; 188:964–968

1371. Su CW, Wu JC, Huang YH et al. Zafirlukast-induced acute hepatitis. Zhonghua Yi Xue Za Zhi (Taipei), 2002; 65:553–556

1372. Davern TJ, Bass NM. Leukotriene antagonists. Clin Liver Dis, 2003; 7:501–512

1373. Danese S, De Vitis I, Gasbarrini A. Severe liver injury associated with zafirlukast. Ann Intern Med, 2001; 135:930

1374. Cocozzella D, Curciarello J, Carallini O et al. Propafenone hepatotoxicity: report of two new cases. Dig Dis Sci, 2003; 48:354–357

1375. Grieco A, Forgione A, Giorgi A et al. Propafenone-related cholestatic hepatitis in an elderly patient. Ital Heart J, 2002; 3:431–434

1376. Fowler R, Imrie K. Thalidomide-associated hepatitis: a case report. Am J Hematol, 2001; 66:300–302

1377. Lewis JH. The rational use of potentially hepatotoxic medications in patients with underlying liver disease. Expert Opin Drug Saf, 2002; 1:159–172

1378. Homberg JC, Abuaf N, Helmi-Khalil S et al. Drug-induced hepatitis with anticytoplasmic organelle antibodies. Hepatology, 1985; 5:722–727

1379. Maria VAJ, Victorino RMM. Diagnostic value of specific T cell reactivity to drugs in 95 cases of drug induced liver injury. Gut, 1997; 41:534–540

1380. Aithal GP, Rawlins MD, Day CP. Clinical diagnostic scale: a useful tool in the evaluation of suspected hepatotoxic adverse drug reactions. J Hepatol, 2000; 33:949–954

1381. Maria VA, Victorino RM. Development and validation of a clinical scale for the diagnosis of drug-induced hepatitis. Hepatology, 1997; 26:664–669

1382. Lee WM. Assessing causality in drug-induced liver injury. J Hepatol, 2000; 33:1003–1005

1383. Zapater P, Such J, Perez-Mateo M, Horga JF. A new Poisson and Bayesian-based method to assign risk and causality in patients with suspected hepatic adverse drug reactions: a report of two new cases of ticlopidine-induced hepatotoxicity. Drug Saf, 2002; 25:735–750

1384. Lucena MI, Camargo R, Andrade RJ et al. Comparison of two clinical scales for causality assessment in hepatotoxicity. Hepatology, 2001; 33:123–130

1385. Andrade RJ, Camargo R, Lucena MI, Gonzalez-Grande R. Causality assessment in drug-induced hepatotoxicity. Expert Opin Drug Saf, 2004; 3:329–344

1386. Larrey D. Epidemiology and individual susceptibility to adverse drug reactions affecting the liver. Semin Liver Dis, 2002; 22:145–155

Tumours and tumour-like lesions of the liver

15

Zachary D. Goodman   Luigi M. Terracciano

Mass lesions in the liver represent a number of disease processes that frequently prompt patients to seek medical attention. Rapidly growing tumours produce abdominal symptoms and even slowly growing tumours, both benign and malignant, may outgrow their blood supply with subsequent infarction and haemorrhage into the tumour or the peritoneal cavity. Some lesions, particularly small benign tumours, may be clinically silent and are only discovered when the patient is evaluated for some other reason. Small tumours may also be detected in asymptomatic patients in screening programs because of increased risk of hepatic malignancy; for example those with chronic viral hepatitis at risk for hepatocellular carcinoma (HCC), or those with primary sclerosing cholangitis at risk for cholangiocarcinoma. This chapter deals with the principal neoplasms and other mass lesions that may occur in the liver. The classification (Table 15.1) follows that of the World Heath Organization Classification of Tumours[1] and the Armed Forces Institute of Pathology Atlas of Tumour Pathology,[2] rearranged to emphasize the histogenesis of the lesions. Although the emphasis is on primary liver tumours, it is important to remember that metastases far outnumber primary tumours, and so these are always considered in differential diagnosis.

The clinical scenario is an important feature in the differential diagnosis of any mass lesion in the liver. Age, gender and predisposing factors such as underlying liver disease or exposure to drugs, chemicals, or parasites influence the likelihood of development of many tumours (Table 15.2). Consequently, one should be very circumspect about diagnosing a tumour of infancy, such as hepatoblastoma, in an adult or a tumour such as hepatocellular adenoma that is strongly associated with oral contraceptive steroids in an elderly male. Rare cases may occur in atypical hosts, but such diagnoses should be questioned and verified. Some tumours, especially HCC, have a striking geographic distribution, due primarily to its association with chronic hepatitis B infection and other chronic liver diseases.

Detection and evaluation of hepatic mass lesions nearly always involves radiological imaging techniques.[3,4] These have evolved rapidly over the past three decades, and the technology continues to advance. The major modalities used to identify and characterize mass lesions are variations of ultrasound (US),[5,6] computed tomography (CT),[7,8] and magnetic resonance imaging (MRI) (Chapter 1).[9,10] When combined with various contrast media, these can provide images to characterize both the lesions and the blood supply to the lesions. The images may be sufficiently characteristic to provide firm diagnosis of some tumours, especially cavernous haemangiomas, or strongly suggest the diagnosis of others, such as focal nodular hyperplasia. In most instances, however, a biopsy is required for definitive diagnosis.

In some cases, clinical information can support imaging studies to give a strong presumptive diagnosis; for example, a mass shown to enlarge on sequential imaging studies over several months in a patient with chronic viral hepatitis and cirrhosis and rising serum α-fetoprotein is almost certainly HCC. Consequently, patients at risk for developing HCC because of chronic liver disease may undergo periodic surveillance with imaging, most often ultrasound, and serum tumour markers, most often α-fetoprotein, in an attempt to detect tumours at a curative stage. It has been suggested that

Table 15.1 Abbreviated classification of primary tumours and tumour-like lesions of the liver

	Benign	Malignant
Hepatocellular tumours	Hepatocellular adenoma Focal nodular hyperplasia Dysplastic nodule	Hepatocellular carcinoma Fibrolamellar hepatocellular carcinoma Combined hepatocellular-cholangiocarcinoma Carcinosarcoma Hepatoblastoma
Biliary tumours	Von Meyenburg complex Bile duct cyst Ciliated foregut cyst Peribiliary gland hamartoma Biliary papillomatosis Biliary cystadenoma	Biliary cystadenocarcinoma Cholangiocarcinoma
Vascular tumours	Haemangioma Infantile haemangioendothelioma	Angiosarcoma Epithelioid haemangioendothelioma
Other tumours	Angiomyolipoma Mesenchymal hamartoma Inflammatory pseudotumour	Primary lymphomas Other sarcomas and rare tumours

Table 15.2 Clinical features of liver tumours

Tumours of infancy and young children	Infantile haemangioendothelioma Mesenchymal hamartoma Hepatoblastoma
Tumours of older children and young adults	Fibrolamellar hepatocellular carcinoma Embryonal sarcoma
Tumours much more frequent in men	Hepatocellular carcinoma
Tumours much more frequent in women	Hepatocellular adenoma Biliary cystadenoma
Tumours associated with chronic liver disease and cirrhosis	Hepatocellular carcinoma
Tumours associated with chemical or drug exposure	Hepatocellular adenoma Hepatocellular carcinoma Angiosarcoma
Tumours associated with parasitic infections and inflammatory diseases of the biliary tract	Cholangiocarcinoma
Tumours associated with congenital anomalies and metabolic diseases	Hepatocellular carcinoma Cholangiocarcinoma

criteria such as two compatible imaging studies can be used in such cases for definitive diagnosis without biopsy, but this remains controversial.[11,12] Clinical considerations determine the need for obtaining tissue but, in general, a definitive diagnosis of a liver tumour requires pathological examination.

Benign hepatocellular tumours and tumour-like lesions

Hepatocellular adenoma and adenomatosis

Hepatocellular adenoma (HCA) is a benign neoplasm that arises in a normal liver composed of cells that closely resemble normal hepatocytes. When multiple (usually more than 10) adenomas are present, the condition is called 'liver adenomatosis'.

Aetiology

HCA typically develops in women in the reproductive age group (15 to 45 years), nearly always associated with oral contraceptive steroid use. Although the absolute risk has always been very low, epidemiological case–control studies conducted in the 1970's found an annual incidence of about 3 to 4 per 100 000 long-term (>5 year) oral contraceptive users, but only 1 per million in non-users or women with less than 2 year's exposure.[13,14] The incidence appears to have decreased in recent decades with the introduction of lower-dose oral contraceptive preparations.[15] The exact mechanism by which adenomas are produced is not known, but experimental evidence suggests that sex hormones are promoters rather than initiators of hepatocellular neoplasms.[16,17] This is supported by the observation that in several cases, unresectable adenomas have been observed to regress after contraceptive steroid use was stopped.[18,19] Furthermore, other steroid hormones, including non-contraceptive oestrogens[20] and anabolic/androgenic steroids,[21] have been associated with HCA. Since hepatocellular adenomas nearly always occur in long-term users of oral contraceptives, any cases outside this setting are highly suspect, and may actually be a different benign lesion such as focal nodular hyperplasia (FNH) or a well-differentiated hepatocellular carcinoma. Cases of HCA have been reported rarely in men, children, and women not taking oral contraceptives, but at least some of these are probably misdiagnoses. Older reports of so-called hepatocellular adenomas in cirrhotic livers are undoubtedly examples of macroregenerative nodules.

HCA has been reported in association with conditions and drug exposures other than steroid hormones, but these are so rare that they are probably coincidental, with two exceptions. One of these is in the inherited glycogen storage diseases, especially Type Ia but also Types III and IV.[22,23] Patients with these disorders may develop multiple adenomas. The other exception is a form of autosomal dominant familial diabetes mellitus, termed 'maturity-onset diabetes of the young, type 3' or MODY3.[24–26] Patients with this disorder also develop multiple adenomas, and they have been found to have a germline mutation of the *TCF1* gene, which codes hepatocyte factor 1a (HNF1a), a transcription factor that controls numerous liver genes. Somatic mutations with HNF1a inactivation are also found in 60% of sporadic or contraceptive steroid-associated HCA, suggesting that it may be important in pathogenesis.

Clinical features

There is very little recent literature on the subject, and it is quite possible that the decreasing incidence of contraceptive steroid-associated HCA may have altered the conventional view. Nevertheless, in two large series compiled in the 1970's, the mean age was 30, and most patients were between 20 and 39.[14,27] Patients usually come to medical attention when symptoms develop, with only 5–10% found incidentally; 25–35% were aware of an abdominal mass; 20–25% had chronic or mild episodic abdominal pain; and 30–40% had acute abdominal pain, due to haemorrhage into the tumour or into the peritoneal cavity. Intraperitoneal haemorrhage, the most serious complication of HCA, regardless of aetiology, often requires emergency surgery and causes circulatory collapse and death in 20% of patients.

Surgical excision is usually advised for HCA to avoid possible rupture and haemorrhage, and because of the risk of malignant transformation. Steroid-associated tumours often regress if the patient stops taking the exogenous hormones,[28] while those associated with glycogen storage disease may regress with dietary therapy.[29] Unresectable tumours or multiple tumours in liver adenomatosis may be treated by liver transplantation. Malignant transformation is rare, since most hepatocellular adenomas are resected when discovered, but there are documented cases of HCC arising in unresected solitary as well as multiple adenomas.[30]

Pathology

HCA, by definition, always arises in a non-cirrhotic liver. A similar-appearing lesion in a cirrhotic liver would be considered a macroregenerative or low-grade dysplastic nodule. Hepatocellular adenoma is a solitary nodule, although

occasional patients may have more than one, and those with glycogen storage disease or other forms of adenomatosis have multiple nodules. The tumours often bulge from the surface of the liver and occasionally are pedunculated. They may measure up to 30 cm in diameter, although the majority are 5–15 cm. They are usually unencapsulated, but on cut section they are well demarcated from the surrounding liver. The colour varies from yellow or tan to brown, and there may be green areas of bile production as well as areas of necrosis or haemorrhage (Fig. 15.1) and sometimes irregular scars from previous necrosis.

Microscopically, HCA is composed of benign hepatocytes arranged in sheets and cords without acinar architecture (Figs 15.2 and 15.3). The tumour cells are usually, but not always, larger and paler than non-tumour hepatocytes in the surrounding tissue (Fig. 15.2), due to increased cytoplasmic glycogen and/or fat. The fat may be quite abundant, simulating fatty liver (Fig. 15.4). Other features that are variably present include bile production (Fig. 15.5), occasionally with pseudogland formation around dilated canaliculi, cytoplasmic lipofuscin granules, Dubin–Johnson

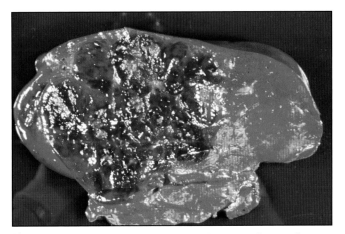

Fig. 15.1 • Hepatocellular adenoma. A resected tumour with areas of necrosis and haemorrhage.

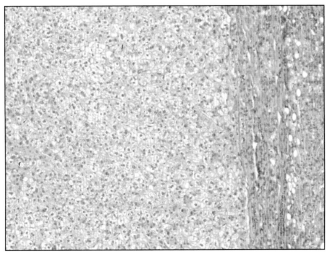

Fig. 15.2 • Hepatocellular adenoma. The tumour (left) is composed of sheets of hepatocytes that are larger and paler than those of the surrounding liver, which shows some compression and mild steatosis. H&E.

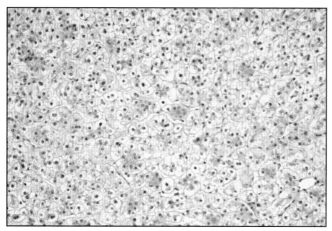

Fig. 15.3 • Hepatocellular adenoma. The tumour has no focally acinar architecture. The cells are large and pale, due to cytoplasmic glycogen. H&E.

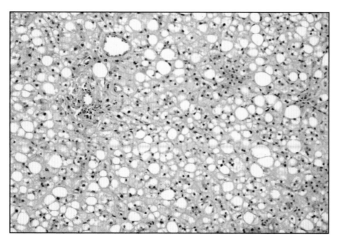

Fig. 15.4 • Hepatocellular adenoma. The tumour has unpaired arteries but no portal areas. Some tumour cells have cytoplasmic fat, simulating hepatic steatosis. H&E.

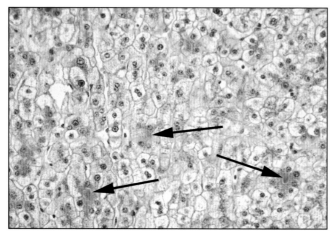

Fig. 15.5 • Hepatocellular adenoma. Bile production by the tumour cells with canalicular bile plugs (arrows). H&E.

pigment and rarely Mallory bodies. The nuclei of the tumour cells are typically uniform and regular, the nuclear–cytoplasmic ratio is low, and mitoses are almost never seen. Nucleoli are seldom prominent. Occasional tumours, especially in patients with long exposure to contraceptive ste-

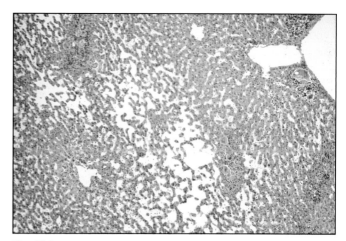

Fig. 15.6 • Hepatocellular adenoma. There is sinusoidal dilatation as well as inflammation and focal ductular proliferation, which has led such tumours to be misdiagnosed as telangiectatic focal nodular hyperplasia. H&E.

roids, may have a few pleomorphic nuclei, resembling large-cell change in non-neoplastic chronic liver disease.

HCA lacks the central scar and large arteries of focal nodular hyperplasia, but areas of fibrosis and septum formation may be present, especially in those associated with glycogen storage disease, presumably reflecting long duration. A well developed reticulin framework is usually present in the tumour. The sinusoids, with flattened endothelial lining cells, are usually compressed, thus contributing to the sheet-like appearance. Sometimes the sinusoids are dilated, a finding which can be mistaken for peliosis hepatis. Bile ducts are not found in HCA, but ductules and progenitor cells may be present.[31] The presence of dilated sinusoids and ductules (Fig. 15.6) have caused some tumours to be classified as a telangiectatic variant of focal nodular hyperplasia, but molecular studies have shown these to be HCA.[32] Thin-walled vascular channels and small arteries are scattered throughout the tumours, but large arteries are only seen around the periphery. Kupffer cells are present though usually inconspicuous, stellate cells are occasionally seen. Haematopoietic elements are noted in the sinusoidal lumen of some tumours, and rare cases have had non-caseating granulomas in the tumour.[33] Areas of haemorrhage may be present as well as recent or old infarcts, and areas of scarring containing haemosiderin-laden macrophages from old haemorrhages.

Differential diagnosis

Among benign lesions, focal nodular hyperplasia can sometimes be difficult to distinguish from HCA, especially in small biopsies. The finding of areas of scarring that contain large arteries and the presence of chronic cholestatic features in the hepatocytes of the lesion favour the diagnosis of focal nodular hyperplasia. Distinction of HCA from well-differentiated HCC can be difficult and sometimes impossible, but can usually be made on histological grounds. Recognition of a trabecular growth pattern and cytological features of malignancy, including high nuclear/cytoplasmic ratios and nuclear irregularities, are most helpful. When a lesion with all the features of HCA has a moderate degree of nuclear irregularity and hyperchromatism, one may wish to take the history into account. If the patient had been taking oral contraceptives or other sex steroids, then the tumour is best regarded as an atypical HCA; but if it is certain that there is no such history, it is probably a well-differentiated HCC. Histochemical and immunohistochemical stains add little to the differential diagnosis of HCA from HCC in the difficult cases. Reticulin fibres are generally decreased in the trabeculae of HCC compared to benign lesions, but well-differentiated carcinomas may have abundant reticulin. Markers of proliferation, such as Ki67, are much more frequent in malignant than benign hepatocellular tumours, but some clearly malignant tumours are negative for these. Markers of endothelial differentiation such as CD34 are expressed only in periportal or periseptal sinusoids in non-neoplastic liver. Although they are usually strongly expressed in HCC, HCA can sometimes have an identical staining pattern.[34]

Focal nodular hyperplasia

Focal nodular hyperplasia (FNH) is a tumour-like malformation composed of hyperplastic nodules of hepatocytes, separated by fibrous septa which often form typical stellate scars. FNH usually occurs in a liver that is otherwise histologically normal, although rare examples of such lesions have also been described in cirrhotic livers. Thick-walled arteries are present in the scars and septa, and ductules (but not ducts) are typically located within the fibrous tissue and at the junction with the parenchymal component. Focal nodular hyperplasia occurs in both sexes and all ages, but they are most commonly found in adult women.[2] Occasional patients present because of a palpable mass but the vast majority are discovered incidentally at surgery, usually for diseases of the gallbladder, or in imaging studies performed for evaluation of abdominal symptoms, most of which are unrelated to the FNH. Lesions discovered during laparoscopic cholecystectomy or by imaging are often not excised, but rather undergo needle biopsy, which may pose a diagnostic challenge. If imaging has demonstrated a central scar, and the suspicion of FNH is high, then the patient may be followed without biopsy.

Despite the fact that FNH is most common in women, contraceptive steroids are not thought to play an aetiological role, unlike HCA. Most evidence points to abnormal blood flow as the key component in pathogenesis, although the exact sequence is unclear. The hepatocellular component is polyclonal,[35] whereas HCA is monoclonal. The blood flow is predominantly arterial through arteries that are abnormally large for the region of the liver that they perfuse,[36,37] while the extracellular matrix of both the septa and sinusoids is similar to that of cirrhotic liver.[38] Furthermore, angiopoietin gene expression is up-regulated in the lesions.[39]

Pathology

FNH can be large, at times occupying an entire lobe of the liver, but over 85% are less than 5 cm in diameter.[2]

Approximately 20% of patients have more than one FNH in the liver, and there is a frequent association with hepatic haemangiomas. The gross appearance is highly characteristic (Figs 15.7 and 15.8). The lesions are usually well circumscribed but non-encapsulated. They frequently bulge from one of the surfaces of the liver and often have a depressed centre, resembling a metastasis. The colour is lighter than that of the adjacent normal liver. On cut section, the lesion is subdivided into smaller nodules by fibrous septa that often run into a stellate scar that may be central or eccentric, or in large lesions there may be several large scars. Microscopically, the lesions invariably have fibrous septa, often with the large central scar (Figs 15.9–15.11). These contain numerous vessels, both arteries and to a lesser extent veins, that course through the septa and the large scars (Fig. 15.12). The large arteries often show eccentric thickening due to intimal proliferation, fibromuscular hyperplasia and disruption of the elastic lamina. The septa are often infiltrated by varying numbers of inflammatory cells, and numerous ductules (Fig. 15.13), but not true bile ducts, are present at the junction of the fibrous septa with the hepatocellular component. The hepatocellular

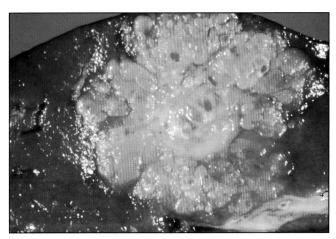

Fig. 15.7 • Focal nodular hyperplasia. On cut section, the lesion has a typical central scar with surrounding nodules that bulge from the cut surface of this fresh specimen.

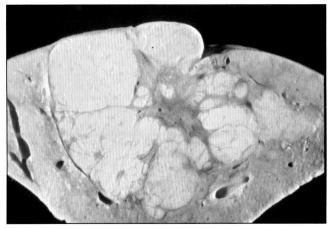

Fig. 15.8 • Focal nodular hyperplasia. This wedge resection was sectioned after fixation, showing the umbilicated central scar, radiating fibrous septa and pale parenchymal nodules.

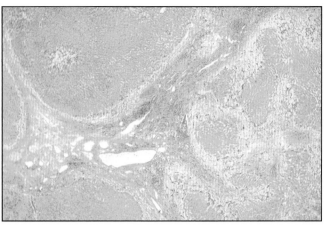

Fig. 15.9 • Focal nodular hyperplasia. The large central scar contains blood vessels and fibrous septa radiating from the scar, separating cirrhosis-like nodules of hepatocytes. H&E.

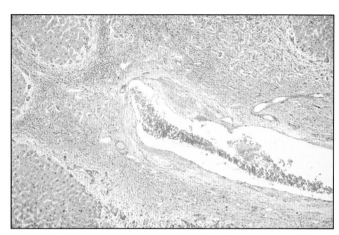

Fig. 15.12 • Focal nodular hyperplasia. There is a large artery in the centre of the central scar. H&E.

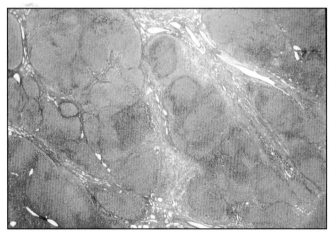

Fig. 15.10 • Focal nodular hyperplasia. The Masson trichrome stain shows the fibrous septa radiating from the central scar. H&E.

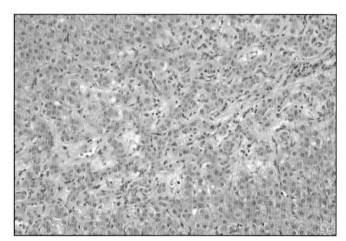

Fig. 15.13 • Focal nodular hyperplasia. Ductules and cholate stasis at the junction between a septum and the parenchyma. H&E.

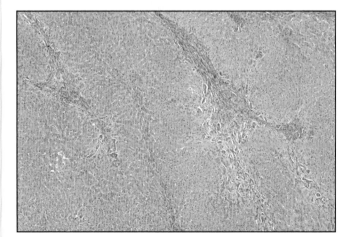

Fig. 15.11 • Focal nodular hyperplasia. Fibrous septa become thin in the periphery of the lesions. Ductules are present at the junction of the septa and parenchyma. Masson trichrome stain.

component is arranged in liver cell plates that are generally two cells thick and supported by a well-developed reticulin framework. They are separated by sinusoidal spaces lined by inconspicuous endothelial cells. The liver cells resemble normal hepatocytes in the adjacent parenchyma, but they may be slightly larger and paler. They may contain fat, especially if the rest of the liver is fatty, and even Mallory bodies if the patient has steatohepatitis. Liver cells adjacent to the fibrous septa of the lesion often show features of chronic cholestasis, with cholate stasis ('pseudoxanthomatous transformation') and copper storage, demonstrable with special stains. These features of chronic cholestasis are present in almost all cases of FNH and can be very helpful in differential diagnosis.[40] The absence of true bile ducts and a connection to the biliary outflow tract in part explains the cholestatic features.

Differential diagnosis

When the entire lesion is excised, together with a rim of normal adjacent parenchyma, the diagnosis is not difficult. The central stellate scar, fibrous septa, ductules and hepatocellular nodules all serve to distinguish FNH from other benign hepatocellular lesions, especially HCA. Needle biopsies may cause difficulty, but if the pathologist is aware that the biopsy is from a mass lesion, then the recognition of scars and septa, ductules and chronic cholestatic features in the hepatocytes all serve to distinguish FNH from other benign hepatocellular lesions, especially HCA. In difficult cases, the constellation of findings should be used as diagnostic criteria rather than any one individual histological feature. As noted earlier, HCA can sometimes have a few septa and ductules, but not all of the features of FNH. Lesions classified as 'telangiectatic FNH' because of the presence of ductules have been shown to be HCA,[32] and it seems likely that other lesions reported to be atypical variants of FNH[41] may also have been misclassified. Distinction from cirrhosis, especially a biliary cirrhosis, may be more difficult, but if part of the specimen shows normal acinar architecture, while part appears cirrhotic, one should suspect FNH. The presence of large, abnormal arteries in the septa is also a valuable clue in distinguishing FNH from cirrhosis.

Dysplastic nodules and putative premalignant lesions

The terminology of these lesions has undergone change in the past decade and remains somewhat confusing.[2,42–45] There may be further changes but, at present, dysplastic nodule (DN) has come to encompass lesions previously called 'adenomatous hyperplasia', 'macroregenerative nodule' and a variety of less popular terms. These are nodules in a cirrhotic liver that are macroscopically distinct from the surrounding cirrhotic nodules. They are usually larger than surrounding nodules and may be detected by imaging studies. They may also differ in colour or texture and may bulge from the surface of the liver. Histological examination is required to distinguish a DN from a small HCC, and they are further classified as low-grade or high-grade, based on morphological features.

Hepatocellular changes associated with the development of HCC are of two types, large-cell change and small-cell change. Large-cell change, originally called 'liver cell dysplasia'[46] refers to cellular enlargement, bizarre nuclear pleomorphism and hyperchromatism with occasional multinucleation of liver cells occurring in groups or sometimes occupying whole cirrhotic nodules. Although associated with the development of HCC, hepatocytes with large-cell change have a low proliferation rate but a greater degree of apoptosis than normal hepatocytes, suggesting a derangements of the normal process of hepatocyte polyploidization.[47] This could possibly be due to chronic inflammation-induced DNA damage, yielding a population of enlarged liver cells with characteristic nuclear changes but, while it may be a habitual feature of cirrhosis and a regular accompaniment of HCC, the preponderance of evidence suggests that it is not a direct precursor of malignancy.

Small-cell change is less readily recognized than large-cell change. It refers to clusters of cells, often forming small nodules within a cirrhotic nodule, with increased nuclear/cytoplasmic ratios and cytoplasmic basophilia. In contrast to large-cell change, hepatocytes with small-cell change have increased proliferative activity and seem more likely to be a direct precursor of HCC.[48,49]

Low-grade dysplastic nodules contain portal areas within the nodule, and are composed of liver cells that are minimally abnormal, although large-cell change may be present (Fig. 15.14) The nuclear/cytoplasmic ratio is normal or slightly increased. Nuclear atypia is minimal and there are no mitoses. Steatosis may be present and there may be Mallory bodies. Iron may be increased or decreased compared to the surrounding cirrhotic liver.

High-grade dysplastic nodules are characterized by small-cell change and features that suggest increased cellular proliferation—plates more than two cells thick, pseudogland formation, cytoplasmic basophilia, high nuclear/cytoplasmic ratio, nuclear hyperchromasia or an irregular nuclear contour. These features are often confined to one or more foci within the nodule, giving the appearance of 'nodule-in-nodule' formation (Fig. 15.15).

It is generally accepted that high-grade DN are precursors of HCC based on several lines of evidence, including morphological features intermediate between low-grade nodules and HCC, the presence of foci of HCC in otherwise high-grade dysplastic nodules (Fig. 15.16) and follow-up showing progression to malignancy in a few cases.[2,43–45, 50,51] Whether low-grade DN can also progress is less clear.

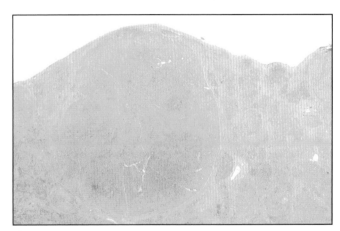

Fig. 15.14 • Low-grade dysplastic nodule. The nodule is much larger than the surrounding cirrhotic nodules. It contains portal areas and is cytologically normal. H&E.

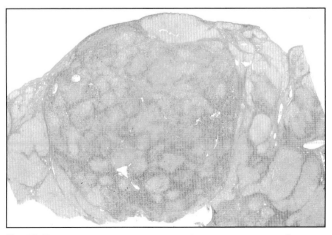

Fig. 15.15 • High-grade dysplastic nodule. There are numerous smaller nodules within the large dysplastic nodule (nodule-in-nodule). H&E.

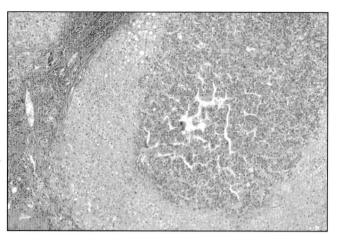

Fig. 15.16 • Hepatocellular carcinoma arising in a high-grade dysplastic nodule. H&E.

Nodular regenerative hyperplasia

Nodular regenerative hyperplasia (NRH) is usually considered a reaction to heterogeneous blood flow within the liver which can be of many causes (Chapter 13).[52] The usual case, a cirrhosis-like micronodular transformation of the liver that mimics cirrhosis but without the scarring typical of that condition, is not likely to be confused with a neoplasm. Occasionally, however, as in cirrhosis, there may be large regenerative nodules among the small cirrhosis-like nodules, causing confusion with hepatocellular adenoma. Furthermore, some cases of liver adenomatosis have been confused with NRH, and sometimes the terms have been used synonymously. The key to recognizing cases of NRH with adenoma-like nodules is in sampling the tissue that surrounds the large nodules. If it shows features of NRH with diffuse nodularity and no intervening normal parenchyma, then the diagnosis is NRH. If the intervening parenchyma is normal or only compressed by the large nodules, then it is adenomatosis.[2]

Malignant hepatocellular tumours

Hepatoblastoma

Hepatoblastoma is the most frequent liver tumour in children, with an annual incidence of approximately 1 per million in children under 15 years of age.[53] It mimics the developing fetal or embryonal liver histologically and may contain other heterologous mesenchymal or epithelial elements. At least 90% occur before the age of 5 years, and the diagnosis in cases reported in older children and adults is always suspect.

Aetiology

As in many other tumours of early childhood, genetic abnormalities appear to play a very strong role. Congenital anomalies are present in approximately 5% of patients and there are strong associations with Beckwith–Wiedemann syndrome and familial adenomatous polyposis coli (APC),

along with a number of other rare syndromes. Numerous chromosomal abnormalities have been found in the tumours and sometimes germline mutations in the patients. Gains of chromosomes 2 and X are common, and loss of heterozygosity of 11p15 is especially important in Beckwith–Wiedemann syndrome-associated hepatoblastoma.[54–56] Cytogenetic studies and comparative genomic hybridization have revealed that tumour cells usually harbour a limited number of chromosomal abnormalities with a mean of three changes per tumour.[57] Recurrent genetic alterations involve chromosomes 2, 20, 1, 8 and X.[55,58] Frequent trisomies 2q and 20, often seen as the only abnormality, have also been observed in other embryonic tumours such as embryonal rhabdomyosarcoma. The DNA content is frequently diploid in the fetal type and aneuploid in half the embryonal and small anaplastic cell types. Microsatellite analysis revealed regions with allelic loss of chromosomes 1 and 11.[59]

Abnormalities of the Wnt signalling pathway involving mutations of the *β-catenin* and *APC* genes play a central role, as in a number of other tumours.[60,61] Several studies revealed that genes encoding components of the wingless/Wnt signal transduction pathway, including the *APC, AXIN1* and *β-catenin genes*, are mutated in a large proportion of cases.[62–65] These mutations lead to abnormal activation and induction of growth-promoting genes. The central molecule of this pathway is β-catenin, which carries mutations in more than half of hepatoblastoma cases. β-catenin is a multifunctional protein that affects cell adhesion and gene expression, and has a pivotal role in cell adhesion through its participation in the cadherin–catenin complex of adherens junction. Activation of insulin-like growth factor 2 (IGF-2) and altered expression of members of the IGF-axis have also been involved, but mutations or allelic deletions of p53 are infrequent in hepatoblastoma.

Clinical features

Approximately 75% of children with hepatoblastoma are male. They usually present because of abdominal enlargement noted by a parent. Weight loss, anorexia, nausea, vomiting, abdominal pain and jaundice are seen less frequently. A right upper quadrant mass is often palpable in the abdomen on physical examination. Serum α-fetoprotein (AFP) is elevated at the time of diagnosis in up to 90% of patients. Radiological studies may be suggestive, but biopsy is usually recommended for definitive diagnosis.

Pathology

Hepatoblastomas usually present as a single mass that may be up to 25 cm in diameter. They are typically lobulated on cut surface and may be yellow, brown, green or variegated, depending on the differentiation of the tumour and whether a mesenchymal component is present (Figs 15.17 and 15.18).

Histologically, hepatoblastoma may be classified as epithelial type, with four subtypes, or mixed epithelial and mesenchymal, with two subtypes.[2] In the Armed Forces

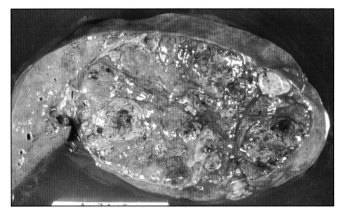

Fig. 15.17 • Hepatoblastoma. The tumour occupies the entire right lobe and has a typically lobulated appearance.

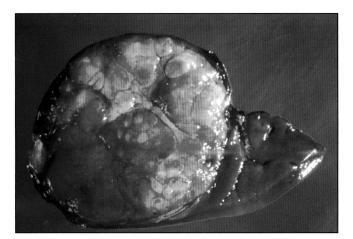

Fig. 15.18 • Hepatoblastoma. A lobectomy specimen, showing a tumour mass bulging from the surface with lobulations on cut section.

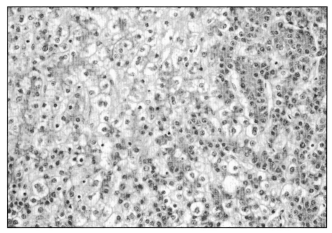

Fig. 15.19 • Hepatoblastoma, fetal epithelial type. The tumour has a characteristic 'light and dark' appearance at low magnification. H&E.

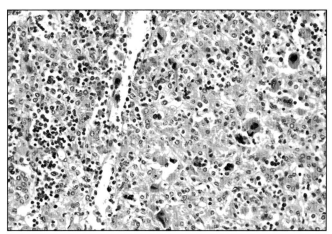

Fig. 15.20 • Hepatoblastoma, fetal epithelial type with abundant extramedullary haematopoiesis. H&E.

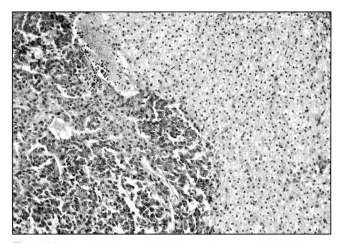

Fig. 15.21 • Hepatoblastoma, epithelial type with embryonal epithelium (left) and fetal epithelium (right). H&E.

Institute of Pathology (AFIP) series,[2,66,67] slightly more than half of tumours were epithelial. These were subdivided into those with a pure fetal epithelial pattern (31% of all cases) and those with fetal mixed with embryonal (19%), macrotrabecular (3%) and/or small cell undifferentiated (3%) components. The fetal epithelial pattern is composed of sheets and thin trabeculae of cells resembling fetal hepatocytes with a small round nucleus and clear to finely granular cytoplasm with variable amounts of cytoplasmic glycogen and lipid giving a 'light and dark' pattern to the tumour when viewed at low power magnification (Fig. 15.19). Haematopoietic cells are almost always present, mimicking the typical extramedullary haematopoiesis of normal fetal liver (Fig. 15.20). The embryonal pattern, when present along with fetal, consists of sheets, clusters or single small, angulated, hyperchromatic cells with a high nuclear:cytoplasmic ratio. Embryonal cells often cluster into glandular, acinar or pseudorosette formations (Fig. 15.21). The macrotrabecular pattern refers to tumours in which a significant proportion is composed of trabeculae more than 10 cells in thickness with either fetal or embryonal type cells or even larger cells that resemble those of hepatocellular carcinoma. The small-cell undifferentiated pattern is composed of noncohesive sheets of small cells similar to those of other 'small blue cell' paediatric neoplasms. In both macrotrabecular

and small-cell undifferentiated tumours, at least part of the mass must resemble more conventional epithelial hepatoblastoma to establish the diagnosis.

The mixed epithelial and mesenchymal pattern of hepatoblastoma contains areas of fetal and embryonal epithelial cells along with primitive mesenchyme and various mesenchymally derived tissues (Figs 15.22–15.25). In approximately three-quarters of mixed tumours, the mesenchymal component consists of immature and mature fibrous tissue and frequently osteoid-like tissue and cartilage. The cells in the osteoid-like areas express cytokeratin and other epithelial markers, indicating that they are metaplastic rather than of truly mesenchymal origin. The remainder of the mixed hepatoblastomas are considered teratoid and may contain a variety of tissues including striated muscle, bone, cartilage, stratified squamous epithelium, mucinous epithelium and melanin-containing epithelium. Tumours that are resected following chemotherapy may show extensive necrosis, while the amount of osteoid-like tissue is frequently increased.[68]

Staging

Several staging systems have been proposed, but the one most widely used is that of the Children's Cancer Study Group (CCSG) and Paediatric Oncology Group (POG), which classifies the tumours postoperatively by their resectability.[57] This classifies tumours as Stage I (complete resection), Stage II (microscopic residual disease), Stage III (macroscopic residual tumour), or Stage IV (distant metastases). At presentation, approximately 38% of hepatoblastomas are Stage I, 9% are Stage II, 24% Stage III and 29% Stage IV.[67,69] With preoperative chemotherapy and liver transplantation, as noted above, the majority of the 53% 'unresectable' (Stages III and IV) cases can be rendered 'resectable'.

Treatment and prognosis

Surgery is the mainstay of treatment of hepatoblastoma, and complete resection is the only chance for cure. Preoperative chemotherapy to shrink the tumour has resulted in improved resectability and has improved the overall 5-year survival rate to 75% from 35% in the 1970s.[57] Liver transplantation has been used in children whose tumours remain unresectable after chemotherapy. Multivariate analyses have shown that the stage of the tumour at the time of initial resection is the key prognostic factor in determining survival.[2,57,67,69] The histological pattern does not independently affect survival when adjusted for age, sex and stage, except perhaps for the small-cell undifferentiated variant, which has a high mortality, even if the initial resection appears complete.[67,70]

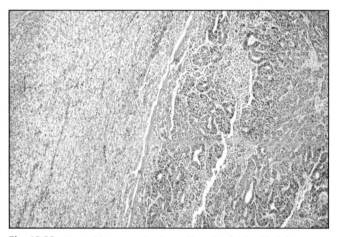

Fig. 15.22 • Hepatoblastoma, mixed type. There is a fetal epithelial component (right) and an embryonal component mixed with primitive mesenchyme (left). H&E.

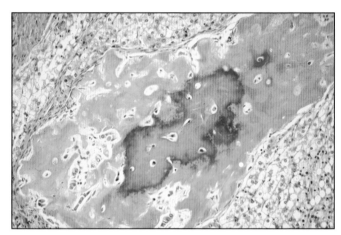

Fig. 15.24 • Hepatoblastoma, mixed type. Partially calcified osteoid in the midst of a fetal epithelial component. H&E.

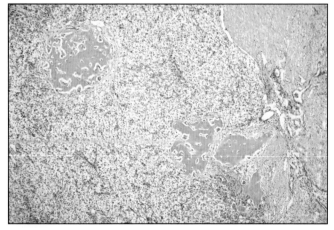

Fig. 15.23 • Hepatoblastoma, mixed type, with osteoid. H&E.

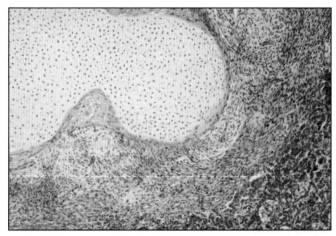

Fig. 15.25 • Hepatoblastoma, mixed type. An area with primitive mesenchyme and cartilage. H&E.

Hepatocellular carcinoma

Hepatocellular carcinoma (HCC) is the most common primary hepatic malignancy of adults. It is a malignant neoplasm composed of cells that differentiate in some way in the manner of hepatocytes. HCC is a tumour that is of interest to investigators in many fields, especially to those interested in the pathogenesis of human cancer. There is striking geographic variation in the incidence of HCC, and its association with viral infections and exposure to chemical agents and other forms of chronic liver injury have provided important clues to carcinogenetic mechanisms. Furthermore, the association of HCC with underlying chronic liver disease is so strong that development of cancer is frequently the terminal event for many patients with chronic liver disease.

Epidemiology and aetiology

One of the most striking features of HCC is the wide variation in its incidence in different parts of the world (Table 15.3).[71] Overall, HCC is the fifth most common malignancy among men and the eighth most common among women worldwide, but east Asia and Subsaharan Africa have by far the greatest number of cases, and in the countries of those regions HCC is among the leading causes of death. In areas of low incidence, such as the United States, carcinoma of the liver (primarily HCC) accounts for only 2.3% of cancer deaths in recent years, with an annual incidence of approximately 4.1 per 100 000.[71,72] It is currently the seventh leading cause of cancer deaths in the US, but the incidence has been

Table 15.3	Relative incidence of primary liver cancer in men in different parts of the world; age adjusted rates per 100 000[71]
High	
Eastern Asia	35.5
Central Africa	24.2
Southeast Asia	18.3
Pacific Islands	18.3
Medium	
East Africa	14.4
West Africa	13.5
Southern Europe	9.8
Caribbean	7.6
Low	
South Africa	6.2
Eastern Europe	5.8
Western Europe	5.8
Western Asia	5.6
North Africa	4.9
South America	4.8
North America	4.1
Australia/New Zealand	3.6
South Central Asia	2.8
Northern Europe	2.6
Central America	2.1

rising, more than doubling between 1975 and 1998.[73] In general, regions of the world with a high incidence of HCC are those that have a high prevalence of chronic hepatitis B infection, but even within these areas there is geographic variability; for example in western Africa the country of Gambia has nearly 5 times the incidence of Nigeria, suggesting that environmental cofactors such as aflatoxin exposure may also be important. Hepatitis C infection is associated with many cases in countries such as Japan where the prevalence of hepatitis B is intermediate but the incidence of HCC is relatively high.

The incidence of HCC generally increases with age, although there are geographic differences.[71] In Europe and the United States, the peak age of incidence is in the seventh decade, while in Qidong province in China, which has the highest incidence in the world, the peak is in the fifth decade. In South Africa, the average age of patients with HCC is 35 years, and 40% are 30 or younger, whereas in Taiwan (another area of high incidence), the majority of patients are 40–60 years old with a peak incidence in the eighth decade.[74] Nevertheless, HCC can occur in younger individuals and even young children.[54] Regardless of geographic location, HCC occurs more frequently in men than women, with male : female ratios in various countries ranging from 2 : 1 to 5 : 1. The precise reason is not known, but it has been shown that many tumours have androgen receptors,[75] raising the possibility that androgens may promote tumour development and growth. There is also a male predominance in risk factors, such as chronic viral hepatitis, alcoholism and smoking, which undoubtedly also play a role.

Cirrhosis. The majority of patients who develop HCC have underlying cirrhosis and, consequently, cirrhosis is a major risk factor for HCC. Macronodular cirrhosis has always been more strongly associated with HCC than micronodular cirrhosis, and cirrhosis of virtually any cause may be complicated by the development of HCC.[76] This also shows geographic variation, so that in Japan and other Asian countries, approximately 90% of patients have underlying cirrhosis,[77] whereas in some parts of Africa only 50–63% are cirrhotic, although most have precirrhotic forms of chronic viral hepatitis.[78] Series from North America have reported 46–91% with cirrhosis.[79] Nevertheless, every series includes some patients without cirrhosis, and some with no evidence of any underlying liver disease.

Viral hepatitis. The majority of cases of HCC in the world are due to hepatitis B virus (HBV), with the number of hepatitis C (HCV)-associated cases increasing in the Western world. HBV and HCV are the main causal agents of chronic hepatitis. Approximately 5–10% of HBV and 75% of HCV infections become chronic.[71,76,80] The epidemiological association of chronic HBV or HCV infection with HCC is well established.[71,72,74,76,81–89] The two viruses are different and the precise mechanisms by which they can cause cancer are not yet well clarified. Besides a direct effect of the virus on the genome, HCC could arise also as indirect result of the cycle of inflammation–necrosis–regeneration that occurs in the setting of chronic hepatitis.[90,91] On the other hand, it has been shown that in many instances the cause of HCC may be accurately determined on the basis of its 'molecular signature'.[92-94]

Hepatitis B. Of all risk factors, HBV infection has the strongest association with the development of HCC. The relative risk of HCC in patients serologically positive for hepatitis B surface antigen (HBsAg) is 98 times that of patients who are negative.[74] Those who are also positive for e antigen (HBeAg), indicating active viral replication, have 3.6 times the risk of those who are surface antigen positive but e antigen negative, suggesting that the activity of the disease plays a role in pathogenesis.[95] Even patients with occult HBV infection (surface antigen negative, with hepatitis B DNA demonstrable in tissue by PCR) may develop HCC, although the incidence and relative risk are not known.[96]

HBV is the prototype member of a virus family called 'hepadnaviridae', which also includes the woodchuck hepatitis virus (WHV), ground squirrel hepatitis virus (GSHV), duck hepatitis B virus (DHBV) and heron hepatitis B virus (HHBV).[97,98] There are biological and genetic similarities between these viruses,[80,97-100] such as a narrow host range, hepatotropism and tendency to chronicity. Among them, WHV infection is most often associated with the development of HCC.[101]

HBV consists of a partially double-stranded DNA genome of 3.2 kb enclosed by envelope proteins (HBsAg) (Chapter 8). The genome is packaged with a core protein (HBcAg) and a DNA polymerase. After penetration of the virus in the cell, its genome becomes a covalently closed, totally double-stranded molecule that can eventually integrate into the host genome. Protein synthesis proceeds from four open reading frames: envelope proteins from the *S* gene, pre-S1 and pre-S2; HBeAg and HBcAg from the *C* gene and pre-C gene sequence; the DNA polymerase from the *P* gene; and X protein from the *X* gene.[80,99,102] DNA replication depends upon reverse transcription of a RNA intermediate in the nucleus. The virions are then built in the cytoplasm and released by the hepatocyte.[103,104]

The integration of HBV in sites within the host genome has been seen as a possible carcinogenetic mechanism. In WHV-induced HCC, WHV DNA integrates adjacent to cellular N-*myc* genes[101] and studies with transgenic mice have shown that this could interfere with the p53 axis.[105] In man the integration is, however, not specific and only rarely associated with activation of cellular oncogenes.[106-111] In a minority of HCC cases, integration of DNA sequences into the host cell genome can activate cellular genes through a mechanism of modification of its expression (i.e. cis-acting mechanism).[112] Moreover, 20% of patients with HCC associated with HBV do not integrate the DNA of the virus. On the other hand, integrated HBV-DNA can generate chromosomal instability and integration can also target the telomerase gene.[92]

Several *HBV* genes have been found in infected tissues more frequently than others, including truncated pre-S2/S, *hepatitis Bx gene (HBx)* and a novel spliced transcript of HBV, named hepatitis B spliced protein (HBSP).[113] The proteins expressed from these integrated genes have been shown to have intracellular effects that may account for their association with HCC, including effects on cellular growth and apoptosis. Among these genes, *HBx* seems to play a pivotal role in hepatocarcinogenesis. *HBx* gene, indeed, harbours weak transcriptional transactivation activity. The 154-amino-acid viral product 'X' (HBx) has been shown to be essential for HBV and WHV infection 'in vivo'.[80,99,114,115] It may be a prime candidate for mediating HBV pathological effects. With regard to oncogenesis, it can directly inactivate the tumour suppressor p53 and the negative growth regulator p55sen,[102,116-118] both involved in the pathway of senescence, and can transcriptionally downregulate p21 and sui1, both of which inhibit hepatocellular growth.[102] Other biological effects of HBx can be summarized as follows:

1. HBx transactivates several cellular promoters by protein–protein interactions, interacting with proliferation, apoptosis, and response to DNA damage.[119-121]
2. HBx influence proteasome function, interfering with the degradation of viral and cellular proteins.[122]
3. HBx may inhibit the DNA repair system.[99,102]
4. HBx influence the mitochondria function and interacts with calcium homeostasis.[123-125]
5. HBx has also been implicated in DNA repair.[99,102]

The real functional consequences in hepatocarcinogenesis of these effects are, however, still unclear.[92,99] One model is that HBx acts (through its effect on calcium homeostasis and consequent activation of calcium-dependent kinases) on NFkB, a transcription factor involved in the control of immune response[126] that has also been associated with HCV polypeptides.

Other HBV proteins have been suggested to enhance the risk for development of HCC. Studies with transgenic mice have shown association between various envelope proteins (namely L and M) and hepatocellular carcinoma, although a real 'cause–effect' relationship could not be demonstrated. The risk enhancement could be indirectly mediated via envelope-induced cellular stress.[127-129]

Hepatitis C. Hepatitis C rivals hepatitis B in importance as an aetiological factor in HCC, and it appears to be largely responsible for the rising incidence of liver cancer in the United States, where 21% of cases are associated with HCV, and it is also believed to be responsible for the relatively high incidence of HCC in Japan and some other countries.[76,82,130,131] Most cases of HCC associated with hepatitis C have occurred after the development of cirrhosis, and the risk is multiplied in the presence of other factors, such as male gender, advanced age, coinfection with other viruses (HBV and/or HIV), alcohol, diabetes or hepatic steatosis. Patients infected with both HBV and HCC have a much greater risk of HCC than with either virus alone.[76]

HCV is a positive strand RNA virus belonging to the Hepaciviridae genus (Flaviviridae family) (Chapter 8). The genome is 9-kb-long single-stranded, linear RNA. Its replication occurs in the rough endoplasmic reticulum (RER), without reverse transcriptase activity.[132-134] The RNA is translated by ribosomes of RER and the resulting polyprotein is modified and cleaved giving rise to 10 polypeptides, including three structural (core, E1 and E2) and multiple non-structural (NS1 to NS5).[135-137] The non-structural proteins associate with ER membrane to form the viral replicase.[138-140]

The mechanism of liver damage in HCV infection is the result of immune response and direct cytopathic effect.[141,142] The continuous process of necrosis and regeneration may make the cells prone to the action of various procarcinogenic substances (HCV proteins?) with genetic instability and subsequent malignant transformation. Based largely on experimental 'in vitro' results, an oncogenic role has been reported for three HCV proteins: core protein, NS3 and NS5a.[99,141] Core protein intervenes in several cellular functions as apoptosis, signal transduction and transformation.[99,141] It modulates p21WAF1 expression, and physically interacts with p53,[143-145] promoting apoptosis and cell proliferation. Moreover, core protein stimulates NFkB, increasing its levels and DNA binding activity and modifying the response to TNF-α.[119] In summary, by modulating the activity of transcription factors and cytokines, it could promote cellular transformation.[99] Also NS3 protein represses the transcription of p21WAF1, both acting on the promoter and via p53.[146-148] NS5a is part of the viral replicase complex, although no defined role in virus replication has been revealed.[80] It has effects on cell-cycle-regulatory kinases and transcription activation machinery (p21 WAF1, p53, cyclins), blocking apoptosis in HCV infection, so contributing to hepatocarcinogenesis.

In general, a possible mechanism of viral-induced hepatocarcinogenesis may involve endoplasmic reticulum (ER) and oxidative stress. ER stress is a homeostatic mechanism that controls cellular metabolism in response to perturbations in protein biosynthesis.[149] Extreme or prolonged ER stress can lead to apoptosis.[150] Non-cytopathic viruses, such as HCV and HBV, inducing ER stress at sublethal levels, can produce alterations in cells that may lead to transformation. On the other side, ER stress is strictly linked to intracellular redox state, so that its ultimate consequence is oxidative stress.[99,151] This is linked to changes in cellular proliferation and to DNA damage; therefore several studies have implicated oxidative stress in the development of HCC in HCV hepatitis.[152,153] Oxidative stress activates intracellular signalling pathways that may promote transformation, such as mitogen-activated protein kinases (MAPKs) pathway.[154] MAPKs are a group of enzymes that include extracellular signal-regulated protein kinase (ERK), c-JUN N-terminal kinase/stress-activated protein kinase (JNK/SAPK) and p38 subfamilies.[99] They respond to various stimuli in different ways; for instance ERK is stimulated by mitogens and endorses survival, while JNK/SAPK and p38 are stimulated by various stresses and promote apoptosis.[155,156]

Aflatoxin B1. Aflatoxins, a family of mycotoxins produced by fungi of the *Aspergillus* genus, are powerful carcinogens in experimental animals. Contamination of food, particularly grains and peanuts, by these toxins is common in the very same parts of the world where HCC is most common, namely China and southern Africa,[157,158] and indeed, before the association with hepatitis B was recognized, aflatoxin B1 was thought to be a principal cause of HCC.[159] Aflatoxin

is converted by cytochrome P450 to 8,9-exo-epoxide, that damages DNA. Aflatoxin B1 (AFB1) binding to guanine residues of DNA can produce G to T mutations,[160,161] that are not found in human HCC in areas with low AFB1 exposure.[162,163] Such mutations in codon 249 of the *p53* tumour suppressor gene are thought to play an important role in carcinogenesis in parts of the world with a high incidence of HCC.[160] There is a synergistic cooperation between HBV and AFB1 in hepatocarcinogenesis, and the combination of chronic hepatitis B infection with dietary aflatoxin exposure more than triples the risk of developing HCC.[164,165]

Alcohol. There is very little evidence that alcohol is directly carcinogenic or genotoxic, but alcoholic cirrhosis is the single most frequent risk factor in the United States and many Western countries.[72,166] Non-genotoxic mechanisms are most probably related to causation. Alcohol is metabolized to acetaldehyde by alcohol dehydrogenase and cytochrome P450 2E1 (CYP2E1), that is associated with microsomes. CYP2E1 produces reactive oxygen species that can lead to DNA damage and transformation.[167] Moreover, polymorphism in alcohol dehydrogenase and CYP2E1 may influence the risk of hepatocarcinogenesis.[166,168] In alcohol-induced cirrhosis, the reserve of S-adenosylmethionine, the methyl donor for DNA methylation, is decreased.[166,169] The effect could be hypomethylation of DNA, with consequent DNA instability, that could be associated with the development of cancer. Alcohol may be synergistic with other risk factors, however, increasing the likelihood of HCC in patients with hepatitis B or C, diabetes, obesity or smoking.[166,170-172] Heavy alcohol consumption is associated with a six-fold increase in risk of HCC in cirrhotic patients.[172]

Diabetes, obesity and fatty liver disease. Diabetes mellitus is associated with a two to three-fold increase in risk of HCC, regardless of other risk factors,[173-175] while obesity is associated with a two to four-fold increased risk.[175-178] Most patients with diabetes or obesity who develop HCC have cirrhosis, and since both diabetes and obesity can lead to cirrhosis through non-alcoholic steatohepatitis (Chapter 7); this presumably accounts for most of the cases. When viral hepatitis, alcohol, or other risk factors are present, the fatty liver disease may be synergistic.[171,172] Approximately one-third of cases of HCC that occur in the United States have no known aetiology, and it is possible that non-alcoholic fatty liver disease (NAFLD)-related cirrhosis is a predisposing factor in may of these.[72,175,179] This hypothesis is supported not only by epidemiological data, but also by the suspected pathogenesis and molecular 'lesions' of NAFLD. Lipid peroxidation with production of free oxygen radicals is thought to be a central event in the pathogenesis of steatohepatitis.[180] This oxidative stress may lead to proliferation of oval cells, in man as in experimental models.[181] The reactive oxygen species (ROS) can induce mutations, for instance, in the *p53* gene. The progression of the neoplastic cells can to be facilitated by the numerous alterations in growth factors and cytokines (TGF or TNF), which have been shown to stimulate oval cell proliferation.[182]

Metabolic diseases. Cases of HCC have occurred in a number of metabolic diseases, but the strongest associations are with genetic haemochromatosis (GH), tyrosinaemia and α_1-antitrypsin deficiency.[183–185] Development of HCC is a frequent terminal event following the development of cirrhosis in GH (approximately 20%), hereditary tyrosinaemia (37%) and α_1-antitrypsin deficiency (15%). Prevention of cirrhosis by phlebotomy in GH and diet with NTBC (2-(2nitro-4-trifluoromethylbenzoyl)-1,3-cyclohexanedione) therapy in tyrosinaemia can prevent HCC in all but a few cases. There is also an increased incidence of HCC in patients with porphyria cutanea tarda, but since that disease is frequently associated with alcohol use and chronic hepatitis C infection, the role of the porphyria is unclear. A few cases of HCC have been reported in patients with glycogen storage diseases, types I and III, in association with hepatocellular adenomas and presumably representing malignant transformation of an adenoma. HCC has also rarely been reported in patients with other forms of porphyria, hypercitrullinaemia, fructosaemia, Wilson disease, Byler disease and Alagille syndrome.

Because of its relative frequency, GH is the metabolic disease that is the most important risk factor in development of HCC, and conversely HCC is recognized as one of the most important complications of GH. The risk of developing HCC in GH individuals is significantly higher (up to 200 times) than the risk of the general population.[186–188] It is not completely clear if this is due to the iron overload in itself or to the development of cirrhosis that invariably occurs in untreated hereditary haemochromatosis (HH) patients.[184] An important role of iron overload in hepatocarcinogenesis, however, has also been demonstrated in patients with iron excess without HH as thalassaemia or the so-called 'African overload'.[189–190] Several studies (in vivo and in vitro) point to a causative role for iron excess in hepatocarcinogenesis.[184] Iron can act directly on cellular proliferation, for instance by inactivating p53. It can also act indirectly, for example by influencing lipid peroxidation and production of reactive oxygen radicals. Iron is, in fact, a substrate for cell proliferation and could initiate the process of carcinogenesis.[191,192] The effect of free iron could be due both to direct damage to chromosomes and to mutation, via the increased production of ROS.[193,194] Interestingly, in patients with HH a particular type of mutation of p53 has been described (A220G) in the DNA binding site of the protein.[195,196] At the same time, it has been hypothesized that the formations of adduct due to lipid peroxidation may lead to DNA damage in patients with GH.

Anabolic and contraceptive steroids. A number of hepatocellular tumours have been reported in patients taking anabolic steroids.[197] Some have been classified as hepatocellular adenoma, others as HCC, based on histological features, but even those called HCC regress when the drug is discontinued, and none has been reported to metastasize. Contraceptive steroids are clearly associated with hepatocellular adenoma. Several case–control series have reported an association with HCC, but others have found a protective effect of contraceptive steroid use as well as other factors that lead to high oestrogen exposure, including multiple pregnancies and early menarche, so the matter remains unresolved.[198,199]

Molecular pathology

During the last 25 years, molecular genetic and phenotypic cellular changes have been extensively studied in human and experimental hepatocarcinogenesis.[92,101,141,165,200–206] A variety of genetic and epigenetic alterations (point mutations, deletions, amplifications, methylations), which may result in the distortion of either gene expression or the biochemical function of genes, have been detected. As in tumours of other sites, the majority of genes and proteins affected have a physiological role (control of differentiation, proliferation, apoptosis, etc.), but their dysregulation is involved in carcinogenesis and they are therefore been called proto-oncogene or tumour suppressor genes.[207–209] Although a number of general pathways have been discovered,[102,210] the type of genetic alterations and their sequence of occurrence may be very variable,[211] reflecting under this aspect the wide range of aetiological factors of HCC. Each HCC has probably its own profile and this heterogeneity can be found also within a given tumour.[212–214] Moreover, while many discrepancies have been observed in molecular genetic changes that appear during hepatocarcinogenesis triggered by various oncogenic agents in different species, similarities in specific phenotypic cellular changes are evident.[215–220]

At the present stage of knowledge, two main 'pathways' regarding hepatocarcinogenesis have been proposed:

1. malignant cell clones arise from hepatocytes by mutations and clonal selections (dedifferentiation hypothesis)
2. activation of hepatic progenitor cells defective in maturation lead to malignant clones (maturation arrest hypothesis)

Of course, these two 'pathways' are not mutually exclusive, and could simultaneously be involved during hepatocarcinogenesis. An intriguing current hypothesis is the possible role of hepatic progenitor cells as target cells for hepatocarcinogenesis, since these cell type are prevalent in early dysplastic foci of human livers affected with the most prevalent carcinogenic conditions, such as viral hepatitis and alcoholic liver disease.

Molecular genetic alterations in HCC

As noted above, most HCCs develop in the setting of chronic hepatopathy as a multistep process.[42,102] Its evolution may take up to 30 years.[94] Foci of dysplastic hepatocytes (DH), low-grade dysplastic nodules (LG-DN) and high-grade dysplastic nodules (HG-DN) have been identified as possible preneoplastic lesions. A minority of HCC arises, however, in the absence of underlying hepatopathy or in children.[71] That underlines the importance of a genetic predisposition in the development of this neoplasm.

Epigenetic alterations in preneoplastic lesions. In preneoplastic lesions, an elevated expression of transforming-growth factor alpha (TGF-α) and insulin-like growth factor 2 (IGF-2) is observed, that is responsible for enhanced hepatocyte proliferation.[205,206,218] This up-regulation is due to the action of cytokines, viral transactivation and altered methylation of the corresponding genes.[92,93,205] Expression of methyltransferases is high in many HCCs,[221] increasing the pool of methyl groups available for methylation reactions.

Genomic alterations in preneoplastic lesions. Loss of heterozygosity (LOH) and microsatellite instability are detected in preneoplastic lesions, with a progression from cirrhosis to HCC. One of the most frequent deletions occurs at 8p, shared by HG–DN and HCCs.[91,222–226] Both microsatellite instability at identical loci and identical allelic deletion or gene mutations have been described in cirrhotic and dysplastic nodules and adjacent HCCs, supporting the hypothesis that HCC often develops as clonal growth from dysplastic nodules.[94,165,205,212,218,222,227] Recently, studies with cDNA array technique have shown that more than 50 genes are dysregulated in dysplastic nodules. They include oncogenes (v-akt homolog 2), Tumour suppressor genes (TSGs) (*WT1*, *Rb1*), DNA repair genes, growth factor and cytokines (*EGFR*, *IGFBP3*), adhesion proteins, signal transduction proteins, transcription factors and housekeeping genes.[228,229]

A probable early event in hepatocarcinogenesis is mutation of β-catenin, an essential component of the Wnt signalling pathway.[230,231] β-catenin is a submembranous protein involved in cell-to-cell adhesion. After phosphorylation and ubiquitination, it is normally degraded by the proteasome complex. Activation of the Wnt pathway leads to overload of β-catenin, that subsequently translocates in to the nucleus, activating *c-myc*, *c-jun*, cyclin D1, fibronectin and matrix metalloproteinases (MMPs).[230] In early stages of HCC, mutation of β-catenin and of other components of the Wnt pathway has been shown.[230,231] Up-regulation of MMPs expression is a feature of the first stages of HCC, but is absent from advanced stages.[232] This could suggest that early HCC could grow by destroying the extracellular matrix and that this feature is at least partially controlled by β-catenin.[233,234]

Epigenetic alterations in HCC. Several events can cause structural genomic aberrations in HCC.[94,205] For instance, *c-myc* amplification is a well-known phenomenon in HCC.[9,1,97,105,226,231,235] This is, however, a relatively late phenomenon, preceded by promoter hypomethylation.[94,205] Reduced expression of *p16INK4A* is due to promoter hypermethylation, LOH, biallelic loss or mutation.[227,231,236–240] HBV and AFB may provoke structural changes in the genome that may lead to mutations or genomic rearrangements.[92,141,169,227] Microsatellite instability has been observed in HCC and could be due to the action of molecular products of HBV and HCV on DNA repair enzymes (see above).[92,94,141] Telomerase activity is impaired by hypermethylation and mutation.[241] In HCC, shortening of telomeres has been consistently observed.[241–244] That results in mitotic non-disjunction and chromosome breaks that eventually lead to chromosomal instability, particularly if an impairment of p53 has occurred.[245]

Genomic alterations in HCC. Most HCCs are aneuploid and show several different genetic alterations, ranging from gains and loss of entire chromosomal arms to point mutations.[205] It is interesting to note that, while alterations in cirrhosis or chronic hepatitis are significantly different from those observed in HCC, dysplastic nodules show a profile that is quite similar to well-differentiated HCCs.[205,206] New aberrations develop as the tumour evolves to large, poorly differentiated.[91,205,206,225,246,247] Most frequent losses have been observed at 1p, 4q, 5q, 6q, 8p, 9p, 13q, 16p, 16q, 17p and gains at 1q, 6p, 8q and 17q by comparative genomic hybridization (CGH).[91,203,205,206,210,224–226,245–250] However, each genomic alteration rarely affect more than half of HCCs, also when cases are stratified according to stage, size or histological grade.[94,205] This heterogeneity could reflect the actions of different causative agents. It has been shown, in some studies, that loss at 10q is preferentially associated with HCV-positive cases, while loss of 4q and 16q and gain of 11q is observed in most cases in HBV-related HCC.[249,251] On the other hand, most chromosomal alterations are observed in HCC independent of aetiology.[165,206] Recently, it has been shown that the Rb1, p53 and Wnt pathways are commonly affected in HCC by different aetiologies.[231] It is now generally accepted that each metabolic pathway involved in control of proliferation, apoptosis or differentiation may be altered in HCC: these molecular circuits are redundant, forming a network in which some molecules (for instance p53 or cyclin D1) are found in nodes interconnecting several pathways. Alterations in genes coding for such proteins may therefore affect multiple pathways.[205]

The frequently deleted chromosomal regions in HCC contain many TSGs, such as *p53*, *Rb*, *p16*, *PTEN*, *DLC1*, *IGF-2R* and the gains involve known oncogenes such as *c-myc*.[94,227] However, it is also possible that other still unidentified genes are involved (an example is 8p23.3 and 8p11.2 deletions, that are frequently observed in HCCs).[223]

Molecular alterations in late stages of hepatocarcinogenesis and in metastasis. In fully developed HCC a frequent deletion is observed at 13q12–14 locus, that contains *RB1*, *LEU1* and *BRCA1*, three well-known oncogenes.[225,245,249] As recalled above, *Rb* is inactivated by several mechanisms: hyperphosphorilation,[252] enhanced degradation via proteasomes[253] and LOH. Another possible mechanism of inactivation of *Rb1* involves *p16INK4*, located on 9p21. The gene is frequently hypermethylated in advanced HCC, but LOH at its locus is also frequently observed.[225,254] Normally, p16INK4, inhibits the cyclin dependent kinases (CDK) 4 and 6, which block the cell cycle through dephosphorylation of *RB1*. Interestingly, p16INK4 shares the promoter with p14ARF, that stabilizes p53 by binding to mdm-2.[255] p14ARF is indeed the product of an alternate reading frame from the same gene that codes for p16INK4.[102] Down-regulation of p16INK4 may therefore inactivate *Rb*, while down-regulation of p14ARF destabilizes p53.[102] Increased expression of oncogenes such as *c-myc* and c-N-*ras* has been related to invasiveness and metastases.[256,257] High levels of MET, the receptor for hepatocyte growth factor (HGF) are probably associated with metastasis.[258] Elevated levels of various growth factors and cytokines (epidermal growth factor, HGF, TNF-α, etc.) are probably causally related to up-regulation of MET.[259,260]

DNA microarrays. The recently developed high-throughput gene expression analysis has allowed a global analysis of molecular alterations in HCC.[261–276] In most cases, transcripts associated with cell proliferation are up-regulated and those related to growth inhibition are down-regulated.[99,165] Dysregulated genes are for example those coding for MMP14, Rho, dynein, PCNA, cyclins, CDC20, CDK4, Wnt, b-catenin, GST and cytochromes. Some of these genes have been subsequently reported as possible therapeutic targets or predictive/prognostic markers.[99,165] However, the statistical methods used in these studies and the real meaning of these results need still to be completely validated. For instance, there is considerable variation in up- and down-regulated genes reported in microarray analysis, still underlining that the molecular pathways involved in hepatocarcinogenesis are different and that the same histopathological changes can correspond to different molecular alteration.

In summary, hepatocarcinogenesis is a multistep process involving different molecular pathways (Fig. 15.26). The differences are probably partly due to the aetiology and partly to the genetic constitution of the host. Some of them are also a consequence of the methodology used. Moreover, the precise sequence of morphological events that lead to the development of HCC is not yet completely elucidated.[42,94,205,206] For instance, the precise relationship between HG–DN and HCC and LG–DN and large regenerative nodule (LRN) is surely not completely clear. On the other hand, although still incomplete and fragmentary, a comprehensive picture is beginning to emerge, both from the genetic and from the functional point of view. The combined action of alterations in the Wnt pathway, the IGF-axis and in the control of cell cycle (CDK, Rb, p53) could lead to the development of dysplastic foci (nodules). The subsequent genetic and epigenetic changes (activation of MMPs, for instance) contribute to the acquisition of the complete malignant phenotype (possibility of infiltration and metastasis) and therefore to the full development if HCC. In this process the additional role of oxidative stress is surely important, at least in alcoholic and NAFLD-related cirrhosis. In a fraction of HCC that do not develop in the setting of cirrhosis and in childhood, c-met and HGF probably have an important function. The challenge for the future is the identification of those changes that are really relevant for HCC development

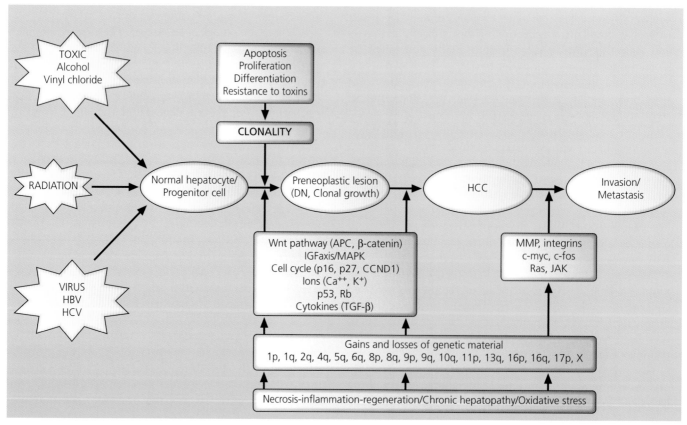

Fig. 15.26 • Pathways of hepatocarcinogenesis.

and that could be diagnostic or prognostic markers or—most importantly—possible targets for therapy.

Clinical features

HCC is clinically silent for most of its course, and the majority of patients present with advanced disease that has little chance of effective treatment. Signs and symptoms usually point to a malignancy in the liver. Upper abdominal pain, weight loss, abdominal enlargement, hepatomegaly with or without a palpable mass, and signs of decompensated liver disease, such as jaundice or ascites, are frequent at presentation. The tumours can invade portal and hepatic veins and bile ducts and can destroy and replace functioning parenchyma in livers that are usually already compromised by cirrhosis, so that some patients present primarily with hepatic decompensation manifested by rapidly accumulating ascites, variceal haemorrhage, hepatic encephalopathy or obstructive jaundice. Rare patients present with distant metastases or paraneoplastic syndromes, such as hypoglycaemia, erythrocytosis, hypercholestrolaemia, hypercalcaemia, isosexual precocious puberty (in children), gynaecomastia (in the absence of cirrhosis), carcinoid syndrome, hypertrophic pulmonary osteoarthropathy, osteoporosis, hypertension, hyperthyroidism, dysfibinogenaemias, porphyria cutanea tarda and a variety of other cutaneous changes.[277,278]

Patients who present with clinically evident disease are rarely candidates for any form of curative therapy. For such patients the median survival is 1 to 3 months, and survival beyond 1 year is unusual.[279–281] There have been advances in palliative therapy, but the most encouraging trends in recent years have been in surveillance and early diagnosis of HCC in high-risk populations combined with advances in surgical and other forms of definitive therapy. In developed countries with advanced health care, it is recommended that patients known to have cirrhosis undergo periodic screening, usually every 6 months, with serum tumour markers and imaging studies.[282,283] Serum α-fetoprotein, an oncofetal antigen that can be produced by HCC, has been widely used for screening in high-risk populations, but its low sensitivity and specificity has limited its usefulness.[284] Other serum markers, such as desgamma-carboxy prothrombin, are becoming available, but their usefulness remains to be proven.

Radiographic imaging is virtually always used in the evaluation of a patient with a suspected liver tumour, and in symptomatic or advanced cases the tumours are easily detected by ultrasound, CT, MRI or angiography.[3,285] For surveillance and detection of early, potentially curable tumours in high-risk patients, however, ultrasonography has become the method of choice.[6,282,283] Skilled sonographers using specialized techniques, such as carbon dioxide enhanced ultrasonography can sometimes detect tumours as small as 8 mm in diameter,[286] although these cannot be reliably distinguished from benign macroregenerative or dysplastic nodules in a cirrhotic liver. Tumours measuring 2 to 3 cm, however, are detected in over 80% of cases. CT and MRI may improve on this in cases where HCC is highly

suspect, and tumours measuring 1 cm are routinely detected, although it is still difficult to distinguish these from benign nodules and, consequently, these are generally used to confirm the presence of suspect nodules.[8,10]

Pathology

Advanced HCC, unsuitable for curative treatment, is generally examined in its entirety only at autopsy.[287–289] The tumour may form a single large mass that replaces an entire lobe, there may be multiple discrete nodules scattered throughout the liver (Fig. 15.27), or there may be numerous cirrhosis-like nodules. Some tumours form an expanding mass well-demarcated from the surrounding liver, with or without a capsule, while others appear to infiltrate the surrounding liver tissue at the tumour margin. Tumours that appear encapsulated (Fig. 15.28) almost always arise in a cirrhotic liver, with the expanding tumour causing compression atrophy of the surrounding cirrhotic nodules and incorporation of cirrhotic scars to form the fibrous capsule. HCC is almost always a soft tumour, often with areas of necrosis, except for the uncommon fibrolamellar variant and even rarer classified histologically as 'scirrhous'. They vary in colour from tan or yellow to greyish-white or, if they produce bile, to green. Vascular invasion is common, and

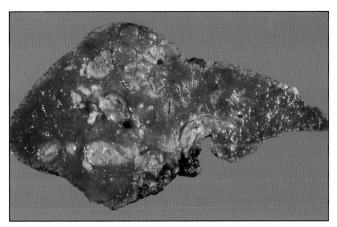

Fig. 15.27 • Hepatocellular carcinoma. A cirrhotic liver with multiple tumour nodules scattered throughout.

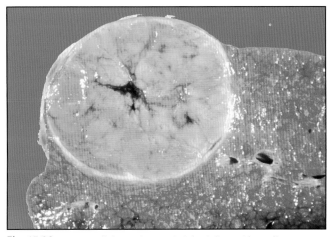

Fig. 15.28 • Hepatocellular carcinoma. A cirrhotic liver with a solitary encapsulated tumour.

both the portal vein and hepatic veins as well as the vena cava may be involved. Invasion of major bile ducts is uncommon but may cause biliary obstruction.

Of greater interest are small tumours that can be examined in resection specimens and in explanted livers removed prior to liver transplantation. The term 'small HCC' has been variably used for tumours up to 2, 3 or even 5 cm in diameter. These are usually detected through surveillance of patients with chronic liver disease, are more likely to be resectable than larger tumours and have a greater likelihood of long-term survival following surgery or other attempts at curative therapy.[282,290] Like dysplastic (or macroregenerative) nodules, they are larger than the surrounding cirrhotic nodules and they may differ in colour (frequently green, yellow or mottled) or they may bulge from the cut surface and, like dysplastic nodules, microscopic examination is needed for correct classification. In one series of 86 resected tumours 2 cm or less in diameter, approximately one-third were encapsulated while another third had indistinct margins, making them difficult to distinguish from the surrounding liver tissue.[291] Smaller tumours were more likely to have indistinct margins but were better differentiated histologically. In another series of 149 resected tumours 3 cm or less in diameter, 87% were encapsulated, but 19% had satellite lesions up to 2 cm from the main tumour mass.[292] Small nodules are easily overlooked in explanted livers unless the specimen is thinly sectioned and examined in detail.[293]

Microscopically, the cells of HCC resemble normal liver cells to a variable extent, depending on the degree of differentiation.[2] Nuclei are usually prominent with prominent nucleoli and a high nuclear : cytoplasmic ratio, and there is usually some hyperchromatism and nuclear irregularity, although this is quite variable. The tumour cells usually have distinct cell membranes and a moderate amount of eosinophilic, finely granular cytoplasm. They may contain a variety of cellular products, mimicking normal and pathological liver cell function. Bile canaliculi are nearly always present between cells and can often be seen by light microscopy (Fig. 15.29), and demonstrated immunohistochemically with polyclonal antiserum to carcinoembryonic

antigen (CEA) (Fig. 15.30) due to the presence of cross-reacting biliary glycoprotein I. Bile pigment may be found in tumour cells or in dilated canaliculi in about 50% of tumours (Figs 15.30–15.32). Cytoplasmic fat (Fig. 15.33) is present in at least some cells in about two-thirds of tumours,

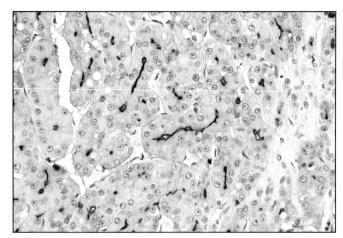

Fig. 15.30 • Hepatocellular carcinoma. An immunostain using polyclonal antiserum to CEA demonstrates bile canaliculi between tumour cells, due to the presence of cross-reacting biliary glycoprotein I.

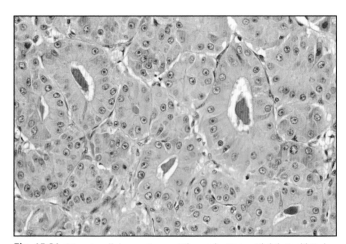

Fig. 15.31 • Hepatocellular carcinoma. Bile production, with bile in dilated canaliculi. H&E.

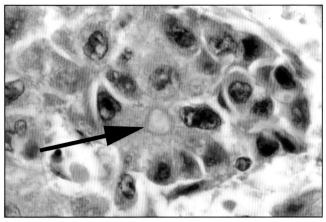

Fig. 15.29 • Hepatocellular carcinoma. The tumour cells resemble liver cells with prominent nuclei and nucleoli, granular eosinophilic cytoplasm and intercellular canaliculi (arrow). H&E.

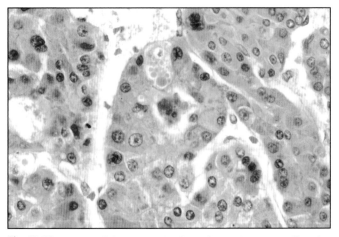

Fig. 15.32 • Hepatocellular carcinoma. Bile production in tumour cells and a dilated canaliculus. H&E.

and is abundant in about 10%. Large amounts of cytoplasmic fat and/or glycogen can cause the cytoplasm to appear white in routine sections, producing a clear-cell appearance (Fig. 15.34). Cytoplasmic Mallory bodies are present in approximately 20% of tumours and hyaline globules (Fig. 15.35) in another 20%, sometimes representing α_1-antitrypsin storage, while fibrinogen and other plasma proteins can be demonstrated by immunostains and sometimes form lightly eosinophilic ground-glass-like cytoplasmic inclusions.

The cells of HCC generally try to grow in ways that mimic the cell plates of normal liver, producing well-recognized growth patterns. In the earliest stages (so-called 'early HCC'), the tumour cells grow within pre-existing liver cell plates of a cirrhotic nodule, retaining the reticulin framework and sometimes preserving portal tracts.[291,294–296] Even though such tumours are very well differentiated, the cells have high nuclear : cytoplasmic ratios, giving an appearance of nuclear crowding, while the proliferation of malignant cells produces abnormal patterns with thin trabeculae and/or pseudoglands (Fig. 15.36). With progression of the tumour, normal structures are lost and the entire nodule is replaced by HCC. Most often the tumour grows in a *trabecular* pattern with thickened cords of cells separated by vascular sinusoids, mimicking the cell plates and sinusoids of normal liver (Figs 15.37–15.39). Rapid growth of the tumour cells causes the plates to become thickened and contorted, producing the trabeculae that are surrounded by endothelial cells which phenotypically resemble capillary

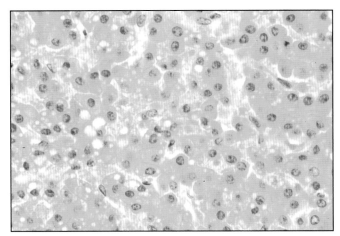

Fig. 15.33 • Hepatocellular carcinoma. A well-differentiated tumour with fat in some tumour cells. H&E.

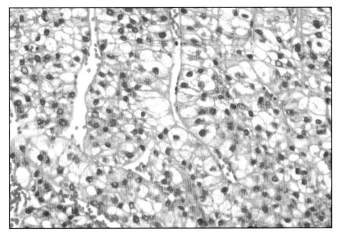

Fig. 15.34 • Hepatocellular carcinoma. A tumour whose cells have abundant glycogen and/or fat, producing a 'clear cell' appearance. H&E.

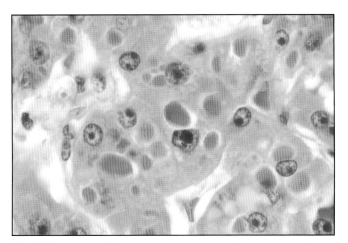

Fig. 15.35 • Hepatocellular carcinoma. A tumour with cytoplasmic hyaline globules. H&E.

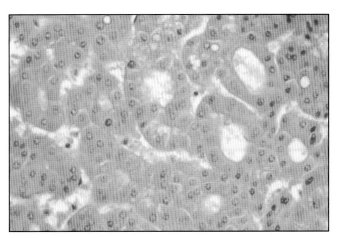

Fig. 15.36 • Hepatocellular carcinoma. An early, well-differentiated tumour in which the cells have a high nuclear : cytoplasmic ratio and are forming pseudoglands within pre-existing liver cell plates. H&E.

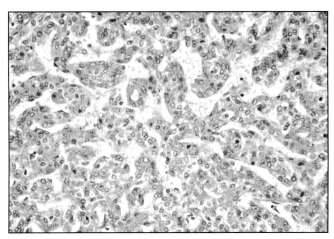

Fig. 15.37 • Hepatocellular carcinoma. A trabecular pattern with very thin trabeculae separated by blood sinusoids. H&E.

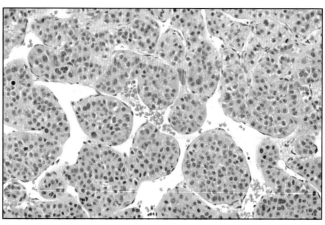

Fig. 15.38 • Hepatocellular carcinoma. A trabecular pattern in which the trabeculae are seen in cross section with masses of tumour cells surrounded by endothelial cells. H&E.

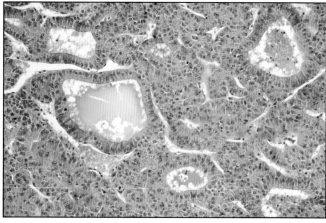

Fig. 15.40 • Hepatocellular carcinoma. A pseudoglandular pattern with a dilated canaliculus in the centres of several trabeculae. H&E.

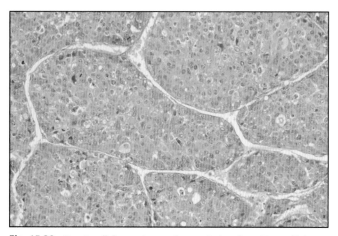

Fig. 15.39 • Hepatocellular carcinoma. A macrotrabecular pattern with large masses of tumour cells forming thick trabeculae. H&E.

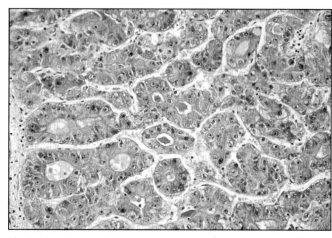

Fig. 15.41 • Hepatocellular carcinoma. A pseudoglandular pattern with bile production. H&E.

endothelium (CD34 positive) rather than normal hepatic sinusoidal endothelium (CD34 negative). The centres of the trabeculae may contain a very dilated canaliculus, producing a *pseudoglandular* pattern (Figs 15.40 and 15.41), or the trabeculae may grow together, compressing the sinusoids and forming sheets of tumour cells, producing a *compact* pattern (Fig. 15.42). Connective tissue stroma is typically sparse and reticulin fibres are absent or reduced, being found only at the periphery of trabeculae. The lack of a desmoplastic stroma is a helpful diagnostic clue and explains why, in contrast to most other malignant epithelial neoplasms, HCC is soft, with a few exceptions. Rarely, tumours with cytological and phenotypic features of otherwise typical HCC will produce abundant stroma, producing the *scirrhous* pattern of HCC (Fig. 15.43). There is also a subset of tumours that has been named *fibrolamellar* HCC, in which the cells have abundant granular eosinophilic cytoplasm as well as abundant stroma composed of lamellae of collagen. This subset, which differs from other types of HCC in clinical features and prognosis, is discussed further in the next section. Other rare variants include: occasional tumours that are otherwise trabecular but develop large vascular lakes within the tumour, mimicking peliosis hepatis, producing the *pelioid* pattern of HCC; tumours with solid or

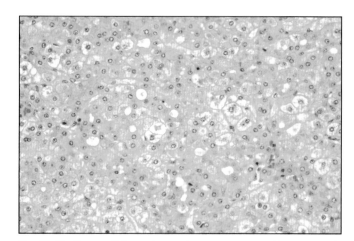

Fig. 15.42 • Hepatocellular carcinoma. A compact pattern with compressed sinusoids. H&E.

trabecular growth but a predominance of clear cells (so-called 'clear cell carcinoma') (Fig. 15.34); tumours that have prominent extramedullary haematopoiesis or a marked lymphocytic or neutrophilic inflammatory infiltrate in the tumour; tumours with osteoclast-like giant cells; and tumours with prominent spindle cell metaplasia, producing a sarcomatoid pattern (Fig. 15.44). In general, with the

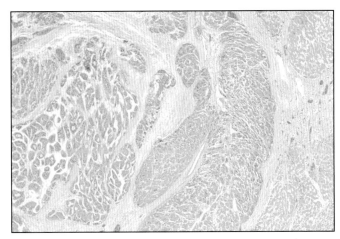

Fig. 15.43 • Hepatocellular carcinoma. A desmoplastic stroma, producing a scirrhous pattern with areas that are trabecular. H&E.

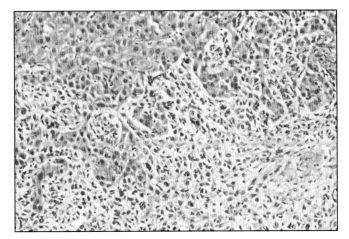

Fig. 15.44 • Hepatocellular carcinoma. Spindle cell metaplasia, producing a sarcomatoid pattern. H&E.

Table 15.4	Antigens that may be demonstrable in HCC by immunohistochemical techniques

Tumour cells

α_1-antitrypsin	Matrix metalloproteinase
α_1-antichymotrypsin	Midkine
α-fetoprotein	Metastatic tumour antigen 1
α-human chorionic gonadotropin	Metastasis suppressor gene products
α-, β- and γ-catenin	Nm23-H1
β2-microglobulin	KAI1
ABH blood group substance	Nuclear factor κB
Albumin	p18
Angiopoietin-1 and -2	p21
Annexin I	p27
Bcl-2	p53
Biliary glycoprotein I	p62
C-fos	P-glycoprotein
C-jun	PIVKA-II
C-kit	Proliferating cell nuclear antigen
C-myc	(PCNA)
C-reactive protein	Prothymosin
Caspase-3	Ras oncogene
Cathepsin B	RECK gene product
CD10	Retinoblastoma gene product
CD44	Somatostatin receptor
CEA (polyclonal)	Survivin
Clusterin	Telomerase
Cyclin D1	Thrombospondin
Cyclooxygenase-2	Tissue inhibitor of
Cytokeratin	metalloproteinase I & II
Clone AE1	Transferrin receptor
Clone AE3	Transforming growth factor-α
Clone Cam 5.2	Transforming growth factor-β1
Cytokeratin 7	Transcription factor ets-1
Cytokeratin 8	Transcription factor mdm2
Cytokeratin 18	Ubiquitin
Cytokeratin 19	Vascular endothelial growth factor
Cytokeratin 20	Vimentin
E-cadherin	
Ephrin-1	*Endothelial cells*
Epidermal growth factor	CD 31
Epithelial membrane antigen (EMA)	CD 34
Erythropoeisis associated antigen (ERY-1)	Factor VIII related antigen
	Fibroblast growth factor
Extracellular signal-regulated protein kinase	*Ulex europaeus* lectin
Factor XIIIa	*Other mesenchymal cells*
FAS	α-smooth muscle actin
Ferritin	(stellate cells)
Fibrinogen	CD68 (Kupffer cells)
Focal adhesion kinase	Calponin
Fragile histidine triad (FHIT) protein	Vimentin
Glypican-3	*Stroma*
Hepatitis B surface, core and X antigens	Collagen IV
	Fibronectin
Hep Par 1	Integrin
Ki-67	Intercellular adhesion
Metallothionein	molecule-1 (ICAM-1)
Lewis^x blood group substance	Laminin
Lewis^y blood group substance	
Macrophage metalloelastase	
MAGE (melanoma antigens) 1–12	

exception of the fibrolamellar type, these have no particular clinical or pathogenetic significance.

Immunostains have been extensively used to study HCC (Table 15.4; see also Chapter 3). Genes that play roles in growth and carcinogenesis are often activated and their products demonstrable by immunohistochemistry. Some, such as proliferating cell nuclear antigen (PCNA), have been reported to correlate with degree of differentiation, rapidity of tumour growth and inversely with length of survival, but since survival in general is so poor, none of these is routinely used in diagnosis or assessment of HCC. Since the cells of HCC mimic normal liver cells, they may produce any of the cellular products that can be found in hepatocytes, both in health and in disease, and, if present, these are readily demonstrated by immunostaining. Many of these can also be found in tumours other than HCC, and so are of little use in differential diagnosis. There are no stains that can consistently distinguish well-differentiated HCC from benign lesions, such as hepatocellular adenoma or dysplastic nodules and, similarly, no single stain can always distinguish poorly differentiated HCC from poorly differentiated cholangiocarcinoma or metastatic adenocarcinoma. However, selected immunostains, taken in the context of other morphological features, can be very helpful in establishing the diagnosis of HCC in difficult cases.[297] *Polyclonal antiserum to carcinoembryonic antigen (pCEA)* is useful in demonstrating bile canaliculi, both in normal liver and in hepatocellular carcinoma, due to the presence of a CEA-like cross-reactive substance called biliary glycoprotein I, one of the most useful of all positive findings in distinguishing HCC from other malignancies (Figs 15.30 and 15.45). Antibodies to CD10 may also be used to outline canaliculi. *Hepatocyte Paraffin 1 (HepPar-1)* is a monoclonal antibody that reacts with an epitope of liver mitochondria, with a typical granular pattern in most liver specimens.[298,299] It also sometimes reacts with renal tubules and intestinal epithelium as well as with intestinal metaplasia in the stomach and oesophagus, so it is not completely specific for hepatocytes. It produces positive staining in approximately 90% of cases of HCC (Fig. 15.46) and only 4% of other tumours, including some cholangiocarcinomas and metastatic adenocarcinomas of the stomach and other sites,[299] and when used in the context of morphology, clinical setting and other stains, HepPar-1 is very useful in distinguishing HCC from other malignancies. Approximately 10% of HCC are negative for HepPar-1, and the degree of positive staining varies from case-to-case; some tumours have a very patchy distribution of positive cells, which can be easily missed in a small biopsy. Nearly all other benign and malignant tumours that we have studied to date have been completely negative, with the exception of a few adenocarcinomas of the stomach and, rarely, cholangiocarcinoma. The pattern of staining for these few exceptions, however, is different from HCC, with a finer and paler cytoplasmic positivity. In some patients we have also observed positive staining in normal kidney tubules (although renal cell carcinomas have all been negative) and in normal intestinal epithelium and intestinal metaplasia of the stomach. Nevertheless, this antibody appears very promising for differentiating HCC from other tumours.

α-fetoprotein (AFP) is frequently elevated in the serum of patients with HCC, even when the tumour is negative by immunostaining. In most published series it has been found in no more than 50% of tumours (with a wide range). It may only be focally present in tumour cell cytoplasm and, in general, it is less useful than pCEA for diagnostic purposes. *Cytokeratins* are sometimes suggested as a means of tumour classification, especially cytokeratin (CK) 7 and 20, but there are many cases where the tumours display aberrant keratin expression, so staining patterns must be interpreted with caution. Normal liver cells have exclusively CD8 and CK18, while biliary epithelium has CK7, CK8, CK18 and CK19, and intestinal epithelium has CK20. HCC usually has CK8 and CK18, and there is a common misconception that it is always negative for CK7, CK19 and CK20. In fact, CK7 is present in about 50% of HCC, while CK20 can be found in about 20% of tumours, and it has been found that tumours with biliary type keratin expression tend to be more poorly differentiated and have a more rapid course than those that do not.[300–302] Consequently, cytokeratin profiles are not very useful in the diagnosis of HCC. *CD34* is present and demonstrable in endothelial cells of large blood vessels and most capillary beds throughout the body with the exception of normal hepatic sinusoidal endothelium. The endothelial cells that surround the trabeculae of HCC are usually positive for CD34 (Fig. 15.47). Benign hepatocellular lesions may have CD34-positive sinusoids in areas that receive increased arterial blood, so that cirrhotic nodules tend to be positive only around the periphery and focal nodular hyperplasia in sinusoids near the fibrous septa; thus, diffuse, regular CD34 positivity of sinusoids can be helpful in distinguishing a cirrhotic nodule from a well-differentiated hepatocellular carcinoma. Staining in hepatocellular adenomas is variable, so that a positive stain does not necessarily indicate malignancy.[297,303]

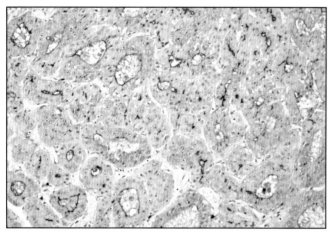

Fig. 15.45 • Hepatocellular carcinoma. Immunostain with polyclonal antiserum to CEA shows staining of canalicular membranes.

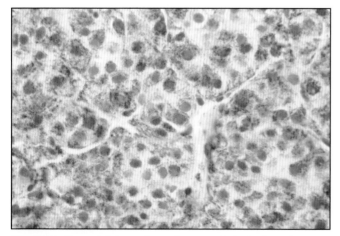

Fig. 15.46 • Hepatocellular carcinoma. Immunostain for HepPar-1 shows granular staining of cytoplasm.

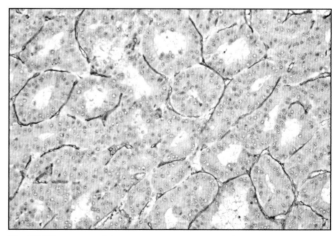

Fig. 15.47 • Hepatocellular carcinoma. Immunostain for CD34 shows staining of endothelial cells surrounding the trabeculae.

Grading and staging

Histological grading of malignant tumours is based on the premise that those that look worse, based on lack of differentiation, degree of anaplasia, or number of mitoses, will grow faster and progress more rapidly to cause the death of the patient. Edmondson and Steiner[304] proposed grading HCC on a scale of I to IV, with increasing nuclear irregularity, hyperchromatism and nuclear/cytoplasmic ratio, associated with decreasing cytological differentiation for each successively higher grade. They placed great emphasis on the amount and appearance of the cytoplasm and the nuclear/cytoplasmic ratio, so that their grade IV tumours had very scant cytoplasm even though the nuclei might be minimally anaplastic. A correlation between the grade and prognosis has been reported by some[305,306] but disputed by others.[307] It is not clear that the Edmondson–Steiner grading system has been uniformly applied, and it has never been widely used. Grading of HCC can be done on the basis of nuclear features alone,[2,308] or nuclear features combined with microvascular invasion.[306] A series of 1063 cases from the AFIP[308] used a modified four-category grading system, based primarily on nuclear features (Fig. 15.48) and found a statistically significant correlation of survival with tumour grade. In this system, illustrated in the AFIP fascicle,[2] grade 1 tumours are composed of cells with abundant cytoplasm and minimal nuclear irregularity, and are impossible to distinguish from hepatocellular adenoma cytologically, so that the diagnosis must be made on the basis of trabecular or pseudoglandular growth, vascular invasion or metastasis. Grade 2 has prominent nucleoli, hyperchromatism and some degree of irregularity of the nuclear membrane. Grade 3 has even greater nuclear pleomorphism and angulated nuclei. Grade 4 has marked pleomorphism, hyperchromatism and usually anaplastic giant cells. There was a statistically significant shortening of survival with higher nuclear grade, but overall survival was very poor with 2.4% living 5 years from diagnosis. In a series of 425 patients undergoing curative resections, nuclear grade and the absence of microvascular invasion were found to be independent predictors of survival, and a combination of these could be used to identify two groups of patients, one with 5-year post-resection survival of approximately 50% and the other approximately 25%.[306] Although it has been recommended

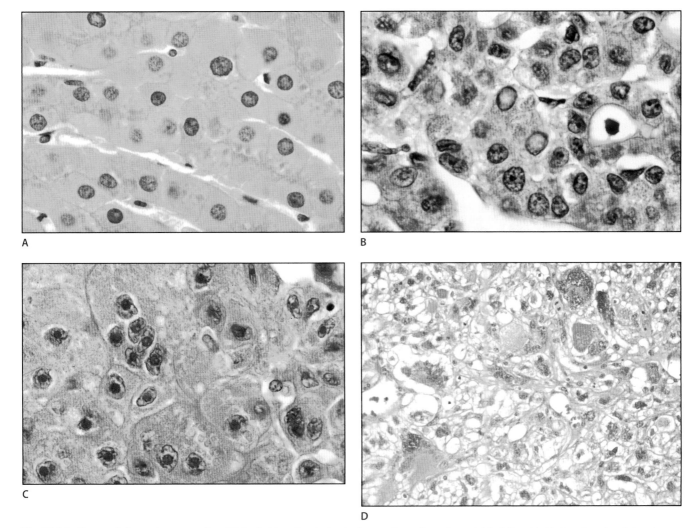

Fig. 15.48 • Hepatocellular carcinoma, grading. **(A)** Grade 1 has abundant cytoplasm and round, regular nuclei, indistinguishable from hepatocellular adenoma. **(B)** Grade 2 has round, regular nuclei, but there is some hyperchromatism, nucleoli, and high nuclear:cytoplasmic ratios. **(C)** Grade 3 has pronounced nuclear irregularity, hyperchromatism, and very prominent nucleoli. **(D)** Grade 4 has marked nuclear pleomorphism with anaplastic giant cells. H&E.

that the grade be reported in resection specimens of HCC,[309] it is not evident how this is clinically relevant in an individual case.

Staging of a malignant tumour is a measure of how far it has progressed in its natural history. A number of staging systems have been proposed to stratify patients by likelihood of survival and to identify those with the best chance of cure,[310-318] but there is still considerable controversy as to which is the best staging method, and what elements constitute the appropriate components of such a system. This is due partly to the fact that HCC often arises in a liver already badly damaged by chronic liver disease and cirrhosis, partly to the fact that most tumours are incurable when discovered, and partly to the recent advances in early diagnosis and treatment which have altered the perceived natural history of HCC in those selected cases. Furthermore, the presence of chronic liver disease or cirrhosis complicates therapy and also leaves the patient at risk for developing new tumours, even if the current HCC is successfully eradicated. Consequently, many staging systems incorporate clinical and laboratory features as well as characteristics of the tumour itself.

TNM (tumour, nodes, metastases) staging, as codified by the International Union against Cancer (UICC), is widely used for many malignancies and is available for HCC (Table 15.5).[129] Most clinical series, however, have used one of the other staging systems (Table 15.6) that incorporate features related to the nature of the underlying liver disease, the functional state of the liver and the size of the tumour in formulating an approach to treatment. One study compared five different staging systems in a series of 187 patients[319] and another compared seven staging systems in 244 patients;[320] both found that the Barcelona Clinic Liver Cancer Staging Classification,[313,318] which incorporates tumour extent, liver function and overall patient performance status was best at identifying treatable patients and predicting survival.

Table 15.5	TNM staging of liver tumours[310]

T1	Single nodule without vascular invasion
T2	Single nodule with vascular invasion or multiple nodules, none more than 5 cm in greatest dimension
T3	Multiple tumours more than 5 cm or tumour involving a major branch of the portal or hepatic vein
T4	Tumour with direct invasion of adjacent organ other than gallbladder or perforation of visceral peritoneum
N0	No regional lymph node metastases
N1	Regional lymph node metastases
M0	No distant metastases
M1	Distant metastases
Stage I	T1 N0 M0
Stage II	T2 N0 M0
Stage IIIA	T3 N0 M0
Stage IIIB	T4 N0 M0
Stage IIIC	Any T N1 M0
Stage IV	Any T or N M1

Differential diagnosis

The difficulties in distinguishing well-differentiated HCC from benign hepatocellular lesions are discussed earlier in this chapter in the sections on hepatocellular adenoma, focal nodular hyperplasia and dysplastic nodules. High nuclear : cytoplasmic ratio of the tumour cells is the most reliable sign of malignancy, even when the nuclei are not atypical, while trabecular or pseudoglandular growth patterns also distinguish well-differentiated HCC from benign hepatocellular lesions. Another benign tumour that can be mistake for HCC is angiomyolipoma, which is discussed later in the chapter.

A frequent problem in differential diagnosis is in distinguishing poorly differentiated HCC from other malignancies, especially metastases but also from poorly differentiated cholangiocarcinoma. A large-cell carcinoma with eosinophilic cytoplasm, prominent nuclei and nucleoli may well be HCC but that diagnosis should not be made without definite evidence of hepatocellular differentiation. Bile canaliculi recognizable on haematoxylin and eosin, polyclonal CEA or CD10 stain, a positive stain for AFP, a granular staining pattern with HepPar-1, or a trabecular growth pattern allows a diagnosis of HCC with more or less certainty, except for the very rare cases of liver metastasis from

Table 15.6	Staging systems for HCC; components of the different systems	
Staging system	**Tumour characteristics**	**Clinical and laboratory features**
Okuda[311]	Tumour size	Ascites Albumin Bilirubin
CLIP[312]	Tumour size Number of nodules Portal vein thrombosis	Child–Turcotte–Pugh score* α-fetoprotein
BCLC[312,318]	Tumour size Number of nodules Portal vein thrombosis	Child–Turcotte–Pugh score* ECOG performance status** Portal hypertension
GRETCH[314]	Vascular invasion	ECOG performance status** Bilirubin Alkaline phosphatase α-fetoprotein
CUPI[315]	TNM stage	Symptoms Ascites Bilirubin Alkaline phosphatase α-fetoprotein
JIS[316]	TNM stage	Child–Turcotte–Pugh score*
Tokyo score[317]	Tumour size Tumour number	Albumin Bilirubin

* Includes bilirubin, albumin, prothrombin time, ascites, encephalopathy.
** Six-grade scale of patient's clinical status ranging from 0 (fully active) to 5 (dead).
ECOG: Eastern Cooperative Oncology Group performance status.

a gastrointestinal adenocarcinoma with hepatoid features. If no such evidence of hepatocellular differentiation is found, the tumour is more likely to be metastatic than primary in the liver. Cholangiocarcinomas and metastatic adenocarcinomas typically have a desmoplastic stroma, in contrast to HCC, and so a tumour with abundant stroma is almost always an adenocarcinoma, with the exception of the rare fibrolamellar type and even rarer scirrhous type of HCC. Metastatic melanomas (especially amelanotic), as well as carcinoids and some more poorly differentiated neuroendocrine tumours, and also renal cell carcinomas may also be confused with HCC, as these all typically have large tumour cells with abundant cytoplasm. If definite features of HCC are not present, these should all be considered and evaluated with a battery of immunostains (S-100 and HMB45 for melanoma, chromogranin and synaptophysin for carcinoids and neuroendocrine tumours, leu-M1 and RCC antigen for renal cell carcinoma).

Spread and metastases

Small untreated tumours followed by imaging studies have been shown to double in volume anywhere from 27 to 605 days, with an average doubling time of approximately five to six months.[321-323] In the early stages, most tumours appear to grow as an expanding, often encapsulated, mass. As tumours enlarge, they infiltrate the surrounding liver tissue and form satellite nodules.[291,292] Microvascular invasion is common, being found in approximately 50% of tumours,[306,308] and intrahepatic metastases, presumably via haematogenous spread, are present in 60% of tumours less than 5 cm in diameter and over 95% of those greater than 5 cm.[323] Thrombosis of the portal vein or its branches occurs in 65–75% and the hepatic veins in 20–25% of advanced tumours.[323,324] Invasion of large bile ducts with obstructive jaundice occurs in approximately 5%. Advanced tumours often invade the diaphragm and occasionally the gallbladder, and peritoneal dissemination can occur. Most patients with HCC die of liver failure due to replacement by the tumour, but extrahepatic metastases are common, being found at autopsy in over one-half of cases,[323,324] with lung and regional lymph nodes as the most frequent sites of metastasis.

Treatment and prognosis

Treatment of HCC has advanced considerably in the past decade, and high cure rates can be obtained for patients with small tumours detected while still asymptomatic. In general, these are patients with known chronic liver disease and cirrhosis, living in developed countries and receiving careful surveillance, usually with semiannual or quarterly screening with serum α-fetoprotein levels and ultrasound examination to detect tumour development. Most patients worldwide, however, present with advanced disease and survive for only a short time.

A number of forms of curative and palliative therapy have been attempted with varying success, and optimal treatment strategies are still controversial.[282,325] Surgical resec-

tion works best for small tumours in patients with no underlying liver disease. For patients with multiple small tumours and compensated cirrhosis, liver transplantation offers the possibility of curing the underlying liver disease as well as the tumour. Since transplantation is not readily available for many patients, percutaneous ablation has become the treatment of choice for early but unresectable tumours. Injection of ethanol directly into the HCC under ultrasound guidance causes necrosis of the tumour and surrounding liver tissue. Several types of thermal ablation have been used similarly, with a device inserted into the lesions, and radiofrequency waves, microwaves, laser or cryoablation are used to destroy the tumour and a rim of surrounding normal tissue. Of these, ethanol injection and radiofrequency ablation have become the most widely used and have been shown to cure small lesions and prolong survival as a temporary treatment for patients awaiting definitive therapy by resection or transplantation. Radiation, chemotherapy and hormonal therapy have proven of little benefit in patients with HCC. Since HCC receives its blood supply from the hepatic artery rather than the portal vein, angiographic embolization of the artery has been used to produce tumour necrosis and prolong survival. The embolic material may be combined with lipiodol and antineoplastic drugs, such as doxorubicin, and this chemoembolization may provide further therapeutic efficacy. Current Barcelona Clinic Liver Cancer (BCLC) recommendations for therapy of HCC, using the BCLC staging classification (Table 15.7), are that stage 0 and A (very early and early HCC) receive curative treatment; surgical resection is advocated for stages A2, A3 or A4; and transplantation or ablation for stages B and C (intermediate or advanced HCC), with chemoembolization for stage B and chemoembolization or enrolment in a clinical trial for newer agents for stage C. Patients with stage D (end-stage HCC) receive symptomatic treatment.[282]

Fibrolamellar hepatocellular carcinoma

This variant of hepatocellular carcinoma has distinctive histological and clinical features and a natural history that justify its separation from other types of hepatocellular carcinoma. Although examples had been noted previously, it was two series published in 1980 that established this as an entity distinct from other types of HCC.[326,327] Of the first 80 cases reported, the mean age was 23,[328] considerably younger than patients with other types of HCC. There are reports of cases in older adults, but verified cases over the age of 40 are rare. Unlike other types of HCC, there are approximately equal numbers of males and females, and no association with chronic liver disease, cirrhosis or any other known risk factor. The tumours tend to be slow-growing compared to other types of HCC and are frequently surgically resectable. Since the tumour occurs in patients without risk factors, they are nearly always symptomatic when detected but, even so, over one-half are judged to be resectable when discovered. Those that are not resectable may be cured by liver transplantation. The first 80 reported cases[328] had a 5-year survival of 56%, compared to less than 5% expected

Stage	ECOG performance status	Tumour	Okuda stage	Liver functional status
0 (Very early HCC)	0	Single, <2 cm	I	Child–Turcotte–Pugh class A No portal hypertension Normal bilirubin
A (Early HCC)				
A1	0	Single, any size	I	No portal hypertension Normal bilirubin
A2	0	Single, any size	I	Portal hypertension present Normal bilirubin
A3	0	Single, any size	I	Portal hypertension Elevated bilirubin
A4	0	2 or 3 tumours, all <3 cm	I–II	Child–Turcotte–Pugh class A or B
B (Intermediate)	0	Large, multinodular	I–II	Child–Turcotte–Pugh class A or B
C (Advanced HCC)	1–2*	Vascular invasion* or extrahepatic spread	I–II	Child–Turcotte–Pugh class A or B
D (End-stage HCC)	3–4**	Any	III**	Child–Turcotte–Pugh class C**

Table 15.7 The Barcelona Clinic Liver Cancer (BCLC) Staging Classification[312,318]

* Stage C = either performance status 1–2 or vascular invasion or extrahepatic spread
** Stage D = either performance status 3–4 or Okuda stage III or Child–Turcotte–Pugh class C
ECOG: Eastern Cooperative Oncology Group performance status.

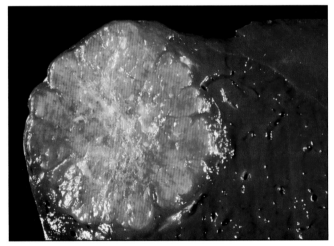

Fig. 15.49 • Fibrolamellar hepatocellular carcinoma. The tumour is hard and yellow to tan with areas of fibrosis. The cut surface stands out above the surrounding non-cirrhotic liver.

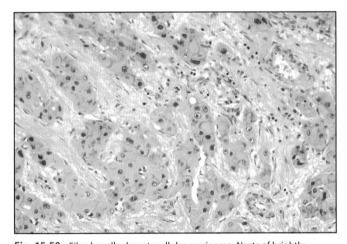

Fig. 15.50 • Fibrolamellar hepatocellular carcinoma. Nests of brightly eosinophilic tumour cells in a fibrous stroma. H&E.

for other types of HCC at that time. The largest reported series of patients treated by surgery (28 patients) or transplantation (13 patients) had 5-year survival of 66%, even though 90% had TNM stage IV disease with extrahepatic metastases at the time of surgery.[329] Thus, fibrolamellar HCC is clearly a different biological entity from other types of HCC.

Pathology

Unlike other types of HCC, fibrolamellar tumours are typically hard, due to the presence of fibrous stroma. Strands of white fibrous tissue are often grossly visible in the tumour, which is otherwise brown, tan or occasionally green. There may even be fibrous septa linked to a central area of scar-

ring, giving the tumour a lobulated appearance reminiscent of focal nodular hyperplasia (Fig. 15.49). For unknown reasons, two-thirds of fibrolamellar HCC arise in the left lobe of the liver, even though it is smaller than the right lobe and, indeed, this the only liver tumour that is more frequent in the left lobe.

Microscopically, fibrolamellar HCC is characterized by distinctive cytological features and the fibrous stroma that give the lesion its name (Fig. 15.50).[2,326,327] The stroma consists of thick, hyalinized bundles of collagen as well as thinner collagen and reticulin fibres that support individual and small groups of tumour cells which may form pseudoglands around dilated canaliculi. The bundles of collagen tend to be arranged in parallel lamellae of varied thickness (Fig. 15.51), hence the name fibrolamellar. Characteristically, the cells are larger that normal liver cells, are polyhedral or

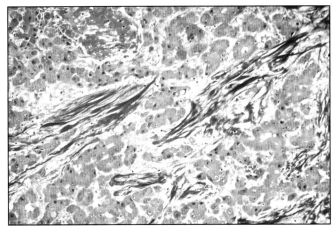

Fig. 15.51 • Fibrolamellar hepatocellular carcinoma. The fibrous stroma is composed of bundles of collagen arranged in parallel lamellae. H&E.

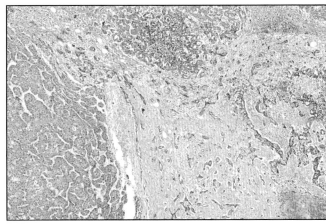

Fig. 15.53 • Combined hepatocellular–cholangiocarcinoma. There is an area of trabecular hepatocellular carcinoma on the left and desmoplastic tubuloglandular cholangiocarcinoma on the right. H&E.

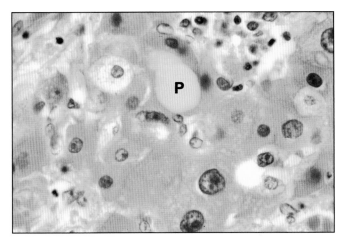

Fig. 15.52 • Fibrolamellar hepatocellular carcinoma. The tumour cells have abundant, granular, deeply eosinophilic cytoplasm, and occasional pale bodies (P) that represent fibrinogen inclusions. H&E.

rounded and have a deeply eosinophilic, coarsely granular cytoplasm (Fig. 15.52) due to the presence of a large number of mitochondria. Bile production may be present and occasional tumours produce mucin. There may be Mallory bodies or hyaline globular cytoplasmic inclusions, usually PAS positive and composed of α_1-antitrypsin. Approximately 50% of tumours have ground glass-like cytoplasmic inclusions or 'pale bodies' (Fig. 15.52) composed of cytoplasmic fibrinogen. The nuclei of the tumour cells are large, hyperchromatic and vesicular, and have prominent, often eosinophilic, nucleoli. Mitoses and multinucleation are infrequent.

Mixed tumours

Combined hepatocellular–cholangiocarcinoma is the term used for tumours with elements of both HCC and cholangiocarcinoma (CC). These account for less than 1% of primary liver malignancies. Some have considered these to be a subtype of HCC,[330–333] while others have suggested that they are actually more closely related to CC.[334–337] In most series, the clinical behaviour has been more like that of HCC, and so they are often considered a special subtype of HCC rather

than a separate tumour.[2] A study of chromosomal changes, however, found similar loss of heterozygosity at 3p and 14p in both CC and combined HCC–CC but not in HCC, suggesting that the combined tumours are closer to CC in pathogenesis.[337]

To be considered combined hepatocellular–cholangiocarcinoma, a tumour should have unequivocal areas of HCC with trabecular growth, bile production or bile canaliculi, as well as unequivocal cholangiocarcinoma with gland formation by biliary-type cells in a desmoplastic stroma or mucin production (Fig. 15.53). HCC with a pseudoglandular pattern may be mistaken for combined hepatocellular–cholangiocarcinomas, but it can be distinguished by the fact that the cells surrounding the pseudoglands resemble hepatocytes and may produce bile but not mucin. Immunostains can be used to supplement the diagnosis, so that HepPar-1 and polyclonal CEA are useful in demonstrating an hepatocellular component, and in situ hybridization for albumin mRNA has also been suggested as a marker of an hepatocellular component.[335] Cytokeratins are not especially useful, since some hepatocellular carcinomas contain biliary-type keratins (CK7 and CK19), but apomucins have been suggested to be another indication of biliary differentiation.[334]

Some tumours that fit the definition of combined hepatocellular–cholangiocarcinoma are 'collision tumours' with coincidental but separate HCC and CC in the same liver. The majority, however, appear to have areas of both HCC and CC, as well as areas of apparent transition from typical HCC to adenocarcinoma or to a mixed hepatocellular and glandular tumour, indicating that there is dual differentiation in the same malignancy. There are reports of occasional poorly differentiated tumours thought to be of intermediate or hepatic progenitor cell phenotype, and it has been suggested that these give rise to the dual differentiation of HCC–CC.[338,339] As noted in the previous section, some fibrolamellar hepatocellular carcinomas produce mucin, and by that definition they could be considered combined HCC–CC. However, like other fibrolamellar carcinomas, they occur in a different clinical setting and have different biological behaviour, and consequently are not usually considered to be HCC–CC.

Carcinosarcoma that has an element of HCC is extremely rare. Most reported cases are actually HCC with spindle-cell change[340] or a combined hepatocellular–cholangiocarcinoma with spindle-cell metaplasia of the cholangiocarcinoma element, whereas a true carcinosarcoma has HCC or combined HCC-CC along with differentiated sarcomatous elements, such as chondrosarcoma, osteosarcoma, leiomyosarcoma or malignant schwannoma.[2,341–344]

Benign biliary tumours and tumour-like lesions

Von Meyenburg complex (biliary microhamartoma)

The von Meyenburg complex is a developmental malformation that is thought to represent persistence of the embryonic ductal plate.[345] They are relatively common, being found in 5.6% of adult autopsies.[346] They may be multiple, and there is an association with solitary bile duct cysts as well as with polycystic liver and kidney disease. The histological appearance is quite characteristic. Individual lesions are seldom larger than 5 mm. They are typically adjacent to a portal area and consist of a fibrous stroma that contains irregularly shaped duct-like structures lined by a low cuboidal epithelium (Fig. 15.54). The ducts are usually somewhat dilated and often U-shaped or branching. They may contain proteinaceous or bile-stained secretions. In occasional lesions, one of the ducts may dilate sufficiently to form a macroscopic cyst. Multiple von Meyenburg complexes are to considered to be part of the spectrum of hepatic fibropolycystic disease (Chapter 4). It is generally believed that both solitary bile duct cyst and the cysts of polycystic disease arise from dilatation of von Meyenburg complexes.[345] There are rare reports of associated cholangiocarcinoma.[347,348]

Bile duct cyst

Bile duct cysts are unilocular and lined by a single layer of columnar or low cuboidal epithelium resting on a basement membrane and a layer of fibrous tissue. They usually contain clear fluid, but if there is secondary trauma or infection, the fluid may be haemorrhagic, purulent or bile-stained. Most solitary cysts are small and asymptomatic, but occasionally they may become large enough to cause abdominal swelling or pain, especially if there is secondary trauma. Patients with polycystic disease are most likely to be symptomatic, and occasionally develop adenocarcinoma in a cyst. Malignancy in a solitary cyst is extremely rare.

Ciliated hepatic foregut cyst

Ciliated foregut cysts are rare lesions believed to arise from the embryonic foregut and to differentiate toward bronchial structures in the liver, analogous to a brochogenic cyst of the mediastinum.[349,350] The cysts are typically subcapsular, small (<4 cm in diameter), usually unilocular, rarely multilocular and contain clear fluid. At least part of the cyst is lined by ciliated, pseudostratified columnar epithelium (Fig. 15.55), although in part the epithelium may be cuboidal or have squamous metaplasia. The epithelium rests on a basement membrane and the cyst is usually surrounded by bundles of smooth muscle and an outer fibrous capsule. As with the bile duct cyst, malignancy is very rare.[351]

Peribiliary gland hamartoma (bile duct adenoma)

This lesion, traditionally called bile duct adenoma, is a small, well-circumscribed mass composed of small acini and tubules set in fibrous stroma. The term peribiliary gland hamartoma was proposed by Bhathal et al.[352] who showed that its cells actually have the phenotype of normal peribiliary glands rather than bile ducts. The largest published series was 152 cases studied at AFIP,[353] with 89 (58.6%)

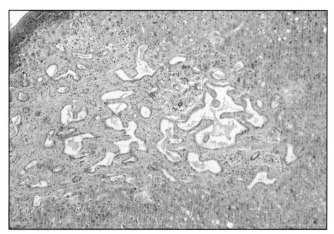

Fig. 15.54 • Von Meyenburg complex. Irregular branching glands with low, columnar epithelium in a fibrous stroma. H&E.

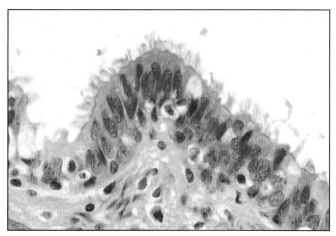

Fig. 15.55 • Ciliated hepatic foregut cyst. The lining is a pseudostratified columnar epithelium with cilia, similar to bronchial epithelium. H&E.

males and 63 (41.4%) females. All were asymptomatic and discovered incidentally during abdominal surgery or at autopsy. As with cysts and von Meyenburg complexes, development of malignancy is extremely rare. In the AFIP series, 82.9% of the lesions were solitary; 6.6% of patients had two lesions and 10.5% had multiple lesions. They were 10 mm or less in diameter in 92.8% of cases. They are typically well-demarcated subcapsular gray or white, firm masses, and when encountered at surgery, they are biopsied because of the clinical suspicion of metastatic carcinoma. Microscopically, peribiliary gland hamartoma is composed of small tubules and acini lined by a single layer of cuboidal to columnar cells resting on a basement membrane (Figs 15.56 and 15.57) Nuclei are basally-placed and show no hyperchromasia, atypia or mitoses. Acidic mucin (alcian blue positive) is usually present in some cells of the lesion. The stroma is fibrous and may be loose and scanty, or dense and hyalinized. There is usually some inflammation, which occasionally is considerable, and normal portal tracts are often identified in the lesion. Large bile ducts are sometimes found adjacent to the lesions (Fig. 15.56), strengthening the theory that these are related to peribiliary glands. The major importance of peribiliary gland hamartoma is its possible confusion with intrahepatic cholangiocarcinoma or meta-static adenocarcinoma. Awareness of the entity along with the presence of pre-existing portal areas, the absence of pleomorphism and mitoses and the configuration of the glands and tubule (round rather than angulated) are all helpful in distinguishing peribiliary gland hamartoma from adenocarcinoma.

Biliary papillomatosis

Biliary papillomatosis is a rare disease characterized by multiple, benign papillary tumours that are typically located in the intra- and extrahepatic bile ducts, and sometimes involving the gallbladder or pancreatic duct. Most cases occur in adults, but a few cases have been reported in children. Symptoms result from biliary obstruction and its complications, and because of the multifocality of the disease, curative resection is difficult, recurrence is frequent, and invasive adenocarcinoma may develop.[354] The affected bile ducts are variably dilated and contain papillary or villous growths of columnar epithelial cells supported by delicate fibrovascular stalks (Fig. 15.58). The epithelial cells may resemble biliary epithelium or there may be foveolar or colonic metaplasia. Mucin production may be present, with or without goblet cells, and there may be varying degrees of dysplasia with 'carcinoma in situ' or even invasive adenocarcinoma.

Hepatobiliary cystadenoma

Hepatobiliary cystadenoma is a solitary, multilocular cystic neoplasm that can arise within the liver, extrahepatic bile ducts or gallbladder, and it is very similar to mucinous cystadenoma of the pancreas.[355] It is almost exclusively a tumour of adult women with only a few cases reported in men or children. Cases usually come to clinical attention because of an enlarging mass that may be painful. Radiological findings are often diagnostic, showing large multilocular cysts with internal septations and sometimes calcifications and other secondary changes, but distinction from cystadenocarcinoma is often not possible.[356] Complete excision is recommended for both cystadenoma and

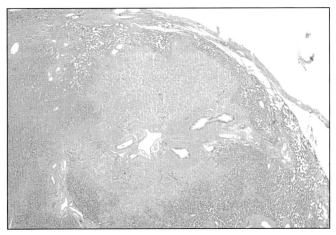

Fig. 15.56 • Peribiliary gland hamartoma (bile duct adenoma). The lesion surrounds a large bile duct. H&E.

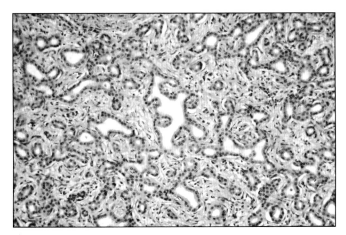

Fig. 15.57 • Peribiliary gland hamartoma (bile duct adenoma). Small tubules and acini with a cuboidal epithelium. H&E.

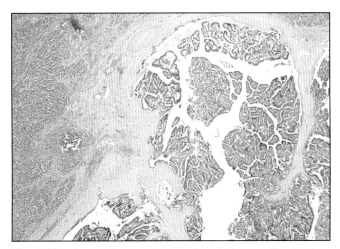

Fig. 15.58 • Biliary papillomatosis. The intrahepatic ducts are dilated and contain papillary tumours on fibrovascular stalks. H&E.

cystadenocarcinoma, since benign tumours that are incompletely excised may recur or undergo malignant transformation.

Most hepatobiliary cystadenomas arise within the liver itself. They may be as large as 28 cm in diameter. There are multiple communicating locules of varied size that generally have a smooth and glistening lining. The locules contain fluid that is usually clear and thin but may be turbid, purulent or bloody. Microscopically, cystadenomas are nearly always mucinous, with only one reported serous variety that was similar to the serous microcystic cystadenoma of the pancreas.[355] The locules of cystadenomas are lined by a predominantly columnar epithelium (Fig. 15.59) which may become cuboidal or flattened in some areas or rarely may be papillary. The epithelial cells usually resemble biliary or foveolar epithelium with mucicarmine and alcian blue positive cytoplasmic mucin. Intestinal metaplasia with goblet cells may also be present. A typical feature, present in over 80% of tumours, is the presence of areas of highly cellular mesenchymal tissue resembling ovarian stroma (Fig 15.59 and 15.60), which has prompted the name 'cystadenoma with mesenchymal stroma'.[357] The ovarian-like stroma is only found in females, and at least some cases have been reported to have oestrogen receptors and progesterone receptors in the stromal cells detected by immunohistochemistry.[358] The epithelium of the locules may become ulcerated with extravasation of cyst fluid into the stroma or wall, or the lesions may be traumatized secondary to their large size, so that inflammation, xanthogranulomatous reaction, scarring, and sometimes calcifications are frequently present in the tumours. The epithelium of cystadenoma may have varying degrees of dysplasia. When high-grade dysplasia or invasive carcinoma is present, then the lesion is considered to have evolved into a cystadenocarcinoma.

The histogenesis as well as the pathogenesis of these unusual tumours remains speculative. The female predominance and ovarian-like stroma has suggested that the tumours arise from ectopic ovarian tissue. Alternatively, it has been suggested that the mesenchymal stroma resembles the primitive mesenchyme of the embryonic gallbladder and large bile ducts, raising the possibility of origin of the tumour from embryonic foregut rests.[359]

Malignant biliary tumours

Hepatobiliary cystadenocarcinoma

Hepatobiliary cystadenocarcinoma is a rare tumour that is multilocular, cystic and contains adenocarcinoma.[355] The majority of these are adenocarcinomas that have arisen in a pre-existing cystadenoma, but there are some that appear to be peculiar cystic adenocarcinomas that are more probably a cystic variant of cholangiocarcinoma, and there are also some, as noted above, that represent adenocarcinomas arising in benign bile duct cysts. This mixed pathogenesis results in more varied clinical and pathological features than in benign cystadenomas. Thus, approximately half of the reported cystadenocarcinomas have occurred in men. The tumours in women frequently have ovarian-type stroma, indicating origin from a benign cystadenoma, while those in men do not. The malignant component may be papillary, tubular, squamous, spindled or some combination of these (Fig. 15.61).

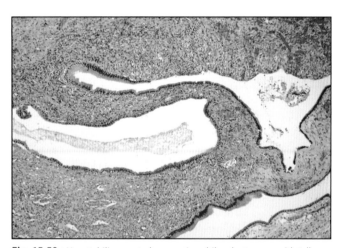

Fig. 15.59 • Hepatobiliary cystadenoma. A multilocular tumour with tall columnar mucinous epithelium overlying a compact ovarian-like stroma. H&E.

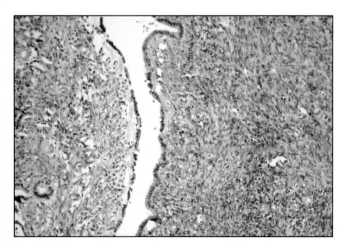

Fig. 15.60 • Hepatobiliary cystadenoma. An area with abundant mesenchymal stroma. H&E.

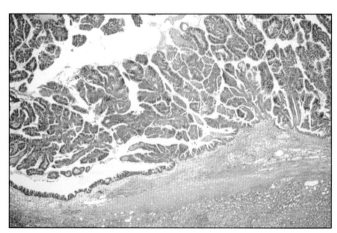

Fig. 15.61 • Hepatobiliary cystadenocarcinoma. A multilocular cystic neoplasm lined with papillary adenocarcinoma. H&E.

Cholangiocarcinoma

Cholangiocarcinoma (CC) is an adenocarcinoma arising from a bile duct. Distinction is often made between those that arise within the liver (intrahepatic or peripheral CC), those that arise at the confluence of the right and left hepatic ducts (hilar CC) and those that arise between the ampulla of Vater and the hepatic hilum (extrahepatic CC). This is justified since the clinical presentations differ. Hilar cholangiocarcinomas, often called 'Klatskin tumours,' produce obstructive jaundice very early in their course and are typically small when they come to clinical attention.[360] Tumours of the extraheptic ducts may be somewhat larger, but they still present while relatively small. Tumours within the liver, however, may become quite large before they are detected. Histologically, however, the features are very similar among tumours arising in any of the sites, and there is close resemblance to ductal adenocarcinoma of the pancreas.

The incidence of intrahepatic cholangiocarcinoma (ICC), based on evidence from national health statistics and surveys of cancer diagnoses, is reported to be rising in several parts of the world, including North America, Europe, Australia and Japan, whereas extrahepatic CC has declined slightly.[361-364] In the United States, the SEER (Surveillance Epidemiology and End Results) program, which gathers data from population-based tumour registries in 11 parts of the United States, found a nearly three-fold increase in the diagnosis of ICC between 1975 and 1999.[363] No cause is apparent, and it remains to be determined whether this is a true increase or merely a change in diagnostic trends brought on by advances in imaging techniques. Thus, in 1975, a patient discovered to have adenocarcinoma in the liver would probably have been given the diagnosis of metastatic adenocarcinoma of unknown primary. In the 21st century, most such patients still are diagnosed as metastatic adenocarcinoma of unknown primary, but an increasing proportion, having no extrahepatic primary demonstrated by extensive imaging studies, receives a diagnosis of ICC. The rarity of the diagnosis of CC in previous years could easily account for its apparent three-fold increase.

It is estimated that CC accounts for approximately 3% of all gastrointestinal cancers worldwide and that ICC comprises 10 to 20% of all primary liver cancer.[364] There is considerable geographic variation in the reported incidence of ICC, ranging from a high of 96 per 100 000 in men in north-eastern Thailand, where the tumour is associated with parasitic infestation of the bile ducts, to a low of 0.1 per 100 000 in Australian women.[364] Some of this may be due to trends in pathological diagnoses, but some is undoubtedly real. In the United States, it is estimated that there are approximately 5000 CC per year, 40% intrahepatic, 7% hilar, and the remainder extrahepatic. In most series, CC is more frequent in men than women (60 to 70%), and while occasional cases occur in young people, the mean age is in the seventh decade.

Aetiology

Possible aetiological factors are much less well established than for HCC, and most cases have no known aetiology, but it is clear that disorders that cause chronic inflammation of the biliary tract are associated with an increased incidence of CC. Most cases of ICC arise in a non-cirrhotic liver, but there does appear to be an increased risk in cirrhosis, so that in Japan approximately 5% of cases occur in cirrhosis caused by viral hepatitis, and patients with cirrhosis due to hepatitis C have approximately 1000-fold increase in risk of ICC compared to the general population.[365,366] Parasitic infections of the biliary tract by *Clonorchis sinensis* and *Opisthorchis viverrini* cause chronic inflammation with adenomatous hyperplasia of the biliary epithelium. These parasites are endemic in south-east Asia and appear to account for the very high incidence of CC in Thailand and adjacent countries.[364] Hepatolithiasis or the formation of stones in the biliary tract, often with recurrent pyogenic cholangitis, is also much more common in east Asia than in other parts of the world and may account for the relatively high incidence of CC in Japan, where biliary parasites are not highly prevalent. The biliary stones cause chronic inflammation and proliferative epithelial changes, and approximately 10% of patients develop CC. Adenocarcinomas can arise in solitary cysts of the liver, and ICC has been reported in congenital hepatic fibrosis, Caroli disease, von Meyenburg complexes and polycystic liver disease. Overall, approximately 3% of patients with various forms of cystic dilatations of the bile ducts, including choledochal cyst, will develop CCs.[367] Primary sclerosing cholangitis, with or without associated inflammatory bowel disease, is strongly associated with the development of CC. In a large series of 394 patients, 12.2% developed CC.[368] Other reported associations with less definite pathogenetic significance include alcohol consumption, anabolic and contraceptive steroid use, genetic haemochromatosis, α_1-antitrypsin deficiency, extrahepatic biliary atresia and Thorotrast exposure.[2]

Molecular pathology

A number of important changes in the regulation of cell growth have been found to be present in CC. For example, down-regulation of β-catenin is reported to be associated with high-grade, high-stage and rapid progression in a number of malignancies.[369] In the majority of ICCs, the expression of β-catenin is rather reduced relative to that in non-cancerous bile ducts in which β-catenin is clearly expressed in the cell membrane of normal intrahepatic ducts.[370,371] The down-regulation of this molecule is correlated with high-grade CC.[271] Immunohistochemical analysis have revealed that the membranous expression of β-catenin is frequently reduced and aberrant nuclear expression has occasionally been found in ICCs. Reduced membranous expression of β-catenin is associated with non-papillary ICCs, which have a more malignant behaviour, and the nuclear translocation of β-catenin results in oncogenic events.[370]

Unregulated proliferation. There is evidence that the epidermal growth factor (EGF) superfamily of transmembrane receptors is involved in the pathogenesis of CC, since normal, reactive and neoplastic biliary epithelial cells express the EGF receptor (EGFR).[372,373] The c-erb-B2/HER-2 protein, a 185-kD transmembrane tyrosine kinase activated in many human tumour types, appears to be functional in CC as well.[374] This molecule is a homologue of EGFR, capable of forming homodimers or heterodimers with other EGF family members, resulting in an unregulated proliferative signal. Transformed cholangiocytes, but not normal biliary epithelial cells, over-express c-erb-B2 as determined by immunohistochemical staining of tumour specimens.[375–377] A transgenic mouse model that over-expresses c-erb-B2 was found to rapidly develop gallbladder adenocarcinomas in the context of elevated cyclooxygenase-2 (COX-2) and EGFR levels.[378] However, c-erbB-2 over-expression, although used as a phenotypic marker for neoplastic transformation, does not appear to correlate with the Ki-67 labelling index or p53 expression in ICC.[379] This finding suggests that the c-erbB-2 oncogene may not be important in the aggressive behaviour and stage of ICC.[213]

COX-2 is up-regulated in a variety of gastrointestinal tumours.[380,381] COX-2 is induced by a variety of cytokines and mitogens under certain pathological conditions.[382] COX-2 over-expression has been observed in chronic cholangitis and in CC cells but not in normal biliary epithelial cells, suggesting that this enzyme may play an important role in bile duct carcinogenesis and tumour progression.[383–385] Expression of COX-2 appears to be related to mitogenic stimulation, while selective inhibition of COX-2 results in reduced tumour cell proliferation.[386] The mechanism by which COX-2 expression leads to increased cell proliferation is not clear; however recent evidence suggests it may be due, at least in part, to inhibition of pathways involved in programmed cell death.[374] In addition, COX-2 may promote bile duct carcinogenesis by modifying or altering DNA bases of biliary epithelial cells thus resulting in DNA damage. Hayashi et al.[383] reported that a higher level of COX-2 is necessary for carcinogenesis in biliary epithelial cells, and that just a moderate level of COX-2 expression would not be sufficient.

Antigrowth control. Antigrowth signalling is a critical mechanism to negatively regulate cell proliferation. Central to this regulatory control is the *p53* gene, which has been found to be mutated in 50% of all human cancers. The *p53* gene regulates proteins that affect the cells ability both to enter the cell cycle and to undergo apoptosis. With respect to cell cycle control, the p21/WAF1/Cip1 protein, regulated by the *p53* gene, binds to the cell division kinase (CDK)1: cyclin D complex and prevents it from phosphorylating Rb, thus preventing the release of transcription factors that regulate genes encoding for proteins critical to entrance into the S phase of the cell cycle. The *p53* gene also regulates Bax, a protein that binds Bcl-2 and antagonizes its antiapoptotic effect on the mitochondrial membrane. In general, p53 function becomes altered because of either a missence mutation in the gene leading to functional inactivation of the p53 protein or the up-regulation of an inhibitor of p53, such as mdm-2. Loss of p53, therefore, results in unrestrained progression through the cell cycle as well as an increase in the relative abundance of antiapoptotic regulatory proteins.

In CC, p53 protein is immunohistochemically detectable in 20 to 80% of the cases.[387–389] However, mutations in the *p53* gene do not correlate with apoptotic rates.[390] Therefore, alteration of the p53 pathway leading to the loss of cell cycle control may be critical to the cellular pathogenesis of CC. In addition, there may be some epigenetic phenomena that stabilize p53 protein. That is, wild-type p53 may be stabilized and then made detectable by forming complexes with other molecules of p53 downstream effector genes, such as WAF-1 and mdm-2.[391,392] Momoi et al.[393] showed that the incidence of *mdm-2* gene amplification in ICC was 31.8%. Alteration of mdm-2 may contribute to later stages of ICC with *mdm-2* amplification. Della Torre et al.[394] reported that *p53* gene mutations occurred in only two of 13 cases of ICC, while high levels of mdm-2 protein were found in 61% of ICC cases and in 70% of the cases displaying stabilized p53 protein. The finding of coexpressed p53 and mdm-2 in ICCs indicates that there is up-regulation of the mdm-2 protein to a level sufficient for binding and accumulating p53 in an inactive complex form.

Recent studies have reported that the expression of cell cycle modulating proteins, such as p16, p21, and p27, is associated with aggressive tumour behaviour in several human malignancies. For example, p27, a cyclin-dependent kinase inhibitor, has an inhibitory effect on the G1-to-S phase transition in the cell cycle through its negative effects on cyclin E/CDK2 and cyclin A/CDK2. Taguchi et al.[395] found that the low expression of nuclear p27 was correlated with vascular invasion in ICC. Fiorentino et al.[396] found that the p27 labelling index was significantly higher in patients without lymph node metastasis, but it decreased greatly in patients with lymph node metastasis. ICC patients with low or absent p27 expression had poor survival compared with the high expression group. Immunohistochemical detection of p27 on routine sections may provide the first biological prognostic marker for ICC, thus influencing therapeutic strategies for these patients. The CDK4:cyclin D complex is also influenced by p16 inhibitory protein, which appears to be a common cellular target in the transformation process. Mutations in this gene are reported in 25% to 83% of resected CC specimens.[397,398] In addition, the p16 labelling index showed a relationship with lymph node metastasis, but not with the Ki-67 labelling index. The p21 labelling index was higher in poorly differentiated cases and showed a direct relationship with the Ki-67 labelling index, although it is a negative regulator of the cell cycle.[399]

Activation of ras and inactivation of p53 are associated with increased and continuous cell proliferation and failure to activate apoptosis, permitting the survival of mutated cells.[222,225] Activation of K-ras occurs by point mutation at codon 12, with changes from glycine to aspartic acid or, less often, valine, which is detected in ICC.[400,401] The incidence of K-ras mutations in ICC ranges from 0% to 100% and shows geographic and ethnic variations.[402,403]

Apoptosis. Apoptosis is an essential component in the regulation of normal tissue development as well as unchecked cell proliferation (Chapter 2). Such pathways are essential for protection against mutational events and accumulation of aberrant cellular processes. Usually, genotoxic events result in either DNA repair or, if the damage is beyond repair, deletion of the cells by apoptosis. Apoptosis is initiated by a series of proteins, called caspases, following ligand activation of CD95/Fas/TRAIL/TNF receptor family or release of cytochrome c by the mitochondria.[404] Under conditions of cellular stress and genomic damage, apoptosis serves to remove such cells and particularly those at risk for malignant transformation. Loss of this protective mechanism allows for selection of cells with a growth advantage and promotes the development of cancer.

Biliary epithelial cells express Fas receptor (FasR) and respond to exogenous Fas ligand (FasL) to undergo programmed cell death. Transformed cells generally retain FasR expression but have a decreased responsiveness to apoptotic signalling and eventually lose receptor expression in the late stages of dedifferentiation.[405] Recently, it has been shown that a frequent and strong expression of FasL in biliary dysplasia and well-differentiated ICCs enables them to escape from immune surveillance by counterattacking Fas-bearing, tumour infiltrating lymphocytes. In fact, down-regulation of Fas expression in ICC cells was significantly correlated with histological dedifferentiation, vascular invasion, perineural invasion, the size of tumour and short survival of ICC patients.[405]

Immunohistochemical studies of CCs support a relative abundance of antiapoptotic mediators, including bcl-2 family members.[405,406] Over-expression of bcl-2 occurs in a wide variety of human cancers, and may contribute to neoplastic expansion by prolonging cell survival. The *bcl-2* gene is generally expressed in bile duct cells and also in ICC[407] and a high content of bcl-2 mRNA was also found in all cases of ICC.[379] In addition, dysregulation of bcl-2 expression in ICCs may be due to inactivation of the *p53* gene, which is known to suppress bcl-2 expression.[408] In fact, in ICC, the expression of bcl-2 was inversely related to lymph node metastasis, vascular invasion, perineural invasion, the Ki-67 labelling index, aberrant p53 expression and the incidence of apoptotic cells. Down-regulation of bcl-2 expression is strongly linked to highly biologically aggressive phenotypes of ICC.[409] Furthermore, participation of other members of bcl-2 family protein has been also reported. Okaro et al.[410] reported that Mcl-1 and bcl-X are involved in the survival of neoplastic biliary epithelial cells. Moreover, in neoplastic biliary cells, other molecular changes, such as K-ras mutation, and/or p53 dysregulation, may inhibit apoptosis after the non-reparable genotoxic event, followed by survival of the mutated cell, and further genetic alterations may lead to malignant transformation of biliary epithelial cells and progression through a multistep process.[388,407]

As previously described, COX-2 is up-regulated by mitogenic stimulation, inflammatory cytokines and exposure to bile acids. Increased levels of COX-2 inhibit FasL-mediated apoptosis by increasing levels of the inhibitory protein myeloid cell leukaemia protein 1 (Mcl-1).[411] It has been shown that bile acids and inflammatory mediators up-regulate Mcl-1, which stabilizes the mitochondrial membrane, prevents cytochrome c release and protects the cells from apoptosis.[374,412]

Pathology

Peripheral ICCs may be quite large when discovered (Fig. 15.62), while tumours that occur near the hepatic hilum are usually small but cause obstructive jaundice in the remainder of the liver. The tumours are usually firm or hard, and vary from white to tan (Figs 15.62 and 15.63). Microscopically, CC may resemble any adenocarcinoma of extrahepatic origin, so that a confident diagnosis depends on the exclusion of other primary sites. The tumour cells are most often arranged in tubules and glands, which may be cribriform, but they can also form nests, solid cords or papillary structures (Figs 15.64–15.66). There is typically a fibrous stroma, in contrast to most hepatocellular carcinomas. It has been noted that patients with scirrhous tumours that have desmoplastic stroma comprising more than 70% of the tissue have significantly worse prognosis following surgery than those with lesser amounts of stroma.[413] Most CCs tend to be well-differentiated although poorly differentiated tumours are not infrequent. The well-differentiated CCs are composed of columnar to cuboidal epithelial cells with a moderate amount of clear or slightly granular, lightly eosinophilic cytoplasm. Nuclei are usually small, and typically lack the prominent, eosinophilic nucleoli of cells of

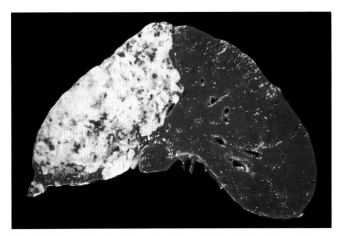

Fig. 15.62 • Intrahepatic cholangiocarcinoma. This peripheral tumour has replaced the entire left lobe.

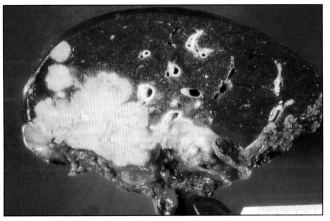

Fig. 15.63 • Intrahepatic cholangiocarcinoma. This lobectomy specimen contains a hard, yellow-white tumour that arose near the hilum and spread peripherally.

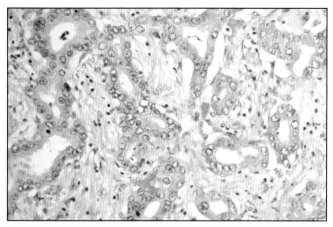

Fig. 15.64 • Cholangiocarcinoma. A tubular adenocarcinoma with glands that resemble biliary epithelium. H&E.

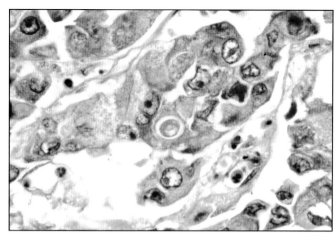

Fig. 15.67 • Cholangiocarcinoma. Focal mucin production, shown with the mucicarmine stain.

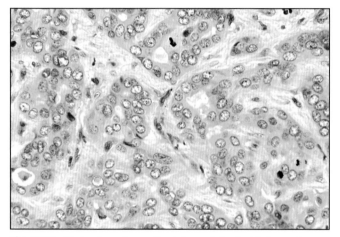

Fig. 15.65 • Cholangiocarcinoma. Poorly formed glands with frequent mitoses. H&E.

Table 15.8	Antigens and genetic markers that have been reported to be present or modified in cholangiocarcinoma	
AFP	Fas ligand	MUC5/6
A, B, H blood group substance	Galectin	Osteopontin
	Gastrin	P16
AgNOR	G-CSF	P27*
Amylase	GM-CSF	P53
Bcl-2	HCG	PCNA
E-cadherin	HLA-DR*	PKR
α-catenin	hTERT	PTH-RP
β-catenin	Interleukin-6	Rb
CD44	Keratin 903*	REG1
CDX1	Ki-67	RTK
CDX2	K-ras	Secretory component
CEA	Lewis a,b,y	Smad4
CA 19-9	Lipase	Telomerase
CK7	LOH (multiple chromosomes)	Tenascin*
CK8		TFF1
CK18	Met	Thrombospondin-1
CK19	MSI	TP1
CK20	Midkine	TPA
COX-2	MMP-7	TRAIL
Cyclin D1	MUC1*	Trypsinogen/trypsin
Decorin	MUC2*	WISP-1v
EMA	MUC3	
ErbB-2	MUC4*	

* Reported to have prognostic significance.

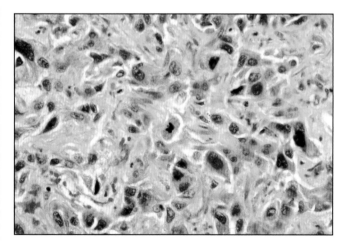

Fig. 15.66 • Cholangiocarcinoma. A poorly differentiated, pleomorphic tumour. H&E.

hepatocellular carcinoma. The tumour cells can grow along sinusoids and spread intravascularly throughout the liver. Mucin, which may be demonstrable with special stains (Fig. 15.67), is seldom abundant, but occasional tumours are mucinous with copious cytoplasmic and extracellular mucin. Other uncommon variants include adenosquamous, clear cell carcinomas and spindle cell or sarcomatoid carcinomas.

Numerous antigens and genetic alterations have been found in CCs (Table 15.8). Many of these play significant roles in carcinogenesis and tumour progression, as noted previously, but none specifically can be used to distinguish CC from metastatic adenocarcinoma. Some have been reported to have prognostic significance, although overall survival is still quite poor. The presence of HLA-DR, MUC2 and the absence of MUC1, MUC4, keratin 903, p27, tenascin and matrix metallopreoteinase-7 have been reported to be associated with better survival following resection.[414–419]

Differential diagnosis

Often the most difficult task is in distinguishing CC from benign reactive ductular proliferation, particularly when there is inflammation, producing reactive atypia. Similarly, peribiliary glands around the major ducts can be quite atypical when there is inflammation and benign von Meyenburg complexes, and peribiliary gland hamartomas (bile duct adenomas) can have considerable cytological atypia when inflamed. Histological features that are helpful in distinguishing well-differentiated CC from benign lesions are nuclear size variation and irregularity, mitoses and cribriform growth pattern.[420] As noted, metastatic adenocarcinoma, especially from foregut derived tissues (lung, oesophagus, stomach, pancreas), is histologically indistinguishable from CC, and must be differentiated on clinical grounds. Hepatocellular carcinoma may grow in a pseudoglandular pattern, but unlike the true glands of CC, there is no mucin production by the cells lining the pseudoglands. Bile may be present in the pseudogland lumen, which is actually a dilated bile canaliculus that can be demonstrated immunohistochemically by a polyclonal CEA or CD10 immunostain. Cells of CC show cytoplasmic staining for CEA and are usually strongly positive for cytokeratin but negative for HepPar-1. Epithelioid haemangioendothelioma can mimic CC, since it produces a desmoplastic stroma and its vascular lumina may suggest gland formation. It can be differentiated from CC by lack of mucin production and by the expression of endothelial cell markers such as Factor VIII-related antigen, CD34 and CD31.

Natural history

CC spreads by direct invasion of surrounding tissue and by infiltrating blood vessels and lymphatics. Extrahepatic metastases are found at autopsy in about three-quarters of patients, with lymph nodes and lungs (74%), peritoneum and adrenals (20%), kidney (15%) and bone (13%) as the most common sites.[2] The median survival is approximately 6 months, with 5-year survival of less than 5% for intrahepatic and 10 to 15% for extrahepatic CC.[364] Surgical resection offers the only hope of cure, but many of the patients present with unresectable tumours. Of those deemed operative candidates, resection with clear margins results in 5-year survival of 20–40% for extrahepatic and 29–36% for ICC.[421]

Benign vascular tumours

Haemangioma

Small benign vascular tumours are common in many areas of the body, including the liver. Only occasionally do they become large enough to be clinically important. Cavernous haemangioma, sclerosing haemangioma, solitary necrotic nodule and various other synonyms have been used to describe different stages of development and involution of this lesion.

Haemangiomas of the liver are the most common benign liver tumour. Their reported incidence depends on how vigorously they are sought. Various series report figures ranging from less than 1% up to 20% for incidental hepatic haemangiomas found at autopsy.[422,423] Haemangiomas occur at all ages, although they are most often diagnosed in adults. Most series have reported a greater frequency in women than in men, but it may be that haemangiomas tend to be larger in women and therefore more often symptomatic and more often diagnosed. A role of sex hormones in the pathogenesis of this tumour has been suggested, but there is little evidence to support this.[2,424] Haemangiomas less than 4 cm in diameter are rarely symptomatic. About 40% of those 4 cm or larger are associated with symptoms.[425] Pain or discomfort, abdominal enlargement, mass and/or hepatomegaly are most frequent. The pain is rarely severe, and its exact cause is seldom apparent. Since surgically resected hepatic haemangiomas frequently contain organizing thrombi, it may be that recurrent or intermittent thromboses cause the tumours to swell, producing stretching of Glisson's capsule and causing the pain. Rare reported cases have presented with spontaneous or traumatic rupture of the haemangioma, but the true incidence of this complication is not known.[426,427] Even rarer is the dramatic syndrome of consumptive coagulopathy, thrombocytopenia and hypofibrinogenaemia (Kasabach–Merritt syndrome) occasionally associated with large hepatic haemangiomas.[428]

The various imaging modalities have all been reported to have useful roles in the detection and diagnosis of hepatic haemangiomas. This is especially important because needle biopsy of haemangiomas with large bore needles may lead to severe haemorrhage.[425] Characteristic findings are described by sonography, CT and arteriography. Magnetic resonance imaging is virtually diagnostic, obviating the need for many biopsies. If any doubt remains, scintigraphy or single photon emission computed tomography (SPECT) with radioisotope-tagged red blood cells can provide a definitive diagnosis.[285]

Pathology

Hepatic haemangiomas are usually solitary. Only about 10% are multiple, and there are only rare reports of diffuse hepatic haemangiomatosis.[429] The vast majority are less than 4 cm in diameter, but occasional tumours may be as large as 30 cm. They may occur anywhere in the liver and are sometimes present on the capsular surface. When viewed through the capsule, they appear as red or purple blotches on the surface. On cut section, they are spongy with relatively little tissue and a great deal of dark, venous blood. Haemangiomas sometimes undergo regressive changes. Areas of thrombosis (recent or old), scarring and, occasionally, calcification may be present in older haemangiomas. They sometimes reach the end stage of this process and resemble a localized fibrous scar, or 'sclerosed haemangioma,' and may even become entirely calcified. Microscopically, these are cavernous haemangiomas with varying-sized vascular channels lined by flattened endothelial cells (Fig. 15.68). They are usually discrete and

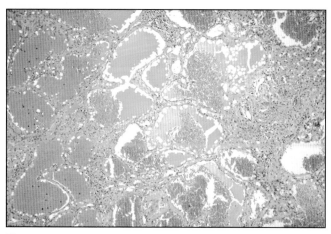

Fig. 15.68 • Cavernous haemangioma. Varying-sized blood-filled spaces are lined by a flattened endothelium overlying a fibrous stroma. H&E.

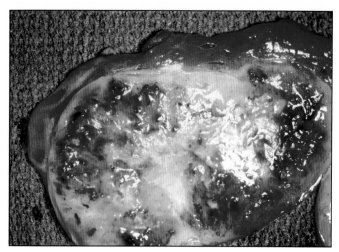

Fig. 15.69 • Infantile haemangioendothelioma. The resected tumour appears variegated with white areas of necrosis and scarring reddish-brown areas of vascularity.

well-demarcated from the surrounding liver, although an occasional haemangioma may contain trapped bile ducts or foci of parenchyma, and occasionally vascular channels may extend into the adjacent parenchyma. Variable amounts of fibrous tissue usually separate the vascular channels. Many consist of thin, delicate strands, while others have large areas of scarring. Fresh and organizing thrombi may be found in the vascular channels. The dynamics of these thrombi are not known, but they are commonly observed in surgically resected haemangiomas. Because of the sluggish blood flow through these tumours, small thrombi are probably constantly forming and lysing, contributing to the typically heterogeneous appearance by MRI. Fibroblasts can be found growing into a few thrombi and are probably the source of the scarring that results in the 'sclerosing haemangioma,' and mast cells may also play a role.[430] In end-stage sclerosed and/or calcified haemangiomas, an underlying vascular pattern can usually still be discerned, providing the clue to the diagnosis.

Infantile haemangioendothelioma

These tumours are similar to the capillary haemangiomas of infancy that are relatively common in the skin and mucous membranes. They are rarely diagnosed in the viscera. As in other sites, hepatic haemangioendotheliomas typically undergo stages of proliferation, maturation and involution, and will eventually disappear if the patient does not develop a fatal complication.

The true incidence of this tumour is impossible to determine, as many small lesions could be asymptomatic and remain undiagnosed. Cutaneous capillary haemangiomas, most of which are clinically insignificant, occur in about 0.5% of neonates; it is conceivable that small hepatic haemangioendotheliomas remain clinically occult and regress without attracting attention. Of those that come to clinical attention, 90% are diagnosed in the first 6 months of life and 33% in the first month.[2,431-433] A few cases have been reported in adults, but these are extraordinary. Females outnumber males by 2:1. Hepatomegaly and/or abdominal mass is a frequent mode of presentation. Coincidental cutaneous haemangiomas are frequent, being reported in anywhere from 11 to 87% of patients. Some patients, and in some series the majority of symptomatic patients, present with high output congestive heart failure due to arteriovenous shunting through the tumour. The natural history of this tumour is variable and belies its histologically benign nature. Up to two-thirds of symptomatic patients may die as a result of the tumour. Causes of death include congestive heart failure, hepatic failure or tumour rupture with haemorrhage. Surgical resection may be possible, but is often not, since the tumour is frequently multicentric, and so hepatic artery ligation or embolization, radiation and corticosteroids have been suggested as alternative therapies. If life-threatening complications can be avoided, most tumours probably regress, and the patients usually do well. A few tumours diagnosed as infantile haemangioendothelioma have pursued an aggressive course with metastasis and death from disseminated disease. Dehner and Ishak noted that these appeared histologically more aggressive and termed them type II haemangioendothelioma.[431] Other cases have been reported as angiosarcoma arising in infantile haemangioendothelioma,[434] but the distinction between cases such as these and type II haemangioendotheliomas is often unclear. Consequently, these are now classified as angiosarcoma, and the term infantile haemangioendothelioma is reserved for the so-called type I tumours.

Pathology

The tumours may be single or multicentric and may occur anywhere in the liver. Individual tumour nodules range from barely visible up to 15 cm in diameter. They are usually well demarcated from the surrounding liver and appear red, brown or white, depending on the degree of vascularity and involutional change. Some tumours appear laminated with yellowish-white areas of necrosis and scarring in the centre and a reddish, well-vascularized periphery (Fig. 15.69). Microscopically, the periphery of the tumour is composed of proliferating small vascular channels (capillary-like), irregularly-shaped, lined by plump endothelial cells (Fig. 15.70) which stain positively for endothelial markers such as factor VIII related antigen and CD34.[435] There is relatively little fibrous stroma, but basement membrane components such as laminen and type IV collagen are present. Bile ducts and hepatocytes are often trapped within the advancing edge of the tumour. Toward the centre of the tumour the amount of stroma increases and number of vascular channels decreases (Fig. 15.71). In many cases, the more centrally located vascular spaces are larger and 'cavernous' with a flattened endothelium. Irregular zones of infarction, necrosis, haemorrhage, scarring and foci of dystrophic calcification are usually present, accounting for the regression of the tumour. The endothelial cells of the proliferating vascular channels at the periphery constitute the neoplastic element. They are typically cytologically bland and form a single layer around the vascular channels. The very rare infantile angiosarcomas (type II haemangioendotheliomas of Dehner and Ishak[431]) have pleomorphic and hyperchromatic endothelial cells with intravascular budding

and branching and often a Kaposiform spindle cell component.[2]

Malignant vascular tumours

Epithelioid haemangioendothelioma

This is an uncommon vascular tumour that has been recognized as a distinct clinicopathological entity in the early 1980's. It was first recognized in the lung and soft tissue, often in a large blood vessel where the epithelioid appearance of the tumour cells caused it to be frequently mistaken for metastatic carcinoma.[436,437] Those that arose in the liver were usually though to be sclerosing cholangiocarcinomas or angiosarcomas, and because of the peculiar histological features, many were thought to be a non-neoplastic fibrosing disorder rather than a neoplasm. Ultrastructural and immunohistochemical studies eventually led to the recognition of these as a distinctive vascular tumour with the clinical behaviour of a low-grade malignancy.[436,438–440]

Clinical aspects

Hepatic epithelioid haemangioendothelioma is a tumour of adults and should not be confused with infantile haemangioendothelioma, despite the similarity of names. The aetiology is unknown. There have been a few cases reported in vinyl chloride workers, in women who had taken oral contraceptive steroids, in patients with hepatitis B and hepatitis C, and following trauma to the liver, but the significance of these is not known. In most cases, no potential aetiological factor can be identified. Reported cases have ranged from 12 to 86 years with the average age in the fifth decade.[438,439] Approximately two-thirds of the cases occur in women. In most cases the disease produces symptoms and signs suggesting a tumour in the liver. Presentation is most often due to abdominal pain, but hepatosplenomegaly, nausea and vomiting, or jaundice may draw attention to the liver. In about 10% of cases, the tumour is discovered incidentally, usually in a patient undergoing abdominal surgery for some other reason. Imaging studies frequently show multiple nodular lesions with or without calcification. Epithelioid haemangioendothelioma of the liver tends to behave like a low-grade malignancy, although the outcome is variable. Most cases are slowly progressive. Some patients have died of hepatic failure or disseminated tumour within a few months of presentation, while others have had a prolonged survival. The longest known patient survival without definitive therapy was 28 years after initial presentation and death in that case was from apparently unrelated causes.[438] Several cases have been successfully treated by surgical excision of the tumour, but because the tumour is so often multifocal and therefore unresectable, liver transplantation is the treatment of choice.[441,442] Interestingly, since it is usually slow-growing, the presence of extrahepatic metastases at the time of transplantation does not affect survival.[441] Overall, and irrespective of therapy, 5-year survival is 43 to 55%, significantly better than most primary hepatic malignancies.[439,440]

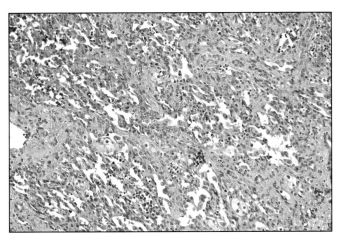

Fig. 15.70 • Infantile haemangioendothelioma. There are variably-sized vascular channels with foci of extramedullary haematopoiesis and a few trapped bile ducts. H&E.

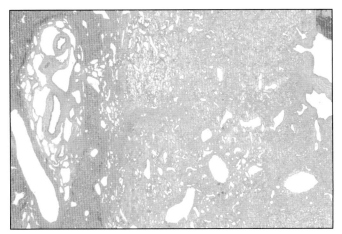

Fig. 15.71 • Infantile haemangioendothelioma. The tumour encroaches on the surrounding normal liver (left) with numerous small vessels at the periphery of the tumour and a few larger, cavernous vessels and fibrosis toward the centre of the tumour (right). H&E.

Pathology

The histological features of hepatic epithelioid haemangio-endothelioma are quite distinctive. It is multifocal in over 70% of cases, usually with multiple nodules of variable size (Figs 15.72 and 15.73). Individual lesions range from smaller than a single hepatic acinus to several centimetres. At its growing margin the tumour tends to infiltrate hepatic sinusoids and small vessels, preserving the underlying acinar architecture. At the centre of a lesion, there is typically dense, often hyalinized fibrous tissue. The tumour produces an abundant stromal matrix, which initially is rich in mucopolysaccharides and appears cartilaginous. In older lesions, there is progressive fibrosis and sometimes calcification. Small groups of tumour cells are scattered throughout the stroma. The cells tend to form lumina within individual cells and between cells (Fig. 15.74), mimicking signet-ring cells and glands of an adenocarcinoma, but mucin stains are invariably negative. Blood cells may occasionally be found in the lumina, providing a clue to the vascular nature of the tumour. Weibel–Palade bodies can sometimes be found by electron microscopy, but immunostains for CD34, CD31 and Factor VIII antigen are nearly always positive to some degree and are the best proof of the endothelial origin of the tumour (Fig. 15.75). Some cases have papillary growths of epithelioid cells, simulating carcinoma (Fig. 15.76), while in others there is prominent growth of the tumour within terminal hepatic venules, portal vein branches, and larger vessels, causing occlusion of the affected vessel by the tumour stroma. Older lesions may

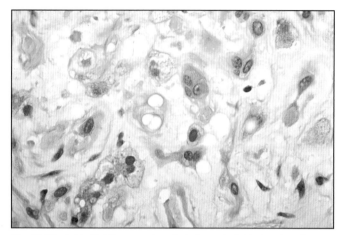

Fig. 15.74 • Epithelioid haemangioendothelioma. Individual and small groups of tumour cells in a mucopolysaccharide-rich stroma. Some tumour cells are epithelioid and some form capillary lumina. H&E.

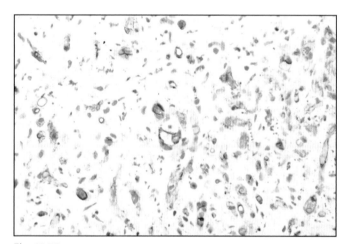

Fig. 15.75 • Epithelioid haemangioendothelioma. Immunostain for CD34 demonstrates that the tumour cells are of endothelial origin.

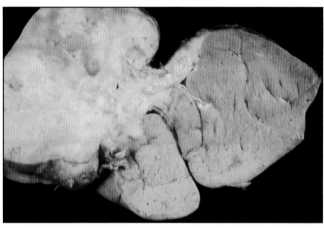

Fig. 15.72 • Epithelioid haemangioendothelioma. Multiple confluent tumour nodules replacing the entire right lobe of the liver.

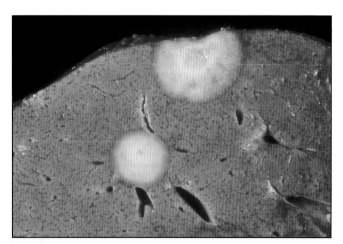

Fig. 15.73 • Epithelioid haemangioendothelioma. Multifocal tumour nodules are hard and white, mimicking metastatic carcinoma.

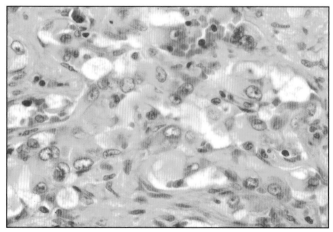

Fig. 15.76 • Epithelioid haemangioendothelioma. Pale, epithelioid tumour cells grow in sinusoids, and form papillary tufts, mimicking metastatic carcinoma. H&E.

consist predominantly of fibrotic stroma and can be difficult to recognize as a neoplasm.

Angiosarcoma

Angiosarcoma of the liver is a rare tumour, but it is the most common primary sarcoma of the liver.[2] It has been estimated that 10 to 20 cases of hepatic angiosarcoma occur per year in the United States and up to 10 cases per year in Great Britain.[443,444]

Aetiology

Hepatic angiosarcoma has been the subject of great interest because of its relationship to environmental carcinogens. Historically, about 25% of cases have been associated with one of four recognized agents: vinyl chloride monomer, Thorotrast, arsenic, or anabolic steroids.[443] Vinyl chloride is a gas that is used to make the plastic polyvinyl chloride. Several cases of hepatic angiosarcoma as well as hepatocellular carcinoma were noted to occur in workers with prolonged exposure to the vinyl chloride monomer during the manufacturing process.[445] Both angiosarcoma and hepatocellular carcinoma have been produced in animals exposed experimentally to vinyl chloride, further strengthening the relationship, and p53 mutations have been found in some human cases associated with vinyl chloride, but not in sporadic angiosarcoma or those related to Thorotrast, suggesting a possible mechanism.[446] Angiosarcomas have also developed in persons exposed to inorganic arsenic. These tumours were found in the 1950's in German vineyard workers and others exposed to arsenical insecticides, in persons who consumed Fowler's solution (potassium arsenite) medicinally for prolonged periods for asthma or psoriasis, and in a few persons exposed to arsenic through drinking water.[443,447] Thorotrast (colloidal thorium dioxide) was used as a radiographic contrast medium from the 1930's to the 1950's. Once injected, nearly all the material remains permanently in the body, accumulating in the liver and to lesser degrees in the spleen, lymph nodes and bone marrow. Thorium is weakly radioactive and emits predominantly alpha and beta particles. The first hepatic angiosarcoma in a person who had received Thorotrast was reported in 1947. Subsequently, numerous other Thorotrast-associated angiosarcomas, as well as hepatocellular carcinomas and cholangiocarcinomas, have been reported.[448-450] The interval between receiving Thorotrast and developing angiosarcoma may be as short as 12 years and as long as 40 years. Thorotrast-related angiosarcomas often develop in a background of chronic liver disease with fibrosis and/or cirrhosis. Angiosarcomas have also developed in several patients taking anabolic androgenic steroids[451] and there are individual reports of a few taking oestrogenic and contraceptive steroids, as well as other drugs, although the significance of these is not known.

Clinical aspects

Hepatic angiosarcoma is predominantly a tumour of older individuals. The peak incidence in various series is in the sixth and seventh decades, although rare cases occur in younger individuals, and a few have occurred in children.[2,446,452] Men are affected more often than women in a ratio as high as 3 to 1. The symptoms and signs of angiosarcoma are non-specific but usually point to a problem in the liver.[446,452] Approximately half of the patients present because of abdominal pain. Weakness, fatigue, weight loss, anorexia and abdominal enlargement are other frequent symptoms. Hepatomegaly is a common finding, being present in 58% to 70% of patients at presentation. Ascites and jaundice are often present. Splenomegaly is a frequent finding in vinyl chloride-associated angiosarcoma. Laboratory findings in patients with angiosarcoma are also non-specific. Anaemia, leukocytosis, and thrombocytopenia are frequent. Nearly all patients show some abnormality in results of liver tests. Mild elevations of serum alkaline phosphatase, AST and bilirubin levels are common. One-half to three-fourths of patients have decreased serum albumin concentration or prolonged prothrombin time. α-fetoprotein and carcinoembryonic antigen, however, are not elevated. Radiological studies are frequently abnormal but seldom suggest a specific diagnosis.[453] Radionuclide scans show distinct filling defects in about 70% of cases, while nearly all the rest are abnormal due to non-homogeneous isotope uptake. Hepatic angiography is almost always abnormal and may suggest the diagnosis of angiosarcoma in the appropriate clinical setting. Especially helpful are the findings of dilated sinusoids and a tumour with peripheral vascularity and central hypovascularity. In patients with Thorotrast-associated angiosarcoma, plain films of the abdomen or chest may show radiopaque accumulations of Thorotrast in the liver, and sometimes in the spleen or lymph nodes. The course of the disease is one of progressive deterioration, often aggravated by catastrophic events related to the vascular nature of the tumours. Intra-abdominal and gastrointestinal haemorrhage are frequent terminal events. Some patients develop problems due to vascular shunting through the tumour, including congestive heart failure, microangiopathic haemolytic anaemia and consumptive coagulopathy. Favourable responses and prolongation of survival have been reported with chemotherapy, but most patients die in hepatic failure within a year. At autopsy, metastases are quite common (60%), most common sites include lung, bone and spleen. Sometimes, however, the distinction between metastasizing hepatic angiosarcoma and extrahepatic multicentric growth may be very difficult or impossible.

Pathology

Angiosarcoma of the liver may form a single tumour nodule, but usually the tumours are multicentric.[2] Typically, multiple nodules are scattered throughout both lobes, varying in size from barely visible up to several centimetres in diameter. On cut section the nodules are red or brown and often appear haemorrhagic. Livers containing angiosarcoma are usually enlarged and may be massive, weighing over 3 kg by the time of death. Microscopically, a wide range of appearances may be seen. Areas of early involvement show dilated hepatic sinusoids lined by hypertrophied

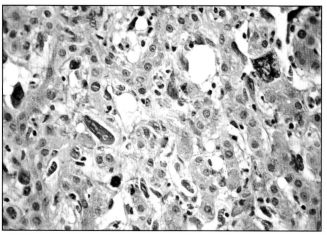

Fig. 15.77 • Angiosarcoma. Large, hyperchromatic, atypical endothelial cells in hepatic sinusoids. H&E.

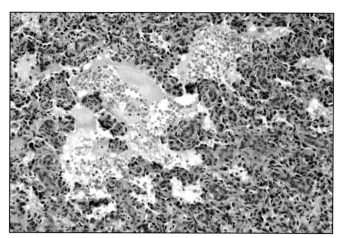

Fig. 15.79 • Angiosarcoma. Loss of hepatocytes, producing cavernous areas lined by malignant endothelial cells. H&E.

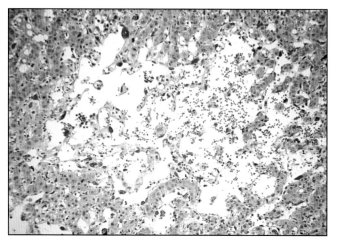

Fig. 15.78 • Angiosarcoma. Atrophy of liver cell plates with sinusoids lined by malignant endothelial cells. H&E.

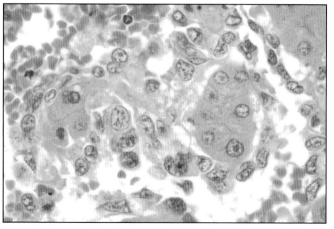

Fig. 15.80 • Angiosarcoma. Epithelioid-appearing tumour cells, mimicking carcinoma. In contrast to epithelioid haemangioendothelioma, there is no stroma. H&E.

endothelial cells with atypical, hyperchromatic nuclei (Fig. 15.77). With progressive involvement, the sinusoids dilate and fill with malignant endothelial cells, while the liver cell plates atrophy (Fig. 15.78). Areas in which the hepatocytes have entirely disappeared develop a cavernous appearance with numerous vascular channels lined by malignant cells (Fig. 15.79). Many tumours also contain more solid areas where the cells have an epithelioid appearance that may be difficult to distinguish from poorly differentiated carcinoma (Fig. 15.80), or epithelioid haemangioendothelioma or a spindled appearance simulating fibrosarcoma. Immunostains for endothelial markers, such as Factor VIII, CD31 or CD34, are frequently, but not invariably, positive. When positive, they may confirm the diagnosis.

Other benign tumours and tumour-like lesions

Mesenchymal hamartoma

Mesenchymal hamartoma is a rare benign lesion, presumably congenital, that is usually diagnosed in the first 2 years

of life and nearly always by the age of 5,[2] most often in male patients (70%). The exact pathogenesis is unknown and several theories on its aetiology, including a peculiar form of ductal plate malformation, an ischaemic origin, and a genuine neoplastic lesion, have been proposed. The lesions may become quite large due to cystic degeneration of the mesenchymal component, and they typically present as an enlarging abdominal mass. They are benign and do not recur after surgical excision, but there are rare reports of embryonal sarcoma arising in association with a previously undiagnosed mesenchymal hamartoma.[454]

The lesions can vary in size from a few centimetres to over 30 cm in diameter, and they typically contain multiple cysts of varying size. The cysts contain clear, yellow or gelatinous fluid and are separated by firm tissue that varies from white to yellow to tan. Microscopically, the lesions consist of disorganized arrangements of primitive mesenchyme, bile ducts and hepatic parenchyma (Fig. 15.81). The mesenchymal element consists of a mixture of spindled cells and collagen in a loose, myxoid stroma. In some areas the stroma undergoes cystic degeneration, producing the grossly visible cysts and giving rise to areas that resemble lymphangioma (Fig. 15.82). In other areas, the mesenchyme surrounds bile

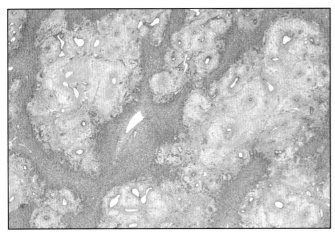

Fig. 15.81 • Mesenchymal hamartoma. Disorganized hepatic parenchyma, bile ducts and primitive mesenchyme. H&E.

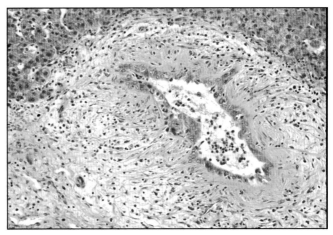

Fig. 15.83 • Mesenchymal hamartoma. Abnormal, inflamed bile duct surrounded by primitive mesenchyme. H&E.

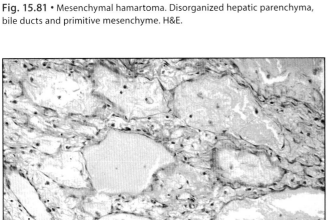

Fig. 15.82 • Mesenchymal hamartoma. Cystic degeneration of primitive mesenchyme, producing lymphangioma-like areas. H&E.

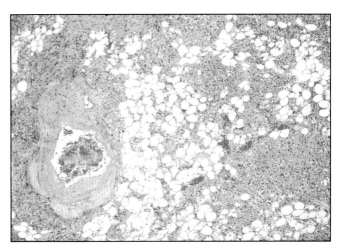

Fig. 15.84 • Angiomyolipoma. A typical lesion with large, abnormal arteries, smooth muscle and adipose tissue. H&E.

ducts that often appear abnormal, irregular and inflamed (Fig. 15.83). Variable numbers of normal-appearing hepatocytes are present in the lesions, but acinar architecture is not present.

Angiomyolipoma

Angiomyolipoma is another presumably hamartomatous benign lesion. It is only rarely diagnosed in children, however, and the mean age at diagnosis in the fifth to sixth decades. It is more common in women than men, 68% to 83% female in large series.[455,456] Unlike angiomyolipoma of the kidney, there are only a few cases associated with tuberous sclerosis.[455] The tumours may become quite large and can present with rupture and haemorrhage, but although over 100 cases have been reported, malignant degeneration is extremely rare and difficult to prove.[457] In fact, the presence of tumour cell nests in abdominal lymph nodes does not necessarily prove a malignant lesion as multicentric lesions of angiomylipoma have been also reported.

The lesions are usually solitary, except occasionally in patients with tuberous sclerosis. The background liver is normal. They can be up to 36 cm in diameter. The colour and consistency depends on the relative proportions of fat

(yellow and soft) and smooth muscle (tan-white and firm) and whether there has been haemorrhage in the tumour. Microscopically, the appearance can be quite variable.[2,456] There is typically an admixture of mature adipose tissue, thick-walled, often hyalinized arteries and smooth muscle (Fig. 15.84), and, unlike the similar tumours of the kidney, nearly all hepatic angiomyolipomas also have an element of haematopoietic cells (Fig. 15.85). The proportion of these elements varies greatly from case to case. Those with a predominance of one element may be difficult to recognize. The smooth muscle component may be spindled or epithelioid and can have irregular, hyperchromatic nuclei and grow in a trabecular pattern, so that many cases with spindle cells have been mistaken for sarcomas and epithelioid smooth muscle for hepatocellular carcinoma (Fig. 15.86).[2,456] Immunostains have been found to be quite helpful in the diagnosis. The smooth muscle cells are usually positive with antibodies to smooth muscle actin, but, remarkably, they are also positive for melanoma-related antigens. HMB-45 is positive in nearly all tumours, and Melan-A, microphthalmia transcription factor and tyrosinase in a sizable proportion.[456,458] CD117 (c-Kit) is also positive in most cases.[459] Histogenetically, angiomyolipomas of all sites are thought

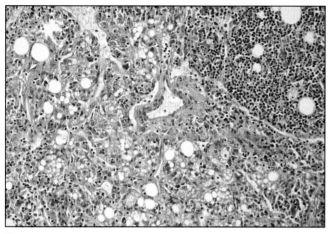

Fig. 15.85 • Angiomyolipoma. A tumour with a large amount of haematopoietic tissue in addition to the other components. H&E.

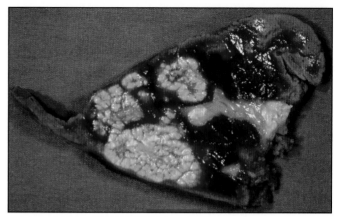

Fig. 15.87 • Inflammatory pseudotumour. Multifocal yellowish-white tissue with areas of necrosis, probably following the course of a bile duct or blood vessel.

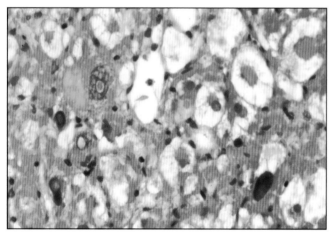

Fig. 15.86 • Angiomyolipoma. A tumour with bizarre, epithelioid smooth muscle cells that might be mistaken for malignancy. H&E.

to be part of the spectrum of tumours of perivascular epithelioid cells that includes such things as clear-cell tumours of the lung and pancreas and several other lesions in different parts of the body.[460]

Inflammatory pseudotumour

Inflammatory pseudotumour is a heterogeneous group of disorders occurring in many body sites and known under many different names including inflammatory myofibroblastic tumour, plasma cell granuloma, inflammatory fibrosarcoma, inflammatory myofibrohistiocytic proliferation and inflammatory fibromyxoid tumour. The inflammatory pseudotumour of the liver is an uncommon, benign, tumour-like lesion that often appears to arise from a healing abscess or other inflammatory condition with rupture of bile ducts and extravasation of bile into the tissue, provoking a xanthogranulomatous inflammatory response that heals with scarring.[2] Similar lesions occur in many body sites, and at least some of these pursue an aggressive course and have been considered to be true neoplasms, most often called inflammatory myofibroblastic tumours.[461] A variety of chromosomal changes, ALK-1 protein over-expression

and clonal proliferations of dendritic and fibroblastic reticulum cells expressing Epstin–Barr virus have supported a neoplastic origin of some lesions.[462] However, despite the histological similarity, it is clear that many of these are inflammatory or infectious in origin.[462,463] In particular, in the liver, some inflammatory pseudotumours are clearly related to bacterial infections such as *Actinomyces*, *Escherichia coli*, *Klebsiella pneumoniae*, *Eikenella corrodens*, and *Proteus*. Since the majority of hepatic lesions seem to be of this type, rather than true neoplasms, the term inflammatory pseudotumour is preferred for this site.

Hepatic inflammatory pseudotumours have been described in patients of all ages from infancy to the eighth decade.[2,464,465] Over 70% are male. Fever, right upper quadrant pain, weight loss and leukocytosis are frequent at presentation. Many lesions are excised on discovery, and the majority recover unless there are complications of surgery or underlying diseases; some lesions not resected have responded to antibiotic therapy with complete resolution.[2,464,465]

Antecedent diseases have been reported in a minority of cases and they include Caroli disease, diverticulitis, gastric ulcers, choledocholithiasis and pneumonia. Furthermore, there are several case reports of hepatic inflammatory pseudotumours associated with sclerosing cholangitis, in which the latter is considered either as the condition preceding or associated with hepatic inflammatory pseudotumour. It has been recently proposed that some of these cases of hepatic inflammatory pseudotumour associated with sclerosing cholangitis might belong to a spectrum of sclerosing pancreatitis and therefore amenable of steroid therapy.[464]

Inflammatory pseudotumours may be solitary or multiple, and can be any size up to an entire lobe of the liver.[465,466] They are usually well-circumscribed, firm and tan or yellow-white, but areas of necrosis may be present (Fig. 15.87). Microscopically the lesions contain a mixture of inflammatory cells with predominance of polyclonal plasma cells (Fig. 15.88), but lymphocytes, sometimes with lymphoid follicles, neutrophils and eosinophils may also be present. The inflammatory cells infiltrate a stroma composed of interlacing bundles of myofibroblasts, fibroblasts and

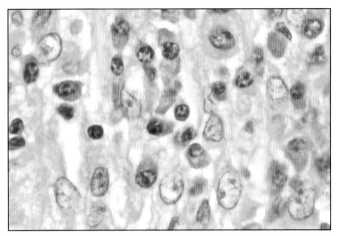

Fig. 15.88 • Inflammatory pseudotumour. Plasma cells and histiocytes are prominent in the inflammatory infiltrate. H&E.

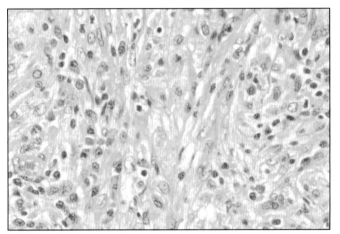

Fig. 15.89 • Inflammatory pseudotumour. Fibroxanthomatous inflammation in addition to plasma cells. H&E.

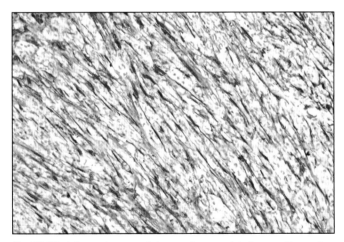

Fig. 15.90 • Inflammatory pseudotumour. Immunostain for smooth muscle actin shows that many of the spindled cells are myofibroblasts.

collagen bundles (Figs 15.89 and 15.90), and dense areas of fibrosis may also be seen. Occluded blood vessels, usually portal vein or hepatic vein branches, are frequently present near the edges of the lesions. A xanthogranulomatous inflammatory response with foamy histiocytes is often be present in areas, and there may be occasional areas of sup-

puration, supporting the notion that the lesions evolve from organizing liver abscesses.

Miscellaneous

Other benign tumours and pseudotumours that are more common in extrahepatic sites but that have occurred in the liver in rare instances include solitary fibrous tumour, leiomyoma, teratoma, schwannoma, neurofibroma, chondroma, myxoma, multicystic mesothelioma and adrenal rest tumour.[2]

Other malignant tumours

Embryonal sarcoma

Embryonal sarcoma of the liver is a rare primitive neoplasm, unique to the liver, with characteristic clinical and histological features. Other terms that have been used for this tumour include undifferentiated sarcoma, mesenchymal sarcoma and malignant mesenchymoma, but embryonal sarcoma is now preferred.[2]

Embryonal sarcoma is predominantly a disease of children and teenagers. More than half the patients are between 6 and 10 years of age, although rare cases have occurred in adults up to the age of 73 years.[2,467] The tumours grow rapidly and become quite large with areas of cystic degeneration and necrosis, so that abdominal swelling, with or without a palpable mass, and pain are the usual presenting findings. Radiological findings reveal a spectrum of solid and cystic features characteristic of the tumour,[468] so that the diagnosis can be strongly suspected in the clinical setting of a child with a large, rapidly growing cystic liver mass. In the older literature, most patients died rapidly of the disease, but in recent years there has been considerable improvement with combinations of surgery and chemotherapy.[469]

Embryonal sarcomas are typically large, measuring 10–20 cm in diameter, with an average weight of 1310 g.[467] The cut surface is variegated, with glistening, grey-white tumour tissue, alternating with cystic gelatinous areas, and/or red and yellow areas of haemorrhage and necrosis (Fig. 15.91). A fibrous pseudocapsule may separate the tumour from the adjacent compressed parenchyma. Microscopically, there are usually large areas of necrosis with patches of viable tumour that tend to be near the edges of the mass. In viable areas, the tumour cells are stellate or spindle-shaped and have ill-defined outlines (Fig. 15.92). They may be compactly or loosely arranged, in an abundant myxoid matrix or fibrous stroma. Tumour cells often have irregular, hyperchromatic nuclei, numerous mitoses and often bizarre giant cells. A characteristic feature is the presence of multiple, varying-sized eosinophilic globules in the tumour cell cytoplasm (Fig. 15.92). The globules are PAS-positive and diastase resistant. By immunohistochemistry, they may contain α_1-antitrypsin, α_1-antichymotrypsin, vimentin, immunoglobulins and/or albumin, but their exact nature remains obscure. Haematopoietic activity is observed in half the

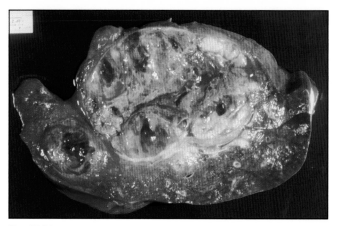

Fig. 15.91 • Embryonal sarcoma. The tumour is gelatinous and fish-flesh in consistency with areas of necrosis.

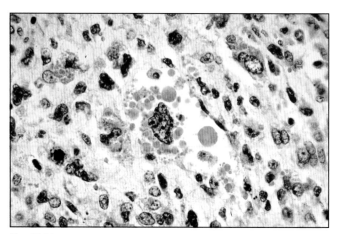

Fig. 15.92 • Embryonal sarcoma. Undifferentiated tumour cells in a myxoid matrix. Some tumour cells contain eosinophilic globules. H&E.

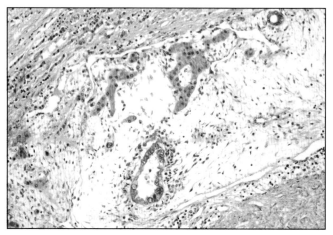

Fig. 15.93 • Embryonal sarcoma. Bizarre, trapped bile ducts and hepatocytes at the periphery of a tumour. H&E.

tumours. The more peripheral areas of the tumours typically contain entrapped bile ducts, which can be dilated, and sometimes clusters of hepatocytes (Fig. 15.93). The histogenesis of the lesion remains unknown. Despite the name, it does not resemble embryonal liver. The resemblance to mesenchymal hamartoma and the occurrence of several cases of embryonal sarcoma apparently arising from

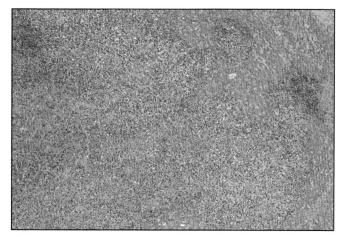

Fig. 15.94 • Diffuse large B cell lymphoma. The tumour causes irregular destruction of hepatic parenchyma. H&E.

mesenchymal hamartomas suggests that it is the malignant counterpart of that tumour.[454]

Primary hepatic lymphoma

The liver is frequently involved in disseminated lymphoma, but primary lymphomas of the liver are relatively rare. Since the spleen is often involved at the time of detection, the term hepatosplenic lymphoma is used synonymously with primary hepatic lymphoma. Primary lymphomas have occurred in patients of all ages. In most cases the aetiology is unknown, but some have been associated with hepatitis C, hepatitis B, HIV and Epstein–Barr virus in patients with post-transplant lymphoproliferative disorder.[2] Most patients present with abdominal pain, swelling and sometimes fever and are found to have a liver mass that reveals lymphoma on biopsy or resection,[470] while some have presented with acute liver failure.[471] Diffuse large B-cell lymphoma (Fig. 15.94) is the most common type, accounting for 80 to 90%. The following have all been reported: extranodal marginal B-cell lymphoma of mucosa-associated lymphoid tissue type (MALT); small lymphocytic B-cell lymphoma; Burkitt lymphoma; T-cell rich B-cell lymphoma; anaplastic large-cell lymphoma of B, T or null cell type; and peripheral T-cell lymphoma.[2,472–475] T-cell lymphomas and T-cell rich (or histiocyte rich) B-cell lymphomas can diffusely involve hepatic sinusoids or primarily involve portal areas, mimicking inflammatory liver diseases and making them difficult to recognize as a lymphoma.[476–478]

Primary hepatic MALT lymphoma is rare, with about 20 cases reported at present.[479,480] In most cases, it is asymptomatic, its clinical course is indolent without extrahepatic involvement and outcome is good after surgical resection without additional chemotherapy or irradiation. Transformation into a high-grade, large-cell, non-Hodgkin lymphoma has been reported in an isolated case.[481] Tumoural nodules are usually single, and very occasionally multiple. Hepatic MALT lymphoma is histologically characterized by: (i) a diffuse infiltration of small or medium-sized B-lymphoid cells with numerous monocytoid cells with a clear cytoplasm; (ii) the presence of lymphoepithelial lesions with bile duct epithelium destruction by tumour cells; and (iii) the persistence of reactive lymphoid follicles that are partially or totally infiltrated by tumour cells. Tumour cells express B-cell markers such as CD20 and CD79a and do not express CD5. Small CD5-positive cells are reactive T lymphocytes. This phenotype allows the distinction with other small B-cell non-Hodgkin lymphomas, that is lymphocytic lymphoma in which cells express CD5 and CD23, and mantle cell lymphoma in which tumour cells express CD5 and cyclin D1.

Miscellaneous malignant lesions

Other malignant tumours that have occurred in the liver on rare occasions include non-hepatocytic malignant mixed tumour, yolk sac tumour, malignant rhabdoid tumour, primary carcinoid, solid-pseudopapillary tumour, ossifying stromal-epithelial tumour, malignant cystic mesothelioma, osteoclastoma-like giant cell tumour, extramedullary plasmacytoma, primary pheochromocytoma, lymphoepithelioma-like carcinoma, embryonal rhabdomyosarcoma, Kaposi sarcoma, fibrosarcoma, leiomyosarcoma, malignant fibrous histiocytoma, osteosarcoma and malignant schwannoma.[2]

References

1. Hamilton SR, Aaltonen LA, eds. World Heath Organization classification of tumours. Pathology and genetics of tumours of the digestive system. Lyon: IARC Press, 2000
2. Ishak KG, Goodman ZD, Stocker JT. Tumors of the liver and intrahepatic bile ducts. Atlas of tumor pathology, 3rd Series, Fascicle 31. Washington: Armed Forces Institute of Pathology, 2001
3. Ros PR, Davis GL. The incidental focal liver lesion. Photon, proton, or needle? Hepatology, 1998; 27:1183–1190
4. Platt JF, Peterson MS, Baron RL. Noninvasive imaging of the liver and biliary system. In: Schiff ER, Sorrell MF, Maddrey WC, eds. Schiff's Diseases of the Liver, 9th edn. Philadelphia: Lippincott Williams & Wilkins, 2003; pp 287–342
5. Wilson SR, Burns PN. Liver mass evaluation with ultrasound: The impact of microbubble contrast agents and pulse inversion imaging. Sem Liver Dis, 2001; 21:147–160
6. Daniele B, Bencivenga A, Megna AS, Tinessa V. Alpha-fetoprotein and ultrasonography screening for hepatocellular carcinoma. Gastroenterology, 2004; 127:S108–S112
7. Federle MP, Blachar A. CT evaluation of the liver: Principles and techniques. Sem Liver Dis, 2001; 21:135–146
8. Baron RL, Brancatelli G. Computed tomographic imaging of hepatocellular carcinoma. Gastroenterology, 2004; 127:S133–S143
9. Beavers KL, Semelka RC. MRI evaluation of the liver. Sem Liver Dis, 2001; 21:161–178
10. Taouli B, Losada M, Holland A, Krinsky G. Magnetic resonance imaging of hepatocellular carcinoma. Gastroenterology, 2004; 127: S144–S152
11. Bruix J, Sherman M, Llovet JM, Beaugrand M, Lencioni R, Burroughs AK, Christensen E, Pagliaro L, Colombo M, Rodes J. Clinical management of hepatocellular carcinoma. Conclusions of the Barcelona-2000 EASL conference. J Hepatol, 2001; 35:421–430
12. Talwalkar JA, Gores GJ. Diagnosis and staging of hepatocellular carcinoma. Gastroenterology, 2004; 127:S126–S132
13. Edmondson HA, Henderson B, Benton B. Liver-cell adenomas associated with use of oral contraceptives. N Engl J Med, 1976; 294:470–472
14. Rooks JB, Ory HW, Ishak KG et al. Epidemiology of hepatocellular adenoma. The role of oral contraceptive use. JAMA, 1979; 242:644–648
15. Lindgren A, Olsson R. Liver damage from low-dose oral contraceptives. J Intern Med, 1993; 234:287–292
16. Porter LE, Van Thiel D, Eagon PK. Estrogens and progestins as tumor inducers. Semin Liv Dis, 1987; 7:24–31
17. Wanless IR, Medline A. Role of estrogens as promoters of hepatic neoplasia. Lab Invest, 1982; 46:313–320
18. Edmondson HA, Reynolds TB, Henderson B, Benton B. Regression of liver cell adenomas associated with oral contraceptives. Ann Intern Med, 1977; 86:180–182
19. Buhler H, Pirovino M, Akovbiantz A et al. Regression of liver cell adenoma. A follow-up study of three consecutive patients after discontinuation of oral contraceptive use. Gastroenterology, 1982; 82:775–782
20. Bork K, Pitton M, Harten P, Koch P. Hepatocellular adenomas in patients taking danazol for hereditary angio-oedema. Lancet, 1999; 353:1066–1067
21. See KL, See M, Gluud C. Liver pathology associated with the use of anabolic-androgenic steroids. Liver, 1992; 12:73–79
22. Labrune P, Trioche P, Duvaltier I, Chevalier P, Odièvre M. Hepatocellular adenomas in glycogen storage disease type I and type III. J Pediatr Gastroenterol Nutr, 1997; 24:276–279
23. Alshak NS, Cocjin J, Podesta L et al. Hepatocellular adenoma in glycogen storage disease type IV. Arch Pathol Lab Med, 1994; 118:88–91
24. Foster JH, Donahue TA, Berman MM. Familial liver-cell adenomas and diabetes mellitus. N Engl J Med, 1978; 299:239–241
25. Bacq Y, Jacquemin E, Balabaud C et al. Familial liver adenomatosis associated with hepatocyte factor 1a inactivation. Gastroenterology, 2003; 125:1470–1475
26. Zucman-Rossi J. Genetic alterations in hepatocellular adenomas: Recent findings and new challenges. J Hepatol, 2004; 40:1036–1039
27. Christopherson WM, Mays ET, Barrows GH. Liver tumors in young women: A clinical pathologic study of 201 cases in the Louisville Registry. In: Fenoglio CM, Wolff M, eds. Progress in surgical pathology, Vol. 2. New York: Masson Publishing, 1980; 187–205
28. Edmondson HA, Reynolds TB, Henderson B, Benton B. Regression of liver cell adenomas associated with oral contraceptives. Ann Intern Med, 1977; 86:180–182
29. Parker P, Burr I, Slonim A, Grishan FK, Greene H. Regression of hepatic adenomas in type Ia glycogen storage disease with dietary therapy. Gastroenterology, 1981; 81:534–536
30. Foster JH, Berman MM. The malignant transformation of liver cell adenomas. Arch Surg, 1994; 129:712–717
31. Libbrecht L, De Vos R, Cassiman D, Desmet V, Aerts R, Roskams T. Hepatic progenitor cells in hepatocellular adenomas. Am J Surg Pathol, 2001; 25:1388–1396
32. Paradis V, Benzekri A, Dargere D, Bieche I, Laurendeau I, Vilgrain V, Belghiti J, Vidaud M, Degott C, Bedossa P. Telangiectatic focal nodular hyperplasia: A variant of hepatocellular adenoma. Gastroenterol, 2004; 126:1323–1329
33. LeBail B, Jouhanole H, Deugnier Y, Salame G, Pellegrin J-L, Saric J, Balabaud C, Bioulac-Sage P. Liver adenomatosis with granulomas in two patients on long-term oral contraceptives. Am J Surg Pathol, 1992; 16:982–987
34. Gouysse G, Frachon S, Hervieu V, Fiorentino M, d'Errico A, Dumortier J, Boillot O, Partensky C, Grigioni WF, Scoazec JY. Endothelial cell differentiation in hepatocellular adenomas: implications for histopathological diagnosis. J Hepatol, 2004; 41:259–266
35. Paradis V, Lauvent A, Flejou J-F, Vidaud M, Bedossa P. Evidence for the polyclonal nature of focal nodular hyperplasia of the liver by the study of X-chromosome inactivation. Hepatology, 1997; 26:891–895
36. Wanless IR, Mawdsley C, Adams R. On the pathogenesis of focal nodular hyperplasia of the liver. Hepatology, 1985; 5:1194–1200
37. Fukukura Y, Nakashima O, Kusaba A, Kage M, Kojiro M. Angioarchitecture and blood circulation in focal nodular hyperplasia of the liver. J Hepatol, 1998; 29:470–475
38. Scoazec J-Y, Flejou J-F, D'Errico A, Couvelard A, Kozyraki R, Fiorention M, Grigioni WF, Feldmann G. Focal nodular hyperplasia of the liver: Composition of the extracellular matrix and expression of cell-cell and adhesion molecules. Hum Pathol, 1995; 26:1114–1115
39. Paradis V, Bieche I, Dargere D, Laurendeau I, Nectous J, Degott C, Belghiti J, Vidaud M, Bedossa P. A quantitative gene expression study suggests a role for angiopoietins in focal nodular hyperplasia. Gastroenterology, 2003; 124:651–659
40. Butron Vila MM, Haot J, Desmet VJ. Cholestatic features in focal nodular hyperplasia of the liver. Liver, 1984; 4:387–395
41. Nguyen BN, Flejou JF, Terris B, Belghiti J, Degott C. Focal nodular hyperplasia of the liver: A comprehensive pathologic study of 305 lesions and recognition of new histologic forms. Am J Surg Pathol, 1999; 23:1441–1454
42. International Working Party. Terminology of nodular hepatocellular lesions. Hepatology, 1995; 22:983–993

43. Theise ND, Park YN, Kokiro M. Dysplastic nodules and hepatocarcinogenesis. Clin Liver Dis, 2002; 6:497–512

44. Hytiroglou P. Morphological changes of early human hepatocarcinogenesis. Semin Liver Dis, 2004; 24:65–75

45. Libbrecht L, Desmet V, Roskams T. Preneoplastic lesions in human hepatocarcinogenesis. Liver Int, 2005; 25:16–27

46. Anthony PP, Vogel CL, Barker LF. Liver cell dysplasia: A premalignant condition. J Clin Pathol, 1973; 26:217–223

47. Lee R, Tsamandas AC, Demetris AJ. Large cell change (liver cell dysplasia) and hepatocellular carcinoma in cirrhosis: Matched case-control study, pathological analysis, and pathogenetic hypothesis. Hepatology, 1997; 26:1415–1422

48. Watanabe S, Okita K, Harada T, Kodama T, Numa Y, Takemoto T, Takahashi T. Morphologic studies of the liver cell dysplasia. Cancer, 1983; 51:2197–2205

49. Le Bail B, Belleannée G, Bernard F-H, Saric J, Balabaud C, Bioulac-Sage P. Adenomatous hyperplasia in cirrhotic livers: histological evaluation, cellular density and proliferative activity of 35 macronodular lesions in the cirrhotic explants of 10 adult French patients. Hum Pathol, 1995; 26:897–906

50. Takayama T, Makuuchi M, Hirohashi S, Sakamoto M, Okazaki N, Takayasu K, Kosuge T, Motoo Y, Yamazaki S, Hasegawa H. Malignant transformation of adenomatous hyperplasia to hepatocellular carcinoma. Lancet, 1990; 336:1150–1153

51. Kojiro M, Nakashima O. Histopathological evaluation of hepatocellular carcinoma with special reference to small early stage tumors. Semin Liver Dis, 1999; 19:287–296

52. Wanless IR. Micronodular transformation (nodular regenerative hyperplasia) of the liver: A report of 64 cases among 2,500 autopsies and a new classification of benign hepatocellular nodules. Hepatology, 1990; 11:789–797

53. Stocker J, Conran R, Selby D. Tumour and pseudotumors of the liver. In: Stocker J, Askin F, eds. Pathology of solid tumors in children. London: Chapman & Hall, 1998; pp 83–110

54. Fletcher JA, Kozakewich HP, Pavelka K, Grier HE, Shamberger RC, Korf B, Morton CC. Consistent cytogenetic aberrations in hepatoblastoma: a common pathway of genetic alterations in embryonal liver and skeletal muscle malignancies? Genes Chromosomes Cancer, 1991; 3:37–43

55. Terracciano LM, Bernasconi B, Ruck P, Stallmach T, Briner J, Sauter G, Moch H, Vecchione R, Pollice L, Pettinato G, Gurtl B, Ratschek M, De Krijger R, Tornillo L, Bruder E. Comparative genomic hybridization analysis of hepatoblastoma reveals high frequency of X-chromosome gains and similarities between epithelial and stromal components. Hum Pathol, 2003; 34:864–871

56. Fukuzawa R, Hata J, Hayashi Y, Ikeda H, Reeve AE. Beckwith-Wiedemann syndrome-associated hepatoblastoma: wnt signal activation occurs later in tumourigenesis in patients with 11p15.5 uniparental disomy. Pediatr Dev Pathol, 2003; 6:299–306

57. Buendia MA. Genetic alterations in hepatoblastoma and hepatocellular carcinoma: common and distinctive aspects. Med Pediatr Oncol, 2002; 39:530–535

58. Weber RG, Pietsch T, von Schweinitz D, Lichter P. Characterization of genomic alterations in hepatoblastomas. A role for gains on chromosomes 8q and 20 as predictors of poor outcome. Am J Pathol, 2000; 157:571–578

59. Albrecht S, von Schweinitz D, Waha A, Kraus JA, von Deimling A, Pietsch T. Loss of maternal alleles on chromosome arm 11p in hepatoblastoma. Cancer Res, 1994; 54:5041–5044

60. Schnater JM, Kohler SE, Lamers WH, von Schweinitz D, Aronson DC. Where do we stand with hepatoblastoma? A review. Cancer, 2003; 98:668–678

61. Ilyas M. Wnt signaling and the mechanistic basis of tumor development. J Pathol, 2005; 205:130–144

62. Koch A, Denkhaus D, Albrecht S, Leuschner I, von Schweinitz D, Pietsch T. Childhood hepatoblastomas frequently carry a mutated degradation targeting box of the beta-catenin gene. Cancer Res, 1999; 59:269–273

63. Taniguchi K, Roberts LR, Aderca IN et al. Mutational spectrum of beta-catenin, AXIN1, and AXIN2 in hepatocellular carcinomas and hepatoblastomas. Oncogene, 2002; 21:4863–4871

64. Wei Y, Fabre M, Branchereau S, Gauthier F, Perilongo G, Buendia MA. Activation of beta-catenin in epithelial and mesenchymal hepatoblastomas. Oncogene, 2000; 19:498–504

65. Wirths O, Waha A, Weggen S et al. Overexpression of human Dickkopf-1, an antagonist of wingless/WNT signaling, in human hepatoblastomas and Wilms' tumors. Lab Invest, 2003; 83:429–434

66. Ishak KG, Glunz PR. Hepatoblastoma and hepatocarcinoma: A report of 47 cases. Cancer, 1967; 20:396–422

67. Conran RM, Hitchcock CL, Waclawiw MA, Stocker JT, Ishak KG. Hepatoblastoma: the prognostic significance of histologic type. Pediatr Pathol, 1992; 12:167–183

68. Saxena R, Leake JL, Shafford EA, Davenport M, Mowat AP, Pritchard J, Mieli-Vergani G, Howard ER, Spitz L, Malone M et al. Chemotherapy effects on hepatoblastoma. A histological study. Am J Surg Pathol, 1993; 17:1266–1271

69. Haas JE, Muczynski KA, Krailo M, Krailo M, Ablin A, Land V, Vietti TJ, Hammond GD. Histopathology and prognosis in childhood hepatoblastoma and hepatocarcinoma. Cancer, 1989; 64:1082–1095

70. Haas JE, Feusner JH, Finegold MJ. Small cell undifferentiated histology in hepatoblastoma may be unfavorable. Cancer, 2001; 92:3130–3134

71. Bosch FX, Ribes J, Diaz M, Cleries R. Primary liver cancer: Worldwide incidence and trends. Gastroenterology, 2004; 127: S5–S16

72. El-Sarag HB. Hepatocellular carcinoma: Recent trends in the United States. Gastroenterology, 2004; 127:S27–S34

73. El-Serag HB, Davila JA, Petersen NJ, McGlynn KA. The continuing increase in the incidence of hepatocellular carcinoma in the United States: an update. Ann Intern Med, 2003; 139:817–823

74. Beasley RP. Hepatitis B virus: The major etiology of hepatocellular carcinoma. Cancer, 1988; 61:1942–1956

75. Nagasue N, Ito A, Yukaya H, Ogawa Y. Androgen receptors in hepatocellular carcinoma and surrounding parenchyma. Gastroenterology, 1985; 89:643–647

76. Fattovich G, Stroffolini T, Zagni I, Donato F. Hepatocellular carcinoma in cirrhosis: incidence and risk factors. Gastroenterology, 2004; 127(5 Suppl 1):S35–50

77. Okuda K. Clinical presentation and natural history of hepatocellular carcinoma and other liver cancers. In: Okuda K, Tabor E, eds. Liver cancer. New York: Churchill Livingstone, 1997; pp1–12

78. Kew MC. Hepatocellular carcinoma with and without cirrhosis: A comparison of South African blacks. Gastroenterology, 1989; 97:136–139

79. Nzeako UC, Goodman ZD, Ishak KG. Hepatocellular carcinoma in cirrhotic and noncirrhotic livers: A clinico-histopathologic study of 804 North American patients. Am J Clin Pathol, 1996; 105:65–75

80. Anzola M. Hepatocellular carcinoma: role of hepatitis B and hepatitis C viruses proteins in hepatocarcinogenesis. J Viral Hepat, 2004; 11:383–393

81. Chiaramonte M, Stroffolini T, Vian A et al. Rate of incidence of hepatocellular carcinoma in patients with compensated viral cirrhosis. Cancer, 1999; 85:2132–2137

82. Davila JA, Morgan RO, Shaib Y, McGlynn KA, El-Serag HB. Hepatitis C infection and the increasing incidence of hepatocellular carcinoma: a population-based study. Gastroenterology, 2004; 127:1372–1380

83. Fattovich G, Pantalena M, Zagni I, Realdi G, Schalm SW, Christensen E. Effect of hepatitis B and C virus infections on the natural history of compensated cirrhosis: a cohort study of 297 patients. Am J Gastroenterol, 2002; 97:2886–2895

84. Hassan MM, Zaghloul AS, El-Serag HB et al. The role of hepatitis C in hepatocellular carcinoma: a case control study among Egyptian patients. J Clin Gastroenterol, 2001; 33:123–126

85. Kiyosawa K, Umemura T, Ichijo T et al. Hepatocellular carcinoma: recent trends in Japan. Gastroenterology, 2004; 127(5 Suppl 1): S17–26

86. Mazzella G, Accogli E, Sottili S et al. Alpha interferon treatment may prevent hepatocellular carcinoma in HCV-related liver cirrhosis. J Hepatol, 1996; 24:141–147

87. Stroffolini T, Chiaramonte M, Tiribelli C et al. Hepatitis C virus infection, HBsAg carrier state and hepatocellular carcinoma: relative risk and population attributable risk from a case-control study in Italy. J Hepatol, 1992; 16:360–363

88. Sun CA, Wu DM, Lin CC et al. Incidence and cofactors of hepatitis C virus-related hepatocellular carcinoma: a prospective study of 12,008 men in Taiwan. Am J Epidemiol, 2003; 157:674–682

89. Takano S, Yokosuka O, Imazeki F, Tagawa M, Omata M. Incidence of hepatocellular carcinoma in chronic hepatitis B and C: a prospective study of 251 patients. Hepatology, 1995; 21:650–655

90. Terracciano L, Tornillo L. Cytogenetic alterations in liver cell tumors as detected by comparative genomic hybridization. Pathologica, 2003; 95:71–82

91. Tornillo L, Carafa V, Richter J et al. Marked genetic similarities between hepatitis B virus-positive and hepatitis C virus-positive hepatocellular carcinomas. J Pathol, 2000; 192:307–312

92. Brechot C. Pathogenesis of hepatitis B virus-related hepatocellular carcinoma: old and new paradigms. Gastroenterology, 2004; 127(5 Suppl 1):S56–61

93. Brechot C. Molecular mechanisms of hepatitis B and C viruses related to liver carcinogenesis. Hepatogastroenterology, 1998; 45 (Suppl 3):1189–1196

94. Grisham JW. Molecular genetic alterations in primary hepatocellular neoplasms: hepatocellular adenoma, hepatocellular carcinoma and hepatoblastoma. In: Coleman WB, Tsongalis GJ, eds. The molecular basis of human cancer. Totowa, New Jersey: Humana Press, 2001; pp 269–346

95. Yang HI, Lu SN, Liaw YF, You SL, Sun CA, Wang LY, Hsiao CK, Chen PJ, Chen DS, Chen CJ. Hepatitis B e antigen and the risk of hepatocellular carcinoma. N Engl J Med, 2002; 347:168–174

96. Pollicino T, Squadrito G, Cerenzia G, Cacciola I, Raffa G, Craxi A, Farinati F, Missale G, Smedile A, Tiribelli C, Villa E, Raimondo G. Hepatitis B virus maintains its pro-oncogenic properties in the case of occult HBV infection. Gastroenterology, 2004; 126:102–110

97. Buendia MA. Hepatitis B viruses and hepatocellular carcinoma. Adv Cancer Res, 1992; 59:167–226

98. Pineau P, Tiollais P. Animal hepadnavirus as a model of carcinogenesis. In: Okuda K, Tabor E, eds. Liver cancer. New York: Chrchill Livingstone, 1997; pp 189–199

99. Block TM, Mehta AS, Fimmel CJ, Jordan R. Molecular viral oncology of hepatocellular carcinoma. Oncogene, 2003; 22:5093–5107

100. Menne S, Tennant BC. Unraveling hepatitis B virus infection of mice and men (and woodchucks and ducks). Nat Med, 1999; 5:1125–1126

101. Tennant BC, Toshkov IA, Peek SF et al. Hepatocellular carcinoma in the woodchuck model of hepatitis B virus infection. Gastroenterology, 2004; 127(5 Suppl 1):S283–293

102. Feitelson MA, Sun B, Satiroglu Tufan NL, Liu J, Pan J, Lian Z. Genetic mechanisms of hepatocarcinogenesis. Oncogene, 2002; 21:2593–2604

103. Pugh JC, Bassendine MF. Molecular biology of hepadnavirus replication. Br Med Bull, 1990; 46:329–353

104. Tiollais P, Pourcel C, Dejean A. The hepatitis B virus. Nature, 1985; 317:489–495

105. Renard CA, Fourel G, Bralet MP et al. Hepatocellular carcinoma in WHV/N-myc2 transgenic mice: oncogenic mutations of beta-catenin and synergistic effect of p53 null alleles. Oncogene, 2000; 19:2678–2686

106. Brechot C, Gozuacik D, Murakami Y, Paterlini-Brechot P. Molecular bases for the development of hepatitis B virus (HBV)-related hepatocellular carcinoma (HCC). Semin Cancer Biol, 2000; 10:211–231

107. Chami M, Gozuacik D, Saigo K et al. Hepatitis B virus-related insertional mutagenesis implicates SERCA1 gene in the control of apoptosis. Oncogene, 2000; 19:2877–2886

108. Gozuacik D, Murakami Y, Saigo K et al. Identification of human cancer-related genes by naturally occurring Hepatitis B Virus DNA tagging. Oncogene, 2001; 20:6233–6240

109. Matsubara K, Tokino T. Integration of hepatitis B virus DNA and its implications for hepatocarcinogenesis. Mol Biol Med, 1990; 7:243–260

110. Paterlini P, Brechot C. The detection of hepatitis B virus (HBV) in HBsAG negative individuals with primary liver cancer. Dig Dis Sci, 1991; 36:1122–1129

111. Wang J, Chenivesse X, Henglein B, Brechot C. Hepatitis B virus integration in a cyclin A gene in a hepatocellular carcinoma. Nature, 1990; 343:555–557

112. Levy L, Renard CA, Wei Y, Buendia MA. Genetic alterations and oncogenic pathways in hepatocellular carcinoma. Ann N Y Acad Sci, 2002; 963:21–36

113. Soussan P, Garreau F, Zylberberg H, Ferray C, Brechot C, Kremsdorf D. In vivo expression of a new hepatitis B virus protein encoded by a spliced RNA. J Clin Invest, 2000; 105:55–60

114. Chen HS, Kaneko S, Girones R et al. The woodchuck hepatitis virus X gene is important for establishment of virus infection in woodchucks. J Virol, 1993; 67:1218–1226

115. Zoulim F, Saputelli J, Seeger C. Woodchuck hepatitis virus X protein is required for viral infection in vivo. J Virol, 1994; 68:2026–2030

116. Huo TI, Wang XW, Forgues M et al. Hepatitis B virus X mutants derived from human hepatocellular carcinoma retain the ability to abrogate p53-induced apoptosis. Oncogene, 2001; 20:3620–3628

117. Ueda H, Ullrich SJ, Gangemi JD et al. Functional inactivation but not structural mutation of p53 causes liver cancer. Nat Genet, 1995; 9:41–47

118. Wang XW, Forrester K, Yeh H, Feitelson MA, Gu JR, Harris CC. Hepatitis B virus X protein inhibits p53 sequence-specific DNA binding, transcriptional activity, and association with transcription factor ERCC3. Proc Natl Acad Sci USA, 1994; 91:2230–2234

119. Tai DI, Tsai SL, Chen YM et al. Activation of nuclear factor kappaB in hepatitis C virus infection: implications for pathogenesis and hepatocarcinogenesis. Hepatology, 2000; 31:656–664

120. Wu CG, Forgues M, Siddique S, Farnsworth J, Valerie K, Wang XW. SAGE transcript profiles of normal primary human hepatocytes expressing oncogenic hepatitis B virus X protein. Faseb J, 2002; 16:1665–1667

121. Yeh CT. Hepatitis B virus X protein: searching for a role in hepatocarcinogenesis. J Gastroenterol Hepatol, 2000; 15:339–341

122. Hu Z, Zhang Z, Doo E, Coux O, Goldberg AL, Liang TJ. Hepatitis B virus X protein is both a substrate and a potential inhibitor of the proteasome complex. J Virol, 1999; 73:7231–7240

123. Bouchard MJ, Wang LH, Schneider RJ. Calcium signaling by HBx protein in hepatitis B virus DNA replication. Science, 2001; 294:2376–2378

124. Chami M, Ferrari D, Nicotera P, Paterlini-Brechot P, Rizzuto R. Caspase-dependent alterations of Ca2+ signaling in the induction of apoptosis by hepatitis B virus X protein. J Biol Chem, 2003; 278:31745–31755

125. Rahmani Z, Huh KW, Lasher R, Siddiqui A. Hepatitis B virus X protein colocalizes to mitochondria with a human voltage-dependent anion channel, HVDAC3, and alters its transmembrane potential. J Virol, 2000; 74:2840–2846

126. Baldwin AS, Jr. The NF-kappa B and I kappa B proteins: new discoveries and insights. Annu Rev Immunol, 1996; 14:649–683

127. Chisari FV, Ferrari C. Hepatitis B virus immunopathology. Springer Semin Immunopathol, 1995; 17:261–281

128. Tai PC, Suk FM, Gerlich WH, Neurath AR, Shih C. Hypermodification and immune escape of an internally deleted middle-envelope (M) protein of frequent and predominant hepatitis B virus variants. Virology, 2002; 292:44–58

129. Xu Z, Jensen G, Yen TS. Activation of hepatitis B virus S promoter by the viral large surface protein via induction of stress in the endoplasmic reticulum. J Virol, 1997; 71:7387–7392

130. Okuda K. Hepatitis C virus and hepatocellular carcinoma. In: Okuda K, Tabor E, eds. Liver cancer. New York: Churchill Livingstone, 1997; pp 39–50

131. Di Bisceglie AM, Lyra AC, Schwartz M, Reddy RK, Martin P, Gores G, Lok AS, Hussain KB, Gish R, Van Thiel DH, Younossi Z, Tong M, Hassanein T, Balart L, Fleckenstein J, Flamm S, Blei A, Befeler AS. Hepatitis C-related hepatocellular carcinoma in the United States: influence of ethnic status. Am J Gastroenterol, 2003; 98:2060–2063

132. Weiland F, Weiland E, Unger G, Saalmuller A, Thiel HJ. Localization of pestiviral envelope proteins E(rns) and E2 at the cell surface and on isolated particles. J Gen Virol, 1999; 80:1157–1165

133. Westaway EG, Mackenzie JM, Kenney MT, Jones MK, Khromykh AA. Ultrastructure of Kunjin virus-infected cells: colocalization of NS1 and NS3 with double-stranded RNA, and of NS2B with NS3, in virus-induced membrane structures. J Virol, 1997; 71:6650–6661

134. Bartenschlager R, Lohmann V. Replication of hepatitis C virus. J Gen Virol, 2000; 81:1631–1648

135. Choo QL, Kuo G, Weiner AJ, Overby LR, Bradley DW, Houghton M. Isolation of a cDNA clone derived from a blood-borne non-A, non-B viral hepatitis genome. Science, 1989; 244:359–362

136. Takamizawa A, Mori C, Fuke I et al. Structure and organization of the hepatitis C virus genome isolated from human carriers. J Virol, 1991; 65:1105–1113

137. Egger D, Wolk B, Gosert R et al. Expression of hepatitis C virus proteins induces distinct membrane alterations including a candidate viral replication complex. J Virol, 2002; 76:5974–5984

138. Hugle T, Fehrmann F, Bieck E et al. The hepatitis C virus nonstructural protein 4B is an integral endoplasmic reticulum membrane protein. Virology, 2001; 284:70–81

139. Pietschmann T, Bartenschlager R. The hepatitis C virus replicon system and its application to molecular studies. Curr Opin Drug Discov Devel, 2001; 4:657–664

140. Wolk B, Sansonno D, Krausslich HG et al. Subcellular localization, stability, and trans-cleavage competence of the hepatitis C virus NS3-NS4A complex expressed in tetracycline-regulated cell lines. J Virol, 2000; 74:2293–2304

141. Liang TJ, Heller T. Pathogenesis of hepatitis C-associated hepatocellular carcinoma. Gastroenterology, 2004; 127(5 Suppl 1): S62–71

142. Sung VM, Shimodaira S, Doughty AL et al. Establishment of B-cell lymphoma cell lines persistently infected with hepatitis C virus in vivo and in vitro: the apoptotic effects of virus infection. J Virol, 2003; 77:2134–2146

143. Kwun HJ, Jang KL. Dual effects of hepatitis C virus Core protein on the transcription of cyclin-dependent kinase inhibitor p21 gene. J Viral Hepat, 2003; 10:249–255

144. Lan KH, Sheu ML, Hwang SJ et al. HCV NS5A interacts with p53 and inhibits p53-mediated apoptosis. Oncogene, 2002; 21:4801–4811

145. Lee MN, Jung EY, Kwun HJ et al. Hepatitis C virus core protein represses the p21 promoter through inhibition of a TGF-beta pathway. J Gen Virol, 2002; 83:2145–2151

146. Ishido S, Muramatsu S, Fujita T et al. Wild-type, but not mutant-type, p53 enhances nuclear accumulation of the NS3 protein of hepatitis C virus. Biochem Biophys Res Commun, 1997; 230:431–436

147. Kwun HJ, Jung EY, Ahn JY, Lee MN, Jang KL. p53-dependent transcriptional repression of p21(waf1) by hepatitis C virus NS3. J Gen Virol, 2001; 82:2235–2241

148. Muramatsu S, Ishido S, Fujita T, Itoh M, Hotta H. Nuclear localization of the NS3 protein of hepatitis C virus and factors affecting the localization. J Virol, 1997; 71:4954–4961

149. Ma Y, Hendershot LM. The unfolding tale of the unfolded protein response. Cell, 2001; 107:827–830

150. Kaufman RJ. Stress signaling from the lumen of the endoplasmic reticulum: coordination of gene transcriptional and translational controls. Genes Dev, 1999; 13:1211–1233

151. McCullough KD, Martindale JL, Klotz LO, Aw TY, Holbrook NJ. Gadd153 sensitizes cells to endoplasmic reticulum stress by down-regulating Bcl2 and perturbing the cellular redox state. Mol Cell Biol, 2001; 21:1249–1259

152. Sumida Y, Nakashima T, Yoh T et al. Serum thioredoxin levels as an indicator of oxidative stress in patients with hepatitis C virus infection. J Hepatol, 2000; 33:616–622

153. Gong G, Waris G, Tanveer R, Siddiqui A. Human hepatitis C virus NS5A protein alters intracellular calcium levels, induces oxidative stress, and activates STAT-3 and NF-kappa B. Proc Natl Acad Sci USA, 2001; 98:9599–9604

154. Finkel T, Holbrook NJ. Oxidants, oxidative stress and the biology of ageing. Nature, 2000; 408:239–247

155. Robinson MJ, Cobb MH. Mitogen-activated protein kinase pathways. Curr Opin Cell Biol, 1997; 9:180–186

156. Wang X, Martindale JL, Liu Y, Holbrook NJ. The cellular response to oxidative stress: influences of mitogen-activated protein kinase signalling pathways on cell survival. Biochem J, 1998; 333:291–300

157. Qian GS, Ross RK, Yu MC et al. A follow-up study of urinary markers of aflatoxin exposure and liver cancer risk in Shanghai, People's Republic of China. Cancer Epidemiol Biomarkers Prev, 1994; 3:3–10

158. Ross RK, Yuan JM, Yu MC et al. Urinary aflatoxin biomarkers and risk of hepatocellular carcinoma. Lancet, 1992; 339:943–946

159. Wogan GN. Aflatoxins as risk factors for hepatocellular carcinoma in humans. Cancer Res (Suppl), 1992; 52:2114s–2118s

160. Tabor E. The role of tumor suppressor genes in the development of hepatocellular carcinoma. In: Tabor E, DiBisceglie AM, Purcell RH, eds. Etiology, pathology, and treatment of hepatocellular carcinoma in North America. Houston: Gulf Publishing Co, 1991; pp 89–96

161. Smela ME, Hamm ML, Henderson PT, Harris CM, Harris TM, Essigmann JM. The aflatoxin B(1) formamidopyrimidine adduct plays a major role in causing the types of mutations observed in human hepatocellular carcinoma. Proc Natl Acad Sci USA, 2002; 99:6655–6660

162. Aguilar F, Harris CC, Sun T, Hollstein M, Cerutti P. Geographic variation of p53 mutational profile in nonmalignant human liver. Science, 1994; 264:1317–1319

163. Kress S, Jahn UR, Buchmann A, Bannasch P, Schwarz M. p53 Mutations in human hepatocellular carcinomas from Germany. Cancer Res, 1992; 52:3220–3223

164. Ming L, Thorgeirsson SS, Gail MH, Lu P, Harris CC, Wang N, Shao Y, Wu Z, Liu G, Wang X, Sun Z. Dominant role of hepatitis B virus and cofactor role of aflatoxin in hepatocarcinogenesis in Qidong, China. Hepatology, 2002; 36:1214–1220

165. Suriawinata A, Xu R. An update on the molecular genetics of hepatocellular carcinoma. Semin Liver Dis, 2004; 24:77–88

166. Morgan TR, Mandayam S, Jamal MM. Alcohol and hepatocellular carcinoma. Gastroenterology, 2004; 127:S87–S96

167. Nair J, Sone H, Nagao M, Barbin A, Bartsch H. Copper-dependent formation of miscoding etheno-DNA adducts in the liver of Long Evans cinnamon (LEC) rats developing hereditary hepatitis and hepatocellular carcinoma. Cancer Res, 1996; 56:1267–1271

168. Ladero JM, Agundez JA, Rodriguez-Lescure A, Diaz-Rubio M, Benitez J. RsaI polymorphism at the cytochrome P4502E1 locus and risk of hepatocellular carcinoma. Gut, 1996; 39:330–333

169. Lieber CS. Alcohol and the liver: 1994 update. Gastroenterology, 1994; 106:1085–1105

170. Stickel F, Schuppan D, Hahn EG, Seitz HK. Cocarcinogenic effects of alcohol in hepatocarcinogenesis. Gut, 2002; 51:132–139

171. Hassan MM, Hwang LY, Hatten CJ, Swaim M, Li D, Abbruzzese JL, Beasley P, Patt YZ. Risk factors for hepatocellular carcinoma: synergism of alcohol with viral hepatitis and diabetes mellitus. Hepatology, 2002; 36:1206–1213

172. Marrero JA, Fontana RJ, Fu S, Conjeevaram HS, Su GL, Lok AS. Alcohol, tobacco and obesity are synergistic risk factors for hepatocellular carcinoma. J Hepatol, 2005; 42:218–224

173. El-Serag HB, Tran T, Everhart JE. Diabetes increases the risk of chronic liver disease and hepatocellular carcinoma. Gastroenterology, 2004; 126:460–468

174. Davila JA, Morgan RO, Shaib Y, McGlynn KA, El-Serag HB. Diabetes increases the risk of hepatocellular carcinoma in the United States: a population based case control study. Gut, 2005; 54:533–539

175. Caldwell SH, Crespo DM, Kang HS, Al-Osaimi AM. Obesity and hepatocellular carcinoma. Gastroenterology, 2004; 127:S97–103

176. Calle EE, Rodriguez C, Walker-Thurmond K, Thun MJ. Overweight, obesity, and mortality from cancer in a prospectively studied cohort of U.S. adults. N Engl J Med, 2003; 348:1625–1638

177. Moller H, Mellemgaard A, Lindvig K, Olsen JH. Obesity and cancer risk: a Danish record-linkage study. Eur J Cancer, 1994; 30A:344–350

178. Nair S, Mason A, Eason J, Loss G, Perrillo RP. Is obesity an independent risk factor for hepatocellular carcinoma in cirrhosis? Hepatology, 2002; 36:150–155

179. Marrero JA, Fontana RJ, Su GL, Conjeevaram HS, Emick DM, Lok AS. NAFLD may be a common underlying liver disease in patients with hepatocellular carcinoma in the United States. Hepatology, 2002; 36:1349–1354

180. Neuschwander-Tetri BA, Caldwell SH. Nonalcoholic steatohepatitis: summary of an AASLD Single Topic Conference. Hepatology, 2003; 37:1202–1219

181. Roskams T, Yang SQ, Koteish A et al. Oxidative stress and oval cell accumulation in mice and humans with alcoholic and nonalcoholic fatty liver disease. Am J Pathol, 2003; 163:1301–1311

182. Leng J, Han C, Demetris AJ, Michalopoulos GK, Wu T. Cyclooxygenase-2 promotes hepatocellular carcinoma cell growth through Akt activation: evidence for Akt inhibition in celecoxib-induced apoptosis. Hepatology, 2003; 38:756–768

183. Ishak KG. Hepatocellular carcinoma associated with the inherited metabolic diseases. In: Tabor E, DiBisceglie AM, Purcell RH, eds. Etiology, pathology, and treatment of hepatocellular carcinoma in North America. Houston: Gulf Publishing Co, 1991; pp 91–106

184. Kowdley KV. Iron, hemochromatosis, and hepatocellular carcinoma. Gastroenterology, 2004; 127:S79–86

185. Russo PA, Mitchell GA, Tanguay RM. Tyrosinemia: A review. Ped Dev Pathol, 2001; 4:212–221

186. Bradbear RA, Bain C, Siskind V et al. Cohort study of internal malignancy in genetic hemochromatosis and other chronic nonalcoholic liver diseases. J Natl Cancer Inst, 1985; 75:81–84

187. Niederau C, Fischer R, Sonnenberg A, Stremmel W, Trampisch HJ, Strohmeyer G. Survival and causes of death in cirrhotic and in noncirrhotic patients with primary hemochromatosis. N Engl J Med, 1985; 313:1256–1262

188. Strohmeyer G, Niederau C, Stremmel W. Survival and causes of death in hemochromatosis. Observations in 163 patients. Ann N Y Acad Sci, 1988; 526:245–257

189. Borgna-Pignatti C, Vergine G, Lombardo T et al. Hepatocellular carcinoma in the thalassaemia syndromes. Br J Haematol, 2004; 124:114–117

190. Mandishona E, MacPhail AP, Gordeuk VR et al. Dietary iron overload as a risk factor for hepatocellular carcinoma in Black Africans. Hepatology, 1998; 27:1563–1566

191. Chenoufi N, Loreal O, Drenou B et al. Iron may induce both DNA synthesis and repair in rat hepatocytes stimulated by EGF/pyruvate. J Hepatol, 1997; 26:650–658

192. Ioannou GN, Kowdley KV. Iron, HFE mutations, and hepatocellular carcinoma: is hepatic iron a carcinogen? Clin Gastroenterol Hepatol, 2003; 1:246–248

193. Loeb LA, James EA, Waltersdorph AM, Klebanoff SJ. Mutagenesis by the autoxidation of iron with isolated DNA. Proc Natl Acad Sci US A, 1988; 85:3918–3922

194. Meneghini R. Iron homeostasis, oxidative stress, and DNA damage. Free Radic Biol Med, 1997; 23:783–792

195. Cho Y, Gorina S, Jeffrey PD, Pavletich NP. Crystal structure of a p53 tumor suppressor-DNA complex: understanding tumourigenic mutations. Science, 1994; 265:346–355

196. Vautier G, Bomford AB, Portmann BC, Metivier E, Williams R, Ryder SD. p53 mutations in british patients with hepatocellular carcinoma: clustering in genetic hemochromatosis. Gastroenterology, 1999; 117:154–160

197. Ishak KG, Zimmerman HJ. Hepatotoxic effects of the anabolic/androgenic steroids. Sem Liver Dis, 1987; 7:230–236

198. Thomas D. Exogenous steroid hormones and hepatocellular carcinoma. In: Tabor E, DiBisceglie AM, Purcell RH, eds. Etiology,

pathology, and treatment of hepatocellular carcinoma in North America. Houston: Gulf Publishing Co, 1991; pp 77–89

199. Yu MW, Chang HC, Chang SC, Liaw YF, Lin SM, Liu CJ, Lee SD, Lin CL, Chen PJ, Lin SC, Chen CJ. Role of reproductive factors in hepatocellular carcinoma: Impact on hepatitis B- and C-related risk. Hepatology, 2003; 38:1393–1400

200. Bergsland EK. Molecular mechanisms underlying the development of hepatocellular carcinoma. Semin Oncol, 2001; 28:521–531

201. Kountouras J, Zavos C, Chatzopoulos D. Apoptosis in hepatocellular carcinoma. Hepatogastroenterology, 2003; 50:242–249

202. Lee JS, Thorgeirsson SS. Genome-scale profiling of gene expression in hepatocellular carcinoma: classification, survival prediction, and identification of therapeutic targets. Gastroenterology, 2004; 127(5 Suppl 1):S51–55

203. Lee JS, Thorgeirsson SS. Genetic profiling of human hepatocellular carcinoma. Semin Liver Dis, 2005; 25:125–132

204. Libbrecht L, Desmet V, Roskams T. Preneoplastic lesions in human hepatocarcinogenesis. Liver Int, 2005; 25:16–27

205. Thorgeirsson SS, Grisham JW. Molecular pathogenesis of human hepatocellular carcinoma. Nat Genet, 2002; 31:339–346

206. Terracciano L, Tornillo L. Cytogenetic alterations in liver cell tumors as detected by comparative genomic hybridization. Pathologica, 2003; 95:71–82

207. Bishop JM. Molecular themes in oncogenesis. Cell, 1991; 64:235–248

208. Stanbridge EJ. Identifying tumor suppressor genes in human colorectal cancer. Science, 1990; 247:12–13

209. Stanbridge EJ. Human tumour suppressor genes. Annu Rev Genet, 1990; 24:615–657

210. Laurent-Puig P, Legoix P, Bluteau O et al. Genetic alterations associated with hepatocellular carcinomas define distinct pathways of hepatocarcinogenesis. Gastroenterology, 2001; 120:1763–1773

211. Pitot HC. Pathways of progression in hepatocarcinogenesis. Lancet, 2001; 358:859–860

212. Chen YJ, Yeh SH, Chen JT et al. Chromosomal changes and clonality relationship between primary and recurrent hepatocellular carcinoma. Gastroenterology, 2000; 119:431–440

213. Cheung ST, Chen X, Guan XY et al. Identify metastasis-associated genes in hepatocellular carcinoma through clonality delineation for multinodular tumor. Cancer Res, 2002; 62:4711–4721

214. Saeki R, Nagai H, Kaneko S et al. Intratumoural genomic heterogeneity in human hepatocellular carcinoma detected by restriction landmark genomic scanning. J Hepatol, 2000; 33:99–105

215. Bannasch P. Pathogenesis of hepatocellular carcinoma: sequential cellular, molecular, and metabolic changes. Prog Liver Dis, 1996; 14:161–197

216. Bannasch P, Haertel T, Su Q. Significance of hepatic preneoplasia in risk identification and early detection of neoplasia. Toxicol Pathol, 2003; 31:134–139

217. Bannasch P, Klimek F, Mayer D. Early bioenergetic changes in hepatocarcinogenesis: preneoplastic phenotypes mimic responses to insulin and thyroid hormone. J Bioenerg Biomembr, 1997; 29:303–313

218. Grisham JW. Interspecies comparison of liver carcinogenesis: implications for cancer risk assessment. Carcinogenesis, 1997; 18:59–81

219. Su Q, Bannasch P. Relevance of hepatic preneoplasia for human hepatocarcinogenesis. Toxicol Pathol, 2003; 31:126–133

220. Su Q, Benner A, Hofmann WJ, Otto G, Pichlmayr R, Bannasch P. Human hepatic preneoplasia: phenotypes and proliferation kinetics of foci and nodules of altered hepatocytes and their relationship to liver cell dysplasia. Virchows Arch, 1997; 431:391–406

221. Saito Y, Kanai Y, Sakamoto M, Saito H, Ishii H, Hirohashi S. Overexpression of a splice variant of DNA methyltransferase 3b, DNMT3b4, associated with DNA hypomethylation on pericentromeric satellite regions during human hepatocarcinogenesis. Proc Natl Acad Sci USA, 2002; 99:10060–10065

222. Maggioni M, Coggi G, Cassani B et al. Molecular changes in hepatocellular dysplastic nodules on microdissected liver biopsies. Hepatology, 2000; 32:942–946

223. Nagai H, Pineau P, Tiollais P, Buendia MA, Dejean A. Comprehensive allelotyping of human hepatocellular carcinoma. Oncogene, 1997; 14:2927–2933

224. Tornillo L, Carafa V, Sauter G et al. Chromosomal alterations in hepatocellular nodules by comparative genomic hybridization: high-grade dysplastic nodules represent early stages of hepatocellular carcinoma. Lab Invest, 2002; 82:547–553

225. Wong N, Lai P, Lee SW et al. Assessment of genetic changes in hepatocellular carcinoma by comparative genomic hybridization

analysis: relationship to disease stage, tumour size, and cirrhosis. Am J Pathol, 1999; 154:37–43

226. Zondervan PE, Wink J, Alers JC et al. Molecular cytogenetic evaluation of virus-associated and non-viral hepatocellular carcinoma: analysis of 26 carcinomas and 12 concurrent dysplasias. J Pathol, 2000; 192:207–215

227. Buendia MA. Genetics of hepatocellular carcinoma. Semin Cancer Biol, 2000; 10:185–200

228. Anders RA, Yerian LM, Tretiakova M et al. cDNA microarray analysis of macroregenerative and dysplastic nodules in end-stage hepatitis C virus-induced cirrhosis. Am J Pathol, 2003; 162:991–1000

229. Kim JW, Sime J, Forgues M. Molecular characterization of preneoplastic liver disease by cDNA microarray. In: 93rd Meeting of the American Association for Cancer Research; April 6–10, 2002. San Francisco, CA, 2003; pp 461–462

230. Doucas H, Garcea G, Neal CP, Manson MM, Berry DP. Changes in the Wnt signalling pathway in gastrointestinal cancers and their prognostic significance. Eur J Can, 2005; 41:365–379

231. Edamoto Y, Hara A, Biernat W et al. Alterations of RB1, p53 and Wnt pathways in hepatocellular carcinomas associated with hepatitis C, hepatitis B and alcoholic liver cirrhosis. Int J Cancer, 2003; 106:334–341

232. Ozaki I, Mizuta T, Zhao G et al. Involvement of the Ets-1 gene in overexpression of matrilysin in human hepatocellular carcinoma. Cancer Res, 2000; 60:6519–6525

233. Lee YI, Lee S, Das GC, Park US, Park SM, Lee YI. Activation of the insulin-like growth factor II transcription by aflatoxin B1 induced p53 mutant 249 is caused by activation of transcription complexes; implications for a gain-of-function during the formation of hepatocellular carcinoma. Oncogene, 2000; 19:3717–3726

234. Park US, Park SK, Lee YI, Park JG, Lee YI. Hepatitis B virus-X protein upregulates the expression of p21waf1/cip1 and prolongs G1→S transition via a p53-independent pathway in human hepatoma cells. Oncogene, 2000; 19:3384–3394

235. Takeo S, Arai H, Kusano N et al. Examination of oncogene amplification by genomic DNA microarray in hepatocellular carcinomas: comparison with comparative genomic hybridization analysis. Cancer Genet Cytogenet, 2001; 130:127–132

236. Esteller M, Herman JG. Cancer as an epigenetic disease: DNA methylation and chromatin alterations in human tumours. J Pathol, 2002; 196:1–7

237. Piao Z, Park C, Park JH, Kim H. Allelotype analysis of hepatocellular carcinoma. Int J Cancer, 1998; 75:29–33

238. Roncalli M, Bianchi P, Bruni B et al. Methylation framework of cell cycle gene inhibitors in cirrhosis and associated hepatocellular carcinoma. Hepatology, 2002; 36:427–432

239. Shim YH, Yoon GS, Choi HJ, Chung YH, Yu E. p16 hypermethylation in the early stage of hepatitis B virus-associated hepatocarcinogenesis. Cancer Lett, 2003; 190:213–219

240. Yang B, Guo M, Herman JG, Clark DP. Aberrant promoter methylation profiles of tumor suppressor genes in hepatocellular carcinoma. Am J Pathol, 2003; 163:1101–1107

241. Satyanarayana A, Manns MP, Rudolph L. Telomeres and telomerase: a Dual Role in Hepatocarcinogenesis. Hepatology, 2004; 40:276–283

242. Miura N, Horikawa I, Nishimoto A, Ohmura H, Hirohashi S. Progressive telomere shortening and telomerase reactivation during hepatocellular carcinogenesis. Cancer Genet Cytogenet, 1997; 93:56–62

243. Paterlini-Brechot P, Saigo K, Murakami Y et al. Hepatitis B virus-related insertional mutagenesis occurs frequently in human liver cancers and recurrently targets human telomerase gene. Oncogene, 2003; 22:3911–3916

244. Yokota T, Suda T, Igarashi M, Kuroiwa T, Waguri N, Kawai H. Telomere length variation and maintenance in hepatocarcinogenesis. Cancer, 2003; 98:110–118

245. Niketeghad F, Decker HJ, Caselmann WH, Lund P, Geissler F, Dienes HP. Frequent genomic imbalances suggest commonly altered tumour genes in human hepatocarcinogenesis. Br J Cancer, 2001; 85:697–704

246. Marchio A, Meddeb M, Pineau P et al. Recurrent chromosomal abnormalities in hepatocellular carcinoma detected by comparative genomic hybridization. Genes Chromosomes Cancer, 1997; 18:59–65

247. Marchio A, Pineau P, Meddeb M et al. Distinct chromosomal abnormality pattern in primary liver cancer of non-B, non-C patients. Oncogene, 2000; 19:3733–3738

248. Boige V, Laurent-Puig P, Fouchet P et al. Concerted nonsyntenic allelic losses in hyperploid hepatocellular carcinoma as determined by a high-resolution allelotype. Cancer Res, 1997; 57:1986–1890

249. Kusano N, Shiraishi K, Kubo K, Oga A, Okita K, Sasaki K. Genetic aberrations detected by comparative genomic hybridization in

hepatocellular carcinomas: their relationship to clinicopathological features. Hepatology, 1999; 29:1858–1862

250. Lerebours F, Olschwang S, Thuille B et al. Fine deletion mapping of chromosome 8p in non-small-cell lung carcinoma. Int J Cancer, 1999; 81:854–858

251. Nishida N, Nishimura T, Ito T, Komeda T, Fukuda Y, Nakao K. Chromosomal instability and human hepatocarcinogenesis. Histol Histopathol, 2003; 18:897–909

252. Sirma H, Weil R, Rosmorduc O et al. Cytosol is the prime compartment of hepatitis B virus X protein where it colocalizes with the proteasome. Oncogene, 1998; 16:2051–2063

253. Higashitsuji H, Itoh K, Nagao T et al. Reduced stability of retinoblastoma protein by gankyrin, an oncogenic ankyrin-repeat protein overexpressed in hepatomas. Nat Med, 2000; 6:96–99

254. Wang G, Zhao Y, Liu X et al. Allelic loss and gain, but not genomic instability, as the major somatic mutation in primary hepatocellular carcinoma. Genes Chromosomes Cancer, 2001; 31:221–227

255. Weber JD, Taylor LJ, Roussel MF, Sherr CJ, Bar-Sagi D. Nucleolar Arf sequesters Mdm2 and activates p53. Nat Cell Biol, 1999; 1:20–26

256. Pascale RM, Simile MM, Feo F. Genomic abnormalities in hepatocarcinogenesis. Implications for a chemopreventive strategy. Anticancer Res, 1993; 13:1341–1356

257. Shen L, Ahuja N, Shen Y et al. DNA methylation and environmental exposures in human hepatocellular carcinoma. J Natl Cancer Inst, 2002; 94:755–761

258. Ueki T, Fujimoto J, Suzuki T, Yamamoto H, Okamoto E. Expression of hepatocyte growth factor and its receptor, the c-met proto-oncogene, in hepatocellular carcinoma. Hepatology, 1997; 25:619–623

259. Chen Q, Seol DW, Carr B, Zarnegar R. Co-expression and regulation of Met and Ron proto-oncogenes in human hepatocellular carcinoma tissues and cell lines. Hepatology, 1997; 26:59–66

260. Jiang JG, Chen Q, Bell A, Zarnegar R. Transcriptional regulation of the hepatocyte growth factor (HGF) gene by the Sp family of transcription factors. Oncogene, 1997; 14:3039–3049

261. Chen X, Higgins J, Cheung ST et al. Novel endothelial cell markers in hepatocellular carcinoma. Mod Pathol, 2004; 17:1198–1210

262. Chung EJ, Sung YK, Farooq M et al. Gene expression profile analysis in human hepatocellular carcinoma by cDNA microarray. Mol Cells, 2002; 14:382–387

263. Fukai K, Yokosuka O, Chiba T et al. Hepatocyte growth factor activator inhibitor 2/placental bikunin (HAI-2/PB) gene is frequently hypermethylated in human hepatocellular carcinoma. Cancer Res, 2003; 63:8674–8679

264. Iizuka N, Oka M, Tamesa T, Hamamoto Y, Yamada-Okabe H. Imbalance in expression levels of insulin-like growth factor 2 and H19 transcripts linked to progression of hepatocellular carcinoma. Anticancer Res, 2004; 24:4085–4089

265. Kurokawa Y, Matoba R, Takemasa I et al. Molecular features of non-B, non-C hepatocellular carcinoma: a PCR-array gene expression profiling study. J Hepatol, 2003; 39:1004–1012

266. Lau WY, Lai PB, Leung MF et al. Differential gene expression of hepatocellular carcinoma using cDNA microarray analysis. Oncol Res, 2000; 12:59–69

267. Liu LX, Jiang HC, Liu ZH et al. Expression of cell cycle/growth regulator genes in human hepatocellular carcinoma and adjacent normal liver tissues. Oncol Rep, 2003; 10:1771–1775

268. Mao HJ, Li HN, Zhou XM, Zhao JL, Wan DF. Monitoring microarray-based gene expression profile changes in hepatocellular carcinoma. World J Gastroenterol, 2005; 11:2811–2816

269. Pan W, Zhang Q, Xi QS, Gan RB, Li TP. FUP1, a gene associated with hepatocellular carcinoma, stimulates NIH3T3 cell proliferation and tumor formation in nude mice. Biochem Biophys Res Commun, 2001; 286:1033–1338

270. Pang E, Hu Y, Chan KY et al. Karyotypic imbalances and differential gene expressions in the acquired doxorubicin resistance of hepatocellular carcinoma cells. Lab Invest, 2005; 85:664–674

271. Qiu W, David D, Zhou B et al. Down-regulation of growth arrest DNA damage-inducible gene 45beta expression is associated with human hepatocellular carcinoma. Am J Pathol, 2003; 162:1961–1974

272. Scandurro AB, Weldon CW, Figueroa YG, Alam J, Beckman BS. Gene microarray analysis reveals a novel hypoxia signal transduction pathway in human hepatocellular carcinoma cells. Int J Oncol, 2001; 19:129–135

273. Shirota Y, Kaneko S, Honda M, Kawai HF, Kobayashi K. Identification of differentially expressed genes in hepatocellular carcinoma with cDNA microarrays. Hepatology, 2001; 33:832–840

274. Tsai CC, Chung YD, Lee HJ et al. Large-scale sequencing analysis of the full-length cDNA library of human hepatocellular carcinoma. J Biomed Sci, 2003; 10:636–643

275. Wang Y, Wu MC, Sham JS, Zhang W, Wu WQ, Guan XY. Prognostic significance of c-myc and AIB1 amplification in hepatocellular carcinoma. A broad survey using high-throughput tissue microarray. Cancer, 2002; 95:2346–2352

276. Zindy P, Andrieux L, Bonnier D et al. Upregulation of DNA repair genes in active cirrhosis associated with hepatocellular carcinoma. FEBS Lett, 2005; 579:95–99

277. Kassianides C, Kew MC. The clinical manfestations and natural history of hepatocellular carcinoma. Gastroenterol Clin N Am, 1987; 16:553–562

278. Kew MC. Clinical and non-imaging diagnosis of hepatocellular carcinoma. In: Okuda K, Tabor E, eds. Liver cancer. Edinburgh: Churchill Livingstone, 1997; pp 315–329

279. Lai CL, Lam KC, Wong KP, Wu PC, Todd D. Clinical features of hepatocellular carcinoma: review of 211 patients in Hong Kong. Cancer, 1981; 47:2746–2755

280. Kew MC, Geddes EW. Hepatocellular carcinoma in rural southern African blacks. Medicine, 1982; 61:98–108

281. Okuda K, Obata H, Nakajima Y, Ohtsuki T, Okazaki N, Ohnishi K. Prognosis of primary hepatocellular carcinoma. Hepatology, 1984; 4:3S–6S

282. Llovet JM, Burroughs A, Bruix J. Hepatocellular carcinoma. Lancet, 2003; 362:1907–1917

283. Bolondi L. Screening for hepatocellular carcinoma in cirrhosis. J Hepatol, 2003; 39:1076–1084

284. Sherman M. Alphafetoprotein: an obituary. J Hepatol, 2001; 34:603–605

285. Friedman AC, Frazier S, Hendrix TM, Ros PR. Focal diseases. In: Friedman AC, Dachman AH, eds. Radiology of the liver, biliary tract, and pancreas. St Louis: Mosby, 1994; pp 169–327

286. Ikeda K, Saitoh S, Koida I, Tsubota A, Arase Y, Chayama K, Kumada H. Imaging diagnosis of small hepatocellular carcinoma. Hepatology, 1994; 20:82–87

287. Eggel H. Über das primäre Carcinom der Leber. Beitr Path Anat Allg Path, 1910; 30:506–604

288. Okuda K, Peters RL, Simpson IW. Gross anatomic features of hepatocellular carcinoma from three disparate geographic areas: Proposal of a new classification. Cancer, 1984; 54:2165–2173

289. Nakashima T, Kojiro M. Hepatocellular carcinoma. An atlas of its pathology. Tokyo: Springer-Verlag, 1987

290. Zhou XD, Tang ZY, Yang BH, Lin ZY, Ma ZC, Ye SL, Wu ZQ, Fan J, Qin LX, Zheng BH. Experience of 1000 patients who underwent hepatectomy for small hepatocellular carcinoma. Cancer, 2001; 91:1479–1486

291. Nakashima O, Sugihara S, Kage M, Kojiro M. Pathomorphologic characteristics of small hepatocellular carcinoma: a special reference to small hepatocellular carcinoma with indistinct margins. Hepatology, 1995; 22:101–105

292. Okusaka T, Okada S, Ueno H, Ikeda M, Shimada K, Yamamoto J, Kosuge T, Yamasaki S, Fukushima N, Sakamoto M. Satellite lesions in patients with small hepatocellular carcinoma with reference to clinicopathologic features. Cancer, 2002; 95:1931–1937

293. Bhattacharya S, Dhillon AP, Rees J, Savage K, Saada J, Burroughs A, Rolles K, Davidson B. Small hepatocellular carcinomas in cirrhotic explant livers: identification by macroscopic examination and lipiodol localization. Hepatology, 1997; 25:613–618

294. Kondo F, Wada K, Nagato Y, Nakajima T, Kondo Y, Hirooka N, Ebara M, Okuda K. Biopsy diagnosis of well-differentiated hepatocellular carcinoma based on new morphologic criteria. Hepatology, 1989; 9:751–755

295. Kondo F, Kondo Y, Nagato Y, Tomizawa M, Wada K. Interstitial tumour cell invasion in small hepatocellular carcinoma. Evaluation in microscopic and low magnification views. J Gastroenterol Hepatol, 1994; 9:604–612

296. Oikawa T, Ojima H, Yamasaki S, Takayama T, Hirohashi S, Sakamoto M. Multistep and multicentric development of hepatocellular carcinoma: histological analysis of 980 resected nodules. J Hepatol, 2005; 42:225–229

297. Varma V, Cohen C. Immunohistochemical and molecular markers in the diagnosis of hepatocellular carcinoma. Adv Anat Pathol, 2004; 11:239–249

298. Minervini MI, Demetris AJ, Lee RG, Carr BI, Madariaga J, Nalesnik MA. Utilization of hepatocyte-specific antibody in the immunocytochemical evaluation of liver tumours. Mod Pathol, 1997; 10:686–692

299. Lugli A, Tornillo L, Mirlacher M, Bundi M, Sauter G, Terracciano LM. Hepatocyte paraffin 1 expression in human normal and neoplastic tissues: tissue microarray analysis on 3,940 tissue samples. Am J Clin Pathol, 2004; 122:721–727

300. Wu PC, Fang JW, Lau VK, Lai CL, Lo CK, Lau JY. Classification of hepatocellular carcinoma according to hepatocellular and biliary differentiation markers. Clinical and biological implications. Am J Pathol, 1996; 149:1167–1175

301. Uenishi T, Kubo S, Yamamoto T, Shuto T, Ogawa M, Tanaka H, Tanaka S, Kaneda K, Hirohashi K. Cytokeratin 19 expression in hepatocellular carcinoma predicts early postoperative recurrence. Cancer Sci, 2003; 94:851–857

302. Auerbach A, Ishak KG, Goodman ZD. A longstanding misconception: Cytokeratin 7 and cytokeratin 20 expression in hepatocellular carcinoma. Mod Pathol, 2004; 17:295A

303. Gouysse G, Frachon S, Hervieu V, Fiorentino M, d'Errico A, Dumortier J, Boillot O, Partensky C, Grigioni WF, Scoazec JY. Endothelial cell differentiation in hepatocellular adenomas: implications for histopathological diagnosis. J Hepatol, 2004; 41:259–266

304. Edmondson HA, Steiner PE. Primary carcinoma of the liver: A study of 100 cases among 48 900 necropsies. Cancer, 1954; 7:462–503

305. Haratake J, Takeda S, Kasai T, Nakano S, Tokui N. Predictable factors for estimating prognosis of patients after resection of hepatocellular carcinoma. Cancer, 1993; 72:1178–1183

306. Lauwers GY, Terris B, Balis UJ, Batts KP, Regimbeau JM, Chang Y, Graeme-Cook F, Yamabe H, Ikai I, Cleary KR, Fujita S, Flejou JF, Zukerberg LR, Nagorney DM, Belghiti J, Yamaoka Y, Vauthey JN. Prognostic histologic indicators of curatively resected hepatocellular carcinomas: a multi-institutional analysis of 425 patients with definition of a histologic prognostic index. Am J Surg Pathol, 2002; 26:25–34

307. Lai CL, Wu PC, Lam KC, Todd D. Histologic prognostic indicators in hepatocellular carcinoma. Cancer, 1979; 44:1677–1683

308. Nzeako UC, Goodman ZD, Ishak KG. Comparison of tumor pathology with duration of survival of North American patients with hepatocellular carcinoma. Cancer, 1995; 76:579–588

309. Dabbs DJ, Geisinger KR, Ruggiero F, Raab SS, Nalesnik M, Silverman JF. Recommendations for the reporting of tissues removed as part of the surgical treatment of malignant liver tumours. Hum Pathol, 2004; 35:1315–1323

310. Sobin L, Wittekind C, eds. UICC TNM classification of malignant tumours, 6th edn. New York: Wiley-Liss, 2002

311. Okuda K, Ohtsuki T, Obata H, Tomimatsu M, Okazaki N, Hasegawa H, Nakajima Y, Ohnishi K. Natural history of hepatocellular carcinoma and prognosis in relation to treatment. Study of 850 patients. Cancer, 1985; 56:918–928

312. The Cancer of the Liver Italian Program (CLIP) Investigators: A new prognostic system for hepatocellular carcinoma: a retrospective study of 435 patients. Hepatology, 1998; 28:751–755

313. Llovet JM, Bru C, Bruix J. Prognosis of hepatocellular carcinoma: the BCLC staging classification. Semin Liver Dis, 1999; 19:329–338

314. Chevret S, Trinchet JC, Mathieu D, Rached AA, Beaugrand M, Chastang C. A new prognostic classification for predicting survival in patients with hepatocellular carcinoma. Groupe d'Etude et de Traitement du Carcinome Hepatocellulaire. J Hepatol, 1999; 31:133–141

315. Leung TW, Tang AM, Zee B, Lau WY, Lai PB, Leung KL, Lau JT, Yu SC, Johnson PJ. Construction of the Chinese University Prognostic Index for hepatocellular carcinoma and comparison with the TNM staging system, the Okuda staging system, and the Cancer of the Liver Italian Program staging system: a study based on 926 patients. Cancer, 2002; 94:1760–1769

316. Kudo M, Chung H, Haji S, Osaki Y, Oka H, Seki T, Kasugai H, Sasaki Y, Matsunaga T. Validation of a new prognostic staging system for hepatocellular carcinoma: the JIS score compared with the CLIP score. Hepatology, 2004; 40:1396–1405

317. Tateishi R, Yoshida H, Shiina S, Imamura H, Hasegawa K, Teratani T, Obi S, Sato S, Koike Y, Fujishima T, Makuuchi M, Omata M. Proposal of a new prognostic model for hepatocellular carcinoma: an analysis of 403 patients. Gut, 2005; 54:419–425

318. Sala M, Forner A, Varela M, Bruix J. Prognostic prediction in patients with hepatocellular carcinoma. Semin Liver Dis, 2005; 25:171–180

319. Cillo U, Bassanello M, Vitale A, Grigoletto FA, Burra P, Fagiuoli S, D'Amico F, Ciarleglio FA, Boccagni P, Brolese A, Zanus G, D'Amico DF. The critical issue of hepatocellular carcinoma prognostic classification: which is the best tool available? J Hepatol, 2004; 40:124–131

320. Marrero JA, Fontana RJ, Barrat A, Askari F, Conjeevaram HS, Su GL, Lok AS. Prognosis of hepatocellular carcinoma: comparison of 7 staging systems in an American cohort. Hepatology, 2005; 41:707–716

321. Sheu JC, Sung JL, Chen DS, Yang PM, Lai MY, Lee CS, Hsu HC, Chuang CN, Yang PC, Wang TH, Lin JT, Lee CZ. Growth rate of asymptomatic hepatocellular carcinoma and its clinical implications. Gastroenterology, 1985; 89:259–266

322. Barbara L, Benzi G, Gaiani S, Fusconi F, Zironi G, Siringo S, Rigamonti A, Barbara C, Grigioni W, Mazziotti A, Bolondi L. Natural history of small untreated hepatocellular carcinoma in cirrhosis: a multivariate analysis of prognostic factors of tumor growth rate and patient survival. Hepatology, 1992; 16:132–137

323. Yuki K, Hirohashi S, Sakamoto M, Kanai T, Shimosato Y. Growth and spread of hepatocellular carcinoma: A review of 240 autopsy cases. Cancer, 1990; 66:2174–2179

324. Nakashima T, Okuda K, Kojiro M, Jimi A, Yamaguchi R, Sakamoto K, Ikari T. Pathology of hepatocellular carcinoma in Japan: 232 consecutive cases autopsied in ten years. Cancer, 1983; 51:863–877

325. Carr BI. Hepatocellular carcinoma: Current management and future trends. Gastroenterology, 2004; 127:S218–S224

326. Craig JR, Peters RL, Edmondson HA, Omata M. Fibrolamellar carcinoma of the liver. Cancer, 1980; 46:372–379

327. Berman MM, Libbey NP, Foster JH. Hepatocellular carcinoma: Polygonal cell type with fibrous stroma—An atypical variant with a favorable prognosis. Cancer, 1980; 46:1448–1455

328. Soreide O, Czerniak A, Bradpiece H, Bloom S, Blumgart L. Characteristics of fibrolamellar hepatocellular carcinoma: A study of nine cases and a review of the literature. Am J Surg, 1986; 151:518–523

329. Pinna AD, Iwatsuki S, Lee RG, Todo S, Madariaga JR, Marsh JW, Casavilla A, Dvorchik I, Fung JJ, Starzl TE. Treatment of fibrolamellar hepatoma with subtotal hepatectomy or transplantation. Hepatology, 1997; 26:877–883

330. Goodman ZD, Ishak KG, Langloss JM, Sesterhenn IA, Rabin L. Combined hepatocellular-cholangiocarcinoma: A histologic and immunohistochemical study. Cancer, 1985; 55:124–135

331. Aoki K, Takayasu K, Kawano T, Muramatsu Y, Moriyama N, Wakao F, Yamamoto J, Shimada K, Takayama T, Kosuge T et al. Combined hepatocellular carcinoma and cholangiocarcinoma: clinical features and computed tomographic findings. Hepatology, 1993; 18:1090–1095

332. Maeda T, Adachi E, Kajiyama K, Sugimachi K, Tsuneyoshi M. Combined hepatocellular and cholangiocarcinoma: proposed criteria according to cytokeratin expression and analysis of clinicopathologic features. Hum Pathol, 1995; 26:956–964

333. Fujii H, Zhu XG, Matsumoto T, Inagaki M, Tokusashi Y, Miyokawa N, Fukusato T, Uekusa T, Takagaki T, Kadowaki N, Shirai T. Genetic classification of combined hepatocellular-cholangiocarcinoma. Hum Pathol, 2000; 31:1011–1017

334. Sasaki M, Nakanuma Y, Ho SB, Kim YS. Cholangiocarcinomas arising in cirrhosis and combined hepatocellular-cholangiocellular carcinomas share apomucin profiles. Am J Clin Pathol, 1998; 109:302–308

335. Tickoo SK, Zee SY, Obiekwe S, Xiao H, Koea J, Robiou C, Blumgart LH, Jarnagin W, Ladanyi M, Klimstra DS. Combined hepatocellular-cholangiocarcinoma: a histopathologic, immunohistochemical, and in situ hybridization study. Am J Surg Pathol, 2002; 26:989–997

336. Jarnagin WR, Weber S, Tickoo SK, Koea JB, Obiekwe S, Fong Y, DeMatteo RP, Blumgart LH, Klimstra D. Combined hepatocellular and cholangiocarcinoma: demographic, clinical, and prognostic factors. Cancer, 2002; 94:2040–2046

337. Cazals-Hatem D, Rebouissou S, Bioulac-Sage P, Bluteau O, Blanche H, Franco D, Monges G, Belghiti J, Sa Cunha A, Laurent-Puig P, Degott C, Zucman-Rossi J. Clinical and molecular analysis of combined hepatocellular-cholangiocarcinomas. J Hepatol, 2004; 41:292–298

338. Theise ND, Yao JL, Harada K, Hytiroglou P, Portmann B, Thung SN, Tsui W, Ohta H, Nakanuma Y. Hepatic 'stem cell' malignancies in adults: four cases. Histopathology, 2003; 43:263–271

339. Kim H, Park C, Han KH, Choi J, Kim YB, Kim JK, Park YN. Primary liver carcinoma of intermediate (hepatocyte-cholangiocyte) phenotype. J Hepatol, 2004; 40:298–304

340. Maeda T, Adachi E, Kajiyama K, Takenaka K, Sugimachi K, Tsuneyoshi M. Spindle cell hepatocellular carcinoma. A clinicopathologic and immunohistochemical analysis of 15 cases. Cancer, 1996; 77:51–57

341. Kishimoto Y, Hijiya S, Nagasako R. Malignant mixed tumor of the liver in adults. Am J Gastroenterol, 1984; 79:229–235

342. Nakajima T, Kubosawa H, Kondo Y, Konno A, Iwama S. Combined hepatocellular-cholangiocarcinoma with variable sarcomatous transformation. Am J Clin Pathol, 1988; 90:309–312

343. Leger-Ravet MB, Borgonovo G, Amato A, Lemaigre G, Franco D. Carcinosarcoma of the liver with mesenchymal differentiation: A case report. Hepatogastroenterology, 1996; 43:255–259

344. Papotti M, Sambataro D, Marchesa P, Negro F. A combined hepatocellular/cholangiocellular carcinoma with sarcomatoid features. Liver, 1997; 17:47–52

345. Desmet VJ. Congenital disease of intrahepatic bile ducts: Variations on the theme 'ductal plate malformation' Hepatology, 1992; 16:1069–1083

346. Redston MS, Wanless IR. The hepatic von Meyenburg complex with hepatic and renal cyst. Modern Pathol, 1996; 9:233–237

347. Jain D, Sarode UR, Abdul-Karim FW, Homer R, Robert ME. Evidence for the neoplastic transformation of von Meyenburg complexes. Am J Surg Pathol, 2000; 24:1131–1139

348. Röcken C, Pross M, Brucks U, Ridweiski K, Roessner A. Cholangiocarcinoma occurring in the liver with multiple bile duct hamartomas. Arch Pathol Lab Med, 2000; 124:1704–1706

349. Terada T, Nakanuma Y, Kono N, Ueda K, Kadoya M, Matsui O. Ciliated hepatic foregut cyst. A mucus histochemical, immunohistochemical, and ultrastructural study in three cases in comparison with normal bronchi and intrahepatic bile ducts. Am J Surg Pathol, 1990; 14:356–363

350. Vick, DJ, Goodman ZD, Deavers MT, Cain J, Ishak KG. Ciliated hepatic foregut cyst: A study of 6 cases and review of the literature. Am J Surg Pathol, 1999; 23:671–677

351. Vick DJ, Goodman ZD, Ishak KG. Squamous cell carcinoma in a ciliated hepatic foregut cyst. Arch Pathol Lab Med, 1999; 123:1115–1117

352. Bhathal PS, Hughes NR, Goodman ZD. The so-called bile duct adenoma is a peribiliary gland hamartoma. Am J Surg Pathol, 1996; 20:858–864

353. Allaire GS, Rabin L, Ishak KG, Sesterhenn IA. Bile duct adenoma. A study of 152 cases. Am J Surg Pathol, 1988; 12:708–715

354. Lee SS, Kim MH, Lee SK, Jang SJ, Song MH, Kim KP, Kim HJ, Seo DW, Song DE, Yu E, Lee SG, Min YI. Clinicopathologic review of 58 patients with biliary papillomatosis. Cancer, 2004; 100:783–793

355. Devaney K, Goodman ZD, Ishak KG. Hepatobiliary cystadenoma and cystadenocarcinoma. A light microscopic and immunohistochemical study of 70 patients. Am J Surg Pathol, 1994; 18:1078–1091

356. Buetow PC, Buck JL, Pantongrag-Brown L, Ros PR, Devaney K, Goodman ZD, Cruess DF: Biliary cystadenoma and cystadenocarcinoma: Clinical-imaging-pathologic correlation with emphasis on the importance of ovarian stroma. Radiology, 1995; 196:805–810

357. Wheeler DA, Edmondson HA. Cystadenoma with mesenchymal stroma (CMS) in the liver and bile ducts: a clinicopathologic study of 17 cases, 4 with malignant change. Cancer, 1985; 56:1434–1445

358. Weihing RR, Shintaku IP, Geller SA, Petrovic LM. Hepatobiliary and pancreatic mucinous cystadenocarcinomas with mesenchymal stroma: Analysis of estrogen receptors/progesterone receptors and expression of tumor-associated antigens. Mod Pathol, 1997; 10:372–379

359. Subramony C, Herrera GA, Turbat-Herrera EA. Hepatobiliary cystadenoma. A study of 5 cases with reference to histogenesis. Arch Pathol Lab Med, 1993; 117:1036–1042

360. Klatskin G. Adenocarcinoma of the hepatic duct at its bifurcation within the porta hepatis. Am J Med, 1965; 38:241–256

361. Patel T. Increasing incidence and mortality of primary intrahepatic cholangiocarcinoma in the United States. Hepatology, 2001; 33:1353–1357

362. Khan SA, Taylor-Robinson SD, Toledano MB, Beck A, Elliott P, Thomas HC. Changing international trends in mortality rates for liver, biliary and pancreatic tumours. J Hepatol, 2002; 37:806–813

363. Shaib YH, Davila JA, McGlynn K, El-Serag HB. Rising incidence of intrahepatic cholangiocarcinoma in the United States: a true increase? J Hepatol, 2004; 40:472–477

364. Shahip Y, El-Sarag HB. The epidemiology of cholangiocarcinoma. Sem Liver Dis, 2004; 24:115–124

365. Terada T, Kida T, Nakanuma Y, Kurumaya H, Doishita K, Takayanagi N. Intrahepatic cholangiocarcinomas associated with nonbiliary cirrhosis. J Clin Gastroenterol, 1994; 18:335–342

366. Kobayashi M, Ikeda K, Saitoh S, Suzuki F, Tsubota A, Suzuki Y, Arase Y, Murashima N, Chayama K, Kumada H. Incidence of primary cholangiocellular carcinoma of the liver in Japanese patients with hepatitis C virus-related cirrhosis. Cancer, 2000; 88:2471–2477

367. Kagawa Y, Kashihara S, Kuramoto S, Maetani S. Carcinoma arising in a congenitally dilated biliary tract. Report of a case and review of the literature. Gastroenterology, 1978; 74:1286–1294

368. Boberg KM, Bergquist A, Mitchell S, Pares A, Rosina F, Broome U, Chapman R, Fausa O, Egeland T, Rocca G, Schrumpf E. Cholangiocarcinoma in primary sclerosing cholangitis: risk factors and clinical presentation. Scand J Gastroenterol, 2002; 37:1205–1211

369. Charpin C, Garcia S, Bouvier C et al. E-cadherin quantitative immunocytochemical assays in breast carcinomas. J Pathol, 1997; 18:294–300

370. Ashida K, Terada T, Kitamura Y, Kaibara N. Expression of E-cadherin, alpha-catenin, beta-catenin, and CD44 (standard and variant isoforms) in human cholangiocarcinoma: an immunohistochemical study. Hepatology, 1998; 27:974–982

371. Sugimachi K, Taguchi K, Aishima S et al. Altered expression of beta-catenin without genetic mutation in intrahepatic cholangiocarcinoma. Mod Pathol, 2001; 14:900–905

372. Harada K, Terada T, Nakanuma Y. Detection of transforming growth factor-alpha protein and messenger RNA in hepatobiliary diseases by immunohistochemical and in situ hybridization techniques. Hum Pathol, 1996; 27:787–792

373. Ito Y, Takeda T, Sasaki Y et al. Expression and clinical significance of the erbB family in intrahepatic cholangiocellular carcinoma. Pathol Res Pract, 2001; 197:95–100

374. Berthiaume EP, Wands J. The molecular pathogenesis of cholangiocarcinoma. Semin Liver Dis, 2004; 24:127–137

375. Radaeva S, Ferreira-Gonzalez A, Sirica AE. Overexpression of C-NEU and C-MET during rat liver cholangiocarcinogenesis: A link between biliary intestinal metaplasia and mucin-producing cholangiocarcinoma. Hepatology, 1999; 29:1453–1462

376. Aishima SI, Taguchi KI, Sugimachi K, Shimada M, Sugimachi K, Tsuneyoshi M. c-erbB-2 and c-Met expression relates to cholangiocarcinogenesis and progression of intrahepatic cholangiocarcinoma. Histopathology, 2002; 40:269–278

377. Terada T, Ashida K, Endo K et al. c-erbB-2 protein is expressed in hepatolithiasis and cholangiocarcinoma. Histopathology, 1998; 33:325–331

378. Kiguchi K, Carbajal S, Chan K et al. Constitutive expression of ErbB-2 in gallbladder epithelium results in development of adenocarcinoma. Cancer Res, 2001; 61:6971–6976

379. Nakanuma Y, Harada K, Ishikawa A, Zen Y, Sasaki M. Anatomic and molecular pathology of intrahepatic cholangiocarcinoma. J Hepatobiliary Pancreat Surg, 2003; 10:265–281

380. DuBois RN, Radhika A, Reddy BS, Entingh AJ. Increased cyclooxygenase-2 levels in carcinogen-induced rat colonic tumors. Gastroenterology, 1996; 110:1259–1262

381. Shirvani VN, Ouatu-Lascar R, Kaur BS, Omary MB, Triadafilopoulos G. Cyclooxygenase 2 expression in Barrett's esophagus and adenocarcinoma: Ex vivo induction by bile salts and acid exposure. Gastroenterology, 2000; 118:487–496

382. Williams CS, Mann M, DuBois RN. The role of cyclooxygenases in inflammation, cancer, and development. Oncogene, 1999; 18:7908–7916

383. Hayashi N, Yamamoto H, Hiraoka N et al. Differential expression of cyclooxygenase-2 (COX-2) in human bile duct epithelial cells and bile duct neoplasm. Hepatology, 2001; 34:638–650

384. Chariyalertsak S, Sirikulchayanonta V, Mayer D et al. Aberrant cyclooxygenase isozyme expression in human intrahepatic cholangiocarcinoma. Gut, 2001; 48:80–86

385. Endo K, Yoon BI, Pairojkul C, Demetris AJ, Sirica AE. ERBB-2 overexpression and cyclooxygenase-2 up-regulation in human cholangiocarcinoma and risk conditions. Hepatology, 2002; 36:439–450

386. Sirica AE, Lai GH, Endo K, Zhang Z, Yoon BI. Cyclooxygenase-2 and ERBB-2 in cholangiocarcinoma: potential therapeutic targets. Semin Liver Dis, 2002; 22:303–313

387. Diamantis I, Karamitopoulou E, Perentes E, Zimmermann A. p53 protein immunoreactivity in extrahepatic bile duct and gallbladder cancer: correlation with tumor grade and survival. Hepatology, 1995; 22:774–779

388. Kang YK, Kim WH, Lee HW, Lee HK, Kim YI. Mutation of p53 and K-ras, and loss of heterozygosity of APC in intrahepatic cholangiocarcinoma. Lab Invest, 1999; 79:477–483

389. Ohashi K, Nakajima Y, Kanehiro H et al. Ki-ras mutations and p53 protein expressions in intrahepatic cholangiocarcinomas: relation to gross tumor morphology. Gastroenterology, 1995; 109:1612–1617

390. Tannapfel A, Weinans L, Geissler F et al. Mutations of p53 tumor suppressor gene, apoptosis, and proliferation in intrahepatic cholangiocellular carcinoma of the liver. Dig Dis Sci, 2000; 45:317–324

391. Furubo S, Harada K, Shimonishi T, Katayanagi K, Tsui W, Nakanuma Y. Protein expression and genetic alterations of p53 and ras in intrahepatic cholangiocarcinoma. Histopathology, 1999; 35:230–240

392. Horie S, Endo K, Kawasaki H, Terada T. Overexpression of MDM2 protein in intrahepatic cholangiocarcinoma: relationship with p53 overexpression, Ki-67 labeling, and clinicopathological features. Virchows Arch, 2000; 437:25–30

393. Momoi H, Itoh T, Nozaki Y et al. Microsatellite instability and alternative genetic pathway in intrahepatic cholangiocarcinoma. J Hepatol, 2001; 35:235–244

394. Della Torre G, Pasquini G, Pilotti S et al. TP53 mutations and mdm2 protein overexpression in cholangiocarcinomas. Diagn Mol Pathol, 2000; 9:41–46

395. Taguchi K, Aishima S, Asayama Y et al. The role of p27kip1 protein expression on the biological behavior of intrahepatic cholangiocarcinoma. Hepatology, 2001; 33:1118–1123

396. Fiorentino M, D'Errico A, Altimari A, Barozzi C, Grigioni WF. High levels of BCL-2 messenger RNA detected by in situ hybridization in human hepatocellular and cholangiocellular carcinomas. Diagn Mol Pathol, 1999; 8:189–194

397. Taniai M, Higuchi H, Burgart LJ, Gores GJ. p16INK4a promoter mutations are frequent in primary sclerosing cholangitis (PSC) and PSC-associated cholangiocarcinoma. Gastroenterology, 2002; 123:1090–1098

398. Tannapfel A, Sommerer F, Benicke M et al. Genetic and epigenetic alterations of the INK4a-ARF pathway in cholangiocarcinoma. J Pathol, 2002; 197:624–631

399. Sugimachi K, Aishima S, Taguchi K et al. The role of overexpression and gene amplification of cyclin D1 in intrahepatic cholangiocarcinoma. J Hepatol, 2001; 35:74–79

400. Watanabe M, Asaka M, Tanaka J, Kurosawa M, Kasai M, Miyazaki T. Point mutation of K-ras gene codon 12 in biliary tract tumors. Gastroenterology, 1994; 107:1147–1153

401. Tada M, Omata M, Ohto M. High incidence of ras gene mutation in intrahepatic cholangiocarcinoma. Cancer, 1992; 69:1115–1118

402. Levi S, Urbano-Ispizua A, Gill R et al. Multiple K-ras codon 12 mutations in cholangiocarcinomas demonstrated with a sensitive polymerase chain reaction technique. Cancer Res, 1991; 51:3497–3502

403. Tsuda H, Satarug S, Bhudhisawasdi V, Kihana T, Sugimura T, Hirohashi S. Cholangiocarcinomas in Japanese and Thai patients: difference in etiology and incidence of point mutation of the c-Ki-ras proto-oncogene. Mol Carcinog, 1992; 6:266–269

404. Hengartner MO. The biochemistry of apoptosis. Nature, 2000; 407:770–776

405. Shimonishi T, Isse K, Shibata F et al. Up-regulation of fas ligand at early stages and down-regulation of Fas at progressed stages of intrahepatic cholangiocarcinoma reflect evasion from immune surveillance. Hepatology, 2000; 32:761–769

406. Charlotte F, L'Hermine A, Martin N et al. Immunohistochemical detection of bcl-2 protein in normal and pathological human liver. Am J Pathol, 1994; 144:460–465

407. Harnois DM, Que FG, Celli A, LaRusso NF, Gores GJ. Bcl-2 is overexpressed and alters the threshold for apoptosis in a cholangiocarcinoma cell line. Hepatology, 1997; 26:884–890

408. Arora DS, Ramsdale J, Lodge JP, Wyatt JI. p53 but not bcl-2 is expressed by most cholangiocarcinomas: a study of 28 cases. Histopathology, 1999; 34:497–501

409. Ito Y, Takeda T, Sasaki Y et al. Bcl-2 expression in cholangiocellular carcinoma is inversely correlated with biologically aggressive phenotypes. Oncology, 2000; 59:63–67

410. Okaro AC, Deery AR, Hutchins RR, Davidson BR. The expression of antiapoptotic proteins Bcl-2, Bcl-X(L), and Mcl-1 in benign, dysplastic, and malignant biliary epithelium. J Clin Pathol, 2001; 54:927–932

411. Nzeako UC, Guicciardi ME, Yoon JH, Bronk SF, Gores GJ. COX-2 inhibits Fas-mediated apoptosis in cholangiocarcinoma cells. Hepatology, 2002; 35:552–559

412. Gores GJ. Cholangiocarcinoma: current concepts and insights. Hepatology, 2003; 37:961–969

413. Kajiyama K, Maeda T, Takenaka K, Sugimachi K, Tsuneyoshi M. The significance of stromal desmoplasia in intrahepatic cholangiocarcinoma. A special reference of 'scirrhous-type' and 'nonscirrhuous-type' growth. Am J Surg Pathol, 1999; 23:892–902

414. Higashi M, Yonezawa S, Ho JJ, Tanaka S, Irimura T, Kim YS, Sato E. Expression of MUC1 and MUC2 mucin antigens in intrahepatic bile duct tumors: its relationship with a new morphological classification of cholangiocarcinoma. Hepatology, 1999; 30:1347–1355

415. Taguchi K, Aishima S, Asayama Y, Kajiyama K, Kinukawa N, Shimada M, Sugimachi K, Tsuneyoshi M. The role of p27kip1 protein expression on the biological behavior of intrahepatic cholangiocarcinoma. Hepatology, 2001; 33:1118–1123

416. Miwa S, Miyagawa S, Soeda J, Kawasaki S. Matrix metalloproteinase-7 expression and biologic aggressiveness of cholangiocellular carcinoma. Cancer, 2002; 94:428–434

417. Aishima S, Asayama Y, Taguchi K, Sugimachi K, Shirabe K, Shimada M, Sugimachi K, Tsuneyoshi M. The utility of keratin 903

418. as a new prognostic marker in mass-forming-type intrahepatic cholangiocarcinoma. Mod Pathol, 2002; 15:1181–1190

418. Matsumura N, Yamamoto M, Aruga A, Takasaki K, Nakano M. Correlation between expression of MUC1 core protein and outcome after surgery in mass-forming intrahepatic cholangiocarcinoma. Cancer, 2002; 94:1770–1776

419. Aishima S, Taguchi K, Terashi T, Matsuura S, Shimada M, Tsuneyoshi M. Tenascin expression at the invasive front is associated with poor prognosis in intrahepatic cholangiocarcinoma. Mod Pathol, 2003; 16:1019–1027

420. Nakajima T, Kondo Y. Well differentiated cholangiocarcinoma. Diagnostic significance of morphologic and immunohistochemical parameters. Am J Surg Pathol, 1989; 13:569–573

421. Lazardidis KN, Gores GJ. Cholangiocarcinoma. Gastroenterology, 2005; 128:1655–1667

422. Craig JR, Peters RL, Edmondson HA. Tumours of the Liver and Intrahepatic Bile Ducts. Atlas of Tumor Pathology, Second Series, Fascicle 26. Washington D.C.: Armed Forces Institute of Pathology, 1989

423. Karhunen PJ. Benign hepatic tumors and tumor-like conditions in men. J Clin Pathol, 1986; 39:183–188

424. Glinkova V, Shevah O, Boaz M, Levine A, Shirin H. Hepatic hemangiomas: Possible association with female sex hormones. Gut, 2004; 53:1352–1355

425. Trastek VF, van Heerden JA, Sheedy PF 2nd, Adson MA. Cavernous hemangiomas of the liver: resect or observe? Am J Surg, 1983; 145:49–53

426. Yamamoto T, Kawarada Y, Yano T, Noguchi T, Mizumoto R. Spontaneous rupture of hemangioma of the liver: treatment with transcatheter hepatic arterial embolization. Am J Gastroenterol, 1991; 86:1645–1649

427. Hotokezaka M, Kojima M, Nakamura K, Hidaka H, Nakano Y, Tsuneyoshi M, Jimi M. Traumatic rupture of hepatic hemangioma. J Clin Gastroenterol, 1996; 23:69–71

428. Shimizu M, Miura J, Itoh H, Saitoh Y. Hepatic giant cavernous hemangioma with microangiopathic hemolytic anemia and consumption coagulopathy. Am J Gastroenterol, 1990; 85:1411–1413

429. Lehmann FS, Beglinger C, Schnabel K, Terracciano L. Progressive development of diffuse liver hemangiomatosis. J Hepatol, 1999; 30:951–954

430. Makhlouf HR, Ishak KG. Sclerosed hemangioma and sclerosing cavernous hemangioma of the liver: a comparative clinicopathologic and immunohistochemical study with emphasis on the role of mast cells in their histogenesis. Liver, 2002; 22:70–78

431. Dehner LP, Ishak KG. Vascular tumours of the liver in infants and children. A study of 30 cases and review of the literature. Arch Pathol, 1971; 92:101–111

432. Selby DM, Stocker JT, Waclawiw MA, Hitchcock CL, Ishak KG. Infantile hemanioendothelioma of the liver. Hepatology, 1994; 20:39–45

433. Boon LM et al. Hepatic vascular anomalies in infancy: A twenty-seven-year experience. J Pediatr, 1996; 129:346–354

434. Kirchner SG, Heller RM, Kasselberg AG, Greene HL. Infantile hepatic hemangioendothelioma with subsequent malignant degeneration. Pediatr Radiol, 1981; 11:42–45

435. Cerar A, Dolenc-Strazar Z, Bartenjev D. Infantile hemangioendothelioma of the liver in a neonate: Immunohistochemical observations. Am J Surg Pathol, 1996; 20:871–876

436. Weiss SW, Enzinger FM. Epithelioid hemangioendothelioma: A vascular tumor often mistaken for carcinoma. Cancer, 1982; 50:970–981

437. Weiss SW, Ishak KG, Dail DH, Sweet DE, Enzinger FM. Epithelioid hemangioendotheliama and related lesions. Sem Diagnostic Pathol, 1986; 3:259–287

438. Ishak KG, Sesterhenn IA, Goodman ZD, Rabin L, Stromeyer FW. Epithelioid hemangioendothelioma of the liver: A clinicopathologic and follow up study of 32 cases. Human Pathol, 1984; 15:839–852

439. Makhlouf HR, Ishak KG, Goodman ZD. Epithelioid hemangioendothelioma of the liver: A clinicopathologic study of 137 cases. Cancer, 1999; 85:562–582

440. Lauffer JM, Zimmermann A, Krahenbuhl L, Triller J, Baer HU. Epithelioid hemangioendothelioma of the liver: A rare hepatic tumor. Cancer, 1996; 78:2318–2327

441. Kelleher MB, Iwatsuki S, Sheahan DG. Epithelioid hemangioendothelioma of the liver. Clinicopathologic correlation of 10 cases treated by orthotopic liver transplantation. Am J Surg Pathol, 1989; 13:999–1008

442. Ben-Haim M, Roayaie S, Ye MQ, Thung SN, Emre S, Fishbein TA, Sheiner PM, Miller CM, Schwartz ME. Hepatic epithelioid hemangioendothelioma: resection or transplantation, which and when? Liver Transpl Surg, 1999; 5:526–531

443. Falk H, Herbert J, Crowley S, Ishak KG, Thomas LB, Popper H, Caldwell GG. Epidimiology of hepatic angiosarcoma in the United States: 1964–1974. Environ Health Persp, 1981; 41:107–113

444. Baxter PJ, Anthony PP, MacSween RNM et al. Angiosarcoma of the liver: annual occurrence and aetiology in Great Britain. Br J Int Med, 1980; 37:213–221

445. Hollstein M, Marion MJ, Lehman T, Welsh J, Harris CC, Martel-Planche G, Kusters I, Montesano R: p53 mutations at A: T base pairs in angiosarcoma of vinyl chloride-exposed factory workers. Carcinogenesis, 1994; 15:1–3

446. Dannaher CL, Tamburro CH, Yam LT. Occupational carcinogenesis: the Louisville experience with vinyl chloride associated hepatic angiosarcoma. Am J Med, 1981; 70:279–287

447. Falk H, Caldwell GG, Ishak KG et al. Arsenic related hepatic angiosarcoma. Am J Indust Med, 1981; 2:43–50

448. Battifora HA. Thorotrast and tumors of the liver. In: Okuda K, Peters RL, eds. Hepatocellular carcinoma. New York: John Wiley and Sons, 1976; pp 83–93

449. Kojiro M, Nakashima T, Ito Y, Ikezaki H, Mori T, Kido C. Thorium dioxide related angiosarcoma of the liver: Pathomorphologic study of 29 autopsy cases. Arch Pathol Lab Med, 1985; 109:853–857

450. Ito Y, Kojiro M, Nakashima T, Mori T. Pathomorphologic characteristics of 102 cases of Thorotrast related hepatocellular carcinoma, cholangiocarcinomas, and hepatic angiosarcoma. Cancer, 1988; 62:1153–1162

451. Falk H, Thomas LB, Popper H, Ishak KG. Hepatic angiosarcoma associated with androgenic-anabolic steroids. Lancet, 1979; 2:1120–1123

452. Locker GY, Doroshow JH, Zwelling LA, Chabner BA. The clinical features of hepatic angiosarcoma: A report of four cases and a review of the English Literature. Medicine, 1979; 58:48–64

453. Buetow PC, Buck JL, Ros PR, Goodman ZD. Malignant vascular tumors of the liver: Radiologic–pathologic correlation. Radiographics, 1994; 14:153–166

454. O'Sullivan MJ, Swanson PE, Knoll J, Taboada EM, Dehner LP. Undifferentiated embryonal sarcoma with unusual features arising within mesenchymal hamartoma of the liver: Report of a case and review of the literature. Pediatr Dev Pathol, 2001; 4:482–489

455. Nonomura A, Mizukami Y, Kadoya M, Matsui O, Shimizu K, Izumi R. Angiomyolipoma of the liver: Its clinical and pathological diversity. Hepato-Biliary-Pancreatic Surgery, 1996; 3:122–132

456. Tsui WM, Colombari R, Portmann BC, Bonetti F, Thung SN, Ferrell LD, Nakanuma Y, Snover DC, Bioulac-Sage P, Dhillon AP. Hepatic angiomyolipoma: a clinicopathologic study of 30 cases and delineation of unusual morphologic variants. Am J Surg Pathol, 1999; 23:34–48

457. Dalle I, Sciot R, de Vos R, Aerts R, van Damme B, Desmet V, Roskams T. Malignant angiomyolipoma of the liver: a hitherto unreported variant. Histopathology, 2000; 36:443–450

458. Makhlouf HR, Ishak KG, Shekar R, Sesterhenn IA, Young DY, Fanburg-Smith JC. Melanoma markers in angiomyolipoma of the liver and kidney: a comparative study. Arch Pathol Lab Med, 2002; 126:49–55

459. Makhlouf HR, Remotti HE, Ishak KG. Expression of KIT (CD117) in angiomyolipoma. Am J Surg Pathol, 2002; 26:493–497

460. Bonetti F, Pea M, Martignoni G, Doglioni C, Zamboni G, Capelli P, Rimondi P, Andrion A. Clear cell ('sugar') tumour of the lung is a lesion strictly related to angiomyolipoma—the concept of a family of lesions characterized by the presence of the perivascular epithelioid cells (PEC). Pathology, 1994; 26:230–236

461. Coffin CM, Humphrey PA, Dehner LP. Extrapulmonary inflammatory myofibroblastic tumour: A clinical and pathological survey. Semin Diag Pathol, 1998; 15:85–101

462. Dehner LP. Inflammatory myofibroblastic tumor: The continued definition of one type of so-called inflammatory pseudotumor. Am J Surg Pathol, 2004; 28:1652–1654

463. Chan J. Inflammatory pseudotumor: A family of lesions of diverse nature and etiologies. Adv Anat Pathol, 1996; 3: 156–171

464. Zen Y, Harada K, Sasaki M, Sato Y, Tsuneyama K, Haratake J, Kurumaya H, Katayanagi K, Masuda S, Niwa H, Morimoto H, Miwa A, Uchiyama A, Portmann BC, Nakanuma Y. IgG4-related sclerosing cholangitis with and without hepatic inflammatory pseudotumor, and sclerosing pancreatitis-associated sclerosing cholangitis: do they belong to a spectrum of sclerosing pancreatitis? Am J Surg Pathol, 2004; 28:1193–1203

465. Dunkelberg J, Goodman Z, Brewer T, Ishak K. Hepatic inflammatory pseudotumor (HIP): Clinicopathologic correlation in 31 cases. Gastroenterology, 1991; 100:A738

466. Shek TWH, Ng IOL, Chan KW. Inflammatory pseudotumor of the liver. Report of four cases and review of the literature. Am J Surg Pathol, 1993; 17:231–238

467. Stocker JT, Ishak KG. Undifferentiated (embryonal) sarcoma of the liver. Cancer, 1978; 42:336–348

468. Buetow PC, Buck JL, Pantongrag-Brown L, Marshall WH, Ros PR, Levine MS, Goodman ZD. Undifferentiated (embryonal) sarcoma of the liver: Pathologic basis of imaging findings in 28 cases. Radiology, 1997; 203:779–783

469. Bisogno G, Pilz T, Perilongo G, Ferrari A, Harms D, Ninfo V, Treuner J, Carli M. Undifferentiated sarcoma of the liver in childhood: a curable disease. Cancer, 2002; 94:252–257

470. Lei KIK. Primary non-Hodgkin's lymphoma of the liver. Leuk Lymphoma, 1998; 29:293–299

471. Lettieri CJ, Berg BW. Clinical features of non-Hodgkin's lymphoma presenting with acute liver failure: A report of five cases and review of published experience. M J Gastroenterol, 2003; 98:1641–1646

472. Page RD, Romaguera JE, Osborne B, Medeiros LJ, Rodriguez J, North L, Sanz-Rodriguez C, Cabanillas F. Primary hepatic lymphoma: favorable outcome after combination chemotherapy. Cancer, 2001; 92:2023–2029

473. Baschinsky DY, Weidner N, Baker PB, Frankel WL. Primary hepatic anaplastic large-cell lymphoma of T-cell phenotype in acquired immunodeficiency syndrome: a report of an autopsy case and review of the literature. Am J Gastroenterol, 2001; 96:227–232

474. Stancu M, Jones D, Vega F, Medeiros LJ. Peripheral T-cell lymphoma arising in the liver. Am J Clin Pathol, 2002; 118:574–581

475. Bronowicki JP, Bineau C, Feugier P, Hermine O, Brousse N, Oberti F, Rousselet MC, Dharancy S, Gaulard P, Flejou JF, Cazals-Hatem D, Labouyrie E. Primary lymphoma of the liver: clinical-pathological features and relationship with HCV infection in French patients. Hepatology, 2003; 37:781–787

476. Khan SM, Cottrell BJ, Millward-Sadler GH, Wright DH. T-cell-rich B-cell lymphoma presenting as liver disease. Histopathology, 1993; 23:217–224

477. Weidmann E. Hepatosplenic T cell lymphoma. A review on 45 cases since the first report describing the disease as a distinct lymphoma entity in 1990. Leukemia, 2000; 14: 991–997

478. Macon WR, Levy NB, Kurtin PJ, Salhany KE, Elkhalifa MY, Casey TT, Craig FE, Vnencak-Jones CL, Gulley ML, Park JP, Cousar JB. Hepatosplenic αβ T-cell lymphomas: a report of 14 cases and comparison with hepatosplenic T-cell lymphomas. Am J Surg Pathol, 2001; 25:285–296

479. Isaacson PG, Banks PM, Best PV, McLure SP, Muller-Hermelink HK, Wyatt JI. Primary low-grade hepatic B-cell lymphoma of mucosa-associated lymphoid tissue (MALT)-type. Am J Surg Pathol, 1995; 19:571–575

480. Ye MQ, Suriawinata A, Black C, Min AD, Strauchen J, Thung SN. Primary hepatic marginal zone B-cell lymphoma of mucosa-associated lymphoid tissue type in a patient with primary biliary cirrhosis. Arch Pathol Lab Med, 2000; 124:604–608

481. Bouron D, Léger-Ravet MB, Gaulard P, Franco D, Capron F. Tumeur hépatique inhabituelle. Ann Pathol, 1999; 19:547–548

Transplantation pathology

Stefan G. Hübscher   Bernard C. Portmann

16

General aspects of liver transplantation

Historical overview and survival following liver transplantation

The first successful human liver transplant was carried out in 1967.[1] Results were poor during the first decade of clinical liver transplantation, with fewer than 30% of patients surviving more than one year.[2,3] Transplant activity during this period was confined to a small number of centres. Subsequent improvements in preservation of donor organs, surgical technique and immunosuppressive drug therapy have greatly improved the outcome following liver transplantation, and one year survival figures in excess of 80% are now achieved in most large centres[4]. For 'good risk' candidates (e.g. patients with end-stage primary biliary cirrhosis) more than 90% can be expected to be alive after one year. Furthermore, because most of the more serious complications of liver transplantation occur during the first year post-transplant, 3 and 5 year survival figures in excess of 70% are now also widely achieved.[4] As a consequence of these improvements, there has been a dramatic world-wide increase in transplant activity.

By the end of December 2001, more than 46 000 liver transplant operations had been carried out in 124 centres in Europe.[4] After an exponential increase in the 1980s and early 1990s transplant activity is plateauing due to a lack of donor organs. This has led to extending the use of cadaveric organs, including splitting livers for use in two recipients (one adult, one paediatric) and using donor livers previously considered unsuitable (e.g transplanting HCV positive livers into HCV-infected recipients). There has also been increased use of living-related liver transplantation (LRLT), particularly in countries such as Japan where there are problems with obtaining cadaveric organs. These alternative strategies may be associated with increased complications compared with standard liver transplant operations. Examples include a higher rate of biliary and vascular complications in split livers and living related donor specimens, and more aggressive recurrent hepatitis C infection following LRLT. Currently approximately 4000 transplants per year are carried out in Europe and nearly 6000 per year in the USA.

Indications for liver transplantation

Liver transplantation is now well established as a treatment for many otherwise incurable liver diseases. The indications for liver transplantation can be divided into three main groups: end-stage chronic liver disease, acute liver failure and hepatic neoplasms (Table 16.1).

Table 16.1	Indications for liver transplantation in 39 136 allograft recipients (European Liver Transplant Registry)[4]

Indication	% of cases
Chronic liver disease	**72.6**
Alcohol	17.8
Hepatitis C	15.3
Hepatitis B (+/− hepatitis D)	7.8
Primary biliary cirrhosis	7.6
Biliary atresia	5.0
Primary sclerosing cholangitis	4.4
Autoimmune hepatitis	2.5
Hepatitis B + C	1.0
Wilson disease	0.9
Alpha-1-antitrypsin deficiency	0.7
Secondary biliary cirrhosis	0.7
Haemochromatosis	0.6
Others	8.2
Acute liver failure	**9.5**
Viral	2.1
Drug/toxic	1.7
Other/unknown	5.7
Hepatic neoplasms	**11.3**
Hepatocellular carcinoma	8.5
Cholangiocarcinoma	1.0
Metastatic tumours	0.8
Other	1.0
Other indications	**6.6**
Familial amyloid polyneuropathy	1.4
Budd–Chiari syndrome	1.0
Polycystic liver disease	0.6
Other	3.7

The commonest indication for liver transplantation is end-stage chronic liver disease, which accounts for 70–80% of all transplant operations. Within this large group, the relative proportions of specific disease types vary from centre to centre. In countries such as the UK, where primary biliary cirrhosis is prevalent, this has been amongst the commonest diseases for which liver transplantation is carried out. In many other centres elsewhere in Europe and in the USA, chronic viral hepatitis (especially hepatitis C) is now the commonest indication for liver transplantation. Approximately 35% of transplants carried out in Europe since 1997 were done for cirrhosis due to hepatitis C and/or hepatitis B.[5] Problems with disease recurrence mean that pathological assessments of post-transplant biopsies are particularly important in this group of patients. Until recently, alcoholic liver disease was a relatively uncommon indication for liver transplantation. However, despite the fact that most centres require a period of at least 6 months' abstinence from alcohol before transplantation is carried out, an increasing proportion of transplant operations are carried out for alcoholic cirrhosis—this is now the second commonest indication for liver transplantation, accounting for approximately 25% of transplant operations.[5,6] In the paediatric population, the commonest indication for liver transplantation continues to be extrahepatic biliary atresia. Transplantation for cirrhosis related to metabolic diseases is also frequently carried out in this group.

Approximately 10% of liver transplant operations are carried out for acute or subacute hepatic failure. The two commonly identified causes within this group are viral agents (mainly hepatitis A and B) and drugs. A small number of cases may represent an acute presentation of autoimmune hepatitis. However, in a large proportion of cases undergoing liver transplantation for acute liver failure no obvious cause can be identified. These cases are often labelled clinically as 'fulminant non-A, non-B, non-C hepatitis' or 'fulminant seronegative hepatitis'.[7–9]

Liver transplantation has also been used in the treatment of primary hepatic neoplasms. For cirrhotic patients the development of a small hepatocellular carcinoma (HCC) represents an important indication for transplantation.[10–11] Because of problems with high rates of tumour recurrence, cases with larger single tumours (>5 cm diameter) or multiple HCCs are no longer considered to be suitable candidates for transplantation.

In addition to transplantation for metabolic diseases associated with liver damage (e.g. alpha-1-antitrypsin deficiency, haemochromatosis, tyrosinaemia, Wilson disease), liver transplantation has also been carried out to correct metabolic defects in which the liver itself shows little or no signs of damage. Examples of the latter include ornithine carbamoyltransferase deficiency, C-protein deficiency, familial hypercholesterolaemia, type 1 hyperoxaluria and familial amyloid polyneuropathy.[12]

Approximately 10–20% of patients who have received a liver allograft require re-transplantation for graft failure related to complications of liver transplantation[13–15] (Table 16.2). The main indications for re-transplantation during the first month relate to problems with poor graft preservation ('primary non function') or graft ischaemia. Rare cases of severe humoral (hyperacute) rejection also occur during this period. Beyond the first month common indications for re-transplantation include chronic rejection and ischaemic biliary complications.[16] In patients surviving more than 1 year following transplantation complications relating to recurrent disease, particularly viral hepatitis, are becoming increasingly common indications for re-transplantation.[13] The overall rate of retransplantation has declined, mainly due to a reduction in the frequency of rejection and ischaemic complications.[14]

Complications of liver transplantation

The main complications of liver transplantation include:

1. problems with the preservation and reperfusion of the donor organ (preservation/reperfusion injury);
2. technical/surgical complications involving vascular and/or biliary structures;
3. rejection;
4. complications of immunosuppressive therapy (e.g. opportunistic infections, post-transplant lymphoproliferative diseases and other solid malignancies and drug toxicity);

| Table 16.2 | Indications for liver retransplantation, frequency and timing | |

Indication	Frequency	Timing after transplantation
Primary non-function	Up to 5–10%	Immediately
Graft ischaemia/infarction — occlusive (hepatic aretery thrombosis) — non-occlusive	Up to 5%	First month
Massive haemorrhagic necrosis — hypercacute (humoral) rejection — 'idiopathic'	Now very rare (<< 1%)	1–3 weeks
Biliary complications (ischaemic cholangitis)	Uncommon (<1%)	1–6 months
Chronic rejection	Incidence declining (now <2%)	Typically during first 12 months Late cases (>12 months) becoming more common
Recurrent disease — HCV	Increasingly frequent (commonest indication for late retransplantation)	From 2–3 years
— HBV	Now very rare (due to prophylactic treatment)	From 2–3 years
— PSC	Rare	Few years
— PBC	Very rare (<1%)	Late (>10 years)
— Autoimmune hepatitis	Rare	>1 year
— NASH	Very rare	From 2–3 years
Other late complications — De novo autoimmune hepatitis	Very rare	>1 year
— 'idiopathic' chronic hepatitis	Rare	>5 years

5. recurrence of the original disease for which transplantation was carried out;

6. acquired liver disease (e.g. 'de novo' autoimmune hepatitis or fatty liver disease).

Many of the complications listed above result in morphological changes within the liver allograft itself, and these will be discussed in the following pages. People undergoing liver transplantation frequently also have complications involving other organs. These can be related both to the original liver disease and to complications of liver transplantation.

Pathological assessments in liver transplantation

Histopathological assessments have an important role to play at all stages in the management of people undergoing liver transplantation. The starting point is an examination of the native (host) liver removed at transplantation. The protocol used for obtaining post-transplant biopsies varies from centre to centre. In many centres a biopsy of the donor liver is carried out immediately after reperfusion. This 'time zero' biopsy is used as a baseline assessment to detect pre-existing disease in the donor liver and to identify changes related to organ preservation and reperfusion. Until fairly recently, protocol biopsies were frequently taken on or around day 7 post-transplantation. This was done because the end of the first week was recognized to be the time when morphological changes of acute cellular rejection were generally first manifest. However, the discovery that histological features of rejection are commonly present in patients with stable graft function, and that such cases do not require additional immunosuppression,[17–20] has led to protocol day 7 biopsies being discontinued in many centres. In some centres protocol biopsies are also obtained in long-term survivors as part of an annual review. These specimens frequently show histological abnormalities, which are present in people who are clinically well with normal or near-normal liver biochemistry.[21–25]

For some conditions where liver biopsy is taken to investigate graft dysfunction, histology can be regarded as the 'gold standard' for diagnosis. The best example is liver allograft rejection, for which no other reliable diagnostic marker currently exists. For other conditions (e.g. hepatitis B or C infection) the cause of graft dysfunction may have been identified using other methods, but liver biopsy provides important additional information regarding morphological changes in the liver (e.g. severity of necroinflammatory activity and fibrosis) and may point to the presence of other co-existing causes of graft dysfunction. In some cases liver biopsy may provide the first clue to a biliary or vascular problem, which is subsequently confirmed radiologically. Fine needle aspiration (FNA) cytology has also been used as an adjunct to liver biopsy in the post-operative assessment of liver allograft recipients. A summary of the main pathological changes which may be seen at different times following liver transplantation is presented in Table 16.3.

Table 16.3 Main pathological changes occurring in the liver allograft

Time	Main diagnoses	Comments/examples
'Time-zero' (post-reperfusion)	Pre-existing donor disease	Macrovesicular steatosis
		Haemochromatosis
	Preservation/reperfusion injury	Changes generally mild at this stage
First month	Rejection	Hyperacute (very rare)
		Acute (common)
		Chronic (uncommon)
	Preservation/reperfusion injury Ischaemia	
1–12 months	Rejection	Acute
		Chronic
	Biliary complications	
	Opportunistic infection	CMV hepatitis (other organisms rarely seen in liver biopsy specimens)
	Recurrent disease	Hepatitis B and C
>12 months	Recurrent disease	Hepatitis C (common)
		PBC, autoimmune hepatitis, PSC (less common)
		Others eg. alcohol, hepatitis B, (uncommon)
	'Idiopathic' chronic hepatitis	
	Rejection	Rare
	Biliary complications	

Examination of native hepatectomy specimens

In most cases examination of hepatectomy specimens obtained at liver transplantation confirms diagnoses which have been made previously. However, detailed pathological studies of these specimens have provided valuable additional information. In particular the opportunity to examine entire livers in a well-preserved state has provided a better understanding of the way in which liver diseases are distributed within the liver as a whole.

For many chronic liver diseases, particularly those associated with bile duct damage, the severity of fibrosis may be very variable, and it is possible to see areas of advanced cirrhosis alongside areas in which a normal architecture is still clearly retained. Examples include primary biliary cirrhosis,[26] primary sclerosing cholangitis (PSC),[27] biliary atresia and liver disease related to cystic fibrosis (Fig. 16.1). These observations raise concerns regarding the use of histological staging in small needle biopsy specimens.

Another example of patchy disease distribution occurs in cases of fulminant hepatic failure associated with submassive hepatic necrosis. Large areas of panacinar necrosis may be seen alongside areas of nodular regeneration in which there is often pronounced cholestasis with little or no inflammation (see Fig. 8.1). A liver biopsy taken from an area of panacinar necrosis may overestimate the severity of disease present in the liver as a whole, whereas a biopsy taken from a cholestatic regeneration nodule may provide no clues either to the nature or the severity of liver injury present. These observations explain why needle biopsies have been found to be unreliable in assessing the severity of liver damage in patients with acute hepatic failure.[28]

For some liver diseases the removal of the whole liver allows a study of larger biliary or vascular structures, which would not normally be sampled in needle biopsy specimens. Examples of this include primary sclerosing cholangitis, in which a spectrum of bile duct lesions affecting ducts of all sizes can be seen,[27] and Budd–Chiari syndrome in which lesions can be seen in hepatic vein branches of varying sizes.

A small proportion of livers removed from patients with chronic liver disease may contain previously unsuspected hepatic neoplasms. The commonest example is hepatocellular carcinoma (HCC) arising in a background of cirrhosis. The incidence varies according to the underlying condition, but is highest in children with tyrosinaemia and adults with chronic viral infection. Most of these incidental hepatocellular carcinomas are solitary small lesions which are cured by transplantation.[29] However, in a small proportion of cases there may be adverse prognostic features such as vascular invasion and occasional cases of recurrent 'incidental' HCC have been documented.[30,31] The possibility of clinically undetected malignancy should also be considered in patients undergoing liver transplantation for primary sclerosing cholangitis. In early studies, up to 10% of PSC livers contained previously undiagnosed cholangiocarcinoma.[32] These tumours were usually hilar in location, often incompletely excised, and were thus associated with a high risk of recurrence. The incidence of cholangiocarcinoma incidentally discovered at liver transplantation appears to be declining for two main reasons. First, there is a tendency to carry out transplantation earlier for PSC, before neoplastic transformation has had time to occur. Secondly, improved methods for detecting small biliary neoplasms radiologically may exclude some patients with PSC-associated cholangiocarcinoma who otherwise might have been trans-

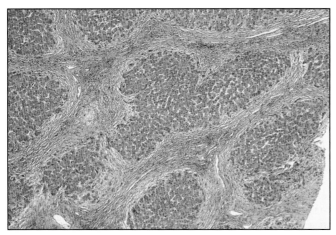

A

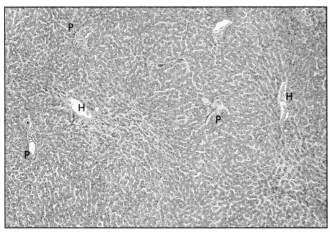

B

Fig. 16.1 • Variation in the severity of fibrosis in chronic biliary disease. These two slides are taken from a single block of liver obtained at transplantation from a patient with primary biliary cirrhosis. One area shows established cirrhosis **(A).** In an adjacent area there is preservation of normal vascular relationships with no evidence of fibrosis **(B).** (P = portal tract, H = hepatic venule). H&E.

planted. A potential protective effect of ursodeoxycholic acid therapy can only be speculated about at the moment. In a recent Scandinavian study, 5% of patients undergoing liver transplantation for PSC had previously unsuspected biliary neoplasms in their explanted livers.[33]

Pathological changes in post-reperfusion biopsies of donor liver and preservation/reperfusion injury

Pre-existing donor lesions

Macrovesicular steatosis is a fairly common finding in donor liver biopsies, the reported prevalence ranging from 13% to 50%.[34–39] A number of donor factors have been implicated including age, weight and alcohol consumption, but in many cases no definite cause can be found. The severity of steatosis is graded according to the proportion of hepatocytes involved: <30% is defined as mild, 30–60% as moderate and >60% as severe. Severe macrovesicular steatosis

has been associated with a high risk of graft non-function in the immediate post-transplant period—'primary non-function'.[40,41] It is thought that large fat droplets may cause mechanical obstruction to the sinusoidal microvasculature resulting in problems with reperfusion of the donor liver at retrieval and subsequent reperfusion in the recipient.[38,42,43] Release of free lipid from hepatocytes as a consequence of ischaemia and/or mechanical forces further compromises sinusoidal blood flow and provides a substrate for enhanced lipid peroxidation during re-oxygenation of the liver, with formation of free radicals resulting in further injury to sinusoidal endothelial cells.[40] Histological studies of failed liver allografts with severe fatty change have shown large extracellular fatty aggregates associated with areas of hepatocyte necrosis, haemorrhage and disruption of the sinusoidal framework.[40,44] Other consequences of fatty change on graft function include an increased susceptibility of sinusoidal endothelial cells to cold and warm ischaemic damage,[45,46] depletion in glycogen content and mitochondrial abnormalities in hepatocytes,[47–49] a shift to necrosis as the main mechanism for cell death after reperfusion (compared with apoptosis as the predominant pathway in non-fatty livers)[50] and an impaired regenerative capacity following cell loss due to preservation/reperfusion injury.[51]

Most transplant surgeons will not use donor livers with severe fatty change.[52] In the USA, many transplant surgeons reject donor livers with lesser degrees of steatosis (>30% of hepatocytes involved).[53] Because macroscopic appearances may not be reliable in assessing the severity of steatosis, a frozen section of the donor liver is often obtained in cases where fatty change is suspected clinically.[38] Fatty change is distributed reasonably uniformly within the liver and one or two needle biopsies should be sufficient to grade the severity of steatosis.[54] The use of specific fat stains such as Oil red O generally increases the amount of fat visualized; however, these methods are prone to considerable technical variation. There are also potential problems with the subjective assessment of steatosis and the use of image analysis may help to provide more objective and reproducible findings.[55]

Although livers with less severe degrees of fatty change can usually be transplanted safely, they are often associated with graft dysfunction in the early post-transplant period, usually manifest as elevation of serum transaminases, sometimes also with prolongation of prothrombin times,[34,56–58] and may result in reduced graft survival.[59] The release of fat droplets from necrotic hepatocytes may be associated with the formation of cystic lesions resembling peliosis hepatitis (lipopeliosis) (Fig. 16.2).[60] The majority of fat is probably cleared during the first week following transplantation.[38]

Microvesicular steatosis is also seen commonly in donor liver biopsies. This may be present both as multiple small droplets filling the hepatocyte without displacing the nucleus or as fewer fat droplets present in only part of the hepatocyte cytoplasm. Small fat droplets are difficult to detect in conventional haematoxylin and eosin stained sections and the incidence and severity of microvesicular steatosis increases if special stains for fat (e.g. Sudan stain)

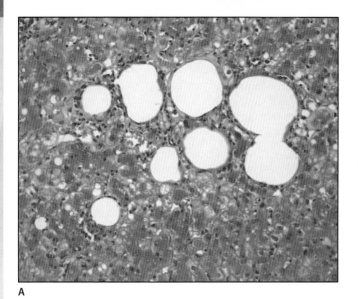

A

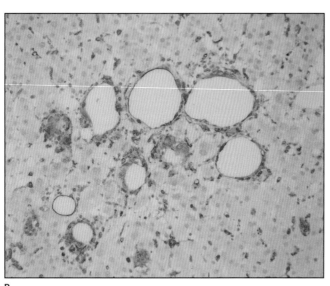

B

Fig. 16.2 • Lipopeliosis. Centrilobular fat microcysts are surrounded by macrophages in this biopsy specimen taken ten days following insertion of a steatotic donor liver. Subsequent biopsy specimens have shown resorption of the fat with only minimal residual perisinusoidal fibrosis. **(A)** H&E; **(B)** immunostaining for CD68.

are used on frozen sections.[61] Although microvesicular steatosis is well recognized as a rare cause of liver failure in the non-transplanted liver (e.g. Reye syndrome), its presence in donor livers, even to a marked degree, is not generally associated with poor graft function.[52,58,62]

A number of other factors may cause damage to the donor liver before its removal for transplantation, without necessarily resulting in abnormalities that are recognizable morphologically. These include episodes of hypotension (leading to ischaemic graft injury), poor nutritional state (resulting in depletion of hepatic glycogen stores) and endotoxaemia, possibly related to mucosal injury of the gut.[63–65]

Moderate or severe hepatocellular siderosis, presumably related to genetic haemochromatosis, has been reported as an incidental finding in a small number donor liver biopsies.[66–71] Donor HFE mutations have been demonstrated in a few cases.[71] In most cases siderosis diminishes following transplantation, suggesting an extrahepatic mechanism for iron overload. However, in many cases iron stores are slow to mobilize and there have been occasional cases in which severe siderosis has persisted for some years following transplantation, suggesting that the liver itself may be abnormal.[68,69,71]

Preservation/reperfusion injury

Time zero biopsies frequently have other morphological abnormalities, which are believed to be related to damage sustained during the process of graft preservation and reperfusion. These include hepatocyte ballooning, spotty necrosis/acidophil body formation, neutrophil polymorph aggregates, and cholestasis.[72–76] Similar changes may be seen, generally to a lesser degree, in biopsies obtained from donor livers prior to reperfusion.[73] Neutrophilic infiltration appears to be largely related to reperfusion injury, and is rarely conspicuous in pre-implantation donor liver biopsies. Changes seen in time zero biopsies are generally mild and tend to be most marked in the centrilobular regions. Occasionally there are larger areas of confluent necrosis.

Two main phases of preservation injury are recognized: an initial phase of cold ischaemia, which typically lasts for several hours, and a much shorter phase of warm ischaemia, immediately prior to graft implantation. The damage occurring during graft preservation is further aggravated during reperfusion, initially via the portal vein and subsequently the hepatic artery.[64,74,77–81]

Ultrastructural studies and experimental models suggest that sinusoidal endothelial cells are most susceptible to the effects of cold ischaemia.[82] Changes seen in sinusoidal endothelial cells include vacuolization of the cytoplasm, enlargement of fenestrae and blebs in sinusoidal lumen. Following reperfusion of the liver, injury is aggravated with death of and detachment of sinusoidal endothelial cells, adherence and activation of neutrophils, lymphocytes and platelets, activation of the complement system and of procoagulant factors resulting in a hypercoagualable state.[64,81,83–87] Kupffer cell activation which occurs at reperfusion is associated with the release of reactive oxygen species (ROS) and cytokines such as tumour necrosis factor (TNF) alpha, interferon-gamma and platelet activating factor,[78,88] further aggravating endothelial cell injury and subsequent damage to hepatocytes.[78,89] Sinusoidal endothelial cell activation results in the upregulation of adhesion molecules (e.g. ICAM-1) and chemokines (e.g. interleukin-8) which are involved in mediating the adhesion and transmigration of neutrophils.[90,91] Other inflammatory cells including T lymphocytes may also be recruited by similar mechanisms and have also been implicated in the pathogenesis of preservation/reperfusion injury (PRI).[88]

Hepatocytes are less susceptible than sinusoidal cells to the effects of cold ischaemia, but are more readily affected by warm ischaemia.[82,92] In addition, the microcirculatory disturbances and recruitment of inflammatory cells caused by sinusoidal endothelial cell injury result in secondary damage to hepatocytes, with liver cell death occurring both by apoptosis and necrosis.[80,81,93] Extrusion of dead hepatocytes into sinusoidal spaces and loss of the extracellular matrix may also further impair sinusoidal blood flow.[94] One morphometric study of post-reperfusion biopsies showed severe PRI to be associated with expansion in the surface volume of hepatocytes exposed to sinusoidal spaces, rendering hepatocytes more susceptible to toxins formed within sinusoids.[95] Other structures which may be susceptible to the effects of preservation injury include hepatocyte tight junctions,[96] biliary canaliculi,[97] and bile duct epithelial cells.[89,98]

Clinical manifestations of PRI mainly relate to hepatocellular dysfunction and there is characteristically a lag period of 12–48 hours between graft reperfusion and the clinical diagnosis of graft dysfunction caused by PRI.[74] Given the fact that changes seen in 'time zero' biopsies reflect a relatively short period of liver injury, it is not surprising that changes seen at this stage are relatively mild. However, in many instances they appear to represent the earliest stages of more severe damage that can be observed in the first few days or weeks following liver transplantation (Fig. 16.3). A number of clinicopathological syndromes which may be attributed to PRI have been described. These include primary graft dysfunction, initial poor function, primary non-function, hepatocyte ballooning, and 'functional' cholestasis.

Primary graft dysfunction (PDF), initial poor function (IPF) and primary non-function (PNF) are related terms which are used to describe grafts which function poorly in the immediate post-transplant period.[41,99] A number of donor and recipient factors have been implicated, but damage related to preservation/reperfusion injury is likely to be a major factor in most cases. It has been suggested that these terms should not be used to describe cases in which there are other peri- or post-operative factors such as vascular occlusion or primary humoral rejection, which can also result in graft dysfunction or failure in the immediate post-transplant period. Clinical features include marked elevation of transaminases (>2000 u/l), hypoglycaemia, haemostatic problems, hyperkalaemia, metabolic acidosis and renal failure. The diagnosis is usually made in the first 24–48 hours following transplantation. There are problems with establishing precise diagnostic criteria for these three syndromes, which probably accounts for the wide variation in their reported frequency. IPF can be regarded as a less severe form in which there is potentially reversible graft dysfunction, whereas PNF is a more severe form in which there is graft failure incompatible with recipient survival. PDF has been suggested as a term to describe all grafts that function poorly in the immediate post-transplant period (IPF and PNF). The reported frequency of PNF ranges from 2% to 23%.[74] Histological studies of grafts obtained at retransplantation have shown areas of coagulative hepatocyte necrosis, either zone 3 or panacinar in distribution,[100,101] suggesting an ischaemic mechanism.

In addition to macrovesicular steatosis, which is generally considered to be a pre-existing donor lesion, a number of the other histological changes that have been observed in 'time zero' biopsies may be of prognostic value in predicting subsequent poor graft function. These include centrilobular necrosis and/or haemorrhage, hepatocyte ballooning, neutrophilic infiltration and numbers of apoptotic bodies.[73,75,76,102] However, because there are problems with grading the severity of many of these features, they are not used routinely as prognostic factors for graft function following transplantation. Caution should also be advised when subcapsular wedge biopsies are taken as a baseline assessment. These may contain large areas of zonal necrosis, presumably reflecting the susceptibility of the subcapsular region to ischaemic damage, with no apparent bearing on subsequent graft function.

Hepatocyte ballooning is a common finding in the early post-transplant period.[57,103–105] It tends to be most marked in peripheral acinar zones (zone 3), but in severe cases can extend to a panacinar distribution. In most cases this lesion can be attributed to the effects of PRI. The finding that severe ballooning is associated with high serum transaminase levels during the first 48 hours following transplantation would support this hypothesis. In cases where ballooning persists beyond the first 2 weeks post-transplant other possible causes should be considered particularly if ballooning is associated with areas of zone 3 necrosis.[103,106]

Cholestasis is also a common finding in early post-transplant biopsies. The cholestatic changes are most often seen in zone 3, but in severe cases of PRI, cholangiolar cholestasis (similar to that seen in sepsis) may also be present in addition to the lobular cholestasis. There are many possible causes including PRI, rejection, viral infection, sepsis, biliary obstruction and drug toxicity.[105,107] A syndrome of 'pure' cholestasis, sometimes also referred to as 'functional' cholestasis, has been reported to occur in the absence of any obvious cause.[101,105,108,109] Some of these cases probably represent a delayed manifestation of preservation/reperfusion injury and cholestasis gradually resolves, sometimes over a period of several weeks.

Although fatty change is mainly considered to be a pre-existing donor lesion, there is some evidence to suggest that graft ischaemia/reperfusion injury may lead to the development of steatosis in the early post-transplant period.[57,62]

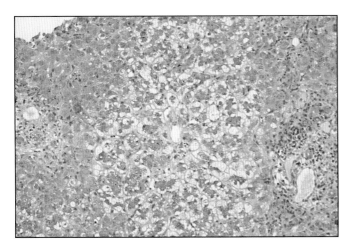

Fig. 16.3 • Preservation /reperfusion injury in liver allograft. This liver biopsy specimen, obtained seven days post-transplantation, shows severe cholestasis and ballooning affecting centrilobular and midzonal hepatocytes. These changes are frequently seen in the absence of rejection and can be ascribed to preservation/reperfusion injury. H&E.

PRI may be involved in the pathogenesis of a number of other post-transplant complications. There is upregulation in the expression of adhesion molecules such as ICAM-1 and E-selectin and co-stimulatory molecules such as CD80 and CD86, not only on sinusoidal cells, but also on hepatocytes, Kupffer cells and hepatic venules.[110-114] These changes may set the scene for the subsequent development of graft rejection. Prolonged cold ischaemia and PRI have also been implicated in the pathogenesis of ischaemic bile duct complications occurring in the liver allograft[115] and other later complications of liver transplantation.[116]

Liver allograft rejection

Definition and classification of rejection

Rejection can be defined as an immunological response to foreign antigens in the donor organ which has the potential to result in graft damage.[117] A degree of immune activation would be expected to occur in all allograft recipients, although this will be modified by immunosuppressive drugs. In the context of liver transplantation, an important distinction has to be made between morphological changes which are seen in the absence of any significant clinical or biochemical abnormalities ('biological' or 'subclinical' rejection) and those which are accompanied by clinical signs of graft dysfunction ('clinical' rejection).[17-20]

Three main patterns of rejection are recognized: hyperacute, acute and chronic.[117] This subdivision is based partly on time of occurrence (hyperacute = immediate, acute = early, chronic = late), but also on pathophysiological mechanisms and clinicopathological features.

Hyperacute (humoral) rejection

Definition and related terms

Hyperacute rejection is defined as graft dysfunction and failure occurring immediately after reperfusion in a recipient harbouring preformed antidonor antibodies. Because clinical presentation in liver allograft recipients is frequently delayed for a period of a few days (see below) the term primary humoral rejection has been suggested as an alternative. Other related terms are acute humoral rejection and antibody mediated rejection.

Although early graft failure due to humoral rejection is very rarely seen now, humoral mechanisms have been implicated in the pathogenesis of the other two main types of liver allograft rejection.[118-122] This is in line with the concepts which have been developed for antibody-mediated rejection in the renal allograft, where hyperacute, acute and chronic forms of humoral rejection are believed to occur.[123]

Incidence

The incidence of hyperacute rejection is difficult to determine, due to problems with establishing a definite diagnosis. For many years, it was considered not to occur at all,

even when ABO incompatible livers were used for transplantation. Subsequent studies identified an accelerated form of humoral rejection occurring in up to 33% of patients receiving ABO incompatible grafts.[124-126] Occasional cases of hyperacute rejection have also been reported in ABO compatible grafts.[118,119] In these cases anti-lymphocyte antibodies or more rarely, anti-endothelial antibodies may be responsible for graft damage.

Clinical features

Most cases present with severe graft dysfunction occurring within the first two weeks of transplantation. In contrast to renal allografts, where signs of hyperacute rejection are visible within a few minutes of reperfusion, changes in liver allografts may take several hours or even days to become manifest. An initial period of stable graft function is followed by a rapid rise in serum transaminases and prothrombin time associated with signs of acute liver failure. Decreased platelet counts and total serum complement activity also occur and are indirect signs of humoral mediated injury.

Humoral rejection is poorly responsive to conventional anti T-cell based immunosuppressive therapy. Alternative approaches which have been employed with some success in ABO-incompatible grafts include plasmapheresis, splenectomy and aggressive quadruple immunosuppression.[121,127] In cases with severe hyperacute humoral rejection urgent re-transplantation offers the only hope for survival.

Histological features

Hyperacute humoral rejection

Histopathological findings vary according to the severity of the humoral reaction and the time at which tissue samples are obtained. In clinical liver transplantation, severe coagulopathy precludes liver biopsy in most cases. In cases where liver biopsy has been feasible, a typical sequence of events has been observed.[124,128] The earliest changes seen in biopsies obtained 2–6 hours following implantation involve deposition of fibrin, platelets, neutrophils and red blood cells in small vessels and hepatic sinusoids. As a consequence of endothelial injury there is widespread neutrophilic exudation, congestion and coagulative hepatocyte necrosis which can be seen in biopsies obtained 1–2 days post implantation. In severe cases this results in a characteristic picture of massive haemorrhagic necrosis throughout the liver (Fig. 16.4). Lack of lymphocyte infiltration, or other typical features of cellular rejection, is another characteristic feature.

Immunohistological studies have shown deposition of immunoglobulins (IgG and IgM), complement (C1q, C3, C4) and fibrinogen in vascular and sinusoidal endothelium.[124,126,128] These deposits tend to be most marked during the earlier stages of hyperacute rejection, between two hours and two days after graft insertion, and rapidly diminish thereafter. Examination of failed allografts reveals more focal deposits of IgM and C1q, mostly confined to arteries.[124,128]

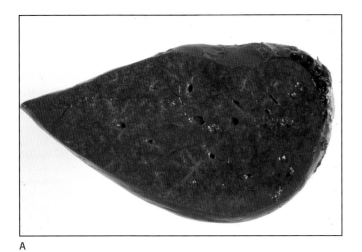

A

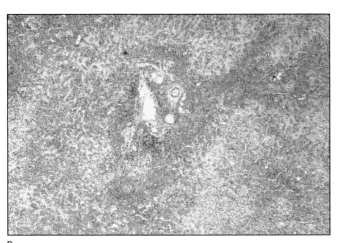

B

Fig. 16.4 • Hyperacute (humoral) rejection of liver allograft. Hepatectomy specimen obtained at re-transplantation showing massive haemorrhagic necrosis **(A)**. Histology shows panacinar haemorrhage and hepatocyte necrosis without an accompanying inflammatory reaction **(B)** H&E.

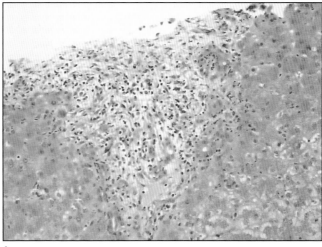

A

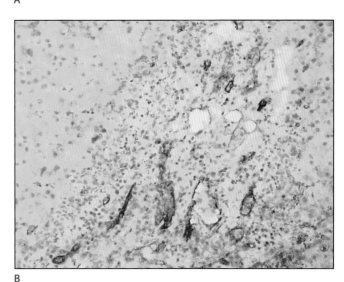

B

Fig. 16.5 • Humoral rejection. Liver biopsy 13 days post-transplant from a patient with a lymphocytotoxic positive cross-match. **(A)** Portal tract is oedematous with a mixed infiltrate of inflammatory cells. Marginal ductular reaction is also present. **(B)** Immunostaining reveals C4d in small portal vessels (Slides courtesy of Dr C Bellamy, University of Edinburgh).

Acute humoral rejection

The presence of pre-formed anti-donor antibodies has been associated with a higher incidence and greater severity of acute rejection. Importantly there may also be atypical histological features—these include portal/periportal oedema, neutrophil-rich inflammatory infiltration in portal tracts and prominent ductular reaction, producing changes resembling those seen in biliary obstruction (Fig. 16.5(A)).[118,119,121] Centrilobular changes of hepatocellular swelling and cholestasis have also been described. Immunostaining for the complement component C4d, which can be carried out on routinely processed tissues, is increasingly used as a marker of humoral rejection in the renal allograft.[123,129] Recent immunohistochemical studies have demonstrated the deposition of C4d in small portal vessels in liver biopsies from ABO-incompatible grafts with features suggestive of humoral rejection[121] (Fig. 16.5(B)). However, similar observations have also been made in cases of otherwise typical acute rejection[122] and the functional significance of C4d deposition in the liver allograft is thus currently uncertain.

Other humoral-mediated lesions in the liver allograft

Anti-donor antibodies have also been implicated in the pathogenesis of early centrilobular changes of hepatocyte ballooning and cholestasis, resembling changes seen in a severe form of preservation/reperfusion injury. Humoral mechanisms may also be involved in the pathogenesis of the bile duct loss and arteriopathy which characterize chronic rejection and with ischaemic bile duct injury and other vascular complications in the liver allograft.[130]

Differential diagnosis

The clinical and histological features described above cannot be regarded as specific for hyperacute rejection. A clinical diagnosis of hyperacute rejection requires exclusion of other causes of graft failure occurring in the early post-operative period, in particular those associated with the syndrome of primary non-function. In contrast to PNF, most cases of hyperacute rejection are associated with an initial period of graft function.

Cases of acute graft failure in the earlier post-transplant period associated with the histological picture of massive haemorrhagic graft necrosis have also been described in the absence of any demonstrable humoral mechanism.[131-134] Non-humoral factors which have been implicated in this setting include ischaemia related to hepatic arterial kinking, gram negative sepsis, a number of opportunistic viral infections including herpes simplex, herpes zoster, adenovirus and enterovirus, recurrent infection with togavirus-like particles and a single organ Schwartzmann reaction. Massive haemorrhagic graft necrosis now occurs very infrequently.

Demetris et al. identified a tetrad of changes, which in combination were considered to be characteristic of primary humoral rejection.[124]

1. Early graft failure with no alternative clinical or pathological explanation.
2. Consistent light and immunofluorescent microscopic findings.
3. Demonstration of a pre-sensitization state in the recipient.
4. Presence of donor-specific antibodies in an eluate from the failed graft.

Immunopathogenetic mechanisms

Hyperacute rejection occurs when a donor organ is transplanted into a recipient with preformed anti-donor antibodies. Endothelial cells in the graft are the main targets for humoral mediated damage. In the case of ABO-incompatibility, naturally occurring antibodies bind to ABO antigens expressed on endothelial cells of the graft resulting in complement activation, thrombosis, neutrophil exudation and haemorrhage. Antibodies to other antigens expressed on graft endothelial cells (e.g. lymphocytotoxic antibodies binding to MHC Class I antigens, or other anti-endothelial antibodies) can also result in similar changes.

In comparison with other organs such as the kidney, the liver is unusually resistant to antibody-mediated rejection, as evidenced by the ability to carry out transplantation successfully in the face of positive anti-donor cross-matching, including ABO-incompatibility. A number of reasons for the reduced susceptibility of the liver to humoral rejection have been postulated.[118,130,135] These include: (i) the presence of a dual blood supply, which may protect the organ from ischaemic damage; (ii) release of soluble class I MHC antigens into the circulation, which can bind to preformed anti-donor antibodies; and (iii) Kupffer cell binding of preformed antibodies and/or removal of immune complexes. Further evidence for the liver having a privileged immunological status in the context of organ transplantation has come from studies showing that transplantation of liver allografts into sensitized recipients is able to protect kidneys transplanted into the same individuals from developing hyperacute rejection.[136,137]

Acute rejection
Definition and related terms

Acute rejection can be defined as immune mediated damage to the liver allograft characterized by cellular infiltrates, principally present in portal areas and associated with damage to bile ducts and vascular structures. Inflammatory changes are also commonly seen in the liver parenchyma, mainly around terminal hepatic venules. Most cases occur in the early post-operative period and are responsive to immunosuppression. Because the diagnosis is principally based on the histopathological finding of cellular infiltrates in the liver, cellular rejection is widely used as an alternative term to acute rejection. Other terms, which have been used, include non-ductopenic rejection, rejection without duct loss, early rejection and reversible rejection.

Incidence and risk factors

Acute rejection is the commonest form of liver allograft rejection. The incidence varies according to whether it is defined on the basis of clinically significant rejection (i.e. rejection accompanied by graft dysfunction requiring additional immunosuppression) or whether it is defined simply on the basis of histological abnormalities. Clinically significant rejection occurs in approximately 20–40% of patients, whereas histological abnormalities can be seen in up to 80% of protocol biopsies obtained around the end of the first week following transplantation.[17-20,138] The incidence of clinically significant rejection appears to be declining, probably related to improvements in immunosuppressive therapy. A higher incidence of acute rejection has been noted in patients undergoing transplantation for autoimmune liver diseases[139,140-144] and in those transplanted for hepatitis C.[145] The latter may reflect different approaches to the use of immunosuppression and the assessment of post-transplant biopsies in HCV positive cases. Conversely, a lower incidence of acute rejection has been documented in patients undergoing transplantation for alcoholic liver disease and chronic hepatitis B infection and in recipients of HLA-mismatched grafts.[139,141,146-148]

Clinical features

The majority of acute rejection episodes occur within the first month of transplantation. Clinical manifestations of acute rejection include pyrexia, graft enlargement and tenderness and reduced bile flow.[149,150] Biochemical abnormalities typically have a predominantly cholestatic pattern. A sudden rise in serum transaminases may be a manifestation of parenchymal-based rejection changes.[151,152] Peripheral blood leukocytosis and eosinophilia are also commonly present. Clinical and biochemical abnormalities are non-specific and the diagnosis therefore requires histological confirmation.

Histological features

Liver biopsy specimens show various combinations of a diagnostic portal-based triad, first observed by Snover et al.,[100] and subsequently confirmed in other studies of post-transplant liver biopsies.[101,153–159] In recent years, there has been increased interest in a spectrum of changes involving terminal hepatic venules and the surrounding liver parenchyma.

Portal tract lesions in acute rejection

The three components of the diagnostic triad are portal inflammation, bile duct damage and venular endothelial inflammation (also known as endothelitis, endotheliitis or endothelialitis). At least two of these three features are required for a diagnosis of acute rejection.[117] The inflammatory lesions which occur in acute rejection can show considerable variation in intensity in different parts of a single biopsy specimen. For this reason it is recommended that sections are obtained from a series of levels and that a minimum of five portal tracts are available for examination.[159]

Portal inflammation begins as a lymphocytic infiltrate.[158] By the time that rejection presents clinically there is typically a mixed infiltrate of cells including lymphocytes (mostly T cells), large activated 'blast' cells, macrophages, neutrophils and eosinophils (Fig. 16.6(A)). All of these cell types are also involved in mediating damage to bile ducts and endothelial cells. The presence of large numbers of eosinophils may be helpful in identifying a more severe form of rejection, which is less likely to respond to additional immunosuppressive therapy.[160,161] The presence of prominent interface hepatitis may also be regarded as a feature of more severe cellular rejection.[159,162] Portal tract granulomas are rarely seen in acute rejection.[163]

The initial damage to bile ducts is probably mediated by lymphocytes, but by the time that rejection is clinically evident there is usually a mixed infiltrate, in many cases including a prominent component of neutrophils[153] (Fig. 16.6(B)). Bile ducts are typically cuffed and focally infiltrated by inflammatory cells, and may show degenerative changes in the form of cytoplasmic vacuolation, pyknosis and focal disruption of the basement membrane. In cases where portal inflammation is particularly intense bile ducts can be effaced by inflammatory cells, and are difficult to identify in routinely stained sections. Immunoperoxidase staining for bile duct cytokeratins is useful in demonstrating that bile ducts are still present in this situation.[164] In some cases the presence of large numbers of neutrophils, including luminal aggregates of pus cells, may mimic

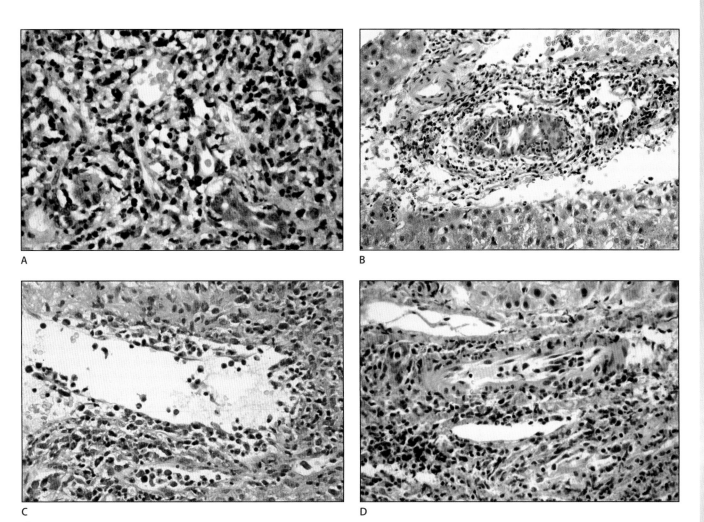

Fig. 16.6 • Portal tract lesions in acute liver allograft rejection. **(A)** Portal tract contains a dense mixed inflammatory infiltrate including lymphocytes, blast cells, neutrophils and eosinophils. **(B)** An interlobular bile duct shows prominent inflammatory infiltration, mainly with neutrophils. **(C)** Portal venule shows subendothelial inflammatory infiltration associated with lifting and focal disruption of the endothelium. **(D)** Inflammatory infiltration of a small arterial branch. Arterial lesions are rarely seen in needle biopsy specimens. H&E.

changes seen in ascending infective cholangitis. Large numbers of neutrophils can also be identified in samples of bile obtained from patients with acute cellular rejection.[165,166]

Venular inflammatory changes are seen in portal and hepatic vein branches. In early or mild cases there is focal lymphoid attachment to the luminal surface of endothelial cells. In more advanced or severe cases there is subendothelial infiltration, associated with lifting and sometimes disruption of endothelial cells (Fig. 16.6(C)). Cells associated with endothelial damage are mostly lymphocytes. However, a mixed infiltrate resembling that seen in bile ducts may also be present. In most cases endothelial inflammation only affects a small segment of the vessel. Involvement of the entire circumference of the venule is generally confined to cases with severe rejection. Venular endothelial inflammation has generally been regarded as the most specific feature of liver allograft rejection. However, it is not invariably present, particularly in cases of acute rejection occurring beyond the early post-transplant period.[158,167] Furthermore, venular endothelial inflammation can be seen in many other conditions in which there is inflammatory infiltration of portal tracts or the liver parenchyma, including viral hepatitis, primary biliary cirrhosis and lymphoproliferative diseases.[168,169]

Arterial lesions including endothelial inflammation and fibrinoid necrosis have been reported, but are rarely seen in small needle biopsy specimens (Fig. 16.6(D)). When present, they have been regarded as a sign of severe damage.[104,158,170] Angiographic studies demonstrating attenuation of large and medium-sized arteries suggest that these vessels may also be affected in acute rejection.[171]

Bile ductular reaction is commonly seen in biopsies showing features of acute rejection[100,172] and may in part be a response to other portal tract changes, especially bile duct damage.[164] Bile ductular reaction may also be a delayed effect of preservation-reperfusion injury.[72]

Parenchymal changes in acute rejection

Lobular inflammatory lesions comprise a spectrum of changes, principally involving hepatic venules and the surrounding liver parenchyma.[151,152,173–175] In some cases there may be a more diffuse lobular hepatitis.[176,177] Other terms which have been used to describe these changes include 'central venulitis', 'centrilobular necrosis', 'centrilobular alterations' and 'hepatitic phase' of rejection. At one end of the spectrum, usually seen in early post-transplant biopsies, hepatic venular endothelial inflammation is a prominent feature (Fig. 16.7(A)). Typical portal tract changes of acute rejection are also present, usually at least moderate in severity. The diagnosis and grading of acute rejection in these cases is relatively straightforward. However, in other cases, usually occurring later post-transplant, centrilobular necroinflammatory lesions are present without conspicuous hepatic vein inflammation (Fig16.7(B)) and sometimes also with minimal or mild portal inflammatory changes. A diagnosis of rejection in such cases is less easily established and other causes of centrilobular damage also need to be considered (discussed later). In some cases hepatic venular

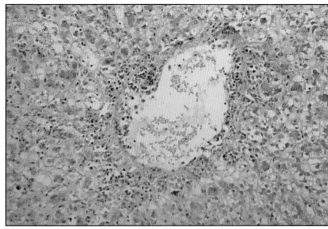

A

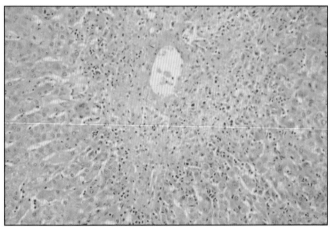

B

Fig. 16.7 • Centrilobular lesions in acute liver allograft rejection. **(A)** Hepatic venule shows subendothelial inflammation. Inflammatory cells extend into the surrounding liver parenchyma where there is a narrow zone of hepatocyte dropout. **(B)** Perivenular necro-inflammatory lesion with normal hepatic venule. H&E.

endothelial inflammation may be associated with veno-occlusive lesions,[178–181] resulting in foci of perivenular necrosis and congestion (Fig. 16.8). Perivenular necroinflammatory lesions and/or associated hepatic veno-occlusive lesions may be associated with the development of parenchymal fibrosis.[181,182]

There is increasing evidence to suggest that the presence of perivenular necroinflammatory lesions indicates a more severe form of acute rejection, which is less likely to respond to immunosuppression and are more likely to progress to chronic rejection. In many cases they appear to be present at an early stage, before bile duct loss is evident: recognition of this process and instigation of appropriate immunosuppressive therapy may prevent progression to irreversible changes of chronic rejection.

Other parenchymal changes frequently seen in association with acute rejection include cholestasis, hepatocyte ballooning, fatty change and spotty acidophil body formation. These lesions tend to be most marked in perivenular regions and in some cases may be causally related to acute rejection; one study has shown an association between the severity of cholestasis and the severity of bile duct damage

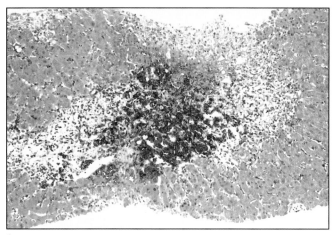

A

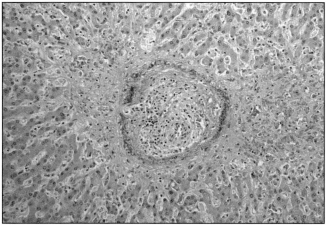

B

Fig. 16.8 • Rejection related veno-occlusive disease. **(A)** Severe congestion and hepatocyte loss are present in the centrilobular region, mimicking the changes seen in venous outflow obstruction. **(B)** Hepatic vein is occluded by a mixture of inflammatory cells and immature fibrous tissue (Haematoxylin van Gieson).

in early post-transplant biopsies.[157] However, particularly in the early post-transplant period, much of the parenchymal damage is more likely to be related to preservation/reperfusion injury than rejection.[57,103,105] In cases where there is zone 3 necrosis and inflammation, it is likely that parenchymal damage is rejection related, even if typical portal tract changes are not conspicuous.[57,175]

Differential diagnosis

The diagnosis of acute rejection rarely poses problems during the first month post-transplant as other causes of graft inflammation are rarely seen during this period. Greater problems exist beyond the early post-transplant period when other causes of graft inflammation become more common. Particularly important in this respect is recurrent hepatitis C infection, which is discussed later. Other diseases associated with a predominantly portal-based inflammatory infiltrate include autoimmune hepatitis (recurrent or acquired) and Epstein–Barr virus associated post-transplant lymphoproliferative disease. In addition to the combination of changes seen in the typical diagnostic

triad, a useful feature pointing to a diagnosis of acute rejection is the presence of a mixed population of inflammatory cells, which is rarely seen to a marked degree in any of the other allograft conditions associated with portal inflammation. Another problem with the assessment of late rejection is that rejection itself may have different features, including less prominent venular endothelial inflammation and more conspicuous lobular changes, including hepatitis-like features.[167,183]

In cases where bile ductular reaction appears unduly prominent, the possibility of biliary tract pathology should be considered, particularly if there is also portal oedema and an infiltrate disproportionately rich in neutrophil polymorphs. Large bile duct obstruction should be relatively easy to exclude radiologically. However, in some cases subtle biliary features may represent the early stages of ischaemic bile duct damage, in which the radiological diagnosis is less straightforward. Biliary features may also be a manifestation of a humoral component in acute rejection.

Response to treatment

There is increasing evidence to suggest that mild (often subclinical) acute rejection may resolve spontaneously without the need for additional immunosuppression.[18–20,138] The development of mild rejection in the early post-transplant period may have a beneficial effect in inducing long-term graft tolerance.[184] A small number of patients with more severe forms of acute rejection (including clinical and biochemical signs of graft dysfunction) have resolved spontaneously without additional immunosuppression.[185] The concept of self-limiting rejection is well recognized in animal models of liver transplantation[186,187] and may also be relevant to human liver transplantation.

In the majority of cases where histological features of acute rejection are accompanied by clinical/biochemical signs of graft dysfunction the administration of additional immunosuppression results in resolution and there is no adverse impact on long-term graft function.[188] In early studies where follow-up biopsies were obtained following treatment for acute rejection,[100] these showed bile duct atypia and features resembling those seen in large bile duct obstruction. Repeat biopsies are now rarely obtained if there is adequate biochemical response to additional immunosuppression. In cases where features of cellular rejection persist despite treatment with corticosteroids (steroid resistant rejection) treatment with other drugs such as OKT3 or Tacrolimus may result in resolution of rejection. A small proportion of cases are unresponsive to all forms of immunosuppression (intractable rejection) and many of these either have or will develop features of chronic rejection.

Chronic rejection

Definition and related terms

Chronic rejection can be defined as immune mediated damage to the liver allograft which is characterized histologically by two main features: loss of small bile ducts and an obliterative vasculopathy affecting large and medium-sized arteries. Chronic rejection occurs later than acute rejection and most cases are unresponsive to immunosuppression. Because bile duct loss is generally considered to be the most important diagnostic feature in needle biopsy specimens, the term ductopenic rejection has been most widely used as an alternative to chronic rejection. Other terms which have been used include late rejection, irreversible rejection, vanishing bile duct syndrome, rejection with bile duct loss, and vascular rejection.

Incidence and risk factors

Chronic rejection is considerably less common than acute rejection. The incidence in series reporting patients transplanted before 1991 ranged from 2% to 20%.[189] This wide variation may partly reflect different criteria used to define chronic rejection. The incidence of chronic rejection is declining, presumably as a consequence of more effective immunosuppression, and now results in graft failure in no more than 2–3% of cases.[190–192]

Risk factors which have been identified for chronic rejection can be divided into two main categories. (i) Donor/recipient factors include transplantation for autoimmune liver disease, male-to-female sex mismatching of donor to recipient, non-European recipient ethnic origin, young recipient age and old donor age.[141,142,193–199] The role of histocompatibility differences is controversial.[200–204] A lower rate of chronic rejection has been observed in recipients of living-related grafts than in those with cadaveric donor organs.[197] (ii) Post-transplant factors include the severity and number of episodes of acute rejection, late presentation of acute rejection (more than 1 month post-transplant), cytomegalovirus infection, hepatitis B and C infection, interferon therapy for viral hepatitis and alcohol abstinence.[140,162,183,192,197,204–213] People undergoing re-transplantation for chronic rejection have an increased risk of developing chronic rejection in subsequent grafts.[149,214]

Clinical features

Chronic rejection typically occurs as a consequence of repeated episodes of acute rejection which are unresponsive to immunosuppression. The peak incidence of graft failure from chronic rejection in studies carried out during the 1980s and early 1990s was 2–6 months post-transplantation.[215] In some cases there was a more acute presentation with rapid progression to graft failure within a few weeks of transplantation ('acute vanishing bile duct syndrome').[216]

Clinically chronic rejection is characterized by progressive jaundice accompanied by cholestatic liver biochemistry.[150,190] The transition from acute to chronic rejection may be associated with an elevation in AST levels.[151,175,217] In common with acute rejection, the clinical and biochemical manifestations of chronic rejection are non-specific and the diagnosis therefore also requires histological confirmation.

Classical cases of chronic rejection presenting with graft failure during the first year post-transplant are now much less common, presumably reflecting improvements in immunosuppression. Instead more cases are diagnosed later; these may have different clinical features including a more insidious presentation and more slowly progressive graft damage. Histological features may also be different and, in some cases, are further modified by interaction with other graft complications (e.g. recurrent HCV infection) making liver biopsy assessment difficult.

Histological features

The two main diagnostic abnormalities seen in chronic rejection are *loss of bile ducts* and an *obliterative arteriopathy* affecting large and medium-sized arteries.[217] Characteristic, but less specific, changes are also present in the liver parenchyma. Some cases of late chronic rejection may have different histological features including *chronic hepatitis-like changes*.[218–220]

During the early stages of chronic rejection bile ducts show inflammatory infiltration, which is indistinguishable from that seen during potentially reversible acute cellular rejection. In cases where there has been an incomplete biochemical response to additional immunosuppression, there may be a reduction in the overall degree of inflammation in portal tracts. However, bile ducts show continued lymphocytic infiltration associated with nuclear pleomorphism, disordered polarity and focal attenuation and/or disruption of biliary epithelium producing a 'dysplastic-like' or atrophic appearance (Fig. 16.9(A)). These changes are associated with features of replicative senescence (e.g. nuclear p21 expression)[221] and are widely regarded as an early sign of impending bile duct loss.[217] As the disease progresses, there is loss of bile ducts, typically associated with a diminishing cellular infiltrate, eventually producing a characteristic 'burnt out' appearance in end-stage livers (Fig. 16.9(B)). Bile duct loss principally affects small (interlobular) bile ducts and is thus readily diagnosed in needle biopsy specimens. It is generally accepted that bile duct loss should be present in more than 50% of portal tracts in order to make a firm diagnosis of chronic rejection. However, there are problems in counting bile ducts accurately, particularly in small needle biopsy specimens. An adequate sample, preferably containing at least 20 portal tracts[216] and/or the demonstration of ductopenia in several biopsies is therefore generally required before a confident diagnosis of bile duct loss can be made. In hepatectomy specimens obtained at re-transplantation there may be loss of epithelium from medium-sized (septal) and large (hilar) ducts. The latter sometimes show a distinctive pattern of luminal obliteration by fibrous tissue and inflammatory cells (Fig. 16.9(C)).

A notable feature is the absence of bile ductular reaction or periportal fibrous expansion in the majority of cases, the exception being when a distal biliary stricture is associated. This is in contrast to other diseases associated with loss of bile ducts, in which these secondary changes are nearly always present. One possible reason for the lack of ductular

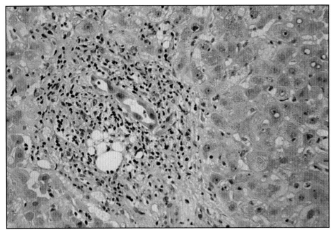

A

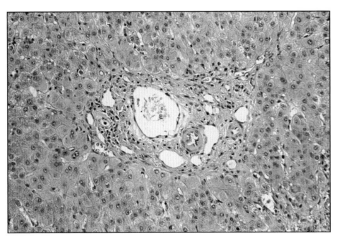

B

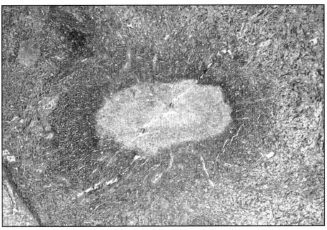

C

Fig. 16.9 • Bile duct lesions in chronic rejection. **(A)** Early chronic rejection. Liver biopsy obtained 5 months post-transplant following unsuccessful treatment of an acute rejection episode. An interlobular bile duct shows nuclear pleomorphism and disordered polarity, producing a 'dysplastic' appearance. **(B)** Late-stage chronic rejection. Portal tract has a characteristic 'burnt-out' appearance with no recognizable bile duct branch. Only mild inflammatory changes are present. **(C)** Large bile duct lesion in end-stage chronic rejection. In this hepatectomy specimen obtained at re-transplantation, the lumen of a large bile duct is occluded by immature fibrous tissue. No residual biliary epithelium is identified. ((A) and (B) H&E. (C) Haematoxylin van Gieson.)

reaction in typical cases of chronic rejection is loss of the vagal innervation, which is thought to be important in progenitor cell activation.[222] The fact that ductular reaction can be seen in cases of late chronic rejection (>1 year post-transplant),[223] a time at which re-innervation of the liver allograft is known to occur,[224,225] would also be in keeping with this hypothesis. However, ductular reaction is seen within the first post-transplant year in cases of biliary tract complications, which would suggest that in this situation they might not arise from progenitor cells. Other studies have attributed the lack of ductular reaction in chronic rejection to an increase in apoptosis[226] or a reduction in proliferative activity[172] within the ductular compartment.

The characteristic vascular lesions of chronic rejection are seen in large and medium-sized arteries and are typically manifest as intimal aggregates of lipid-laden foamy macrophages (Fig. 16.10(A)) although other layers of the arterial wall can also be affected. These occlusive arterial foam cell lesions may produce abnormalities that can be detected angiographically.[171] In some cases with a more acute presentation, there is a prominent infiltrate of inflammatory cells (Fig. 16.10(B)),[227] mainly T lymphocytes, suggesting an overlap with acute cellular rejection. Conversely, in cases with a more prolonged course, there are increasing numbers of myofibroblasts associated with varying degrees of intimal fibrosis. However, advanced fibromuscular intimal thickening of the type classically seen in end-stage chronic rejection affecting renal or cardiac allografts, is rarely found in liver allograft rejection (Fig. 16.10(C)). Macrophages and mesenchymal cells in arterial lesions are of recipient origin.[228] Because these arterial lesions rarely affect small vessels of the size sampled in needle biopsy specimens, the definitive diagnosis of chronic vascular rejection is usually only made when the whole liver is available for examination (Fig. 16.10(D)). However, smaller portal tracts may show a reduced number of small arterial branches and other microvascular channels.[151,229,230] These changes appear to occur during the early stages of chronic rejection, before bile duct loss is present.

Inflammatory and/or foam cell lesions are also seen in portal and hepatic venules in some cases of chronic rejection, particularly those associated with a more acute presentation, again suggesting that there are areas of overlap with acute cellular rejection.[227,231] Inflammatory lesions in hepatic venules may also result in fibrous luminal obliteration, producing changes similar to those seen in hepatic veno-occlusive disease.[180,181] Similar changes can also occur in small portal vein branches (Fig. 16.11). A combination of veno-occlusive lesions involving portal and hepatic veins appears to be important in the pathogenesis of the parenchymal fibrosis in chronic rejection, in some cases resulting in a cirrhosis-like appearance.[223] A similar mechanism has been postulated for the development of fibrosis and cirrhosis in non-transplant liver.[232,233]

In the majority of cases of chronic rejection, bile duct loss and occlusive arteriopathy are both present. Morphometric studies have demonstrated a parallelism between the severity of these two components of chronic rejection,[229] and have suggested that ischaemia may be a factor contributing

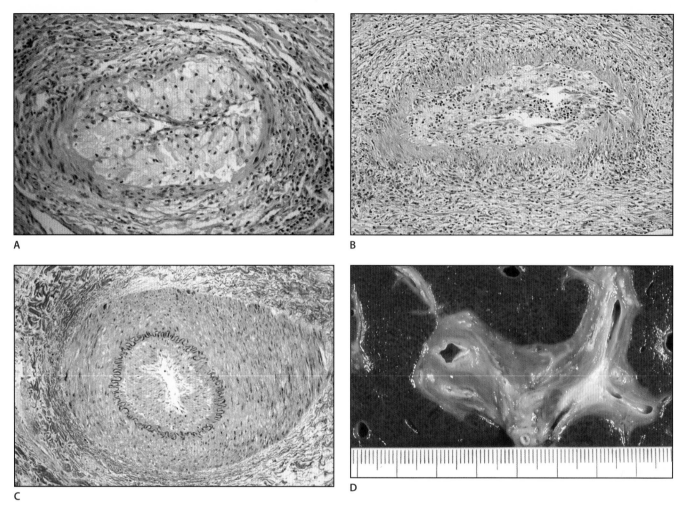

Fig. 16.10 • Arterial lesions in chronic rejection. **(A)** A medium-sized muscular artery contains an intimal foam cell lesion resulting in luminal occlusion. **(B)** A medium-sized muscular artery shows prominent inflammatory infiltration involving all layers of the vessel wall. The majority of infiltrating cells are T lymphocytes. **(C)** Fibromuscular intimal thickening in chronic liver allograft rejection. These lesions are less commonly seen than intimal foam cell lesions. When present, they probably reflect long-standing damage. (a) and (b) H&E. (c) Elastic haematoxylin van Gieson. **(D)** Bi-sected liver allograft removed 4 months after transplantation. Occluded arterial branches stand up as yellow cords or nodules within large perihilar portal tracts. One well-opened portal vein branch to the left shows yellow thickening of its wall.

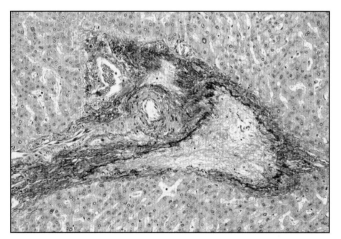

Fig. 16.11 • Portal veno-occlusive disease in chronic rejection. A portal vein branch shows occlusion by fibrous tissue. The presence of this lesion in combination with hepatic veno-occlusive lesions may be important in the pathogenesis of parenchymal fibrosis in chronic rejection. Elastic haematoxylin van Gieson.

to bile duct loss in the liver allograft. However, there are well-documented cases with a purely ductopenic or a purely vascular form of chronic rejection. In a combined series of 72 cases from 3 centres,[234–236] 51 (71%) had both lesions, 10 (14%) had ductopenia alone and 11 (15%) had a purely vascular form of chronic rejection.

Perivenular bilirubinostasis is a prominent finding in chronic rejection and, in most cases, is presumably related to bile duct loss. Cholestasis can also be seen with the purely vascular form of chronic rejection, suggesting that ischaemia may also be a factor in some cases. It must be pointed out that ductopenia affecting the fine terminal branches of the bile ducts may easily be overlooked. In addition, bile duct strictures at the hilum, which are not uncommonly associated, are difficult to demonstrate on explanted graft and could at times contribute to the cholestasis. Sinusoidal foam cells are commonly seen and are probably also a response to cholestasis.

Perivenular necrosis is also a common finding in chronic rejection (Fig. 16.12(A)) and typically occurs as a sequela to

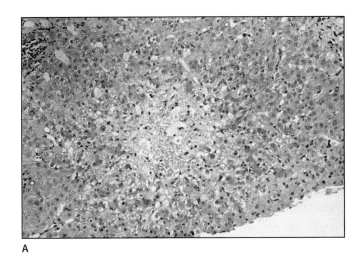

A

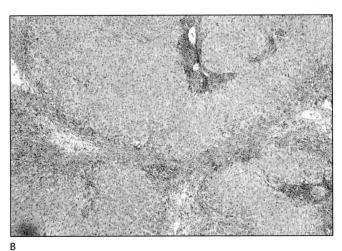

B

Fig. 16.12 • (A) Parenchymal damage in chronic rejection. There is an area of lytic necrosis involving acinar zone 3. Mild congestion is also present in this area along with severe cholestasis. **(B)** More extensive parenchymal damage with areas of bridging necrosis accompanied by a moderately dense infiltrate of inflammatory cells. H&E.

the necroinflammatory lesions, which are seen during the preceding phase of acute rejection.[151] Humoral mechanisms may also be involved. In cases where there is incomplete biochemical response to additional immunosuppression the cellular infiltration in perivenular regions often subsides, but hepatocellular dropout persists. Necrosis typically has a lytic pattern and is accompanied by reticulin collapse and immature collagen fibre deposition. In some cases there may be more extensive necrosis with bridging and nodule formation (Fig. 16.12(B)). Even in cases where zonal necrosis has been detected in serial biopsies over a period of several months the lesions frequently retain an appearance suggesting acute damage, without the formation of mature collagen or elastic fibres, suggesting a dynamic equilibrium between hepatocyte loss and regeneration in perivenular regions. However, in some cases there is development of more mature fibrous lesions, which may ultimately progress to cirrhosis-like changes.[182,223,237] A range of rejection-related ischaemic mechanisms have also been implicated in the pathogenesis of parenchymal necrosis and fibrosis; these include occlusive lesions in large and medium-sized arteries, loss of small arterial branches and occlusive lesions

involving portal and/or hepatic veins. Although centrilobular necrosis has been regarded as a 'surrogate marker' of rejection-related arteriopathy, a definite association between these two processes has not been convincingly demonstrated.[151]

In addition to the two main patterns of chronic rejection described above (ductopenic and vascular), the possibility of a chronic hepatitis-like pattern of chronic rejection has been postulated. A number of studies have suggested that late cellular rejection may have different histological features from typical early acute rejection including less conspicuous bile duct damage and venular endothelial inflammation, more periportal necrosis and more prominent lobular inflammation, producing a chronic hepatitis-like appearance.[167,183,218] Others have noted problems in distinguishing chronic rejection from chronic hepatitis.[183,219] Many biopsies obtained more than 12 months post-transplant have histological features of chronic hepatitis, for which no obvious cause is apparent. By a process of exclusion, some of these cases may represent a late form of rejection.

Differential diagnosis of chronic rejection

A number of diseases in the liver allograft may be associated with portal inflammatory infiltration, bile duct damage and in some cases bile duct loss. These include recurrent viral hepatitis (in particular hepatitis C), recurrent biliary disease (primary biliary cirrhosis, primary sclerosing cholangitis) and ischaemic cholangiopathy which, as discussed later, has histological features closely resembling those seen in PSC.

The relationship between recurrent hepatitis C infection and liver allograft rejection is considered in more detail later. Cases with combined features of hepatitis C and chronic rejection pose particular problems for diagnosis and management. Although chronic rejection is similar to PBC and PSC (and ischaemic cholangiopathy) in that all three are vanishing bile duct diseases, there are important histological differences. The granulomatous bile duct lesions which occur in PBC and the sclerosing duct lesions which occur in PSC are different to the 'dysplastic-like' bile duct lesions which are seen during the early stages of chronic rejection. Perhaps the most useful feature which distinguishes typical cases of chronic rejection from other diseases with bile duct loss in the liver allograft is the absence of secondary biliary features such as ductular reaction, periportal fibrosis and deposition of copper-associated protein. However, these secondary biliary features may be seen in some cases of late chronic rejection, developing several years post-transplant.[223] Bilirubinostasis is rarely prominent in other biliary tract diseases unless there is advanced fibrosis/cirrhosis, severe ductopenia or, in the case of PSC, a major bile duct stricture associated with features of large duct obstruction. The finding of severe unexplained cholestasis occurring beyond the early post-transplant period unaccompanied by portal tract changes suggesting biliary obstruction should therefore prompt a careful search for subtle bile duct lesions which might suggest a diagnosis of early chronic rejection.

The differential diagnosis of the centrilobular (zone 3) lesions which occur in chronic (and acute) rejection is more difficult.[106,179,238,239] Whilst many cases are rejection-related, a number of other factors including vascular problems, viral hepatitis, autoimmune hepatitis (recurrent or acquired) and drug toxicity may also be implicated in the pathogenesis of centrilobular lesions in the liver allograft (Table 16.4).

Amongst the vascular causes of centrilobular necrosis (CLN), preservation/reperfusion injury is unlikely to result in lesions persisting beyond the early post-operative period. Even in biopsy specimens obtained around the first week following transplantation, CLN is most likely to be rejection-related,[57] particularly if it is accompanied by a lymphocytic inflammatory infiltrate. Rejection-associated changes resulting in hepatic veno-occlusive lesions and surrounding congestion and necrosis may be indistinguishable from other causes of venous outflow obstruction. In many cases, the presence of rejection-related inflammatory changes either in association with or preceding histological features suggesting venous outflow obstruction is helpful in pointing to rejection as a likely cause for centrilobular congestion and necrosis.[178,180,240,241]

Centrilobular inflammation and necrosis may be seen in association with recurrent or, more rarely, acquired viral or autoimmune hepatitis. Parenchymal features which favour a diagnosis of rejection in this context include prominent hepatic venular endothelial inflammation together with prominent bilirubinostasis and/or ballooning in surrounding viable hepatocytes.[106] The presence of conspicuous bile duct injury and/or bile duct loss and portal venular endothelial inflammation and the lack of prominent interface activity are also features which favour a diagnosis of rejection rather than hepatitis.[106]

Centrilobular necrosis and hepatic veno-occlusive lesions can also be seen as a toxic injury related to use of the immunosuppressive drugs azathioprine and Tacrolimus (FK506) and as a manifestation of 'idiopathic' post-transplant chronic hepatitis.

Table 16.4	Possible causes of centrilobular (acinar zone 3) necrosis in the liver allograft
Ischaemia	— preservation/reperfusion injury
	— vascular occlusion (hepatic artery, portal vein, hepatic vein)
Rejection	— acute
	— chronic
Viral hepatitis (recurrent or acquired)	— hepatitis B
	— hepatitis C
Autoimmune hepatitis	— recurrent
	— acquired
Drugs	— azathioprine
	— Tacrolimus (FK 506)
Other	— 'idiopathic' chronic hepatitis

Response to treatment and outcome

The treatment of chronic rejection is dependent on the stage at which the disease is diagnosed. Cases of early chronic rejection, in which bile duct atypia is present with little or no duct loss, may respond to the use of potent immunosuppressive agents such as Tacrolimus,[190,242] OKT3,[243] Mycophenolate mofetil,[244] Rapamycin,[245] or Sirolimus.[246] By contrast, advanced chronic rejection, typically associated with severe biochemical cholestasis and advanced bile duct loss, is generally unresponsive to immunosuppression and re-transplantation is required. A small number of cases with apparently advanced chronic rejection (including bile duct loss in more than 50% of portal tracts) have recovered spontaneously, or with the use of additional immunosuppression.[170,247,248] Interestingly, some of these patients have had follow-up liver biopsies showing a persistent paucity of bile ducts without other histological features of chronic rejection.[247] Ductopenia has also been noted as an incidental finding in protocol biopsies taken at annual review from patients who are clinically well with no previous biopsies suggesting chronic rejection.[249,250] Other cases may have gradual bile duct loss taking place over a period of 5–10 years without progressing to graft failure.[251] These observations suggest that some patients may suffer permanent duct loss as a result of rejection, but that sufficient ducts remain to allow the graft to function well. Because of these observations, and the risks associated with undertaking a second transplant operation, the decision to re-transplant should only be made when a confident diagnosis of irreversible graft damage can be established.

Relationship between acute and chronic rejection

The subdivision of liver allograft rejection into acute and chronic forms is based on three main diagnostic features: time of onset, behaviour and histological changes (Table 16.5). Whilst this approach is useful clinically, areas of overlap exist for each of these three features. Acute and chronic rejection are thus best regarded as different ends of a spectrum of immune-mediated damage occurring within the liver allograft. Histologically, a broad spectrum of

Table 16.5	Main criteria used for the diagnosis of acute and chronic liver allograft rejection	
	Acute	**Chronic**
Time of onset	Early	Late
Response to treatment	Reversible	Irreversible
Histological features	Cellular infiltrates	Bile duct loss
	— portal tracts	Obliterative arteriopathy
	— bile ducts	
	— portal and hepatic venules	
	— liver parenchyma	

changes exists between the cellular infiltrates which characterize early acute rejection and the ductopenia and obliterative vasculopathy which is seen in end stage chronic rejection. Most cases of chronic rejection are preceded by episodes of acute rejection. Many biopsies obtained during the evolution of chronic rejection have features of ongoing cellular rejection, and these features may also be seen in hepatectomy specimens obtained at re-transplantation.

Grading and staging of liver allograft rejection

In line with the concepts underlying the systems devised for the semi-quantitative scoring of histological features in chronic hepatitis, 'grading' of liver allograft rejection refers to necro-inflammatory activity, mainly seen in acute rejection, whereas 'staging' is more appropriately applied to features indicating progressive liver injury in chronic rejection.

A number of systems have been proposed for grading acute liver allograft rejection.[18,104,158,252] The Banff schema is a consensus document devised by an international panel of liver transplant pathologists, physicians, surgeons and scientists.[159] The schema incorporates two components (Tables 16.6 and 16.7). The first is a global assessment of the overall rejection grade (Table 16.6). This represents a modification of the National Institute of Diabetes and Digestive and Kidney Diseases (NIDDK) system for grading liver allograft rejection, devised by a group of US pathologists.[162] The second component of the Banff schema involves scoring the three main features of liver allograft rejection semiquantitatively on a scale of 0 (absent) to 3 (severe) to produce an overall rejection activity index (RAI) (Table 16.7). This closely resembles the scoring systems which have been used in several European centres, and is analogous to the histological activity index used to grade necroinflammatory activity in cases of chronic hepatitis.[253,254] A number of studies have shown that the the Banff schema is simple to use, reproducible and clinically useful in making decisions regarding therapy and prognosis.[195,255,256] In one study of 575 acute rejection episodes, the presence of moderate/severe rejection correlated with higher transaminase levels, the development of perivenular fibrosis and an increased

Table 16.6	Banff schema for grading liver allograft rejection—global assessment of overall rejection grade[159]
Global assessment*	**Criteria**
Indeterminate	Portal inflammatory infiltrate that fails to meet the criteria for the diagnosis of acute rejection
Mild	Rejection infiltrate in a minority of the triads, that is generally mild, and confined within the portal spaces
Moderate	Rejection infiltrate, expanding most or all of the triads
Severe	As above for moderate, with spillover into periportal areas and moderate to severe perivenular inflammation that extends into the hepatic parenchyma and is associated with perivenular hepatocyte necrosis

Note: Global assessment of rejection grade made on a review of the biopsy and after the diagnosis of rejection has been established

* Verbal description of mild, moderate, or severe acute rejection could also be labelled as Grade I, II and III respectively

Table 16.7	Banff schema for grading liver allograft rejection—rejection activity index[159]	
Category	**Criteria**	**Score**
Portal inflammation	Mostly lymphocytic inflammation involving, but not noticeably expanding, a minority of the triads.	1
	Expansion of most or all of the triads, by a mixed infiltrate containing lymphocytes with occasional blasts, neutrophils and eosinophils.	2
	Marked expansion of most or all of the triads by a mixed infiltrate containing numerous blasts and eosinophils with inflammatory spillover into the periportal parenchyma.	3
Bile duct inflammation/damage	A minority of the ducts are cuffed and infiltrated by inflammatory cells and show only mild reactive changes such as increased nuclear : cytoplasmic ratio of the epithelial cells.	1
	Most or all of the ducts infiltrated by inflammatory cells. More than an occasional duct shows degenerative changes such as nuclear pleomorphism, disordered polarity and cytoplasmic vacuolization of the epithelium.	2
	As above for 2, with most or all of the ducts showing degenerative changes or focal lumenal disruption.	3
Venous endothelial inflammation	Subendothelial lymphocytic infiltration involving some, but not a majority of the portal and/or hepatic venules.	1
	Subendothelial infiltration involving most or all of the portal and/or hepatic venules.	2
	As above for 2, with moderate or severe perivenular inflammation that extends into the perivenular parenchyma and is associated with perivenular hepatocyte necrosis.	3

NOTE: Total Score = Sum of components

risk for developing chronic rejection.[256] The venous endothelial component of the RAI was also predictive for the development of graft failure from chronic rejection. Grade 3 venous endothelial inflammation is defined on the basis of centrilobular necroinflammatory lesions (Table 16.7), emphasizing the predictive value of these changes in identifying the transition to chronic rejection.

The Banff schema is now widely used and has improved the consistency in the diagnosis and grading of acute rejection between different centres involved in liver transplantation. Problems may still be encountered when biopsies are taken beyond the early post-transplant period—partly because the histological features at this stage may be different, but also because there are other potential causes for cellular infiltration in the liver allograft. This particularly applies to biopsies obtained from hepatitis C positive individuals (discussed later). In cases where there is any uncertainty regarding the overall diagnosis of rejection, grading should not be carried out.

More recently the Banff schema has been modified by an international panel to incorporate features relating to the staging of chronic rejection[217] (Table 16.8). This was based on the results of several studies analysing histological changes in serial post-transplant biopsies and hepatectomy specimens obtained at retransplantation for chronic rejection.[151,174,223,243] A distinction is made between changes occurring during the early stages of chronic rejection, when the disease is potentially still reversible, from those indicating advanced or irreversible disease, for which retransplantation is the only therapeutic option. In the liver biopsy diagnosis of early chronic rejection, particular emphasis is placed on the recognition of bile duct atypia, which can be seen before bile duct loss has occurred, and zone 3 necroinflammatory lesions, which also occur at an early stage in the disease process. Application of the modified Banff criteria has been shown to greatly improve the sensitivity of needle biopsies for diagnosing chronic rejection at an early stage.[177] More importantly, the use of powerful immunosuppressive agents at an early stage in the disease process may prevent the development of irreversible graft damage. Although bile duct loss has been the most widely used feature indicating progression to late (irreversible) chronic rejection, it should be noted that there are problems in counting bile ducts accurately in needle biopsy specimens, particularly concerning sampling variation. Examination of hepatectomy specimens with end-stage disease sometimes reveals marked variation in the degree of bile duct loss from one part of the liver to another. Perivenular fibrosis with bridging may also be indicative of irreversible graft damage,[243] although this is not always a reliable criterion.[182] Because histological features in needle biopsy specimens are not reliable in identifying irreversible graft damage due to chronic rejection, clinical features and biochemical markers are also used to determine the point at which retransplantation is required. As discussed earlier, areas of overlap exist between acute and chronic rejection, and an individual biopsy many show features of ongoing inflammatory activity, which can be graded, as well as signs of progressive liver injury (e.g. bile duct loss), which can be staged.

Some of the other features listed in Table 16.8 (e.g. lesions affecting large arteries and bile ducts) can only be diagnosed reliably in hepatectomy specimens—for these lesions the distinction between 'early' and 'late' chronic rejection is based on theoretical concepts, which cannot be applied to needle biopsy assessment. Other features (e.g. cholestasis, sinusoidal foam cells) are non-specific findings which can be seen in a variety of other conditions.

Table 16.8 Histopathological features characteristically seen during the early and late stages of chronic liver allograft rejection[217]

Structure	Early CR	Late CR
Small bile ducts (<60 μm)	Degenerative changes involving a majority of ducts: eosinophilic transformation of the cytoplasm; increased N : C ratio; nuclear hyperchromasia; uneven nuclear spacing; ducts only partially lined by biliary epithelial cells	Degenerative changes in remaining bile ducts
	Bile duct loss in <50% of portal tracts	Loss in ≥50% of portal tracts
Terminal hepatic venules and zone 3 hepatocytes	Intimal/luminal inflammation	Focal obliteration
	Lytic zone 3 necrosis and inflammation	Variable inflammation
	Mild perivenular fibrosis	Severe (bridging) fibrosis
Portal tract hepatic arterioles	Occasional loss involving < 25% of portal tracts	Loss involving >25% of portal tracts
Other	So-called 'transition' hepatitis with spotty necrosis of hepatocytes	Sinusoidal foam cell accumulation: marked cholestasis
Large perihilar hepatic artery branches	Intimal inflammation, focal foam cell deposition without lumenal compromise	Lumenal narrowing by subintimal foam cells
		Fibrointimal proliferation
Large perihilar bile ducts	Inflammation damage and focal foam cell deposition	Mural fibrosis

Reprinted with permission of Wiley-Liss, Inc., a subsidary of John Wiley & Sons, Inc.

Immunopathogenesis of acute and chronic rejection

Targets for immune damage in the liver allograft

All of the normal cells of the liver are potential targets for immune mediated damage in acute and chronic rejection. Histological studies have demonstrated lesions involving bile ducts, vascular endothelial cells and hepatocytes (mainly in the centrilobular zones). Kupffer cells and other sinusoidal cells may also be destroyed in liver allograft rejection and replaced by cells of recipient phenotype.[257–260]

Stages in allograft rejection

There are three main stages in allograft rejection.[261,262] The first stage, or afferent arm, involves the presentation of graft alloantigens and the recognition of these antigens by recipient T lymphocytes. There is then a phase of T cell activation and cytokine release. In the final stage, or efferent arm, there is recruitment and activation of effector cells which mediate damage to target structures within the allograft.

The afferent arm of the immune response

This involves the processing and presentation of graft allo-antigens and the recognition of these antigens by recipient T cells. Central to this process is the antigen-specific interaction between the T cell receptor expressed on the surface of T lymphocytes and MHC molecules expressed on the surface of graft antigen presenting cells (Fig. 16.13). The main MHC class II antigen presenting cells in the normal liver are dendritic cells which are located in portal areas and, to a lesser extent, in acinar zone 3 of the liver parenchyma.[263–265] Two main pathways of antigen presentation are involved.[266,267] In the first or direct pathway, dendritic cells migrate to regional lymph nodes where they present MHC antigens to alloreactive T lymphocytes.[266] This is the main pathway involved in early post-transplant period. Later on, the donor antigen presenting cell population is replaced by host APCs but these can still process and present other donor alloantigens. This indirect pathway appears to be important in sustaining an ongoing persistent immune response. Interactions involving CD4 and class II MHC antigens expressed by 'professional' antigen presenting cells are primarily involved in the initial stages of graft recognition. Kupffer cells also constitutively express MHC class II antigens and may also be involved in antigen presentation to CD4 positive T cells.

The interaction between T cells and graft cells involves other important signalling pathways including adhesion molecules, which enable T cells to bind to graft cells, and co-stimulatory molecules, which are required for T cell activation (Fig. 16.13). These other factors are not antigen specific. Two important costimulatory molecule-ligand pairs are CD28/B7[268] and CD40/CD154.[269] In the absence of appropriate co-stimulatory signals, T cells do not become fully activated and either become unresponsive to further antigenic stimuli (anergic) or undergo apoptosis.

Cells in the normal liver have a limited expression of MHC antigens, adhesion molecules and other molecules involved in the alloimmune response. Following liver transplantation there is cytokine mediated upregulation of many of these molecules on bile ducts, hepatocytes and endothelial cells.[112,257,264,270–276] The functional significance these changes is uncertain but they are involved both in enhancing antigen presentation and in promoting T cell activation and effector mechanisms.

T-cell activation and cytokine release

The binding of the T-cell receptor to MHC antigens triggers a cascade of intracellular signalling events leading to the activation and proliferation of responding T cells and the subsequent migration of these cells to the liver allograft. Here they secrete cytokines that promote effector functions not only of T lymphocytes themselves but also of other effector cells, including macrophages, NK cells and other inflammatory cells.

Two main subsets of activated CD4 positive T cells are recognized: Th1 and Th2 cells.[266] Th1 cells are induced by IL-12 and interferon gamma (IFN-gamma) to secrete IL-2, tumour necrosis factor β (TNF-β) and IFN-gamma. These cytokines have a variety of proinflammatory effects including the generation of cytotoxic T lymphocytes (CTLs), activation of macrophages, and upregulation of B7 costimulatory molecules resulting in further T cell activation. Th2 cells are stimulated by IL-4 to secrete IL-4, IL-5, IL-6, IL-10 and IL-13. Th2 cytokines stimulate antibody production by B cells and also activate eosinophils and mast cells. The Th1

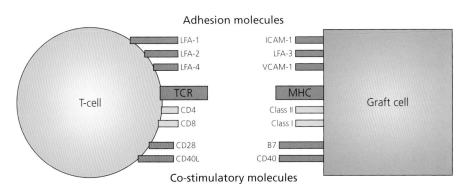

Adhesion molecules

LFA-1 ICAM-1
LFA-2 LFA-3
LFA-4 VCAM-1

T-cell

TCR MHC
CD4 Class II
CD8 Class I

CD28 B7
CD40L CD40

Graft cell

Co-stimulatory molecules

Fig. 16.13 • Interaction between T cells and graft cells. Three main components are illustrated. The first involves the interaction between T-cell receptor (TCR) and MHC molecules on donor liver cells. Additional factors are adhesion molecules and co-stimulatory molecules.

cytokine IFN-gamma has an inhibitory effect on Th2 cell proliferation and cytokine secretion. Conversely, the Th2 cytokine IL10 inhibits Th1 cell proliferation and cytokine secretion. This reciprocal relationship leads to a dynamic balance between Th1 and Th2 cytokines in allograft rejection. Expression of Th1 cytokines within allografts is typically associated with rejection, whereas Th2 cytokines appear to be involved with allograft acceptance. However the specificity and functional significance of Th1 versus Th2 responses in the context of human liver transplantation is uncertain.[266,277,278]

Effector mechanisms in liver allograft rejection

The main effector mechanisms in liver allograft rejection are summarized in Table 16.9.

Antigen-specific damage to graft cells is mediated by T lymphocytes. Immunohistochemical studies have shown that T cells predominate in graft infiltrates. A mixed population of CD4 and CD8 positive cells has been identified in varying proportions.[279] CD8 positive cells appear to be particularly involved with mediating damage to bile ducts and vascular endothelium[270] and are also the predominant cell found in parenchymal infiltrates, particularly in perivenular regions in cases of chronic rejection.[279] Activated CD8+ cytotoxic T lymphoctes can interact directly with MHC class 1 molecules expressed on graft cells resulting in death of graft cells by apoptosis. Two main pathways for T cell mediated apoptosis have been identified.[262] The first involves the synthesis and secretion of cytolytic granules which contain perforin, granzymes and granulysin. Upon binding to the target cell, these granules move to the site of contact and fuse with the target cell membrane. This results in the formation of pores, produced by polymerization of perforin, and the influx or cytolytic proteins (granzymes and granulysin), which activate caspases and trigger apoptosis of the target cell. The second pathway involves the interaction between Fas ligand (Fas-L) which is upregulated on the surface of CTLs and Fas expressed on the surface of target cells. Upregulation of Fas expression, most likely induced by cytokines released from activated T cells, has been demonstrated on hepatocytes, bile ducts and endothelial cells (sinusoidal and vascular) in rejecting liver allografts.[275,280] These changes are associated with graft infiltration by Fas-L

positive T lymphocyes and result in increased apoptosis of hepatocytes and biliary epithelial cells.[280-285] Interactions involving CD40, expressed on target cells, and CD40 ligand, expressed on effector cells, have also been implicated in the pathogenesis of Fas-mediated apoptosis of hepatocytes and biliary epithelial cells in rejecting liver allografts.[275,276] CD40-L positive macrophages appear to play an important role in this process and may also be involved in other aspects of immune activation in the liver allograft.[286,287]

Some of the cytokines released by activated T cells (e.g. interferon gamma and TNFα) may result in damage to adjacent structures in a non-antigen specific manner. In addition, T cell derived cytokines result in the recruitment and activation of a number of other inflammatory cells including neutrophils, eosinophils, macrophages, and NK cells. All of these cells can also augment T cell mediated damage to target structures in a non-antigen-specific manner.[261,288] Mast cells have been implicated in the pathogenesis of bile duct injury in chronic rejection.[289]

Humoral factors have also been implicated in mediating damage to bile ducts and vascular endothelial cells in chronic liver allograft rejection. An association has been reported between positive lymphocyte cross-match and chronic rejection.[290] Donor-specific class 1 antibodies have also been documented in chronic rejection and it has been suggested that these could bind to class 1 antigens expressed on biliary epithelium.[291] Antibody deposition has also been demonstrated immunohistochemically in bile ducts and arteries of chronically rejecting liver allografts.[292,293] As discussed earlier, humoral mechanisms have also been implicated in the development of a modified form of acute rejection in the early post-transplant period.

Ischaemia may also be important in mediating damage to bile ducts and other structures in liver allograft rejection. Bile ducts, which only have a single arterial supply from the hepatic arterial system, are particularly susceptible to ischaemic damage. Vascular lesions that have been implicated in mediating bile duct loss in chronic rejection include occlusive lesions in large and medium-sized arteries, loss of terminal hepatic arterioles and destruction of portal tract microvasculature.[151,229,230] Morphometric studies have shown that the severity of arterial lesions correlates with the degree of bile duct loss and that the loss of portal tract vessels precedes bile duct loss in liver allograft rejection. The possible role of vascular lesions in mediating damage to perivenular hepatocytes in liver allograft rejection has been discussed earlier.

Table 16.9	Effector mechanisms in liver allograft rejection

1. T-cell mediated cell lysis
   direct (T-cell binding to target cell)
   indirect (cytokine-mediated)

2. Innate immune response
   NK T cells
   Other non-antigen specific inflammatory
   cells (eosinophils, neutrophils, macrophages)

3. Antibody-mediated damage

4. Ischaemia

Response to rejection-induced liver injury

The liver has a considerable capacity for regeneration. Increased hepatocyte proliferation occurs within the early post-transplant period in response to preservation/reperfusion injury.[294] In cases of chronic rejection, increased proliferative activity can be seen in surviving hepatocytes surrounding perivenular zones of hepatocyte necrosis (Fig. 16.14). Proliferation of biliary epithelial cells can also be seen in liver allograft rejection. The final outcome of rejection in the liver allograft thus depends on the balance

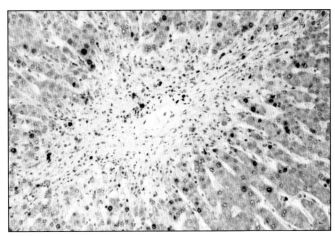

Fig. 16.14 • Hepatocyte proliferation in chronic rejection. Ki67 immunostaining shows numerous proliferating hepatocytes surrounding an area of perivenular necrosis.

between factors leading to cell death and the capacity for a compensatory proliferative response.

Several studies have suggested that bone-marrow-derived progenitor cells may be recruited to the liver and have the potential to differentiate into the various cell types present in the liver.[259,260,295–301] This process may represent an important response to liver allograft damage, particularly in cases where the regenerative capacity of the liver allograft is impaired (e.g. severe recurrent hepatitis C infection), and has also been implicated in the development of tolerance. However, with the exception of Kupffer cells and, at a seemingly lower rate, endothelial cells, which are extensively replaced by cells of recipient origin, the majority of other cells in the liver allograft retain a donor phenotype.

Development of graft tolerance

Compared with other solid organs, the liver appears to have a reduced susceptibility to the development of rejection and an increased potential for the development of tolerance.[262,266,302,303] Spontaneous acceptance of MHC-incompatible liver allografts is well recognized in animal models and transplantation of the liver induces tolerance for other organ grafts which would otherwise be rejected. The development of early cellular infiltrates in allogeneic rodent livers and the subsequent spontaneous resolution of these inflammatory changes supports the idea that early immune activation is an important stage in the development of graft tolerance. Similar observations have also been made in the setting of human liver transplantation. In some patients with stable graft function immunosuppression can be considerably reduced or even withdrawn completely.[304,305] Factors which may promote the process of tolerance include clonal deletion of alloreactive T cells by soluble class 1 MHC molecules,[266] the unique anatomy of the sinusoidal microenvironment which promotes intrasinusoidal T cell apoptosis[306–308] and the establishment of a donor-derived population of haemopoietic stem cells in the recipient (microchimerism).[309,310] Kupffer cells are also involved in regulating T cell responses and mediating T cell apoptosis.[311] Donor

leukocytes transplanted with the liver also appear to be important in the induction of tolerance and may be associated with the development of a mild rejection response that subsequently resolves.[266] Although dendritic cells (DCs) are principally involved in antigen presentation, subpopulations of immature dendritic cells have been implicated in the induction of regulatory T cell responses. Regulatory T cells (Treg) are a subset of CD4+, CD25+ cells, which have a range of immunosuppressive actions designed mainly as a mechanism of self-tolerance, but also believed to be important in transplant tolerance.[312,313] The process of T cell apoptosis within the liver leads to the release of anti-inflammatory molecules such as TGF-beta and IL-10.[312] Expression on biliary epithelial cells of HLA-G, which suppresses CD4+ T cell proliferation and promotes Th2-type responses, has been associated with allograft acceptance.[314]

Infections

General aspects

Infections are very common in liver allograft recipients. They include the usual infections which occur after major abdominal surgery as well as a broad spectrum of opportunistic infections arising as a consequence of immunosuppression. In addition, the liver allograft is the prime target of infection (recurrent or de novo) by the hepatotropic viruses.

Opportunistic viral infections

Cytomegalovirus

Cytomegalovirus (CMV) is the commonest opportunistic organism to be seen in liver allograft biopsies. The peak time of occurrence is between 4 and 12 weeks following transplantation. About 30–50% of liver allograft recipients develop serological signs of CMV infection.[315] Many of these do not have any accompanying symptoms and liver biopsies are rarely obtained from people in this group. A smaller proportion of cases develop symptomatic CMV infection associated with fever, myalgia, malaise, leukopenia and thrombocytopenia.[316,317]

The liver is the commonest site of organ involvement by CMV in liver allograft recipients.[318] The incidence of CMV hepatitis appears to be declining, presumably as a result of more effective antiviral prophylaxis and treatment, and in a recent study was only 2.1%.[319] Cases of CMV are also presenting later than previously, in some cases associated with discontinuation of antiviral prophylaxis.[320] Other manifestations of CMV disease which occur less frequently include pneumonia, gastrointestinal disease, neurological complications and chorioretinitis.[321] The main risk factor for the development of CMV disease is the insertion of a liver from a CMV seropositive donor into a CMV seronegative recipient.[315,317,319] Other risk factors include liver transplantation for acute fulminant hepatitis, acute rejection, the amount and type of immunosuppressive therapy given, hepatic artery thrombosis, hepatitis C infection, HLA-DR matching and infection with human herpes viruses 6 and 7.[315,317,319,322–327]

The characteristic histological finding in CMV hepatitis is the presence of scattered neutrophilic aggregates (microabscesses) within the liver parenchyma (Fig. 16.15(A)). Parenchymal microgranulomas are also commonly seen. There is occasionally a picture of spotty lobular inflammation and lobular disarray, which is indistinguishable from other forms of viral hepatitis. Other features which have been reported include mild portal inflammation—sometimes associated with mild inflammation of bile duct and portal venules, suggesting mild cellular rejection—Kupffer cell enlargement and hepatocellular changes including anisocytosis, anisokaryosis, nuclear hyperchromatism and increased numbers of mitoses.[328,329] Viral inclusions are mostly seen within the cytoplasm and/or nucleus of infected hepatocytes, usually in the vicinity of inflammatory lesions, and to a lesser degree in bile ducts, sinusoidal lining cells and vascular endothelial cells.[330] In one study of serial post-transplant liver biopsies CMV infection was first detected within sinusoidal cells, several days before typical histological features of CMV hepatitis became apparent.[331] Immunohistochemical staining for CMV antigens is useful in confirming the presence of the virus, particularly in cases where there are suggestive inflammatory lesions but no obvious inclusions[331,332] (Fig. 16.15(B)). In situ hybridization techniques have also been used but do not appear to be more sensitive than immunohistochemistry.[328,333]

Although parenchymal neutrophil microabscesses are highly suggestive of CMV hepatitis, these lesions may also occur in cases with no evidence of CMV infection e.g. other infections (bacterial, viral or fungal), graft ischaemia and biliary obstruction/cholangitis. In some cases no obvious disease association can be found.[334,335] Neutrophil aggregates in CMV negative cases tend to be smaller and more numerous than those occurring in association with CMV infection (mini microabscesses).[334]

CMV infection has been implicated as a risk factor for the development of chronic rejection,[204,212] possibly via cytokine-mediated upregulation of MHC molecules or other immunogenic molecules, although this remains controversial.[319,336] Alternatively, the high-dose immunosuppression used to treat patients who develop chronic rejection may predispose to opportunistic infections including CMV. CMV infection has also been implicated as a risk factor for the development of hepatic artery thrombosis, portal vein thrombosis and biliary complications after liver transplantation.[319,337–340] These complications may relate to the capacity of the virus to infect vascular endothelial cells and biliary epithelium. CMV infection of vascular endothelial cells is associated with a rapid procoagulant response.[337]

Epstein–Barr virus

Epstein–Barr virus is associated with a broad spectrum of lymphoproliferative diseases in immunocompromised individuals. The great majority are B cell proliferations and are related to the normal T cell mediated control of EBV infection being impaired as a consequence of immunosuppression. The clinicopathological spectrum ranges from simple lymphoid hyperplasia through to high-grade malignant lymphoma.[341–345] A small number of cases of EBV associated T cell lymphoma have also been documented in liver allograft recipients.[346–348]

In the World Health Organization classification of neoplastic lymphoid diseases, three main categories of post-transplant lymphoproliferative disorder (PTLD) have been recognized:[349] early lesions (reactive plasmacytic hyperplasia or infectious mononucleosis like); polymorphic PTLD (polyclonal or monoclonal); and monomorphic PTLD. The polymorphic PTLD is considered to be a distinctive form of lymphoproliferation which is only seen in immunocompromised individuals. By contrast, cases classified as monomorphic PTLD have essentially the same features as lymphomas occurring in immunocompetent individuals. Although EBV is the major risk factor for the development of lymphoproliferative diseases in immunocompromised individuals, there is also an increased risk for developing

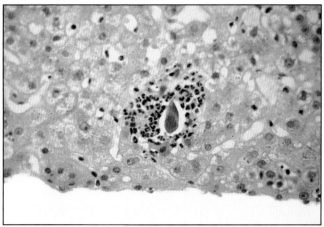

A

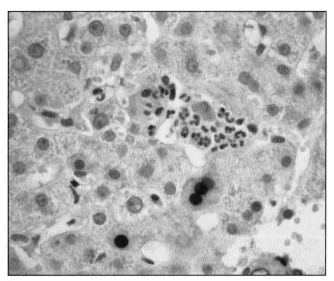

B

Fig. 16.15 • CMV hepatitis in the liver allograft. **(A)** A dense aggregate of neutrophils (microabscess) surrounds a cell containing a characteristic eosinophilic inclusion. H&E. **(B)** Immunostaining with antibodies reacting with early CMV antigens detects positive nuclei in absence of obvious inclusions.

non-EBV related lymphomas. The latter tend to occur at a later time than EBV-associated PTLD.[350,351] The majority of PTLDs occurring in liver allograft recipients are derived from recipient lymphoid cells. However, a few cases of donor origin have been described.[352-355]

The main risk factors for EBV related PTLD include primary infection (most commonly seen in paediatric patients) and the amount and type of immunosuppression used.[356-360] Other risk factors include CMV infection, HCV infection and (within the paediatric population) young age at transplantation.[356,359-361] The insertion of an EBV-positive organ into an EBV negative recipient is associated with an increased risk of primary EBV infections[362] and this also appears to be a risk factor for the development of donor-derived PTLD. Measurement of viral load using PCR techniques may be useful in the diagnosis and management of EBV-associated PTLD.[363-365]

The reported incidence of EBV-associated PTLD in liver allograft recipients ranges from 1% to 12%.[344,359,360,366] Most cases present during the first year following transplantation. During the early stages where there is a polyclonal B cell proliferation, the disease is frequently reversible with a reduction in immunosuppression. Treatment with antiviral agents may also be of benefit at this stage. Progression to monoclonal B cell proliferation indicates more aggressive disease, which is less likely to be responsive to changes in immunosuppression and requires alternative forms of treatment including combination chemotherapy, anti B cell monoclonal antibodies and adoptive immunotherapy with virus-specific T cells.[343,344,366-368]

Hepatic infiltration is commonly seen in association with EBV-related PTLD. In some cases, particularly those in which PTLD is donor-derived, the infiltrate is confined to the liver itself. In these cases there may be formation of localized masses, particularly in the porta hepatis, which can present with features of biliary obstruction.[344,354,355,369] In other cases there is more diffuse hepatic involvement, frequently associated with extrahepatic disease. Infiltrates are predominantly portal in location, with variable involvement of the liver parenchyma, where there may be a mononucleosis-like pattern of sinusoidal infiltration. Distinction from other causes of portal inflammation, particularly rejection, may be difficult and in some cases EBV related PTLD may coexist with rejection.[370] Helpful pointers to a diagnosis of EBV related lymphoid infiltration are the presence of a pleomorphic infiltrate including a high proportion of plasmacytoid cells, immunoblasts and frequent mitoses[371] (Fig. 6.16(A)). Immunohistochemical demonstration that the majority of cells are B cells, in contrast to rejection where the infiltrate is predominantly composed of T cells is also helpful. Immunohistochemistry can also be used to demonstrate light or heavy chain restriction, which indicates the presence of monoclonal B cell proliferation.[372] Immunoglobulin gene rearrangement analysis is a more sensitive method for demonstrating clonal proliferation of B cells in PTLD.[342,373] Immunohistochemical staining for virus-associated proteins (e.g. latent membrane protein 1) and in situ hybridization (ISH) for nucleic acids or virus encoded nuclear RNAs (EBERs) can also be used to detect

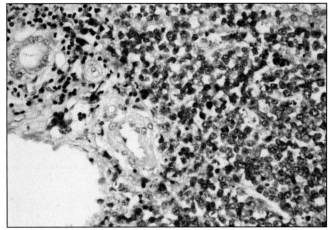
A

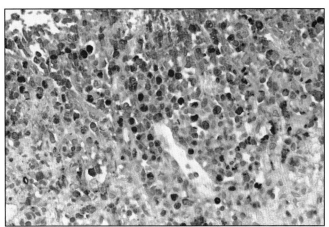
B

Fig. 16.16 • EBV associated post-transplant lymphoproliferative disease. **(A)** Portal tract contains a dense infiltrate of lymphoid cells. These include numerous blast cells, a feature which is helpful in distinguishing lymphoproliferative disease from other causes of portal infiltration including rejection. **(B)** In situ hybridization for Epstein–Barr virus encoded nuclear RNAs (EBERs) confirms that a large proportion of infiltrating lymphoid cells are EBV positive.

the virus in tissue sections (Fig. 6.16(B)), ISH is the more sensitive.[374]

A small number of EBV positive cells may be found amongst portal inflammatory cells in other conditions, including acute and chronic rejection and in inflammatory diseases occurring in a non-transplanted liver.[375] Lymphoid infiltration should therefore only be ascribed to EBV infection if a substantial proportion of the cells can be shown to contain the virus.[376,377] Cases with mixed features of EBV hepatitis and rejection also pose problems for diagnosis and management.[370]

Other rare opportunistic viruses

Adenovirus is mainly seen in paediatric liver transplant recipients.[378,379] However, a few cases have also been described in adults.[380,381] In the early stages there may be parenchymal inflammatory lesions resembling those seen in CMV hepatitis.[379,380] In more severe cases there are small or larger areas of confluent parenchymal necrosis. In some

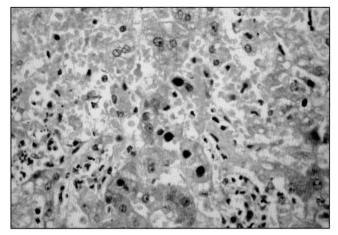

Fig. 16.17 • Adenovirus hepatitis in the liver allograft. Several hepatocytes have characteristic basophilic nuclear inclusions ('smudge cells'). Adjacent to these there is an irregular area of haemorrhage and hepatocyte necrosis. H&E.

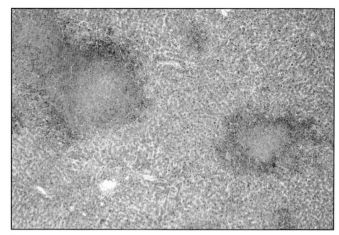

A

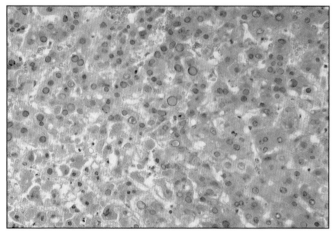

B

Fig. 16.18 • Herpes simplex virus hepatitis. **(A)** Two sharply circumscribed areas of coagulative necrosis are surrounded by a zone of haemorrhage. **(B)** Many surviving hepatocytes surrounding an area of necrosis contain characteristic eosinophilic nuclear inclusions. H&E.

cases this may have a prominent haemorrhagic picture. The characteristic nuclear inclusions have an irregular contour producing a 'smudge cell' effect (Fig. 16.17). Immunohistochemistry using an anti-adenovirus group antibody is useful to confirm the diagnosis. Adenovirus infection can also involve the biliary tree with necrotizing cholangitis and loss of interlobular bile ducts.[382]

Herpes simplex is a rare cause of allograft hepatitis.[383,384] It is characterized by foci of parenchymal necrosis containing neutrophils and macrophages (Fig. 16.18(A)). These may develop into more extensive areas of confluent necrosis associated with a high mortality. Similar changes have also been observed with Varicella Zoster virus.[385] Dense nuclear inclusions are seen in viable cells at the edge of necrotic areas (Fig. 16.18B), but these are rarely detected in liver biopsy specimens.

The human herpesviruses (HHV) 6 and 7 are relatively recently recognized members of the beta-herpesvirus family and are closely related to CMV. HHV-6 infection, occurs in up to 80% of liver allograft recipients, usually between 2 and 8 weeks post-transplant.[386] Most cases represent reactivation and result in a mild febrile illness or subclinical disease.[387] Hepatic involvement may be associated with a mild degree of graft dysfunction. Histological features attributed to HHV-6 hepatitis are mild/moderate portal lymphocytic inflammation (without damage to bile ducts or portal vessels) and foci of parenchymal inflammation, including neutrophil aggregates similar to those seen in CMV hepatitis.[388,389] HHV-6 antigens can also be demonstrated immunohistochemically in portal inflammatory cells. Although direct effects of HHV-6 infection on the liver allograft appear fairly mild, it has been implicated as a risk factor for other graft complications including CMV disease, invasive fungal infection, more aggressive recurrent HCV infection and rejection.[327,386,390-394] HHV-6 induced upregulation of adhesion molecules and lymphocyte activation may be important in the pathogenesis of liver allograft rejection.[389] HHV-7 infection has been implicated in the pathogenesis of CMV infection,[326,327,394] but does not appear to have any direct effects on the liver allograft itself.

Bacterial infections

Although bacterial infections are very common in liver allograft recipients, it is very uncommon to see direct morphological evidence of bacterial infection in liver biopsy specimens. Gram negative sepsis is associated with a characteristic picture of severe cholestasis with cholangiolar proliferation and bile plugging at the periphery of portal tracts and this needs to be considered in the differential diagnosis of intrahepatic cholestasis in the early post-operative period. Ascending cholangitis should be suspected if signs of biliary obstruction are combined with pus cells in the lumina of interlobular bile ducts. Luminal pus cells are also seen in acute rejection (see above) but the presence of other portal inflammatory changes helps to distinguish this from ascending infection. Ischaemic necrosis of bile ducts (see below) is frequently associated with bile sludging and superadded bacterial infection is commonly seen in these areas.

Fungal infections

The commonest opportunistic fungal infections observed in liver allograft recipients are Aspergillus and Candida.[395-397]

Although the liver may be involved in systemic infection with these organisms, it is extremely rare to observe fungi in post-transplant needle biopsies. Superadded fungal infection is quite commonly seen in association with necrotic bile ducts in hepatectomy specimens removed for ischaemic bile duct necrosis.[398] Fungal infection of the hepatic artery may result in thrombosis[399] or pseudoaneurysm formation and rupture.[400]

Vascular problems

Liver transplantation involves three sets of vascular anastomoses: hepatic artery, portal vein and vena cava. All three may be associated with technical complications (e.g. anastomotic stricture or kinking) and/or thrombosis resulting in vascular occlusion. The effects of vascular occlusion in the liver allograft are broadly similar to those occurring in the non-transplanted liver, and only those aspects which have particular relevance to liver transplant pathology will be considered here. Because of their small size, paediatric liver allograft recipients, have a higher risk of vascular complications, particularly hepatic artery thrombosis.[337,401] An increased risk of vascular complications has also been reported with segmental liver grafts, which are increasingly used in living donor liver transplantation.[402,403]

Ischaemia has been an important cause of graft failure in the early post-operative period.[404] In early studies up to 50% of failed allografts removed within the first month following transplantation had morphological evidence of ischaemic damage.[405] Factors predisposing to graft ischaemia in the early post-operative period include problems with graft preservation, technical problems during the operation, anatomy and size of donor vessels and general factors such as hypotension and excessive bleeding. Many cases have a multifactorial aetiology. In some cases thrombi can be detected in hepatic arteries and/or portal vein branches. However, in many instances there is no demonstrable vascular occlusion.[404] Improvements in patient selection, graft preservation and surgical technique have probably all contributed to a reduced incidence of non-occlusive infarction in the early post-transplant period.

Graft ischaemia in the early post-transplant period is characterized by irregular 'geographical' areas of infarction with surrounding haemorrhagic borders (Fig. 16.19(A)). Histology shows coagulative necrosis of the liver parenchyma with variable infiltration by neutrophil polymorphs (Fig. 16.19(B)). There is relative sparing of portal tracts and, in less severe cases, necrosis may be confined to peripheral acinar regions. Post-transplant biopsies may be useful in establishing that ischaemic damage is present, but are not reliable in determining the severity as there is considerable sampling variation. Small peripheral infarcts are commonly seen in liver allografts which are otherwise functioning well and can give rise to concern if they are inadvertently biopsied.[406] Conversely, even livers showing extensive infarction frequently contain large areas in which hepatocytes are well preserved. Changes seen in graft ischaemia occurring in the immediate post-operative period merge with those observed

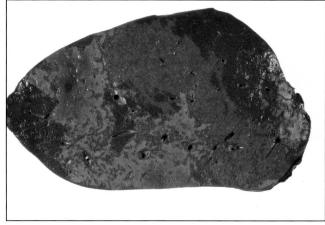

A

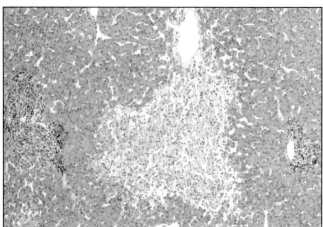

B

Fig. 16.19 • Ischaemic necrosis in the liver allograft. **(A)** Hepatectomy specimen obtained at re-transplantation contains characteristic irregular geographical areas of infarction with a surrounding haemorrhagic border. **(B)** In a less severely affected area there is a small area of coagulative necrosis next to a hepatic venule. H&E.

in cases of severe preservation/reperfusion injury, 'primary non-function' and also unexplained massive haemorrhagic graft necrosis.

Hepatic artery thrombosis (HAT) occurs in 1–8% of patients following liver transplantation, in many cases resulting in the need for retransplantation.[407–412] Predisposing factors include technical problems with the arterial anastomosis, abnormal arterial anatomy, a small-for-size graft, CMV infection, a thrombotic tendency and previous episodes of rejection.[337,338,402,408,411–413] HAT occurring in the early post-transplant period is often associated with ischaemic graft necrosis. An important complication of later hepatic artery thrombosis is ischaemic bile duct necrosis, typically affecting large intrahepatic bile ducts.[338] In cases undergoing re-transplantation for ischaemic biliary complications, there is usually little damage to the liver parenchyma.

The three main forms of rejection may all be associated with graft ischaemia. Changes are most marked in hyperacute (humoral) rejection which produces a picture resembling non-thrombotic infarction of the liver. Alterations in blood flow have also been noted in acute rejection, although it is not clear if these changes produce lesions that are detected histologically.[171] Occlusive lesions involving hepatic arteries, portal veins and hepatic veins have been implicated in the pathogenesis of bile duct loss, perivenular hepatocyte necrosis and parenchymal fibrosis in chronic rejection.

Occlusion of the suprahepatic vena cava as a consequence of anastomotic stricture, kinking or thrombosis may result in the Budd–Chiari syndrome. Budd–Chiari syndrome has also been described as a rare complication of using the 'piggy back' technique for hepatic venous anastomosis.[414] This histological diagnosis of venous outflow obstruction in the liver allograft is problematic, as congestive changes indistinguishable from those occurring in Budd–Chiari syndrome can be also seen as a consequence of rejection or drug-related hepatic venos-occlusive lesions.

Biliary complications

Biliary complications occur at two main sites in the liver allograft. Anastomotic complications develop at the site of the surgical anastomosis between donor and recipient bile ducts. There are also non-anastomotic complications which involve large bile ducts within the liver allograft itself. The overall incidence of biliary complications ranges from 5% to 25%.[415–417]

Anastomotic complications

Historically, complications related to the biliary anastomosis were a major cause of morbidity and mortality following liver transplantation and biliary reconstruction was considered to be the 'technical Achilles heel' of liver transplantation.[418] Refinements in surgical technique, including the widespread use of duct to duct anastomosis, have significantly reduced the rate of biliary complications. A higher incidence has been noted in children, presumably reflecting the small size of the bile ducts and/or their vascular supply.[419]

Anastomotic complications present either as bile leaks, usually occurring in the early post-operative period, or as bile duct strictures which present somewhat later, usually during the first 6 months. Histological features of biliary obstruction are similar to those seen in a non-transplanted liver. Acute biliary obstruction is characterized by portal changes of oedema, bile ductular reaction and neutrophilic infiltration accompanied by variable cholestasis. Several of these features can also be seen in acute rejection.[416] Changes which would favour a diagnosis of acute rejection rather than simple biliary obstruction include a prominent mononuclear portal infiltrate, conspicuous bile duct damage and the presence of venular endothelial inflammation. In some cases biliary obstruction in the liver allograft may remain asymptomatic for a considerable period of time. In such cases biopsies may show signs of chronic cholestasis, including deposition of copper associated protein and progressive periportal fibrosis resulting eventually in biliary cirrhosis. Liver biopsy may be useful in determining the severity of biliary fibrosis in this setting, in addition to identifying

non-biliary causes for graft dysfunction.[420] Rare cases of late biliary obstruction have been attributed to the development of traumatic neuroma at the liver hilum.[421,422]

Non-anastomotic complications

These have become increasingly recognized as an important complication of liver transplantation.[423] Most are thought to have an ischaemic basis.[424] Recognized risk factors include hepatic artery thrombosis, the obliterative vasculopathy of chronic rejection, use of ABO incompatible grafts and preservation/reperfusion injury associated with prolonged cold ischaemia.[102,126,216,229,424–427]

Ischaemic biliary complications present either as strictures or as dilatations involving one or more large intrahepatic bile ducts. Most cases present between 1 and 6 months following transplantation.[428,429] Radiological appearances may resemble those seen in primary sclerosing cholangitis.[429,430] Superadded infection frequently leads to the formation of one or more intrahepatic abscesses, for which re-transplantation is frequently required.[409]

Liver biopsies obtained from patients with ischaemic biliary complications typically show features of biliary obstruction. However, changes seen are frequently patchy in distribution, and only minor histological abnormalities may be present in patients who have gross radiological abnormalities in the hilum. Interlobular bile ducts may show cytological atypia with an atrophic appearance resembling change seen during the early stages of chronic rejection.[217,385] Perivenular hepatocyte dropout, ballooning and cholestasis, also features of chronic rejection, have been documented in cases of ischaemic cholangitis.[105,424] However, chronic rejection is characterized by lesions predominantly affecting small bile ducts, occurring in the absence of secondary biliary features such as bile ductular reaction or periportal fibrosis. By contrast, large ducts are mostly affected in ischaemic cholangitis, with changes in smaller portal areas occurring as a secondary event.

Examination of failed allografts at re-transplantation typically shows irregular collections of bile stained material centred on necrotic, ulcerated and inflamed large and medium-sized bile ducts. These often contain biliary sludge or bile casts[431] (Fig. 16.20). There is frequently superadded bacterial or fungal infection. Bile extravasation may extend for some distance into surrounding tissue, accompanied by necrosis and inflammation. There may also be fibro-obliterative lesions involving medium-sized ducts, disappearance of small interlobular ducts and secondary changes of ductular reaction and biliary fibrosis resembling changes seen in primary sclerosing cholangitis.[429]

Disease recurrence

General aspects

With improved long-term survival following transplantation, problems related to disease recurrence are becoming increasingly important. Most of the common diseases for

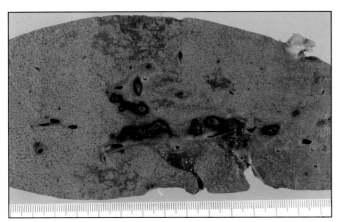

A

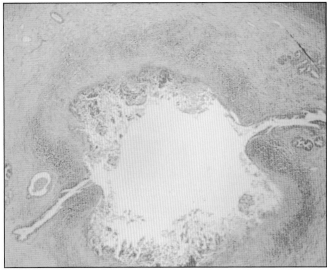

B

Fig. 16.20 • Ischaemic bile duct necrosis. **(A)** Necrotic, deeply bile stained areas are centred on portal tracts. The surrounding liver parenchyma shows centrilobular cholestasis and patchy areas of bile stained ischaemic necrosis (upper part of the liver, up to the Glisson's capsule). **(B)** A large bile duct shows a marked segmental dilatation due to extensive mucosal ulceration with inspissated biliary sludge. Note near normal duct segments on both sides. Such changes closely resemble large bile duct lesions seen in sclerosing cholangitis. H&E.

which liver transplantation is done can recur. The clinical consequences of disease recurrence vary considerably. Some conditions (e.g. malignant hepatic neoplasms) recur fairly early, usually within the first 2 years, resulting in a high mortality. Other diseases (e.g. primary biliary cirrhosis) recur in a mild, often sub-clinical form, with no obvious impact on graft or patient survival.

The histological diagnosis of recurrent disease is influenced by a number of transplant-related factors. There may be similarities between the histological features of the primary disease which is suspected to recur and other complications of liver transplantation. Examples of these include similarities between: hepatitis C and acute cellular rejection; primary biliary cirrhosis and chronic rejection; and primary sclerosing cholangitis and ischaemic cholangitis. Interactions between recurrent disease and other graft complications (e.g. hepatitis C and chronic rejection) can sometimes produce complex changes which are difficult to

interpret. Immunosuppressive therapy may also have an effect—diseases which are thought to be immune-mediated (e.g. autoimmune hepatitis or PBC) are likely to be prevented from recurring or progress more slowly as a consequence of immunosuppression. Conversely, viral infections behave in a more aggressive manner in an immunocompromised individual.

Although it is widely accepted that some autoimmune diseases (e.g. PBC and autoimmune hepatitis) recur following transplantation, there are conceptual problems with making this diagnosis. As MHC matching is not carried out routinely following liver transplantation, it is likely that immune responses are being directed against foreign antigens rather than self antigens (i.e. **allo**immune disease rather than **auto**immune disease). The recognition that classical serological and histological features of autoimmune hepatitis may develop in patients transplanted for non-immunological diseases[432–437] raises further questions regarding the concept of recurrent autoimmune disease. It is possible that viral agents, which have been postulated in the pathogenesis of autoimmune disease in the native liver, may trigger the development of recurrent autoimmune disease in the liver allograft.[438,439]

Hepatitis B

Incidence and risk factors

During the 1980s and early 1990s recurrence of HBV infection was a common and important complication of liver transplantation. In a large combined European series of 372 patients, the overall actuarial risk of recurrent infection 3 years following transplantation was 50%.[440] This was associated with a marked reduction in overall graft survival—less than 50% at 5 years. The most important risk factor for recurrent infection is the presence of active viral replication at the time of transplantation, which in turn is affected by the clinical presentation (acute or chronic disease) and the presence of co-infection with hepatitis delta virus (HDV). The highest incidence of recurrent HBV infection (>80%) occurred in cirrhotic patients who were HBV-DNA positive. Conversely, fulminant hepatitis B infection was associated with a much lower risk of re-infection (<20%) because a massive immune response usually results in the elimination of viral antigens. Coinfection with hepatitis delta virus (HDV) was likewise associated with a lower risk of recurrent HBV infection, due to the inhibitory effect of HDV on HBV replication. Other risk factors which have been associated with more frequent or more severe recurrent disease, include Asian descent, the presence of pre-core or pre-S mutations, coexistent hepatocellular carcinoma, HBV genotype 4 and previous transplantation for HBV infection.[441–447]

The use of anti-viral therapy pre- and post-transplant has resulted in a marked reduction in both incidence and severity of recurrent HBV infection in recent years.[448–452] Pre-transplant treatment with lamivudine (LAM) and, more recently adefovir, is mainly directed at reducing viral DNA levels at the time of transplant. Post-transplant combination prophylaxis with LAM and anti HBs immunoglobulin

(HBIg) is then used to prevent recurrence. The risk of developing recurrent HBV infection is now less than 10% and survival in this group of patients is now comparable to that seen in other cirrhotic patients undergoing liver transplantation. However, even in patients with no histological or serological evidence of recurrent HBV infection small amounts of HBV-DNA can be detected by PCR in serum, liver or peripheral blood mononuclear cells, providing a potential source for recurrent disease if anti-viral therapy is discontinued.[450,453]

Histopathological features and natural history

Histopathological findings in HBV infection of the liver allograft can be divided into two main categories. Typical features of HBV infection, as seen in the non-transplanted liver, occur in the majority of cases. More rarely there are atypical patterns of liver damage, presumably related to other factors present in liver allograft recipients.

Typical features of recurrent HBV infection

Three main phases of re-infection have been identified.[454,455] In the initial *'incubation phase'* (first 3 months post-transplant) biopsies may show changes related to acute rejection or other early post-transplant complications of liver transplantation. Histological changes directly attributable to HBV are rarely present during this phase, although a slight disarray of hepatocytes is sometimes seen.[456] Positive immunohistochemical staining for HBV-associated antigens is usually the first sign of recurrent infection, typically in the form of focal cytoplasmic or nuclear staining for core antigen[457,458] (Fig. 16.21). During the second phase of *'early re-infection'* (usually 1–6 months post-transplant) biopsies typically show features of a mild lobular hepatitis. Varying degrees of portal inflammation may also be present. Portal and periportal inflammatory changes generally become more prominent as the disease progresses to the third stage of *'established (chronic) infection'* (more than 6 months post-transplant) and resemble those which are seen in chronic hepatitis B involving the non-transplanted liver. The severity and speed of progression have been considerably greater in the liver allograft than in the native liver. In a combined series of 42 patients re-infected with HBV prior to 1991, 41 developed acute hepatitis, 20 progressed to chronic hepatitis and 8 had become cirrhotic within a period ranging from 7 to 70 months.[441,459]

Atypical features of recurrent HBV infection

Three main atypical patterns of re-infection have been identified: hepatocyte ballooning, fatty change and a distinctive cholestatic syndrome ('fibrosing cholestatic hepatitis').[455] These frequently occur in combination and appear to be part of a spectrum of HBV infection occurring in immuno-compromised individuals. The use of anti-viral strategies, which reduce viral levels even in cases where recurrent infection occurs, has prevented these atypical manifestations of recurrent HBV infection from occurring.

Hepatocyte ballooning typically occurs without significant accompanying inflammation and is associated with

diffuse, often panacinar, cytoplasmic and nuclear immunostaining for HBcAg (Fig. 16.21(B), (C)). A similar pattern of immunostaining has also been described for HbeAg.[460] These observations suggest that massive viral replication can result in direct cytopathic damage to hepatocytes. Hepatocyte ballooning may be accompanied by varying degrees of fatty change. In cases where steatosis is particularly prominent the term 'steatoviral hepatitis' has been used.[456]

The term 'fibrosing cholestatic hepatitis' (FCH) has been widely used to describe a distinctive pattern of graft damage associated with rapidly progressive graft failure. Most cases presented during the first few months following transplantation.[441,455–457,460] FCH is characterized histologically by periportal fibrosis extending as thin perisinusoidal strands for varying distances into the liver lobule, accompanied by flat ductular structures without an identifiable lumen (Fig. 16.21(D), (E) and (F)). Liver parenchyma shows prominent hepatocyte ballooning, cholestasis and widespread immunoreactivity for HBcAg (nuclear and cytoplasmic) and to a variable degree for HBsAg. (Also see Fig 8.25, 8.26.) Inflammatory changes are generally mild or absent. Prior to the availability of preventive measures and specific therapy, this unique type of injury rapidly progressed to liver failure in the face of limited hepatocyte necrosis and, would, in the case of re-tranplantation, recur and progress even more rapidly than in the first graft.[453]

Pathogenetic mechanisms

HBV-associated nucleic acids have been identified in peripheral blood mononuclear cells and several extrahepatic sites and these are presumed to be the source of re-infection in the liver allograft.[461,462] Two main pathways have been implicated in causing graft damage following re-infection with HBV: (i) Immune-mediated mechanisms, as seen in the non-transplanted liver, mainly involve HLA class 1-restricted viral recognition by HBV-specific CD8 T-cells and are probably responsible for producing the more typical inflammatory changes seen in recurrent HBV infection.[463] (ii) Direct cytopathic damage related to uncontrolled viral replication occurring in the setting of immunosuppression is the more likely mechanism for producing atypical patterns of recurrent HBV infection.

The immunosuppressive agents used in liver transplantation may have a direct effect in promoting HBV replication: corticosteroids can activate a steroid responsive promoter in the HBV genome[464] and azathioprine may also directly promote viral replication.[465] HLA-matching is not carried out routinely in liver transplantation and host-viral interactions involving recognition of class I MHC molecules by cytotoxic T lymphocytes are thus likely to be impaired in most cases. HLA class 1 independent HBcAg-specific T cell responses have been demonstrated in liver allograft recipients with recurrent HBV infection.[466] The development of mutations in the HBV genome may also be important in enabling the virus to escape from immune recognition or antiviral therapy. Examples include the pre-core mutant, which is associated with more severe disease in the liver

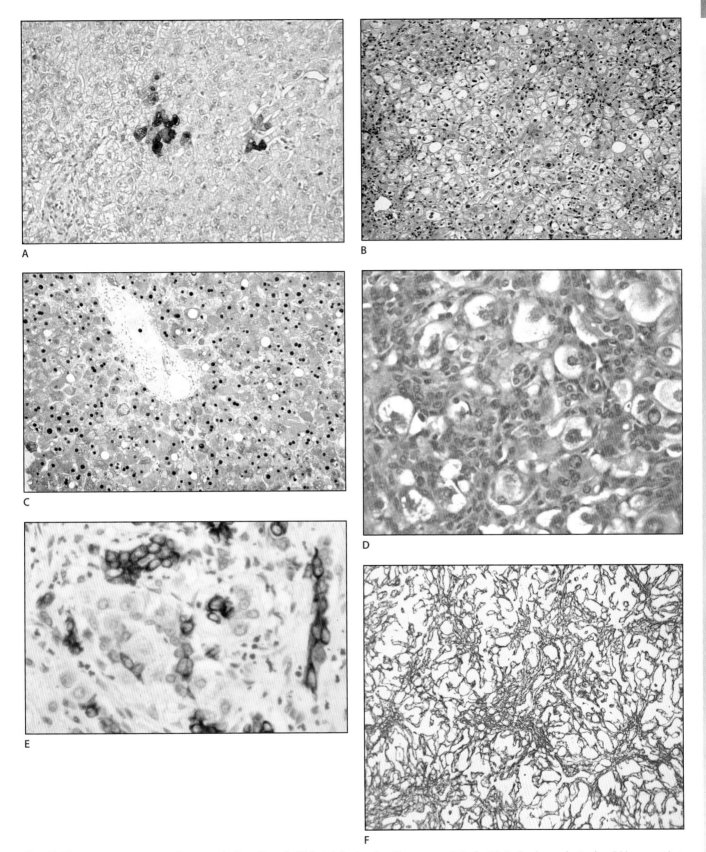

Fig. 16.21 • Recurrent hepatitis B infection in the liver allograft. **(A)** Early infection. Focal immunoreactivity for HBcAg (nuclear and cytoplasmic) is present in a liver biopsy which otherwise appears normal. **(B)** Diffuse hepatocyte ballooning and mild fatty change are present, without an accompanying inflammatory reaction. **(C)** Diffuse immunoreactivity for HBcAg (nuclear and cytoplasmic) is present (same case as fig 16.21b). These changes suggest that there is massive viral replication resulting in direct cytopathic damage to hepatocytes. **(D)** Fibrosing cholestatic hepatitis B infection. Ballooned or 'ground glass' hepatocytes are shown intermingled with small ductular structures (H&E), the latter highlighted by immunostaining for biliary cytokeratin (CK7) in **(E)**. **(F)** Lower magnification to show widespread perisinusoidal fibrosis.

allograft and mutations in the YMDD locus of the HBV polymerase gene, which have been identified in cases where viral 'escape' occurs on lamivudine therapy.[443,467] In fibrosing cholestatic hepatitis B the massive viral burden is likely to interfere with basic cell function, in particular regeneration, one possible explanation for the extensive and widespread ductular reaction observed in this situation.

Hepatitis C

Incidence and risk factors

More than 90% of patients with chronic hepatitis C virus infection who undergo liver transplantation have virological markers of recurrent infection post-transplant.[468–470] Graft re-infection probably begins during reperfusion and viral replication commences within a few hours thereafter.[471] Viral levels typically decrease in the immediate postoperative period, but rapidly return to pre-transplant levels, often within a few days.[471,472] The levels of HCV-RNA subsequently increase, typically reaching up to 100 times pretransplant levels 2–3 months post-transplant.[472,473]

About 50% of patients remain asymptomatic during the first 12 months post-transplant,[474] but the majority (70–95%) will eventually develop histological features of graft hepatitis.[475–478] Risk factors predisposing to more severe liver disease, usually defined according to severity of necroinflammatory activity, presence of atypical cholestatic features or the development of fibrosis in post-transplant biopsies, are summarized in Table 16.10.[468,469,472,479–500] The most important risk factors relate to the use of immunosuppression, either as baseline therapy or to treat episodes of acute rejection. The increased viral replication that occurs in the setting of immunosuppression predisposes to more severe HCV-related graft damage, which may be aggravated when the immune system is reconstituted following tapering of immunosuppression. Levels of viraemia are also important and appear to correlate with both the onset of clinical episodes of acute graft hepatitis and the subsequent progression to chronic liver disease or graft failure.

Histological features seen in early post-transplant biopsies may also be predictive of more aggressive disease behaviour. These include the severity of necroinflammatory activity (periportal and/or lobular), presence and/or severity of macrovesicular steatosis and the presence of prominent hepatocyte ballooning and/or cholestasis.[62,476,483,501–505] For example, the presence and severity of macrovesicular steatosis in biopsy specimens taken during the first month has been shown to correlate with the subsequent development of persistent transaminitis and fibrosis.[503] Likewise the histological activity index (HAI) in first post-transplant biopsies with features of recurrent HCV (within 4–6 months after OLT) correlated with subsequent progression to fibrosis and cirrhosis.[504,505] Severe steatosis may be the initial histologic manifestation of recurrent hepatitis in cases of HCV genotype 3.[506] Other aetiological factors, particularly those related to NAFLD, should also be considered in the differential diagnosis of fatty change in post-transplant biopsies from HCV positive patients.[507] Replicative senes-

Table 16.10	Risk factors for severe/progressive disease in recurrent hepatitis C infection
Early acute rejection	— severity of rejection — number of rejection episodes — amount/type of immunosuppression
Viral factors (HCV-related)	— HCV genotype (genotype 1b or 4) — HCV-RNA levels(pre- and post-transplant) — viral divergence
Viral factors (other)	— CMV — HHV-6 — absence of HBV/HDV
Early time of first presentation with graft hepatitis	
Recent year of transplantation	
HLA-matching	
Donor age	
Previous transplantation for HCV	
Non-white race	
Warm ischaemic time	
Living donor transplantation	
Donor hepatic iron concentration	
Histological findings in early post-transplant biopsies	— fatty change — necroinflammatory activity — cholestasis

cence in early post-transplant biopsies has also been implicated as a risk factor for fibrosis progression in recurrent HCV infection.[508]

Histological features and natural history

Distinction between recurrent HCV and other graft complications such as rejection cannot be made on the basis of clinical or biochemical changes alone and liver biopsy is thus important in establishing a diagnosis of HCV infection in the liver allograft.[468] Liver biopsy is also useful in assessing the severity of necroinflammatory activity and fibrosis. Typical features of HCV infection, as seen in the nontransplanted liver, occur in the majority of cases. More rarely there are atypical patterns of liver damage, presumably related to other factors present in liver allograft recipients.

Typical features of recurrent HCV infection

Three main phases can be identified.[476,501,505,509] During the initial stage of *graft re-infection* (0–2 months posttransplant), when viral RNA levels are already high, the assessment of HCV-related changes is difficult, due to the frequent presence of other causes of graft damage such as preservation-reperfusion injury and acute rejection. HCV-related inflammation is rarely seen at this stage. Instead, there is typically a picture of lobular disarray associated with hepatocyte ballooning, acidophil bodies and sometimes increased mitotic activity. Fatty change may also be seen at this stage.[501,503,510] The second stage of *established graft infection* (2–4 months post-transplant) is characterized by more typical features of acute hepatitis. Inflammation is

generally mild, predominantly lobular in location and is associated with minor degrees of lobular disarray, hepatocellular ballooning, acidophil bodies and Kupffer cell enlargement (Fig. 16.22(A)). Sinusoidal lymphocytosis is sometimes a feature. Varying degrees of portal inflammation may also be seen at this stage. The third stage of *progressive liver damage* (>6 months post-transplant) is characterized by histological features of chronic hepatitis resembling

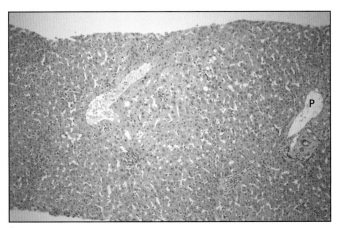

A

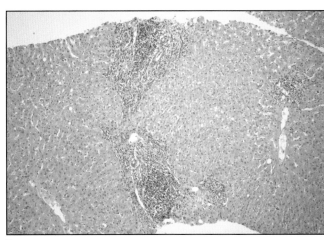

B

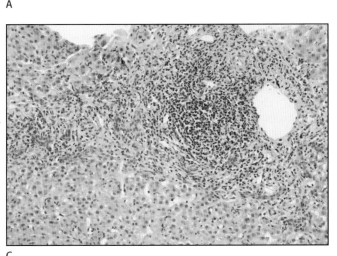

C

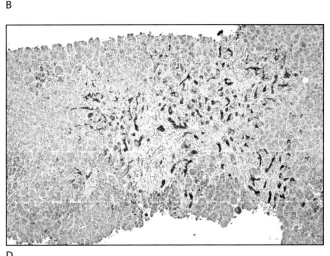

D

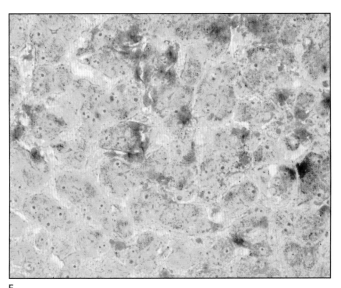

E

Fig. 16.22 • Recurrent hepatitis C infection. **(A)** Early recurrent HCV. Biopsy obtained three months post-transplantation showing spotty parenchymal inflammation. Occasional fat droplets are also identified. A portal tract (P) appears normal. H&E. **(B)** Chronic hepatitis C infection in the liver allograft. This biopsy obtained six months post-transplant shows typical histological features of chronic hepatitis C, including portal inflammation with lymphoid aggregates, mild interface hepatitis, spotty parenchymal inflammation and mild fatty change. H&E. **(C)** Recurrent hepatitis C infection with cholestatic features. This portal tract contains a moderately dense lymphoid infiltrate including a lymphoid aggregate. However, there is also extensive marginal ductular reaction, a feature not typically seen in chronic hepatitis C infection involving the non-transplanted liver. H&E. **(D)** Immunoperoxidase staining for biliary cytokeratins (AE1) confirms the presence of extensive ductular reaction (same case as figure 16.22c). **(E)** Rapidly progressive recurrent hepatitis C. Marked granular staining of hepatocyte cytoplasm treated with an anti-HCV core antibody. Double immunostaining for HCV core antigen (grey-brown) and CD8 antigen (blue).

those seen in chronic HCV infection of the non-transplanted liver (Fig. 16.22(B)). There is a predominantly mononuclear portal inflammatory infiltrate, typically associated with lymphoid aggregates and focal lymphocytic infiltration of bile ducts. In cases where bile duct damage is conspicuous, distinction from acute cellular rejection can be difficult (see below). Variable interface hepatitis is seen. There is also commonly spotty lobular inflammation, fatty change (usually macrovesicular) and focal acidophil body formation. Approximately 50% of patients have histological evidence of chronic hepatitis at one year post-transplant, this figure rising with longer periods of follow up.

There is increasing evidence that HCV infection behaves more aggressively in the liver allograft than in the non-transplanted liver. Histologically, more severe degrees of necroinflammatory activity have been noted, including areas of confluent and bridging necrosis, which are very rarely, if at all seen in non-immunocompromised individuals.[476,505] There is also more rapid progression to fibrosis and cirrhosis.[476,478,483,511,512] Fibrosis is commonly present in biopsies obtained 1 year after transplantation and the fibrosis stage at this time predicts the subsequent development of severe fibrosis or cirrhosis.[513,514] A small number of cases progress to cirrhosis within 1–2 years of transplantation, approximately 10–30% are cirrhotic 5 years post-transplant, and 50% by 7–10 years. A case of de novo hepatocellular carcinoma occurring in association with recurrent HCV cirrhosis, 7 years after transplantation, has also been reported, again supporting the concept of accelerated disease progression in the liver allograft.[515] Recurrent HCV is now recognized as a major cause of late graft failure and in some centres is now the leading indication for retransplantation in patients surviving more than 12 months post-transplant.[516]

A number of immunohistochemical studies of post-transplant biopsies from HCV-positive individuals have been carried out.[476,509,517–520] These have shown that HCV antigens can be detected in liver biopsies within a few days of liver transplantation and 30–50% of cases become positive within the first month of transplantation. Similar observations have been made using in situ polymerase chain reaction methods, which appear to be more sensitive than immunohistochemistry.[519] The appearance of HCV antigens correlates with peak serum HCV RNA levels and extensive staining for HCV may be seen in biopsies showing hepatocyte ballooning and lobular disarray with little or no accompanying inflammation. The appearance and extent of expression of HCV antigens has also been shown to correlate with the onset and histological severity of hepatitis. Others histological features correlating with intrahepatic viral load are bile duct damage, lymphoid aggregates and cholestasis.[519] Expression of HCV antigens may be increased following corticosteroid therapy for acute cellular rejection and reduced or abolished by antiviral therapy.[520] The proportion of positively stained hepatocytes tends to diminish as disease progresses from acute to chronic hepatitis. The availability of reliable antibodies which work on paraffin sections might increase the utility of immunohistoche-

mistry in the routine assessment of post-transplant biopsies.[520]

Atypical features of recurrent HCV infection

A number of atypical histological manifestations of recurrent HCV infection have been recognized. These are probably related to HCV infection occurring in a setting of immunosuppression and resemble those which have been seen in cases of atypical recurrent hepatitis B infection.

Diffuse hepatocyte ballooning sometimes occurs without a conspicuous inflammatory reaction, raising the possibility of direct cytopathic damage.[474] In cases where ballooning is confined to perivenular regions, distinction from other causes of centrilobular ballooning may be difficult. A small proportion of cases develop a severe cholestatic syndrome, which resembles fibrosing cholestatic hepatitis (FCH) B infection.[474,482,521–527] This typically occurs in the early post-transplant period (1–3 months) and is associated with high serum and intrahepatic HCV RNA levels and with an impaired HCV immune response, suggesting that it may represent a form of severe hepatocellular injury related to direct cytopathic effects of HCV. In addition to severe bilirubinostasis, the liver parenchyma often shows prominent hepatocyte ballooning, which may be the earliest histological manifestation of this condition. There is also portal tract expansion with prominent marginal zones of ductular reaction, mimicking changes seen in biliary obstruction (Fig. 16.22(C), (D)). In contrast to classical fibrosing cholestatic hepatitis B infection, where inflammation is minimal or absent, most cases of cholestatic recurrent HCV are seen in conjunction with more typical hepatitic lesions. Other causes of cholestasis (e.g. biliary obstruction, drug toxicity) should be excluded before attributing cholestasis to HCV infection alone.[528] Most cases of cholestatic HCV progress rapidly to graft failure or death within a few months of diagnosis. Examination of failed allografts obtained at retransplantation has shown varying histological changes including persistent severe cholestasis and hepatocyte ballooning, multiacinar necrosis, bridging fibrosis and cirrhosis.[521,522] In some cases biochemical and histological recovery has been achieved by reducing immunosuppression.

An unusual pattern of recurrent HCV infection with granulomatous bile duct destruction, closely resembling changes seen in primary biliary cirrhosis, was noted in a single biopsy obtained 18 months post-transplant from a woman with recurrent HCV hepatitis.[529] Granulomatous bile duct lesions have subsequently been reported in association with HCV infection in the non-transplanted liver.[530] One case of post-transplant granulomatous hepatitis has been attributed to recurrent HCV infection.[531]

Distinction between hepatitis C infection and acute rejection

The distinction between recurrent HCV infection and acute rejection (AR) is one of the most common problems in the assessment of post-transplant biopsies. Both conditions are characterized by predominantly portal-based inflammation, which may involve bile ducts and portal venous endothelium. Features which are helpful in distinguishing recurrent HCV hepatitis from acute rejection are summarized in Table 16.11. Whilst none of these features can be regarded as absolutely specific for either condition, a careful assessment of the pattern of inflammation and associated changes listed in Table 16.11 should enable the main cause of graft damage to be identified with a reasonable degree of confidence in the majority of cases. The timing of events is also helpful in deciding if cellular infiltrates in the liver are due to rejection or hepatitis C. The majority of acute rejection episodes occur in the first month post-transplant. HCV-related inflammatory changes, particularly in portal tracts, should not be present during this period. Conversely, acute rejection is rare more than 12 months post-transplant, whereas this is a time at which portal inflammatory changes related to recurrent HCV infection are likely to be present. Serum HCV-RNA levels tend to be higher in HCV patients with recurrent disease than in those with pure rejection, but there is considerable overlap between the two groups.[532,533] In a small proportion of biopsies distinction between hepatitis C and cellular rejection may be difficult or impossible. It is likely that the changes present in many such cases reflect a combination of HCV and rejection-related graft damage.[533-535] In the majority of instances where a dual pathology is suspected, the rejection-related changes are at worst mild in severity. Additional immunosuppression is not indicated in this situation and recurrent HCV is best regarded as the primary diagnosis.[533] Increased immunosuppression should only be considered as a treatment option if features of cellular rejection are at least moderate in severity, or if there are features suggestive of progression to chronic rejection.

Recurrent HCV and chronic rejection

A higher than expected incidence of chronic (ductopenic) rejection has been reported in a number of studies of recurrent HCV infection.[208,209,536,537] This may reflect shared immunopathogenetic mechanisms of liver damage. Lymphocytic infiltration of bile ducts is a typical feature of chronic HCV infection and may be associated with upregulation of MHC antigens, adhesion molecules and chemokines on biliary epithelium. HCV-induced changes could thus augment immune-mediated bile duct damage in the liver allograft. An alternative mechanism in patients developing rejection (acute or chronic) following interferon therapy for recurrent HCV infection relates to non-specific stimulation of the immune system by interferon.[206,538-541] In some patients responding favourably to anti-HCV therapy, viral clearance has been associated with improvement in hepatocellular microsomal function, resulting in increased metabolism of immunosuppressive drugs, which may further predispose to rejection.[542]

Pathogenetic mechanisms

In common with recurrent HBV infection, re-infection of the liver allograft with hepatitis C virus probably takes place via peripheral blood leukocytes.[543] Graft re-infection and viral replication occur within a few hours of reperfusion.[471]

Table 16.11	Comparison of histological changes occurring in hepatitis C infection and acute cellular rejection of the liver allograft

(A) Portal and periportal changes

	Hepatitis C	Rejection
Portal inflammation	mononuclear cells (lymphoid aggregates)	mixed infiltrate (lymphocytes, macrophages, blast cells, neutrophils, eosinophils)
Interface hepatitis	variable	mild
Bile duct inflammation	mild (lymphocytes)	prominent (mixed infiltrate)
Bile duct loss	none	variable (in cases progressing to chronic rejection)
Venous endothelial inflammation	none/mild	yes
Fibrosis	yes	no

(B) Parenchymal changes

	Hepatitis C	Rejection
Parenchymal inflammation	generally mild	variable
pattern	spotty	confluent
distribution	random	perivenular
associated features	lobular disarray	hepatic vein endothelial inflammation
Cholestasis	rare (except FCH-like cases)	common
Fatty change	yes (macrovesicular)	no
Acidophil bodies	common	less numerous

During the next 2–4 months there is continued viral replication associated with rising serum viral RNA levels. Large amounts of viral antigen can also be detected immmunohistochemically during this period. Hepatocellular proliferation is frequently a prominent finding in early post-transplant biopsies, probably reflecting a response to preservation/reperfusion injury, and is a factor which may favour viral replication during the initial phase of graft re-infection.

There is a delay of 2–4 months before biochemical and histological features of acute hepatitis become manifest. This stage coincides with peak serum HCV-RNA levels and is associated with a vigorous immune response, including HCV-specific CD4+ and CD8+ cells, both of which are important in viral elimination.[544–547] Lobular infiltrates rich in CD8+ T cells and CD57+ natural killer cells can also be seen at this stage.[509] The upregulation of Fas antigen expression on hepatocytes induced by HCV replication appears to be important in the pathogenesis of lobular inflammation and apoptosis in recurrent HCV infection.[548,549]

RNA levels tend to decline as recurrent HCV infection progresses to the stage of chronic hepatitis, 6–12 months post-transplant. This phase is characterized by a relatively low-level anti-HCV CD4 response, similar to that seen with chronic HCV infection in the non-transplanted liver. However, compared with the non-transplanted liver, HCV infection in the liver allograft is still associated with higher viral RNA levels, greater degrees of hepatocellular proliferation and apoptosis and a more prominent Th1/interferon-gamma inflammatory response.[278,470,509,543] These differences may partly explain why chronic HCV infection behaves more aggressively in the liver allograft compared with the native liver. Other factors which may predispose to more aggressive HCV infection in the liver allograft include the presence of a co-existent alloimmune response and an increase in body mass index (BMI), which is known to be a risk factor for more severe HCV-associated disease in non-transplanted individuals.[470] The presence of replicative senescence in hepatocytes in early post-transplant biopsies has been associated with an increased risk of developing progressive fibrosis[508]—this could account for the more severe disease associated with the use of older donor livers.

Atypical cholestatic patterns of recurrent HCV infection have been associated with high viral RNA levels in liver and serum, absence of an HCV-specific CD4 response and a shift from a Th1 to a Th2 cytokine profile.[523,524,527,550,551] These observations suggest the possibility of direct cytopathic injury to hepatocytes caused by the virus itself.[470,543] A similar mechanism has also been proposed for aggressive cholestatic HCV infection occurring in the setting of cardiac transplantation.[552] However, in contrast to classical fibrosing cholestatic HBV infection, where inflammation is minimal and massive hepatocellular expression of viral antigens is universal, features of cholestatic recurrent HCV infection are more complex and variable. As discussed earlier, features of ballooning and cholestasis frequently co-exist with more typical hepatitic changes. In addition hepatocellular expression of viral antigens is variable, but

generally prominent in those exhibiting a rapid progression (Fig. 16.22(E)).

Hepatitis B and C co-infection

A small proportion of patients undergoing liver transplantation for chronic viral hepatitis are co-infected with HBV and HCV.[448,480,485,511,553] A few cases have also been reported in which liver transplantation was carried out for HBV or HCV disease alone and co-infection with the other virus occurred following transplantation.[554]

HBV positive patients co-infected with HCV appear to have less severe disease than patients with HBV infection alone,[448,554] probably related to HCV-induced inhibition of HBV replication, which has also been described in the non-transplanted liver.[555] In co-infected patients treated with HBIg immunoprophylaxis the predominant histological changes in post-transplant biopsies appear to be HCV-related, suggesting effective inhibition of HBV replication. The severity of HCV hepatitis in these cases also appears to be less than those with HCV infection alone, possibly due to the presence of anti-HCV antibodies in the immunoglobulins used for HBV immunoprophylaxis.[480,511] Co-infection with HDV as well as HBV is also associated with suppression of viral replication and less severe inflammatory activity.[485]

Hepatitis delta

Patients co-infected with HDV are at lower risk of developing recurrent HBV infection following liver transplantation than those infected with HBV alone,[440,556] presumably related to inhibitory effects of HDV on HBV replication. In the absence of immunoprophylaxis, patients coinfected with HBV and HDV still frequently used to develop recurrent HBV-related disease following liver transplantation.[557–559] However, the use of anti-viral therapies pre- and post-transplant has largely eliminated problems of recurrent HBV infection, including cases co-infected with HDV.[448]

A number of early studies suggested that re-infection with HDV could occur without HBV infection.[458,557–559] HDV was identified immunohistochemically in post-transplant biopsies as early as one week post-transplant.[558] HDV-RNA was also identified in serum in the early post-transplant period in the absence of detectable markers of HBV infection.[559] HDV re-infection alone was not associated with clinically significant graft dysfunction or with histological signs of hepatitis and markers of HDV infection eventually disappeared. The use of more sensitive polymerase chain reaction (PCR)-based techniques to detect HBV and HDV viraemia has shown that cases with HDV infection previously characterized as isolated also have low levels of HBV viremia.[560]

In cases where conventional serum markers of HBV infection become positive, there are usually biochemical and histological signs of graft hepatitis. Recurrent hepatitis is generally less severe with combined HBV/HDV infection than with HBV infection alone. HBV-DNA levels are lower,[561] there is a lower risk of progression to cirrhosis and fibrosing cholestatic hepatitis is very uncommon.[562] Rare cases where fulminant recurrent HBV infection has occurred despite co-infection with HDV have been associated with markers of active HBV replication at the time of transplantation.[563]

Other hepatitis viruses

There have been occasional reports describing recurrent hepatitis A infection as the likely cause of an acute hepatitic illness following liver transplantation.[564,565] There is no evidence to suggest that infection with HEV recurs following transplantation. A togavirus-like particle detected in the nuclei of hepatocytes was implicated in the pathogenesis of liver damage in nine patients undergoing liver transplantation for fulminant hepatitis of unknown aetiology and in the development of recurrent acute liver failure in 5 of these patients during the first week following transplantation.[566]

Hepatitis G virus (HGV) is present in the serum of 10–25% of patients undergoing liver transplantation[567-570] and has been observed both in association with chronic viral infection (HBV and HCV) and in patients undergoing liver transplantation for non-viral causes of liver disease. Prevalence rates between 12% and 64% have been found in post-transplant samples.[567-571] Many of these cases presumably represent acquired infection. In cases with presumed recurrence of HGV infection post-transplant RNA levels are persistently lower than those observed prior to transplantation.[572] There is no evidence that HGV infection (recurrent or acquired) has any effect on graft function, histological changes or overall survival.[569,570,573,574]

Primary biliary cirrhosis

It is now generally accepted that primary biliary cirrhosis (PBC) recurs following liver transplantation.[250,575-580] Occasional cases have developed histological features suggestive of recurrent PBC during the first few months,[581] but the majority occur between one and ten years following transplantation. The reported rates of recurrent PBC range from 8–75%, but an overall prevalence in the region of 20–30% at 10 years can be anticipated.[579,580,582]

Risk factors for recurrent PBC include reduction or withdrawal of immunosuppression, treatment with azathioprine or Tacrolimus (FK506), recipient and/or donor age and cold and warm ischaemic times.[249,581-587] Genetic factors have been implicated in the pathogenesis of PBC recurring in patients undergoing living donor transplantation, but the number of such cases studied is small.[588]

An important problem with the diagnosis of recurrent PBC relates to the lack of a specific diagnostic marker. There are difficulties with applying the standard biochemical, serological and histological criteria for the diagnosis of PBC to the patient who has undergone liver transplantation. There are many other causes of cholestasis in the liver allograft including rejection, other biliary complications and drug toxicity.[107,589] Antimitochondrial antibodies (including anti-M$_2$) and elevations in serum IgM levels persist in the majority of patients following liver transplan-

tation, but the diagnostic significance of these findings is uncertain. There are also potential problems with interpreting histological findings, particularly as liver allograft rejection may also be associated with bile duct inflammation and bile duct loss. However, in most cases distinction between PBC and rejection is not a problem as the pattern of bile duct damage in these two conditions is quite different. In addition, features of chronic cholestasis including marginal ductular reaction, cholate stasis, and copper-associated protein deposition, which are typically seen in PBC, occur much less commonly in liver allograft rejection.

The application of rigid histological criteria, including the presence of granulomatous destructive cholangitis, has a high diagnostic specificity for recurrent PBC (Fig. 16.23(A)). Whilst there have been occasional reported cases of portal granulomas in acute cellular rejection[163] and granulomatous cholangitis in recurrent HCV infection,[529] the presence of granulomatous bile duct lesions should still be regarded as presumptive evidence of PBC recurrence. However, as florid duct lesions are only seen in approximately 30% of liver biopsies from non-transplanted patients with PBC,[590] this kind of approach may under-estimate the true incidence of recurrent disease.[250,591] Aberrant expres-

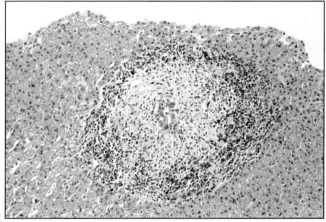

A

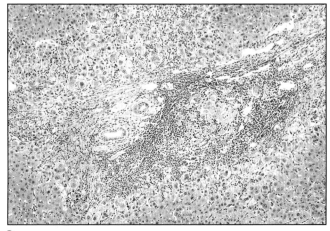

B

Fig. 16.23 • Recurrent primary biliary cirrhosis. **(A)** Portal tract contains a granulomatous bile duct lesion. **(B)** Cirrhotic liver obtained at re-transplantation. Severe fibrosis is rarely seen in patients with histological features of PBC. H&E.

sion of the mitochondrial antigen, pyruvate dehydrogenase complex (PDC)-E2 on bile ducts, has been implicated in the pathogenesis of antibody-mediated bile duct damage in the non-transplanted liver.[592] However, immunohistochemical studies of E2 expression in liver allografts have produced conflicting results.[593,594]

Most patients are asymptomatic with normal or mildly deranged liver biochemistry. Liver biopsies mostly show minimal or mild periportal fibrosis and portal tract lesions suggestive of recurrent PBC are typically patchy in distribution. A solitary florid inflammatory bile duct lesion is not uncommonly present in a biopsy which otherwise appears normal. This contrasts with portal inflammatory lesions in rejection, which are usually more diffuse. In other cases features of chronic hepatitis precede or occur in conjunction with diagnostic bile duct lesions—this process may be associated with a plasma-cell-rich infiltrate or other features suggestive of autoimmune hepatitis.[578,584,595] A small proportion of cases have developed more severe disease with recurrent symptoms and progressive fibrosis, and in occasional cases this had led to an established cirrhosis and the need for re-transplantation (Fig. 16.23(B)).[582,596] However, such cases are unusual and overall there is no evidence that PBC recurrence has any significant impact on graft or patient survival.

Primary sclerosing cholangitis

Many studies have documented radiological and/or histological features of sclerosing cholangitis in patients undergoing liver transplantation for PSC, with prevalence rates ranging from 6–37%.[597-602] Overall, 20–25% of patients transplanted for PSC will develop features compatible with recurrent disease during the first 5 years post-transplant.[589,603] Possible risk factors for recurrent PSC include CMV infection, male sex, immunosuppression with OKT3 and recipient-donor gender mismatch.[600,603-605] By contrast, previous colectomy for inflammatory bowel disease is associated with a lower risk of developing recurrent PSC,[604] possibly due to interruption of the pathway of immune trafficking between gut and liver which has been suggested as an important mechanism in the pathogenesis of PSC.[606,607]

Clinical manifestations of recurrent PSC include recurrent episodes of cholangitis and other problems related to the development of biliary strictures. In the majority of cases the impact of recurrent PSC is relatively mild, with no significant reduction in graft or patient survival.[589,602,608] However, up to 5–10% of patients eventually develop graft failure requiring retransplantation.[597,609] The presence of hilar xanthogranulomatous cholangiopathy in the native liver has been identified as an adverse prognostic feature following liver transplantation, although this was not related to disease recurrence.[605,610]

As in the native liver, histological features of fibrous cholangitis are infrequently seen in liver allograft biopsies from cases of recurrent PSC (Fig. 16.24). Instead the diagnosis is more often based on findings of chronic cholestasis, ductopenia, ductular reaction and biliary fibrosis. Patients transplanted for PSC have an increased risk of developing chronic

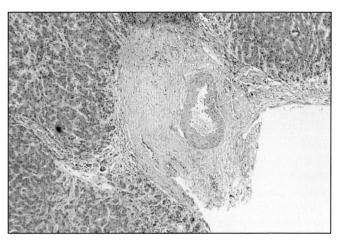

Fig. 16.24 • Recurrent sclerosing cholangitis. In this hepatectomy specimen obtained at re-transplantation, a bile duct is replaced by a characteristic fibro-obliterative scar. H&E.

rejection[611] and in some cases distinction between these two disease processes has proved to be difficult.[600] Approximately 25% of patients with recurrent PSC develop bridging fibrosis or cirrhosis during the first 5 years post-transplant.[601] There has been a single case report of de novo cholangiocarcinoma in the setting of recurrent PSC, 8 years post-transplant.[612]

A major diagnostic problem concerns the distinction between recurrent PSC and ischaemic biliary complications, which can be associated with very similar radiological and histological abnormalities.[429,598,613] Ischaemic biliary complications present generally during the first 6 months following transplantation, whereas most cases of presumed PSC recurrence have been diagnosed more than 12 months post-transplant. Furthermore a number of studies (including two where assessments were made 'blinded' to the original diagnosis) have shown that histological and/or radiological features of sclerosing cholangitis are seen significantly more frequently in patients transplanted for PSC (20–27%) than in those transplanted for other diseases (1–6%).[597,598,601] Whilst these studies provide good evidence that PSC does recur, the diagnosis in individual cases cannot be made with certainty on the basis of histological and/or radiological features alone and other causes of biliary tract disease, particularly ischaemic cholangitis, should be excluded.

Autoimmune hepatitis

The reported incidence of recurrent autoimmune hepatitis after liver transplantation ranges from 11–83%, giving an average recurrence rate of 20–30%.[575,614-624] The most important risk factor for recurrent AIH is suboptimal immunosuppression. Other risk factors include type 1 AIH, HLA-DR3 recipient positivity and severity of necroinflammatory activity in the native hepatectomy specimen.

Most cases present between 1 and 6 years post-transplant, although features attributed to recurrent AIH have been seen as early as 35 days post-transplant.[618] The criteria that have been used in the diagnosis of recurrent AIH include biochemical, serological and histological changes and response to immunosuppressive therapy. In the absence of a single specific diagnostic feature, the diagnosis is best made using a combination of these features.[620,625]

Histological features are typically those of a chronic hepatitis, as seen in the non-transplanted liver, with a predominantly portal-based plasma-cell-rich mononuclear inflammatory infiltrate associated with prominent interface hepatitis. There is a suggestion that these changes may be less well developed in the setting of immunosuppression.[626] In some cases histological features of recurrent AIH may precede clinical and biochemical recurrence by several years.[623] There are many other possible causes of chronic hepatitis in the liver allograft, including recurrent and acquired viral infection, which should be excluded. Varying degrees of lobular inflammation are frequently present, in more severe cases including areas of confluent or bridging necrosis. Lobular inflammatory changes may sometimes occur as the first manifestation of recurrent disease, before typical portal inflammatory changes are present.[618,627]

There is a complex relationship between AIH and liver allograft rejection. Patients undergoing liver transplantation for AIH have an increased risk for developing acute and chronic rejection, possibly reflecting a general state of increased immune responsiveness. Recurrent AIH has also been identified as a further risk factor for progression to chronic rejection.[196] There are areas of overlap in the histological features of AIH and acute cellular rejection—this particularly applies to cases of late cellular rejection, which may have chronic-hepatitis-like features. Autoantibodies arising de novo after transplantation have developed in association with episodes of acute cellular rejection.[628,629] HLA-matching is not carried out routinely for liver allograft recipients and the immune responses occurring in patients transplanted for AIH are thus not HLA-restricted in the way which characterizes autoimmune disease in the non-transplanted individual. These observations suggest that so-called recurrent *auto*immune hepatitis may in fact represent an *allo*immune response, possibly a form of cellular rejection.[622] However, there are a number of ways in which autoimmune responses in the liver allograft could bypass the usual pathway of MHC restriction, suggesting that the concept of recurrent autoimmune hepatitis is still tenable.[436,437]

For most cases of recurrent autoimmune hepatitis occurring in a setting of suboptimal immunosuppression, biochemical and histological features rapidly resolve once adequate immunosuppression is restored. However, up to 30–40% of patients have more aggressive disease resulting in cirrhosis and graft failure.[615,617–619,630] A higher re-recurrence rate, in the region of 70%, has been observed after retransplantation.[615,617,619,630]

Alcoholic liver disease

Alcoholic liver disease is now one of the commonest indications for liver transplantation.[4,6] Approximately 10–30% of patients return to drinking following liver transplantation, but this is rarely associated with serious graft complications.[631–637] The presence of steatohepatitis in the native

hepatectomy specimen suggests recent alcohol consumption and has been suggested as a risk factor for recidivism,[638] but this has not been confirmed by other studies.[634,639] Occasional alcohol-dependent patients have developed rejection-related problems due to non-compliance with immunosuppression, infrequently resulting in graft failure.[640,641]

Post-transplant biopsies obtained from patients who return to excess alcohol consumption have shown mostly minor abnormalities.[237,631,633–635,638,642] Fatty change is the commonest finding, being present in more than 60% of heavy drinkers post-transplant.[641] There have also been reports of more severe abnormalities including steatohepatitis and pericellular fibrosis, rarely leading to cirrhosis or graft failure.[237,635,638,641]

Hepatic neoplasms

Hepatocellular carcinoma

In early studies of liver transplantation for HCC, recurrence rates in the region of 30–50% were observed, resulting in an overall survival in the region of 25–30% at 5 years.[643] The most important factors influencing outcome are tumour size and number. Other prognostic factors are pre-transplant alpha fetoprotein levels, lymph node involvement, bilobar spread, vascular invasion (gross and microscopic), presence of satellite nodules (closely related to microvascular invasion), histological grade, mitotic activity, proliferation index and the concomitant presence of cirrhosis.[644–654] Immunostaining for CD34 may be useful as an adjunct to detect microscopic vascular invasion.[655] In recent years liver transplantation for HCC has been restricted to patients with solitary tumours less than 5 cm diameter or up to 3 lesions no more than 3 cm diameter; this has resulted in considerably lower recurrence rates, with survival figures in excess of 70% at 3 and 5 years.[31,656–659]

Small, previously undetected HCCs are not infrequently identified when hepatectomy specimens are obtained from patients undergoing liver transplantation for cirrhosis, particularly of viral aetiology. The majority of these incidental tumours are solitary small lesions, usually less than 2 cm diameter, which appear to be cured by liver transplantation.[29] However, some cases of recurrent HCC in this situation have been documented.[30,31,660]

In most cases disease recurrence is detected either by the finding of rising serum alpha fetoprotein levels, or by the radiological detection of tumour nodules. The latter are most commonly seen in the liver and lungs.[661,662] Multifocal disease is frequently present. Histological confirmation of disease recurrence is rarely required. There has been a single case report describing an adult patient transplanted for alcoholic cirrhosis and multifocal HCC, who developed recurrent tumour in the form of a mixed hepatoblastoma.[663]

Cholangiocarcinoma

Outcome following liver transplantation for cholangiocarcinoma has been poor, with recurrence rates as high as 90%

having been documented in some studies.[643,664–666] Hilar neoplasms are particularly problematic, as the extent of spread is difficult to identify macroscopically, and microscopic spread of tumour is commonly seen at the hilar resection margin, frequently in a perineural distribution. Lymph node metastases are also commonly present. These findings are associated with early tumour recurrence, frequently intrahepatic, usually within the first few months following transplantation.[667] Perineural invasion has also been identified as an adverse prognostic feature when liver transplantation is carried out for peripheral cholangiocarcinoma.[668] In cases where tumour can be resected with clear surgical margins and absence of lymph node metastases, a more favourable outcome has been observed.[669,670]

Other primary neoplasms

Liver transplantation has been carried out for various other primary hepatic neoplasms including fibrolamellar carcinoma, hepatoblastoma, epithelioid haemangioendothelioma and haemangiosarcoma. Many of these tumours have also recurred. Patients transplanted for fibrolamellar HCC have a lower risk of recurrence and an improved survival compared with those transplanted for conventional HCC, even when the latter occurs in absence of any underlying chronic liver disease.[671] However, for the other primary hepatic neoplasms listed above the numbers are too small to provide meaningful statistical data.

Metastatic neoplasms

Liver transplantation has been carried out for a number of metastatic hepatic neoplasms. Again, the numbers are generally too small to provide meaningful statistical data, but the results have been generally poor. However, a favourable outcome has been reported for some patients transplanted for metastatic neuroendocrine neoplasms.[672,673] A case of peripheral T cell lymphoma presenting as acute liver failure and reappearing in the liver allograft has been reported.[674]

Haemochromatosis (and other causes of iron overload)

Genetic haemochromatosis (GH) is an uncommon indication for liver transplantation.[71,675] Post-transplant survival is poor compared with patients undergoing transplantation for other causes of cirrhosis—this has been attributed to various factors including an increased risk of infections, recurrence of co-incidental hepatocellular carcinoma and cardiac complications. There is little evidence to suggest that significant iron re-accumulation occurs, during the first 2–10 years following transplantation, particularly if other causes of iron overload, such as blood transfusion, are excluded.[69,71,675–677] A single case of severe hepatic siderosis 4 years post-transplant has been seen following transplantation of C282Y heterozygous donor liver into a recipient heterozygous for a novel pathogenic HFE mutation.[678] In view of the fact that iron accumulation in the native liver appears to be a very slow process in genetic haemochroma-

tosis, a considerably longer follow-up period will be required to determine the incidence and clinical significance of iron re-accumulation in the liver allograft.

Many patients undergoing liver transplantation for other causes of cirrhosis have non-HFE related secondary iron overload, in some cases to a degree resembling that seen in GH.[679–682] The presence of severe pre-transplant siderosis has been associated with a greater frequency of iron accumulation in late post-transplant biopsies.[682]

Giant cell hepatitis

Occasional cases of recurrent giant cell hepatitis have been reported in paediatric and adult patients.[683–687] Possible aetiological factors are viral agents (including human papilloma virus type 6 and hepatitis C) and autoimmune liver disease. An aggressive course with rapid progression to cirrhosis and/or graft failure has been documented in several cases;[683,686,687] in particular giant cell hepatitis associated with Coombs positive anaemia invariably recurs and is now considered a contraindication for liver transplantation.[688]

Non-alcoholic steatohepatitis (NASH)

In recent years NASH has been recognized as an increasingly important cause of chronic liver disease, in some cases leading to cirrhosis and the need for liver transplantation.[689] Recurrence of fatty liver disease has been reported in many studies.[689–695] Many cases were initially labelled as cryptogenic but were subsequently found to have histological features of—and/or—risk factors for fatty liver disease. Fatty change is seen in 60–100% of cases, usually within a few months of transplantation. Approximately 10–40% of them develop features of steatohepatitis, usually fairly mild, and up to 12% progress to cirrhosis. In occasional cases disease progression is unusually rapid, resulting in graft failure within 2–3 years of transplantation.[689]

Most cases of NASH are associated with factors related to the metabolic syndrome, such as obesity, hyperlipidaemia, hypertension and diabetes mellitus. These factors frequently persist following liver transplantation, predisposing to NASH recurring in the liver allograft. Liver transplantation itself predisposes to several components of the metabolic syndrome and distinction between recurrent and de novo NASH may therefore be difficult.[696]

Budd–Chiari syndrome

Recurrence of Budd–Chiari syndrome has been described in a number of cases, presumably reflecting persistence of the underlying thrombotic tendency that exists in the majority of these patients.[697–701]

Other recurrent diseases

A number of other diseases have been suspected to recur on rare occasions. These include hepatic and/or portal veno-occlusive disease,[702] erythropoietic protoporphyria,[703] granulomatous hepatitis of unknown aetiology,[167] sarcoidosis,[704] and alveolar echinococcosis.[705]

De novo disease

Acquired viral hepatitis (HBV and HCV)

Infection with these two viruses may be acquired from the donor liver, from blood products or rarely from other sources. Many cases of de novo HBV infection have occurred as a consequence of immunosuppresion-related reactivation of latent virus in donors with previous HBV infection (anti-HBs and/or anti-HBc positive), who were thought to be immune to HBV at the time of transplantation.[706–710] The risk of developing de novo HBV infection from anti-HBc positive donors appears to be less in recipients who also have markers of previous HBV infection than in those who are HBV naïve. The use of antiviral prophylaxis has reduced the incidence of donor-derived HBV infection.[711] Cases of apparent acquired hepatitis B infection have also been described as a result of reactivation of latent virus in the recipient liver.[706,712] However, symptomatic hepatitis B infection is relatively uncommon in these cases.[713]

The incidence of acquired HCV infection has greatly diminished since screening of donors for HCV was introduced in the early 1990s.[714] However, some seronegative donors may contain small amounts of HCV-RNA, which can only be detected by PCR techniques, and have the potential to infect recipients.[715] Because of the shortage of donor organs HCV-positive organs are sometimes used for transplantation in HCV-positive recipients—the outcome in such cases is similar to that seen in HCV-positive individuals receiving HCV-negative grafts.[716]

Histological features of acquired HBV and HCV infection are similar to those seen with recurrent viral infection (discussed earlier). Acquired disease generally behaves less aggressively, with less rapid progression to fibrosis or cirrhosis.[475,251,706,712] However, some cases of acquired HBV infection have a more severe course including progression to cirrhosis or presentation with acute liver failure.[717,718]

Acquired autoimmune hepatitis

Several studies have shown that classical biochemical, serological and histological features of autoimmune hepatitis may develop in patients transplanted for diseases other than AIH[432–437,719,720] (p. 843). A higher incidence, in the region of 5–10%, has been reported in children, possibly related to immunosuppressive drugs interfering with normal T cell maturation. In adults, the most common underlying diseases are PBC and PSC. Occasionally features of de novo AIH and recurrent PBC may be seen concurrently.[595] Donor and/or recipient HLA alleles (HLA-DR4/DR3) known to confer susceptibility to AIH in the native liver also appear to predispose to de novo AIH. Other risk factors include donor/recipient Glutathione S-Transferase (GST) mismatch, with the development of donor-specific anti-GST antibodies, and previous episodes of rejection.[721,722a–c] Autoantibodies

arising de novo following liver transplantation have also been noted in association with episodes of rejection,[628,629] suggesting that so-called de novo AIH may in fact represent a form of late cellular rejection. The alternative term 'Graft dysfunction mimicking autoimmune hepatitis' has been proposed.[435]

Histological features closely resemble those of naturally occurring and recurrent AIH. They include predominantly mononuclear infiltrates in portal tracts associated with interface hepatitis (Fig. 16.25). Parenchymal inflammation is also commonly present and in severe cases may be associated with confluent and bridging necrosis. Ductular reaction may also be prominent in some cases.[434] Most cases respond well to additional immunosuppression, but some have a more aggressive course leading to cirrhosis or graft failure.

Acquired non-alcoholic steatohepatitis (NASH)

Cases of NASH, apparently arising de novo following liver transplantation have been reported.[692] Many of these have developed following liver transplantation for 'cryptogenic' cirrhosis[693,694] or have other pre-transplant risk factors for NASH, and might thus be better regarded as recurrent rather than acquired disease. The liver transplant patient is at risk of several components of the insulin resistance syndrome, such as diabetes mellitus, hypertension, hyperlipidaemia and obesity,[696] which may exacerbate other pre-transplant risk factors. Some cases of post-transplant NASH may arise without any obvious predisposing factors.[723]

De novo neoplasia

There have been two case reports of de novo hepatic neoplasia occurring post-transplant—one case of hepatocellular carcinoma arising on a background of cirrhosis due to recurrent hepatitis C infection[515] and another of cholangiocarcinoma complicating recurrent sclerosing cholangitis.[612] Liver transplant patients are also at risk of developing a number of extrahepatic neoplasms, including EBV-

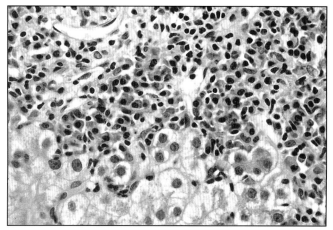

Fig. 16.25 • 'Acquired' autoimmune hepatitis 3.5 years after transplantation for PSC and cholangiocarcinoma. Note the dense plasma-cell rich interface hepatitis. Serum ANA and SMA titres were 1:80 and 1:640, respectively. H&E.

associated PTLD, other lymphomas and tumours of the skin and gastrointestinal tract.[724] Some of these may also spread to involve the liver allograft.

Giant cell hepatitis

Two cases of de novo giant cell hepatitis occurring after liver transplantation have been documented.[683]

Other histological findings in post-transplant biopsy specimens

Biopsies obtained from adult and paediatric patients surviving long term following liver transplantation often show histological abnormalities, for which no definite cause can be identified.[21–25,106,167,199,251,725–727] Many of the biopsies studied have been protocol specimens obtained from patients who are clinically well, with good graft function and normal or near-normal liver biochemistry. In three large series only 7–30% of patients had biopsies showing either normal histology or minimal/mild non-specific changes.[23,250,251]

Unexplained ('idiopathic') chronic hepatitis

10–40% of patients biopsied as part of routine annual review have histological features of chronic hepatitis, the cause of which is uncertain.[21–25,250,725,727,728] The frequency may vary depending on definition, in particular the cut-off point between non-specific inflammation and chronic hepatitis, and the extent to which potential causes have been excluded. Most are clinically asymptomatic with good graft function. Minor abnormalities of serum biochemistry are frequently detected, principally in the form of a mild transaminitis.

The predominant histological finding is a mononuclear portal inflammatory infiltrate associated with variable interface hepatitis (Fig. 16.26(A)). Bile duct damage and venous endothelial inflammation are not conspicuous. Inflammatory changes are commonly present in the liver parenchyma and tend to be most marked in zone 3 where there are also sometimes foci of confluent necrosis[106] (Fig. 16.26(B)). Necroinflammatory activity is generally mild, but in some cases there may be prominent interface hepatitis and/or areas of confluent/bridging necrosis. Widespread multiacinar necrosis associated with acute graft failure has also been seen in a few cases. In two cases the picture closely resembled changes seen in the original liver removed at transplantation.[729] About 10–15% of patients followed up for a minimum of 10 years have developed progressive periportal fibrosis resulting in an established cirrhosis (Hübscher SG, unpublished) (Fig. 16.26(C)).[729a]

Possible causes for chronic hepatitis in the liver allograft include viral agents (recurrent or acquired), autoimmune disease (recurrent or acquired) drugs or a modified form of rejection. (Table 16.12). Known viral agents including hepatitis B, C and G cannot be identified in the great majority of patients developing chronic hepatitis after transplanta-

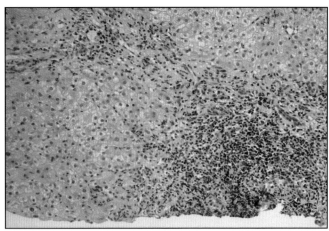

A

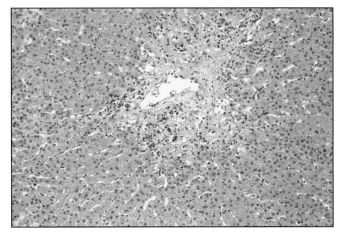

B

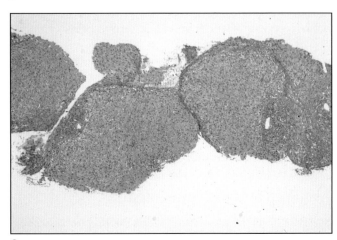

C

Fig. 16.26 • Unexplained chronic hepatitis in the liver allograft. **(A)** Portal tract contains a dense infiltrate of lymphoid cells associated with prominent interface hepatitis. **(B)** An area of zone 3 parenchymal inflammation is associated with confluent hepatocyte necrosis. **(C)** In this biopsy there has been progressive fibrosis, leading to an established cirrhosis, five years post-transplant (Haematoxylin van Gieson).

tion for non-viral causes of liver disease. Features of chronic hepatitis are also seen in autoimmune hepatitis and biliary diseases (PBC, PSC), which have the potential to recur in 20–30% of patients. In some cases features of a non-specific chronic hepatitis have preceded the development of more typical histological features or other diagnostic markers of

Table 16.12	Causes of chronic hepatitis in the liver allograft

Viral disease (recurrent or acquired)
— Hepatitis B
— Hepatitis C
— Other

Recurrent autoimmune disease
— Autoimmune hepatitis
— Primary biliary cirrhosis
— Primary sclerosing cholangitis

Drugs

'De novo' autoimmune hepatitis

Rejection (chronic or recurrent late cellular rejection)

'Idiopathic'

recurrent autoimmune disease.[578,584,623] In an increasing number of cases histological findings of post-transplant hepatitis are associated with the development of autoantibodies, suggesting a diagnosis of acquired autoimmune hepatitis. In one study drug toxicity was considered as the most likely aetiology in 7 of 31 cases with otherwise unexplained post-transplant hepatitis.[728]

By a process of exclusion, in those cases where no other cause for chronic hepatitis can be identified, it is possible that this represents a modified form of rejection.[620] Whilst typical features of acute or chronic rejection are not seen, some biopsies with predominantly hepatitic features have other changes raising the possibility of rejection. It has also been suggested that late cellular rejection may have features which differ from those typically seen in early acute rejection and more closely resemble those occurring in chronic viral or autoimumune hepatitis.[104,167,183,218] Admitted or suspected non-compliance with the immunosuppressive regimen often provide circumstantial evidence to underpin this interpretation. In our experience non-compliance may produce a form of recurrent cellular rejection leading to progressive fibrosis with architectural distortion. In that respect a detailed clinical history is important; drug levels in the serum may be misleading as the patients are bound to have resumed therapy before coming to the hospital.

Other miscellaneous findings in post-transplant liver biopsies

A number of other histological findings of uncertain pathogenesis and functional significance have been documented in reviews of post-transplant liver pathology.[23,167,199,251,385] Subtle architectural abnormalities are a common finding and include thickening of cell plates, minor degrees of lobular disarray, sinusoidal dilatation/congestion and sinusoidal fibrosis. It is possible that some of these changes reflect disorders of blood clotting and/or drug toxicity.

The transient development of alpha-1-antitrypsin globules has been seen in post-transplant biopsies on rare occasions.[730] Aggregates of haemopoietic stem cells are commonly found in post-transplant liver biopsies.[731,732] Donor age has been identified as a risk factor for the development of fibrosis in the liver allograft irrespective of the underlying disease process.[199]

Drug toxicity in liver allograft recipients

Many of the drugs administered to liver transplant patients, including the immunosuppressive agents, are potentially hepatotoxic (see Chapter 14). The diagnosis of drug toxicity in liver allograft recipients is difficult due to problems in distinguishing it from other complications of liver transplantation. Much of the best evidence for hepatotoxicity related to immunosuppressive drugs has come from studies of recipients of non-liver allografts. In addition to direct effects of hepatotoxicity, immunosuppressive drugs also have important effects in modulating other graft complications including recurrent and acquired viral and autoimmune diseases.

Cyclosporin A (CsA)

Studies of CsA carried out mainly on animals have shown predominantly centrilobular (zone 3) lesions including hepatocyte ballooning, cholestasis and spotty hepatocellular necrosis.[733,734] Similar changes have also been reported in occasional human subjects.[735] Possible mechanisms of CsA induced hepatotoxicity include impairment of hepatocellular antioxidant enzyme activities[736] or disorganization of the canalicular bile salt export pump transporter mechanism.[737] CsA has been shown experimentally to enhance hepatocyte regeneration[738] and has been postulated as a possible cause of otherwise unexplained nodular changes in late post-transplant biopsies.[23]

Azathioprine

Azathioprine has been associated with a range of lesions related to vascular and/or sinusoidal endothelial cell injury.[23,739,740] These include sinusoidal dilatation and peliosis hepatis, veno-occlusive disease, centrilobular necrosis and nodular regenerative hyperplasia (Fig. 16.27). In some cases reversal of liver injury has occurred following withdrawal of the drug.[739,740] There is some evidence to suggest that azathioprine may also be directly toxic to hepatocytes.[741] Other liver lesions which have been attributed to azathioprine include cholestasis and mild hepatitic changes.[739,742]

Corticosteroids

Corticosteroids have been associated with the development of nodular regenerative hyperplasia (NRH) in the liver[743] and have been implicated in the pathogenesis of NRH occurring in renal and bone marrow allograft recipients.[744]

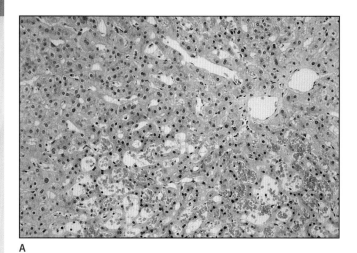

A

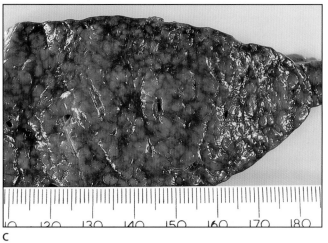

B

C

Fig. 16.27 • Presumed azathioprine-related liver injury. **(A)** Early changes showing sinusoidal dilatation and congestion with thinning of intervening liver cell plates at nine months after transplantation. H&E. **(B)** Nodular regenerative hyperplasia in a needle biopsy specimen taken 2.5 years after liver transplantation. Silver method for reticulin. **(C)** Cut section of an allograft removed 6.5 years after orthotopic liver transplantation showing multiple yellow-tan nodules, which stand up on a background of dark red congested parenchyma devoid of significant fibrosis, a pattern characteristic of nodular regenerative hyperplasia.

Tacrolimus (FK506)

Tacrolimus has hepatotrophic effects[745] and has been suggested as a possible cause of nodular changes in late post-transplant biopsies.[23] It has also been implicated in the pathology of centrilobular necrosis in the liver allograft,[746] although this is controversial.[173]

Other immunosuppressive agents

Sirolimus (rapamycin) has been reported to cause abnormalities of liver enzymes[747] and in one study was implicated as a risk factor for hepatic artery thrombosis.[748]

Cytological monitoring of liver allografts

Several studies have suggested that fine needle aspiration (FNA) cytology may be useful as an adjunct to conventional histology in the post-operative assessment of liver allograft recipients, the main application being in the diagnosis of acute rejection.[749–757]

The cytological diagnosis of rejection is based on comparing differential white cell counts in liver aspirates with those in peripheral blood, in a manner similar to that previously described for renal allografts.[758] Correction factors are applied to give increased weighting to cells which are thought to have the greatest significance for the cytological diagnosis of rejection: these are activated lymphoid cells and lymphoid blast cells, which are characteristically seen during the early stages of acute rejection and mononuclear phagocytes which predominate during the later stages of acute rejection and may also be a feature of chronic rejection.[750,751,759,760] The corrected scores for individual cell types are then added to produce a total inflammatory score. Hepatocytes obtained from rejecting liver allografts may also show a number of changes including swelling and vacuolation, accumulation of bile pigment and individual cell necrosis, although these are not specific for rejection.[749,750] Although the presence of large numbers of monocytes/macrophages suggests the development of chronic rejection, this finding lacks diagnostic specificity, and needle biopsy histology is required to make a definitive diagnosis of chronic rejection.[761]

A good correlation between the cytological and histological diagnosis of rejection has generally been observed.[17,751–753] The main theoretical advantage of the FNA technique is its low invasiveness, thus enabling frequent samples to be obtained and an early diagnosis of acute rejection to be made, before other clinical or biochemical signs are present.[755] Subsequent therapeutic responses can also be monitored closely. However, as additional immunosuppression is only required when cellular infiltrates in the liver are accompanied by other signs of graft dysfunction, the facility which FNA provides for frequent sampling has little clinical importance and most centres do not carry out cytological monitoring of liver allografts.

Cytology is less useful in the diagnosis of other complications of liver transplantation. Bacterial infections may be associated with neutrophilia in liver aspirates.[762] Viral infections, including cytomegalovirus, hepatitis B and hepatitis C, are typically associated with increased numbers of lymphoid cells in liver aspirates.[763,764] This may give rise to problems with the differential diagnosis of rejection. However, in viral infection the infiltrate is composed mainly of small lymphocytes with fewer activated cells or blast cells and total inflammatory scores are thus typically lower than those occurring in acute rejection.[763] Isometric vacuolation of hepatocytes has been described as a manifestation of cyclosporin A toxicity.[750]

Samples of bile have also been used for the cytological assessment of rejection and other complications of liver transplantation.[166,765] High cellularity has been noted during episodes of primary non-function, sepsis and rejection. A predominance of neutrophils is a feature of acute rejection and sepsis.

Liver disease after bone marrow transplantation

General aspects

Liver disease occurs in up to 80% of patients undergoing bone marrow transplantation (BMT)[766-768] and is the main cause of death following BMT.[769] The most serious hepatic complication in the first few weeks following BMT is veno-occlusive disease (VOD) related to the use of chemotherapy and total body irradiation to ablate recipient bone marrow prior to donor bone marrow infusion.[770,771] Recent studies have suggested that the primary site of toxic injury is sinusoidal endothelial cells and the term 'sinusoidal obstruction syndrome' has been proposed as an alternative to VOD.[772] Chemoradiation has also been implicated in the pathogenesis of nodular regenerative hyperplasia following BMT.[744] These vascular complications are discussed elsewhere (see Chapter 13). Bone marrow allograft recipients are also susceptible to a number of opportunistic infections, some of which may involve the liver.[773] Common causes of chronic liver disease post-BMT are chronic viral hepatitis (mainly hepatitis C), iron overload and chronic graft versus host disease (GVHD). In many cases liver disease has a mulifactorial aetiology.[774]

Graft versus host disease

GVHD is most commonly seen as a complication of bone marrow transplantation, where it occurs as a result of infusion of allogeneic donor lymphoid cells into an immunocompromised recipient. It can also occur rarely following infusion of autologous haempoietic cell transplantation.[775] GVHD has also been seen less frequently in other groups of immunocompromised individuals. These include immunosuppressed patients transfused with non-irradiated blood products, premature or low birth weight neonates due to transplacental transfer of maternal T cells and recipients of

solid organ grafts due to transplantation of lymphoid tissues contained in the donor organs.[776-780] GVHD is an important complication of small bowel transplantation due to the large amount of native lymphoid tissue contained in the donor organ. It has also been seen as a rare complication of liver transplantation.[781]

GVHD develops in approximately 30–60% of BMT patients.[780] Liver involvement typically occurs as part of a multisystem disorder associated with cutaneous and gastrointestinal complications. However, hepatic GVHD can rarely occur in the absence of any other obvious organ involvement.[768,782,783]

GVHD is divided into acute and chronic forms.[784,785] Acute GVHD occurs during the first few weeks following BMT and mainly affects the skin, liver and gastrointestinal tract. Chronic GVHD is usually defined as disease occurring more than 100 days following BMT and tends to involve a greater range of tissues including not only the three sites affected in acute GVHD, but also salivary glands, lymph nodes, mouth, eyes, lungs and the musculoskeletal system.

Hepatic involvement in GVHD is characterized by jaundice and cholestatic liver biochemistry. Serum alkaline phosphatase and bilirubin levels may reach up to 20 times the upper limit of normal.[768] Transaminitis is typically mild. In a small proportion of cases, GVHD presents with features of acute hepatitis,[786-791] in which case peak transaminase levels frequently exceed 1000 U/L. In most cases presentation with features of acute hepatitis appears to be related to recent reduction in immunosuppressive therapy. Neither the cholestatic nor the hepatitic biochemical changes seen in classical and hepatitic variants of GVHD respectively are sufficiently specific to make a definite diagnosis and histological confirmation is therefore required.

GVHD is typically associated with a predominantly mononuclear portal inflammatory infiltrate. Immunohistochemical studies have shown that the infiltrate is rich in CD8 positive cytotoxic T lymphocytes and CD57 positive natural killer cells.[792-794] The majority of infiltrating T cells have the memory phenotype and show alpha/beta expression.[795] In contrast to liver allograft rejection where portal inflammatory infiltrates are frequently dense, the portal infiltrate in GVHD is typically mild.[796]

Bile duct damage is the most characteristic histological feature of GVHD. During the early stages there is bile duct atypia characterized by nuclear pleomorphism, cytoplasmic vacuolation and disordered polarity resembling the 'dysplastic'-like changes which occur during the early stages of chronic liver allograft rejection (Fig. 16.28(A)). Oncocytic metaplasia of biliary epithelium has also been reported as a feature of hepatic GVHD.[797] Immunohistochemial studies have shown increased expression of class II MHC antigens on bile ducts in GVHD,[793,798] which may enhance their susceptibility to immune-mediated damage. Other studies have suggested that hepatic dendritic cells may be the main targets for immune responses in GVHD and that bile ducts, present in close proximity to portal dendritic cells, may be damaged as innocent bystanders.[799-800] In some cases there is progressive destruction of interlobular bile ducts, possibly

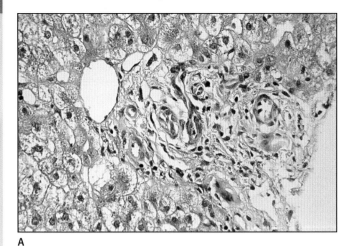

A

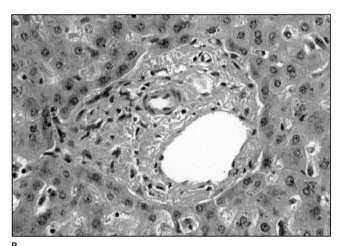

B

Fig. 16.28 • Bile duct lesions in graft versus host disease. **(A)** Early GVHD. Bile duct shows nuclear pleomorphism and disordered polarity producing a 'dysplastic' appearance, closely resembling the changes seen in early chronic liver allograft rejection (see Fig. 16.9(a)). Portal inflammatory changes are only mild. **(B)** Chronic graft versus host disease associated with a vanishing bile duct syndrome. In this hepatectomy specimen obtained at liver transplantation, the majority of portal tracts lacked recognisable bile ducts. In common with chronic liver allograft rejection there is a lack of ductular reaction or periportal fibrosis. H&E.

related to Fas mediated apoptosis.[801] In common with chronic liver allograft rejection, bile duct loss is not generally accompanied by bile ductular reaction or periportal fibrosis[802] (Fig. 16.28(B)). However, occasional cases of chronic GVHD with a biliary pattern of cirrhosis have been described.[803–805]

Mild spotty parenchymal inflammation and hepatocyte apoptosis are also commonly seen in typical cases of graft versus host disease.[806] More prominent lobular inflammatory changes are seen in cases presenting with hepatitic features and closely resemble changes occurring in acute viral hepatitis.[786] In some cases these may also be perivenular areas of confluent necrosis. Cases with hepatitic features also have characteristic portal features of GVHD, including degenerative changes in bile ducts.[786–791] Early diagnosis and distinction from acute viral hepatitis is important as delay in increasing immunosuppression may lead to the development of progressive cholestasis with loss of bile ducts, despite resolution of hepatitic features. Venous endothelial

inflammation has also been reported as a feature of acute hepatic graft versus host disease,[785,807] but in most cases is not prominent.

Hepatitis B and C infections in bone marrow transplantation

Hepatitis B infection behaves more aggressively following bone marrow transplantation, presumably related to immunosuppression. Cases of fulminant hepatic failure and fibrosing cholestatic hepatitis have been described in the context.[808–810]

Hepatitis C infection has a high prevalence in bone marrow allograft patients, probably related to previous blood transfusion, and is a common cause for liver disease following bone marrow transplantation and is the major cause of cirrhosis in long-term survivors.[769,774,811,812] There may be problems in the clinical distinction between viral hepatitis and other hepatic complications of bone marrow transplantation, particularly GVHD, and liver biopsy is helpful in this situation. The role of HBV and HCV as risk factors for the development of VOD and GVHD post-BMT is uncertain.[813–815]

Iron overload

Siderosis is a common finding in liver biopsies obtained from BMT patients and in the great majority of cases can be attributed to previous blood transfusions. Reversal of iron-induced cirrhosis has been reported in some thalassaemic patients following BMT and iron depletion therapy.[816] There is some evidence to suggest that iron overload may be a factor contributing to liver dysfunction following bone marrow transplantation, including fibrosis progression in hepatitis C positive cases.[817,818] Hepatic GVHD may exacerbate hepatic siderosis in susceptible individuals with HFE mutations, although the mechanism is unclear.[816]

Liver pathology after transplantation of other solid organs

Liver disease is commonly seen in the recipients of other solid organ allografts, principally kidneys and hearts.[819] Pathogenetic factors include pre-existing liver disease (e.g. chronic viral hepatitis related to haemodialysis in renal allograft recipients), the effects of immunosuppression and side effects related to drug toxicity. The spectrum of changes related to immunosuppression in renal and cardiac allograft recipients is broadly similar to that seen following liver transplantation.

Opportunistic Infections

Cytomegalovirus and adenovirus may result in liver damage similar to that seen in liver allograft recipients. Rare cases of fatal adenovirus hepatitis have been reported in renal allograft recipients, including one occurring as a complication of fibrosing cholestatic hepatitis B infection.[820,821]

Herpes simplex hepatitis appears to be much more common in renal or cardiac allograft recipients, and may present during the first 3 weeks after transplantation.[822] Diffuse hepatic involvement is associated with a high mortality.[383]

Human Herpesvirus 6 (HHV-6) infection has been associated with hepatitis in renal and cardiac allograft recipients;[823,824] in one case this was associated with giant cell transformation of biliary epithelium. Single cases of hepatic (visceral) bacillary epithelioid angiomatosis[825] and hepatic cryptococcosis[826] have been documented in cardiac allograft recipients.

Hepatitis B and C are important causes of liver disease in renal allograft recipients. Advanced liver disease at the time of transplant is an important predictor for subsequent liver-related mortality and the presence of established cirrhosis with active viral infection is considered a relative contraindication to renal transplantation.[827] Up to 20% of cardiac allograft recipients may also be infected with HBV or HCV.[828] As the liver is the main site of replication of HBV and HCV, one might expect immunosuppressed patients in whom the liver is retained to have more severe disease than those in whom it is removed. However, this effect is counterbalanced by the retention of an organ with complete MHC matching, which means that MHC-restricted T cell responses are less severely inhibited in renal or cardiac allograft recipients than in liver allograft recipients.

The histological severity of HBV-related liver disease increases following renal transplantation and is associated with more rapid progression to cirrhosis and an increased mortality from liver failure.[829–831] There have been a number of cases of fibrosing cholestatic hepatitis B (FCH) in renal allograft recipients.[832,833] Histological appearances and clinical outcome are similar to those seen in FCH involving liver allografts. Liver disease related to acquired HBV infection in non-liver transplant recipients has also been documented.[834] The incidence and severity appear to be less than in liver allograft recipients, probably because transplanted kidneys and hearts have a much lower viral load than transplanted livers. Reactivation of latent HBV infection has been reported as a rare complication of renal transplantation.[835]

A high prevalence of HCV infection exists among patients undergoing renal transplantation, with rates ranging from 10% to 60%.[836,837] Most cases are related to long-term haemodialysis. HCV is the most common cause of chronic liver dysfunction in renal transplant patients. HCV infection is less commonly seen in cardiac allograft recipients.[838] In most cases disease is mild and resembles that seen in the non-transplanted liver.[836,839] However, some cases develop more aggressive disease with prominent necroinflammatory activity,[840] more prominent fibrosis[841] or rapid progression to cirrhosis.[842] There have also been occasional reports of a severe cholestatic form of HCV infection resembling FCH occurring in cardiac and renal allograft recipients.[552,843,844] A cholestatic syndrome with bile duct damage and loss has been observed in four renal transplant recipients with HCV infection, although the mechanism underlying this association is uncertain.[845] Occasional renal transplant patients have developed features resembling those seen in fibrosing cholestatic hepatitis, in the absence of HBV or HCV infection.[846,847]

References

1. Starzl TE, Groth CG, Brettschneider L, Penn I, Fulginiti VA, Moon JB et al. Orthotopic homotransplantation of the human liver. Ann Surg, 1968; 168:392–415
2. Starzl TE, Koep LJ, Halgrimson CG, Hood J, Schroter GP, Porter KA et al. Fifteen years of clinical liver transplantation. Gastroenterology, 1979; 77:375–388
3. Starzl TE, Iwatsuki S, Van Thiel DH, Gartner JC, Zitelli BJ, Malatack JJ et al. Evolution of liver transplantation. Hepatology, 1982; 2:614–636
4. Adam R, McMaster P, O'Grady JG, Castaing D, Klempnauer JL, Jamieson N et al. Evolution of liver transplantation in Europe: report of the European Liver Transplant Registry. Liver Transpl, 2003; 9:1231–1243
5. Neuberger J. Developments in liver transplantation. Gut, 2004; 53:759–768
6. McMaster P. Transplantation for alcoholic liver disease in an era of organ shortage. Lancet, 2000; 355:424–425
7. Mutimer D, Shaw J, Neuberger J, Skidmore S, Martin B, Hubscher S et al. Failure to incriminate hepatitis B, hepatitis C, and hepatitis E viruses in the aetiology of fulminant non-A non-B hepatitis. Gut, 1995; 36:433–436
8. Ferraz ML, Silva AE, Macdonald GA, Tsarev SA, Di Bisceglie AM, Lucey MR. Fulminant hepatitis in patients undergoing liver transplantation: evidence for a non-A, non-B, non-C, non-D, and non-E syndrome. Liver Transpl Surg, 1996; 2:60–66
9. Ben Ari Z, Samuel D, Zemel R, Baruch Y, Gigou M, Sikuler E et al. Fulminant non-A-G viral hepatitis leading to liver transplantation. Arch Intern Med, 2000; 160:388–392
10. Mazzaferro V, Regalia E, Doci R, Andreola S, Pulvirenti A, Bozzetti F et al. Liver transplantation for the treatment of small hepatocellular carcinomas in patients with cirrhosis. N Engl J Med, 1996; 334:693–699
11. Yao FY, Ferrell L, Bass NM, Bacchetti P, Ascher NL, Roberts JP. Liver transplantation for hepatocellular carcinoma: comparison of the proposed UCSF criteria with the Milan criteria and the Pittsburgh modified TNM criteria. Liver Transpl, 2002; 8:765–774
12. Starzl TE, Demetris AJ, Van Thiel D. Liver transplantation (1). N Engl J Med, 1989; 321:1014–1022
13. Facciuto M, Heidt D, Guarrera J, Bodian CA, Miller CM, Emre S et al. Retransplantation for late liver graft failure: predictors of mortality. Liver Transpl, 2000; 6:174–179
14. Kashyap R, Jain A, Reyes J, Demetris AJ, Elmagd KA, Dodson SF et al. Causes of retransplantation after primary liver transplantation in 4000 consecutive patients: 2 to 19 years follow-up. Transplant Proc, 2001; 33:1486–1487
15. Yoo HY, Maheshwari A, Thuluvath PJ. Retransplantation of liver: primary graft nonfunction and hepatitis C virus are associated with worse outcome. Liver Transpl, 2003; 9:897–904
16. Kim WR, Wiesner RH, Poterucha JJ, Therneau TM, Malinchoc M, Benson JT et al. Hepatic retransplantation in cholestatic liver disease: impact of the interval to retransplantation on survival and resource utilization. Hepatology, 1999; 30:395–400
17. Schlitt HJ, Nashan B, Krick P, Ringe B, Wittekind C, Wonigeit K et al. Intragraft immune events after human liver transplantation. Correlation with clinical signs of acute rejection and influence of immunosuppression. Transplantation, 1992; 54:273–278
18. Hubscher S. Diagnosis and grading of liver allograft rejection: a European perspective. Transplant Proc, 1996; 28:504–507
19. Tippner C, Nashan B, Hoshino K, Schmidt-Sandte E, Akimaru K, Boker KH et al. Clinical and subclinical acute rejection early after liver transplantation: contributing factors and relevance for the long-term course. Transplantation, 2001; 72:1122–1128
20. Bartlett AS, Ramadas R, Furness S, Gane E, McCall JL. The natural history of acute histologic rejection without biochemical graft dysfunction in orthotopic liver transplantation: a systematic review. Liver Transpl, 2002; 8:1147–1153
21. Nakhleh RE, Schwarzenberg SJ, Bloomer J, Payne W, Snover DC. The pathology of liver allografts surviving longer than one year. Hepatology, 1990; 11:465–470
22. Hubscher SG. Chronic hepatitis in liver allografts. Hepatology, 1990; 12:1257–1258
23. Slapak GI, Saxena R, Portmann B, Gane E, Devlin J, Calne R et al. Graft and systemic disease in long-term survivors of liver transplantation. Hepatology, 1997; 25:195–202

24. Pessoa MG, Terrault NA, Ferrell LD, Detmer J, Kolberg J, Collins ML et al. Hepatitis after liver transplantation: the role of the known and unknown viruses. Liver Transpl Surg, 1998; 4:461–468

25. Davison SM, Skidmore SJ, Collingham KE, Irving WL, Hubscher SG, Kelly DA. Chronic hepatitis in children after liver transplantation: role of hepatitis C virus and hepatitis G virus infections. J Hepatol, 1998; 28:764–770

26. Garrido MC, Hubscher SG. Accuracy of staging in primary biliary cirrhosis. J Clin Pathol, 1996; 49:556–559

27. Harrison RF, Hubscher SG. The spectrum of bile duct lesions in end-stage primary sclerosing cholangitis. Histopathology, 1991; 19:321–327

28. Hanau C, Munoz SJ, Rubin R. Histopathological heterogeneity in fulminant hepatic failure. Hepatology, 1995; 21:345–351

29. Choi SH, Lee HH, Lee DS, Choi JH, Heo JS, Lee KW et al. Clinicopathological features of incidental hepatocellular carcinoma in liver transplantation. Transplant Proc, 2004; 36:2293–2294

30. Achkar JP, Araya V, Baron RL, Marsh JW, Dvorchik I, Rakela J. Undetected hepatocellular carcinoma: clinical features and outcome after liver transplantation. Liver Transpl Surg, 1998; 4:477–482

31. Gonzalez-Uriarte J, Valdivieso A, Gastaca M, Errasti G, Campo M, Hernandez MJ et al. Liver transplantation for hepatocellular carcinoma in cirrhotic patients. Transplant Proc, 2003; 35:1827–1829

32. Marsh JW, Jr., Iwatsuki S, Makowka L, Esquivel CO, Gordon RD, Todo S et al. Orthotopic liver transplantation for primary sclerosing cholangitis. Ann Surg, 1988; 207:21–25

33. Brandsaeter B, Isoniemi H, Broome U, Olausson M, Backman L, Hansen B et al. Liver transplantation for primary sclerosing cholangitis; predictors and consequences of hepatobiliary malignancy. J Hepatol, 2004; 40:815–822

34. Markin RS, Wisecarver JL, Radio SJ, Stratta RJ, Langnas AN, Hirst K et al. Frozen section evaluation of donor livers before transplantation. Transplantation, 1993; 56:1403–1409

35. Trevisani F, Colantoni A, Caraceni P, Van Thiel DH. The use of donor fatty liver for liver transplantation: a challenge or a quagmire? J Hepatol, 1996; 24:114–121

36. Rinella ME, Alonso E, Rao S, Whitington P, Fryer J, Abecassis M et al. Body mass index as a predictor of hepatic steatosis in living liver donors. Liver Transpl, 2001; 7:409–414

37. Ryan CK, Johnson LA, Germin BI, Marcos A. One hundred consecutive hepatic biopsies in the workup of living donors for right lobe liver transplantation. Liver Transpl, 2002; 8:1114–1122

38. Koneru B, Dikdan G. Hepatic steatosis and liver transplantation current clinical and experimental perspectives. Transplantation, 2002; 73:325–330

39. Verran D, Kusyk T, Painter D, Fisher J, Koorey D, Strasser S et al. Clinical experience gained from the use of 120 steatotic donor livers for orthotopic liver transplantation. Liver Transpl, 2003; 9:500–505

40. Todo S, Demetris AJ, Makowka L, Teperman L, Podesta L, Shaver T et al. Primary nonfunction of hepatic allografts with preexisting fatty infiltration. Transplantation, 1989; 47:903–905

41. Ploeg RJ, D'Alessandro AM, Knechtle SJ, Stegall MD, Pirsch JD, Hoffmann RM et al. Risk factors for primary dysfunction after liver transplantation–a multivariate analysis. Transplantation, 1993; 55:807–813

42. Seifalian AM, Piasecki C, Agarwal A, Davidson BR. The effect of graded steatosis on flow in the hepatic parenchymal microcirculation. Transplantation, 1999; 68:780–784

43. Ijaz S, Yang W, Winslet MC, Seifalian AM. Impairment of hepatic microcirculation in fatty liver. Microcirculation 2003; 10:447–456

44. Birsner JH, Wan C, Cheng G, Evans ZP, Polito CC, Fiorini RN et al. Steatotic liver transplantation in the mouse: a model of primary nonfunction. J Surg Res, 2004; 120:97–101

45. Fukumori T, Ohkohchi N, Tsukamoto S, Satomi S. The mechanism of injury in a steatotic liver graft during cold preservation. Transplantation, 1999; 67:195–200

46. Hayashi M, Fujii K, Kiuchi T, Uryuhara K, Kasahara M, Takatsuki M et al. Effects of fatty infiltration of the graft on the outcome of living-related liver transplantation. Transplant Proc, 1999; 31:403

47. Nadig SN, Periyasamy B, Shafizadeh SF, Polito C, Fiorini RN, Rodwell D et al. Hepatocellular ultrastructure after ischemia/reperfusion injury in human orthotopic liver transplantation. J Gastrointest Surg, 2004; 8:695–700

48. Peralta C, Rosello-Catafau J. The future of fatty livers. J Hepatol, 2004; 41:149–151

49. Caraceni P, Bianchi C, Domenicali M, Maria PA, Maiolini E, Parenti CG et al. Impairment of mitochondrial oxidative phosphorylation in rat fatty liver exposed to preservation-reperfusion injury. J Hepatol, 2004; 41:82–88

50. Selzner M, Rudiger HA, Sindram D, Madden J, Clavien PA. Mechanisms of ischemic injury are different in the steatotic and normal rat liver. Hepatology, 2000; 32:1280–1288

51. Selzner M, Clavien PA. Failure of regeneration of the steatotic rat liver: disruption at two different levels in the regeneration pathway. Hepatology, 2000; 31:35–42

52. Urena MA, Moreno GE, Romero CJ, Ruiz-Delgado FC, Moreno SC. An approach to the rational use of steatotic donor livers in liver transplantation. Hepatogastroenterology, 1999; 46:1164–1173

53. Imber CJ, St Peter SD, Lopez I, Guiver L, Friend PJ. Current practice regarding the use of fatty livers: a trans-Atlantic survey. Liver Transpl, 2002; 8:545–549

54. Frankel WL, Tranovich JG, Salter L, Bumgardner G, Baker P. The optimal number of donor biopsy sites to evaluate liver histology for transplantation. Liver Transpl, 2002; 8:1044–1050

55. Marsman H, Matsushita T, Dierkhising R, Kremers W, Rosen C, Burgart L et al. Assessment of donor liver steatosis: pathologist or automated software? Hum Pathol, 2004; 35:430–435

56. Adam R, Reynes M, Johann M, Morino M, Astarcioglu I, Kafetzis I et al. The outcome of steatotic grafts in liver transplantation. Transplant Proc, 1991; 23:1538–1540

57. Neil DA, Hubscher SG. Are parenchymal changes in early post-transplant biopsies related to preservation-reperfusion injury or rejection? Transplantation, 2001; 71:1566–1572

58. Imber CJ, St Peter SD, Handa A, Friend PJ. Hepatic steatosis and its relationship to transplantation. Liver Transpl, 2002; 8:415–423

59. Marsman WA, Wiesner RH, Rodriguez L, Batts KP, Porayko MK, Hay JE et al. Use of fatty donor liver is associated with diminished early patient and graft survival. Transplantation, 1996; 62:1246–1251

60. Ferrell L, Bass N, Roberts J, Ascher N. Lipopeliosis: fat induced sinusoidal dilatation in transplanted liver mimicking peliosis hepatis. J Clin Pathol, 1992; 45:1109–1110

61. Garcia Urena MA, Colina Ruiz-Delgado F, Moreno GE, Jimenez RC, Garcia G, I, Loinzaz SC et al. Hepatic steatosis in liver transplant donors: common feature of donor population? World J Surg, 1998; 22:837–844

62. Crowley H, Lewis WD, Gordon F, Jenkins R, Khettry U. Steatosis in donor and transplant liver biopsies. Hum Pathol, 2000; 31:1209–1213

63. Yokoyama I, Todo S, Miyata T, Selby R, Tzakis AG, Starzl TE. Endotoxemia and human liver transplantation. Transplant Proc, 1989; 21:3833–3841

64. Clavien PA, Harvey PR, Strasberg SM. Preservation and reperfusion injuries in liver allografts. An overview and synthesis of current studies. Transplantation, 1992; 53:957–978

65. Adam R, Astarcioglu I, Gigou M, Isaac J, Bismuth H. The influence of the glycogen content of the donor liver on subsequent graft function and survival in rat liver transplantation. Transplantation, 1992; 54:753–756

66. Dietze O, Vogel W, Braunsperger B, Margreiter R. Liver transplantation in idiopathic hemochromatosis. Transplant Proc, 1990; 22:1512–1513

67. Adams PC, Ghent CN, Grant DR, Frei JV, Wall WJ. Transplantation of a donor liver with haemochromatosis: evidence against an inherited intrahepatic defect. Gut, 1991; 32:1082–1083

68. Koskinas J, Portmann B, Lombard M, Smith T, Williams R. Persistent iron overload 4 years after inadvertent transplantation of a haemochromatotic liver in a patient with primary biliary cirrhosis. J Hepatol, 1992; 16:351–354

69. Powell LW. Does transplantation of the liver cure genetic hemochromatosis? J Hepatol, 1992; 16:259–261

70. Dabkowski PL, Angus PW, Smallwood RA, Ireton J, Jones RM. Site of principal metabolic defect in idiopathic haemochromatosis: insights from transplantation of an affected organ. BMJ, 1993; 306:1726

71. Crawford DH, Fletcher LM, Hubscher SG, Stuart KA, Gane E, Angus PW et al. Patient and graft survival after liver transplantation for hereditary hemochromatosis: Implications for pathogenesis. Hepatology, 2004; 39:1655–1662

72. Tillery W, Demetris J, Watkins D, Goldstein R, Poplawski S, Husberg B et al. Pathologic recognition of preservation injury in hepatic allografts with six months follow-up. Transplant Proc, 1989; 21:1330–1331

73. Kakizoe S, Yanaga K, Starzl TE, Demetris AJ. Evaluation of protocol before transplantation and after reperfusion biopsies from human orthotopic liver allografts: considerations of preservation and early immunological injury. Hepatology, 1990; 11:932–941

74. Chazouilleres O, Calmus Y, Vaubourdolle M, Ballet F. Preservation-induced liver injury. Clinical aspects, mechanisms and therapeutic approaches. J Hepatol, 1993; 18:123–134

75. Abraham S, Furth EE. Quantitative evaluation of histological features in 'time-zero' liver allograft biopsies as predictors of rejection or graft failure: receiver-operating characteristic analysis application. Hum Pathol, 1996; 27:1077–1084

76. Gaffey MJ, Boyd JC, Traweek ST, Ali MA, Rezeig M, Caldwell SH et al. Predictive value of intraoperative biopsies and liver function tests for preservation injury in orthotopic liver transplantation. Hepatology, 1997; 25:184–189

77. Clavien PA. Sinusoidal endothelial cell injury during hepatic preservation and reperfusion. Hepatology, 1998; 28:281–285

78. Bilzer M, Gerbes AL. Preservation injury of the liver: mechanisms and novel therapeutic strategies. J Hepatol, 2000; 32:508–515

79. Kang KJ. Mechanism of hepatic ischemia/reperfusion injury and protection against reperfusion injury. Transplant Proc, 2002; 34:2659–2661

80. Jaeschke H, Lemasters JJ. Apoptosis versus oncotic necrosis in hepatic ischemia/reperfusion injury. Gastroenterology, 2003; 125:1246–1257

81. Jaeschke H. Molecular mechanisms of hepatic ischemia-reperfusion injury and preconditioning. Am J Physiol Gastrointest Liver Physiol, 2003; 284:G15–G26

82. Schon MR, Kollmar O, Akkoc N, Matthes M, Wolf S, Schrem H et al. Cold ischemia affects sinusoidal endothelial cells while warm ischemia affects hepatocytes in liver transplantation. Transplant Proc, 1998; 30:2318–2320

83. Sindram D, Porte RJ, Hoffman MR, Bentley RC, Clavien PA. Platelets induce sinusoidal endothelial cell apoptosis upon reperfusion of the cold ischemic rat liver. Gastroenterology, 2000; 118:183–191

84. Straatsburg IH, Boermeester MA, Wolbink GJ, van Gulik TM, Gouma DJ, Frederiks WM et al. Complement activation induced by ischemia-reperfusion in humans: a study in patients undergoing partial hepatectomy. J Hepatol, 2000; 32:783–791

85. Upadhya GA, Strasberg SM. Platelet adherence to isolated rat hepatic sinusoidal endothelial cells after cold preservation. Transplantation, 2002; 73:1764–1770

86. Bellamy MC, Gedney JA, Buglass H, Gooi JH. Complement membrane attack complex and hemodynamic changes during human orthotopic liver transplantation. Liver Transpl, 2004; 10:273–278

87. Balabaud C, Cunha AS, Bioulac-Sage P. Microvascular graft dysfunction. J Hepatol, 2004; 41:340–343

88. Le Moine O, Louis H, Demols A, Desalle F, Demoor F, Quertinmont E et al. Cold liver ischemia-reperfusion injury critically depends on liver T cells and is improved by donor pretreatment with interleukin 10 in mice. Hepatology, 2000; 31:1266–1274

89. Kukan M, Haddad PS. Role of hepatocytes and bile duct cells in preservation-reperfusion injury of liver grafts. Liver Transpl, 2001; 7:381–400

90. Lentsch AB, Kato A, Yoshidome H, McMasters KM, Edwards MJ. Inflammatory mechanisms and therapeutic strategies for warm hepatic ischemia/reperfusion injury. Hepatology, 2000; 32:169–173

91. Benkoel L, Dodero F, Hardwigsen J, Benoliel AM, Bongrand P, Botta-Fridlund D et al. Expression of intercellular adhesion molecule-1. Dig Dis Sci, 2003; 48:2167–2172

92. Ikeda T, Yanaga K, Kishikawa K, Kakizoe S, Shimada M, Sugimachi K. Ischemic injury in liver transplantation: difference in injury sites between warm and cold ischemia in rats. Hepatology, 1992; 16:454–461

93. Patel T, Gores GJ. Apoptosis in liver transplantation: a mechanism contributing to immune modulation, preservation injury, neoplasia, and viral disease. Liver Transpl Surg, 1998; 4:42–50

94. Huet PM, Nagaoka MR, Desbiens G, Tarrab E, Brault A, Bralet MP et al. Sinusoidal endothelial cell and hepatocyte death following cold ischemia-warm reperfusion of the rat liver. Hepatology, 2004; 39:1110–1119

95. Vertemati M, Sabatella G, Minola E, Gambacorta M, Goffredi M, Vizzotto L. Morphometric analysis of primary graft non-function in liver transplantation. Histopathology, 2005; 46:451–459

96. Konno H, Lowe PJ, Hardison WG, Miyai K, Nakamura S, Baba S. Breakdown of hepatic tight junctions during reoxygenation injury. Transplantation, 1992; 53:1211–1214

97. Cutrin JC, Cantino D, Biasi F, Chiarpotto E, Salizzoni M, Andorno E et al. Reperfusion damage to the bile canaliculi in transplanted human liver. Hepatology, 1996; 24:1053–1057

98. Xu WH, Ye QF, Xia SS. Apoptosis and proliferation of intrahepatic bile duct after ischemia-reperfusion injury. Hepatobiliary Pancreat Dis Int, 2004; 3:428–432

99. Strasberg SM, Howard TK, Molmenti EP, Hertl M. Selecting the donor liver: risk factors for poor function after orthotopic liver transplantation. Hepatology, 1994; 20:829–838

100. Snover DC, Sibley RK, Freese DK, Sharp HL, Bloomer JR, Najarian JS et al. Orthotopic liver transplantation: a pathological study of 63 serial liver biopsies from 17 patients with special reference to the diagnostic features and natural history of rejection. Hepatology, 1984; 4:1212–1222

101. Demetris AJ, Lasky S, Van Thiel DH, Starzl TE, Dekker A. Pathology of hepatic transplantation: A review of 62 adult allograft recipients immunosuppressed with a cyclosporine/steroid regimen. Am J Pathol, 1985; 118:151–161

102. Busquets J, Figueras J, Serrano T, Torras J, Ramos E, Rafecas A et al. Postreperfusion biopsies are useful in predicting complications after liver transplantation. Liver Transpl, 2001; 7:432–435

103. Hubscher SG. Histological findings in liver allograft rejection— new insights into the pathogenesis of hepatocellular damage in liver allografts. Histopathology, 1991; 18:377–383

104. Snover DC, Freese DK, Sharp HL, Bloomer JR, Najarian JS, Ascher NL. Liver allograft rejection. An analysis of the use of biopsy in determining outcome of rejection. Am J Surg Pathol, 1987; 11:1–10

105. Khettry U, Backer A, Ayata G, Lewis WD, Jenkins RL, Gordon FD. Centrilobular histopathologic changes in liver transplant biopsies. Hum Pathol, 2002; 33:270–276

106. Nakazawa Y, Walker NI, Kerlin P, Steadman C, Lynch SV, Strong RW et al. Clinicopathological analysis of liver allograft biopsies with late centrilobular necrosis: a comparative study in 54 patients. Transplantation, 2000; 69:1599–1608

107. Ben Ari Z, Pappo O, Mor E. Intrahepatic cholestasis after liver transplantation. Liver Transpl, 2003; 9:1005–1018

108. Williams JW, Vera S, Peters TG, Van Voorst S, Britt LG, Dean PJ et al. Cholestatic jaundice after hepatic transplantation. A nonimmunologically mediated event. Am J Surg, 1986; 151:65–70

109. Adler M, Deprez C, Rickaert F, Gulbis B, Vandestadt J, Lambilliotte JP et al. Cholestatic syndrome due to preservation injury after liver transplantation. Transplant Proc, 1988; 20:644–645

110. Mueller AR, Platz KP, Haak M, Undi H, Muller C, Kottgen E et al. The release of cytokines, adhesion molecules, and extracellular matrix parameters during and after reperfusion in human liver transplantation. Transplantation, 1996; 62:1118–1126

111. el Wahsh M, Fuller F, Sreekumar NS, Burroughs A, Dhillon P, Rolles K et al. Effect of reperfusion on human allograft ICAM-1 expression and its correlation with histological evidence of reperfusion changes. Transplant Proc, 1997; 29:3000–3001

112. Kojima N, Sato M, Suzuki A, Sato T, Satoh S, Kato T et al. Enhanced expression of B7-1, B7-2, and intercellular adhesion molecule 1 in sinusoidal endothelial cells by warm ischemia/ reperfusion injury in rat liver. Hepatology, 2001; 34:751–757

113. Ohkohchi N, Hirano T, Satake M, Satomi S. Immunological reactions in liver graft perireperfusion in living donor liver transplantation—change of expression of adhesion molecules, deposition of immunoglobulins and cytokine level. Hepatogastroenterology, 2003; 50:1090–1096

114. Kwekkeboom J, Kuijpers MA, Bruyneel B, Mancham S, Baar-Heesakkers E, Ijzermans JN et al. Expression of CD80 on Kupffer cells is enhanced in cadaveric liver transplants. Clin Exp Immunol, 2003; 132:345–351

115. Busquets J, Figueras J, Serrano T, Torras J, Ramos E, Rafecas A et al. Postreperfusion biopsy changes predict biliary complications after liver transplantation. Transplant Proc, 2002; 34:256–258

116. Lee YM, O'Brien CB, Yamashiki N, Behro M, Weppler D, Tzakis AG et al. Preservation injury patterns in liver transplantation associated with poor prognosis. Transplant Proc, 2003; 35:2964–2966

117. International Working Party. Terminology for hepatic allograft rejection. International Working Party. Hepatology, 1995; 22:648–654

118. Demetris AJ, Murase N, Nakamura K, Iwaki Y, Yagihashi A, Valdivia L et al. Immunopathology of antibodies as effectors of orthotopic liver allograft rejection. Semin Liver Dis, 1992; 12:51–59

119. Demetris AJ, Nakamura K, Yagihashi A, Iwaki Y, Takaya S, Hartman GG et al. A clinicopathological study of human liver allograft recipients harboring preformed IgG lymphocytotoxic antibodies. Hepatology, 1992; 16:671–681

120. Ge X, Ericzon BG, Nowak G, oHrstrom H, Broome U, Sumitran-Holgersson S. Are preformed antibodies to biliary epithelial cells of clinical importance in liver transplantation? Liver Transpl, 2003; 9:1191–1198

121. Haga H, Egawa H, Shirase T, Miyagawa A, Sakurai T, Minamiguchi S et al. Periportal edema and necrosis as diagnostic histological features of early humoral rejection in ABO-incompatible liver transplantation. Liver Transpl, 2004; 10:16–27

122. Krukemeyer MG, Moeller J, Morawietz L, Rudolph B, Neumann U, Theruvath T et al. Description of B lymphocytes and plasma cells, complement, and chemokines/receptors in acute liver allograft rejection. Transplantation, 2004; 78:65–70

123. Montgomery RA, Hardy MA, Jordan SC, Racusen LC, Ratner LE, Tyan DB et al. Consensus opinion from the antibody working group on the diagnosis, reporting, and risk assessment for antibody-mediated rejection and desensitization protocols. Transplantation, 2004; 78:181–185

124. Demetris AJ, Jaffe R, Tzakis A, Ramsey G, Todo S, Belle S et al. Antibody-mediated rejection of human orthotopic liver allografts. A study of liver transplantation across ABO blood group barriers. Am J Pathol, 1988; 132:489–502

125. Gugenheim J, Samuel D, Fabiani B, Saliba F, Castaing D, Reynes M et al. Rejection of ABO incompatible liver allografts in man. Transplant Proc, 1989; 21:2223–2224

126. Gugenheim J, Samuel D, Reynes M, Bismuth H. Liver transplantation across ABO blood group barriers. Lancet, 1990; 336:519–523

127. Hanto DW, Fecteau AH, Alonso MH, Valente JF, Whiting JF. ABO-incompatible liver transplantation with no immunological graft losses using total plasma exchange, splenectomy, and quadruple immunosuppression: evidence for accommodation. Liver Transpl, 2003; 9:22–30

128. Demetris AJ, Jaffe R, Tzakis A, Ramsey G, Todo S, Belle S et al. Antibody mediated rejection of human liver allografts: transplantation across ABO blood group barriers. Transplant Proc, 1989; 21:2217–2220

129. Nickeleit V, Mihatsch MJ. Kidney transplants, antibodies and rejection: is C4d a magic marker? Nephrol Dial Transplant, 2003; 18:2232–2239

130. Takaya S, Bronsther O, Iwaki Y, Nakamura K, Abu-Elmagd K, Yagihashi A et al. The adverse impact on liver transplantation of using positive cytotoxic crossmatch donors. Transplantation, 1992; 53:400–406

131. Hubscher SG, Adams DH, Buckels JA, McMaster P, Neuberger J, Elias E. Massive haemorrhagic necrosis of the liver after liver transplantation. J Clin Pathol, 1989; 42:360–370

132. McCaughan GW, Huynh JC, Feller R, Painter D, Waugh R, Sheil AG. Fulminant hepatic failure post liver transplantation: clinical syndromes, correlations and outcomes. Transpl Int, 1995; 8:20–26

133. Zimmermann A, Lerut J. Early fulminant graft failure in orthotopic liver transplantation with massive haemorrhagic necrosis. Ital J Gastroenterol, 1995; 27:501–505

134. Burke GW, Cirocco R, Viciana A, Ruiz P, Markou M, Allouch M et al. Early graft loss secondary to massive hemorrhagic necrosis following orthotopic liver transplantation. Evidence for cytokine-mediated univisceral Shwartzman reaction. Transplantation, 1996; 61:1370–1376

135. Astarcioglu I, Gugenheim J, Crafa F, Saint Paul MC, Reynes M. Hyperacute rejection of liver allografts in sensitized rats: role of nonparenchymal liver cells. J Surg Res, 1995; 58:182–188

136. Fung J, Makowka L, Tzakis A, Klintmalm G, Duquesnoy R, Gordon R et al. Combined liver-kidney transplantation: analysis of patients with preformed lymphocytotoxic antibodies. Transplant Proc, 1988; 20:88–91

137. Flye MW, Duffy BF, Phelan DL, Ratner LE, Mohanakumar T. Protective effects of liver transplantation on a simultaneously transplanted kidney in a highly sensitized patient. Transplantation, 1990; 50:1051–1054

138. Therapondos G, Hayes PC. Is this the end for protocol early posttransplant liver biopsies? Liver Transpl, 2002; 8:1154–1155

139. Neuberger J. Incidence, timing, and risk factors for acute and chronic rejection. Liver Transpl Surg, 1999; 5:S30–S36

140. Wiesner RH, Demetris AJ, Belle SH, Seaberg EC, Lake JR, Zetterman RK et al. Acute hepatic allograft rejection: incidence, risk factors, and impact on outcome. Hepatology, 1998; 28:638–645

141. Berlakovich GA, Imhof M, Karner-Hanusch J, Gotzinger P, Gollackner B, Gnant M et al. The importance of the effect of underlying disease on rejection outcomes following orthotopic liver transplantation. Transplantation, 1996; 61:554–560

142. Hayashi M, Keeffe EB, Krams SM, Martinez OM, Ojogho ON, So SK et al. Allograft rejection after liver transplantation for autoimmune liver diseases. Liver Transpl Surg, 1998; 4:208–214

143. Seiler CA, Dufour JF, Renner EL, Schilling M, Buchler MW, Bischoff P et al. Primary liver disease as a determinant for acute rejection after liver transplantation. Langenbecks Arch Surg, 1999; 384:259–263

144. Florman S, Schiano T, Kim L, Maman D, Levay A, Gondolesi G et al. The incidence and significance of late acute cellular rejection (>1000 days) after liver transplantation. Clin Transplant, 2004; 18:152–155

145. McTaggart RA, Terrault NA, Vardanian AJ, Bostrom A, Feng S. Hepatitis C etiology of liver disease is strongly associated with early acute rejection following liver transplantation. Liver Transpl, 2004; 10:975–985

146. Farges O, Saliba F, Farhamant H, Samuel D, Bismuth A, Reynes M et al. Incidence of rejection and infection after liver transplantation as a function of the primary disease: possible influence of alcohol and polyclonal immunoglobulins. Hepatology, 1996; 23:240–248

147. Sugawara Y, Mizuta K, Kawarasaki H, Takayama T, Imamura H, Makuuchi M. Risk factors for acute rejection in pediatric living related liver transplantation: the impact of HLA matching. Liver Transpl, 2001; 7:769–773

148. Sugawara Y, Makuuchi M, Kaneko J, Saiura A, Imamura H, Kokudo N. Risk factors for acute rejection in living donor liver transplantation. Clin Transplant, 2003; 17:347–352

149. Adams DH, Neuberger JM. Patterns of graft rejection following liver transplantation. J Hepatol, 1990; 10:113–119

150. Neuberger J. Liver allograft rejection—current concepts on diagnosis and treatment. J Hepatol, 1995; 23 Suppl 1:54–61

151. Neil DA, Hubscher SG. Histologic and biochemical changes during the evolution of chronic rejection of liver allografts. Hepatology, 2002; 35:639–651

152. Hassoun Z, Shah V, Lohse CM, Pankratz VS, Petrovic LM. Centrilobular necrosis after orthotopic liver transplantation: association with acute cellular rejection and impact on outcome. Liver Transpl, 2004; 10:480–487

153. Hubscher SG, Clements D, Elias E, McMaster P. Biopsy findings in cases of rejection of liver allograft. J Clin Pathol, 1985; 38:1366–1373

154. Williams JW, Peters TG, Vera SR, Britt LG, Van Voorst SJ, Haggitt RC. Biopsy-directed immunosuppression following hepatic transplantation in man. Transplantation, 1985; 39:589–596

155. Eggink HF, Hofstee N, Gips CH, Krom RA, Houthoff HJ. Histopathology of serial graft biopsies from liver transplant recipients. Am J Pathol, 1984; 114:18–31

156. Vierling JM, Fennell RH, Jr. Histopathology of early and late human hepatic allograft rejection: evidence of progressive destruction of interlobular bile ducts. Hepatology, 1985; 5:1076–1082

157. Kemnitz J, Ringe B, Cohnert TR, Gubernatis G, Choritz H, Georgii A. Bile duct injury as a part of diagnostic criteria for liver allograft rejection. Hum Pathol, 1989; 20:132–143

158. Demetris AJ, Qian SG, Sun H, Fung JJ. Liver allograft rejection: an overview of morphologic findings. Am J Surg Pathol, 1990; 14 Suppl 1:49–63

159. International Panel. Banff schema for grading liver allograft rejection: an international consensus document. Hepatology, 1997; 25:658–663

160. Ben Ari Z, Dhillon AP, Garwood L, Rolles K, Davidson B, Burroughs AK. Prognostic value of eosinophils for therapeutic response in severe acute hepatic allograft rejection. Transplant Proc, 1996; 28:3624–3628

161. Nagral A, Ben Ari Z, Dhillon AP, Burroughs AK. Eosinophils in acute cellular rejection in liver allografts. Liver Transpl Surg, 1998; 4:355–362

162. Demetris AJ, Seaberg EC, Batts KP, Ferrell LD, Ludwig J, Markin RS et al. Reliability and predictive value of the National Institute of Diabetes and Digestive and Kidney Diseases Liver Transplantation Database nomenclature and grading system for cellular rejection of liver allografts. Hepatology, 1995; 21:408–416

163. Ferrell LD, Lee R, Brixko C, Bass NM, Lake JR, Roberts JP et al. Hepatic granulomas following liver transplantation. Clinicopathologic features in 42 patients. Transplantation, 1995; 60:926–933

164. Harrison RF, Patsiaoura K, Hubscher SG. Cytokeratin immunostaining for detection of biliary epithelium: its use in counting bile ducts in cases of liver allograft rejection. J Clin Pathol, 1994; 47:303–308

165. Adams DH, Burnett D, Stockley RA, Elias E. Patterns of leukocyte chemotaxis to bile after liver transplantation. Gastroenterology, 1989; 97:433–438

166. Carrasco L, Sanchez-Bueno F, Sola J, Robles R, Rodriguez JM, Ramirez P et al. Use of bile cytology for early diagnosis of complications in orthotopic liver transplantation. Cytopathology, 1998; 9:406–414

167. Pappo O, Ramos H, Starzl TE, Fung JJ, Demetris AJ. Structural integrity and identification of causes of liver allograft dysfunction occurring more than 5 years after transplantation. Am J Surg Pathol, 1995; 19:192–206

168. Nonomura A, Mizukami Y, Matsubara F, Kobayashi K. Clinicopathological study of lymphocyte attachment to endothelial cells (endotheliitis) in various liver diseases. Liver, 1991; 11:78–88

169. Lory J, Zimmermann A. Endotheliitis-like changes in chronic hepatitis C. Histol Histopathol, 1997; 12:359–366

170. Freese DK, Snover DC, Sharp HL, Gross CR, Savick SK, Payne WD. Chronic rejection after liver transplantation: a study of clinical, histopathological and immunological features. Hepatology, 1991; 13:882–891

171. Devlin J, Page AC, O'Grady J, Portmann B, Karani J, Williams R. Angiographically determined arteriopathy in liver graft dysfunction and survival. J Hepatol, 1993; 18:68–73

172. van den Heuvel MC, de Jong KP, van der Horst ML, Poppema S, Slooff MJ, Gouw AS. Impaired regeneration of biliary cells in human chronic liver allograft rejection. Special emphasis on the role of the finest branches of the biliary tree. Liver Transpl, 2004; 10:28–35

173. Krasinskas AM, Ruchelli ED, Rand EB, Chittams JL, Furth EE. Central venulitis in pediatric liver allografts. Hepatology, 2001; 33:1141–1147

174. Gouw AS, van den Heuvel MC, van den Berg AP, Slooff MJ, de Jong KP, Poppema S. The significance of parenchymal changes of acute cellular rejection in predicting chronic liver graft rejection. Transplantation, 2002; 73:243–247

175. Lovell MO, Speeg KV, Halff GA, Molina DK, Sharkey FE. Acute hepatic allograft rejection: a comparison of patients with and without centrilobular alterations during first rejection episode. Liver Transpl, 2004; 10:369–373

176. Quaglia AF, Del Vecchio BG, Greaves R, Burroughs AK, Dhillon AP. Development of ductopaenic liver allograft rejection includes a 'hepatitic' phase prior to duct loss. J Hepatol, 2000; 33:773–780

177. Sebagh M, Blakolmer K, Falissard B, Roche B, Emile JF, Bismuth H et al. Accuracy of bile duct changes for the diagnosis of chronic liver allograft rejection: reliability of the 1999 Banff schema. Hepatology, 2002; 35:117–125

178. Dhillon AP, Burroughs AK, Hudson M, Shah N, Rolles K, Scheuer PJ. Hepatic venular stenosis after orthotopic liver transplantation. Hepatology, 1994; 19:106–111

179. Ludwig J, Gross JB, Jr., Perkins JD, Moore SB. Persistent centrilobular necroses in hepatic allografts. Hum Pathol, 1990; 21:656–661

180. Sebagh M, Debette M, Samuel D, Emile JF, Falissard B, Cailliez V et al. 'Silent' presentation of veno-occlusive disease after liver transplantation as part of the process of cellular rejection with endothelial predilection. Hepatology, 1999; 30:1144–1150

181. Nakazawa Y, Chisuwa H, Mita A, Ikegami T, Hashikura Y, Terada M et al. Life-threatening veno-occlusive disease after living-related liver transplantation. Transplantation, 2003; 75:727–730

182. Martin SR, Russo P, Dubois J, Alvarez F. Centrilobular fibrosis in long-term follow-up of pediatric liver transplant recipients. Transplantation, 2002; 74:828–836

183. Cakaloglu Y, Devlin J, O'Grady J, Sutherland S, Portmann BC, Heaton N et al. Importance of concomitant viral infection during late acute liver allograft rejection. Transplantation, 1995; 59:40–45

184. Farges O, Nocci KA, Sebagh M, Reynes M, Bismuth H. Low incidence of chronic rejection in patients experiencing histological acute rejection without simultaneous impairment in liver function tests. Transplant Proc, 1995; 27:1142–1143

185. Dousset B, Hubscher SG, Padbury RT, Gunson BK, Buckels JA, Mayer AD et al. Acute liver allograft rejection—is treatment always necessary? Transplantation, 1993; 55:529–534

186. Calne RY, White HJ, Yoffa DE, Binns RM, Maginn RR, Herbertson RM et al. Prolonged survival of liver transplants in the pig. Br Med J, 1967; 4:645–648

187. Kamada N, Davies HS, Wight D, Culank L, Roser B. Liver transplantation in the rat. Biochemical and histological evidence of complete tolerance induction in non-rejector strains. Transplantation, 1983; 35:304–311

188. Dousset B, Conti F, Cherruau B, Louvel A, Soubrane O, Houssin D et al. Is acute rejection deleterious to long-term liver allograft function? J Hepatol, 1998; 29:660–668

189. Wiesner RH, Ludwig J, van Hoek B, Krom RA. Current concepts in cell-mediated hepatic allograft rejection leading to ductopenia and liver failure. Hepatology, 1991; 14:721–729

190. Wiesner RH, Batts KP, Krom RA. Evolving concepts in the diagnosis, pathogenesis, and treatment of chronic hepatic allograft rejection. Liver Transpl Surg, 1999; 5:388–400

191. Ludwig J, Hashimoto E, Porayko MK, Therneau TM. Failed allografts and causes of death after orthotopic liver transplantation from 1985 to 1995: decreasing prevalence of irreversible hepatic allograft rejection. Liver Transpl Surg, 1996; 2:185–191

192. Jain A, Demetris AJ, Kashyap R, Blakomer K, Ruppert K, Khan A et al. Does tacrolimus offer virtual freedom from chronic rejection after primary liver transplantation? Risk and prognostic factors in 1048 liver transplantations with a mean follow-up of 6 years. Liver Transpl, 2001; 7:623–630

193. Devlin JJ, O'Grady JG, Tan KC, Calne RY, Williams R. Ethnic variations in patient and graft survival after liver transplantation. Identification of a new risk factor for chronic allograft rejection. Transplantation, 1993; 56:1381–1384

194. Candinas D, Gunson BK, Nightingale P, Hubscher S, McMaster P, Neuberger JM. Sex mismatch as a risk factor for chronic rejection of liver allografts. Lancet, 1995; 346:1117–1121

195. Blakolmer K, Jain A, Ruppert K, Gray E, Duquesnoy R, Murase N et al. Chronic liver allograft rejection in a population treated primarily with tacrolimus as baseline immunosuppression: long-term follow-up and evaluation of features for histopathological staging. Transplantation, 2000; 69:2330–2336

196. Milkiewicz P, Gunson B, Saksena S, Hathaway M, Hubscher SG, Elias E. Increased incidence of chronic rejection in adult patients transplanted for autoimmune hepatitis: assessment of risk factors. Transplantation, 2000; 70:477–480

197. Gupta P, Hart J, Cronin D, Kelly S, Millis JM, Brady L. Risk factors for chronic rejection after pediatric liver transplantation. Transplantation, 2001; 72:1098–1102

198. Nair S, Eustace J, Thuluvath PJ. Effect of race on outcome of orthotopic liver transplantation: a cohort study. Lancet, 2002; 359:287–293

199. Rifai K, Sebagh M, Karam V, Saliba F, Azoulay D, Adam R et al. Donor age influences 10-year liver graft histology independently of hepatitis C virus infection. J Hepatol, 2004; 41:446–453

200. Neuberger JM, Adams DH. Is HLA matching important for liver transplantation? J Hepatol, 1990; 11:1–4

201. Donaldson P, Underhill J, Doherty D, Hayllar K, Calne R, Tan KC et al. Influence of human leukocyte antigen matching on liver allograft survival and rejection: 'the dualistic effect.' Hepatology, 1993; 17:1008–1015

202. Donaldson PT, Thomson LJ, Heads A, Underhill JA, Vaughan RW, Rolando N et al. IgG donor-specific crossmatches are not associated with graft rejection or poor graft survival after liver transplantation. An assessment by cytotoxicity and flow cytometry. Transplantation, 1995; 60:1016–1023

203. Charco R, Vargas V, Balsells J, Lazaro JL, Murio E, Jaurrieta E et al. Influence of anti-HLA antibodies and positive T-lymphocytotoxic crossmatch on survival and graft rejection in human liver transplantation. J Hepatol, 1996; 24:452–459

204. Evans PC, Smith S, Hirschfield G, Rigopoulou E, Wreghitt TG, Wight DG et al. Recipient HLA-DR3, tumour necrosis factor-alpha promoter allele-2 (tumour necrosis factor-2) and cytomegalovirus infection are interrelated risk factors for chronic rejection of liver grafts. J Hepatol, 2001; 34:711–715

205. Dousset B, Conti F, Houssin D, Calmus Y. Acute vanishing bile duct syndrome after interferon therapy for recurrent HCV infection in liver-transplant recipients. N Engl J Med, 1994; 330:1160–1161

206. Feray C, Samuel D, Gigou M, Paradis V, David MF, Lemonnier C et al. An open trial of interferon alfa recombinant for hepatitis C after liver transplantation: antiviral effects and risk of rejection. Hepatology, 1995; 22:1084–1089

207. Van Thiel DH, Bonet H, Gavaler J, Wright HI. Effect of alcohol use on allograft rejection rates after liver transplantation for alcoholic liver disease. Alcohol Clin Exp Res, 1995; 19:1151–1155

208. Hoffmann RM, Gunther C, Diepolder HM, Zachoval R, Eissner HJ, Forst H et al. Hepatitis C virus infection as a possible risk factor for ductopenic rejection (vanishing bile duct syndrome) after liver transplantation. Transpl Int, 1995; 8:353–359

209. Loinaz C, Lumbreras C, Gonzalez-Pinto I, Colina F, Gomez R, Fuertes A et al. High incidence of posttransplant hepatitis and chronic rejection associated with hepatitis C virus infection in liver transplant recipients. Transplant Proc, 1995; 27:1217–1218

210. Soin AS, Rasmussen A, Jamieson NV, Watson CJ, Friend PJ, Wight DG et al. CsA levels in the early posttransplant period—predictive of chronic rejection in liver transplantation? Transplantation, 1995; 59:1119–1123

211. Anand AC, Hubscher SG, Gunson BK, McMaster P, Neuberger JM. Timing, significance, and prognosis of late acute liver allograft rejection. Transplantation, 1995; 60:1098–1103

212. Lautenschlager I, Hockerstedt K, Jalanko H, Loginov R, Salmela K, Taskinen E et al. Persistent cytomegalovirus in liver allografts with chronic rejection. Hepatology, 1997; 25:190–194

213. Gao LH, Zheng SS. Cytomegalovirus and chronic allograft rejection in liver transplantation. World J Gastroenterol, 2004; 10:1857–1861

214. van Hoek B, Wiesner RH, Ludwig J, Paya C. Recurrence of ductopenic rejection in liver allografts after retransplantation for vanishing bile duct syndrome. Transplant Proc, 1991; 23:1442–1443

215. Lowes JR, Hubscher SG, Neuberger JM. Chronic rejection of the liver allograft. Gastroenterol Clin North Am, 1993; 22:401–420

216. Ludwig J, Wiesner RH, Batts KP, Perkins JD, Krom RA. The acute vanishing bile duct syndrome (acute irreversible rejection) after orthotopic liver transplantation. Hepatology, 1987; 7:476–483

217. Demetris A, Adams D, Bellamy C, Blakolmer K, Clouston A, Dhillon AP et al. Update of the International Banff Schema for Liver Allograft Rejection: working recommendations for the histopathologic staging and reporting of chronic rejection. An International Panel. Hepatology, 2000; 31:792–799

218. Kemnitz J, Gubernatis G, Bunzendahl H, Ringe B, Pichlmayr R, Georgii A. Criteria for the histopathological classification of liver allograft rejection and their clinical relevance. Transplant Proc, 1989; 21:2208–2210

219. Demetris AJ, Fung JJ, Todo S, McCauley J, Jain A, Takaya S et al. Conversion of liver allograft recipients from cyclosporine to FK506 immunosuppressive therapy—a clinicopathologic study of 96 patients. Transplantation, 1992; 53:1056–1062

220. Kemnitz J, Mogilevski G, Erhard J, Gubernatis G. Post-transplant livers. Am J Surg, Pathol, 1996; 20:510–513

221. Lunz JG, III, Contrucci S, Ruppert K, Murase N, Fung JJ, Starzl TE et al. Replicative senescence of biliary epithelial cells precedes bile duct loss in chronic liver allograft rejection: increased expression of p21(WAF1/Cip1) as a disease marker and the influence of immunosuppressive drugs. Am J Pathol, 2001; 158:1379–1390

222. Cassiman D, Libbrecht L, Sinelli N, Desmet V, Denef C, Roskams T. The vagal nerve stimulates activation of the hepatic progenitor cell compartment via muscarinic acetylcholine receptor type 3. Am J Pathol, 2002; 161:521–530

223. Nakazawa Y, Jonsson JR, Walker NI, Kerlin P, Steadman C, Lynch SV et al. Fibrous obliterative lesions of veins contribute to progressive fibrosis in chronic liver allograft rejection. Hepatology, 2000; 32:1240–1247

224. Boon AP, Hubscher SG, Lee JA, Hines JE, Burt AD. Hepatic reinnervation following orthotopic liver transplantation in man. J Pathol, 1992; 167:217–222

225. Dhillon AP, Sankey EA, Wang JH, Wightman AK, Mathur S, Burroughs AK et al. Immunohistochemical studies on the innervation of human transplanted liver. J Pathol, 1992; 167:211–216

226. Koukoulis GK, Shen J, Karademir S, Jensen D, Williams J. Cholangiocytic apoptosis in chronic ductopenic rejection. Hum Pathol, 2001; 32:823–827

227. Liu G, Butany J, Wanless IR, Cameron R, Greig P, Levy G. The vascular pathology of human hepatic allografts. Hum Pathol, 1993; 24:182–188

228. Miyagawa-Hayashino A, Tsuruyama T, Haga H, Oike F, Il-Deok K, Egawa H et al. Arteriopathy in chronic allograft rejection in liver transplantation. Liver Transpl, 2004; 10:513–519

229. Oguma S, Belle S, Starzl TE, Demetris AJ. A histometric analysis of chronically rejected human liver allografts: insights into the mechanisms of bile duct loss: direct immunologic and ischemic factors. Hepatology, 1989; 9:204–209

230. Matsumoto Y, McCaughan GW, Painter DM, Bishop GA. Evidence that portal tract microvascular destruction precedes bile duct loss in human liver allograft rejection. Transplantation, 1993; 56:69–75

231. Jain D, Robert ME, Navarro V, Friedman AL, Crawford JM. Total fibrous obliteration of main portal vein and portal foam cell venopathy in chronic hepatic allograft rejection. Arch Pathol Lab Med, 2004; 128:64–67

232. Wanless IR, Wong F, Blendis LM, Greig P, Heathcote EJ, Levy G. Hepatic and portal vein thrombosis in cirrhosis: possible role in development of parenchymal extinction and portal hypertension. Hepatology, 1995; 21:1238–1247

233. Tanaka M, Wanless IR. Pathology of the liver in Budd–Chiari syndrome: portal vein thrombosis and the histogenesis of veno-centric cirrhosis, veno-portal cirrhosis, and large regenerative nodules. Hepatology, 1998; 27:488–496

234. van Hoek B, Wiesner RH, Krom RA, Ludwig J, Moore SB. Severe ductopenic rejection following liver transplantation: incidence, time of onset, risk factors, treatment, and outcome. Semin Liver Dis, 1992; 12:41–50

235. Deligeorgi-Politi H, Wight DG, Calne RY, White DG. Chronic rejection of liver transplants revisited. Transpl Int, 1994; 7:442–447

236. Neil DA, Adams DH, Gunson B, Hubscher SG. Is chronic rejection of liver transplants different from graft arteriosclerosis of kidney and heart transplants? Transplant Proc, 1997; 29:2539–2540

237. Tabatabai L, Lewis WD, Gordon F, Jenkins R, Khettry U. Fibrosis/cirrhosis after orthotopic liver transplantation. Hum Pathol, 1999; 30:39–47

238. Gomez R, Colina F, Moreno E, Gonzalez I, Loinaz C, Garcia I et al. Etiopathogenesis and prognosis of centrilobular necrosis in hepatic grafts. J Hepatol, 1994; 21:441–446

239. Turlin B, Slapak GI, Hayllar KM, Heaton N, Williams R, Portmann B. Centrilobular necrosis after orthotopic liver transplantation: a longitudinal clinicopathologic study in 71 patients. Liver Transpl Surg, 1995; 1:285–289

240. Tsamandas AC, Jain AB, Felekouras ES, Fung JJ, Demetris AJ, Lee RG. Central venulitis in the allograft liver: a clinicopathologic study. Transplantation, 1997; 64:252–257

241. Allen KJ, Rand EB, Hart J, Whitington PF. Prognostic implications of centrilobular necrosis in pediatric liver transplant recipients. Transplantation, 1998; 65:692–698

242. Sher LS, Cosenza CA, Michel J, Makowka L, Miller CM, Schwartz ME et al. Efficacy of tacrolimus as rescue therapy for chronic rejection in orthotopic liver transplantation: a report of the U.S. Multicenter Liver Study Group. Transplantation, 1997; 64:258–263

243. Blakolmer K, Seaberg EC, Batts K, Ferrell L, Markin R, Wiesner R et al. Analysis of the reversibility of chronic liver allograft rejection implications for a staging schema. Am J Surg Pathol, 1999; 23:1328–1339

244. Pfitzmann R, Klupp J, Langrehr JM, Uhl M, Neuhaus R, Settmacher U et al. Mycophenolate mofetil for immunosuppression after liver transplantation: a follow-up study of 191 patients. Transplantation, 2003; 76:130–136

245. Markiewicz M, Kalicinski P, Teisseyre J, Ismail H, Kaminski A, Teisseyre M. Rapamycin in children after liver transplantation. Transplant Proc, 2003; 35:2284–2286

246. Neff GW, Montalbano M, Slapak-Green G, Berney T, Bejarano PA, Joshi A et al. A retrospective review of sirolimus (Rapamune) therapy in orthotopic liver transplant recipients diagnosed with chronic rejection. Liver Transpl, 2003; 9:477–483

247. Hubscher SG, Buckels JA, Elias E, McMaster P, Neuberger J. Vanishing bile-duct syndrome following liver transplantation—is it reversible? Transplantation, 1991; 51:1004–1010

248. Noack KB, Wiesner RH, Batts K, van Hoek B, Ludwig J. Severe ductopenic rejection with features of vanishing bile duct syndrome: clinical, biochemical, and histologic evidence for spontaneous resolution. Transplant Proc, 1991; 23:1448–1451

249. Padbury RT, Gunson BK, Dousset B, Hubscher SG, Buckels JA, Neuberger JM et al. Steroid withdrawal from long-term immunosuppression in liver allograft recipients. Transplantation, 1993; 55:789–794

250. Hubscher SG, Elias E, Buckels JA, Mayer AD, McMaster P, Neuberger JM. Primary biliary cirrhosis. Histological evidence of disease recurrence after liver transplantation. J Hepatol, 1993; 18:173–184

251. Sebagh M, Rifai K, Feray C, Yilmaz F, Falissard B, Roche B et al. All liver recipients benefit from the protocol 10-year liver biopsies. Hepatology, 2003; 37:1293–1301

252. Datta GS, Hudson M, Burroughs AK, Morris R, Rolles K, Amlot P et al. Grading of cellular rejection after orthotopic liver transplantation. Hepatology, 1995; 21:46–57

253. Knodell RG, Ishak KG, Black WC, Chen TS, Craig R, Kaplowitz N et al. Formulation and application of a numerical scoring system for assessing histological activity in asymptomatic chronic active hepatitis. Hepatology, 1981; 1:431–435

254. Ishak K, Baptista A, Bianchi L, Callea F, De Groote J, Gudat F et al. Histological grading and staging of chronic hepatitis. J Hepatol, 1995; 22:696–699

255. Ormonde DG, de Boer WB, Kierath A, Bell R, Shilkin KB, House AK et al. Banff schema for grading liver allograft rejection: utility in clinical practice. Liver Transpl Surg, 1999; 5:261–268

256. Demetris AJ, Ruppert K, Dvorchik I, Jain A, Minervini M, Nalesnik MA et al. Real-time monitoring of acute liver-allograft rejection using the Banff schema. Transplantation, 2002; 74:1290–1296

257. Gouw AS, Houthoff HJ, Huitema S, Beelen JM, Gips CH, Poppema S. Expression of major histocompatibility complex antigens and replacement of donor cells by recipient ones in human liver grafts. Transplantation, 1987; 43:291–296

258. Steinhoff G, Wonigeit K, Sorg C, Behrend M, Mues B, Pichlmayr R. Patterns of macrophage immigration and differentiation in human liver grafts. Transplant Proc, 1989; 21:398–400

259. Ng IO, Chan KL, Shek WH, Lee JM, Fong DY, Lo CM et al. High frequency of chimerism in transplanted livers. Hepatology, 2003; 38:989–998

260. Grassi A, Susca M, Ravaioli M, Grazi GL, D'Errico A, Bontadini A et al. Detection of recipient's cells in liver graft using antibodies to mismatched HLA class I antigens. Liver Transpl, 2004; 10:1406–1414

261. Vierling JM. Immunology of acute and chronic hepatic allograft rejection. Liver Transpl Surg, 1999; 5:S1–S20

262. Martinez OM, Rosen HR. Basic concepts in transplant immunology. Liver Transpl, 2005; 11:370–381

263. Barbatis C, Kelly P, Greveson J, Heryet A, McGee JO. Immunocytochemical analysis of HLA class II (DR) antigens in liver disease in man. J Clin Pathol, 1987; 40:879–884

264. Hubscher SG, Adams DH, Elias E. Changes in the expression of major histocompatibility complex class II antigens in liver allograft rejection. J Pathol, 1990; 162:165–171

265. Demetris AJ, Qian S, Sun H, Fung JJ, Yagihashi A, Murase N et al. Early events in liver allograft rejection. Delineation of sites of simultaneous intragraft and recipient lymphoid tissue sensitization. Am J Pathol, 1991; 138:609–618

266. Bishop GA, McCaughan GW. Immune activation is required for the induction of liver allograft tolerance: implications for immunosuppressive therapy. Liver Transpl, 2001; 7:161–172

267. Briscoe DM, Sayegh MH. A rendezvous before rejection: where do T cells meet transplant antigens? Nat Med, 2002; 8:220–222

268. Carreno BM, Collins M. The B7 family of ligands and its receptors: new pathways for costimulation and inhibition of immune responses. Annu Rev Immunol, 2002; 20:29–53

269. Quezada SA, Jarvinen LZ, Lind EF, Noelle RJ. CD40/CD154 interactions at the interface of tolerance and immunity. Annu Rev Immunol, 2004; 22:307–328

270. Demetris AJ, Lasky S, Van Thiel DH, Starzl TE, Whiteside T. Induction of DR/IA antigens in human liver allografts. An immunocytochemical and clinicopathologic analysis of twenty failed grafts. Transplantation, 1985; 40:504–509

271. Hubscher SG, Adams DH, Elias E. Beta-2-microglobulin expression in the liver after liver transplantation. J Clin Pathol, 1988; 41:1049–1057

272. Adams DH, Hubscher SG, Shaw J, Rothlein R, Neuberger JM. Intercellular adhesion molecule 1 on liver allografts during rejection. Lancet, 1989; 2:1122–1125

273. Steinhoff G. Major histocompatibility complex antigens in human liver transplants. J Hepatol, 1990; 11:9–15

274. Steinhoff G, Behrend M, Schrader B, Pichlmayr R. Intercellular immune adhesion molecules in human liver transplants: overview on expression patterns of leukocyte receptor and ligand molecules. Hepatology, 1993; 18:440–453

275. Afford SC, Randhawa S, Eliopoulos AG, Hubscher SG, Young LS, Adams DH. CD40 activation induces apoptosis in cultured human hepatocytes via induction of cell surface fas ligand expression and amplifies fas-mediated hepatocyte death during allograft rejection. J Exp Med, 1999; 189:441–446

276. Afford SC, Ahmed-Choudhury J, Randhawa S, Russell C, Youster J, Crosby HA et al. CD40 activation-induced, Fas-dependent apoptosis and NF-kappaB/AP-1 signaling in human intrahepatic biliary epithelial cells. FASEB J 2001; 15:2345–2354

277. Conti F, Calmus Y, Rouer E, Gaulard P, Louvel A, Houssin D et al. Increased expression of interleukin-4 during liver allograft rejection. J Hepatol, 1999; 30:935–943

278. Schirren CA, Jung M, Worzfeld T, Mamin M, Baretton GB, Gruener NH et al. Cytokine profile of liver- and blood-derived nonspecific T cells after liver transplantation: T helper cells type 1/0 lymphokines dominate in recurrent hepatitis C virus infection and rejection. Liver Transpl, 2000; 6:222–228

279. McCaughan GW, Davies JS, Waugh JA, Bishop GA, Hall BM, Gallagher ND et al. A quantitative analysis of T lymphocyte populations in human liver allografts undergoing rejection: the use of monoclonal antibodies and double immunolabeling. Hepatology, 1990; 12:1305–1313

280. Rivero M, Crespo J, Mayorga M, Fabrega E, Casafont F, Pons-Romero F. Involvement of the Fas system in liver allograft rejection. Am J Gastroenterol 2002; 97:1501–1506

281. Nawaz S, Fennell RH. Apoptosis of bile duct epithelial cells in hepatic allograft rejection. Histopathology, 1994; 25:137–142

282. Krams SM, Egawa H, Quinn MB, Martinez OM. Apoptosis as a mechanism of cell death in a rat model of liver allograft rejection. Transplant Proc, 1995; 27:466–467

283. Afford SC, Hubscher S, Strain AJ, Adams DH, Neuberger JM. Apoptosis in the human liver during allograft rejection and end-stage liver disease. J Pathol, 1995; 176:373–380

284. Gapany C, Zhao M, Zimmermann A. The apoptosis protector, bcl-2 protein, is downregulated in bile duct epithelial cells of human liver allografts. J Hepatol, 1997; 26:535–542

285. Tannapfel A, Kohlhaw K, Ebelt J, Hauss J, Liebert U, Berr F et al. Apoptosis and the expression of Fas and Fas ligand (FasL) antigen

286. Goddard S, Williams A, Morland C, Qin S, Gladue R, Hubscher SG et al. Differential expression of chemokines and chemokine receptors shapes the inflammatory response in rejecting human liver transplants. Transplantation, 2001; 72:1957–1967

287. Yang ZF, Ho DW, Chu AC, Wang YQ, Fan ST. Linking inflammation to acute rejection in small-for-size liver allografts: the potential role of early macrophage activation. Am J Transplant, 2004; 4:196–209

288. Hsieh CL, Obara H, Ogura Y, Martinez OM, Krams SM. NK cells and transplantation. Transpl Immunol, 2002; 9:111–114

289. O'Keeffe C, Baird AW, Nolan N, McCormick PA. Mast cell hyperplasia in chronic rejection after liver transplantation. Liver Transpl, 2002; 8:50–57

290. Batts KP, Moore SB, Perkins JD, Wiesner RH, Grambsch PM, Krom RA. Influence of positive lymphocyte crossmatch and HLA mismatching on vanishing bile duct syndrome in human liver allografts. Transplantation, 1988; 45:376–379

291. Donaldson PT, Alexander GJ, O'Grady J, Neuberger J, Portmann B, Thick M et al. Evidence for an immune response to HLA class I antigens in the vanishing-bileduct syndrome after liver transplantation. Lancet, 1987; 1:945–951

292. Demetris AJ, Markus BH, Burnham J, Nalesnik M, Gordon RD, Makowka L et al. Antibody deposition in liver allografts with chronic rejection. Transplant Proc, 1987; 19:121–125

293. Adams DH, Hubscher SG, Burnett D, Elias E. Immunoglobulins in liver allograft rejection: evidence for deposition and secretion within the liver. Transplant Proc, 1990; 22:1834–1835

294. Harrison RF, Reynolds GM, Rowlands DC. Immunohistochemical evidence for the expression of proliferating cell nuclear antigen (PCNA) by non-proliferating hepatocytes adjacent to metastatic tumours and in inflammatory conditions. J Pathol, 1993; 171:115–122

295. Theise ND, Nimmakayalu M, Gardner R, Illei PB, Morgan G, Teperman L et al. Liver from bone marrow in humans. Hepatology, 2000; 32:11–16

296. Avital I, Feraresso C, Aoki T, Hui T, Rozga J, Demetriou A et al. Bone marrow-derived liver stem cell and mature hepatocyte engraftment in livers undergoing rejection. Surgery 2002; 132:384–390

297. Fogt F, Beyser KH, Poremba C, Zimmerman RL, Khettry U, Ruschoff J. Recipient-derived hepatocytes in liver transplants: a rare event in sex-mismatched transplants. Hepatology, 2002; 36:173–176

298. Gao Z, McAlister VC, Williams GM. Repopulation of liver endothelium by bone-marrow-derived cells. Lancet, 2001; 357:932–933

299. Kleeberger W, Rothamel T, Glockner S, Flemming P, Lehmann U, Kreipe H. High frequency of epithelial chimerism in liver transplants demonstrated by microdissection and STR-analysis. Hepatology, 2002; 35:110–116

300. Hove WR, van Hoek B, Bajema IM, Ringers J, van Krieken JH, Lagaaij EL. Extensive chimerism in liver transplants: vascular endothelium, bile duct epithelium, and hepatocytes. Liver Transpl, 2003; 9:552–556

301. Wu T, Cieply K, Nalesnik MA, Randhawa PS, Sonzogni A, Bellamy C et al. Minimal evidence of transdifferentiation from recipient bone marrow to parenchymal cells in regenerating and long-surviving human allografts. Am J Transplant, 2003; 3:1173–1181

302. Starzl TE, Murase N, Demetris A, Trucco M, Fung J. The mystique of hepatic tolerogenicity. Semin Liver Dis, 2000; 20:497–510

303. Reding R, Davies HF. Revisiting liver transplant immunology: from the concept of immune engagement to the dualistic pathway paradigm. Liver Transpl, 2004; 10:1081–1086

304. Mazariegos GV, Reyes J, Marino IR, Demetris AJ, Flynn B, Irish W et al. Weaning of immunosuppression in liver transplant recipients. Transplantation, 1997; 63:243–249

305. Devlin J, Doherty D, Thomson L, Wong T, Donaldson P, Portmann B et al. Defining the outcome of immunosuppression withdrawal after liver transplantation. Hepatology, 1998; 27:926–933

306. Knolle PA, Limmer A. Neighborhood politics: the immunoregulatory function of organ-resident liver endothelial cells. Trends Immunol 2001; 22:432–437

307. Clouston AD, Jonsson JR, Balderson GA, Fawcett J, Lynch SV, Kelso A et al. Lymphocyte apoptosis and cell replacement in human liver allografts. Transplantation, 2002; 73:1828–1834

308. Crispe IN. Hepatic T cells and liver tolerance. Nat Rev Immunol, 2003; 3:51–62

309. Starzl TE, Demetris AJ, Murase N, Ildstad S, Ricordi C, Trucco M. Cell migration, chimerism, and graft acceptance. Lancet, 1992; 339:1579–1582

in rejection and reinfection in liver allograft specimens. Transplantation, 1999; 67:1079–1083

310. Starzl TE, Murase N, Thomson A, Demetris AJ. Liver transplants contribute to their own success. Nat Med, 1996; 2:163–165

311. Sun Z, Wada T, Maemura K, Uchikura K, Hoshino S, Diehl AM et al. Hepatic allograft-derived Kupffer cells regulate T cell response in rats. Liver Transpl, 2003; 9:489–497

312. Lau AH, De Creus A, Lu L, Thomson AW. Liver tolerance mediated by antigen presenting cells: fact or fiction? Gut, 2003; 52:1075–1078

313. Wood KJ, Sakaguchi S. Regulatory T cells in transplantation tolerance. Nat Rev Immunol, 2003; 3:199–210

314. Creput C, Durrbach A, Menier C, Guettier C, Samuel D, Dausset J et al. Human leukocyte antigen-G (HLA-G) expression in biliary epithelial cells is associated with allograft acceptance in liver-kidney transplantation. J Hepatol, 2003; 39:587–594

315. Mutimer D. CMV infection of transplant recipients. J Hepatol, 1996; 25:259–269

316. Kanj SS, Sharara AI, Clavien PA, Hamilton JD. Cytomegalovirus infection following liver transplantation: review of the literature. Clin Infect Dis, 1996; 22:537–549

317. Sampathkumar P, Paya CV. Management of cytomegalovirus infection after liver transplantation. Liver Transpl, 2000; 6:144–156

318. Paya CV, Hermans PE, Wiesner RH, Ludwig J, Smith TF, Rakela J et al. Cytomegalovirus hepatitis in liver transplantation: prospective analysis of 93 consecutive orthotopic liver transplantations. J Infect Dis, 1989; 160:752–758

319. Seehofer D, Rayes N, Tullius SG, Schmidt CA, Neumann UP, Radke C et al. CMV hepatitis after liver transplantation: incidence, clinical course, and long-term follow-up. Liver Transpl, 2002; 8:1138–1146

320. Shibolet O, Ilan Y, Kalish Y, Safadi R, Ashur Y, Eid A et al. Late cytomegalovirus disease following liver transplantation. Transpl Int, 2003; 16:861–865

321. Emery VC. Investigation of CMV disease in immunocompromised patients. J Clin Pathol, 2001; 54:84–88

322. Paya CV, Wiesner RH, Hermans PE, Larson-Keller JJ, Ilstrup DM, Krom RA et al. Risk factors for cytomegalovirus and severe bacterial infections following liver transplantation: a prospective multivariate time-dependent analysis. J Hepatol, 1993; 18:185–195

323. Mutimer DJ, Shaw J, O'Donnell K, Elias E. Enhanced (cytomegalovirus) viral replication after transplantation for fulminant hepatic failure. Liver Transpl Surg, 1997; 3:506–512

324. Humar A, Malkan G, Moussa G, Greig P, Levy G, Mazzulli T. Human herpesvirus-6 is associated with cytomegalovirus reactivation in liver transplant recipients. J Infect Dis, 2000; 181:1450–1453

325. DesJardin JA, Cho E, Supran S, Gibbons L, Werner BG, Snydman DR. Association of human herpesvirus 6 reactivation with severe cytomegalovirus-associated disease in orthotopic liver transplant recipients. Clin Infect Dis, 2001; 33:1358–1362

326. Mendez JC, Dockrell DH, Espy MJ, Smith TF, Wilson JA, Harmsen WS et al. Human beta-herpesvirus interactions in solid organ transplant recipients. J Infect Dis, 2001; 183:179–184

327. Lautenschlager I, Lappalainen M, Linnavuori K, Suni J, Hockerstedt K. CMV infection is usually associated with concurrent HHV-6 and HHV-7 antigenemia in liver transplant patients. J Clin Virol, 2002; 25:S57–S61

328. Colina F, Juca NT, Moreno E, Ballestin C, Farina J, Nevado M et al. Histological diagnosis of cytomegalovirus hepatitis in liver allografts. J Clin Pathol, 1995; 48:351–357

329. Lautenschlager I, Hockerstedt K, Taskinen E. Histologic findings associated with CMV infection in liver transplantation. Transplant Proc, 2003; 35:819

330. Evans PC, Coleman N, Wreghitt TG, Wight DG, Alexander GJ. Cytomegalovirus infection of bile duct epithelial cells, hepatic artery and portal venous endothelium in relation to chronic rejection of liver grafts. J Hepatol, 1999; 31:913–920

331. Theise ND, Conn M, Thung SN. Localization of cytomegalovirus antigens in liver allografts over time. Hum Pathol, 1993; 24:103–108

332. Barkholt LM, Ehrnst A, Veress B. Clinical use of immunohistopathologic methods for the diagnosis of cytomegalovirus hepatitis in human liver allograft biopsy specimens. Scand J Gastroenterol, 1994; 29:553–560

333. Paya CV, Holley KE, Wiesner RH, Balasubramaniam K, Smith TF, Espy MJ et al. Early diagnosis of cytomegalovirus hepatitis in liver transplant recipients: role of immunostaining, DNA hybridization and culture of hepatic tissue. Hepatology, 1990; 12:119–126

334. Macdonald GA, Greenson JK, DelBuono EA, Grady WM, Merion RM, Frank TS et al. Mini-microabscess syndrome in liver transplant recipients. Hepatology, 1997; 26:192–197

335. Lamps LW, Pinson CW, Raiford DS, Shyr Y, Scott MA, Washington MK. The significance of microabscesses in liver transplant biopsies: a clinicopathological study. Hepatology, 1998; 28:1532–1537

336. Paya CV, Wiesner RH, Hermans PE, Larson-Keller JJ, Ilstrup DM, Krom RA et al. Lack of association between cytomegalovirus infection, HLA matching and the vanishing bile duct syndrome after liver transplantation. Hepatology, 1992; 16:66–70

337. Pastacaldi S, Teixeira R, Montalto P, Rolles K, Burroughs AK. Hepatic artery thrombosis after orthotopic liver transplantation: a review of nonsurgical causes. Liver Transpl, 2001; 7:75–81

338. Gunsar F, Rolando N, Pastacaldi S, Patch D, Raimondo ML, Davidson B et al. Late hepatic artery thrombosis after orthotopic liver transplantation. Liver Transpl, 2003; 9:605–611

339. Halme L, Hockerstedt K, Lautenschlager I. Cytomegalovirus infection and development of biliary complications after liver transplantation. Transplantation, 2003; 75:1853–1858

340. Vivarelli M, Cucchetti A, La Barba G, Bellusci R, De Vivo A, Nardo B et al. Ischemic arterial complications after liver transplantation in the adult: multivariate analysis of risk factors. Arch Surg, 2004; 139:1069–1074

341. Rustgi VK. Epstein–Barr viral infection and posttransplantation lymphoproliferative disorders. Liver Transpl Surg, 1995; 1:100–108

342. Knowles DM, Cesarman E, Chadburn A, Frizzera G, Chen J, Rose EA et al. Correlative morphologic and molecular genetic analysis demonstrates three distinct categories of posttransplantation lymphoproliferative disorders. Blood, 1995; 85:552–565

343. McCarthy M, Ramage J, McNair A, Gane E, Portmann B, Pagliuca A et al. The clinical diversity and role of chemotherapy in lymphoproliferative disorder in liver transplant recipients. J Hepatol, 1997; 27:1015–1021

344. Ben Ari Z, Amlot P, Lachmanan SR, Tur-Kaspa R, Rolles K, Burroughs AK. Posttransplantation lymphoproliferative disorder in liver recipients: characteristics, management, and outcome. Liver Transpl Surg, 1999; 5:184–191

345. Hopwood P, Crawford DH. The role of EBV in post-transplant malignancies: a review. J Clin Pathol, 2000; 53:248–254

346. Dockrell DH, Strickler JG, Paya CV. Epstein–Barr virus-induced T cell lymphoma in solid organ transplant recipients. Clin Infect Dis, 1998; 26:180–182

347. George TI, Jeng M, Berquist W, Cherry AM, Link MP, Arber DA. Epstein–Barr virus-associated peripheral T-cell lymphoma and hemophagocytic syndrome arising after liver transplantation: case report and review of the literature. Pediatr Blood Cancer, 2005; 44:270–276

348. Lundell R, Elenitoba-Johnson KS, Lim MS. T-cell posttransplant lymphoproliferative disorder occurring in a pediatric solid-organ transplant patient. Am J Surg Pathol, 2004; 28:967–973

349. Harris NL, Jaffe ES, Diebold J, Flandrin G, Muller-Hermelink HK, Vardiman J et al. The World Health Organization classification of neoplastic diseases of the haematopoietic and lymphoid tissues: Report of the Clinical Advisory Committee Meeting, Airlie House, Virginia, November 1997. Histopathology, 2000; 36:69–86

350. Leblond V, Davi F, Charlotte F, Dorent R, Bitker MO, Sutton L et al. Posttransplant lymphoproliferative disorders not associated with Epstein–Barr virus: a distinct entity? J Clin Oncol, 1998; 16:2052–2059

351. Dotti G, Fiocchi R, Motta T, Gamba A, Gotti E, Gridelli B et al. Epstein–Barr virus-negative lymphoproliferate disorders in long-term survivors after heart, kidney, and liver transplant. Transplantation, 2000; 69:827–833

352. Lones MA, Lopez-Terrada D, Weiss LM, Shintaku IP, Said JW. Donor origin of posttransplant lymphoproliferative disorder localized to a liver allograft: demonstration by fluorescence in situ hybridization. Arch Pathol Lab Med, 1997; 121:701–706

353. Strazzabosco M, Corneo B, Iemmolo RM, Menin C, Gerunda G, Bonaldi L et al. Epstein–Barr virus-associated post-transplant lympho-proliferative disease of donor origin in liver transplant recipients. J Hepatol, 1997; 26:926–934

354. Nuckols JD, Baron PW, Stenzel TT, Olatidoye BA, Tuttle-Newhall JE, Clavien PA et al. The pathology of liver-localized post-transplant lymphoproliferative disease: a report of three cases and a review of the literature. Am J Surg Pathol, 2000; 24:733–741

355. Baron PW, Heneghan MA, Suhocki PV, Nuckols JD, Tuttle-Newhall JE, Howell DN et al. Biliary stricture secondary to donor B-cell lymphoma after orthotopic liver transplantation. Liver Transpl, 2001; 7:62–67

356. Walker RC, Marshall WF, Strickler JG, Wiesner RH, Velosa JA, Habermann TM et al. Pretransplantation assessment of the risk of lymphoproliferative disorder. Clin Infect Dis, 1995; 20:1346–1353

357. Sokal EM, Antunes H, Beguin C, Bodeus M, Wallemacq P, de Ville DG et al. Early signs and risk factors for the increased incidence of

Epstein–Barr virus-related posttransplant lymphoproliferative diseases in pediatric liver transplant recipients treated with tacrolimus. Transplantation, 1997; 64:1438–1442

358. Younes BS, McDiarmid SV, Martin MG, Vargas JH, Goss JA, Busuttil RW et al. The effect of immunosuppression on posttransplant lymphoproliferative disease in pediatric liver transplant patients. Transplantation, 2000; 70:94–99

359. Guthery SL, Heubi JE, Bucuvalas JC, Gross TG, Ryckman FC, Alonso MH et al. Determination of risk factors for Epstein–Barr virus-associated posttransplant lymphoproliferative disorder in pediatric liver transplant recipients using objective case ascertainment. Transplantation, 2003; 75:987–993

360. Heo JS, Park JW, Lee KW, Lee SK, Joh JW, Kim SJ et al. Posttransplantation lymphoproliferative disorder in pediatric liver transplantation. Transplant Proc, 2004; 36:2307–2308

361. McLaughlin K, Wajstaub S, Marotta P, Adams P, Grant DR, Wall WJ et al. Increased risk for posttransplant lymphoproliferative disease in recipients of liver transplants with hepatitis C. Liver Transpl, 2000; 6:570–574

362. Smets F, Bodeus M, Goubau P, Reding R, Otte JB, Buts JP et al. Characteristics of Epstein–Barr virus primary infection in pediatric liver transplant recipients. J Hepatol, 2000; 32:100–104

363. Mutimer D, Kaur N, Tang H, Singhal S, Shaw J, Whitehead L et al. Quantitation of Epstein–Barr virus DNA in the blood of adult liver transplant recipients. Transplantation, 2000; 69:954–959

364. Holmes RD, Sokol RJ. Epstein–Barr virus and post-transplant lymphoproliferative disease. Pediatr Transplant, 2002; 6:456–464

365. Tsai DE, Nearey M, Hardy CL, Tomaszewski JE, Kotloff RM, Grossman RA et al. Use of EBV PCR for the diagnosis and monitoring of post-transplant lymphoproliferative disorder in adult solid organ transplant patients. Am J Transplant, 2002; 2:946–954

366. Leblond V, Choquet S. Lymphoproliferative disorders after liver transplantation. J Hepatol, 2004; 40:728–735

367. Serinet MO, Jacquemin E, Habes D, Debray D, Fabre M, Bernard O. Anti-CD20 monoclonal antibody (Rituximab) treatment for Epstein–Barr virus-associated, B-cell lymphoproliferative disease in pediatric liver transplant recipients. J Pediatr Gastroenterol Nutr, 2002; 34:389–393

368. Yedibela S, Reck T, Niedobitek G, Gramatzki M, Repp R, Hohenberger W et al. Anti-CD20 monoclonal antibody treatment of Epstein–Barr virus-induced intrahepatic lymphoproliferative disorder following liver transplantation. Transpl Int, 2003; 16:197–201

369. Raymond E, Tricottet V, Samuel D, Reynes M, Bismuth H, Misset JL. Epstein–Barr virus-related localized hepatic lymphoproliferative disorders after liver transplantation. Cancer, 1995; 76:1344–1351

370. Randhawa P, Blakolmer K, Kashyap R, Raikow R, Nalesnik M, Demetris AJ et al. Allograft liver biopsy in patients with Epstein–Barr virus-associated posttransplant lymphoproliferative disease. Am J Surg Pathol, 2001; 25:324–330

371. Rizkalla KS, Asfar SK, McLean CA, Garcia BM, Wall WJ, Grant DR. Key features distinguishing post-transplantation lymphoproliferative disorders and acute liver rejection. Mod Pathol, 1997; 10:708–715

372. Nalesnik MA. Posttransplantation lymphoproliferative disorders (PTLD): current perspectives. Semin Thorac Cardiovasc Surg, 1996; 8:139–148

373. Cleary ML, Nalesnik MA, Shearer WT, Sklar J. Clonal analysis of transplant-associated lymphoproliferations based on the structure of the genomic termini of the Epstein–Barr virus. Blood, 1988; 72:349–352

374. Lones MA, Shintaku IP, Weiss LM, Thung SN, Nichols WS, Geller SA. Posttransplant lymphoproliferative disorder in liver allograft biopsies: a comparison of three methods for the demonstration of Epstein–Barr virus. Hum Pathol, 1997; 28:533–539

375. Hubscher SG, Williams A, Davison SM, Young LS, Niedobitek G. Epstein–Barr virus in inflammatory diseases of the liver and liver allografts: an in situ hybridization study. Hepatology, 1994; 20:899–907

376. Randhawa PS, Jaffe R, Demetris AJ, Nalesnik M, Starzl TE, Chen YY et al. Expression of Epstein–Barr virus-encoded small RNA (by the EBER-1 gene) in liver specimens from transplant recipients with post-transplantation lymphoproliferative disease. N Engl J Med, 1992; 327:1710–1714

377. Niedobitek G, Mutimer DJ, Williams A, Whitehead L, Wilson P, Rooney N et al. Epstein–Barr virus infection and malignant lymphomas in liver transplant recipients. Int J Cancer, 1997; 73:514–520

378. Koneru B, Jaffe R, Esquivel CO, Kunz R, Todo S, Iwatsuki S et al. Adenoviral infections in pediatric liver transplant recipients. JAMA, 1987; 258:489–492

379. Michaels MG, Green M, Wald ER, Starzl TE. Adenovirus infection in pediatric liver transplant recipients. J Infect Dis, 1992; 165:170–174

380. Saad RS, Demetris AJ, Lee RG, Kusne S, Randhawa PS. Adenovirus hepatitis in the adult allograft liver. Transplantation, 1997; 64:1483–1485

381. McGrath D, Falagas ME, Freeman R, Rohrer R, Fairchild R, Colbach C et al. Adenovirus infection in adult orthotopic liver transplant recipients: incidence and clinical significance. J Infect Dis, 1998; 177:459–462

382. Brundler MA, Rodriguez-Baez N, Jaffe R, Weinberg AG, Rogers BB. Adenovirus ascending cholangiohepatitis. Pediatr Dev Pathol, 2003; 6:156–159

383. Kusne S, Schwartz M, Breinig MK, Dummer JS, Lee RE, Selby R et al. Herpes simplex virus hepatitis after solid organ transplantation in adults. J Infect Dis, 1991; 163:1001–1007

384. Bissig KD, Zimmermann A, Bernasch D, Furrer H, Dufour JF. Herpes simplex virus hepatitis 4 years after liver transplantation. J Gastroenterol, 2003; 38:1005–1008

385. Demetris AJ, Jaffe R, Starzl TE. A review of adult and pediatric post-transplant liver pathology. Pathol Annu, 1987; 22:347–386

386. Razonable RR, Paya CV. The impact of human herpesvirus-6 and -7 infection on the outcome of liver transplantation. Liver Transpl, 2002; 8:651–658

387. Schlitt HJ, Shi L. Human herpesvirus-6 and liver transplantation. J Hepatol, 2002; 37:681–683

388. Lautenschlager I, Linnavuori K, Hockerstedt K. Human herpesvirus-6 antigenemia after liver transplantation. Transplantation, 2000; 69:2561–2566

389. Lautenschlager I, Harma M, Hockerstedt K, Linnavuori K, Loginov R, Taskinen E. Human herpesvirus-6 infection is associated with adhesion molecule induction and lymphocyte infiltration in liver allografts. J Hepatol, 2002; 37:648–654

390. Rogers J, Rohal S, Carrigan DR, Kusne S, Knox KK, Gayowski T et al. Human herpesvirus-6 in liver transplant recipients: role in pathogenesis of fungal infections, neurologic complications, and outcome. Transplantation, 2000; 69:2566–2573

391. Humar A, Kumar D, Raboud J, Caliendo AM, Moussa G, Levy G et al. Interactions between cytomegalovirus, human herpesvirus-6, and the recurrence of hepatitis C after liver transplantation. Am J Transplant, 2002; 2:461–466

392. Singh N, Husain S, Carrigan DR, Knox KK, Weck KE, Wagener MM et al. Impact of human herpesvirus-6 on the frequency and severity of recurrent hepatitis C virus hepatitis in liver transplant recipients. Clin Transplant, 2002; 16:92–96

393. Feldstein AE, Razonable RR, Boyce TG, Freese DK, El Youssef M, Perrault J et al. Prevalence and clinical significance of human herpesviruses 6 and 7 active infection in pediatric liver transplant patients. Pediatr Transplant, 2003; 7:125–129

394. Yoshikawa T. Human herpesvirus-6 and -7 infections in transplantation. Pediatr Transplant, 2003; 7:11–17

395. Wade JJ, Rolando N, Hayllar K, Philpott-Howard J, Casewell MW, Williams R. Bacterial and fungal infections after liver transplantation: an analysis of 284 patients. Hepatology, 1995; 21:1328–1336

396. Singh N. The changing face of invasive aspergillosis in liver transplant recipients. Liver Transpl, 2002; 8:1071–1072

397. Fung JJ. Fungal infection in liver transplantation. Transpl Infect Dis, 2002; 4:18–23

398. Said A, Safdar N, Lucey MR, Knechtle SJ, D'Alessandro A, Musat A et al. Infected bilomas in liver transplant recipients, incidence, risk factors and implications for prevention. Am J Transplant, 2004; 4:574–582

399. Marco DP, De Cicco L, Gallo G, Llera J, De Santibanez E, D'agostino D. Hepatic arterial thrombosis due to Mucor species in a child following orthotopic liver transplantation. Transpl Infect Dis, 2000; 2:33–35

400. Lowell JA, Coopersmith CM, Shenoy S, Howard TK. Unusual presentations of nonmycotic hepatic artery pseudoaneurysms after liver transplantation. Liver Transpl Surg, 1999; 5:200–203

401. Rela M, Muiesan P, Bhatnagar V, Baker A, Mowat AP, Mieli-Vergani G et al. Hepatic artery thrombosis after liver transplantation in children under 5 years of age. Transplantation, 1996; 61:1355–1357

402. Sieders E, Peeters PM, TenVergert EM, de Jong KP, Porte RJ, Zwaveling JH et al. Early vascular complications after pediatric liver transplantation. Liver Transpl, 2000; 6:326–332

403. Broelsch CE, Frilling A, Testa G, Cicinnati V, Nadalin S, Paul A et al. Early and late complications in the recipient of an adult living donor liver. Liver Transpl, 2003; 9:S50–S53

404. Quiroga J, Colina I, Demetris AJ, Starzl TE, Van Thiel DH. Cause and timing of first allograft failure in orthotopic liver transplantation: a study of 177 consecutive patients. Hepatology, 1991; 14:1054–1062

405. Hubscher SG. Transplant pathology of the liver. Currrent Diagnostic Pathology, 1994; 11:59–69

406. Feld R, Wechsler RJ, Dumsha JZ, Westerberg S, Munoz S, Boiskin I et al. Significance of the computed tomography finding of subcapsular hepatic necrosis in liver transplantation. Abdom Imaging, 1996; 21:161–165

407. Bhattacharjya S, Gunson BK, Mirza DF, Mayer DA, Buckels JA, McMaster P et al. Delayed hepatic artery thrombosis in adult orthotopic liver transplantation–a 12-year experience. Transplantation, 2001; 71:1592–1596

408. Oh CK, Pelletier SJ, Sawyer RG, Dacus AR, McCullough CS, Pruett TL et al. Uni- and multi-variate analysis of risk factors for early and late hepatic artery thrombosis after liver transplantation. Transplantation, 2001; 71:767–772

409. Stange BJ, Glanemann M, Nuessler NC, Settmacher U, Steinmuller T, Neuhaus P. Hepatic artery thrombosis after adult liver transplantation. Liver Transpl, 2003; 9:612–620

410. Heffron TG, Pillen T, Welch D, Smallwood GA, Redd D, Romero R. Hepatic artery thrombosis in pediatric liver transplantation. Transplant Proc, 2003; 35:1447–1448

411. Mas VR, Fisher RA, Maluf DG, Wilkinson DS, Garrett CT, Ferreira-Gonzalez A. Hepatic artery thrombosis after liver transplantation and genetic factors: prothrombin G20210A polymorphism. Transplantation, 2003; 76:247–249

412. Ishigami K, Zhang Y, Rayhill S, Katz D, Stolpen A. Does variant hepatic artery anatomy in a liver transplant recipient increase the risk of hepatic artery complications after transplantation? AJR Am J Roentgenol, 2004; 183:1577–1584

413. Emre S, Soejima Y, Altaca G, Facciuto M, Fishbein TM, Sheiner PA et al. Safety and risk of using pediatric donor livers in adult liver transplantation. Liver Transpl, 2001; 7:41–47

414. Parrilla P, Sanchez-Bueno F, Figueras J, Jaurrieta E, Mir J, Margarit C et al. Analysis of the complications of the piggy-back technique in 1112 liver transplants. Transplantation, 1999; 67:1214–1217

415. Moser MA, Wall WJ. Management of biliary problems after liver transplantation. Liver Transpl, 2001; 7:S46–S52

416. Jagannath S, Kalloo AN. Biliary Complications After Liver Transplantation. Curr Treat Options Gastroenterol 2002; 5:101–112

417. Patkowski W, Nyckowski P, Zieniewicz K, Pawlak J, Michalowicz B, Kotulski M et al. Biliary tract complications following liver transplantation. Transplant Proc, 2003; 35:2316–2317

418. Calne RY. A new technique for biliary drainage in orthotopic liver transplantation utilizing the gall bladder as a pedicle graft conduit between the donor and recipient common bile ducts. Ann Surg, 1976; 184:605–609

419. Heffron TG, Emond JC, Whitington PF, Thistlethwaite JR, Jr., Stevens L, Piper J et al. Biliary complications in pediatric liver transplantation. A comparison of reduced-size and whole grafts. Transplantation, 1992; 53:391–395

420. Sutcliffe R, Maguire D, Mroz A, Portmann B, O'Grady J, Bowles M et al. Bile duct strictures after adult liver transplantation: a role for biliary reconstructive surgery? Liver Transpl, 2004; 10:928–934

421. Colina F, Garcia-Prats MD, Moreno E, Garcia-Munoz H, Ballestin C, Mayordomo JI et al. Amputation neuroma of the hepatic hilum after orthotopic liver transplantation. Histopathology, 1994; 25:151–157

422. Mentha G, Rubbia-Brandt L, Orci L, Becker C, Giostra E, Majno P et al. Traumatic neuroma with biliary duct obstruction after orthotopic liver transplantation. Transplantation, 1999; 67:177–179

423. Sanchez-Urdazpal L, Gores GJ, Ward EM, Maus TP, Buckel EG, Steers JL et al. Diagnostic features and clinical outcome of ischemic-type biliary complications after liver transplantation. Hepatology, 1993; 17:605–609

424. Ludwig J, Batts KP, MacCarty RL. Ischemic cholangitis in hepatic allografts. Mayo Clin Proc, 1992; 67:519–526

425. Sanchez-Urdazpal L, Batts KP, Gores GJ, Moore SB, Sterioff S, Wiesner RH et al. Increased bile duct complications in liver transplantation across the ABO barrier. Ann Surg, 1993; 218:152–158

426. Scotte M, Dousset B, Calmus Y, Conti F, Houssin D, Chapuis Y. The influence of cold ischemia time on biliary complications following liver transplantation. J Hepatol, 1994; 21:340–346

427. Guichelaar MM, Benson JT, Malinchoc M, Krom RA, Wiesner RH, Charlton MR. Risk factors for and clinical course of non-anastomotic biliary strictures after liver transplantation. Am J Transplant, 2003; 3:885–890

428. Sanchez-Urdazpal L, Gores GJ, Ward EM, Maus TP, Wahlstrom HE, Moore SB et al. Ischemic-type biliary complications after orthotopic liver transplantation. Hepatology, 1992; 16:49–53

429. Sebagh M, Farges O, Kalil A, Samuel D, Bismuth H, Reynes M. Sclerosing cholangitis following human orthotopic liver transplantation. Am J Surg Pathol, 1995; 19:81–90

430. Sheng R, Zajko AB, Campbell WL, Abu-Elmagd K. Biliary strictures in hepatic transplants: prevalence and types in patients with primary sclerosing cholangitis vs those with other liver diseases. AJR Am J Roentgenol, 1993; 161:297–300

431. Shah JN, Haigh WG, Lee SP, Lucey MR, Brensinger CM, Kochman ML et al. Biliary casts after orthotopic liver transplantation: clinical factors, treatment, biochemical analysis. Am J Gastroenterol, 2003; 98:1861–1867

432. Kerkar N, Hadzic N, Davies ET, Portmann B, Donaldson PT, Rela M et al. De-novo autoimmune hepatitis after liver transplantation. Lancet, 1998; 351:409–413

433. Jones DE, James OF, Portmann B, Burt AD, Williams R, Hudson M. Development of autoimmune hepatitis following liver transplantation for primary biliary cirrhosis. Hepatology, 1999; 30:53–57

434. Gupta P, Hart J, Millis JM, Cronin D, Brady L. De novo hepatitis with autoimmune antibodies and atypical histology: a rare cause of late graft dysfunction after pediatric liver transplantation. Transplantation, 2001; 71:664–668

435. Heneghan MA, Portmann BC, Norris SM, Williams R, Muiesan P, Rela M et al. Graft dysfunction mimicking autoimmune hepatitis following liver transplantation in adults. Hepatology, 2001; 34:464–470

436. Czaja AJ. Autoimmune hepatitis after liver transplantation and other lessons of self-intolerance. Liver Transpl, 2002; 8:505–513

437. Vergani D, Mieli-Vergani G. Autoimmunity after liver transplantation. Hepatology, 2002; 36:271–276

438. Poupon R, Poupon RE. Retrovirus infection as a trigger for primary biliary cirrhosis? Lancet, 2004; 363:260–261

439. Vento S, Cainelli F. Is there a role for viruses in triggering autoimmune hepatitis? Autoimmun Rev, 2004; 3:61–69

440. Samuel D, Muller R, Alexander G, Fassati L, Ducot B, Benhamou JP et al. Liver transplantation in European patients with the hepatitis B surface antigen. N Engl J Med, 1993; 329:1842–1847

441. Todo S, Demetris AJ, Van Thiel D, Teperman L, Fung JJ, Starzl TE. Orthotopic liver transplantation for patients with hepatitis B virus-related liver disease. Hepatology, 1991; 13:619–626

442. Jurim O, Martin P, Shaked A, Goldstein L, Millis JM, Calquhoun SD et al. Liver transplantation for chronic hepatitis B in Asians. Transplantation, 1994; 57:1393–1395

443. McMillan JS, Bowden DS, Angus PW, McCaughan GW, Locarnini SA. Mutations in the hepatitis B virus precore/core gene and core promoter in patients with severe recurrent disease following liver transplantation. Hepatology, 1996; 24:1371–1378

444. Roche B, Samuel D, Feray C, Majno P, Gigou M, Reynes M et al. Retransplantation of the liver for recurrent hepatitis B virus infection: the Paul Brousse experience. Liver Transpl Surg, 1999; 5:166–174

445. Grottola A, Buttafoco P, Del Buono MG, Cremonini C, Colantoni A, Gelmini R et al. Pretransplantation pre-S2 and S protein heterogeneity predisposes to hepatitis B virus recurrence after liver transplantation. Liver Transpl, 2002; 8:443–448

446. Wong PY, McPeake JR, Portmann B, Tan KC, Naoumov NV, Williams R. Clinical course and survival after liver transplantation for hepatitis B virus infection complicated by hepatocellular carcinoma. Am J Gastroenterol, 1995; 90:29–34

447. Devarbhavi HC, Cohen AJ, Patel R, Wiesner RH, Dickson RC, Ishitani MB. Preliminary results: outcome of liver transplantation for hepatitis B virus varies by hepatitis B virus genotype. Liver Transpl, 2002; 8:550–555

448. Steinmuller T, Seehofer D, Rayes N, Muller AR, Settmacher U, Jonas S et al. Increasing applicability of liver transplantation for patients with hepatitis B-related liver disease. Hepatology, 2002; 35:1528–1535

449. Villamil FG. Prophylaxis with anti-HBs immune globulins and nucleoside analogues after liver transplantation for HBV infection. J Hepatol, 2003; 39:466–474

450. Roche B, Samuel D. Liver transplantation for hepatitis B virus-related liver disease: indications, prevention of recurrence and results. J Hepatol, 2003; 39:S181–S189

451. Roche B, Samuel D. Evolving strategies to prevent HBV recurrence. Liver Transpl, 2004; 10:S74–S85

452. Kim WR, Poterucha JJ, Kremers WK, Ishitani MB, Dickson ER. Outcome of liver transplantation for hepatitis B in the USA. Liver Transpl, 2004; 10:968–974

453. Samuel D. Liver transplantation and hepatitis B virus infection: the situation seems to be under control, but the virus is still there. J Hepatol, 2001; 34:943–945

454. Demetris AJ, Jaffe R, Sheahan DG, Burnham J, Spero J, Iwatsuki S et al. Recurrent hepatitis B in liver allograft recipients. Differentiation between viral hepatitis B and rejection. Am J Pathol, 1986; 125:161–172

455. Davies SE, Portmann BC, O'Grady JG, Aldis PM, Chaggar K, Alexander GJ et al. Hepatic histological findings after transplantation for chronic hepatitis B virus infection, including a unique pattern of fibrosing cholestatic hepatitis. Hepatology, 1991; 13:150–157

456. Phillips MJ, Cameron R, Flowers MA, Blendis LM, Greig PD, Wanless I et al. Post-transplant recurrent hepatitis B viral liver disease. Viral-burden, steatoviral, and fibroviral hepatitis B. Am J Pathol, 1992; 140:1295–1308

457. Demetris AJ, Todo S, Van Thiel DH, Fung JJ, Iwaki Y, Sysyn G et al. Evolution of hepatitis B virus liver disease after hepatic replacement. Practical and theoretical considerations. Am J Pathol, 1990; 137:667–676

458. Hopf U, Neuhaus P, Lobeck H, Konig V, Kuther S, Bauditz J et al. Follow-up of recurrent hepatitis B and delta infection in liver allograft recipients after treatment with recombinant interferon-alpha. J Hepatol, 1991; 13:339–346

459. Samuel D, Bismuth A, Mathieu D, Arulnaden JL, Reynes M, Benhamou JP et al. Passive immunoprophylaxis after liver transplantation in HBsAg-positive patients. Lancet, 1991; 337:813–815

460. Harrison RF, Davies MH, Goldin RD, Hubscher SG. Recurrent hepatitis B in liver allografts: a distinctive form of rapidly developing cirrhosis. Histopathology, 1993; 23:21–28

461. Davison F, Alexander GJ, Trowbridge R, Fagan EA, Williams R. Detection of hepatitis B virus DNA in spermatozoa, urine, saliva and leucocytes, of chronic HBsAg carriers. A lack of relationship with serum markers of replication. J Hepatol, 1987; 4:37–44

462. Feray C, Zignego AL, Samuel D, Bismuth A, Reynes M, Tiollais P et al. Persistent hepatitis B virus infection of mononuclear blood cells without concomitant liver infection. The liver transplantation model. Transplantation, 1990; 49:1155–1158

463. Malacarne F, Webster GJ, Reignat S, Gotto J, Behboudi S, Burroughs AK et al. Tracking the source of the hepatitis B virus-specific CD8 T cells during lamivudine treatment. J Infect Dis, 2003; 187:679–682

464. Tur-Kaspa R, Burk RD, Shaul Y, Shafritz DA. Hepatitis B virus DNA contains a glucocorticoid-responsive element. Proc Natl Acad Sci USA, 1986; 83:1627–1631

465. McMillan JS, Shaw T, Angus PW, Locarnini SA. Effect of immunosuppressive and antiviral agents on hepatitis B virus replication in vitro. Hepatology, 1995; 22:36–43

466. Marinos G, Rossol S, Carucci P, Wong PY, Donaldson P, Hussain MJ et al. Immunopathogenesis of hepatitis B virus recurrence after liver transplantation. Transplantation, 2000; 69:559–568

467. Ling R, Mutimer D, Ahmed M, Boxall EH, Elias E, Dusheiko GM et al. Selection of mutations in the hepatitis B virus polymerase during therapy of transplant recipients with lamivudine. Hepatology, 1996; 24:711–713

468. Berenguer M, Lopez-Labrador FX, Wright TL. Hepatitis C and liver transplantation. J Hepatol, 2001; 35:666–678

469. Berenguer M. Outcome of posttransplantation hepatitis C virus disease—is it the host, the virus, or how we modify the host and/or the virus? Liver Transpl, 2002; 8:889–891

470. McCaughan GW, Zekry A. Pathogenesis of hepatitis C virus recurrence in the liver allograft. Liver Transpl, 2002; 8:S7–S13

471. Garcia-Retortillo M, Forns X, Feliu A, Moitinho E, Costa J, Navasa M et al. Hepatitis C virus kinetics during and immediately after liver transplantation. Hepatology, 2002; 35:680–687

472. Gane EJ, Naoumov NV, Qian KP, Mondelli MU, Maertens G, Portmann BC et al. A longitudinal analysis of hepatitis C virus replication following liver transplantation. Gastroenterology, 1996; 110:167–177

473. Chazouilleres O, Kim M, Combs C, Ferrell L, Bacchetti P, Roberts J et al. Quantitation of hepatitis C virus RNA in liver transplant recipients. Gastroenterology, 1994; 106:994–999

474. Ferrell LD, Wright TL, Roberts J, Ascher N, Lake J. Hepatitis C viral infection in liver transplant recipients. Hepatology, 1992; 16:865–876

475. Feray C, Gigou M, Samuel D, Paradis V, Wilber J, David MF et al. The course of hepatitis C virus infection after liver transplantation. Hepatology, 1994; 20:1137–1143

476. Gane EJ, Portmann BC, Naoumov NV, Smith HM, Underhill JA, Donaldson PT et al. Long-term outcome of hepatitis C infection after liver transplantation. N Engl J Med, 1996; 334:815–820

477. Sanchez-Fueyo A, Restrepo JC, Quinto L, Bruguera M, Grande L, Sanchez-Tapias JM et al. Impact of the recurrence of hepatitis C virus infection after liver transplantation on the long-term viability of the graft. Transplantation, 2002; 73:56–63

478. Gane E. The natural history and outcome of liver transplantation in hepatitis C virus–infected recipients. Liver Transpl, 2003; 9: S28–S34

479. Charlton M, Seaberg E, Wiesner R, Everhart J, Zetterman R, Lake J et al. Predictors of patient and graft survival following liver transplantation for hepatitis C. Hepatology, 1998; 28:823–830

480. Feray C, Gigou M, Samuel D, Ducot B, Maisonneuve P, Reynes M et al. Incidence of hepatitis C in patients receiving different preparations of hepatitis B immunoglobulins after liver transplantation. Ann Intern Med, 1998; 128:810–816

481. Cotler SJ, Gaur LK, Gretch DR, Wile M, Strong DM, Bronner MP et al. Donor-recipient sharing of HLA class II alleles predicts earlier recurrence and accelerated progression of hepatitis C following liver transplantation. Tissue Antigens, 1998; 52:435–443

482. Pessoa MG, Bzowej N, Berenguer M, Phung Y, Kim M, Ferrell L et al. Evolution of hepatitis C virus quasispecies in patients with severe cholestatic hepatitis after liver transplantation. Hepatology, 1999; 30:1513–1520

483. Prieto M, Berenguer M, Rayon JM, Cordoba J, Arguello L, Carrasco D et al. High incidence of allograft cirrhosis in hepatitis C virus genotype 1b infection following transplantation: relationship with rejection episodes. Hepatology, 1999; 29:250–256

484. Papatheodoridis GV, Patch D, Dusheiko GM, Burroughs AK. The outcome of hepatitis C virus infection after liver transplantation—is it influenced by the type of immunosuppression? J Hepatol, 1999; 30:731–738

485. Taniguchi M, Shakil AO, Vargas HE, Laskus T, Demetris AJ, Gayowski T et al. Clinical and virologic outcomes of hepatitis B and C viral coinfection after liver transplantation: effect of viral hepatitis D. Liver Transpl, 2000; 6:92–96

486. Testa G, Crippin JS, Netto GJ, Goldstein RM, Jennings LW, Brkic BS et al. Liver transplantation for hepatitis C: recurrence and disease progression in 300 patients. Liver Transpl, 2000; 6:553–561

487. Ghobrial RM, Steadman R, Gornbein J, Lassman C, Holt CD, Chen P et al. A 10-year experience of liver transplantation for hepatitis C: analysis of factors determining outcome in over 500 patients. Ann Surg, 2001; 234:384–393

488. Wali M, Harrison RF, Gow PJ, Mutimer D. Advancing donor liver age and rapid fibrosis progression following transplantation for hepatitis C. Gut, 2002; 51:248–252

489. Everson GT. Impact of immunosuppressive therapy on recurrence of hepatitis C. Liver Transpl, 2002; 8:S19–S27

490. Berenguer M, Prieto M, San Juan F, Rayon JM, Martinez F, Carrasco D et al. Contribution of donor age to the recent decrease in patient survival among HCV-infected liver transplant recipients. Hepatology, 2002; 36:202–210

491. Berenguer M, Prieto M, Palau A, Rayon JM, Carrasco D, Juan FS et al. Severe recurrent hepatitis C after liver retransplantation for hepatitis C virus-related graft cirrhosis. Liver Transpl, 2003; 9:228–235

492. Wali MH, Heydtmann M, Harrison RF, Gunson BK, Mutimer DJ. Outcome of liver transplantation for patients infected by hepatitis C, including those infected by genotype 4. Liver Transpl, 2003; 9:796–804

493. Everson GT, Trotter J. Role of adult living donor liver transplantation in patients with hepatitis C. Liver Transpl, 2003; 9: S64–S68

494. Lake JR. The role of immunosuppression in recurrence of hepatitis C. Liver Transpl, 2003; 9:S63–S66

495. Shiffman ML, Vargas HE, Everson GT. Controversies in the management of hepatitis C virus infection after liver transplantation. Liver Transpl, 2003; 9:1129–1144

496. Zimmerman MA, Trotter JF. Living donor liver transplantation in patients with hepatitis C. Liver Transpl, 2003; 9:S52–S57

497. Machicao VI, Bonatti H, Krishna M, Aqel BA, Lukens FJ, Nguyen JH et al. Donor age affects fibrosis progression and graft survival after liver transplantation for hepatitis C. Transplantation, 2004; 77:84–92

498. Toniutto P, Fabris C, Bortolotti N, Minisini R, Avellini C, Fumo E et al. Evaluation of donor hepatic iron concentration as a factor of early fibrotic progression after liver transplantation. J Hepatol, 2004; 41:307–311

499. Garcia-Retortillo M, Forns X, Llovet JM, Navasa M, Feliu A, Massaguer A et al. Hepatitis C recurrence is more severe after living donor compared to cadaveric liver transplantation. Hepatology, 2004; 40:699–707

500. Berenguer M. What determines the natural history of recurrent hepatitis C after liver transplantation? J Hepatol, 2005; 42:448–456

501. Greenson JK, Svoboda-Newman SM, Merion RM, Frank TS. Histologic progression of recurrent hepatitis C in liver transplant allografts. Am J Surg Pathol, 1996; 20:731–738

502. Rosen HR, Gretch DR, Oehlke M, Flora KD, Benner KG, Rabkin JM et al. Timing and severity of initial hepatitis C recurrence as predictors of long-term liver allograft injury. Transplantation, 1998; 65:1178–1182

503. Pelletier SJ, Iezzoni JC, Crabtree TD, Hahn YS, Sawyer RG, Pruett TL. Prediction of liver allograft fibrosis after transplantation for hepatitis C virus: persistent elevation of serum transaminase levels versus necroinflammatory activity. Liver Transpl, 2000; 6:44–53

504. Sreekumar R, Gonzalez-Koch A, Maor-Kendler Y, Batts K, Moreno-Luna L, Poterucha J et al. Early identification of recipients with progressive histologic recurrence of hepatitis C after liver transplantation. Hepatology, 2000; 32:1125–1130

505. Guido M, Fagiuoli S, Tessari G, Burra P, Leandro G, Boccagni P et al. Histology predicts cirrhotic evolution of post transplant hepatitis C. Gut, 2002; 50:697–700

506. Gordon FD, Pomfret EA, Pomposelli JJ, Lewis WD, Jenkins RL, Khettry U. Severe steatosis as the initial histologic manifestation of recurrent hepatitis C genotype 3. Hum Pathol, 2004; 35:636–638

507. Machicao VI, Krishna M, Bonatti H, Aqel BA, Nguyen JH, Weigand SD et al. Hepatitis C recurrence is not associated with allograft steatosis within the first year after liver transplantation. Liver Transpl, 2004; 10:599–606

508. Trak-Smayra V, Contreras J, Dondero F, Durand F, Dubois S, Sommacale D et al. Role of replicative senescence in the progression of fibrosis in hepatitis C virus (HCV) recurrence after liver transplantation. Transplantation, 2004; 77:1755–1760

509. Ballardini G, De Raffele E, Groff P, Bioulac-Sage P, Grassi A, Ghetti S et al. Timing of reinfection and mechanisms of hepatocellular damage in transplanted hepatitis C virus-reinfected liver. Liver Transpl, 2002; 8:10–20

510. Baiocchi L, Tisone G, Palmieri G, Rapicetta M, Pisani F, Orlando G et al. Hepatic steatosis: a specific sign of hepatitis C reinfection after liver transplantation. Liver Transpl Surg, 1998; 4:441–447

511. Feray C, Caccamo L, Alexander GJ, Ducot B, Gugenheim J, Casanovas T et al. European collaborative study on factors influencing outcome after liver transplantation for hepatitis C. European Concerted Action on Viral Hepatitis (EUROHEP) Group. Gastroenterology, 1999; 117:619–625

512. Charlton M. The impact of advancing donor age on histologic recurrence of hepatitis C infection: the perils of ignored maternal advice. Liver Transpl, 2003; 9:535–537

513. Berenguer M, Aguilera V, Prieto M, Carrasco D, Rayon M, San Juan F et al. Delayed onset of severe hepatitis C-related liver damage following liver transplantation: a matter of concern? Liver Transpl, 2003; 9:1152–1158

514. Firpi RJ, Abdelmalek MF, Soldevila-Pico C, Cabrera R, Shuster JJ, Theriaque D et al. One-year protocol liver biopsy can stratify fibrosis progression in liver transplant recipients with recurrent hepatitis C infection. Liver Transpl, 2004; 10:1240–1247

515. Saxena R, Ye MQ, Emre S, Klion F, Nalesnik MA, Thung SN. De novo hepatocellular carcinoma in a hepatic allograft with recurrent hepatitis C cirrhosis. Liver Transpl Surg, 1999; 5:81–82

516. Rosen HR. Hepatitis B and C in the liver transplant recipient: current understanding and treatment. Liver Transpl, 2001; 7:S87–S98

517. Gretch DR, Bacchi CE, Corey L, dela RC, Lesniewski RR, Kowdley K et al. Persistent hepatitis C virus infection after liver transplantation: clinical and virological features. Hepatology, 1995; 22:1–9

518. Vargas V, Krawczynski K, Castells L, Martinez N, Esteban J, Allende H et al. Recurrent hepatitis C virus infection after liver transplantation: immunohistochemical assessment of the viral antigen. Liver Transpl Surg, 1998; 4:320–327

519. Nuovo GJ, Holly A, Wakely P, Jr., Frankel W. Correlation of histology, viral load, and in situ viral detection in hepatic biopsies from patients with liver transplants secondary to hepatitis C infection. Hum Pathol, 2002; 33:277–284

520. Verslype C, Nevens F, Sinelli N, Clarysse C, Pirenne J, Depla E et al. Hepatic immunohistochemical staining with a monoclonal antibody against HCV-E2 to evaluate antiviral therapy and reinfection of liver grafts in hepatitis C viral infection. J Hepatol, 2003; 38:208–214

521. Schluger LK, Sheiner PA, Thung SN, Lau JY, Min A, Wolf DC et al. Severe recurrent cholestatic hepatitis C following orthotopic liver transplantation. Hepatology, 1996; 23:971–976

522. Dickson RC, Caldwell SH, Ishitani MB, Lau JY, Driscoll CJ, Stevenson WC et al. Clinical and histologic patterns of early graft failure due to recurrnet hepatitis C in four patients after liver transplantation. Transplantation, 1996; 61:701–705

523. Taga SA, Washington MK, Terrault N, Wright TL, Somberg KA, Ferrell LD. Cholestatic hepatitis C in liver allografts. Liver Transpl Surg, 1998; 4:304–310

524. Doughty AL, Spencer JD, Cossart YE, McCaughan GW. Cholestatic hepatitis after liver transplantation is associated with persistently high serum hepatitis C virus RNA levels. Liver Transpl Surg, 1998; 4:15–21

525. Doughty AL, Painter DM, McCaughan GW. Post-transplant quasispecies pattern remains stable over time in patients with recurrent cholestatic hepatitis due to hepatitis C virus. J Hepatol, 2000; 32:126–134

526. Deshpande V, Burd E, Aardema KL, Ma CK, Moonka DK, Brown KA et al. High levels of hepatitis C virus RNA in native livers correlate with the development of cholestatic hepatitis in liver allografts and a poor outcome. Liver Transpl, 2001; 7:118–124

527. Zekry A, Bishop GA, Bowen DG, Gleeson MM, Guney S, Painter DM et al. Intrahepatic cytokine profiles associated with posttransplantation hepatitis C virus-related liver injury. Liver Transpl, 2002; 8:292–301

528. Cotler SJ, Taylor SL, Gretch DR, Bronner MP, Rizk R, Perkins JD et al. Hyperbilirubinemia and cholestatic liver injury in hepatitis C-infected liver transplant recipients. Am J Gastroenterol, 2000; 95:753–759

529. Sebagh M, Farges O, Emile JF, Bismuth H, Reynes M. An unusual pattern of hepatitis C virus infection in a liver allograft. Histopathology, 1995; 27:190–192

530. Hoso M, Nakanuma Y, Kawano M, Oda K, Tsuneyama K, van de WJ et al. Granulomatous cholangitis in chronic hepatitis C: a new diagnostic problem in liver pathology. Pathol Int, 1996; 46:301–305

531. Barcena R, SanRoman AL, Del Campo S, Garcia M, Moreno A, De Vicente E et al. Posttransplant liver granulomatosis associated with hepatitis C? Transplantation, 1998; 65:1494–1495

532. Gottschlich MJ, Aardema KL, Burd EM, Nakhleh RE, Brown KA, Abouljoud MS et al. The use of hepatitis C viral RNA levels in liver tissue to distinguish rejection from recurrent hepatitis C. Liver Transpl, 2001; 7:436–441

533. Demetris AJ, Eghtesad B, Marcos A, Ruppert K, Nalesnik MA, Randhawa P et al. Recurrent hepatitis C in liver allografts: prospective assessment of diagnostic accuracy, identification of pitfalls, and observations about pathogenesis. Am J Surg Pathol, 2004; 28:658–669

534. Younossi ZM, Boparai N, Gramlich T, Goldblum J, George P, Mayes J. Agreement in pathologic interpretation of liver biopsy specimens in posttransplant hepatitis C infection. Arch Pathol Lab Med, 1999; 123:143–145

535. Regev A, Molina E, Moura R, Bejarano PA, Khaled A, Ruiz P et al. Reliability of histopathologic assessment for the differentiation of recurrent hepatitis C from acute rejection after liver transplantation. Liver Transpl, 2004; 10:1233–1239

536. Charco R, Vargas V, Allende H, Edo A, Balsells J, Murio E et al. Is hepatitis C virus recurrence a risk factor for chronic liver allograft rejection? Transpl, Int, 1996; 9:S195–S197

537. Lumbreras C, Colina F, Loinaz C, Domingo MJ, Fuertes A, Dominguez P et al. Clinical, virological, and histologic evolution of hepatitis C virus infection in liver transplant recipients. Clin Infect Dis, 1998; 26:48–55

538. Saab S, Kalmaz D, Gajjar NA, Hiatt J, Durazo F, Han S et al. Outcomes of acute rejection after interferon therapy in liver transplant recipients. Liver Transpl, 2004; 10:859–867

539. Samuel D. Hepatitis C, interferon, and risk of rejection after liver transplantation. Liver Transpl, 2004; 10:868–871

540. Stravitz RT, Shiffman ML, Sanyal AJ, Luketic VA, Sterling RK, Heuman DM et al. Effects of interferon treatment on liver histology and allograft rejection in patients with recurrent hepatitis C following liver transplantation. Liver Transpl, 2004; 10:850–858

541. Garcia-Retortillo M, Forns X. Prevention and treatment of hepatitis C virus recurrence after liver transplantation. J Hepatol, 2004; 41:2–10

542. Kugelmas M, Osgood MJ, Trotter JF, Bak T, Wachs M, Forman L et al. Hepatitis C virus therapy, hepatocyte drug metabolism, and risk for acute cellular rejection. Liver Transpl, 2003; 9:1159–1165

543. McCaughan GW, Zekry A. Mechanisms of HCV reinfection and allograft damage after liver transplantation. J Hepatol, 2004; 40:368–374

544. Schirren CA, Jung MC, Worzfeld T, Mamin M, Baretton G, Gerlach JT et al. Hepatitis C virus-specific CD4+ T cell response after liver transplantation occurs early, is multispecific, compartmentalizes to the liver, and does not correlate with recurrent disease. J Infect Dis, 2001; 183:1187–1194

545. Schirren CA, Zachoval R, Gerlach JT, Ulsenheimer A, Gruener NH, Diepolder HM et al. Antiviral treatment of recurrent hepatitis C virus (HCV) infection after liver transplantation: association of a strong, multispecific, and long-lasting CD4+ T cell response with HCV-elimination. J Hepatol, 2003; 39:397–404

546. Gruener NH, Jung MC, Ulsenheimer A, Gerlach JT, Zachoval R, Diepolder HM et al. Analysis of a successful HCV-specific CD8+ T cell response in patients with recurrent HCV-infection after orthotopic liver transplantation. Liver Transpl, 2004; 10:1487–1496

547. Weston SJ, Leistikow RL, Reddy KR, Torres M, Wertheimer AM, Lewinsohn DM et al. Reconstitution of hepatitis C virus-specific T-cellmediated immunity after liver transplantation. Hepatology, 2005; 41:72–81

548. Crespo J, Rivero M, Mayorga M, Fabrega E, Casafont F, Gomez-Fleitas M et al. Involvement of the fas system in hepatitis C virus recurrence after liver transplantation. Liver Transpl, 2000; 6:562–569

549. Di MV, Brenot C, Samuel D, Saurini F, Paradis V, Reynes M et al. Influence of liver hepatitis C virus RNA and hepatitis C virus genotype on FAS-mediated apoptosis after liver transplantation for hepatitis C. Transplantation, 2000; 70:1390–1396

550. Rosen HR, Hinrichs DJ, Gretch DR, Koziel MJ, Chou S, Houghton M et al. Association of multispecific CD4(+) response to hepatitis C and severity of recurrence after liver transplantation. Gastroenterology, 1999; 117:926–932

551. Rosen HR. Hepatitis C virus in the human liver transplantation model. Clin Liver Dis 2003; 7:107–125

552. Lim HL, Lau GK, Davis GL, Dolson DJ, Lau JY. Cholestatic hepatitis leading to hepatic failure in a patient with organ-transmitted hepatitis C virus infection. Gastroenterology, 1994; 106:248–251

553. Khettry U, Anand N, Gordon FD, Jenkins RL, Tahan SR, Loda M et al. Recurrent hepatitis B, hepatitis C, and combined hepatitis B and C in liver allografts: a comparative pathological study. Hum Pathol, 2000; 31:101–108

554. Huang EJ, Wright TL, Lake JR, Combs C, Ferrell LD. Hepatitis B and C coinfections and persistent hepatitis B infections: clinical outcome and liver pathology after transplantation. Hepatology, 1996; 23:396–404

555. Sato S, Fujiyama S, Tanaka M, Yamasaki K, Kuramoto I, Kawano S et al. Coinfection of hepatitis C virus in patients with chronic hepatitis B infection. J Hepatol, 1994; 21:159–166

556. Lok AS. Prevention of recurrent hepatitis B post-liver transplantation. Liver Transpl, 2002; 8:S67–S73

557. Ottobrelli A, Marzano A, Smedile A, Recchia S, Salizzoni M, Cornu C et al. Patterns of hepatitis delta virus reinfection and disease in liver transplantation. Gastroenterology, 1991; 101:1649–1655

558. Davies SE, Lau JY, O'Grady JG, Portmann BC, Alexander GJ, Williams R. Evidence that hepatitis D virus needs hepatitis B virus to cause hepatocellular damage. Am J Clin Pathol, 1992; 98:554–558

559. Samuel D, Zignego AL, Reynes M, Feray C, Arulnaden JL, David MF et al. Long-term clinical and virological outcome after liver transplantation for cirrhosis caused by chronic delta hepatitis. Hepatology, 1995; 21:333–339

560. Smedile A, Casey JL, Cote PJ, Durazzo M, Lavezzo B, Purcell RH et al. Hepatitis D viremia following orthotopic liver transplantation involves a typical HDV virion with a hepatitis B surface antigen envelope. Hepatology, 1998; 27:1723–1729

561. O'Grady JG, Smith HM, Davies SE, Daniels HM, Donaldson PT, Tan KC et al. Hepatitis B virus reinfection after orthotopic liver transplantation. Serological and clinical implications. J Hepatol, 1992; 14:104–111

562. Pons JA. Role of liver transplantation in viral hepatitis. J Hepatol, 1995; 22:146–153

563. Marsman WA, Wiesner RH, Batts KP, Poterucha JJ, Porayko MK, Niesters HG et al. Fulminant hepatitis B virus: recurrence after liver transplantation in two patients also infected with hepatitis delta virus. Hepatology, 1997; 25:434–438

564. Fagan E, Yousef G, Brahm J, Garelick H, Mann G, Wolstenholme A et al. Persistence of hepatitis A virus in fulminant hepatitis and after liver transplantation. J Med Virol, 1990; 30:131–136

565. Gane E, Sallie R, Saleh M, Portmann B, Williams R. Clinical recurrence of hepatitis A following liver transplantation for acute liver failure. J Med Virol, 1995; 45:35–39

566. Fagan EA, Ellis DS, Tovey GM, Lloyd G, Smith HM, Portmann B et al. Toga virus-like particles in acute liver failure attributed to sporadic non-A, non-B hepatitis and recurrence after liver transplantation. J Med Virol, 1992; 38:71–77

567. Berenguer M, Terrault NA, Piatak M, Yun A, Kim JP, Lau JY et al. Hepatitis G virus infection in patients with hepatitis C virus infection undergoing liver transplantation. Gastroenterology, 1996; 111:1569–1575

568. Fried MW, Khudyakov YE, Smallwood GA, Cong M, Nichols B, Diaz E et al. Hepatitis G virus co-infection in liver transplantation recipients with chronic hepatitis C and nonviral chronic liver disease. Hepatology, 1997; 25:1271–1275

569. Haagsma EB, Cuypers HT, Gouw AS, Sjerps MC, Huizenga JR, Slooff MJ et al. High prevalence of hepatitis G virus after liver transplantation without apparent influence on long-term graft function. J Hepatol, 1997; 26:921–925

570. Kallinowski B, Seipp S, Dengler T, Klar E, Theilmann L, Stremmel W. Clinical impact of hepatitis G virus infection in heart and liver transplant recipients. Transplant Proc, 2002; 34:2288–2291

571. Dickson RC, Qian KP, Lau JY. High prevalence of GB virus-C/hepatitis G virus infection in liver transplant recipients. Transplantation, 1997; 63:1695–1697

572. Berg T, Muller AR, Platz KP, Hohne M, Bechstein WO, Hopf U et al. Dynamics of GB virus C viremia early after orthotopic liver transplantation indicates extrahepatic tissues as the predominant site of GB virus C replication. Hepatology, 1999; 29:245–249

573. Cotler SJ, Gretch DR, Bronner MP, Tateyama H, Emond MJ, dela RC et al. Hepatitis G virus co-infection does not alter the course of recurrent hepatitis C virus infection in liver transplantation recipients. Hepatology, 1997; 26:432–436

574. Karayiannis P, Brind AM, Pickering J, Mathew J, Burt AD, Hess G et al. Hepatitis G virus does not cause significant liver disease after liver transplantation. J Viral Hepatol, 1998; 5:35–42

575. Neuberger J, Portmann B, Macdougall BR, Calne RY, Williams R. Recurrence of primary biliary cirrhosis after liver transplantation. N Engl J Med, 1982; 306:1–4

576. Polson RJ, Portmann B, Neuberger J, Calne RY, Williams R. Evidence for disease recurrence after liver transplantation for primary biliary cirrhosis. Clinical and histologic follow-up studies. Gastroenterology, 1989; 97:715–725

577. Balan V, Batts KP, Porayko MK, Krom RA, Ludwig J, Wiesner RH. Histological evidence for recurrence of primary biliary cirrhosis after liver transplantation. Hepatology, 1993; 18:1392–1398

578. Sebagh M, Farges O, Dubel L, Samuel D, Bismuth H, Reynes M. Histological features predictive of recurrence of primary biliary cirrhosis after liver transplantation. Transplantation, 1998; 65:1328–1333

579. Neuberger J. Liver transplantation for primary biliary cirrhosis: indications and risk of recurrence. J Hepatol, 2003; 39:142–148

580. Neuberger J. Recurrent primary biliary cirrhosis. Liver Transpl, 2003; 9:539–546

581. Wong PY, Portmann B, O'Grady JG, Devlin JJ, Hegarty JE, Tan KC et al. Recurrence of primary biliary cirrhosis after liver transplantation following FK506-based immunosuppression. J Hepatol, 1993; 17:284–287

582. Liermann Garcia RF, Evangelista GC, McMaster P, Neuberger J. Transplantation for primary biliary cirrhosis: retrospective analysis of 400 patients in a single center. Hepatology, 2001; 33:22–27

583. Ramos HC, Reyes J, Abu-Elmagd K, Zeevi A, Reinsmoen N, Tzakis A et al. Weaning of immunosuppression in long-term liver transplant recipients. Transplantation, 1995; 59:212–217

584. Khettry U, Anand N, Faul PN, Lewis WD, Pomfret EA, Pomposelli J et al. Liver transplantation for primary biliary cirrhosis: a long-term pathologic study. Liver Transpl, 2003; 9:87–96

585. Dmitrewski J, Hubscher SG, Mayer AD, Neuberger JM. Recurrence of primary biliary cirrhosis in the liver allograft: the effect of immunosuppression. J Hepatol, 1996; 24:253–257

586. Sanchez EQ, Levy MF, Goldstein RM, Fasola CG, Tillery GW, Netto GJ et al. The changing clinical presentation of recurrent primary biliary cirrhosis after liver transplantation. Transplantation, 2003; 76:1583–1588

587. Neuberger J, Gunson B, Hubscher S, Nightingale P. Immunosuppression affects the rate of recurrent primary biliary cirrhosis after liver transplantation. Liver Transpl, 2004; 10:488–491

588. Hashimoto E, Shimada M, Noguchi S, Taniai M, Tokushige K, Hayashi N et al. Disease recurrence after living liver transplantation for primary biliary cirrhosis: a clinical and histological follow-up study. Liver Transpl, 2001; 7:588–595

589. Faust TW. Recurrent primary biliary cirrhosis, primary sclerosing cholangitis, and autoimmune hepatitis after transplantation. Liver Transpl, 2001; 7:S99–108

590. Wiesner RH, LaRusso NF, Ludwig J, Dickson ER. Comparison of the clinicopathologic features of primary sclerosing cholangitis and primary biliary cirrhosis. Gastroenterology, 1985; 88:108–114

591. Sylvestre PB, Batts KP, Burgart LJ, Poterucha JJ, Wiesner RH. Recurrence of primary biliary cirrhosis after liver transplantation: Histologic estimate of incidence and natural history. Liver Transpl, 2003; 9:1086–1093

592. Joplin R, Lindsay JG, Hubscher SG, Johnson GD, Shaw JC, Strain AJ et al. Distribution of dihydrolipoamide acetyltransferase (E2) in the liver and portal lymph nodes of patients with primary biliary

cirrhosis: an immunohistochemical study. Hepatology, 1991; 14:442–447

593. Neuberger J, Wallace L, Joplin R, Hubscher S. Hepatic distribution of E2 component of pyruvate dehydrogenase complex after transplantation. Hepatology, 1995; 22:798–801

594. van de WJ, Gerson LB, Ferrell LD, Lake JR, Coppel RL, Batts KP et al. Immunohistochemical evidence of disease recurrence after liver transplantation for primary biliary cirrhosis. Hepatology, 1996; 24:1079–1084

595. Tan CK, Sian Ho JM. Concurrent de novo autoimmune hepatitis and recurrence of primary biliary cirrhosis post-liver transplantation. Liver Transpl, 2001; 7:461–465

596. Kurdow R, Marks HG, Kraemer-Hansen H, Luttges J, Kremer B, Henne-Bruns D. Recurrence of primary biliary cirrhosis after orthotopic liver transplantation. Hepatogastroenterology, 2003; 50:322–325

597. Harrison RF, Davies MH, Neuberger JM, Hubscher SG. Fibrous and obliterative cholangitis in liver allografts: evidence of recurrent primary sclerosing cholangitis? Hepatology, 1994; 20:356–361

598. Sheng R, Campbell WL, Zajko AB, Baron RL. Cholangiographic features of biliary strictures after liver transplantation for primary sclerosing cholangitis: evidence of recurrent disease. AJR Am J Roentgenol, 1996; 166:1109–1113

599. Goss JA, Shackleton CR, Farmer DG, Arnaout WS, Seu P, Markowitz JS et al. Orthotopic liver transplantation for primary sclerosing cholangitis. A 12-year single center experience. Ann Surg, 1997; 225:472–481

600. Jeyarajah DR, Netto GJ, Lee SP, Testa G, Abbasoglu O, Husberg BS et al. Recurrent primary sclerosing cholangitis after orthotopic liver transplantation: is chronic rejection part of the disease process? Transplantation, 1998; 66:1300–1306

601. Graziadei IW, Wiesner RH, Batts KP, Marotta PJ, LaRusso NF, Porayko MK et al. Recurrence of primary sclerosing cholangitis following liver transplantation. Hepatology, 1999; 29:1050–1056

602. Bjoro K, Schrumpf E. Liver transplantation for primary sclerosing cholangitis. J Hepatol, 2004; 40:570–577

603. Kugelmas M, Spiegelman P, Osgood MJ, Young DA, Trotter JF, Steinberg T et al. Different immunosuppressive regimens and recurrence of primary sclerosing cholangitis after liver transplantation. Liver Transpl, 2003; 9:727–732

604. Vera A, Moledina S, Gunson B, Hubscher S, Mirza D, Olliff S et al. Risk factors for recurrence of primary sclerosing cholangitis of liver allograft. Lancet, 2002; 360:1943–1944

605. Khettry U, Keaveny A, Goldar-Najafi A, Lewis WD, Pomfret EA, Pomposelli JJ et al. Liver transplantation for primary sclerosing cholangitis: a long-term clinicopathologic study. Hum Pathol, 2003; 34:1127–1136

606. Grant AJ, Lalor PF, Hubscher SG, Briskin M, Adams DH. MAdCAM-1 expressed in chronic inflammatory liver disease supports mucosal lymphocyte adhesion to hepatic endothelium (MAdCAM-1 in chronic inflammatory liver disease). Hepatology, 2001; 33:1065–1072

607. Eksteen B, Grant AJ, Miles A, Curbishley SM, Lalor PF, Hubscher SG et al. Hepatic endothelial CCL25 mediates the recruitment of CCR9+ gut-homing lymphocytes to the liver in primary sclerosing cholangitis. J Exp Med, 2004; 200:1511–1517

608. Graziadei IW. Recurrence of primary sclerosing cholangitis after liver transplant. Liver Transpl, 2002; 8:575–581

609. Solano E, Khakhar A, Bloch M, Quan D, McAlister V, Ghent C et al. Liver transplantation for primary sclerosing cholangitis. Transplant Proc, 2003; 35:2431–2434

610. Keaveny AP, Gordon FD, Goldar-Najafi A, Lewis WD, Pomfret EA, Pomposelli JJ et al. Native liver xanthogranulomatous cholangiopathy in primary sclerosing cholangitis: impact on posttransplant outcome. Liver Transpl, 2004; 10:115–122

611. Graziadei IW, Wiesner RH, Marotta PJ, Porayko MK, Hay JE, Charlton MR et al. Long-term results of patients undergoing liver transplantation for primary sclerosing cholangitis. Hepatology, 1999; 30:1121–1127

612. Heneghan MA, Tuttle-Newhall JE, Suhocki PV, Muir AJ, Morse M, Bornstein JD et al. De-novo cholangiocarcinoma in the setting of recurrent primary sclerosing cholangitis following liver transplant. Am J Transplant, 2003; 3:634–638

613. Brandsaeter B, Schrumpf E, Clausen OP, Abildgaard A, Hafsahl G, Bjoro K. Recurrent sclerosing cholangitis or ischemic bile duct lesions—a diagnostic challenge? Liver Transpl, 2004; 10:1073–1074

614. Wright HL, Bou-Abboud CF, Hassanein T, Block GD, Demetris AJ, Starzl TE et al. Disease recurrence and rejection following liver transplantation for autoimmune chronic active liver disease. Transplantation, 1992; 53:136–139

615. Birnbaum AH, Benkov KJ, Pittman NS, McFarlane-Ferreira Y, Rosh JR, LeLeiko NS. Recurrence of autoimmune hepatitis in children after liver transplantation. J Pediatr Gastroenterol Nutr, 1997; 25:20–25

616. Prados E, Cuervas-Mons V, de la MM, Fraga E, Rimola A, Prieto M et al. Outcome of autoimmune hepatitis after liver transplantation. Transplantation, 1998; 66:1645–1650

617. Ratziu V, Samuel D, Sebagh M, Farges O, Saliba F, Ichai P et al. Long-term follow-up after liver transplantation for autoimmune hepatitis: evidence of recurrence of primary disease. J Hepatol, 1999; 30:131–141

618. Ayata G, Gordon FD, Lewis WD, Pomfret E, Pomposelli JJ, Jenkins RL et al. Liver transplantation for autoimmune hepatitis: a long-term pathologic study. Hepatology, 2000; 32:185–192

619. Reich DJ, Fiel I, Guarrera JV, Emre S, Guy SR, Schwartz ME et al. Liver transplantation for autoimmune hepatitis. Hepatology, 2000; 32:693–700

620. Hubscher SG. Recurrent autoimmune hepatitis after liver transplantation: diagnostic criteria, risk factors, and outcome. Liver Transpl, 2001; 7:285–291

621. Gonzalez-Koch A, Czaja AJ, Carpenter HA, Roberts SK, Charlton MR, Porayko MK et al. Recurrent autoimmune hepatitis after orthotopic liver transplantation. Liver Transpl, 2001; 7:302–310

622. Molmenti EP, Netto GJ, Murray NG, Smith DM, Molmenti H, Crippin JS et al. Incidence and recurrence of autoimmune/alloimmune hepatitis in liver transplant recipients. Liver Transpl, 2002; 8:519–526

623. Duclos-Vallee JC, Sebagh M, Rifai K, Johanet C, Ballot E, Guettier C et al. A 10 year follow up study of patients transplanted for autoimmune hepatitis: histological recurrence precedes clinical and biochemical recurrence. Gut, 2003; 52:893–897

624. Vogel A, Heinrich E, Bahr MJ, Rifai K, Flemming P, Melter M et al. Long-term outcome of liver transplantation for autoimmune hepatitis. Clin Transplant, 2004; 18:62–69

625. Manns MP, Bahr MJ. Recurrent autoimmune hepatitis after liver transplantation-when non-self becomes self. Hepatology, 2000; 32:868–870

626. Czaja AJ. Behavior and significance of autoantibodies in type 1 autoimmune hepatitis. J Hepatol, 1999; 30:394–401

627. Sempoux C, Horsmans Y, Lerut J, Rahier J, Geubel A. Acute lobular hepatitis as the first manifestation of recurrent autoimmune hepatitis after orthotopic liver transplantation. Liver, 1997; 17:311–315

628. Duclos-Vallee JC, Johanet C, Bach JF, Yamamoto AM. Autoantibodies associated with acute rejection after liver transplantation for type-2 autoimmune hepatitis. J Hepatol, 2000; 33:163–166

629. Lohse AW, Obermayer-Straub P, Gerken G, Brunner S, Altes U, Dienes HP et al. Development of cytochrome P450 2D6-specific LKM-autoantibodies following liver transplantation in Wilson's disease—possible association with a steroid-resistant transplant rejection episode. J Hepatol, 1999; 31:149–155

630. Milkiewicz P, Hubscher SG, Skiba G, Hathaway M, Elias E. Recurrence of autoimmune hepatitis after liver transplantation. Transplantation, 1999; 68:253–256

631. Lucey MR, Carr K, Beresford TP, Fisher LR, Shieck V, Brown KA et al. Alcohol use after liver transplantation in alcoholics: a clinical cohort follow-up study. Hepatology, 1997; 25:1223–1227

632. Lucey MR, Weinrieb RM. Liver transplantation and alcoholics: is the glass half full or half empty? Gut, 1999; 45:326–327

633. Pageaux GP, Michel J, Coste V, Perney P, Possoz P, Perrigault PF et al. Alcoholic cirrhosis is a good indication for liver transplantation, even for cases of recidivism. Gut, 1999; 45:421–426

634. Bellamy CO, DiMartini AM, Ruppert K, Jain A, Dodson F, Torbenson M et al. Liver transplantation for alcoholic cirrhosis: long term follow-up and impact of disease recurrence. Transplantation, 2001; 72:619–626

635. Burra P, Mioni D, Cecchetto A, Cillo U, Zanus G, Fagiuoli S et al. Histological features after liver transplantation in alcoholic cirrhotics. J Hepatol, 2001; 34:716–722

636. Neuberger J, Schulz KH, Day C, Fleig W, Berlakovich GA, Berenguer M et al. Transplantation for alcoholic liver disease. J Hepatol, 2002; 36:130–137

637. Lim JK, Keeffe EB. Liver transplantation for alcoholic liver disease: current concepts and length of sobriety. Liver Transpl, 2004; 10:S31–S38

638. Conjeevaram HS, Hart J, Lissoos TW, Schiano TD, Dasgupta K, Befeler AS et al. Rapidly progressive liver injury and fatal alcoholic hepatitis occurring after liver transplantation in alcoholic patients. Transplantation, 1999; 67:1562–1568

639. Tome S, Martinez-Rey C, Gonzalez-Quintela A, Gude F, Brage A, Otero E et al. Influence of superimposed alcoholic hepatitis on the outcome of liver transplantation for end-stage alcoholic liver disease. J Hepatol, 2002; 36:793–798

640. Lucey MR. Alcohol injury in the transplanted liver. Liver Transpl Surg, 1997; 3:S26–S31

641. Pageaux GP, Bismuth M, Perney P, Costes V, Jaber S, Possoz P et al. Alcohol relapse after liver transplantation for alcoholic liver disease: does it matter? J Hepatol, 2003; 38:629–634

642. Tang H, Boulton R, Gunson B, Hubscher S, Neuberger J. Patterns of alcohol consumption after liver transplantation. Gut, 1998; 43:140–145

643. Pichlmayr R, Weimann A, Ringe B. Indications for liver transplantation in hepatobiliary malignancy. Hepatology, 1994; 20:33S–40S

644. Bismuth H, Majno PE, Adam R. Liver transplantation for hepatocellular carcinoma. Semin Liver Dis, 1999; 19:311–322

645. Marsh JW, Dvorchik I, Bonham CA, Iwatsuki S. Is the pathologic TNM staging system for patients with hepatoma predictive of outcome? Cancer, 2000; 88:538–543

646. Figueras J, Ibanez L, Ramos E, Jaurrieta E, Ortiz-de-Urbina J, Pardo F et al. Selection criteria for liver transplantation in early-stage hepatocellular carcinoma with cirrhosis: results of a multicenter study. Liver Transpl, 2001; 7:877–883

647. Kirimlioglu H, Dvorchick I, Ruppert K, Finkelstein S, Marsh JW, Iwatsuki S et al. Hepatocellular carcinomas in native livers from patients treated with orthotopic liver transplantation: biologic and therapeutic implications. Hepatology, 2001; 34:502–510

648. Molmenti EP, Klintmalm GB. Liver transplantation in association with hepatocellular carcinoma: an update of the International Tumor Registry. Liver Transpl, 2002; 8:736–748

649. Moya A, Berenguer M, Aguilera V, Juan FS, Nicolas D, Pastor M et al. Hepatocellular carcinoma: Can it be considered a controversial indication for liver transplantation in centers with high rates of hepatitis C? Liver Transpl, 2002; 8:1020–1027

650. Adam R, Del Gaudio M. Evolution of liver transplantation for hepatocellular carcinoma. J Hepatol, 2003; 39:888–895

651. Fiorentino M, Altimari A, Ravaioli M, Gruppioni E, Gabusi E, Corti B et al. Predictive value of biological markers for hepatocellular carcinoma patients treated with orthotopic liver transplantation. Clin Cancer Res, 2004; 10:1789–1795

652. Plessier A, Codes L, Consigny Y, Sommacale D, Dondero F, Cortes A et al. Underestimation of the influence of satellite nodules as a risk factor for post-transplantation recurrence in patients with small hepatocellular carcinoma. Liver Transpl, 2004; 10:S86–S90

653. Roayaie S, Schwartz JD, Sung MW, Emre SH, Miller CM, Gondolesi GE et al. Recurrence of hepatocellular carcinoma after liver transplant: patterns and prognosis. Liver Transpl, 2004; 10:534–540

654. Shetty K, Timmins K, Brensinger C, Furth EE, Rattan S, Sun W et al. Liver transplantation for hepatocellular carcinoma validation of present selection criteria in predicting outcome. Liver Transpl, 2004; 10:911–918

655. Salizzoni M, Romagnoli R, Lupo F, David E, Mirabella S, Cerutti E et al. Microscopic vascular invasion detected by anti-CD34 immunohistochemistry as a predictor of recurrence of hepatocellular carcinoma after liver transplantation. Transplantation, 2003; 76:844–848

656. Bechstein WO, Guckelberger O, Kling N, Rayes N, Tullius SG, Lobeck H et al. Recurrence-free survival after liver transplantation for small hepatocellular carcinoma. Transpl Int, 1998; 11:S189–S192

657. Heneghan MA, O'Grady JG. Liver transplantation for malignant disease. Baillieres Best Pract Res Clin Gastroenterol, 1999; 13:575–591

658. Ho MC, Wu YM, Hu RH, Ko WJ, Yang PM, Lai MY et al. Liver transplantation for patients with hepatocellular carcinoma. Transplant Proc, 2004; 36:2291–2292

659. Bhattacharjya S, Bhattacharjya T, Quaglia A, Dhillon AP, Burroughs AK, Patch DW et al. Liver transplantation in cirrhotic patients with small hepatocellular carcinoma: an analysis of pre-operative imaging, explant histology and prognostic histologic indicators. Dig Surg, 2004; 21:152–159

660. Cho CS, Knechtle SJ, Heisey DM, Hermina M, Armbrust M, D'Alessandro AM et al. Analysis of tumor characteristics and survival in liver transplant recipients with incidentally diagnosed hepatocellular carcinoma. J Gastrointest Surg, 2001; 5:594–601

661. Klintmalm GB. Liver transplantation for hepatocellular carcinoma: a registry report of the impact of tumor characteristics on outcome. Ann Surg, 1998; 228:479–490

662. Schlitt HJ, Neipp M, Weimann A, Oldhafer KJ, Schmoll E, Boeker K et al. Recurrence patterns of hepatocellular and fibrolamellar carcinoma after liver transplantation. J Clin Oncol, 1999; 17:324–331

663. Dumortier J, Bizollon T, Chevallier M, Ducerf C, Baulieux J, Scoazec JY et al. Recurrence of hepatocellular carcinoma as a mixed hepatoblastoma after liver transplantation. Gut, 1999; 45:622–625

664. Haug CE, Jenkins RL, Rohrer RJ, Auchincloss H, Delmonico FL, Freeman RB et al. Liver transplantation for primary hepatic cancer. Transplantation, 1992; 53:376–382

665. O'Grady JG, Polson RJ, Rolles K, Calne RY, Williams R. Liver transplantation for malignant disease. Results in 93 consecutive patients. Ann Surg, 1988; 207:373–379

666. Wall WJ. Liver transplantation for hepatic and biliary malignancy. Semin Liver Dis, 2000; 20:425–436

667. Meyer CG, Penn I, James L. Liver transplantation for cholangiocarcinoma: results in 207 patients. Transplantation, 2000; 69:1633–1637

668. Robles R, Figueras J, Turrion VS, Margarit C, Moya A, Varo E et al. Liver transplantation for peripheral cholangiocarcinoma: Spanish experience. Transplant Proc, 2003; 35:1823–1824

669. Iwatsuki S, Todo S, Marsh JW, Madariaga JR, Lee RG, Dvorchik I et al. Treatment of hilar cholangiocarcinoma (Klatskin tumors) with hepatic resection or transplantation. J Am Coll Surg, 1998; 187:358–364

670. Heimbach JK, Gores GJ, Haddock MG, Alberts SR, Nyberg SL, Ishitani MB et al. Liver transplantation for unresectable perihilar cholangiocarcinoma. Semin Liver Dis, 2004; 24:201–207

671. Houben KW, McCall JL. Liver transplantation for hepatocellular carcinoma in patients without underlying liver disease: a systematic review. Liver Transpl Surg, 1999; 5:91–95

672. Lehnert T. Liver transplantation for metastatic neuroendocrine carcinoma: an analysis of 103 patients. Transplantation, 1998; 66:1307–1312

673. Fernandez JA, Robles R, Marin C, Hernandez Q, Sanchez BF, Ramirez P et al. Role of liver transplantation in the management of metastatic neuroendocrine tumors. Transplant Proc, 2003; 35:1832–1833

674. Blakolmer K, Gaulard P, Mannhalter C, Swerdlow S, Fassati LR, Rossi G et al. Unusual peripheral T cell lymphoma presenting as acute liver failure and reappearing in the liver allograft. Transplantation, 2000; 70:1802–1805

675. Brandhagen DJ. Liver transplantation for hereditary hemochromatosis. Liver Transpl, 2001; 7:663–672

676. Farrell FJ, Nguyen M, Woodley S, Imperial JC, Garcia-Kennedy R, Man K et al. Outcome of liver transplantation in patients with hemochromatosis. Hepatology, 1994; 20:404–410

677. Bralet MP, Duclos-Vallee JC, Castaing D, Samuel D, Guettier C. No hepatic iron overload 12 years after liver transplantation for hereditary hemochromatosis. Hepatology, 2004; 40:762

678. Wigg AJ, Harley H, Casey G. Heterozygous recipient and donor HFE mutations associated with a hereditary haemochromatosis phenotype after liver transplantation. Gut, 2003; 52:433–435

679. Fiel MI, Schiano TD, Bodenheimer HC, Thung SN, King TW, Varma CR et al. Hereditary hemochromatosis in liver transplantation. Liver Transpl Surg, 1999; 5:50–56

680. Brandhagen DJ, Alvarez W, Therneau TM, Kruckeberg KE, Thibodeau SN, Ludwig J et al. Iron overload in cirrhosis-HFE genotypes and outcome after liver transplantation. Hepatology, 2000; 31:456–460

681. Stuart KA, Fletcher LM, Clouston AD, Lynch SV, Purdie DM, Kerlin P et al. Increased hepatic iron and cirrhosis: no evidence for an adverse effect on patient outcome following liver transplantation. Hepatology, 2000; 32:1200–1207

682. Parolin MB, Batts KP, Wiesner RH, Bernstein PS, Zinsmeister AR, Harmsen WS et al. Liver allograft iron accumulation in patients with and without pretransplantation hepatic hemosiderosis. Liver Transpl, 2002; 8:331–339

683. Pappo O, Yunis E, Jordan JA, Jaffe R, Mateo R, Fung J et al. Recurrent and de novo giant cell hepatitis after orthotopic liver transplantation. Am J Surg Pathol, 1994; 18:804–813

684. Durand F, Degott C, Sauvanet A, Molas G, Sicot C, Marcellin P et al. Subfulminant syncytial giant cell hepatitis: recurrence after liver transplantation treated with ribavirin. J Hepatol, 1997; 26:722–726

685. Lerut JP, Claeys N, Ciccarelli O, Pisa R, Galant C, Laterre PF et al. Recurrent postinfantile syncytial giant cell hepatitis after orthotopic liver transplantation. Transpl Int, 1998; 11:320–322

686. Hassoun Z, N'Guyen B, Cote J, Marleau D, Willems B, Roy A et al. A case of giant cell hepatitis recurring after liver transplantation and treated with ribavirin. Can J Gastroenterol, 2000; 14:729–731

687. Nair S, Baisden B, Boitnott J, Klein A, Thuluvath PJ. Recurrent, progressive giant cell hepatitis in two consecutive liver allografts in a middle-aged woman. J Clin Gastroenterol, 2001; 32:454–456

688. Melendez HV, Rela M, Baker AJ, Ball C, Portmann B, Mieli-Vergani G et al. Liver transplant for giant cell hepatitis with autoimmune haemolytic anaemia. Arch Dis Child, 1997; 77:249–251

689. Charlton M, Kasparova P, Weston S, Lindor K, Maor-Kendler Y, Wiesner RH et al. Frequency of nonalcoholic steatohepatitis as a cause of advanced liver disease. Liver Transpl, 2001; 7:608–614

690. Kim WR, Poterucha JJ, Porayko MK, Dickson ER, Steers JL, Wiesner RH. Recurrence of nonalcoholic steatohepatitis following liver transplantation. Transplantation, 1996; 62:1802–1805

691. Molloy RM, Komorowski R, Varma RR. Recurrent nonalcoholic steatohepatitis and cirrhosis after liver transplantation. Liver Transpl Surg, 1997; 3:177–178

692. Garcia RF, Morales E, Garcia CE, Saksena S, Hubscher SG, Elias E. Recurrent and de novo non-alcoholic steatohepatitis following orthotopic liver transplantation. Arq Gastroenterol, 2001; 38:247–253

693. Ong J, Younossi ZM, Reddy V, Price LL, Gramlich T, Mayes J et al. Cryptogenic cirrhosis and posttransplantation nonalcoholic fatty liver disease. Liver Transpl, 2001; 7:797–801

694. Ayata G, Gordon FD, Lewis WD, Pomfret E, Pomposelli JJ, Jenkins RL et al. Cryptogenic cirrhosis: clinicopathologic findings at and after liver transplantation. Hum Pathol, 2002; 33:1098–1104

695. Sanjeevi A, Lyden E, Sunderman B, Weseman R, Ashwathnarayan R, Mukherjee S. Outcomes of liver transplantation for cryptogenic cirrhosis: a single-center study of 71 patients. Transplant Proc, 2003; 35:2977–2980

696. Burke A, Lucey MR. Non-alcoholic fatty liver disease, non-alcoholic steatohepatitis and orthotopic liver transplantation. Am J Transplant, 2004; 4:686–693

697. Seltman HJ, Dekker A, Van Thiel DH, Boggs DR, Starzl TE. Budd–Chiari syndrome recurring in a transplanted liver. Gastroenterology, 1983; 84:640–643

698. Ruckert JC, Ruckert RI, Rudolph B, Muller JM. Recurrence of the Budd–Chiari syndrome after orthotopic liver transplantation. Hepatogastroenterology, 1999; 46:867–871

699. Settmacher U, Nussler NC, Glanemann M, Haase R, Heise M, Bechstein WO et al. Venous complications after orthotopic liver transplantation. Clin Transplant, 2000; 14:235–241

700. Srinivasan P, Rela M, Prachalias A, Muiesan P, Portmann B, Mufti GJ et al. Liver transplantation for Budd–Chiari syndrome. Transplantation, 2002; 73:973–977

701. Bahr MJ, Schubert J, Bleck JS, Tietge UJ, Boozari B, Schmidt RE et al. Recurrence of Budd–Chiari syndrome after liver transplantation in paroxysmal nocturnal hemoglobinuria. Transpl Int, 2003; 16:890–894

702. Fiel MI, Schiano TD, Klion FM, Emre S, Hytiroglou P, Ishak KG et al. Recurring fibro-obliterative venopathy in liver allografts. Am J Surg Pathol, 1999; 23:734–737

703. de Torres I, Demetris AJ, Randhawa PS. Recurrent hepatic allograft injury in erythropoietic protoporphyria. Transplantation, 1996; 61:1412–1413

704. Fidler HM, Hadziyannis SJ, Dhillon AP, Sherlock S, Burroughs AK. Recurrent hepatic sarcoidosis following liver transplantation. Transplant Proc, 1997; 29:2509–2510

705. Bresson-Hadni S, Koch S, Beurton I, Vuitton DA, Bartholomot B, Hrusovsky S et al. Primary disease recurrence after liver transplantation for alveolar echinococcosis: long-term evaluation in 15 patients. Hepatology, 1999; 30:857–864

706. Chazouilleres O, Mamish D, Kim M, Carey K, Ferrell L, Roberts JP et al. 'Occult' hepatitis B virus as source of infection in liver transplant recipients. Lancet, 1994; 343:142–146

707. Dickson RC, Everhart JE, Lake JR, Wei Y, Seaberg EC, Wiesner RH et al. Transmission of hepatitis B by transplantation of livers from donors positive for antibody to hepatitis B core antigen. The National Institute of Diabetes and Digestive and Kidney Diseases Liver Transplantation Database. Gastroenterology, 1997; 113:1668–1674

708. Marusawa H, Uemoto S, Hijikata M, Ueda Y, Tanaka K, Shimotohno K et al. Latent hepatitis B virus infection in healthy individuals with antibodies to hepatitis B core antigen. Hepatology, 2000; 31:488–495

709. Prieto M, Gomez MD, Berenguer M, Cordoba J, Rayon JM, Pastor M et al. De novo hepatitis B after liver transplantation from hepatitis B core antibody-positive donors in an area with high prevalence of anti-HBc positivity in the donor population. Liver Transpl, 2001; 7:51–58

710. Roque-Afonso AM, Feray C, Samuel D, Simoneau D, Roche B, Emile JF et al. Antibodies to hepatitis B surface antigen prevent viral reactivation in recipients of liver grafts from anti-HBC positive donors. Gut, 2002; 50:95–99

711. Lee KW, Lee DS, Lee HH, Kim SJ, Joh JW, Seo JM et al. Prevention of de novo hepatitis B infection from HbcAb-positive donors in

living donor liver transplantation. Transplant Proc, 2004; 36:2311–2312

712. Roche B, Samuel D, Gigou M, Feray C, Virot V, Schmets L et al. De novo and apparent de novo hepatitis B virus infection after liver transplantation. J Hepatol, 1997; 26:517–526

713. Abdelmalek MF, Pasha TM, Zein NN, Persing DH, Wiesner RH, Douglas DD. Subclinical reactivation of hepatitis B virus in liver transplant recipients with past exposure. Liver Transpl, 2003; 9:1253–1257

714. Everhart JE, Wei Y, Eng H, Charlton MR, Persing DH, Wiesner RH et al. Recurrent and new hepatitis C virus infection after liver transplantation. Hepatology, 1999; 29:1220–1226

715. Challine D, Pellegrin B, Bouvier-Alias M, Rigot P, Laperche L, Pawlotsky JM. HIV and hepatitis C virus RNA in seronegative organ and tissue donors. Lancet, 2004; 364:1611–1612

716. Gallegos-Orozco JF, Vargas HE, Rakela J. Virologically compromised donor grafts in liver transplantation. J Hepatol, 2004; 41:512–521

717. Crespo J, Fabrega E, Casafont F, Rivero M, Heras G, de la PJ et al. Severe clinical course of de novo hepatitis B infection after liver transplantation. Liver Transpl Surg, 1999; 5:175–183

718. Segovia R, Sanchez-Fueyo A, Rimola A, Grande L, Bruguera M, Costa J et al. Evidence of serious graft damage induced by de novo hepatitis B virus infection after liver transplantation. Liver Transpl, 2001; 7:106–112

719. Salcedo M, Vaquero J, Banares R, Rodriguez-Mahou M, Alvarez E, Vicario JL et al. Response to steroids in de novo autoimmune hepatitis after liver transplantation. Hepatology, 2002; 35:349–356

720. Mieli-Vergani G, Vergani D. De novo autoimmune hepatitis after liver transplantation. J Hepatol, 2004; 40:3–7

721. D'Antiga L, Dhawan A, Portmann B, Francavilla R, Rela M, Heaton N et al. Late cellular rejection in paediatric liver transplantation: aetiology and outcome. Transplantation, 2002; 73:80–84

722a. Miyagawa-Hayashino A, Haga H, Egawa H, Hayashino Y, Sakurai T, Minamiguchi S et al. Outcome and risk factors of de novo autoimmune hepatitis in living-donor liver transplantation. Transplantation, 2004; 78:128–135

722b. Aguilera I, Wichmann I, Sousa JM, Bernardos A, Franco E, Garcia-Lozano JR et al. Antibodies against glutathione S-transferase T1 (GSTT1) in patients with de novo immune hepatitis following liver transplantation. Clin Exp Immunol, 2001; 126:535–539

722c. Aguilera I, Sousa JM, Gavilan F, Bernardos A, Wichmann I, Nunez-Roldan A. Glutathione S-transferase T1 mismatch constitutes a risk factor for de novo immune hepatitis after liver transplantation. Liver Transpl, 2004; 10:1166–1172

723. Poordad F, Gish R, Wakil A, Garcia-Kennedy R, Martin P, Yao FY. De novo non-alcoholic fatty liver disease following orthotopic liver transplantation. Am J Transplant, 2003; 3:1413–1417

724. Fung JJ, Jain A, Kwak EJ, Kusne S, Dvorchik I, Eghtesad B. De novo malignancies after liver transplantation: a major cause of late death. Liver Transpl, 2001; 7:S109–S118

725. Rosenthal P, Emond JC, Heyman MB, Snyder J, Roberts J, Ascher N et al. Pathological changes in yearly protocol liver biopsy specimens from healthy pediatric liver recipients. Liver Transpl Surg, 1997; 3:559–562

726. Berenguer M, Rayon JM, Prieto M, Aguilera V, Nicolas D, Ortiz V et al. Are posttransplantation protocol liver biopsies useful in the long term? Liver Transpl, 2001; 7:790–796

727. Heneghan MA, Zolfino T, Muiesan P, Portmann BC, Rela M, Heaton ND et al. An evaluation of long-term outcomes after liver transplantation for cryptogenic cirrhosis. Liver Transpl, 2003; 9:921–928

728. Nakhleh RE, Krishna M, Keaveny AP, Dickson RC, Rosser B, Nguyen JH et al. Review of 31 cases of morphologic hepatitis in liver transplant patients not related to disease recurrence. Transplant Proc, 2005; 37:1240–1242

729. Mohamed R, Hubscher SG, Mirza DF, Gunson BK, Mutimer DJ. Posttransplantation chronic hepatitis in fulminant hepatic failure. Hepatology, 1997; 25:1003–1007

729a. Evans HM, Kelly DA, McKiernan PJ, Hübscher SG. Progressive histological damage in liver allografts following paediatric liver transplantation. Hepatology, 2006; in press

730. Combs C, Brunt EM, Solomon H, Bacon BR, Brantly M, Di Bisceglie AM. Rapid development of hepatic alpha1-antitrypsin globules after liver transplantation for chronic hepatitis C. Gastroenterology, 1997; 112:1372–1375

731. Schlitt HJ, Schafers S, Deiwick A, Eckardt KU, Pietsch T, Ebell W et al. Extramedullary erythropoiesis in human liver grafts. Hepatology, 1995; 21:689–696

732. Tsamandas AC, Jain AB, Raikow RB, Demetris AJ, Nalesnik MA, Randhawa PS. Extramedullary hematopoiesis in the allograft liver. Mod Pathol, 1995; 8:671–674

733. Farthing MJ, Clark ML. Nature of the toxicity of cyclosporin A in the rat. Biochem Pharmacol, 1981; 30:3311–3316

734. Ryffel B, Donatsch P, Madorin M, Matter BE, Ruttimann G, Schon H et al. Toxicological evaluation of cyclosporin A. Arch Toxicol, 1983; 53:107–141

735. Bluhm RE, Rodgers WH, Black DL, Wilkinson GR, Branch R. Cholestasis in transplant patients—what is the role of cyclosporin? Aliment Pharmacol Ther, 1992; 6:207–219

736. Durak I, Kacmaz M, Cimen MY, Buyukkocak S, Elgun S, Ozturk HS. The effects of cyclosporine on antioxidant enzyme activities and malondialdehyde levels in rabbit hepatic tissues. Transpl Immunol, 2002; 10:255–258

737. Roman ID, Fernandez-Moreno MD, Fueyo JA, Roma MG, Coleman R. Cyclosporin A induced internalization of the bile salt export pump in isolated rat hepatocyte couplets. Toxicol Sci, 2003; 71:276–281

738. Mazzaferro V, Porter KA, Scotti-Foglieni CL, Venkataramanan R, Makowka L, Rossaro L et al. The hepatotropic influence of cyclosporine. Surgery, 1990; 107:533–539

739. Sterneck M, Wiesner R, Ascher N, Roberts J, Ferrell L, Ludwig J et al. Azathioprine hepatotoxicity after liver transplantation. Hepatology, 1991; 14:806–810

740. Gane E, Portmann B, Saxena R, Wong P, Ramage J, Williams R. Nodular regenerative hyperplasia of the liver graft after liver transplantation. Hepatology, 1994; 20:88–94

741. Lee AU, Farrell GC. Mechanism of azathioprine-induced injury to hepatocytes: roles of glutathione depletion and mitochondrial injury. J Hepatol, 2001; 35:756–764

742. Sparberg M, Simon N, del Greco F. Intrahepatic cholestasis due to azathioprine. Gastroenterology, 1969; 57:439–441

743. Stromeyer FW, Ishak KG. Nodular transformation (nodular 'regenerative' hyperplasia) of the liver. A clinicopathologic study of 30 cases. Hum Pathol, 1981; 12:60–71

744. Snover DC, Weisdorf S, Bloomer J, McGlave P, Weisdorf D. Nodular regenerative hyperplasia of the liver following bone marrow transplantation. Hepatology, 1989; 9:443–448

745. Francavilla A, Barone M, Todo S, Zeng Q, Porter KA, Starzl TE. Augmentation of rat liver regeneration by FK 506 compared with cyclosporin. Lancet, 1989; 2:1248–1249

746. Hytiroglou P, Lee R, Sharma K, Theise ND, Schwartz M, Miller C et al. FK506 versus cyclosporine as primary immunosuppressive agent for orthotopic liver allograft recipients. Histologic and immunopathologic observations. Transplantation, 1993; 56:1389–1394

747. Groth CG, Backman L, Morales JM, Calne R, Kreis H, Lang P et al. Sirolimus (rapamycin)-based therapy in human renal transplantation: similar efficacy and different toxicity compared with cyclosporine. Sirolimus European Renal Transplant Study Group. Transplantation, 1999; 67:1036–1042

748. Conti F, Morelon E, Calmus Y. Immunosuppressive therapy in liver transplantation. J Hepatol, 2003; 39:664–678

749. Hockerstedt K, Lautenschlager I, Ahonen J, Eklund B, Isoniemi H, Korsback C et al. Diagnosis of acute rejection in liver transplantation. J Hepatol, 1988; 6:217–221

750. Lautenschlager I, Hockerstedt K, Ahonen J, Eklund B, Isoniemi H, Korsback C et al. Fine-needle aspiration biopsy in the monitoring of liver allografts. II. Applications to human liver allografts. Transplantation, 1988; 46:47–53

751. Kirby RM, Young JA, Hubscher SG, Elias E, McMaster P. The accuracy of aspiration cytology in the diagnosis of rejection following orthotopic liver transplantation. Transpl Int, 1988; 1:119–126

752. Carbonnel F, Samuel D, Reynes M, Benhamou JP, Bismuth H, Bach JF et al. Fine-needle aspiration biopsy of human liver allografts. Correlation with liver histology for the diagnosis of acute rejection. Transplantation, 1990; 50:704–707

753. Kubota K, Ericzon BG, Reinholt FP. Comparison of fine-needle aspiration biopsy and histology in human liver transplants. Transplantation, 1991; 51:1010–1013

754. Schlitt HJ, Nashan B, Ringe B, Wonigeit K, Pichlmayr R. Routine monitoring of liver grafts by transplant aspiration cytology: clinical experience with 3000 TACs. Transplant Proc, 1993; 25:1970–1971

755. Their M, Lautenschlager I, von Willebrand E, Hockerstedt K, Holmberg C, Jalanko H. The use of fine-needle aspiration biopsy in detection of acute rejection in children after liver transplantation. Transpl Int, 2002; 15:240–247

756. Kuijf ML, Kwekkeboom J, Kuijpers MA, Willems M, Zondervan PE, Niesters HG et al. Granzyme expression in fine-needle aspirates from liver allografts is increased during acute rejection. Liver Transpl, 2002; 8:952–956

757. Kwekkeboom J, Zondervan PE, Kuijpers MA, Tilanus HW, Metselaar HJ. Fine-needle aspiration cytology in the diagnosis of acute rejection after liver transplantation. Br J Surg, 2003; 90:246–247

758. Hayry P, von Willebrand E. Practical guidelines for fine needle aspiration biopsy of human renal allografts. Ann Clin Res, 1981; 13:288–306

759. Lautenschlager I, Hockerstedt K, von Willebrand E, Scheinin TM, Ahonen J, Scheinin B et al. Aspiration cytology of a human liver allograft. Transplant Proc, 1984; 16:1243–1246

760. Lautenschlager I, Hockerstedt K, Taskinen E, Korsback C, Makisalo H, Hayry P. Fine-needle aspiration biopsy in the monitoring of liver allografts. I. Correlation between aspiration biopsy and core biopsy in experimental pig liver allografts. Transplantation, 1988; 46:41–46

761. Hayry P, Lautenschlager I. Fine-needle aspiration biopsy in transplantation pathology. Semin Diagn Pathol, 1992; 9:232–237

762. Von Willebrand E, Lautenschlager I. Organ Transplantation. In: Gray W, editor. Diagnostic Cytopathology. Edinburgh: Churchill Livingstone, 1995:529–541

763. Lautenschlager I, Nashan B, Schlitt HJ, Hoshino K, Ringe B, Tillmann HL et al. Different cellular patterns associated with hepatitis C virus reactivation, cytomegalovirus infection, and acute rejection in liver transplant patients monitored with transplant aspiration cytology. Transplantation, 1994; 58:1339–1345

764. Lautenschlager I, Nashan B, Schlitt HJ, Ringe B, Wonigeit K, Pichlmayr R. Early intragraft inflammatory events of liver allografts leading to chronic rejection. Transpl Int, 1995; 8:446–451

765. Topalidis T, Bechstein WO, Bohmann C, Stockmann K, Neuhaus P. New preparation method for bile cytology in liver transplantation: diagnosis of rejection. Transplant Proc, 1993; 25:1979

766. McDonald GB, Shulman HM, Sullivan KM, Spencer GD. Intestinal and hepatic complications of human bone marrow transplantation. Part I. Gastroenterology, 1986; 90:460–477

767. McDonald GB, Shulman HM, Sullivan KM, Spencer GD. Intestinal and hepatic complications of human bone marrow transplantation. Part II. Gastroenterology, 1986; 90:770–784

768. McDonald GB, Shulman HM, Wolford JL, Spencer GD. Liver disease after human marrow transplantation. Semin Liver Dis, 1987; 7:210–229

769. El Sayed MH, El Haddad A, Fahmy OA, Salama II, Mahmoud HK. Liver disease is a major cause of mortality following allogeneic bone-marrow transplantation. Eur J Gastroenterol Hepatol, 2004; 16:1347–1354

770. McDonald GB, Sharma P, Matthews DE, Shulman HM, Thomas ED. Venocclusive disease of the liver after bone marrow transplantation: diagnosis, incidence, and predisposing factors. Hepatology, 1984; 4:116–122

771. Shulman HM, Fisher LB, Schoch HG, Henne KW, McDonald GB. Veno-occlusive disease of the liver after marrow transplantation: histological correlates of clinical signs and symptoms. Hepatology, 1994; 19:1171–1181

772. DeLeve LD, Shulman HM, McDonald GB. Toxic injury to hepatic sinusoids: sinusoidal obstruction syndrome (veno-occlusive disease). Semin Liver Dis, 2002; 22:27–42

773. Wang WH, Wang HL. Fulminant adenovirus hepatitis following bone marrow transplantation. A case report and brief review of the literature. Arch Pathol Lab Med, 2003; 127:e246–e248

774. Tomas JF, Pinilla I, Garcia-Buey ML, Garcia A, Figuera A, Gomez-Garcia de Soria VGG et al. Long-term liver dysfunction after allogeneic bone marrow transplantation: clinical features and course in 61 patients. Bone Marrow Transplant, 2000; 26:649–655

775. Saunders MD, Shulman HM, Murakami CS, Chauncey TR, Bensinger WI, McDonald GB. Bile duct apoptosis and cholestasis resembling acute graft-versus-host disease after autologous hematopoietic cell transplantation. Am J Surg Pathol, 2000; 24:1004–1008

776. Decoste SD, Boudreaux C, Dover JS. Transfusion-associated graft-vs-host disease in patients with malignancies. Report of two cases and review of the literature. Arch Dermatol, 1990; 126:1324–1329

777. Funkhouser AW, Vogelsang G, Zehnbauer B, Tunnessen WW, Beschorner WE, Sanders M et al. Graft versus host disease after blood transfusions in a premature infant. Pediatrics, 1991; 87:247–250

778. Flidel O, Barak Y, Lifschitz-Mercer B, Frumkin A, Mogilner BM. Graft versus host disease in extremely low birth weight neonate. Pediatrics, 1992; 89:689–690

779. Jamieson NV, Joysey V, Friend PJ, Marcus R, Ramsbottom S, Baglin T et al. Graft-versus-host disease in solid organ transplantation. Transpl Int, 1991; 4:67–71

780. Appleton AL, Sviland L. Current thoughts on the pathogenesis of graft versus host disease. J Clin Pathol, 1993; 46:785–789

781. Taylor AL, Gibbs P, Bradley JA. Acute graft versus host disease following liver transplantation: the enemy within. Am J Transplant, 2004; 4:466–474

782. Gholson CF, Yau JC, LeMaistre CF, Cleary KR. Steroid-responsive chronic hepatic graft-versus-host disease without extrahepatic graft-versus-host disease. Am J Gastroenterol, 1989; 84:1306–1309

783. Yeh KH, Hsieh HC, Tang JL, Lin MT, Yang CH, Chen YC. Severe isolated acute hepatic graft-versus-host disease with vanishing bile duct syndrome. Bone Marrow Transplant, 1994; 14:319–321

784. Shulman HM, Sullivan KM, Weiden PL, McDonald GB, Striker GE, Sale GE et al. Chronic graft-versus-host syndrome in man. A long-term clinicopathologic study of 20 Seattle patients. Am J Med, 1980; 69:204–217

785. Snover DC. Acute and chronic graft versus host disease: histopathological evidence for two distinct pathogenetic mechanisms. Hum Pathol, 1984; 15:202–205

786. Strasser SI, Shulman HM, Flowers ME, Reddy R, Margolis DA, Prumbaum M et al. Chronic graft-versus-host disease of the liver: presentation as an acute hepatitis. Hepatology, 2000; 32:1265–1271

787. Fujii N, Takenaka K, Shinagawa K, Ikeda K, Maeda Y, Sunami K et al. Hepatic graft-versus-host disease presenting as an acute hepatitis after allogeneic peripheral blood stem cell transplantation. Bone Marrow Transplant, 2001; 27:1007–1010

788. Malik AH, Collins RH, Jr., Saboorian MH, Lee WM. Chronic graft-versus-host disease after hematopoietic cell transplantation presenting as an acute hepatitis. Am J Gastroenterol, 2001; 96:588–590

789. Chiba T, Yokosuka O, Kanda T, Fukai K, Imazeki F, Saisho H et al. Hepatic graft-versus-host disease resembling acute hepatitis: additional treatment with ursodeoxycholic acid. Liver, 2002; 22:514–517

790. Ma SY, Au WY, Ng IO, Lie AK, Leung AY, Liang R et al. Hepatitic graft-versus-host disease after hematopoietic stem cell transplantation: clinicopathologic features and prognostic implication. Transplantation, 2004; 77:1252–1259

791. Maeng H, Lee JH, Cheong JW, Lee ST, Hahn JS, Ko YW et al. Chronic graft-versus-host disease of the liver presenting as an acute hepatitis following nonmyeloablative hematopoietic stem cell transplantation. Int J Hematol, 2004; 79:501–504

792. Sloane JP, Norton J. The pathology of bone marrow transplantation. Histopathology, 1993; 22:201–209

793. Tanaka M, Umihara J, Shimmoto K, Cui SJ, Sata H, Ishikawa T et al. The pathogenesis of graft-versus-host reaction in the intrahepatic bile duct. An immunohistochemical study. Acta Pathol Jpn, 1989; 39:648–655

794. Dilly SA, Sloane JP. An immunohistological study of human hepatic graft-versus-host disease. Clin Exp Immunol, 1985; 62:545–553

795. Diamond DJ, Chang KL, Jenkins KA, Forman SJ. Immunohistochemical analysis of T cell phenotypes in patients with graft-versus-host disease following allogeneic bone marrow transplantation. Transplantation, 1995; 59:1436–1444

796. Sloane JP, Farthing MJ, Powles RL. Histopathological changes in the liver after allogeneic bone marrow transplantation. J Clin Pathol, 1980; 33:344–350

797. Bligh J, Morton J, Durrant S, Walker N. Oncocytic metaplasia of bile duct epithelium in hepatic GVHD. Bone Marrow Transplant, 1995; 16:317–319

798. Norton J, al Saffar N, Sloane JP. Adhesion molecule expression in human hepatic graft-versus-host disease. Bone Marrow Transplant. 1992; 10:153–156

799. Hardy CL, Morahan G, Bhathal PS. A study of graft versus host disease using bile duct implants under the kidney capsule. Liver, 2000; 20:16–26

800. Zhang Y, Shlomchik WD, Joe G, Louboutin JP, Zhu J, Rivera A et al. APCs in the liver and spleen recruit activated allogeneic CD8+ T cells to elicit hepatic graft-versus-host disease. J Immunol, 2002; 169:7111–7118

801. Ueno Y, Ishii M, Yahagi K, Mano Y, Kisara N, Nakamura N et al. Fas-mediated cholangiopathy in the murine model of graft versus host disease. Hepatology, 2000; 31:966–974

802. Marks DI, Dousset B, Robson A, Imvrios G, Buckels JA, Elias E et al. Orthotopic liver transplantation for hepatic GVHD following allogeneic BMT for chronic myeloid leukaemia. Bone Marrow Transplant, 1992; 10:463–466

803. Rhodes DF, Lee WM, Wingard JR, Pavy MD, Santos GW, Shaw BW et al. Orthotopic liver transplantation for graft-versus-host disease following bone marrow transplantation. Gastroenterology, 1990; 99:536–538

804. Stechschulte DJ, Jr., Fishback JL, Emami A, Bhatia P. Secondary biliary cirrhosis as a consequence of graft-versus-host disease. Gastroenterology, 1990; 98:223–225

805. Knapp AB, Crawford JM, Rappeport JM, Gollan JL. Cirrhosis as a consequence of graft-versus-host disease. Gastroenterology, 1987; 92:513–519

806. Shulman HM, Sharma P, Amos D, Fenster LF, McDonald GB. A coded histologic study of hepatic graft-versus-host disease after human bone marrow transplantation. Hepatology, 1988; 8:463–470

807. Andersen CB, Horn T, Sehested M, Junge J, Jacobsen N. Graft-versus-host disease: liver morphology and pheno/genotypes of inflammatory cells and target cells in sex-mismatched allogeneic bone marrow transplant patients. Transplant Proc, 1993; 25:1250–1254

808. McIvor C, Morton J, Bryant A, Cooksley WG, Durrant S, Walker N. Fatal reactivation of precore mutant hepatitis B virus associated with fibrosing cholestatic hepatitis after bone marrow transplantation. Ann Intern Med, 1994; 121:274–275

809. Cooksley WG, McIvor CA. Fibrosing cholestatic hepatitis and HBV after bone marrow transplantation. Biomed Pharmacother 1995; 49:117–124

810. Caselitz M, Link H, Hein R, Maschek H, Boker K, Poliwoda H et al. Hepatitis B associated liver failure following bone marrow transplantation. J Hepatol, 1997; 27:572–577

811. Ribas A, Gale RP. Should people with hepatitis C virus infection receive a bone marrow transplant? Bone Marrow Transplant, 1997; 19:97–99

812. Strasser SI, Sullivan KM, Myerson D, Spurgeon CL, Storer B, Schoch HG et al. Cirrhosis of the liver in long-term marrow transplant survivors. Blood, 1999; 93:3259–3266

813. Norol F, Roche B, Girardin MF, Kuentz M, Desforges L, Cordonnier C et al. Hepatitis C virus infection and allogeneic bone marrow transplantation. Transplantation, 1994; 57:393–397

814. Lau GK, Liang R, Chiu EK, Lee CK, Lam SK. Hepatic events after bone marrow transplantation in patients with hepatitis B infection: a case controlled study. Bone Marrow Transplant, 1997; 19:795–799

815. Strasser SI, Myerson D, Spurgeon CL, Sullivan KM, Storer B, Schoch HG et al. Hepatitis C virus infection and bone marrow transplantation: a cohort study with 10-year follow-up. Hepatology, 1999; 29:1893–1899

816. Muretto P, Angelucci E, Lucarelli G. Reversibility of cirrhosis in patients cured of thalassemia by bone marrow transplantation. Ann Intern Med, 2002; 136:667–672

817. McKay PJ, Murphy JA, Cameron S, Burnett AK, Campbell M, Tansey P et al. Iron overload and liver dysfunction after allogeneic or autologous bone marrow transplantation. Bone Marrow Transplant, 1996; 17:63–66

818. Angelucci E, Muretto P, Nicolucci A, Baronciani D, Erer B, Gaziev J et al. Effects of iron overload and hepatitis C virus positivity in determining progression of liver fibrosis in thalassemia following bone marrow transplantation. Blood, 2002; 100:17–21

819. Ahsan N, Rao KV. Hepatobiliary diseases after kidney transplantation unrelated to classic hepatitis virus. Semin Dial 2002; 15:358–365

820. Norris SH, Butler TC, Glass N, Tran R. Fatal hepatic necrosis caused by disseminated type 5 adenovirus infection in a renal transplant recipient. Am J Nephrol, 1989; 9:101–105

821. Longerich T, Haferkamp K, Tox U, Schirmacher P. Acute liver failure in a renal transplant patient caused by adenoviral hepatitis superimposed on a fibrosing cholestatic hepatitis B. Hum Pathol, 2004; 35:894–897

822. Ludwig J, Batts KP. Transplantation Pathology. In: MacSween RNM, Anthony PP, Scheuer PJ, Burt AD, Portmann BC, editors. Pathology of the Liver. Edinburgh: Churchill Livingstone, 1994:766–786

823. Rossi C, Delforge ML, Jacobs F, Wissing M, Pradier O, Remmelink M et al. Fatal primary infection due to human herpesvirus 6 variant A in a renal transplant recipient. Transplantation, 2001; 71:288–292

824. Randhawa PS, Jenkins FJ, Nalesnik MA, Martens J, Williams PA, Ries A et al. Herpesvirus 6 variant A infection after heart transplantation with giant cell transformation in bile ductular and gastroduodenal epithelium. Am J Surg Pathol, 1997; 21:847–853

825. Kemper CA, Lombard CM, Deresinski SC, Tompkins LS. Visceral bacillary epithelioid angiomatosis: possible manifestations of disseminated cat scratch disease in the immunocompromised host: a report of two cases. Am J Med, 1990; 89:216–222

826. Utili R, Tripodi MF, Ragone E, Casillo R, Pasquale G, De Santo L et al. Hepatic cryptococcosis in a heart transplant recipient. Transpl Infect Dis, 2004; 6:33–36

827. Gane E, Pilmore H. Management of chronic viral hepatitis before and after renal transplantation. Transplantation, 2002; 74:427–437

828. Cadranel JF, Di M, V, Dorent R, Bernard B, Hoang C, Myara A et al. Effects of ursodeoxycholic acid (ursodiol) treatment on chronic viral hepatitis in heart transplant patients: results of a prospective, double-blind, placebo-randomized study. Transplantation, 2003; 75:977–982

829. Fairley CK, Mijch A, Gust ID, Nichilson S, Dimitrakakis M, Lucas CR. The increased risk of fatal liver disease in renal transplant patients who are hepatitis Be antigen and/or HBV DNA positive. Transplantation, 1991; 52:497–500

830. Goffin E, Pirson Y, van Ypersele dS. Implications of chronic hepatitis B or hepatitis C infection for renal transplant candidates. Nephrol Dial Transplant, 1995; 10:88–92

831. Fornairon S, Pol S, Legendre C, Carnot F, Mamzer-Bruneel MF, Brechot C et al. The long-term virologic and pathologic impact of renal transplantation on chronic hepatitis B virus infection. Transplantation, 1996; 62:297–299

832. Lam PW, Wachs ME, Somberg KA, Vincenti F, Lake JR, Ferrell LD. Fibrosing cholestatic hepatitis in renal transplant recipients. Transplantation, 1996; 61:378–381

833. Jung S, Lee HC, Han JM, Lee YJ, Chung YH, Lee YS et al. Four cases of hepatitis B virus-related fibrosing cholestatic hepatitis treated with lamivudine. J Gastroenterol Hepatol, 2002; 17:345–350

834. Wachs ME, Amend WJ, Ascher NL, Bretan PN, Emond J, Lake JR et al. The risk of transmission of hepatitis B from HBsAg(-), HBcAb(+), HBIgM(-) organ donors. Transplantation, 1995; 59:230–234

835. Berger A, Preiser W, Kachel HG, Sturmer M, Doerr HW. HBV reactivation after kidney transplantation. J Clin Virol, 2005; 32:162–165

836. Berthoux F, Berthoux P, Mosnier JF, El Deeb S, Cecillon S, Haem J. Systematic evaluation of liver disease in hepatitis C virus-infected renal transplant recipients: clinical and pathological study. Nephrol Dial Transplant 2000; 15 Suppl 8:55–59

837. Van Thiel D, Nadir A, Shah N. Hepatitis C and renal disease. Transplant Proc, 2002; 34:2429–2431

838. Zein NN, McGreger CG, Wendt NK, Schwab K, Mitchell PS, Persing DH et al. Prevalence and outcome of hepatitis C infection among heart transplant recipients. J Heart Lung Transplant 1995; 14:865–869

839. Alric L, Di Martino V, Selves J, Cacoub P, Charlotte F, Reynaud D et al. Long-term impact of renal transplantation on liver fibrosis during hepatitis C virus infection. Gastroenterology, 2002; 123:1494–1499

840. Cisterne JM, Rostaing L, Izopet J, Chabannier MH, Baron E, Duffaut M et al. Epidemiology of HCV infection: disease and renal transplantation. Nephrol Dial Transplant, 1996; 11 Suppl 4:46–47

841. Toz H, Ok E, Yilmaz F, Akarca US, Erensoy S, Zeytinoglu A et al. Clinicopathological features of hepatitis C virus infection in dialysis and renal transplantation. J Nephrol, 2002; 15:308–312

842. Brunson ME, Lau JY, Davis GL, Scornik J, Howard RJ, Pfaff WW. Non-A, non-B hepatitis and elevated serum aminotransferases in renal transplant patients. Correlation with hepatitis C infection. Transplantation, 1993; 56:1364–1367

843. Zylberberg H, Carnot F, Mamzer MF, Blancho G, Legendre C, Pol S. Hepatitis C virus-related fibrosing cholestatic hepatitis after renal transplantation. Transplantation, 1997; 63:158–160

844. Delladetsima JK, Boletis JN, Makris F, Psichogiou M, Kostakis A, Hatzakis A. Fibrosing cholestatic hepatitis in renal transplant recipients with hepatitis C virus infection. Liver Transpl Surg, 1999; 5:294–300

845. Delladetsima JK, Makris F, Psichogiou M, Kostakis A, Hatzakis A, Boletis JN. Cholestatic syndrome with bile duct damage and loss in renal transplant recipients with HCV infection. Liver, 2001; 21:81–88

846. Munoz dB, Benito A, Colina F, Andres A, Dominguez-Gil B, Munoz MA et al. Fibrosing cholestatic hepatitis-like syndrome in hepatitis B virus-negative and hepatitis C virus-negative renal transplant recipients. Am J Kidney Dis, 2001; 38:640–645

847. Duseja A, Nada R, Kalra N, Acharya SK, Minz M, Joshi K et al. Fibrosing cholestatic hepatitis-like syndrome in a hepatitis B virus and hepatitis C virus-negative renal transplant recipient: a case report with autopsy findings. Trop Gastroenterol, 2003; 24:31–34

Liver pathology associated with diseases of other organs or systems

17

Alastair D. Burt

The preceding chapters have dealt chiefly with the diversity of diseases in which the hepatic involvement has been primary. A group remains in which the primary disease is predominantly extrahepatic, but in which liver dysfunction may develop and sometimes be of clinical and morphological significance. These diseases will be dealt with in turn on a systemic basis, but three morphological entities which represent a response to a variety of causes will be described first. These are:

- *non-specific reactive hepatitis*, an ill-defined morphological entity which reflects the general and non-specific response of the liver to a wide variety of systemic processes;
- hepatic *granulomatous conditions*, which may arise as part of generalized granulomatous disease, may be a component of certain primary liver diseases or may also represent a non-specific response to extrahepatic disease; and
- *steatosis* (or fatty liver) which may develop in a wide diversity of disorders and which, depending on the aetiology or the presence of associated inflammatory change, may result in both acute and chronic hepatic dysfunction.

Non-specific reactive hepatitis

This description was first applied by Popper & Schaffner.[1] They succinctly defined a morphological entity which may be widespread within the liver, representing either the residuum of previous inflammatory intrahepatic disease or a response to a variety of extrahepatic disease processes, especially febrile illnesses and inflammation somewhere in the splanchnic bed. The changes may also be localized within the liver, representing a response to a variety of focal liver injuries such as vascular lesions or space-occupying lesions.

There are no specific clinical manifestations and although there may be mild increases in serum aminotransferase levels there is no specific disturbance of liver function tests. Such symptoms or abnormalities of function as may be present can usually be attributed to the underlying or associated disease.

The morphological features which characterize non-specific reactive hepatitis are outlined below. They may exist in various combinations, and may show varying degrees of severity; the essential feature in making the diagnosis is that, even when the changes are widespread, they still tend to be 'focal'. Thus, only some portal tracts are involved, and the parenchymal changes do not demonstrate a uniform zonal distribution.

Portal tract changes

The medium-sized and smaller portal tracts are affected and there may also be focal periportal inflammation. The portal tracts contain a variable chronic inflammatory cell infiltrate but an entirely normal portal tract may be seen in the same microscopic field, emphasizing the focal nature of these reactive changes (Fig. 17.1A,B). Lymphocytes usually predominate but ceroid-containing macrophages may also be present and, rarely, a few plasma cells and eosinophils; neutrophil polymorphs are hardly ever seen. The cellular infiltrate within the portal tract is diffuse. The limiting plate is intact, but where the infiltrate is more intense, some irregular spillover into the periportal parenchyma may occur without any liver-cell necrosis. In a few instances, especially in older age groups, lymphoid follicles may be present.

Parenchymal changes

These comprise foci of liver-cell necrosis and Kupffer-cell prominence. The foci of necrosis may be very small, involving only a few hepatocytes, or may be larger involving several liver-cell plates and producing focal reticulin collapse or condensation. In relation to these foci, lymphocytes and macrophages accumulate (Fig. 17.1C), and are best demonstrated on a periodic acid-Schiff (PAS) diastase preparation. The larger foci, comprising small macrophage aggregates, are sometimes referred to as microgranulomas, although the term granulomatoid reaction is a more accurate description in that epithelioid cells are only poorly developed and giant cells are not seen (Fig. 17.1D). Kupffer-cell hyperplasia occurs near foci of liver-cell necrosis, and in addition generalized Kupffer-cell prominence may be evident, particularly in the perivenular zones. Increased lipofuscin and ceroid pigment deposits are present; there may be irregular focal steatosis and some variation in hepatocyte and nuclear size.

The major differential diagnoses are mild chronic hepatitis C virus (HCV) infection and residual acute hepatitis of varied aetiologies (see Ch. 8). In chronic HCV infection lymphoid follicles, focal hepatocyte necrosis and reactive Kupffer-cell hyperplasia are also seen. In addition, low-grade interface hepatitis is often present and acidophil bodies may be evident. In non-specific reactive hepatitis,

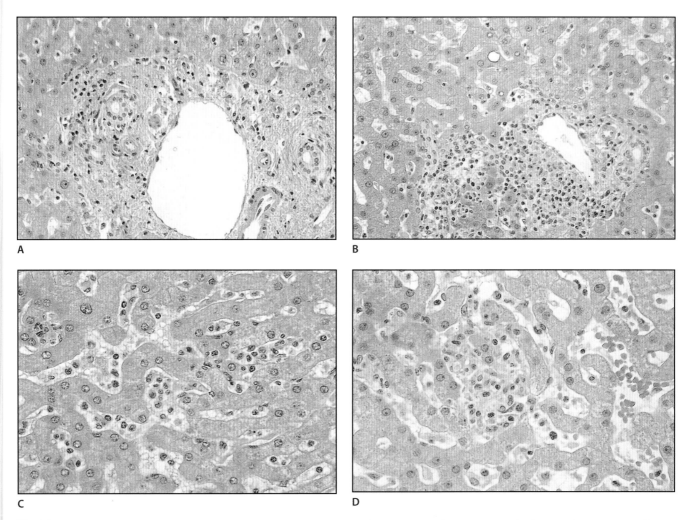

Fig. 17.1 • Non-specific reactive hepatitis: these illustrations are from a biopsy taken from a patient with a carcinoma in the ileo-caecal region. **(A)** Portal tract showing a very light chronic inflammatory cell infiltrate; **(B)** portal tract showing a mixed lymphocyte and macrophage infiltrate with some periportal spillover; **(C)** sinusoidal infiltrate of inflammatory cells with reactive Kupffer-cell hyperplasia; **(D)** granulomatoid aggregate of lymphocytes and macrophages. H & E.

macrophages predominate around foci of liver-cell necrosis. In many instances it is not possible to distinguish between the two on the histological features and circulating anti-HCV antibodies or HCV RNA should be sought. In residual viral hepatitis there is usually a more generalized portal tract involvement, slight portal tract fibrosis with some septum formation may be present, parenchymal changes are predominantly perivenular, some single-cell acidophilic necrosis may be found, and a Prussian blue (Perls') reaction will often show mild Kupffer-cell siderosis.

Space-occupying lesions in the liver

Tumour deposits and other focal lesions may produce both obstructive and pressure effects and liver biopsies undertaken in the investigation of these may show fairly distinctive features.[2,3] Non-specific reactive changes are usually present. The portal tracts show some oedema; there is irregularity, sometimes focal, of the limiting plates with a cholangiolitis, comprising prominence of the marginal bile ductules and an infiltrate of neutrophil polymorphs (Fig. 17.2A,B); periductal neutrophils are sometimes conspicuous particularly around the smallest terminal bile ducts and around isolated ductules within the parenchyma (Fig. 17.2C). The portal tract changes may develop due to local interference with bile flow. In addition, however, sinusoidal dilatation and congestion may occur due to pressure on hepatic venules. The hepatic veins are normal and hepatocytes within zones of dilatation rarely show atrophy. The sinusoidal dilatation is most striking in the perivenular areas but in some instances the changes are more extensive (Fig. 17.2C).

Hepatic granulomas

Granulomas may occur in the liver in a wide variety of disorders, some of which are primary in the liver, but most are part of a generalized disease process. The use of the term *epithelioid cell granulomas* serves to distinguish them from *lipogranulomas*, which are seen in steatotic livers, particularly in alcoholic liver disease.[4] The latter comprise loose aggregates of lymphocytes and macrophages, sometimes with a few poorly developed epithelioid cells and, rarely, one or two multinucleated giant cells (Fig. 17.3A). They occur against a background of steatosis and lipid material is usually demonstrable around the lesions and within the constituent macrophages.

A number of reports have drawn attention to lipogranulomas which may occur in non-fatty liver and which tend to be more common in portal tracts than in the parenchyma.[5–7] They are frequently perivenular and appear as a cluster of variably sized lipid droplets surrounded by a light infiltrate of lymphocytes and macrophages; there is some local increase in fibrous tissue (Fig. 17.3B). Spleen and lymph nodes may also be involved. They are thought to be the result of mineral oil deposition and such oils are widely used in the food industry.[6,7] These lesions are generally of little consequence and are most often seen as incidental

findings on liver biopsy or at autopsy. However, Keen et al.[8] described two cases in which extensive mineral oil lipogranulomatosis led to venous outflow obstruction. Rarely, they may be seen as part of a disseminated process following self-administration of mineral oil injections.[9]

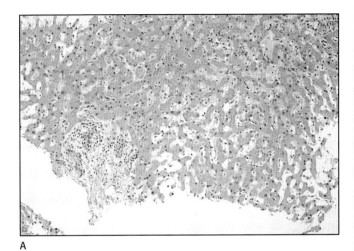

A

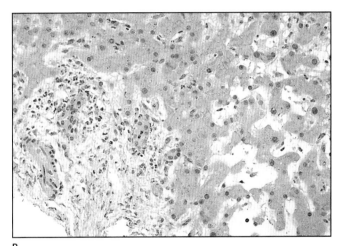

B

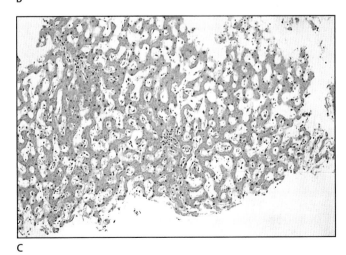

C

Fig. 17.2 • Liver biopsy from a patient suspected of having metastatic tumour. **(A)** There is some sinusoidal dilatation and the portal tract shows oedema and inflammation which in **(B)** is associated with an acute cholangiolitis. **(C)** There is more marked sinusoidal dilatation evident in this area of the biopsy. H & E.

Bernstein et al.[10] drew attention to a peculiar appearance of the hepatic granulomas in Q fever. These show a distinctive ring pattern (Fig. 17.3C) in which fibrin is deposited circumferentially within or at the margin of the granulomas; a central fat vacuole may be present. The association between these so-called fibrin-ring or doughnut granulomas and Q fever has been confirmed.[11] It is now apparent, however, that they are not pathognomonic for this disease.[12] Their occurrence in a variety of conditions including Boutonneuse fever,[13] allopurinol hypersensitivity,[14] cytomegalovirus (CMV) infection,[15] leishmaniasis,[16] hepatitis A,[17] staphylococcal infection,[18] Epstein–Barr virus (EBV) infection,[19] systemic lupus erythematosus[20] and giant-cell arteritis[21] suggests that the granulomas may represent a relatively non-specific but uncommon response to injury.[12,20–23]

The following account is confined to a discussion of epithelioid cell granulomas. These represent in part focal collections of macrophages which have undergone phenotypic modulation to predominantly secretory (as opposed to phagocytic) cells in response to antigenic stimulation; recruitment of circulating dendritic cell precursors are thought to contribute to the epithelioid cell population.[24,25] This is normally an example of delayed type hypersensitivity which is under the regulation of Th1 lymphocytes and a variety of associated cytokines and chemokines including interleukin (IL)-1, interferon γ, tumour necrosis factor and Rantes. Th2 cells play an important role in the formation of granulomas associated with parasites (e.g. *Schistosoma mansoni*).[26] There is recent evidence suggesting that the tetraspanin molecule CD9 plays a central role in granuloma formation.[27] Osteopontin is also involved, acting as a mediator for the recruitment of cells into developing granulomas and a stimulus for their persistence.[28]

Granulomas may be found in up to 10% of liver biopsies.[29,30] The list of causes of hepatic granulomas (Table 17.1) is a long one and many are rare.[31–50] For the histopathologist few distinguishing morphological features are found in most cases.[51,52] Four distinct clinicopathological correlates are observed:[52,53] (i) cases in which the cause can be identified on the basis of the histopathology; (ii) those in which the cause is known but is not morphologically apparent; (iii) those in which the cause is suspected; and (iv) those in which it is unknown. In establishing a diagnosis there is a need for a detailed clinical history, appropriate skin testing and careful microbiological, serological and biochemical screening; assays for angiotensin converting enzyme may be helpful in the case of sarcoidosis. The PAS stain is most useful for defining the number and distribution of granulomas. Involvement of bile ducts with associated ductal damage suggests primary biliary cirrhosis but may also be associated with drug injury and sarcoidosis; periductal bile granulomas may occur in large-duct obstruction but there is usually an accompanying acute cholangitis.

A non-portal distribution of granulomas is said to be characteristic of tuberculosis;[1] in biopsies, caseation is an infrequent feature and acid-fast bacilli are demonstrated in less than 10% of proven cases; these findings are much more common in autopsy material. In miliary tuberculosis

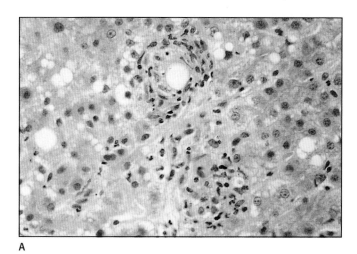

A

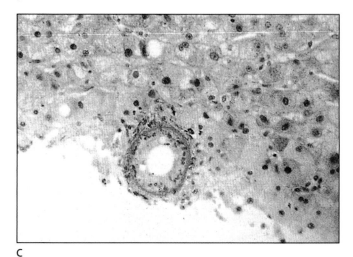

B

C

Fig. 17.3 • Hepatic granulomas. **(A)** Lipogranuloma in a fatty liver; the larger one above comprises a central fat globule surrounded by a cuff of inflammatory cells. H & E. **(B)** Mineral oil granulomas, found incidentally at autopsy, are present both in a portal tract and in the perivenular zone; there is also chronic inflammation of the portal tract, and some increase in fibrous tissue is present around the parenchymal collection of lipid-laden macrophages. Haematoxylin-phloxine-saffron. Courtesy of Dr I R Wanless. **(C)** Fibrin ring granuloma from a patient with Q fever; there is a cuff of inflammatory cells in which neutrophils are prominent. MSB. Courtesy of Dr A Sherwood.

Table 17.1	Hepatic granulomas—reported causes

INFECTIOUS DISEASES

Bacterial
  Actinomycosis
  Bartonella henselae[31]
  Borrelia (Lyme disease)[32]
  Botryomycosis
  Brucellosis
  Cat-scratch disease
  Granuloma inguinale
  Listeriosis
  Melioidosis
  Nocardiosis
  Proprioniosis
  Staphylococcal infections
  Syphilis (primary and secondary)
  Tularaemia[33]
  Typhoid
  Whipple disease
  Yersinia enterocolitica[34]

Mycobacterial
  Tuberculosis
  Atypical mycobacteria (e.g. *M. avium intracellulare*)
  BCG immunization and immunotherapy[35]
  Leprosy (lepromatous and tuberculoid)

Rickettsial
  Boutonneuse fever
  Q fever
  Rickettsia conorii infection

Chlamydial
  Lymphopathia venereum
  Psittacosis

Fungal
  Aspergillosis
  Blastomycosis (North and South American)
  Candidiasis
  Coccidioidomycosis
  Cryptococcus
  Histoplasmosis
  Mucormycosis
  Paracoccidioidomycosis

Viral
  CMV infection
  EBV—infectious mononucleosis[19]
  Hepatitis A[17]
  Hepatitis B[36]
  Hepatitis C[37]
  Varicella[38]

Parasitic
  Amoebiasis
  Ancylostomiasis
  Capillariasis
  Enterobius vermicularis infection[39]
  Fascioliasis
  Giardiasis
  Linguatula serrata[40]
  Paragonimiasis
  Opisthorchiasis
  Pentastomiasis
  Schistosomiasis
  Strongyloidiasis
  Toxocariasis
  Visceral leishmaniasis (kala-azar)

HYPERSENSITIVITY
  Drugs (see Ch 14)
  Metals—beryllium, copper, gold

IMMUNOLOGICAL DISEASES
  Common variable immunodeficiency[41]
  Chronic granulomatous disease of childhood[42]
  Hypogammaglobulinaemia
  Polymyalgia rheumatica
  Primary biliary cirrhosis
  Primary sclerosing cholangitis
  Rheumatic fever[43]
  Systemic lupus erythematosus
  Vascular diseases
    allergic granulomatosis
    necrotizing angiitis in drug abuse[44]
    polyarteritis nodosa
    temporal arteritis
  Wegener granulomatosis

FOREIGN MATERIALS
  Anthracotic pigments
  Barium
  Cement and mica dust
  Mineral oil—radiocontrast media, food additives
  Polyvinyl pyrrolidone
  Silica
  Silicone rubber—renal dialysis tubing[45]
  Starch
  Suture material
  Talc
  Thorotrast

NEOPLASMS
  Extrahepatic malignancy[46]
  Hepatocellular adenoma and liver adenomatosis[47]
  Hodgkin disease
  Non-Hodgkin lymphoma

MISCELLANEOUS
  Biliary tract obstruction—bile granulomas
  Chronic inflammatory bowel disease
  Eosinophilic enteritis[48]
  Jejuno-ileal bypass surgery
  Porphyria cutanea tarda[49]
  Sarcoidosis
  Lipiodolized neocarzinostatin[50]

This table is based on several excellent reviews;[21,22,23,29,30] additional references are given where appropriate

well-formed giant-cell granulomas are infrequent in biopsies and the characteristic features are a marked generalized Kupffer-cell hyperplasia with small macrophage 'microgranulomas'.

Particulate material such as schistosome ova may be seen on routine stains or may be identified on phase-contrast or polarizing microscopy. Serial sectioning may be necessary to show that the lesion is primarily vascular. Special microbial stains including immunohistochemistry are applied when infectious agents are suspected[30,53] and polymerase chain reaction (PCR) for microbial DNA or RNA using liver tissue may also be of value.[54] Eosinophil–rich granulomas should raise the possibility of toxacariasis (visceral larva migrans).[55]

In an early study of over 6000 biopsies,[29] 74% were associated with generalized granulomatous disease, 4% with primary hepatic disease, and in the remaining 22% no definite diagnosis was reached. This failure to establish a cause for hepatic granulomas in 20–25% of patients has been reported by others[56] and in some series the figure has been as high as 50%.[57] Prospective follow-up may result in the aetiology of the granuloma declaring itself in a further 15%.[57,58] In a recent retrospective study of 1662 consecutive biopsies, Gaya et al.[59] found 63 cases with hepatic granulomas; in this group the commonest underlying diagnoses were primary biliary cirrhosis (23.8%), sarcoidosis (11.1%), drugs (9.5%), HCV (9.5%), autoimmune overlap syndrome (6.3%) and Hodgkin disease (6.3%). In some 5–10% of patients no specific diagnosis is reached and they may be regarded as having *idiopathic granulomatous hepatitis*.[56,59] Such patients characteristically have a prolonged or recurrent pyrexial illness with weight loss, myalgia, arthralgia and vague abdominal pain.[56] They fail to benefit from a trial of antituberculous drugs[58] but may improve in response to administration of corticosteroids or methotrexate;[60] in some patients the condition resolves spontaneously.[61] It should be stressed that the diagnosis of idiopathic granulomatous hepatitis is one of exclusion and should be made only after exhaustive investigation has failed to identify a specific aetiology. The term is in some respects a misnomer, in that there is seldom any significant hepatocellular damage,[56] and it has been suggested that it may represent a form of sarcoidosis confined to the liver.[56]

A study by Collins et al.[62] of 23 cases of hepatic granulomas in children showed that the yield of specific diagnoses is increased when molecular approaches are included. They identified an aetiology in 87%; histoplasma was incriminated in 65% of their cases by PCR.

There is one report of familial granulomatous hepatitis in which two parents and three of their seven children were affected.[63] There are also occasional reports of hepatocellular carcinoma developing in patients with chronic granulomatous hepatitis.[64,65]

Sarcoidosis and the liver

Sarcoidosis, a disease of unknown aetiology,[66] is one of the most common causes of non-caseating hepatic granulomas. The disease most commonly affects young adults but may occasionally be seen in children.[67] The incidence of hepatic involvement in published series ranges from 17 to 90%.[68–73] The liver follows lymph nodes and lung in frequency of involvement. Klatskin[29] estimated that the affected liver may contain as many as 75 million granulomas but, despite this, the large majority of patients show minimal evidence of clinical or biochemical hepatic dysfunction. In some patients a diagnosis of sarcoidosis has been established on liver biopsy where there was no radiological evidence of pulmonary involvement.[74]

The histopathology of hepatic sarcoidosis was reviewed by Ishak.[72] Sarcoid granulomas occur diffusely in the liver but tend to be more frequent in portal tracts or in the periportal area. They consist of a compact aggregate of irregularly arranged large epithelioid cells, sometimes with multinucleated giant cells, and with a surrounding rim of lymphocytes and macrophages; occasional eosinophils may also be present (Fig. 17.4A). The peripheral mantle of lymphocytes is a mixed population of CD4- and CD8- positive cells. Schaumann and asteroid bodies tend to be infrequent in hepatic granulomas of sarcoidosis. Central granular eosinophilic fibrinoid necrosis may occur but caseation is never found. Reticulin fibres are abundant within the granulomas, particularly in older lesions, when a surrounding cuff of fibrous tissue becomes prominent and dense scars taking on some of the staining reactions of amyloid may develop. In the majority of cases resolution is complete, but giant cells may persist for some time in the fibrous scars. Confluent granulomas may result in extensive irregular scarring. A non-specific reactive hepatitis often accompanies the granulomas, and lobular hepatitis may be a prominent feature when there is active clinical disease.[68–70] Damage to bile ducts (Fig. 17.4B) may be seen in some portal tracts, the lesions resembling those seen in primary biliary cirrhosis.[69,72]

In a few patients with sarcoidosis, progressive liver disease with portal hypertension, ascites and hepatic encephalopathy ensues.[68,69,71,75,76] Maddrey et al.,[68] in a review of 300 patients described 20 in whom there was clinical and/or biochemical evidence of liver disease; of these, 10 showed severe functional hepatic impairment with or without portal hypertension. In some, progressive portal and parenchymal fibrosis developed. The fibrosis was in part related to the presence of granulomas, but extensive fibrosis unrelated to granulomas also occurred and contributed to the development of cirrhosis. The histological appearances in a similar patient who died of hepatic failure are shown in Figures 17.4C and D. In their study of 100 cases of hepatic sarcoidosis, Devaney et al.[69] found fibrosis in 21 and cirrhosis in 6 patients.

Portal hypertension may develop in the absence of cirrhosis.[68,75–77] Valla et al.[77] described patients with sarcoidosis in whom portal hypertension was the predominant clinical feature. In these 32 patients the portal hypertension was due to a presinusoidal block, the result of a pressure effect by portal tract granulomas, and sometimes a superimposed sinusoidal block due to fibrosis. Nodular regenerative hyperplasia may contribute in some cases.[69] Obstruction of hepatic vein branches by sarcoid granulomas is a rare cause of Budd–Chiari syndrome.[78]

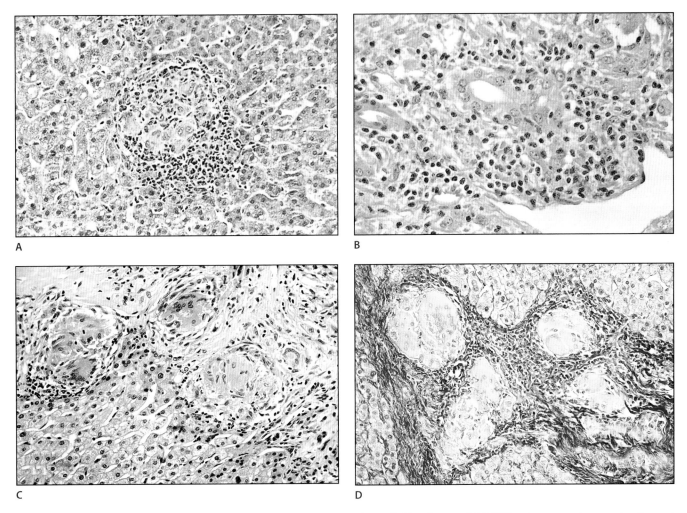

Fig. 17.4 • Liver in sarcoidosis. **(A)** Typical parenchymal granuloma with a surrounding cuff of lymphocytes. H & E. **(B)** Portal tract granuloma causing damage to the bile duct. H & E. **(C)** Diffuse hepatic involvement in sarcoidosis with a confluent aggregate of giant-cell granulomas. H & E. **(D)** The extensive scarring is shown here on a van Gieson stain.

A chronic prolonged cholestatic syndrome with progression to biliary cirrhosis may rarely occur in sarcoidosis and this must be considered in the differential diagnosis of chronic cholestatic disease.[79–81] Histologically there is ductopenia which correlates with the amount of fibrosis. Rudzki and his colleagues[82] reviewed 21 such cases and reported five of their own; clinically and biochemically these patients expressed many of the features of primary biliary cirrhosis but anti-mitochondrial antibody was not found and their five additional cases were males. Devaney et al.[69] described bile-duct lesions similar to primary biliary cirrhosis in 19% of their patients with sarcoidosis and in 13% there were lesions resembling primary sclerosing cholangitis.

Murphy et al.[83] emphasized the progressive bile-duct loss which was a feature in their five patients, three of whom were male and all of whom were black. The similarities between sarcoidosis and primary biliary cirrhosis have been reviewed in a number of studies.[79,80,83–85] In the 'overlap' patients, pulmonary symptoms were the principal initial manifestations with cholestatic liver disease developing subsequently.[76] In general, anti-mitochondrial antibody is not present in sarcoidosis and the Kveim–Siltzbach test is negative in primary biliary cirrhosis (although the latter is no longer in routine clinical use). There are very rare cases in which both tests are positive[86] and it remains speculative whether these patients have two co-existing disorders.[85]

Occasional cases of cholestasis in sarcoidosis are the result of a mass effect of sarcoid nodules at the hilum of the liver with bile-duct obstruction.[72,87] Hepatic sarcoidosis does not appear to respond well to therapeutic intervention. Although frequently used, there is no evidence that corticosteroids prevent disease progression in asymptomatic patients.[88] A variety of agents including methotrexate have been used in cases with advanced liver disease[71] but in some transplantation may be indicated; the disease may recur in the allograft.[89]

In the recent study of Lipson et al.,[90] sarcoidosis was the indication for hepatic transplantation in 0.3% of adult patients in their centre. Graft and patient survival rates were comparable to other disease groups; hepatic granulomas were seen in the allograft of one patient after five years follow up.

Steatosis

Steatosis or fatty liver is characterized by the accumulation of lipid within the cytoplasm of hepatocytes. It is a common finding in liver biopsy specimens.[91] The significance of small amounts is uncertain; it is often a non-specific finding and may be a manifestation of the aging liver.[92] More extensive fat accumulation occurs in a large number of primary hepatic disorders (see Chapters 6 and 7) and in a variety of systemic conditions.

In normal liver, lipid accounts for approximately 5% of total wet weight.[93] This can increase to as much as 50% in steatosis resulting in marked hepatomegaly (up to 5 kg). On cut section at autopsy or in explant specimens, the liver has a pale yellow appearance and a greasy consistency (Fig. 17.5A); the colour is largely due to retained carotenes. Histologically, in routine-fixed material the fat in hepatocytes is seen as cytoplasmic vacuoles since the lipid is lost during processing. Lipid can be demonstrated in cryostat sections using oil red O or Sudan black or in tissue that has been post-fixed in osmium tetroxide.[94]

Two major patterns of steatosis are recognized on light microscopy: *macrovesicular* and *microvesicular* (see also Chapter 2).[91,95] In the former the hepatocytes are distended by a single droplet which displaces the nucleus (Fig. 17.5B). Uncomplicated macrovesicular steatosis has generally been regarded a benign and fully reversible condition although the notion has been challenged recently.[96] In some cases this form of steatosis may be accompanied by additional features of cell injury including ballooning degeneration, cytoskeletal abnormalities and accompanying necroinflammation—*steatohepatitis*.[95,97] Microvesicular steatosis (Fig. 17.5C and D) is generally a serious condition with hepatic dysfunction and coma and one which is often associated with impaired β-oxidation of lipids. Factors that may be involved in the pathogenesis of both forms of steatosis are outlined in Table 17.2.

The distinction between macrovesicular and microvesicular steatosis is not absolute and in some biopsies one may see a mixed pattern; this may be of prognostic importance in alcoholic liver disease.[98] In animal models, there is a gradual transition from a microvesicular form to large droplet steatosis by coalescence of the cytoplasmic lipid

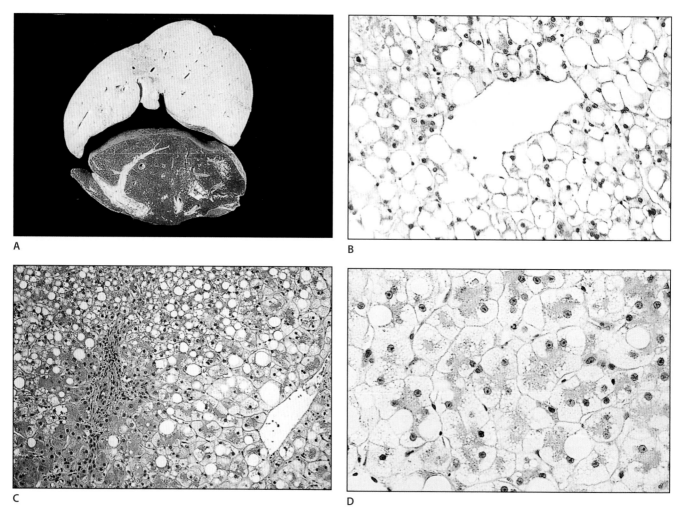

Fig. 17.5 • Fatty liver. **(A)** Gross appearance showing the yellow colour contrasting with a normal liver. **(B)** Macrovesicular perivenular steatosis in an alcoholic patient; there is no fibrosis. Masson trichrome. **(C)** Alcoholic foamy degeneration in which both macrovesicular and microvesicular steatosis is present in the perivenular and mid-zones. H & E. **(D)** Note that the nucleus remains in a central position in the microvesicular pattern, whereas it is displaced when a macrovesicle is present; there is also canalicular and intracellular bilirubinostasis. PAS-diastase.

Table 17.2	Mechanisms which may be involved in causing fatty liver

A. Increased triglyceride synthesis
   1. Excessive availability of fatty acids
       Dietary intake
       Adipose tissue, e.g. obesity, diabetes mellitus, corticosteroid therapy
       Parenteral nutrition
   2. Increased availability of fatty acid precursors
       Carbohydrate-rich dietary intake
       Alcohol
   3. Reduced fatty acid oxidation
       Mitochondrial dysfunction, e.g. drugs/toxins; Reye syndrome
       Acyl-CoA dehydrogenase deficiency

B. Reduced triglyceride excretion
   1. Reduced apoprotein synthesis
       Protein malnutrition, e.g. kwashiorkor, gastrointestinal malabsorption
       Metabolic diseases (Ch. 5)
       Drug/toxin-induced injury, e.g. tetracycline, carbon tetrachloride, alcohol

C. Cryptogenic

Table 17.3	Causes of microvesicular steatosis

Acute fatty liver of pregnancy

Reye syndrome

Drugs
   Salicylate toxicity
   Sodium valproate toxicity[101]
   Tetracycline toxicity
   2-arylpropionic acids (e.g. ketoprofen)[102]
   Amineptine[103]
   MDMA (ecstasy)[104]
   Didanosine[105]
   Fialuridine[106]
   Stavudine[107]

Acute iron toxicity[108]

Aflatoxins

Jamaican vomiting disease[109]

Multiple hornet stings[110]

Alcoholic foamy degeneration[111]

Inherited urea cycle disorders[112]

Inherited disorders of fatty acid metabolism[113]

Mitochondrial cytopathies[114]

Wolman disease

Cholesterol ester storage disease[115]

Hepatitis D infection in Amazonian Indians (Labrea fever)[116]

Bacillus cereus toxins[117]

Navajo neuropathy[118]

Pearson's syndrome[119]

vacuoles.[99] An autopsy study of adults with no history of liver disease has suggested that the prevalence of microvesicular steatosis may be underestimated.[100]

Macrovesicular steatosis is the commoner form and the causes are discussed in Chapter 7. The distribution of fat is variable. In alcoholic steatosis, the fat is generally first seen in perivenular zones while that seen in wasting disease (such as AIDS) and following steroid therapy commences in the periportal zones. In our experience however, there may be no apparent zonality in these conditions.[95]

The causes of microvesicular steatosis are listed in Table 17.3.[101–117] The first to be recognized was acute fatty liver of pregnancy (p. 898). It was subsequently recognized to be a key feature in Reye syndrome and more recently it has been described with a variety of therapeutic agents.[102] Recent evidence suggests that a feature common to all forms of microvesicular steatosis is impairment of mitochondrial β-oxidation.[118] This is the process by which acyl-coenzyme A (CoA) derived from long-, medium- and short-chain fatty acids is progressively cleaved into acetyl-CoA units. The process leads to the generation of reducing equivalents for oxidative phosphorylation and involves five complexes found within the inner mitochondrial membranes; some of the subunits of these complexes are encoded by mitochondrial DNA. Some inherited metabolic conditions associated with microvesicular steatosis, notably some of the mitochondrial cytopathies,[112] are associated with mitochondrial DNA mutations or deletions. Drug-induced microvesicular steatosis may involve direct inhibition of β-oxidation by drug metabolites.[102] Chronic alcohol abuse may lead to acquired mitochondrial DNA deletions and may be associated with so-called alcoholic foamy degeneration[119] (Ch. 6).

The classical form of steatohepatitis is that associated with alcohol abuse. However, identical histological changes can be seen in non-alcoholic patients. The term *non-alcoholic steatohepatitis* (NASH) is now widely accepted for this entity.[97] It is a disease of increasing prevalence and importance and is discussed in detail in Chapter 7.

Focal fatty change

This was first described in 1980, since then it has become increasingly recognized in that it is picked up by imaging techniques including ultrasound or computed tomography, and may simulate metastatic disease.[120,121] The lesions may be single or multiple,[122] they may sometimes be nodular, and they have occasionally been associated with other hepatic abnormalities such as cirrhosis.[123] The basic architecture of the liver, however, is usually preserved and while some patients have been identified in whom factors predisposing to generalized macrovesicular steatosis were present, the mechanisms leading to a non-homogeneous distribution of fat are not clear, although local hypoxia has been postulated to play a role.[121] The lesion must be distinguished from other intrahepatic lipid-rich lesions such as lipoma, angiolipoma, myelolipoma and coelomic fat ectopia. Focal steatosis may also occur in hepatic adenomas and focal nodular hyperplasia.[124]

Nutritional liver disease

Malnutrition may be the cause of, or may be a contributory factor in certain liver diseases and conversely disturbances of nutrition occur in liver disease and are significant factors in the clinical syndromes which accompany hepatic dysfunction.[125,126]

The liver in protein-energy malnutrition

Steatosis is an almost invariable feature of kwashiorkor although it is less frequently encountered in marasmus.[127,128] The steatosis of kwashiorkor is first seen as small droplets in periportal hepatocytes. These lipid globules later coalesce and the changes progress to involve the entire lobule.[127–129] Following refeeding, lipid first clears from the perivenular hepatocytes. In the vast majority of cases, the steatosis of kwashiorkor is manifest by asymptomatic hepatomegaly. Biochemical tests of liver function are often normal although occasional cases of severe cholestasis have been described.[130] Histologically, there is little hepatocyte necrosis or inflammation. Mallory body-like material has been described in some cases[128] but a true steatohepatitis does not develop.

It was previously thought that fibrosis and cirrhosis were long-term consequences of the hepatic involvement in kwashiorkor. This concept of so-called nutritional liver disease developed from observations in experimental models where animals developed cirrhosis when fed nutritionally deficient diets and from epidemiological studies which demonstrated a high incidence of cirrhosis in populations in whom protein-energy malnutrition was a major problem. The concept was further applied to other forms of chronic liver disease and it was at one time suggested that alcoholic cirrhosis might be the result of dietary insufficiency.[131] It is now clear that the observations made in choline- or protein-deficient rats are not relevant to the pathogenesis of human liver disease and that the steatosis of kwashiorkor per se does not lead to cirrhosis.[132] Liver dysfunction is not a significant cause of mortality in protein-energy malnutrition. When fibrosis and/or necroinflammation is present in patients with kwashiorkor it is likely to be related to another factor such as chronic hepatitis B virus (HBV) infection.[127]

The pathogenesis of steatosis in kwashiorkor remains controversial. Although aflatoxin ingestion may be a contributory factor in some parts of the world,[133] most evidence suggests that the lipid accumulation results from an imbalance in hepatic carbohydrate, protein and lipid metabolism.[127] Several studies have demonstrated abnormal plasma lipid profiles resulting in an increased delivery of non-esterified fatty acids to hepatocytes.[134] There is also evidence that apolipoprotein deficiency occurs, leading to decreased

mobilization of triglycerides from liver cells.[135] Doherty and co-workers[136] have shown that hepatocytes in kwashiorkor lack peroxisomes and they have postulated that this may lead to altered β-oxidation of fat, thereby contributing to the development of steatosis.

Fatty liver is not a feature of the other major form of malnutrition, marasmus. Steatosis, if present, is mild and focal with no particular zonal distribution. The hepatocytes tend to be atrophic and the sinusoids are dilated but there is no parenchymal inflammation and no fibrosis. Peliosis hepatis has been reported in a patient with marasmus.[137]

Total parenteral nutrition

Total parenteral nutrition (TPN) by the intravenous route (also referred to as intravenous alimentation) has become an accepted treatment modality over the past 30 years. Peden et al.[138] first drew attention to hepatic complications in infants treated with TPN and such complications are now well recognized in both infants and adults. However, it is difficult to define precisely the contribution which TPN might make to liver dysfunction in these patients in that, in many instances, the primary disease for which TPN is indicated and the clinical complications, sepsis for example, which subsequently develop, might themselves cause liver injury.[139] The hepatic complications associated with TPN have been reviewed in detail[140–142] and, although the same mechanisms may operate in producing some of the liver injuries, the effects in infancy and adults differ. In both infants and adults biliary sludging, cholelithiasis and acalculous cholecystitis are common and this may result in biliary obstruction.

Hepatic disease in infants

The incidence of TPN-associated cholestasis in infants correlates inversely with the gestational age and birth weight and is also related to the duration of treatment.[141] The diagnosis is one of exclusion, and 'physiological' cholestasis, the numerous other causes of neonatal cholestasis (see Chapter 4) and sepsis have also to be considered.

Morphologically, the changes are not specific and are extremely variable.[138,140,143,144] Bilirubinostasis affecting liver cells and canaliculi is consistently present and may develop in a matter of days; cholestatic rosettes are frequently observed; bile plugs may also be present in interlobular bile ducts. Steatosis is infrequent. The portal tracts show a variable mixed inflammatory cell infiltrate and, with prolonged therapy, a periportal ductular reaction and progressive fibrosis may lead to a biliary cirrhosis (Fig. 17.6).[142] Where treatment is prolonged serial liver biopsy is indicated to assess any liver injury.[145] There is evidence to suggest that progressive disease with fibrosis may be less frequent than previously feared in children on long-term TPN.[146] A recent autopsy study detailed findings in 24 neonates that had been treated with TPN. The severity of liver injury was related to the length of therapy. Those with a duration of TPN administration of greater than 6 weeks were more likely to have significant fibrosis and cholestasis than those on shorter courses.[147]

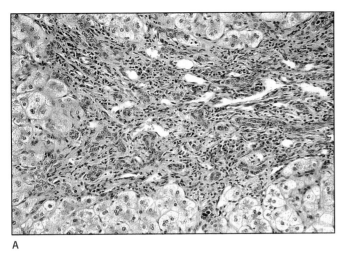 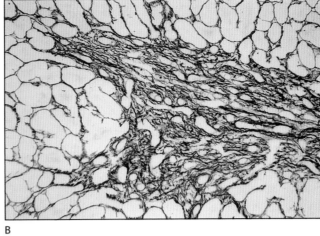

Fig. 17.6 • Severe liver injury associated with long-standing TPN in a 13-month-old child with necrotizing enterocolitis. Prominent portal tract expansion with fibrosis, ductular reaction and mild inflammatory cell infiltration including pigmented macrophages. **(A)** H & E. **(B)** Gordon and Sweets reticulin.

The pathogenetic mechanisms involved in TPN-associated cholestasis are not clear. Physiological immaturity of hepatic excretory function, including bile acid metabolism and transport, the absence of enteral nutrition with disturbances of the normal enterohepatic circulation, suppression of trophic or secretion-stimulating hormones and the composition of the infusate, including specific unidentified deficiencies, have been suggested.[148]

Hepatic disease in adults

Hepatic abnormalities are common following parenteral nutrition in older children and adults but the incidence is difficult to establish and, in most cases, evidence of hepatic dysfunction is transient. High-calorie dextrose-based TPN was used initially, but lower calorie infusions containing fat are now more common and have been associated with a lower incidence of hepatic dysfunction. However, whereas increases in serum bilirubin are mild and relatively uncommon when compared with that in infants, increases in the serum levels of transaminases, alkaline phosphatase and β-glutamyltranspeptidase are found in 20–60% of patients, may develop within 5–20 days of commencing treatment, and may persist in 15–25% of patients who receive long-term TPN.[140,149] When conservative management of TPN-related liver disease fails, isolated intestinal or intestine/liver transplantation may be required.[150]

The morphological lesions in the liver (Fig. 17.7) include intrahepatic cholestasis, macrovesicular steatosis and portal and periportal fibrosis.[140,151,152] Intrahepatic perivenular bilirubinostasis develops after 2–3 weeks on TPN and may be accompanied by periportal inflammation and portal fibrosis which persists after discontinuation of treatment. Forrest et al.[153] demonstrated clinical improvement in a patient treated with anti-TNFα monoclonal antibody suggesting that this cytokine plays a role in the process. Chronic cholestasis in TPN-associated liver disease is associated with significant secondary copper overload.[154] The macrovesicular steatosis is predominantly periportal and is thought to be due to imbalance in the rate of fat deposition and removal, although carnitine and choline deficiency have both been postulated.[155,156]

Non-alcoholic steatohepatitis may also occur but the true incidence of progression to cirrhosis is not clear.[140,157] In the study of 60 patients by Bowyer et al.[157] who had been treated with long-term TPN, nine (15%) had persistently abnormal liver function tests; biopsy in eight of the patients showed steatohepatitis in all, with perivenular fibrosis in three and nodular regeneration in one.

The liver in gastrointestinal diseases

Hepatic involvement in diseases of the gastrointestinal tract is not uncommon, the portal vein affording a means whereby toxins, microorganisms and tumour emboli may gain direct access to the organ. Non-specific reactive hepatitis, intrahepatic sepsis and disseminated intrahepatic metastases result. However, there are specific hepatobiliary disorders which may accompany chronic inflammatory bowel disease (IBD) and a few other miscellaneous associations are also outlined below.

Chronic inflammatory bowel disease

Liver disease in ulcerative colitis was first reported by Thomas[158] in 1873 who described an enlarged fatty liver in a young male. The hepatic lesions in Crohn disease were subsequently found to resemble those described in ulcerative colitis; with some exceptions, the spectrum of the liver disease in each is essentially similar. Hepatic dysfunction in Crohn disease is more frequently associated with colonic involvement and is usually coincident with other extra-intestinal systemic complications.[159] The association between liver dysfunction and chronic IBD is now well recognized and a number of detailed clinicopathological reviews have been published.[160–163]

The classic studies by Mistilis and his colleagues[164,165] drew attention to so-called pericholangitis associated with

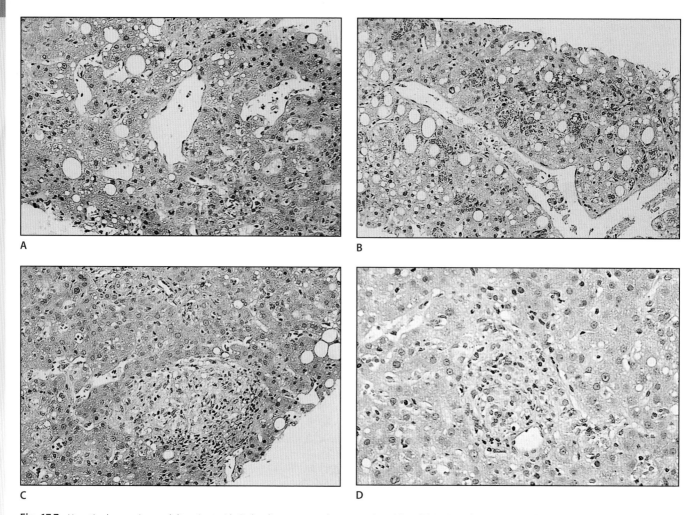

Fig. 17.7 • Hepatic changes in an adult patient with Crohn disease on total parenteral nutrition. **(A)** Perivenular macrovesicular and microvesicular steatosis and bilirubinostasis. H & E. **(B)** Prominent aggregates of ceroid-containing macrophages. PAS-diastase. **(C)** A granulomatoid aggregate of foamy macrophages with some lymphocytes and plasma cells. H & E. **(D)** Portal tract inflammation with prominent macrophages, lymphocytes and occasional eosinophils. H & E.

ulcerative colitis, and they found this liver lesion in 5.4% of 441 ulcerative colitis patients. They emphasized injury to intrahepatic bile ducts as part of this disease entity, which could pursue a chronic course sometimes leading to cirrhosis. In subsequent studies the term pericholangitis became synonymous with the liver involvement in chronic IBD.[166,167] The development of endoscopic retrograde cholangiopancreatography (ERCP), however, served to draw attention to those patients in whom there were obliterative lesions in the biliary system, to which the term primary sclerosing cholangitis (PSC) was applied. It now seems highly unlikely that pericholangitis exists as a disease entity separate from PSC[168] and histopathologists should no longer use the term as a morphological diagnosis.[169] The development of PSC in inflammatory bowel disease may reflect a common or overlapping autoimmune process;[170] atypical forms of p-anti-neutrophil cytoplasmic antibodies (pANCA) are seen in PSC and IBD.[171]

Abnormalities of liver function tests have been reported in approximately 50% of patients with chronic IBD.[172,173] However, the frequency of histologically proven significant liver disease is considered to be much lower, although there are no prospective studies on patients from the time of first presentation. Estimated frequencies have ranged from 5 to 17%[174] in ulcerative colitis and from 10 to 30% in Crohn disease.[159,174] These may be underestimates in that abnormalities of liver function tests do not necessarily correlate with morphological evidence of liver disease. However, if the liver function tests are normal, Broome and his colleagues[175] have reported that less than 3% develop biopsy-proven liver disease on follow-up. In a patient with chronic IBD and persistently abnormal liver function tests, PSC is the most likely diagnosis. Interestingly, Vadstrup[176] has shown that subnormal ALT levels may be seen in patients with Crohn disease.

The approximate frequency of the other hepatic lesions which occur in chronic IBD is summarized in Table 17.4.

Steatosis

This is the commonest histological abnormality in the liver in this setting. It is clinically asymptomatic and hepatomegaly is unusual. It is of a macrovesicular pattern and although its extent seems to be related to the severity of

Table 17.4	Liver involvement in chronic inflammatory bowel disease	
	Approximate frequency
Fatty liver	50%
Primary sclerosing cholangitis	3–5%
Chronic hepatitis	1–2%
Cirrhosis	2–5%
Bile-duct carcinoma[(a)]	Risk of tumour increased 10-fold
Gallstones[(b)]	Increased 5–10 fold
Epithelioid granulomas[(c)]	5%
Amyloidosis[(c)]	Rare
Pylephlebitis and pyogenic inflammation	Very rare

[(a)] Ulcerative colitis only
[(b)] Crohn disease only
[(c)] Probably more common in Crohn disease

the bowel disease it may persist after colectomy.[167] The development of steatosis is probably a non-specific manifestation of the accompanying toxaemia, malnutrition and anaemia.

Chronic hepatitis

Prevalence rates up to 10% have previously been reported, but these may have been overestimates due to difficulties in distinguishing between autoimmune hepatitis and sclerosing cholangitis. In addition, chronic hepatitis due to post-transfusional chronic HCV infection was not excluded in earlier studies. An estimate of 1–2% seems likely for ulcerative colitis, but there is little evidence of an increased incidence in association with Crohn disease.[161] A diagnosis of chronic hepatitis should not be made unless the ERCP is normal. The difficulties in establishing the diagnosis have been emphasized by Rabinovitz et al.[177] in a report of the simultaneous occurrence of PSC and autoimmune hepatitis in a patient with ulcerative colitis. Primary biliary cirrhosis has also been described in ulcerative colitis.[178]

Cirrhosis

The overall prevalence of cirrhosis is about 2–5%.[161,162,172] Edwards & Truelove[179] reported that cirrhosis was present in 2.5% of patients with ulcerative colitis and accounted for 10% of all deaths in a follow-up period of over 20 years. Cirrhosis is 12–50 times commoner in patients with chronic IBD when compared with controls,[179,180] and is usually associated with extensive disease of the colon. Cirrhosis may develop as a sequel to PSC where it will show a biliary pattern, or less commonly as a sequel to chronic hepatitis

(viral or autoimmune) where the pattern will often be macronodular. In post-colectomy patients with cirrhosis, bleeding may occur from varices at the ileostomy stoma or at the ileo-rectal anastomosis.[172,181] Biliary cirrhosis due to PSC in patients with inflammatory bowel disease may necessitate liver transplantation; colonic disease may be exacerbated in the post-transplant period.[182]

Cholangiocarcinoma

This tumour shows a 10–30-fold increase in incidence in patients with ulcerative colitis,[183,184] but in Crohn disease the association appears to be uncommon.[185] Conversely, in carcinoma of the proximal bile ducts ulcerative colitis is present in 8–20% of patients.[186,187] The clinical and pathological evidence, reviewed by Rosen & Nagorney,[187] suggests that the carcinoma develops as a complication of PSC (Fig. 17.8) and, indeed, that PSC may be a premalignant condition[188] in which this tumour develops in 10–15% of cases.[188–190] Carcinoma usually develops in patients with long-standing (15 years or more), extensive and severe ulcerative colitis. On average, the patients are 20 years younger than other patients with cholangiocarcinoma. The tumour may arise some years after total colectomy[183,184] and may involve intra- or extrahepatic ducts and gallbladder. The differential diagnosis from sclerosing cholangitis is difficult and many tumours are not diagnosed until liver resection at transplantation or at autopsy. The prognosis is dismal, with a mean survival time of approximately 6–18 months. Liver transplantation is of limited value and tumours found incidentally at the time of operation may recur in the allograft.[191]

Miscellaneous

Gallstones

Gallstones have a 5–10-fold increased frequency in patients with Crohn disease of the terminal ileum.[192] This is related to the extent and duration of the ileal disease and the length of bowel which may have to be resected. This complication

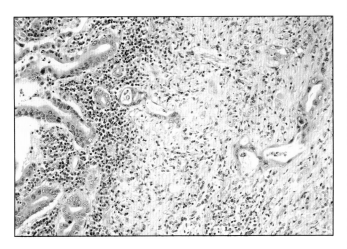

Fig. 17.8 • Biliary epithelial dysplasia and invasive cholangiocarcinoma in primary sclerosing cholangitis associated with ulcerative colitis. H & E.

is thought to be due to bile acid malabsorption and possibly changes in bile acid composition[193] causing cholesterol saturation in the bile. The gallbladder may itself be affected by Crohn disease.[194]

Amyloidosis

Amyloidosis of AA type may develop in both ulcerative colitis and Crohn disease but is more common in the latter.[195] Liver involvement is very uncommon, however.[196] Regression of amyloidosis following colectomy has been reported.[197]

Granulomas

Granulomas are found in the liver in approximately 5% of patients, predominantly in Crohn disease,[159,160,166,180] and may resolve quickly after colectomy.

Pylephlebitis and pyogenic abscess

Pylephlebitis and pyogenic abscess of the liver are now rare and potentially avoidable complications[198–200] but may sometimes be the initial presenting feature.[201] Disseminated aseptic abscesses have been described in Crohn disease.[202] Inflammatory pseudotumour has also been seen in two patients.[203]

Portal vein thrombosis

Portal vein thrombosis may occur in both ulcerative colitis and Crohn disease.[158,161] *Venous outflow obstruction* due to thrombosis has also been reported[204,205] in two cases in association with anti-cardiolipin antibodies.[205,206] However, although both thrombotic events and anti-cardiolipin antibodies are prevalent in IBD a correlation between the two is not evident.[206]

Iatrogenic hepatic disease

Iatrogenic hepatic disease may also be seen in IBD. TPN is frequently used in severe Crohn disease; liver complications of this therapy are outlined in p. 890. Some of the therapeutic agents used in the treatment of IBD may be associated with hepatotoxicity.[207] Liver dysfunction may occur as part of multiorgan failure when there is toxic megacolon.[208] Hepatic angiomyolipoma has been described in a patient with ulcerative colitis.[209]

Miscellaneous bowel diseases with liver involvement

Coeliac disease

Hagander et al.[210] found increased serum levels of aminotransferases and alkaline phosphatase in 39% of 74 adult patients and noted improvement in these indices on a gluten-free diet. Liver biopsy in 13 showed non-specific reactive hepatitis in five, cirrhosis and/or chronic hepatitis in seven, and in one case cirrhosis was complicated by a hepatocellular carcinoma. In a retrospective survey of 132 adult patients, abnormalities of liver function tests were found in 47%, 11% having increased alkaline phosphatase

levels and 36% increased aminotransferases.[211] Significant improvement in aminotransferases levels on a gluten-free diet was seen in 18 of 32 patients studied prospectively; liver biopsies in 37 patients showed non-specific changes in 26, chronic hepatitis in five, normal appearances in five and primary sclerosing cholangitis in one (also accompanied by ulcerative colitis). Mitchison et al.[212] noted abnormalities of liver function tests responsive to a gluten-free diet in three patients, one of whom had steatosis and two of whom had non-specific reactive hepatitis.

Lindberg et al.[213] reported elevated serum aminotransferases levels in children with coeliac disease, a finding which they also observed in gastrointestinal allergies and which led them to suggest that the liver dysfunction was non-specific and secondary to mucosal injury. This is supported by a large retrospective study which showed a strong correlation between elevated serum aminotransferases and intestinal permeability.[214] In a retrospective autopsy study of 19 cases of malabsorption, Pollock[215] noted that in the five patients with a confirmed diagnosis of coeliac disease, two had chronic hepatitis, in one of whom cirrhosis and a hepatocellular carcinoma had developed. Autoimmune hepatitis was described in two cases of coeliac disease[216] and Demir et al. found cirrhosis in five children with the disorder.[217]

Logan et al.[218] reported the co-existence of adult coeliac disease in four patients with primary biliary cirrhosis. This association has been confirmed in several subsequent studies.[219,220] Other forms of autoimmune cholestatic liver disease including autoimmune cholangitis and PSC have been described in patients with coeliac disease.[221–225] Rarely, hepatic T-cell lymphoma may occur.[226] Nodular regenerative hyperplasia has been described in three patients with coeliac disease.[227,228]

Further details of liver abnormalities in this condition can be found in a recent systemic review.[229]

Whipple disease

Whipple disease (see also Ch. 9) may frequently show widespread systemic involvement. The PAS-positive-diastase-resistant foamy macrophages which characterize the intestinal involvement may also be found in the liver (Fig. 17.9).[230,231] The 'sickle-form' bacilli seen in these macrophages have also been described in Kupffer cells.[232] Non-caseating epithelioid cell granulomas also occur in the liver in Whipple disease and may precede the onset of intestinal symptoms;[233] these granulomas, however, do not contain identifiable bacilli.[234] PCR for *Tropheryma whippelii* may be used to demonstrate the presence of organisms.[235] Massive steatosis has been described in one patient.[236]

Eosinophilic gastroenteritis

Hepatic granulomas with a prominent eosinophil infiltrate have been reported in two patients,[48] and in a patient with systemic involvement an intense eosinophilic infiltrate was present in the portal tracts.[237] Sclerosing cholangitis has been described in the hypereosinophilic syndrome (p. 906) in which there was intestinal involvement.[238]

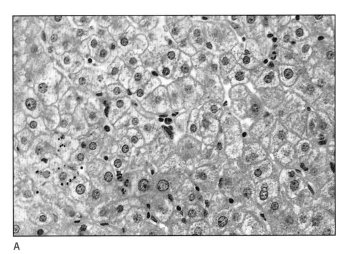
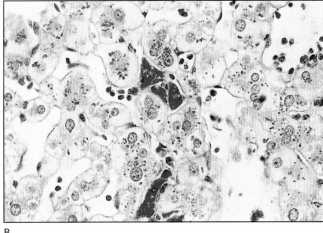

Fig. 17.9 • Liver biopsy in a patient with Whipple disease. **(A)** There is Kupffer-cell hyperplasia with some large intrasinusoidal cells. H & E. **(B)** These are strongly PAS-positive. PAS-diastase. Courtesy of Dr Carole D Kooijman.

The liver in pancreatic diseases

Exocrine pancreas

Cystic fibrosis is associated with liver disease; this topic is discussed in Chapter 5.

Extrahepatic obstruction may occur very rarely as a result of annular pancreas but this should be a diagnosis of exclusion.[239] Jaundice is the initial presenting symptom in 60–70% of patients with carcinoma of the head of pancreas and ampullary region, and eventually develops in 80% of patients.[240] Jaundice, often transient, may develop in 15–75% of patients with acute pancreatitis and may be the result of bile-duct obstruction due to inflammation, or it may result from a common aetiology such as alcohol abuse or gallstones.[241] Obstructive jaundice is rare in chronic pancreatitis, but it may occur in an acute exacerbation[241] or from pressure due to a pancreatic pseudocyst.[242] Steatosis, portal tract inflammation, ductular reaction and fibrosis and cirrhosis are not uncommon associations of chronic pancreatitis, but seem most likely to be due to alcohol abuse or cholelithiasis, common aetiological factors in pancreatitis.

Liver abnormalities may be seen in patients with autoimmune pancreatitis, in particular there is an association with primary sclerosing cholangitis.[243] It has been suggested that the bile duct and pancreatic abnormalities in such individuals are both part of a multisystem IgG4-related autoimmune process.[244] Hepatic inflammatory pseudotumour has been described in autoimmune pancreatitis.[245]

Pancreatic pseudocysts have been described within the liver.[246] Fulminant hepatic failure may occur in severe acute pancreatitis.[247] Segmental or localized portal hypertension occurs in some patients with chronic hepatitis on a background of pancreatitis, most probably as a consequence of splenic vein occlusion or stenosis.[248]

The converse relationships between liver and exocrine pancreas are worth noting. Evidence of acute haemorrhagic pancreatitis has been found in a third of patients with panacinar liver cell necrosis;[249] it may also occur in acute fatty liver of pregnancy[250] and with acute hepatitis A[251] and C.[252]

Endocrine pancreas

The liver has a key role in carbohydrate metabolism. The possible 'hepatotropic' effects of pancreatic hormones were first investigated by Starzl and his colleagues[253] and it is now clear that insulin, glucagon and insulin-like growth factors together with several other hormones and hepatic growth factors, modulate hepatic function in normal circumstances and regulate hepatic regeneration after liver injury. Only in diabetes mellitus, however, is there evidence of significant liver disease in association with islet-cell dysfunction.

Diabetes mellitus

The role of type II diabetes in the development of NAFLD is discussed in Chapter 7. Here we consider only the liver abnormalities in insulin-dependent type I diabetes. The metabolic disturbances which involve the liver have been reviewed elsewhere.[254]

In type I diabetes, resulting from a lack of insulin, the liver contributes to the disturbances in carbohydrate metabolism. The hyperglycaemia results from breakdown of glycogen and over-production of glucose by the liver together with a decreased uptake of glucose from the portal vein blood. The activity of glucose 6-phosphatase is increased with resulting increased glycogenolysis and decreased phosphorylation in the liver. Over-production of glucose also occurs due to a loss of the normal feedback inhibition of gluconeogenesis by plasma glucose levels.[255] The uptake of glucose from portal vein blood is considerably reduced and may fall from 60% extraction to as low as 25%.[255] This is the result of low levels of hepatic glucokinase, the enzyme responsible for glucose trapping. The ketoacidosis of severe and prolonged diabetes is due to increased lipolysis, a release of free fatty acids into the circulation and a failure to inhibit their oxidation in the liver because of insulin lack, and increased β-oxidation of the fatty acids.[256] Increased levels of glucagon may enhance adipose tissue lipolysis.[257] Disturbances of lipid metabolism also occur. Hyper-triglyceridaemia results from increased production of very-low-density lipoprotein (VLDL) by the liver combined with a decreased peripheral clearance due to a deficiency of lipo-protein lipase.

Lorenz and Barenwald[258] first drew attention to the presence of marked glycogenosis in the livers of children with type I diabetes. This phenomenon can be associated with grossly elevated serum transaminases.[259] It is a feature seen particularly in patients with the so-called Mauriac syndrome characterized by poor glycaemic control, growth retardation and pubertal delay.[260] The glycogenosis may give rise to hepatomegaly but the changes are reversible and not thought to lead to chronic liver injury.

Chatila and West[261] described adult cases with similar features in which there was hepatomegaly and elevated liver enzymes in the context of poor diabetic control (Fig. 17.10). The phenomenon has been observed in recently diagnosed patients and disappears when the patients become euglycaemic on insulin therapy.[262]

This pattern of liver injury has also been described in *anorexia nervosa* where the glycogenosis is though to represent an adaptive response to starvation.[263]

Collagenization of the space of Disse together with deposition of basement membrane components has been reported in diabetes[264,265] and it has been suggested that this lesion might represent liver involvement as part of diabetic microangiopathy.[265]

There are case reports of liver-cell adenoma,[266] of nodular regenerative hyperplasia,[267] of xanthomatous neuropathy affecting unmyelinated nerve fibres in the hilum and in large portal tracts,[268] of intrahepatic[269] and perihepatic[270] abscess and of PSC[271] occurring in patients with diabetes.

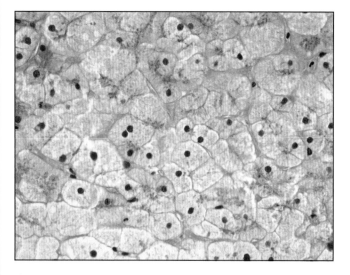

Fig. 17.10 • Liver in type I diabetes mellitus. Hepatocytes are enlarged due to glycogenosis; the appearances resemble those seen in inherited glycogen storage diseases. H & E.

Giant mitochondria, sometimes a feature of alcoholic liver disease, may also be seen in diabetes.[272]

The liver in endocrine diseases

The effects of gonadal steroids on the liver occur principally in relation to their therapeutic administration; they have been reviewed elsewhere[273] and are dealt with in Chapter 14.

Thyroid

The liver is an 'end-organ' in which thyroid hormones modify various hepatocellular synthetic activities and modulate bilirubin and bile acid metabolism; in turn the liver metabolizes these hormones and is the principal site for conversion of T4 to T3. The liver synthesizes the major thyroid-hormone-binding proteins.[274] Some thyroid hormones are conjugated as glucuronides and sulphates in the liver, and very small amounts of T3 and T4 are excreted in the bile. Altered thyroid hormone metabolism is found in a variety of acute and chronic liver diseases[275,276] and the serum levels of the hormone metabolites may reflect prognosis.[277] There is a well-recognized clinical association between autoimmune thyroid disease and primary biliary cirrhosis (see Chapter 11); occasional cases of Graves disease with autoimmune hepatitis and primary sclerosing cholangitis are also described.[278–280]

Hyperthyroidism

Abnormal liver function tests have been variously reported in 15–75% of patients with hyperthyroidism.[281–283] Increased serum alkaline phosphatase is the most common abnormality; aminotransferases and bilirubin may also be increased but this usually resolves when patients become euthyroid.[284] Unexplained clinical jaundice[285] may sometimes develop with liver failure.[286] Although in early studies on fatal, thyrotoxic crisis cases it was a feature in 20% of patients, in some of these coincidental cardiac failure may have been contributory.[287] Post-infantile giant cell hepatitis (Chapter 4) has been documented in one patient with Graves disease.[288]

In autopsy studies of patients dying of thyrotoxicosis and its complications, abnormalities were reported in the liver in a significant majority and comprised fatty liver, focal necrosis, venous congestion, parenchymal atrophy and cirrhosis. In biopsy studies, however, only mild non-specific changes were found, comprising mild steatosis, reduced hepatocyte glycogen, cytoplasmic vacuolization, parenchymal inflammation and Kupffer-cell hyperplasia, some nuclear irregularity and hyperchromatism and a minimal increase in portal tract inflammatory cells.[289,290] Ultrastructural studies have shown hypertrophy of the smooth endoplasmic reticulum, mitochondrial enlargement and glycogen depletion.[291]

Hypothyroidism

No constant or specific abnormalities of liver function tests have been reported.[281] There is impaired bile acid synthesis and, experimentally, a reduction in bile flow has been demonstrated due to a reduction in the bile salt-independent component of bile.[292] Increased serum bilirubin levels are common in severe myxoedema, and there is a single case report of cholestasis in association with hypothyroidism.[293] There is growing evidence that hypothyroidism may be a risk factor for NAFLD.[294]

There are occasional reports of ascites with accumulation of fluid of a high protein content, occurring in the absence of congestive cardiac failure and clearing in response to hormone replacement therapy.[295] Baker et al.[295] reported concentric thickening of the walls of central venules, perivenular hepatocyte loss and perivenular fibrosis. Ono & Ishizaki[296] reported a case of nodular regenerative hyperplasia in association with Hashimoto's disease.

In *congenital cretinism*, jaundice due to an unconjugated hyperbilirubinaemia may persist for several weeks, the mechanisms for an apparent failure of hepatocyte uptake being uncertain.[297]

Adrenal cortex

Features of Cushing syndrome, abdominal striae, facial mooning and acne, may develop in autoimmune hepatitis but without evident adrenal dysfunction.[298,299] Secondary hyperaldosteronism is a feature of hepatic decompensation (Chapter 1). Furthermore there is increasing awareness of adrenal insufficiency in patients with liver failure—so-called hepatoadrenal syndrome.[300,301] Steatosis is a frequent finding in Cushing syndrome[302] and fatty liver develops after a 4-week course of corticosteroid therapy. Fatal fat embolism, of presumed fatty liver origin, has been reported after corticosteroid treatment.[303]

Olsson et al.[304] reported corticosteroid-responsive elevation of serum aminotransferases in four patients with Addison disease; liver biopsy in one showed a lymphocytic infiltrate of the portal tracts. There is a case report of Addison disease with hypertension and renal and hepatic microthrombosis in the primary antiphospholipid syndrome.[305] Focal nodular hyperplasia is described in association with small adrenocortical tumours[306] and in the setting of primary aldosteronism.[307] Both intrahepatic cholestasis and chronic hepatitis have been reported as paraneoplastic phenomena in phaeochromocytoma.[308,309]

Pituitary

The interactions between the liver and the pituitary in health and disease have been reviewed in a number of studies;[310] the central role of the liver in the growth hormone/insulin like growth factor axis has recently been highlighted by Baruch.[311] Hepatomegaly is frequently found in acromegaly and is accompanied by increased excretion capacity, the mechanisms for which are uncertain.[312] Liver dysfunction is described in hypopituitarism;[313] these patients develop a phenotype similar to metabolic syndrome with central obesity and diabetes and the whole spectrum of NAFLD may be seen, including cirrhosis.[314,315]

Neonatal (giant cell) hepatitis is recorded in congenital hypopituitarism.[316]

Miscellaneous

Orloff reported a syndrome of hyperparathyroidism, cirrhosis and portocaval shunt.[317] Refractory ascites has been reported in POEMS syndrome,[318] in which there is polyneuropathy (P), organomegaly (O), endocrinopathy (E) M (M) protein band and skin (S) changes. Chronic cholestasis is described in Turner syndrome[319] and by MRI some patients have been shown to have fatty liver.[320] Roulot et al. described the histopathological features in 27 patients with Turner syndrome. This confirmed NAFLD as a complication but also drew attention to a high frequency of vascular abnormalities and associated nodular lesions with nodular regenerative hyperplasia in six and multiple focal nodular hyperplasia in two cases.[321] Liver enzyme abnormalities are recorded in severe ovarian hyperstimulation syndrome.[322]

The liver in pregnancy

In the following account the changes which occur in the liver in normal pregnancy and the liver diseases which are peculiar to pregnancy are outlined. In addition, liver disease may develop and complicate pregnancy, and, conversely, established liver diseases may be complicated by pregnancy. For an account of the effects of pregnancy on acute and chronic liver disease the reader is referred to medical and obstetrical texts and to several excellent reviews and case studies.[323–328]

Normal pregnancy

In general, the liver functions normally in pregnancy.[329] There is no increase in liver size. Although total blood volume and cardiac output are increased by 50%, hepatic blood flow remains unchanged resulting, in the third trimester, in a relative decrease of 25–30% in the proportion of the cardiac output which passes through the liver.[330] Consequently, drugs that are cleared by the liver in a blood-flow-dependent manner have a reduced clearance rate in pregnancy.

Conventional liver function tests are altered in the course of pregnancy.[331] The total increase in alkaline phosphatase is in part due to the placental isoenzyme, but the hepatic isoenzyme also increases; the level may remain elevated for 4–6 weeks post-partum. The serum aminotransferases, γ-glutamyl transferase, 5-nucleotidase and the prothrombin time remain normal, and in suspected hepatic dysfunction during pregnancy these indices are of most diagnostic help.

Light-microscopic examination of the liver shows minor non-specific changes. These have included cellular and nuclear pleomorphism, increased numbers of binucleate cells, steatosis, increased cellular and nuclear glycogen, mild reactive Kupffer-cell hyperplasia and some lymphocytic infiltration of portal tracts—features which, however, do not constitute a 'liver of pregnancy'. Electron-microscopic examination shows features which are considered to be adaptive responses to the hormonal changes; they comprise proliferation of the smooth endoplasmic reticulum, giant mitochondria with increase in crystalline inclusions, and increased numbers of peroxisomes.[332,333]

Liver disease in pregnancy

Liver disease in pregnancy has been the subject of a number of reviews.[323,324,334] The estimated frequency of jaundice in pregnancy is 1 per 1500 gestations, and it has been subdivided into jaundice in pregnancy and jaundice of pregnancy. *Jaundice in pregnancy* includes any disease which is normally accompanied by icterus, and of these acute viral hepatitis is the most common (40% of all cases of jaundice during pregnancy). Various medical complications in pregnancy (10%) and large-duct obstruction (6%) also contribute significantly.

Jaundice of pregnancy comprises:

(i)   intrahepatic cholestasis of pregnancy;
(ii) acute fatty liver of pregnancy;
(iii) jaundice in toxaemia of pregnancy;
(iv) a miscellaneous group associated with hyperemesis gravidarum, haemolytic and megaloblastic anaemias of pregnancy, and hydatidiform mole; and an unclassifiable group in which the jaundice is mild and where no specific hepatic disease is identified.

Intrahepatic cholestasis of pregnancy

This has been recently reviewed by Riely and Bacq[335] and is dealt with in Chapter 5. Pregnant women with this condition have pruritus and/or jaundice with elevated fasting serum bile acid levels.[334] Histologically the liver shows a marked bilirubinostasis (Fig. 17.11). The changes revert following delivery but frequently recur during subsequent pregnancies. There is a significant risk of fetal loss. It is now recognised that the disorder is associated with a transporter

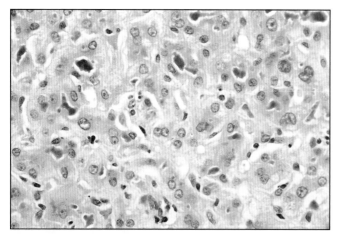

Fig. 17.11 • Cholestasis of pregnancy. Note marked bilirubinostasis with minimal accompanying inflammation—'bland cholestasis'. H & E.

protein defect; MDR3 gene mutations have been identified in some patients with this condition.[335–337]

Acute fatty liver of pregnancy

This was first defined by Sheehan in 1940,[338] who termed it obstetric acute yellow atrophy; his classic description of the clinical and histological features has not been improved upon. The clinical features are reviewed in a number of papers.[250,339–343] It is a rare disease, but the diagnosis is now being made earlier suggesting that it may be more common than previously thought.[344]

The large majority of patients are primigravidae, frequently there is a twin pregnancy, the disease occurs at any age in the child-bearing period, and male births are more common than female. Characteristically, it develops in the last 10 weeks and usually in the last 4 weeks of pregnancy. Occasional cases are described in the second trimester. After a mild prodromal illness, severe vomiting and jaundice develop in a few days with rapidly progressive acute liver failure. Many patients have hypertension and proteinuria suggesting toxaemia of pregnancy, a differential diagnosis which has to be considered.[345]

Biochemically, the hyperbilirubinaemia is moderate, 100 μmol/l (5.8 mg/100 ml); there is mild elevation of the aminotransferases, 1200 iu/l; the prothrombin time is prolonged to 2–4 times normal; hypoglycaemia may be marked and is a contributory factor in the early coma. Serum immunoglobulins are not increased and this contrasts with the findings in acute hepatitis; serum amylase and lipase may be elevated because of an associated pancreatitis.[250] The presence of circulating normoblasts, noted by Sheehan,[346] has been emphasized by Burroughs et al.[339] who found them in the blood film in 10 of 11 patients.

The mortality rate for both mother and fetus was as high as 80–85% in early series. However, Pockros and his colleagues[340] reported a maternal mortality of 2/18 (11%) and a fetal mortality of 5/20 (25%), an improved survival which they attributed to better supportive therapy. A more recent study of 28 consecutive cases reported zero maternal mortality.[343] Early diagnosis and delivery and the occurrence of milder forms of the disease improve the outlook for mother and child.[340,343,347] Liver transplantation has been carried out for this condition.[348]

In surviving cases there is no report of progression to chronic liver disease and subsequent uncomplicated pregnancy has been reported.[339,343,349] There are however case reports of recurrent fatty liver of pregnancy,[350] and one case in which intrahepatic cholestasis of pregnancy was later complicated by acute fatty liver of pregnancy.[351]

Macroscopically, the liver is usually smaller than normal and has a distinctive pale yellow colour. Sheehan[338] wrote '. . . there was a gross fatty change affecting the entire lobule except a sharply defined rim of normal cells around the portal tracts. The affected cells were bloated by a fine foam of tiny white vacuoles throughout the cytoplasm so that they resembled the cells of suprarenal cortex. The nuclei were normal and there was an entire absence of necrobiotic change.' These features are shown in Fig. 17.12. In some cases the steatosis may be diffuse without periportal sparing.[339,341] Canalicular and hepatocellular bilirubinostasis are present. There is Kupffer-cell hyperplasia, aggregates of ceroid-laden macrophages are conspicuous, and there is usually only a mild, predominantly mononuclear cell infiltrate of the parenchyma and portal tracts, sometimes with a number of eosinophils and occasional plasma cells.

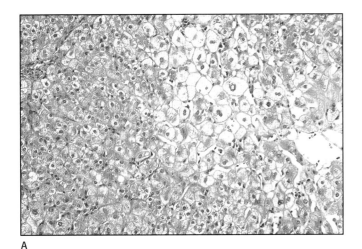

A

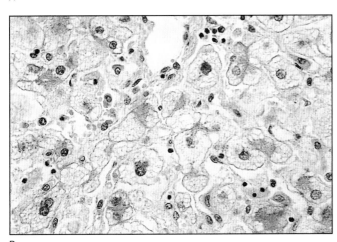

B

C

Fig. 17.12 • Acute fatty liver of pregnancy **(A)** Microvesicular steatosis involving perivenular and mid-zones. H & E. **(B)** At a higher power note the swollen hepatocytes and the microvesicular fatty accumulation, H & E, shown in **(C)** with an oil red O stain.

Intrasinusoidal fibrin deposits have been reported, occasionally associated with microhaemorrhages.[339,341]

The reduced liver weight at autopsy despite the presence of steatosis indicates that there has been liver-cell loss,[339,341] and morphologically this is best seen with a reticulin stain. Joske et al.[352] noted mid-zonal necrosis in one case. Serial biopsies in survivors show progressive disappearance of fat from the periportal to the perivenular zone and, in our experience, this happens within days of parturition.

Ultrastructurally[339,353] the fat is not membrane bound; there is dilatation of the rough endoplasmic reticulum and some cells show cytoplasmic degeneration with autophagic vacuoles; the mitochondria show considerable variation in size and shape.

Extrahepatic complications include gastrointestinal haemorrhage, renal failure, sometimes with fatty infiltration of renal tubules,[354] intravascular haemolysis,[352] pancreatitis and peripancreatic bleeding[341] and disseminated intravascular coagulation.[355] The coagulation defect accounts for many of the complications, and it may be temporarily aggravated by delivery.[340]

This condition forms part of the spectrum of diseases characterized by microvesicular steatosis (p. 889). The pathogenesis remains uncertain but it is likely that there is an acquired β-oxidation defect. A contribution of nonsteroidal anti-inflammatory drugs (including aspirin) has been postulated.[356] Inherited defects of fatty acid oxidation including carnitine palmitoyl transferases may be important in some cases.[357] Some authors have suggested that acute fatty liver of pregnancy is part of the spectrum of pre-eclampsia. Minakami et al.[358] produced evidence supportive of this, finding microvesicular steatosis in all 41 liver biopsies from cases of pre-eclampsia. However, Rolfes & Ishak[341] were of the opinion that there was no similarity between acute fatty liver and the liver changes in pre-eclampsia and eclampsia, a view to which the present author also subscribes.

The liver in toxaemia of pregnancy

If jaundice occurs in the early stages of toxaemia of pregnancy it is usually haemolytic in type and mild with serum bilirubin levels of less than 100 μmol/l (5.8 mg/dl). Occasional cases may present with severe jaundice.[359,360] The serum alkaline phosphatase is also abnormally elevated and aminotransferase levels may be in the range of 100–1000 iu/l.

The overall incidence of liver dysfunction in toxaemia is less than 50%. In Barron's[361] experience, pre-eclampsia is the commonest cause of hepatic tenderness and disturbed liver function tests in pregnancy, hepatic involvement also being an indicator of severe maternal disease. Liver biopsy has been normal in many jaundiced patients or may show only mild non-specific reactive changes with some hepatocellular pleomorphism.[362] Arias & Mancilla-Jimenez[363] reported intrasinusoidal fibrin deposition in all of their series of 12 biopsies, a pattern similar to that which affects renal glomerular capillaries.

In severe and fatal cases the distinctive liver lesion comprises periportal intrasinusoidal fibrin deposition with irregular areas of liver-cell necrosis exciting a minimal inflammatory reaction (Fig. 17.13A). The hepatic arteries and arterioles in the adjacent portal tract show plasmatic vasculosis with seepage of fibrin into and through their walls (Fig. 17.13B). The vascular changes are similar to those occurring in other organs in severe toxaemia and are the result of endothelial cell damage and activation of intravascular coagulation. Sheehan[338] found periportal lesions in 90% of fatal cases, but Antia et al.[362] reported them in only 5 of 15 cases.

HELLP syndrome

It is estimated that 2–12% of patients with toxaemia of pregnancy develop the HELLP syndrome which comprises haemolysis (H), elevated liver enzymes (EL) and a low platelet count (LP).[364,365] It occurs predominantly in multiparous women over 25 years of age. Some cases occur a few hours to 6 days post-partum.[366] Maternal complications include placental abruption, acute renal failure and hepatic rupture, with a maternal mortality rate of 3%. Recurrence

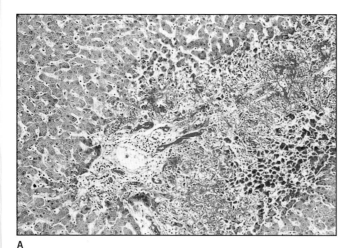

A

B

Fig. 17.13 • Liver in toxaemia of pregnancy. **(A)** Area of periportal necrosis with intrasinusoidal fibrin deposition. **(B)** Hepatic arterioles showing plasmatic vasculosis; intrasinusoidal fibrin deposition is also present. Masson trichrome.

of the syndrome has been reported in only one instance.[367] It has been described in a single case in association with embryonal sarcoma of the liver.[368]

There is now strong evidence that HELLP forms part of a disease spectrum which includes pre-eclampsia.[369,370] Liver biopsies show features of a non-specific reactive hepatitis with a mild portal tract chronic inflammatory cell infiltrate. However, in some cases periportal or focal parenchymal necrosis with a fibrin exudate has been reported, similar to that described in eclampsia. Intrahepatic haemorrhage and subcapsular haematomas with rupture may occur, on occasions necessitating transplantation.[366,371,372] The liver injury may be mediated by CD95 signaling.[373]

Miscellaneous liver lesions in pregnancy

Hyperemesis gravidarum

When jaundice occurs in hyperemesis gravidarum it is usually mild[374,375] but there may be marked elevation of aminotransferases.[374] Histological examination of the liver in a small number of cases showed non-specific reactive changes.[376]

Spontaneous rupture of the liver

Spontaneous rupture of the liver has now been reported in over 100 cases and there have been recent extended reviews.[377,378] The clinical presentation is usually acute with profound collapse, sometimes out of proportion to the amount of blood in the peritoneal cavity.[379] The rupture is thought to occur from subcapsular haematomas and there may be a history of minor trauma. These haematomas may be found without peritoneal leakage,[380] and they are usually sharply circumscribed.

Spontaneous rupture occurs most commonly in association with toxaemia and in the last trimester of pregnancy. In 15–20% of cases there is no associated hypertension and it sometimes occurs immediately postpartum.[381]

Liver pregnancy

A number of extrauterine pregnancies with placental attachment to the liver are recorded,[382–385] and in one of these the pregnancy went to term but with eventual maternal and fetal death.[385]

Abscess

Liver abscess due to *Listeria monocytogenes* arising during pregnancy has been described in a single case.[386]

Hepatic infarction

This has been reported during pregnancy in a patient with underlying anti-phospholipid syndrome.[387]

The liver in haematological and lymphoreticular diseases

Liver involvement in the histiocytoses and the haemophagocytic syndromes is discussed in Chapter 4.

Anaemias

Fatty liver is a frequent accompaniment of anaemia from any cause. In the haemolytic anaemias and in refractory anaemias, secondary iron overload may develop; in the former there is also an increased risk of hepatic or portal vein thrombosis.[388] The increased incidence of cholelithiasis in haemolytic syndromes predisposes to biliary obstruction. Morphological changes in *sickle cell anaemia* are common,[389] resulting from a combination of anoxia and impaired sinusoidal blood flow; secondary iron overload is also present.[390,391] Aggregations of red cells and thrombi are prominent in the perivenular zones producing sinusoidal congestion, which in addition, and in contrast to passive venous congestion, may become equally pronounced in all zones. Hepatic vein thrombosis may occur.[389,392] Crescent-shaped red cells can be readily identified in the sinusoids and in Kupffer cells, which also contain haemosiderin and ceroid pigment (Fig. 17.14). Ultrastructural studies show collagenization in the space of Disse. In patients dying in sickle cell crisis the liver is enlarged and purplish in colour and, in addition to the severe sinusoidal distension and obstruction, focal liver-cell necrosis may be a prominent feature. Focal nodular hyperplasia, possibly related to local ischaemia, has been reported in children[393] and there is a case report of an hepatic biloma.[394]

Spherocytes in *congenital spherocytosis* and acanthocytes in *abetalipoproteinaemia*[395] may also be recognized within sinusoids on light microscopy.

Hepatic vein, splenic vein and portal vein thrombosis have been reported in patients with *paroxysmal nocturnal haemoglobinuria*.[396,397]

Leukaemias

Hepatic involvement in acute leukaemia is not usually a significant clinical feature but hepatomegaly and cholestasis may occur. In *acute lymphoblastic leukaemia* the infiltrate is usually in the portal tracts whereas both portal tracts and sinusoids are involved in *acute myeloid leukaemia*.[398] Massive blastic infiltration of the liver producing fulminant liver failure, probably secondary to hepatocellular ischaemia, has been reported in acute leukaemia and also in patients with non-Hodgkin lymphomas.[399–402]

In *hairy cell leukaemia*, clinical hepatomegaly is present in 30–40% of patients; there may be mild disturbances of liver function tests but infiltration of the liver sinusoids and portal tracts is present in all cases and may produce a characteristic lesion.[403,404] The sinusoidal infiltrate is linear (Fig. 17.15A); there may be peliosis-like lesions, congestion and occasionally granulomas.[405] Nanba et al.[406] reported splenic 'pseudosinuses' in all of 14 patients and also noted hepatic 'angiomatous lesions' in three of five liver biopsies. Roquet et al.[407] found these angiomatous lesions in 9 of 14 patients (Fig. 17.15B). They comprise dilated blood-filled spaces to the walls of which the tumour cells are attached. The lesions are multifocal, may involve portal tracts and sometimes occur in clusters; they resemble haemangiomas or peliosis hepatis. The leukaemic cells have a clear cytoplasm and may be easily overlooked in haematoxylin and eosin (H&E)-stained sections but are identified by their content of tartrate-resistant acid phosphatase[403,408] or by immunohistochemical methods.[409]

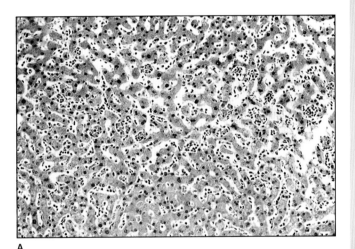

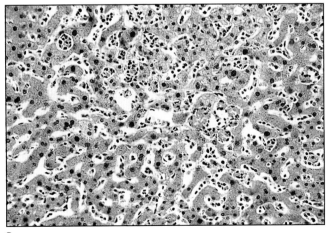

Fig. 17.15 • Liver in hairy cell leukaemia. **(A)** Sinusoidal dilatation and diffuse intrasinusoidal infiltration by leukaemic cells. **(B)** Angiomatous lesions comprising congested sinusoids surrounded by a ring of leukaemic cells. H & E. Courtesy of Dr H Tavadia.

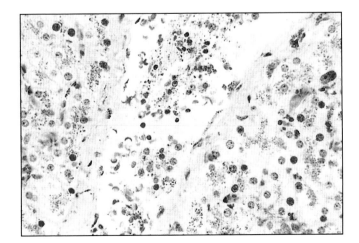

Fig. 17.14 • Liver in sickle cell anaemia. Note the sickled red cells in the hepatic venule and congested sinusoids: there is also abundant haemosiderin in perivenular hepatocytes and Kupffer cells. Martius Scarlet Blue.

An ultrastructural study of the peliotic lesions demonstrated loss of continuity of sinusoidal lining cells with the hairy cells coming into direct contact with hepatocytes and extravasation of blood into the space of Disse.[404] These changes resemble those seen in peliosis hepatis[410] and Zafrani and his colleagues suggested that the hairy cells cause endothelial damage.

In *chronic lymphoblastic leukaemias*, liver dysfunction is a late clinical feature and the hepatic infiltrate is predominantly within portal tracts.[398] Nodular regenerative hyperplasia with portal hypertension has been reported.[411] More than 50% of patients with *chronic myeloid leukaemia* have clinical hepatomegaly on presentation and in acute blastic crises sinusoidal infiltration by leukaemic cells is present.[398]

Chronic liver disease, affecting over 65% of children with acute leukaemias in long-term remission from acute leukaemia, was reported by Locasculli et al.[412] Some of this was probably drug-related (Ch. 14), but the authors noted that all of 20 children who had had acute hepatitis developed chronic liver disease. Conversely, there are sporadic reports of a beneficial effect of acute hepatitis in patients with various forms of leukaemia.[413,414] Hepatic venous outflow obstruction has been recorded in chronic lymphocytic leukaemia due to tumour cell infiltration.[415,416] Hepatocellular carcinoma may arise in children previously treated for acute lymphoblastic leukaemia.[417]

Chronic myeloproliferative disorders and myelodysplastic syndromes

These myeloproliferative disorders include primary polycythaemia (polycythaemia vera), myelofibrosis and essential thrombocythaemia. The hepatic complications in these disorders comprise: (i) venous outflow obstruction with thrombosis; (ii) non-cirrhotic portal hypertension which may develop because of perisinusoidal fibrosis, hepatic infiltration and increased blood flow,[418] nodular regenerative hyperplasia or portal vein thrombosis; (iii) extramedullary haemopoiesis and sinusoidal dilatation; (iv) iron overload; and (v) viral- and drug-induced hepatitis.

Cases are described in which venous outflow obstruction has arisen on the basis of concomitant myeloproliferative disease and factor V Leiden mutations.[419,420]

Extramedullary haemopoiesis may be found in the liver, and is usually a feature in over 90% of patients with myelofibrosis.[421–423] Histologically (Fig. 17.16), pleomorphic clumps of erythroid and myeloid precursors together with megakaryocytes are present in the sinusoids and the space of Disse, and portal tract involvement develops as a late feature. In some cases megakaryocytes may be found on their own.[424] The pleomorphism helps to distinguish extramedullary haemopoiesis from the hepatic infiltration in leukaemia, infectious mononucleosis, Felty syndrome and the tropical splenomegaly syndrome. Extramedullary haemopoiesis is a normal feature in the fetal liver and in the neonatal liver up to 5 weeks of age. It may persist for longer in the presence of neonatal hepatitis or anaemia from any cause. In the adult it may also occur in aplastic anaemia

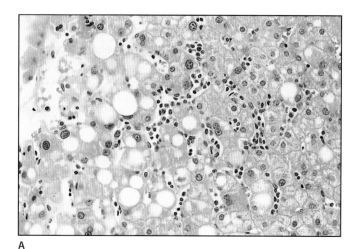

Fig. 17.16 • Extramedullary haemopoiesis in the liver. **(A)** Pleomorphic intrasinusoidal infiltrate and **(B)** megakaryocyte. H & E.

and in a variety of so-called marrow-replacement syndromes including tumour metastases, myelomatosis and osteopetrosis.

The sinusoidal dilatation found in 50% of patients with myelofibrosis, is thought to be due to obstruction by the extramedullary haemopoiesis.[423] Perisinusoidal fibrosis[425–427] has been attributed to stellate cell activation by platelet-derived growth factor or other cytokines released by megakaryocytes and activated macrophages.[426,427]

Myelodysplastic syndromes

Haemosiderosis is frequent in the refractory and sideroblastic anaemia categories, and leukaemic infiltration develops when blast transformation occurs.

Myelomatosis

Portal tract and sinusoidal infiltration by extramedullary myeloma is not uncommon[428] and may manifest as large focal deposits.[429] In a series of 64 autopsies, hepatic involvement was seen in 40% and in the absence of plasma cell leukaemia.[430] Multiple myeloma has been associated with acute cholestatic hepatitis.[431]

In Waldenström macroglobulinaemia portal hypertension due to hepatic infiltration by tumour cells[432] and to nodular regenerative hyperplasia has been reported;[433] macroglobulin deposition in the space of Disse has been observed, and light chain deposition with peliosis hepatis and nodular regenerative hyperplasia has also been reported in one patient.[434]

Lymphoreticular neoplasms

These are subdivided into Hodgkin disease and non-Hodgkin lymphoma. The former is always a secondary tumour in the liver but a number of hepatic lesions may occur in the absence of tumour involvement. Imaging techniques, in particular CT scanning, and changes in patient management have meant that staging laparotomy with liver biopsy is now less frequently carried out in these diseases.[435]

Hodgkin disease

Clinical manifestations of hepatic involvement include fever, hepatomegaly and jaundice. Severe cholestatic hepatitis with liver failure and widespread liver involvement by Hodgkin disease has been reported[436] and occasional patients present with acute liver failure.[437] Rapidly progressive NASH was described in a single case by Kosmidou et al.[438]

Liver involvement in Hodgkin disease is found in about 55% of patients at autopsy. The frequency of diagnostic hepatic lesions on liver biopsy ranges from 5 to 10% depending on whether percutaneous needle biopsy or wedge biopsy at laparotomy has been examined.[439–441] Deposits in the liver vary considerably in size, in some instances showing a diffuse distribution of uniform small nodules, whilst in others large masses or a combination of these patterns may be present. Hepatic involvement is more common in the lymphocyte depleted and mixed cellularity subtypes and, with the exception of very rare cases,[442] has not been found in the absence of splenic involvement.[443]

Microscopically, the diagnosis is often straightforward, but problems arise in the interpretation of possible early hepatic involvement. Tumour deposits almost invariably involve portal tracts and caution should be exercised in interpreting infiltrates confined to the parenchyma. Non-specific portal tract inflammation—comprising lymphocytes, plasma cells and eosinophils—may frequently be found. Reed–Sternberg cells should be identified before making a definite diagnosis and atypical histiocytes should be regarded only as suggestive evidence.[441,443] Chronic inflammatory cell infiltration of portal tracts must not be regarded as evidence of liver involvement.[443,444] In our experience mitotic activity within the portal tract infiltrate and perivascular 'cushioning' by portal tract lymphoid aggregates should be regarded with suspicion. The bile ducts may be obliterated by neoplastic cells which may sometimes strikingly surround and extend into the duct epithelium.[445] Parenchymal lymphoid aggregates (Fig. 17.17A), sometimes

with cytological atypia, may be found in 10% of biopsy specimens.[446]

Epithelioid cell granulomas are found in 8–12% of patients.[439,447] They tend to occur in portal tracts, but may also involve the parenchyma and may be present diffusely (Fig. 17.17B–D). Similar granulomas may be found in bone marrow, lymph nodes and spleen.[448] In some instances they are related to previous lymphangiography,[449] and lipid deposits may be present; in the others the aetiology is uncertain but is possibly related to the altered immunity in patients with Hodgkin disease. They should not be regarded as evidence of organ involvement by Hodgkin disease, but they have been associated with a better prognosis.[448] Granulomatous hepatitis may precede clinical expression of Hodgkin disease.[450]

Peliosis hepatis and sinusoidal dilatation (Fig. 17.17E) involving the perivenular and mid zones[451] have been reported in patients who were not receiving androgenic steroids. The frequency of sinusoidal dilatation in these studies ranged from 40 to 50% and its presence did not correlate with hepatic involvement or with histological type. Bruguera et al.[451] noted its association with the presence of systemic symptoms.

Clinical jaundice develops in up to 15% of patients with Hodgkin disease. It may be mild and of a haemolytic nature, may be obstructive[452] and severe when there are extensive hepatic metastases, or may be treatment-related.[453] Cases of unexplained intrahepatic cholestasis have also been reported.[454] Hübscher and his colleagues[455] reported three patients with intrahepatic cholestasis in whom liver biopsy showed loss of intrahepatic bile ducts. They suggested that a vanishing bile-duct syndrome was a possible explanation for the intrahepatic cholestasis. These observations have been confirmed in other studies[456] and the author has also seen similar cases (Fig. 17.17F).

There is a report of three patients with primary sclerosing cholangitis in whom Hodgkin disease developed.[457] Massive necrosis with fulminant hepatic failure has been described as a paraneoplastic syndrome in a single case.[458]

Non-Hodgkin lymphoma

Macroscopic liver involvement in generalized non-Hodgkin lymphoma occurs at autopsy with about the same frequency as in Hodgkin disease. The liver is the organ most commonly involved after lymph nodes, spleen and bone marrow. Liver involvement was found in 15–20% of biopsy specimens taken during staging laparotomy[435] and was almost invariably associated with clinical hepatomegaly and splenic involvement.

The clinicopathological correlations in the non-Hodgkin lymphomas are not so well defined as in Hodgkin disease. Epithelioid cell granulomas occur in about 10% of cases and may sometimes be extensive;[459,460] their presence does not indicate hepatic involvement by tumour. Jaundice may occur in the absence of intrahepatic metastases.[461] Patients with concurrent cirrhosis and non-Hodgkin lymphoma have been reported;[462] in some the cirrhosis was complicated by hepatocellular carcinoma.[463]

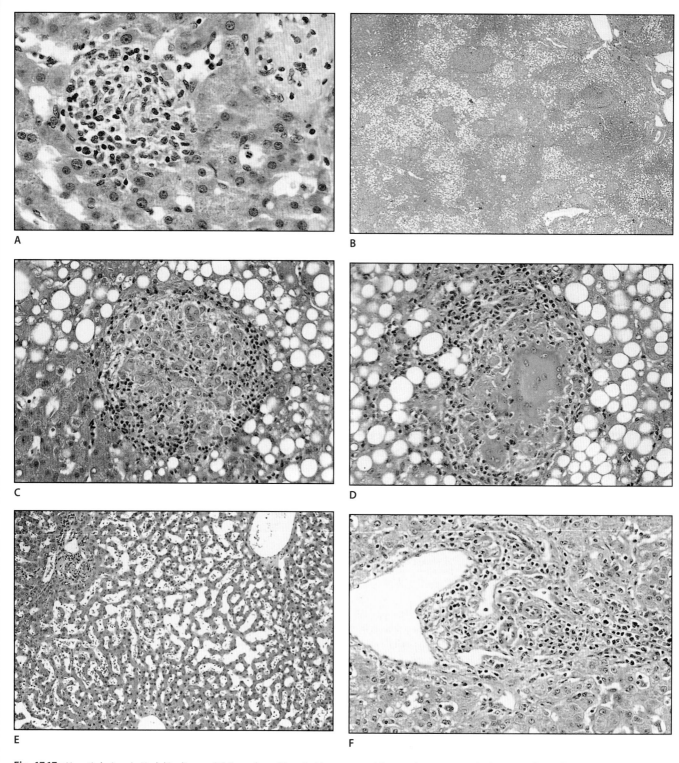

Fig. 17.17 • Hepatic lesions in Hodgkin disease. (A) Parenchymal lymphoid aggregate: this comprises some atypical mononuclear cells and lymphocytes but there are no Reed–Sternberg cells; **(B)** diffuse granulomatous involvement and fatty liver but with no tumour deposits; these granulomas show variegated appearances **(C and D). (E)** Sinusoidal dilatation involving periportal and mid-zones. **(F)** Cholestatic syndrome in a middle-aged male; there is a diffuse chronic inflammatory cell infiltrate of the portal tract in which no bile duct can be identified. H & E.

B-cell lymphomas

The patterns of infiltration by non-Hodgkin lymphoma are well described by Dargent & DeWolf Peters.[464] The better differentiated low-grade lymphocytic and follicular lymphomas, mantle-cell and marginal-zone lymphomas and lymphoid leukaemias tend to produce multiple small nodular deposits, predominantly in portal tracts and some-

times with sinusoidal permeation, whereas the less well-differentiated high-grade lymphomas produce large irregular deposits which destructively involve both portal tracts and parenchyma.

The microscopic features in the liver usually resemble those in involved lymph nodes, although regional and organ diversity in histological appearances is well recognized.[464] The differential diagnosis from non-specific inflammation depends on the abnormal cytological features, the more extensive, total or near-total involvement of portal tracts, and the tendency to extend beyond the portal tracts and spill over into the periportal parenchyma.[441] We have seen lympho-epithelial lesions of the bile ducts in one case but this is unusual other than in primary mucosal associated lymphoid tissue lymphomas (MALTomas). True follicle formation may very occasionally be seen in follicular lymphomas. Immunophenotyping with the demonstration of light chain restriction may be helpful in establishing a diagnosis of malignancy.[465]

Burkitt lymphoma

In Burkitt lymphoma, hepatic deposits have been reported in 50–70% of cases,[466,467] sometimes with predominant liver involvement and sometimes with subcapsular involvement only, suggesting direct spread from the peritoneum.

T-cell lymphomas

In peripheral T-cell lymphomas liver involvement is present in about 50% of cases and patients may sometimes present with liver disease.[468] In addition to focal portal tract and parenchymal involvement (Fig. 17.18), there may sometimes be a predominant pattern of intrasinusoidal permeation. This appears to be particularly the case for Tγ/δ lymphomas (see below).[469,470] In adult T-cell leukaemia where liver involvement is common,[471] the infiltrate is usually sinusoidal.[472]

In tropical splenomegaly and non-tropical idiopathic splenomegaly, intrasinusoidal permeation by mononuclear cells is present. The infiltrate in the tropical form consists of T-cells and there may also be portal fibrosis.[473] In the non-tropical form this pattern of liver involvement was seen in patients who subsequently developed lymphoma.[474]

Hepatic involvement has been reported in *Sezary syndrome* and in *mycosis fungoides* both in biopsy material and also in 17 of a series of 45 patients examined post-mortem.[475–478] In *angiocentric lymphomas*, focal intrahepatic deposits and intrasinusoidal infiltration may be seen, sometimes accompanied by Kupffer-cell erythrophagocytosis.[441] Liver involvement has also been reported in *angioimmunoblastic lymphadenopathy*[441] and there is a case report in which the liver showed nodular regenerative hyperplasia, peliosis hepatitis and perisinusoidal fibrosis.[479]

Primary hepatic lymphomas

It is now recognized that in some patients with malignant lymphoma the disease is either confined to the liver or the presenting symptoms are related to liver involvement—so-called primary lymphoma of liver (see Chapter 15). These cases are relatively rare; their clinical behaviour and association with hepatitis C and primary biliary cirrhosis are reviewed in several recent articles.[480–483]

Hepatosplenic T-cell lymphoma

Hepatosplenic T-cell lymphoma is associated with the consistent presence of isochromosome 7q.[469,470] It is usually confined to the liver and spleen where there is sinusoidal permeation by small lymphoid cells (Fig. 17.19); bone marrow involvement may however be overlooked. The cells normally show clonal Tγ/δ receptor gene rearrangement[469] although occasional cases with similar clinical and histological features show α/β clonal expansion.[484] It may develop on a background of immunosuppression.[485]

T-cell or histiocyte rich B-cell lymphoma

T-cell or histiocyte rich B-cell lymphoma may also be confined to the liver. This may mimic Hodgkin disease.[486] There are frequently B symptoms at the time of presentation and marked liver dysfunction may be apparent.[487] Histologically, this tumour is characterized by a florid reactive stromal response which includes macrophages and small T-lymphocytes; this may obscure the CD20+ve malignant cells which can be present in small numbers (Fig. 17.20).[486]

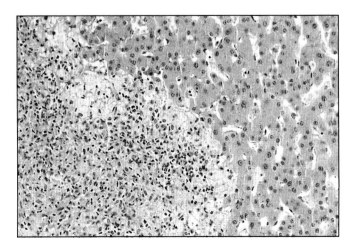

Fig. 17.18 • Peripheral T-cell lymphoma in liver; there is a granulomatoid appearance to the tumour deposit and the hepatocytes at the parenchymal tumour interface show a vacuolated appearance. H & E.

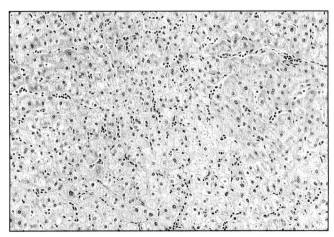

Fig. 17.19 • T γ/δ lymphoma: infiltration of the hepatic sinusoids by small lymphocytes; note irregular outline of lymphoid cells. There is no evidence of significant liver cell injury. H & E.

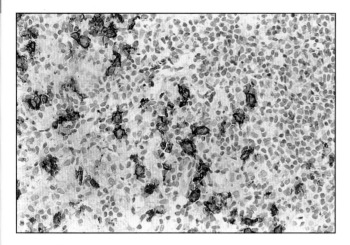

Fig. 17.20 • T cell rich B-cell lymphoma. The malignant cells are set amidst a background of reactive lymphocytes. Immunoreactivity for CD20.

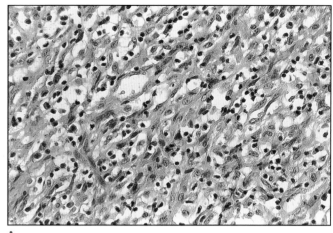

A

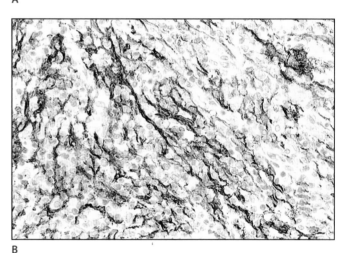

B

Fig. 17.21 • Follicular dendritic cell tumour. **(A)** Inflammatory pseudotumour-like appearance; note accompanying inflammatory cells including plasma cells. H & E. **(B)** Immunoreactivity for CD21.

Follicular dendritic cell tumours

Follicular dendritic cell tumours of the liver are uncommon.[488–490] They are characterized by an inflammatory pseudotumour-like histological appearance with fascicles of bland spindle cells and often only occasional pleomorphic cells (Fig. 17.21). The tumour cells are positive for CD21, CD35 and with R4/23 and KiM4 antibodies. There is evidence that this is an EBV-driven clonal proliferation. The tumour may show local infiltration but does not appear to metastasize.

Other primary hepatic lymphomas that have been described include: *MALToma*,[491–494] *plasmacytoma*[495] and *angiocentric lymphoma*.[496] Post-transplant lymphoproliferative disease (PTLD) may occur as a localized lesion in the liver.

Autoimmune lymphoproliferative disease

This disorder is characterized by generalized lymphadenopathy, elevated serum aminotransferases, lymphocytosis, splenomegaly and autoimmune phenomena.[497] The underlying defect appears to be impaired lymphocyte apoptosis due to an inherited mutation of the CD95 (Fas) gene.[498] In a study of 10 patients, Lim et al.[499] reported abnormalities in liver biopsies of two cases. In one, there was a mild lymphocytic infiltrate of CD3+ T-cells (CD4–/CD8–) with periportal fibrosis and extramedullary haemopoiesis. In the other, there was a chronic hepatitis with features consistent with an autoimmune hepatitis.

Miscellaneous haematological diseases with liver involvement

Thrombocytopenic purpura

Perisinusoidal fibrosis was reported in 10 patients undergoing splenectomy for thrombocytopenic purpura, in eight of whom the disease was idiopathic.[500] It was postulated that platelet-derived growth factor and activated macrophages were causal factors in producing the fibrosis, analogous to the similar lesion which has been reported in myelofibrosis.[426] Phagocytosis of platelets by Kupffer cells may be seen in autoimmune thrombocytopenia.[501] Veno-occlusive disease has been described in a case of thrombocytopenic purpura with polymyositis.[502]

Hypereosinophilic syndrome

This is a rare condition characterized by persistent and marked eosinophilia combined with organ dysfunction.[503] Chronic hepatitis has been described in five patients with idiopathic hypereosinophilic syndrome.[504,505] In their patient, Foong et al.[505] demonstrated activated eosinophils in a liver biopsy, with deposition of eosinophil major basic protein in areas of hepatocyte injury. Focal necrosis was observed in the case of Ung et al.[506] and a mass effect of the eosinophilic infiltrate has been described.[507] Fauci et al.[508] noted that 30% of patients with the hypereosinophilic syndrome demonstrated mild hepatomegaly and/or minor disturbances of liver function tests; sinusoidal congestion, hepatitis and periportal inflammation were present in some cases.

Familial hypofibrinogenaemia/dysfibrinogenaemia

Familial cases of hypofibrinogenaemia have been reported in which hepatocytes contain intracytoplasmic PAS-negative (or weakly positive) globular inclusions which on immunohistochemistry react specifically with anti-fibrinogen antisera.[509-512] Brennan et al.[512] described the molecular and functional basis for abnormal storage of the protein in cirrhosis associated with fibrinogen Brescia (Fig. 17.22). A single mutation at codon 284 of the gamma chain gene has also been demonstrated in association with an increase in this portion of the disialo isoforms suggesting that misfolding of the variant protein may cause its hepatic retention.[513] Similar perivenular globular inclusions have been shown to contain C3 and C4 components of complement[514,515] (Fig. 17.23); these patients had normal serum complement levels. These disorders have now been categorized as endoplasmic reticulum storage diseases (Ch. 5).[512]

Marucci et al. have suggested that fibrinogen inclusions in hepatocytes may occasionally arise in patients who do not have an underlying genetic abnormality but in whom there is an acquired endoplasmic reticulin storage disease during the course of an infection disease.[516]

The liver in the rheumatoid and connective tissue diseases

The liver is rarely affected in the collagen diseases.[517-520] With the exception of secondary amyloidosis (type AA), now most commonly seen in rheumatoid arthritis, evidence for any significant hepatic dysfunction is scant and few specific morphological abnormalities have been described. A generalized necrotizing arteritis may complicate many of the rheumatoid and connective tissue diseases and hepatic involvement may be part of this; nodular regenerative hyperplasia,[433] haematoma[521] and spontaneous hepatic rupture may then develop.[522,523] Many of the therapeutic

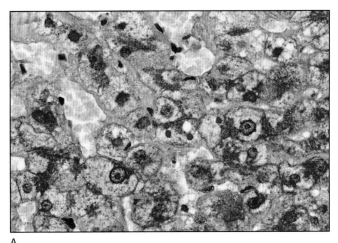

A

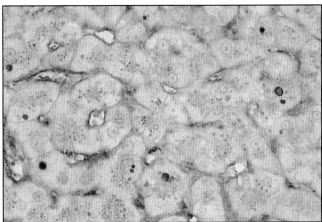

B

Fig. 17.23 • Complement protein accumulation in hepatocytes. **(A)** Intracytoplasmic globular inclusions showing an intense red staining on a Masson's trichrome. **(B)** They contain the C4 component of complement and were also weakly positive for C3; there is some perisinusoidal positivity. Immunoperoxidase stain.

agents used in the rheumatoid and connective tissue diseases are potentially hepatotoxic and may be responsible for some of the hepatic abnormalities seen in these conditions; of particular note is the potential risk of fibrosis following methotrexate therapy in rheumatoid arthritis[524] and of hepatitis in relation to the use of newer disease modifying agents.[525]

Rheumatoid diseases

Rheumatoid arthritis (RA)

Based on the evidence provided by the frequency of abnormal liver function tests in RA, in particular raised serum alkaline phosphatase levels, Kendall et al. postulated the existence of a 'rheumatoid liver'.[526,527] Increased serum levels of γ-glutamyl-transpeptidase and alkaline phosphatase have been reported in a number of studies, increased levels being found in up to 80% of patients in some series.[528,529] The liver isoenzyme of alkaline phosphatase is predominantly raised;[528] the increases in enzyme levels have been correlated with the clinical activity of RA. However, while clinical or imaging evidence of hepatomegaly may be found in

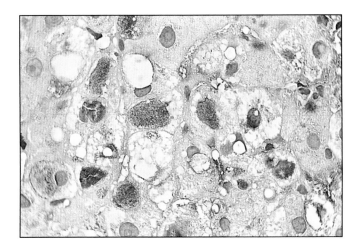

Fig. 17.22 • Fibrinogen Brescia: cytoplasmic inclusions are identified by immunohistochemistry. Courtesy of Professor F Callea.

10–20% of patients,[530,531] other clinical signs of chronic liver disease are usually lacking. Liver biopsy and autopsy studies have not revealed any consistent or specific findings, the main abnormalities being non-specific reactive hepatitis, steatosis and minimal portal fibrosis;[532–537] chronic hepatitis and sinusoidal dilatation have occasionally been reported.[538,539] In an autopsy series of 188 cases, Ruderman et al.[540] found diffuse fibrosis in 15 but severe fibrotic disease was rare. Diseases such as primary biliary cirrhosis or α_1-antitrypsin deficiency may occur coincidentally with RA.[541–544]

Nodular regenerative hyperplasia (Fig. 17.24A) frequently associated with Felty syndrome, has been reported in a small number of patients with RA and its pathogenesis has been associated with rheumatoid vasculitis.[543–545] Spontaneous rupture of the liver may complicate the vasculitis.[523] There is a single case report of rheumatoid nodules in the liver (Fig. 17.24B).[546] In a study by Landas and co-workers, lipogranulomas were found in the livers of 56% of their patients with severe RA.[547] The lesions contained pigment which was shown by spectroscopy to be gold particles, thought to be related to therapy.

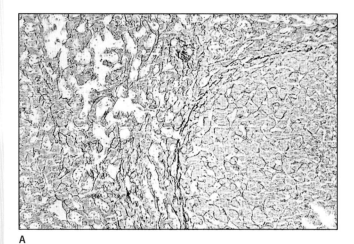

A

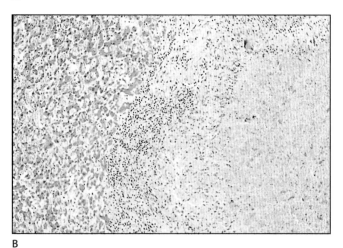

B

Fig. 17.24 • Liver in rheumatoid arthritis. **(A)** Nodular regenerative hyperplasia in a patient with Felty syndrome. Gordon & Sweets reticulin stain. **(B)** Rheumatoid nodule. Courtesy of Dr Carole D Kooijman.

Sjögren syndrome

There is a strong association between the sicca complex and RA. Hepatomegaly and abnormal liver function tests are documented in approximately one quarter of patients with Sjögren syndrome.[530,548] As with RA, there are no consistent changes seen in liver biopsies. In most cases non-specific reactive changes are found.[530] A form of Sjögren syndrome, which clinically and immunopathologically resembles that associated with RA, is seen in patients with primary biliary cirrhosis;[549] clinical symptoms of the sicca complex occur in almost 50% of patients and histological changes diagnostic of Sjögren syndrome in over 25%— features which suggest that there may be an overlap between the two conditions. Furthermore, an earlier study demonstrated anti-mitochondrial antibodies (AMA) in 11% of patients with Sjögren disease, although this was based on an immunofluorescent test and PBC-specific AMAs were not sought.[530] Two cases are recorded with concomitant Sjögren syndrome and type I autoimmune hepatitis.[550] Montefusco et al.[551] reported an association between sclerosing cholangitis, chronic pancreatitis and Sjögren syndrome. There is also a relationship between Sjögren syndrome and hepatitis C; over 15% of patients have anti-HCV antibodies and there is some evidence that the virus may be the initiating event in some patients.[552] Primary hepatic lymphoma has been described in Sjögren syndrome.[553]

Felty syndrome

In Felty syndrome, in which rheumatoid arthritis is accompanied by splenomegaly and neutropenia, mononuclear sinusoidal infiltration may occur[554,555] and the syndrome is frequently complicated by portal hypertension associated with nodular regenerative hyperplasia.[556–558] In their review of 26 patients with Felty syndrome and evidence of hepatic dysfunction, Blendis et al.[556] reported that 13 had portal hypertension with oesophageal varices, and in nine of these there was histological evidence of nodular regenerative hyperplasia. On the basis of a further prospective study, Blendis and his colleagues reported that abnormalities of liver architecture may develop in two-thirds of patients with Felty syndrome and, in at least half of these, nodular regenerative hyperplasia and portal hypertension will be present.[557] The pathogenesis of nodular regenerative hyperplasia in RA and Felty syndrome is not fully established but evidence suggests that rheumatoid vasculitis affecting intrahepatic arterial radicles may play a role (Chapter 13).[545]

Juvenile rheumatoid arthritis (Still disease)

Minor abnormalities of liver function tests have been noted in patients with the febrile systemic type of Still disease but, in the small number of liver biopsies examined, only non-specific reactive changes were found.[558,559] The hepatic manifestations of the adult-onset form of Still disease (seronegative arthritis) are similar, with hepatomegaly and raised aminotransferases being found in up to 76% of patients.[560,561] However, life-threatening hepatic failure, possibly drug-induced, has been noted with a fatal outcome in some.[561–563] There is a single case report in which there was severe hepatitis which responded to immunosuppression.[564]

Connective tissue diseases

Systemic lupus erythematosus (SLE)

Dubois et al.[565] reported jaundice of a predominantly hae-molytic type in 3.8% of 520 patients, and death from hepatic failure of unspecified aetiology in 4% of 249 patients with SLE. Runyon et al.,[566] in a retrospective survey of 206 cases, found severe chronic liver disease in 9 (4.4%); these included cirrhosis, chronic hepatitis and primary biliary cirrhosis. In contrast, Gibson and Myers[567] found no significant liver disease in their series of 81 patients, and in another prospective study, no clinical or biochemical abnormalities of liver function were found in 76% of 260 SLE patients.[568] However, persistent and unexplained increases in serum aminotransferase levels were found in 15 (8%) patients and, in 12 of these, the enzyme changes matched the SLE activity. This suggests that subclinical liver disease may be a manifestation of SLE in a small minority of patients. In a retrospective review of 1468 cases, Matsumoto and colleagues[569] noted a history of chronic hepatitis in 36 patients (2.5%), in eight of whom it was reported to be 'active'; cirrhosis was present in 17 (1.2%).

The commonest histological finding is macrovesicular steatosis;[569] this may in part be due to corticosteroid therapy. Mild periportal inflammation is often present[567] but a true chronic hepatitis is rare. Hepatic granulomas have been described in several cases[566] and Murphy et al.[20] reported a case in whom the granulomas were of fibrin-ring type; this patient, however, had concomitant cytomegalovirus and staphylococcal infections.

The relationship between 'lupoid' or autoimmune hepa-titis and SLE has been reviewed in detail by Mackay.[570] Although both diseases are characterized by the presence of circulating antinuclear antibodies, the specificities of these antibodies differ. The immunogenetic and pathogenetic mechanisms of autoimmune hepatitis and SLE are also dis-similar.[570] Patients in whom both entities are present, such as those described by Runyon et al.,[566] probably represent co-existent diseases rather than an 'overlap' syndrome. Occasional cases of co-existing SLE and primary biliary cir-rhosis are described.[571]

Nodular regenerative hyperplasia has been described in SLE.[572] In the autopsy study of Matsumoto et al.,[569] three of 52 cases of SLE had nodular regenerative hyperplasia sug-gesting that this may be a relatively common, but clinically silent, complication. The anti-phospholipid syndrome, in which there are anti-phospholipid antibodies and which is found in a proportion of patients with SLE, is associated with a thrombotic tendency.[573] It has been suggested that by interfering with intrahepatic blood flow, thrombotic occlu-sion may play a role in the pathogenesis of nodular regen-erative hyperplasia in some cases.[574] These antibodies have also been implicated in cases of veno-occlusive disease and Budd–Chiari syndrome occurring in SLE or 'lupus-like' disease.[575,576]

Peliosis hepatis was found in six of the cases reported by Matsumoto et al.;[569] arteritis, complicated by hepatic infarction in one instance, was a feature in 20% of their patients and might have been of causal significance in the nodular regenerative hyperplasia. Other common findings in their series were sinusoidal congestion and bilirubinostasis which were attributed to the terminal ill-nesses, rather than SLE per se. Hepatic infarction[577,578] and spontaneous rupture of the liver[579] has been reported, each in two patients. There is a single case report of mala-coplakia[580] occurring in SLE. Laxer et al.,[581] in reporting four cases, suggested that neonatal hepatitis may occur as a complication of neonatal lupus erythematosus with the presence of maternal auto-antibodies; in occasional cases it may be the sole clinical manifestation of the disease.[582] Viral and protozoal infection of the liver such as *cryptococcus* are seen with increased frequency in SLE patients.[583]

Hepatobiliary disease is seen in neonatal lupus erythae-matosis; Scleroderma and progressive systemic sclerosis have infrequently been associated with hepatic disease. Bartholomew et al.[584] reported liver involvement in 8 of 727 patients with scleroderma, and D'Angelo et al.[585] in an autopsy study found cirrhosis in 5 of 57 patients, a lower incidence than in their carefully matched control group. In a study of four scleroderma patients with portal hyperten-sion, Morris et al.[586] reported that one had cirrhosis, two had chronic hepatitis, and in the fourth patient the liver was normal apart from some granulomas. Extrahepatic biliary disease associated with fibrosis of the gallbladder[587] and large-duct obstruction due to vasculitis and ulceration[588] have been reported. PSC associated with systemic sclerosis was reported by Fraile et al.[589]

An association of primary biliary cirrhosis with the cal-cinosis, Raynaud phenomenon, oesophageal dysfunction, sclerodactyly and telangiectasis (CREST) syndrome was first suggested by Murray-Lyon et al. in 1970[590] and subse-quently confirmed in numerous reports. Anti-mitochon-drial antibodies are found in up to one quarter of patients with the CREST syndrome although the histological changes of primary biliary cirrhosis are present in only 3–4%.[591] Nodular regenerative hyperplasia has been reported in progressive systemic sclerosis[592] as has hepatic infarction.[593]

Mixed connective tissue disease

This syndrome is characterized by an overlap of the clinical features of SLE, progressive systemic sclerosis and polymyo-sitis and by high titres of antibodies to the ribonucleopro-tein fraction of extractable nuclear antigens. In a study of 61 patients, only four had clinical evidence of liver disease,[594] and liver biopsy in one showed chronic hepatitis with cir-rhosis. A further three patients with mixed connective tissue disease and chronic hepatitis have subsequently been reported.[595,596] Non-specific reactive hepatitis was noted in an autopsy study by Singsen et al.[597] of three children with this disease. Venous outflow obstruction with thrombosis has been reported in association with mixed connective tissue disease.[598]

Miscellaneous musculoskeletal and multisystem disorders

Polymyalgia rheumatica

Increased levels of serum alkaline phosphatase are found in over a third of patients and the levels may parallel disease activity.[599] Sattar et al.[600] reported anti-mitochondrial antibodies in 11 of 36 patients with co-existing primary biliary cirrhosis in some cases. Morphological changes in the liver have comprised non-specific reactive hepatitis, steatosis and granulomas; there may sometimes be a moderately intense portal tract inflammation with lymphoid follicles.[601,602] There is an increased frequency of nodular regenerative hyperplasia.[433]

Polymyositis and dermatomyositis

An association between primary biliary cirrhosis and polymyositis has been reported in a small number of cases.[603–605] Unexplained hepatosplenomegaly and minor abnormalities of liver function tests may occur in children with dermatomyositis[606] and there are case reports of patients with polymyositis who were subsequently found to have a hepatocellular carcinoma.[607,608]

Weber-Christian disease

In Weber-Christian disease, Oram and Cochrane[609] reported severe hepatomegaly due to fatty liver. Inflammation of intrahepatic fat may occur, similar to the panniculitis which characterizes this disease (Fig. 17.25). In a case described by Kimura et al.[610] there was steatohepatitis and abundant Mallory bodies were seen. The changes were predominantly in periportal zones; the patient had no other known risk factor for non-alcoholic steatohepatitis.

Systemic vasculitides

Liver involvement in these disorders is discussed in Chapter 13. The liver may be affected in over 40% of cases of *polyarteritis nodosa* (Fig. 17.26) producing infarction in many instances.[611] Hepatic infarction has also been described in *Churg–Strauss syndrome*.[612] Intrahepatic arterial vasculitis has also been noted with *temporal arteritis*[613] and the liver may be involved in *Takayasu arteritis*.[614] Goritsas et al. reported a case of *polyarteritis nodosa* in which there was both nodular regenerative hyperplasia and injury of intrahepatic bile ducts.[615] In the vascular subtype of *Behçets disease*, venous outflow obstruction[616–618] has been reported as has nodular regenerative hyperplasia.[616–619]

The liver in renal diseases

Hepatic dysfunction is well recognized in patients with chronic renal disease. This is true in patients maintained on haemodialysis and in patients receiving allografts, and in both these groups chronic viral infection is the most common cause of hepatic injury. A number of less common causes of liver dysfunction are also reviewed in this section; the hepatotoxic effects of immunosuppressant therapy in allograft recipients are discussed in Chapter 16.

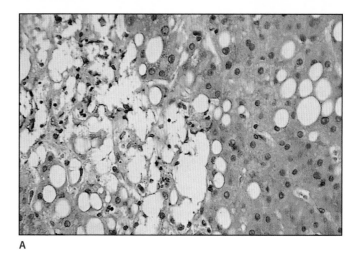

A

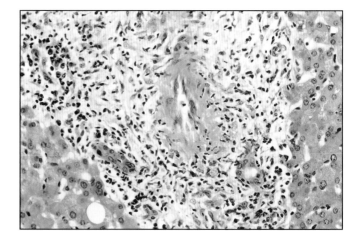

B

Fig. 17.25 • Liver in Weber–Christian disease. **(A)** There is macrovesicular steatosis and in the accumulation on the left there is inflammation. **(B)** A mixed mononuclear and neutrophil polymorph infiltrate is present in the inflamed fat. H & E.

Fig. 17.26 • Involvement of hepatic artery branch by polyarteritis nodosa. H & E.

Viral hepatitis

Viral hepatitis is a recognized major complication of hae-modialysis. There is no evidence that hepatitis A contributes to the problem.[620–622] In early studies on hepatitis B, sero-logical evidence of infection in haemodialysis patients was found in up to 40%, and chronic HBs antigenaemia was found in 10–15%.[621,623] However, careful screening strate-gies have resulted in a considerable reduction in these figures and Alter et al.[624] reported that whereas the preva-lence rate of HBs antigenaemia in haemodialysis units in the USA was 7.8% in 1976, the corresponding figure in the following decade was 0.6%; current prevalence remains less than 1%. In both haemodialysis and transplant patients who develop acute hepatitis B the illness is mild[625] and, indeed, in many the acute infection is asymptomatic, although fulminant hepatic failure can occur.[620,626,627] However, acquired HBV infection in these patients is associ-ated with a high risk of chronic infection, a major cause of morbidity and mortality in many transplant centres.[625–628]

The incidence of HBV-associated chronic hepatitis in hae-modialysis patients may be as high as 5% and the disease is usually more rapidly progressive, presumably due to the immunosuppressant effects of the patients' azotaemia.[629] Similarly, histological evidence of more rapidly progressive chronic hepatitis has been found in renal transplant patients.[627,630,631] Cases of fibrosing cholestatic hepatitis akin to that seen with recurrent HBV in liver transplantation have also been described in renal allograft recipients.[632] It is worth mentioning that in haemodialysis patients only 40–60% have an adequate response to hepatitis B vaccine.[633,634] There is little evidence that persistent HBs antigenaemia jeopar-dizes the survival of the renal allograft.[633]

The role of HCV in causing liver disease in haemodialysis and transplant patients has been intensely investigated.[635,636] There is a high prevalence of HCV antibody in patients maintained on haemodialysis; early studies, using the first generation antibody tests, suggested prevalence rates of 35% in unselected patients[636,637] and 12% in transplant recipi-ents.[638] A study from Hong Kong combining RNA and antibody assays reported 25% and 30% positivity rates respectively in a series of 51 patients.[639] In a study of 37 transplant patients with biopsy proven liver disease 12 of 15 patients with chronic hepatitis were HCV antibody-positive using a second generation RIBA assay.[628] A study following renal transplant recipients for 21 years showed those with HBV and HCV to have a high rate of viral replica-tion and a higher overall mortality than non-infected patients.[636] Patients are described in which there is a rapidly progressive HCV hepatitis resembling the fibrosing choles-tatic hepatitis of HBV.[640] There is however no evidence that HCV has any adverse effect on renal graft survival.[641]

Cytomegalovirus (CMV) infection is very common in patients being treated for chronic renal disease[620] and acute infection or reactivation may occur in up to 50% of patients undergoing renal transplantation.[642] Clinically, episodes of CMV hepatitis are apparently not modified in these patients. However, the widespread infection in renal transplant recip-ients makes it difficult to assess a causal role for CMV; the absence of histological evidence of infection argues against its having an important role in producing chronic liver dys-function. Epstein–Barr virus (EBV) and adenovirus infec-tion of the liver in renal patients is relatively rare although more than 80% of allograft recipients harbour EBV in their oropharynx.[643] Herpes simplex (and herpes zoster) serocon-version occurs in a significant proportion of transplant recipients; disseminated infection with hepatic involvement has been reported.[644]

Peliosis hepatis and nodular regenerative hyperplasia

Peliosis hepatis has been reported in two patients on chronic haemodialysis,[645,646] and has also been noted in a number of renal allograft recipients,[647,648] occurring as a complica-tion in 2% of one series of 500 patients.[647] In some cases it was associated with nodular regenerative hyperplasia, a lesion which may also occur on its own in allograft recipi-ents. Allison et al.,[628] in reporting nodular regenerative hyperplasia in 5 of 27 transplant patients who had under-gone biopsy, estimated that there were 38 previously reported cases in some of whom portal hypertension and hepatic failure had developed.[649–652] Veno-occlusive disease[653,654] and hepatic sinusoidal dilatation, sometimes with portal hypertension,[655] have also been reported in transplant patients. Nataf et al.[656] reported two transplant recipients with idiopathic portal hypertension in whose biopsies perisinusoidal fibrosis was present. The aetiology of these vascular complications in the liver remains uncer-tain. Current evidence suggests that they are related to the use of azathioprine[655] although sinusoidal endothelial cell disease due to CMV infection has also been postulated.[648]

Miscellaneous liver diseases

Haemosiderosis

Moderate or severe secondary iron overload develops in patients who receive blood transfusion while on dialysis and may cause hepatic dysfunction after transplanta-tion.[657,658] Pahl et al.[659] noted haemosiderosis at autopsy in 13 of 78 patients maintained on haemodialysis. Rao & Anderson[658] noted that significant, and sometimes unex-plained haemosiderosis (grade 3 to 4+) was more frequent after renal transplantation and was associated with cirrho-sis in a number of patients.

Neoplasms and infiltrates

Hepatocellular carcinoma has been reported in a number of patients[660–662] and, of 1436 neoplasms that developed in 1348 patients reported in the Denver Transplant Tumour Registry, 14 were hepatocellular carcinomas.[663]

Intrahepatic haematomas may occur in haemodialysis patients who have developed a bleeding diathesis.[664]

The presence in the liver of silicone particles from dialysis tubing, evoking a *granulomatous reaction* in some cases, has been reported[665,666] and may sometimes lead to scarring.[667] Multiple aluminium-containing epithelioid cell granulomas were found at autopsy in the liver, spleen and lymph nodes of two patients on long-term haemodialysis.[668]

There is a case report of diffuse microscopic hepatic *calcification* in a patient on haemodialysis.[669] In *dialysis-related amyloidosis*, in which β2-microglobulin is the precursor protein, vascular deposition in the liver has been reported in a few cases.[670,671]

The liver in amyloidosis and light chain deposition disease

Amyloidosis

Since the first description by Rokitansky[672] in 1842, amyloid and amyloidosis have continued to intrigue pathologist and clinician alike. Amyloidosis is now classified on the basis of the chemical composition of the amyloid fibrils and their precursor protein.[673–675] Current nomenclature includes 25 human proteins; the most common of these are documented in Table 17.5. Systemic amyloidosis may occur:

1. as *primary or myeloma-related (AL)*:
   a. in association with plasma cell dyscrasias, multiple myeloma, B-cell malignancies and Waldenström disease; the amyloid (A) fibril contains light chains (AL), and the precursor protein is the amino-terminal variable region of kappa or lambda chains, and
   b. in association with heavy chain disease in which the fibril contains heavy chain (AH) and the precursor protein is IgG$_1$;
2. as *secondary or reactive (AA)* in association with long-standing chronic inflammatory processes, e.g. rheumatoid arthritis and bronchiectasis, Hodgkin disease, and occasionally non-lymphoid malignancies such as gastric and renal carcinoma and benign tumours including liver-cell adenomas;[677] the fibril is amyloid A (AA) and the precursor protein, serum AA,

is an apolipoprotein which is an acute phase protein (Chapter 1);

3. in *heredofamilial forms* which, with the exception of familial Mediterranean fever, are all of autosomal dominant inheritance, show varying geographical or ethnic distribution, affect different organs; and whose precursor proteins include various transthyretins, fibrinogen α chain, apolipoprotein AI and AII, lyzozyme and gelsolin;[675–679] and
4. in patients on *long-term renal dialysis* in which the precursor protein is β2-microglobulin and where liver involvement is rare.

Hepatic involvement in the three major forms of systemic amyloidosis is common. One autopsy study showed hepatic deposits in 70% of cases.[678] Clinical evidence of liver dysfunction is often not significant.[680–684] Hepatomegaly is present in up to 80% of patients and may be associated with pain when there is a rapid increase in size;[685,686] calcification was a feature in one case.[687] Mild jaundice may occur in 5–10% and, rarely, there may be severe cholestasis.[688] It may be the presenting feature, however, and this carries a poor prognosis.[689–692] The mechanisms of the jaundice are not clear. Portal hypertension may develop[693] and there are case reports of co-existent nodular regenerative hyperplasia[694] and of spontaneous rupture of the liver.[695] Percutaneous liver biopsy causes haemorrhage in approximately 5% of patients—sometimes this is massive.[696] Serum amyloid P scintigraphy is now being used in place of liver biopsy in some centres.

Macroscopically, the liver may be markedly enlarged, weighing up to 9 kg. It is pale, of rubbery consistency and, if amyloid is present in large amounts, it may show the classic waxy lardaceous appearance. Microscopically, the amyloid is demonstrable by conventional stains including Congo red and Sirius red. The AL and AA forms can be distinguished histologically in that pretreatment with potassium permanganate abolishes the Congo red affinity of the AA fibrils, whereas AL fibrils are resistant to this treatment.[697] In addition, immunohistochemical methods[698] may be applied to show the presence of the pentraxin P component,[699] which is synthesized by the liver, circulates as serum amyloid P (SAP) and is present in all types of amyloid. Fibrils can also be identified using transmission electronic microscopy and with atomic force microscopy.[700] There are several patterns of intrahepatic deposition. The amyloid may be deposited in blood vessels—vascular pattern; perisinusoidally in the space of Disse in linear or globular pattern—sinusoidal pattern; in perivascular portal tract fibrous tissue; and in large intrahepatic bile ducts and peribiliary glands.

In the vascular pattern of distribution, hepatic arteries and arterioles are mainly involved (Fig. 17.27A,B) but deposition can also occur in portal veins and, occasionally, in hepatic veins. In the sinusoidal pattern the accumulation is in the space of Disse producing compression atrophy of the liver-cell plates (Fig. 17.27C). A round globular form, 3–40 μm in diameter (Fig. 17.27D,E), may be found involving the space of Disse and portal tracts in patients

Table 17.5	Classification of amyloidosis
Type	**Fibril protein precursor**
AA	Serum amyloid A
AL	Ig light chains
ATTR	Normal or variant transthyretin
Aβ$_2$M	β2-microglobulin
Aβ	β protein precursor
AapoAI	Apolipoprotein AI
AFib	Fibrinogen α chain
ALys	Lysozyme
ACys	Cystatin C
AGel	Gelsolin
AIAAP	Islet amyloid polypeptide

who are clinically identical to others with amyloidosis;[701-703] some of the globules may be phagocytosed by Kupffer cells. The sinusoidal pattern usually occurs alone, although patients have been noted with coincidental sinusoidal and globular deposition.[681] A pattern of predominantly portal tract deposition (Fig. 17.27F) is sometimes seen (Bruguera; personal communication). Sasaki and his col-leagues[704] noted amyloid deposition (both of AA and AL type) under the lining epithelium of large intrahepatic bile ducts and in the peribiliary glands; they suggested that massive deposition in these sites might cause biliary obstruction.

There may be zonal variation in the amount of amyloid deposited and there is a tendency for the perivenular areas

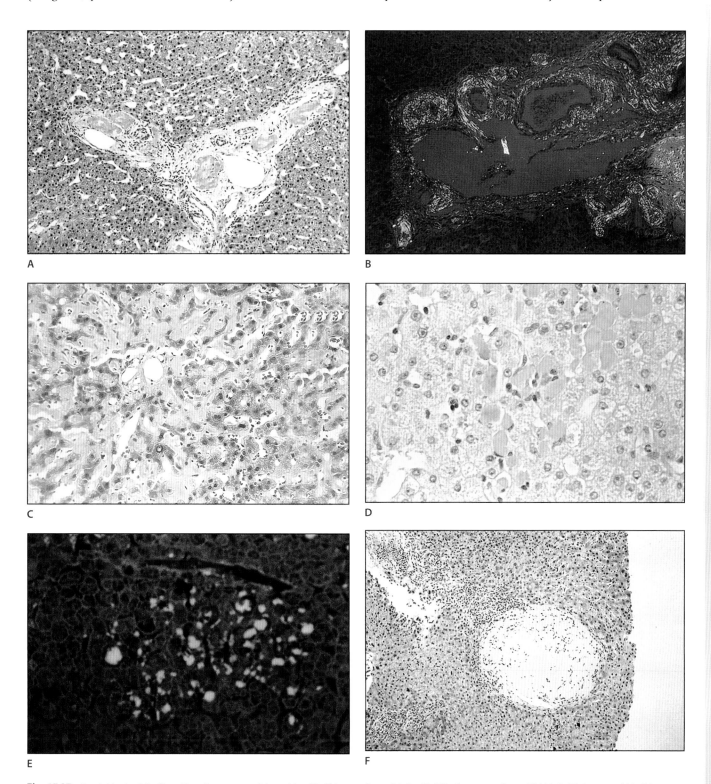

A

B

C

D

E

F

Fig. 17.27 • Amyloidosis of the liver. Vascular pattern of deposition (**A, B**) in a patient with familial Mediterranean fever. (**A**) H & E. (**B**) Congo red birefringence. Courtesy of Dr J Lough. (**C**) Linear sinusoidal pattern of deposition, predominantly perivenular and producing compression atrophy of liver-cell plates. H & E. (**D, E**) Globular sinusoidal pattern. Sirius red and fluorescence microscopy after thioflavine T stain. (**F**) Predominantly portal tract deposition. H & E. Courtesy of Dr H Tavadia.

to be less affected. The distribution pattern in the liver cannot be used to distinguish with certainty between the various forms of systemic amyloidosis. Whereas previously it was considered that the vascular pattern was predominant in AL and the sinusoidal pattern in AA, Chopra et al.[681] found sinusoidal involvement a consistent feature in the AL form and vascular involvement a consistent feature in the AA form, an observation which was confirmed by Looi & Sumithran.[682] Chopra et al.[681] found exclusive parenchymal involvement only in AL and, correspondingly, exclusive vascular involvement only in AA cases.

Liver transplantation has been used in the treatment of patients with hepatic failure due to amyloidosis.[675] In cases where the deposition was due to a hereditary form, transplantation also serves as 'surgical gene therapy'. Explants from patients with familial amyloidotic polyneuropathy appear macroscopically and microscopically normal except for amyloid deposition in nerve branches and occasionally within portal vein and bile-duct walls at the hilum.[676] The livers can be used for so-called domino transplantation.[675,705]

Light chain deposition disease

In 1976 Randall and his colleagues[706] first described *non-amyloid light chain disease* in which a plasma cell dyscrasia was associated with tissue deposition of light chains. Presenting with renal failure, their two patients also had hepatic involvement with deposition of light chains in the space of Disse. The disease mainly affects the kidney,[707,708] but skin,[709] pulmonary[710] and vascular involvement[711] have also been reported. Liver involvement is usually incidental, and in only a very few patients has there been significant hepatic dysfunction.[712–718] The clinical manifestations have included hepatomegaly, disturbance of liver function tests and one case of severe unexplained cholestasis.[718]

The striking abnormality in the liver is the deposition of light chains in the space of Disse and in the portal tracts accompanied by sinusoidal dilatation and sometimes peliosis hepatis. These deposits do not contain component P and do not stain with Congo red; they are intensely chromophilic with trichrome stains (Fig. 17.28A) and are PAS-positive diastase-resistant. The light chain nature of the deposits can be confirmed by immunohistochemistry (Fig. 17.28B). However, in some cases the deposits have been shown to also contain heavy chains[719,720] and there may be increased deposition of type I and type IV collagen and of fibronectin.[715,716,718] On electron microscopy the deposits appear as granular non-fibrillar material in the space of Disse and in the pericellular spaces (Fig. 17.28C).

There have been a number of recent reports in which light chain deposition and AL amyloid deposits have both been found in the kidney and in the liver.[717,719,721,722] In addition, Faa et al.[718] noted that, at the ultrastructural level, fibrillar material was present in the perisinusoidal deposits in their case of light chain deposition disease. These observations have suggested that light chain deposition disease and amyloidosis of the AL type represent different stages or different patterns of expression in a disease spectrum.

The liver in cardiovascular diseases

Congestive cardiac failure

In prolonged right-sided heart failure the liver is usually enlarged, firm and tender. At autopsy there is a so-called nutmeg pattern on the cut surface in which dark, congested and haemorrhagic perivenular areas alternate with paler mid-zone areas, which may show fatty change, and light periportal areas.[723] Microscopically, there is venous congestion and perivenular sinusoidal congestion, compression atrophy of liver-cell plates, and the hepatocytes contain increased amounts of lipofuscin pigment and, occasionally, hyaline globules.[724] With increasing congestion, bridging liver-cell necrosis may link hepatic vein branches[723] and a light inflammatory infiltrate, predominantly neutrophil polymorph, is noted. Perivenular fibrosis develops in the areas of necrosis, and fibrous septa form and extend to link with portal tracts producing the lesion of so-called *cardiac sclerosis* which resembles a micronodular cirrhosis. The basic liver architecture, however, is preserved and a true cardiac cirrhosis rarely, if ever, develops. There is some evidence that the liver injury associated with long-standing cardiac disease may, at least in part, be reversible; liver function has been shown to improve following cardiac transplantation.[725]

Cardiac sclerosis of varying severity is seen in up to 50% of patients with congestive cardiac failure.[723] Nodular regenerative hyperplasia develops in the periportal zones and it is of interest, historically, that this lesion was first described by Steiner[726] in patients with cardiac failure.

Acute circulatory failure

Hepatic injury in acute heart failure and peripheral circulatory shock are thought to be the result of hypoperfusion. They comprise necrosis of hepatocytes initially in the perivenular areas (the so-called microcirculatory periphery of the acinus). In severe cases there is also involvement of the mid-zone[723,727] and, in some instances, this zone may be selectively damaged.[728] A similar syndrome, to which the term ischaemic or hypoxic hepatitis has been applied, may develop in many other conditions in which there is systemic hypotension—severe trauma, burns, surgical operation, haemorrhage, pulmonary embolism and peritonitis, for example.[727,729–732] The syndrome may also occur in children[733] The severity of the liver injury can, in some patients, be related to the degree of hypotension and the duration of the shock state.[734,735] However, in others systemic hypotension may not have been a feature although there was evidence of left ventricular failure.[729]

In ischaemic hepatitis there may be mild jaundice, and there is a dramatic and rapid rise in serum aminotransferases with an equally rapid resolution on clinical recovery.[729,732] Rarely, jaundice may be the presenting clinical feature in cardiac failure.[736] Acute liver failure may develop, but this is usually seen when there is acute-on-

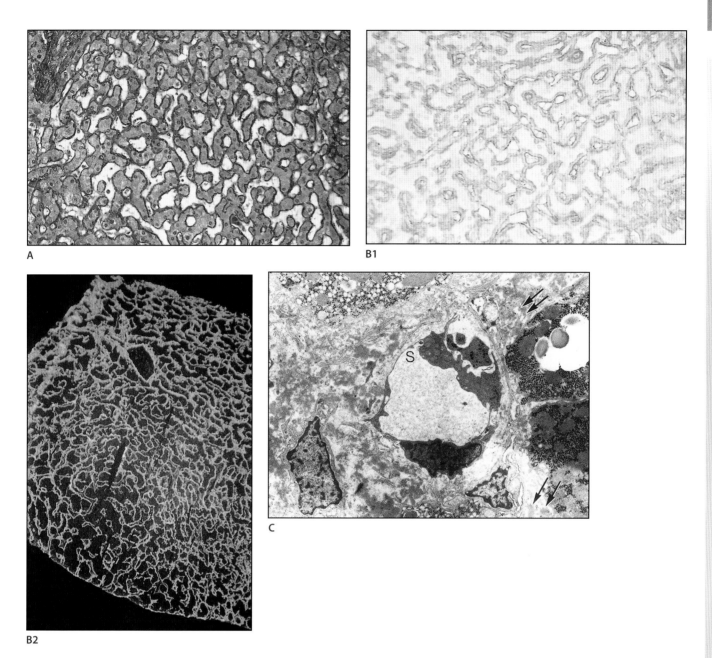

Fig. 17.28 • Light chain deposition disease. Perisinusoidal deposition of lambda light chains shown by: **(A)** Mallory trichrome stain; **(B1)** Immunoperoxidase and **(B2)** immunoflourescent staining; **(C)** electron micrograph showing granular deposits in the space of Disse and in the intercellular space (double arrows). s = sinusoidal lumen. ×4500. Panels **(B2)** and **(C)** from Droz et al.[715]

chronic cardiac failure.[737,738] Shibayama et al.,[739] on the basis of experimental work in rodents, postulated that severe hypotensive episodes caused an increased diffusion of endotoxin from the gastrointestinal tract, with aggravation of the liver injury.

Histologically, there is coagulative necrosis of hepatocytes (Fig. 17.29A), sinusoidal congestion and, sometimes, canalicular bilirubinostasis at the periphery of the necrotic areas. Inflammation is minimal and usually comprises neutrophil polymorphs. Loss of liver cells may cause focal collapse with corresponding condensation of the perivenular reticulin framework (Fig. 17.29B). With resolution, prominent aggregates of ceroid-containing macrophages

are present. Dystrophic calcification may develop (Fig. 17.30).[740]

Hyperpyrexia

Hyperpyrexia of sufficient severity and duration may be fatal. In such patients Gore & Isaacson[741] found an enlarged liver with a mottled appearance. Histologically, the hepatocytes contained small vacuoles, probably microvesicular steatosis, a phenomenon which developed early and was followed approximately 16 hours post-hyperthermia by perivenular necrosis. Similar changes have been observed with the 'recreational' drug ecstasy (Chapter 14).[742]

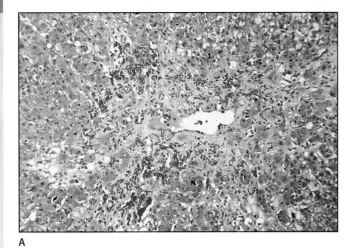

A

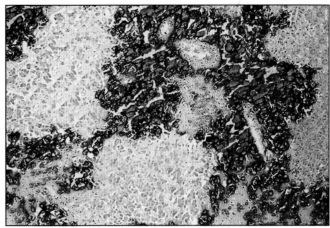

Fig. 17.30 • Dystrophic calcification in the autopsy liver of a child aged 6 years who had had episodes of ischaemic hepatitis related to surgical treatment of congenital heart disease. H & E. Courtesy of Dr A Howatson.

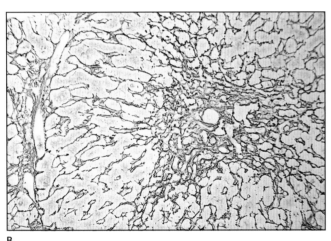

B

Fig. 17.29 • Ischaemic hepatitis following myocardial infarction. There is coagulative necrosis involving the perivenular areas with collapse of the liver cell plates. (A) H & E. (B) Reticulin.

Heat stroke

Heat stroke also leads to hepatocellular degeneration with necrosis and congestion in the perivenular area. Bianchi et al.[743] studied two cases of heat stroke; in both patients the blood pressure had at one time dropped to unrecordable levels. Serial liver biopsies were performed. The patients became icteric on the third day and there was a dramatic increase in serum aminotransferases. At 9 days, the histopathological changes comprised confluent perivenular necrosis, hydropic swelling of hepatocytes, cholestasis, and proliferation of marginal bile ducts with a cholangiolitis. Cholestasis was still present after 4 weeks but there was progressive improvement with complete resolution after one year.

Rubel & Ishak[744] studied the liver in the successive stages of fatal exertional heat stroke in 50 young men, most of them military recruits. In those five who died 'on the spot' the liver showed microvesicular steatosis, haemosiderosis, congestion, hepatocellular degeneration and extramedullary haemopoiesis. In those who survived up to 8 days microvesicular steatosis was present together with bile stasis (sometimes ductal) and an acute cholangitis and cholangiolitis. The possible mechanisms of the liver injury included, in addition to the hyperthermia, hypoxia (shock, heart failure), coagulopathy, sepsis and endotoxaemia, and in some patients haemolysis. In some cases the hepatic injury due to heat stroke can lead to liver failure[745] and cause a fatal outcome a week or more after the initial insult; hepatic transplantation may be indicated when progressive clinical decompensation develops.[746] Clinical liver disease has been seen to recur in a single case.[747]

Miscellaneous

Severe steatosis has been reported in three siblings associated with *patent ductus venosus*.[748]

Ischaemic hepatitis has been described in obese individuals with *obstructive sleep apnoea*; NAFLD is a common feature in patients with this condition, probably through insulin resistance.[749] Ghaferi and Hutchins[750] have reported on long-term hepatic injury in patients who have undergone the Fontan procedure for *congenital ventricular defects*. Cardiac sclerosis was a common complication; hepatic adenoma and hepatocellular carcinoma were seen in individual patients.

Miscellaneous liver involvement in other diseases

Skin diseases

Liver involvement in mycosis fungoides and Sézary syndrome has already been noted.

Systemic mastocytosis

Mast cells are very scanty in the normal liver, and although increased numbers are occasionally seen in acute and chronic hepatitis and in end-stage fibrosis, particularly biliary cirrhosis,[751–753] the numbers present are considerably less than those encountered in mastocytosis.

Systemic mastocytosis may be confined to the skin in 90% of patients—classic urticaria pigmentosa, whereas in 10% of patients other organs, notably bone marrow, spleen, lymph nodes and liver are involved—generalized mastocytosis.[754,755] There is also a rare malignant mastocytosis in which there is no skin involvement and which follows a rapidly fatal course.

The liver abnormalities in generalized mastocytosis have been reviewed.[756-758] Hepatomegaly is found in 60–80% of patients with liver involvement and mast cell infiltrates, predominantly involving portal tracts but also within sinusoids, are present in 40–50% of patients; in only rare cases is the sinusoidal infiltrate predominant; mast cells may also be found within endothelium and subendothelially. Cirrhosis and hepatic fibrosis are found in 4% and 14% of cases respectively. Non-cirrhotic portal hypertension has also been reported,[759-761] accompanied by intractable ascites in some patients[762,763] Cholestasis may also develop.[764] The mechanisms of the portal hypertension are uncertain and have been variously attributed to portal fibrosis, perisinusoidal fibrosis and increased splenic blood flow; Bonnet et al.[762] noted obstruction of portal and hepatic venules with sinusoidal dilatation and peliosis in their patient. The clinicopathological features were found to mimic autoimmune cholangitis in a recent report of four cases.[765]

Lichen planus

Korkij et al.,[766] in a retrospective study, found abnormalities of liver function tests in 52% of a series of 73 patients with lichen planus, compared with 36% in 272 control patients with other cutaneous diseases. Liver biopsy in eight patients showed three cases each of chronic hepatitis and cirrhosis, the others showing alcoholic hepatitis and metastatic lung carcinoma. In prospective studies Cottoni and colleagues[767] reported chronic liver disease in 16 of 62 patients and del Olmo et al.,[768] in a study of patients with lichen planus of the mouth, found abnormal liver function tests in 22 of 65 patients with biopsy-proven chronic liver disease in 12 of these. Recent reports suggest a causal association between HCV infection and lichen planus.[769] Two cases of hepatocellular carcinoma and lichen planus have been reported.[770]

Other skin disorders

von Recklinghausen disease
In this disorder liver complications reported include obstructive jaundice due to a periampullary tumour,[771] a primary neurilemmoma of the liver[772] and hepatic neurofibromas from which a mixed malignant schwannoma and angiosarcoma developed.[773]

Pityriasis rotunda
Pityriasis rotunda has been shown to be a useful cutaneous marker of hepatocellular carcinoma in South African blacks[774,775] and pityriasis rubra pilaris has been described as the presenting feature in one case.[776]

Psoriasis
There is no good evidence that psoriasis itself has any specific effects on the liver but the hepatotoxic effects of methotrexate therapy have to be carefully monitored (Ch. 14). Liver transplantation has been performed in three patients with psoriasis in whom methotrexate-induced cirrhosis developed.[777]

Miscellaneous other associations include reports of acute hepatitis[778] and chronic hepatitis[779] in patients with febrile panniculitis, of autoimmune hepatitis in association with pyoderma gangrenosum[780] and in Sweets syndrome.[781] Liver involvement may occur in lipoid proteinosis, an inherited disorder of collagen metabolism in which hyalinized extracellular matrix glycoproteins are deposited mainly in the skin, oral cavity and larynx.[782,783] The weakly PAS-positive material accumulates in portal tracts (Fig. 17.31) producing compression of the bile ducts.

There are reported associations between porphyria and hepatocellular carcinoma[784,785] and prurigo and hepatocellular adenomatosis.[786] Spontaneous rupture of the liver has been described in Ehlers Danlos disease type IV.[787]

Neuromuscular and neurodegenerative diseases

Nodular regenerative hyperplasia has been reported in a patient with myasthenia gravis.[788] In patients with myotonic dystrophy elevation of the serum levels of γ-glutamyl-transpeptidase and alkaline phosphatase[789,790] and of serum deoxycholic acid[791] have been reported. Liver biopsy of an affected mother and daughter showed enlargement of hepatic stellate cells.[790] Histological changes in the liver are seen in neuroferritinopathy, a dominantly inherited movement disorder.[792] Unusual iron-containing intranuclear inclusions in hepatocytes have been identified in a single case (personal observation; Fig 17.32).

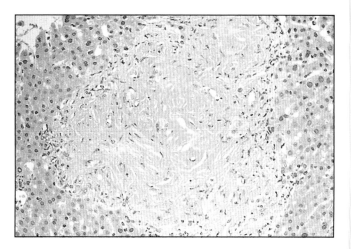

Fig. 17.31 • Liver involvement in lipoid proteinosis; hyalinized matrix glycoprotein deposits have accumulated in the portal tract. H & E. Courtesy of Dr Judy Mäkinen.

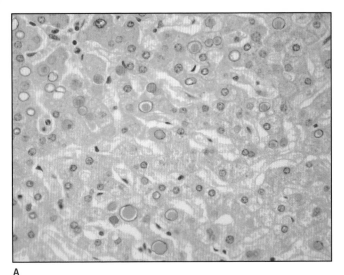
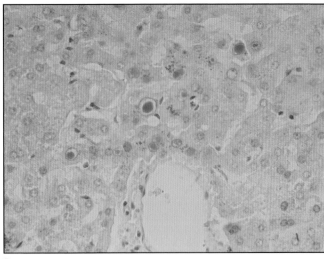

Fig. 17.32 • Iron-containing intranuclear inclusions in neuroferritinopathy. **(A)** H & E. **(B)** Perl's stain.

References

1. Popper H, Schaffner F. Liver: structure and function. New York: McGraw-Hill, 1957
2. Gerber MA, Thung SN, Bodenheimer HC, Kapelman B, Schaffner F. Characteristic histological triad in liver adjacent to metastatic neoplasm. Liver, 1986; 6:85–88
3. Jenkins D, Gilmore IT, Doel C, Gallwan S. Liver biopsy in the diagnosis of malignancy. Q J Med, 1995; 88:819–825
4. Christoffersen P, Braendstrup O, Juhl E, Poulsen H. Lipogranulomas in human liver biopsies with fatty change. Acta Pathol Microbiol Scand (A), 1971; 79:150–158
5. Dincsoy HP, Weesner RE, MacGee J. Lipogranulomas in non-fatty human liver. A mineral oil-induced environmental disease. Am J Clin Pathol, 1982; 78:35–41
6. Wanless IR, Geddie WR. Mineral oil lipogranulomata in liver and spleen. Arch Pathol Lab Med, 1985; 109:283–286
7. Delladetsima JK, Hom T, Poulsen H. Portal tract lipogranulomas in liver biopsies. Liver, 1987; 7:9–17
8. Keen ME, Engstrand DA, Hafez GR. Hepatic lipogranulomatosis simulating veno-occlusive disease of the liver. Arch Pathol Lab Med, 1985; 109:70–72
9. Rollins CE, Reiber G, Guinee DG, Lie JT. Disseminated lipogranulomas and sudden death from self administered mineral oil injection. Am J Forens Med Pathol, 1997; 18:199–103
10. Bernstein M, Edmondson HA, Barbour BH. The liver lesion in Q-fever. Arch Int Med, 1965; 116:491–498
11. Hofmann CE, Heaton JW. Q fever hepatitis: clinical manifestations and pathological findings. Gastroenterology, 1982; 83:474–479
12. Marazulea M, Moreno A, Yebra M, Cerezo E, Gomez-Gesto C, Vargas JA. Hepatic fibrin-ring granulomas: a clinicopathologic study of 23 patients. Hum Pathol, 1991; 22:607–613
13. Beorchia S, Rouhier D, Woehrle R et al. Anomalies hépatiques au cours de la fièvre boutonneuse méditerranéenne. Ann Gastroenterol Hepatol, 1986; 22:87–90
14. Vanderstigel M, Zafrani ES, Lejonc JL, Schaeffer A, Portos JL. Allopurinol hypersensitivity syndrome as a cause of hepatic fibrinring granulomas. Gastroenterology, 1985; 90:188–190
15. Lobdell DH. 'Ring' granulomas in cytomegalovirus hepatitis. Arch Pathol Lab Med, 1987; 111:881–882
16. Moreno A, Marazuela M, Yebra M et al. Hepatic fibrin-ring granulomas in visceral leishmaniasis. Gastroenterology, 1988; 95:1123–1126
17. Ponz E, Garcia-Pagan JC, Bruguera M, Bruix J, Rodes J. Hepatic fibrin-ring granulomas in a patient with hepatitis A. Gastroenterology, 1991; 100:268–270
18. Font J, Bruguera M, Perez-Villa F, Ingelmo M. Hepatic fibrin-ring granulomas caused by *Staphylococcus epidermidis* generalized infection. Gastroenterology, 1987; 93:1449–1451
19. Nenert M, Mavier P, Dubuc N, Deforges J, Zafrani ES. Epstein-Barr virus infection and hepatic fibrin-ring granulomas. Hum Pathol, 1988; 19:608–610
20. Murphy E, Griffiths MR, Hunter JA, Burt AD. Fibrin-ring granulomas: a non-specific reaction to liver injury. Histopathology, 1991; 19:91–93
21. Lefkowitch JH. Hepatic granulomas. J Hepatol, 1999; 30:40–45
22. James DG, Scheuer PJ. Hepatic granulomas. In: Bircher J, Benhamou J-P, McIntyre N, eds. Oxford textbook of clinical hepatology, 2nd edn. Oxford: OUP, 1999: pp 1099–1108
23. Valla DC, Benhamou JP. Hepatic granulomas and hepatic sarcoidosis. Clin Liver Dis. 2000; 4:269–285
24. Thomson AW, O'Connell PJ, Steptoe RJ, Lu L. Immunobiology of liver dendritic cells. Immunol Cell Biol, 2002; 80:65–73
25. Yoneyama H, Ichida T. Recruitment of dendritic cells to pathological niches in inflamed liver. Med Mol Morphol, 2005 Sep; 38:136–141
26. Kaplan MH, Whitfield JR, Boros DL, Grusby MJ. Th2 cells are required for the *Schistosoma mansoni* egg-induced granulomatous response. J Immunol, 1998; 160:1850–1856
27. Yamane H, Tachibana I, Takeda Y et al. Propionibacterium acnes-induced hepatic granuloma formation is impaired in mice lacking tetraspanin CD9. J Pathol. 2005 Aug; 206(4):486–492
28. Morimoto J, Inobe M, Kimura C et al. Osteopontin affects the persistence of beta-glucan-induced hepatic granuloma formation and tissue injury through two distinct mechanisms. Int Immunol, 2004 Mar; 16(3):477–488
29. Klatskin G. Hepatic granulomata: problems in interpretation. Mount Sinai J Med, 1977; 44:798–812
30. Ishak KG. Granulomas of the liver. In: Ioachim HL, ed. Pathology of granulomas. New York: Raven Press, 1983: pp 307–369
31. Murano I, Yoshii H, Kurashige H, Sugio Y, Tsukahara M. Giant hepatic granuloma caused by Bartonella henselae. Pediatr Infect Dis J. 2001; 20:319–320
32. Chavanet P, Dillon D, Lancot JP et al. Granulomatous hepatitis associated with Lyme disease. Lancet, 1987; ii:623–624
33. Lamps LW, Havens JM, Sjostedt A, Page DL, Scott MA. Histologic and molecular diagnosis of tularemia: a potential bioterrorism agent endemic to North America. Mod Pathol, 2004; 17:489–495
34. Stjernberg U, Jilseth C, Ritland S. Granulomatous hepatitis in *Yersinia enterocolitica* infection. Hepatogastroenterology, 1987; 34:56–57
35. Van Outryve SM, Francque SM, Gentens PA et al. Bacillus Calmette–Guerin-induced granulomatous hepatitis in a patient with a superficial bladder carcinoma. Eur J Gastroenterol Hepatol, 2004; 16:1027–1032
36. Tahan V, Ozaras R, Lacevic N et al. Prevalence of hepatic granulomas in chronic hepatitis B. Dig Dis Sci, 2004; 49:1575–1577

37. Ozaras R, Tahan V, Mert A et al. The prevalence of hepatic granulomas in chronic hepatitis C. J Clin Gastroenterol. 2004; 38:449–452

38. Eshchar J, Reif L, Warou M, Alkan WJ. Hepatic lesion in chickenpox: a case report. Gastroenterology, 1973; 64:462–466

39. Mondou EN, Gnepp DR. Hepatic granuloma resulting from *Enterobius vermicularis*. Am J Clin Pathol, 1989; 91:97–100

40. Mendeloff J. Healed granulomas of the liver due to tongue worm infection. Am J Clin Pathol, 1965; 43:433–437

41. Morimoto Y, Routes JM Granulomatous disease in common variable immunodeficiency. Curr Allergy Asthma Rep, 2005; 5:370–375

42. Nakhleh RE, Glock M, Snover DC. Hepatic pathology of chronic granulomatous disease of childhood. Arch Pathol Lab Med, 1992; 116:71–75

43. Kuntz HC, Oellig WP, Thiel H et al. Leberveränderungen bei akuten rheumatischen Fieber. Med Klin, 1981; 76:504–506

44. Citron BP, Halpern M, McCarron M et al. Necrotizing angiitis associated with drug abusers. N Engl J Med, 1970; 283:1003–1011

45. Leong ASY, Disney APS, Gove DW. Spallation and migration of silicone from blood-pumping tubing in patients on hemodialysis. N Engl J Med, 1982; 306:135–140

46. Chagnac A, Gal R, Kimche D, Zevin D, Machtey I, Levi J. Liver granulomas: a possible paraneoplastic manifestation of hypernephroma. Am J Gastroenterol, 1985; 80:989–992

47. Le Bail B, Jouhauole H, Deugnier Y et al. Liver adenomatosis with granulomas in two patients on long term oral contraceptives. Am J Surg Pathol, 1992; 16:982–987

48. Everett GD, Mitros FA. Eosinophilic gastroenteritis with hepatic eosinophilic granulomas. Am J Gastroenterol, 1980; 74:519–521

49. Cortes JM, Oliva H, Paradinas FJ et al. The pathology of the liver in porphyria cutanea tarda. Histopathology, 1980; 4:471–485

50. Ichikawa T, Takagi H, Yamada T et al. Granulomas in hepatocellular carcinoma induced by lipiodolized SMANCS, a polymer-conjugated derivative of neocarzinostatin. Histopathology. 2002; 40:579–580

51. McCluggage WG, Sloan JM. Hepatic granulomas in Northern Ireland: a thirteen year review. Histopathology, 1994; 25:219–228

52. Denk H, Scheuer PJ, Baptista A et al. Guidelines for the diagnosis and interpretation of hepatic granulomas. Histopathology, 1994; 25:209–218

53. Ferrell LD. Hepatic granulomas: a morphologic approach to diagnosis. Surg Pathol, 1990; 3:87–106

54. Alcantra-Payawal DE, Matsumura M, Shiratori Y et al. Direct detection of *Myocbacterium tuberculosis* using polymerase chain reaction assay among patients with hepatic granuloma. J Hepatol, 1997; 27:620–627

55. Kaplan KJ, Goodman ZD, Ishak KG. Eosinophilic granuloma of the liver: a characteristic lesion with relationship to visceral larva migrans. Am J Surg Pathol, 2001; 25:1316–1321

56. Simon HB, Wolff SM. Granulomatous hepatitis and prolonged fever of unknown origin: a study of 13 patients. Medicine, 1973; 52:1–21

57. Sartin JS, Walker RC. Granulomatous hepatitis: a retrospective review of 88 cases at the Mayo Clinic. Mayo Clin Proc, 1991; 66:914–918

58. Cunningham D, Mills PR, Quigley EMM et al. Hepatic granulomas: experience over a 10-year period in the West of Scotland. Q J Med, 1982; 202:162–170

59. Gaya DR, Thorburn D, Oien KA, Morris AJ, Stanley AJ. Hepatic granulomas: a 10 year single centre experience. J Clin Pathol, 2003 Nov; 56(11):850–853

60. Knox TA, Kaplan MM, Geffand JA, Wolff SM. Methotrexate treatment of idiopathic granulomatous hepatitis. Ann Intern Med, 1995; 122:592–595

61. Zoutman DE, Ralph ED, Frei JV. Granulomatous hepatitis and fever of unknown origin. An 11-year experience of 23 cases with three year's follow up. J Clin Gastroenterol, 1991; 13:69–75

62. Collins MH, Jiang B, Goffie JM, Chong SK, Lee CH. Hepatic granulomas in children. A clinicopathologic analysis of 23 cases including polymerase chain rection for histoplasma. Am J Surg Pathol, 1996; 20:332–338

63. Mahida Y, Palmer KR, Lovell D, Silk DBA. Familial granulomatous hepatitis: a hitherto unrecognized entity. Am J Gastroenterol, 1988; 83:42–45

64. Melia WM, Calvey H, Portmann B, Williams R. Hepatocellular carcinoma complicating chronic granulomatous hepatitis. J Clin Pathol, 1983; 36:1062–1066

65. Wong VS, Adab N, Young GR, Sturgess R. Hepatic sarcoidosis complicated by hepatocellular carcinoma. Eur J Gastroenterol Hepatol, 1999; 11:353–355

66. Zumla A, James DG. Granulomatous infections: etiology and classification. Clin Infect Dis, 1996; 23:146–158

67. Fauroux B, Clement A. Paediatric sarcoidosis. Paediatr Respir Rev, 2005; 6:128–133

68. Maddrey WC, Johns CJ, Boittnott JK, Iber FL. Sarcoidosis and chronic hepatic disease: a clinical and pathologic study of 20 patients. Medicine, 1970; 40:375–395

69. Devaney K, Goodman ZD, Epstein MS, Zimmerman HJ, Ishak KG. Hepatic sarcoidosis: clinicopathological features in 100 patients. Am J Surg Pathol, 1993; 17:1272–1280

70. Hercules H de C, Bethlem NM. Value of liver biopsy in sarcoidosis. Arch Pathol Lab Med, 1984; 108:831–834

71. Layden TJ, Kulik L. Hepatic manifestations of pulmonary diseases. Clin Liver Dis, 2002; 6:969–979, ix

72. Ishak KG. Sarcoidosis of the liver and bile ducts. Mayo Clin Proc, 1998; 73:467–472

73. Lehmuskallio E, Hannuksela M, Halme H. The liver in sarcoidosis. Acta Med Scand, 1977; 202:289–293

74. Israel HL, Margolis ML, Rose LJ. Hepatic granulomatosis and sarcoidosis. Further observations. Dig Dis Sci, 1984; 29:353–356

75. Moreno-Merlo F, Wanless IR, Shimamatsu K, Sherman M, Greig P, Chiasson D. The role of granulomatous phlebitis and thrombosis in the pathogenesis of cirrhosis and portal hypertension in sarcoidosis. Hepatology, 1997; 26:554–560

76. Wanless IR. Noncirrhotic portal hypertension: recent concepts. Prog Liver Dis, 1996; 14:265–278

77. Valla D, Pessegueiro-Miranda H, Degott C et al. Hepatic sarcoidosis with portal hypertension. A report of seven cases with a review of the literature. Q J Med, 1987; 63:531–554

78. Russi EW, Bansky G, Pfaltz M, Spinas G, Hammer B, Senning A. Budd–Chiari syndrome in sarcoidosis. Am J Gastroenterol, 1986; 81:71–75

79. Qureshi WA. Intrahepatic cholestatic syndromes: pathogenesis, clinical features and management. Dig Dis, 1999; 17:49–59

80. Kim WR, Ludwig J, Lindor KD. Variant forms of cholestatic diseases involving small bile ducts in adults. Am J Gastroenterol, 2000; 95:1130–1138

81. Bass NM, Burroughs AK, Scheuer PJ, James DG, Sherlock S. Chronic intrahepatic cholestasis due to sarcoidosis. Gut, 1982; 23:417–421

82. Rudzki C, Ishak KG, Zimmerman HJ. Chronic intrahepatic cholestasis of sarcoidosis. Am J Med, 1975; 59:373–387

83. Murphy JR, Sjogren MH, Kikendall JW, Peura DA, Goodman Z. Small bile duct abnormalities in sarcoidosis. J Clin Gastroenterol, 1990; 12:555–561

84. Stanley NN, Fox RA, Whimster WF, Sherlock S, James DG. Primary biliary cirrhosis or sarcoidosis—or both? N Engl J Med, 1972; 287:1282–1284

85. Maddrey WC. Sarcoidosis and primary biliary cirrhosis. Associated disorders? N Engl J Med, 1983; 308:588–590

86. Stanca CM, Fiel MI, Allina J, Caracta CF, Odin JA. Liver failure in an antimitochondrial antibody-positive patient with sarcoidosis: primary biliary cirrhosis or hepatic sarcoidosis? Semin Liver Dis, 2005; 25:364–370

87. Reteigm MA, Fashir BM. Biliary tract obstruction due to sarcoidosis: a case report. Am J Gastroenterol, 1997; 92:527–528

88. Vatti R, Sharma OP. Course of asymptomatic liver involvement in sarcoidosis: role of therapy in selected cases. Sarcoidosis Vasc Diffuse Lung Dis, 1997; 14:73–76

89. Hunt J, Gordon FD, Jenkins RL, Lewis WD, Khettry U. Sarcoidosis with selective involvement of a second liver allograft: report of a case and review of the literature. Mod Pathol, 1999; 12:325–328

90. Lipson EJ, Fiel MI, Florman SS, Korenblat KM. Patient and graft outcomes following liver transplantation for sarcoidosis Clin Transplant. 2005; 19:487–491

91. Burt AD, MacSween RNM, Peters TJ, Simpson KJ: Non-alcoholic fatty liver: causes and complications In: McIntyre N, Bemhamou J-P, Bircher J, Rizzetto M, Rodes J, eds. Oxford: OUP, Oxford textbook of clinical hepatology, 1991:pp 863–872

92. Findor J, Perez V, Bruch Igartua E, Giovanetti M, Fioravantti N. Structure and ultrastructure of the liver in aged persons. Acta Hepatogastroenterol, 1973; 20:200–204

93. Cairns SR, Peters TJ. Biochemical analysis of hepatic lipid in alcoholic and diabetic and control subjects. Clin Sci, 1983; 65:645–652

94. Hall P, Gormley BM, Jarvis LR et al. A staining method for the detection and measurement of fat droplets in hepatic tissue. Pathology, 1980; 12:605–608

95. Burt AD, Mutton A, Day CP. Diagnosis and interpretation of steatosis and steatohepatitis. Semin Diagn Pathol, 1998; 15:246–258

96. Day CP, James OFW. Hepatic steatosis—innocent bystander or guilty party? Hepatology, 1998; 27:1463–1466

97. Ludwig J, Viggiano TR, McGill DB et al. Non-alcoholic steatohepatitis—Mayo Clinic experiences with a hitherto unnamed disease. Mayo Clin Proc, 1980; 55:434–438

98. Teli MR, Day CP, Burt AD et al. Determinants of progression to cirrhosis or fibrosis in pure alcoholic fatty liver. Lancet, 1995; 346:987–990

99. Sabesin SM, Frase S, Ragland JB. Accumulation of nascent lipoproteins in rat hepatic Golgi during induction of fatty liver by orotic acid. Lab Invest, 1977; 37:127–135

100. Fraser JL, Antonioli DA, Chopra S et al. Prevalence and non-specificity of microvesicular fatty change in the liver. Mod Pathol, 1995; 8:65–70

101. Zimmermann HJ, Ishak KG. Valproate-induced hepatic injury: analyses of 23 fatal cases. Hepatology, 1982; 2:591–597

102. Fromenty B, Pessayre D. Impaired mitochondrial function in microvesicular steatosis. Effects of drugs, ethanol, hormones and cytokines. J Hepatol, 1997; 26 (suppl 2):43–54

103. Milroy CM, Clark JC, Forrest ARW. Pathology of deaths associated with 'ecstasy' and 'eve' misuse. J Clin Pathol, 1996; 49:149–153

104. Hu B, French SW. 2′,3′-dideoxyinosine induced Mallory bodies in patients with HIV. Am J Clin Pathol, 1997; 108:280–283

105. Miller KD, Cameron M, Wood LV, Dalakas MC, Kovacs JA. Lactic acidosis and hepatic steatosis associated with use of stavudine: report of four cases. Ann Intern Med, 2000; 133:192–196

106. Luongo MA, Bjornson SS. The liver in ferrous sulphate poisoning. A report of three fatal cases in children and an experimental study. N Engl J Med, 1954; 251:995–999

107. Tanaka K, Kean EA, Johnson B. Jamaican vomiting sickness. Biochemical investigation of two cases. N Engl J Med, 1976; 295:461–467

108. Weizman Z, Mussafi H, Ishay JS et al. Multiple hornet stings with features of Reye's syndrome. Gastroenterology, 1985; 89:1407–1410

109. Uchida T, Kao H, Quispe Sjogren M et al. Alcoholic foamy degeneration—a pattern of acute alcoholic injury of the liver. Gastroenterology, 1983; 84:683–692

110. Badizadegan K, Perez-Atayde AR. Focal glycogenosis of the liver in disorders of ureagenesis: its occurrence and diagnostic significance. Hepatology, 1997; 26:365–373

111. Taubman B, Hale DE, Kelley RI. Familial Reye-like syndrome: a presentation of medium-chain acyl-coenzyme A dehydrogenase deficiency. Pediatrics, 1987; 79:382–385

112. Morris AA. Mitochondrial respiratory chain disorders and the liver. Liver, 1999; 5:357–368

113. Schiff L, Schubert WK, McAdams A et al. Hepatic cholesterol ester storage disease, a familial disorder. 1. Clinical aspects. Am J Med, 1968; 44:538–546

114. Popper H, Thung SN, Gerber MA et al. Histologic studies of severe delta agent infection in Venezuelan Indians. Hepatology, 1983; 3:906–912

115. Mahler H, Pasi A, Kramer JM et al. Fulminant liver failure in association with the emetic toxin Bacillus cereus. N Engl J Med, 1997; 336:1142–1148

116. Holve S, Hu D, Shub M, Tyson RW, Sokol RJ. Liver disease in Navajo neuropathy. J Pediatr, 1999; 135:482–493

117. Krahenbuhl S, Kleinle S, Henz S et al. Microvesicular steatosis, hemosiderosis and rapid development of liver cirrhosis in a patient with Pearson's syndrome. J Hepatol, 1999; 31:550–555

118. Fromenty B, Berson A, Pessayre D. Microvesicular steatosis and steatohepatitis: role of mitochondrial dysfunction and lipid peroxidation. J Hepatol, 1997; 26(suppl 1):13–22

119. Mansouri A, Fromenty B, Berson A et al. Multiple hepatic mitochondrial deletions suggest premature oxidative ageing in alcoholic patients. J Hepatol, 1997; 27:96–102

120. Browner MK, Austin GE, Lewin KJ. Focal fatty change of the liver; a hitherto poorly recognised entity. Gastroenterology, 1980; 78:247–252

121. Grove A, Vyberg B, Vyberg M. Focal fatty change of the liver. A review and a case associated with continuous ambulatory peritoneal dialysis. Virchows Arch (A), 1991; 419:69–75

122. Sterling RK, Herbener TE, Jacobs GH et al. Multifocal hepatic lesions in AIDS: an unusual presentation of steatosis. Am J Gastroenterol, 1997; 92:1934–1936

123. Terada T, Nakanuma Y, Hoso M, Saito K, Sasaki M, Nonomura A. Fatty macroregenerative nodule in non-steatotic liver cirrhosis. A morphologic study. Virchows Arch (A), 1989; 415:131–136

124. Mortele KJ, Stubbe J, Praet M, Van Langenhove P, De Bock G, Kunnen M. Intratumoral steatosis in focal nodular hyperplasia coinciding with diffuse hepatic steatosis: CT and MRI findings with histologic correlation. Abdom Imaging, 2000; 25:179–181

125. Siriboonkoom W, Gramlich L. Nutrition and chronic liver disease. Can J Gastroenterol, 1998; 12:201–207

126. Riordan SM, Williams R. Nutrition and liver transplantation. J Hepatol, 1999; 31:955–962

127. Quigley EM, Zetterman RK. Hepatobiliary complications of malabsorption and malnutrition. Semin Liver Dis, 1988; 8:218–228

128. Webber BL, Freiman I. The liver in kwashiorkor. A clinical and electron microscopic study. Arch Pathol, 1974; 98:400–408

129. Praharaj KC, Choudhury U. The liver in kwashiorkor. A clinicohistopathological study. J Ind Med Assoc, 1977; 69:77–80

130. McLean AEN. Hepatic failure in malnutrition. Lancet, 1962; ii:1292–1294

131. Himsworth HP. Lectures on the liver and its diseases, 2nd edn. Oxford: Blackwell, 1950:p 91

132. McLaren DS, Faris R, Zekian B. The liver during recovery from protein-calorie malnutrition. J Trop Med Hyg, 1968; 71:271–281

133. Reid GM. Kwashiorkor. Med Hypotheses, 1984; 14:401–406

134. Truswell AS, Hansen JDL, Watson CE, Wannenburg P. Relation of serum lipids and lipoproteins to fatty liver in kwashiorkor. Am J Clin Nutr, 1969; 22:568–576

135. Sidransky H. Nutritional disturbances of protein metabolism in the liver. Am J Pathol, 1976; 84:649–668

136. Doherty JF, Golden MHN, Brooks SEH. Peroxisomes and the fatty liver of malnutrition: an hypothesis. Am J Clin Nutr, 1991; 54:674–677

137. Simon DM, Krause R, Galambos JT. Peliosis hepatis in a patient with marasmus. Gastroenterology, 1988; 95:805–809

138. Peden VH, Witzleben CL, Skelton MA. Total parenteral nutrition. J Pediat, 1971; 78:180–181

139. Faust TW, Reddy KR. Postoperative jaundice. Clin Liver Dis, 2004; 8:151–166

140. Klein S, Nealon WH. Hepatobiliary abnormalities associated with total parenteral nutrition. Semin Liver Dis, 1988; 8:237–246

141. Kaufman SS, Gondolesi GE, Fishbein TM. Parenteral nutrition associated liver disease. Semin Neonatol, 2003; 8:375–381

142. Chung C, Buchman AL. Postoperative jaundice and total parenteral nutrition-associated hepatic dysfunction. Clin Liver Dis, 2002; 6:1067–1084

143. Body JJ, Bleiberg H, Bron D et al. Total parenteral nutrition-induced cholestasis mimicking large bile duct obstruction. Histopathology, 1982; 6:787–792

144. Benjamin D. Hepatobiliary dysfunction in infants and children associated with long-term total parenteral nutrition. A clinicopathologic study. Am J Clin Pathol, 1981; 76:276–283

145. Dahms BB, Halpin TC Jr. Serial liver biopsies in parenteral nutrition-associated cholestasis of early infancy. Gastroenterology, 1981; 81:136–144

146. Misra S, Ament ME, Vargas JH, Skoff C, Reyen L, Herzog F. Chronic liver disease in children on long-term parenteral nutrition. J Gastroenterol Hepatol, 1996; 11:S4–S6

147. Zambrano E, El-Hennawy M, Ehrenkranz RA, Zelterman D, Reyes-Mugica Total parenteral nutrition induced liver pathology: an autopsy series of 24 newborn cases. Pediatr Dev Pathol, 2004; 7:425–432.

148. Moss RL, Amii LA. New approaches to understanding the etiology and treatment of total parenteral nutrition-associated cholestasis. Semin Pediatr Surg, 1999; 8:140–147

149. Grant JP, Cox CE, Kleinman LM et al. Serum hepatic enzyme and bilirubin elevations during parenteral nutrition. Surg Gynecol Obstet, 1977; 145:573–580

150. Buchman AL, Iyer K, Fryer J. Parenteral nutrition-associated liver disease and the role for isolated intestine and intestine/liver transplantation. Hepatology, 2005; 43:9–19

151. Stanko KT, Nathan G, Mendelow H, Adibi SA. Development of hepatic cholestasis and fibrosis in patients with massive loss of intestine supported by prolonged parenteral nutrition. Gastroenterology, 1987; 92:197–202

152. Wolfe BM, Walker BK, Shaul DB, Wong L, Ruebner BH. Effect of total parenteral nutrition on hepatic histology. Arch Surg, 1988; 123:1084–1090

153. Forrest EH, Oien KA, Dickson S, Galloway D, Mills PR. Improvement in cholestasis associated with total parenteral nutrition after treatment with an antibody against tumour necrosis factor alpha. Liver, 2002; 22:317–320

154. Blaszyk H, Wild PJ, Oliveira A, Kelly DG, Burgart LJ. Hepatic copper in patients receiving long-term total parenteral nutrition. J Clin Gastroenterol, 2005; 39:318–320

155. Palombo JD, Schnure F, Bistrian BR et al. Improvement of liver function tests by administration of L-carnitine to a carnitine-deficient patient receiving home parenteral nutrition: A case report. JPEN, 1987; 11:88–92

156. Buchman AL, Ament ME, Sohel M et al. Choline deficiency causes reversible hepatic abnormalities in patients receiving parenteral nutrition: proof of a human choline requirement:

a placebo-controlled trial. JPEN J Parenter Enteral Nutr. 2001; 25:260–268

157. Bowyer BA, Fleming CR, Ludwig J, Petz J, McGill DB. Does long-term home parenteral nutrition in adult patients cause chronic liver disease? JPEN, 1985; 9:11–17

158. Thomas CH. Ulceration of the colon with a much enlarged fatty liver. Trans Path Soc Phil, 1873; 4:87–88

159. Perrett AD, Higgins G, Johnston HH, Massarella GR, Truelove SC, Wright R. The liver in Crohn's disease. Q J Med, 1971; 40:187–209

160. Schrumpf E, Fausa O, Elgjo K, Kolmannskog F. Hepato-biliary complications of inflammatory bowel disease. Semin Liver Dis, 1988; 8:201–209

161. Raj V, Lichtenstein DR. Hepatobiliary manifestations of inflammatory bowel disease. Gastroenterol Clin North Am, 1999; 28:491–513

162. Balistreri WF. Hepatobiliary complications of inflammatory bowel disease: overview of the issues. Inflamm Bowel Dis, 1998; 4:220–224

163. Smyth C, Kelleher D, Keeling PW. Hepatic manifestations of gastrointestinal diseases. Inflammatory bowel disease, celiac disease, and Whipple's disease. Clin Liver Dis, 2002; 6:1013–1032

164. Mistilis SP. Pericholangitis and ulcerative colitis. I. Pathology, etiology and pathogenesis. Ann Intern Med, 1965; 63:1–16

165. Mistilis SP, Skyring AP, Goulston SJM. Pericholangitis and ulcerative colitis. II. Clinical aspects. Ann Intern Med, 1965; 63:17–26

166. Dordal E, Glasgov S, Kirsner JB. Hepatic lesions in chronic inflammatory bowel disease. I. Clinical correlations with liver biopsy diagnoses in 103 patients. Gastroenterology, 1967; 52:239–253

167. Eade MN. Liver disease in ulcerative colitis. I. Analysis of operative liver biopsy in 138 consecutive patients having colectomy. Ann Intern Med, 1970; 72:475–487

168. Wee A, Ludwig J. Pericholangitis in chronic ulcerative colitis: Primary sclerosing cholangitis of the small bile ducts? Ann Intern Med, 1985; 102:581–587

169. Desmet VJ, Geboes K. Liver lesions in inflammatory bowel disorders. J Pathol, 1987; 151:247–255

170. Das KM. Relationship of extraintestinal involvement in inflammatory bowel disease: new insights into autoimmune pathogenesis. Dig Dis Sci, 1999; 44:1–13

171. Terjung B, Spengler U, Sauerbruch T, Worman HJ. 'Atypical p-ANCA' in IBD and hepatobiliary disorders react with a 50-kilodalton nuclear envelope protein of neutrophils and myeloid cell lines. Gastroenterology, 2000; 119:310–322

172. Dew MJ, Thompson H, Allan RN. The spectrum of hepatic dysfunction in inflammatory bowel disease. Q J Med, 1979; 48:113–135

173. Schrumpf E, Gjone E. Hepatobiliary disease in ulcerative colitis. Scand J Gastroenterol, 1982; 17:961–964

174. Wewer V, Gluud C, Schlichting P, Burcharth F, Binder V. Prevalence of hepatobiliary dysfunction in a regional group of patients with chronic inflammatory bowel disease. Scand J Gastroenterol, 1991; 26:97–102

175. Broome U, Glaumann H, Hultcrantz R. Liver histology and follow-up of 68 patients with ulcerative colitis and normal liver function tests. Gut, 1990; 31:468–472

176. Vadstrup S. Subnormal alanine aminotransferase values in blood of patients with Crohn disease. Scand J Gastroenterol, 2004; 39:554–556

177. Rabinovitz M, Demetris AJ, Bou-Abboud CF, Van Thiel DH. Simultaneous occurrence of primary sclerosing cholangitis and autoimmune chronic active hepatitis in a patient with ulcerative colitis. Dig Dis Sci, 1992; 37:1606–1611

178. Konlentaki M, Koutroubakis IE, Petinaki E et al. Ulcerative colitis associated with primary biliary cirrhosis. Dig Dis Sci, 1999; 44:1953–1956

179. Edwards PC, Truelove SC. The course and prognosis of ulcerative colitis. Gut, 1963; 4:299–315

180. Kem F. Hepatobiliary disorders in inflammatory bowel disease. In: Schiff L, Schiff ER, eds. Diseases of the liver, 4th edn. Philadelphia: Lippincott, 1987: pp 1450–1460

181. Wiesner RH, LaRusso NF, Dozois RR, Beaver SJ. Peristomal varices after proctocolectomy in patients with primary sclerosing cholangitis. Gastroenterology, 1986; 90:316–322

182. Gow PJ, Chapman RW. Liver transplantation for primary sclerosing cholangitis. Liver, 2000; 20:97–103

183. Ritchie JK, Allan RN, MacCartney J et al. Biliary tract carcinoma associated with ulcerative colitis. Q J Med, 1974; 43:263–279

184. Mir-Jadjlessi SH, Farmer RG, Sivak MV. Bile duct carcinoma in patients with ulcerative colitis. Dig Dis Sci, 1987; 32:145–154

185. Berman MD, Falchuk KR, Trey C. Carcinoma of the biliary tree complicating Crohn's disease. Dig Dis Sci, 1980; 25:795–797

186. Ross AP, Braasch JW. Ulcerative colitis and carcinoma of the proximal bile ducts. Gut, 1973; 14:94–97

187. Rosen CB, Nagorney DM. Cholangiocarcinoma complicating primary sclerosing cholangitis. Semin Liver Dis, 1991; 11:26–30

188. Bergquist A, Glaumann H, Persson B, Broome U. Risk factors and clinical presentation of hepatobiliary carcinoma in patients with primary sclerosing cholangitis: a case control study. Hepatology, 1998; 27:311–316

189. Wee A, Ludwig J, Coffey RJ, LaRusso NF, Wiesner RH. Hepatobiliary carcinoma associated with primary sclerosing cholangitis and chronic ulcerative colitis. Hum Pathol, 1985; 16:719–726

190. Broome U, Loftberg R, Veress B, Eriksson LS. Primary sclerosing cholangitis and ulcerative colitis: evidence for increased neoplastic potential. Hepatology, 1995; 22:1404–1408

191. Stieber AC, Marino IR, Iwatsuki S, Starzl TE. Cholangiocarcinoma in sclerosing cholangitis: the role of liver transplantation. Int Surg, 1989; 74:1–3

192. Baker A, Kaplan M, Norton RA, Patterson JF. Gallstones in inflammatory bowel disease. Am J Dig Dis Sci, 1974; 19:109–112

193. Lapidus A, Einasson K. Effects of ileal resection on biliary lipids and bile acid composition in patients with Crohn's disease. Gut, 1991; 32:1488–1491

194. McClure J, Banerjee SS, Schofield PS. Crohn's disease of the gallbladder. J Clin Pathol, 1984; 37:516–518

195. Gitkind MJ, Wright SC. Amyloidosis complicating inflammatory bowel disease: a case report and review of the literature. Dig Dis Sci, 1990; 35:906–908

196. Mandelstam P, Simmons DE, Mitchell B. Regression of amyloid in Crohn's disease after bowel resection: a 19 year follow-up. J Clin Gastroenterol, 1989; 11:324–326

197. Fitchen JH. Amyloidosis and granulomatous ileocolitis: Regression after surgical removal of the involved bowel. N Engl J Med, 1975; 292:352–353

198. Mir-Madjlessi SH, McHenry MC, Farmer RG. Liver abscess in Crohn's disease: report of four cases and review of the literature. Gastroenterology, 1986; 91:987–993

199. Margalit M, Elinav H, Ilan Y, Shalit M. Liver abscess in inflammatory bowel disease: report of two cases and review of the literature. J Gastroenterol Hepatol, 2004; 19:1338–1342

200. Inoue T, Hirata I, Egashira Y et al. Refractory ulcerative colitis accompanied with cytomegalovirus colitis and multiple liver abscesses: a case report. World J Gastroenterol, 2005; 11:5241–5244

201. Song J, Swekla M, Colorado P, Reddy R, Hoffmann S, Fine S. Liver abscess and diarrhea as initial manifestations of ulcerative colitis: case report and review of the literature. Dig Dis Sci, 2003; 48:417–421

202. Andre M, Aumaitre O, Papo T et al. Disseminated aseptic abscesses associated with Crohn's disease: a new entity? Dig Dis Sci, 1998; 43:420–428

203. Papachristou GI, Wu T, Marsh W, Plevy SE. Inflammatory pseudotumour of the liver associated with Crohn's disease. J Clin Gastroenterol, 2004; 38:818–822

204. Kraut J, Berman JH, Gunasekaran TS et al. Hepatic vein thrombosis (Budd–Chiari syndrome) in an adolescent with ulcerative colitis. J Pediatr Gastroenterol Nutr, 1997; 25:417–420

205. Junge U, Wienke J, Schuler A. Acute Budd–Chiari syndrome, portal and splenic vein thrombosis in a patient with ulcerative colitis associated with antiphospholipid antibodies and protein C deficiency. Z Gastroenterol, 2001; 39:845–852

206. Praderio L, Dagna L, Longhi P, Rubin G, Sabbadini MG. Budd–Chiari syndrome in a patient with ulcerative colitis: association with anticardiolipin antibodies. J Clin Gastroenterol, 2000; 30:203–204

207. Bashir RM, Lewis JH. Hepatotoxicity of drugs used in the treatment of gastrointestinal disorders. Gastroenterol Clin North Am, 1995; 24:937–967

208. Caprilli R, Latella G, Vernia P, Frieri G. Multiple organ dysfunction in ulcerative colitis. Am J Gastroenterol, 2000; 95:1258–1262

209. Suzuki S, Nakamura S, Ishida H et al. Hepatic angiomyolipoma developing during the follow-up of ulcerative colitis: report of a case and review of the literature. Surg Today, 1996; 26:635–639

210. Hagander B, Brandt L, Sjolund K et al. Hepatic injury in adult coeliac disease. Lancet, 1977; ii:270–272

211. Jacobsen MB, Fausa O, Elgjo K, Schrumpf E. Hepatic lesions in adult coeliac disease. Scand J Gastroenterol, 1990; 25:656–662

212. Mitchison HC, Record CO, Bateson MC, Cobden I. Hepatic abnormalities in coeliac disease: three cases of delayed diagnosis. Postgrad Med J, 1989; 65:920–922

213. Lindberg T, Berg NO, Borulf S, Jakobsson I. Liver damage in coeliac disease and other food intolerances in childhood. Lancet, 1978; i:390–391

214. Novacek G, Miehsler W, Wrba F, Ferenci P, Penner E, Vogelsang H. Prevalence and clinical importance of hypertransaminasaemia in coeliac disease. Eur J Gastroenterol Hepatol, 1999; 11:283–288

215. Pollock DJ. The liver in coeliac disease. Histopathology, 1977; 1:421–430

216. Leonardi S, Pavone P, Rotolo N, Spina M, La Rosa M. Autoimmune hepatitis associated with celiac disease in childhood: report of two cases. J Gastroenterol Hepatol, 2003; 18:1324–1327

217. Demir H, Yuce A, Caglar M et al. Cirrhosis in children with celiac disease. J Clin Gastroenterol, 2005; 39:630–633

218. Logan RFA, Ferguson A, Finlayson NDC, Weir DG. Primary biliary cirrhosis and coeliac disease. Lancet, 1978; i:230–233

219. Sorensen HT, Thulstrup AM, Blomqvist P, Norgaard B, Fonager K, Ekbom A. Risk of primary biliary liver cirrhosis in patients with coeliac disease: Danish and Swedish cohort data. Gut, 1999; 44:736–738

220. Floreani A, Betterle C, Baragiotta A et al. Prevalence of coeliac disease in primary biliary cirrhosis and of antimitochondrial antibodies in adult coeliac disease patients in Italy. Dig Liver Dis. 2002 Apr; 34(4):258–261

221. Volta U, Rodrigo L, Granito A et al. Celiac disease in autoimmune cholestatic liver disorders. Am J Gastroenterol, 2002; 97:2609–2613

222. Gogos CA, Nikolopoulou V, Zolota V, Siampi V, Vagenakis A. Autoimmune cholangitis in a patient with celiac disease: a case report and review of the literature. J Hepatol, 1999; 30:321–324

223. Hay JE, Wiesner RH, Shorter RG et al. Primary sclerosing cholangitis and celiac disease: a novel association. Gastroenterology, 1988; 94:A545

224. Venturini I, Cosenza R, Miglioli L et al. Adult celiac disease and primary sclerosing cholangitis: two case reports. Hepatogastroenterology, 1998; 45:2344–2347

225. Sedlack RE, Smyrk TC, Czaja AJ, Talwalkar JA. Celiac disease-associated autoimmune cholangitis. Am J Gastroenterol, 2002; 97:3196–3198

226. Freeman HJ. Hepatobiliary tract and pancreatic disorders in celiac disease. Can J Gastroenterol, 1997; 11:77–81

227. Riestra S, Dominguez F, Rodrigo L. Nodular regenerative hyperplasia of the liver in a patient with celiac disease. J Clin Gastroenterol, 2001; 33:323–326

228. Austin A, Campbell E, Lane P, Elias E. Nodular regenerative hyperplasia of the liver and coeliac disease: potential role of IgA anticardiolipin antibody. Gut, 2004; 53:1032–1034

229. Duggan JM, Duggan AE. Systematic review: the liver in coeliac disease. Aliment Pharmacol Ther, 2005; 21:515–518

230. Enzinger FM, Helwig EB. Whipple's disease. A review of the literature and report of fifteen cases. Virchows Arch (A), 1963; 336:238–269

231. Misra PS, Lebwohl P, Laufer H. Hepatic and appendiceal Whipple's disease with negative jejunal biopsies. Am J Gastroenterol, 1981; 75:302–306

232. Sieracki C, Fine G. Whipple's disease: observations on systemic involvement. II. Gross and histologic observations. Arch Pathol, 1959; 67:81–93

233. Cho C, Linscheer WG, Hirschkorn MA, Ashutosh K. Sarcoid-like granulomas as an early manifestation of Whipple's disease. Gastroenterology, 1984; 87:941–947

234. Saint-Marc Girardin M-F, Zafrani ES et al. Hepatic granulomas in Whipple's disease. Gastroenterology, 1984; 86:753–756

235. Petrides PE, Muller-Hocker J, Fredricks DN, Relman DA. PCR analysis of T. Whippelii DNA in a case of Whipple's disease: effect of antibiotics and correlation with histology. Petrides PE, Muller-Hocker J, Fredricks DN, Relman DA. Am J Gastroenterol, 1998; 93:1579–1582

236. Schultz M, Hartmann A, Dietmaier W et al. Massive steatosis hepatis: an unusual manifestation of Whipple's disease. Am J Gastroenterol, 2002; 97:771–772

237. Robert F, Omura E, Durant JR. Mucosal eosinophilic gastroenteritis with systemic involvement. Am J Med, 1977; 62:139–143

238. Ichikawa N, Taniguchi A, Akama et al. Sclerosing cholangitis associated with hypereosinophilic syndrome. Intern Med, 1997; 36:561–564

239. Benger JR, Thompson MH. Annular pancreas and obstructive jaundice. Am J Gastroenterol, 1997; 92:713–714

240. Braganza JM, Howat HT. Cancer of the pancreas. Clin Gastroenterol, 1972; 1:219–237

241. Frieden JH. The significance of jaundice in acute pancreatitis. Arch Surg, 1965; 90:422–426

242. Masih B, Lowenfels AB, Pendse PD, Rohman M. Jaundice from pancreatic pseudocyst. NY State J Med, 1971; 71:2312–2313

243. Ichimura T, Kondo S, Ambo Y et al. Primary sclerosing cholangitis associated with autoimmune pancreatitis. Hepatogastroenterology, 2002; 49:1221–1224

244. Kamisawa T, Funata N, Hayashi Y et al. A new clinicopathological entity of IgG4-related autoimmune disease. J Gastroenterol, 2003; 38(10):982–984

245. Sato Y, Harada K, Nakanuma Y. Hepatic inflammatory pseudotumour related to autoimmune pancreatitis. Histopathology, 2004; 45:418–419

246. Mofredj A, Cadranel JF, Dautreaux M et al. Pancreatic pseudocyst located in the liver: a case report and literature review. J Clin Gastsroenterol, 2000; 30:83–83

247. Kuo PC, Plotkin JS, Johnson LB. Acute pancreatitis and fulminant hepatic failure. J Am Coll Surg, 1998; 187:522–528

248. Takase M, Suda K, Suzuki F, Nakamura T, Futagawa S. A histopathologic study of localized portal hypertension as a consequence of chronic pancreatitis. Arch Pathol Lab Med, 1997; 121:612–614

249. Parbhoo SP, Welch J, Sherlock S. Acute pancreatitis in patients with fulminant hepatic failure. Gut, 1973; 14:428

250. Riely CA. Acute fatty liver of pregnancy. Semin Liver Dis, 1987; 7:47–54

251. Agarwal KS, Puliyel JM, Mathew A, Lahoti D, Gupta R. Acute pancreatitis with cholestatic hepatitis: an unusual manifestation of hepatitis A. Ann Trop Paediatr, 1999; 19:391–394

252. Alvares-Da-Silva MR, Francisconi CF, Waechter FL. Acute hepatitis C complicated by pancreatitis: another extrahepatic manifestation of hepatitis C virus? J Viral Hepat, 2000; 7:84–86

253. Starzl TE, Watanabe K, Porter KA, Putnam CA. Effects of insulin, glucagon and insulin/glucagon infusion on liver morphology and cell division after complete portocaval shunt in dogs. Lancet, 1976; i:821–825

254. Ferrell FJ, Keeffe EB. Diabetes and the hepatobiliary system. Clin Liver Dis, 1998; 2:119–131

255. Wahren J, Felig P, Cerasi E, Luft R. Splanchnic and peripheral glucose and amino acid metabolism in diabetes mellitus. J Clin Invest, 1972; 51:1870–1878

256. McGarry JD, Foster DW. Regulation of ketogenesis and clinical aspects of the ketotic state. Metabolism, 1972; 21:471–489

257. Gerich JE, Lorenzi M, Bier DM et al. Prevention of human diabetic keto-acidosis by somatostatin. N Engl J Med, 1975; 292:985–989

258. Lorenz G, Barenwald G. Histologic and electron-microscopic liver changes in diabetic children. Acta Hepatogastroenterol, 1979; 26:435–438

259. Ledesma S, Nubiola A, Tito L, Lopez D, Torres M. Hepatic dysfunction caused by the accumulation of hepatocellular glycogen in diabetes mellitus. J Gastroenterol Hepatol, 2000; 23:456–457

260. Van Steenbergen W, Lanckmans S. Liver disturbances in obesity and diabetes mellitus. Int J Obes Relat Metab Disord, 1995; 19:S27–36

261. Chatila R, West AB. Hepatomegaly and abnormal liver tests due to glygenosis in adults with diabetes. Medicine, 1996; 75:327–333

262. Carcione L, Lombardo F, Messina MF, Rosano M, De Luca F. Liver glycogenosis as early manifestation in type I diabetes mellitus. Diabetes Nutr Metab, 2003; 16:182–184

263. Komuta M, Harada M, Ueno T et al. Unusual accumulation of glycogen in liver parenchymal cells in a patient with anorexia nervosa. Intern Med, 1998; 37:678–682

264. Bernuau D, Guillot R, Durand AM et al. Ultrastructural aspects of the liver perisinusoidal space in diabetic patients with and without microangiopathy. Diabetes, 1982; 31:1061–1067

265. Latry P, Bioulac-Sage P, Echinard E et al. Perisinusoidal fibrosis and basement membrane-like material in the livers of diabetic patients. Hum Pathol, 1987; 18:775–780

266. Foster JH, Donohue TA, Berman MM. Familial liver cell adenomas and diabetes mellitus. N Engl J Med, 1978; 299:239–241

267. Thung SN, Gerber MA, Bodenheimer HC Jr. Nodular regenerative hyperplasia of the liver in a patient with diabetes mellitus. Cancer, 1982; 49:543–546

268. Ludwig J, Dyck J, LaRusso FN. Xanthomatous neuropathy of liver. Hum Pathol, 1982; 13:1049–1051

269. Saccente M. Klebsiella pneumoniae liver abscess, endophthalmitis, and meningitis in a man with newly recognized diabetes mellitus. Clin Infect Dis, 1999; 29:1570–1571

270. Forbes LE, Bajaj M, McGinn T, Berlin A. Perihepatic abscess formation in diabetes: a complication of silent gallstones. Am J Gastroenterol, 1996; 91:786–788

271. Alberti-Flor JJ, Jeffers L, Schiff ER. Primary sclerosing cholangitis occurring in a patient with systemic lupus erythematosus and diabetes mellitus. Am J Gastroenterol, 1984; 79:889–891

272. Bruguera M, Bertran A, Bombi JA, Rodes J. Giant mitochondria in hepatocytes. A diagnostic hint for alcoholic liver disease. Gastroenterology, 1977; 73:1383–1387

273. Ishak KG, Zimmerman HJ. Hepatotoxic effects of the anabolic/androgenic steroids. Semin Liver Dis, 1987; 7:230–236

274. Salata R, Klein I, Levey GS. Thyroid hormone homeostasis and the liver. Semin Liver Dis, 1985; 5:29–34

275. Menon KV, Kamath PS. Managing the complications of cirrhosis. Mayo Clin Proc, 2000; 75:501–509

276. Malik R, Hodgson H. The relationship between the thyroid gland and the liver. QJM, 2002; 95:559–569

277. Van Thiel DH, Udani M, Schade RR, Sanghvi A, Starzl TE. Prognostic value of thyroid hormone levels in patients evaluated for liver transplantation. Hepatology, 1985; 5:862–866

278. Inoue K, Okajima T, Tanaka E et al. A case of Graves' disease associated with autoimmune hepatitis and mixed connective tissue disease. Endocr J, 1999; 46:173–177

279. Janssen HLA, Smelt AHM, van Hoek B. Graves' hyperthyroidism in a patient with primary sclerosing cholangitis. Coincidence or combined pathogenesis? Eur J Gastroenterol Hepatol, 1998; 10:269–271

280. Cui B, Abe M, Hidata S et al. Autoimmune hepatitis associated with Graves' disease. Intern Med, 2003; 42:331–335

281. Bayraktar M, van Thiel DH. Abnormalities in measures of liver function and injury in thyroid disorders. Hepatogastroenterology, 1997; 44:1614–1618

282. Gurlek A, Cobankara V, Bayraktar M. Liver tests in hyperthyroidism: effect of antithyroid therapy. J Clin Gastroenterol, 1997; 24:180–183

283. Biscoveanu M, Hasinski S. Abnormal results of liver function tests in patients with Graves' disease. Endocr Pract, 2000; 6:367–369

284. Bader AA, August GP, Austin A. Hypertransaminasemia in two children with hyperthyroidism. J Pediatr Gastroenterol Nutr. 2001 Apr; 32(4):484–486

285. Barnes SC, Wicking JM, Johnston JD. Graves' disease presenting with cholestatic jaundice. Ann Clin Biochem, 1999; 36:677–679

286. Choudhary AM, Roberts I. Thyroid storm presenting with liver failure. J Clin Gastroenterol, 1999; 29:318–321

287. Greenberger NJ, Milligan FD, De Groot LJ, Isselbacher KJ. Jaundice and thyrotoxicosis in the absence of congestive cardiac failure. Am J Med, 1964; 36:840–846

288. Harrison RA, Bahar A, Payne MM. Postinfantile giant cell hepatitis associated with long-term elevated transaminase levels in treated Graves' disease. Am J Med, 2002; 112:326–327

289. Movitt ER, Gerstl B, Davis AE. Needle liver biopsy in thyrotoxicosis. Arch Intern Med, 1953; 91:729–739

290. Sola J, Pardo-Mindan FJ, Zozaya J, Quiroga J, Sangro B, Prieto J. Liver changes in patients with hyperthyroidism. Liver, 1991; 11:193–197

291. Klion FM, Segal R, Schaffner F. The effect of altered thyroid function on the ultrastructure of the human liver. Am J Med, 1971; 50:317–324

292. Van Steenbergen W, Fevery J, De Vos R et al. Thyroid hormone and the hepatic handling of bilirubin. I. Effects of hypothyroidism and hyperparathyroidism on the hepatic transport of bilirubin mono- and diconjugates in the Wistar rat. Hepatology, 1989; 9:314–321

293. Ariza CR, Frate AC, Sierra I. Hypothyroidism-associated cholestasis. JAMA, 1984; 252:2392

294. Liangpunsakul S, Chalasani N. Is hypothyroidism a risk factor for non-alcoholic steatohepatitis? J Clin Gastroenterol, 2003; 37:340–343

295. Baker A, Kaplan M, Wolfe H. Central congestive fibrosis of the liver in myxoedema ascites. Ann Intern Med, 1972; 77:927–929

296. Ono M, Ishizaki T. A case of nodular regenerative hyperplasia of the liver in Hashimoto's struma. Acta Hepatol Jpn, 1984; 25:682–687

297. Weldon AP, Danks DM. Congenital hypothyroidism and neonatal jaundice. Arch Dis Child, 1972; 47:469–471

298. McCann VJ, Fulton TT. Cortisol metabolism in chronic liver disease. J Clin Endocrinol Metab, 1975; 40:1038–1044

299. Soffer LJ, Iannaccone A, Gabrilove JL. Cushing's syndrome: a study of 50 patients. Am J Med, 1961; 30:129–146

300. Harry R, Auzinger G, Wendon J. The clinical importance of adrenal insufficiency in acute hepatic dysfunction. Hepatology, 2002; 36:395–402

301. Marik PE, Gayowski T, Starzl TE. Hepatic Cortisol Research and Adrenal Pathophysiology Study Group. The hepatoadrenal syndrome: a common yet unrecognized clinical condition. Crit Care Med, 2005; 33:1254–1259

302. Rockall AG, Sohaib SA, Evans D et al. Hepatic steatosis in Cushing's syndrome: a radiological assessment using computed tomography. Eur J Endocrinol, 2003; 149:543–548

303. Hill RB Jr. Fatal fat embolism from steroid-induced fatty liver. N Engl J Med, 1961; 265:318–320

304. Olsson RG, Lindgren A, Zettergren L. Liver involvement in Addison's disease. Am J Gastroenterol, 1990; 85:435–438

305. Iram S, Sidki K, Al-Marshedy A-R, Judzewitsch R. Addison's disease, hypertension, renal and hepatic microthrombosis in primary antiphospholipid syndrome. Postgrad Med J, 1991; 67:385–388

306. Cameron FJ, Sohaib SA, Scheimberg I, Dicks-Mireaux C. The significance of hepatic lesions associated with small adrenocortical tumours in childhood. Br J Radiol, 1997; 70:852–855

307. Karagiannis A, Tziomalos K, Patsiaoura K et al. Focal nodular hyperplasia of the liver in a patient with primary aldosteronism. J Gastroenterol Hepatol, 2004; 19:480–481

308. Chung CH, Wang CH, Tzen CY, Liu CP. Intrahepatic cholestasis as a paraneoplastic syndrome associated with pheochromocytoma. J Endocrinol Invest, 2005; 28:175–179

309. Kang JM, Lee WJ, Kim WB et al. Systemic inflammatory syndrome and hepatic inflammatory cell infiltration caused by an interleukin-6 producing pheochromocytoma. Endocr J. 2005; 52:193–198

310. van Thiel DH, Gabeler JS, Schade RR. Liver disease and the hypothalamic pituitary axis. Semin Liver Dis, 1985; 5:35–45

311. Baruch Y. The liver: a large endocrine gland. J Hepatol, 2000; 32:505–507

312. Preisig R, Morris TQ, Shaver JC, Christy NP. Volumetric haemodynamic and excretory characteristics of the liver in acromegaly. J Clin Invest, 1966; 45:1379–1387

313. Arrigo T, Wasniewska M, Ghizzoni L, Messina MF, Crisafulli G, De Luca F. Liver dysfunction associated with congenital hypopituitarism. J Endocrinol Invest, 2000; 23:215–216

314. Adams LA, Feldstein A, Lindor KD, Angulo P. Nonalcoholic fatty liver disease among patients with hypothalamic and pituitary dysfunction. Hepatology, 2004; 39:909–914

315. Nakajima K, Hashimoto E, Kaneda H et al. Pediatric nonalcoholic steatohepatitis associated with hypopituitarism. J Gastroenterol, 2005; 40:312–315

316. Reiterer EE, Zenz W, Deutsch J, Preisegger KH, Simbrunner J, Borkenstein MH. [Congenital hypopituitarism and giant cell hepatitis in a three month old girl] Klin Padiatr. 2002; 214:136–139

317. Orloff MJ. Hyperparathyroidism, cirrhosis and portacaval shunt. A new clinical syndrome. An J Surg, 1988; 155:76–81

318. Loeb JM, Hauger PH, Carney JD, Cooper AD. Refractory ascites due to POEMS syndrome. Gastroenterology, 1989; 96:247–249

319. Wardi J, Knobel B, Shahmurov M, Melamud E, Avni Y, Shirin H. Chronic cholestasis associated with Turner's syndrome: 12 years of clinical and histopathological follow-up. Digestion, 2003; 67:96–99

320. Ostberg JE, Thomas EL, Hamilton G, Attar MJ, Bell JD, Conway GS. Excess visceral and hepatic adipose tissue in Turner syndrome determined by magnetic resonance imaging: estrogen deficiency associated with hepatic adipose content. J Clin Endocrinol Metab, 2005; 90:2631–2635.

321. Roulot D, Degott C, Chazouilleres O et al. Vascular involvement of the liver in Turner's syndrome. Hepatology, 2004; 39:239–247

322. Obrzut B, Kuczynski W, Grygoruk C, Putowski L, Kluz S, Skret A. Liver dysfunction in severe ovarian hyperstimulation syndrome. Gynecol Endocrinol, 2005; 21:45–49

323. Guntupalli SR, Steingrub J. Hepatic disease and pregnancy: an overview of diagnosis and management. Crit Care Med, 2005; 33(10 Suppl):S332–339

324. Benjaminov FS, Heathcote J. Liver disease in pregnancy. Am J Gastroenterol. 2004; 99:2479–2488

325. Aggarwal N, Sawnhey H, Suril V, Vasishta K, Jha M, Dhiman RK. Pregnancy and cirrhosis of the liver. Aus NZJ Obstet Gynaecol, 1999; 39:503–506

326. Casele HL, Laifer SA. Pregnancy after liver transplantation. Semin Perinatol, 1998; 22:149–155

327. Colle I, Hautekete M. Remission of autoimmune hepatitis during pregnancy: a report of two cases. Liver, 1999; 19:55–57

328. Varma R. Course and prognosis of pregnancy in women with liver disease. Semin Liver Dis, 1987; 7:59–66

329. Seymour CA, Chadwick VS. Liver and gastrointestinal function in pregnancy. Postgrad Med J, 1979; 55:343–352

330. Robson SC, Mutch E, Boys RJ, Woodhouse KW. Apparent liver blood flow during pregnancy: a serial study using

indocyanine green clearance. Br J Obstet Gynaecol, 1990; 97:720–724

331. Krejs GJ. Jaundice during pregnancy. Semin Liver Dis, 1983; 3:73–82

332. Gonzalez-Angulo A, Aznar-Ramos R, Marquez-Monter H, Bierzwinsky GS, Martinez-Manautou J. The ultrastructure of liver cells in women under steroid therapy. I. Normal pregnancy and trophoblastic growth. Acta Endocrinol, 1970; 65:193–206

333. Perez V, Gorodisch S, Casavilla F, Maruffo C. Ultrastructure of the human liver at the end of normal pregnancy. Am J Obstet Gynaecol, 1971; 110:428–431

334. Knox TA, Olans LB. Liver disease in pregnancy. N Engl J Med, 1996; 22:569–576

335. Riely CA, Bacq Y. Intrahepatic cholestasis of pregnancy. Clin Liver Dis, 2004; 8:167–176

336. Dixon PH, Weerasekera N, Linton KJ et al. Heterozygous MDR3 missense mutation associated with intrahepatic cholestasis of pregnancy: evidence for a defect in protein trafficking. Hum Mol Genet, 2000; 9:1209–1217

337. Lucena JF, Herrero JI, Quiroga J et al. A multidrug resistance 3 gene mutation causing cholelithiasis, cholestasis of pregnancy, and adulthood biliary cirrhosis. Gastroenterology, 2003; 124:1037–1042

338. Sheehan HL. The pathology of hyperemesis and vomiting of late pregnancy. J Obstet Gynaecol, 1940; 46:658–699

339. Burroughs AK, Seong NH, Dojcinov DM et al. Idiopathic acute fatty liver of pregnancy in twelve patients. Q J Med, 1982; 204:481–497

340. Pockros PJ, Peters RL, Reynolds TB. Idiopathic fatty liver of pregnancy: findings in ten cases. Medicine, 1984; 63:1–11

341. Rolfes DB, Ishak KG. Acute fatty liver of pregnancy: a clinicopathologic study of 35 cases. Hepatology, 1985; 5:1149–1158

342. Mabie WC. Acute fatty liver of pregnancy. Gastroenterol Clin North Am, 1992; 21:951–960

343. Castro MA, Fasset MJ, Reynolds RB, Shaw KJ, Goodwin TM. Reversible peripartum liver failure: a new perspective on the diagnosis, treatment, and cause of acute fatty liver of pregnancy, based on 28 consecutive cases. Am J Obstet Gynecol, 1999; 181:389–396

344. Monga M, Katz AR. Acute fatty liver in the second trimester. Obstet Gynecol, 1999; 93:811–813

345. Rolfes DB, Ishak KG. Liver disease in pregnancy. Histopathology, 1986; 10:555–570

346. Sheehan HL. Jaundice in pregnancy. Am J Obstet Gynecol, 1961; 81:427–440

347. Pereira SP, O'Donohue J, Wendon J, Williams R. Maternal and perinatal outcome in severe pregnancy-related liver disease. Hepatology, 1997; 26:1258–1262

348. Ockner SA, Brunt EM, Cohn SM et al. Fulminant hepatic failure caused by acute fatty liver of pregnancy treated by orthotopic liver transplantation. Hepatology, 1990; 11:59–64

349. Jenkins WF, Darling MR. Idiopathic acute fatty liver of pregnancy: subsequent uncomplicated pregnancy. J Obstet Gynaecol, 1980; 1:100–101

350. Barton JR, Sibai BM, Mabie WC et al. Recurrent acute fatty liver of pregnancy. Am J Obstet Gynecol, 1990; 163:534–538

351. Vanjak D, Moreau R, Roche-Sicot J, Soulier A, Sicot C. Intrahepatic cholestasis of pregnancy and acute fatty liver of pregnancy: an unusual but favourable association. Gastroenterology, 1991; 100:1123–1125

352. Joske RA, McCully DJ, Mastaglia FL. Acute fatty liver of pregnancy. Gut, 1968; 9:489–493

353. Weber FL, Snodgrass PJ, Powell DE et al. Abnormalities of hepatic mitochondrial urea-cycle enzyme activities and hepatic ultrastructure in acute fatty liver of pregnancy. J Lab Clin Med, 1979; 94:27–41

354. Slater DN, Hague WM. Renal morphological changes in idiopathic acute fatty liver of pregnancy. Histopathology, 1984; 8:567–581

355. Liebman HA, McGhee WG, Patch MJ, Feinstein DI. Severe depression of antithrombin III associated with disseminated intravascular coagulation in women with fatty liver of pregnancy. Ann Intern Med, 1983; 98:330–333

356. Baldwin GS. Do NSAIDs contribute to acute fatty liver of pregnancy? Med Hypotheses, 2000; 54:846–849

357. Innes AM, Seargeant LE, Balachandra K et al. Hepatic carnitine palmitoyltransferase I deficiency presenting as maternal illness in pregnancy. Pediatr Res, 2000; 47:43–45

358. Minakami H, Oka N, Sato T et al. Pre-eclampsia: a microvesicular fat disease of the liver? Am J Obstet Gynecol, 1988; 159:1043–1047

359. Killam AP, Dillard SH, Patton RC, Pedersen PR. Pregnancy-induced hypertension complicated by acute liver disease and disseminated

intravascular coagulation. Am J Obstet Gynecol, 1975; 123:823–828

360. Long RG, Scheuer PJ, Sherlock S. Pre-eclampsia presenting with deep jaundice. J Clin Pathol, 1977; 30:212–215

361. Barron WM. The syndrome of pre-eclampsia. Gastroenterol Clin North Am, 1992; 21:851–872

362. Antia FP, Bharadwaj TP, Watsa MC, Master J. Liver in normal pregnancy, pre-eclampsia and eclampsia. Lancet, 1958; ii:776–778

363. Arias F, Mancilla-Jimenez R. Hepatic fibrinogen deposits in pre-eclampsia. Immunofluorescent evidence. N Engl J Med, 1976; 295:578–582

364. Stone JH. HELLP syndrome: hemolysis, elevated liver enzymes, and low platelets. JAMA, 1998; 280:559–562

365. Curtin WM, Weinstein L. A review of HELLP syndrome. J Perinatol, 1999; 19:138–143

366. Barton JR, Sibai BM. Care of the pregnancy complicated by HELLP syndrome. Gastroenterol Clin North Am, 1992; 21: 937–950

367. Sibai BM, Taslimi MM, El-Nazer A et al. Maternal-perinatal outcome associated with the syndrome of hemolysis, elevated liver enzymes, and low platelets in severe pre-eclampsia-eclampsia. Am J Obstet Gynecol, 1986; 155:501–509

368. Akerboom-Straberger BM, Lotgering FK. Embryonal sarcoma of the liver in pregnancy, associated with HELLP syndrome. Am J Obstet Gynecol, 2004; 190:556–557

369. Sibai BM. The HELLP syndrome (hemolysis, elevated liver enzymes and low platelets): Much ado about nothing? Am J Obstet Gynecol, 1990; 162:311–316

370. Smulian J, Shen-Schwarz S, Scorza W, Kinzler W, Vintzileos A. A clinicohistopathologic comparison between HELLP syndrome and severe preeclampsia. J Matern Fetal Neonatal Med. 2004; 16:287–293

371. Sheikh RA, Yasmeen S, Pauly MP, Riegler JL. Spontaneous intrahepatic hemorrhage and hepatic rupture in the HELLP syndrome: four cases and a review. J Clin Gastroenterol, 1999; 28:323–328

372. Shames BD, Fernandez LA, Sollinger HW et al. Liver transplantation for HELLP syndrome. Liver Transpl, 2005; 11:224–228

373. Strand S, Strand D, Seufert R et al. Placenta-derived CD95 ligand causes liver damage in hemolysis, elevated liver enzymes, and low platelet count syndrome. Gastroenterology, 2004; 126:849–858

374. Abell TL, Riely CA. Hyperemesis gravidarum. Gastroenterol Clin North Am, 1992; 21:835–849

375. Wallstedt A, Riely CA, Shaver D et al. Prevalence and characteristics of liver dysfunction in hyperemesis gravidarum. Clin Res, 1990; 38:970–976

376. Adams RH, Gordon J, Combes B. Hyperemesis gravidarum. I. Evidence of hepatic dysfunction. Obstet Gynecol, 1968; 31:659–664

377. Neerhoff MG, Zelman W, Sullivan T. Hepatic rupture in pregnancy: a review. Obstet Gynecol Surg, 1989; 44:407–409

378. Ralston SJ, Schwaitzberg SD. Liver hematoma and rupture in pregnancy. Semin Perinatol, 1998; 22:141–148

379. Golan A, White RG. Spontaneous rupture of the liver associated with pregnancy. A report of 5 cases. S Afr Med J, 1979; 133–136

380. Manas KJ, Welsh JD, Rankin RA, Miller DD. Hepatic haemorrhage without rupture in pre-eclampsia. N Engl J Med, 1985; 312:424–426

381. Shaw C, Fattah N, Lynch D, Stokes M. Spontaneous rupture of the liver following a normal pregnancy and delivery. Ir Med J, 2005; 98:27–28

382. Morley AHG. Liver pregnancies. Lancet, 1956; i:994–995

383. Delabrousse E, Site O, Le Mouel A, Riethmuller D, Kastler B. Intrahepatic pregnancy: sonography and CT findings. Am J Roentgenol, 1999; 173:1377–1378

384. De Almeida Barbosa A Jr, Rodriguez de Freitas LA, Andrade Mota M. Primary pregnancy in the liver. A case report. Pathol Res Prac, 1991; 187:329–331

385. Meare Y, Ekna JB, Raolison S. Un cas de grossesse à implantation hépatique avec enfant vivant. Sem des Hôpitaux de Paris, 1965; 41:1430–1433

386. Lindgren P, Pla JC, Hogberg U, Tarnvik A. Listeria monocytogenes-induced liver abscess in pregnancy. Acta Obstet Gynecol, Scand, 1997; 76:486–488

387. Khong SY, James M, Smith P. Diagnosis of liver infarction postpartum. Obstet Gynecol, 2005; 105:1271–1273

388. Edwards CQ. Anemia and the liver. Hepatobiliary manifestations of anemia. Clin Liver Dis, 2002; 6:891–907, viii

389. Banerjee S, Owen C, Chopra S. Sickle cell hepatopathy. Hepatology, 2001; 33:1021–1028

390. Song YS. Hepatic lesions in sickle cell anemia. Am J Pathol, 1957; 33:331–351

391. Mills LR, Mwakyusa D, Milner PF. Histopathologic features of liver biopsy specimens in sickle cell disease. Arch Path Lab Med, 1988; 112:290–294

392. Sty JR. Hepatic vein thrombosis in sickle cell anaemia. Amer J Ped Haematol Oncol, 1982; 4:213–215

393. Heaton ND, Pain J, Cowan NC, Salisbury J, Howard ER. Focal nodular hyperplasia of the liver: a link with sickle cell disease. Arch Dis Chil, 1991; 66:1073–1074

394. Middleton JP, Wolper JC. Hepatic biloma complicating sickle cell disease. A case report and a review of the literature. Gastroenterology, 1984; 86:743–744

395. Avigan MI, Ishak KG, Gregg RE, Hoofnagle JH. Morphologic features of the liver in abetalipoproteinemia. Hepatology, 1984; 4:1223–1226

396. Grossman JA, McDermott WV. Paroxysmal nocturnal haemoglobinuria associated with hepatic and portal vein thrombosis. Am J Surg, 1974; 127:733–736

397. Liebowitz AI, Hartman RC. The Budd–Chiari syndrome and paroxysmal nocturnal haemoglobinuria. Br J Haematol, 1981; 48:1–6

398. Walz-Mattmuller R, Horny HP, Ruck P, Kaiserling E. Incidence and pattern of liver involvement in haematological malignancies. Pathol Res Pract, 1998; 194:781–789

399. Shelab TM, Kaminski MS, Lok AS. Acute liver failure due to hepatic involvement by haematologic malignancy. Dig Dis Sci, 1997; 42:1400–1405

400. Smith BC, James OF. The failing malignant liver. Gut, 1998; 42:454–455

401. Zafrani ES, Leclercq B, Vernan J-P, Pinaudeau Y, Chomette G, Dhumeaux D. Massive blastic infiltrations of the liver: a cause of fulminant hepatic failure. Hepatology, 1983; 3:428–432

402. Nizalik E, Zayed E, Foyle A. Malignant lymphoma presenting as fulminant hepatic failure. Can J Gastroenterol, 1989; 3:111–114

403. Yam LT, Janckila AJ, Chan CH, Chin-Yang LI. Hepatic involvement in hairy cell leukaemia. Cancer, 1983; 51:1497–1504

404. Zafrani ES, Degos F, Guigui B et al. The hepatic sinusoid in hairy cell leukemia: an ultrastructural study of 12 cases. Hum Pathol, 1987; 18:801–807

405. Bendix-Hansen K, Bayer Kristensen I. Granulomas of spleen and liver in hairy cell leukaemia. APMIS, 1984; 92:157–160

406. Nanba K, Soban EJ, Bowling MC, Berard CW. Splenic pseudosinuses and hepatic angiomatous lesions. Distinctive features of hairy cell leukaemia. Am J Clin Pathol, 1977; 67:415–526

407. Roquet M-L, Zafrani E-S, Farcet J-P, Reyes F, Pinaudeau Y. Histopathological lesions of the liver in hairy cell leukemia: a report of 14 cases. Hepatology, 1985; 5:496–500

408. Grouls V, Stiers R. Hepatic involvement in hairy cell leukaemia: diagnosis by tartrate resistant acid phosphatase enzyme histochemistry on formalin-fixed and paraffin-embedded liver biopsy specimens. Path Res Pract, 1984; 178:332–334

409. Falini B, Schwarting R, Enber W et al. The differential diagnosis of hairy cell leukemia with a panel of monoclonal antibodies. Am J Clin Pathol, 1985; 83:289–300

410. Zafrani ES, Cazier A, Baudelot AM et al. Ultrastructural lesions of the liver in human peliosis. A report of 12 cases. Am J Pathol, 1984; 114:349–359

411. Rozman M. Chronic lymphatic leukaemia and portal hypertension. Med Clinics Barcelona, 1989; 92:26–28

412. Locasculli A, Vergani GM, Uderzo C et al. Chronic liver disease in children with leukaemia in long-term remission. Cancer, 1983; 52:1080–1087

413. Barton JC, Conrad ME. Beneficial effects of hepatitis in patients with acute myelogenous leukemia. Ann Intern Med, 1979; 90:188–190

414. Brody SA, Russell WG, Krantz SB, Graber E. Beneficial effect of hepatitis in leukemic reticulo-endotheliosis. Arch Intern Med, 1981; 141:1080–1081

415. Costa F, Choy CG, Seiter K, Hann L, Thung SN, Michaeli J. Hepatic outflow obstruction and liver failure due to leukemic cell infiltration in chronic lymphocytic leukemia. Leuk Lymphoma, 1998; 30:403–410

416. Picardi M, Muretto P, Luciano L. Budd–Chiari syndrome in chronic myeloid leukemia. Haematologica, 2000; 85:429

417. Kumari TP, Shanvas A, Mathews A, Kusumakumary P. Hepatocellular carcinoma: a rare late event in childhood acute lymphoblastic leukemia. J Pediatr Hematol Oncol, 2000; 22:289–290

418. Dubois A, Dauzat M, Pignodel C et al. Portal hypertension in lymphoproliferative and myeloproliferative disorders: hemodynamic and histological correlations. Hepatology, 1993; 17:246–250

419. Hoffman R, Nimer A, Lanir N, Brenner B, Baruch Y. Budd–Chiari syndrome associated with factor V Leiden mutation: a report of 6 patients. Liver Transpl Surg, 1999; 5:96–100

420. Simsek S, Verheesen RV, Haagsma EB, Lourens J. Subacute Budd–Chiari syndrome associated with polycythemia vera and factor V Leiden mutation. Neth J Med, 2000; 57:62–67

421. Amos JA, Goodbody RA. Lymph node and liver biopsy in the myeloproliferative disorders. Br J Cancer, 1959; 13:173–180

422. Ligumski M, Polliak A, Benbassat J. Nature and incidence of liver involvement in agnogenic myeloid metaplasia. Scand J Haematol, 1978; 21:81–93

423. Pereira A, Bruguera M, Cervantes F, Rozman C. Liver involvement at diagnosis of primary myelofibrosis: a clinicopathological study of twenty-two cases. Eur J Haematol, 1988; 40:355–361

424. Scheuer PJ. Liver biopsy interpretation, 4th edn. London: Bailliere Tindall, 1988; p 243

425. Degott C, Capron JP, Bettan L et al. Myeloid metaplasia, perisinusoidal fibrosis, and nodular regenerative hyperplasia of the liver. Liver, 1985; 5:276–281

426. Bioulac-Sage P, Roux D, Quinton A, Lamouliatte H, Balabaud C. Ultrastructure of sinusoids in patients with agnogenic myeloid metaplasia. J Submicrosc Cytol, 1986; 14:815–821

427. Roux D, Merlio JP, Quinton A, Lamouliatte H, Balabaud C, Bioulac-Sage P. Agnogenic myeloid metaplasia, portal hypertension and sinusoidal abnormalities. Gastroenterology, 1987; 92:1067–1072

428. Hayes LW, Bennett WH, Hech FJ. Extra-medullary lesions in multiple myeloma; review of literature and pathologic studies. Arch Pathol, 1952; 53:262–272

429. Thiruvengadam R, Penetranti R, Grolsky HJ et al. Multiple myeloma presenting as space-occupying lesions of the liver. Cancer, 1990; 65:2784–2786

430. Thomas FB, Clausen KP, Greenberger NJ. Liver disease in multiple myeloma. Arch Intern Med, 1973; 132:195–202

431. Barth C, Bosse A, Andus T. Severe acute cholestatic hepatitis by infiltration of monoclonal plasma cells in multiple myeloma. Z Gastroenterol, 2005; 43:1129–1132

432. Brooks AP. Portal hypertension in Waldenström's macroglobulinaemia. Br Med J, 1976; 1:689–690

433. Wanless IR. Micronodular transformation (nodular regenerative hyperplasia) of the liver: a report of 64 cases among 2500 autopsies and a new classification of benign hepatocellular nodules. Hepatology, 1990; 11:787–797

434. Voinchet O, Degott C, Scoazec J-Y, Feldmann G, Benhamou J-P. Peliosis hepatis, nodular regenerative hyperplasia of the liver, and light chain deposition in a patient with Waldenström's macroglobulinemia. Gastroenterology, 1988; 95:482–486

435. Kim H, Dorfman RF. Morphological studies of 84 untreated patients subjected to laparotomy for the staging of non-Hodgkin's lymphomas. Cancer, 1974; 33:657–674

436. Lefkowitch JH, Falkow S, Whitlock RT. Hepatic Hodgkin's disease simulating cholestatic hepatitis with liver failure. Arch Path Lab Med, 1985; 109:424–426

437. Gunasekaran TS, Hassall E, Dimmick JE, Chan KW. Hodgkin's disease presenting with fulminant liver disease. J Pediatr Gastroenterol Nutr, 1992; 15:189–193

438. Kosmidou IS, Aggarwal A, Ross JJ, Worthington MG. Hodgkin's disease with fulminant non-alcoholic steatohepatitis. Dig Liver Dis, 2004; 36:691–693

439. Abt AB, Kirschner RH, Belliveau RE et al. Hepatic pathology associated with Hodgkin's disease. Cancer, 1974; 33:1564–1571

440. Kaplan HS. Hodgkin's disease: unfolding concepts concerning its nature, management and prognosis. Cancer, 1980; 45:2439–2474

441. Jaffe ES. Malignant lymphomas: pathology of hepatic involvement. Semin Liver Dis, 1987; 7:257–268

442. Gordon CD, Sidawy MK, Talarico L, Kondi E. Hodgkin's disease in the liver without splenic involvement. Arch Intern Med, 1984; 144:2277–2278

443. Rappaport H, Bernard CW, Butler JJ, Dorfman RF, Lukes RJ, Thomas LB. Report of the committees on histopathological criteria contributing to staging of Hodgkin's disease. Cancer Res, 1971; 31:1864–1865

444. Skovsgaard T, Brinckmeyer LM, Vesterager L et al. The liver in Hodgkin's disease. II. Histopathologic findings. Eur J Cancer Clin Oncol, 1982; 18:429–435

445. Cavalli G, Casali AM, Lambertini F, Busachi C. Changes in the small biliary passages in the hepatic localization of Hodgkin's disease. Virchows Arch (A), 1979; 384:295–306

446. Leslie KO, Colby TV. Hepatic parenchymal lymphoid aggregates in Hodgkin's disease. Hum Pathol, 1984; 15:808–809

447. Kadin ME, Donaldson SS, Dorfman RF. Isolated granulomas in Hodgkin's disease. N Engl J Med, 1970; 283:859–861

448. Sacks EL, Donaldson SS, Gordon J, Dorfman RF. Epithelioid granulomas associated with Hodgkin's disease. Cancer, 1978; 41:562–567

449. Pak HY, Friedman NB. Pseudosarcoid granulomas in Hodgkin's disease. Hum Pathol, 1981; 12:832–837

450. Bergter W, Fetzer I-C, Sattler B, Ramadori G. Granulomatous hepatitis preceding Hodgkin's disease. Pathol Oncol Res, 1996; 2:177–180

451. Bruguera M, Caballero T, Carreras E et al. Hepatic sinusoidal dilatation in Hodgkin's disease. Liver, 1987; 7:76–80

452. Abe H, Kubota K, Makkuuchi M. Obstructive jaundice secondary to Hodgkin's disease. Am J Gastroenterol, 1977; 92:526–527

453. Birrer MJ, Young RC. Differential diagnosis of jaundice in lymphoma patients. Semin Liver Dis, 1987; 7:269–277

454. Yalcin S, Kars A, Sokmensuer C, Atahan L. Extrahepatic Hodgkin's disease with intrahepatic cholestasis: report of two cases. Oncology, 1999; 57:83–85

455. Hubscher SG, Lumley MA, Elias E. Vanishing bile duct syndrome: a possible mechanism for intrahepatic cholestasis in Hodgkin's lymphoma. Hepatology, 1993; 17:70–77

456. de Medeiros BC, Lacerda MA, Telles JE, da Silva JA, de Medeiros CR. Cholestasis secondary to Hodgkin's disease: report of 2 cases of vanishing bile duct syndrome. Haematologica, 1998; 83:1038–1040

457. Man KM, Drejet A, Keefe EB. Primary sclerosing cholangitis and Hodgkin's disease. Hepatology, 1993; 18:1127–1131

458. Dourakis SP, Tzemanakis E, Deutsch M, Kafiri G, Hadziyannis SJ. Fulminant hepatic failure as a presenting paraneoplastic manifestation of Hodgkin's disease. Eur J Gastroenterol Hepatol, 1999; 11:1055–1058

459. Kahn LB, King H, Jacobs P. Florid epithelioid cell and sarcoid-type reaction associated with non-Hodgkin's lymphoma. S Afr Med J, 1977; 51:341–347

460. Saito K, Nakanuma Y, Ogawa S, Arai Y, Hayashi M. Extensive hepatic granulomas associated with peripheral T-cell lymphoma. Am J Gastroenterol, 1991; 86:1243–1246

461. Watterson J, Priest JR. Jaundice as a paraneoplastic phenomenon in a T-cell lymphoma. Gastroenterology, 1989; 97:1319–1322

462. Cozzolino G, Lonardo A, Fracica G, Cacciatore L. Three more cases of concurrent liver cirrhosis and non-Hodgkin's lymphoma. Ital J Gastroenterol, 1984; 16:235–237

463. Di Stasi M, Cavanna L, Fornari F et al. Association of non-Hodgkin's lymphoma and hepatocellular carcinoma. Oncology, 1990; 47:80–83

464. Dargent JL, De Wolf-Peeters C. Liver involvement by lymphoma: identification of a distinctive pattern of infiltration related to T-cell/ histiocyte-rich B-cell lymphoma. Ann Diagn Pathol, 1998; 2:363–369

465. Voigt JJ, Vinel JP, Caveriviere P et al. Diagnostique immunohistochimique des localisations hépatiques des hémopathies lymphoides malignes; étude de 80 cas. Gastroenterol Clin Biol, 1989; 13:343–352

466. Wright DH, Burkitt's tumour. A post-mortem study of 50 cases. Br J Surg, 1964; 51:245–251

467. Banks PM, Arseneau JC, Gralnick HR et al. American Burkitt's lymphoma: a clinicopathologic study of 30 cases. Am J Med, 1975; 58:322–329

468. Gaulard P, Zafrani ES, Mavier P et al. Peripheral T-cell lymphoma presenting as predominant liver disease: a report of three cases. Hepatology, 1986; 6:864–868

469. Weidmann E. Hepatosplenic T cell lymphoma. A review on 45 cases since the first report describing the disease as a distinct lymphoma entity in 1990. Leukemia, 2000; 14:991–997

470. de Wolf-Peeters C, Achten R. γδT-cell lymphomas: a homogenous entity? Histopathology, 2000; 36:294–305

471. Yamada Y, Kamihira S, Murata K et al. Frequent hepatic involvement in adult T-cell leukaemia: comparison with non-Hodgkin's lymphoma. Leuk Lymphoma, 1977; 26:327–335

472. Blayney D, Jaffe E, Blattner W et al. The human T-cell leukemia/lymphoma virus (HTLV) associated with American adult T-cell leukemia/lymphoma (ATL). Blood, 1983; 62:401–405

473. Fakunle YM, Greenwood BM. The nature of hepatic lymphocytic infiltrates in the tropical splenomegaly syndrome. Clin Exp Immunol, 1982; 48:546–550

474. Dacie JV, Brain MC, Harrison CV, Lewis SM, Worlledge SM. Non-tropical idiopathic splenomegaly (primary hypersplenism): a review of ten cases and their relationship to malignant lymphoma. Br J Haematol, 1982; 17:317–333

475. Paradinas FJ, Harrison KM. Visceral lesions in an unusual case of Sezary's syndrome. Cancer, 1974; 33:1068–1074

476. Variakojis D, Rosas-Uribe A, Rappaport H. Mycosis fungoides. Pathologic findings in staging laparotomies. Cancer, 1974; 33:1589–1600

477. Rappaport H, Thomas L. Mycosis fungoides. The pathology of extracutaneous involvement. Cancer, 1974; 34:1198–1292

478. Madsen JA, Tallini G, Glusac EJ, Salem RR, Braverman I, Robert ME. Biliary tract obstruction secondary to mycosis fungoides: a case report. J Clin Gastroenterol, 1999; 28:56–60

479. Cadranel J-F, Cadranel J, Buffet C et al. Nodular regenerative hyperplasia of the liver, peliosis hepatis, and perisinusoidal fibrosis. Association with angioimmunoblastic lymphadenopathy and severe hypoxemia. Gastroenterology, 1990; 99:268–273

480. Memeo L, Pecorello I, Ciardi A, Aiello E, De Quarto A, Di Tondo U. Primary non-Hodgkin's lymphoma of the liver. Acta Oncol, 1999; 38:655–658

481. Manns MP, Rambusch EG. Autoimmunity and extrahepatic manifestations in hepatitis C virus infection. J Hepatol, 1999; 31(suppl 1):39–42

482. Lei KI. Primary non-Hodgkin's lymphoma of the liver. Leuk Lymphoma, 1998; 29:293–299

483. Bronowicki JP, Bineau C, Feugier P et al. Primary lymphoma of the liver: clinical-pathological features and relationship with HCV infection in French patients. Hepatology, 2003; 37:781–787

484. Suarez F, Wlodarska I, Rigal-Huguet F et al. Hepatosplenic alphabeta T-cell lymphoma: an unusual case with clinical, histologic, and cytogenetic features of gammadelta hepatosplenic T-cell lymphoma. Am J Surg Pathol, 2000; 24:1027–1032

485. Francois A, Lesesve JF, Stamatoullas A et al. Hepatosplenic gamma/delta T-cell lymphoma: a report of two cases in immunocompromised patients, associated with isochomosome 7q. Am J Surg Pathol, 1997; 21:781–790

486. De Wolf-Peeters C, Pittaluga S. T-cell rich B-cell lymphoma: a morphological variant of a variety of non-Hodgkin's lymphomas or a clinicopathological entity? Histopathology, 1995; 26:383–385

487. Khan SM, Cottrell BJ, Millward-Sadler GH, Wright DH. T-cell-rich B-cell lymphoma presenting as liver disease. Histopathology, 1993; 23:217–224

488. Selves J, Meggato F, Brousset P et al. Inflammatory pseudotumor of the liver. Evidence for follicular dendritic reticulum cell proliferation associated with clonal Epstein-Barr virus. Am J Surg Pathol, 1996; 20:747–753

489. Shek TW, Ho FC, Ng IO, Chan AC, Ma L, Srivastava G. Follicular dendritic cell tumor of the liver. Evidence for an Epstein-Barr virus-related clonal proliferation of follicular dendritic cells. Am J Surg Pathol, 1996; 20:313–324

490. Perez-Ordonez B, Rosai J. Follicular dendritic cell tumor: review of the entity. Semin Diagn Pathol, 1998; 15:144–154

491. Ye MQ, Suriawinata A, Black C, Min AD, Strauchen J, Thung SN. Primary hepatic marginal zone B-cell lymphoma of mucosa-associated lymphoid tissue type in a patient with primary biliary cirrhosis. Arch Pathol Lab Med, 2000; 124:604–608

492. Kirk CM, Lewin D, Lazarchick J. Primary hepatic B-cell lymphoma of mucosa-associated lymphoid tissue. Arch Pathol Lab Med, 1999; 123:716–719

493. Prabhu RM, Medeiros IJ, Kumar D. Primary hepatic low-grade B-cell lymphoma of mucosa-associated lymphoid tissue (MALT) associated with primary biliary cirrhosis. Mod Pathol, 1998; 11:404–410

494. Maes M, Depardieu C, Dargent JL et al. Primary low-grade B-cell lymphoma of MALT-type occurring in the liver: a study of two cases. J Hepatol, 1997; 27:922–927

495. Demirhan B, Sokmensuer C, Karakayali H, Gungen Y, Dogan A, Haberal M. Primary extramedullary plasmacytoma of the liver. J Clin Pathol, 1997; 50:74–76

496. O'Brien CB, Pollack BJ, Furth EE, Fox K, Schnall MD. Primary hepatic angiocentric lymphoma. Dig Dis Sci, 1997; 42:427–430

497. Sneller MC, Straus SE, Jaffe ES et al. A novel lymphoproliferative/autoimmune syndrome resembling murine lip/gld disease. J Clin Invest, 1992; 90:334–341

498. Fisher GH, Rosenberg FJ, Straus SE et al. Dominant interfering Fas gene mutations impair apoptosis in a human autoimmune lymphoproliferative syndrome. Cell, 1995; 81:935–946

499. Lim MS, Straus SE, Dale JK et al. Pathological findings in human autoimmune lymphoproliferative syndrome. Am J Pathol, 1998; 153:1541–1550

500. Lafon ME, Bioulac-Sage P, Grimaud JA et al. Perisinusoidal fibrosis of the liver in patients with thrombocytopenic purpura. Virchows Arch (A), 1987; 411:553–559

501. Neiman JC, Mant MJ, Shnitka TK. Phagocytosis of platelets by Kupffer cells in immune thrombocytopenia. Arch Pathol Lab Med, 1987; 111:563–565

502. Ishida Y, Utikoshi M, Kurosaki M et al. Hepatic veno-occlusive disease in a case of polymyositis associated with thrombotic thrombocytopenic purpura/hemolytic uremic syndrome. Intern Med, 1998; 37:694–699

503. Wilkins HJ, Crane MM, Copeland K, Williams WV. Hypereosinophilic syndrome: an update. Am J Hematol, 2005; 80:148–157

504. Croffy B, Kopelman R, Kaplan M. Hypereosinophilic syndrome. Association with chronic active hepatitis. Dig Dis Sci, 1988; 33:233–239

505. Foong A, Scholes JV, Gleich GJ, Kephart GM, Holt PR. Eosinophil-induced chronic active hepatitis in the idiopathic hypereosinophilic syndrome. Hepatology, 1991; 13:1090–1094

506. Ung KA, Remotti H, Olsson R. Eosinophilic hepatic necrosis in hypereosinophilic syndrome. J Clin Gastroenterol, 2000; 31:323–327

507. Reyes M, Abraham C, Abedi M, Carucci LR, Schwartz LB. Hypereosinophilic syndrome with hepatobiliary masses and obstructive jaundice. Ann Allergy Asthma Immunol, 2005; 94:25–28

508. Fauci AS, Harley JB, Roberts WC et al. The idiopathic hypereosinophilic syndrome. Clinical, pathophysiologic and therapeutic considerations. Ann Intem Med, 1982; 97:78–92

509. Pfeifer U, Ormanns W, Klinge O. Hepatocellular fibrinogen storage in familial hypofibrinogenemia. Virchows Arch (A), 1981; 36:247–255

510. Callea F, de Vos R, Togni R et al. Fibrinogen inclusions in liver cells: a new type of ground-glass hepatocyte: immune, light and electron microscopic characterisation. Histopathology, 1986; 10:65–74

511. Callea F, Brisigoth M, Fabbretti G, Bonino F, Desmet VJ. Hepatic endoplasmic reticulin storage diseases. Liver, 1992; 12:357–362

512. Brennan SO, Wyatt J, Medicina D, Callea F, George PM. Fibrinogen Brescia: hepatic endoplasmic reticulum storage and hypofibrinogenemia because of a γ284 gly → arg mutation. Am J Pathol, 2000; 157:189–196

513. Duga S, Assetta R, Sautagostine E et al. Missense mutations in the human beta fibrinogen gene cause congenital afibrinogenemia by impairing fibrinogen secretion. Blood, 2000; 95:1336–1341

514. Storch W, Riedel H, Trautmann B, Justus J, Hiemann D. Storage of the complement components C4, C3 and C3-activator in the human liver as PAS-negative globular hyaline bodies. Exp Pathol, 1982; 21:199–203

515. Storch W. Immunohistological investigation of PAS-negative intracisternal hyalin in human liver biopsy specimens. Virchows Arch (A), 1985; 48:155–165

516. Marucci G, Morandi L, Macchia S et al. Fibrinogen storage disease without hypofibrinogenaemia associated with acute infection. Histopathology, 2003; 42:22–25

517. Mills PR, Sturrock RD. Clinical associations between arthritis and liver disease. Ann Rheum Dis, 1982; 41:295–307

518. Asherson RA, Hughes GRV. Musculoskeletal diseases and the liver. In: McIntyre N, Benhamou J-P, Bircher J, Rizzetto M, Rodes J, eds. Oxford textbook of clinical hepatology. Oxford: OUP, 1991: pp 1196–1201

519. Walker NJ, Zurier RB. Liver abnormalities in rheumatic diseases. Clin Liver Dis, 2002; 6:933–946

520. Abraham S, Begum S, Isenberg D. Hepatic manifestations of autoimmune rheumatic diseases. Ann Rheum Dis, 2004; 63:123–129

521. Ayers AB, Fitchett DH. Hepatic haematoma in polyarteritis. Br J Radiol, 1976; 49:184–185

522. Haslock I. Spontaneous rupture of the liver in systemic lupus erythematosus. Ann Rheum Dis, 1974; 33:482–484

523. Pettersson T, Lepantalo M, Friman C, Ahonen J. Spontaneous rupture of the liver in rheumatoid arthritis. Scand J Rheumatol, 1986; 15:348–349

524. Richard S, Guerret S, Gerard F, Tebib JG, Vignon E. Hepatic fibrosis in rheumatoid arthritis patients treated with methotrexate: application of a new semi-quantitative scoring system. Rheumatology (Oxford), 2000; 39:50–54

525. Suissa S, Ernst P, Hudson M, Bitton A, Kezouh A. Newer disease-modifying antirheumatic drugs and the risk of serious hepatic adverse events in patients with rheumatoid arthritis. Am J Med. 2004 15; 117:87–92

526. Kendall MJ, Cockel R, Becker J, Hawkins CF. Raised serum alkaline phosphatase in rheumatoid disease. Ann Rheum Dis, 1970; 29:537–540

527. Kendall MJ, Cockel R, Becker J, Hawkins CF. Rheumatoid liver. Br Med J, 1970; i:221

528. Fermandes L, Sullivan SN, McFarlane IG et al. Studies on the frequency and pathogenesis of liver involvement in rheumatoid arthritis. Ann Rheum Dis, 1975; 34:198–199

529. Spooner RJ, Smith DH, Bedford D, Beck PR. Serum gamma-glutamyltransferase and alkaline phosphatase in rheumatoid arthritis. J Clin Pathol, 1982; 35:638–641

530. Webb J, Whaley K, MacSween RNM, Nuki G, Dick WC, Buchanan WW. Liver disease in rheumatoid arthritis and Sjögren's syndrome. Ann Rheum Dis, 1975; 34:70–81

531. Tiger LH, Gorden MH, Ehrlich GE, Shapiro B. Liver enlargement demonstrated by scintigraphy in rheumatoid arthritis. J Rheumatol, 1976; 3:15–20

532. Rau R, Pfenninger K, Boni A. Liver function tests and liver biopsies in patients with rheumatoid arthritis. Ann Rheum Dis, 1975; 34:198–199

533. Van den Bogaerde J, Benyou HLC. Musculoskeletal disease and the liver In: Bircher J, Benhamou, J-P, McIntgre N eds Oxford Texbtook of Clinical Hepatology, 1999 OUP; Oxford pp 1727–1733

534. Dietrichson O, From A, Christofferson P, Juhl E. Morphological changes in liver biopsies from patients with rheumatoid arthritis. Scand J Rheumatol, 1976; 5:65–69

535. Whaley K, Webb J. Liver and kidney disease in rheumatoid arthritis. Clin Rheum Dis, 1977; 3:527–547

536. Mills PR, MacSween RNM, Dick WC, More IA, Watkinson G. Liver disease in rheumatoid arthritis. Scott Med J, 1980; 25: 18–22

537. Rau R, Karger T, Herborn G, Frenzel H. Liver biopsy findings in patients with rheumatoid arthritis undergoing longterm treatment with methotrexate. J Rheumatol, 1989; 16:489–493

538. Job-Deslandre C, Feldmann JL, Diyan Y, Meukes CJ. Chronic hepatitis during rheumatoid arthritis. Clin Exp Rheumatol 1991; 9:507–510

539. Laffon A, Moreno A, Gutierrez-Bucero A et al. Hepatic sinusoidal dilatation in rheumatoid arthritis. J Clin Gastroenterol, 1989; 11:653–657

540. Ruderman EM, Crawford JM, Maier A, Liu JJ, Gravallese EM, Weinblatt ME. Histologic liver abnormalities in an autopsy series of patients with rheumatoid arthritis. Br J Rheumatol, 1977; 36:210–213

541. The LG, Steven MM, Cappell HA. Alpha-1-antitrypsin associated liver disease in rheumatoid arthritis. Postgrad Med J, 1985; 61:171–172

542. Sherlock S, Scheuer PJ. The presentation and diagnosis of 100 patients with primary biliary cirrhosis. N Engl J Med, 1973; 289:674–678

543. Harris M, Rash RM, Dymock IW. Nodular non-cirrhotic liver associated with portal hypertension in a patient with rheumatoid arthritis. J Clin Pathol, 1974; 27:963–966

544. Stomeyer FW, Ishak K. Nodular transformation (nodular 'regenerative' hyperplasia) of the liver. Hum Pathol, 1981; 12:60–71

545. Reynolds WJ, Wanless IR. Nodular regenerative hyperplasia of the liver in a patient with rheumatoid vasculitis: a morphometric study suggesting a role for hepatic arteritis in the pathogenesis. J Rheumatol, 1984; 11:838–842

546. Smits JG, Kooijman CD. Rheumatoid nodules in liver (letter). Histopathology, 1986; 10:1211–1212

547. Landas SK, Mitros FA, Furst DE, La Brecque DR. Lipogranulomas and gold in the liver in rheumatoid arthritis. Am J Surg Pathol, 1992; 16:171–174

548. Bloch KJ, Buchanan WW, Wohl MJ, Bunin JJ. Sjögren's syndrome. A clinical, pathological and serological study of 62 cases. Medicine, 1965; 44:187–231

549. Tsianos EV, Hoofnagle JH, Fox PC et al. Sjögrens syndrome in patients with primary biliary cirrhosis. Hepatology, 1990; 11:730–734

550. Biasi D, Caramasch P, Carletto A et al. Sjögren's syndrome associated with autoimmune hepatitis. A case report. Clin Rheumatol, 1997; 16:409–412

551. Montefusco PP, Geiss AC, Bronzo RL et al. Sclerosing cholangitis, chronic pancreatitis and Sjögren's syndrome: a syndrome complex. Am J Surg, 1984; 147:822–826

552. Ramos-Casals M, Garcia-Carrasco M, Cervera R, Font J. Sjögren's syndrome and hepatitis C virus. Clin Rheumatol, 1999; 18:93–100

553. Tsuruta S, Enjoji M, Nakamuta M et al. Primary hepatic lymphoma in a patient with Sjogren's syndrome. J Gastroenterol, 2002; 37:129–132

554. Blendis LM, Ansell ID, Lloyd-Jones K, Hamilton E, Williams R. Liver in Felty's syndrome. Br Med J, 1970; 1:131–135

555. Cohen ML, Mamier JW, Bredfeldt JE. Sinusoidal lymphocytosis of the liver in Felty's syndrome with a review of the liver involvement in Felty's syndrome. J Clin Gastroenterol, 1989; 11:92–94

556. Blendis LM, Parkinson MC, Shilkin KB, Williams R. Nodular regenerative hyperplasia of the liver in Felty's syndrome. Q J Med, 1974; 43:25–32

557. Blendis LM, Lovell D, Barris CG, Ritland S, Catton D, Vesia P. Esophageal variceal bleeding associated with nodular regenerative hyperplasia. Ann Rheum Dis, 1978; 37:183–186

558. Schaller J, Beckwith B, Wedgwood RJ. Hepatic involvement in juvenile rheumatoid arthritis. J Pediatr, 1970; 77:203–210

559. Korneich H, Malouf NN, Hanson V. Acute hepatic dysfunction in juvenile rheumatoid arthritis. J Pediatr, 1971; 79:27–35

560. Andres E, Kurtz JE, Perrin AE et al. Retrospective monocentric study of 17 patients with adult Still's disease, with special focus on liver abnormalities. Hepatogastroenterology, 2003; 50:192–195

561. Esdaile JM, Tannenbaum J, Hawkins D. Adult Still's disease. Am J Med, 1980; 68:825–830

562. Baker DG, Shumacher HR, Reginato AJ. Fifteen patients with adult onset Still's disease: life threatening liver failure in two. Arch Rheum, 1979; 22:590

563. Dino O, Provenzano G, Giannuoli G, Sciarrino E, Pouyet M, Pagliaro L. Fulminant hepatic failure in adult onset Still's disease. J Rheumatol, 1996; 213:784–785

564. Janssen HL, van Laar JM, van Hoek B, den Ottolander GJ, van Krieken JH, Breedveld FC. Severe hepatitis and pure red cell aplasia in adult Stills' disease: good response to immunosuppressive therapy. Dig Dis Sci, 1999; 44:1639–1642

565. Dubois EL, Wierzchowiecki M, Cox MB, Weirner JM. Duration and death in systemic lupus erythematosus. An analysis of 249 cases. JAMA, 1974; 227:1399–1402

566. Runyon BA, LaBrecque DR, Anuras S. The spectrum of liver disease in systemic lupus erythematosus: report of 33 histologically-proved cases and review of the literature. Am J Med, 1980; 69:187–194

567. Gibson T, Myers AR. Subclinical liver disease in systemic lupus erythematosus. J Rheumatol, 1981; 8:752–759

568. Miller MH, Urowitz MB, Gladman DD, Blendis LM. The liver in systemic lupus erythematosus. Q J Med, 1984; 211:401–409

569. Matsumoto T, Yoshimme T, Shimouchi K et al. The liver in systemic lupus erythematosis: pathologic analysis of 52 cases and review of Japanese autopsy registry data. Hum Pathol, 1992; 23:1151–1158

570. Mackay IR. The hepatitis-lupus connection. Semin Liver Dis, 1991; 11:234–240

571. Schifter T, Lewinski UH. Primary biliary cirrhosis and systemic lupus erythematosus. A rare association. Clin Exp Rheumatol, 1997; 15:313–314

572. Colin AF, Alberti N, Solis JA et al. Diffuse nodular regenerative hyperplasia of the liver (DNRH). A clinicopathologic study of 24 cases. Liver, 1989; 9:253–265

573. Hughes GRV. The antiphospholipid syndrome: ten years on. Lancet, 1993; 342:342–344

574. Morla RM, Ramos-Casals M, Garcia-Carrasco M et al. Nodular regenerative hyperplasia of the liver and antiphospholipid antibodies: report of two cases and review of the literature. Lupus, 1999; 8:160–163

575. Asherson RA, Thompson RP, MacLachlan N, Baguley E, Hicks P, Hughes GR. Visceral arterial occlusions, Budd–Chiari syndrome, recurrent fetal loss and the 'lupus anticoagulant' in systemic lupus erythematosus. J Rheumatol, 1989; 16:219–224

576. Pelletier S, Landi B, Piette JC et al. Antiphospholipid syndrome as the second cause of non-tumorous Budd–Chiari syndrome. J Hepatol, 1994; 21:76–80

577. Khoury G, Tohi M, Oren M, Traub YM. Massive hepatic infarction in systemic lupus erythematosus. Dig Dis Sci, 1990; 35:1557–1560

578. Kaplan B, Cooper J, Lager D, Abecassis M. Hepatic infarction in a hemodialysis patient with systemic lupus erythematosus. Am J Kidney Dis, 1995; 26:785–787

579. Haslock I. Spontaneous rupture of the liver in systemic lupus erythematosus. Ann Rheum Dis, 1974; 33:482–484

580. Robertson SJ, Higgins RB, Powell C. Malakoplakia of liver: a case report. Hum Pathol, 1992; 22:1294–1295

581. Laxer RM, Roberts EA, Gross KR et al. Liver disease in neonatal lupus erythematosus. J Paed, 1990; 116:238–242

582. Lee LA, Sokol RJ, Buyon JP. Hepatobiliary disease in neonatal lupus: prevalence and clinical characteristics in cases enrolled in a national registry. Pediatrics, 2002; 109:E11

583. van Hoek B. The spectrum of liver disease in systemic lupus erythematosus. Neth J Med, 1996; 48:244–253

584. Bartholomew LG, Cain JC, Winkelmann RK, Baggenstoss AH. Chronic disease of the liver associated with systemic scleroderma. Am J Dig Dis, 1964; 9:43–55

585. D'Angelo WA, Fries JF, Masi AT, Shulman LE. Pathologic observations in systemic sclerosis (scleroderma). Am J Med, 1969; 46:428–440

586. Morris JS, Htut T, Read AE. Scleroderma and portal hypertension. Ann Rheum Dis, 1972; 31:316–318

587. Copeman PNM, Medd WD. Diffuse systemic sclerosis with abnormal liver and gallbladder. Br Med J, 1967; ii:353–354

588. Wildenthal K, Schenker S, Smiley JD, Ford KL. Obstructive jaundice and gastrointestinal haemorrhage in progressive systemic sclerosis. Arch Int Med, 1968; 121:365–368

589. Fraile G, Rodriguez-Garcia JL, Morena A. Primary sclerosing cholangitis associated with systemic sclerosis. Postgrad Med J, 1991; 67:189–192

590. Murray-Lyon IM, Thompson RPH, Ansell ID, Williams R. Scleroderma and primary biliary cirrhosis. Br Med J, 1970; ii:258–259

591. Barnett AJ. The systemic involvement in scleroderma. Med J Aust, 1977; 2:659–662

592. Lurie B, Novis B, Banks J et al. CRST syndrome and nodular transformation of the liver. A case report. Gastroenterology, 1973; 64:457–461

593. McMahon HE. Systemic scleroderma and massive infarction of intestine and liver. Surg Gynecol Obstet, 1972; 134:10–14

594. Marshall JB, Ravendhran N, Sharp GC. Liver disease in mixed connective tissue disease. Arch Intern Med, 1983; 143:1817–1818

595. Rolny P, Goobar J, Zettergren L. HBsAg-negative chronic active hepatitis and mixed connective tissue disease syndrome. An unusual association observed in two patients. Acta Med Scand, 1984; 215:391–395

596. Maeda M, Kanayama M, Hasumura Y, Takeuchi J, Uchida T. Case of mixed connective tissue disease associated with autoimmune hepatitis. Dig Dis Sci, 1988; 33:1487–1490

597. Singsen BH, Swanson VL, Bernstein BH et al. A histologic evaluation of mixed connective tissue disease in childhood. Am J Med, 1980; 68:710–717

598. Cosnes J, Robert A, Levy VG, Darnis F. Budd–Chiari syndrome in a patient with mixed connective tissue disease. Dig Dis Sci, 1980; 25:467–469

599. von Knorring J, Wasastjerna C. Liver involvement in polymyalgia rheumatica. Scand J Rheumatol, 1976; 5:179–204

600. Sattar MA, Cawley MID, Hamblin TJ, Robertson JC. Polymyalgia rheumatica and antimitochondrial antibodies. Ann Rheum Dis, 1984; 43:264–266

601. Thompson K, Roberts PF. Chronic hepatitis in polymyalgia rheumatica. Postgrad Med J, 1976; 52:236–238

602. Leong AS-Y, Alp MH. Hepatocellular disease in the giant cell arteritis/polymyalgia rheumatica. Scand J Rheumatol, 1981; 5:179–204

603. James O, Macklon AF, Watson AJ. Primary biliary cirrhosis—a revised clinical spectrum. Lancet, 1978; i:1278–1281

604. Epstein O, Burroughs AK, Sherlock S. Polymyositis and acute onset systemic sclerosis in a patient with primary biliary cirrhosis: a clinical syndrome similar to the mixed connective tissue disease. J Roy Soc Med, 1981; 74:456–458

605. Bondeson J, Veress B, Lindroth Y, Lindgren S. Polymyositis associated with asymptomatic primary biliary cirrhosis. Clin Exp Rheumatol, 1998; 26:172–174

606. Bitnum S, Daeschner CW, Travis LB, Dodge WF, Hopps H. Dermatomyositis. J Pediatr, 1974; 64:101–131

607. Sattar MA, Guindi RT, Khan RA, Tungekar MF. Polymyositis and hepatocellular carcinoma. Clin Rheumatol, 1988; 7:538–542

608. Leaute-Labreze C, Perel Y, Trieb A. Childhood dermatomyositis associated with hepatocarcinoma. N Engl J Med, 1995; 333:1083

609. Oram S, Cochrane GM. Weber-Christian disease with visceral involvement. An example with hepatic enlargement. Br Med J, 1958; 2:281–284

610. Kimura H, Kayo M, Iyok et al. Alcoholic hyaline (Mallory bodies) in a case of Weber-Christian disease: electron microscopic observations of liver involvement. Gastroenterology, 1986; 78:807–812

611. Bailey M, Chapin W, Licht H, Reynolds JC. The effects of vasculitis on the gastrointestinal tract and liver. Gastroenterol Clin North Am, 1998; 27:747–782

612. Otani Y, Anzai S, Shibuya H et al. Churg-Strauss syndrome (CSS) manifested as necrosis of fingers and toes and liver infarction. J Dermatol, 2003; 30:810–815

613. Rousselet M-Ch, Kettani S, Rohmer V, Saint-Andre J-P. A case of temporal arteritis with intrahepatic arterial involvement. Path Res Pract, 1989; 185:329–331

614. Lankisch MR, Scolapio JS, Thistle JL, Witzig TE, McBane RD. Elevated liver enzymes preceding vessel involvement in Takayasu's arteritis. J Hepatol, 1999; 30:349–350

615. Goritsas CP, Repanti M, Papadaki E, Lazarou N, Andonopoulos AP. Intrahepatic bile duct injury and nodular regenerative hyperplasia of the liver in a patient with polyarteritis nodosa. J Hepatol, 1997; 26:727–730

616. Matsumoto T, Uekusa T, Fukuda Y. Vasculo-Behcet's disease: a pathologic study of eight cases. Hum Pathol, 1991; 22:45–51

617. Bayraktar Y, Ozaslan E, Van Thiel DH. Gastrointestinal manifestations of Behcet's disease. J Clin Gastroenterol, 2000; 30:144–154

618. Bayraktar Y, Balkanci F, bayraktar M, Calguneri M. Budd–Chiari syndrome: a common complication of Behcet's disease. Am J Gastroenterol, 1997; 92:858–862

619. Bloxham C, Henderson DC, Hampson J, Burt AD. Nodular regenerative hyperplasia in Behcet's disease. Histopathology, 1992; 20:452–454

620. Ware AJ, Luby JP, Hollinger B et al. Etiology of liver disease in renal transplant patients. Ann Int Med, 1979; 91:364–371

621. Ware AJ, Gorder NL, Gurian LE et al. Value of screening for markers of hepatitis in dialysis units. Hepatology, 1983; 3:513–518

622. Rodes J, Arroyo V. The liver in urogenital diseases In: Bircher J, Benhamou J-P, McIntyre N, eds. Oxford textbook of clinical hepatology, 2nd edn Oxford: OUP, 1999; pp 1701–1708

623. Chan MK, Moorhead JF. Hepatitis B and the dialysis and renal transplantation unit. Nephron, 1981; 27:229–232

624. Alter MJ, Favero MS, Maynard JE. Impact of infection control strategies on the incidence of dialysis associated hepatitis in the US. J Infect Dis, 1986; 153:1149–1151

625. Briggs WA, Lazarus JM, Birch AG, Hampers CL, Hager EB, Merrill JP. Hepatitis affecting haemodialysis and transplant patients. Its considerations and consequences. Arch Intern Med, 1973; 132:21–28

626. Dusheiko G, Song E, Bowyer S et al. Natural history of hepatitis B virus infection in renal transplant recipients—a fifteen year follow-up. Hepatology, 1983; 3:330–336

627. Pol S, Debure A, Degott C et al. Chronic hepatitis in kidney allograft recipients. Lancet, 1990; ii:878–880

628. Allison MC, Mowat A, McCruden EAB et al. The spectrum of chronic liver disease in renal transplant recipients. Q J Med, 1992; 301:355–367

629. Degott C, Degos F, Jungers P et al. Relationship between liver histopathological changes and HBsAg in 111 patients treated by long-term hemodialysis. Liver, 1983; 3:377–384

630. Parfrey PS, Forbes RDC, Hutchinson TA et al. The clinical and pathological course of hepatitis B liver disease in renal transplant recipients. Transplantation, 1984; 37:461–466

631. Debure A, Degos F, Pol S et al. Liver diseases and hepatic complications in renal transplant patients. Adv Nephrol, 1988; 17:375–400

632. Brind AM, Bennett MK, Bassendine MF. Nucleoside analogue therapy in fibrosing cholestatic hepatitis—a case report in an HBsAg positive renal transplant recipient. Liver, 1998; 18:134–139

633. Crosnier J, Jungers P, Courouce AM et al. Randomised placebo-controlled trial of hepatitis B surface antigen vaccine in French haemodialysis units. I. Haemodialysis patients. Lancet, 1981; i:797–800

634. Carreno V, Mora I, Escuin F et al. Vaccination against hepatitis B in renal dialysis units: short or normal vaccination schedule? Clin Nephrol, 1985; 24:215–220

635. Huang CC. Hepatitis in patients with end-stage renal disease. J Gastroenterol Hepatol, 1997; 12:S236–241

636. Younossi ZM, Braun WE, Protiva DA, Gifford RW, Straffon RA. Chronic viral hepatitis in renal transplant recipients with allografts functioning for more than 20 years. Transplantation, 1999; 67:272–275

637. Schlipkoter U, Roggendorf M, Ernst G et al. Hepatitis C virus antibodies in haemodialysis patients. Lancet, 1990; 335:1409

638. Kallinowski B, Theilmann L, Gmelin K et al. Incidence and prevalence of antibodies to hepatitis C virus in kidney transplanted patients. J Hepatol, 1991; 12:404–405

639. Chan TM, Lok ASF, Cheng IKP, Chan RT. Prevalence of hepatitis C virus infection in haemodialysis patients: a longitudinal study comparing the results of RNA and antibody assays. Hepatology, 1990; 11:5–8

640. Zylberberg H, Carnot F, Mamzer MF, Blancho G, Legendre C, Pol S. Hepatitis C virus-related fibrosing cholestatic hepatitis after renal transplantation. Transplantation, 1997; 63:158–160

641. Morales JM, Campistol JM, Andres A, Rodicio JL. Hepatitis C virus and renal transplantation. Curr Opin Nephrol Hypertens, 1998; 7:177–183

642. Glen J. Cytomegalovirus infection following renal transplantation. Rev Infect Dis, 1981; 3:1151–1178

643. Shiman-Chang R, Lewis JP, Reynolds RD, Sullivan MJ, Neuman J. Oropharyngeal secretion of Epstein-Barr virus by patients with lymphoproliferative disorders and by recipients of renal homografts. Ann Intern Med, 1978; 88:36–40

644. Anuras S, Summers R. Fulminant herpes simplex hepatitis in an adult. Report of a case in renal transplant recipient. Gastroenterology, 1976; 70:425–428

645. Taxy JB. Peliosis: a morphologic curiosity becomes an iatrogenic problem. Hum Pathol, 1978; 9:331–340

646. Hillion D, De Viel E, Bergue A et al. Peliosis hepatis in a chronic haemodialysis patient. Nephron, 1983; 35:205–206

647. Degott C, Rueff B, Kreis H et al. Peliosis hepatitis in recipients of renal transplants. Gut, 1978; 19:748–753

648. Mourad G, Bories P, Berthelemy C, Barneon G, Michel H, Mion C. Peliosis hepatis and nodular regenerative hyperplasia of the liver in renal transplants. Is cytomegalovirus the cause of this severe disease? Transplant Proc, 1987; 19:3697–3698

649. Buffet C, Cantarovitch M, Pelletier G et al. Three cases of nodular regenerative hyperplasia of the liver following renal transplantation. Nephrol Dial Transplant, 1988; 3:327–330

650. Morales JM, Prieto C, Mestre MJ et al. Nodular regenerative hyperplasia of the liver in renal transplantation. Transplant Proc, 1987; 19:3694–3696

651. Naber AHJ, Van Haelst U, Yap SH. Nodular regenerative hyperplasia of the liver: an important cause of portal hypertension in non-cirrhotic patients. J Hepatol, 1991; 12:94–99

652. Colina F, Alberti N, Solis JA, Martinez-Tello FJ. Diffuse nodular regenerative hyperplasia of the liver (DNRH). A clinicopathologic study of 24 cases. Liver, 1989; 9:253–265

653. Marubbio AT, Danielson B. Hepatic veno-occlusive disease in a renal transplant patient receiving azathioprine. Gastroenterology, 1975; 69:739–743

654. Read AE, Wiesner RH, LaBrecque DR et al. Hepatic veno-occlusive disease associated with renal transplantation and azathioprine therapy. Ann Intern Med, 1986; 104:651–655

655. Gerlag PGG, Van Hoof JP. Hepatic sinusoidal dilatation with portal hypertension during azathioprine treatment: a cause of chronic liver disease after kidney transplantation. Transplant Proc, 1987; 19:3699–3703

656. Nataf C, Feldman G, Lebrec D et al. Idiopathic portal hypertension (perisinusoidal fibrosis) after renal transplantation. Gut, 1979; 20:531–537

657. Sidi Y, Boner G, Bergamen D et al. Haemochromatosis in a renal transplant recipient. Clin Nephrol, 1980; 13:197–200

658. Rao KV, Anderson WR. Hemosiderosis and hemochromatosis in renal transplant recipients. Am J Nephrol, 1985; 5:419–430

659. Pahl MV, Vaziri ND, Dure-Smith B et al. Hepatobiliary pathology in hemodialysis patients: an autopsy study of 78 cases. Am J Gastroenterol, 1986; 81:783–787

660. Pritzker K. Neoplasia in renal transplant recipients. Can Med Ass J, 1972; 107:1059

661. Schroter GPJ, Weil IR, Penn I, Speers WC, Waddell WR. Hepatocellular carcinoma associated with chronic hepatitis B virus infection after kidney transplantation. Lancet, 1982; ii:381–382

662. Gardner BP, Evans DB. Primary hepatocellular carcinoma arising in a renal transplant recipient with polycystic disease. Postgrad Med J, 1983; 59:120–121

663. Penn I. The occurrence of cancer in immune deficiencies. Curr Probl Cancer, 1982; 6:1–64

664. Boraa S, Kleinfeld M. Subcapsular liver hematomas in a patient on chronic haemodialysis. Ann Intern Med, 1980; 93:574–575

665. Leong AS-Y, Gove DW. Foreign material in the tissues of patients on recurrent haemodialysis. Ultrastructure Pathol, 1981; 2:401–403

666. Parfrey PS, O'Driscoll JP, Paradinas FJ. Refractile material in the liver of haemodialysis patients. Lancet, 1981; i:1101–1102

667. Hunt J, Farthing MJG, Baker LRI, Crocker PR, Levison DA. Silicone in the liver: possible late effects. Gut, 1989; 30:239–242

668. Kurumaya H, Kono N, Nakanuma Y, Tomoda F, Takazakura E. Hepatic granulomata in long-term hemodialysis patients with hyperaluminaemia. Arch Path Lab Med, 1989; 113:1132–1134

669. Sugiura H, Yoshida K, Nakanuma Y et al. Hepatic calcification in the course of hemodialysis. Am J Gastroenterol, 1987; 82:786–789

670. Campistol JM, Sole M, Munoz-Gomez J, Lopez-Pedret J, Revert L. Systemic involvement in dialysis-amyloidosis. Am J Nephrol, 1990; 10:389–396

671. Koch KM. Dialysis-related amyloidosis. Kidney Int, 1992; 41:1416–1429

672. Rokitansky C. Handbuch der Pathologischen Anatomie, 1842; 3:311

673. Westermark P, Benson MD, Buxbaum JN et al. Nomenclature Committee of the International Society of Amyloidosis. Amyloid: toward terminology clarification. Report from the Nomenclature Committee of the International Society of Amyloidosis. Amyloid, 2005; 12:1–4

674. Kyle RA, Gertz MA. Systemic amyloidosis. Clin Rev Oncol Haematol, 1990; 10:49–87

675. Gillmore JD, Lovat LB, Hawkins PN. Amyloidosis and the liver. J Hepatol, 1999; 30 (suppl I):17–33

676. Monteiro E, Freire A, Barroso E. Familial amyloid polyneuropathy and liver transplantation. J Hepatol, 2004; 41:188–194

677. Cosme A, Horcajada JP, Vidair F et al. Systemic AA amyloidosis induced by oral contraceptive-associated hepatocellular adenoma: a 13 year follow up. Liver, 1995; 15:164–167

678. Buck FS, Koss MN. Hepatic amyloidosis: morphologic differences between systemic AL and AA types. Hum Pathol, 1991; 22:904–907

679. Obici L, Palladini G, Giorgetti S et al. Liver biopsy discloses a new apolipoprotein A-I hereditary amyloidosis in several unrelated Italian families. Gastroenterology, 2004; 126:1416–1422

680. Gertz MA, Kyle RA. Hepatic amyloidosis: clinical appraisal in 77 patients. Hepatology, 1997; 25:118–121

681. Chopra S, Rubinow A, Koff RS, Cohen AS. Hepatic amyloidosis. A histopathologic analysis of primary (AL) and secondary (AA) forms. Am J Pathol, 1984; 115:186–193

682. Looi L-M, Sumithran E. Morphologic differences in the pattern of liver infiltration between systemic AL and AA amyloidosis. Hum Pathol, 1988; 19:732–735

683. Kyle RA, Bayrd ED. Amyloidosis: a review of 236 cases. Medicine, 1975; 54:271–299

684. Melato M, Manconi R, Magris D et al. Different morphologic aspects and clinical features in massive hepatic amyloidosis. Digestion, 1984; 29:138–145

685. Levy-Lehad E, Steiner-Salz D, Berkman N et al. Reversible functional aplasia and sub-capsular liver haematoma: two distinctive manifestations of amyloidosis. Klin Wschr, 1987; 65:1104–1107

686. Park MA, Mueller PS, Kyle RA, Larson DR, Plevak MF, Gertz MA. Primary (AL) hepatic amyloidosis: clinical features and natural history in 98 patients. Medicine (Baltimore), 2003; 82:291–298

687. Kennan NM, Evans C. Case report: hepatic and splenic calcification due to amyloid. Clin Radiol, 1991; 44:60–61

688. Oliai A, Koff RS. Case report: primary amyloidosis presenting as 'sicca complex' and severe intrahepatic cholestasis. Am J Dig Dis, 1972; 17:1033–1036

689. Rockey DC. Striking cholestatic liver disease: a distinct manifestation of advanced primary amyloidosis. South Med J, 1999; 92:236–241

690. Rubinow A, Koff RS, Cohen AS. Severe intrahepatic cholestasis in primary amyloidosis. A report of a few cases and a review of the literature. Am J Med, 1978; 64:937–946

691. Sandberg-Gertzen H, Ericzon BG, Blomberg B. Primary amyloidosis with spontaneous splenic rupture, cholestasis, and liver failure treated with emergency liver transplantation. Am J Gastroenterol, 1998; 93:2254–2256

692. Hoffman MS, Stein BE, Davidian MM, Rosenthal WS. Hepatic amyloidosis presenting as severe intrahepatic cholestasis: a case report and review of the literature. Am J Gastroenterol, 1988; 83:783–785

693. Itescu S. Hepatic amyloidosis: an unusual case of ascites and portal hypertension. Arch Intern Med, 1984; 144:2257–2259

694. Kitazono M, Saito Y, Kinoshita M et al. Nodular regenerative hyperplasia of the liver in a patient with multiple myeloma and systemic amyloidosis. Arch Pathol Jpn, 1985; 35:961–967

695. Bujanda L. Beguiristain A, Alberdi F et al. Spontaneous rupture of the liver in amyloidosis. Am J Gastroenterol, 1997; 92:1385–1386

696. Harrison RF, Hawkins PN, Roche WR, MacMahon RF, Hubscher SG, Buckels JA. 'Fragile' liver and massive hepatic haemorrhage due to hereditary amyloidosis. Gut, 1996; 38:151–152

697. Wright JR, Calkins E, Humphrey RL. Potassium permanganate reaction in amyloidosis: a histologic method to assist in differentiating forms of the disease. Lab Invest, 1977; 36:274–279

698. Shirahama T, Skinner M, Sipe JD, Cohen AS. Widespread occurrence of A P in amyloidotic tissues: an immunohistochemical observation. Virchows Arch (B), 1985; 48:197–206

699. Garlanda C, Bottazzi B, Bastone A, Mantovani A. Pentraxins at the crossroads between innate immunity, inflammation, matrix deposition, and female fertility. Annu Rev Immunol, 2005; 23:337–366

700. Melling M, Karimian-Teherani D, Mostler S, Behnam M, Hochmeister S. 3-D morphological characterization of the liver parenchyma by atomic force microscopy and by scanning electron microscopy. Microsc Res Tech, 2004; 64:1–9

701. French SW, Schloss GT, Stillman AE. Unusual amyloid bodies in human liver. Am J Clin Pathol, 1981; 75:400–402

702. Kanel GC, Uchida T, Peters RL. Globular hepatic amyloid—an unusual morphologic presentation. Hepatology, 1981; 1:647–652

703. Agaram N, Shia J, Klimstra DS et al. Globular hepatic amyloid: a diagnostic peculiarity that bears clinical significance. Hum Pathol, 2005; 36:845–849

704. Sasaki M, Nakanuma Y, Terada T et al. Amyloid deposition in intrahepatic large bile ducts and peribiliary glands in systemic amyloidosis. Hepatology, 1990; 12:743–746

705. Schmidt HH, Nashan B, Propsting MJ et al. Familian amyloidotic polyneuropathy: domino liver transplantation. J Hepatol, 1999; 30:293–298

706. Randall RE, Williamson WC, Mullinax F, Tung MY, Still WJS. Manifestations of systemic light chain deposition. Am J Med, 1976; 60:293–299

707. Silver MM, Hearn SA, Ritchie S et al. Renal and systemic kappa light chain deposits and their plasma cell origin identified by immunoelectron microscopy. Am J Pathol, 1986; 122:17–27

708. Confalonieri R, Barbiano di Belgioioso G, Banfi G et al. Light chain nephropathy: histological and clinical aspects in 15 cases. Nephrol Dial Transplant, 1988; 3:150–156

709. Maury CPJ, Teppo AM. Massive cutaneous hyalinosis. Am J Clin Pathol, 1984; 82:543–551

710. Kijner CH, Yousem SY. Systemic light chain deposition disease presenting as multiple pulmonary nodules. Am J Surg Pathol, 1988; 12:405–413

711. Stone GC, Wall BA, Oppliger IR et al. A vasculopathy with deposition of lambda light chain crystals. Ann Int Med, 1989; 110:275–278

712. Pozzi C, Locatelli F. Kidney and liver involvement in monoclonal light chain disorders. Semin Nephrol, 2002; 22:319–330

713. Preud'homme JL, Morel-Maroger L, Brouet JC et al. Synthesis of abnormal immunoglobulins in lymphoplasmacytic disorders with visceral light chain deposition. Am J Med, 1980; 69:703–710

714. Girelli CM, Lodi G, Rocca F. Kappa light chain deposition disease of the liver. Eur J Gastroenterol Hepatol, 1998; 10:429–430

715. Droz D, Noel LH, Carnot F, Degos F, Ganeval D, Grunfeld JP. Liver involvement in non-amyloid light chain deposits disease. Lab Invest, 1984; 50:683–689

716. Bedossa P, Fabre M, Paraf F, Martin E, Lemaigre G. Light chain deposition disease with liver dysfunction. Hum Pathol, 1988; 19:1008–1014

717. Pelletier G, Fabre M, Attali P et al. Light chain deposition disease presenting with hepatomegaly: an association with amyloid-like fibrils. Postgrad Med J, 1988; 64:804–808

718. Faa G, Van Eyken P, De Vos R et al. Light chain deposition disease of the liver associated with AL-type amyloidosis and severe cholestasis. A case report and literature review. J Hepatol, 1991; 12:75–82

719. Feiner HD. Pathology of dysproteinemia: light chain amyloidosis, non-amyloid immunoglobulin deposition disease, cryoglobulinemia syndromes and macroglobulinemia of Waldenström. Hum Pathol, 1988; 19:1255–1272

720. Ganeval D, Noel LH, Droz D, Leibowitch J. Systemic lambda light chain deposition in a patient with myeloma. Br Med J, 1981; 282:681–683

721. Kirkpatrick CJ, Curry A, Galle J, Melzner I. Systemic kappa light chain deposition and amyloidosis in multiple myeloma: novel morphological observations. Histopathology, 1986; 10:1065–1076

722. Casiraghi MA, De Paoli A, Assi A et al. Hepatic amyloidosis with light chain deposition disease. A rare association. Dig Liver Dis, 2000; 32:795–798

723. Lefkowitch JH, Mendez L. Morphological features of hepatic injury in cardiac disease and shock. J Hepatol, 1986; 2:313–327

724. Klatt EC, Koss MN, Young TS, MacAuley L, Martin SE. Hepatic hyaline globules associated with passive congestion. Arch Pathol Lab Med, 1988; 112:510–513

725. Dichtl W, Vogel W, Dunst KM et al. Cardiac hepatopathy before and after heart transplantation. Transpl Int, 2005; 18:697–702

726. Steiner PE. Nodular regenerative hyperplasia of the liver. Am J Pathol, 1959; 35:943–953

727. Ellenberg M, Osserman KE. Role of shock in production of central liver cell necrosis. Am J Med, 1951; 11:170–178

728. de la Monte SM, Arcide JM, Moore GW, Hutchins GM. Midzonal necrosis as a pattern of hepatocellular injury after shock. Gastroenterology, 1984; 86:627–631

729. Henrion J, Schapira M, Luwaert R, Colin L, Delannoy A, Heller FR. Hypoxic hepatitis: clinical and hemodynamic study in 142 consecutive cases. Medicine (Baltimore), 2003; 82:392–406

730. Gibson PR, Dudley FJ. Ischaemic hepatitis: clinical features, diagnosis and prognosis. Aust NZ J Med, 1984; 14:822–825

731. Gitlin N, Serio KM. Ischemic hepatitis: widening horizons. Am J Gastroenterol, 1992; 87:831–836

732. Fuchs S, Bogomolskiyahalom V, Paltiel O, Ackerman Z. Ischemic hepatitis: Clinical and laboratory observations of 34 patients. J Clin Gastroenterol, 1998; 26:183–186

733. Garland JS, Werlin SL, Rice TB. Ischemic hepatitis in children: diagnosis and clinical course. Crit Care Med, 1988; 16:1209–1212

734. Sherlock S. The liver in heart failure. Relation of anatomical, functional and circulatory changes. Br Heart J, 1951; 13:273–293

735. Arcidi JR, Moore GW, Hutchins GM. Hepatic morphology in cardiac dysfunction. A clinicopathologic study of 1000 subjects at autopsy. Am J Pathol, 1981; 104:159–166

736. van Lingen R, Warshow U, Dalton HR, Hussaini SH. Jaundice as a presentation of heart failure. J R Soc Med, 2005; 98:357–359

737. Nouel O, Herrion J, Degott C et al. Fulminant hepatic failure due to transient circulatory failure in patients with chronic heart disease. Dig Dis Sci, 1980; 25:49–52

738. Giallourakis CC, Rosenberg PM, Friedman LS. The liver in heart failure. Clin Liver Dis, 2002; 6:947–967, viii–ix

739. Shibayama Y. The role of hepatic venous congestion and endotoxaemia in the production of fulminant hepatic failure secondary to congestive heart failure. J Pathol, 1987; 151:133–138

740. Shibuya A, Unuma T, Sugimoto T et al. Diffuse hepatic calcification as a sequela to shock liver. Gastroenterology, 1985; 89:196–201

741. Gore I, Isaacson NH. Pathology of hyperpyrexia; observations at autopsy in 17 cases of fever therapy. Am J Pathol, 1949; 25:1029–1046

742. Milroy CM. Ten years of 'ecstasy'. J Roy Soc Med, 1999; 92:68–71

743. Bianchi L, Ohnacker H, Beck K, Zimmerli-Ning M. Liver damage in heatstroke and its regression. Hum Pathol, 1972; 3:237–248

744. Rubel LR, Ishak KG. The liver in fatal exertional heatstroke. Liver, 1983; 3:249–260

745. Gierchsky T, Boberg KM, Farstad IN, Halvorsen S, Schrumpf E. Severe liver failure in exertional heat stroke. Scand J Gastroenterol, 1999; 34:824–827

746. Hassanein T, Razack A, Gavaler JS, Van Thiel DH. Heat stroke; its clinical and pathological presentation, with particular attention to the liver. Am J Gastroenterol, 1992; 87:1382–1389

747. Sort P, Mas A, Salmerson JM, Bruguera M, Rodes J. Recurrent liver involvement in heatstroke. Liver, 1996; 16:335–337

748. Uchino T, Endo F, Ikeda S, Shiraki K, Sera Y, Matsuda I. Three brothers with progressive hepatic dysfunction and severe hepatic steatosis due to a patent ductus venosus. Gastroenterology, 1996; 110:1964–1968

749. Tanne F, Gagnadoux F, Chazouilleres O et al. Chronic liver injury during obstructive sleep apnea. Hepatology, 2005; 41:1290–1296

750. Ghaferi AA, Hutchins GM. Progression of liver pathology in patients undergoing the Fontan procedure: Chronic passive congestion, cardiac cirrhosis, hepatic adenoma, and hepatocellular carcinoma. J Thorac Cardiovasc Surg, 2005; 129:1348–1352

751. Murata K, Okudaira M, Akashio K. Mast cells in human liver tissue. Acta Derm Venereol Suppl (Stockh), 1973; 73:157–178

752. Bardadin KA, Scheuer PJ. Mast cells in acute hepatitis. J Pathol, 1986; 149:315–325

753. Farrell DJ, Hines JE, Walls AF, Kelly PJ, Bennett MK, Burt AD. Intrahepatic mast cells in chronic liver diseases. Hepatology, 1995; 22:1175–1181

754. Lennert K, Parwaresch MR. Mast cells and mast cell neoplasia: a review. Histopathology, 1979; 3:349–365

755. Akin C, Metcalfe DD. Systemic mastocytosis. Annu Rev Med, 2004; 55:419–432

756. Webb TA, Li CY, Yam LT. Systemic mast cell disease: A clinical and hematopathologic study of 26 cases. Cancer, 1982; 49:927–938

757. Yam LT, Chan CH, Li CY. Hepatic involvement in systemic mast cell disease. Am J Med, 1986; 80:819–826

758. Horny H-P, Kaiserling E, Campbell M, Parwaresch MR, Lennert K. Liver findings in generalized mastocytosis. A clinicopathologic study. Cancer, 1989; 63:532–538

759. Capron J-P, Lebrec D, Degott C, Chirrac D, Coevoet B, Delobel J. Portal hypertension in systemic mastocytosis. Gastroenterology, 1978; 74:595–597

760. Grundfest S, Cooperman AM, Ferguson R, Benjamin S. Portal hypertension associated with systemic mastocytosis and splenomegaly. Gastroenterology, 1980; 78:370–373

761. Ghandur-Mnaymneh L, Gould E. Systemic mastocytosis with portal hypertension. Autopsy findings and ultrastructural study of the liver. Arch Path Lab Med, 1985; 109:76–78

762. Bonnet P, Smadja C, Szekely A-M et al. Intractable ascites in systemic mastocytosis treated by portal diversion. Dig Dis Sci, 1987; 32:209–213

763. Narayanan MN, Liu Yin JA, Azzawi S, Warnes TW, Turck WPG. Portal hypertension and ascites in systemic mastocytosis. Postgrad Med J, 1989; 65:394–396

764. Safyan EL, Veerabagu MP, Swerdlow SH, Lee RG, Rakela J. Intrahepatic cholestasis due to systemic mastocytosis: a case report and review of literature. Am J Gastroenterol, 1997; 92:1197–1200

765. Kyriakou D, Kouroumalis E, Konsolas J et al. Systemic mastocytosis: A rare cause of noncirhotic portal hypertension simulating autoimmune cholangitis—Report of four cases. Am J Gastroenterol, 1998; 93:106–108

766. Korkij W, Chuang T-Y, Soltani K. Liver abnormalities in patients with lichen planus. A retrospective case-control study. J Am Acad Dermatol, 1984; 11:609–615

767. Cottoni F, Solinas A, Piga MR, Tocco A, Lissia M, Cerimele D. Lichen planus, chronic liver diseases, and immunologic involvement. Dermatol Res, 1988; 280:S55–S60

768. del Olmo JA, Almenar E, Bagan JV et al. Liver abnormalities in patients with lichen planus of the oral cavity. Eur J Gastroenterol Hepatol, 1990; 2:479–481

769. Mignogna MD, Lo Muzio L, Lo Russo L, Fedele S, Ruoppo E, Bucci E. Oral lichen planus: different clinical features in HCV-positive and HCV-negative patients. Int J Dermatol, 2000; 39:134–139

770. Virgili A, Robert E, Rebora A. Hepatocellular carcinoma and lichen planus: report of two cases. Dermatology, 1992; 184:137–138

771. Meyer GW, Griffiths WJ, Welsh J, Cohen L, Johnson L, Weaver MJ. Brief reports: Hepatobiliary involvement in von Recklinghausen's disease. Ann Intern Med, 1982; 97:722–723

772. Young SJ. Primary malignant neurilemmoma (Schwannoma) of the liver in a case of neurofibromatosis. J Pathol, 1975; 117:151–153

773. Lederman SM, Martin EG, Laffey KT, Lefkowitch JH. Hepatic neurofibromatosis, malignant schwannoma and angiosarcoma in von Recklinghausen's disease. Gastroenterology, 1987; 92:234–239

774. Di Bisceglie AM, Hodkinson HJ, Berkowitz I, Kew MC. Pityriasis rotunda. A cutaneous marker of hepatocellular carcinoma in South African Blacks. Arch Dermatol, 1986; 122:802–804

775. Berkowitz I, Hodgkinson HJ, Kew MC, Di Bisceglie AM. Pityriasis rotunda as a cutaneous marker of hepatocellular carcinoma: a comparison with its prevalence in other diseases. Br J Dermatol, 1989; 120:545–549

776. Sharma S, Weiss GR, Paulger B. Pityriasis rubra pilaris is an initial presentation of hepatocellular carcinoma. Dermatology, 1997; 194:166–167

777. Gilbert SC, Klintmalm G, Menter A, Silverman A. Methotrexate-induced cirrhosis requiring liver transplantation in three patients with psoriasis. Arch Intern Med, 1990; 150:889–891

778. Pascual M, Widmann J-J, Schifferli JA. Recurrent febrile panniculitis and hepatitis in two patients with acquired complement deficiency and paraproteinemia. Am J Med, 1987; 83:959–962

779. Banerjee AK, Grainger SL, Davies DR, Thompson RPH. Active chronic hepatitis and febrile panniculitis. Gut, 1989; 30:1018–1019

780. Langley JM, Roberts EA, Ipp M, Laxer RM, Boxall L, Phillips MJ. Pyoderma gangrenosum and autoimmune chronic active hepatitis in a 17 year old female. Can J Gastroenterol, 1988; 2:137–139

781. Kumar A, Helwig K, Komar MJ. Sweet's syndrome in association with probable autoimmune hepatitis. J Clin Gastroenterol, 1999; 29:349–350

782. Caplan RM. Visceral involvement in lipoid proteinosis. Arch Dermatol, 1967; 95:149–155

783. Weedon D. Cutaneous deposits in the skin. In: Weedon D, ed. Systemic pathology, 3rd edn, vol 9. Symmers W St C. (Gen. Ed.) Edinburgh: Churchill Livingstone, 1993: pp 412–443

784. Dean G, Freestone M, van den Berg JP, Coenen JL. Primary liver cancer in two sisters in Holland with intermittent acute porphyria. S Afr Med J, 1997; 87:731–732

785. Audant C, Puy H, Deybach JC, Soule JG, Nordmann Y. Occurrence of hepatocellular carcinoma in a case of hereditary coproporphyria. Am J Gastroenterol, 1997; 92:1389–1390

786. Loze I, Tessier MH, Jumbou O, Dreno B. Hepatocellular adenomatosis presenting as prurigo. Br J Dermatol, 2000; 142:384–386

787. Gelbmann CM, Kollinger M, Gmeinwieser J, Leser HG, Holstege A, Scholmerich J. Spontaneous rupture of liver in a patient with Ehlers Danlos disease type IV. Dig Dis Sci, 1997; 42:1724–1730

788. Eliakim R, Ligumsky M, Jurim O, Shouval D. Nodular regenerative hyperplasia with portal hypertension in a patient with myasthenia gravis. Am J Gastroenterol, 1987; 82:674–676

789. Theodore C, Cornud F, Mendez J et al. Cholestasis and myotonic dystrophy. N Engl J Med, 1979; 301:329–430

790. Poynard T, Bedossa P, Naveau S et al. Perisinusoidal cells (Ito cells) enlargement in a family with myotonic dystrophy. Liver, 1989; 9:276–278

791. Soderhall S, Gustafsson J, Bjorkhem I. Deoxycholic acid in myotonic dystrophy. Lancet, 1982; i:1046–1069

792. Crompton DE, Chinnery PF, Fey C et al. Neuroferritinopathy: a window on the role of iron in neurodegeneration. Blood Cells Mol Dis, 2002; 29:522–531

Subject Index

Notes: Page numbers in *italics* indicate figures and those in **bold** indicate tables